Diseases

Second Edition

Diseases

Second Edition

Springhouse Corporation
Springhouse, Pennsylvania

STAFF

Executive Director
Matthew Cahill

Editorial Director
June Norris

Clinical Manager
Judith Schilling McCann, RN, MSN

Art Director
John Hubbard

Clinical Project Manager
Beverly Ann Tscheschlog, RN

Editors
Margaret Eckman, Nancy Priff

Copy Editors
Cynthia C. Breuninger (manager), Christine Cunniffe, Brenna Mayer, Christina P. Ponczek, Doris Weinstock, Pamela Wingrod

Designers
Arlene Putterman (associate art director), Elaine Ezrow, Jacalyn Facciolo, Linda Franklin, Susan Hopkins, Ann Raphun, Jeff Sklarow

Illustrators
John Carlance, Kevin Curry, Jacalyn Facciolo, Darcy Feralio, Jean Gardner, Bob Jackson, Phyllis Carol Nathans, Bob Neumann, Judy Newhouse

Typography
Diane E. Paluba (manager), Joyce Rossi Biletz, Phyllis Marron, Valerie Rosenberger

Manufacturing
Deborah Meiris (director), Pat Dorshaw (manager), T.A. Landis

Production Coordination
Margaret A. Rastiello

Editorial Assistants
Beverly Lane, Mary Madden

The authors and publisher gratefully acknowledge the following individuals and organizations who provided photographs: Evelina Bernardino, p. 1167; Centers for Disease Control and Prevention, pp. 130, 136; *Consultant* magazine, p. 273; Robert Ford, p. 697; Fran Heyl Associates (© Herb Charles Ohlmeyer), p. 1095; Tom McHugh Photo Researchers, p. 272; Christopher Papa, p. 1169; Reed and Carnrick Pharmaceuticals, p. 1172.

Printed in the United States of America.
DIS2-030498

 A member of the Reed Elsevier plc group

Library of Congress Cataloging-in-Publication Data

Diseases. — 2nd ed.
    p. cm.
    Includes bibliographical references and index.
    1. Diseases — Handbooks, manuals, etc.   2. Nursing — Handbooks, manuals, etc.   I. Springhouse Corporation.
    [DNLM: 1. Nursing Care.   2. Nursing Process.
    3. Disease — nurses' instruction WY 100 D6112 1997]
RC55.D558 1997
616 — dc20
DNLM/DLC
                                  96-19799
ISBN 0-87434-839-0 (alk. paper)   CIP

CONTENTS

CONTRIBUTORS AND CONSULTANTS

Mary Ann Cali-Ascani, RN, MSN, OCN
 Oncology Nurse Manager
 Easton (Pa.) Hospital

Kerry H. Cheever, RN, MSN, CCRN, CEN
 Williams-Brice College of Nursing
 University of South Carolina
 Columbia

Patricia L. Clutter, RN, MEd, CEN
 Staff Nurse, Emergency Trauma Center
 St. John's Regional Health Center
 Springfield, Mo.

Ellen Digan, MA, MT (ASCP)
 Professor and Coordinator of
 Medical Laboratory Technician
 Program
 Manchester (Conn.) Community
 Technical College

Nancy G. Evans, RN, BSN, CGRN
 Nurse Manager, Gastroenterology Department
 Daniel Freeman Memorial and Marina Hospital
 Inglewood, Calif.

Marilyn A. Folcik, RN, MPH, ONC
 Assistant Director, Department of Surgery
 Hartford (Conn.) Hospital

Susan Fralick, RN, MSN
 Instructor
 Roxborough Memorial Hospital School of Nursing
 Philadelphia

Ellie Franges, RN, MSN, CNRN, CCRN
 Director of Neuroscience Services
 Sacred Heart Hospital
 Allentown, Pa.

Karen Alyce Graf, RN, BSN, CURN
 Urology Nurse Coordinator
 New York University Medical Center
 Rusk Institute of Rehabilitation Medicine
 New York

Linda B. Haas, RN, CDE
 Clinical Nurse Specialist, Endocrinology
 Puget Sound Veterans Health Care System
 Seattle

Sande Jones, RN,C, CS, MSN, MSEd
 Clinical Nurse Specialist, Special Immunology
 Mount Sinai Medical Center
 Miami

Karen Landis, RN, MS, CCRN
 Pulmonary Clinical Nurse Specialist
 Lehigh Valley Hospital
 Allentown, Pa.

Amanda Keller Martin, RN, BSN, MEd, CNOR
 Clinical Educator
 Ochsner Foundation Hospital
 New Orleans

Margaret Massoni, RN, MS, CS
 Assistant Professor
 College of the University of New York
 The College of Staten Island (N.Y.)

Linda Rae Merrow, RN,C, MS, CNSN
 Medical Clinical Nurse Specialist
 Greater Baltimore Medical Center

Cheryl Milford, RN, MS, MBA, CCRN
 Staff Development Specialist
 Ohio State University Medical Center
 Columbus

Patricia L. Radzewicz, RN, BSN
 Associate Claims Manager
 University of Illinois
 Chicago

Linda E. Reese, RN, MA
 Associate Professor, Deputy Chairperson
 Department of Nursing
 College of Staten Island (N.Y.)

Lynne Rosenberg, RN, MSN
 Instructor
 Montgomery County Community College
 Blue Bell, Pa.

Nancy V. Runta, RN,C, BSN, CCRN
 Medical-Surgical Staff Development Educator
 North Penn Hospital
 Lansdale, Pa.

Steven J. Schweon, RN,C, BSN, CCRN
    Assistant Epidemiologist
    Hahnemann University Hospital
    Philadelphia

Regina Shannon-Bodnar, RN, MSN, OCN
    Director of Patient Care Services
    Hospital of Baltimore

Brenda K. Shelton, RN, MS, CCRN, OCN
    Critical Care Clinical Nurse Specialist
    Johns Hopkins Oncology Center
    Baltimore

Johanna K. Stiesmeyer, RN, MS, CCRN
    Clinical Consultant
    Nursing Educational Services
    Placitas, N.Mex.

Donald A. St. Onge, RN, MSN
    Pulmonary Clinical Nurse Specialist
    Allegheny General Hospital
    Pittsburgh

Rosemary Theroux, RN,C, MS
    Independent Women's Health Nurse Practitioner
    Framingham, Mass.

Joseph B. Warren, RN, BSN, CNRN
    Administrator, Clinical Research
    Kinetic Concepts, Inc.
    San Antonio, Tex.

Patti Zuzelo, RN, MSN, CCRN
    Medical-Surgical Coordinator
    Roxborough Memorial Hospital School of Nursing
    Philadelphia

FOREWORD

Drug-resistant bacteria. Hantavirus pulmonary syndrome and other newly identified diseases. Genetically engineered drugs. Developments in diseases and their treatments are occurring at a tremendous rate. How do you keep pace with this ever-expanding body of information? Where can you learn—quickly and easily—about the latest drug or technology that changes the accepted treatment for a disease? How do you keep track of the most recent drug-resistant strains of bacteria?

Diseases, Second Edition, has the answers you need, and more. This invaluable reference contains current information on virtually every disease you're likely to encounter. Besides containing new entries on such exotic emerging diseases as Ebola virus, this new edition of *Diseases* gives you detailed coverage of disorders that are on the rise, such as cryptosporidiosis and attention deficit hyperactivity disorder. It includes the latest guidelines for treatment. And it has the most up-to-date information on new tests, drugs, and procedures—all presented in one well-organized, clearly written volume.

The book opens with a chapter on mental and emotional disorders, which includes the most recent diagnostic criteria from the *Diagnostic and Statistical Manual IV.* The next three chapters focus on infection, trauma, and neoplasms. The following chapters cover disorders of every major body system, from the immune system to the skin. Altogether, *Diseases,* Second Edition, presents more than 500 diseases and disorders.

At the beginning of each chapter, you'll find an overview of anatomy and physiology, nursing assessment, and diagnostic tests. Next, you'll see separate entries for each disease.

Each entry starts with a brief description of the disease. Major *Causes* of the disorder and possible *Complications* follow. The next section, *Assessment findings,* focuses on patient history and physical assessment findings. It's followed by a section on *Diagnostic tests,* which covers laboratory findings associated with the disease. *Treatment* discusses the methods used to manage the disease. Following this,

a list of relevant, current *Nursing diagnoses* helps you plan your care. Finally, a comprehensive section on *Nursing interventions* suggests ways to put your plan of care into action and includes *Patient teaching* instructions to help you give your patient and his family information and skills they need for home care.

Throughout *Diseases,* Second Edition, many new illustrations and photographs appear. Also, special graphic devices, or logos, highlight important information. New to this edition, the *Home care* logo identifies guidelines you can use to help you and your patient manage his disease at home. The *Pathophysiology* logo clarifies the disease process. The *Assessment tips* logo signals useful, often timesaving techniques for assessing your patient. The *Warning* logo draws your attention to critical information that can help you manage potentially dangerous situations. At the *Plan of care* logo, you'll find a case study that illustrates how to apply the nursing process in clinical practice.

With the rapid development of new technologies and new ways to treat diseases, and with the continuing emergence of new diseases, wouldn't you like to have an expert on hand whenever you need one? Packed with vital information, *Diseases,* Second Edition, is the "expert" you've been looking for. For virtually every disease, it puts the information you need right at your fingertips—so you can give your patients the best care possible.

Joseph T. Catalano, RN, PhD, CCRN
Professor of Nursing
East Central University
Ada, Okla.

Diseases

Second Edition

1 MENTAL AND EMOTIONAL DISORDERS

INTRODUCTION

In recent years, a convergence of social, economic, and professional forces has dramatically changed the mental health field. Community and professional organizations, for instance, have established family advocacy programs, substance abuse rehabilitation programs, stress management workshops, bereavement groups, victim assistance programs, and violence shelters. The public education system has established widespread information programs about mental health issues. The proliferation of self-help and coping books, media attention to mental and emotional disorders, and an increased interest in maintaining wellness through nutrition and exercise reflect the growing public acceptance of personal responsibility for wellness.

Social changes

In today's society, more people than ever before experience mental health problems. Some researchers blame social changes for the rise in mental and emotional disorders. These changes have altered the traditional family structure and contributed to the loss of the extended family. The result: an increased number of single parents, dysfunctional families, troubled children, and homeless people.

The loss of effective support systems strains a person's ability to cope with even minor problems. For example, a working mother may lack the necessary support to meet the demands of her job, her home, her spouse, and her children. When she views herself as ineffective in these roles, her self-esteem falters and her level of stress intensifies.

Women aren't the only members of society who face an increased risk of mental disorders—the problem affects all ages and socioeconomic levels. For example, the rate of teenage depression and suicide has more than tripled in the past 20 years. Alcohol and substance abuse are proliferating and their victims are becoming younger. Isolation, fear of violent crime, and loneliness have contributed to a similar rise in depression among elderly people. Combat veterans, rape victims, and child abuse victims struggle to cope with the trauma they've experienced.

Economic forces

Recent cuts in federal funding of mental health programs place future control of mental health services at the state and local community levels and drastically reduce the funds available for training new professionals. This funding squeeze has forced increased collaboration between community psychiatric facilities (short-term inpatient, outpatient, and auxiliary services) and long-term inpatient state facilities.

Professional changes

Mental health professionals have experienced enormous changes in perspective, focus, and direction. These changes—documented in the American Psychiatric Association's *Diagnostic and Statistical Manual of Mental Disorders,* 4th edition *(DSM-IV)*—provide a unified system of classifying mental disorders. This system requires the clinician to consider many aspects of the patient's behavior, mental performance, history, and culture, emphasizing observable data rather than subjective and theoretical impressions.

The *DSM-IV* defines a mental disorder as a clinically significant behavioral or psychological syndrome or pattern that's associated with current distress (a painful symptom) or disability (impairment in one or more important areas of functioning) or with a significantly greater risk of suffering, death, pain, disability, or an important loss of freedom. This syndrome or pattern mustn't be merely an expected, culturally sanctioned response, such as grief over the death of a loved one. Whatever its original cause, it must currently be considered a sign of a behavioral, psychological, or biological dysfunction.

To add diagnostic detail, the *DSM-IV* uses a multiaxial approach. This approach specifies that every patient be evaluated on each of five axes, as follows:
• *Axis I:* clinical disorders—the diagnosis (or diagnoses) that best describes the presenting complaint
• *Axis II:* personality disorders and mental retardation
• *Axis III:* general medical conditions—a description of any concurrent medical conditions or disorders
• *Axis IV:* psychosocial and environmental problems that may affect the diagnosis, treatment, and prognosis of the mental disorder
• *Axis V:* global assessment of functioning (GAF), based on a scale of 1 to 100. The GAF scale allows evaluation of the patient's overall psychological, social, and occupational function.

The first three axes, which constitute the official diagnostic assessment, encompass the entire spectrum of mental and physical disorders, ensuring consideration of disorders that frequently are overlooked. This system requires multiple diagnoses whenever necessary. For example, on Axis I, a patient may have both a psychoactive substance use disorder and a mood disorder. He may even have multiple diagnoses within the same class, as in major depression superimposed on cyclothymic disorders. A patient also may have a disorder on Axes I, II, and III simultaneously.

Axis IV identifies psychosocial and environmental problems that affect the patient's condition. Such problems can stem from the patient's primary support group, social environment, education, occupation, housing conditions, economic status, access to health care, contact with the legal system, or involvement in crime as well as from other sources.

Axis V uses the GAF scale to measure how well the patient has functioned over the past year. It also encompasses his current level of functioning.

A patient's diagnosis after being evaluated on these five axes may look like this:
Axis I: adjustment disorder with anxious mood
Axis II: obsessive-compulsive personality
Axis III: Crohn's disease, acute bleeding episode
Axis IV: recent remarriage, death of father
Axis V: GAF = 83.

Related professional forces

A new emphasis on holistic care has promoted a closer relationship between psychiatry and medicine. Increasing numbers of hospitalized patients benefit from psychiatric consultations, reflecting a growing recognition of the emotional basis of physical disorders. Conversely, advances in neurobiology have revolutionized our understanding of the physiologic basis of mental function. These advances have improved the diagnosis and treatment of mental disorders.

Psychosocial assessment

In all clinical areas and settings, you'll encounter patients with mental and emotional problems. Begin your care of these patients with a psychosocial assessment. For this assessment to be effective, you need to establish a therapeutic relationship based on trust. To develop such a relationship, your words and actions must communicate to the patient that his thoughts and behaviors are important to you. Effective communication involves both sending and receiving messages. It doesn't depend entirely on the spoken word. Nonverbal communication—eye contact, posture, facial expression, gestures, clothing, affect, even silence—can convey a powerful message. (For more information, see *Communication barriers.*)

Choose a quiet, private setting for the assessment interview. Interruptions and distractions threaten confidentiality and interfere with effective listening. If you're meeting the patient for the first time, introduce yourself and explain the interview's purpose. Sit at a comfortable distance from the patient, and give him your undivided attention.

During the interview, adopt a professional but friendly attitude, and maintain good eye contact. A calm, nonthreatening tone of voice will encourage the patient to talk more openly. Avoid value judgments. Don't rush through the interview; building a trusting therapeutic relationship takes time.

Patient history

Obtaining a patient history helps establish a baseline for future assessments and gives clues to the underlying or precipitating cause of the current problem. When gathering the history, keep in mind that the patient may not be a reliable source of information, particularly if he's mentally ill. If possible, verify his responses with family members, friends, or health care personnel. Also check hospital records from previous admissions, if possible, and compare his past behavior, symptoms, and circumstances with the current situation.

When taking the patient's history, explore the following information: chief complaint, current symptoms, psychiatric history, demographic data, socioeconomic data, cultural and religious beliefs, medication history, and physical illnesses.
• *Chief complaint.* The patient may not voice his chief complaint directly. Instead, you, another nurse, family members, or friends may note that the patient is having difficulty coping or is exhibiting unusual behavior. If this occurs, determine whether the patient is aware of the problem. When documenting the patient's response, write it verbatim, and enclose it in quotation marks.
• *Current symptoms.* Find out about the onset of symptoms, their severity and persistence, and whether they occurred abruptly or insidiously. Compare the patient's condition with his normal level of function.
• *Psychiatric history.* Discuss past psychiatric disturbances, such as episodes of delusions, violence, attempted suicides, drug or alcohol abuse, or depression, and previous psychiatric treatment.
• *Demographic data.* Determine the patient's age, sex, ethnic origin, primary language, birthplace, religion, and marital status. Use this information to establish a baseline and validate the patient's record.
• *Socioeconomic data.* Patients who are experiencing economic or personal hardships are more likely to show symptoms of distress during an illness. Information about your patient's educational level, housing

COMMUNICATION BARRIERS

Ineffective communication can prevent a successful interview.

Language difficulties or differences
If the patient speaks English, try to use language that's appropriate to his educational level. Avoid medical terms that he may not understand.

If the patient speaks a foreign language or an ethnic dialect, an interpreter can help you communicate. But remember that the presence of a third person may make the patient less willing to share his feelings.

Be aware of words that can have more than one meaning. For instance, the word "bad" also can be used as slang to mean "good."

Inappropriate responses
Inadvertently, your responses to the patient could suggest disinterest, anxiety, or annoyance. Or they could imply value judgments. Examples include abruptly changing the subject or discounting the patient's feelings.

Hearing loss
If the patient can't hear you clearly, he may misinterpret your responses. If you're interviewing a patient with impaired hearing, check whether he's wearing a hearing aid. If so, is it turned on? If not, can he read lips? If possible, face him and speak clearly and slowly, using common words and keeping your questions short, simple, and direct.

If the patient is elderly, use a low tone of voice. With aging, the ability to hear high-pitched tones deteriorates first. If the patient's hearing impairment is severe, he may have to communicate by writing, or you may need to collect information from his family or friends.

Thought disorders
If the patient's thought patterns are incoherent or irrelevant, he may be unable to interpret messages correctly, focus on the interview, or provide appropriate responses.

When assessing such a patient, ask simple questions about concrete topics and clarify his responses. Encourage him to express himself clearly.

Paranoid thinking
When dealing with a paranoid patient, approach him in a nonthreatening way. Avoid touching him because he may misinterpret your touch as an attempt to harm him. Also, keep in mind that he may not mean the things he says.

Hallucinations
A hallucinating patient experiences imaginary sensory perceptions with no basis in reality. These distortions prevent him from hearing and responding appropriately.

Show concern if the patient is hallucinating, but don't reinforce his perceptions. Be as specific as possible when you give him commands. For instance, if he says he's hearing voices, tell him to stop listening to the voices and listen to you instead.

Delusions
A deluded patient defends irrational beliefs or ideas despite factual evidence to the contrary. Some delusions may be so bizarre that you'll immediately recognize them; others may be difficult to identify.

Don't condemn or agree with a patient's delusional beliefs, and don't dismiss a statement because you think it's delusional. Instead, gently emphasize reality without being argumentative.

Delirium
A delirious patient experiences disorientation, hallucinations, and confusion. Misinterpretation and inappropriate responses often result.

Talk directly to such a patient and ask simple questions. Offer frequent reassurance.

Dementia
The patient who suffers dementia—an irreversible deterioration of mental capacity—may experience changes in memory and thought patterns, and his language may become distorted or slurred.

When interviewing such a patient, minimize distractions. Use simple and concise language. Avoid making any statements that could be easily misinterpreted.

conditions, income, current employment status, and family may provide clues to his current problem.
• *Cultural and religious beliefs.* Determine the patient's background and values because they will affect his response to illness and his adaptation to hospital care. Remember that certain questions and behaviors considered inappropriate in one culture may be sanctioned in another.

• *Medication history.* Certain drugs can cause symptoms of mental illness. Review any medications the patient may be taking, including over-the-counter drugs, and check for interactions. If he's taking an antipsychotic, antidepressant, anxiolytic, or antimanic, ask if his symptoms have improved, if he's taking the medication as prescribed, and if he has experienced any adverse reactions.

COPING MECHANISMS DEFINED

Coping, or defense, mechanisms help to relieve anxiety. The most common ones are defined in the glossary below.
• *Denial.* Refusal to admit truth or reality.
• *Displacement.* Transference of an emotion from its original object to a substitute.
• *Fantasy.* Creation of unrealistic or improbable images to escape from daily pressures and responsibilities.
• *Identification.* Unconscious adoption of the personality characteristics, attitudes, values, and behavior of another person.
• *Projection.* Displacement of negative feelings onto another person.
• *Rationalization.* Substitution of acceptable reasons for the real or actual reasons motivating behavior.
• *Reaction formation.* Conduct in a manner opposite from the way the person feels.
• *Regression.* Return to behavior of an earlier, more comfortable time in life.
• *Repression.* Exclusion of unacceptable thoughts and feelings from the conscious mind, leaving them to operate in the subconscious.

• *Physical illnesses.* Find out if the patient has a history of medical disorders that may cause disorientation, distorted thought processes, depression, or other symptoms of mental illness. For instance, does he have a history of renal or hepatic failure, infection, thyroid disease, increased intracranial pressure, or a metabolic disorder?

Patient appearance, behavior, and mental status

Observe and record your assessment of the patient's appearance, behavior, mood, thought processes, cognitive function, coping mechanisms, and potential for self-destructive behavior.
• *General appearance.* The patient's appearance helps to indicate his emotional and mental status. Specifically, note his dress and grooming. Is his appearance clean and appropriate to his age, sex, and situation?

Is the patient's posture erect or slouched? Is his head lowered? What about his gait? Is it brisk, slow, shuffling, or unsteady? Does he walk normally? Note his facial expression. Does he look alert or does he stare blankly? Does he appear sad or angry? Does the patient maintain direct eye contact? Does he stare at you for long periods?
• *Behavior.* Note the patient's demeanor and overall attitude as well as any extraordinary behavior, such as

speaking to a person who isn't present. Also record mannerisms. Does he bite his nails, fidget, or pace? Does he display any tics or tremors? How does he respond to the interviewer? Is he cooperative, friendly, hostile, or indifferent?
• *Mood.* Does the patient appear excited or depressed? Is he crying, sweating, breathing heavily, or trembling? Ask him to describe his current feelings in concrete terms and to suggest possible reasons for these feelings. Note inconsistencies between body language and mood (such as smiling when discussing an anger-provoking situation).
• *Thought processes and cognitive function.* Evaluate the patient's orientation to time, place, and person, noting any confusion or disorientation. Look for delusions, hallucinations, obsessions, compulsions, fantasies, and daydreams.

Check the patient's attention span and ability to recall events, both distant and recent past. For example, to assess immediate recall, ask him to repeat a series of five or six names of objects. Test his intellectual functioning by asking him to add a series of numbers and his sensory perception and coordination by having him copy a simple drawing. Inappropriate responses to a hypothetical situation ("What would you do if you won the lottery?") can indicate impaired judgment. Keep in mind that the patient's cultural background and personal values will influence his answer.

Finally, assess the patient's degree of insight by asking if he understands the significance of his illness, the proposed treatment plan, and the effect it will have on his life.

Note any speech characteristics that may indicate altered thought processes, including minimal monosyllabic responses, irrelevant or illogical replies to questions, convoluted or excessively detailed speech, repetitive speech patterns, a flight of ideas, and sudden silence without an obvious reason.
• *Coping mechanisms.* The patient who's faced with a stressful situation may adopt coping or defense mechanisms—behaviors that operate on an unconscious level to protect the ego. Examples include denial, regression, displacement, projection, reaction formation, and fantasy (see *Coping mechanisms defined*). Look for an excessive reliance on these coping mechanisms.
• *Potential for self-destructive behavior.* Mentally healthy people may intentionally take death-defying risks, such as participating in dangerous sports. The risks taken by self-destructive patients, however, are not death-defying, but death-seeking.

Not all self-destructive behavior is suicidal in intent. Some patients engage in self-destructive behavior because it helps them feel alive. A patient who has lost touch with reality may cut or mutilate body parts to focus on physical pain, which may be less overwhelming than emotional distress.

Assess the patient for suicidal tendencies (see *Suicide's warning signs*), particularly if he reports signs and symptoms of depression. Not all such patients want to die; however, the incidence of suicide is higher in depressed patients than in patients with other diagnoses. Schizophrenic patients also may attempt suicide, responding to voices that command them to kill themselves. Unfortunately, recognizing suicide potential in these patients may be difficult.

Diagnostic tests
The laboratory tests, psychological tests, and EEG and brain imaging studies summarized below provide information about the patient's mental status and possible physical causes of his signs and symptoms.

Laboratory tests
Urinalysis, hemoglobin and hematocrit levels, serum electrolyte and serum glucose levels, and liver, kidney, and thyroid function tests screen for physical disorders that can cause psychiatric signs and symptoms. Toxicologic studies of blood and urine can detect the presence of many drugs, and current laboratory methods can quantify the blood levels of these drugs. Patients undergoing treatment with psychotherapeutic drugs may need routine toxicology screening to ensure that they aren't receiving a toxic dose (see *Toxicology screening,* page 8).

Psychological and mental status tests
These tests evaluate the patient's mood, personality, and mental status. Frequently used tests include the following:
• The *Mini–Mental State Examination* measures orientation, registration, recall, calculation, language, and graphomotor function.
• The *Cognitive Capacity Screening Examination* measures orientation, memory, calculation, and language.
• The *Cognitive Assessment Scale* measures orientation, general knowledge, mental ability, and psychomotor function.
• The *Global Deterioration Scale* assesses and stages primary degenerative dementia, based on orientation, memory, and neurologic function.

SUICIDE'S WARNING SIGNS

During the patient interview, be alert for the following signs of suicidal behavior:
• withdrawal and social isolation
• signs and symptoms of depression, which may include crying, fatigue, helplessness, poor concentration, reduced interest in sex and other activities, sadness, constipation, and weight loss
• farewells to friends and family
• putting affairs in order
• giving away prized possessions
• covert suicide messages and death wishes
• obvious suicide messages, such as "I'd be better off dead."

• The *Functional Dementia Scale* measures orientation, affect, and the ability to perform activities of daily living.
• The *Beck Depression Inventory* helps diagnose depression and determine its severity. This test may provide objective evidence of the need for treatment; it's also used to monitor the patient's response during treatment.
• The *Eating Attitudes Test* detects patterns that suggest an eating disorder.
• The *Minnesota Multiphasic Personality Inventory* helps assess personality traits and ego function in adolescents and adults. Test results include information on coping strategies, defenses, strengths, gender identification, and self-esteem. The test pattern may strongly suggest a diagnostic category, point to a suicide risk, or indicate the potential for violence.

EEG and brain imaging studies
To screen for brain abnormalities, the doctor may order tests that visualize electrical brain wave pattern disturbances or anatomic alterations.
• An *EEG* graphically records the brain's electrical activity. Abnormal results may indicate organic disease, psychotropic drug use, or certain psychological disorders.
• A *computed tomography (CT) scan* combines radiologic and computer analysis of tissue density to produce images of intracranial structures not readily seen on standard X-rays. This test can help detect brain contusions or calcifications, cerebral atrophy, hydrocephalus, inflammation, space-occupying lesions, and vascular abnormalities.
• A *magnetic resonance imaging (MRI) scan* is a noninvasive imaging technique. MRI localizes atomic nu-

TOXICOLOGY SCREENING

Toxic levels of certain drugs can be detected in blood, urine, or both.

Blood
- alcohol (ethyl, isopropyl, and methyl)
- ethchlorvynol (Placidyl)

Urine
- chlorpromazine (Thorazine)
- cocaine
- desmethyldoxepin (metabolite of doxepin)
- heroin (metabolized to and detected as morphine)
- imipramine (Tofranil)
- methadone
- morphine
- phencyclidine

Blood and urine
- acetaminophen
- amitriptyline (Elavil)
- amobarbital (Amytal)
- butabarbital (Butisol)
- butalbital (one component in Fiorinal)
- caffeine
- carisoprodol (Soma)

- chlordiazepoxide (Librium)
- codeine
- desipramine (Pertofrane)
- desmethyldiazepam (metabolite of diazepam)
- diazepam (Valium)
- diphenhydramine (Benadryl)
- doxepin (Sinequan)
- flurazepam (Dalmane)
- glutethimide (Doriden)
- ibuprofen (Motrin, Medipren)
- meperidine (Demerol)
- mephobarbital (Mebaral)
- meprobamate (Miltown, Equanil)
- methapyrilene
- methaqualone (Quaalude)
- methyprylon (Noludar)
- norpropoxyphene (metabolite of propoxyphene)
- nortriptyline (Aventyl)
- oxazepam (Serax)
- pentazocine (Talwin)
- pentobarbital (Nembutal)
- phenobarbital (Luminal)
- propoxyphene (Darvon)
- salicylates and their conjugates
- secobarbital (Seconal)
- talbutal (Lotusate)

clei that magnetically align and then fall out of alignment in response to a radio frequency pulse. In a process called precession, the MRI scanner records signals from nuclei as they realign; it then translates the signals into detailed pictures of body structures. Compared with conventional X-rays and CT scans, the MRI scan provides superior contrast of soft tissues and sharper differentiation of normal and abnormal tissues. The MRI scan also provides images of multiple planes, including sagittal and coronal views, in regions where bones usually interface.

• A *positron emission tomography (PET) scan* provides colorimetric information about the brain's metabolic activity by detecting how quickly tissues consume radioactive isotopes. PET scanning is a technique that's used mainly for diagnosing neuropsychiatric problems, such as Alzheimer's disease, and some mental illnesses.

DISORDERS OF INFANCY, CHILDHOOD, AND ADOLESCENCE

The disorders in this section include mental retardation and Down's syndrome, which are transmitted genetically; bulimia nervosa and anorexia nervosa, which mainly affect adolescents; tic disorders, which begin before age 21; and autism, a disorder that usually becomes apparent before age 3.

MENTAL RETARDATION

The American Association on Mental Retardation (AAMR) defines mental retardation as "significantly subaverage general intellectual function existing concurrently with deficits in adaptive behavior manifesting itself during the developmental period (before age 18)." An estimated 1% to 3% of the population is mentally retarded, demonstrating an IQ below 70 and an associated deficit in carrying out tasks required for personal independence.

Retardation commonly is accompanied by additional physical and emotional disorders that may constitute handicaps in themselves. Mental retardation places a significant burden on patients and their families, resulting in stress, frustration, and family problems.

Causes

The AAMR has grouped the causes of mental retardation into ten categories (see *Causes of mental retardation*). But a specific cause is identifiable in only 25% of retarded people and, of these, only 10% have the potential for cure through medical or surgical intervention. In the remaining 75%, predisposing factors, such as deficient prenatal or perinatal care, inadequate nutrition, poor social environment, and poor child-rearing practices, contribute significantly to mental retardation.

Prenatal screening for genetic defects (such as Tay-Sachs disease) and genetic counseling for families at risk for specific defects have reduced the incidence of genetically transmitted mental retardation.

Complications

Mental retardation poses a risk to patient safety and family integrity. For example, mentally retarded people are vulnerable to physical and mental abuse by others. The birth of a mentally retarded child can precipitate dysfunctional behaviors within the family, depending on the severity of the retardation, the amount of physical care required, and the family's financial resources and coping skills.

Assessment findings

The observable effects of mental retardation are deviations from normal adaptive behaviors, ranging from learning disabilities and uncontrollable behavior to severe cognitive and motor skill impairment. Such deviations may be present during infancy and early childhood or, in mild retardation, not until school age or later. The earlier a child's adaptive deficit is recognized and he's placed in a special learning program, the more likely he is to achieve age-appropriate adaptive behaviors.

If the patient is older, review his adaptation to his environment, especially if he's in a group-living situation.

The family of a mentally retarded patient may report a multitude of problems, stemming from frustration, fear, and exhaustion. These problems, such as finan-

CAUSES OF MENTAL RETARDATION

Possible causative factors in mental retardation include the following:
• chromosomal abnormalities (Down's syndrome, Klinefelter's syndrome)
• disorders resulting from unknown prenatal influences (hydrocephalus, hydranencephaly, microcephaly)
• disorders of metabolism or nutrition (phenylketonuria, hypothyroidism, Hurler syndrome, galactosemia, Tay-Sachs disease)
• environmental influences (cultural-familial retardation, poor nutrition, lack of medical care)
• gestational disorders (prematurity)
• gross brain disorders that develop after birth (neurofibromatosis, intracranial neoplasm)
• infection and intoxication (congenital rubella, syphilis, lead poisoning, meningitis, encephalitis, insecticides, drugs, maternal viral infection, toxins)
• psychiatric disorders (autism)
• trauma or physical agents (mechanical injury, asphyxia, hyperpyrexia).

cial difficulties, abuse, and divorce, can compromise the child's care. Examination may reveal signs of abuse or neglect.

Mentally retarded people may exhibit signs and symptoms of other disorders, such as cleft lip, congenital heart defects, and cerebral palsy, as well as a lowered resistance to infection.

Diagnostic tests

A score below 70 on a standardized IQ test confirms mental retardation. The recognized levels of mental retardation are as follows:
• mild retardation, IQ 55 to 69
• moderate retardation, IQ 40 to 54
• severe retardation, IQ 25 to 39
• profound retardation, IQ less than 25.
These ranges of IQ scores may differ slightly, depending on the IQ test used. The IQ test primarily predicts school performance and must be supplemented by other diagnostic evaluations.

For example, the Adaptive Behavior Scale, a test that deals with behaviors important to activities of daily living, determines the patient's adaptive profile. This test evaluates self-help skills (toileting and eating), physical and social development, language, socialization, and time and number concepts. It also examines inappropriate behaviors (such as violent or destructive acts, withdrawal, and self-abusive or sexually aberrant behavior).

Age-appropriate adaptive behaviors are assessed by the use of developmental screening tests, such as the Denver Developmental Screening test. These tests compare the subject's functional level with the normal level for the same chronologic age. The greater the discrepancy between chronologic and developmental age, the more severe the retardation.

In children, the functional level rests on sensory motor skills, self-help skills, and socialization. In adolescents and adults, it rests on academic skills, reasoning and judgment skills, and social skills. Continuing assessment and review of development are essential for effective management.

Treatment
Effective management of a mentally retarded patient requires an interdisciplinary team approach that provides complete, continuous, and coordinated services. A primary goal is to develop the patient's strengths as fully as possible, taking into account his interests, personal experiences, and resources. Another major goal is the development of social adaptive skills to help the patient function as normally as possible.

Mentally retarded children require special education and training, ideally beginning in infancy. An individualized, effective education program can optimize the quality of life for even the profoundly retarded.

The prognosis for people with mental retardation is related more to timing and aggressive treatment, personal motivation, training opportunities, and associated conditions than to the mental retardation itself. With good support systems, many mentally retarded people become productive members of society. Successful management leads to independent functioning and occupational skills for some and a sheltered environment for others.

Nursing diagnoses
• Altered growth and development
• Altered health maintenance
• Family coping: Potential for growth
• Functional incontinence
• Knowledge deficit
• Powerlessness
• Risk for injury
• Self-care deficit

Nursing interventions
• Support the parents of a child diagnosed with mental retardation. Not only may they be overwhelmed by caretaking and financial concerns, but they also may have difficulty accepting and bonding with their child.
• Remember that the mentally retarded child has all the ordinary needs of a normal child plus those created by his handicap. The child especially needs affection, acceptance, stimulation, and prudent, consistent discipline; he is less able to cope if rejected, overprotected, or forced beyond his abilities.
• When caring for a hospitalized retarded patient, promote continuity of care by acting as a liaison for parents and other health care professionals involved in his care.
• During hospitalization, continue training programs already in place, but remember that illness may bring on some regression in behavior and skills.
• For the severely retarded child, suggest ways for parents to cope with the guilt, frustration, and exhaustion that often accompany caring for such a child. In particular, parents of a severely retarded child need an extensive teaching and discharge planning program, including physical care procedures, stress reduction techniques, support services, and referral to developmental programs. As needed, request a social service consultation to investigate community resources available to assist the family.

Patient teaching
• Teach parents how to care for the special needs of the retarded child. Suggest that they contact the AAMR and the Association for Retarded Citizens for more information and referral to sources of community support.
• Teach retarded adolescents how to deal with physical changes and sexual maturation. Encourage participation in appropriate sex education classes. Keep in mind that the retarded person may experience difficulty in expressing his sexual concerns because of limited verbal skills.

DOWN'S SYNDROME
The first disorder attributed to a chromosomal aberration, Down's syndrome (also known as mongolism and trisomy 21 syndrome) characteristically produces mental retardation, abnormal facial features, and other distinctive physical abnormalities. It's commonly associated with heart defects and other congenital disorders.

Life expectancy and quality for patients with Down's syndrome have increased significantly because of improved treatment of related complications and better developmental education programs. Nevertheless, up to 44% of patients who have congenital heart disease die before they're 1 year old.

Overall, Down's syndrome occurs in 1 per 800 to 1,000 live births, but the incidence increases with maternal age, especially after age 35. For instance, at age 20, a mother has about one chance in 2,000 of having a child with Down's syndrome; by age 49, she has one chance in 12. Although women over age 35 account for fewer than 8% of all births, they bear 20% of all children with Down's syndrome.

Causes

Down's syndrome usually results from trisomy 21, an aberration in which chromosome 21 has three copies instead of the normal two because of faulty meiosis (nondisjunction) of the ovum or, sometimes, the sperm. This results in a karyotype of 47 chromosomes instead of the normal 46.

Although the incidence of nondisjunction increases with maternal age, the extra chromosome originates from the mother only 80% of the time. Studies suggest that in some cases, the chromosomal abnormality results from deterioration of the oocyte. Such degeneration can be caused by age or the cumulative effects of environmental factors, such as radiation and viruses. About 4% of the time, Down's syndrome results from an unbalanced translocation in which the long arm of chromosome 21 breaks and attaches to another chromosome.

Complications

Mortality is high in the fetus and neonate. Early death usually results from complications precipitated by associated congenital heart defects. If the patient survives to adulthood, premature senile dementia, similar to Alzheimer's disease, usually occurs in the fourth decade. An increased incidence of leukemia, acute and chronic infections, diabetes mellitus, and thyroid disorders is common.

Assessment findings

The physical signs of Down's syndrome are readily apparent at birth. The neonate is lethargic and a poor feeder. Inspection reveals craniofacial anomalies, such as slanting, almond-shaped eyes (epicanthal folds); a protruding tongue; a small, open mouth; a single transverse palmar crease (simian crease); small white spots (Brushfield's spots) on the iris; a small skull; a flat bridge across the nose; a flattened face; small external ears; and a short neck with excess skin.

Other physical abnormalities include dry, sensitive skin with decreased elasticity, umbilical hernia, short stature, and short extremities with broad, flat, and squarish hands and feet. The patient's hands have a dysplastic middle phalanx of the fifth finger, and his feet have a wide space between the first and second toes. Fingerprints and footprints are abnormal. Hypotonic limb muscles impair reflex development.

Examination reveals an absent Moro reflex and hyperextensible joints. The patient's posture, coordination, and balance are impaired. In many cases, a child with Down's syndrome also has congenital heart disease (septal defects or pulmonary or aortic stenosis), duodenal obstruction (from atresia, stenosis, or annular pancreas), clubfoot, imperforate anus, cleft lip and palate, Hirschsprung's disease, meningomyelocele, and pelvic bone abnormalities.

As the child grows, dental development is slow, with abnormal or absent teeth. He also exhibits strabismus and, occasionally, cataracts. The genitalia develop poorly, and puberty is delayed. The female with Down's syndrome may menstruate and be fertile. The male is infertile with low serum testosterone levels; in many, the testes fail to descend.

Patients with Down's syndrome have an IQ between 30 and 50; however, social performance usually is beyond that expected for their mental age. Intellectual development slows with age.

Diagnostic tests

A karyotype showing the chromosomal abnormality confirms the diagnosis of Down's syndrome. Other tests can reveal Down's syndrome before birth. For example, prenatal ultrasonography can suggest Down's syndrome if a duodenal obstruction or an atrioventricular canal defect is present. Reduced levels of alpha-fetoprotein may indicate Down's syndrome. A simple blood test for alpha-fetoprotein is routinely offered to most pregnant women.

Amniocentesis also allows prenatal diagnosis; 80% of all amniocenteses are done for this purpose and are recommended for pregnant women past age 35. Amniocentesis is indicated for a pregnant woman of any age when either she or the father carries a translocated chromosome.

Additional medical tests confirm the presence of associated conditions. Developmental screening tests, such as the Denver Developmental Screening test, determine the severity of retardation and chart the patient's progress in response to intervention or education programs.

Treatment

Surgery to correct cardiac defects and other related congenital abnormalities, antibiotic therapy for recurrent infections, and thyroid hormone replacement for hypothyroidism have improved life expectancy considerably for patients with Down's syndrome. Plastic surgery may correct the characteristic facial traits, especially the protruding tongue, cleft lip, and cleft palate. Benefits beyond improved appearance may include improved speech, reduced susceptibility to dental caries, and fewer orthodontic problems later.

Parents of Down's syndrome children are encouraged to keep their children at home whenever possible. Early intervention (such as infant stimulation programs) increases sensory awareness and has proved helpful with some patients. Special education programs, mandated in most communities, permit the child to maximize his potential and promote self-esteem. His physical condition and self-image also can benefit from special athletic programs. As adults, many Down's syndrome patients have become productive workers at jobs that match their intellectual abilities.

Nursing diagnoses

• Altered family processes
• Altered growth and development
• Altered parenting
• Ineffective family coping
• Knowledge deficit
• Risk for injury
• Self-care deficit
• Self-esteem disturbance

Nursing interventions

• Establish a trusting relationship with the child's parents, and encourage communication during the difficult period soon after diagnosis. Recognize signs of grieving.
• Encourage the parents to hold and nurture their child.
• Refer the parents and older siblings for genetic and psychological counseling, as appropriate, to help them evaluate future risks and develop coping skills.
• Refer the parents to national Down's syndrome organizations and other community resources.

Patient teaching

• Emphasize the importance of adequate exercise and maximal environmental stimulation. Refer the parents to infant stimulation classes, which may begin in the early months of life.
• Assist the parents in setting realistic goals for their child. Although his mental development may seem normal at first, warn the parents not to view this early development as a sign of future progress. By the time the child is 1 year old, his development clearly will lag behind that of normal children. Help the parents view their child's achievements in a positive light.
• Teach the parents the importance of a balanced diet. Stress the need for patience while feeding their child, who may have more difficulty sucking, be less demanding, and seem less eager to eat than normal babies.
• Advise the parents to remember the emotional needs of other children in the family.

BULIMIA NERVOSA

The essential features of bulimia nervosa include eating binges followed by feelings of guilt, humiliation, and self-deprecation. These feelings precipitate the patient's engaging in self-induced vomiting, the use of laxatives or diuretics, or strict dieting or fasting to overcome the effects of the binges. Unless the patient devotes an excessive amount of time to binging and purging, bulimia nervosa seldom is incapacitating.

Bulimia nervosa usually begins in adolescence or early adulthood and can occur simultaneously with anorexia nervosa. It affects nine females for every one male. Between 1% and 3% of adolescent and young women meet the diagnostic criteria for bulimia nervosa; 5% to 15% have some symptoms of the disorder.

Causes

The exact cause of bulimia is unknown, but various psychosocial factors are thought to contribute to its development. Such factors include family disturbance or conflict, sexual abuse, maladaptive learned behavior, struggle for control or self-identity, cultural overemphasis on physical appearance, and parental obesity. Bulimia nervosa is strongly associated with depression.

Complications

The repetitive vomiting in bulimia nervosa can result in dental caries, erosion of tooth enamel, and gum infections. Electrolyte imbalances (including metabolic alkalosis, hypochloremia, and hypokalemia) or dehydration can occur, increasing the risk of serious physical complications—such as arrhythmias—or even sudden death. Ipecac syrup intoxication can cause cardiac failure in patients who rely on this drug to induce vomiting. Rare complications include esophageal tears and gastric ruptures.

Suicide is a potential psychiatric complication of bulimia nervosa. In addition, bulimic patients are more prone to psychoactive substance use disorders.

Assessment findings

The history of a patient with bulimia nervosa is characterized by episodic binge eating that may occur up to several times a day. The patient commonly reports a binge-eating episode during which she continues eating until abdominal pain, sleep, or the presence of another person interrupts it. The preferred food usually is sweet, soft, and high in calories and carbohydrate content.

The bulimic patient may appear thin or slightly overweight. Typically, however, although the patient's weight frequently fluctuates, it usually stays within the normal range—through the use of diuretics, laxatives, vomiting, and exercise. So, unlike the anorexic patient, the bulimic patient usually can keep her eating disorder hidden.

Overt clues to this disorder include hyperactivity, peculiar eating habits or rituals, frequent weighing, and a distorted body image (see *Characteristics of bulimic patients*).

The patient may complain of abdominal and epigastric pain caused by acute gastric dilation. Amenorrhea also may be present. Repetitive vomiting may cause painless swelling of the salivary glands, hoarseness, throat irritation or lacerations, and dental erosion. In addition, the patient may exhibit calluses of the knuckles or abrasions and scars on the dorsum of the hand, resulting from tooth injury during self-induced vomiting.

A bulimic patient commonly is perceived by others as a "perfect" student, mother, or career woman; an adolescent may be distinguished for participation in competitive activities, such as gymnastics, sports, or ballet. However, the patient's psychosocial history may reveal an exaggerated sense of guilt, symptoms of depression, childhood trauma (especially sexual abuse), parental obesity, or a history of unsatisfactory sexual relationships.

CHARACTERISTICS OF BULIMIC PATIENTS

Recognizing the bulimic patient isn't always easy. Unlike anorexic patients, bulimic patients don't deny that their eating habits are abnormal, but they commonly conceal their behavior out of shame and humiliation. If you suspect bulimia nervosa, be on the lookout for the following psychological features:
• difficulties with impulse control
• chronic depression
• exaggerated sense of guilt
• low tolerance for frustration
• recurrent anxiety
• feelings of alienation
• self-consciousness
• difficulty expressing feelings, such as anger
• impaired social or occupational adjustment.

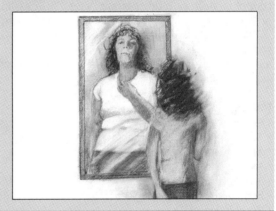

Diagnostic criteria

Diagnosis of bulimia nervosa can be confirmed when the patient meets the *DSM-IV* criteria for this disorder: recurrent episodes of binge eating (rapid consumption of a large amount of food in a discrete period of time) and repeated inappropriate behaviors to prevent weight gain (such as self-induced vomiting, laxative abuse, and fasting) that occur, on average, twice a week for 3 months.

The Beck Depression Inventory may identify coexisting depression.

Laboratory tests can help determine the presence and severity of complications. Serum electrolyte studies may show elevated bicarbonate, decreased potassium, and decreased sodium levels.

A baseline electrocardiogram may be done if tricyclic antidepressants will be prescribed.

Treatment

Treatment of bulimia nervosa may continue for several years. Interrelated physical and psychological symptoms must be treated simultaneously. Merely promoting weight gain isn't sufficient to guarantee long-term recovery. A patient whose physical status is severely compromised by inadequate or chaotic eating patterns is difficult to engage in the psychotherapeutic process.

Psychotherapy focuses on breaking the binge-purge cycle and helping the patient regain control over eating behavior. Treatment may occur in either an inpatient or outpatient setting. It includes behavior modification therapy, possibly in highly structured psychoeducational group meetings. Individual psychotherapy and family therapy, which address the eating disorder as a symptom of unresolved conflict, may help the patient understand the basis of her behavior and teach her self-control strategies. Antidepressant drugs, such as imipramine, may be used to supplement psychotherapy.

The patient also may benefit from participation in self-help groups, such as Overeaters Anonymous, or in a drug rehabilitation program if she has a concurrent substance abuse problem.

Nursing diagnoses

- Altered family processes
- Altered nutrition: Less than body requirements
- Altered oral mucous membrane
- Altered parenting
- Anxiety
- Body image disturbance
- Chronic low self-esteem
- Constipation
- Denial
- Fluid volume deficit
- Hyperthermia
- Impaired social interaction
- Ineffective family coping
- Ineffective individual coping
- Powerlessness
- Sleep pattern disturbance
- Social isolation

Nursing interventions

- Supervise the patient during mealtimes and for a specified period after meals, usually 1 hour. Set a time limit for each meal. Provide a pleasant, relaxed environment for eating.
- Using behavior modification techniques, reward the patient for satisfactory weight gain.

- Establish a contract with the patient, specifying the amount and type of food to be eaten at each meal.
- Encourage the patient to recognize and verbalize her feelings about her eating behavior. Provide an accepting and nonjudgmental atmosphere, controlling your reactions to her behavior and feelings.
- Encourage the patient to talk about stressful issues, such as achievement, independence, socialization, sexuality, family problems, and control.
- Identify the patient's elimination patterns.
- Assess the patient's suicide potential.
- Refer the patient and her family to the American Anorexia/Bulimia Association and to Anorexia Nervosa and Related Eating Disorders as sources of additional information and support.

Patient teaching

- Teach the patient how to keep a food journal to monitor treatment progress.
- Outline the risks of laxative, emetic, and diuretic abuse for the patient.
- Provide assertiveness training to help the patient gain control over her behavior and achieve a realistic and positive self-image.
- If the patient is taking a prescribed tricyclic antidepressant, instruct her to take the drug with food. Warn her to avoid consuming alcoholic beverages; exposing herself to sunlight, heat lamps, or tanning beds; and discontinuing the medication unless she has notified the doctor.

ANOREXIA NERVOSA

The key feature of anorexia nervosa is self-imposed starvation resulting from a distorted body image and an intense and irrational fear of gaining weight, even when the patient is obviously emaciated. An anorexic patient is preoccupied with her body size, describes herself as "fat," and commonly expresses dissatisfaction with a particular aspect of her physical appearance. Although the term *anorexia* suggests that the patient's weight loss is associated with a loss of appetite, this is rare.

Anorexia nervosa and bulimia nervosa can occur simultaneously. In anorexia nervosa, the refusal to eat may be accompanied by compulsive exercising, self-induced vomiting, or abuse of laxatives or diuretics.

Anorexia occurs in 5% to 10% of the population; over 90% of those affected are females. This disorder occurs primarily in adolescents and young adults but also may affect older women and, occasionally, males.

The prognosis varies but improves if the patient is diagnosed early or if she wants to overcome the disorder and seeks help voluntarily. Mortality ranges from 5% to 15% — the highest mortality associated with a psychiatric disturbance. One-third of these deaths can be attributed to suicide.

Causes

No one knows exactly what causes anorexia nervosa. Researchers in neuroendocrinology are seeking a physiologic cause but have found nothing definite. Clearly, social attitudes that equate slimness with beauty play some role in provoking this disorder; family factors also are implicated. Most theorists believe that refusing to eat is a subconscious effort to exert personal control over life.

Complications

Serious medical complications can result from the malnutrition, dehydration, and electrolyte imbalances caused by prolonged starvation, vomiting, or laxative abuse. For example, malnutrition may cause hypoalbuminemia and subsequent edema or hypokalemia, leading to ventricular arrhythmias and renal failure. Poor nutrition and dehydration, coupled with laxative abuse, produce changes in the bowel similar to those in chronic inflammatory bowel disease. Frequent vomiting can cause esophageal erosion, ulcers, tears, and bleeding, as well as tooth and gum erosion and dental caries.

Cardiovascular complications can be life-threatening and include decreased left ventricular muscle mass, chamber size, and myocardial oxygen uptake; reduced cardiac output; hypotension; bradycardia; electrocardiographic changes, such as nonspecific ST interval, T-wave changes, and prolonged PR interval; heart failure; and sudden death, possibly caused by ventricular arrhythmias. Anorexia nervosa also may increase susceptibility to infection.

Amenorrhea may occur when the patient loses about 25% of her normal body weight. It usually is associated with anemia. Possible complications of prolonged amenorrhea include estrogen deficiency (increasing the risk of calcium deficiency and osteoporosis) and infertility. Normal menses usually return when the patient weighs at least 95% of her normal weight.

Assessment findings

The patient's history usually reveals a 15% or greater weight loss for no organic reason, coupled with a morbid dread of being fat and a compulsion to be thin. The anorexic patient tends to be angry and ritualistic. She may report amenorrhea, infertility, loss of libido, fatigue, sleep alterations, intolerance to cold, and constipation.

Hypotension and bradycardia may be present. Inspection may reveal an emaciated appearance, with skeletal muscle atrophy, loss of fatty tissue, atrophy of breast tissue, blotchy or sallow skin, lanugo on the face and body, and dryness or loss of scalp hair. Calluses of the knuckles and abrasions and scars on the dorsum of the hand may result from tooth injury during self-induced vomiting. Other signs of vomiting include dental caries and oral or pharyngeal abrasions.

Palpation may disclose painless salivary gland enlargement and bowel distention. Slowed reflexes may occur on percussion. Oddly, the patient usually demonstrates restless activity and vigor (despite undernourishment) and may exercise avidly without apparent fatigue.

During psychosocial assessment, the anorexic patient may express a morbid fear of gaining weight and an obsession with her physical appearance. Paradoxically, she also may be obsessed with food, preparing elaborate meals for others. Social regression, including poor sexual adjustment and fear of failure, is common. Like bulimia nervosa, anorexia nervosa often is associated with depression. The patient may report feelings of despair, hopelessness, and worthlessness as well as suicidal thoughts.

Diagnostic criteria

A diagnosis of anorexia nervosa is confirmed when the patient meets the following criteria documented in the *DSM-IV*:
• refusal to maintain body weight over a minimal normal weight for age and height (for instance, weight loss leading to maintenance of body weight 15% below that expected); or failure to achieve expected weight gain during a period of growth, leading to body weight 15% below that expected
• intense fear of gaining weight or becoming fat, even though underweight
• disturbance in perception of body weight, size, or shape (that is, the person claims to feel fat even when emaciated or believes that one body area is too fat even when obviously underweight)
• in females, absence of at least three consecutive menstrual cycles when otherwise expected to occur.

In addition, laboratory tests reveal clinical status and help to rule out endocrine, metabolic, and central nervous system abnormalities; cancer; malabsorption

CRITERIA FOR HOSPITALIZING ANOREXIC PATIENTS

Anorexic patients can be successfully treated on an outpatient basis. But if the patient displays any of the signs listed below, hospitalization is mandatory:
• rapid weight loss equal to 15% or more of normal body mass
• persistent bradycardia (50 beats/minute or less)
• hypotension with a systolic reading less than or equal to 90 mm Hg
• hypothermia (core body temperature less than or equal to 97° F [36.1° C])
• presence of medical complications
• suicidal ideation
• persistent sabotage or disruption of outpatient treatment
• resolute denial of condition and the need for treatment.

syndrome; and other disorders that cause physical wasting.

Abnormal findings that may accompany a weight loss greater than 30% of normal body weight include:
• low hemoglobin level, platelet count, and white blood cell count
• prolonged bleeding time due to thrombocytopenia
• decreased erythrocyte sedimentation rate
• decreased levels of serum creatinine, blood urea nitrogen, uric acid, cholesterol, total protein, albumin, sodium, potassium, chloride, calcium, and fasting blood glucose (resulting from malnutrition)
• elevated levels of alanine aminotransferase (formerly SGPT) and aspartate aminotransferase (formerly SGOT) in severe starvation states
• elevated serum amylase levels when pancreatitis is not present
• in females, decreased levels of serum luteinizing hormone and follicle-stimulating hormone
• decreased triiodothyronine levels, resulting from a lower basal metabolic rate
• dilute urine caused by an impairment in the kidneys' ability to concentrate urine
• nonspecific ST interval, T-wave changes, and prolonged PR interval on the electrocardiogram. Ventricular arrhythmias also may be present.

Treatment

Appropriate treatment aims to promote weight gain or control the patient's compulsive binge eating and purg-

ing and to correct malnutrition and the underlying psychological dysfunction. Hospitalization in a medical or psychiatric unit may be required to improve the patient's precarious physical state. (See *Criteria for hospitalizing anorexic patients*.) Hospitalization may be as brief as 2 weeks or may stretch from a few months to 2 years or longer.

A team approach to care—combining aggressive medical management, nutritional counseling, and individual, group, or family psychotherapy or behavior modification therapy—is the best approach. Treatment is difficult and results may be discouraging. Many clinical centers are now developing inpatient and outpatient programs specifically for managing eating disorders.

Treatment may include behavior modification (privileges depend on weight gain); curtailed activity for physical reasons (such as arrhythmias); vitamin and mineral supplements; a reasonable diet, with or without liquid supplements; subclavian, peripheral, or enteral hyperalimentation (enteral and peripheral routes carry less risk of infection); and group, family, or individual psychotherapy. (See *Planning effective care in anorexia nervosa*.)

All forms of psychotherapy, from psychoanalysis to hypnotherapy, have been used in treating anorexia nervosa, with varying success. To be successful, psychotherapy should address the underlying problems of low self-esteem, guilt, and anxiety; feelings of hopelessness and helplessness; and depression.

Nursing diagnoses
• Activity intolerance
• Altered family processes
• Altered growth and development
• Altered nutrition: Less than body requirements
• Altered oral mucous membrane
• Altered parenting
• Anxiety
• Body image disturbance
• Chronic low self-esteem
• Constipation
• Denial
• Fluid volume deficit
• Hyperthermia
• Ineffective family coping
• Ineffective individual coping
• Noncompliance
• Powerlessness
• Social isolation

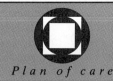

Plan of care

PLANNING EFFECTIVE CARE IN ANOREXIA NERVOSA

How would you go about identifying nursing diagnoses and planning, implementing, and evaluating care for an anorexic patient? To prepare for such a challenge, consider that you're caring for Ruth Howard, a 17-year-old high school junior.

Ruth has lived with her mother since her parents' divorce 3 years ago. An honor student, she is also a member of the track team.

Ruth's father often neglects to send child support payments. To make ends meet, her mother took on a second job 6 months ago. She depends on Ruth to help care for her younger brothers, clean the house, and prepare meals.

Three days ago, Ruth fainted in class. Today, she has come for an examination to determine why.

Patient history
Mrs. Howard is frantic. "I don't know what I'll do if there's anything wrong with Ruthie," she tells you. "I couldn't manage without her." But for all her concern, she has failed to notice that her daughter has lost 22 lb (10 kg) over the past 2 months.

Ruth downplays the fainting episode. "I feel fine now," she insists. "I was just up too late studying." She appears anxious and upset. Despite her recent weight loss, she describes herself as "fat" and asks if you can recommend a diet. "When I'm home with the kids I just pig out, but I don't have time to exercise enough," she says.

Physical assessment
You examine Ruth and find that she's 5'8" and weighs only 102 lb (46.3 kg). Her skin is sallow, and her hair dry and limp. Her blood

pressure is 90/65 mm Hg; her pulse rate, 32 beats/minute.

Ruth reveals that she hasn't menstruated for 2 months. Although easily fatigued, she has trouble falling asleep.

Nursing diagnoses
From your assessment, you've learned that Ruth is extremely concerned about being overweight, despite a recent loss of more than 20 lb (9 kg). When considered along with her physical condition, this obsession points to anorexia nervosa. Her considerable stress has probably worsened her eating problems.

Based on your assessment findings, you arrive at the following nursing diagnoses:
• Altered nutrition: Less than body requirements, related to morbid fear of gaining weight
• Body image disturbance related to false perception of body fat
• Self-esteem disturbance related to inability to meet perceived responsibilities
• Ineffective individual coping related to situational crisis.

Expected outcomes
To improve Ruth's nutritional status, help her identify unresolved problems, and develop more effective coping skills, you set the following goals. She must:
• increase her food intake to adequate levels while reducing her caloric expenditure
• regain normal body weight
• learn the complications of malnutrition and their prevention
• improve her self-esteem
• eliminate the association between food, stress, and anger
• use more effective coping skills, such as talking things over with a favorite teacher.

Implementation
To implement the care plan, you'll take the following steps:
• During Ruth's hospital stay, monitor her vital signs, intake and output, and laboratory test results. Assess for dehydration and metabolic and nutritional alterations.
• Set up a strict eating plan for Ruth. Weigh her daily in the same clothes, on the same scale, at the same time, and before she voids. Allow only supervised exercise.
• Emphasize consequences of Ruth's failure to follow her eating plan (such as not being able to make phone calls).
• Encourage Ruth to express her feelings. Discuss ways to alleviate stress. Praise her accomplishments.
• Review Ruth's coping strategies, and teach her methods for working out her problems.
• Assess the need for family intervention. Explore Ruth's feelings about family members.
• Observe how Ruth and her mother interact. Identify any deficits in parenting skills.
• Discuss the need for family therapy with the doctor or psychiatric clinical nurse specialist.

Evaluation
Ruth will resume healthy eating patterns and regain the weight she has lost. She'll describe the medical consequences of self-enforced starvation and outline her plans for preventing them through adequate nutrition balanced with moderate amounts of exercise. She'll discuss methods for relieving anxiety and solving personal problems that don't involve food or excessive weight loss.

Further measures
Later, evaluate Ruth's adherence to the treatment plan. Encourage her to verbalize her concerns about her family life and her future.

CLASSIFYING TICS

According to the *DSM-IV*, motor and vocal tics are classified as simple or complex. However, the boundaries of these categories remain unclear. In addition, combinations of tics may occur simultaneously.

Motor tics
Simple motor tics include eye blinking, neck jerking, shoulder shrugging, head banging, head turning, tongue protrusion, lip or tongue biting, nail biting, hair pulling, and facial grimacing.
    Some examples of *complex motor tics* are facial gestures, grooming behaviors, hitting or biting oneself, jumping, hopping, touching, squatting, deep knee bends, retracing steps, twirling when walking, stamping, smelling an object, and imitating the movements of someone who is being observed (echopraxia).

Vocal tics
Examples of *simple vocal tics* include coughing, throat clearing, grunting, sniffing, snorting, hissing, clicking, yelping, and barking.
    Complex vocal tics may involve repeating words out of context; using socially unacceptable words, many of which are obscene (coprolalia); or repeating the last-heard sound, word, or phase of another person (echolalia).

Nursing interventions
• During hospitalization, regularly monitor vital signs, nutritional status, and intake and output. Weigh the patient daily—before breakfast if possible. Because the patient fears being weighed, vary the weighing routine. Keep in mind that weight should increase from morning to night.
• Help the patient establish a target weight, and support her efforts to achieve this goal.
• Negotiate an adequate food intake with the patient. Be sure that she understands that she'll need to comply with this contract or lose privileges. Frequently offer small portions of food or drinks if the patient wants them. Allow the patient to maintain control over the types and amounts of food eaten, if possible.
• Maintain one-on-one supervision of the patient during meals and for 1 hour afterward to ensure compliance with the dietary treatment program. For the hospitalized anorexic patient, food is considered a medication.
• During an acute anorexic episode, nutritionally complete liquids are more acceptable because they eliminate the need to choose between foods—something the anorexic patient often finds difficult. If tube feedings or other special feeding measures become necessary, fully explain these measures to the patient and be ready to discuss her fears or reluctance; limit the discussion about food itself.
• Anticipate a weight gain of about 1 lb/week.
• If edema or bloating occurs after the patient has returned to normal eating behavior, reassure her that this phenomenon is temporary. She may fear that she is becoming fat and stop complying with the treatment plan.
• Encourage the patient to recognize and assert her feelings freely. If she understands that she can be assertive, she gradually may learn that expressing her true feelings will not result in her losing control or love.
• If a patient receiving outpatient treatment must be hospitalized, maintain contact with her treatment team to facilitate a smooth return to the outpatient setting.
• Remember that the anorexic patient uses exercise, preoccupation with food, ritualism, manipulation, and lying as mechanisms to preserve the only control she thinks that she has in her life.
• Because the patient and her family may need therapy to uncover and correct dysfunctional patterns, refer them to Anorexia Nervosa and Related Eating Disorders, a national information and support organization. This organization may help them understand what anorexia is, convince them that they need help, and help them find a psychotherapist or medical doctor who is experienced in treating this disorder.

Patient teaching
• Emphasize to the patient how improved nutrition can reverse the effects of starvation and prevent complications.
• Teach the patient how to keep a food journal, including the types of food eaten, eating frequency, and feelings associated with eating and exercise.
• Advise family members to avoid discussing food with the patient.

TIC DISORDERS
This group of three disorders includes Tourette syndrome, chronic motor or vocal tic disorder, and transient tic disorder. Although they're similar pathophysiologically, these disorders differ in severity and prognosis. (For information about related stress dis-

orders, see *Stress disorders with physical manifestations*, page 20.)

All tic disorders, commonly known simply as "tics," are involuntary, spasmodic, recurrent, and purposeless motor movements or vocalizations. These disorders are classified as motor or vocal and as simple or complex (see *Classifying tics*). Tics begin before age 18. The median age of onset for Tourette syndrome is age 7, but this disorder can occur as early as age 2. All tic disorders are three times more common in males than in females.

Transient tics usually are self-limiting, but Tourette syndrome follows a chronic course characterized by remissions and exacerbations.

Causes
Although their exact cause is unknown, tic disorders occur more frequently in certain families, suggesting a genetic cause. Tics commonly develop when a child experiences overwhelming anxiety, usually associated with normal maturation. Tics may be precipitated or exacerbated by the use of phenothiazines and central nervous system (CNS) stimulants or by head trauma.

Complications
The severe compulsive movements associated with Tourette syndrome can result in physical injury, including blindness subsequent to retinal detachment, orthopedic disorders, and dermatologic complications, or even self-mutilation. The patient also may experience impaired social, academic, or occupational functioning because of rejection by others or anxiety about the tics in social situations.

Assessment findings
Assessment findings vary according to the type of tic disorder. Inspection, coupled with the patient's history, may reveal the specific motor or vocal patterns that characterize the tic, as well as the frequency, complexity, and precipitating causes. The patient or his family may report that the tics occur sporadically many times a day.

Note whether certain situations exacerbate the tics. All tic disorders may be exacerbated by stress, and they usually diminish markedly during sleep. The patient also may report that they occur during activities that require concentration, such as reading or sewing.

Determine if the patient can control the tics. Although he may experience the tic as irresistible, most patients can, with conscious effort, control them for short periods.

Psychosocial assessment may reveal the underlying stressful factors that trigger the tic. In addition, problems with social adjustment, lack of self-esteem, and depression may be identified.

Diagnostic criteria
The diagnosis of a tic disorder is based on fulfillment of the criteria documented in the *DSM-IV*.

For *Tourette syndrome:*
• Both multiple motor and one or more vocal tics have been present at some time during the illness, although not necessarily concurrently.
• The tics occur many times over the course of a day (usually in bouts) nearly every day or intermittently for more than 1 year.
• Onset occurs before age 18.
• Occurrence is not exclusively during psychoactive substance intoxication or known CNS disease.

For *chronic motor or vocal tic disorder:*
• Either motor or vocal tics, but not both, have been present at some time during the illness.
• The tics occur many times a day nearly every day or intermittently for more than 1 year.
• Onset occurs before age 18.
• Occurrence is not exclusively during psychoactive substance intoxication or known CNS disease.

For *transient tic disorder:*
• Single or multiple motor or vocal tics, or both, are present.
• The tics occur many times a day nearly every day for at least 4 weeks, but for no longer than 12 consecutive months.
• The patient has no history of Tourette syndrome or chronic motor or vocal tic disorder.
• Onset occurs before age 18.
• Occurrence is not exclusively during psychoactive substance intoxication or known CNS disease.

All tic disorders cause marked distress or significant impairment in social, occupational, or other important areas of functioning.

Treatment
Effective treatment requires correction of the underlying psychopathology by identifying and resolving the sources of the patient's anxiety, stress, and intrapsychic conflict. Without correction of the underlying psychopathology, pressuring the patient to control the tics will be unsuccessful; he can do so only briefly, and then only with intense effort. Behavior modification techniques and operant conditioning have been suc-

STRESS DISORDERS WITH PHYSICAL MANIFESTATIONS

In addition to tic disorders, other stress-related disorders that produce physical signs in children include stuttering, functional enuresis, functional encopresis, sleepwalking, and sleep terrors.

Stuttering
This disorder, characterized by abnormalities of speech rhythms with repetitions and hesitations at the beginning of words, also may involve movements of the respiratory muscles, shoulders, and face.

Stuttering may be associated with mental dullness, poor social background, and a history of birth trauma. This disorder most commonly occurs in children of average or superior intelligence who fear they can't meet the expectations of socially striving, success-oriented families.

Related problems may include low self-esteem, tension, anxiety, humiliation, and withdrawal from social situations because of fear of stuttering.

About 80% of stutterers recover after age 16. Evaluation and treatment by a speech pathologist teaches the stutterer to place equal weight on each syllable in a sentence, to breathe properly, and to control anxiety.

Functional enuresis
This disorder is characterized by intentional or involuntary voiding of urine, usually during the night (nocturnal enuresis).

Considered normal in children until age 3 or 4, functional enuresis occurs in about 40% of children at this age and persists in 10% to age 5, in 5% to age 10, and in 1% of males to age 18. The disorder persists longer in males.

Causes may be related to stress in the child's life, such as the birth of a sibling, the move to a new home, divorce, separation, hospitalization, faulty toilet training (inconsistent, demanding, or punitive), and unrealistic responsibilities that are not age-appropriate.

Associated problems include low self-esteem, social withdrawal from peers because of ostracism and ridicule, and anger, rejection, and punishment by caregivers.

Advise parents to avoid punitive reactions that burden the child with additional stress and guilt. A matter-of-fact attitude helps the child learn to control his bladder function without undue stress.

If enuresis persists into late childhood, treatment with imipramine (Tofranil) may help. *Caution:* Tofranil can cause schizophrenia-like symptoms in young children. Dry-bed therapy may include the use of an alarm apparatus (wet bell pad), social motivation, self-correction of accidents, and positive reinforcement.

Functional encopresis
Denoted by evacuation of feces into the child's clothes or inappropriate receptacles, functional encopresis is associated with low intelligence, cerebral dysfunction, or other developmental symptoms, such as language lag.

Predisposing factors may include psychosocial stress as well as inadequate or inconsistent toilet training.

Related problems may include repressed anger, withdrawal from peers in social relationships, and loss of self-esteem.

Treatment involves encouraging the child to come to his parents whenever he has an "accident." Encourage the parents to help the child by giving him clean clothes without criticism or punishment. A medical examination should be performed to rule out any physical disorder. Child, adult, and family therapy may be needed to help reduce anger and disappointment over the child's development and to correct parenting techniques.

Sleepwalking and sleep terrors
In sleepwalking, the child calmly rises from bed in a state of altered consciousness and walks about with no subsequent recollection of any dream content. In sleep terrors, he awakes terrified, in a state of clouded consciousness, often unable to recognize parents and familiar surroundings. Visual hallucinations are common.

Sleep terrors are a normal developmental event in 2- and 3-year-old children, usually occurring within 30 minutes to 3½ hours of sleep onset. Tachycardia, tachypnea, diaphoresis, dilated pupils, and piloerection are associated with sleep terrors. The child also may fear being alone.

Tell parents to make sure the child has access to them at night. Sleep terrors usually are self-limiting and subside within a few weeks.

cessful when the patient experiences tics that are mild.

No medications are helpful in treating transient tics. Haloperidol is considered the drug of choice if the patient has Tourette syndrome. Pimozide, an oral dopamine-blocking drug, may be substituted in patients who can't tolerate or don't respond well to haloperidol. Alternatively, clonazepam or clonidine may be prescribed.

Nursing diagnoses
• Anxiety
• Body image disturbance
• Chronic low self-esteem
• Impaired social interaction
• Ineffective individual coping
• Powerlessness
• Risk for injury
• Social isolation

Nursing interventions
• Offer emotional support and help the patient prevent fatigue.
• Suggest that the patient with Tourette syndrome contact the Tourette Syndrome Association for information and support.

Patient teaching
• Help the patient to identify and eliminate any avoidable stress and to learn positive new ways to deal with anxiety.
• Encourage the patient to verbalize his feelings about his illness. Help him understand that the movements are involuntary and that he shouldn't feel guilty or blame himself.

AUTISTIC DISORDER
A severe, pervasive developmental disorder, autistic disorder is marked by unresponsiveness to social contact, gross deficits in intelligence and language development, ritualistic and compulsive behaviors, restricted capacity for developmentally appropriate activities and interests, and bizarre responses to the environment. (For information about similar disorders in this class, see *Other pervasive developmental disorders*.)

The disorder usually becomes apparent before the child reaches age 3, but in some children the actual onset is difficult to determine. Occasionally, autistic disorder isn't recognized until the child enters school, when his abnormal social development becomes obvious.

Autistic disorder is rare, affecting 4 to 5 children per 10,000 births. It affects four to five times more males than females, usually the firstborn male. Although the degree of impairment varies, the prognosis is poor and most patients require a structured environment throughout life.

OTHER PERVASIVE DEVELOPMENTAL DISORDERS

Although autistic disorder is the most severe and most typical of the pervasive developmental disorders, recent evidence points to other, similar disorders in this class.

For example, the *DSM-IV* category *pervasive developmental disorder not otherwise specified* refers to those patients who don't meet the criteria for autistic disorder but who *do* exhibit impaired development of reciprocal social interaction and of verbal and nonverbal communication skills.

Some patients with this diagnosis exhibit a markedly restricted repertoire of activities and interests, but others don't. Research suggests that these disorders are more common than autistic disorder, occurring in 6 to 10 of every 10,000 children.

Causes
The causes of autistic disorder remain unclear but are thought to include psychological, physiologic, and sociological factors. Previously, it was thought that most parents of autistic children were intelligent, educated people of high socioeconomic status; recent studies suggest that this may not be true.

The parents of an autistic child may appear distant and unaffectionate toward the child. However, because autistic children are clearly different from birth, and because they are unresponsive or respond with rigid, screaming resistance to touch and attention, parental remoteness may be merely a frustrated, helpless reaction to this disorder, not its cause.

Some theorists consider autistic disorder related to early understimulation that causes the child to seek contact with the world through self-stimulating behaviors; or to overwhelming overstimulation that leads to regression, muteness, and unresponsiveness to external stimuli. Controlled studies haven't confirmed this etiology.

Recent studies have pointed to an association between neurobiological factors and autism. Defects in the central nervous system that may arise from prenatal complications (such as rubella or phenylketonuria), high maternal stress in the first trimester, and genetic factors appear to play a role in the development of autism.

Complications

Autistic disorder may be complicated by epileptic seizures. Seizures usually begin before adolescence and occur most commonly in patients whose IQ is below 50. Depression is common in adolescence and early adulthood, especially in patients with normal or above-average IQs. The onset of depression usually is triggered by the patient's recognition of the extent of his handicap.

During periods of stress, catatonic phenomena, such as excitement or posturing, or an undifferentiated psychotic state with delusions and hallucinations may occur. These symptoms usually resolve quickly when the stress is relieved.

Assessment findings

A primary characteristic of infantile autistic disorder is unresponsiveness to people. Infants with this disorder won't cuddle, avoid eye contact and facial expression, and are indifferent to affection and physical contact. Parents may report that the child becomes rigid or flaccid when held, cries when touched, and shows little or no interest in human contact.

As the infant grows older, his smiling response is delayed or absent. He doesn't lift his arms in anticipation of being picked up or form an attachment to a specific caregiver. Nor does he show the anxiety about strangers that's typical in the 8-month-old infant.

The autistic child fails to learn the usual socialization games (peek-a-boo, pat-a-cake, or bye-bye). He's likely to relate to others only to fill a physical need and then without eye contact or speech (for example, by dragging the adult to the sink when he's thirsty). The autistic child is said to "look right through" a person as though he were not physically present. The end result may be mutual withdrawal between parents and child.

Severe language impairment and lack of imaginative play are characteristic. The child may be mute or may use immature speech patterns. For example, he may use a single word to express a series of activities; he may say "ground" when referring to any step in using a playground slide.

His speech commonly shows echolalia (meaningless repetition of words or phrases addressed to him) and pronoun reversal ("you go walk" when he means "I want to go for a walk"). When answering a question, he may simply repeat the question to mean yes and remain silent to mean no.

He shows little imagination, seldom acting out adult roles or engaging in fantasy play. In fact, he may insist on lining up an exact number of toys in the same manner over and over or repetitively mimic the actions of someone else.

The autistic child shows characteristically bizarre behavior patterns, such as screaming fits, rituals, rhythmic rocking, arm flapping, and crying without tears, and disturbed sleeping and eating patterns. His behavior may be self-destructive (hand biting, eye gouging, hair pulling, or head banging) or self-stimulating (playing with his own saliva, feces, and urine).

His bizarre responses to his environment include an extreme compulsion for sameness—for example, the slightest change in the arrangement of furniture can cause the child to return it immediately to its original place or, if he's unsuccessful, to fall into a panic state, marked by head banging, screaming, or biting himself.

In response to sensory stimuli, the autistic child may underreact or overreact; he may ignore objects—dropping those he is given or not looking at them—or he may become excessively absorbed in them—continually watching the objects or the movement of his own fingers over the objects. He commonly responds to stimuli by head banging, rocking, whirling, and hand flapping. He appears to rely more on smell, taste, and touch, which don't require him to reach out to the environment, and tends to avoid using sight and hearing to respond to or interact with the environment.

The autistic child may exhibit additional behavioral abnormalities, such as:
• cognitive impairment (most have an IQ of 35 to 49)
• eating, drinking, and sleeping problems, for example, limiting his diet to just a few foods, excessive drinking, or repeatedly waking during the night and rocking
• mood disorders, including labile mood, giggling or crying without reason, lack of emotional responses, no fear of real danger but excessive fear of harmless objects, and generalized anxiety.

Diagnostic criteria

A diagnosis of autistic disorder is confirmed when the patient meets the criteria set forth in the *DSM-IV*. At least 6 of the following 12 characteristics must be present, including at least 2 items from the first section, 1 from the second, and 1 from the third.
• Qualitative impairment in social interaction as manifested by the following:
– marked impairment in the use of multiple nonverbal behaviors (for example, eye contact, facial expression, body posture, and gestures) to regulate social interaction

—failure to develop peer relationships appropriate to developmental level
—a lack of spontaneous seeking to share enjoyment, interests, or achievements with others
—a lack of social or emotional reciprocity.
• Qualitative impairments in communication as manifested by the following:
—a delay in or a total lack of development of spoken language (with no attempt to compensate for inadequate language skills nonverbally through gestures or mime)
—in those with adequate speech, marked impairment in the ability to initiate or sustain conversation with others
—stereotyped and repetitive use of language or idiosyncratic language
—lack of varied, spontaneous make-believe play or social imitative play appropriate to developmental level.
• Restricted repetitive and stereotyped patterns of behavior, interests, and activities as manifested by the following:
—encompassing preoccupation with one or more stereotyped and restricted patterns of interest that is abnormal either in intensity or focus
—apparently inflexible adherence to specific, nonfunctional routines or rituals
—stereotyped and repetitive motor mannerisms, such as hand or finger flapping or complex whole-body movements
—persistent preoccupation with parts of objects.
The diagnosistic criteria also include delays or abnormal functioning in at least one of the following areas before age 3:
—social interaction
—language skills
—symbolic or imaginative play.

Treatment
The difficult and prolonged treatment of autistic disorder must begin early, continue for years (through adolescence), and involve the child, parents, teachers, and therapists in coordinated efforts to encourage social adjustment and speech development and to reduce self-destructive behavior.

Behavioral techniques are used to decrease symptoms and increase the child's ability to respond. Positive reinforcement, using food and other rewards, can enhance language and social skills. Providing pleasurable sensory and motor stimulation (jogging, playing with a ball) encourages appropriate behavior and

helps eliminate inappropriate behavior. Pharmacologic intervention may be helpful. Haloperidol often mitigates withdrawn and stereotypical behavior patterns, making the child more amenable to behavior modification therapies.

Treatment may take place in a psychiatric institution, in a specialized school, or in a day-care program, but the current trend is toward home treatment. Helping family members to develop strong one-on-one relationships with the autistic child commonly initiates responsive, imitative behavior. Because family members tend to feel inadequate and guilty, they may need counseling. Until the causes of infantile autism are known, prevention is not possible.

Nursing diagnoses
• Altered family processes
• Altered growth and development
• Altered thought processes
• Anxiety
• Impaired adjustment
• Impaired verbal communication
• Ineffective family coping
• Personal identity disturbance
• Risk for injury
• Risk for violence
• Self-care deficit
• Social isolation

Nursing interventions
• Reduce self-destructive behaviors. Physically stop the child from harming himself, while firmly saying "no." When he responds to your voice, first give a primary reward (such as food); later, substitute verbal or physical reinforcement (such as "good" or a hug or a pat on the back).
• Foster appropriate use of language. Provide positive reinforcement when the child indicates his needs correctly. Give verbal reinforcement at first (such as "good" or "great"); later, give physical reinforcement (such as a hug or a pat on the hand or shoulder).
• Encourage development of self-esteem. Show the child that he's acceptable as a person. If he sits on the floor, sit on the floor with him.
• Encourage self-care. For example, place a brush in the child's hand and guide his hand to brush his hair. Similarly, teach him to wash his hands and face.
• Encourage acceptance of minor environmental changes. Prepare the child for the change by telling him about it. Make the change minor: For example, change the color of his bedspread or the placement of

food on his plate. When he has accepted minor changes, move on to bigger ones.

• Provide emotional support to the parents. Refer them to the Autism Society of America in Washington, D.C., for further assistance.

Patient teaching

• Teach the parents how to physically care for the child's needs.

• Teach the parents how to identify signs of excessive stress and coping skills to use under these circumstances. Emphasize that they'll be ineffective caregivers if they don't take the time to meet their own needs in addition to those of their child.

• Help the parents understand that they aren't responsible for the child's condition.

ATTENTION-DEFICIT HYPERACTIVITY DISORDER

The patient with attention-deficit hyperactivity disorder has difficulty focusing his attention, engaging in quiet passive activities, or both. Some patients have an attention deficit without hyperactivity; they are less likely to be diagnosed and receive treatment.

Although attention-deficit hyperactivity disorder is present at birth, diagnosis before age 4 or 5 is difficult unless the child exhibits severe symptoms. Some patients, however, aren't diagnosed until they reach adulthood.

This disorder occurs in roughly 3% to 5% of school-age children. Males are three times more likely to be affected than females.

Causes

Attention-deficit hyperactivity disorder is thought to be a physiologic brain disorder with a familial tendency. Some studies indicate that it may result from altered neurotransmitter levels in the brain.

Complications

Emotional and social complications can result from the child's impulsive behavior, inattentiveness, and disorganization in school. Hyperactivity can also lead to poor nutrition.

Assessment findings

The patient is usually characterized as a fidgeter and a daydreamer. He also may be described as inattentive and lazy. The parents may state that their child is intelligent but that his school or work performance is sporadic. They may also report that he has a tendency to jump quickly from one partly completed project, thought, or task to another.

If the child is younger, the parents may note that he has difficulty waiting in line, remaining in his seat, waiting his turn, or concentrating on one activity long enough to complete it.

An older child or an adult may be described as impulsive and easily distracted by irrelevant thoughts, sights, or sounds. He may also be characterized as emotionally labile, inattentive, or prone to daydreaming. His disorganization becomes apparent as he has difficulty meeting deadlines and keeping track of school or work tools and materials.

Diagnostic criteria

Commonly, the child with attention-deficit hyperactivity disorder is referred for evaluation by the school. Accurate diagnosis of this disorder usually begins by obtaining information from several sources, such as the parents, the teachers, and the child himself.

Complete psychological, medical, and neurologic evaluations are then performed on the child to rule out other problems. Next, the child undergoes tests that measure impulsiveness, attention, and the ability to sustain a task. The findings portray a clear picture of attention-deficit hyperactivity disorder and of the specific areas of support the child will need.

For characteristic findings in patients with this condition, see *Diagnosing attention-deficit hyperactivity disorder*.

Treatment

Education is the first step in effective treatment of attention-deficit hyperactivity disorder. The entire treatment team (which ideally includes parents, teachers, and therapists as well as the patient and the doctor) must fully understand the nature of this disorder as well as the disorder's effect on the individual's ability to function.

Specific treatments vary, depending on the severity of signs and symptoms and their effects on the patient's ability to function adequately. Behavior modification, coaching, external structure, use of planning and organizing systems, and supportive psychotherapy can all help the patient more effectively cope with the disorder.

Some patients benefit from medication to relieve symptoms. Ideally, the treatment team identifies the symptoms to be managed, selects appropriate medication, and then tracks the patient's symptoms care-

DIAGNOSING ATTENTION-DEFICIT HYPERACTIVITY DISORDER

The *DSM-IV* groups selected symptoms into inattention and hyperactivity-impulsivity categories. Diagnosis of attention-deficit hyperactivity disorder is based on the person demonstrating at least six symptoms from one or both of these categories. A patient with symptoms mainly from the inattention category is classified as a predominantly inattentive type; a patient with mainly hyperactivity-impulsivity symptoms is diagnosed as a predominantly hyperactive-impulsive type. Someone with at least six symptoms from both groups has combined-type attention-deficit hyperactivity disorder—the most common type. The symptoms must have persisted for at least 6 months to a degree that they are maladaptive and inconsistent with the person's developmental level.

Symptoms of inattention
The person manifesting *inattention*:
• often fails to pay close attention to details or makes careless mistakes in schoolwork, work, or other activities
• often has difficulty sustaining attention in tasks or play activities
• often does not seem to listen when spoken to directly
• often does not follow through on instructions and fails to finish schoolwork, chores, or duties in the workplace (not because of oppositional behavior or failure to understand instructions)
• often has difficulty organizing tasks and activities
• often avoids, dislikes, or is reluctant to engage in tasks that require sustained mental effort, such as schoolwork or homework
• often loses things necessary for tasks or activities

(for example, toys, school assignments, pencils, books, or tools)
• often becomes distracted by extraneous stimuli
• often demonstrates forgetfulness in daily activities.

Symptoms of hyperactivity-impulsivity
The person manifesting *hyperactivity*:
• often fidgets with hands or feet or squirms in his seat
• often leaves his seat in the classroom or in other situations in which remaining seated is expected
• often runs about or climbs excessively in situations in which remaining seated is expected
• often has difficulty playing or engaging in leisure activities quietly
• often is characterized as "on the go" or acts as if "driven by a motor"
• often talks excessively.
   The person manifesting *impulsivity*:
• often blurts out answers before questions have been completed
• often has difficulty awaiting his turn
• often interrupts or intrudes on others.

Additional features
• Some symptoms that caused impairment were evident before age 7.
• Some impairment from the symptoms is present in two or more settings (for example, at school, at work, and at home).
• Clinically significant impairment in social, academic, or occupational functioning must be clearly evident.
• The symptoms do not occur exclusively during the course of a pervasive developmental disorder, schizophrenia, or another psychotic disorder and are not better accounted for by another mental disorder.

---

fully to determine the effectiveness of the medication. Stimulants, such as methylphenidate and dextroamphetamine, are the most commonly used agents. However, other drugs, including tricyclic antidepressants (such as desipramine and nortriptyline), mood stabilizers, and beta blockers, sometimes help control symptoms.

Nursing diagnoses
• Altered family processes
• Altered nutrition: Less than body requirements
• Impaired social interaction
• Ineffective family coping: Compromised
• Ineffective management of therapeutic regimen: Families

• Risk for altered parenting
• Risk for loneliness

Nursing interventions
• Set realistic expectations and limits because the patient with attention-deficit hyperactivity disorder is easily frustrated (which, in turn, results in decreased self-control).
• Always remain calm and consistent with the child. Your calm manner will help him to maintain his self-control.
• Try to keep all your instructions to the child short and simple.
• Provide praise, rewards, and positive feedback whenever possible.

• Help the child's parents and other family members develop planning and organizing systems to help them cope more effectively with the child's short attention span.
• Make certain that the parents fully understand the child's prescribed medication regimen. Teach them about any adverse reactions that may occur, emphasizing those that may require immediate medical attention.
• Provide the patient with diversional activities suited to his short attention span.
• Encourage the parents to provide the child with nutritious snacks, such as fruit, to supplement his dietary intake.
• Refer the parents to appropriate support groups and community organizations.

PSYCHOACTIVE SUBSTANCE USE DISORDERS

This section includes disorders, such as alcoholism and psychoactive drug abuse and dependence, that affect the central nervous system and cause physical and mental harm.

ALCOHOLISM

A chronic disorder, alcoholism most often is described as the uncontrolled intake of alcoholic beverages that interferes with physical and mental health, social and familial relationships, and occupational responsibilities. Alcoholism cuts across all social and economic groups, involves both sexes, and occurs at all stages of the life cycle, beginning as early as elementary school age.

Most adults in the United States are light drinkers; a minority—about 10% of the population—account for 50% of all alcohol consumption. About 13% of all adults over age 18 have suffered from alcohol abuse or dependence at some time in their lives. The prevalence of drinking is highest between the ages of 21 and 34, but current statistics show that up to 19% of 12- to 17-year-olds have a serious drinking problem. Males are two to five times more likely to abuse alcohol than are females. According to some statistics, alcohol abuse is a factor in 60% of all automobile accidents. Alcoholism has no known cure.

Causes

Numerous biological, psychological, and sociocultural factors may cause alcohol addiction, but no clear evidence confirms the influence of any of these factors. Family background may play a significant part: An offspring of one alcoholic parent is seven to eight times more likely to become an alcoholic than is a peer without such a parent. Biological factors may include genetic or biochemical abnormalities, nutritional deficiencies, endocrine imbalances, and allergic responses.

Psychological factors may include the urge to drink alcohol to reduce anxiety or symptoms of mental illness; the desire to avoid responsibility in familial, social, and work relationships; and the need to bolster self-esteem.

Sociocultural factors include the availability of alcoholic beverages, group or peer pressure, an excessively stressful life-style, and social attitudes that approve frequent imbibing. Advertising supports society's message that alcohol consumption is part of a healthy life-style. Paradoxically, many alcoholics come from families in which alcohol is forbidden.

Complications

Most body tissues can be adversely affected by the heavy intake of alcohol (see *Complications of alcohol use*).

Assessment findings

Because alcoholics may hide or deny their addiction and may temporarily manage to maintain a functional life, assessing for alcoholism can be difficult. Note physical and psychosocial symptoms that suggest alcoholism. For example, the patient's history may suggest a need for daily or episodic alcohol use for adequate function, an inability to discontinue or reduce alcohol intake, episodes of anesthesia or amnesia during intoxication (blackouts), episodes of violence during intoxication, and interference with social and familial relationships and occupational responsibilities.

Many minor complaints may be alcohol-related. The patient may report malaise, dyspepsia, mood swings or depression, and an increased incidence of infection. Observe the patient for poor personal hygiene and untreated injuries, such as cigarette burns, fractures, and bruises, which he can't fully explain. Note any evidence of an unusually high tolerance for sedatives and narcotics.

Watch for secretive behavior, which may be an attempt to hide the disorder or the patient's stock of al-

COMPLICATIONS OF ALCOHOL USE

Alcohol can damage body tissues by its direct irritating effects, by changes that take place in the body during its metabolism, by aggravation of existing disease, by accidents occurring during intoxication, and by interactions between the substance and drugs. Such tissue damage can cause the following complications.

Cardiopulmonary complications
• Cardiac arrhythmias
• Cardiomyopathy
• Chronic obstructive pulmonary disease
• Essential hypertension
• Increased risk of tuberculosis
• Pneumonia

Hepatic complications
• Alcoholic hepatitis
• Cirrhosis
• Fatty liver

GI complications
• Chronic diarrhea
• Esophageal cancer
• Esophageal varices
• Esophagitis
• Gastric ulcers
• Gastritis
• GI bleeding
• Malabsorption
• Pancreatitis

Neurologic complications
• Alcoholic dementia
• Alcoholic hallucinosis
• Alcohol withdrawal delirium
• Korsakoff's syndrome
• Peripheral neuropathy
• Seizure disorders
• Subdural hematoma
• Wernicke's encephalopathy

Psychiatric complications
• Amotivational syndrome
• Depression
• Fetal alcohol syndrome
• Impaired social and occupational functioning
• Multiple substance abuse
• Suicide

Other complications
• Beriberi
• Hypoglycemia
• Leg and foot ulcers
• Prostatitis

cohol. Suspect alcoholism if the patient uses inordinate amounts of after-shave lotion or mouthwash. Deprived of his usual supply of alcohol, an alcoholic may consume it in any form he can find.

When confronted about his drinking, the patient may deny or rationalize the problem. Alternatively, he may be guarded or hostile in his response and may even sign out of the hospital against medical advice. He also may project his anger or feelings of guilt or inadequacy onto others to avoid confronting his illness.

In addition to these progressive signs of psychological deterioration, chronic alcohol abuse brings with it a vast array of physical complications. Assess for these complications in a patient with an alcohol-related disorder.

After abstinence or reduction of alcohol intake, manifestations of withdrawal may vary (see *Signs and symptoms of alcohol withdrawal,* page 28). Withdrawal signs and symptoms begin shortly after drinking has stopped and last for 5 to 7 days. The patient initially experiences anorexia, nausea, anxiety, fever, insomnia, diaphoresis, and tremor, progressing to severe tremulousness, agitation and, possibly, hallucinations and violent behavior. Major motor seizures, also known as "rum fits," can occur during withdrawal. Suspect alcoholism in any patient with unexplained seizure activity.

Diagnostic criteria
The diagnosis of alcohol dependence is confirmed when the patient meets the following criteria documented in the *DSM-IV.*
• At least three of the following signs and symptoms must be present:
— alcohol often taken in larger amounts or for a longer time than the person intended
— persistent desire or one or more unsuccessful efforts to cut down or control alcohol use
— excessive time spent in activities necessary to obtain alcohol
— frequent intoxication or withdrawal symptoms when expected to fulfill major obligations at work, school, or home, or when alcohol consumption is physically hazardous
— important social, occupational, or recreational activities given up or reduced because of alcohol consumption

SIGNS AND SYMPTOMS OF ALCOHOL WITHDRAWAL

Withdrawal signs and symptoms may vary in degree from mild (morning hangover) to severe (alcohol withdrawal delirium). Formerly known as delirium tremens or DTs, alcohol withdrawal delirium is marked by acute distress following abrupt withdrawal after prolonged or massive use.

Signs and symptoms	Mild withdrawal	Moderate withdrawal	Severe withdrawal
Motor impairment	Inner tremulousness with hand tremor	Visible tremors	Gross, uncontrollable bodily shaking
Anxiety	Mild restlessness	Obvious motor restlessness and painful anxiety	Extreme restlessness and agitation with intense fearfulness
Sleep disturbance	Restless sleep or insomnia	Marked insomnia and nightmares	Total wakefulness
Appetite	Impaired appetite	Marked anorexia	Rejection of all food and fluid except alcohol
GI symptoms	Nausea	Nausea and vomiting	Dry heaves and vomiting
Confusion	None	Variable	Marked confusion and disorientation
Hallucinations	None	Vague, transient visual and auditory hallucinations and illusions; commonly nocturnal; often with meaning	Visual and occasional auditory hallucinations, usually of fearful or threatening content; misidentification of people and frightening delusions related to hallucinatory experiences
Pulse rate	Tachycardia	Pulse rate of 100 to 120 beats/minute	Pulse rate of 120 to 140 beats/minute
Blood pressure	Normal or slightly elevated systolic	Usually elevated systolic	Elevated systolic and diastolic
Sweating	Slight	Obvious	Marked hyperhidrosis
Seizures	None	Possible	Common

—continued alcohol consumption despite knowledge of having a persistent or recurrent social, psychological, or physical problem that is caused or exacerbated by alcohol use

—marked tolerance: need for markedly increased amounts of alcohol to achieve intoxication or desired effect, or markedly diminished effect with continued use of the same amount

—characteristic withdrawal symptoms

—alcohol often consumed to relieve or avoid withdrawal symptoms

• Some symptoms must have persisted for at least 1 month or have occurred repeatedly over a longer time.

In addition to a psychiatric examination, laboratory tests can confirm alcohol use and the presence of complications. For example, laboratory data can document recent alcohol ingestion. A blood alcohol level of 0.10% weight/volume (200 mg/dl) is accepted as the level of intoxication. Serum electrolyte levels may identify electrolyte abnormalities (in severe hepatic disease, the blood urea nitrogen level is increased and the serum glucose level is decreased).

Further testing may reveal increased serum ammonia and serum amylase levels. Urine toxicology may help to determine if the alcoholic with alcohol withdrawal delirium or another acute complication abuses other drugs as well.

Liver function studies, revealing increased levels of serum cholesterol, lactate dehydrogenase, alanine aminotransferase (formerly SGPT), aspartate aminotransferase (formerly SGOT), and creatine phosphokinase, may all point to liver damage, and elevated serum amylase and lipase levels point to acute pancreatitis. A hematologic workup can identify anemia, thrombocytopenia, increased prothrombin time, and increased partial thromboplastin time.

Treatment

Total abstinence is the only effective treatment. Supportive programs that offer detoxification, rehabilitation, and aftercare, including continued involvement in Alcoholics Anonymous (AA), may produce long-term results.

Acute intoxication is treated symptomatically by supporting respiration, preventing aspiration of vomitus, replacing fluids, administering I.V. glucose to prevent hypoglycemia, correcting hypothermia or acidosis, and initiating emergency treatment for trauma, infection, or GI bleeding.

Treatment of chronic alcoholism relies on medications to deter alcohol use and treat effects of withdrawal; psychotherapy, using behavior modification techniques, group therapy, and family therapy; and appropriate measures to relieve associated physical problems.

Aversion, or deterrent, therapy uses a daily oral dose of disulfiram to prevent compulsive drinking. This drug interferes with alcohol metabolism and allows toxic levels of acetaldehyde to accumulate in the patient's blood, producing immediate and potentially fatal distress if the patient consumes alcohol up to 2 weeks after taking it.

Disulfiram is contraindicated during pregnancy and in patients with diabetes, heart disease, severe hepatic disease, or any disorder in which such a reaction could be especially dangerous. Another form of aversion therapy attempts to induce aversion by administering alcohol with an emetic.

For long-term success with aversion, or deterrent, therapy, the sober alcoholic must learn to fill the place alcohol once occupied in his life with something constructive. Indeed, for patients with abnormal dependence or for those who also abuse other drugs, aversion therapy with disulfiram may only substitute one drug dependence for another; so it should be used prudently.

Tranquilizers, particularly the benzodiazepines, occasionally are used to relieve overwhelming anxiety during rehabilitation. However, these drugs have addictive potential (substituting one substance abuse problem for another), and they can precipitate coma or even death when combined with alcohol. Phenothiazines and other antipsychotics are prescribed to control hyperactivity and psychosis. Anticonvulsants, antiemetics, and antidiarrheals also are used to treat symptoms of alcohol withdrawal.

Supportive counseling or individual, group, or family psychotherapy may improve the alcoholic's ability to cope with stress, anxiety, and frustration and help him gain insight into the personal problems and conflicts that may have led him to alcohol abuse. Ongoing support groups also can help him overcome his dependence on alcohol. In AA, a self-help group with more than a million members worldwide, the alcoholic finds emotional support from others with similar problems. About 40% of AA's members stay sober as long as 5 years, and 30% stay sober longer than 5 years.

Nursing diagnoses
• Altered protection
• Altered role performance
• Altered thought processes
• Anxiety
• Defensive coping
• Functional incontinence
• Hopelessness
• Impaired physical mobility
• Impaired social interaction
• Impaired tissue integrity
• Ineffective denial
• Ineffective family coping
• Ineffective individual coping
• Noncompliance
• Personal identity disturbance
• Powerlessness
• Risk for injury
• Risk for violence
• Self-care deficit
• Sensory or perceptual alterations
• Sleep pattern disturbance
• Spiritual distress

Nursing interventions
• During acute intoxication or withdrawal, carefully monitor the patient's mental status, heart rate, breath

sounds, blood pressure, and temperature every 30 minutes to 6 hours, depending on the severity of his signs and symptoms.
• Assess the patient for signs of inadequate nutrition and dehydration. Institute seizure precautions and administer drugs, as ordered, to treat the signs and symptoms of withdrawal in chronic alcohol abuse.
• During withdrawal in chronic alcohol abuse, orient the patient to reality because he may have hallucinations and may try to harm himself or others. Maintain a calm environment, minimizing noise and shadows to reduce the incidence of delusions and hallucinations. Avoid restraining the patient unless necessary to protect him or others.
• Approach the patient in a nonthreatening way. Limit sustained eye contact, which can be perceived as threatening. Even if he's verbally abusive, listen attentively and respond with empathy. Explain all procedures.
• Monitor the patient for signs of depression or impending suicide.
• In chronic alcoholism, help the patient accept his drinking problem and the necessity for abstinence. Confront his behavior, urging him to examine his actions more realistically.
• Refer the patient to AA and offer to arrange a visit from an AA member. Stress how this organization can provide the support he'll need to abstain from alcohol. A concerned religious advisor also can provide the motivation for a personal conversion to sobriety.
• For alcoholics who have lost all contact with family and friends and who have a long history of unemployment, trouble with the law, or other problems associated with alcohol abuse, rehabilitation may involve job training, sheltered workshops, halfway houses, and other supervised facilities.
• Refer spouses of alcoholics to Al-Anon and children, to Alateen. By participating in these self-help groups, family members learn to relinquish responsibility for the alcoholic's drinking so that they can live meaningful and productive lives. Point out that family involvement in rehabilitation can reduce family tensions.
• Refer adult children of alcoholics to the National Association for Children of Alcoholics. This organization may provide support in understanding and coping with their past.

Patient teaching
• Educate the patient and his family about his illness. Warn them that the patient will be tempted to drink again and will be unable to control himself after the first drink. Therefore, he must abstain from alcohol for the rest of his life.
• Explain to the patient and family that relapses may occur. Help them negotiate a plan to help the patient if he does experience a relapse.
• If the patient is taking disulfiram (or has taken it within the previous 2 weeks), warn him of the effects of alcohol ingestion, which may last from 30 minutes to 3 hours or longer. The reaction includes nausea, vomiting, facial flushing, headache, shortness of breath, red eyes, blurred vision, sweating, tachycardia, hypotension, and fainting. Emphasize that even a small amount of alcohol will induce this adverse reaction and that the longer he takes the drug, the greater will be his sensitivity to alcohol. Because of this, he must avoid even medicinal sources of alcohol, such as mouthwash, cough syrups, liquid vitamins, and cold remedies.
• Inform the patient that paraldehyde, a sedative, is chemically similar to alcohol and may provoke a disulfiram-type reaction.
• Advise the patient that aversion therapy may continue for months or years and that he should remain under medical supervision during that time.

PSYCHOACTIVE DRUG ABUSE AND DEPENDENCE

The National Institute on Drug Abuse defines this condition as the use of a legal or an illegal drug that causes physical, mental, emotional, or social harm. Examples of commonly abused drugs include narcotics, stimulants, depressants, antianxiety agents, and hallucinogens. Drug abuse is a major public health problem in today's society.

Psychoactive drug abuse can occur at any age. Experimentation with drugs commonly begins in adolescence; recent statistics, however, document a trend toward drug use among preadolescents. Drug abuse often leads to addiction, which may involve physical or psychological dependence, or both. The most dangerous form of abuse occurs when users mix several drugs simultaneously—including alcohol. The resultant interactions can complicate assessment, precipitate life-threatening complications, and delay withdrawal.

Causes
Psychoactive drug abuse commonly results from a combination of low self-esteem, peer pressure, inadequate coping skills, and curiosity. Most people who are

predisposed to drug abuse have few mental or emotional resources against stress, an excessive dependence on others, and a low tolerance for frustration. Often anxious, angry, or depressed, they demand immediate relief of tension or distress. Taking the drug gives them pleasure by relieving tension, abolishing loneliness, achieving a temporarily peaceful or euphoric state, or simply relieving boredom.

Drug dependence may follow experimentation with drugs in response to peer pressure. It also may follow the use of drugs to relieve physical pain, but this is uncommon.

Complications

Chronic drug abuse, especially I.V. use, can lead to life-threatening complications, such as cardiac and respiratory arrest, intracranial hemorrhage, acquired immunodeficiency syndrome, tetanus, subacute bacterial endocarditis, hepatitis, vasculitis, septicemia, thrombophlebitis, pulmonary emboli, gangrene, malaria, malnutrition and GI disturbances, respiratory infections, musculoskeletal dysfunction, trauma, depression, increased risk of suicide, and psychosis.

Materials used to "cut" street drugs also can cause toxic or allergic reactions. The specific effects of the street drug vary according to the substance used, its duration of action, and the dosage (see *Understanding commonly abused substances,* pages 32 to 34).

Impaired social and occupational functioning also result from chronic drug use, creating personal, professional, and financial problems. When drug use begins in early adolescence, it may lead to behavioral problems and a failure to complete school.

Assessment findings

The signs and symptoms of acute drug intoxication vary, depending on the drug. The drug user seldom seeks treatment specifically for his drug problem. Instead, he may seek emergency treatment for drug-related injuries or complications, such as a motor vehicle accident, burns from free-basing, an overdose, physical deterioration from illness or malnutrition, or withdrawal. Friends, family members, or law enforcement officials may bring the patient to the hospital because of respiratory depression, unconsciousness, acute injury, or a psychiatric crisis.

Examine the patient for signs and symptoms of drug use or drug-related complications, as well as for clues to the type of drug ingested. For example, fever can result from stimulant or hallucinogen intoxication, from withdrawal, or from infection from I.V. drug use.

Inspect the eyes for lacrimation from opiate withdrawal, nystagmus from central nervous system (CNS) depressants and phencyclidine (PCP) intoxication, and drooping eyelids from opiate or CNS depressant use. Constricted pupils occur with opiate use or withdrawal; dilated pupils, with the use of hallucinogens or amphetamines.

Examine the nose for rhinorrhea from opiate withdrawal and the oral and nasal mucosa for signs of drug-induced irritation. Drug sniffing can cause inflammation, atrophy, or perforation of the nasal mucosa. Dental conditions commonly result from the poor oral hygiene associated with chronic drug use. Also inspect under the tongue for evidence of I.V. drug injection.

Inspect the skin. Sweating, a common sign of intoxication with opiates or CNS stimulants, also accompanies most drug withdrawal syndromes. Drug use may induce a sensation of bugs crawling on the skin, known as formication; as a result, the skin may be excoriated from scratching.

Needle marks or tracks are an obvious sign of I.V. drug abuse. Note that the patient may attempt to conceal or disguise injection sites with tattoos or by selecting an inconspicuous site, such as under the nails. In addition, self-injection can sometimes cause cellulitis or abscesses, especially in patients who also are chronic alcoholics. Puffy hands can be a late sign of thrombophlebitis or of fascial infection caused by self-injection on the hands or arms.

Auscultation may disclose bilateral crackles and rhonchi caused by smoking and inhaling drugs or by opiate overdose. Other cardiopulmonary signs of overdose include pulmonary edema, respiratory depression, aspiration pneumonia, and hypotension. CNS stimulants and some hallucinogens may precipitate refractory acute-onset hypertension or cardiac arrhythmias. Withdrawal from opiates or depressants also can provoke arrhythmias and, occasionally, hypotension.

During opiate withdrawal, the patient may report abdominal pain, nausea, or vomiting. Opiate abusers also commonly complain of hemorrhoids, a consequence of the constipating effects of these drugs. Palpation of an enlarged liver, with or without tenderness, may indicate hepatitis.

Neurologic symptoms of drug abuse include tremors, hyperreflexia, hyporeflexia, and seizures. Abrupt withdrawal may precipitate signs of CNS depression ranging from lethargy to coma, hallucinations, or signs of overstimulation, including euphoria and violent behavior.

(Text continues on page 35.)

UNDERSTANDING COMMONLY ABUSED SUBSTANCES

Substance	Signs and symptoms	Interventions
Stimulants		
Cocaine • *Street names:* coke, flake, snow, nose candy, hits, crack (hardened form), rock, crank • *Routes:* ingestion, injection, sniffing, smoking • *Dependence:* psychological • *Duration of effect:* 15 minutes to 2 hours; with crack, rapid high of short duration followed by down feeling • *Medical uses:* local anesthetic	• *Of use:* abdominal pain; alternating euphoria and fear; anorexia; cardiotoxicity, such as ventricular fibrillation or cardiac arrest; coma; confusion; diaphoresis; dilated pupils; excitability; fever; grandiosity; hyperpnea; hypotension or hypertension; insomnia; irritability; nausea and vomiting; pallor or cyanosis; perforated nasal septum with prolonged use; pressured speech; psychotic behavior with large doses; respiratory arrest; seizures; spasms; tachycardia; tachypnea; visual, auditory, and olfactory hallucinations; weight loss • *Of withdrawal:* anxiety, depression, fatigue	• Place the patient in a quiet room. • If cocaine was ingested, induce vomiting or perform gastric lavage. Follow with activated charcoal and a saline cathartic. • If cocaine was sniffed, remove residual drug from mucous membranes. • Monitor vital signs. • Give propranolol for tachycardia. • Perform cardiopulmonary resuscitation for ventricular fibrillation and cardiac arrest, as indicated. • Give a tepid sponge bath for fever. • Administer an anticonvulsant, as ordered, for seizures.
Amphetamines • *Street names:* for amphetamine sulfate—bennies, grennies, cartwheels; for methamphetamine—speed, meth, crystal; for dextroamphetamine sulfate—dexies, hearts, oranges • *Routes:* ingestion, injection • *Dependence:* psychological • *Duration of effect:* 1 to 4 hours • *Medical uses:* hyperkinesis, narcolepsy, weight control	• *Of use:* altered mental status (from confusion to paranoia), coma, diaphoresis, dilated reactive pupils, dry mouth, exhaustion, hallucinations, hyperactive tendon reflexes, hypertension, hyperthermia, paradoxical reaction in children, psychotic behavior with prolonged use, seizures, shallow respirations, tachycardia, tremors • *Of withdrawal:* abdominal tenderness, apathy, depression, disorientation, irritability, long periods of sleep, muscle aches, suicide (with sudden withdrawal)	• Place the patient in a quiet room. • If the drug was ingested, induce vomiting or perform gastric lavage; give activated charcoal and a saline or magnesium sulfate cathartic. • Add ammonium chloride or ascorbic acid to I.V. solution to acidify urine to a pH of 5. Also, administer mannitol to induce diuresis, as ordered. • Monitor vital signs. • As ordered, give a short-acting barbiturate, such as pentobarbital, for seizures; haloperidol for assaultive behavior; phentolamine for hypertension; propranolol for tachyarrhythmias; and lidocaine for ventricular arrhythmias. • Restrain the patient if he's experiencing hallucinations or paranoia. • Give a tepid sponge bath for fever. • Institute suicide precautions.
Hallucinogens		
Lysergic acid diethylamide (LSD) • *Street names:* acid, microdot, sugar, big D • *Routes:* ingestion, smoking • *Dependence:* possibly psychological • *Duration of effect:* 8 to 12 hours • *Medical uses:* none	• *Of use:* abdominal cramps, arrhythmias, chills, depersonalization, diaphoresis, diarrhea, distorted visual perception and perception of time and space, dizziness, dry mouth, fever, grandiosity, hallucinations, heightened sense of awareness, hyperpnea, hypertension, illusions, increased salivation, muscle aches, mystical experiences, nausea, palpitations, seizures, tachycardia, vomiting • *Of withdrawal:* none	• Place the patient in a quiet room. • If the drug was ingested, induce vomiting or perform gastric lavage. Follow with activated charcoal and a cathartic. • Monitor vital signs, and give diazepam for seizures, as ordered. • Reorient the patient to time, place, and person, and restrain him, as necessary.

UNDERSTANDING COMMONLY ABUSED SUBSTANCES *(continued)*

Substance	Signs and symptoms	Intervention
Hallucinogens *(continued)*		
Phencyclidine • *Street names:* PCP, hog, angel dust, peace pill, crystal superjoint, elephant tranquilizer, rocket fuel • *Routes:* ingestion, injection, smoking • *Dependence:* possibly psychological • *Duration of effect:* 30 minutes to several days • *Medical uses:* veterinary anesthetic	• *Of use:* amnesia; blank stare; cardiac arrest; decreased awareness of surroundings; delusions; distorted body image; distorted sense of sight, hearing, and touch; drooling; euphoria; excitation and psychoses; fever; gait ataxia; hallucinations; hyperactivity; hypertensive crisis; individualized unpredictable effects; muscle rigidity; nystagmus; panic; poor perception of time and distance; possible chromosomal damage; psychotic behavior; recurrent coma; renal failure; seizures; sudden behavioral changes; tachycardia; violent behavior • *Of withdrawal:* none	• Place the patient in a quiet room. • If the drug was ingested, induce vomiting or perform gastric lavage. Follow with activated charcoal. • Add ascorbic acid to I.V. solution to acidify urine. • Monitor vital signs and urine output. • If ordered, give a diuretic; propranolol for hypertension or tachycardia; nitroprusside for severe hypertensive crisis; diazepam for seizures; diazepam or haloperidol for agitation or psychotic behavior; and physostigmine salicylate, diazepam, chlordiazepoxide, or chlorpromazine for a "bad trip."
Depressants		
Alcohol • *Found in:* beer, wine, distilled spirits; also contained in cough syrup, aftershave, and mouthwash • *Route:* ingestion • *Dependence:* physical, psychological • *Duration of effect:* varies according to the individual and the amount ingested; metabolized at rate of 10 ml/hour • *Medical uses:* neurolysis (absolute alcohol); emergency tocolytic; treatment of ethylene glycol and methanol poisoning	• *Of acute use:* coma, decreased inhibitions, euphoria followed by depression or hostility, impaired judgment, incoordination, respiratory depression, slurred speech, unconsciousness, vomiting • *Of withdrawal:* delirium, hallucinations, tremors, seizures	• Place the patient in a quiet room. • If alcohol was ingested within 4 hours, induce vomiting or perform gastric lavage; give activated charcoal and saline cathartic. • Monitor vital signs. • As ordered, give diazepam for seizures and chlordiazepoxide, chloral hydrate, or paraldehyde for hallucinations and delirium. • Institute seizure precautions. • Provide I.V. fluid replacement as well as dextrose, thiamine, B-complex vitamins, and vitamin C to treat dehydration, hypoglycemia, and nutritional deficiencies. • Assess for aspiration pneumonia. • Prepare the patient for dialysis if his vital functions are severely depressed.
Benzodiazepines (alprazolam, chlordiazepoxide, clonazepam, clorazepate, diazepam, flurazepam, halazepam, lorazepam, midazolam, oxazepam, prazepam, quazepam, temazepam, triazolam) • *Street names:* dolls, green and whites, roaches, yellow jackets • *Routes:* ingestion, injection • *Dependence:* physical, psychological • *Duration of effect:* 4 to 8 hours • *Medical uses:* antianxiety agent, anticonvulsant, sedative, hypnotic	• *Of use:* ataxia, drowsiness, hypotension, increased self-confidence, relaxation, slurred speech • *Of overdose:* confusion, coma, drowsiness, respiratory depression • *Of withdrawal:* abdominal cramps, agitation, anxiety, diaphoresis, hypertension, tachycardia, tonic-clonic seizures, tremors, vomiting	• If the drug was ingested, induce vomiting or perform gastric lavage. Follow with activated charcoal and a cathartic. • Monitor the patient's vital signs. • Give supplemental oxygen for hypoxia-induced seizures. • As ordered, give I.V. fluids for hypertension and physostigmine salicylate for respiratory or central nervous system (CNS) depression.

(continued)

UNDERSTANDING COMMONLY ABUSED SUBSTANCES *(continued)*

Substance	Signs and symptoms	Intervention
Depressants *(continued)*		

Barbiturates
(amobarbital, phenobarbital, secobarbital)
• *Street names:* for barbiturates—downers, barbs; for amobarbital—blue angels, blue devils; for phenobarbital—purple hearts, goofballs; for secobarbital—reds, red devils
• *Routes:* ingestion, injection
• *Dependence:* physical, psychological
• *Duration:* 1 to 16 hours
• *Medical uses:* anesthetic, anticonvulsant, sedative, hypnotic

Signs and symptoms:
• *Of use:* absent reflexes, blisters or bullous lesions, cyanosis, depressed level of consciousness (from confusion to coma), fever, flaccid muscles, hypotension, hypothermia, nystagmus, paradoxical reaction in children and elderly people, poor pupil reaction to light, respiratory depression
• *Of withdrawal:* agitation, anxiety, fever, insomnia, orthostatic hypotension, tachycardia, tremors
• *Of rapid withdrawal:* anorexia, apprehension, hallucinations, orthostatic hypotension, tonic-clonic seizures, tremors, weakness

Intervention:
• If ingestion was recent, induce vomiting or perform gastric lavage. Follow with activated charcoal.
• Monitor vital signs, and perform frequent neurologic assessments.
• As ordered, give an I.V. fluid bolus for hypotension and alkalinize urine.
• Use seizure precautions; relieve withdrawal symptoms, as ordered.
• Use a hypothermia or hyperthermia blanket for temperature alterations.

Opiates
(codeine, heroin, morphine, meperidine, opium)
• *Street names:* for heroin—junk, horse, H, smack; for morphine—morph, M
• *Routes:* for codeine, meperidine, morphine—ingestion, injection, smoking; for heroin—ingestion, injection, inhalation, smoking; for opium—ingestion, smoking
• *Dependence:* physical, psychological
• *Duration of effect:* 3 to 6 hours
• *Medical uses:* for codeine—analgesia, antitussive; for heroin—none; for morphine, meperidine—analgesia; for opium—analgesia, antidiarrheal

Signs and symptoms:
• *Of use:* anorexia, arrhythmias, clammy skin, constipation, constricted pupils, decreased level of consciousness, detachment from reality, drowsiness, euphoria, hypotension, impaired judgment, increased pigmentation over veins, lack of concern, lethargy, nausea, needle marks, respiratory depression, seizures, shallow or slow respirations, skin lesions or abscesses, slurred speech, swollen or perforated nasal mucosa, thrombosed veins, urine retention, vomiting
• *Of withdrawal:* abdominal cramps, anorexia, chills, diaphoresis, dilated pupils, hyperactive bowel sounds, irritability, nausea, panic, piloerection, runny nose, sweating, tremors, watery eyes, yawning

Intervention:
• If the drug was ingested, induce vomiting or perform gastric lavage.
• As ordered, give naloxone until CNS effects are reversed.
• Give I.V. fluids to increase circulatory volume.
• Use extra blankets for hypothermia; if ineffective, use a hyperthermia blanket.
• Reorient the patient to time, place, and person.
• Assess breath sounds to monitor for pulmonary edema.
• Monitor for signs and symptoms of withdrawal.

| **Cannabinoids** | | |

Marijuana
• *Street names:* pot, grass, weed, Mary Jane, roach, reefer, joint, THC
• *Routes:* ingestion, smoking
• *Dependence:* psychological
• *Duration of effect:* 2 to 3 hours
• *Medical uses:* antiemetic for chemotherapy

Signs and symptoms:
• *Of use:* acute psychosis; agitation; amotivational syndrome; anxiety; asthma; bronchitis; conjunctival reddening; decreased muscle strength; delusions; distorted sense of time and self-perception; dry mouth; euphoria; hallucinations; impaired cognition, short-term memory, and mood; incoordination; increased hunger; increased systolic pressure when supine; orthostatic hypotension; paranoia; spontaneous laughter; tachycardia; vivid visual imagery
• *Of withdrawal:* chills, decreased appetite, increased rapid-eye-movement (REM) sleep, insomnia, irritability, nervousness, restlessness, tremors, weight loss

Intervention:
• Place the patient in a quiet room.
• Monitor vital signs.
• Give supplemental oxygen for respiratory depression and I.V. fluids for hypotension.
• Give diazepam, as ordered, for extreme agitation and acute psychosis.

Carefully review the patient's medical history. Suspect drug abuse if he reports a painful injury or chronic illness but refuses a diagnostic workup. In his attempt to obtain drugs, the dependent patient may feign illnesses, such as migraine headaches, myocardial infarction, and renal colic; claim an allergy to over-the-counter analgesics; or even request a specific medication. Also be alert for a previous history of overdose or a high tolerance to potentially addictive drugs. I.V. drug users may have a history of hepatitis or human immunodeficiency virus (HIV) infection because they often share dirty needles. Female drug users may report a history of amenorrhea.

The psychiatric history of a patient who abuses drugs may reveal suggestive behavior patterns or the presence of known risk factors. For example, the patient may give a fictitious name and address, display a reluctance to discuss previous hospitalizations, or seek treatment at a medical facility across town rather than in his own neighborhood. If possible, interview family members to verify his responses.

If the patient admits to drug use, try to determine the extent to which this behavior interferes in his life. Note whether he expresses a desire to overcome his dependence on drugs. If possible, obtain a drug history consisting of substances ingested, amount, frequency, and last dose. Expect incomplete or inaccurate responses. Drug-induced amnesia, a depressed level of consciousness, or ignorance may distort the patient's recollection of the facts; he also may deliberately fabricate answers to avoid arrest or to downplay a suicide attempt.

The hospitalized drug abuser is likely to be uncooperative, disruptive, or even violent. He may experience mood swings, anxiety, impaired memory, sleep disturbances, flashbacks, slurred speech, depression, and thought disorders. Some patients resort to plays on sympathy, bribery, or threats to obtain drugs, or try to manipulate caregivers by pitting one staff member against another.

Diagnostic criteria

The diagnosis of psychoactive substance dependence is confirmed when the patient meets the criteria documented in the *DSM-IV*.
• At least three of the following must be present:
— substance often taken in larger amounts or for a longer time than the patient intended
— persistent desire or one or more unsuccessful efforts to cut down or control substance use

— excessive time devoted to activities necessary to obtain the substance
— frequent intoxication or withdrawal symptoms when expected to fulfill major obligations at work, school, or home, or when substance use is physically hazardous
— important social, occupational, or recreational activities given up or reduced because of substance use
— continued substance use despite the recognition of a persistent or recurrent social, psychological, or physical problem that is caused or exacerbated by the use of the substance
— marked tolerance: need for markedly increased amounts of the substance to achieve intoxication or the desired effect, or markedly diminished effect with continued use of the same amount
— characteristic withdrawal symptoms
— substance often taken to relieve or avoid withdrawal symptoms.
• Some symptoms must have persisted for at least 1 month or have occurred repeatedly over a longer time.

Additional tests can confirm drug use, determine the amount and type of drug taken, and reveal complications. For example, a serum or urine drug screen can detect substances that were ingested recently. Characteristic findings in other tests include elevated serum globulin levels, hypoglycemia, leukocytosis, liver function abnormalities, positive Venereal Disease Research Laboratory (VDRL) or rapid plasma reagin test results due to elevated protein fractions, elevated mean corpuscular hemoglobin levels, elevated uric acid levels, and reduced blood urea nitrogen levels.

Treatment

The patient with acute drug intoxication should receive symptomatic treatment based on the drug ingested. Measures include fluid replacement therapy and nutritional and vitamin supplements, if indicated; detoxification with the same drug or a pharmacologically similar drug (exceptions include cocaine, hallucinogens, and marijuana, which are not used for detoxification); sedatives to induce sleep; anticholinergics and antidiarrheal agents to relieve GI distress; antianxiety drugs for severe agitation, especially in cocaine abusers; and symptomatic treatment of complications. Depending on the dosage and time elapsed before admission, additional treatment may include gastric lavage, induced emesis, activated charcoal, forced diuresis and, possibly, hemoperfusion or hemodialysis.

Treatment of drug dependence commonly involves a triad of care: detoxification, short- and long-term rehabilitation, and aftercare; the latter means a lifetime of abstinence, usually aided by participation in Narcotics Anonymous or a similar self-help group.

Detoxification, the controlled and gradual withdrawal of an abused drug, is achieved through substitution of a drug with similar action. Such gradual replacement of the abused drug controls the effects of withdrawal, reducing the patient's discomfort and associated risks.

Depending on which drug the patient has abused, detoxification may be managed on an inpatient or outpatient basis. For example, withdrawal from depressants can produce hazardous effects, such as generalized tonic-clonic seizures, status epilepticus, and hypotension; the severity of these effects determines whether the patient can be safely treated as an outpatient or requires hospitalization. Withdrawal from depressants usually doesn't require detoxification. Opioid withdrawal causes severe physical discomfort and can even be life-threatening. To minimize these effects, chronic opioid abusers commonly are detoxified with methadone.

To ease withdrawal from opioids, depressants, and other drugs, useful nonchemical measures may include psychotherapy, exercise, relaxation techniques, and nutritional support. Sedatives and tranquilizers may be administered temporarily to help the patient cope with insomnia, anxiety, and depression.

After withdrawal, rehabilitation is needed to prevent recurrence of drug abuse. Rehabilitation programs are available for both inpatients and outpatients; they usually last a month or longer and may include individual, group, and family psychotherapy. During and after rehabilitation, participation in a drug-oriented self-help group may be helpful. The largest such group is Narcotics Anonymous.

Nursing diagnoses
• Altered protection
• Altered role performance
• Altered thought processes
• Anxiety
• Defensive coping
• Functional incontinence
• Hopelessness
• Impaired physical mobility
• Impaired social interaction
• Impaired tissue integrity
• Ineffective denial
• Ineffective family coping

• Ineffective individual coping
• Noncompliance
• Personal identity disturbance
• Powerlessness
• Risk for injury
• Risk for violence
• Self-care deficit
• Sensory or perceptual alterations
• Sleep pattern disturbance
• Spiritual distress

Nursing interventions
• Focus on restoring physical health, educating the patient and his family about drug abuse and dependence, providing support, and encouraging participation in drug treatment programs and self-help groups.

During an acute episode:
• Continuously monitor the patient's vital signs, and observe for complications of overdose and withdrawal, such as cardiopulmonary arrest, seizures, and aspiration.
• Based on standard hospital policy, institute appropriate measures to prevent suicide attempts.
• Give medications, as ordered, to decrease withdrawal symptoms; monitor and record their effectiveness.
• Maintain a quiet, safe environment during withdrawal from any drug because excessive noise may agitate the patient. Remove harmful objects from the room, and use restraints only if you suspect that he might harm himself or others. Institute seizure precautions.

When the acute episode has resolved:
• Develop self-awareness and an understanding and positive attitude toward the patient; control your reactions to his undesirable behaviors—commonly, psychological dependency, manipulation, anger, frustration, and alienation.
• Set limits for dealing with demanding, manipulative behavior.
• Carefully monitor and promote adequate nutrition.
• Administer medications carefully to prevent hoarding by the patient. Check the patient's mouth to ensure that the medication has been swallowed. Closely monitor visitors who might supply the patient with drugs.
• Refer the patient for detoxification and rehabilitation, as appropriate. Give him a list of available resources.
• Encourage family members to seek help whether or not the abuser seeks it. You can suggest private therapy or community mental health clinics.

FIVE TYPES OF SCHIZOPHRENIA

The *DSM-IV* recognizes five types of schizophrenia based on the patient's signs and symptoms. Here are the distinguishing characteristics.

Catatonic schizophrenia

The catatonic patient may be unable to move around or take care of his personal needs. Commonly, he doesn't feed himself or talk and may show bizarre, stereotypic mannerisms, such as facial grimacing and sucking mouth movements. Rarely, he may also exhibit waxy flexibility, in which the body (especially the extremities) will rigidly hold any placed position for prolonged periods.

Diminished sensitivity to painful stimuli and rapid swings between excitement and stupor may be observed. An excitement phase may include extreme psychomotor agitation with excessive, senseless, or incoherent talking or shouting and with increased potential for destructive, violent behavior.

Paranoid schizophrenia

Persecutory or grandiose delusional thought content and possibly delusional jealousy characterize paranoid schizophrenia. This condition may be associated with unfocused anxiety, anger, argumentativeness, and violence. It may also involve gender-identity problems, including fears of being thought of as homosexual or of being approached by homosexuals.

Although the patient frequently experiences auditory hallucinations related to a single theme, he typically doesn't display some of the symptoms common to other types of schizophrenia, including incoherence, marked loosening of associations, flat or grossly inappropriate affect, catatonic behavior, and grossly disorganized behavior.

Paranoid schizophrenia may cause only minimal impairment of function if the patient doesn't act on the delusional thoughts. His affective responsiveness may remain intact, but interactions with others commonly show stilted formality or intensity.

Disorganized schizophrenia

Characteristics of disorganized schizophrenia include marked loosening of associations; grossly disorganized behavior; blunted, silly, flat, or inappropriate affect; incoherence; grimacing; unsystematic delusions; social withdrawal; and hypochondriacal complaints.

This type of schizophrenia may begin early and insidiously with no significant remissions. The patient usually exhibits extreme social impairment.

Residual schizophrenia

Residual schizophrenia is distinguished by emotional blunting, social withdrawal, eccentric behavior, illogical thinking, and mild loosening of associations following resolution of an acute psychotic episode. The patient has no prominent delusions, hallucinations, incoherence, or grossly disorganized behavior.

Undifferentiated schizophrenia

This type is characterized by atypical symptoms or a mixture of symptoms associated with several subtypes, such as delusions, incoherence, hallucinations, or grossly disorganized behavior.

Patient teaching

If the patient refuses to participate in a rehabilitation program, teach him how to minimize the risk of drug-related complications, as follows:
• Review measures for preventing HIV infection and hepatitis. Stress that these infections are readily transmitted by sharing needles with other drug users and by unprotected sexual intercourse.
• Advise the patient to use a new needle for every injection or to clean needles with a solution of chlorine bleach and water.
• Emphasize the importance of using a condom during intercourse to prevent disease transmission and pregnancy. If necessary, teach the female drug abuser about other methods of birth control. Explain the devastating effects of drugs on the developing fetus.

SCHIZOPHRENIC DISORDERS

Characterized by disordered thinking, schizophrenic disorders include schizophrenia and delusional disorders.

SCHIZOPHRENIA

This disorder is characterized by disturbances (for at least 6 months) in thought content and form, perception, affect, sense of self, volition, interpersonal relationships, and psychomotor behavior. The *DSM-IV* recognizes catatonic, paranoid, disorganized, residual, and undifferentiated schizophrenia (see *Five types of schizophrenia*). Schizophrenia affects approximately 1% to 2% of the U.S. population and appears to be equally prevalent among males and females. Onset of symp-

DIAGNOSING SCHIZOPHRENIA

The following criteria described in the *DSM-IV* are used to diagnose a person with schizophrenia.

Characteristic symptoms

A person with schizophrenia has two or more of the following signs and symptoms, each present for a significant portion of time during a 1-month period (or less, if successfully treated):
- delusions
- prominent hallucinations (throughout the day for several days or several times a week for several weeks, with each hallucinatory experience lasting more than a few moments)
- disorganized speech (for example, frequent derailment or incoherence)
- grossly disorganized or catatonic behavior
- negative symptoms (for example, flat affect, inability to make decisions, or inability to speak).

The diagnosis requires only one of these characteristic signs or symptoms if the person's delusions are bizarre (that is, involving a phenomenon that the person's culture would regard as implausible) or if hallucinations consist of a voice issuing a running commentary on the person's behavior or thoughts, or consist of two or more voices conversing with each other.

Social and occupational dysfunction

For a significant period during the course of the disturbance, one or more major areas of functioning (such as work, interpersonal relationships, or self-care) are markedly below the level achieved before the onset of the disturbance.

When the disturbance begins in childhood or adolescence, the dysfunction takes the form of failure to achieve the expected level of interpersonal, academic, or occupational development.

Duration

Continuous signs and symptoms of the disturbance persist for at least 6 months. The 6-month period must include at least 1 month of symptoms that match the characteristic, active-phase signs and symptoms (or less if signs and symptoms have been successfully treated) and may include periods of prodromal or residual symptoms.

During the prodromal or residual periods, signs of the disturbance may be manifested by only negative symptoms or by two or more characteristic symptoms in a less severe form (for example, odd beliefs or unusual perceptual experiences).

Schizoaffective and mood disorder exclusion

Schizoaffective disorder and mood disorder with psychotic features have been ruled out for these reasons: Either no major depressive, manic, or mixed episodes have occurred concurrently with the active-phase signs and symptoms *or,* if mood disorder episodes have occurred during active-phase signs and symptoms, their total duration has been relatively brief in comparison with the duration of the active and residual periods.

Substance and general medical condition exclusion

The disturbance is not due to the direct physiologic effects of a substance or a general medical condition.

Relationship to a pervasive developmental disorder

If the person has a history of autistic disorder or another pervasive developmental disorder, the additional diagnosis of schizophrenia is appropriate only if prominent delusions or hallucinations also are present for at least 1 month (or less if successfully treated).

---

toms usually occurs during adolescence or early adulthood.

This disorder produces varying degrees of impairment. As many as one-third of schizophrenic patients have just one psychotic episode and no more after that. Some patients have no disability between periods of exacerbation; other patients need continuous institutional care. The prognosis worsens with each acute episode.

Causes

Schizophrenia may result from a combination of genetic, biological, cultural, and psychological factors. For example, some evidence supports a genetic predisposition to this disorder. Close relatives of schizophrenic patients are up to 50 times more likely to develop schizophrenia; the closer the degree of biological relatedness, the higher the risk.

The most widely accepted biochemical hypothesis holds that schizophrenia results from excessive activity at dopaminergic synapses. Other neurotransmitter alterations may also contribute to schizophrenic symptoms. Schizophrenic patients also have structural abnormalities of both the frontal and temporolimbic systems.

Numerous psychological and sociocultural causes, such as disturbed family and interpersonal patterns, also have been proposed as possible causes. Schizophrenia has a higher incidence among lower socioeconomic groups, possibly related to downward social drift or lack of upward socioeconomic mobility, and to high stress levels, possibly induced by poverty, social failure, illness, and inadequate social resources. Higher incidence also is linked to low birth weight and congenital deafness.

Complications
Because of disordered thought processes, the schizophrenic patient often neglects personal hygiene or ignores health needs. As a result, the patient has a shorter life expectancy than the general population. He also presents a high suicide risk.

Assessment findings
Schizophrenia is associated with a wide variety of abnormal behaviors; therefore, assessment findings vary greatly, depending on both the type and phase of the illness.

Although behaviors and functional deficiencies can vary widely among patients and even in the same patient at different times, watch for the following characteristic signs and symptoms during the assessment interview:
• ambivalence — coexisting strong positive and negative feelings, leading to emotional conflict
• apathy
• clang associations — words that rhyme or sound alike used in an illogical, nonsensical manner — for instance, "It's the rain, train, pain"
• concrete thinking — inability to form or understand abstract thoughts
• delusions — false ideas or beliefs accepted as real by the patient. Delusions of grandeur, persecution, and reference (distorted belief regarding the relation between events and one's self; for example, a belief that television programs address the patient on a personal level) are common in schizophrenia. Also common are feelings of being controlled, somatic illness, and depersonalization.
• echolalia — meaningless repetition of words or phrases
• echopraxia — involuntary repetition of movements observed in others
• flight of ideas — rapid succession of incomplete and unconnected ideas
• hallucinations — false sensory perceptions with no basis in reality. Usually visual or auditory, hallucinations also may be olfactory (smell), gustatory (taste), or tactile (touch).

• illusions — false sensory perceptions with some basis in reality; for example, a car backfiring mistaken for a gunshot
• loose associations — rapid shifts among unrelated ideas
• magical thinking — belief that thoughts or wishes can control other people or events
• neologisms — bizarre words that have meaning only for the patient
• poor interpersonal relationships
• regression — return to an earlier developmental stage
• thought blocking — sudden interruption in the patient's train of thought
• withdrawal — disinterest in objects, people, or surroundings
• word salad — illogical word groupings; for example, "She had a star, barn, plant."

Diagnostic criteria
Complete physical and psychiatric examinations rule out an organic cause of schizophrenic symptoms, such as an amphetamine-induced psychosis. Diagnosis rests on fulfilling the criteria in the *DSM-IV*. (See *Diagnosing schizophrenia*.)

Several tests — including brain imaging studies, tissue studies, functional and metabolic studies, and psychological tests — can be helpful in the diagnosis of schizophrenia.

Treatment
In schizophrenia, treatment focuses on meeting both the physical and psychosocial needs of the patient, based on his previous level of adjustment and his response to medical and nursing interventions. Treatment typically includes a combination of drug therapy, long-term psychotherapy for the patient and his family, vocational counseling, and the use of community resources.

The primary treatment (for more than 30 years), antipsychotic drugs (sometimes called neuroleptic drugs) appear to work by blocking postsynaptic dopamine receptors. These antipsychotic drugs reduce the incidence of psychotic symptoms, such as hallucinations and delusions, as well as relieve anxiety and agitation. Other psychiatric drugs, such as antidepressants and anxiolytics, may also be prescribed to control associated signs and symptoms.

Some antipsychotic drugs cause numerous adverse reactions, several of which are irreversible (see *Reviewing adverse effects of antipsychotic drugs*, page 40). Most experts admit that patients who are withdrawn,

REVIEWING ADVERSE EFFECTS OF ANTIPSYCHOTIC DRUGS

Antipsychotic drugs (sometimes known as neuroleptic drugs) can cause sedative, anticholinergic, or extrapyramidal effects; orthostatic hypotension; and, rarely, neuroleptic malignant syndrome.

Sedative, anticholinergic, and extrapyramidal effects
High-potency drugs (such as haloperidol) are minimally sedative and minimally anticholinergic but result in a high incidence of extrapyramidal adverse effects. Intermediate-potency agents (such as molindone) are associated with a moderate incidence of adverse effects, whereas low-potency drugs (such as chlorpromazine) are highly sedative and anticholinergic but elicit few extrapyramidal adverse effects.

The most common extrapyramidal effects are dystonia, parkinsonism, and akathisia. Dystonia most frequently occurs in young males, usually within the first few days of treatment. Characterized by anguished tonic contractions of the muscles in the neck, mouth, and tongue, dystonia may be misdiagnosed as a psychotic symptom. Diphenhydramine hydrochloride (Benadryl) or benztropine (Cogentin) administered I.M. or I.V. provides rapid relief.

Drug-induced parkinsonism results in bradykinesia, muscle rigidity, shuffling or propulsive gait, stooped posture, flat facial affect, tremors, and drooling. Parkinsonism may occur from 1 week to several months after the initiation of drug treatment. Drugs prescribed to reverse or prevent this syndrome include benztropine, trihexyphenidyl (Artane), and amantadine (Symmetrel).

Signs and symptoms of akathisia include restlessness, pacing, and an inability to rest or sit still. Propranolol relieves this adverse effect.

Orthostatic hypotension
Low-potency neuroleptics can also cause orthostatic hypotension because they block alpha-adrenergic receptors. If severe, place the patient in the supine position and give I.V. fluids for hypovolemia. If further treatment is necessary, an alpha-adrenergic agonist, such as norepinephrine (Levophed) or metaraminol (Aramine), may be ordered to relieve hypotension. Mixed alpha- and beta-adrenergic drugs, such as epinephrine, or beta-adrenergic drugs, such as isoproterenol, should not be given because they can produce further reduction in blood pressure.

Neuroleptic malignant syndrome
In up to 1% of patients, antipsychotic drugs produce this life-threatening syndrome. Signs and symptoms include elevated body temperature, muscle rigidity, and altered consciousness, occurring hours to months after the initiation of drug therapy or increasing the dose. Treatment is symptomatic, largely consisting of dantrolene and other measures to counter muscle rigidity associated with hyperthermia. You'll need to continuously monitor the patient's vital signs and mental status.

isolated, or apathetic show little improvement after this drug treatment.

High-potency antipsychotics include fluphenazine, haloperidol, thiothixene, and trifluoperazine. Loxapine, molindone, and perphenazine are intermediate in potency, and chlorpromazine and thioridazine are low in potency. Haloperidol decanoate, fluphenazine decanoate, and fluphenazine enanthate are depot formulations that are implanted I.M., resulting in gradual release over a 30-day period, thus improving compliance.

Clozapine, which differs chemically from other antipsychotic drugs, may be prescribed for severely ill patients who fail to respond to standard treatment. This agent effectively controls a wider range of signs and symptoms without the usual adverse effects. However, clozapine can cause drowsiness, sedation, excessive salivation, tachycardia, dizziness, and seizures, as well as agranulocytosis, a potentially fatal blood disorder characterized by a low white blood cell count and pronounced neutropenia.

Routine blood monitoring is essential to detect the estimated 1% to 2% of all patients taking clozapine who will develop agranulocytosis. If the disorder is caught in the early stages, agranulocytosis is reversible.

Clinicians disagree about the effectiveness of psychotherapy in treating schizophrenia. Although a patient who has experienced a single acute psychotic episode may respond, psychotherapy is often futile in a patient with a long history of chronic disease. Nonetheless, some doctors use it as an adjunct to reduce loneliness, isolation, and withdrawal and enhance productivity.

Other studies suggest that psychoeducation and social skills training are more productive approaches for the chronic schizophrenic. Besides improving understanding of the disorder, these methods teach the patient and his family coping strategies, effective communication techniques, and social skills, such as grocery shopping.

Because schizophrenia is so disruptive to the family, all members may require psychotherapy. Family therapy can reduce guilt and disappointment as well as improve acceptance of the patient and his bizarre behavior.

Nursing diagnoses
• Altered nutrition: Less than body requirements
• Altered role performance
• Altered thought processes
• Anxiety
• Body image disturbance
• Fear
• Fluid volume deficit
• Hopelessness
• Impaired home maintenance management
• Impaired social interaction
• Impaired verbal communication
• Ineffective family coping
• Ineffective individual coping
• Personal identity disturbance
• Powerlessness
• Risk for injury
• Risk for violence: Self-directed or directed at others
• Self-care deficit
• Sensory or perceptual alterations
• Sleep pattern disturbance
• Social isolation

Nursing interventions
• Assess the patient's ability to carry out the activities of daily living, paying special attention to his nutritional status. Monitor his weight if he isn't eating. If he thinks that his food is poisoned, allow him to fix his own food when possible, or offer him foods in closed containers that he can open. If you give liquid medication in a unit-dose container, allow the patient to open the container.
• Maintain a safe environment, minimizing stimuli. Administer medication to decrease symptoms and anxiety. Use physical restraints according to your hospital's policy to ensure the patient's safety and that of others.
• Adopt an accepting and consistent approach with the patient. Don't avoid or overwhelm him. Keep in mind that short, repeated contacts are best until trust has been established.
• Avoid promoting dependence. Meet the patient's needs, but only do for the patient what he can't do for himself.

Reward positive behavior to help the patient improve his level of functioning.
• Engage the patient in reality-oriented activities that involve human contact: inpatient social skills training groups, outpatient day care, and sheltered workshops. Provide reality-based explanations for distorted body images or hypochondriacal complaints. Clarify private language, autistic inventions, or neologisms, explaining to the patient that what he says is not understood by others. If necessary, set limits on inappropriate behavior.
• If the patient is hallucinating, explore the content of the hallucinations. If he hears voices, find out if he believes that he must do what they command. Tell the patient you don't hear the voices but you know they're real to him. Avoid arguing about the hallucinations; if possible, change the subject.
• Don't tease or joke with the patient. Choose words and phrases that are unambiguous and clearly understood. For instance, a patient who's told, "That procedure will be done on the floor," may become frightened, thinking he is being told to lie down on the floor.
• If the patient is expressing suicidal thoughts, institute suicide precautions. Document his behavior and your precautions.
• If the patient is expressing homicidal thoughts (for example, "I have to kill my mother"), institute homicidal precautions. Notify the doctor and the potential victim. Document the patient's comments and who was notified.
• Don't touch the patient without telling him first exactly what you're going to do. For example, clearly explain to him, "I'm going to put this cuff on your arm so I can take your blood pressure." If necessary, postpone procedures that require physical contact with hospital personnel until the patient is less suspicious or agitated.
• Remember, institutionalization may produce new symptoms and handicaps in the patient that are not part of his diagnosed illness, so evaluate symptoms carefully.
• Mobilize community resources to provide a support system for the patient and reduce his vulnerability to stress. Ongoing support is essential to his mastery of social skills.
• Encourage compliance with the medication regimen to prevent relapse. Also monitor the patient carefully for adverse effects of drug therapy, including drug-induced parkinsonism, acute dystonia, akathisia, tar-

dive dyskinesia, and malignant neuroleptic syndrome. Make sure you document and report such effects promptly.

In addition, for *catatonic schizophrenia:*
• Assess the patient for physical illness. Remember that the mute patient won't complain of pain or physical symptoms; if he's in a bizarre posture, he's at increased risk for pressure ulcers or decreased circulation to a body area.
• Meet physical needs for adequate food, fluid, exercise, and elimination; follow orders with respect to nutrition, urinary catheterization, and enema.
• Provide range-of-motion exercises or ambulate the patient every 2 hours.
• Prevent physical exhaustion and injury during periods of hyperactivity.
• Tell the patient directly, specifically, and concisely what needs to be done. Don't offer the negativistic patient a choice. For example, you might say, "It's time to go for a walk. Let's go."
• Spend some time with the patient even if he's mute and unresponsive. He's acutely aware of his environment even though he seems not to be. Your presence can be calming and reassuring. Avoid mutual withdrawal.
• Verbalize for the patient the message his nonverbal behavior seems to convey, and encourage him to do so as well.
• Offer reality orientation. You might say: "The leaves on the trees are turning colors and the air is cooler. It's fall!" Emphasize reality in all contacts to reduce distorted perceptions.
• Stay alert for violent outbursts from the patient; get help promptly to intervene safely for yourself and the patient.

For *paranoid schizophrenia:*
• When the patient is newly admitted, minimize his contact with the staff.
• Don't crowd the patient physically or psychologically; he may strike out to protect himself.
• Be flexible; allow the patient some control. Approach him in a calm and unhurried manner. Let him talk about anything he wishes initially, but keep conversation light and social, and avoid entering into power struggles.
• Respond to the patient's condescending attitudes (arrogance, put-downs, sarcasm, or open hostility) with neutral remarks.
• Don't let the patient put you on the defensive and don't take his remarks personally. If he tells you to leave

him alone, do leave, but make sure you return soon. Brief contacts with the patient may be most useful at first.
• Don't try to combat the patient's delusions with logic. Instead, respond to feelings, themes, or underlying needs – for example, "It seems you feel you've been treated unfairly" (persecution).
• Build trust; be honest and dependable. Don't threaten, and don't promise what you can't fulfill.
• Don't tease, joke, argue with, or confront the patient. Remember, his distorted perception will cause him to misinterpret such action in a way that's derogatory to himself.

Patient teaching
• If the patient is taking clozapine, stress the importance of returning weekly to the hospital or outpatient setting to have his blood monitored.
• Teach the patient the importance of complying with the medication regimen. Tell him that he should report any adverse effects, but that he shouldn't just stop taking the drug. If he takes a slow-release formulation, make sure he understands when to return to the doctor for his next dose of medication.
• Involve the patient's family in his treatment, particularly because his altered thought processes and sensory and perceptual alterations often make teaching difficult or impossible. Teach family members how to recognize an impending relapse and suggest ways to manage symptoms, such as tension, nervousness, insomnia, decreased concentration ability, and loss of interest.

DELUSIONAL DISORDERS
According to the *DSM-IV,* delusional disorders are characterized by false beliefs with a plausible basis in reality. Formerly referred to as paranoid disorders, delusional disorders are known to involve erotomanic, grandiose, jealous, or somatic themes as well as persecutory delusions (for more information, see *Delusional disorder or paranoid schizophrenia?*). Some patients experience several types of delusions, whereas other patients experience unspecified delusions that have no dominant theme (see *Delusional themes,* page 44).

Delusional disorders commonly begin in middle or late adulthood, usually between ages 40 and 55, but they can occur at a younger age. These uncommon illnesses affect less than 1% of the population; the incidence is about equal in men and women. Typically chronic, these disorders often interfere with social and marital relationships but seldom impair intellectual or occupational functioning significantly.

Causes

Delusional disorders of later life strongly suggest a hereditary predisposition. At least one study has linked the development of delusional disorders to inferiority feelings in the family. Some researchers suggest that delusional disorders are the product of specific early childhood experiences with an authoritarian family structure. Others hold that anyone with a sensitive personality is particularly vulnerable to developing a delusional disorder.

Certain medical conditions are known to exaggerate the risks of delusional disorders: head injury, chronic alcoholism, deafness, and aging. Predisposing factors linked to aging include isolation, lack of stimulating interpersonal relationships, physical illness, and diminished hearing and vision. In addition, severe stress (such as a move to a foreign country) may precipitate a delusional disorder.

Complications

The delusional patient who acts on his irrational beliefs may pose a threat to himself or others. The more extreme the patient's rage, the greater the risk of violent behavior or suicide.

Assessment findings

The psychiatric history of a delusional patient may be unremarkable, aside from behavior related to his delusions. He's likely to report problems with social and marital relationships, including depressive symptoms or sexual dysfunction. In fact, about one-third of delusional patients are widowed, divorced, or separated at the time of first admission. Others describe a life marked by social isolation or hostility. Such patients may deny feeling lonely, relentlessly criticizing or placing unreasonable demands on others.

Gathering accurate information from a delusional patient may prove difficult. He may deny his feelings, disregard the circumstances leading to hospitalization, and refuse treatment. However, the patient's responses and behavior during the assessment interview provide clues that can help to identify his disorder. Family members may confirm your observations, often reporting that the patient is chronically jealous or suspicious.

For example, note how effectively the patient communicates. He may be evasive or reluctant to answer

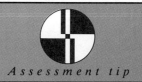

Assessment tip

DELUSIONAL DISORDER OR PARANOID SCHIZOPHRENIA?

To distinguish between these two disorders, consider the following characteristics.

Delusional disorder

In a delusional disorder, the patient's delusions reflect reality and are arranged into a coherent system. They're based on misinterpretations of or elaborations on reality.

The patient doesn't experience hallucinations, and his affect and behavior are normal.

Paranoid schizophrenia

In paranoid schizophrenia, the patient's delusions are scattered, illogical, and incoherently arranged with no relation to reality.

The patient may have hallucinations, his affect is inappropriate and inconsistent, and his behavior is bizarre.

questions. Alternatively, he may be overly talkative, explaining events in great detail and emphasizing what he has achieved, prominent people he knows, or places he has traveled. Statements that first seem logical may later prove irrelevant. Some of his answers may be contradictory, jumbled, or irrational.

Be alert for expressions of denial, projection, and rationalization. Once delusions become firmly entrenched, the patient will no longer seek to justify his beliefs. However, if he's still struggling to maintain his delusional defenses, he may make statements that reveal his condition, such as "People at work won't talk to me because I'm smarter than them." Accusatory statements are also characteristic of the patient with a delusional disorder. A patient who's chronically late for work, for example, may insist that he lost his job because his supervisor was incompetent. Record pervasive delusional themes (for example, grandiose or persecutory).

Also watch for nonverbal cues, indicating suspiciousness or mistrust, such as excessive vigilance or obvious apprehension on entering the room. During questions, the patient may listen intently, reacting defensively to imagined slights or insults. He may sit at

DELUSIONAL THEMES

In a patient with a delusional disorder, the delusions are well systematized and follow a predominant theme. Common delusional themes are listed below.

Erotomanic delusions
A prevalent delusional theme, erotomanic delusions concern romantic or spiritual love. The patient believes that he shares in an idealized (rather than sexual) relationship with someone of higher status — a superior at work, a celebrity, or an anonymous stranger.

The patient may hold this delusion in secret but more commonly will try to contact the object of his delusion through calls, letters, gifts, or even spying. He may attempt to rescue his beloved from imagined danger. The patient with erotomanic delusions frequently harasses public figures and often comes to the attention of the police.

Grandiose delusions
The patient with grandiose delusions believes that he has great, unrecognized talent, special insight, or prophetic power, or has made an important discovery. To achieve recognition, he may contact government agencies, such as the Federal Bureau of Investigation. The patient with a religiously oriented delusion of grandeur may become a cult leader. Less commonly, he believes that he shares a special relationship with some well-known personality, such as a rock star or a world leader. The patient may believe himself to be a famous person, his identity usurped by an imposter.

Jealous delusions
These delusions focus on infidelity. For example, a patient may insist that his spouse or lover has acted unfaithfully and search for evidence to justify the delusion, such as spots on bed sheets. He may confront his partner, try to control her movements, follow her, or track down her suspected lover. He may physically assault her or, less likely, his perceived rival.

Persecutory delusions
The patient suffering from persecutory delusions, the most common delusional theme, believes that he's being followed, harassed, plotted against, poisoned, mocked, or deliberately prevented from achieving his long-term goals. These delusions may evolve into a

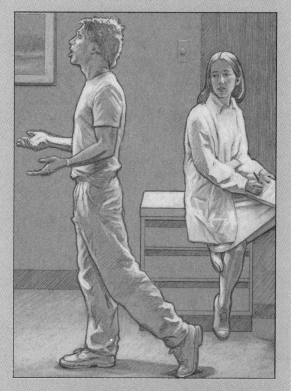

simple or complex persecution scheme, in which even the slightest injustice is interpreted as part of the scheme.

Such a patient may file numerous lawsuits or seek redress from government agencies (querulous paranoia). A patient who becomes resentful and angry may lash out violently against the alleged offender.

Somatic delusions
This delusional theme centers on an imagined physical defect or deformity. The patient may perceive a foul odor coming from his skin, mouth, rectum, or other body part. Other delusions involve skin-crawling insects, internal parasites, or physical illness.

the edge of his seat or fold his arms as if to shield himself. If he carries papers or money, he may clutch them firmly.

Diagnostic criteria
Psychiatric examination confirms the presence of the following diagnostic criteria in the *DSM-IV*:

• Nonbizzare delusions of at least 1 month's duration are present, involving real-life situations, such as being followed, poisoned, infected, loved at a distance, or deceived by one's spouse or lover.
• Auditory or visual hallucinations, if present, are not prominent.

• Apart from the delusion or its ramifications, behavior is not obviously odd or bizarre.

• If a major depressive or manic syndrome has been present during the delusional disturbance, the total duration of all episodes of the mood syndrome has been brief relative to the total duration of the delusional disturbance.

• The patient has never met diagnostic criteria for schizophrenia (presence of characteristic psychotic symptoms in the active phase for at least 1 week), and it cannot be established that an organic factor initiated and maintained the disturbance.

In addition, blood and urine tests, psychological tests, and a neurologic evaluation rule out organic causes of the delusions, such as amphetamine-induced psychoses and Alzheimer's disease. Endocrine function tests are performed to rule out hyperadrenalism, pernicious anemia, and thyroid disorders such as "myxedemic madness."

Treatment

Effective treatment of delusional disorders, consisting of a combination of drug therapy and psychotherapy, must correct the behavior and mood disturbances that result from the patient's mistaken belief system. Treatment also may include mobilizing a support system for the isolated, aged patient.

Drug treatment with antipsychotic agents is similar to that used in schizophrenic disorders. Antipsychotics appear to work by blocking postsynaptic dopamine receptors. These drugs reduce the incidence of psychotic symptoms, such as hallucinations and delusions, and relieve anxiety and agitation. Other psychiatric drugs, such as antidepressants and anxiolytics, may be prescribed to control associated symptoms.

High-potency antipsychotics include fluphenazine, haloperidol, thiothixene, and trifluoperazine. Loxapine succinate, molindone, and perphenazine are intermediate in potency, and chlorpromazine and thioridazine are low-potency agents. Haloperidol decanoate, fluphenazine decanoate, and fluphenazine enanthate are depot formulations that are implanted I.M. and release the drug gradually over a 30-day period, improving compliance.

Clozapine, which differs chemically from other antipsychotic drugs, may be prescribed for severely ill patients who fail to respond to standard neuroleptic treatment. This agent effectively controls a wider range of psychotic symptoms without the usual adverse effects.

However, clozapine can cause drowsiness, sedation, excessive salivation, tachycardia, dizziness, and seizures, as well as agranulocytosis, a potentially fatal blood disorder characterized by a low white blood cell count and pronounced neutropenia. Routine blood monitoring is essential to detect the estimated 1% to 2% of all patients taking clozapine who develop agranulocytosis. If caught in the early stages, the disorder is reversible.

Nursing diagnoses

• Altered nutrition: Less than body requirements
• Altered thought processes
• Anxiety
• Fear
• Impaired home maintenance management
• Impaired social interaction
• Ineffective family coping
• Ineffective individual coping
• Noncompliance
• Personal identity disturbance
• Powerlessness
• Risk for injury
• Risk for violence: Self-directed or directed at others
• Sensory or perceptual alterations
• Social isolation

Nursing interventions

• In dealing with the patient, be direct, straightforward, and dependable. Whenever possible, elicit his feedback. Move slowly, with a matter-of-fact manner and respond without anger or defensiveness to his hostile remarks.

• Respect the patient's privacy and space needs. Avoid touching him unnecessarily.

• Take steps to reduce social isolation, if the patient allows. Gradually increase social contacts after he has become comfortable with the staff.

• Watch for refusal of medication or food, resulting from the patient's irrational fear of poisoning.

• Monitor the patient carefully for adverse effects of neuroleptic drugs: drug-induced parkinsonism, acute dystonia, akathisia, tardive dyskinesia, and malignant neuroleptic syndrome.

Patient teaching

• If the patient is taking clozapine, stress the importance of returning weekly to the hospital or outpatient setting to have his blood monitored.

• Emphasize the importance of complying with the prescribed medication treatment. Instruct the patient to report any adverse effects instead of stopping the drug. If he's taking a slow-release formulation, be sure he understands when to return to the doctor for his next dose.

• Involve the family in treatment. Teach them how to recognize an impending relapse and suggest ways to manage symptoms. These include tension, nervousness, insomnia, decreased concentration ability, and loss of interest.

MOOD DISORDERS

In these disorders, a person's mood becomes so intense and persistent that it interferes with his social and psychological function. Mood disorders include bipolar disorder and major depression.

BIPOLAR DISORDER

This affective disorder is marked by severe pathologic mood swings from hyperactivity and euphoria to sadness and depression. Either the manic or the depressive episodes may predominate, or the two moods can be mixed.

In cyclothymia, a variant of bipolar disorder, numerous episodes of hypomania and depressive symptoms are too mild to meet the criteria for major depression or bipolar illness (see *Cyclothymic disorder*). In some patients, bipolar disorder assumes a seasonal pattern, characterized by a cyclic relation between the onset of the mood episode and a particular 60-day period of the year.

The American Psychiatric Association estimates that 0.4% to 1.6% of adults experience bipolar disorder. This disorder is equally common in women and men, more common in higher socioeconomic groups, and associated with high levels of creativity. It can begin any time after adolescence, but onset usually occurs between ages 20 and 35; about 35% of patients experience onset between ages 35 and 60. Before the onset of overt symptoms, many patients with bipolar disorder have an energetic and outgoing personality with a history of wide mood swings.

Bipolar disorder recurs in 80% of patients; as they grow older, the attacks recur more frequently and last longer. This illness is associated with a significant mortality; 20% of patients are victims of suicide, many just as the depression lifts.

Causes and pathophysiology

The cause of bipolar disorder is unclear, but hereditary, biological, and psychological factors may play a part. For example, the incidence of bipolar disorder among relatives of affected patients is higher than in the general population and highest among maternal relatives. The closer the relationship, the greater the susceptibility. A child with one affected parent has a 25% chance of developing bipolar disorder; a child with two affected parents, a 50% chance. The incidence of this illness in siblings is 20% to 25%; 66% to 96% in identical twins.

Although certain biochemical changes accompany mood swings, it's not clear whether these changes cause the mood swings or result from them. In both mania and depression, intracellular sodium concentration increases during illness and returns to normal with recovery.

Most experts agree that patients with mood disorders have a defect in the way the brain handles certain neurotransmitters—chemical messengers that shuttle nerve impulses between neurons. Low levels of dopamine and norepinephrine, for example, have been

CYCLOTHYMIC DISORDER

A chronic mood disturbance of at least 2 years' duration, cyclothymic disorder involves numerous episodes of hypomania or depressive symptoms that are not of sufficient severity or duration to qualify as a major depressive episode.

Cyclothymia commonly starts in adolescence or early adulthood. Beginning insidiously, this disorder leads to persistent social and occupational dysfunction.

In the hypomanic phase, the patient may experience insomnia; hyperactivity; inflated self-esteem; increased productivity and creativity; overinvolvement in pleasurable activities, including an increased sexual drive; physical restlessness; and rapid speech. Depressive symptoms may include insomnia, feelings of inadequacy, decreased productivity, social withdrawal, loss of libido, loss of interest in pleasurable activities, lethargy, depressed speech, and crying.

A number of medical disorders (for example, endocrinopathies, such as Cushing's disease; stroke; brain tumors; head trauma; and drug overdose) can produce a similar pattern of mood alteration. These organic causes must be ruled out before making a diagnosis of cyclothymic disorder.

linked to depression, whereas excessively high levels of these chemicals are associated with mania.

Changes in the concentration of acetylcholine and serotonin also may play a role. Although neurobiologists have yet to prove that these chemical shifts cause bipolar disorder, it's widely assumed that most antidepressant medications work by modifying these neurotransmitter systems.

New data suggest that changes in the circadian rhythms that control hormone secretion, body temperature, and appetite may contribute to the development of bipolar disorder.

Emotional or physical trauma, such as bereavement, disruption of an important relationship, or severe accidental injury, may precede the onset of bipolar disorder; however, bipolar disorder often appears without identifiable predisposing factors.

Manic episodes may follow a stressful event but are also associated with antidepressant therapy and childbirth. Major depressive episodes may be precipitated by chronic physical illness, psychoactive drug dependence, psychosocial stressors, and childbirth. Other familial influences, especially the early loss of a parent, parental depression, incest, or abuse, may predispose to depressive illness.

Complications

The impulsive behavior characteristic of manic episodes may have far-reaching emotional and social consequences, such as bankruptcy, child abuse, and divorce. Exhaustion and poor nutrition may result from hyperactivity and sleep disturbances. A patient with bipolar disorder also represents a substantial suicide risk. Suicide can occur impulsively during a manic episode or after the resolution of a depressive episode.

Assessment findings

Widely varying assessment findings depend on whether the patient is experiencing a manic or a depressive episode.

During the assessment interview, the *manic* patient typically appears euphoric, expansive, or irritable with little control over his activities and responses. He may describe hyperactive or excessive behavior, including elaborate plans for numerous social events, efforts to renew old acquaintances by telephoning friends at all hours of the night, buying sprees, or promiscuous sexual activity. He seldom hesitates to start projects for which he has little aptitude.

The patient's activities may have a bizarre quality, such as dressing in colorful or strange garments, wearing excessive makeup, or giving advice to passing strangers. He often expresses an inflated sense of self-esteem, ranging from uncritical self-confidence to marked grandiosity, which may be delusional. For example, grandiose beliefs involving a special relationship with God or some well-known figure are common.

Note the patient's speech patterns and concentration level. Accelerated speech, frequent changes of topic, and flight of ideas are common features of the manic phase. He's easily distracted and rapidly responds to external stimuli, such as background noise or a ringing telephone.

Physical examination of the manic patient may reveal signs of malnutrition and poor personal hygiene. He may report sleeping and eating less than usual.

Hypomania, more common than acute mania, can be recognized during the assessment interview by three classic symptoms: elated but unstable mood, pressured speech, and increased motor activity. The hypomanic patient may appear elated, hyperactive, easily distracted, talkative, irritable, impatient, impulsive, and full of energy, but seldom exhibits flight of ideas, delusions, or an absence of discretion and self-control.

The patient who experiences a *depressive episode* may report a loss of self-esteem, overwhelming inertia, social withdrawal, and feelings of hopelessness, apathy, or self-reproach. He may believe that he is wicked and deserves to be punished. His growing sadness, guilt, negativity, and fatigue place extraordinary burdens on his family.

During the assessment interview, the depressed patient may speak and respond slowly. He may complain of difficulty concentrating or thinking clearly but usually is not obviously disoriented or intellectually impaired.

Physical examination may reveal psychomotor retardation, lethargy, low muscle tonus, weight loss, slowed gait, and constipation. The patient also may report sleep disturbances (falling asleep, staying asleep, or early morning awakening), sexual dysfunction, headaches, chest pains, and a heaviness in the limbs. Typically, symptoms are worse in the morning and gradually subside as the day goes on.

His concerns about his health may become hypochondriacal: He may worry excessively about having cancer or some other severe illness. In an elderly patient, physical symptoms may be the only clues to depression.

Suicide is an ever-present risk, especially as the depression begins to lift. Then, a rising energy level may strengthen the patient's resolve to carry out suicidal plans.

The suicidal patient may also harbor homicidal ideas, thinking, for example, of killing his family either in anger or to spare them pain and disgrace.

Diagnostic criteria

A diagnosis of bipolar I or II disorder is confirmed when the patient meets the criteria established in the *DSM-IV*.

Bipolar I disorders can be classified as one of six types: single manic, hypomanic, manic, depressed, mixed, or unspecified. Bipolar II disorder is present when the patient has a history of one or more major depressive and hypomanic episodes, but no history of manic episodes.

For a *manic or hypomanic episode:*
• The patient experiences a distinct period of abnormally and persistently elevated, expansive, or irritable mood.
• During the mood disturbance, at least three of these symptoms must persist (four, if the mood is only irritable) and be present to a significant degree:
— inflated self-esteem or grandiosity
— decreased need for sleep
— increased talkativeness or pressure to keep talking
— flight of ideas or subjective experience that thoughts are racing
— distractibility
— increased goal-directed activity or psychomotor agitation
— excessive involvement in pleasurable activities that have a high potential for painful consequences.

For a *manic episode* only:
• The mood disturbance is sufficiently severe to cause marked impairment in occupational function, usual social activities, or relations with others, or to require hospitalization to prevent harm to self or others.
• At no time during the disturbance have delusions or hallucinations persisted for as long as 2 weeks in the absence of prominent mood symptoms.
• The disturbance isn't superimposed on schizophrenia, schizophreniform disorder, delusional disorder, or psychotic disorder not otherwise specified.
• No organic factor has initiated and maintained the disturbance.

For a *depressive episode:*
• At least five of the following symptoms must have been present during the same 2-week period and represent a change from previous function; one of these symptoms must be either a depressed mood or a loss of interest in previously pleasurable activities:
— depressed mood (irritable mood in children and adolescents) most of the day, nearly every day, as indicated by subjective account or observation by others
— markedly diminished interest or pleasure in all, or almost all, activities most of the day, nearly every day
— significant weight loss or weight gain when not dieting or a change in appetite nearly every day
— insomnia or hypersomnia nearly every day
— psychomotor agitation or retardation nearly every day
— fatigue or loss of energy nearly every day
— feelings of worthlessness and excessive or inappropriate guilt nearly every day
— diminished ability to think or concentrate, or indecisiveness, nearly every day
— recurrent thoughts of death, recurrent suicidal ideation without a specific plan, or suicide attempt or a specific plan for committing suicide.
• No organic factor initiated and maintained the disturbance.
• The disturbance isn't a normal reaction to the death of a loved one.
• At no time during the disturbance have delusions or hallucinations persisted for as long as 2 weeks in the absence of prominent mood symptoms.
• The disturbance isn't superimposed on schizophrenia, schizophreniform disorder, delusional disorder, or psychotic disorder not otherwise specified.

For a *mixed episode:*
• The current or most recent episode involves the full symptomatic picture of both manic and major depressive episodes intermixed or rapidly alternating every few days.
• Prominent depressive symptoms last at least a full day.

A physical examination and laboratory tests, such as endocrine function studies, rule out medical causes of the mood disturbances, including intra-abdominal neoplasm, hypothyroidism, heart failure, cerebral arteriosclerosis, parkinsonism, psychoactive drug abuse, brain tumor, and uremia. In addition, a review of medications prescribed for other disorders may point to drug-induced depression or mania.

Treatment

Widely used to treat bipolar disorder, lithium proves highly effective in relieving and preventing manic episodes. The drug curbs the accelerated thought processes and hyperactive behavior without the sedating effect of antipsychotic drugs. In addition, it may prevent the recurrence of depressive episodes; however, it's ineffective in treating acute depression.

Lithium has a narrow therapeutic range, so treatment must be initiated cautiously and the dosage adjusted slowly. Therapeutic blood levels must be maintained for 7 to 10 days before effects appear; therefore, antipsychotic drugs often are used in the interim for sedation and symptomatic relief. Because lithium is excreted by the kidneys, any renal impairment necessitates withdrawal of the drug.

Anticonvulsants, such as carbamazepine, valproic acid, and clonazepam, are used to treat mood disorders either alone or along with lithium. Carbamazepine, a potent antimanic, often is effective in lithium-resistant patients.

Antidepressants occasionally are used to treat depressive symptoms. However, these drugs may trigger a manic episode.

Nursing diagnoses
For the *manic phase:*
- Altered health maintenance
- Altered nutrition: Less than body requirements
- Altered thought processes
- Chronic low self-esteem
- Impaired home maintenance management
- Impaired physical mobility
- Impaired verbal communication
- Ineffective denial
- Ineffective individual coping
- Risk for violence: Self-directed or directed at others
- Self-care deficit
- Sensory or perceptual alterations
- Sexual dysfunction
- Sleep pattern disturbance
- Social isolation
    For the *depressive phase:*
- Altered health maintenance
- Altered nutrition: Less than body requirements
- Altered thought processes
- Altered urinary elimination
- Chronic low self-esteem
- Constipation
- Hopelessness
- Impaired home maintenance management
- Impaired physical mobility
- Impaired verbal communication
- Ineffective denial
- Ineffective individual coping
- Powerlessness
- Risk for violence: Self-directed or directed at others
- Self-care deficit
- Sensory or perceptual alterations
- Sexual dysfunction
- Sleep pattern disturbance
- Social isolation

Nursing interventions
For the *manic patient:*
- Remember the manic patient's physical needs. Encourage him to eat; he may jump up and walk around the room after every mouthful but will sit down again if you remind him. Offer high-calorie finger foods, sandwiches, and cheese and crackers to supplement his diet if he can't remain seated long enough to complete a meal.
- Suggest short daytime naps, and help with personal hygiene. As the patient's symptoms subside, encourage him to assume responsibility for personal care.
- Provide emotional support, maintain a calm environment, and set realistic goals for behavior.
- Provide diversional activities suited to a short attention span; firmly discourage the patient if he tries to overextend himself.
- When necessary, reorient the patient to reality, and tactfully divert conversations when they become intimately involved with other patients or staff members.
- In a calm, clear, and self-confident manner, set limits for the manic patient's demanding, hyperactive, manipulative, and acting-out behaviors. Setting limits lets the patient know that you'll provide security and protection by refusing inappropriate and possibly harmful requests. Avoid leaving an opening for the patient to test or argue.
- Listen to requests attentively and with a neutral attitude, but avoid power struggles if the patient tries to put you on the spot for an immediate answer. Explain that you'll seriously consider the request and will respond later.
- Collaborate with other staff members to provide consistent responses to the patient's manipulations or acting out.
- Watch for early signs of frustration (when the patient's anger escalates from verbal threats to hitting an object). Tell the patient firmly that threats and hitting are unacceptable and that these behaviors show that he needs help to control his behavior. Then tell him

that the staff will help him move to a quiet area and will help him control his behavior so he won't hurt himself or others. Staff members who have practiced as a team can work effectively to prevent acting-out behavior or to remove and confine a patient.

• Alert the staff team promptly when acting-out behavior escalates. It's safer to have help available before you need it than to try controlling an anxious or frightened patient by yourself.

• Once the incident is over and the patient is calm and in control, discuss his feelings with him and offer suggestions to prevent recurrence.

For the *depressed patient:*

• The depressed patient needs continual positive reinforcement to improve his self-esteem. Provide a structured routine, including activities to boost confidence and promote interaction with others (for instance, group therapy), and keep reassuring him that his depression will lift.

• Encourage the patient to talk or to write down his feelings if he's having trouble expressing them. Listen attentively and respectfully, and allow him time to formulate his thoughts if he seems sluggish. Record your observations and conversations to assist in the evaluation of his condition.

• To prevent possible self-injury or suicide, remove harmful objects from the patient's environment (glass, belts, rope, bobby pins), observe him closely, and strictly supervise his medications. Institute suicide precautions as dictated by hospital policy.

• Don't forget the patient's physical needs. If he's too depressed to take care of himself, help him with personal hygiene. Encourage him to eat, or feed him, if necessary. If he's constipated, add high-fiber foods to his diet; offer small, frequent meals; and encourage physical activity. To help him sleep, give back rubs or warm milk at bedtime.

• If the patient is taking an antidepressant, watch for signs of mania.

Patient teaching

• If the patient is taking lithium, teach him and his family to discontinue the drug and notify the doctor if signs of toxicity, such as diarrhea, abdominal cramps, vomiting, unsteadiness, drowsiness, muscle weakness, polyuria, and tremors, occur.

• Advise the patient to take lithium with food or after meals to avoid stomach upset.

• Because restricting sodium intake increases lithium toxicity, instruct the patient to maintain a normal diet and normal salt and water intake.

• Lithium may impair mental and physical function; caution against driving or operating dangerous equipment while taking the drug.

MAJOR DEPRESSION

Also known as unipolar disorder, major depression is a syndrome of persistent sad, dysphoric mood accompanied by disturbances in sleep and appetite, lethargy, and an inability to experience pleasure (anhedonia). Major depression occurs in 10% to 15% of adults, affecting all racial, ethnic, and socioeconomic groups. It affects both sexes but is more common in women.

About half of all depressed patients experience a single episode and recover completely; the rest have at least one recurrence. Recurrences may follow a protracted symptom-free period, or they may occur sporadically, increasing in frequency as the patient grows older, or as clusters of episodes. Depression is difficult to treat, especially in children, adolescents, elderly patients, and those with a history of chronic disease.

Causes

The multiple causes of depression are controversial and not completely understood. Current research suggests possible genetic, familial, biochemical, physical, psychological, and social causes. Psychological causes (the focus of many nursing interventions) may include feelings of helplessness and vulnerability, anger, hopelessness and pessimism, and low self-esteem; they may be related to abnormal character and behavior patterns and troubled personal relations. In many patients, the history identifies a specific personal loss or severe stress that probably interacts with a person's predisposition to provoke major depression.

The term *primary depression* describes unipolar disorder with no known cause other than family history. Patients with primary depression have no history of a significant personality disturbance before the first depressive episode.

Secondary depression refers to symptoms that occur in response to a specific event or that have a recognizable organic basis. For example, many physical disorders are associated with secondary depression. Among the most prominent are metabolic disturbances, such as hypoxia and hypercalcemia; endocrine disorders, such as diabetes and Cushing's disease; neurologic diseases, such as Parkinson's and Alzheimer's disease; cancer (especially of the pancreas); viral and bacterial infections, such as influenza and pneumonia; cardiovascular disorders, such as conges-

SUICIDE PREVENTION GUIDELINES

To help deter potential suicide in the patient with major depression, keep in mind the following guidelines.

Assess for clues to suicide
Watch for such clues as communicating suicidal thoughts, threats, and messages; hoarding medication; talking about death and feelings of futility; giving away prized possessions; describing a suicide plan; and changing behavior, especially as depression begins to lift.

Provide a safe environment
Check patient areas and correct dangerous conditions, such as exposed pipes, windows without safety glass, and access to the roof or open balconies.

Remove dangerous objects
Remove such objects as belts, razors, suspenders, light cords, glass, knives, nail files, and clippers from the patient's environment.

Consult with staff
Recognize and document both verbal and nonverbal suicidal behaviors; keep the doctor informed; share data with all staff; clarify the patient's specific restrictions; assess risk and plan for observation; clarify day and night staff responsibilities and frequency of consultation.

Observe the suicidal patient
Be alert when the patient is using a sharp object (shaving); taking medication; or using the bathroom (to prevent hanging or other injury). Assign the patient to a room near the nurses' station and with another patient. Continuously observe the acutely suicidal patient.

Maintain personal contact
Help the suicidal patient feel that he's not alone or without resources or hope. Encourage continuity of care and consistency of primary nurses. Building emotional ties to others is the ultimate technique for preventing suicide.

tive heart failure; pulmonary disorders, such as chronic obstructive lung disease; musculoskeletal disorders, such as degenerative arthritis; GI disorders, such as irritable bowel syndrome; genitourinary problems, such as incontinence; collagen vascular diseases, such as lupus; and anemias.

Drugs prescribed for medical and psychiatric conditions, as well as many commonly abused substances, also can precipitate secondary depression. Examples include antihypertensives, psychotropics, antiparkinsonian drugs, narcotic and nonnarcotic analgesics, numerous cardiovascular medications, oral antidiabetics, antimicrobials, steroids, chemotherapeutic agents, cimetidine, and alcohol.

Complications
Major depression can profoundly alter social, family, and occupational functioning. However, suicide is the most serious complication of major depression, resulting when the patient's feelings of worthlessness, guilt, and hopelessness are so overwhelming that he no longer considers life worth living. Nearly twice as many women as men attempt suicide, but men are far more likely to succeed. (See *Suicide prevention guidelines.*)

Assessment findings
The primary features of major depression are a predominantly sad mood and a loss of interest or pleasure in daily activities. During the assessment interview, the patient may complain of feeling "down in the dumps," may express doubts about his self-worth or ability to cope, or may simply appear unhappy and apathetic. He also may report feeling angry or anxious. Other common symptoms include difficulty concentrating or thinking clearly, distractibility, and indecisiveness. Take special note if the patient reveals suicidal thoughts, a preoccupation with death, or previous suicide attempts.

The psychosocial history may reveal life problems or losses that can account for the depression. Alternatively, the patient's medical history may implicate a physical disorder or the use of prescription, nonprescription, or illegal drugs that can cause depression.

The patient may report an increase or a decrease in appetite, sleep disturbances (for example, insomnia or early awakening), a lack of interest in sex, constipation, or diarrhea. Other signs you may note during a physical examination include agitation (such as hand wringing or restlessness) and psychomotor retardation (for example, slowed speech). (To distinguish major depression from dysthymia, a disorder with similar symptoms, see *Dysthymia: A chronic affective disorder,* page 52.)

DYSTHYMIA: A CHRONIC AFFECTIVE DISORDER

Formerly known as depressive neurosis, this disorder is characterized by a chronic dysphoric mood (irritable mood in children) that persists at least 2 years in adults and 1 year in children and adolescents. During periods of depression, the patient also may experience poor appetite or overeating, insomnia or hypersomnia, low energy or fatigue, low self-esteem, poor concentration, difficulty making decisions, and feelings of hopelessness.

A diagnosis of dysthymia is confirmed when the patient exhibits at least two of the symptoms listed above nearly every day, with intervening normal moods lasting no more than 2 months during a 2-year period.

The disorder typically begins in childhood, adolescence, or early adulthood and causes only mild social or occupational impairment. In adults, it's more common in females; in children and adolescents, it's equally common in both sexes.

Diagnostic criteria

A patient is diagnosed with major depression when he fulfills the criteria documented in the *DSM-IV.*

For a *single major depressive episode:*

• At least five of the following symptoms must have been present during the same 2-week period and represent a change from previous functioning; one of these symptoms must be either depressed mood or loss of interest in previously pleasurable activities:

— depressed mood (irritable mood in children and adolescents) most of the day, nearly every day, as indicated by either subjective account or observation by others

— a markedly diminished interest or pleasure in all, or almost all, activities most of the day, nearly every day

— significant weight loss or weight gain when not dieting or a change in appetite nearly every day

— insomnia or hypersomnia nearly every day

— psychomotor agitation or retardation nearly every day

— fatigue or loss of energy nearly every day

— feelings of worthlessness and excessive or inappropriate guilt nearly every day

— diminished ability to think or concentrate, or indecisiveness, nearly every day

— recurrent thoughts of death, recurrent suicidal ideation without a specific plan, or suicide attempt or a specific plan for committing suicide.

• It cannot be established that an organic factor initiated and maintained the disturbance.

• The disturbance is not a normal reaction to a loved one's death, or it persists for more than 2 months after such a loss.

• The symptoms cause clinically significant distress or impairment in social, occupational, or other important areas of functioning.

• The disorder is not superimposed on schizophrenia, schizophreniform disorder, delusional disorder, or psychotic disorder not otherwise specified.

• The patient has never had a manic episode or an unequivocal hypomanic episode.

For a *recurrent major depressive episode,* the patient must meet the criteria outlined earlier for a single major depressive episode. In addition, he should have experienced two or more major depressive episodes, each separated by at least 2 months of return to more or less usual functioning.

Psychological tests, such as the Beck Depression Inventory, can be used to determine the onset, severity, duration, and progression of depressive symptoms. The dexamethasone-suppression test may show a failure to suppress cortisol secretion; however, this test has a high false-negative rate. Toxicology screening may suggest a drug-induced depression.

Treatment

The primary treatment methods are drug therapy, electroconvulsive therapy (ECT), and psychotherapy. They aim to relieve the depressive symptoms.

Drug therapy, which includes tricyclic antidepressants (such as amitriptyline), monoamine oxidase inhibitors (for example, isocarboxazid), maprotiline, trazodone, bupropion, sertraline, or fluoxetine, modifies the activity of relevant neurotransmitter pathways.

Tricyclic antidepressants (TCAs), the most widely used of the antidepressant drugs, prevent the reuptake of norepinephrine or serotonin or both into the presynaptic nerve endings, resulting in increased synaptic concentrations of these neurotransmitters. They also cause a gradual loss in the number of beta-adrenergic receptors.

Monoamine oxidase (MAO) inhibitors block the enzymatic degradation of norepinephrine and serotonin. These agents often are prescribed for patients with atypical depression (for example, depression marked by an increase in appetite and the need for sleep, rather than anorexia and insomnia) and for some patients who fail to respond to TCAs. The MAO inhibitors are associated with a high risk of toxicity; patients treated with one of these drugs must be able to comply with the necessary dietary restrictions. Conservative doses of a MAO inhibitor may be combined with a TCA for patients refractory to either drug alone.

Maprotiline is a potent blocker of norepinephrine uptake, whereas trazodone, fluoxetine, and sertraline are selective serotonin uptake blockers. These drugs are especially useful in patients who are unable to tolerate the adverse effects of TCAs or MAO inhibitors. The mechanism of action of bupropion is unknown.

When a depressed patient is incapacitated, actively suicidal, or psychotically depressed, or when antidepressants are contraindicated or ineffective, ECT often is the treatment of choice. Six to 12 treatments usually are required, although improvement often is evident after only a few treatments. Although researchers don't know exactly why ECT works, they hypothesize that the treatment somehow affects the same receptor sites as antidepressant medications. The unilateral method of administration (where the seizure is induced in the nondominant hemisphere of the brain) appears to decrease confusion and memory loss associated with ECT.

Short-term psychotherapy also is effective in the treatment of major depression. Many psychiatrists believe that the best results are achieved with a combination of individual, family, or group psychotherapy and medication. After resolution of the acute episode, patients with a history of recurrent depression may be maintained on low doses of antidepressant drugs as a preventive measure.

Nursing diagnoses
• Altered nutrition: Less than body requirements
• Altered nutrition: More than body requirements
• Altered parenting
• Altered thought processes
• Anxiety
• Chronic low self-esteem
• Constipation
• Diversional activity deficit
• Dysfunctional grieving
• Fatigue
• Hopelessness
• Impaired home maintenance management
• Impaired social interaction
• Ineffective denial
• Ineffective individual coping
• Personal identity disturbance

• Powerlessness
• Risk for injury
• Risk for violence: Self-directed or directed at others
• Self-care deficit
• Sensory or perceptual alterations
• Sexual dysfunction
• Sleep pattern disturbance
• Social isolation
• Spiritual distress

Nursing interventions
• To prevent the patient from becoming isolated, try to spend some time with him each day. Avoid long periods of silence, which tend to increase anxiety.
• Share your observations of the patient's behavior with him. For instance, you might say, "You're sitting all by yourself, looking very sad. Is that how you feel?" Because the patient may think and react sluggishly, try to speak slowly and allow ample time for him to respond. Avoid feigned cheerfulness, but don't hesitate to laugh with the patient and point out the value of humor.
• Encourage the patient to talk about and write down his feelings. Show him he's important by listening attentively and respectfully, preventing interruptions, and avoiding judgmental responses.
• Provide a structured routine, including noncompetitive activities, to build the patient's self-confidence and encourage interaction with others. Urge him to join group activities and to socialize.
• Reassure the patient that he can help ease his depression by expressing his feelings, participating in pleasurable activities, and improving grooming and hygiene.
• Ask the patient if he thinks of death or suicide. Such thoughts signal an immediate need for consultation and assessment. Failure to detect suicidal thoughts early may encourage the patient to attempt suicide. The risk of suicide increases as the depression lifts.
• Record all observations of and conversations with the patient because they are valuable for evaluating his response to treatment.
• While caring for the patient's psychological needs, don't forget his physical needs. If he's too depressed to take care of himself, help him with personal hygiene. Encourage him to eat, or feed him, if necessary. If he's constipated, add high-fiber foods to his diet; offer small, frequent feedings; and encourage physical activity and fluid intake. Offer warm milk or back rubs at bedtime to improve sleep.

• If the patient has been prescribed an antidepressant, monitor for evidence of seizures. Some antidepressants significantly lower the seizure threshold.
• Recognize that it may take several weeks for the antidepressants to produce an effect.

Patient teaching
• Teach the patient about his depression. Emphasize that effective methods are available to relieve his symptoms. Help him to recognize distorted perceptions and link them to his depression. Once the patient learns to recognize depressive thought patterns, he can consciously begin to substitute self-affirming thoughts.
• If the patient has been prescribed an antidepressant, stress the need for compliance and review adverse reactions. For drugs that produce strong anticholinergic effects, such as amitriptyline and amoxapine, suggest sugarless gum or hard candy to relieve dry mouth. Many antidepressants are sedating (for example, amitriptyline and trazodone); warn the patient to avoid activities that require alertness, including driving and operating mechanical equipment.
• Caution the patient taking a TCA to avoid drinking alcoholic beverages or taking other central nervous system depressants during therapy.
• If the patient is taking a MAO inhibitor, emphasize that he must avoid foods that contain tyramine, caffeine, or tryptophan. Emphasize that the ingestion of tyramine can cause a hypertensive crisis. Examples of foods that contain these substances are cheese; sour cream; beer, chianti, or sherry; pickled herring; liver; canned figs; raisins; bananas; avocados; chocolate; soy sauce; fava beans; yeast extracts; meat tenderizers; coffee; and colas.

ANXIETY DISORDERS

A component of most psychological disorders and many organic disorders, anxiety is a common complaint of most hospitalized patients. Diagnosed anxiety disorders are classified into six basic types: phobias, generalized anxiety disorders, panic disorders, obsessive-compulsive disorders, posttraumatic stress disorder, and acute stress disorders.

PHOBIAS
Defined as a persistent and irrational fear of a specific object, activity, or situation, a phobia results in a compelling desire to avoid the perceived hazard. The patient recognizes that his fear is out of proportion to any actual danger, but he can't control it or explain it away. Three types of phobias exist: *agoraphobia*, the fear of being alone or of open space; *social*, the fear of embarrassing oneself in public; and *specific*, the fear of a single specific object, such as animals or heights (see *Common specific phobias*).

About 7% of all Americans suffer from a phobic disorder. In fact, phobias are the most common psychiatric disorders in women and the second most common in men. Social phobias are more common in men, whereas agoraphobia and specific phobias are more common in women. Social phobias typically begin in late childhood or early adolescence; specific phobias usually begin in childhood. Most phobic patients have no family history of phobias or other psychiatric illnesses.

Both agoraphobia and social phobia tend to be chronic and resistant to treatment. Therefore, the prognosis for these subtypes is only fair. A specific phobia usually resolves spontaneously as the child matures.

Causes
A phobia develops when anxiety about an object or a situation compels the patient to avoid it.

The precise cause of most phobias is unknown, but they may result from drug withdrawal, drug abuse, and anxiety-related behaviors, such as the inability to cope with anger and dependence.

Complications
Agoraphobia can dominate a patient's life, restricting his normal activities and even confining him to his home. A patient with social phobia may lose a job promotion because of his fear of speaking in public, or he may be continually inconvenienced by his fear of using a public lavatory. The phobic patient is at risk for other mental disorders, such as episodic abuse of alcohol, barbiturates, and anxiolytics.

Agoraphobia may include panic disorder, and severe social or occupational impairment may lead to depression.

Assessment findings
The phobic patient typically reports signs of severe anxiety when confronted with the feared object or situation. A patient with agoraphobia, for example, may complain of dizziness, a sensation of falling, deper-

sonalization or a feeling of unreality, loss of bladder or bowel control, vomiting, or cardiac distress when he leaves home or crosses a bridge. Similarly, a patient who fears flying may report that he begins to sweat, his heart pounds, and he feels panicky and short of breath when he's on an airplane.

A patient who routinely avoids the object of his phobia may report a loss of self-esteem and feelings of weakness, cowardice, or ineffectiveness. If he hasn't mastered the phobia, he also may exhibit signs of mild depression.

Diagnostic criteria

The diagnosis of all three types of phobias is based on fulfillment of the relevant criteria documented in the *DSM-IV*.

For *agoraphobia without panic disorder:*
• The patient has a fear of being in places or situations from which escape might be difficult or embarrassing or in which help might not be available if he suddenly develops symptoms that could be incapacitating or extremely embarrassing. As a result of this fear, he either restricts travel or needs a companion when away from home, or endures agoraphobic situations despite intense anxiety.
• The patient has never met the criteria for panic disorder.

For a *social phobia:*
• The patient has a persistent fear of one or more social situations in which he is exposed to possible scrutiny by others and fears that he may do something or act in a way that will be humiliating or embarrassing.
• The fear is not related to an Axis III disorder, if present.
• During some phase of the disturbance, exposure to the specific phobic stimulus almost invariably provokes an immediate anxiety response.
• The patient avoids the phobic situation or endures it with intense anxiety.
• The patient's avoidant behavior interferes with occupational functioning or with usual social activities or relationships with others, or the patient experiences marked distress about having the fear.
• The patient recognizes that his fear is excessive or unreasonable.
• If the patient is under age 18, the disturbance does not meet the criteria for avoidant disorder of childhood or adolescence.

For a *specific phobia:*
• The patient has a persistent fear of an object or a situation other than fear of having a panic attack or of

COMMON SPECIFIC PHOBIAS

Examples of specific phobias include:
• acrophobia—fear of heights
• algophobia—fear of pain
• astraphobia—fear of lightning
• claustrophobia—fear of closed spaces
• erythrophobia—fear of blushing
• hematophobia—fear of blood
• hydrophobia—fear of water
• iatrophobia—fear of doctors
• monophobia—fear of being alone
• myosophobia—fear of dirt and germs
• nyctophobia—fear of night and darkness
• pyrophobia—fear of fire
• senilophobia—fear of growing old
• sitophobia—fear of eating
• xenophobia—fear of strangers
• zoophobia—fear of animals.

humiliation or embarrassment in certain social situations.
• During some phase of the disturbance, exposure to the specific phobic stimulus almost invariably provokes an immediate anxiety response.
• The patient avoids the object or situation or endures it with intense anxiety.
• The patient's fear or his avoidant behavior significantly interferes with his normal routine or his usual social activities or relationships with others, or the patient experiences marked distress about having the fear.
• The patient recognizes that his or her fear is excessive or unreasonable.
• The phobic stimulus is unrelated to the content of the obsessions of obsessive-compulsive disorder or the trauma of posttraumatic stress disorder.

Treatment

The effectiveness of treatment depends on the severity of the patient's phobia. Because phobic behavior may never be completely cured, the goal of treatment is to help the patient function effectively. Although antianxiety drugs may help control phobia, they must be prescribed with caution to prevent addiction. Antidepressants may help relieve symptoms in patients with agoraphobia, but they can't cure it completely.

Systematic desensitization, a behavioral therapy, may be more effective than drugs, especially if it includes encouragement, instruction, and suggestion. Such therapy should help the patient understand that his phobia is symbolic of a more fundamental anxiety and that he must deal with it directly.

In some cities, phobia clinics and group therapy are available. People who have recovered from phobias can often help other phobic patients.

Nursing diagnoses
• Altered thought processes
• Anxiety
• Fear
• Impaired social interaction
• Impaired verbal communication
• Ineffective family coping
• Ineffective individual coping
• Pain
• Personal identity disturbance
• Powerlessness
• Social isolation

Nursing interventions
• Provide for the patient's safety and comfort and monitor fluid and food intake, as needed. Certain phobias may inhibit food or fluid intake, disturb hygiene, and disrupt the patient's ability to rest.
• No matter how illogical the patient's phobia seems, avoid the urge to trivialize his fears. Remember that this behavior represents an essential coping mechanism. A facile pep talk or ridicule may alienate him or increase his loss of self-esteem.
• Ask the patient how he normally copes with the fear. When he's able to face the fear, encourage him to verbalize and explore his personal strengths and resources with you.
• Don't let the patient withdraw completely. If he's being treated as an outpatient, suggest small steps to overcome his fears, such as planning a brief shopping trip with a supportive family member or friend.
• In social phobias, the patient fears criticism. Encourage him to interact with others and provide continuous support and positive reinforcement.
• Support participation in psychotherapy, including desensitization therapy. However, don't force insight. Challenging the patient may aggravate anxiety or lead to panic attacks.

Patient teaching
• To increase self-esteem and reduce anxiety, explain to the patient that his phobia is a way of coping with anxiety, especially if he perceives his behavior as silly or unreasonable.

• Teach the patient specific relaxation techniques, such as listening to music and meditating.
• Suggest ways to channel the patient's energy and relieve stress (such as running and creative activities).
• If the patient is taking an antidepressant or an antianxiety agent, stress the importance of compliance with the prescribed therapy. Teach him to recognize adverse reactions and instruct him to report such reactions to the doctor.

GENERALIZED ANXIETY DISORDER
Anxiety is a feeling of apprehension caused by a threat to a person or his values. Some describe it as an exaggerated feeling of impending doom, dread, or uneasiness. Unlike fear—a reaction to danger from a specific external source—anxiety is a reaction to an internal threat, such as an unacceptable impulse or a repressed thought that's straining to reach a conscious level.

A rational response to a real threat, occasional anxiety is a normal part of life. Overwhelming anxiety, however, can result in generalized anxiety disorder—uncontrollable, unreasonable worry that persists for at least 6 months and narrows perceptions or interferes with normal functioning. Recent evidence shows that the prevalence of generalized anxiety disorder is greater than previously thought and may be even greater than depression.

Generalized anxiety disorder can begin at any age but typically has an onset in the 20s and 30s. It is equally common in men and women.

Causes
Theorists such as Freud, Horney, and Rank describe the cause of anxiety states in different ways, but they all share a common premise: Conflict, whether intrapsychic, sociopersonal, or interpersonal, promotes an anxiety state.

Complications
Anxiety may cause mild impairment in social or occupational functioning. In addition, the anxious patient may attempt to relieve his discomfort by abusing psychoactive drugs, such as alcohol or anxiolytics.

Assessment findings
Psychological or physiologic symptoms of anxiety states vary with the degree of anxiety (for more information, see *Rating anxiety levels*). Mild anxiety mainly causes psychological symptoms, with unusual self-awareness and alertness to the environment. Moderate

anxiety leads to selective inattention, yet with the ability to concentrate on a single task. Severe anxiety causes an inability to concentrate on more than scattered details of a task. A panic state with acute anxiety causes a complete loss of concentration, often with unintelligible speech.

Physical examination of the patient with generalized anxiety disorder may reveal symptoms of motor tension, including trembling, muscle aches and spasms, headaches, and an inability to relax. Autonomic signs and symptoms include shortness of breath, tachycardia, sweating, and abdominal complaints.

In addition, the patient may startle easily and complain of feeling apprehensive, fearful, or angry and of having difficulty concentrating, eating, and sleeping. The medical, psychiatric, and psychosocial histories fail to identify a specific physical or environmental cause of the anxiety.

Diagnostic criteria

When the patient's symptoms match the following criteria documented in the *DSM-IV*, the diagnosis of generalized anxiety disorder is confirmed:
• The patient has an unrealistic or excessive anxiety and worry about two or more life circumstances for 6 months or longer, during which he has been bothered most days by these concerns. In children and adolescents, the anxiety and worry may revolve around academic, athletic, and social performance.
• If another Axis I disorder is present, the focus of the anxiety and worry is unrelated to it.
• The disturbance does not occur only during the course of a mood disorder or a psychotic disorder.
• It cannot be established that an organic factor initiated and maintained the disturbance.
• Anxiety and worry are linked with three or more of the following symptoms (or one or more in a child):
— restlessness or feeling keyed up or on edge
— being easily fatigued
— difficulty concentrating or mind going blank
— irritability
— muscle tension
— sleep disturbance.

Laboratory tests must exclude organic causes, such as hyperthyroidism, pheochromocytoma, coronary artery disease, supraventricular tachycardia, and Ménière's disease. For example, an electrocardiogram can rule out myocardial ischemia in a patient with chest pain. Blood tests, including complete blood count, white blood cell differential, and serum lactate and calcium levels, can rule out hypocalcemia.

RATING ANXIETY LEVELS

Use the following criteria to help you recognize and quantify anxiety in your patient. For example, you may consider a touchy, restless patient with poor concentration moderately anxious. You may describe him as having +2 anxiety.

Mild anxiety (+1)
In mild anxiety, the patient reports slight discomfort. He is alert, asks questions, seeks help, and can solve problems.

Moderate anxiety (+2)
The moderately anxious patient is irritable, may speak rapidly, and appears restless and shaky. He needs help to focus on the presenting problem.

Severe anxiety (+3)
The patient with severe anxiety can't cope with his situation; for example, he may say, "I can't think" or "I don't know what to do." He may not hear or pay attention to directions or information.

Panic (+4)
In this state, the patient's behavior projects great emotional pain and disorganization. He may be unresponsive or run about wildly. He's unable to focus his attention or to solve problems.

Because anxiety is the central feature of other mental disorders, psychiatric evaluation must rule out phobias, obsessive-compulsive disorders, depression, and acute schizophrenia.

Treatment

Drug treatment and psychotherapy may help a patient with this disorder. The benzodiazepine antianxiety drugs may relieve mild anxiety and improve the patient's coping ability. Tricyclic antidepressants or higher doses of benzodiazepines may relieve severe anxiety and panic attacks. Buspirone, an antianxiety drug, causes less sedation and less risk of physical and psychological dependence than the benzodiazepines. These drugs can ease distress and facilitate psychotherapy.

Psychotherapy has two goals: helping the patient identify and deal with the cause of anxiety and eliminating environmental factors that precipitate an anxious reaction. The patient may also learn relaxation techniques, such as deep breathing, progressive muscle relaxation, focused relaxation, and visualization.

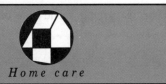

Home care

LIVING WITH GENERALIZED ANXIETY DISORDER

Follow these guidelines to help your patient live with generalized anxiety disorder:
• Make sure the patient (or his caregiver) knows the name, dosage, and adverse effects of the prescribed medications.
• Urge the patient to call the doctor if adverse reactions occur but not to discontinue the drug without his doctor's approval.
• Advise the patient not to drive or perform other hazardous activities until the drug's effects are known and drug tolerance occurs. Also counsel him to avoid alcohol and other central nervous system depressants.
• Teach the patient coping techniques, such as distraction, massage, muscle relaxation, breathing exercises, and imagery.
• Help the patient identify the causes of his anxiety, and review ways to deal with them.
• Suggest ways the patient can modify his environment to eliminate precipitating factors.

Nursing diagnoses
• Anxiety
• Chronic low self-esteem
• Defensive coping
• Diarrhea
• Ineffective community coping
• Ineffective denial
• Ineffective individual coping
• Powerlessness
• Self-esteem disturbance
• Sensory or perceptual alterations
• Sleep pattern disturbance

Nursing interventions
• Help the patient develop effective coping mechanisms to manage his anxiety. (See *Living with generalized anxiety disorder*.)
• Stay with the patient when he's anxious, and encourage him to discuss his feelings. Reduce environmental stimuli and remain calm.
• Suggest activities that distract him from his anxiety.
• Give antianxiety drugs or tricyclic antidepressants as prescribed, and evaluate the patient's response.

Patient teaching
• Warn the patient and his family that antianxiety drugs may cause adverse reactions, such as drowsiness, fatigue, ataxia, blurred vision, slurred speech, tremors, and hypotension.
• Advise the patient to discontinue medications only with the doctor's approval because abrupt withdrawal could cause severe symptoms.

PANIC DISORDER
Characterized by recurrent episodes of intense apprehension, terror, and impending doom, panic disorder represents anxiety in its most severe form. Initially unpredictable, these "panic attacks" may come to be associated with specific situations or tasks. The disorder may exist concurrently with agoraphobia, especially in women. Equal numbers of men and women are affected by panic disorder alone, whereas panic disorder with agoraphobia occurs about twice as often in women compared with men.

Panic disorder typically has an onset in late adolescence or early adulthood, often in response to a sudden loss. It also may be triggered by severe separation anxiety experienced during early childhood. Without treatment, panic disorder can persist for years, with alternating exacerbations and remissions.

Causes
Like other anxiety disorders, panic disorder may stem from a combination of physical and psychological factors. For example, some theorists emphasize the role of stressful events or unconscious conflicts that occur early in childhood.

Recent evidence indicates that alterations in brain biochemistry, especially in norepinephrine, serotonin, and gamma-aminobutyric acid activity, may also contribute to panic disorder.

Complications
Coexistence of panic disorder with agoraphobia may severely compromise the patient's ability to carry out normal daily activities. If possible, the patient may endure anxiety-provoking situations despite intense discomfort. Ultimately, he may become so fearful that he can no longer leave home alone.

The patient with panic disorder also is at high risk for a psychoactive substance use disorder, resorting to alcohol or anxiolytics in an attempt to relieve his fear.

Assessment findings

The patient with panic disorder typically complains of repeated episodes of unexpected apprehension, fear or, rarely, intense discomfort. These panic attacks may last from a few minutes to several hours and may leave the patient shaken, fearful, and exhausted. They occur several times a week, sometimes even daily. Because the attacks occur spontaneously, without exposure to a known anxiety-producing situation, the patient often worries between attacks about when the next episode will occur.

Physical examination of the patient during a panic attack may reveal signs of intense anxiety, such as hyperventilation, tachycardia, trembling, and profuse sweating. He may also complain of difficulty breathing, digestive disturbances, and chest pain.

Diagnostic criteria

The diagnosis of panic disorder is based on fulfillment of the following criteria documented in the *DSM-IV*:
• One or more panic attacks have occurred that were unexpected and were not triggered by situations in which the person was the focus of other people's attention.
• Attacks have been followed by a period of at least a month of persistent fear of having another attack.
• At least four of the following signs and symptoms must have developed during one of the attacks:
— shortness of breath or smothering sensations
— dizziness or faintness
— palpitations or tachycardia
— trembling or shaking
— sweating
— feelings of choking
— nausea or abdominal distress
— depersonalization or derealization
— numbness or tingling sensations (paresthesia)
— hot flashes or chills
— chest pain or discomfort
— fear of dying, going crazy, or doing something uncontrolled during the attack.
• During the attack, at least four of the symptoms above developed suddenly and increased in intensity within 10 minutes of the beginning of the first symptom noticed in the attack.
• It cannot be established that an organic factor initiated and maintained the disturbance.

Because many medical conditions can mimic panic disorder, additional tests may be ordered to rule out an organic basis for the symptoms. For example, serum glucose rules out hypoglycemia, urine catecholamines and vanillylmandelic acid rule out pheochromocytoma, and thyroid function tests rule out hyperthyroidism.

Urine and serum toxicology tests reveal the presence of psychoactive substances that can precipitate panic attacks, including barbiturates, caffeine, and amphetamines.

Treatment

Panic disorder may respond to behavioral therapy, supportive psychotherapy, or drug therapy, singly or in combination. Behavioral therapy works best when agoraphobia accompanies panic disorder because the identification of anxiety-inducing situations is easier.

Psychotherapy commonly uses cognitive techniques to enable the patient to view anxiety-provoking situations more realistically and to recognize panic symptoms as a misinterpretation of essentially harmless physical sensations.

Drug therapy includes antianxiety drugs, such as diazepam, alprazolam, and clonazepam, and beta blockers, such as propranolol, to provide symptomatic relief. Antidepressants, especially imipramine, and antipsychotic medications also are used to treat panic disorder.

Nursing diagnoses

• Altered thought processes
• Anxiety
• Fear
• Ineffective individual coping
• Knowledge deficit
• Powerlessness
• Risk for injury
• Risk for violence: Directed at others
• Self-esteem disturbance
• Sensory or perceptual alterations
• Sleep pattern disturbance

Nursing interventions

• Stay with the patient until the attack subsides. If left alone, he may become even more anxious.
• Maintain a calm, serene approach. Use statements such as "I won't let anything here hurt you," and "I'll stay with you" to assure the patient you are in control of the immediate situation. Avoid insincere expressions of reassurance.
• The patient's perceptual field may be narrowed, and excessive stimuli may cause him to feel overwhelmed. Dim bright lights or raise dim lights as necessary. If

the patient loses control, remove him to a smaller, quieter space.
• The patient may be so overwhelmed that he cannot follow lengthy or complicated processes. Speak in short, simple sentences, and slowly give one direction at a time. Avoid giving lengthy explanations and asking too many questions.
• Allow the patient to pace around the room (provided he isn't belligerent) to help expend energy. Show him how to take slow, deep breaths if he's hyperventilating.
• Avoid touching the patient until you've established rapport. Unless he trusts you, he may be too stimulated or frightened to find touch reassuring.
• Administer antianxiety drugs, as ordered.

Patient teaching
• During and after a panic attack, encourage the patient to express his feelings and to cry, if necessary. Discuss his fears and help him identify situations or events that trigger the attacks.
• Teach the patient relaxation techniques, such as deep-breathing exercises. Point out ways he can use these methods to relieve stress or short-circuit a panic attack.
• Review with the patient any adverse effects of the drugs he'll be taking. Caution him to notify the doctor before discontinuing the medication because abrupt withdrawal could cause severe symptoms.

OBSESSIVE-COMPULSIVE DISORDER

Obsessive thoughts and compulsive behaviors represent recurring efforts to control overwhelming anxiety, guilt, or unacceptable impulses that persistently enter the consciousness.

The word *obsession* refers to a recurrent idea, thought, or image. To reduce the discomfort caused by the obsession, the patient attempts to ignore, suppress, or neutralize these thoughts by substituting a more acceptable mental image or activity.

A *compulsion,* the action used to block an obsession, is a ritualistic, repetitive, and involuntary defensive behavior. Performing a compulsive behavior reduces the patient's anxiety and reinforces the probability that the behavior will recur.

Obsessions and compulsions may be simple or complex and ritualized. Mild forms of the disorder are relatively common in the general population, occurring with equal frequency in both sexes and with typical onset in adolescents or young adults. Generally, an obsessive-compulsive disorder is chronic, often with re-

missions and flare-ups. The prognosis is better when symptoms are quickly identified, diagnosed, and treated, and when the resulting environmental stress is recognized and adjusted.

Causes
The cause of obsessive-compulsive disorder is unknown. Some studies suggest the possibility of brain lesions, but the most useful research and clinical studies base an explanation on psychological theories. (See *Possible causes of obsessive-compulsive disorder.*) In addition, major depression, organic brain syndrome, and schizophrenia may contribute to the onset of obsessive-compulsive disorder.

Complications
Obsessions and compulsions cause significant distress and may severely impair occupational and social functioning. In some cases, the compulsions may become the patient's major activity.

Compulsive behaviors can also endanger the health and safety of the patient or those around him. For example, a person who compulsively washes his hands may develop severe dermatitis or a skin infection. A mother obsessed with thoughts of killing her infant may neglect the child completely rather than risk giving in to violent urges.

Patients with obsessive-compulsive disorder are prone to abuse psychoactive substances, such as alcohol and anxiolytics, in an attempt to relieve their anxiety. In addition, major depression and other anxiety disorders often coexist with obsessive-compulsive states.

Assessment findings
The psychiatric history of a patient with this disorder may reveal the presence of obsessive thoughts, words, or mental images that persistently and involuntarily invade the consciousness. Some common obsessions include thoughts of violence (such as stabbing, shooting, maiming, or hitting), thoughts of contamination (images of dirt, germs, or feces), repetitive doubts and worry about a tragic event, and repeating or counting images, words, or objects in the environment. The patient recognizes that the obsessions are a product of his own mind and that they interfere with normal daily activities.

The patient's history also may reveal the presence of compulsions, irrational and recurring impulses to repeat a certain behavior. Common compulsions include repetitive touching, sometimes combined with count-

POSSIBLE CAUSES OF OBSESSIVE-COMPULSIVE DISORDER

No one knows exactly what causes obsessive-compulsive disorder, but theories abound. Of the major theoretical causes described below, the psychoanalytic theory is accepted by most psychiatrists.

Psychoanalytic theory	Learning theory	Interpersonal theory	Existentialist theory
• Psychodynamic factors (ego defenses), including isolation, undoing, and reaction formation	• Obsession—conditioned stimulus to anxiety	• Irrational coping strategies to handle (inflexible) intense anxiety or guilt	• Inability to live with uncertainty or ambiguity
• Psychogenic factors, including preoccupation with aggression, preoccupation with dirt, disturbed growth and development pattern related to anal-sadistic phase	• Compulsion—reduced anxiety reinforces behavior	• Inflexible self-contempt	• Wish to flee situation of great anxiety
	• Approach avoidance—reduces conflict	• Avoidance of anxiety-laden relationships (withdrawal)	• Threat of nonexistence
• Regression, including fixation at earlier level of development (anal stage), ambivalence, and magical thinking	• Emphasis on cognitive change to alter behavior	• Defenses (sublimation, selective inattention, substitution, dissociation)	• Religious rituals
		• Inferiority feelings (to gain control of others)	• Excessively high morals
		• Threat to autonomy and loss of individuality	
		• Family patterns and coping styles that reinforce obsessions	
		• Inability to enjoy life	

ing; doing and undoing (opening and closing doors, rearranging things); washing (especially hands); and checking (to be sure no tragedy has occurred). The patient's anxiety often is so strong that he will avoid the situation or the object that evokes the impulse.

When the obsessive-compulsive phenomena are mental, observation may reveal no behavioral abnormalities. However, compulsive acts may be observed, although feelings of shame, nervousness, or embarrassment may prompt the patient to try limiting these acts to his own private time.

During the assessment interview, determine the patient's personality type. The obsessional personality usually is rigid and conscientious and has great aspirations. He exhibits a formal, reserved manner, with precise and careful movements and posture; he takes responsibility seriously and finds decision making difficult. He lacks creativity and the ability to find alternate solutions to his problems.

Such a person tends to be painfully accurate and complete—carefully qualifying his statements to avoid making a mistake, and anticipating every move and gesture of the person to whom he speaks. His affect is flat and unemotional, except for controlled anxiety. Self-awareness is intellectual, without accompanying emotion or feeling.

Also evaluate the impact of obsessive-compulsive phenomena on the patient's normal routine. He'll typically report moderate to severe impairment of social and occupational functioning.

Diagnostic criteria

The diagnosis of obsessive-compulsive disorder is confirmed when the patient's signs and symptoms meet the established criteria in the *DSM-IV.*

For an *obsession:*

• The patient experiences, at least initially, recurrent and persistent ideas, thoughts, impulses, or images as intrusive and senseless—for example, a parent has repeated impulses to kill a loved child, or a religious person has recurrent blasphemous thoughts.

BEHAVIORAL THERAPIES

The following behavioral therapies may be used to treat the patient with obsessive-compulsive disorder.

Aversion therapy
Application of a painful stimulus creates an aversion to the obsession that leads to undesirable behavior (compulsion).

Thought stopping
This technique breaks the habit of fear-inducing anticipatory thoughts. The patient learns to stop unwanted thoughts by saying the word "stop" and then focusing his attention on achieving calmness and muscle relaxation.

Thought switching
To replace fear-inducing self-instructions with competent self-instructions, the patient learns to replace negative thoughts with positive ones until the positive thoughts become strong enough to overcome the anxiety-provoking ones.

Flooding
This frequent full-intensity exposure (through the use of imagery) to an object that triggers a symptom must be used with caution because it produces extreme discomfort.

Implosion therapy
A form of desensitization, implosion therapy calls for repeated exposure to a highly feared object.

Response prevention
Preventing compulsive behavior by distraction, persuasion, or redirection of activity, this form of behavior therapy may require hospitalization or involvement of the family to be effective.

• The patient attempts to ignore or suppress such thoughts or impulses or to neutralize them with some other thought or action.
• The patient recognizes that the obsessions are the products of his mind, not externally imposed.
• If another Axis I disorder is present, the content of the obsession is unrelated to it; for example, the ideas, thoughts, or images are not about food in the presence of an eating disorder, about drugs in the presence of a psychoactive substance use disorder, or about guilt thoughts in a major depressive disorder.
For *compulsions:*
• The patient performs repetitive, purposeful, and intentional behaviors in response to an obsession, or according to certain rules or in a stereotypic manner.
• The patient's behavior is designed to neutralize or prevent discomfort or some dreaded event or situation; however, either the activity is not connected in a realistic way with what it is designed to neutralize or prevent, or it is clearly excessive.
• The patient recognizes that his behavior is excessive or unreasonable (this may not be true for young children or for patients whose obsessions have evolved into overvalued ideas).

The obsessions or compulsions, as defined above, must cause marked distress, be time-consuming (take more than an hour a day), or significantly interfere with the person's normal routine, occupational functioning, or usual social activities or relationships.

Treatment
In obsessive-compulsive disorder, treatment aims to reduce anxiety, resolve inner conflicts, relieve depression, and teach more effective ways of dealing with stress. Such treatment (especially during an acute episode) may include antipsychotic or antidepressant drugs. Intensive long-term psychotherapy, brief supportive psychotherapy, or group therapy is the preferred treatment.

Behavioral therapies—aversion therapy, thought stopping, thought switching, flooding, implosion therapy, and response prevention—have also been effective. (See *Behavioral therapies.*)

Nursing diagnoses
• Altered role performance
• Altered thought processes
• Anxiety
• Fear
• Impaired adjustment
• Impaired social interaction
• Ineffective individual coping
• Personal identity disturbance
• Powerlessness
• Risk for impaired skin integrity
• Risk for injury
• Sleep pattern disturbance

Nursing interventions
• Approach the patient unhurriedly.
• Provide an accepting atmosphere; don't show shock, amusement, or criticism of the ritualistic behavior.

• Allow the patient time to carry out the ritualistic behavior (unless it's dangerous) until he can be distracted into some other activity. Blocking this behavior raises anxiety to an intolerable level.

• Keep the patient's physical health in mind. For example, compulsive hand washing may cause skin breakdown, and rituals or preoccupations may cause inadequate food and fluid intake and exhaustion. Provide for basic needs, such as rest, nutrition, and grooming, if the patient becomes involved in ritualistic thoughts and behaviors to the point of self-neglect.

• Let the patient know you're aware of his behavior. For example, you might say, "I noticed you've made your bed three times today; that must be very tiring for you." Help the patient explore feelings associated with the behavior. For example, ask him, "What do you think about while you are performing your chores?"

• Make reasonable demands and set reasonable limits; make their purpose clear. Avoid creating situations that increase frustration and provoke anger, which may interfere with treatment.

• Explore patterns leading to the behavior or recurring problems.

• Listen attentively, offering feedback.

• Encourage the use of appropriate defense mechanisms to relieve loneliness and isolation.

• Engage the patient in activities to create positive accomplishments and raise his self-esteem and confidence.

• Encourage active diversional resources, such as whistling or humming a tune, to divert attention from the unwanted thoughts and to promote a pleasurable experience.

• Assist the patient with new ways to solve problems and to develop more effective coping skills by setting limits on unacceptable behavior (for example, by limiting the number of times per day he may indulge in obsessive behavior). Gradually shorten the time allowed. Help him focus on other feelings or problems for the remainder of the time.

• Identify insight and improved behavior (reduced compulsive behavior and fewer obsessive thoughts). Evaluate behavioral changes by your own and the patient's reports.

• Identify disturbing topics of conversation that reflect underlying anxiety or terror.

• Observe when interventions do not work; reevaluate and recommend alternative strategies.

• Find ways to deal with the anger and frustration the patient may arouse in you.

Patient teaching

• Help the patient identify progress and set realistic expectations of himself and others.

• Explain how to channel emotional energy to relieve stress (for example, through sports and creative endeavors). In addition, teach the patient relaxation and breathing techniques to help reduce anxiety.

POSTTRAUMATIC STRESS DISORDER

Characteristic psychological consequences that develop after exposure to an extremely traumatic event are classified as posttraumatic stress disorder.

This disorder can follow almost any distressing event, including a natural or man-made disaster, physical or sexual abuse, an assault, or a rape. Psychological trauma accompanies the physical trauma and involves intense fear and feelings of helplessness and loss of control. The patient subsequently may experience the event in the form of intrusive memories, nightmares, or dissociative episodes. Such flashbacks often are elicited by situations that resemble or symbolize the original trauma.

Posttraumatic stress disorder can be acute, chronic, or delayed. When the precipitating event is of human design, the disorder is more severe and more persistent. Onset can occur at any age, even during childhood.

Causes

Posttraumatic stress disorder occurs in response to an extremely distressing event, including a serious threat of harm to the patient or his family, such as war, abuse, or violent crime. It may be triggered by sudden destruction of his home or community by a bombing, fire, flood, tornado, earthquake, or similar disaster. It may also follow witnessing the death or serious injury of another person by torture, in a death camp, by natural disaster, or by a motor vehicle or airplane crash.

Preexisting psychopathology can predispose the patient to this disorder. However, this disorder can develop in anyone, especially if the stressor is extreme.

Complications

Impairment may be mild or severe, affecting nearly every aspect of life. Phobic avoidance of situations or activities resembling or symbolizing the original trauma may interfere with interpersonal relationships.

Emotional lability, depression, and guilt may result in self-defeating behavior or even suicide. Anxiety disorders and psychoactive substance use disorders are other common complications of posttraumatic stress disorder.

Assessment findings

The psychosocial history of a patient with posttraumatic stress disorder may reveal early life experiences, interpersonal factors, military experiences, or other incidents that suggest the precipitating event. Typically, the patient may report that his symptoms began immediately or soon after the trauma, although they may not develop until months or years later. In this case, avoidance symptoms usually have been present during the latency period.

Common symptoms include pangs of painful emotion and unwelcome thoughts; a traumatic reexperiencing of the event; difficulty falling or staying asleep, frequent nightmares of the traumatic event, and aggressive outbursts on awakening; emotional numbing—diminished or constricted response; and chronic anxiety or panic attacks (with physical signs and symptoms).

The patient may display rage and survivor guilt, use of violence to solve problems, depression and suicidal thoughts, phobic avoidance of situations that arouse memories of the trauma (for example, hot weather and tall grasses for the Vietnam veteran), memory impairment or difficulty concentrating, and feelings of detachment or estrangement that destroy interpersonal relationships. Some patients experience organic symptoms, fantasies of retaliation, and substance abuse.

Diagnostic criteria

The diagnosis of posttraumatic stress disorder is confirmed when the patient's signs and symptoms meet the following criteria documented in the *DSM-IV*:
• The patient has experienced a traumatic event in which both of the following occurred:
—actual or threatened death or serious injury or threat to the physical integrity of the patient or others
—a response of intense fear, helplessness, or horror (or in a child, a response of disorganization and agitation).
• The patient persistently reexperiences this traumatic event in at least one of the following ways:
—recurrent and intrusive distressing recollections of the event (or in a child, repetitive play that expresses feelings about the event)
—recurrent distressing dreams of the event (or in a child, nightmares unrelated to the event)
—suddenly acting or feeling as if the traumatic event

were recurring, including a sense of reliving the experience, illusions, hallucinations, and dissociative episodes (flashbacks), even those that occur when awakening or intoxicated (or in a child, reenactment of the traumatic event)
—intense psychological distress at exposure to events that symbolize or resemble an aspect of the traumatic event
—physiologic reactivity on exposure to events that symbolize or resemble an aspect of the traumatic event.
• The patient must exhibit persistent avoidance of the stimuli associated with the trauma or numbing of general responsiveness not present before the trauma, as indicated by at least three of the following:
—efforts to avoid thoughts or feelings associated with the trauma
—efforts to avoid activities or situations that arouse recollections of the trauma
—inability to recall an important aspect of the event
—sharply decreased interest in significant activities
—feeling of detachment or estrangement from others
—restricted range of affect, for example, not being able to love others
—sense of foreshortened future, for example, not expecting to be able to have a career, spouse, family, or typical life span.
• Persistent signs of increased arousal (not previously present) as indicated by two or more of the following:
—difficulty falling or staying asleep
—irritability or outbursts of anger
—difficulty concentrating
—hypervigilance
—exaggerated startle response.
• The disturbance must have lasted at least 1 month.
• The disturbance must cause significant distress or impairment of social, occupational, or other important areas of functioning.

Treatment

Goals of treatment include reducing the target symptoms, preventing chronic disability, and promoting occupational and social rehabilitation. Specific treatment may emphasize behavioral techniques (relaxation therapy to decrease anxiety and induce sleep, or progressive desensitization); antianxiety and antidepressant drugs, prescribed with caution to avoid possible dependence; or brief psychotherapy (supportive, insight, or cathartic) to minimize the risks of dependency and chronicity.

Support groups are highly effective and are provided through many Veterans Administration centers and crisis clinics. These groups provide a forum in which victims of this disorder can work through their feelings with others who have had similar conflicts. Group settings are appropriate for most degrees of symptoms presented. Some group programs include spouses and families in their treatment processes. Rehabilitation programs in physical, social, and occupational areas also are available for victims of chronic posttraumatic stress disorder.

Many patients need treatment for depression, alcohol or drug abuse, or medical conditions before psychological healing can take place.

Nursing diagnoses
• Altered role performance
• Altered thought processes
• Anxiety
• Chronic low self-esteem
• Fear
• Hopelessness
• Impaired social interaction
• Ineffective individual coping
• Personal identity disturbance
• Post-trauma response
• Powerlessness
• Risk for violence: Self-directed or directed at others
• Sensory or perceptual alterations
• Sleep pattern disturbance

Nursing interventions
• Encourage the patient to express his grief, complete the mourning process, and gain coping skills to relieve anxiety and desensitize him to memories of the event.
• Keep in mind that such a patient tends to sharply test your commitment and interest. So first examine your feelings about the event (war or other trauma) so you won't react with disdain and shock. Reacting this way hampers your working relationship with the patient and reinforces his poor self-image and sense of guilt.
• Practice crisis intervention techniques as needed.
• Establish trust by accepting the patient's current level of functioning and by assuming a positive, consistent, honest, and nonjudgmental attitude.
• Give approval as the patient shows a commitment to work on his problem.
• Deal constructively with the patient's displays of anger. Encourage joint assessment of angry outbursts (identify how anger escalates and explore preventive measures that family members can take to regain control). Provide a safe, staff-monitored room in which the

patient can safely deal with urges to commit physical violence or self-abuse by displacement (such as pounding and throwing clay or destroying selected items). Encourage him to move from physical to verbal expressions of anger.
• Help the patient relieve shame and guilt precipitated by real actions (such as killing or mutilation) that violated a consciously held moral code. Help him put his behaviors into perspective, recognize his isolation and self-destructive behavior as forms of atonement, and accept forgiveness from himself and others. Refer the patient to clergy as appropriate.
• Provide for or refer the patient to group therapy with other victims for peer support and forgiveness.

Patient teaching
• Carefully review the healing process with the patient. Remind him that setbacks shouldn't be equated with treatment failure.
• Help the patient regain control over angry impulses by identifying situations in which he lost control and by talking about past and precipitating events (conceptual labeling) to help with later problem-solving skills.
• Teach relaxation and breathing techniques to help reduce anxiety.
• Refer the patient to appropriate community resources.

SOMATOFORM DISORDERS

The patient with a somatoform disorder complains of physical signs and symptoms and typically travels from doctor to doctor in search of treatment. Physical examinations and laboratory tests fail to uncover an organic basis for his signs and symptoms. Somatoform disorders include somatization disorder, conversion disorder, somatoform pain disorder, and hypochondriasis.

SOMATIZATION DISORDER
When multiple recurrent signs and symptoms of several years' duration suggest that physical disorders exist without a verifiable disease or pathophysiologic condition to account for them, somatization disorder is present. The typical patient with somatization disorder usually undergoes repeated medical examinations and diagnostic testing that—unlike the symptoms themselves—can be potentially dangerous or debilitating. The patient often "doctor shops" in search of yet

another diagnostic workup. However, unlike the hypochondriac, she's not preoccupied with the belief that she has a specific disease.

Somatization disorder usually is chronic with exacerbations during times of stress. The patient's signs and symptoms are involuntary, and she consciously wants to feel better. Nonetheless, she's seldom entirely symptom-free. Onset of signs and symptoms usually occurs in adolescence or, rarely, in the 20s. This disorder primarily affects women; it's seldom diagnosed in men.

Causes
Both genetic and environmental factors contribute to the development of somatization disorder.

Complications
The patient with somatization disorder constantly consults with doctors—both in and out of the hospital. As a result, she may undergo unnecessary surgery and runs an increased risk of substance abuse disorders that involve prescribed medications. The patient also may experience long periods of incapacitating depression, leading to threatened or attempted suicide. Death from suicide usually is related to psychoactive substance use.

Assessment findings
Examination of a patient with somatization disorder is characterized by physical complaints presented in a dramatic, vague, or exaggerated way, often as part of a complicated medical history in which many physical diagnoses have been considered. An important clue to this disorder is a history of multiple medical evaluations at different institutions, with different doctors—sometimes simultaneously—without significant findings.

The patient usually appears anxious and depressed. Common physical complaints include:
• conversion or pseudoneurologic signs and symptoms (for example, paralysis or blindness)
• GI discomfort (abdominal pain, nausea, or vomiting)
• female reproductive difficulties (such as painful menstruation)
• psychosexual problems (for example, sexual indifference)
• chronic pain (for example, back pain)
• cardiopulmonary symptoms (chest pain, dizziness, or palpitations).

The patient with somatization disorder typically relates her current complaints and previous evaluations in great detail. She may be quite knowledgeable about tests, procedures, and medical jargon. She doesn't discuss other aspects of her life without including her many signs and symptoms. In fact, any attempts to explore areas other than her medical history may cause her noticeable anxiety. She tends to disparage previous health care professionals and previous treatment, often with the comment, "No one seems to understand. Everyone thinks I'm imagining these things."

Ongoing assessment should focus on new signs or symptoms or any change in old ones to avoid missing a developing physical disease.

Diagnostic criteria
The diagnosis of somatization disorder is confirmed when the symptoms meet the following criteria that are documented in the *DSM-IV:*
• The patient has a history of many physical complaints, beginning before age 30 and persisting for several years, that cause her to seek medical treatment or that impair important areas of functioning.
• The patient reports all of the following at some time during the disturbance:
— *Two GI signs or symptoms:* vomiting (other than during pregnancy), abdominal pain (other than during menstruation), nausea (other than motion sickness), bloating, diarrhea, or intolerance of different foods
— *Four pain symptoms:* pain in extremities, back pain, joint pain, rectal pain, menstrual pain, pain during urination, pain during sexual intercourse, other pain (excluding headaches)
— *One conversion or pseudoneurologic sign or symptom:* amnesia, difficulty swallowing, loss of voice, deafness, double vision, blurred vision, blindness, fainting or loss of consciousness, seizures, difficulty walking, paralysis or muscle weakness, urine retention or difficulty urinating
— *One sexual sign or symptom:* burning sensation in sexual organs or rectum (other than during intercourse), sexual indifference, pain during intercourse, impotence, painful menstruation, irregular menstrual periods, excessive menstrual bleeding, vomiting throughout pregnancy.
To identify a symptom as significant:
• No organic abnormality or pathophysiologic mechanism exists to account for the patient's sign or symptom. Or, if a related organic abnormality is present, the complaint or resulting social or occupational impairment grossly exceeds what would be expected from the physical findings.

Diagnostic tests rule out physical disorders that cause vague and confusing somatic symptoms, such as hyperparathyroidism, porphyria, multiple sclerosis, and systemic lupus erythematosus. In addition, multiple physical signs and symptoms that become apparent for the first time late in the patient's life usually are the result of physical disease, rather than somatization disorder.

Treatment
The goal of treatment is to help the patient learn to live with her signs and symptoms. After diagnostic evaluation has ruled out organic causes, the patient should be told that although she has no serious illness, she will continue to receive care to ease her signs and symptoms.

The most important aspect of treatment is a continuing, supportive relationship with a health care provider who acknowledges the patient's signs and symptoms and is willing to help her live with them. The patient should have regularly scheduled appointments to review her signs and symptoms and the effectiveness of her coping strategies. The patient with somatization disorder seldom acknowledges any psychological aspect of her illness and rejects psychiatric treatment.

Nursing diagnoses
• Altered family processes
• Altered health maintenance
• Altered role performance
• Altered thought processes
• Anxiety
• Body image disturbance
• Fear
• Impaired adjustment
• Impaired social interaction
• Ineffective individual coping
• Pain
• Personal identity disturbance
• Sexual dysfunction

Nursing interventions
• Acknowledge the patient's symptoms, and support her efforts to function and cope despite her distress. Be careful not to characterize her signs and symptoms as imaginary. Tell her the results and meanings of any tests she undergoes.
• Emphasize the patient's strengths (for example, "It's good that you can still work, even though you're in

pain. You can be pleased with that accomplishment"). Gently point out to her the time relationship between stress and physical symptoms.
• Help the patient manage stress. Typically, her relationships are linked to her signs and symptoms; relieving them can have an impact on her interactions with others.
• Negotiate a care plan with input from the patient and, if possible, her family. Encourage and help them to understand the patient's need for troublesome signs and symptoms.
• If you develop an attitude that says, "These people don't really want to get better, so why should I waste my time?" acknowledge your feelings honestly. If appropriate, consult a psychiatric clinical nurse specialist to help you develop effective means of dealing with your feelings.

Patient teaching
• Teach the patient coping strategies to help her deal with her discomfort. In particular, relaxation and deep-breathing techniques can do much to ease the patient's signs and symptoms by decreasing her anxiety and stress.

CONVERSION DISORDER
Previously called hysterical neurosis, conversion type, a conversion disorder allows a patient to resolve a psychological conflict through the loss of a specific physical function — for example, by paralysis, blindness, or the inability to swallow. Unlike factitious disorders or malingering (see *Factitious disorders,* page 68), the patient's loss of physical function is involuntary. However, laboratory tests and diagnostic procedures don't disclose an organic cause.

Conversion disorder can occur in either sex at any age. An uncommon disorder, it usually begins in adolescence or early adulthood. The conversion symptom itself is not life-threatening and usually has a short duration.

Causes
The patient suddenly develops the conversion symptom soon after experiencing a traumatic conflict he believes that he cannot handle. Two theories can explain why this occurs. According to the first, the patient achieves a "primary gain" when the symptom keeps a psychological conflict out of conscious awareness. For example, a person may experience blindness after witnessing a violent crime.

FACTITIOUS DISORDERS

Marked by the irrational, repetitious simulation of a physical or mental illness for the purpose of obtaining medical treatment, factitious disorders are severely psychopathologic conditions. The symptoms are intentionally produced and can be either physical or psychological. These disorders are more common in men than in women.

Chronic factitious disorder with physical symptoms

Also called Munchausen syndrome, this is the most common factitious disorder. The patient convincingly presents with intentionally feigned symptoms. These symptoms may be fabricated (acute abdominal pain with no underlying disease); self-inflicted (deliberately infecting an open wound); an exacerbation or exaggeration of a preexisting disorder (taking penicillin despite a known allergy); or a combination of all the above.

The history of a patient with Munchausen syndrome may include:
• multiple admissions to various hospitals, typically across a wide geographic area
• extensive knowledge of medical terminology

• pathologic lying
• evidence of previous treatment, such as surgery
• shifting complaints and signs and symptoms
• eagerness to undergo hazardous and painful procedures
• discharge against medical advice to avoid detection
• poor interpersonal relationships
• refusal of psychiatric examination
• psychoactive substance or analgesic use.

Factitious disorder with psychological symptoms

Causing severely impaired function, this disorder is characterized by intentional feigning of symptoms suggestive of a mental disorder. However, the symptoms represent how the patient views the mental disorder and seldom coincide with any of the diagnostic categories documented in the *DSM-IV.*

This disorder almost always coexists with a severe personality disorder. Most patients have a history of psychoactive substance use, often in an attempt to elicit the desired symptoms.

The second theory suggests that the patient achieves "secondary gain" from the symptom by avoiding a traumatic activity. For example, a soldier may develop a "paralyzed" hand that prevents him from entering into combat.

Complications

Conversion disorder symptoms can severely impede normal activities. Prolonged loss of function may result in real and serious complications, such as contractures, disuse atrophy, and pressure ulcers.

The conversion symptom may encourage the patient with a dependent personality to adopt the role of a chronic invalid. Unnecessary diagnostic or therapeutic medical procedures increase the risk of complications in such a patient.

Assessment findings

The history of a patient with conversion disorder may reveal the sudden onset of a single, debilitating sign or symptom that prevents normal function of the affected body part, such as paralysis of a leg. The patient may describe a recent and severe psychologically stressful event that preceded the symptom. Oddly, the patient doesn't show the affect and concern that such a severe symptom usually elicits.

Assessment findings obtained during a physical examination are inconsistent with the primary symptom. For instance, tendon reflexes may be normal in a "paralyzed" part of the body, loss of function fails to follow anatomic patterns of innervation, or normal pupillary responses and evoked potentials are present in a patient who complains of blindness.

Diagnostic criteria

The diagnosis of conversion disorder is based on fulfillment of the following criteria from the *DSM-IV:*
• The patient exhibits a loss of or alteration in voluntary motor or sensory function that suggests a physical disorder.
• Psychological factors are judged to be associated with the symptom because of a temporal relationship between a psychosocial stressor that is apparently related to a psychological conflict or need and the onset or exacerbation of the symptom.
• The patient is not intentionally producing or feigning the symptom.
• The symptom is not a culturally sanctioned response pattern and cannot, after appropriate investigation, be explained by a known physical disorder.
• The symptom is not limited to pain or a disturbance in sexual functioning.

• The symptom causes clinically significant distress or impairment of social, occupational, or other important areas of functioning.

A thorough physical evaluation must rule out any physical cause, especially diseases with vague physical onsets (such as multiple sclerosis or systemic lupus erythematosus).

Treatment
Psychotherapy, family therapy, relaxation therapy, behavior therapy, or hypnosis may be used alone or in combination (two or more) to treat conversion disorder.

Nursing diagnoses
• Activity intolerance
• Anxiety
• Fear
• Impaired physical mobility
• Impaired social interaction
• Ineffective individual coping
• Risk for impaired skin integrity
• Risk for injury
• Self-care deficit
• Sensory or perceptual alterations

Nursing interventions
• Help the patient maintain integrity of the affected system. Regularly exercise paralyzed limbs to prevent muscle wasting and contractures.
• Frequently change the bedridden patient's position to prevent pressure ulcers.
• Ensure adequate nutrition, even if the patient is complaining of GI distress.
• Provide a supportive environment, and encourage the patient to discuss the stress that provoked the conversion disorder. Don't force the patient to talk, but convey a caring attitude to help him share his feelings.
• Don't insist that the patient use the affected system. This will only anger him and prevent a therapeutic relationship.
• Add your support to the recommendation for psychiatric care.
• Include the patient's family in all care. They may be part of the patient's stress, and they are essential to support the patient and help him regain normal function.

Patient teaching
• Teach the patient effective coping strategies, such as relaxation and deep-breathing techniques, to help him reduce stress and relieve anxiety.

PAIN DISORDER
The striking feature of pain disorder is a persistent complaint of pain. The pain is the patient's major complaint, is sufficiently severe to warrant clinical attention, and significantly impairs social, occupational, or other important areas of functioning. Psychological factors play a significant role in the onset, severity, exacerbation, or maintenance of the pain. The patient does not intentionally produce or feign the pain. Women experience certain forms of pain, such as chronic headaches, more than men.

Causes
The pain may be related to psychological factors, medical conditions, or both. When the pain results from a general medical condition, it is not considered a mental disorder (pain disorder) and is coded on Axis III–general medical conditions.

Complications
The most serious complications of pain disorder are iatrogenic; they include psychoactive substance dependence, multiple surgical interventions, and those complications that are associated with extensive diagnostic evaluations.

Assessment findings
The cardinal feature of pain disorder is a history of chronic, consistent complaints of pain. The patient may relate a long history of evaluations and medical procedures at multiple settings without much noticeable pain relief. Because of frequent hospitalizations, the patient may be familiar with pain medications and tranquilizers. She may even ask for a specific medication and know the correct dosage and route of administration.

When a medical condition is a contributing factor to the pain, physical assessment findings are consistent with that medical condition. A psychosocial assessment may reveal that the patient is angry at health care professionals because they've failed to relieve her pain.

Diagnostic criteria
The diagnosis of pain disorder may be difficult to make because the perception of pain is subjective. The diagnosis is based on fulfillment of the following criteria documented in the *DSM-IV*:
• The patient's chief complaint is pain in one or more anatomic sites, and the pain is sufficient to warrant clinical attention.

• The pain causes clinically significant distress or impairment of social, occupational, or other important areas of functioning.

• Psychological factors are judged to have an important role in the onset, severity, exacerbation, or maintenance of the pain.

• The pain is not intentionally produced or feigned.

• The pain is not accounted for by a mood, anxiety, or psychotic disorder and does not meet the criteria for dyspareunia.

Treatment

In pain disorder, treatment aims to ease the pain and help the patient live with it. Treatment at a comprehensive pain center may be helpful. Supportive measures for pain relief may include hot or cold packs, physical therapy, distraction techniques, and cutaneous stimulation with massage or transcutaneous electrical nerve stimulation. Measures to reduce the patient's anxiety also may help.

A continuing, supportive relationship with an understanding health care professional is essential for effective management; regularly scheduled follow-up appointments are helpful.

Analgesics become an issue because the patient believes that she has to "fight to be taken seriously." The patient should clearly be told which medication she will receive in addition to supportive pain-relief measures. Regularly scheduled analgesic doses can be more effective than scheduling medication as needed. Regular doses combat pain by reducing the patient's anxiety about asking for medication, and they eliminate unnecessary confrontations. The use of placebos will destroy trust when the patient discovers deceit.

Nursing diagnoses

• Altered health maintenance
• Anxiety
• Impaired social interaction
• Ineffective family coping
• Ineffective individual coping
• Pain
• Personal identity disturbance

Nursing interventions

• Observe and record the characteristics of the patient's pain, including severity, duration, and any precipitating factors.

• Provide a caring atmosphere in which the patient's complaints are taken seriously and every effort is made to provide relief. This means communicating to the patient that you'll collaborate with her on a treatment plan, clearly stating the limitations. For example, you might say, "I can stay with you now for 15 minutes, but you can't receive another dose of pain medication until 2 p.m."

• Don't tell the patient that she's imagining the pain or can wait longer for medication that's due. Assess her complaints and help her understand what's contributing to the pain. To elicit contributing perceptions and fears, you might say, "I've noticed you complain of more pain after your doctor visits. What are his visits like for you?"

• Provide other, nonpharmacologic comfort measures, such as repositioning, back massage, or heat application, whenever possible.

• Teach the patient coping strategies to help her deal with the pain. For example, you can teach her to perform progressive muscle relaxation or deep-breathing exercises.

• Encourage the patient to maintain independence despite her pain.

• Offer attention at times other than during the patient's complaints of pain, to weaken the link to secondary gain.

• Consider psychiatric referrals; however, realize that the patient may resist psychiatric intervention, and don't expect psychiatric treatment to replace analgesic measures.

Patient teaching

• Teach the patient noninvasive, drug-free methods of pain control, such as guided imagery, relaxation techniques, and distraction through reading or writing.

HYPOCHONDRIASIS

The dominant feature of hypochondriasis (previously referred to as hypochondriacal neurosis) is an unrealistic misinterpretation of the severity and significance of physical signs or sensations as abnormal. This leads to preoccupation with fear of having a serious disease, which persists despite medical reassurance to the contrary. Hypochondriasis causes severe social and occupational impairment. It is not due to other mental disorders, such as schizophrenia, mood disorder, or somatization disorder.

Hypochondriasis appears to be equally common in men and women. It can begin at any age, but onset most frequently occurs between ages 20 and 30. The course of the disease usually is chronic, although the severity of symptoms may vary.

Causes

Hypochondriasis is not linked to any specific cause. However, this disorder frequently develops in people or the relatives of those who have experienced an organic disease. It allows the patient to assume a dependent sick role to ensure his needs are met. Such a patient is unaware of these unmet needs and does not consciously cause his symptoms. Stress increases the risk of developing hypochondriasis.

Complications

Hypochondriasis entails a danger of overlooking a serious, organic disease, given the patient's previously unfounded complaints. It also has the potential for significant complications or disabilities, resulting from multiple evaluations, tests, and invasive procedures.

This disorder may severely impair social and occupational functioning. Possible psychiatric complications include anxiety, depression, and obsessive-compulsive disorder.

Assessment findings

The dominant feature of hypochondriasis is the misinterpretation of symptoms — usually multiple complaints that involve a single organ system — as signs of serious illness. As medical evaluation proceeds, complaints may shift and change. Symptoms can range from specific to general, vague complaints, and often are associated with a preoccupation with normal body functions.

The hypochondriacal patient will relate a chronic history of waxing and waning symptoms. Commonly, he will have undergone multiple evaluations for similar symptoms or complaints of serious illness. His past contacts with health care professionals make him quite informed and knowledgeable about illness, diagnosis, and treatment.

Diagnostic criteria

A diagnosis of hypochondriasis is confirmed when the patient's symptoms meet the following criteria established in the *DSM-IV*:
• The patient exhibits a preoccupation with the fear of having or the belief that he has a serious disease, based on his interpretation of physical signs or sensations as evidence of physical illness.
• Appropriate physical evaluation does not support the diagnosis of any physical disorder that can account for

the physical signs or sensations or the patient's unwarranted interpretation of them, and the symptoms referred to above are not just symptoms of panic attacks.
• The fear of having or the belief that one has a disease persists despite medical reassurance.
• Duration of the disturbance is at least 6 months.
• The belief that one has a disease is not of delusional intensity, as in delusional disorder, somatic type.

Treatment

The goal of treatment is to help the patient continue to lead a productive life despite distressing symptoms and fears. After medical evaluation is complete, the patient should be told clearly that he doesn't have a serious disease but that continued medical follow-up will help control his symptoms. Providing a diagnosis won't make hypochondriasis disappear, but it may ease the patient's anxiety.

Regular outpatient follow-up can help the patient deal with his symptoms and is necessary to detect organic illness. (Up to 30% of these patients develop an organic disease.) Because the patient can be demanding and irritating, consistent follow-up may be difficult.

Most patients don't acknowledge any psychological influence on their symptoms and resist psychiatric treatment.

Nursing diagnoses

• Anxiety
• Chronic pain
• Impaired adjustment
• Impaired social interaction
• Ineffective individual coping
• Risk for injury
• Self-esteem disturbance

Nursing interventions

• Provide a supportive relationship that lets the patient feel cared for and understood. The patient with hypochondriasis feels real pain and distress, so don't deny his symptoms or challenge his behavior.
• Firmly state that medical test results were negative. Instead of reinforcing his symptoms, encourage him to discuss his other problems, and urge his family to do the same.
• Recognize that the patient will never be symptom-free, and don't become angry when he won't give up his disease. Such anger can drive the patient away to yet another unnecessary medical evaluation.

Patient teaching
• Help the patient and family find new ways to deal with stress other than development of physical symptoms. For example, teaching the patient more effective coping strategies can reduce his need to resort to hypochondriacal behavior.
• If the patient is receiving a tranquilizer, both he and his family should know its dosage, expected effects, and possible adverse effects (for example, drowsiness, fatigue, blurred vision, and hypotension).
• Warn the patient who's taking tranquilizers to avoid alcohol or other central nervous system depressants because they may potentiate tranquilizer action. Warn him to take the drug only as prescribed (larger or more frequent doses may lead to dependence); to avoid hazardous tasks until he has developed a tolerance to the tranquilizer's sedative effects; and to continue the tranquilizer as his doctor directs because abrupt withdrawal may be hazardous.

DISSOCIATIVE AND PERSONALITY DISORDERS

Dissociation refers to an unconscious defense mechanism that keeps troubling thoughts out of a person's awareness. The patient with a dissociative disorder experiences temporary changes in consciousness, identity, and motor function. The patient with a personality disorder suffers chronic, maladaptive behavior patterns. The disorders included in this section are dissociative identity disorder, dissociative fugue, dissociative amnesia, depersonalization disorder, and personality disorders.

DISSOCIATIVE IDENTITY DISORDER
A complex disturbance of identity and memory, dissociative identity disorder is characterized by the existence of two or more distinct, fully integrated personalities in the same person. The personalities alternate in dominance. Each has unique memories, behavior patterns, and social relationships; rigid and flamboyant personalities often are combined. Usually, one personality is unaware of the existence of the others.

Dissociative identity disorder usually begins in childhood, but patients seldom seek treatment until much later in life. The disorder is three to nine times more common in women than in men.

Causes
The cause of dissociative identity disorder is not known. The patient typically has experienced abuse, often sexual, or another form of severe emotional trauma in childhood. Psychiatrists believe that a child exposed to such overwhelming stimuli may evolve multiple personalities to dissociate herself from the traumatic situation. The dissociated contents become linked with one of many possible shaping influences for personality organization.

Complications
Dissociative identity disorder may be complicated by severe social and occupational impairment, depending on the nature of the personalities and their interrelationships. Often, one or more of the personalities have a coexisting mental disorder, such as generalized anxiety disorder, borderline personality disorder, or mood disorder. Suicide attempts, self-mutilation, externally directed violence, and psychoactive drug dependence also may occur.

Assessment findings
The patient with dissociative identity disorder may seek medical treatment for a concurrent psychiatric disorder that's present in one of the personalities. She may have a history of unsuccessful psychiatric treatment, or she may report periods of amnesia and disturbances in time perception. Family members or friends may describe incidents that the patient can't recall, as well as pronounced alterations in facial presentation, voice, and behavior.

The transition from one personality to another often is triggered by stress or idiosyncratically meaningful social or environmental cues. Although usually sudden (seconds to minutes), the transition can occur over hours or days. Hypnosis and amobarbital may facilitate the transition.

Diagnostic criteria
The diagnosis of dissociative identity disorder is based on fulfilling the following criteria from the *DSM-IV*:
• Two or more distinct personalities or personality states (each with its own relatively enduring pattern of perceiving, relating to, and thinking about the environment and self) exist within the person.
• At least two of these personalities or personality states recurrently take control of the person's behavior.
• The person has an inability to recall important personal information that is too extensive to be explained by ordinary forgetfulness.

• The disturbance is not due to the physiologic effects of a substance.

Treatment
Psychotherapy is essential to unite the personalities and prevent the personality from splitting again. The treatment's success is linked to the strength of the therapist's relationship with each of the personalities. All of the personalities, whether disagreeable or congenial, require equal respect and empathetic concern.

Nursing diagnoses
• Altered family processes
• Altered role performance
• Altered thought processes
• Body image disturbance
• Fear
• Impaired adjustment
• Impaired social interaction
• Ineffective denial
• Ineffective individual coping
• Personal identity disturbance
• Post-trauma response
• Powerlessness
• Risk for violence: Self-directed or directed at others
• Sexual dysfunction

Nursing interventions
• Establish an empathetic relationship with each emerging personality.
• Monitor the patient's actions for evidence of self-directed violence or violence directed at others.
• Recognize even small gains.

Patient teaching
• Teach the patient more effective defense mechanisms and coping skills, including use of available social support systems.
• Stress the importance of continuing psychotherapy. Point out that the therapy may be prolonged, with alternating successes and failures, and that one or more of the personalities may resist treatment.

DISSOCIATIVE FUGUE
The patient suffering from dissociative fugue wanders or travels while mentally blocking out a traumatic event. During the fugue state, he usually assumes a different personality; later he can't recall what happened. The degree of impairment varies, depending on the duration of the fugue and the nature of the personality state it invokes. Dissociative fugue may be related to dissociative identity disorder, narcissistic personality disorder, and sleepwalking.

The age of onset varies. Although the fugue state usually is brief (hours to days), it can last for many months and carry the patient far from home. The prognosis for complete recovery is good, and recurrences are rare.

Causes
Dissociative fugue typically follows an extremely stressful event, such as combat experience, a natural disaster, a violent or abusive confrontation, or personal rejection. Heavy alcohol use may constitute a predisposing factor.

Complications
If the patient resorts to violence during the fugue state, he will have to face the legal, social, and personal consequences of his behavior when he returns to his normal state of mind.

Assessment findings
Psychiatric examination of the patient with dissociative fugue may reveal that he has assumed a new, more uninhibited identity. If the new personality is still evolving, he may avoid social contact. On the other hand, he may have traveled to a distant location, set up a new residence, and developed a well-integrated network of social relationships that don't suggest any mental alteration.

The psychosocial history of such a patient may include episodes of violent behavior. After recovery, he typically can't remember these and other events that took place during the fugue state.

Diagnostic criteria
The diagnosis of dissociative fugue is confirmed if the patient's symptoms meet the following criteria documented in the *DSM-IV*:
• The predominant disturbance is sudden, unexpected travel away from home or the patient's customary place of work, with an inability to recall the past.
• The patient assumes a new partial or complete identity or is confused about his personal identity.
• The disturbance is not due to dissociative identity disorder or an organic mental disorder.

Treatment
Psychotherapy aims to help the patient recognize the traumatic event that triggered the fugue state and to

TYPES OF AMNESIA

The *DSM-IV* recognizes five types of amnesia, based on the time period and the amount of information lost to recall:
• *Localized amnesia*—failure to recall all events that occurred during a circumscribed time period
• *Selective amnesia*—failure to recall some of the events that occurred during a circumscribed time period
• *Generalized amnesia*—failure to recall all events over the entire life span
• *Continuous amnesia*—failure to recall events subsequent to a specific time up to and including the present
• *Systematized amnesia*—failure to recall certain categories of information, such as memories of one's family.

develop reality-based strategies for coping with anxiety. A trusting, therapeutic relationship is essential for successful therapy.

Nursing diagnoses
• Altered family processes
• Altered role performance
• Altered thought processes
• Anxiety
• Defensive coping
• Fear
• Impaired social interaction
• Ineffective individual coping
• Personal identity disturbance
• Post-trauma response
• Risk for violence: Self-directed or directed at others

Nursing interventions
• Assist the patient in using reality-based coping strategies under stress, rather than those strategies that distort reality.
• Help the patient recognize and deal with anxiety-producing experiences.
• Establish a therapeutic, nonjudgmental relationship.

Patient teaching
• Teach the patient effective coping strategies to use in stressful situations, rather than those strategies that distort reality.

DISSOCIATIVE AMNESIA

The essential feature of dissociative amnesia is a sudden inability to recall important personal information that cannot be explained by ordinary forgetfulness. The patient typically can't recall all events that occurred during a specific time period, but other types of recall disturbance also are possible. (See *Types of amnesia*.)

This disorder commonly occurs during war and natural disasters. Although it is more common in adolescents and young women, it also is seen in young men after combat experience. The amnesic event typically ends abruptly, and recovery is complete, with rare recurrences.

Causes
Dissociative amnesia follows severe psychosocial stress, often involving a threat of physical injury or death. Amnesia also may occur after thinking about or engaging in unacceptable behavior, such as an extramarital affair.

Complications
Mild to severe social impairment may occur during the amnesic episode.

Assessment findings
During the assessment interview, the amnesic patient may appear perplexed and disoriented, wandering aimlessly. He won't be able to remember the event that precipitated the episode and probably won't recognize his inability to recall information.

After the episode has ended, the patient usually is unaware that he has suffered what is known as a recall disturbance.

Diagnostic criteria
A diagnosis of dissociative amnesia is confirmed when the patient's symptoms meet the following criteria established in the *DSM-IV*:
• The main disturbance is an episode of sudden inability to recall important personal information that is too extensive to be explained by normal forgetfulness.
• The disturbance is not due to dissociative identity disorder or organic mental disorder.
• The symptoms cause clinically significant distress or impairment of social, occupational, or other areas of functioning.

Treatment
Psychotherapy aims to help the patient recognize the traumatic event that triggered the amnesia and the

anxiety it produced. A trusting therapeutic relationship is essential to achieving this goal. The therapist subsequently attempts to teach the patient reality-based coping strategies.

Nursing diagnoses
• Altered family processes
• Altered role performance
• Altered thought processes
• Anxiety
• Defensive coping
• Fear
• Impaired social interaction
• Ineffective individual coping
• Personal identity disturbance
• Post-trauma response
• Powerlessness

Nursing interventions
• Assist the patient in using reality-based coping strategies under stress, rather than those strategies that distort reality.
• Help the patient recognize and deal with anxiety-producing experiences.
• Establish a therapeutic, nonjudgmental relationship.

Patient teaching
• Teach the patient effective coping strategies to use in stressful situations, rather than those strategies that distort reality.

DEPERSONALIZATION DISORDER
Persistent or recurrent episodes of detachment characterize depersonalization disorder. During these episodes, self-awareness is temporarily altered or lost; the patient often perceives this alteration in consciousness as a barrier between himself and the outside world. The sense of depersonalization may be restricted to a single body part, such as a limb, or it may encompass the whole self.

Although the patient seldom loses touch with reality completely, the episodes of depersonalization may cause him severe distress.

Depersonalization disorder usually has a sudden onset in adolescence or early in adult life. It follows a chronic course, with periodic exacerbations and remissions, and resolves gradually.

Causes
Depersonalization disorder typically stems from severe stress, including war experiences, accidents, and natural disasters.

Complications
Hypochondriasis and psychoactive substance use may be associated with depersonalization disorder.

Assessment findings
The patient with depersonalization disorder may complain of feeling detached from his entire being and body, as if he were watching himself from a distance or living in a dream. He also may report sensory anesthesia, a loss of self-control, difficulty speaking, and feelings of derealization and losing touch with reality.

Common findings during the assessment interview include symptoms of depression, obsessive rumination, somatic concerns, anxiety, fear of going insane, a disturbed sense of time, and a prolonged recall time, as well as physical complaints, such as dizziness.

Diagnostic criteria
The depersonalization disorder diagnosis is confirmed by comparing the patient's symptoms with the following criteria established in the *DSM-IV*:
• Persistent or recurrent experiences of depersonalization are indicated by a person's feeling detached from his mind or body (as if he were observing himself from the outside) or feeling like an automaton (as if he were in a dream).
• During the depersonalization experience, reality testing remains intact.
• The depersonalization is sufficiently severe and persistent to cause marked distress.
• The depersonalization experience is the predominant disturbance and is not a symptom of another disorder, such as schizophrenia, panic disorder, or agoraphobia.

Treatment
Psychotherapy aims to establish a trusting therapeutic relationship in which the patient can come to recognize the traumatic event and the anxiety it evoked. The therapist subsequently teaches the patient to use reality-based coping strategies, rather than to detach himself from the situation.

Nursing diagnoses
• Altered family processes
• Altered role performance
• Altered thought processes

- Anxiety
- Defensive coping
- Fear
- Impaired social interaction
- Ineffective individual coping
- Personal identity disturbance
- Post-trauma response
- Powerlessness

Nursing interventions
- Assist the patient in using reality-based coping strategies under stress, rather than those strategies that distort reality.
- Help the patient recognize and deal with anxiety-producing experiences.
- Establish a therapeutic, nonjudgmental relationship.

Patient teaching
- Teach the patient effective coping strategies to use in stressful situations, rather than those strategies that distort reality.

PERSONALITY DISORDERS
Defined as individual traits that reflect chronic, inflexible, and maladaptive patterns of behavior, personality disorders cause social discomfort and impair social and occupational functioning.

Although no statistics exist to quantify personality disorders, they are, nevertheless, widespread. Most patients with personality disorders don't receive treatment; when they do, they're typically managed as outpatients.

Personality disorders fall on Axis II of the *DSM-IV* classification system. Personality notations are appropriate and useful for all patients and help provide a fuller picture of the patient and a more accurate diagnosis. For example, many features that are characteristic of personality disorders are apparent during an episode of another mental disorder (such as a major depressive episode in a patient with compulsive personality features).

The prognosis is variable. Personality disorders typically have an onset before or during adolescence and early adulthood and persist throughout adult life.

Causes
Only recently have personality disorders been categorized in detail, and research continues to identify their causes.

Various theories attempt to explain the origin of personality disorders. Biological theories hold that these disorders may stem from chromosomal and neuronal abnormalities or head trauma. Social theories hold that the disorders reflect learned responses, having much to do with reinforcement, modeling, and aversive stimuli as contributing factors. Psychodynamic theories hold that personality disorders reflect deficiencies in ego and superego development and are related to poor mother-child relationships that are fraught with unresponsiveness, overprotectiveness, or early separation.

Complications
The patient's maladaptive behavior often leads to social and occupational impairment. Personality disorders also increase the risk of mood disturbances, such as anxiety and depression, as well as psychoactive substance use disorders.

Assessment findings
Each specific personality disorder produces characteristic signs and symptoms, which may vary among patients and within the same patient at different times. In general, the history of the patient with a personality disorder will reveal long-standing difficulties in interpersonal relations, ranging from dependency to withdrawal, and in occupational functioning, with effects ranging from compulsive perfectionism to intentional sabotage.

The patient with a personality disorder may show any degree of self-confidence ranging from no self-esteem to arrogance. Convinced that his behavior is normal, he avoids responsibility for the consequences of his behavior, often resorting to projections and blame.

Diagnostic criteria
For diagnostic traits in specific personality disorders, see *Diagnostic criteria for personality disorders.*

Treatment
Personality disorders are difficult to treat. Treatment depends on the patient's symptoms but requires a trusting relationship in which the therapist can use a direct approach.

Drug therapy is ineffective but may be used to relieve severe distress, such as acute anxiety and depression. Family and group therapy usually are effective.

Hospital inpatient milieu therapy in crisis situations and possibly for long-term treatment of borderline per-

DIAGNOSTIC CRITERIA FOR PERSONALITY DISORDERS

The diagnosis of each recognized personality disorder is based on fulfillment of the following relevant diagnostic criteria defined in the *DSM-IV.*

General criteria

All types of personality disorders must meet the general diagnostic criteria for personality disorders. These disorders are characterized by an enduring pattern of behaviors and inner experiences that deviates significantly from the norms and expectations of the patient's culture. This pattern affects two or more of the following:
• cognition (including ways of interpreting and perceiving self, people, and events)
• affectivity (including the degree, range, lability, and appropriateness of emotional responses)
• interpersonal functioning
• impulse control.

This pattern of behaviors and inner experiences is inflexible, extends to a broad range of personal and social situations, and leads to clinically significant distress or impairment of social, occupational, or other important areas of functioning. It is stable and long-lasting, with onset that is traceable to early adulthood or even adolescence. The pattern is not more likely to result from another mental disorder or general medical condition and is not a direct physiologic effect of a medication or another substance.

Paranoid personality disorder

The patient must exhibit a pervasive and unwarranted tendency, beginning by early adulthood and present in a variety of contexts, to interpret the actions of people as deliberately demeaning or threatening, as indicated by at least four of the following:
• expects, without sufficient basis, to be exploited or harmed by others
• questions, without justification, the loyalty and trustworthiness of friends and associates
• finds hostile or evil meanings in benign remarks or events
• bears grudges or is unforgiving of insults or slights
• won't confide in others because of unwarranted fear that the information will be used against him
• is easily slighted and quick to react with anger or to counterattack
• questions, without justification, the fidelity of spouse or sexual partner.

These symptoms must not occur exclusively during the course of schizophrenia or a delusional disorder.

Schizoid personality disorder

The patient must exhibit a pervasive pattern of indifference to social relationships and a restricted range of emotional experience and expression, beginning by early adulthood and present in a variety of contexts, as indicated by at least four of the following:
• neither desires nor enjoys close relationships, including being part of a family
• almost always chooses solitary activities
• seldom, if ever, claims or appears to experience strong emotions, such as anger and joy
• indicates little, if any, desire to have sexual experiences with another person
• is indifferent to the praise and criticism of others
• has no close friends or confidants other than first-degree relatives
• displays constricted affect, coldness, or detachment.

These symptoms must not occur exclusively during the course of schizophrenia or a delusional disorder.

Schizotypal personality disorder

The patient must exhibit a pervasive pattern of deficits in interpersonal relatedness and peculiarities of ideation, appearance, and behavior, beginning by early adulthood and present in a variety of contexts, as indicated by at least five of the following:
• ideas of reference (excluding delusions of reference)
• excessive social anxiety
• odd beliefs or magical thinking, influencing behavior and inconsistent with subcultural norms
• unusual perceptual experiences
• odd or eccentric behavior or appearance
• no close friends or confidants (or only one) other than first-degree relatives
• odd speech and thinking
• inappropriate or constricted affect
• suspiciousness or paranoid ideation.

These symptoms must not occur exclusively during the course of schizophrenia or a pervasive developmental disorder.

Antisocial personality disorder

The patient must be at least 18 years old and must have displayed a pervasive pattern of disregard for and violation of the rights of others since age 15, as indicated by a history of three or more of the following:
• failure to conform to social norms with respect to lawful behaviors, as shown by repeatedly performing acts that are grounds for arrest
• deceitfulness, as shown by repeatedly lying, using aliases, or conning others for personal profit or pleasure
• impulsivity or failure to plan ahead
• irritability and aggressiveness, as indicated by repeated physical fights or assaults
• reckless disregard for own safety or the safety of others
• consistent irresponsibility, as demonstrated by repeated failure to sustain consistent work or honor financial obligations to others
• lack of remorse, as demonstrated by indifference to

(continued)

DIAGNOSTIC CRITERIA FOR PERSONALITY DISORDERS *(continued)*

Antisocial personality disorder *(continued)*
or rationalization of hurting, mistreating, or stealing from another.

None of these symptoms of antisocial behavior should have occurred exclusively during the course of schizophrenia or manic episodes.

The patient must also display some signs of conduct disorder before age 15. The patient with conduct disorder consistently behaves in ways that violate the basic rights of others or major age-appropriate societal norms or rules. Signs and symptoms of conduct disorder include the following:
• aggression toward people and animals
— bullies, threatens, or intimidates others
— frequently initiates physical fights
— has used a weapon that can seriously harm others
— has been physically cruel to people or animals
— has stolen while confronting a victim (for example, mugging, purse snatching, extortion)
— has forced someone into sexual activity
• property destruction
— has deliberately set fires with the intention of causing serious property damage
— has deliberately destroyed others' property in different ways, such as vandalism
• theft or deceitfulness
— has broken into a house, building, or car
— frequently lies to obtain goods or favors or to avoid obligations (conning behavior)
— has stolen items of value without confronting a victim (for instance, by shoplifting or forgery)
• serious rule violations
— frequently stays out at night despite parental prohibitions, beginning before age 13
— has run away from home at least twice while living in parental or parental surrogate home (or once without returning for a lengthy period)
— is often truant from school, beginning before age 13.

Patients with conduct disorder also display clinically significant impairment of social, academic, or occupational functioning because of behavior disturbances.

Borderline personality disorder
The patient must exhibit a pervasive pattern of instability of mood, interpersonal relationships, and self-image, beginning by early adulthood and present in a variety of contexts, as indicated by at least five of the following:
• pattern of unstable and intense interpersonal relationships characterized by alternating between extremes of overidealization and devaluation
• impulsiveness in at least two areas that are potentially self-damaging, such as spending, sex, substance abuse, shoplifting, reckless driving, and binge eating (excluding suicidal or self-mutilating behavior)

• affective instability—marked shifts from baseline mood to depression, irritability, or anxiety, lasting usually a few hours and seldom more than a few days
• inappropriate, intense anger or lack of control of anger
• recurrent suicidal threats, gestures, or behavior, or self-mutilating behavior
• persistent identity disturbance manifested by uncertainty about at least two of the following: self-image, sexual orientation, long-term goals or career choice, type of friends desired, and preferred values
• chronic feelings of emptiness or boredom
• frantic efforts to avoid real or imagined abandonment.

Histrionic personality disorder
The patient must exhibit a pervasive pattern of excessive emotionality and attention-seeking, beginning by early adulthood and present in a variety of contexts, as indicated by at least five of the following:
• constantly seeks or demands reassurance, approval, or praise
• is inappropriately sexually seductive in appearance or behavior
• consistently uses physical appearance to draw attention to self
• expresses emotion with inappropriate exaggeration
• is uncomfortable not being the center of attention
• displays rapidly shifting and shallow expression of emotions
• is easily influenced by others
• has a style of speech that is excessively impressionistic and lacking in detail
• considers relationships to be more intimate than they actually are.

Narcissistic personality disorder
The patient must exhibit a pervasive pattern of grandiosity, lack of empathy, and hypersensitivity to the evaluation of others, beginning by early adulthood and present in a variety of contexts, as indicated by at least five of the following:
• displays arrogant, haughty behaviors or attitudes
• is interpersonally exploitative—takes advantage of others to achieve his own ends
• has a grandiose sense of self-importance
• believes that his problems are unique and can be understood only by other special people
• is preoccupied with fantasies of unlimited success, power, brilliance, beauty, or ideal love
• has a sense of entitlement—unreasonable expectation of especially favorable treatment
• requires constant attention and admiration
• lacks empathy—is unable to recognize and experience how others feel
• is preoccupied with feelings of envy.

(continued)

DIAGNOSTIC CRITERIA FOR PERSONALITY DISORDERS *(continued)*

Avoidant personality disorder

The patient must display a pervasive pattern of social discomfort, fear of negative evaluation, and timidity, beginning by early adulthood and present in a variety of contexts, as indicated by at least four of the following:

• avoids occupational activities that involve significant interpersonal contact because of fears of criticism, disapproval, or rejection
• is unwilling to become involved with people unless certain of being liked
• shows restraint in intimate relationships because of the fear of being shamed or ridiculed
• is preoccupied with being criticized or rejected in social situations
• is inhibited in new interpersonal situations because of feelings of inadequacy
• views self as socially inept, personally unappealing, or inferior to others
• is unusually reluctant to take personal risks or engage in new activities because they may prove embarrassing.

Dependent personality disorder

The patient must demonstrate a pervasive pattern of dependent and submissive behavior, beginning by early adulthood and present in a variety of contexts, as indicated by at least five of the following:

• is unable to make everyday decisions without an excessive amount of advice or reassurance from others
• allows others to make most of his important decisions
• agrees with people even when he believes that they are wrong because of fear of being rejected
• has difficulty initiating projects or doing things on his own
• volunteers to do things that are unpleasant or demeaning to get other people to like him
• feels uncomfortable or helpless when alone, or goes to great lengths to avoid being alone
• feels devastated or helpless when close relationships end
• is frequently preoccupied with fears of being abandoned
• is easily hurt by criticism or disapproval.

Obsessive-compulsive personality disorder

The patient must display a pervasive pattern of perfectionism and inflexibility, beginning by early adulthood and present in a variety of contexts, as indicated by at least five of the following:

• perfectionism that interferes with task completion
• preoccupation with details, rules, lists, order, organization, or schedules until the major point of the activity is lost
• unreasonable insistence that others submit to exactly his way of doing things or unreasonable reluctance to allow others to do things because of the conviction that they will not do them correctly
• excessive devotion to work and productivity to the exclusion of leisure activities and friendships (not accounted for by obvious economic need)
• overconscientiousness, scrupulousness, and inflexibility about matters of morality, ethics, or values (not accounted for by cultural or religious identification)
• lack of generosity in giving time, money, or gifts when no personal gain is likely
• inability to discard worn-out or worthless objects even when they have no sentimental value.

Passive-aggressive personality disorder

The patient must display a pervasive pattern of negative attitudes and passive resistance to demands for adequate social and occupational performance, beginning by early adulthood and present in a variety of contexts, as indicated by at least four of the following:

• passively resists accomplishing and fulfilling routine occupational and social tasks
• complains of being unappreciated and misunderstood by others
• is argumentative and sullen
• expresses resentment and envy of those who are apparently more fortunate
• voices persistent and exaggerated complaints of personal misfortune
• alternates between contrition and hostile defiance.
  These signs and symptoms do not occur exclusively during a major depressive episode and are not better accounted for by dysthymic disorder.

sonality disorders can be effective. Inpatient treatment is controversial, however, because most patients with personality disorders are noncompliant with extended therapeutic regimens; for such patients, outpatient therapy may be more useful.

Nursing diagnoses

• Altered parenting
• Altered role performance
• Altered sexuality patterns
• Altered thought processes
• Anxiety
• Chronic low self-esteem

- Fear
- Impaired adjustment
- Impaired social interaction
- Ineffective individual coping
- Powerlessness
- Sexual dysfunction
- Social isolation

Nursing interventions

- Know your own feelings and reactions as the basis for assessing the patient's overt responses.
- Offer patient, persistent, consistent, and flexible care. Take a direct, involved approach to ensure the patient's trust. Keep in mind that many of these patients don't respond well to interviewing, whereas others are charming and convincing.
- Teach the patient social skills, and reinforce appropriate behavior.
- Encourage expression of feelings, self-analysis of behavior, and accountability for actions.

   Specific care measures vary with the particular personality disorder.

   For *paranoid personality disorder:*
- Avoid situations that threaten the patient's autonomy.
- Approach the patient in a straightforward and candid manner, adopting a professional, rather than a casual or friendly, attitude. Remember that remarks intended to be humorous are easily misinterpreted by the paranoid patient.
- Provide a supportive and nonjudgmental environment in which the patient can safely explore and verbalize his feelings.

   For *schizoid personality disorder:*
- Remember that the schizoid patient needs close human contact but is easily overwhelmed. Respect his need for privacy, and slowly build a trusting therapeutic relationship so that he finds more pleasure than fear in relating to you.
- Give the patient plenty of time to express his feelings. Keep in mind that if you push him to do so before he's ready, he may retreat.

   For *schizotypal personality disorder:*
- Recognize that this type of patient is easily overwhelmed by stress. Allow him plenty of time to make difficult decisions.
- Be aware that the patient may relate unusually well to certain staff members and not at all to others.

   For *antisocial personality disorder:*
- Be clear about your expectations and the consequences of failing to meet them.

- Use a straightforward, matter-of-fact approach to set limits on unacceptable behavior. Encourage and reinforce positive behavior.
- Expect the patient to refuse to cooperate so that he can gain control.

   For *borderline personality disorder:*
- Encourage the patient to take responsibility for himself. Don't attempt to rescue him from the consequences of his actions.
- Don't try to solve problems that the patient can solve himself.
- Maintain a consistent approach in all interactions with the patient; ensure that other team members use the same approach.
- Recognize that the patient may idolize some staff members and devalue others.
- Don't take sides in the patient's disputes with other staff members.

   For *histrionic personality disorder:*
- Recognize that this patient usually functions well as long as he receives attention, flattery, and admiration. As a result, he may never receive appropriate treatment.
- Give the patient choices in care strategies, and incorporate his wishes into the treatment plan as much as possible. By increasing his sense of self-control, you'll reduce anxiety.
- Approach the patient formally. He may be uncomfortable with a casual approach.

   For *narcissistic personality disorder:*
- Respond positively to the patient's sense of entitlement, even when it's unreasonable. A critical attitude may cause him to become even more demanding and difficult.
- Focus on positive traits or on his feelings of pain, loss, or rejection.

   For *avoidant personality disorder:*
- Assess for signs of depression. Social impairment increases the risk of affective disorders in these patients.
- Establish a trusting interpersonal relationship with the patient. Be aware that he may become dependent on the few staff members whom he believes he can trust.
- Be sure that all upcoming procedures are known to the patient in plenty of time for him to adjust. This patient is unable to handle surprises well.
- Inform the patient when you will and will not be available if he needs assistance.

   For *dependent personality disorder:*
- Initially, give the patient explicit directives, rather than ask him to make decisions. Then encourage him

to make easy decisions, such as what to wear or which television program to watch. Continue to provide support and reassurance as his decision-making ability improves.

For *obsessive-compulsive personality disorder:*
• Allow the patient to control his own treatment plan by offering choices whenever possible.
• Adopt a professional approach in your interactions with the patient. Avoid informality; this patient wants strict attention to detail.

For *passive-aggressive personality disorder:*
• Avoid power struggles with the patient.
• Provide the patient with as much opportunity to control his treatment as possible. Offer options and allow the patient to choose, even if he chooses all of them. Verify his approval before initiating specific treatment.

Patient teaching
• When providing care for any patient with a personality disorder, assess the patient's coping skills. As necessary, teach him more effective strategies to alleviate stress and reduce anxiety.

SEXUAL DISORDERS

The disorders in this section affect a person's sexual ability or response, sexual behavior, or gender identity.

FEMALE AROUSAL AND ORGASMIC DISORDER

One of the severest forms of female sexual dysfunction, arousal disorder is an inability to experience sexual pleasure. Orgasmic disorder, the most common type of female sexual dysfunction, is an inability to achieve orgasm. Unlike the woman with arousal disorder, the woman with orgasmic disorder may desire sexual activity and become aroused but feels inhibited as she approaches orgasm.

Arousal and orgasmic disorder are considered primary if they exist in a woman who has never experienced sexual arousal or orgasm; they're considered secondary when some physical, mental, or environmental condition inhibits or obliterates previously normal sexual functioning.

The prognosis is good for temporary or mild dysfunction that results from misinformation or situational stress but guarded for dysfunction that results from intense anxiety, chronically discordant relationships, psychological disturbances, or drug or alcohol abuse in either partner.

Causes
One or more of the following factors may cause arousal or orgasmic disorder:
• drug use—central nervous system depressants, antidepressants, alcohol, illegal drugs and, rarely, oral contraceptives
• disease—general systemic illness, diseases of the endocrine or nervous system, and diseases that impair muscle tone or contractility
• gynecologic factors—chronic vaginal or pelvic infection or pain (from endometriosis), congenital anomalies, and genital cancers
• stress and fatigue
• inadequate or ineffective stimulation
• psychological factors—performance anxiety, guilt, depression, unconscious conflicts about sexuality, or fear of losing control of feelings or behavior
• discordant relationships—poor communication, hostility or ambivalence toward the partner, fear of abandonment or of asserting independence, or boredom with sex.

The likelihood of sexual dysfunction and the type of dysfunction depend on how well the woman copes with the pressures imposed by these factors.

Complications
Sexual dysfunction may impair marital or other sexual relationships.

Assessment findings
The woman with arousal disorder usually reports limited or absent sexual desire and experiences little or no pleasure from sexual stimulation. The patient's history may include:
• a high level of family stress or fatigue, as occurs in many working mothers with children under age 5 who are too exhausted to care about sex
• misinformation about sex and sexuality
• a pattern of dysfunctional sexual response
• conceptual problems in childhood and adolescence about sex in general and, specifically, about masturbation, incest, rape, sexual fantasies, and homosexual or heterosexual practices
• concerns about contraception and reproductive ability
• interpersonal problems in the current sexual relationship, including the partner's attitude toward sex

• poor self-esteem and body image.

Physical signs of arousal disorder include a lack of vaginal lubrication and the absence of signs of genital vasocongestion.

The woman with orgasmic disorder may report an inability to achieve orgasm, either totally or under certain circumstances. Many women experience orgasm through masturbation or other means but not through intercourse alone. Others achieve orgasm with some partners but not with others.

Diagnostic criteria

The diagnosis of sexual dysfunction is based on fulfillment of the criteria established in the *DSM-IV*.

For *female arousal disorder:*
• Persistent or recurrent, partial or complete failure to attain or maintain the lubrication-swelling response of sexual excitement until completion of sexual activity
• Marked distress or interpersonal difficulty as a result of the disturbance.

In addition, the disorder does not occur exclusively during the course of another Axis I disorder, such as major depression.

For *female orgasmic disorder:*
• Persistent or recurrent delay in or absence of orgasm after a normal sexual excitement phase during sexual activity that the clinician judges to be adequate in focus, intensity, and duration. Some women can experience orgasm during noncoital clitoral stimulation, but can't experience it during coitus in the absence of manual clitoral stimulation. In most of these women, this represents a normal variation of the female sexual response and doesn't justify the diagnosis. In some, however, this represents a psychological inhibition that does justify the diagnosis. This difficult judgment is assisted by a thorough sexual evaluation, which may require a trial of treatment.
• Marked distress or interpersonal difficulty as a result of the disturbance.

In addition, the disorder does not occur exclusively during the course of another Axis I disorder, such as major depression.

A thorough physical examination, laboratory tests, and the medical history rule out physical causes of arousal or orgasmic disorder.

Treatment

Arousal disorder is difficult to treat, especially when the woman has never experienced sexual pleasure.

Therapy is designed to help the patient relax, become aware of her feelings about sex, and eliminate guilt and fear of rejection.

Specific measures usually include sensate focus exercises similar to those developed by Masters and Johnson, which emphasize touching and awareness of sensual feelings over the entire body — not just genital sensations — and minimize the importance of intercourse and orgasm.

Psychoanalytic treatment consists of free association, dream analysis, and discussion of life patterns to achieve greater sexual awareness. One behavioral approach attempts to correct maladaptive patterns through systematic desensitization to situations that provoke anxiety, partially by encouraging the patient to fantasize about these situations.

The goal in treating orgasmic disorder is to decrease or eliminate involuntary inhibition of the orgasmic reflex. Treatment may include experiential therapy, psychoanalysis, and behavior modification.

Treatment of primary orgasmic disorder may involve teaching the patient self-stimulation. Also, the therapist may teach distraction techniques, such as focusing attention on fantasies, breathing patterns, or muscle contractions to relieve anxiety. Thus, the patient learns new behavior through exercises she does in the privacy of her home between sessions. The therapist gradually involves the patient's sexual partner in the treatment sessions, although some therapists treat the couple as a unit from the outset.

Treatment of secondary orgasmic disorder aims to decrease anxiety and promote the factors necessary for the patient to experience orgasm. The therapist should communicate an accepting and permissive attitude and help the patient understand that satisfactory sexual experiences don't always require coital orgasm.

Nursing diagnoses

• Altered family processes
• Altered sexuality patterns
• Anxiety
• Self-esteem disturbance
• Sexual dysfunction

Nursing interventions

• Communicate an open, nonjudgmental attitude when caring for a patient with a sexual dysfunction.
• Listen to the patient's problems empathetically.
• Refer the patient to doctors, nurses, psychologists, social workers, or counselors trained in sex therapy.

Patient teaching
• Provide accurate information regarding sexual anatomy and physiology and sexual response patterns.
• As a helpful guideline, inform the patient that the therapist's certification by the American Association of Sex Educators, Counselors, and Therapists or by the American Society for Sex Therapy and Research usually ensures quality treatment. If the therapist is not certified by one of these organizations, advise the patient to inquire about the therapist's training in sex counseling and therapy.

DYSPAREUNIA

The term dyspareunia refers to pain associated with intercourse. It may be mild or severe enough to restrict the enjoyment of intercourse. Dyspareunia may be associated with physical disorders or, less commonly, with psychologically based sexual dysfunctions.

Occurring almost exclusively in women, this disorder typically occurs in the late 20s and early 30s, a few years after the establishment of a sustained sexual relationship. The prognosis is good if the underlying disorder can be treated successfully.

Causes

Physical causes of dyspareunia include an intact hymen; deformities or lesions of the introitus or vagina; retroversion of the uterus; genital, rectal, or pelvic scar tissue; acute or chronic infections of the genitourinary tract; and disorders of the surrounding viscera (including residual effects of pelvic inflammatory disease or disease of the adnexal and broad ligaments).

Among the many other possible physical causes are:
• endometriosis
• benign and malignant growths and tumors
• insufficient lubrication, often due to use of drugs, such as antihistamines, decongestants, and nonsteroidal anti-inflammatory drugs, or to estrogen loss associated with menopause
• radiation to the genital area
• allergic reactions to diaphragms, condoms, or other contraceptives.

Acute onset of dyspareunia is a classic sign of pelvic inflammatory disease caused by *Neisseria gonorrhoeae* or *Chlamydia trachomatis.*

Psychological causes include fear of pain or injury during intercourse, recollection of a previous painful experience, guilty feelings about sex, fear of pregnancy or of injury to the fetus during pregnancy, anxiety caused by a new sexual partner or technique, and mental or physical fatigue.

Complications

Dyspareunia can impair marital or other sexual relationships.

Assessment findings

The patient with dyspareunia usually complains of discomfort ranging from mild aches to severe pain before, during, or after intercourse. Vaginal itching or burning also may be present.

Diagnostic criteria

The diagnosis of dyspareunia is confirmed when symptoms meet the following criteria established in the *DSM-IV:*
• Genital pain is recurrent or persistent before, during, or after sexual intercourse.
• The disturbance is not exclusively caused by lack of lubrication or vaginismus.
• The disturbance causes marked distress or interpersonal difficulty.

Physical examination and laboratory tests help determine the underlying disorder.

Treatment

The treatment of physical causes of dyspareunia may include creams and water-soluble jellies for inadequate lubrication, appropriate medications for infections, excision of hymenal scars, and gentle stretching of painful scars at the vaginal opening with a medium-sized Graves speculum. The patient may be advised to change her coital position to reduce pain on deep penetration.

Methods for treating psychologically based dyspareunia vary. Psychotherapy may uncover hidden conflicts that are creating fears concerning intercourse. Sensate focus exercises de-emphasize intercourse itself and teach appropriate foreplay techniques. Information about appropriate methods of contraception can reduce fear of pregnancy; education concerning sexual activity during pregnancy can relieve fears of harming the fetus.

Nursing diagnoses
• Altered family processes
• Altered sexuality patterns
• Anxiety
• Knowledge deficit
• Sexual dysfunction

Nursing interventions

• Communicate an open, nonjudgmental attitude in caring for a patient with dyspareunia.
• Listen empathetically to the patient's complaints of sex-related pain, and encourage her to express her feelings freely.
• As needed, refer the patient to a doctor, nurse, psychologist, social worker, or counselor trained in sex therapy.

Patient teaching

• Provide instruction concerning anatomy and physiology of the reproductive system, contraception, and the human sexual response cycle.
• When appropriate, give advice and information on drugs that may affect the patient's sexual response and on lubricating jellies and creams.
• As a helpful guideline, inform the patient that a therapist's certification by the American Association of Sex Educators, Counselors, and Therapists or by the American Society for Sex Therapy and Research usually assures quality treatment. If the therapist is not certified by one of these organizations, advise the patient to inquire about the therapist's training in sex counseling and therapy.

VAGINISMUS

An involuntary spastic constriction of the lower vaginal muscles, vaginismus usually stems from the fear of vaginal penetration. If severe, it may prevent intercourse. Vaginismus affects women of all ages and backgrounds. The prognosis is excellent for a motivated patient who has no untreatable organic abnormalities.

Causes

Vaginismus may be physical or psychological in origin. It may occur spontaneously as a protective reflex to pain, or it may result from organic causes, such as abnormalities of the hymen, genital herpes, obstetric trauma, and atrophic vaginitis.

Psychological causes of vaginismus include:
• childhood and adolescent exposure to rigid, punitive, and guilt-ridden attitudes toward sex
• fears resulting from painful or traumatic sexual experiences, such as incest or rape
• early traumatic experience with pelvic examinations
• phobias of pregnancy, venereal disease, or cancer
• dysfunctional childhood experiences and family attitudes toward sex

• concern about contraception and potential pregnancy
• conflicts with the sexual partner.

Complications

Vaginismus can impair marital or other sexual relationships.

Assessment findings

The patient with vaginismus may report muscle spasm with constriction and pain on insertion of any object into the vagina, such as a vaginal tampon, diaphragm, or speculum. She may profess a lack of sexual interest or a normal level of sexual desire (typically characterized by sexual activity without intercourse).

Diagnostic criteria

The diagnosis of vaginismus is based on fulfillment of the following criteria established in the *DSM-IV*:
• The patient experiences recurrent or persistent involuntary spasm of the musculature of the outer third of the vagina, which interferes with coitus.
• The disturbance causes marked distress or interpersonal difficulty.
• The disturbance is not caused exclusively by a physical disorder and is not due to another Axis I disorder.

A carefully performed pelvic examination confirms the diagnosis by demonstrating involuntary constriction of the musculature surrounding the outer portion of the vagina.

Treatment

Appropriate treatment is designed to eliminate maladaptive muscle constriction and underlying psychological problems. In Masters and Johnson therapy, the patient uses a graduated series of plastic dilators, which she inserts into her vagina while tensing and relaxing her pelvic muscles. The patient controls the time the dilator is left in place (if possible, she retains it for several hours) and the movement of the dilator. Together with her sexual partner, she begins sensate focus and counseling therapy to increase sexual responsiveness, improve communications skills, and resolve any underlying conflicts.

Kaplan therapy also uses progressive insertion of dilators or fingers (in vivo desensitization therapy), with behavior therapy (imagining vaginal penetration until it can be tolerated) and, if necessary, psychoanalysis and hypnosis. Both Masters and Johnson and Kaplan report a 100% cure rate; however, Kaplan states that the patient and her partner may show other sexual dysfunctions that necessitate additional therapy.

Nursing diagnoses
• Altered family processes
• Altered sexuality patterns
• Anxiety
• Knowledge deficit
• Sexual dysfunction

Nursing interventions
• Communicate an open, nonjudgmental attitude in caring for a patient with vaginismus.
• Listen empathetically to the patient's complaints of sex-related pain, and encourage her to express her feelings.
• Because a pelvic examination may be painful for the patient, proceed gradually, at the patient's own pace. Support her throughout the pelvic examination, explaining each step beforehand. Encourage her to verbalize her feelings, and take plenty of time to answer her questions.
• As needed, refer the patient to a doctor, nurse, psychologist, social worker, or counselor trained in sex therapy.

Patient teaching
• Provide instruction concerning anatomy and physiology of the reproductive system, contraception, and the human sexual response cycle.
• When appropriate, advise the patient about drugs that may affect sexual response and about lubricating jellies and creams.
• As a helpful guideline, inform the patient that the therapist's certification by the American Association of Sex Educators, Counselors, and Therapists or by the American Society for Sex Therapy and Research usually assures quality treatment. If the therapist is not certified by one of these organizations, advise the patient to inquire about the therapist's training in sex counseling and therapy.

MALE ERECTILE DISORDER
Characterized as primary or secondary, erectile dysfunction (or impotence) refers to the inability of a man to attain or maintain penile erection long enough to complete intercourse. The patient with primary impotence has never achieved sufficient erection. Secondary impotence, which is more common and less serious than the primary form, implies that, despite the current inability, the patient has succeeded in completing intercourse in the past. Transient periods of impotence

are not considered dysfunctional and probably occur in 50% of men.
Three types of secondary erectile disorder occur:
• Partial — The patient is unable to achieve a full erection or to keep his erection long enough to penetrate his partner.
• Intermittent — The patient sometimes is potent with the same partner.
• Selective — The patient is potent only with certain partners.
Erectile disorder affects all age-groups but increases in frequency with age. The prognosis depends on the severity and duration of impotence and on the underlying cause.

Causes
Psychogenic factors are responsible for 50% to 60% of cases of erectile disorder; the rest can be attributed to organic factors. In some patients, psychogenic and organic factors coexist, making isolation of the primary cause difficult.
Psychogenic causes may be intrapersonal, reflecting personal sexual anxieties, or interpersonal, reflecting a disturbed sexual relationship. Intrapersonal factors include guilt, fear, depression, and feelings of inadequacy resulting from a previous traumatic sexual experience, rejection by parents or peers, exaggerated religious orthodoxy, abnormal mother-son intimacy, or homosexual experiences or fantasies.
Interpersonal factors may stem from differences in sexual preferences between partners, lack of communication, insufficient knowledge of sexual function, or nonsexual personal conflicts.
Situational impotence, a temporary condition, may develop in response to stress. Organic causes include chronic diseases, such as cardiopulmonary disease, diabetes mellitus, multiple sclerosis, and renal failure; spinal cord trauma; complications of surgery; drug- or alcohol-induced dysfunction; and, rarely, genital anomalies or central nervous system defects.

Complications
Erectile disorder may seriously disrupt marital or other sexual relationships.

Assessment findings
The history of a patient with erectile disorder may reveal a long-standing inability to achieve erection, a sudden loss of erectile function, or a gradual decline in function. In addition, the patient may describe a his-

tory of medical disorders, drug therapy, or psychological trauma that may contribute to erectile disorder.

If the cause is psychogenic rather than organic, the patient may report that he can achieve erection through masturbation but not with a partner. He may display characteristic signs of anxiety when discussing his condition, such as sweating and palpitations, or appear disinterested. Depression, another common complaint, may be either a cause or a result of the impotence.

Diagnostic criteria
A diagnosis of male erectile disorder is confirmed when the patient's symptoms meet either of the following two criteria, established in the *DSM-IV*:
• The patient experiences a persistent or recurrent partial or complete failure to attain or maintain erection until completion of sexual activity.
• The disturbance causes marked distress or interpersonal difficulty.

In addition, the disorder should not occur exclusively during the course of another Axis I disorder, such as major depression.

Laboratory tests are ordered to rule out chronic diseases, such as diabetes, and other vascular, neurologic, or urogenital problems.

Treatment
Sex therapy, which is designed to reduce performance anxiety, may effectively cure psychogenic impotence. To be most effective, such therapy should include both partners.

The course and content of sex therapy for male erectile disorder depend on the specific cause of the disorder and the nature of the male-female relationship. Treatment usually includes sensate focus therapy, which restricts the couple's sexual activity and encourages them to become more attuned to the physical sensations of touching. Other measures include improving verbal communication skills, eliminating unreasonable guilt, and reevaluating attitudes toward sex and sexual roles.

Treatment of organic impotence focuses on eliminating the cause, if possible. If the cause cannot be eliminated, psychological counseling may help the couple deal realistically with their situation and explore alternatives for sexual expression. Some patients with organic impotence may benefit from a surgically inserted inflatable or semirigid penile prosthesis.

Nursing diagnoses
• Altered family processes
• Altered sexuality patterns
• Anxiety
• Ineffective individual coping
• Knowledge deficit
• Self-esteem disturbance
• Sexual dysfunction

Nursing interventions
• Help the patient feel comfortable about discussing his sexuality.
• As needed, refer the patient to a doctor, nurse, psychologist, social worker, or counselor trained in sex therapy.
After penile prosthesis surgery:
• Apply ice packs to the penis for 24 hours.
• Empty the Jackson-Pratt drain when it is full.
• If the patient has an inflatable prosthesis, instruct him to pull the scrotal pump downward to ensure proper alignment.
• When ordered, have the patient practice inflating and deflating the device.

Patient teaching
• Provide instruction concerning anatomy and physiology of the reproductive system and the human sexual response cycle, as needed.
• After penile implant surgery, instruct the patient to avoid intercourse until the incision heals, usually in 6 weeks. Advise him to report signs of infection to the doctor.
• As a helpful guideline, inform the patient that the therapist's certification by the American Association of Sex Educators, Counselors, and Therapists or by the American Society for Sex Therapy and Research usually assures quality treatment. If the therapist is not certified by one of these organizations, advise the patient to inquire about the therapist's training in sex counseling and therapy.

PREMATURE EJACULATION
One of the most common types of male sexual dysfunction, premature ejaculation describes an inability to control the ejaculatory reflex during intercourse. As a result, ejaculation occurs before or immediately after penetration or before the wishes of both partners. This disorder affects men of all ages.

Causes

Premature ejaculation may result from anxiety and may be linked to immature sexual experiences. Other psychological factors include ambivalence toward or unconscious hatred of women, a negative sexual relationship in which the patient unconsciously denies his partner sexual fulfillment, and guilt feelings about sex.

Psychological factors aren't the only cause of premature ejaculation; this disorder can also occur in emotionally healthy men with stable, positive relationships. Rarely, premature ejaculation may be linked to an underlying degenerative neurologic disorder, such as multiple sclerosis, or an inflammatory process, such as posterior urethritis or prostatitis.

Complications

Premature ejaculation can seriously disrupt marital or other sexual relationships. In addition, the disorder can lead to generalized anxiety disorder, as well as to pervasive feelings of inadequacy, guilt, and self-doubt.

Assessment findings

The patient's history may reveal that he can't prolong foreplay or that he can prolong foreplay but ejaculates as soon as intromission occurs. In some cases, the patient's partner may seek psychiatric treatment, complaining that the patient is indifferent to her sexual needs.

Diagnostic criteria

The diagnosis of premature ejaculation is based on fulfillment of the following criterion established in the *DSM-IV*: persistent or recurrent ejaculation with minimal sexual stimulation before, during, or shortly after penetration and before the person wishes it to occur.

The clinician may take into account factors that affect duration of the excitement phase, such as age, novelty of the sexual partner or situation, and frequency of sexual activity.

Treatment

Masters and Johnson have developed a highly successful, intensive treatment program for premature ejaculation. The program combines insight therapy, behavioral techniques, and experiential sessions that involve both sexual partners. The program is designed to help the patient focus on sensations of impending orgasm. The therapy sessions, which continue for 2 weeks or longer, typically include:

• mutual physical examination, which increases the couple's awareness of anatomy and physiology, while reducing shameful feelings about sexual parts of the body
• sensate focus, which allows each partner, in turn, to caress the other's body without intercourse and to focus on the pleasurable sensations of touch
• the squeeze technique, which helps the patient gain control of ejaculatory tension by having the woman squeeze his penis, with her thumb on the frenulum and her forefinger and middle finger on the dorsal surface, near the coronal ridge. At the patient's direction, she applies and releases pressure every few minutes during a touching exercise to delay ejaculation by keeping him at an earlier phase of the sexual response cycle. (See *The squeeze technique: Position and pressure important,* page 88.)

The stop-and-start technique also helps delay ejaculation. With the woman in the superior position, this method involves pelvic thrusting until orgasmic sensations start and then stopping and restarting to aid control of ejaculation. The couple eventually is allowed to achieve orgasm.

Nursing diagnoses

• Altered family processes
• Altered sexuality patterns
• Anxiety
• Knowledge deficit
• Self-esteem disturbance
• Sexual dysfunction

Nursing interventions

• Convey sympathy and a nonjudgmental attitude when caring for a patient with premature ejaculation.
• Provide expert teaching in a comfortable environment that encourages open discussion of sexuality.
• As needed, refer the patient to a doctor, nurse, psychologist, social worker, or counselor trained in sex therapy.

Patient teaching

• Provide instruction concerning anatomy and physiology of the reproductive system and the human sexual response cycle, as needed.
• Encourage a positive self-image by explaining that premature ejaculation is a common disorder that doesn't reflect on the patient's masculinity.
• Assure the patient that the condition is reversible.
• As a helpful guideline, inform the patient that a therapist's certification by the American Association of Sex

THE SQUEEZE TECHNIQUE: POSITION AND PRESSURE IMPORTANT

To delay ejaculation using the squeeze technique, the patient's partner must position her fingers correctly around the penis and apply the right amount of pressure. When the patient feels the urge to ejaculate, the partner should place her thumb on the frenulum of the penis and her index and middle fingers above and below the coronal ridge, as shown here. Then, tell her to squeeze the penis from front to back. How firmly she should squeeze will depend on the erection's stiffness: more firmly for a stiff penis and less firmly for a partially flaccid one. The patient will feel pressure but no pain.

Anatomic structures

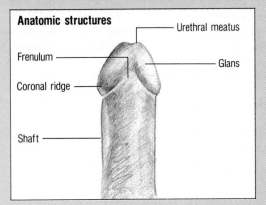

- Urethral meatus
- Frenulum
- Glans
- Coronal ridge
- Shaft

Hand position

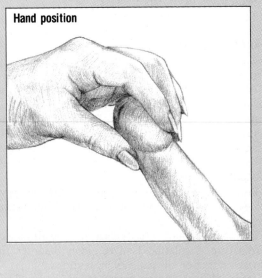

Educators, Counselors, and Therapists or by the American Society for Sex Therapy and Research usually assures quality treatment. If the therapist is not certified by one of these organizations, advise the patient to inquire about the therapist's training in sex counseling and therapy.

GENDER IDENTITY DISORDERS

Sexual disorders that involve gender identity produce persistent feelings of gender discomfort and dissatisfaction. Defined as the intimate personal feeling one has about being male or female, gender identity includes three components: self-concept, perception of an ideal partner, and external presentation of masculinity and femininity through behavior, dress, and mannerisms.

Patients with these disorders typically behave and present themselves as people of the opposite sex, which they intensely desire to become. The disorder affects more men than women and usually begins in childhood. Rare in both children and adults, gender identity disorders should not be confused with the far more common phenomenon of feeling inadequate in fulfilling the expectations normally associated with a particular sex.

Causes

Current theories about the causes of gender identity disorders suggest a combination of predisposing factors: chromosomal anomaly, hormonal imbalance (particularly in utero during brain formation), and pathologic defects in early parent-child bonding and child-rearing practices. For example, parents who deliberately treat their child as a member of the opposite sex significantly contribute to gender identity disorder.

Complications

Many children, particularly boys, are rejected by their peer group; this social conflict may be reflected in poor academic performance. Girls may not experience social difficulties until early adolescence.

Transsexualism may seriously impair social and occupational functioning, partly because of psychopathology and partly because of problems in attempting to live in the desired gender role. Anxiety and depression are common and can lead to suicide attempts. Rarely, men may mutilate their genitalia.

The onset of gender identity disorder after marriage may significantly disrupt the marital relationship.

Assessment findings

During the assessment interview, a child with a gender identity disorder may express the desire to be—or insist that he or she is—the opposite sex. Such a child may express disgust with his genitalia and the belief, often expressed as an ardent hope, that when he grows up, he will become the opposite sex.

Men with a gender identity disorder may describe a lifelong history of feeling feminine and pursuing feminine activities. Women exhibit similar propensities for opposite sex activities and discomfort with the female role. In both instances, the crisis seems especially acute during puberty. Development of secondary sex characteristics (breasts and pubic hair in the female; enlarged penis and testes in the male) may precipitate intense distress or intensify the feeling that one is a misfit.

Diagnostic criteria

The diagnosis of gender identity disorder is confirmed when the patient's signs and symptoms meet the criteria established in the *DSM-IV.*

For gender identity disorder, both a strong and persistent cross-gender identification (not just a desire for perceived cultural advantages of being the other sex) as well as a persistent discomfort with his or her sex or sense of inappropriateness in the gender role of that sex must be present.

In children, this cross-gender identification is manifested by at least four of the following:
• a repeatedly stated desire to be, or insistence that he or she is, the other sex
• in boys, a preference for cross-dressing or simulating female attire; in girls, insistence on wearing only stereotypically masculine clothing
• a strong and persistent preference for cross-sex roles in make-believe play or persistent fantasies of being the other sex
• an intense desire to participate in the stereotypical games of the other sex
• a strong preference for playmates of the other sex.

In adolescents and adults, this cross-gender identification is manifested by such symptoms as a stated desire to be the other sex, frequently posing as the other sex, a desire to live or be treated as the other sex, or the conviction that he or she has the typical feelings and reactions of the other sex.

Discomfort with his or her own sex is manifested by any of the following:
• in boys, an assertion that his penis or testes are disgusting or will disappear or an assertion that it would be better not to have a penis, or an aversion toward rough play and rejection of stereotypically male toys, games, and activities
• in girls, rejection of urinating in a sitting position, an assertion that she wants to grow a penis, an assertion that she does not want to grow breasts or menstruate, or a marked aversion toward normative feminine clothing
• in adolescents and adults, a preoccupation with getting rid of primary and secondary sex characteristics (asking for hormone therapy, surgery, or other procedures to alter sexual characteristics to simulate the other sex) or a belief that he or she was born the wrong sex.

Diagnostic criteria for gender identity disorder also includes the following:
• The disturbance is not concurrent with a physical intersex disorder.
• The disturbance causes clinically significant distress or impairment of social, occupational, or other areas of functioning.

Treatment

Individual and family therapy are indicated for treatment of childhood gender identity disorders. Ideally, a therapist of the same sex may be useful for role modeling purposes. The earlier this problem is diagnosed and treatment begins, the more hopeful the prognosis for the child.

In an adult, individual and couples therapy may help the patient to cope with the decision to live as the opposite sex or to cope with the knowledge that he or she will not be able to live as the opposite sex.

Sex reassignment through hormonal and surgical treatment may be an option; however, surgical sex reassignment has not been as beneficial as first hoped. Severe psychological problems may persist after sex reassignment and sometimes lead to suicide. Furthermore, these patients may have gender disorders as part of a larger pattern of depression and personality disorders, such as a borderline personality disorder.

With or without treatment, female transsexuals have shown stabler patterns of adjustment than male transsexuals have demonstrated.

Appropriate psychiatric management, including hospitalization, may be necessary if the patient displays evidence of the potential for violent behavior, such as suicidal ideation and fantasies of self-mutilation.

Nursing diagnoses
• Altered family processes
• Altered growth and development

- Altered role performance
- Anxiety
- Body image disturbance
- Chronic low self-esteem
- Impaired social interaction
- Ineffective family coping
- Ineffective individual coping
- Personal identity disturbance
- Powerlessness
- Risk for injury
- Sexual dysfunction
- Social isolation

Nursing interventions
- Use a nonjudgmental approach in facial expression, tone of voice, and choice of words to convey your acceptance of the person's choices. By gaining the patient's trust, you'll lessen his discomfort about discussing his sexuality.
- Realize that treating such a patient with empathy doesn't threaten your own sexuality.
- Respect the patient's privacy and sense of modesty, particularly during procedures or examinations.
- Monitor for related or compounded problems, such as suicidal thought or intent, depression, and anxiety.
- As needed, refer the patient to a doctor, nurse, psychologist, social worker, or counselor trained in sex therapy.

Patient teaching
- As a helpful guideline, inform the patient that the therapist's certification by the American Association of Sex Educators, Counselors, and Therapists or by the American Society for Sex Therapy and Research usually assures quality treatment. If the therapist is not certified by one of these organizations, advise the patient to inquire about the therapist's training in sex counseling and therapy.

PARAPHILIAS
Characterized by a dependence on unusual behaviors or fantasies to achieve sexual excitement, paraphilias are complex psychosexual disorders. The imagery or acts may involve the use of inanimate objects (especially clothing), repetitive sexual activity that includes suffering or humiliation, or sexual behavior with nonconsenting partners. The *DSM-IV* recognizes eight types of paraphilias: exhibitionism, fetishism, frotteurism, pedophilia, sexual masochism, sexual sad-

ism, transvestic fetishism, and voyeurism. (See *Types of paraphilias.*)

Some paraphilias that violate social mores or norms are considered sex offenses or sex crimes. However, everyone has sexual fantasies, and sexual behavior between two consenting adults that's not physically or psychologically harmful is not considered a paraphilia.

Little data exist on the prevalence of paraphilias in our society. Most people with paraphilias come to the mental health care system not because of their own distress, but at the behest of their partners or legal authorities.

Causes
The specific cause of paraphilias is not known, although several contributing factors have been identified. Many patients with these disorders come from dysfunctional families, characterized by isolation and sexual, emotional, or physical abuse. Others suffer from other mental disorders, such as psychoactive substance use disorders or a personality disorder.

Complications
Sexual masochism may sometimes result in serious physical injury. Paraphilias that involve another person, particularly voyeurism, exhibitionism, frotteurism, pedophilia, and sexual sadism, commonly lead to arrest and incarceration. Exhibitionists, pedophiles, and voyeurs make up the majority of apprehended sex offenders, and sexual offenses against children constitute a significant proportion of all reported criminal sex acts.

Assessment findings
The patient's history will reveal the particular pattern of abnormal sexual behaviors associated with one of the eight recognized paraphilias.

Diagnostic criteria
The diagnosis of paraphilia is confirmed when the patient's symptoms meet the criteria established in the *DSM-IV*.

For *exhibitionism:*
- Over a period of at least 6 months, the patient has experienced recurrent, intense sexual urges and sexually arousing fantasies involving the exposure of his genitalia to an unsuspecting stranger.
- The fantasies, urges, or behaviors cause clinically significant distress or impairment of social, occupational, or other areas of functioning.

TYPES OF PARAPHILIAS

Some people derive sexual excitement through behaviors or fantasies known as paraphilias. Eight paraphilias, including exhibitionism, fetishism, frotteurism, pedophilia, sexual masochism, sexual sadism, transvestic fetishism, and voyeurism, are described below.

Exhibitionism

The patient with this paraphilia obtains sexual gratification from publicly exposing his genitals to others, principally female passersby. The problem is most common in men (who often achieve erection while exposing themselves). Some masturbate to orgasm at the time.

Fetishism

The term "fetish" describes a recurrent and intense sexual arousal to an inanimate object (most often an article of women's clothing, such as panties or boots) or body parts that are neither primary nor secondary sexual organs. The patient frequently masturbates while holding, rubbing, or smelling the fetish object, or may ask his partner to wear the object during their sexual encounters. Fetishism occurs primarily in men and typically follows a chronic course.

Frotteurism

The patient with this type of paraphilia achieves sexual arousal by touching or rubbing a nonconsenting person. For example, he may rub his genitals against a woman's thigh or fondle her breasts. The behavior frequently occurs in crowded places, where it's easier to avoid detection. It is most common between ages 15 and 25.

Pedophilia

The pedophile (almost always a man) is erotically aroused by, and seeks sexual gratification from, children. This urge forms his preferred or exclusive sexual activity. Prepubertal children are the most common targets, and attraction to girls is almost twice as common as attraction to boys. The pedophile may sexually abuse his own children or those of a friend or relative or, rarely, he may even abduct a child. He may be quite attentive to all of the child's needs to gain the child's loyalty and prevent the child from reporting the encounters. Some pedophiles also are attracted to adults.

Sexual masochism

Sexual masochism refers to the urge to submit to physical or psychological pain, such as being humiliated, beaten, bound, or tortured, to achieve sexual gratification. This disorder is chronic.

Infantilism, a form of sexual masochism, is a desire to be treated as a helpless infant, including wearing diapers. One dangerous form of this paraphilia, sexual hypoxyphilia, relies on oxygen deprivation to induce sexual arousal. The patient uses a noose, mask, plastic bag, or chemical to induce a temporary decrease in brain oxygenation. Equipment malfunction or other mistakes can cause accidental death.

Sexual sadism

The converse of sexual masochism, sadism refers to recurrent, intense sexual urges and fantasies that involve inflicting physical or psychological suffering. The sadist derives sexual gratification from this behavior.

Transvestic fetishism

The transvestite is a heterosexual man who obtains sexual pleasure from cross-dressing (dressing in women's clothing). He may select a single article of apparel, such as a garter or stockings or he may dress entirely as a woman, with a well made-up face and an immaculate feminine coiffure. This behavior often is accompanied by masturbation and mental images of other men being attracted to him as a "woman."

Voyeurism

The voyeur derives sexual pleasure from looking at sexual objects or sexually arousing situations, such as an unsuspecting couple engaged in sexual intercourse. No sexual orgasm may occur during the voyeuristic activity or later in response to the memory of what the person witnessed. Onset of this disorder is before age 15, and it tends to be chronic.

For *fetishism:*
• Over a period of 6 months, the patient has experienced recurrent, intense sexual urges and sexually arousing fantasies involving the use of nonliving objects by himself.
• The fantasies, sexual urges, or behaviors cause clinically significant distress.
• The fetishes are not restricted to articles of female clothing used in cross-dressing or devices designed for the purpose of tactile genital stimulation.

For *frotteurism:*
• Over a period of at least 6 months, the patient has experienced recurrent, intense sexual urges and sexually arousing fantasies involving touching or rubbing

against a nonconsenting person.
• The fantasies, urges, or behaviors cause clinically significant distress.

For *pedophilia:*
• Over a period of at least 6 months, the patient has experienced recurrent, intense sexual urges and sexually arousing fantasies involving sexual activity with a prepubescent child or children (generally age 13 or younger).
• The fantasies, urges, or behaviors cause clinically significant distress.
• The patient is at least 16 years old and at least 5 years older than the child or children involved. The late adolescent involved in an ongoing sexual relationship with a 12- or 13-year-old child should not be included in this group.

For *sexual masochism:*
• Over a period of at least 6 months, the patient has experienced recurrent, intense sexual urges, sexually arousing fantasies, or behaviors involving the act of being humiliated, beaten, bound, or otherwise made to suffer.
• The fantasies, urges, or behaviors cause clinically significant distress.

For *sexual sadism:*
• Over a period of at least 6 months, the patient has experienced recurrent, intense sexual urges, sexually arousing fantasies, or behaviors involving acts in which the psychological or physical suffering of the victim is sexually exciting to the patient.
• The fantasies, urges, or behaviors cause clinically significant distress.

For *transvestic fetishism:*
• Over a period of at least 6 months, the patient (a heterosexual man) has experienced recurrent, intense sexual urges, sexually arousing fantasies, or behaviors involving cross-dressing.
• The fantasies, urges, or behaviors cause clinically significant distress.
• The patient does not meet the *DSM-IV* criteria for gender identity disorder.

For *voyeurism:*
• Over a period of at least 6 months, the patient has experienced recurrent, intense sexual urges, sexually arousing fantasies, or behaviors involving the act of observing an unsuspecting person disrobing or engaging in sexual activity.
• The fantasies, urges, or behaviors cause clinically significant distress.

Treatment
Paraphilias require mandatory treatment when the patient's sexual preferences result in socially unacceptable or harmful behavior. Depending on the paraphilia, treatment may include a combination of psychotherapy, behavior therapy, pharmacotherapy, and surgery. The effectiveness of treatment varies.

Nursing diagnoses
• Altered role performance
• Altered sexuality patterns
• Anxiety
• Chronic low self-esteem
• Impaired social interaction
• Personal identity disturbance
• Risk for injury
• Risk for violence: Directed at others
• Self-esteem disturbance
• Sexual dysfunction

Nursing interventions
• Use a nonjudgmental approach in facial expression, tone of voice, and choice of words to convey your acceptance of the patient's choices.
• Realize that treating such a patient with empathy doesn't threaten your own sexuality.
• Encourage the patient to express his sexual preferences as well as his feelings about them.
• As needed, refer the patient to a doctor, nurse, psychologist, social worker, or counselor trained in sex therapy.

Patient teaching
• As a helpful guideline, inform the patient that a therapist's certification by the American Association of Sex Educators, Counselors, and Therapists or by the American Society for Sex Therapy and Research usually ensures quality treatment. If the therapist is not certified by one of these organizations, advise the patient to inquire about the therapist's training in sex counseling and therapy.

SELECTED REFERENCES
Anai-Otong, D. *Psychiatric Nursing: Biological and Behavioral Concepts.* Philadelphia: W.B. Saunders Co., 1995.
Butler, K.Z., et al. *Clinical Handbook of Psychotropic Drugs,* 4th ed. Seattle: Hogrefe & Huber Publishers, 1994.

Diagnostic and Statistical Manual of Mental Disorders, 4th ed. Washington, D.C.: American Psychiatric Association, 1994.

Fortinash, K.M., and Holoday-Worret, P.A. *Psychiatric Nursing Care Plans,* 2nd ed. St. Louis: Mosby-Year Book, Inc., 1995.

Gulanick, M., et al. *Nursing Care Plans: Nursing Diagnosis and Intervention,* 3rd ed. St. Louis: Mosby-Year Book, Inc., 1994.

Isselbacher, K.J., et al., eds. *Harrison's Principles of Internal Medicine,* 13th ed. New York: McGraw-Hill Book Co., 1994.

Lysaker, P., et al. "Work Performance over Time for People with Schizophrenia," *Psychosocial Rehabilitation Journal* 18(3):141-45, January 1995.

Rakel, R.E., ed. *Conn's Current Therapy 1995.* Philadelphia: W.B. Saunders Co., 1995.

Rich, D. "Relapse in the Major Mental Disorders," *Mental Health Nursing* 3(4):132-44, December 1994.

Smith, L. "Clozapine: Indications and Implications for Treatment," *Nursing Times* 91(30):40-41, July 1995.

Stuart, G.W., and Sundeen, S.J. *Principles and Practice of Psychiatric Nursing,* 5th ed. St. Louis: Mosby-Year Book, Inc., 1995.

Taylor, C.M., and Sparks, S.M. *Nursing Diagnosis Reference Manual,* 3rd ed. Springhouse, Pa.: Springhouse Corp., 1995.

Tierney, L.M., et al. *Current Medical Diagnosis and Treatment 1995.* East Norwalk, Conn.: Appleton & Lange, 1995.

Wilson, H.S., and Kneisl, C.R. *Psychiatric Nursing,* 4th ed. Menlo Park, Calif.: Addison-Wesley Publishing Co., 1992.

2 INFECTION

INTRODUCTION

Despite improved methods of treating and preventing infection — potent antibiotics, rigorous immunizations, and modern sanitation — infection still accounts for much serious illness, even in highly industrialized countries. In developing countries, infection remains one of the most pressing health problems.

What is infection?

Infection is the invasion and multiplication of microorganisms in or on body tissues that produces signs and symptoms as well as an immune response. Such reproduction injures the host by causing cellular damage from microorganism-produced toxins or intracellular multiplication, or by competing with host metabolism. The host's own immune response may compound the tissue damage. The damage may be localized (as in infected pressure ulcers) or systemic. The infection's severity varies with the pathogenicity and number of the invading microorganisms, and the strength of host defenses.

Why are the microorganisms that cause infectious diseases so hard to overcome? Many complex reasons exist:
• Some bacteria — especially gram-negative bacilli — develop resistance to antibiotics.
• Some microorganisms — the influenza virus, for example — have so many strains that a single vaccine can't provide protection against them all.
• Most viruses resist antiviral drugs.
• Some microorganisms localize in areas that make treatment difficult, such as the central nervous system or bone.

Moreover, certain factors contribute to increase the risk of infection. For example, travel can expose people to diseases for which they have little natural immunity. In addition, the expanded use of immunosuppressants, surgery, and other invasive procedures increases the risk of infection. (See *Glossary of epidemiology,* page 96, and *Reportable infectious diseases,* page 97.)

Kinds of infections

A laboratory-verified infection that causes no signs and symptoms is called a *subclinical, silent,* or *asymptomatic infection.* A multiplication of microbes that produces no signs, symptoms, or immune responses is called a *colonization.* A person with a subclinical infection or a colonization may be a carrier and transmit infection to others.

A *latent infection* occurs after a microorganism has been dormant in the host, sometimes for years. An *ex-ogenous infection* results from environmental pathogens; an *endogenous infection,* from the host's normal flora (for instance, *Escherichia coli* displaced from the colon, which may cause urinary tract infection).

The varied forms of microorganisms responsible for infectious diseases include bacteria, spirochetes (a type of bacteria), viruses, rickettsiae, chlamydiae, fungi, and protozoa. Larger organisms, such as helminths (worms), also may cause disease.

Bacteria

Single-cell microorganisms with well-defined cell walls, bacteria can multiply independently on artificial media without the need for other cells. In developing countries, where poor sanitation heightens the risk of infection, bacterial diseases commonly cause death and disability. Even in industrialized countries, they're still the most common fatal infectious diseases.

Bacteria can be classified by shape. Spherical bacterial cells are called *cocci*; rod-shaped bacteria, *bacilli*; and spiral-shaped bacteria, *spirilla.* They also can be classified by their response to staining (gram-positive, gram-negative, or acid-fast bacteria), their motility (motile or nonmotile bacteria), their tendency toward capsulation (encapsulated or nonencapsulated bacteria), their capacity to form spores (sporulating or nonsporulating bacteria), and their oxygen requirements (aerobic bacteria need oxygen to grow; anaerobic bacteria do not).

Spirochetes

A type of bacteria, spirochetes are flexible, slender, undulating spiral rods that have cell walls. Most are anaerobic. The three forms pathogenic in humans include *Treponema, Leptospira,* and *Borrelia.*

Viruses

Viruses are subcellular organisms made up of only a ribonucleic acid (RNA) or a deoxyribonucleic acid (DNA) nucleus covered with proteins. They are the smallest known organisms, so tiny that they're visible only through an electron microscope. Viruses can't replicate independent of host cells. Rather, they invade a host cell and stimulate it to participate in the formation of additional virus particles. The estimated 400 viruses that infect humans are classified according to their size, shape (spherical, rod-shaped, or cubic), or means of transmission (respiratory, fecal, oral, or sexual).

GLOSSARY OF EPIDEMIOLOGY

Epidemiology is the study of the origin, frequency, and distribution of disease in a given population. It also examines disease transmission as well as host and environmental factors that influence disease development.

Several terms describe disease occurrence or frequency. In an *epidemic,* a disease occurs more frequently than normal. An *outbreak,* however, is a sudden appearance of the disease, typically in a small portion of the population. An *endemic disease* is persistently present in a given locale, whereas a *hyperendemic disease* has a high incidence across all age-groups. A *reservoir* refers to the natural habitat of the causative microorganism; a *source,* to the site where the host directly acquired the disease.

Microorganisms can multiply within a source. The source includes a *vector,* a carrier that transmits the disease indirectly from person to person. This usually is an arthropod (for example, a mosquito), but it can be a person who has the disease or was recently exposed to it. Transmission also may occur through a *vehicle,* such as contaminated food or water. Microorganisms can multiply within a vehicle.

Rickettsiae

Relatively uncommon in the United States, these small, gram-negative bacteria-like organisms frequently induce life-threatening infections. Like viruses, they require a host cell for replication. Three genera of rickettsiae include *Rickettsia, Coxiella,* and *Rochalimaea.*

Chlamydiae

Larger than viruses, chlamydiae have recently been found to be intracellular obligate bacteria. Unlike other bacteria, they depend on host cells for replication; unlike viruses, they're susceptible to antibiotics.

Fungi

These single-cell organisms have nuclei enveloped by nuclear membranes. They have rigid cell walls like plant cells but lack chlorophyll, the green matter necessary for photosynthesis. They also show relatively little cellular specialization. Fungi occur as yeasts (single-cell, oval-shaped organisms) or molds (organisms with hyphae, or branching filaments). Depending on the environment, some fungi may occur in both forms. Fungal diseases in humans are called mycoses.

Protozoa

Protozoa are the simplest single-cell organisms of the animal kingdom, but they show a high level of cellular specialization. Like other animal cells, they have cell membranes rather than cell walls, and their nuclei are surrounded by nuclear membranes.

Helminths

The three groups of helminths that invade humans include nematodes, cestodes, and trematodes. Nematodes are cylindrical, unsegmented, elongated helminths that taper at each end; this shape has earned them the designation *roundworm.* Cestodes, better known as *tapeworms,* have bodies that are flattened front to back with distinct, regular segments. Tapeworms also have heads with suckers or sucking grooves. Trematodes have flattened, unsegmented bodies. They are called *blood, intestinal, lung,* or *liver flukes,* depending on their infection site.

Modes of transmission

Most infectious diseases are transmitted in one of four ways.

In *contact transmission,* the susceptible host comes into direct contact (as in sexually transmitted diseases) or indirect contact (contaminated inanimate objects or the close-range spread of respiratory droplets) with the source.

Airborne transmission results from inhalation of contaminated evaporated saliva droplets (as in pulmonary tuberculosis), which sometimes are suspended in airborne dust particles or vapors.

In *enteric* (fecal-oral) *transmission,* the organisms are found in feces and are ingested by susceptible victims, often through fecally contaminated food or water.

Vector-borne transmission occurs when an intermediate carrier (vector), such as a flea or a mosquito, transfers an organism.

Prevention of contagion

The following measures can be taken to prevent the transmission of infectious diseases:
• drug prophylaxis
• universal precautions
• hand washing between patients
• comprehensive immunization (including immunization of travelers to or emigrants from endemic areas)
• improved nutrition, living conditions, and sanitation
• correction of environmental factors.

Although prophylactic antibiotic therapy may prevent certain diseases, the risk of superinfection and the emergence of drug-resistant strains may outweigh the benefits. So prophylactic antibiotics usually are reserved for patients at high risk for exposure to dangerous infection.

Appropriate immunization can now prevent many diseases, including diphtheria, tetanus, pertussis, measles, rubella, some forms of meningitis, poliomyelitis, hepatitis B, pneumococcal pneumonia, influenza, rabies, and tetanus.

Vaccines—which contain live but attenuated (weakened) or killed microorganisms—and toxoids—which contain bacterial exotoxins—induce immunity against bacterial and viral diseases by stimulating the recipient's antibody formation.

Immune serums, which contain previously formed antibodies from hyperimmunized donors or pooled plasma, provide temporary passive immunity. Antitoxins provide immunity to various toxins. Passive immunization is used only when active immunization is perilous or impossible, or when complete protection requires both active and passive immunization. (See *Immunization schedule*, page 98.)

Nosocomial infections

A *nosocomial infection* is one that develops while a patient is in a hospital or another institution. Most infections of this type result from group A *Streptococcus pyogenes, Staphylococcus, E. coli, Klebsiella, Proteus, Pseudomonas, Haemophilus influenzae, Candida albicans,* and hepatitis viruses.

Nosocomial infections usually are transmitted by direct contact. Less often, they're transmitted by inhalation of or wound invasion by airborne organisms, or by contaminated equipment and solutions.

Despite hospital infection-control programs that include surveillance, prevention, and education, an estimated 2 million nosocomial infections occur each year, resulting in approximately 20,000 deaths. Since the 1980s, staphylococcal infections have been increasing, but fungal infections and infections caused by gram-negative bacilli have been steadily decreasing.

Nosocomial infections continue to pose a problem because most hospital patients are older and more debilitated than in the past. The advances in treatment that increase longevity in patients with diseases that alter immune defenses also create a population at high risk for infection. Moreover, the growing use of invasive and surgical procedures, immunosuppressants, and antibiotics predisposes patients to infection and su-

REPORTABLE INFECTIOUS DISEASES

Most states require that certain diseases be reported to local public health authorities. Such reports should include the patient's name, address, age, race, and sex, along with the disease or suspected disease and the means of exposure, if known.

Reportable diseases vary from state to state but may include acute respiratory viral diseases, anthrax, botulism, brucellosis, chancroid, cholera, congenital rubella syndrome, diphtheria, epidemic neonatal diarrhea, gonorrhea, hepatitis (A and B), histoplasmosis, human immunodeficiency virus infection, inclusion conjunctivitis, infectious encephalitis, influenza, keratoconjunctivitis, legionellosis, leprosy, leptospirosis, listeriosis, Lyme disease, malaria, meningococcal meningitis, meningococcemia, mumps, paratyphoid fever, pertussis, plague, poliomyelitis, psittacosis, pulmonary and extrapulmonary tuberculosis, Q fever, rabies, rat-bite fever, relapsing fever, rubella, rubeola, scabies, shigellosis, smallpox, syphilis, tetanus, toxic shock syndrome, trichinosis, typhoid fever, typhus, and yersiniosis.

Some states also require reporting of actinomycosis, amebiasis, lymphocytic choriomeningitis, coccidioidomycosis, acute bacterial conjunctivitis and epidemic hemorrhagic conjunctivitis, granuloma inguinale, hemorrhagic jaundice, impetigo, lymphogranuloma venereum, pediculosis, bacterial and mycoplasmal pneumonia, ringworm, Rocky Mountain spotted fever, staphylococcal infections, streptococcal infections, trachoma, and tularemia.

perinfection and helps create new strains of antibiotic-resistant bacteria. The growing number of personnel that come in contact with each patient increases the risk of exposure.

Preventive measures

Here's how you can help prevent nosocomial infections:
• Follow strict infection-control procedures.
• Document hospital infections as they occur.
• Identify outbreaks early, and take steps to prevent their spread.
• Eliminate unnecessary procedures that contribute to infection.
• Strictly follow necessary isolation techniques. (See *Isolation precautions*, pages 99 and 100.)
• Observe *all* patients for signs of infection, especially patients who are at high risk for infection.

IMMUNIZATION SCHEDULE

Childhood immunizations for normal infants and children usually are given on a fixed schedule. Before each scheduled immunization, ask the parents about the child's health history. Also obtain the child's history of allergies.

After immunization, tell the parents to report a severe reaction, especially to the first dose of pertussis vaccine. Give them an immunization record.

Note: Three Haemophilus b conjugate (HbCV) vaccines are available (only two are licensed for use in children as young as 2 months). In children age 15 months or less, the same vaccine brand and dose should be given for each scheduled dose. Recommended conjugate vaccines include:

• diphtheria CRM_{197} protein conjugate, sometimes called HbOC (HibTITER)
• meningococcal protein conjugate, sometimes called PRP-OMP (PedvaxHIB)
• diphtheria toxoid conjugate, also known as PRP-D (ProHIBit).

Keep in mind that oral polio vaccine (OPV) and diphtheria and tetanus toxoids and pertussis vaccine (DTP) normally are given at age 18 months; however, they may be administered at 15 months instead.

Measles-mumps-rubella (MMR) usually is given at age 15 months, with a booster when the child enters school at age 4 to 6. When the risk of disease is high (as in a local outbreak), children as young as age 1 may be vaccinated. These children should also be vaccinated at age 15 months and on entry into school.

Hepatitis B virus (HBV) is also a recommended universal childhood immunization, with the first dose soon after birth, the second dose between ages 1 and 2 months, and the third dose between 6 and 18 months (or, alternatively, between ages 1 and 2 months, at 4 months, and between 6 and 18 months).

The following chart shows a typical schedule.

Age	Immunization
Birth	HBV
2 months	First dose: DTP; trivalent OPV; HbCV; HbOC or PRP-OMP; second dose: HBV
4 months	Second dose: DTP, OPV, HbCV, and HbOC or PRP-OMP
6 months	Third dose: DTP, OPV (optional), HbCV, HbOC, and HBV
12 months	Tuberculin test and PRP-OMP
15 months	HbOC or PRP-D
18 months	OPV and HbCV
4 to 6 years	DTP, OPV, MMR, and tetanus toxoid
11 to 12 years	MMR, if not received by school entry age
Every 10 years	Tetanus and diphtheria toxoids only

• Follow good hand-washing techniques, and encourage other staff members to do the same.
• Keep staff members and visitors with obvious infection, as well as known carriers, away from susceptible patients.

Universal precautions

Because a medical history and a physical examination can't reliably identify all patients infected with human immunodeficiency virus (HIV) or other blood-borne pathogens, the Centers for Disease Control and Prevention (CDC) replaced its 1983 blood and body fluid precautions with new guidelines. These guidelines, published in 1987, recommend that universal blood and body fluid precautions be used in the care of *all* patients—not just those with known or suspected blood-borne infection. Further isolation precautions should be used as necessary if associated conditions, such as infectious diarrhea or tuberculosis, are diagnosed or suspected.

Specific guidelines

Because blood is the single most important source of HIV, hepatitis B virus (HBV), and other pathogens, universal precautions apply to blood and to other body fluids that contain visible blood. Universal precautions also apply to seminal, vaginal, cerebrospinal, synovial, pleural, peritoneal, pericardial, and amniotic fluids as well as to body tissue.

Universal precautions don't apply to feces, nasal secretions, sputum, sweat, tears, urine, and vomitus (unless they contain visible blood). Nor do they apply to saliva. General infection-control practices already in existence—including the use of gloves for digital examination of mucous membranes and endotracheal

ISOLATION PRECAUTIONS

To prevent the transmission of infectious diseases, the Centers for Disease Control (CDC) has published recommendations for two systems of hospital isolation precautions. The *disease-specific* isolation system stipulates the precautions needed to prevent transmission of a certain disease. The *category-specific* isolation system, covered below, describes six of the seven categories of isolation according to major modes of transmission.

The seventh category, universal precautions, replaces the blood and body fluid precautions published by the CDC in 1983. It's been expanded to cover *all* patients not just those with known or suspected blood-borne diseases. Because of the special concern over the risk of transmitting human immunodeficiency virus, this category is covered separately and in greater detail.

Type of isolation and diseases requiring isolation	Private room	Mask	Gown	Gloves	Special handling of waste or contaminated articles
Strict isolation Prevents transmission of contagious or virulent infections by air or contact. The patient may require a room with special ventilation. *Diseases:* Pharyngeal diphtheria, viral hemorrhagic fevers, pneumonic plague, smallpox, varicella-zoster virus (localized in immunocompromised patient or disseminated)	X with door closed	X	X	X	X
Contact isolation Aims to prevent transmission of epidemiologically important infections that don't require strict isolation. Health care workers should wear masks, gowns, and gloves for direct or close contact, although these guidelines may vary, depending on the infection. *Diseases in any age group:* Group A streptococcal endometritis; impetigo; pediculosis; *Staphylococcus aureus* or *Streptococcus pneumoniae* infection; rabies; rubella; scabies; staphylococcal scalded skin syndrome; major skin, wound, or burn infection (draining and not adequately covered by dressing); vaccinia; primary disseminated herpes simplex; cutaneous diphtheria; and infection or colonization with various bacteria that resist antibiotic therapy *Diseases in infants and young children:* Acute respiratory infections, influenza, infectious pharyngitis, viral pneumonia, group A streptococcal infection *Diseases in neonates:* Gonococcal conjunctivitis, staphylococcal furunculosis, neonatal disseminated herpes simplex	X	0	⊗	⊗	X
Respiratory isolation Aims to prevent transmission of infections spread primarily through the air by droplets. *Diseases: Haemophilus influenzae* epiglottitis, erythema infectiosum, measles, *H. influenzae* or meningococcal meningitis, meningococcal pneumonia, meningococcemia, mumps, pertussis, *H. influenzae* pneumonia in children	X with door closed	0	—	—	X
Acid-fast bacillus isolation Aims to prevent a patient with active pulmonary or laryngeal tuberculosis from transmitting the acid-fast bacillus to other patients. Place the patient in a room with special ventilation. *Disease:* Tuberculosis	X with door closed	0	⊗	—	X

(continued)

ISOLATION PRECAUTIONS *(continued)*

Type of isolation and diseases requiring isolation	Private room	Mask	Gown	Gloves	Special handling of waste or contaminated articles
Enteric precautions Attempt to prevent transmission of infection through direct or indirect contact with feces. *Diseases:* Amebic dysentery; cholera; coxsackievirus disease; acute diarrhea with suspected infection; echovirus disease; encephalitis unless known not to be caused by enteroviruses; *Clostridium difficile* or *Staphylococcus* enterocolitis; enteroviral infection; gastroenteritis caused by *Campylobacter* species, *Cryptosporidium* species, *Dientamoeba fragilis, Escherichia coli, Giardia lamblia,* *Salmonella* species, *Shigella* species, *Vibrio parahaemolyticus,* viruses, or *Yersinia enterocolitica;* hand, foot, and mouth disease; hepatitis A; herpangina; necrotizing enterocolitis; pleurodynia; poliomyelitis; typhoid fever; viral pericarditis, viral myocarditis, or viral meningitis unless known not to be caused by enteroviruses	D	—	⊗	⊗	X
Drainage and secretion precautions Aims to prevent transmission of infection from direct or indirect contact with purulent material or drainage. *Diseases:* Conjunctivitis; minor or limited abscess; minor or limited burn, skin, wound, or pressure ulcer infection	—	—	⊗	⊗	X

Key   X = Always necessary
⊗ = Necessary if soiling of hands or clothing is likely
0 = Necessary for close contact or if patient is coughing and doesn't reliably cover mouth
D = Desirable but optional; necessary only if patient has poor hygiene
— = Unnecessary

suctioning, and hand washing after exposure to saliva—should further minimize the minute risk, if any, of salivary transmission of HIV and HBV.

Gloves are unnecessary when feeding a patient or wiping saliva from the patient's skin. However, special precautions are recommended for dentistry.

Routine precautions
Follow these CDC guidelines when providing patient care:
• Use appropriate barrier precautions to prevent skin and mucous membrane exposure whenever you anticipate contact with the blood or other body fluids of any patient. Wear gloves for touching blood and body fluids, mucous membranes, or nonintact skin of all patients; for handling items or surfaces soiled with blood

or body fluids; and for performing venipuncture and other vascular access procedures. Change your gloves after contact with each patient.
• To prevent exposure of mucous membranes of the mouth, nose, and eyes, wear a mask and protective eyewear or a face shield during procedures that are likely to generate droplets of blood or other body fluids. Wear a gown or an apron during procedures that are likely to generate splashes of blood or other body fluids.
• Wash your hands and other skin surfaces immediately and thoroughly if they become contaminated with blood or other body fluids. Also wash your hands immediately after removing gloves.
• Take precautions to prevent injuries from needles, scalpels, and other sharp instruments or devices dur-

ing procedures. Be careful when cleaning used instruments, disposing of used needles, and handling sharp instruments after procedures.

To prevent needle-stick injuries, don't recap needles, bend or break them by hand, or remove them from disposable syringes. After use, place disposable syringes and needles, scalpel blades, and other sharp items in puncture-resistant containers for disposal. Keep such containers nearby. Place large-bore, reusable needles in a puncture-resistant container for transport to the reprocessing area.
• Although saliva hasn't been implicated in HIV transmission, make sure you keep mouthpieces, resuscitation bags, or other ventilation devices readily available to minimize the need for emergency mouth-to-mouth resuscitation.
• If you have exudative lesions or weeping dermatitis, avoid providing direct patient care or handling patient care equipment until the condition completely resolves.

Precautions for invasive procedures
According to the CDC, invasive procedures include the following:
• surgical entry into tissues, cavities, or organs, and repair of major traumatic injuries in an operating or delivery room, emergency department, or outpatient setting (including a dentist's office)
• cardiac catheterization and angiography
• vaginal and cesarean delivery as well as other invasive obstetric procedures during which bleeding may occur
• manipulation, cutting, or removal of any oral or perioral tissues, including tooth structures, during which bleeding may occur.

For invasive procedures, follow these additional precautions:
• Use barrier precautions with all patients. Always wear gloves and a surgical mask. If a procedure may result in blood or body fluids splashing or bone chips flying, also wear an apron or a gown and protective eyewear or a face shield.
• Wear gloves and a gown when handling the placenta or an infant during vaginal or cesarean delivery until blood and amniotic fluid have been removed from the infant's skin. Wear gloves while caring for the umbilical cord after delivery.
• If your glove tears, remove the old glove and put on a new one as quickly as possible.

Need for accurate assessment
Accurate assessment helps identify infectious diseases and prevents avoidable complications. Complete assessment consists of a patient history, a physical examination, and diagnostic tests.

The history should include the patient's sex, age, address, occupation, and place of work; known exposure to infection; and date of disease onset. It also should detail information about recent hospitalization, blood transfusions, blood donation denial by the Red Cross or other agencies, vaccination, travel or camping trips, and exposure to animals.

If applicable, ask the patient about possible exposure to sexually transmitted diseases and about drug abuse. Also ask him about his usual dietary patterns, unusual fatigue, and factors that may predispose the patient to infection, such as neoplastic disease and alcoholism. Notice if the patient is listless or uneasy, lacks concentration, or has any obvious abnormality of mood or affect.

In suspected infection, a physical examination includes assessment of the skin, mucous membranes, liver, spleen, and lymph nodes. Check for and note the location and type of drainage from skin lesions. Record skin color, temperature, and turgor; ask if the patient has pruritus. Take his temperature, using the same route consistently, and watch for a fever, the best indicator of many infections. Note and record the pattern of temperature change and the effect of antipyretics. Be aware that certain analgesics may contain antipyretics. In a high fever, especially in children, watch for seizures.

Check the patient's pulse rate. Infection commonly increases the pulse rate, but some infections, such as typhoid fever, may decrease it. In severe infection or when complications are possible, monitor the patient for hypotension, hematuria, oliguria, hepatomegaly, jaundice, palpable and painful lymph nodes, bleeding from gums or into joints, and altered level of consciousness. Obtain diagnostic tests and appropriate cultures, as ordered.

GRAM-POSITIVE COCCI

Although most gram-positive cocci cause organ-specific disorders, *Staphylococcus aureus* and group A beta-hemolytic streptococci cause systemic disorders.

GUIDELINES FOR DIAGNOSING TOXIC SHOCK SYNDROME

According to the Centers for Disease Control, a diagnosis of toxic shock syndrome can't be made unless a physical assessment and diagnostic tests reveal at least three of the following:
• GI effects, including vomiting and profuse diarrhea
• muscular effects, with severe myalgia or a fivefold or greater increase in serum creatine phosphokinase levels
• mucous membrane effects, such as frank hyperemia
• renal involvement, with blood urea nitrogen or serum creatinine levels at least double the norm
• hepatocellular damage, with levels of serum bilirubin, alanine aminotransferase (formerly SGPT), and aspartate aminotransferase (formerly SGOT) at least double the norm
• blood involvement, with signs of thrombocytopenia and a platelet count of less than 100,000/mm^3
• central nervous system effects, such as disorientation without focal signs.

TOXIC SHOCK SYNDROME

An acute bacterial infection, toxic shock syndrome most commonly is associated with continuous use of tampons, especially the superabsorbent type, during menstruation. Of the reported cases, 96% involve women, and 92% of these cases begin during menstruation. The incidence of this infection continues to rise, and the recurrence rate is about 30%. Most patients recover fully.

Causes
Toxic shock syndrome is caused by penicillin-resistant *S. aureus*. Although tampons are clearly implicated in this infection, their exact role is uncertain. They may contribute to the infection by:
• introducing *S. aureus* into the vagina during insertion
• absorbing toxin from the vagina
• traumatizing the vaginal mucosa during insertion, thus leading to infection
• providing a favorable environment for growth of *S. aureus*.

When toxic shock syndrome is unrelated to menstruation, it seems to be linked to *S. aureus* infections, such as abscesses, osteomyelitis, and postoperative infections.

Complications
Toxic shock syndrome can lead to persistent neurologic and psychological abnormalities, renal failure, rash, dehydration, and peripheral cyanosis.

Assessment findings
The patient commonly reports that she consistently uses tampons—especially the superabsorbent type—throughout menstruation and changes tampons infrequently. She may complain of intense myalgia, vomiting, diarrhea, and headache. Her temperature may be over 104° F (40° C).

Inspection may reveal rigors, conjunctival hyperemia, vaginal hyperemia, and vaginal discharge. A deep red rash also may develop, especially on the palms and soles. The rash appears within a few hours of the onset of infection and later desquamates. The patient may seem listless and confused.

Palpation may disclose signs of shock—a rapid, thready pulse and hypotension.

Diagnostic tests
Isolation of *S. aureus* from vaginal discharge or lesions helps support the diagnosis, but a confirmed diagnosis must follow the criteria set by the Centers for Disease Control. (See *Guidelines for diagnosing toxic shock syndrome.*) Negative results on blood tests for Rocky Mountain spotted fever, leptospirosis, and measles help rule out these disorders.

Treatment
Appropriate treatment may consist of I.V. antistaphylococcal antibiotics that are beta-lactamase–resistant, such as oxacillin, nafcillin, and methicillin. To reverse shock, the patient will need fluid replacement with saline solution and colloids. Other measures may include supportive treatment for diarrhea, nausea, and vomiting.

Nursing diagnoses
• Altered thought processes
• Diarrhea
• Fluid volume deficit
• Hyperthermia
• Pain

Nursing interventions
• Frequently monitor the patient's vital signs.
• Administer I.V. antibiotics over a 15-minute period to ensure peak levels that destroy microorganisms. Watch for signs of penicillin allergy.

• Check the patient's fluid and electrolyte balance. Replace fluids I.V., as ordered.
• Monitor intake, output, and weight daily to assess fluid balance and to prevent dehydration and renal failure.
• Obtain specimens of vaginal and cervical secretions for culture of *S. aureus.*
• Check neurologic vital signs every 4 to 8 hours. Reorient the patient as needed. Use appropriate safety measures to prevent injury.
• Use universal precautions for any vaginal discharge and lesion drainage.
• Administer analgesics cautiously because of the risk of hypotension and liver failure.

Patient teaching
• Advise the patient to avoid using tampons, particularly the superabsorbent type, because of the risk of recurrence.

SCARLET FEVER
Although scarlet fever (scarlatina) usually follows streptococcal pharyngitis, this disorder also may follow other streptococcal infections, such as wound infections, urosepsis, and puerperal sepsis. It's most common in children ages 3 to 15. The incubation period commonly lasts from 2 to 4 days but may be only 1 day or extend to 7 days.

Causes
Group A beta-hemolytic streptococci cause scarlet fever. The infecting strain produces one of three erythrogenic toxins, which triggers a sensitivity reaction in the patient.

Complications
This disorder can lead to severe disseminated toxic illness, septicemia, rheumatic heart disease, and liver damage.

Assessment findings
The patient may report a sore throat, headache, chills, anorexia, abdominal pain, and malaise. He's likely to have a temperature of 100° to 103° F (37.8° to 39.4° C). In addition, he commonly has had contact with a person with a sore throat.

Inspection of the patient's mouth initially shows an inflamed and heavily coated tongue. As the disease progresses, you'll note a strawberry-like tongue. As it progresses further, the tongue begins to peel and becomes beefy red. It returns to normal by the end of the second week. The uvula, tonsils, and posterior oropharynx appear red and edematous, with mucopurulent exudate.

Inspection of the skin may reveal a fine, erythematous rash that appears first on the upper chest and back. It later spreads to the neck, abdomen, legs, and arms but doesn't appear on the soles and palms. The rash resembles sunburn with goosebumps and blanches when you apply pressure. The patient's face appears flushed, except around the mouth, which remains pale. During convalescence, the skin sheds.

The cervical lymph nodes feel enlarged and tender on palpation. The liver also may feel slightly enlarged and tender, and you may note tachycardia.

Diagnostic tests
A pharyngeal culture is positive for group A beta-hemolytic streptococci. A complete blood count reveals granulocytosis and, possibly, a reduced red blood cell count.

Treatment
Antibiotic therapy with penicillin or erythromycin is administered for 10 days, along with antipyretics.

Nursing diagnoses
• Activity intolerance
• Altered oral mucous membrane
• High risk for infection
• Hyperthermia
• Impaired skin integrity
• Pain

Nursing interventions
• Implement respiratory secretion precautions for 24 hours after starting antibiotic therapy.
• Keep the patient on complete bed rest while he's febrile to prevent complications, promote recovery, and help conserve his energy.
• Offer frequent oral fluids and oral hygiene, and administer antipyretics, as ordered.
• Apply topical anesthetics on the patient's tongue and throat to relieve pain.
• Provide skin care to relieve discomfort from the rash.

Patient teaching
• Instruct the patient (or his parents) to make sure he takes his oral antibiotics for the prescribed length of time.

GRAM-NEGATIVE COCCI

Most gram-negative organisms cause organ-specific disorders. *Neisseria gonorrhoeae,* however, causes gonorrhea—a disorder that can become systemic.

GONORRHEA

A common venereal disease, gonorrhea usually starts as an infection of the genitourinary tract, especially the urethra and cervix. It also can begin in the rectum, pharynx, or eyes. Left untreated, gonorrhea spreads through the blood to the joints, tendons, meninges, and endocardium; in women, it also can lead to chronic pelvic inflammatory disease (PID) and sterility.

Gonorrhea is especially prevalent among people between the ages of 15 and 29, with the highest incidence occurring between ages 20 and 24. It's also prevalent in people with multiple partners. With adequate treatment, the prognosis is excellent, although reinfection is common.

Causes

Transmission of *N. gonorrhoeae,* the organism that causes gonorrhea, occurs almost exclusively through sexual contact with an infected person. A child born of an infected mother, however, can contract gonococcal ophthalmia neonatorum during passage through the birth canal. Also, a person with gonorrhea can contract gonococcal conjunctivitis by touching his eyes with a contaminated hand.

Complications

Gonorrhea can lead to PID, acute epididymitis, septic arthritis, dermatitis, and perihepatitis. Severe gonococcal conjunctivitis can lead to corneal ulceration and, possibly, blindness. Rare complications include meningitis, osteomyelitis, pneumonia, and adult respiratory distress syndrome.

Assessment findings

The patient may report unprotected sexual contact (vaginal, oral, or anal) with an infected person, an unknown partner, or multiple sex partners. He also may have a history of sexually transmitted disease.

After a 3- to 6-day incubation period, a male patient may complain of dysuria, although both sexes can remain asymptomatic. A patient with a rectal infection may complain of anal itching, burning, and tenesmus and pain with defecation, or he may be asymptomatic. A patient with a pharyngeal infection may be asymptomatic or may complain of a sore throat.

Assessment of a patient with gonorrhea reveals a low-grade fever. If the disease has become systemic, or if the patient has developed PID or acute epididymitis, the fever is higher. Other assessment findings vary with the infection site.

Inspection of the male patient's urethral meatus reveals a purulent discharge; such discharge may be expressed from a female patient's urethra, and her meatus may appear red and edematous. Inspection of the cervix with a speculum discloses a greenish yellow discharge, the most common sign in females. Vaginal inspection reveals engorgement, redness, swelling, and a profuse purulent discharge. (The vagina is the most common infection site in female children over age 1.)

If the patient has a rectal infection, inspection may reveal a purulent discharge or rectal bleeding. In an ocular infection, inspection may reveal a purulent discharge from the conjunctiva; in a pharyngeal infection, inspection may reveal redness and a purulent discharge.

If the infection has become systemic, papillary skin lesions—possibly pustular, hemorrhagic, or necrotic—may appear on the hands and feet.

Palpation of the patient with PID reveals tenderness over the lower quadrant, abdominal rigidity and distention, and adnexal tenderness (usually bilateral). In a patient with perihepatitis, palpation discloses right upper quadrant tenderness.

Your assessment of a patient with a systemic infection may reveal pain and a cracking noise when moving an involved joint. Asymmetrical involvement of only a few joints—typically the knees, ankles, and elbows—may differentiate gonococcal arthritis from other forms of arthritis.

Diagnostic tests

A culture from the infection site (the urethra, cervix, rectum, or pharynx), grown on a Thayer-Martin medium, usually establishes the diagnosis. A culture of conjunctival scrapings confirms gonococcal conjunctivitis. In a male patient, a Gram stain that shows gram-negative diplococci may confirm gonorrhea.

Diagnosis of gonococcal arthritis requires identification of gram-negative diplococci on smears made from joint fluid and skin lesions. Complement fixation and immunofluorescent assays of serum reveal antibody titers four times the normal rate.

Treatment

For uncomplicated gonorrhea in adults, the recommended treatment is 250 mg of ceftriaxone given I.M. in a single dose plus 100 mg of doxycycline hyclate given twice a day by mouth for 7 days. As an alternative to the doxycycline—which helps combat gonorrhea and also treats the frequently coexisting chlamydial or mycoplasmal infection—the patient can receive 500 mg of oral tetracycline four times a day for 7 days. For patients who can't take doxycycline or tetracycline, such as pregnant women, treatment consists of 500 mg of oral erythromycin for 7 days.

If the infection was acquired from a person proven to have susceptible nonpenicillinase-producing gonorrhea, the patient can receive 1 g of probenecid by mouth (to block penicillin excretion) plus either 3.5 g of ampicillin by mouth in a single dose or 3 g of amoxicillin by mouth in a single dose. This is followed by a 7-day course of doxycycline or tetracycline.

Disseminated gonococcal infection requires 1 g of ceftriaxone given I.M. or I.V. every 24 hours for 7 days. Adult gonococcal ophthalmia requires 1 g of ceftriaxone given I.M. in a single dose.

Because many strains of antibiotic-resistant gonococci exist, follow-up cultures are necessary 4 to 7 days after treatment and again in 6 months. (For a pregnant patient, final follow-up must occur before delivery.)

Routine instillation of 1% silver nitrate drops or erythromycin ointment into the eyes of neonates has greatly reduced the incidence of gonococcal ophthalmia neonatorum.

Nursing diagnoses

• Altered sexuality patterns
• Knowledge deficit
• Pain
• Risk for infection

Nursing interventions

• Before treatment, determine if the patient has any drug sensitivities. During treatment, watch closely for signs of a drug reaction.
• Use universal precautions when obtaining specimens for laboratory examination and when caring for the patient. Carefully place all soiled articles in containers, and dispose of them according to hospital policy.
• Monitor the patient for complications.
• Isolate the patient with an eye infection.

• If the patient has gonococcal arthritis, apply moist heat to ease pain in affected joints. Administer analgesics, as ordered.
• If the doctor or laboratory hasn't already done so, report all cases of gonorrhea to the local public health authorities so that they can follow up with the patient's sexual partners. Examine and test all people exposed to gonorrhea.
• Report all cases of gonorrhea in children to child abuse authorities.
• Routinely instill prophylactic medications, according to hospital protocol, in the eyes of all neonates on admission to the nursery. Check the neonate of an infected mother for any signs of infection. Take specimens for culture from his eyes, pharynx, and rectum.

Patient teaching

• Urge the patient to inform all sexual partners of the infection so that they can seek treatment.
• Tell the patient to avoid sexual contact until cultures prove negative and infection is eradicated.
• Advise the partner of an infected person to receive treatment even if the partner doesn't have a positive culture. Recommend that the partner avoid sexual contact with anyone until treatment is complete because reinfection is extremely common.
• Counsel the patient and all sexual partners to be tested for human immunodeficiency virus and hepatitis B infection.
• Instruct the patient to be careful when coming into contact with any bodily discharges to avoid contaminating the eyes.
• Tell the patient to take anti-infective drugs for the length of time prescribed.
• To prevent reinfection, tell the patient to avoid sexual contact with anyone *suspected* of being infected, to use condoms during intercourse, to wash genitalia with soap and water before and after intercourse, and to avoid sharing washcloths or douche equipment.
• Advise returning for follow-up testing.

GRAM-POSITIVE BACILLI

These bacilli produce a violet color, using a Gram stain. Examples of infections caused by gram-positive bacilli include diphtheria, listeriosis, tetanus, botulism, gas gangrene, actinomycosis, and nocardiosis.

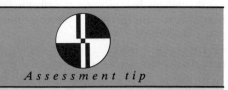

Assessment tip

DISTINGUISHING DIPHTHERIA FROM SIMILAR DISORDERS

When assessing a patient for diphtheria, you can rule out similar disorders by keeping in mind the distinguishing characteristics of each disorder.
• To distinguish diphtheria from mononucleosis, remember that in diphtheria, a pseudomembrane forms over oral and nasal mucous membranes. Attempts to remove this membrane usually cause bleeding—a characteristic that distinguishes diphtheria from mononucleosis. The membrane produced by mononucleosis doesn't cause bleeding when removed.
• To distinguish diphtheria from streptococcal pharyngitis, note the intensity and onset of symptoms. Streptococcal pharyngitis usually produces a more intense local reaction, a higher fever, and more severe dysphagia.
• To differentiate diphtheria from bacterial epiglottitis, remember that the latter disorder typically develops more acutely. Also, indirect laryngoscopy shows an extremely reddened epiglottis without the membrane typical of diphtheria.

DIPHTHERIA

An acute, highly contagious, toxin-mediated infection, diphtheria usually infects the respiratory tract, primarily involving the tonsils, nasopharynx, and larynx. Cutaneous, stool, and wound diphtheria are the most common types in the United States, often resulting from nontoxigenic strains. The GI and urinary tracts, conjunctivae, and ears seldom are involved.

Thanks to effective immunization, diphtheria has become rare in many parts of the world, including the United States. Since 1972, however, the incidence of cutaneous diphtheria has increased, especially in the Pacific Northwest and the Southwest. It's particularly likely to strike in areas where crowding and poor hygienic conditions prevail. Most victims are children under age 15. Mortality from diphtheria is up to 10%.

Causes

Diphtheria is caused by *Corynebacterium diphtheriae,* a gram-positive rod. Transmission usually occurs through intimate contact or by airborne respiratory droplets from apparently healthy carriers or convalesc-ing patients. Many more people carry this disease than contract active infection.

Diphtheria is more prevalent during the colder months because of closer person-to-person contact indoors, but it can be contracted at any time of the year.

Complications

The extensive pseudomembrane formation and swelling that occur during the first few days of the disease may cause respiratory obstruction. Other complications include myocarditis, polyneuritis (primarily affecting motor fibers but possibly also sensory neurons), encephalitis, cerebral infarction, bacteremia, renal failure, pulmonary emboli, and bronchopneumonia caused by *C. diphtheriae* or other superinfecting organisms. Serum sickness may result from antitoxin therapy.

Assessment findings

The patient's history may show inadequate immunization and an exposure period of less than 1 week. The patient may complain of a sore throat (the most common complaint in adults) and dysphagia; a child is more likely to complain of nausea and vomiting. The patient also may complain of chills, a rasping cough, and hoarseness and may have a temperature of 100° to 102° F (37.8° to 38.9° C).

Inspection may reveal a characteristic thick, patchy grayish green membrane over the mucous membranes of the pharynx, larynx, tonsils, soft palate, and nose.

If the patient develops respiratory obstruction, inspection will reveal stridor, suprasternal and substernal retraction and, possibly, cyanosis, restlessness, and tachypnea. In cutaneous diphtheria, you'll note skin lesions that resemble impetigo.

During palpation, you may note enlarged cervical lymph nodes. If the patient has an obstructed airway, auscultation may disclose diminished breath sounds. (See *Distinguishing diphtheria from similar disorders.*)

Your assessment may reveal palatal and pharyngeal paralysis, ocular or ciliary paralysis, progressive muscle weakness, and paresthesia in neurologic involvement. You may observe signs of peripheral neuritis 2 to 3 months after the onset of illness.

Diagnostic tests

Culture of throat swabs or of specimens taken from suspicious lesions that show *C. diphtheriae* confirms the diagnosis. Electrocardiogram (ECG) abnormalities may indicate myocardium involvement.

Treatment

Initial therapy is based on clinical findings and does not wait for a confirmed diagnosis based on culture. Standard treatment includes diphtheria antitoxin administered by I.M. or I.V. infusion. Antibiotics, such as penicillin and erythromycin, eliminate organisms from the upper respiratory tract and elsewhere so that the patient doesn't remain a carrier. Other measures are taken to prevent complications (for example, airway maintenance to prevent possible suffocation).

Nursing diagnoses

- Altered nutrition: Less than body requirements
- Impaired skin integrity
- Ineffective airway clearance
- Ineffective breathing pattern
- Risk for fluid volume deficit
- Risk for infection
- Risk for injury
- Sensory or perceptual alterations

Nursing interventions

- Obtain cultures, as ordered.
- Assess respiratory effort and status. Report stridor, alterations in level of consciousness or oxygen saturation, and cyanosis.
- Administer humidified oxygen, as ordered, and elevate the head of the bed to prevent pressure on the diaphragm and compromised breathing.
- Keep an emergency cricothyrotomy set available in case airway obstruction occurs.
- Offer frequent, small feedings of liquids and soft foods to a patient with mild to moderate dysphagia. Administer parenteral fluids, as ordered, for a patient who can't swallow.
- Administer drugs as ordered. Before giving diphtheria antitoxin, which is made from horse serum, obtain eye and skin tests to determine sensitivity. Although time-consuming and hazardous, desensitization should be attempted if tests are positive because diphtheria antitoxin is the only *specific* treatment available. If sensitivity tests are negative, the antitoxin is given before laboratory confirmation of the diagnosis because mortality increases when antitoxin administration is delayed.
- After giving antitoxin or penicillin, be alert for anaphylaxis. (See *Diphtheria hazards.*) In patients who receive erythromycin, watch for thrombophlebitis.
- Maintain infection and strict isolation precautions until two consecutive negative nasopharyngeal cul-

Warning

DIPHTHERIA HAZARDS

When caring for a patient with diphtheria, be alert for these potentially life-threatening hazards:
- After giving antitoxin, penicillin, or both, monitor for signs of anaphylaxis, and keep epinephrine 1:1,000 and resuscitative equipment handy.
- In a patient who receives erythromycin, watch for thrombophlebitis.
- Assess for symptoms of airway obstruction. Have a tracheostomy tray available.
- Watch for signs of shock, which can develop suddenly as a result of systemic vascular collapse, airway obstruction, or anaphylaxis.
- Be alert for signs of myocarditis, such as a sudden decrease in pulse rate, an irregular heartbeat, and pallor. Also be alert for heart murmurs and ECG changes. Ventricular fibrillation is a common cause of sudden death in diphtheria patients. Be prepared to intervene immediately.

tures are obtained — at least 1 week after drug therapy stops.
- Report all cases of diphtheria to local public health authorities; follow up on others who have been exposed to the patient, if appropriate.
- If paralysis occurs, assist the patient in a rehabilitation program to restore optimal functioning.

Patient teaching

- Teach the patient proper disposal of nasopharyngeal secretions.
- Explain the need for follow-up testing. Advise the patient to expect a prolonged convalescent period.
- Treatment of exposed individuals with antitoxin remains controversial. Suggest that the patient's family members later receive diphtheria toxoid (usually given as combined diphtheria and tetanus toxoids or as a combination including pertussis vaccine for children under age 6) if they haven't been immunized.
- Stress the need for childhood immunizations to all parents.

LISTERIOSIS

Caused by the weakly hemolytic, gram-positive bacillus *Listeria monocytogenes*, listeriosis most often occurs in fetuses, in neonates during the first 3 weeks of life, and in older or immunosuppressed adults. The infected fetus usually is stillborn or born prematurely, almost always with lethal listeriosis. This infection produces a milder illness in pregnant women and varying degrees of illness in older or immunosuppressed patients. The prognosis depends on the severity of the underlying disease.

Causes
The primary method of transmission in neonatal infection is through the placenta in utero or during passage through an infected birth canal. Other modes of transmission include inhaling contaminated dust; drinking contaminated, unpasteurized milk; coming in contact with infected animals, contaminated sewage or mud, or soil contaminated with feces containing *L. monocytogenes*; and, possibly, person-to-person transmission.

Complications
Listeriosis can cause sepsis, diffuse clotting dyscrasias, respiratory insufficiency, circulatory insufficiency, meningitis, cerebritis, granulomatous skin infections, and nonpurulent conjunctivitis.

Assessment findings
The patient's history may be unremarkable, although the patient may report eye or skin exposure to laboratory animals or to animals seen in veterinary practice. An infected pregnant woman—especially if she's in her third trimester—may complain of back pain and malaise. She also may have a fever. The parents of an infected infant may report that he seems acutely ill or simply weak.

Your assessment of an infected pregnant woman may reveal hypotension, although the rest of the assessment may be normal.

You may note that an infant appears acutely ill on inspection. He also may exhibit skin lesions on his trunk or extremities. These may appear as papules and may ulcerate. If he has developed meningitis, you may note irritability, lethargy, seizures, or coma. You'll seldom see fulminant manifestations with coma in an adult unless he develops *Listeria* sepsis.

In an infant, abscesses may make organ masses palpable; palpation also will disclose tense fontanels if the infant has meningitis.

Other assessment findings may include hypotension and vasodilation if the patient has developed sepsis, although these are less profound than in gram-negative

sepsis. You may note diffuse mottling, signs of coagulation abnormalities with septic emboli, and disseminated intravascular coagulation with *Listeria* sepsis.

Diagnostic tests
L. monocytogenes is identified by its tumbling motility on a wet mound of the culture. Other supportive diagnostic test results include positive culture of blood, spinal fluid, drainage from cervical or vaginal lesions, or lochia from a mother with an infected infant; however, isolation of the organism from these specimens often is difficult. The proportion of monocytes in the blood also will increase.

Treatment
The patient usually receives I.V. ampicillin or penicillin for 3 to 6 weeks, possibly with gentamicin to increase its effectiveness. Alternative treatments include erythromycin, chloramphenicol, tetracycline, and cotrimoxazole.

Ampicillin and penicillin G, with or without gentamycin, are best for treating meningitis caused by *L. monocytogenes* because they more easily cross the blood-brain barrier. Pregnant women require prompt, vigorous treatment to combat fetal infection.

Nursing diagnoses
• Altered thought processes
• Dysfunctional grieving
• Impaired skin integrity
• Ineffective family coping
• Risk for infection

Nursing interventions
• Promptly deliver specimens to the laboratory.
• Use secretion precautions until a series of cultures are negative. Take special care when handling lochia from an infected mother and secretions from her infant's eyes, nose, mouth, and rectum, including meconium.
• Use universal precautions when appropriate.
• Infuse I.V. penicillin (not aminoglycosides) over 15 minutes to ensure adequate blood levels.
• Monitor for signs of septic shock and disseminated intravascular coagulation.
• Evaluate neurologic status at least every 2 hours. In an infant, check fontanels for bulging. Maintain adequate I.V. fluid intake; accurately measure intake and output.
• Institute seizure precautions as needed.

• Provide psychological support for the parents of a critically ill neonate or a stillborn infant.

Patient teaching
• Teach the adult patient proper disposal of infectious material.

TETANUS

Also referred to as lockjaw, tetanus is an acute exotoxin-mediated infection caused by the anaerobic, spore-forming, gram-positive bacillus *Clostridium tetani*. The infection usually is systemic, but it may be localized. Tetanus is fatal in up to 60% of nonimmunized people, often within 10 days of onset. The disease's incubation period ranges from 3 to 4 weeks in mild tetanus to under 2 days in severe tetanus. When symptoms develop within 3 days of exposure, the prognosis is poor. In North America, about 75% of all cases occur between April and September.

Tetanus occurs worldwide, but it's more prevalent in agricultural regions and developing countries that lack mass immunization programs. It's one of the most common causes of neonatal deaths in developing countries, where infants of nonimmunized mothers are delivered under unsterile conditions. In such infants, the infection enters through the unhealed umbilical cord.

Once *C. tetani* enters the body, it causes local infection and tissue necrosis. It also produces toxins that enter the bloodstream and lymphatics and eventually spread to central nervous system tissue.

Causes
Transmission occurs through a puncture wound that is contaminated by soil, dust, or animal excreta containing *C. tetani*, or by way of burns or minor wounds.

Complications
Atelectasis, pneumonia, pulmonary emboli, airway obstruction, acute gastric ulcers, seizures, flexion contractures, and cardiac arrhythmias can result from tetanus.

Assessment findings
The patient's history may reveal inadequate immunization, and the patient may report a recent skin wound or burn. He may complain of pain or paresthesia at the site of injury and recall early complaints of difficulty chewing or swallowing food. He usually has a normal body temperature or a slight fever in the early stages, although his fever may rise as the disease progresses.

If the tetanus remains localized, your assessment may disclose signs of spasm and increased muscle tone near the wound.

If the tetanus becomes systemic, your assessment may reveal an irregular heartbeat, marked muscle hypertonicity, hyperactive deep tendon reflexes, tachycardia, profuse sweating, low-grade fever, and painful, involuntary muscle contractions. Specific findings may include:
• rigid neck and facial muscles (especially cheek muscles), resulting in lockjaw (trismus) and a grotesque, grinning expression called risus sardonicus
• rigid somatic muscles, causing arched-back rigidity (opisthotonos); palpation reveals boardlike abdominal rigidity
• intermittent tonic seizures that last for several minutes and may result in cyanosis and sudden death by asphyxiation.

Despite pronounced neuromuscular symptoms, assessment shows normal cerebral and sensory function.

Diagnostic tests
Blood cultures and tetanus antibody tests commonly are negative; only a third of patients have a positive wound culture. Cerebrospinal fluid pressure may rise above normal.

Treatment
Within 72 hours after a puncture wound, a patient with no previous history of tetanus immunization first requires tetanus immune globulin or tetanus antitoxin to confer temporary protection. Next, he needs active immunization with tetanus toxoid. A patient who has not received tetanus immunization within 5 years needs a booster injection of tetanus toxoid.

If tetanus develops despite immediate postinjury treatment, the patient will require airway maintenance and a muscle relaxant, such as diazepam, to decrease muscle rigidity and spasm. If muscle contractions aren't relieved by muscle relaxants, a neuromuscular blocker may be needed.

The patient with tetanus also requires high-dose antibiotics — preferably penicillin administered I.V. if he's not allergic to it. If he is allergic to penicillin, tetracycline can be substituted.

Nursing diagnoses
• Altered nutrition: Less than body requirements
• Altered urinary elimination
• Impaired physical mobility

- Ineffective airway clearance
- Ineffective breathing pattern
- Pain
- Risk for disuse syndrome
- Risk for injury
- Self-care deficit

Nursing interventions

- Before tetanus develops, thoroughly debride and clean the injury site with 3% hydrogen peroxide, and check the patient's immunization history. Record the cause of the injury. If it was caused by an animal bite, report the case to local public health authorities.
- Before giving penicillin and tetanus immune globulin, antitoxin, or toxoid, obtain an accurate history of the patient's allergies to immunizations or penicillin. If the patient has a history of any allergies, keep epinephrine 1:1,000 (for subcutaneous injection) and emergency airway equipment available.
- After tetanus develops, maintain an adequate airway and ventilation to prevent pneumonia and atelectasis. Suction as needed and watch for signs of respiratory distress.
- Keep emergency airway equipment on hand because the patient may require artificial ventilation or oxygen administration. Have endotracheal and tracheotomy equipment on hand. In an emergency, the doctor may perform a tracheotomy if the patient becomes extremely rigid.
- Administer I.V. therapy as prescribed. Monitor intake and output.
- Monitor the patient's electrocardiogram for arrhythmias frequently. Also check vital signs. Be prepared to resuscitate the patient and initiate life support.
- Because even minimal external stimulation provokes muscle spasms, keep the patient's room dark and quiet. Warn visitors not to upset or overly stimulate the patient.
- Turn the patient frequently to prevent contractures, pressure ulcers, and pulmonary stasis. Perform range-of-motion exercises to maintain flexibility.
- Perform all activities of daily living for the sedated patient.
- Give muscle relaxants and sedatives, as ordered, and schedule patient care to coincide with heaviest sedation.
- Check the patient's skin for signs of pressure ulcers. Place the patient on an air mattress, and use other skin protective measures, as warranted.
- If urine retention develops, insert an indwelling urinary catheter.

- Insert an artificial airway, if necessary, to prevent tongue injury, and maintain the airway during spasms.
- Provide adequate nutrition to meet the patient's increased metabolic needs. He may need nasogastric feedings or total parenteral nutrition.

Patient teaching

- During the patient's convalescence, encourage gradual active exercises.
- Institute a bladder retraining program if the patient was catheterized.
- Stress the importance of maintaining active immunization with a booster dose of tetanus toxoid every 10 years.
- Inform the patient with a skin injury or burn that he should receive tetanus prophylaxis.

BOTULISM

This life-threatening paralytic illness results from an exotoxin produced by the gram-positive, anaerobic bacillus *Clostridium botulinum*. It occurs as botulism food poisoning, wound botulism, and infant botulism.

Botulism occurs worldwide and affects adults more often than children. The incidence of botulism in the United States had been declining, but the current trend toward home canning has resulted in an upswing in recent years.

The mortality is about 25%, with death most often caused by respiratory failure during the first week of illness. Onset within 24 hours of ingestion signals critical and potentially fatal illness.

Causes

Botulism usually results from eating improperly preserved foods, such as home-canned fruits and vegetables, sausages, and smoked or preserved fish or meat. Rarely, it results from wound infection with *C. botulinum*.

Honey contaminated with *C. botulinum* spores is a common source of infection in infants. Findings have shown that an infant's GI tract can become colonized with *C. botulinum*, and then the exotoxin is produced within the infant's intestine. (See *Infant botulism*.)

Complications

Botulism can result in respiratory failure and paralytic ileus.

Assessment findings

The patient may report having eaten home-canned food 12 to 36 hours before the onset of symptoms.

The patient may complain of vertigo, dry mouth, sore throat, weakness, nausea, vomiting, constipation, and diarrhea. Concurrently or up to 3 days later, he may report diplopia, blurred vision, dysarthria, and dysphagia from cranial nerve impairment. Later, he may experience dyspnea from muscle weakness or paralysis. His body temperature will remain normal.

The patient may appear alert and oriented on inspection. Ocular signs may include ptosis and dilated, nonreactive pupils. Oral mucous membranes commonly appear dry, red, and crusted.

Palpation may reveal abdominal distention with absent bowel sounds.

Further assessment may disclose descending weakness or paralysis of muscles in the extremities or trunk—the major physical finding in botulism. The patient's deep tendon reflexes may be intact, diminished, or absent. He won't have pathologic reflexes or sensory impairment.

Diagnostic tests

Identification of the exotoxin in the patient's serum, stool, or gastric contents, or in the suspected food, confirms the diagnosis. An electromyogram showing diminished muscle action potential after a single supramaximal nerve stimulus also is diagnostic.

Diagnosis must rule out conditions often confused with botulism, such as Guillain-Barré syndrome, myasthenia gravis, cerebrovascular accident, staphylococcal food poisoning, tick paralysis, chemical intoxication, carbon monoxide poisoning, fish poisoning, trichinosis, and diphtheria.

Treatment

For adults, treatment consists of I.V. or I.M. administration of botulinum antitoxin (available through the Centers for Disease Control).

Early elective tracheotomy and ventilatory assistance can be lifesaving in respiratory failure. The patient will need nasogastric suctioning and total parenteral nutrition (TPN) if he develops significant paralytic ileus.

Nursing diagnoses

• Altered nutrition: Less than body requirements
• Altered oral mucous membrane
• Fear
• Impaired physical mobility

INFANT BOTULISM

Infant botulism, which usually afflicts children between 3 and 20 weeks old, is often associated with a history of honey ingestion. This disorder can produce floppy infant syndrome, which is characterized by constipation, a feeble cry, a depressed gag reflex, and an inability to suck. The infant also exhibits a flaccid facial expression, ptosis, and ophthalmoplegia—the result of cranial nerve deficits.

As the disease progresses, the infant develops generalized weakness, hypotonia, areflexia, and a sometimes striking loss of head control. Respiratory arrest occurs in almost half of affected infants.

Intensive supportive care allows most infants to recover completely. Antitoxin therapy isn't recommended because of the risk of anaphylaxis.

• Impaired swallowing
• Impaired verbal communication
• Ineffective airway clearance
• Ineffective breathing pattern
• Pain
• Self-care deficit
• Sensory alteration

Nursing interventions

• If you suspect the patient ate contaminated food, obtain a careful history of his food intake for the past several days. Determine if other family members exhibit similar symptoms and have eaten the same food.
• Observe the patient carefully for abnormal neurologic signs.
• If the patient ate the food within several hours, induce vomiting, begin gastric lavage, and give a high enema to purge any unabsorbed toxin from the bowel. Family members or friends who have eaten the same food also should receive this treatment.
• If clinical signs of botulism appear, have the patient admitted to the intensive care unit (isolation isn't required).
• Monitor cardiac and respiratory function carefully. Assess vital capacity frequently; report reduced vital capacity, reduced inspiratory effort, or respiratory distress.
• Before giving the antitoxin, obtain an accurate patient history of allergies, especially to horses, and perform a skin test. Then administer botulinum antitoxin, as ordered, to neutralize any circulating toxin. After-

EFFECTS OF *CLOSTRIDIUM PERFRINGENS*

As *C. perfringens* grows in a closed wound, it destroys cell walls and causes hemolysis, local tissue death, and increasing edema.

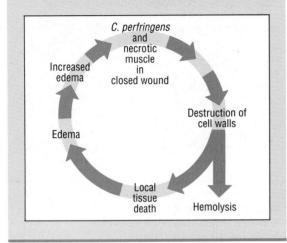

ward, watch for anaphylaxis or other hypersensitivity reactions as well as serum sickness. Keep epinephrine 1:1,000 (for subcutaneous administration) and emergency airway equipment available.

• Closely assess and record the patient's neurologic function, including bilateral motor status (reflexes and ability to move arms and legs). Check the patient's cough and gag reflexes, and suction as needed.

• If the patient has difficulty swallowing, initiate nasogastric tube feedings or TPN, as ordered.

• Administer I.V. fluids, as ordered. Monitor input and output.

• Turn the patient often, and encourage deep-breathing exercises. Position him in proper alignment, and assist with range-of-motion exercises.

• If the patient is on mechanical ventilation, monitor his arterial blood gas levels to detect signs of hyperventilation or hypoventilation.

• If the patient has difficulty speaking, try to anticipate his needs. Assure him that this symptom will pass, and establish an alternative method of communication.

• Because botulism sometimes is fatal, keep the patient and family informed about the course of the disease.

• Immediately report all cases of botulism to local public health authorities.

Patient teaching

• If ingestion of contaminated food is suspected but the patient returns home before neurologic symptoms occur, advise him and his family to watch for such signs as weakness, blurred vision, and slurred speech. Tell them to return the patient to the hospital immediately if such signs appear.

• To help prevent botulism in the future, encourage the patient and his family to use proper techniques in processing and preserving foods. Warn them to avoid even *tasting* food from a bulging can or one with a peculiar odor, and to sterilize by boiling any utensil that contacts suspected food. Explain that eating even a small amount of food contaminated with botulism toxin can prove fatal.

• Tell parents not to feed honey to their infants.

GAS GANGRENE

This rare condition is caused by local infection with the anaerobic, spore-forming, gram-positive, rod-shaped bacillus *Clostridium perfringens* or another clostridial species. It occurs in devitalized tissues and results from compromised arterial circulation after trauma or surgery. The usual incubation period is 1 to 4 days but can vary from 3 hours to 6 weeks or longer.

Gas gangrene carries a high mortality unless therapy begins immediately. With prompt treatment, 80% of patients with gas gangrene of the extremities survive; the prognosis is poorer for gas gangrene in other sites, such as the abdominal wall or the bowel.

Causes

The organism most often responsible, *C. perfringens,* is a normal inhabitant of the GI and female genitourinary tracts; it's also prevalent in soil. Transmission occurs when the organism enters the body during trauma or surgery.

Because *C. perfringens* is anaerobic, gas gangrene occurs most frequently in deep wounds, especially those in which tissue necrosis further reduces the oxygen supply. When *C. perfringens* invades soft tissues, it produces thrombosis of regional blood vessels, tissue necrosis, and localized edema. Such necrosis releases both carbon dioxide and hydrogen subcutaneously, producing interstitial gas bubbles.

Gas gangrene occurs most commonly in the extremities and in abdominal wounds, and less often in the uterus. (See *Effects of Clostridium perfringens.*)

Complications

Possible complications include renal failure, hypotension, shock, hemolytic anemia, and tissue death, requiring amputation of the affected body part.

Assessment findings

The patient's medical history may reveal recent surgery (within 72 hours), traumatic injury, septic abortion, or delivery. The patient typically complains of sudden, severe pain at the wound site.

Your assessment in the early stage may show a normal body temperature, followed by a moderate rise, usually not above 101° F (38.3° C). Other assessment findings may include hypotension, tachycardia, and tachypnea, all signs of toxemia.

Inspection may reveal localized swelling and discoloration (often dusky brown or reddish), with formation of bullae and necrosis within 36 hours from the onset of symptoms. Soon the skin over the wound may rupture, revealing dark red or black necrotic muscle, accompanied by a foul-smelling, watery or frothy discharge. The patient may appear pale, prostrate, and motionless because of systemic toxicity but usually remains alert and oriented and is extremely apprehensive.

Palpation may detect subcutaneous emphysema (the presence of gas in the soft tissues), the hallmark of gas gangrene.

In later stages, the patient's level of consciousness may deteriorate to delirium and coma.

Diagnostic tests

Several tests confirm the diagnosis. Anaerobic cultures of wound drainage show *C. perfringens*; a Gram stain of wound drainage discloses large, gram-positive, rod-shaped bacteria; X-rays reveal gas in tissues; and blood studies show leukocytosis and, later, hemolysis.

Diagnostic tests must rule out synergistic gangrene and necrotizing fasciitis. Unlike gas gangrene, both of these disorders anesthetize the skin around the wound.

Treatment

Appropriate treatment includes careful observation for signs of myositis and cellulitis. The patient needs *immediate treatment* if these signs appear and *immediate* wide surgical excision of all affected tissues and necrotic muscle in myositis. Delayed or inadequate surgical excision is fatal.

The patient also needs I.V. administration of high-dose penicillin and, after adequate debridement, hyperbaric oxygenation, if available. For 1 to 3 hours every 6 to 8 hours, the patient is placed in a hyperbaric chamber and exposed to pressures designed to increase oxygen tension and prevent multiplication of the anaerobic clostridia. Surgery may take place within the hyperbaric chamber if the chamber is large enough.

Nursing diagnoses

- Anxiety
- Decreased cardiac output
- Fear
- Impaired skin integrity
- Impaired tissue integrity
- Pain
- Risk for infection

Nursing interventions

- Throughout the patient's illness, provide adequate fluid replacement. Monitor intake and output and central venous pressure.
- Assess pulmonary and cardiac function often. Maintain the airway and ventilation.
- To prevent skin breakdown and further infection, provide good skin care. Place the patient on an air mattress or an air-fluidized bed.
- After surgery, provide meticulous wound care.
- Before penicillin administration, obtain a patient history of allergies. Afterward, watch closely for signs of a hypersensitivity reaction.
- Deodorize the room to control foul odor from the wound. Prepare the patient emotionally for a large wound after surgical excision and for possible daily debridement. The wound usually is left open and requires frequent dressing changes and soaks.
- Institute wound precautions. Dispose of drainage material properly (double-bag dressings in plastic bags for incineration), and wear sterile gloves when changing dressings. No special cleaning measures are required after the patient is discharged.
- After recovery, refer the patient for physical rehabilitation, as necessary.
- For the patient who won't survive, psychological support is critical. The patient may remain alert until death, knowing that death is imminent and unavoidable.
- To prevent gas gangrene, routinely take precautions to render all wound sites unsuitable for growth of clostridia by attempting to keep granulation tissue viable. Adequate debridement is imperative to reduce anaerobic growth conditions. Be alert for devitalized tissues,

and promptly tell the surgeon if you notice any. Position the patient to facilitate drainage, and eliminate all dead spaces in closed wounds.

Patient teaching
• Tell any patient who reports sudden, severe, and persistent pain at a wound site to consult a doctor at once.
• Teach the patient with a cast or covered wound to report any foul odor or drainage.

ACTINOMYCOSIS

This infection is primarily caused by the gram-positive, anaerobic bacillus *Actinomyces israelii*, which produces granulomatous, suppurative lesions with abscesses. Common infection sites are the head, neck, thorax, and abdomen, but actinomycosis can spread to contiguous tissues, causing multiple draining sinuses. Rare sites of actinomycotic infection are the bones, brain, liver, kidneys, and female reproductive organs.

Occurring sporadically and infrequently, actinomycosis affects twice as many males—usually ages 15 to 35—as females. It is most likely to affect people with dental disease or human immunodeficiency virus infection.

Causes
A. israelii occurs as part of the normal flora of the throat, tonsillar crypts, and mouth, particularly around carious teeth. Infection results from its traumatic introduction into body tissues.

Complications
Diffuse involvement of the maxillofacial subcutaneous tissue and sinuses is the typical complication of actinomycosis. Abscesses and fistulae may involve the brain or be aspirated and cause pneumonia and empyema.

Assessment findings
The patient's signs and symptoms reflect the organ involved. In cervicofacial actinomycosis, a traumatic injury or dental extraction that occurs days to months before the onset of symptoms may be part of the patient history. In GI actinomycosis, abdominal involvement usually is associated with previous surgery, an inflammatory bowel condition, or perforated ulcers or diverticula.

The patient may complain of pain at the infection site and fever. Inspection may reveal edema of the mouth or neck in cervicofacial actinomycosis, a pro-

ductive cough with occasional hemoptysis in pulmonary actinomycosis, and draining sinuses with any form of the disorder. The exudate characteristically contains sulfur granules (yellowish gray masses, which actually are colonies of *A. israelii*).

Palpation may detect tender, indurated swellings in the mouth or neck if that site is infected or possibly a tender mass in the right lower quadrant if ileocecal lesions are present.

Diagnostic tests
Isolation of *A. israelii* in exudate or tissue confirms actinomycosis. Other tests that help identify it are:
• *microscopic examination* of sulfur granules
• *Gram staining* of excised tissue or exudate to reveal branching gram-positive filaments
• *chest X-ray* to show lesions in unusual locations, such as the shaft of a rib.

Treatment
High-dose I.V. penicillin or tetracycline therapy precedes surgical excision and drainage of abscesses in all forms of the disease and continues for 3 to 6 weeks. After parenteral therapy, treatment with oral penicillin or tetracycline may continue for 1 to 6 months. Clindamycin or erythromycin also may be used.

Nursing diagnoses
• Anxiety
• Pain
• Risk for infection

Nursing interventions
• Follow universal precautions when handling secretions.
• After surgery, provide proper aseptic wound management.
• Administer antibiotics, as ordered. Before giving the first dose, obtain an accurate patient history of allergies. Watch for hypersensitivity reactions, such as rash, fever, itching, and signs of anaphylaxis. If the patient has a history of any allergies, keep epinephrine 1:1,000 (for subcutaneous injection) and resuscitative equipment available.
• Administer analgesics, as ordered.

Patient teaching
• Stress the importance of good oral hygiene and proper dental care.

NOCARDIOSIS

An acute, subacute, or chronic bacterial infection, nocardiosis is caused by a weakly gram-positive species of the genus *Nocardia* — usually *Nocardia asteroides*. Nocardiosis is most common in men, especially those with compromised immune defense mechanisms. Its mortality in brain infection exceeds 80%. In other forms, mortality is 50%, even with appropriate therapy.

Causes

Nocardia is a genus of aerobic, gram-positive bacteria with branching filaments similar in appearance to fungi. Normally found in soil, these organisms occasionally cause disease in humans and animals throughout the world. Their incubation period is unknown, but it is probably several weeks. The usual mode of transmission is inhalation of organisms suspended in dust. Less often, transmission occurs by direct inoculation through puncture wounds or abrasions.

Complications

Meningitis, seizures, and cardiac arrhythmias are possible complications.

Assessment findings

The patient history may reveal the coexistence of a debilitating disease, such as diabetes, chronic congestive heart failure, or human immunodeficiency virus infection. The patient may complain of anorexia, weight loss, pleural pain, or dyspnea. With central nervous system (CNS) infection, the patient may report dizziness, headache, and nausea. His body temperature may be as high as 105° F (40.6° C).

You'll note a cough that produces thick, tenacious, mucopurulent and, possibly, blood-tinged sputum. Chills and night sweats also may develop. With CNS infection, the patient may have seizures and become disoriented and confused.

Palpation may detect subcutaneous abscesses that feel more firm than fluctuant and that lack the induration associated with actinomycosis.

Auscultation of the lungs may reveal crackles. Other assessment findings are variable but may include manifestations of tracheitis, bronchitis, pericarditis, endocarditis, peritonitis, mediastinitis, septic arthritis, keratoconjunctivitis, and purulent meningitis.

Diagnostic tests

Identification of *Nocardia* by culture of sputum or discharge is difficult, often requiring special staining techniques in conjunction with a typical clinical picture (usually progressive pneumonia despite antibiotic therapy). Diagnosis occasionally requires biopsy of lung or other tissue. Chest X-rays vary, and may show fluffy or interstitial infiltrates, nodules, or abscesses. Up to 40% of nocardial infections elude diagnosis until postmortem examination.

In brain infection with meningitis, lumbar puncture shows nonspecific changes, such as increased opening pressure. Cerebrospinal fluid shows increased white blood cell and protein levels and decreased glucose levels compared with serum glucose levels.

Treatment

Nocardiosis requires 12 to 18 months of treatment, preferably with co-trimoxazole or with high doses of sulfonamides. If the patient fails to respond to sulfonamide treatment, other drugs, such as ampicillin, amikacin, or erythromycin, may be added. Treatment also includes surgical drainage of abscesses and excision of necrotic tissue. The acute phase requires complete bed rest; as the patient improves, activity can increase.

Nursing diagnoses

• Altered nutrition: Less than body requirements
• Altered thought processes
• Decreased cardiac output
• Hyperthermia
• Impaired gas exchange
• Impaired physical mobility
• Ineffective airway clearance
• Pain
• Risk for injury

Nursing interventions

• Nocardiosis requires no isolation because it's not transmitted from person to person.
• Provide adequate nourishment through total parenteral nutrition, nasogastric tube feedings, or a balanced diet.
• Give tepid sponge baths and antipyretics, as ordered, to reduce fever and analgesics for headache, as needed.
• Monitor for allergic reactions to antibiotics.
• High-dose sulfonamide therapy (especially sulfadiazine) predisposes the patient to crystalluria and oliguria. So assess frequently, force fluids, and alkalinize the urine with sodium bicarbonate, as ordered, to prevent these complications.

• In a patient with pulmonary infection, perform chest physiotherapy. Auscultate the lungs daily, checking for increased crackles or consolidation. Note and record the amount, color, and thickness of sputum.
• In brain infection, regularly assess neurologic function. Watch for signs of increased intracranial pressure, such as decreased level of consciousness and respiratory abnormalities. Use appropriate safety measures to protect the patient from injury.
• In long-term hospitalization, turn the patient often, and assist with range-of-motion exercises.
• Provide support and encouragement to help the patient and his family cope with this long-term illness.

Patient teaching
• Before the patient is discharged, stress the need for a regular medication schedule to maintain therapeutic blood levels, even after symptoms subside. Explain the importance of frequent follow-up examinations.
• Teach the patient how to identify symptoms of recurrent disease by assessing sputum and degree of respiratory difficulty.

GRAM-NEGATIVE BACILLI

Infections caused by gram-negative bacilli may be mild to life-threatening and may have local to systemic effects. Such infections include salmonella infection, shigellosis, *Escherichia coli* and other Enterobacteriaceae infections, *Pseudomonas* infections, and many others.

SALMONELLA INFECTION
One of the most common infections in the United States (more than 2 million new cases appear annually), salmonella infection is caused by gram-negative bacilli of the genus *Salmonella,* a member of the Enterobacteriaceae family. It occurs as enterocolitis, bacteremia, localized infection, typhoid fever, or paratyphoid fever. Nontyphoidal forms of salmonella infection usually produce mild to moderate illness, with low mortality. Enterocolitis and bacteremia are especially common (and more virulent) among infants, elderly people, and people already weakened by other infections, especially human immunodeficiency virus infection. Paratyphoid fever is rare in the United States.

Typhoid fever, the most severe form of salmonella infection, usually lasts from 1 to 4 weeks. Most typhoid patients are under age 30; most carriers are women over age 50. The incidence of typhoid fever in the United States is increasing as a result of travel to endemic areas. Mortality is about 3% in people who are treated and 10% in those who are untreated. An attack of typhoid fever confers lifelong immunity, although the patient may become a carrier.

Causes
The most common species of *Salmonella* include *S. typhi,* which causes typhoid fever; *S. enteritidis,* which usually causes enterocolitis; and *S. choleraesuis,* which commonly causes bacteremia. Of an estimated 1,700 serotypes of *Salmonella,* 10 cause the diseases most common in the United States. All 10 can survive for weeks in water, ice, sewage, and food.

Nontyphoidal salmonella infection usually follows the ingestion of contaminated or inadequately processed foods, especially eggs, chicken, turkey, and duck. Proper cooking reduces the risk of contracting salmonella infection but doesn't eliminate it. Other causes include contact with infected people or animals and ingestion of contaminated dry milk, chocolate bars, or pharmaceuticals of animal origin. Salmonella infection may occur in children under age 5 from fecal-oral spread.

Typhoid fever usually results from drinking water contaminated by excretions of a carrier.

Complications
Salmonella infections may result in complications, such as intestinal perforation or hemorrhage, cerebral thrombosis, pneumonia, endocarditis, myocarditis, meningitis, pyelonephritis, osteomyelitis, cholecystitis, hepatitis, septicemia, and acute circulatory failure.

Assessment findings
Clinical manifestations of salmonella infections vary, depending on the specific clinical syndrome. (See *Assessing for salmonella infection.*)

Assessment findings for paratyphoid fever are the same as for typhoid fever, but the clinical course usually is milder. In localized infections, assessment findings depend on the site.

Diagnostic tests
In most cases, diagnosis requires isolating the organism in a culture, particularly blood (in typhoid or paratyphoid fever and bacteremia) or feces (in typhoid

ASSESSING FOR SALMONELLA INFECTION

Depending on the form of salmonella infection, the patient experiences varying signs and symptoms. Typical findings in three forms of salmonella infection—enterocolitis, bacteremia, and typhoid fever—are discussed below.

Enterocolitis
In this form of salmonella infection, the patient may report having eaten contaminated food 6 to 48 hours before the onset of symptoms. He also may report sudden onset of nausea, vomiting (usually self-limiting), myalgia, headache, and a rise in temperature up to 102° F (38.9° C). The cardinal sign, diarrhea, usually persists for less than 7 days and may be accompanied by mild to severe abdominal cramping.

Inspection may reveal signs of dehydration—dry mucous membranes and decreased skin turgor. Auscultation may detect increased bowel sounds; palpation may detect abdominal tenderness.

Bacteremia
The patient's history commonly reveals immunocompromise, especially acquired immunodeficiency syndrome. Typically, the patient complains of anorexia, weight loss (without GI symptoms), joint pain, and chills. The disorder may follow a severe febrile course, lasting for days or weeks. The patient feels profoundly warm, and inspection may reveal dry skin with poor turgor and rapid, shallow breathing.

Auscultation may disclose normoactive or hypoactive bowel sounds and a systolic murmur if tachycardia develops. Palpation may detect a rapid, thready pulse and varying degrees of peripheral edema.

Typhoid fever
In this infection, the patient's history may reveal ingestion of contaminated food or water, typically 1 to 2 weeks before symptoms developed. Symptoms of enterocolitis occasionally arise within hours of ingesting *Salmonella typhi*.

Signs and symptoms follow a typical course. In the first week, the patient may report the insidious onset of malaise, anorexia, myalgia, and headache. In the second week, he may complain of chills, weakness, cough, increasing abdominal pain, and diarrhea or, more frequently, constipation. In the third week, he may experience worsening fatigue and weakness (which usually subside by the week's end), although relapses or complications can develop.

The patient's temperature may rise to 104° F (40° C), usually in the evening. The patient looks acutely ill, and rose-colored spots that blanch with pressure may appear on the trunk. Delirium, confusion, and coma may occur. Bowel sounds are typically hypoactive; chest auscultation may reveal crackles. Palpation may disclose abdominal distention and tenderness, the characteristic sensation of displacing air- and fluid-filled loops of bowel, an enlarged liver and spleen and, sometimes, cervical lymphadenopathy.

---

or paratyphoid fever and enterocolitis). Other appropriate culture specimens include urine, bone marrow, pus, and vomitus. In endemic areas, clinical symptoms of enterocolitis allow a working diagnosis before the cultures are positive. The presence of *S. typhi* in stools 1 or more years after treatment indicates that the patient is a carrier (about 3% of patients).

Widal's test, an agglutination reaction against somatic and flagellar antigens, may suggest typhoid fever with a fourfold rise in titer. Drug use or liver disease also can increase these titers and invalidate test results. Other supportive laboratory values may include transient leukocytosis during the first week of typhoidal salmonella infection, leukopenia during the third week, and leukocytosis in local infection.

Treatment
The type of antimicrobial agent chosen to treat typhoid fever, paratyphoid fever, or bacteremia depends on organism sensitivity. Choices include ampicillin, amoxicillin, chloramphenicol, ciprofloxacin, ceftriaxone, cefotaxime, and, for the severely toxemic patient, cotrimoxazole. Localized abscesses may require surgical drainage. Enterocolitis requires a short course of antibiotics only if it causes septicemia or prolonged fever.

Symptomatic treatment includes bed rest and fluid and electrolyte replacement. Camphorated opium tincture, kaolin and pectin mixtures, diphenoxylate, codeine, or small doses of morphine can relieve diarrhea and control cramps for patients who remain active.

Nursing diagnoses
• Activity intolerance
• Altered nutrition: Less than body requirements
• Diarrhea
• Hyperthermia
• Pain

Home care

PREVENTING RECURRENCE OF SALMONELLA INFECTION

To prevent salmonella infection from recurring, follow these teaching guidelines:
• Explain the causes of salmonella infection.
• Show the patient how to wash his hands by wetting them under running water, lathering with soap and scrubbing, rinsing under running water with his fingers pointing down, and drying with a clean towel or paper towel.
• Tell the patient to wash his hands after using the bathroom and before eating.
• Tell him to cook foods thoroughly—especially eggs and chicken—and to refrigerate them at once.
• Teach him how to avoid cross-contaminating foods by cleaning preparation surfaces with hot, soapy water and drying them thoroughly after use; cleaning surfaces between foods when preparing more than one food; and washing his hands before and after handling each food.
• Tell the patient with a positive stool culture to avoid handling food and to use a separate bathroom or clean the bathroom after each use.
• Tell the patient to report dehydration, bleeding, or recurrence of signs of salmonella infection.

• Risk for fluid volume deficit
• Risk for infection

Nursing interventions

• Follow enteric precautions. Wash your hands thoroughly before and after any contact with the patient.
• Wear gloves and a gown when disposing of feces or fecally contaminated objects. Continue enteric precautions until three consecutive stool cultures are negative—the first one 48 hours after antibiotic treatment ends, followed by two more at 24-hour intervals.
• Observe the patient closely for signs of bowel perforation: sudden pain in the lower right abdomen and rebound tenderness, one or more rectal bleeding episodes, sudden fall in temperature or blood pressure, orthostatic hypotension, and rising pulse rate.
• During acute infection, promote rest, take safety precautions (because the patient may become delirious), and assign him a room close to the nurses' station so

that you can check on him often. Use a room deodorizer to minimize odor from diarrhea.
• Record intake and output. Maintain adequate I.V. fluid and electrolyte therapy, as ordered. When the patient can tolerate oral feedings, encourage high-calorie fluids, such as milk shakes. Watch for constipation.
• Provide good skin and mouth care. Turn the patient frequently, and perform mild passive exercises, as indicated. Apply mild heat to relieve abdominal cramps.
• *Don't* administer antipyretics. They mask fever and may lead to hypothermia. Instead, promote heat loss by applying tepid, wet towels (don't use alcohol or ice) to the patient's groin and axillae or by wiping wet towels down his arms and legs.
• Report salmonella cases to public health officials.

Patient teaching

• Advise the patient's close contacts to obtain a medical examination and treatment if cultures are positive. (See *Preventing recurrence of salmonella infection.*)
• Urge those at high risk for contracting typhoid fever (laboratory workers and travelers) to be vaccinated.

SHIGELLOSIS

Also called bacillary dysentery, shigellosis is an acute intestinal infection that causes a high fever (especially in children) and acute, self-limiting diarrhea with tenesmus; it also may cause electrolyte imbalance and dehydration. It's most common in children ages 1 to 4, but adults often acquire the illness from children.

Shigellosis is endemic in North America, Europe, and the tropics. In the United States, about 23,000 cases appear annually, usually in children or in elderly, debilitated, or malnourished people. Shigellosis commonly occurs among confined populations, such as those in nursing homes and hospitals.

The prognosis for this infection is good. Mild infections normally subside within 10 days; severe infections may persist for 2 to 6 weeks. With prompt treatment, shigellosis is fatal in only about 1% of cases; in severe *Shigella dysenteriae* epidemics, mortality may reach 8%.

Causes

Shigellosis is caused by *Shigella*, a short, nonmotile, gram-negative, rod-shaped bacterium. Shigella can be classified into four groups, all of which may cause shigellosis: group A, consisting of *S. dysenteriae,* which is most common in Central America and causes particularly severe infection and septicemia; group B, consisting of *S. flexneri;* group C, consisting of *S. boydii;* and group D, consisting of *S. sonnei,* which accounts for most cases reported in the United States.

Transmission is through the fecal-oral route, by direct contact with contaminated objects, or through ingestion of contaminated food or water. The housefly may be a vector.

Complications
Although not common, complications may be fatal in children and debilitated patients. Such complications include electrolyte imbalance (especially hypokalemia), metabolic acidosis, and shock. Less common complications include conjunctivitis, iritis, arthritis, rectal prolapse, secondary bacterial infection, acute blood loss from mucosal ulcers, and toxic neuritis.

Assessment findings
The patient's history commonly reveals crowded living conditions and family members or close contacts with acute diarrhea (the incubation period is 1 to 4 days between cases).

The patient initially may complain of nausea, abdominal pain, and diarrhea. In a day or two, stools usually increase in number but are smaller and contain pus, mucus, and blood (associated with tenesmus). High fever usually is present in children, but not in adults unless it's associated with dehydration.

Inspection may reveal a patient in considerable discomfort, with dehydration, dry mucous membranes, loss of skin turgor, and decreased urine output. Central venous pressure and blood pressure also may fall.

Auscultation may detect hyperactive bowel sounds. Palpation may elicit abdominal tenderness, especially over the lower abdominal quadrants, with accompanying distention. A dehydrated patient may have a rapid, thready pulse.

Diagnostic tests
During acute illness, stool cultures usually are positive. Microscopic examination of a fresh stool specimen may reveal mucus, red blood cells, and polymorphonuclear leukocytes; direct immunofluorescence with specific antisera may reveal *Shigella.* Severe infection increases hemagglutinating antibody levels. Sigmoidoscopy may reveal typical superficial ulcerations.

Diagnosis must rule out other causes of diarrhea, such as enteropathogenic *Escherichia coli* infection, malabsorption diseases, and amoebic or viral diseases.

Treatment
Shigellosis treatment involves enteric precautions and includes a low-residue diet and, most important, replacement of fluids and electrolytes with I.V. infusions of 0.9% sodium chloride solution (with electrolytes) in sufficient quantities to maintain a urine output of 40 to 50 ml/hour.

Antibiotics are of questionable value but may be used in an attempt to eliminate the pathogen and thereby prevent further spread. Ampicillin, tetracycline, or co-trimoxazole may be useful in severe cases, especially in children with overwhelming fluid and electrolyte losses. Ciprofloxacin and norfloxacin usually are effective.

Antidiarrheals that slow intestinal motility are contraindicated in shigellosis because they delay fecal excretion of *Shigella* and prolong fever and diarrhea. An investigational vaccine containing attenuated strains of *Shigella* appears promising in preventing shigellosis.

Nursing diagnoses
• Diarrhea
• Hyperthermia
• Pain
• Risk for fluid volume deficit
• Risk for impaired skin integrity
• Risk for infection

Nursing interventions
• Provide supportive care to minimize complications and increase patient comfort.
• Administer I.V. fluids and electrolytes, as ordered. Measure intake and output, including stools, carefully. Weigh the patient daily. Encourage oral fluids when the patient can tolerate them.
• Correct identification of *Shigella* requires examination and culture of fresh stool specimens. Therefore, hand carry specimens directly to the laboratory. If shigellosis is suspected, include this information on the laboratory slip.
• Use a disposable hot water bottle to relieve abdominal discomfort, and schedule care to conserve patient strength.
• To help prevent spreading this disease, maintain enteric precautions until three stool cultures are negative for *Shigella.* If you're at risk for exposure to the patient's stool, put on a gown and gloves before entering the room. Keep the patient's (and your own) nails short to avoid harboring organisms. Change soiled linens

ENTEROBACTERIAL INFECTIONS

Bacteria of the family Enterobacteriaceae cause enterobacterial infections. These gram-negative bacilli include *Escherichia coli, Arizona, Citrobacter, Enterobacter, Erwinia, Hafnia, Klebsiella, Morganella, Proteus, Providencia, Salmonella, Serratia, Shigella,* and *Yersinia.*

Enterobacterial infections can be exogenous (from other people or the environment), endogenous (from one part of the body to another), or a combination of both. They may cause any of many bacterial diseases: bacterial (gram-negative) pneumonia, empyema, endocarditis, osteomyelitis, septic arthritis, urethritis, cystitis, bacterial prostatitis, urinary tract infection, pyelonephritis, perinephric abscess, abdominal abscess, cellulitis, skin ulcers, appendicitis, gastroenterocolitis, diverticulitis, corneal conjunctivitis, meningitis, bacteremia, and intracranial abscess.

Appropriate antibiotic therapy depends on the results of culture and sensitivity tests. The aminoglycosides, quinolones, cephalosporins, and penicillins — such as ampicillin, mezlocillin, and piperacillin — prove most effective.

promptly and store them in an isolation container.
• Keep the perianal area clean and lubricate it after each episode of diarrhea.
• Provide a room deodorizer to minimize odor from diarrhea.
• Report shigellosis to local health authorities.

Patient teaching
• Instruct the patient to use proper hand-washing technique, especially after defecating and before eating or handling food.
• Inform parents of the signs and symptoms of dehydration in infants and young children, and tell them when they should notify the doctor.

ESCHERICHIA COLI AND OTHER ENTEROBACTERIACEAE INFECTIONS

Enterobacteriaceae — a family of mostly aerobic, gram-negative bacilli — cause local and systemic infections, including an invasive diarrhea that resembles shigellosis and, more often, a noninvasive, toxin-mediated diarrhea that resembles cholera. With other bacilli of this family, *Escherichia coli* causes most nosocomial infections. Noninvasive, enterotoxin-producing *E. coli*

infections may be a major cause of diarrheal illness in children in the United States.

The prognosis in mild to moderate infection is good. But severe infection requires immediate fluid and electrolyte replacement to avoid fatal dehydration, especially among children, in whom the risk of death may be quite high.

The incidence of *E. coli* infection is highest among travelers returning from other countries, particularly Mexico (noninvasive), Southeast Asia (noninvasive), and South America (invasive). *E. coli* infection also causes other diseases, especially in people whose resistance is low. (See *Enterobacterial infections.*)

Causes
Although some strains of *E. coli* exist as part of the normal GI flora, infection usually comes from nonindigenous strains. For example, noninvasive diarrhea results from two toxins produced by enterotoxigenic or enteropathogenic strains of *E. coli.* These toxins interact with intestinal juices and promote excessive loss of chloride and water. In the invasive form, *E. coli* directly invades the intestinal mucosa without producing enterotoxins, thereby causing local irritation, inflammation, and diarrhea. Normal strains can cause infection in immunocompromised patients.

Transmission can occur directly from an infected person or indirectly by ingestion of contaminated food or water or by contact with contaminated utensils. Incubation takes 12 to 72 hours.

Complications
Bacteremia, severe dehydration, life-threatening electrolyte disturbances, acidosis, and shock can result.

Assessment findings
Recent travel to another country, ingestion of contaminated food or water, or recent close contact with a person experiencing diarrhea may be part of the patient history.

The cardinal symptom is diarrhea. In the noninvasive form, watery diarrhea begins abruptly, along with cramping abdominal pain; in infants, the infection begins with loose, watery stools that change from yellow to green and contain little mucus or blood. In the invasive form, abdominal cramps are accompanied by diarrheal stools that may contain blood and pus. The patient may report that vomiting and anorexia precede diarrhea. He also may typically report a low-grade fever that occurs on the first and second days of infection.

In infants, inspection may reveal listlessness and irritability before the onset of diarrhea. With dehydration, especially in children, you'll note dry skin and mucous membranes (with decreased skin turgor), sunken fontanels, and sunken eyes. Expect to see signs and symptoms of hyponatremia, hypokalemia, hypomagnesemia, and hypocalcemia from electrolyte losses caused by vomiting and diarrhea.

In dehydration, auscultation may reveal hyperactive bowel sounds and orthostatic hypotension; palpation may reveal a rapid, thready pulse.

Diagnostic tests

Because certain strains showing *E. coli* normally reside in the GI tract, culturing is of little value. However, blood cultures of *E. coli* point to systemic infection.

A firm diagnosis requires sophisticated identification procedures, such as bioassays, which are expensive, time-consuming and, consequently, not widely available. Diagnosis must rule out salmonella infection and shigellosis, other common infections that produce similar signs and symptoms.

Treatment

Appropriate treatment consists of enteric precautions, correction of fluid and electrolyte imbalances, and, in an infant or immunocompromised patient, I.V. antibiotics based on the organism's drug sensitivity. For severe diarrhea that poses a risk of dehydration, bismuth subsalicylate or tincture of opium may be ordered.

Nursing diagnoses

• Altered nutrition: Less than body requirements
• Decreased cardiac output
• Diarrhea
• Pain
• Risk for fluid volume deficit
• Risk for impaired skin integrity
• Risk for infection

Nursing interventions

• Institute enteric precautions for all patients to prevent transmission of the organism to healthy people.
• Use proper hand-washing technique.
• Keep accurate intake and output records. Measure stool volume and note the presence of blood and pus. Replace fluids and electrolytes as needed, monitoring for decreased serum sodium and chloride levels and signs of gram-negative septic shock.
• Watch for signs of dehydration. Monitor vital signs to detect early indications of circulatory collapse.
• Clean the perianal area and lubricate it after each episode of diarrhea. Provide a room deodorizer.
• Give nothing by mouth; administer antibiotics, as ordered; and maintain body warmth.
• During epidemics, screen all hospital personnel and visitors for diarrhea, and prevent people with the disorder from having direct patient contact.
• Resistant strains of *E. coli* develop in patients on antibiotic therapy. Obtain routine surveillance cultures, and evaluate culture and sensitivity results, as indicated.

Patient teaching

• Explain proper hand-washing technique to hospital personnel, patients, and their families. Stress the importance of washing hands before eating or preparing food and after defecating, changing diapers, or having any contact with feces.
• Advise travelers to other countries to avoid unbottled water, ice, unpeeled fruit, and uncooked vegetables.
• If the patient will be cared for at home, teach him the signs of dehydration, and tell him to seek prompt medical attention if these occur.

PSEUDOMONAS INFECTIONS

A small gram-negative bacillus, *Pseudomonas* primarily produces nosocomial infections, superinfections of various parts of the body, and a rare disease called melioidosis. The most common infections associated with *Pseudomonas* include skin infections (such as burns and pressure ulcers), urinary tract infections, infant epidemic diarrhea and other diarrheal illnesses, bronchitis, pneumonia, bronchiectasis, meningitis, corneal ulcers, mastoiditis, otitis externa, and otitis media. This bacillus is especially associated with bacteremia, endocarditis, and osteomyelitis in drug addicts.

In local *Pseudomonas* infections, treatment usually is successful and complications rare. However, in patients with poor resistance to infection—for example, premature infants, elderly people, and persons with debilitating disease, burns, or wounds—septicemic *Pseudomonas* infections are considered serious. In some patients they may even cause death. (See *Melioidosis*, page 122.)

Causes

The most common species of *Pseudomonas* is *P. aeruginosa*. Other pathogenic species include *P. maltophi-*

MELIOIDOSIS

Wound penetration, inhalation, or ingestion of the gram-negative bacterium *Pseudomonas pseudomallei* causes melioidosis. Once confined to Southeast Asia, Central America, South America, Madagascar, and Guam, incidence in the United States is rising because of the recent influx of Southeast Asian immigrants.

Two forms: Chronic and acute
Melioidosis occurs in two forms: chronic melioidosis, which causes osteomyelitis and lung abscesses; and acute melioidosis (rare), which causes pneumonia, bacteremia, and prostration. Acute melioidosis commonly is fatal. Most infections are chronic, however, and produce clinical symptoms only with accompanying malnutrition, major surgery, or severe burns.

Diagnostic measures consist of isolation of *P. pseudomallei* in a culture of exudate, blood, or sputum; serology tests (complement fixation, passive hemagglutination); and chest X-ray, with findings that resemble tuberculosis.

Treatment includes oral tetracycline as well as co-trimoxazole, abscess drainage, and, in severe cases, chloramphenicol until X-rays show resolution of the primary abscesses.

The prognosis is good because most patients experience mild infections and acquire permanent immunity. The aggressive use of antibiotics and sulfonamides has improved the prognosis in acute melioidosis.

lia, *P. cepacia, P. fluorescens, P. testosteroni, P. acidovorans, P. alcaligenes, P. stutzeri, P. putrefaciens,* and *P. putida.*

These organisms frequently are found in hospital liquids that have been allowed to stand for a long time, such as benzalkonium chloride, hexachlorophene soap, saline solution, water in flower vases, and fluids in incubators, humidifiers, and respiratory therapy equipment. Outside the hospital, *Pseudomonas* skin infections have been associated with the use of contaminated whirlpools, hot tubs, spas, and swimming pools.

In elderly patients, *Pseudomonas* infection usually enters through the genitourinary tract; in infants, through the umbilical cord, skin, or GI tract.

Complications
Septic shock—the most serious complication of *Pseudomonas* infections—can cause death in people who are severely immunocompromised or resistant to an-

tibiotics. *Pseudomonas* produces severe mucopurulent pneumonia, which may be necrotizing.

Assessment findings
The immunocompromised hospital patient is the most vulnerable to *Pseudomonas*. Signs and symptoms vary with the infection site. In respiratory infection, the patient may complain of dyspnea, a cough producing purulent sputum, and chills. In urinary tract infection, he may report urinary urgency and frequency, dysuria, nocturia, low back pain, and malaise. In otitis externa, he may describe a painful or itching ear that is draining.

Although the patient's body temperature may be normal in some local infections, it will be elevated in severe infection, such as bacteremia associated with *Pseudomonas*.

Inspection findings also vary. For example, in a respiratory infection, you may note cyanosis, apprehension, dyspnea and, possibly, mental confusion. In otitis externa, using an otoscope, you may observe a tender, swollen external auditory canal filled with drainage. The drainage has a sickly sweet odor and consists of a greenish blue pus that forms a crust on wounds.

Abscesses may be palpable and tender on the skin surface. In *Pseudomonas* pneumonia, percussion discloses dullness over areas of mucopurulent drainage consolidation, and auscultation of the lungs may reveal crackles in areas of drainage collection.

Diagnostic tests
Diagnosis relies on isolation of the *Pseudomonas* organism in blood, cerebrospinal fluid, urine, exudate, or sputum culture.

Treatment
In the debilitated or otherwise vulnerable patient with clinical evidence of *Pseudomonas* infection, treatment should begin immediately, without waiting for laboratory test results. Antibiotic treatment includes aminoglycosides, such as gentamicin or amikacin, combined with a *Pseudomonas*-sensitive penicillin, such as ceftazidime or imipenem/cilastatin. Such combination therapy is necessary because *Pseudomonas* quickly becomes resistant to penicillin derivatives alone.

In urinary tract infections, carbenicillin indanyl sodium can be used alone if the organism is susceptible and the infection doesn't have systemic effects; the drug is excreted in urine and builds up high urine levels that prevent resistance.

Local *Pseudomonas* infections or septicemia secondary to wound infection requires 1% acetic acid irrigations, topical applications of colistimethate sodium and polymyxin B, and debridement or drainage of the infected wound.

Nursing diagnoses
• Impaired gas exchange
• Impaired skin integrity
• Ineffective airway clearance
• Pain
• Risk for infection

Nursing interventions
• Observe and record the character of wound exudate and sputum.
• Before administering antibiotics, ask the patient about a history of allergies, especially to penicillin.
• Monitor the patient's hearing and renal function (urine output, specific gravity, urinalysis, and blood urea nitrogen and serum creatinine levels) during treatment with aminoglycosides.
• For respiratory infections, maintain a patent airway by suctioning secretions whenever necessary, and provide adequate oxygenation. Perform chest physiotherapy and postural drainage as needed.
• Administer ordered analgesics as needed.
• Protect immunocompromised patients from exposure to this infection. Attention to hand washing and aseptic techniques prevents further spread.
• Use strict sterile technique when changing dressings that involve infected wounds. Clean the wounds with a bactericidal solution and apply local antibiotic ointment, if ordered.
• To prevent *Pseudomonas* infection, maintain proper endotracheal and tracheostomy suctioning technique: Use strict sterile technique when caring for I.V. lines, catheters, and other tubes; properly dispose of suction bottle contents; label and date solution bottles, and change them frequently, according to policy. Change water for fresh flowers daily. Avoid using humidifiers in the patient's room.

Patient teaching
• Reinforce the importance of completing the course of antibiotic therapy as prescribed.
• Teach the immunocompromised patient to avoid having sources of stagnant or contaminated water at home. Advise him to change the water for fresh flowers daily and, if a humidifier is essential, to change its water daily. Whirlpools and swimming pools must be scrupulously clean.
• Educate the patient who wears contact lenses, especially extended-wear soft lenses, to care for them properly and to report any associated eye trauma or other symptoms.
• Tell the patient to avoid drinking water when traveling to endemic areas.

LEGIONNAIRES' DISEASE
An acute bronchopneumonia, Legionnaires' disease is produced by a gram-negative bacillus. This disease was named for 221 persons (34 of whom died) who became ill during an American Legion convention in Philadelphia in July 1976. Outbreaks, usually occurring in late summer and early fall, may be epidemic or confined to a few cases. The disease may range from a mild illness (with or without pneumonitis) to serious multilobar pneumonia with a mortality as high as 15%.

A less severe, self-limiting form of the illness, Pontiac fever subsides within a few days but leaves the patient fatigued for several weeks. This disorder stems from the same organism as Legionnaires' disease but produces few or no respiratory symptoms, no pneumonia, and no fatalities.

Legionnaires' disease is more common in men than in women and is most likely to affect:
• middle-aged or elderly people
• immunocompromised patients (particularly those receiving corticosteroids after transplantation) or those with lymphoma or other disorders associated with impaired humoral immunity
• patients with a chronic underlying disease, such as diabetes, chronic renal failure, or chronic obstructive pulmonary disease
• alcoholics
• cigarette smokers (three to four times more likely to contract Legionnaires' disease than nonsmokers).

Causes
Legionnaires' disease results from infection with *Legionella pneumophila,* an aerobic, gram-negative bacillus that's probably transmitted by air. The organism's natural habitat seems to be water—either hot or cold. In the past, air-conditioning systems were thought to be the main source of transmission. Recently, public health officials have identified water distribution systems as the primary reservoir for the organism.

Complications

Patients in whom pneumonia develops also may experience hypoxia and acute respiratory failure. Other complications include hypotension, delirium, seizures, congestive heart failure, arrhythmias, renal failure, and shock, which usually is fatal.

Assessment findings

The patient history may include presence at a suspected source of infection. Onset of Legionnaires' disease may be gradual or sudden. After a 2- to 10-day incubation period (or a 1- to 2-day incubation period in Pontiac fever), the patient may report nonspecific prodromal symptoms, including diarrhea, anorexia, malaise, diffuse myalgia and generalized weakness, headache, and recurrent chills.

With Legionnaires' disease, the patient typically reports a cough—initially nonproductive, but eventually productive. He also may complain of dyspnea and chest pain or, sometimes, nausea, vomiting, and abdominal pain.

With Pontiac fever, the patient may complain of myalgia, malaise, chills, headache, a nonproductive cough, and nausea. An unremitting fever may develop within 12 to 48 hours, and the patient's temperature may reach 105° F (40.6° C).

Inspection may reveal grayish or rust-colored, nonpurulent and, occasionally, blood-streaked sputum. You also may note tachypnea, bradycardia (in about 50% of patients), and neurologic signs, especially an altered level of consciousness.

Chest percussion may disclose dullness over areas of secretions and consolidation or pleural effusions. Auscultation may reveal fine crackles, developing into coarse crackles as the disease progresses.

Diagnostic tests

• *Chest X-ray* typically shows patchy, localized infiltration, which progresses to multilobar consolidation (usually involving the lower lobes) and pleural effusion. In fulminant disease, chest X-ray reveals opacification of the entire lung.
• *Laboratory tests* include various blood studies and cultures. Blood test findings may include leukocytosis; increased erythrocyte sedimentation rate; a moderate increase in liver enzyme (alkaline phosphatase, alanine aminotransferase [formerly SGPT], and aspartate aminotransferase [formerly SGOT]) levels; and decreased partial pressure of oxygen and, initially, decreased partial pressure of carbon dioxide.

Bronchial washings, blood and pleural fluid cultures, and transtracheal aspirate studies rule out other pulmonary infections.
• Definitive tests include *direct immunofluorescence* of *L. pneumophila* and *indirect fluorescent serum antibody testing*. These tests compare findings from initial blood studies with findings from those done at least 3 weeks later. A convalescent serum sample showing a fourfold or greater rise in antibody titer for *L. pneumophila* confirms the diagnosis.

Treatment

Antibiotic treatment begins as soon as Legionnaires' disease is suspected and diagnostic material is collected. Treatment needn't await test results. Erythromycin is the drug of choice. If erythromycin is ineffective alone, rifampin can be added to the regimen. If erythromycin is contraindicated (for example, if the patient is allergic to the drug), rifampin alone or rifampin with doxycycline or co-trimoxazole may be used.

Supportive therapy includes administration of antipyretics, fluid replacement, circulatory support with pressor drugs if necessary, and oxygen administration by mask or cannula or by mechanical ventilation with positive end-expiratory pressure.

Nursing diagnoses

• Altered thought processes
• Hyperthermia
• Impaired gas exchange
• Ineffective airway clearance
• Ineffective breathing pattern
• Pain
• Risk for fluid volume deficit
• Risk for injury
• Self-care deficit

Nursing interventions

• Monitor the patient's respiratory status. Evaluate chest wall expansion, depth and pattern of respirations, cough, and chest pain. Watch the patient for restlessness, which may indicate hypoxemia. He may need suctioning, repositioning, postural drainage, chest physiotherapy, or aggressive oxygen therapy.
• Provide mechanical ventilation or other respiratory therapy if ordered.
• Continually evaluate vital signs, arterial blood gas levels, hydration, and color of lips and mucous membranes. Be alert for signs of shock (decreased blood

pressure; tachycardia; weak, thready pulse; diaphoresis; and clammy skin).
• Keep the patient comfortable and protected from drafts. Give tepid sponge baths or use cooling blankets to lower his fever.
• Provide mouth care frequently. If necessary, apply soothing cream to irritated nostrils.
• Replace fluids and electrolytes as needed. Nausea and vomiting may require administration of antiemetics, as ordered. If renal failure develops, prepare the patient for dialysis.
• Monitor the patient's level of consciousness for signs of neurologic deterioration. As needed, institute seizure precautions.
• Administer antipyretics and antibiotic therapy, as ordered.
• Administer antianxiety agents as ordered to decrease oxygen requirements and improve tolerance.

Patient teaching
• Provide pulmonary hygiene instructions. Explain the purpose of postural drainage, and tell the patient how to perform coughing and deep-breathing exercises.
• Teach the patient how to dispose of soiled tissues to prevent disease transmission.

CHOLERA
Also called Asiatic cholera and epidemic cholera, this disease is an acute, enterotoxin-mediated GI infection caused by the gram-negative rod *Vibrio cholerae.* Cholera produces profuse diarrhea, vomiting, and fluid and electrolyte losses. A similar bacterium, *Vibrio parahaemolyticus,* causes food poisoning. (See *Vibrio parahaemolyticus food poisoning.*)

Cholera is most common in Africa, southern and Southeast Asia, and the Middle East, although isolated outbreaks have occurred in Japan, Australia, and Europe. It usually occurs during the warmer months and is most prevalent among lower socioeconomic groups. In India, cholera is especially common among children ages 1 to 5, but in other endemic areas, it's equally distributed among all age-groups.

Even with prompt diagnosis and treatment, cholera is fatal in up to 2% of children because of difficulty with fluid replacement. In adults, it is fatal in fewer than 1%. Untreated cholera, however, may be fatal in as many as 50% of its victims. Cholera infection confers only transient immunity. About 3% of patients who recover continue to carry *V. cholerae* in the gall-

VIBRIO PARAHAEMOLYTICUS FOOD POISONING

A common cause of gastroenteritis in Japan, *Vibrio parahaemolyticus* also has caused outbreaks on American cruise ships and in the eastern and southeastern coastal areas of the United States, especially during the summer.

This organism, which thrives in a salty environment, is transmitted by ingesting uncooked or undercooked contaminated shellfish, particularly crabs and shrimp. After an incubation period of 2 to 48 hours, the organism causes watery diarrhea, moderately severe cramps, nausea, vomiting, headache, weakness, chills, and fever.

The food poisoning usually is self-limiting and subsides spontaneously within 2 days. Occasionally, it's more severe and may even be fatal in debilitated or elderly people.

Diagnosis requires bacteriologic examination of vomitus, blood, stool smears, or fecal specimens collected by rectal swab. Diagnosis must rule out other causes of food poisoning and other acute GI disorders.

Supportive treatment consists primarily of bed rest, oral fluid replacement and, sometimes, oral tetracycline. I.V. fluid replacement seldom is necessary.

Thorough cooking of seafood prevents this infection.

bladder; however, most patients are free of the infection after about 2 weeks.

Causes
Humans are the only documented hosts and victims of *V. cholerae,* a motile, aerobic rod. The disease is transmitted directly through food and water contaminated with fecal material from carriers or people with active infections. A deficiency or absence of hydrochloric acid in gastric juices may increase susceptibility to cholera.

Complications
Cholera can lead to hypoglycemia, severe electrolyte depletion, hypovolemic shock, metabolic acidosis, renal failure, liver failure, bowel ischemia, and bowel infarction.

Assessment findings
The patient may reside in or report recent travel to an endemic area. After the incubation period (several hours to 5 days), he may complain of abdominal gur-

gling and fullness, the result of increased peristalsis. He may next report acute, painless, profuse, watery diarrhea and effortless vomiting unaccompanied by nausea.

As the number of stools increases, the patient may report white flecks of mucus in his stools ("rice water stools"). He also may complain of intense thirst, weakness, muscle cramps (especially in the extremities), and oliguria—all from the massive fluid and electrolyte losses that result from diarrhea and vomiting. Fluid loss in adults may reach 1 liter/hour.

If fluid loss is severe, your assessment will reveal fever, tachycardia, and thready or absent peripheral pulses. (You won't note fever if cholera isn't complicated by severe dehydration.) You may note hypotension within an hour of the onset of symptoms.

During inspection, you may observe dry skin and mucous membranes (with loss of skin turgor), cyanosis, a pinched facial expression, sunken eyeballs, and profound weakness. The patient usually has an altered level of consciousness—he's likely to appear apathetic or detached, although oriented to person, place, and time.

Auscultation may reveal inaudible bowel sounds with profuse fluid and electrolyte depletion. Palpation of the abdomen may reveal a distended abdomen but no generalized or focal tenderness.

In children, you may observe unconsciousness or seizures, possibly caused by hypoglycemia.

Diagnostic tests
A culture of *V. cholerae* from feces or vomitus indicates cholera, but definitive diagnosis requires agglutination and other clear reactions to group- and type-specific antisera.

A dark-field microscopic examination of fresh feces showing rapidly moving bacilli (like shooting stars) allows for a quick, tentative diagnosis. Immunofluorescence also allows rapid diagnosis. Diagnosis must rule out *Escherichia coli* infection, salmonella infection, and shigellosis.

Treatment
Travelers to endemic areas can receive the cholera vaccine. Unfortunately, the vaccine now available confers only 60% to 80% immunity and is effective for only 3 to 6 months. Because of this, vaccination is impractical for residents of endemic areas; only an improvement in sanitation can control the disease.

Once the patient has cholera, he requires rehydration by rapid I.V. infusion with large amounts of iso-tonic saline solution, alternating with isotonic sodium bicarbonate or sodium lactate or with glucose. He also may receive potassium, calcium, and magnesium replacements in the I.V. solution.

After the I.V. infusions have corrected hypovolemia, the patient only needs fluid infusions sufficient to maintain normal pulse rate and skin turgor or to replace fluid lost through diarrhea. An oral glucose-electrolyte solution can be substituted for I.V. infusions.

In mild cholera, the patient only needs early oral fluid replacement. A patient who is suspected of having cholera can receive tetracycline. However, with the emergence of bacterial strains that resist traditional antibiotic therapy, he's likely to receive furazolidone or co-trimoxazole instead. Antibiotic therapy shortens the duration of diarrhea, diminishing fluid and electrolyte losses.

Nursing diagnoses
• Altered oral mucous membrane
• Altered thought processes
• Altered tissue perfusion
• Decreased cardiac output
• Diarrhea
• Fatigue
• Fluid volume deficit
• Risk for infection
• Self-care deficit

Nursing interventions
• During the acute phase of the disease, provide enteric precautions and supportive care, and closely observe the patient.
• Accurately measure intake and output (making sure to include stool volume), and assess the patient for other signs of fluid loss. (See *Estimating fluid volume depletion in cholera.*)
• Monitor results of serum electrolyte and glucose tests. Administer replacement fluids and electrolytes, as ordered.
• During therapy, continue to evaluate peripheral and central pulses, central venous pressure, and orthostatic blood pressure. The results help in adjusting infusion rates, particularly when the patient has renal failure. Carefully observe neck veins and auscultate the lungs for indications of fluid overload from cardiac failure.
• Administer tetracycline or other antibiotics to the patient, as ordered.
• Wear a gown and gloves when handling feces-contaminated articles or when a danger of contaminating

ESTIMATING FLUID VOLUME DEPLETION IN CHOLERA

Use this chart to estimate fluid volume loss in a patient with cholera.

Assessment	Depletion (percentage of body weight) 0% to 3%	4% to 8%	8% to 12%
Central pulses (femoral, carotid)	Full	Full	Weak
Peripheral pulses (radial, pedal)	Full	Weak	Absent
Skin turgor	Normal	Decreased	Poor
Eyes	Normal	Slightly sunken	Sunken
Muscles	Normal	Some cramps	Severe cramps
Appearance	Alert; slight thirst	Alert; thirsty	Restless; very thirsty
Urine output	Normal	Reduced	Absent

clothing exists, and wash your hands after leaving the patient's room.

Patient teaching
• Instruct the patient and his family on proper hand-washing technique and the need to wash their hands before eating or preparing food and after bowel movements, changing diapers, or any contact with feces.
• Teach the patient's family how to take the oral antibiotic, if ordered.
• If the family cares for the patient at home, make sure they know how to replace his fluids, salt, and glucose orally.
• Advise any patient traveling to an endemic area to boil all drinking water.
• If the doctor orders a cholera vaccine, tell the patient that he'll need a booster 3 to 6 months later for continuing protection.

HAEMOPHILUS INFLUENZAE INFECTION

Although *Haemophilus influenzae* can affect many organ systems, it most frequently attacks the respiratory system. It's a common cause of epiglottitis, laryngotracheobronchitis, pneumonia, bronchiolitis, otitis media, and meningitis. Less often, it causes bacterial endocarditis, conjunctivitis, facial cellulitis, septic arthritis, and osteomyelitis.

H. influenzae infection predominantly affects children, although it's becoming more common in adults, especially if they have a history of alcoholism and are over age 50. It infects about half of all children before age 1 and virtually all children by age 3, although a vaccine has reduced this number. The vaccine is administered at ages 2, 4, 6, and 15 months.

Causes
A small, gram-negative, pleomorphic aerobic bacillus, *H. influenzae* appears predominantly in coccobacillary exudates. It's usually found in the pharynx and less often in the conjunctiva and genitourinary tract. Transmission occurs by direct contact with secretions or by airborne droplets.

Complications
The microorganism can cause subdural effusions and permanent neurologic sequelae from meningitis; complete upper airway obstruction from epiglottitis; and pericarditis, pleural effusion, and respiratory failure from pneumonia.

Assessment findings
The patient may report a recent viral infection. He commonly complains of a generalized malaise and is

Warning

AVOIDING OBSTRUCTION IN ACUTE EPIGLOTTITIS

If a child develops symptoms of acute epiglottitis, *don't* attempt to examine his throat or obtain a throat culture—either could lead to a fatal respiratory obstruction. Only an experienced professional, such as an anesthetist or anesthesiologist, should perform such a procedure, and only with emergency airway equipment nearby.

likely to have a high fever. Other symptoms vary. For example, with acute epiglottitis, the patient may complain of a sore throat, severe dysphagia, and dyspnea. With pneumonia, he may report a productive cough, dyspnea, and pleuritic chest pain. With meningitis, he may experience headache, vomiting, photophobia, and diplopia.

Your inspection findings will vary with the site of infection. For example, a child with acute epiglottitis appears restless and irritable and may exhibit use of accessory muscles to breathe. Typically, he attempts to relieve severe respiratory distress by hyperextending his neck, sitting up, and leaning forward with his mouth open, tongue protruding, and nostrils flaring.

You also may observe stridor and inspiratory retractions. The trachea appears normal. The pharyngeal mucosa may look reddened (rarely with soft yellow exudate) but usually appears normal or shows only slight, diffuse redness. The epiglottis appears red with considerable edema. Severe pain makes swallowing difficult or impossible. (See *Avoiding obstruction in acute epiglottitis.*)

Your inspection of a patient with pneumonia may reveal shaking chills, tachypnea, a productive cough, and impaired or asymmetrical chest movement caused by pleuritic pain.

With meningitis, you may note an altered level of consciousness (LOC) progressing to seizures and coma as the disease progresses. You also may observe positive Brudzinski's and Kernig's signs and exaggerated and symmetrical deep tendon reflexes. If the patient is a young child, he's less likely to exhibit the nuchal rigidity you may see in other patients. With se-

vere meningeal irritation, you may observe opisthotonos.

If the patient has advanced pneumonia, chest percussion may reveal dullness over areas of lung consolidation.

In epiglottitis or pneumonia, auscultation may detect gurgles; in lung consolidation and upper airway obstruction, decreased breath sounds.

Diagnostic tests

Isolation of the organism, usually with a blood culture, confirms *H. influenzae* infection. A positive nasopharyngeal culture is not diagnostic because this may be a normal finding in healthy people. Other laboratory findings include polymorphonuclear leukocytosis (15,000 to 30,000/mm^3) and, in young children with severe infection, leukopenia (2,000 to 3,000/mm^3).

Treatment

H. influenzae type b infections may be rapidly fatal without prompt, effective treatment. Formerly, ampicillin produced excellent results, but strains of *H. influenzae* resistant to this antibiotic have developed. Because of this, therapy for serious infections must include other agents until the infection's susceptibility to ampicillin is ensured. Many doctors now use cefotaxime or ceftriaxone initially. As an alternative, they may prescribe a combination of chloramphenicol and ampicillin. If the strain proves susceptible to ampicillin, the doctor discontinues chloramphenicol.

The home patient with a less serious infection may receive ampicillin or amoxicillin.

Nursing diagnoses
• Altered nutrition: Less than body requirements
• Altered thought processes
• Anxiety
• Impaired gas exchange
• Impaired swallowing
• Ineffective airway clearance
• Ineffective breathing pattern
• Pain
• Risk for aspiration
• Risk for fluid volume deficit
• Risk for infection
• Sensory or perceptual alterations

Nursing interventions
• Maintain respiratory isolation. Use proper handwashing technique, properly dispose of respiratory se-

cretions, and place soiled tissues in a biohazard container.

• Maintain adequate respiratory function. Provide cool humidification and oxygenation therapy for respiratory infection, as needed; use croup tents for children and face tents for adults. Frequently monitor respiratory status. Watch for increasing restlessness and for tachycardia, cyanosis, dyspnea, and retractions, which may indicate the need for an emergency tracheotomy.

• Keep emergency equipment readily available, especially for the patient with meningitis or epiglottitis. This includes an oral airway, a tracheotomy tray, endotracheal tubes, a hand-held resuscitation bag, suction and oxygen equipment, and a laryngoscope with blades of various sizes. The patient may need a smaller endotracheal tube because of laryngeal edema.

• Monitor pulse oximetry and arterial blood gas levels. Remember to assess the patient's LOC or degree of lethargy to estimate the severity of hypoxemia.

• Suction the patient as needed, using sterile technique.

• Check the patient's history for drug allergies before administering antibiotics. Monitor his complete blood count for signs of bone marrow depression when therapy includes ampicillin or chloramphenicol.

• Give analgesics or antianxiety agents, as ordered.

• Administer racemic epinephrine to the oropharynx.

• Monitor intake (including I.V. infusions) and output. Watch for signs of dehydration, such as decreased skin turgor, parched lips, concentrated urine, decreased urine output, and increased pulse rate. Provide sufficient oral or I.V. fluids, or both, as ordered.

• Provide a quiet, calm environment. Organize your physical care measures, and perform them quickly to avoid disrupting the patient's rest.

• Avoid fluid overload in a patient with meningitis because of the danger of cerebral edema.

• For the patient with meningitis, assess neurologic function often, watching for deterioration. Be alert for a temperature increase up to 102° F (38.9° C), deteriorating LOC, nuchal rigidity, onset of seizures, and altered respirations, all of which may signal an impending crisis.

• Frequently reorient the patient with an altered LOC.

• Maintain adequate nutrition and elimination.

• Position the patient carefully. Elevate the head of the bed, turn him often, and assist with range-of-motion exercises.

Patient teaching

• Inform the parents of a child infected with *H. influenzae* about the high risk of acquiring this infection at day-care centers.

• Encourage parents to have their young children receive the *H. influenzae* vaccine to prevent these infections.

• Ensure that the patient or his parents understand the importance of continuing the prescribed antibiotic until the entire prescription is finished. The patient shouldn't stop taking the drug because he begins feeling better.

• Provide support and a careful explanation of procedures (especially intubation, tracheotomy, and suctioning) to the patient and his family or to the patient's parents.

• If the patient undergoes a tracheotomy, explain to him and his family that this measure typically will be used for 4 to 7 days.

• Teach the patient with pneumonia how to cough and perform deep-breathing exercises to clear secretions.

• To control the spread of infection, teach the patient to dispose of secretions properly and to use proper hand-washing technique.

• For home treatment of a respiratory infection, suggest using a room humidifier or breathing moist air from a shower or bath, as necessary.

PERTUSSIS

Also called whooping cough, pertussis is a highly contagious infection. It characteristically produces an irritating cough that becomes paroxysmal and often ends in a high-pitched, inspiratory whoop.

Pertussis is endemic throughout the world and usually occurs in early spring and late winter. About half the time it strikes nonimmunized children under age 2, probably because women of childbearing age don't usually have high serum levels of *Bordetella pertussis* antibodies to transmit to their offspring.

Since the 1940s, immunization and aggressive diagnosis and treatment have significantly reduced mortality from whooping cough in the United States. Pertussis mortality in children under age 1 usually is a result of pneumonia and other complications. Pertussis also is dangerous in elderly people but tends to be less severe in older children and adults.

Causes

Pertussis usually results from the nonmotile, gram-negative coccobacillus *Bordetella pertussis*; occasion-

BORDETELLA PERTUSSIS

This microscopic enlargement shows *Bordetella pertussis*, the nonmotile, gram-negative coccobacillus that commonly causes whooping cough. After entering the tracheobronchial tree, *B. pertussis* causes mucus to become increasingly tenacious. The classic 6-week course of whooping cough then follows.

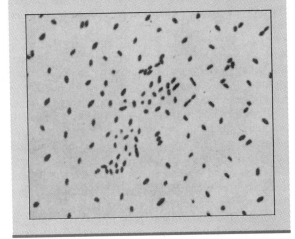

ally, it's caused by the related similar bacteria *B. parapertussis* or *B. bronchiseptica*. (See *Bordetella pertussis*.)

Pertussis usually is transmitted by direct inhalation of contaminated droplets from a patient in the acute stage. It also may be spread indirectly through soiled linen and other articles contaminated by respiratory secretions.

Complications

The paroxysmal coughing that pertussis causes may induce complications, such as increased venous pressure, epistaxis, periorbital edema, conjunctival hemorrhage, hemorrhage of the anterior chamber of the eye, detached retina and blindness, rectal prolapse, inguinal or umbilical hernia, seizures, atelectasis, and pneumonitis.

In infants, choking spells may cause apnea, anoxia, and disturbed acid-base balance. Residual mental retardation or learning disabilities may result. During the paroxysmal stage, patients also are highly vulnerable to fatal secondary bacterial or viral infections.

Assessment findings

The patient's history may reveal a lack of immunization coupled with exposure to pertussis during the previous 3 weeks. Pertussis follows a classic 6-week course that includes three 2-week stages with varying symptoms.
• During the first (catarrhal) stage, the patient experiences a hacking, nocturnal cough, anorexia, sneezing, lacrimation, and rhinorrhea.
• During the second (paroxysmal) stage, he experiences spasmodic and recurrent coughing that may expel tenacious mucus. Each cough characteristically ends in a loud, crowing, inspiratory whoop, and choking on mucus causes vomiting. (If the patient is a very young infant, he may not develop the typical whoop.)
• In the third (convalescent) stage, paroxysmal coughing and vomiting gradually subside. However, for months afterward, even a mild upper respiratory tract infection may trigger paroxysmal coughing.

During your assessment, you may find the patient's temperature normal or low. Inspection in the first stage may reveal mild conjunctivitis and listlessness; in later stages, you may note engorgement of neck veins or epistaxis during paroxysmal coughing, and exhaustion and cyanosis afterward.

During auscultation, you may hear diminished breath sounds in the lung periphery because of hypoventilation. You'll also detect wheezes, particularly after coughing, in the upper airways.

Diagnostic tests

Nasopharyngeal swabs and sputum cultures show *B. pertussis* only in the early stages of pertussis. Although fluorescent antibody screening of nasopharyngeal smears provides quicker results than cultures, it's less reliable.

The white blood cell (WBC) count increases, especially in a child older than 6 months who's in the early paroxysmal stage. The WBC count occasionally reaches 175,000 to 200,000/mm^3, with 60% to 90% lymphocytes.

Treatment

Infants usually require hospitalization and vigorous supportive therapy, often in the intensive care unit, and fluid and electrolyte replacement. Other measures include adequate nutrition, oxygen therapy as warranted, and administration of antitussives and antibiotics, chiefly erythromycin, as ordered.

Nursing diagnoses
- Activity intolerance
- Altered parenting
- Anxiety
- Impaired gas exchange
- Ineffective airway clearance
- Ineffective breathing pattern
- Pain
- Risk for fluid volume deficit
- Risk for infection
- Risk for injury

Nursing interventions
- Pertussis calls for aggressive supportive care and respiratory isolation (masks only) for 5 to 7 days after initiation of antibiotic therapy.
- To decrease exposure to infective organisms, change soiled linen, empty the suction bottle, and change the trash bag at least once each shift.
- Collect nasopharyngeal specimens for laboratory testing.
- Provide oxygen and moist air, and assist respiration, if needed.
- Suction secretions as necessary. Elevate the head of the bed to facilitate breathing.
- Encourage the patient to breathe deeply after receiving antitussives to enhance ventilation.
- Create a quiet environment to decrease coughing stimulation.
- Provide small, frequent meals to ensure adequate nutrition.
- Monitor acid-base, fluid, and electrolyte balance. Administer parenteral fluid therapy, as ordered, if vomiting is severe.
- Assess for complications related to excessive coughing.
- Report pertussis cases to local public health authorities.
- Administer antibiotic therapy promptly, as ordered.

Patient teaching
- Encourage the patient or his parents to inform anyone the patient has contacted to see a doctor promptly.
- Carefully explain all procedures to parents of young children, and offer emotional support.
- Tell the patient or his parents to report complications to the doctor, including a rising fever, abdominal protrusion, seizures, and a return of symptoms.
- Tell the parents of very young infants (who are particularly susceptible to pertussis) that immunization — usually with the diphtheria and tetanus toxoids and pertussis vaccine — should take place at 2, 4, and 6 months. Boosters follow at 18 months and at 4 to 6 years. Inform them that the risk of pertussis is greater than the risk of vaccine complications, such as neurologic damage. However, the vaccination may cause seizures or unusual and persistent crying, a possible sign of a severe neurologic reaction. If this happens, the doctor may not order the other doses. Explain that the vaccine is contraindicated in children over age 6 because it can cause a high fever.
- Direct the parents to report adverse reactions to the vaccine to the doctor.

BRUCELLOSIS
Also called undulant fever, Malta fever, and Mediterranean fever, brucellosis is an acute febrile illness that's transmitted to humans from animals.

Although brucellosis occurs throughout the world, it's most prevalent in the Middle East, Africa, Russia, India, South America, and Europe. Such measures as pasteurization of dairy products and immunization of cattle have reduced the incidence of brucellosis in the U.S. population. Most recently, especially in California and Texas, most cases have been linked to unpasteurized goat's milk cheese from Mexico.

Brucellosis most frequently occurs among farmers, stock handlers, butchers, and veterinarians. Because of such occupational risks, the disease traditionally infects men six times more often than it does women, especially men between ages 20 and 50; it's less common in children. Because hydrochloric acid in gastric juices kills *Brucella* bacteria, people with achlorhydria are particularly susceptible to this disease.

The incubation period usually ranges from 5 to 35 days but sometimes lasts for months. The prognosis is good. With treatment, brucellosis seldom is fatal, although complications can cause permanent disability.

Causes
Brucellosis is caused by the nonmotile, non-sporeforming, gram-negative coccobacillus *Brucella*, notably *B. suis* (found in swine), *B. melitensis* (in goats), *B. abortus* (in cattle), and *B. canis* (in dogs).

The disease is transmitted through the consumption of unpasteurized dairy products or uncooked or undercooked, contaminated meat. It's also passed on through contact with infected animals or their secretions or excretions.

Complications

Brucellosis can result in endocarditis, orchitis, persistent hepatosplenomegaly, and osteoarticular problems, such as arthritis and osteomyelitis. Skin manifestations, such as eczematous rashes, petechiae, and purpura, are possible, as is pulmonary involvement, including pleural effusions and pneumothorax.

Brucellosis can cause abscesses in the testes, ovaries, kidneys, spleen, liver, bone, and brain (meningitis and encephalitis). About 15% of patients with such brain abscesses develop hearing and visual disorders, hemiplegia, and ataxia.

Assessment findings

The patient's history may reveal direct exposure to animals, especially cattle or swine, possibly related to the patient's occupation. Or the patient may report ingestion of unpasteurized dairy products, most notably goat's milk cheese, or recent travel to an endemic area.

Because the disease has an insidious onset, the patient usually won't report symptoms until he reaches the acute phase. Then he may complain of fatigue, headache, backache, weight loss, anorexia, myalgia, and arthralgia. When he reaches the chronic phase, he may report recurrent depression, anxiety, sleep disturbances, fatigue, headache, and malaise.

Despite this disease's common name of undulant fever, your assessment seldom will show a truly intermittent (undulant) fever. The patient is more likely to have a normal temperature or low-grade fever in the morning and an increase in temperature in the afternoon.

On inspection, you may note drenching sweats, chills, and weakness in the acute phase and persistent fatigue in the chronic phase. Palpation may reveal lymphadenopathy and hepatosplenomegaly with tenderness in the left upper quadrant. It also may show abscesses and granuloma formation in subcutaneous tissue.

Diagnostic tests

Multiple agglutination tests help to confirm the diagnosis. About 90% of patients with brucellosis have agglutinin titers of 1:160 or more within 3 weeks of developing this disease. However, elevated agglutination titers also follow a relapse, skin tests, and vaccination against tularemia, *Yersinia* infection, or cholera. Agglutination tests also allow monitoring of treatment effectiveness.

Multiple (three to six) cultures of blood and bone marrow and biopsies of infected tissue (such as the spleen) provide a definitive diagnosis. Culturing is best done during the acute phase.

Blood studies indicate an increased erythrocyte sedimentation rate and a normal or reduced white blood cell count.

Treatment

The World Health Organization recommends a 6-week course of doxycycline plus rifampin. Alternative treatments include chloramphenicol, with or without streptomycin, and co-trimoxazole.

Nursing diagnoses

- Altered nutrition: Less than body requirements
- Anxiety
- Fatigue
- Impaired tissue integrity
- Knowledge deficit
- Pain
- Risk for infection
- Sexual dysfunction
- Sleep pattern disturbance

Nursing interventions

- Keep suppurative granulomas and abscesses dry. Properly dispose of all secretions, soiled dressings, and wet linens.
- Monitor and record the patient's temperature every 4 hours. Use the same route (oral or rectal) every time.
- Assess for enlarged lymph nodes and liver after treatment.
- Provide frequent hygiene, especially after sweating.
- Use soothing mentholated or diphenhydramine lotion to relieve itching. Avoid deodorant soaps, powders, and lotions.
- Ask the dietary department to provide between-meal milk shakes and other supplemental foods to counter weight loss. Determine the patient's food preferences and attempt to obtain these foods. Provide a pleasant environment at mealtime.
- Give antibiotics and analgesics, as ordered.
- Assess the patient for murmurs, weakness, vision loss, and joint inflammation — all may be indications of complications.
- During the chronic phase, watch the patient for signs of depression and disturbed sleep patterns. Administer sedatives as ordered, and plan activities to allow adequate rest. Try to create a quiet environment conducive to sleep.

Patient teaching
• Stress the importance of continuing medication for the prescribed duration. To prevent recurrence, advise the patient to cook meat thoroughly and avoid using unpasteurized dairy products.
• Warn meat packers and other people at risk for occupational exposure to wear rubber gloves and goggles.
• Teach the patient about the risk of fertility problems resulting from brucellosis.

CHANCROID
A sexually transmitted disease, chancroid (or soft chancre) is characterized by painful genital ulcers and inguinal adenitis.

Chancroid occurs worldwide but is particularly common in tropical countries. The infection is on the rise in the United States and is associated with increased risk for human immunodeficiency virus (HIV) infection. It affects males more often than females.

The incubation period varies but typically ranges from 5 to 7 days. Chancroidal lesions may heal spontaneously and usually respond well to treatment when no secondary infections are present.

Causes
Chancroid results from *Haemophilus ducreyi,* a short, nonmotile, gram-negative bacillus. Poor personal hygiene may predispose men—especially those who are uncircumcised—to this disease.

Complications
Phimosis and urethral fistulas may occur in men.

Assessment findings
The patient may report unprotected sexual contact with an infected person or with unknown or multiple partners. He may complain of pain associated with ulcers and lymphadenopathy. He also may experience headaches and malaise (in 50% of patients).

An inspection of the genital area initially reveals single or multiple papules surrounded by erythema. These rapidly become pustular and then ulcerate. The ulcers are nonindurated with ragged edges, have a base of granulation tissue, and bleed easily. They range from 1 to 2 mm in diameter.

You may observe the ulcers on the prepuce, frenulum, coronal sulcus, shaft, or glans penis in a male patient. In a female patient, you may note ulcers on the labia, fourchette, vestibule, clitoris, cervix, or anus, although many women are asymptomatic. Rarely, you'll observe lesions on the tongue, lip, or breast.

When you inspect the inguinal area within 2 to 3 weeks of onset, you're likely to observe unilateral lymphadenopathy with overlying erythema. If the patient hasn't received treatment, you may observe suppuration with bubo formation. Rupture of the abscess may follow.

On palpation, you may note tender, fluctuant inguinal nodes.

Diagnostic tests
Blood agar cultures provide a reliable diagnosis 75% of the time. Gram stains of ulcer exudate or bubo aspirate are 50% reliable. Biopsy confirms the diagnosis but is used only in resistant cases or when cancer is suspected.

Dark-field examination and serologic testing rule out other sexually transmitted diseases (genital herpes, syphilis, lymphogranuloma venereum) that cause similar ulcers.

Treatment
The first choice for treatment is 500 mg of oral erythromycin given four times a day for 7 days, or possibly 250 mg of ceftriaxone given I.M. in a single dose.

Alternatively, the patient can receive 500 mg of oral ciprofloxacin twice a day for 3 days. In areas where resistance to trimethoprim is uncommon, the patient can receive co-trimoxazole (160 mg trimethoprim and 800 mg sulfamethoxazole) twice a day for 7 days.

Aspiration of fluid-filled nodes and careful personal hygiene help prevent the infection from spreading.

Nursing diagnoses
• Altered sexuality patterns
• Body image disturbance
• Impaired skin integrity
• Knowledge deficit
• Pain
• Risk for infection

Nursing interventions
• Use universal precautions whenever you may come into contact with genital secretions—for instance, when collecting specimens and performing a physical examination.
• Administer anti-infectives and, possibly, analgesics, as ordered. Make sure the patient isn't allergic to the medication before giving the first dose, and ask him to rate the pain both before and after intervention.

• Provide topical care by washing the affected area with soap and water, followed by a bactericidal agent. Don't allow the area to remain moist; this can enhance the growth of the organism.
• Report all cases of chancroid to the local board of health, if required in your state.
• Examine the patient's sexual contacts, and refer them for treatment, even if they're asymptomatic.

Patient teaching
• Instruct the patient to take his anti-infective medication for the period prescribed.
• Teach the patient not to apply creams, lotions, or oils on or near his genitalia or on other lesion sites. Doing so may enhance the spread of the disease.
• Advise the patient to abstain from sexual contact until follow-up shows that healing is complete (usually about 2 weeks after treatment begins).
• Instruct the patient to wash his genitalia three times daily with soap and water. If he's uncircumcised, tell him to retract the foreskin to thoroughly clean the glans penis.
• Counsel the patient about HIV infection. Also, recommend HIV testing because of the heightened risk chancroid causes.
• Inform the patient that condoms may provide protection from future infection.

SPIROCHETES AND MYCOBACTERIA

Diseases caused by spirochetes and mycobacteria may advance from mild to incapacitating and life-threatening. Most progress in stages and all affect skin integrity to some extent.

SYPHILIS
A chronic, infectious, sexually transmitted disease, syphilis begins in the mucous membranes and quickly becomes systemic, spreading to nearby lymph nodes and the bloodstream. Untreated, the disease progresses in four stages: primary, secondary, latent, and late (formerly called tertiary).

Incidence is on the rise in the United States and is highest among urban populations, especially in people between ages 15 and 39, drug users, and those infected with the human immunodeficiency virus (HIV).

In 1990, about 134,250 new syphilis cases were reported in the United States; in 1989, about 115,110 cases were reported.

Untreated syphilis can lead to crippling or death. With early treatment, the prognosis is excellent. The incubation period varies but typically lasts about 3 weeks.

Causes
The spirochete *Treponema pallidum* causes syphilis. Transmission occurs primarily through sexual contact during the primary, secondary, and early latent stages of infection. Prenatal transmission (from an infected mother to the fetus) also is possible (see *Understanding congenital syphilis*). Transmission by way of a fresh blood transfusion is rare. After 96 hours in stored blood, the T. *pallidum* spirochete dies.

Complications
Aortic regurgitation or aneurysm, meningitis, and widespread central nervous system damage can result from advanced syphilis.

Assessment findings
The typical patient history will point to unprotected sexual contact with an infected person or with multiple or anonymous sexual partners.

In a patient with *primary syphilis,* you may observe one or more chancres (small, fluid-filled lesions) on the genitalia and others on the anus, fingers, lips, tongue, nipples, tonsils, or eyelids. In female patients, chancres may develop on the cervix or the vaginal wall. These usually painless lesions start as papules and then erode. They have indurated, raised edges and clear bases and typically heal after 3 to 6 weeks, even when untreated. In the primary stage, palpation may reveal enlarged unilateral or bilateral regional lymph nodes (adenopathy).

In *secondary syphilis* (beginning within a few days or up to 8 weeks after the initial chancres appear), the patient may complain of headache, nausea, vomiting, malaise, anorexia, weight loss, sore throat, and a slight fever.

On inspection, you may see symmetrical mucocutaneous lesions. The rash of secondary syphilis may appear macular, papular, pustular, or nodular. Lesions are uniform, well defined, and generalized. Macules typically erupt between rolls of fat on the trunk and, proximally, on the arms, palms, soles, face, and scalp. In warm, moist body areas (the perineum, scrotum, or vulva, for example), the lesions enlarge and erode,

UNDERSTANDING CONGENITAL SYPHILIS

A woman can transmit syphilis transplacentally to the fetus throughout pregnancy. Congenital syphilis may sometimes be called prenatal syphilis because about 50% of infected fetuses die before or shortly after birth. The prognosis improves for infants who develop overt infection after age 2.

Suspicious signs and symptoms

The infant with congenital syphilis may appear healthy at birth, but he usually develops characteristic lesions—vesicular, bullous eruptions on the palms and soles—3 weeks later. Soon thereafter, a maculopapular rash similar to that in secondary syphilis may erupt on the face, mouth, or genitalia.

Condylomata lata typically break out around the anus. Lesions also may erupt on the mucous membranes of the mouth, pharynx, and nose. If lesions affect the larynx, the infant's cry sounds weak and forced. If nasal mucous membranes are involved, a discharge may develop and may be slight and mucopurulent or copious with blood-tinged pus. Visceral and bone lesions, liver or spleen enlargement with ascites, and nephrotic syndrome may develop.

Late congenital syphilis becomes apparent after age 2 and may be identified through blood studies or through unmistakable syphilitic manifestations: screwdriver-shaped central incisors, deformed molars or cusps, thick clavicles, saber shins, bowed tibias, nasal septum perforation, nerve deafness, and neurosyphilis.

Test findings

In the infant with congenital syphilis, the VDRL titer, if reactive at birth, stays the same or rises, indicating active disease. The infant's titer drops in 3 months if the mother received effective prenatal treatment. Absolute diagnosis necessitates dark-field microscopic examination of umbilical vein blood or lesional drainage.

Therapy

An infant with abnormal cerebrospinal fluid (CSF) may receive aqueous crystalline penicillin G, I.M. or I.V. (50,000 units/kg of body weight daily divided in two doses for at least 10 days), or aqueous penicillin G procaine I.M. (50,000 units/kg of body weight daily for at least 10 days).

An infant with normal CSF may receive a single injection of penicillin G benzathine (50,000 units/kg of body weight).

Nursing interventions

When caring for an infant with congenital syphilis, record the extent of the rash, and watch for signs of systemic involvement, especially laryngeal swelling, jaundice, and decreased urine output.

---

producing highly contagious, pink or grayish white lesions (condylomata lata).

Alopecia, which usually is temporary, may occur with or without treatment. The patient also may complain of brittle, pitted nails.

Palpation may disclose generalized lymphadenopathy.

In *latent syphilis,* physical signs and symptoms are absent except for possible recurrence of mucocutaneous lesions that resemble those of secondary syphilis.

In *late syphilis,* the patient's complaints will vary with the involved organ. Late syphilis has three subtypes: neurosyphilis, late benign syphilis, and cardiovascular syphilis.

If *neurosyphilis* affects meningovascular tissues, the patient may report headache, vertigo, insomnia, hemiplegia, seizures, and psychological difficulties. If neurosyphilis affects parenchymal tissue, he may report paresis, alteration in intellect, paranoia, illusions, and hallucinations. Inspection may reveal Argyll Robertson pupil (a small, irregular pupil that is nonreactive to light but accommodates for vision), ataxia, slurred speech, trophic joint changes, positive Romberg's sign, and a facial tremor.

If the patient has *late benign syphilis,* he may complain of gummas—lesions that develop between 1 and 10 years after infection. A single gumma may be a chronic, superficial nodule or a deep, granulomatous lesion that's solitary, asymmetrical, painless, indurated, and large or small. Visible on the skin and mucocutaneous tissues, gummas commonly affect bones and can develop in any organ. If they involve the nasal septum or palate, they may cause perforation and disfigurement.

In *cardiovascular syphilis,* decreased cardiac output may cause decreased urine output and decreased sensorium related to hypoxia. Auscultation may reveal pulmonary congestion.

Diagnostic tests

• *Dark-field microscopy* to identify *T. pallidum* from lesional exudate provides an immediate syphilis diagnosis. This method is most effective when moist lesions are present, as in primary, secondary, and congenital

IDENTIFYING SYPHILIS BY DARK-FIELD MICROSCOPY

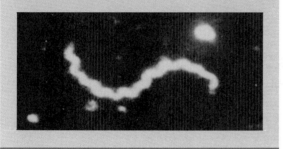

In syphilis, the presence of spiral-shaped bacteria (*Treponema pallidum*) on dark-field examination confirms the diagnosis.

syphilis (see *Identifying syphilis by dark-field microscopy*).

• *Nontreponemal serologic tests* include the Venereal Disease Research Laboratory (VDRL) slide test, the rapid plasma reagin (RPR) test, and the automated reagin (ART) test. These tests can detect nonspecific antibodies, which become reactive within 1 to 2 weeks after the primary syphilis lesion appears or 4 to 5 weeks after the infection begins. Rapid and inexpensive, the tests are used for screening patients and blood products.

• *Treponemal serologic studies* include the fluorescent treponemal antibody absorption (FTA-ABS) test, the *Treponema pallidum* hemagglutination assay (TPHA), and the microhemagglutination assay (MHA-TP). These tests detect the specific antitreponemal antibody and can confirm positive screening results. Once reactive, a patient's blood samples will always be reactive.

• *Cerebrospinal fluid examination* identifies neurosyphilis when the total protein level is above 40 mg/dl, the VDRL slide test is reactive, and the white blood cell count exceeds five mononuclear cells/mm³.

Treatment

Antibiotic therapy—penicillin administered I.M.—is the treatment of choice. For early syphilis, treatment may consist of a single injection of penicillin G benzathine I.M. (2.4 million units). Syphilis of more than 1 year's duration may respond to penicillin G benzathine I.M. (2.4 million units/week for 3 weeks).

Patients who are allergic to penicillin may be successfully treated with tetracycline or erythromycin (in either case, 500 mg by mouth four times a day for 15 days for early syphilis, 30 days for late infections). Tetracycline is contraindicated during pregnancy.

Nursing diagnoses
• Altered sexuality patterns
• Altered thought processes
• Body image disturbance
• Impaired physical mobility
• Impaired skin integrity
• Knowledge deficit
• Risk for infection
• Risk for injury
• Sexual dysfunction

Nursing interventions
• Follow universal precautions when assessing the patient, collecting specimens, and treating lesions.
• Check for a history of drug sensitivity before administering the first dose of medication.
• Promote rest and adequate nutrition.
• In secondary syphilis, keep lesions clean and dry. If they're draining, dispose of contaminated materials properly.
• Assess for complications of late syphilis if the patient's infection is older than 1 year. In late syphilis, provide symptomatic care during prolonged treatment.
• As needed, obtain a physical or occupational therapy consultation. Also consult with a social worker to determine home care needs.
• Report all syphilis cases to the appropriate health authorities.

Patient teaching
• Make sure the patient clearly understands his medication and dosage schedule and knows how to obtain the medication.
• Stress the importance of completing the prescribed course of therapy even after symptoms subside. Evaluate the need for home nursing care.
• Urge the patient to inform sexual partners of his infection and to encourage them to seek testing and treatment.
• Remind the patient to schedule follow-up tests.
• Advise the patient to refrain from sexual activity until he completes treatment and follow-up VDRL and RPR test results are normal.
• Counsel the patient and sexual partners about HIV infection and recommend HIV testing.

TRACKING LYME DISEASE STATE BY STATE

In 1995, U.S. public health authorities received 9,634 reports of Lyme disease—a decrease of 3,309 since 1994. Most cases occurred in the northeastern states, with fewer cases occurring in the western portion of the country (as shown on this map).

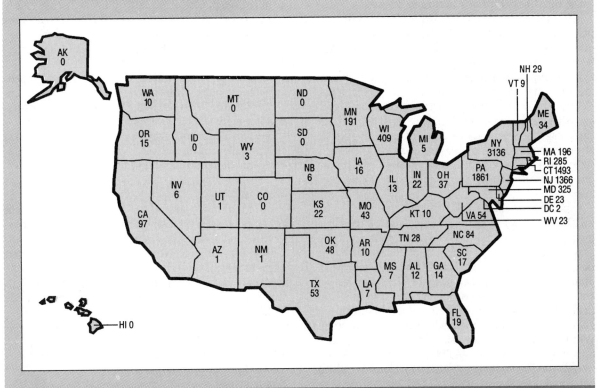

• Inform the patient that using condoms may provide protection against sexually transmitted diseases.

LYME DISEASE

Named for the small Connecticut town in which it was first recognized in 1975, Lyme disease affects multiple body systems. It typically begins in summer or early fall with the classic skin lesion called erythema chronicum migrans. Weeks or months later, cardiac, neurologic, or joint abnormalities develop, possibly followed by arthritis. The incidence has risen in most states over the past 8 years. (See *Tracking Lyme disease state by state*.)

Causes

Lyme disease is caused by the spirochete *Borrelia burgdorferi*. Carried by the minute tick *Ixodes dammini* (or another tick in the Ixodidae family), the disease occurs when a tick injects spirochete-laden saliva into the bloodstream or deposits fecal matter on the skin. After incubating for 3 to 32 days, the spirochetes migrate outward on the skin, causing a rash and disseminating to other skin sites or organs by the bloodstream or lymph system. The spirochetes' life cycle is incompletely understood: They may survive for years in the joints, or they may die after triggering an inflammatory response in the host.

Complications

Myocarditis, pericarditis, arrhythmias, heart block, meningitis, encephalitis, cranial or peripheral neuropathies, and arthritis are among the known complications of Lyme disease.

Assessment findings

Your assessment findings may be deceptive. Patient complaints vary in frequency and severity, probably because the illness typically occurs in stages.

The patient's history may reveal recent exposure to ticks—especially if the patient lives, works, or plays in wooded areas where Lyme disease is endemic. And he may report the onset of symptoms in warmer months. Typically reported symptoms include fatigue, malaise, and migratory myalgias and arthralgias. Nearly 10% of patients report cardiac symptoms, such as palpitations and mild dyspnea, especially in the early stage. Severe headache and stiff neck, suggestive of meningeal irritation, also may occur in the early stage when the rash erupts. At a later stage, the patient may report neurologic symptoms, such as memory loss.

Especially in children, body temperature may rise to 104° F (40° C) in the early stage and be accompanied by chills. You may see erythema chronicum migrans, which begins as a red macule or papule at the tick bite site and may grow as large as 2″ (5 cm) in diameter. The patient may describe the lesion as hot and pruritic. Characteristic lesions (not seen in all patients) have bright red outer rims and white centers. They usually appear on the axilla, thigh, and groin. Within a few days, other lesions may erupt, as may a migratory, ringlike rash and conjunctivitis. In 3 to 4 weeks, the lesions fade to small red blotches, which persist for several more weeks.

Bell's palsy may be seen in the second stage and may occur alone. In the later stage, inspection may disclose signs and symptoms of intermittent arthritis: joint swelling, redness, and limited movement. Typically, the disease affects one or only a few joints, especially large ones, such as the knee.

Palpation of the pulse may detect tachycardia or irregular heartbeat. During the first or second stage, you may detect regional lymphadenopathy as well. The patient may complain of tenderness in the skin lesion site or the posterior cervical area. You'll note generalized lymphadenopathy less commonly.

If the patient has neurologic involvement, Kernig's and Brudzinski's signs usually aren't positive, and neck stiffness usually occurs only with extreme flexion.

Diagnostic tests

Blood tests, including antibody titers to identify *B. burgdorferi,* are the most practical diagnostic tests. Or the enzyme-linked immunosorbent assay (ELISA) may be ordered because of its greater sensitivity and specificity. However, serologic test results don't always confirm the diagnosis—especially in Lyme disease's early stages before the body produces antibodies—or seropositivity for *B. burgdorferi.* Also, the validity of test results depends on laboratory techniques and interpretation.

Mild anemia in addition to elevated erythrocyte sedimentation rate, white blood cell count, serum immunoglobulin M levels, and aspartate aminotransferase (formerly SGOT) levels support the diagnosis.

A lumbar puncture may be ordered if Lyme disease involves the central nervous system. Analysis of cerebrospinal fluid may detect antibodies to *B. burgdorferi.*

Treatment

A 10- to 20-day course of antibiotics is the treatment of choice. Adults typically receive tetracycline or doxycycline; penicillin and erythromycin are alternatives. Children usually receive oral penicillin. Administered early in the disease, these medications can minimize later complications. In later stages, high-dose penicillin, administered I.V., or ceftriaxone, administered I.V. or I.M., may produce good results.

Nursing diagnoses

- Altered thought processes
- Decreased cardiac output
- Fatigue
- Hyperthermia
- Impaired physical mobility
- Pain
- Risk for infection

Nursing interventions

- Plan care to provide adequate rest.
- Ask the patient about possible drug allergies before administering antibiotics.
- Administer analgesics and antipyretics, as ordered.
- If the patient has arthritis, help him with range-of-motion and strengthening exercises, but avoid overexerting him.
- Protect the patient from sensory overload, and reorient him if needed. Also, encourage him to express his feelings and concerns about memory loss, if appropriate.

Patient teaching
• Instruct the patient to take antibiotic medications as prescribed.
• Urge him to return for follow-up care and to report recurrent or new symptoms to the doctor.
• Inform the patient, his family, and other caregivers about ways to prevent Lyme disease. Advise them to avoid tick-infested areas, if possible. If this measure isn't feasible, suggest covering the skin with clothing, using insect repellants, inspecting exposed skin for attached ticks at least every 4 hours, and removing ticks, if present, with tweezers or forceps and firm traction.

RELAPSING FEVER

Whether it's called bilious typhoid or tick, fowl-nest, cabin, or vagabond fever, relapsing fever is an acute infectious disease caused by a species of the *Borrelia* spirochetes. Transmitted by lice or ticks and characterized by relapses and remissions, this disease occurs most often in North and Central Africa, Europe, Asia, and South America. No cases of louse-borne relapsing fever have been reported in the United States since 1900. However, tick-borne relapsing fever does occur in the United States, mostly in Texas and other western states.

The incubation period for relapsing fever is 5 to 15 days (the average is 7 days). With treatment, the prognosis for both louse- and tick-borne relapsing fever is excellent.

Untreated, louse-borne relapsing fever has a mortality over 10%. During an epidemic, the mortality rises to 50%, especially among impoverished, malnourished, debilitated populations.

Causes

The body louse (*Pediculus humanus corporis*) carries the spirochete responsible for relapsing fever (*B. recurrentis*). This louse transmits the disease from person to person. Inoculation occurs when the victim crushes the louse, causing its infected blood or body fluid to seep into the victim's broken skin or mucous membranes. Louse-borne relapsing fever typically erupts epidemically during wars, famines, and mass migrations. Cold weather and crowded living conditions favor the spread of body lice.

Tick-borne relapsing fever is caused by several species of *Borrelia* transmitted to humans by *Ornithodoros* ticks. Outbreaks usually occur during the summer when ticks and their hosts (chipmunks, goats, prairie dogs) are most active. Cold-weather outbreaks may af-

flict people who sleep in tick-infested cabins, such as campers. Because tick bites are painless and *Ornithodoros* ticks frequently feed at night without imbedding themselves in the victim's skin, many people are bitten unknowingly.

Complications

Nephritis, bronchitis, pneumonia, endocarditis, seizures, cranial nerve lesions, paralysis, and coma are complications of this disease. Death may result from hyperpyrexia, massive bleeding, circulatory failure, splenic rupture, or a secondary infection.

Assessment findings

The patient's history may reveal recent travel in an epidemic or a louse-infested area. Or you may find that the patient was recently exposed to ticks or a tick-infested area.

Clinical signs and symptoms of louse- and tick-borne relapsing fever are similar. The patient may relate sudden prostration, headache, severe myalgia, arthralgia, diarrhea, vomiting, coughing, and eye or chest pains.

Palpation commonly discloses splenomegaly and, possibly, hepatomegaly and lymphadenopathy. During febrile periods, when body temperature may rise suddenly to 105° F (40.6° C), the victim's pulse rate and respiratory rate increase, and you may note a transient, macular rash that may spread over his torso.

The first attack usually lasts from 3 to 6 days; then the patient's temperature drops quickly, accompanied by profuse sweating. About 5 to 10 days later, a second febrile, symptomatic period begins. In louse-borne infection, additional relapses are unusual, but in tick-borne disease, a second or third relapse is common. As the afebrile intervals lengthen, relapses become shorter and milder as the body accumulates antibodies to fight the infection.

Diagnostic tests

Blood smears done with Wright's or Giemsa stain may confirm the diagnosis by revealing the infecting spirochete if blood is obtained during a febrile period. *Borrelia* spirochetes may be less detectable in subsequent relapses because their number in the blood declines.

In such cases, a sample of the patient's blood or tissue may be injected into a young rat and incubated there for 1 to 10 days. If the patient has relapsing fever, subsequent testing of the rat's tail blood may disclose large numbers of spirochetes.

Urine and cerebrospinal fluid analyses may uncover spirochete-induced infection. Other abnormal findings include a white blood cell (WBC) count as high as 25,000/mm³, with increases in lymphocyte levels and erythrocyte sedimentation rate. However, the WBC count may be within normal limits. Because the *Borrelia* organism is a spirochete, test findings in relapsing fever may be similar to those in syphilis.

Treatment

An adult usually receives oral antibiotic therapy—tetracycline for 4 to 5 days is the first choice. In children and in seriously ill patients who can't take tetracycline, penicillin G, erythromycin, or ceftriaxone may be administered as an alternative.

Antibiotics should not be given at the height of a severe febrile attack. If they are given, a Jarisch-Herxheimer reaction may occur, causing malaise, rigor, leukopenia, flushing, fever, tachycardia, rising respiratory rate, and hypotension. This reaction, which is caused by toxic by-products from massive spirochete destruction, can mimic septic shock and may prove fatal.

Antimicrobial therapy should be postponed until the patient's fever subsides. Until then, supportive therapy (parenteral fluids and electrolytes) should be given instead.

When tetracycline, penicillin G, erythromycin, or ceftriaxone fails to control relapsing fever, chloramphenicol may be given with caution. A complete blood count should be done regularly during treatment with chloramphenicol because a fatal granulocytopenia, thrombocytopenia, or even aplastic anemia may develop.

Nursing diagnoses

• Altered thought processes
• Diarrhea
• Hyperthermia
• Impaired skin integrity
• Pain
• Risk for fluid volume deficit
• Sensory or perceptual alterations

Nursing interventions

• Monitor the patient's vital signs, level of consciousness (LOC), and temperature every 2 to 4 hours throughout febrile periods. Watch for and immediately report any signs of neurologic complications, such as decreasing LOC and seizures. To reduce fever, give tepid sponge baths or apply a hypothermia blanket, and administer antipyretics, as ordered.
• Administer analgesics, as ordered, to alleviate discomfort during febrile periods.
• Maintain adequate fluid intake to prevent dehydration. Provide I.V. fluids, as ordered. Accurately measure intake and output, especially for the patient with vomiting and diarrhea.
• Give antibiotics carefully. Document and report any hypersensitivity reaction (rash, fever, anaphylaxis), especially a Jarisch-Herxheimer reaction.
• Treat flushing, hypotension, and tachycardia with vasopressors or fluids, as ordered.
• Look for symptoms of relapsing fever in family members and in others who may have been exposed to ticks or lice along with the victim.
• Use proper hand-washing technique. Isolation is unnecessary because the disease isn't transmitted from person to person.
• Report all cases of louse- or tick-borne relapsing fever to the local public health department, as required by law.

Patient teaching

• Teach the patient and caregivers measures to reduce body temperature and prevent dehydration, if patient care will occur at home. Also, demonstrate proper hand-washing technique.
• Advise the patient to plan frequent rest periods.
• Encourage the patient to take antibiotic medications exactly as prescribed.
• Help the patient and caregivers recognize the signs and symptoms of neurologic toxicity: altered memory, hallucinations, and agitation.
• To help prevent relapsing fever, advise anyone traveling to tick-infested areas to wear clothing that covers as much skin as possible. Recommend fastening sleeves and collars and tucking pant legs into boots or socks.

LEPROSY

Sometimes called Hansen's disease, leprosy is a chronic, systemic infection characterized by progressive cutaneous lesions. Most prevalent in underdeveloped areas of Asia (especially India and China), Africa, South America, and the Caribbean and Pacific islands, leprosy affects about 15 million people worldwide. About 4,000 victims are in the United States, mostly in California, Texas, Louisiana, Florida, New

York, and Hawaii. The long incubation period may last between 6 months and 8 years.

With timely and correct treatment, this seldom fatal disease has a good prognosis. Acute episodes may intensify leprosy's slowly progressing course, but whether such exacerbations are part of the disease process or a reaction to therapy remains unclear.

Untreated, leprosy can cause severe disability, blindness, and deformities. Leprosy takes three distinct forms:
• *Lepromatous leprosy,* the most serious form, causes damage to the upper respiratory tract, eyes, testes, nerves, and skin.
• *Tuberculoid leprosy* affects peripheral nerves and sometimes the surrounding skin, especially on the face, arms, legs, and buttocks.
• *Borderline (dimorphous) leprosy* has characteristics of both lepromatous and tuberculoid leprosy. In this form of leprosy, skin lesions appear diffuse and poorly defined.

Causes

Leprosy is caused by *Mycobacterium leprae,* an acid-fast bacillus that attacks cutaneous tissue and peripheral nerves, especially the ulnar, radial, posteropopliteal, anterotibial, and facial nerves. The central nervous system appears highly resistant.

Contrary to popular belief, leprosy isn't highly contagious. Rather, continuous, close contact is needed to transmit it. In fact, 9 out of 10 persons have a natural immunity to leprosy. Susceptibility—highest during childhood—seems to decrease with age. Presumably, transmission occurs through airborne respiratory droplets that contain *M. leprae* or by inoculation through skin breaks (from a contaminated hypodermic or tattoo needle, for example).

Complications

Erythema nodosum leprosum, seen in lepromatous leprosy, may produce fever, malaise, lymphadenopathy, and painful, red skin nodules—usually during antimicrobial treatment, although the skin lesions may occur in untreated people.

In Mexico and other Central American countries, some patients with lepromatous disease develop *Lucio's phenomenon:* generalized reddened lesions with necrotic centers. These ulcers may extend into muscle and fascia.

Leprosy also may be complicated by secondary bacterial infection of skin ulcers, amyloidosis, deformity contractures, ocular disorders that can result in blindness and, rarely, hepatitis and exfoliative dermatitis.

Assessment findings

The patient may report living in close contact with another person who has leprosy. When the bacilli damage the skin's fine nerves, he may notice anesthesia, anhidrosis, and dryness. If the bacilli attack a large nerve trunk, he may experience motor nerve damage, weakness, and pain followed by peripheral anesthesia, muscle paralysis, or atrophy. In later stages, he may seek treatment for clawhand, footdrop, and visual disturbances, such as photophobia and blindness.

Lepromatous and tuberculoid leprosies affect the skin in markedly different ways. In lepromatous disease, early multiple lesions appear symmetrical and erythematous. Sometimes they erupt as macules or papules with smooth surfaces. Later, they enlarge and form plaques or nodules called lepromas on the earlobes, nose, eyebrows, and forehead, giving the patient a characteristic leonine appearance.

In advanced stages, *M. leprae* may infiltrate the entire skin surface. Lepromatous leprosy also causes loss of eyebrows, eyelashes, and sebaceous and sweat gland function, as well as conjunctival and scleral nodules. Upper respiratory tract lesions cause epistaxis, ulcerated uvula and tonsils, septal perforation, and nasal collapse. Lepromatous leprosy can lead to orchitis and resultant testicular atrophy. Fingertips and toes deteriorate as bone resorption follows trauma and infection in these insensitive areas. Injury, ulceration, infection, and disuse of the deformed parts cause scars and contractures.

When tuberculoid leprosy affects the skin (sometimes it affects only the neurologic system), it produces large, raised, erythematous plaques or macules with clearly defined borders. As the lesions progress, they become rough, hairless, and hypopigmented. The patient usually reports numbness in the resultant scars.

In the patient with borderline leprosy, you'll see numerous skin lesions, but they're smaller and less sharply defined than tuberculoid lesions. The patient may report some feeling in the lesions. (Keep in mind that untreated borderline leprosy may deteriorate into lepromatous disease.)

Palpation may detect hepatosplenomegaly in a patient with lepromatous leprosy. Lesions are all superficial and easily palpable.

Diagnostic tests

Identification of acid-fast bacilli in skin and nasal mucosa scrapings confirms a diagnosis of leprosy. A skin biopsy shows the typical histologic pattern of nerve changes. The skin biopsy and scrapings also are evaluated to determine the percentage of fully intact cells (morphologic index) and to measure the amount of bacteria present (bacterial index).

Treatment

Leprosy usually responds to antimicrobial therapy with sulfones, primarily oral dapsone, which may cause hypersensitivity reactions. Especially dangerous — but rare — reactions include hepatitis and exfoliative dermatitis. If these reactions occur, sulfone therapy should stop at once.

If leprosy fails to respond to sulfones or if the patient has respiratory or other complications, an alternative therapy, such as rifampin with clofazimine or ethionamide, may be effective.

Clawhand, wristdrop, or footdrop may necessitate surgical correction.

When leprosy becomes inactive (as determined by morphologic and bacterial studies), the patient with lepromatous leprosy will need lifetime therapy; the patient with tuberculoid leprosy can discontinue treatment after 3 years. The need for ongoing treatment in borderline leprosy depends on the disease's severity, but treatment may continue for up to 10 years.

Because erythema nodosum leprosum is considered a sign that the patient is responding to treatment, antimicrobial therapy should be continued if this reaction occurs.

The National Hansen's Disease Center reports good results using thalidomide and clofazimine to treat erythema nodosum leprosum. Because of the teratogenicity associated with thalidomide, the treatment requires a signed consent form and strict adherence to established protocols. Corticosteroids may be included in the therapy.

Nursing diagnoses

- Body image disturbance
- Impaired physical mobility
- Impaired skin integrity
- Pain
- Risk for infection
- Risk for injury
- Sensory or perceptual alterat
- Sexual dysfunction
- Social isolation

Nursing interventions

- Provide supportive patient care, taking steps to control acute infection, prevent complications, speed recovery and rehabilitation, and provide emotional encouragement.
- Give antipyretics, analgesics, and sedatives, as needed. Watch for and report erythema nodosum leprosum, Lucio's phenomenon, and other complications.
- Take precautions against the possible spread of infection even though leprosy isn't highly contagious. Instruct patients to cover coughs or sneezes with a paper tissue and to dispose of it properly. Take infection precautions when handling clothing or articles that touch open skin lesions.
- Plan care to promote adequate rest and optimal nutrition.
- Give the patient and family opportunities to express their feelings.
- Initiate or participate in consultations with other health team members — especially for the patient with deformities. An interdisciplinary rehabilitation program, including physiotherapy and plastic surgery, may be necessary.
- Inspect the patient's skin, and report observed changes. Assist with general hygiene and comfort measures, and provide a skin care program.

Patient teaching

- Instruct the patient to be careful not to injure an anesthetized leg by putting too much weight on it. Advise him to carefully test bath water to avoid scalding. To prevent ulcerations, suggest wearing sturdy footwear and soaking feet in warm water after any kind of exercise, even a short walk. Advise rubbing the feet with petrolatum, oil, or lanolin.
- Recommend that the patient use a tear substitute twice a day and protect his eyes — especially if he experiences decreased corneal sensation and lacrimation. Tell him to avoid rubbing his eyes and to wear sunglasses. Explain that these measures help prevent the corneal irritation and ulceration that lead to blindness.
- Tell the patient to take antimicrobial medications exactly as prescribed for the entire length of time prescribed — in some cases, for life.
- If appropriate, refer the patient to a regional treatment center or to the Gillis W. Long Hansen's Disease Center in Carville, La. This international research and education center provides diagnostic studies, treatment, and education for patients with leprosy. Patients

are encouraged to return home as soon as their medical condition permits. The federal government pays the full cost of medical and nursing care.

MYCOSES

Caused by such fungi as yeasts and molds, mycotic diseases may be superficial or systemic. Candidiasis, cryptococcosis, histoplasmosis, coccidioidomycosis, and sporotrichosis are among prevalent mycotic diseases.

CANDIDIASIS

Also known as candidosis and moniliasis, this usually mild, superficial fungal infection can lead to severe disseminated infections and fungemia in an immunocompromised patient. In most cases, the causative fungi infect the nails (paronychia), skin (diaper rash), or mucous membranes, especially the oropharynx (thrush), vagina (vaginitis), esophagus, and GI tract.

These fungi may enter the bloodstream and invade the kidneys, lungs, endocardium, brain, or other structures, causing serious systemic infection. Such systemic infection predominates among drug abusers and hospital patients (particularly diabetic and immunosuppressed patients).

The prognosis varies, depending on the patient's resistance. The incidence of candidiasis continues to rise because of increasing use of I.V. antibiotic therapy and increasing numbers of immunocompromised patients in the acute care setting.

Causes
Most cases of candidiasis result from infection with *Candida albicans* or *C. tropicalis,* although eight other potentially disease-causing strains exist among the more than 150 species of *Candida.* One of the normal flora of the GI tract, mouth, vagina, and skin, *C. albicans* causes infection when some change in the body permits their sudden proliferation. The changes may be triggered by rising glucose levels from diabetes mellitus, lowered resistance from such diseases as cancer, immunosuppressant drug therapy, radiation, aging, or irritation from dentures.

The infecting organism may enter the body through I.V. or urinary catheterization, drug abuse, total parenteral nutrition, or surgery. The most common precipitator is the use of broad-spectrum antibiotics, such as tetracycline. These agents decrease the number of normal bacterial flora, which permits the number of fungi, including candidal organisms, to increase.

A mother with vaginitis can transmit the organism (as oral thrush) to the neonate during vaginal delivery.

Complications
The most common complications include *Candida* dissemination with organ failure of the kidneys, brain, GI tract, eyes, lungs, and heart.

Assessment findings
The patient's history may reveal an underlying illness, such as cancer, diabetes, or human immunodeficiency virus infection; a recent course of antibiotic or antineoplastic therapy; or drug abuse.

Depending on the infection site, superficial infection may cause the following signs and symptoms:
• Skin—scaly, erythematous, papular rash, possibly covered with exudate and erupting in breast folds, between fingers, and at the axillae, groin, and umbilicus (in diaper rash, papules appear at the edges of the rash)
• Nails—red, swollen, darkened nailbeds; occasionally, purulent discharge; sometimes the nail separates from the nailbed
• Esophageal mucosa—occasionally, scales in the mouth and throat
• Vaginal mucosa—white or yellow discharge, with local excoriation; white or gray raised patches on vaginal walls, with local inflammation
• Oropharyngeal mucosa—cream-colored or bluish white lacelike patches of exudate on the tongue, mouth, or pharynx that reveal bloody engorgement when scraped. Pain and a burning sensation in the mouth and throat may occur. These lesions may swell, causing respiratory distress in infants. (See *Identifying thrush,* page 144.)

If the patient has systemic disease, he also may report myalgia, arthralgia, chills with a high and spiking fever, prostration, and rash. Other specific complaints vary, depending on the infection site:
• Lungs—hemoptysis, cough; coarse breath sounds in the lung fields infected by *Candida*
• Kidneys—flank pain, dysuria, hematuria, cloudy urine with casts
• Brain—headache, nuchal rigidity, seizures, focal neurologic deficits
• Eyes—blurred vision, orbital or periorbital pain, exudate, floating scotomata, and lesions with a white, cotton-ball appearance seen during ophthalmoscopy

IDENTIFYING THRUSH

Candidiasis of the oropharyngeal mucosa (thrush) causes cream-colored or bluish white pseudomembranous patches on the tongue, mouth, or pharynx (as shown). Fungal invasion may extend to circumoral tissues.

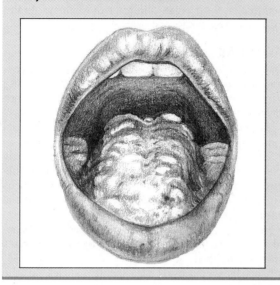

• Endocardium—chest pain and arrhythmias. Auscultation may reveal a systolic or diastolic murmur with endocarditis.

Diagnostic tests

Detection of candidal organisms by a Gram stain of skin, vaginal scrapings, pus, or sputum or on skin scrapings prepared in potassium hydroxide solution confirms the diagnosis.

Tests for systemic infection include blood and tissue cultures.

Treatment

Initial treatment aims to improve the underlying condition that predisposes the patient to candidiasis. For example, measures may be taken to control diabetes or to discontinue antibiotic therapy or catheterization, if possible.

For superficial candidiasis, the doctor may prescribe an antifungal medication, such as nystatin. Amphotericin B and gentian violet are effective for candidiasis of the skin and nails. Rarely used because it stains the skin purple, gentian violet is effective for paronychial

candidiasis, thrush, and vaginitis. Clotrimazole, fluconazole, and miconazole are effective in mucous membrane and vaginal candidiasis. And ketoconazole or fluconazole is the primary choice for chronic candidiasis of the mucous membranes.

Treatment for systemic infection consists mainly of I.V. amphotericin B, but flucytosine or miconazole may be added.

Nursing diagnoses

• Altered oral mucous membrane
• Altered urinary elimination
• Hyperthermia
• Impaired skin integrity
• Impaired swallowing
• Pain
• Risk for aspiration
• Sensory or perceptual alterations
• Sexual dysfunction

Nursing interventions

• Observe universal precautions.
• Swab nystatin on the oral mucosa of an infant with thrush. Have older children and adults swish nystatin in the mouth. Some clinicians believe that oral thrush leads to esophagitis. They suggest swallowing the nystatin after swishing.
• Provide a nonirritating mouthwash to loosen tenacious secretions and a soft toothbrush to avoid irritation.
• Relieve mouth discomfort with a topical anesthetic, such as lidocaine or benzocaine, at least 1 hour before meals. Be cautious, however: Using excessive anesthetic may suppress the gag reflex and lead to aspiration.
• Suggest a soft diet for the patient with severe dysphagia. Advise the patient with mild dysphagia to chew food thoroughly.
• Apply cornstarch, nystatin powder, or dry padding in intertriginous areas of obese patients to prevent irritation and candidal growth.
• Record dates of I.V. catheter insertion, and replace the catheter according to your hospital's policy, to prevent phlebitis.
• Frequently check vital signs of patients with systemic infection. Provide appropriate supportive care. In patients with renal involvement, carefully monitor intake and output. Also monitor blood urea nitrogen, serum creatinine, and urine blood and protein levels.
• Check high-risk patients daily, especially those receiving antibiotics. Watch for patchy areas, irritation,

sore throat, oral and gingival bleeding, and other signs of superinfection. If you note a vaginal discharge, document the color and amount.

• Assess the patient with candidiasis for underlying systemic causes, such as diabetes mellitus. If the patient is receiving amphotericin B for systemic candidiasis, he may have severe chills, fever, anorexia, nausea, vomiting, hypokalemia, and renal impairment. Premedicate him with aspirin, antihistamines, or antiemetics, as ordered, to help reduce adverse reactions.

• Carefully monitor intake and output and potassium levels while the patient is receiving medication.

• Prepare to give a blood transfusion if ordered and if the patient has a low platelet count — from underlying disease or from treatment with amphotericin B, for example.

Patient teaching

• Demonstrate comprehensive oral hygiene practices, and have the patient perform a return demonstration. Recommend that the patient use alkaline mouth care products because increased acidity promotes candidal growth.

• Tell a patient using nystatin solution to swish it around his mouth for several minutes before swallowing. Be sure he knows not to scrape the lesions but to coat them with the medication.

• Encourage a woman in her third trimester of pregnancy to be examined for vaginitis to protect her infant from thrush infection at birth.

• Direct the patient with dyspareunia to take intravaginal medication as prescribed. Listen to her concerns and reassure her that sexual impairment should resolve when her infection subsides. Tell her that her sexual partner usually won't need concomitant treatment.

CRYPTOCOCCOSIS

Usually beginning as a pulmonary infection that produces no signs or symptoms, cryptococcosis (also known as torulosis and European blastomycosis) disseminates to extrapulmonary sites, including the central nervous system (CNS), skin, bones, prostate gland, liver, and kidneys.

With treatment, the prognosis in pulmonary cryptococcosis is good. Without treatment (particularly in immunocompromised patients), the disease can lead to CNS infection and death (invariably within 3 years). Treatment dramatically reduces mortality but

not necessarily neurologic deficits, such as paralysis and hydrocephalus.

Most prevalent in men between ages 30 and 60 and rare in children, cryptococcosis is especially likely to attack immunocompromised patients, particularly those with Hodgkin's disease, sarcoidosis, leukemia, or lymphomas and those taking immunosuppressant drugs. The incidence is rising, especially in patients with acquired immunodeficiency syndrome (AIDS). In these patients, cryptococcosis is the fourth leading life-threatening infection.

In the United States, the disease occurs mostly in the central and western states. It is primarily an urban infection.

Causes

Found in dust particles contaminated by pigeon feces, the airborne fungus *Cryptococcus neoformans* causes cryptococcosis.

Complications

Optic atrophy, ataxia, hydrocephalus, deafness, paralysis, organic mental syndrome, and personality changes are possible complications of cryptococcosis.

Assessment findings

The patient's history may be unremarkable, or you may learn that the patient has human immunodeficiency virus (HIV) infection or another immunosuppressive disorder. The patient with pulmonary cryptococcosis usually is asymptomatic but may complain of dull chest pain and a cough producing a slight amount of white, blood-streaked sputum. He may or may not be febrile.

The onset of CNS involvement (cryptococcal meningitis) is gradual. It causes progressively severe frontal and temporal headache, diplopia, blurred vision, dizziness, ataxia, aphasia, vomiting, tinnitus, memory changes, inappropriate behavior, irritability, and psychosis. Untreated symptoms may progress to coma and death, usually a result of cerebral edema or hydrocephalus.

Other signs and symptoms include facial weakness, seizures (only in the late stage), and papilledema. Nuchal rigidity is typically absent, but you may elicit hyperactive reflexes.

The patient with bone involvement may complain of pain in the long bones, skull, spine, and joints.

With skin involvement, you'll observe red facial papules and other skin abscesses, with or without ulceration.

Rarely, auscultation reveals pleural friction rub or crackles.

Diagnostic tests

Although imaging tests (a routine chest X-ray or a chest computed tomography scan) showing a pulmonary lesion may point to pulmonary cryptococcosis, this infection commonly escapes diagnosis until it disseminates. A definitive diagnosis requires identification of *C. neoformans* by analysis or culture of the sputum, urine, prostatic secretions, or bone marrow aspirate. Other test procedures include tissue or pleural biopsy.

In CNS infection, *C. neoformans* detected in an India ink preparation of cerebrospinal fluid (CSF) is diagnostic. Blood cultures are positive only in severe infection.

Test results that support the diagnosis include elevated antigen titer in serum and CSF in disseminated infection; increased CSF pressure, protein levels, and white blood cell count in CNS infection; and moderately decreased CSF glucose levels in about 50% of patients. Patients with AIDS typically have slight or no CSF abnormalities, although *C. neoformans* usually can be cultured.

Treatment

Cryptococcosis is best treated with a combination of amphotericin B and flucytosine — typically for 6 weeks. Because flucytosine may produce adverse reactions, amphotericin B alone may be used in selected cases.

Intrathecal administration of amphotericin B usually is tried only in patients with CNS infection who relapse, fail to respond to I.V. administration, or develop nephrotoxicity.

Observation and excision of lesions may be sufficient treatment in previously healthy people who have a single focus of infection in the lungs or bone or on the skin and have no evidence of the organism in CSF, urine, or blood.

Nursing diagnoses
• Altered thought processes
• Impaired gas exchange
• Impaired physical mobility
• Ineffective breathing pattern
• Pain
• Risk for injury
• Sensory or perceptual alterations

Nursing interventions
• Although you needn't isolate the patient with cryptococcosis, use strict aseptic technique when administering amphotericin B intrathecally.
• Check the patient's vital signs, and note changes in mental status, orientation, pupillary response, and motor function. Watch for headache and vomiting.
• Assess the patient for phlebitis before giving I.V. amphotericin B. Infuse the drug slowly, and dilute as ordered — rapid infusion may cause circulatory collapse.
• Before therapy, draw serum for testing to determine electrolyte levels and baseline renal status. During drug therapy, watch for decreased urine output, elevated blood urea nitrogen and serum creatinine levels, and hypokalemia. Monitor complete blood count and urinalysis results. Monitor magnesium and potassium levels and hepatic function as well.
• Tell the patient to report hearing loss, tinnitus, or dizziness.
• Monitor blood levels of flucytosine, observing for adverse effects, such as diarrhea. Also be alert for decreased white blood cell and platelet counts.
• Give analgesics, antihistamines, and antiemetics, as ordered, for fever, chills, nausea, and vomiting. Manage shaking chills with small doses of meperidine or morphine sulfate, as ordered. Give these drugs in the early morning or late evening so that they don't sedate the patient for the entire day.
• Evaluate the need for long-term venous access for administering amphotericin B.
• Provide psychological support to help the patient cope with long-term treatment.
• If the patient exhibits altered mental status, reorient him throughout the day, follow a consistent routine, speak slowly and clearly, use safety measures as needed to protect him from injury, and refer him and his family to appropriate resources to plan postdischarge care.
• If the patient has vision loss, provide a safe environment. Modify the environment to maximize retained vision. Provide nonvisual sensory stimulation as possible. Encourage the patient to express his feelings, and refer him and his family to appropriate community services for information and support.

Patient teaching
• Explain medication therapy. Discuss dosage, desired drug actions, adverse effects, and need for long-term treatment.
• Urge the patient to return for follow-up care and evaluation. Typically, he'll need an examination every few

months for 1 year, even if he feels well and has no symptoms.

HISTOPLASMOSIS

This fungal infection has several other names, including Ohio Valley disease, Central Mississippi Valley disease, Appalachian Mountain disease, and Darling's disease. In the United States, histoplasmosis occurs in three forms: primary acute histoplasmosis, progressive disseminated histoplasmosis (acute disseminated or chronic disseminated disease), and chronic pulmonary (cavitary) histoplasmosis. The last form produces cavitations in the lung similar to those seen in pulmonary tuberculosis.

A fourth form, African histoplasmosis, occurs only in Africa and is caused by the fungus *Histoplasma capsulatum* var. *duboisii.*

Histoplasmosis occurs worldwide, especially in the temperate areas of Asia, Africa, Europe, and North and South America. In the United States, it's most prevalent in the central and eastern states, especially in the Mississippi and Ohio river valleys.

Probably because of occupational exposure, histoplasmosis is more common in men than in women. Fatal disseminated disease occurs more frequently in infants and elderly men.

The incubation period ranges from 5 to 18 days, although chronic pulmonary histoplasmosis may progress slowly for many years. The prognosis varies with each form. The primary acute form is benign, but the progressive disseminated form is fatal in about 90% of patients. Without proper chemotherapy, chronic pulmonary histoplasmosis is fatal in about 50% of patients within 5 years.

Causes

Histoplasmosis is caused by *H. capsulatum,* which is found in the feces of birds and bats and in soil contaminated by their feces, such as that near roosts, chicken coops, barns, caves, and underneath bridges.

Transmission occurs through inhalation of *H. capsulatum* or *H. capsulatum* var. *duboisii* spores or through the invasion of spores after minor skin trauma.

Complications

Possible complications include vascular or bronchial obstruction, acute pericarditis, pleural effusion, mediastinal fibrosis or granuloma, intestinal ulceration, Addison's disease, endocarditis, and meningitis.

Assessment findings

The patient may have a history of an immunocompromised condition or exposure to contaminated soil in an endemic area.

The severity of symptoms depends on the size of the inhaled inoculum and the immune condition of the host. Also, symptoms vary with the form of the disease. For example, a patient with *primary acute histoplasmosis* may be asymptomatic, or he may complain of a mild respiratory illness similar to a severe cold or influenza. He also may report malaise, headache, myalgia, anorexia, cough, and chest pain. A patient with *progressive disseminated histoplasmosis* may complain of anorexia, weight loss and, possibly, pain, hoarseness, and dysphagia. A patient with *chronic pulmonary histoplasmosis* may have symptoms that mimic pulmonary tuberculosis. He may complain of a productive cough, dyspnea, and occasional hemoptysis. He'll eventually experience weight loss and breathlessness.

During your assessment, you'll usually note fever, which may rise as high as 105° F (40.6° C), although its severity and duration can vary.

Inspection findings vary with the kind of histoplasmosis. A patient with primary acute histoplasmosis usually won't reveal any characteristic signs. If the patient has disseminated histoplasmosis, though, you may observe ulceration of the oropharynx, tachypnea in later stages, and pallor from anemia. You also may observe jaundice and ascites. In the patient with late-stage chronic pulmonary histoplasmosis, inspection may reveal shortness of breath, extreme weakness, and cyanosis.

Palpation may reveal hepatosplenomegaly and lymphadenopathy, characteristic findings in the progressive disseminated form of the disease.

Diagnostic tests

Miliary calcification in the lung or spleen and a positive histoplasmin skin test indicate exposure to histoplasmosis. Rising complement fixation and agglutination titers (more than 1:32) strongly suggest histoplasmosis.

Diagnosis requires a morphologic examination of tissue biopsy and culture of *H. capsulatum* from sputum in acute primary and chronic pulmonary histoplasmosis. A diagnosis of disseminated histoplasmosis requires biopsy and culture of bone marrow, lymph nodes, blood, and infection sites. Cultures take several weeks to grow these organisms.

Faster diagnosis is possible with stained biopsies, using Gomori's stains (methenamine silver) or periodic acid–Schiff reaction. Findings must rule out tuberculosis and other diseases that produce similar symptoms.

The diagnosis of histoplasmosis caused by *H. capsulatum* var. *duboisii* calls for an examination of tissue biopsy and culture of the affected site.

Treatment

Treatment includes antifungal therapy, surgery, and supportive care.

Antifungal therapy plays the most important role. Except for asymptomatic primary acute histoplasmosis (which resolves spontaneously) and the African form, histoplasmosis requires high-dose or long-term (10-week) therapy with amphotericin B or ketoconazole.

Surgery includes lung resection to remove pulmonary nodules, a shunt for increased intracranial pressure, and cardiac repair for constrictive pericarditis.

Supportive care includes oxygen for respiratory distress, glucocorticoids for adrenal insufficiency, and parenteral fluids for dysphagia caused by oral or laryngeal ulcerations. Histoplasmosis doesn't necessitate isolation.

Nursing diagnoses

- Activity intolerance
- Altered nutrition: Less than body requirements
- Decreased cardiac output
- Impaired swallowing
- Ineffective breathing pattern
- Pain
- Risk for injury

Nursing interventions

- Provide supportive nursing care for the patient with histoplasmosis.
- Administer drugs, as ordered. Because amphotericin B may cause pain, chills, fever, nausea, and vomiting, give appropriate antipyretics, antihistamines, analgesics, and antiemetics, as ordered. Small doses of meperidine or morphine sulfate may help reduce shaking chills. Give these drugs in the early morning or late evening so that they don't sedate the patient for the entire day.
- Perform a respiratory assessment every shift. Note diminished breath sounds or pleural friction rub, and evaluate for effusion.
- Refer to the chest X-ray results to determine if the patient has pulmonary or pleural effusion.

- Provide oxygen therapy if needed. Plan rest periods.
- Assess the patient's cardiovascular status every shift. If you note muffled heart sounds, jugular vein distention, pulsus paradoxus, or other signs of cardiac tamponade, report these signs to the doctor immediately.
- Assess neurologic status every shift and report any changes in level of consciousness or nuchal rigidity.
- Consult with the dietitian and patient concerning food preferences. Provide an appetizing, nutritious diet. The patient may benefit from small, frequent feedings. If he has oropharyngeal ulceration, he may need soft, bland foods. If the ulcerations are severe, he may need I.V. therapy.
- Monitor for signs and symptoms of hypoglycemia and hyperglycemia, which indicate adrenal dysfunction.
- Test all stools for blood and report its presence.
- Make sure a patient with chronic pulmonary or disseminated histoplasmosis receives psychological support to help him cope with long-term treatment. As needed, refer him to a social worker or an occupational therapist. Help the parents of a child with this disease arrange for a visiting teacher.

Patient teaching

- Teach the patient about drug therapy, including adverse effects.
- Inform the patient about the need for follow-up care on a regular basis for at least a year.
- Tell the patient to report to the doctor cardiac and pulmonary signs that could indicate effusions.
- To help prevent histoplasmosis, teach people in endemic areas to watch for early signs of this infection and to seek treatment promptly. Instruct people who risk occupational exposure to contaminated soil to wear face masks.

BLASTOMYCOSIS

Also called North American blastomycosis and Gilchrist's disease, blastomycosis is a fungal infection that usually affects the lungs and produces bronchopneumonia. During the chronic stage of illness, the disease may disseminate through the blood and cause skin disorders (most commonly), osteomyelitis, genitourinary (GU) disorders, and central nervous system (CNS) disorders (rarely). In contrast to other fungal diseases, it seldom acts as an opportunistic infection. (See *How blastomycosis progresses*.)

Blastomycosis is found in North America (where *Blastomyces dermatitidis* normally inhabits the soil)

HOW BLASTOMYCOSIS PROGRESSES

Blastomycosis can follow one of several courses, ranging from asymptomatic pneumonia followed by recovery with no further developments to symptomatic pneumonia that progresses to pulmonary disease with extrapulmonary involvement. It also can pass through both acute and chronic stages. Use the flowchart below to trace the various courses the disease can take.

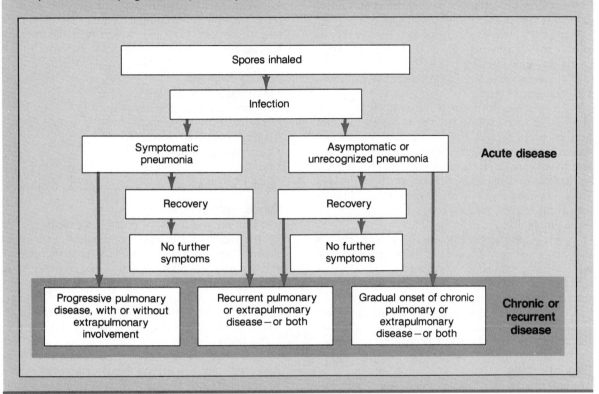

and is endemic to the southeastern United States. Sporadic cases have been reported in Africa.

The incubation period ranges from weeks to months. Untreated blastomycosis is slowly progressive and usually fatal, although spontaneous remission may occur. With antifungal drug therapy and supportive treatment, the prognosis for patients with blastomycosis is good.

Causes

Blastomycosis is caused by the yeastlike fungus *B. dermatitidis*. The fungus is probably inhaled by people whose work or recreation brings them in close contact with the soil. No occupational link has been found.

Complications

Blastomycosis can cause skin abscesses or fistulas, meningitis, cerebral abscesses, Addison's disease, pericarditis, and arthritis.

Assessment findings

The patient may report exposure to soil in a wooded area. Symptoms vary, depending on the involved site. The patient with acute pulmonary blastomycosis may complain of a dry, hacking, or productive cough (occasionally with hemoptysis); pleuritic chest pain; myalgia; and arthralgia—symptoms similar to those of a viral upper respiratory tract infection.

If the disease reaches the chronic stage, the patient may complain of a productive cough accompanied by hemoptysis, anorexia, malaise, weight loss, and pleuritic chest pain.

A patient with bone involvement usually doesn't report pain. But a patient with a GU infection may complain of deep perineal pain; patients with epididymitis, orchitis, or prostatitis also report pain.

Your assessment is likely to reveal fever and chills in the acute stage, although you may detect only a low-grade fever or no fever in the chronic stage.

With CNS involvement, inspection may reveal an altered level of consciousness (LOC), lethargy, and a change in mood or affect.

With pneumonia, inspection may show tachypnea and shortness of breath.

With cutaneous involvement, you may see two types of skin lesions on exposed body parts: small, pustular, gray or white papules that spread and become encrusted and, less frequently, ulcerative lesions.

If the disease disseminates to the bone, you may see soft-tissue swelling and redness over bony lesions. These findings usually occur in the thoracic, lumbar, and sacral regions; the long bones of the legs; and the skull (in children).

As you inspect the patient with GU involvement, you may note swelling in the groin and scrotum. His urine may appear cloudy or show hematuria.

Palpation may reveal warmth and tenderness over involved bones or genital sites.

Auscultation may disclose decreased breath sounds if consolidation occurs. In acute pulmonary infection, the lower lobes are affected most often.

Diagnostic tests
Accurate diagnosis of blastomycosis requires the following:
• a culture of *B. dermatitidis* from skin lesions, pus, sputum, or pulmonary secretions
• microscopic examination of tissue biopsy from the skin or the lungs, or of bronchial washings, sputum, or pus
• complement fixation testing (a high titer in extrapulmonary disease suggests a poor prognosis but is not conclusive)
• immunodiffusion testing to detect antibodies for the A and B antigen of blastomycosis.

Suspected pulmonary blastomycosis also requires a chest X-ray, which may show pulmonary infiltrates.

Other abnormal laboratory findings include an increased white blood cell count, an elevated erythrocyte sedimentation rate, slightly increased serum globulin levels, mild normochromic anemia, and, with bone lesions, increased alkaline phosphatase levels.

Treatment
Although amphotericin B previously was the drug of choice, ketoconazole currently is used to treat mild to moderate blastomycosis. Because ketoconazole doesn't cross the blood-brain barrier, amphotericin B is used for patients with CNS involvement. It's also used for those with life-threatening infection, those who can't tolerate ketoconazole, and those whose disease progresses despite treatment with ketoconazole.

Nursing diagnoses
• Impaired gas exchange
• Impaired physical mobility
• Impaired skin integrity
• Ineffective airway clearance
• Ineffective breathing pattern
• Pain
• Risk for injury

Nursing interventions
• Administer analgesics, as ordered, for pain.
• If the patient is receiving ketoconazole, monitor for elevated liver enzyme levels and nausea that doesn't subside. Also watch for unusual fatigue, jaundice, dark urine, and pale stools.
• If ordered, slowly infuse I.V. amphotericin B. During the infusion, closely monitor the patient's vital signs. His temperature may rise, but it should subside within 1 to 2 hours.
• Watch for adverse effects of amphotericin B, such as decreased urine output, and monitor laboratory results for increased blood urea nitrogen and serum creatinine levels as well as hypokalemia. These may indicate renal toxicity. Report hearing loss, tinnitus, or dizziness immediately.
• To relieve adverse effects of amphotericin B, give antiemetics, antihistamines, and antipyretics, as ordered. Small doses of meperidine or morphine sulfate may help to reduce shaking chills. Make sure that you administer these drugs early in the morning or late in the evening so that they don't sedate the patient for the entire day.
• If the patient has a pulmonary infection, assess his respiratory status frequently, and monitor arterial blood gas levels. Also, administer oxygen and suction the patient's airway as needed, encourage coughing and deep breathing, and observe secretions for changes in character and amount. Watch especially for hemoptysis.

• If the patient experiences joint pain or swelling, elevate the joint and apply heat.
• If CNS infection occurs, watch the patient carefully for decreasing LOC and unequal pupillary response.
• Watch for hematuria in men with disseminated disease.
• If cutaneous involvement occurs, frequently inspect the patient's skin. Also, provide supportive measures, such as assisting with hygiene, using protective skin care devices, and keeping the patient's linen clean, dry, and wrinkle-free.

Patient teaching
• Explain that the disease is infectious, but not contagious.
• Teach the patient about drug therapy, including adverse effects. Stress the importance of completing the prescribed course of treatment, which may take up to 6 months.
• Show the patient how to clean skin lesions with a bactericidal agent to prevent superinfection. Tell him he also can use soothing nondeodorant lotions.
• Inform the patient that he needs regular follow-up treatment.

COCCIDIOIDOMYCOSIS
Also called valley fever and San Joaquin Valley fever, coccidioidomycosis is a fungal infection. It occurs primarily as a respiratory infection, although generalized dissemination may occur. The *primary* pulmonary form usually is self-limiting and seldom fatal. The rare *secondary* (progressive, disseminated) form produces abscesses throughout the body and carries a mortality of up to 60%, even with treatment.

Such dissemination is more common in darkskinned men and pregnant women. Immunosuppressive conditions, especially human immunodeficiency virus infection, Hodgkin's disease, and malignant lymphoma, also are risk factors for disseminated disease.

Coccidioidomycosis is endemic to the southwestern United States, especially between the San Joaquin Valley in California and southwestern Texas. It's also found in Mexico, Guatemala, Honduras, Venezuela, Colombia, Argentina, and Paraguay.

Because of population distribution and an occupational link (it's common in migrant farm laborers), coccidioidomycosis strikes many Philippine Americans, Mexican Americans, Native Americans, and Blacks. In primary infection, the incubation period ranges from 1 to 4 weeks.

Causes
Coccidioidomycosis is caused by the fungus *Coccidioides immitis*. It may result from inhalation of *C. immitis* spores found in the soil in endemic areas, or from inhalation of spores from dressings or plaster casts of infected people. It's most prevalent during warm, dry months.

Complications
This disease can cause bronchiectasis, osteomyelitis, meningitis, hepatosplenomegaly, and liver failure.

Assessment findings
The patient may report living in or travel to an endemic area. If he has primary coccidioidomycosis, he'll usually complain of acute or subacute respiratory symptoms, such as dry cough, pleuritic chest pain, sore throat, chills, malaise, headache, anorexia, and arthralgias.

In rare cases, coccidioidomycosis disseminates to other organs several weeks or months after the primary infection. If this happens, the patient may complain of bone pain if the disease causes skeletal abscesses. He may complain of headache and a stiff neck from meningitis if central nervous system (CNS) abscesses occur. Less frequently, splenic, hepatic, renal, and subcutaneous abscesses develop.

The patient may report hemoptysis, with or without chest pain, in chronic pulmonary cavitation. This can occur in both the primary and the disseminated form.

During your assessment, you'll probably note fever. A fever that persists for weeks may be the sole sign of the disease.

In some patients—particularly white women—you may note tender red nodules (erythema nodosum) on the legs, especially the shins, on inspection. These may develop from 3 days to several weeks after onset. With musculoskeletal involvement, you may see local swelling and redness in involved sites. If the patient develops meningitis, you may note an altered level of consciousness (LOC), sluggishness, and seizures.

On palpation, you may note warmth and tenderness over involved musculoskeletal sites. You also may note nuchal rigidity if the patient has meningitis.

Diagnostic tests
Typical clinical features and skin and serologic studies confirm the diagnosis.

The primary form—and sometimes the disseminated form—produces a positive coccidioidin skin test. In the first week of illness, complement fixation for IgG antibodies, or in the first month, positive serum precipitins (immunoglobulins) also establish the diagnosis. Examination or immunodiffusion testing of sputum, pus from lesions, and a tissue biopsy may show *C. immitis* spores. Antibodies in pleural and joint fluid and a rising serum or body fluid antibody titer indicate dissemination.

Other laboratory findings include an increased white blood cell (WBC) count, an elevated erythrocyte sedimentation rate, and eosinophilia. A chest X-ray shows bilateral diffuse infiltrates.

In coccidioidal meningitis, examination of cerebrospinal fluid shows a WBC count increase to more than $500/mm^3$ (primarily from mononuclear leukocytes), increased protein levels, and decreased glucose levels. Ventricular fluid obtained from the brain may contain complement fixation antibodies.

After diagnosis, the results of serial skin tests, blood cultures, and serologic testing may document the effectiveness of therapy.

Treatment
Mild primary coccidioidomycosis usually requires only bed rest and relief of symptoms. Severe primary disease and dissemination require long-term I.V. infusion of fluids and antifungals, such as amphotericin B.

CNS dissemination calls for intrathecal administration of amphotericin B and, possibly, lesion excision or drainage. Severe pulmonary lesions may require lobectomy. Miconazole and ketoconazole suppress *C. immitis* but seldom eradicate it. Amphotericin B treatment usually lasts for 6 to 18 months, but treatment with miconazole or ketoconazole may be lifelong.

Nursing diagnoses
• Altered thought processes
• Impaired gas exchange
• Impaired skin integrity
• Ineffective breathing pattern
• Pain
• Risk for injury

Nursing interventions
• Don't wash off the circle marked on the skin for serial skin tests because this aids in reading test results.
• In mild primary disease, encourage bed rest and adequate fluid intake. Record the amount and color of sputum. Watch for shortness of breath, which may point to pleural effusion. Provide analgesics, as ordered, for a patient with arthralgia or headache.
• In the patient with pneumonia, frequently assess respiratory status, including arterial blood gas results. Administer oxygen, if needed, and encourage coughing and deep breathing.
• Coccidioidomycosis requires strict secretion precautions if the patient has draining lesions. Sterile dressing technique and careful hand washing are essential.
• If the patient has CNS dissemination, carefully monitor him for a decreased LOC, a change in mood or affect, or muscle twitching.
• Before intrathecal administration of amphotericin B, explain the procedure to the patient, and reassure him that he'll receive analgesics before a lumbar puncture. If he needs an I.V. infusion of amphotericin B, administer it slowly, as ordered. Rapid infusion may cause circulatory collapse.

During infusion, monitor the patient's vital signs. His temperature may rise but should return to normal within 1 to 2 hours. Watch for decreased urine output, and monitor laboratory test results for elevated blood urea nitrogen and creatinine levels and for hypokalemia. Tell the patient to immediately report hearing loss, tinnitus, dizziness, and all symptoms of toxicity.

To ease the adverse effects of amphotericin B, give antiemetics, antihistamines, and antipyretics, as ordered. Small doses of meperidine or morphine sulfate may help reduce shaking chills. Give these drugs in the early morning or late evening so that they don't sedate the patient for the entire day.

Patient teaching
• Teach the patient that the illness is infectious, but not contagious.
• Instruct the patient about drug therapy, including adverse effects.
• Inform the patient about the need for continued follow-up care and long-term medication management.

SPOROTRICHOSIS
A chronic fungal disease, sporotrichosis occurs in two forms: cutaneous lymphatic, the most common form, and extracutaneous. The second form includes osteoarticular sporotrichosis and the rarely occurring pulmonary sporotrichosis.

Sporotrichosis most frequently occurs among horticulturists, agricultural workers, and home gardeners.

The incubation period usually lasts from 1 week to 3 months. The prognosis for cutaneous lymphatic sporotrichosis is good, and fatalities are rare. Extracutaneous sporotrichosis is more difficult to treat and has a guarded prognosis.

Causes

Sporotrichosis is caused by the fungus *Sporothrix schenckii*, which is found in soil, wood, sphagnum moss, and decaying vegetation throughout the world. The fungus usually enters through broken skin or through inhalation (pulmonary form).

Complications

Sporotrichosis can lead to arthritis, osteomyelitis and, rarely, pneumonitis.

Assessment findings

The patient's history may reveal exposure through occupation or hobbies, such as farming or gardening.

A patient with osteoarticular sporotrichosis may complain of pain, especially in the knees, wrists, ankles, and elbows. A patient with pulmonary sporotrichosis may report a productive cough, anorexia, fatigue, weight loss and, possibly, dyspnea and hemoptysis.

During your assessment, you may note low-grade fever in a patient with either extracutaneous form.

During inspection, look for characteristic skin lesions on the patient with cutaneous lymphatic sporotrichosis, usually on the hands or fingers. Each lesion begins as a small, painless, movable, subcutaneous nodule. It then grows progressively larger, discolors and, eventually, ulcerates. Later, more lesions form along the adjacent lymph node chain. (See *Viewing cutaneous lymphatic sporotrichosis.*)

In the patient with osteoarticular sporotrichosis, you may observe edema and decreased mobility in involved joints.

Diagnostic tests

Typical clinical findings and culture of *S. schenckii* in sputum, pus, or bone drainage confirm the diagnosis. Histologic identification is difficult. Despite pulmonary symptoms, few definitive abnormalities appear on a chest X-ray.

Treatment

The cutaneous lymphatic form of the disease usually responds to application of a saturated solution of potassium iodide, usually continued for 1 to 2 months

VIEWING CUTANEOUS LYMPHATIC SPOROTRICHOSIS

Ulceration, swelling, and crusting of nodules on fingers is characteristic of cutaneous lymphatic sporotrichosis.

after lesions heal. Occasionally, cutaneous lesions must be excised or drained.

The extracutaneous form responds to I.V. amphotericin B but may require several weeks of treatment. Cavitary pulmonary lesions may require surgery.

Sporotrichosis doesn't necessitate isolation.

Nursing diagnoses

- Altered nutrition: Less than body requirements
- Fatigue
- Impaired physical mobility
- Impaired skin integrity
- Pain
- Risk for injury

Nursing interventions

- Keep lesions clean, and carefully dispose of contaminated dressings.
- Keep the patient as comfortable as possible, and apply heat to affected joints to relieve pain, if ordered.
- Administer anti-inflammatory agents, as ordered.
- If the patient is receiving I.V. amphotericin B, infuse it slowly. Rapid infusion may cause circulatory collapse.

Monitor vital signs during the infusion. Watch for decreased urine output, and check laboratory test results for elevated blood urea nitrogen, serum creatinine, and potassium levels.

If the patient reports hearing loss, tinnitus, dizziness, or other signs of toxicity, give antiemetics, antihistamines, and antipyretics, as ordered. Small doses of meperidine or morphine sulfate may help reduce shaking chills. Give these drugs in the early morning or late evening so that they don't sedate the patient for the entire day.
• If joint involvement impairs the patient's mobility, encourage warm soaks, progressive movement, and range-of-motion exercises, unless contraindicated. Refer the patient to a physical therapist, if needed.

Patient teaching
• Inform the patient that the illness is infectious but not contagious.
• Teach the patient about drug therapy, and tell him to immediately report adverse effects.
• To help prevent sporotrichosis, advise horticulturists, agricultural workers, and home gardeners to wear gloves while working.
• Encourage the patient to return for follow-up appointments.

VIRUSES

Several hundred different viruses may infect humans and are spread chiefly by humans themselves. Diagnosis often remains difficult. Viral diseases are not susceptible to antibiotics, but sometimes antibiotics are used to prevent complications.

COMMON COLD
An acute, usually afebrile viral infection, the common cold causes inflammation of the upper respiratory tract. The most common infectious disease, it's more prevalent in children, adolescent boys, and women. In temperate climates, it occurs more often in the colder months; in the tropics, during the rainy season. Colds usually are benign and self-limiting, but they cause more lost time from school or work than any other illness.

Causes
About 90% of colds stem from a viral infection of the upper respiratory tract passages and consequent mucous membrane inflammation. Some colds result from mycoplasma. More than 100 viruses can cause the common cold. Major offenders include rhinoviruses, coronaviruses, myxoviruses, adenoviruses, coxsackieviruses, and echoviruses.

A cold is communicable for 2 to 3 days after the onset of symptoms. Transmission occurs through airborne respiratory droplets or through contact with contaminated objects, including hands. Children acquire new strains from their schoolmates and pass them on to family members. Contrary to popular belief, fatigue or drafts don't increase susceptibility.

Complications
Secondary bacterial infection may occur, causing sinusitis, otitis media, pharyngitis, or lower respiratory tract infection.

Assessment findings
The patient's history may reveal exposure to others with the common cold. After an incubation period of 1 to 4 days, the patient initially complains of nasal congestion, headache, and burning, watery eyes. He also may report chills, myalgia, arthralgia, malaise, lethargy, and a hacking, nonproductive, or nocturnal cough. Most patients are afebrile, although fever may occur, especially in children.

Clinical features develop more fully as the cold progresses. By the second day (in addition to initial symptoms), the patient may report a copious nasal discharge that often irritates the nose, adding to his discomfort. About 3 days after onset, major symptoms diminish, but the "stuffed up" feeling often persists for a week. Reinfection (with productive cough) is common, but complications are rare.

Inspection may reveal a reddened nose and eyes and nasal discharge. The nasal and pharyngeal mucous membranes may exhibit increased erythema, and the patient's voice may have a nasal quality. The skin around the nose may be excoriated because of frequent nose blowing.

Diagnostic tests
No explicit diagnostic test exists to isolate the specific organism responsible for the common cold. Despite infection, white blood cell count and differential are within normal limits. Diagnosis must rule out allergic rhinitis, measles, rubella, and other disorders that pro-

duce similar early symptoms. A temperature higher than 100° F (37.8° C), severe malaise, anorexia, tachycardia, exudate on the tonsils or throat, petechiae, and tender lymph glands may point to a more serious disorder and require additional diagnostic tests.

Treatment

Because the common cold has no cure, the primary treatment — aspirin or acetaminophen, fluids, and rest — is purely symptomatic. Aspirin and acetaminophen ease myalgia and headache; fluids help loosen accumulated respiratory secretions and maintain hydration; and rest combats fatigue and weakness. Because aspirin has been associated with Reye's syndrome in children, acetaminophen is the drug of choice for a child with a cold and fever.

Decongestants can relieve nasal congestion. Throat lozenges relieve soreness, and steam encourages expectoration. Nasal douching, sinus drainage, and antibiotics aren't necessary except in complications or chronic illness. Pure antitussives relieve severe coughs but are contraindicated with productive coughs when cough suppression is harmful. The role of vitamin C remains controversial. In infants, saline nose drops and mucus aspiration with a bulb syringe may be beneficial.

No preventive measures currently are available. Vitamin therapy, interferon administration, and ultraviolet irradiation are under investigation.

Nursing diagnoses
• Fatigue
• Impaired skin integrity
• Knowledge deficit
• Pain

Nursing interventions
• Administer antipyretics and analgesics, as ordered.
• Refer the patient for medical care if he has a persistent high fever, changes in level of consciousness, or significant respiratory symptoms.

Patient teaching
• Emphasize that antibiotics don't cure the common cold.
• Tell the patient to stay in bed for the first few days; to use a lubricant on his nostrils to decrease irritation; to relieve throat irritation with sugarless hard candy or cough drops; to increase fluid intake; and to eat light meals.

• A warm bath or heating pad can reduce aches and pains but won't hasten a cure. Suggest a hot or cold steam vaporizer to relieve nasal congestion. Commercial expectorants are available, but their effectiveness is questionable.
• Advise against overuse of nose drops or sprays because these may cause rebound congestion.
• To help prevent colds, warn the patient to minimize contact with people who have them. To avoid spreading colds, tell him to wash his hands often, to cover his mouth and nose when he coughs or sneezes, to avoid sharing towels and drinking glasses, and to properly dispose of used tissues.

RESPIRATORY SYNCYTIAL VIRUS INFECTION

Occurring almost exclusively in infants and young children, respiratory syncytial virus infection is the leading cause of lower respiratory tract infections, pneumonia, tracheobronchitis, and bronchiolitis in this age-group. It's also a suspected cause of the fatal respiratory diseases of infancy.

Antibody titers suggest that most children under age 4 have contracted some, often mild, form of respiratory syncytial virus infection. In fact, bronchiolitis associated with this disorder peaks at age 2 months, making it the only viral disease that has its maximum impact during the first few months of life.

This virus creates annual epidemics during the late winter and early spring in temperate climates and during the rainy season in the tropics.

Causes

Respiratory syncytial virus infection results from a subgroup of the myxoviruses that resemble paramyxovirus. The organism is transmitted from person to person by respiratory secretions and has an incubation period of 4 to 5 days.

Reinfection is common, producing milder symptoms than the primary infection. School-age children, adolescents, and young adults with mild reinfections are probably the source of infection for infants and young children.

Complications

Young children, especially infants, are at increased risk for severe infection. Common complications include pneumonia, bronchiolitis, tracheobronchitis, and otitis media. Acute complications include apnea and respiratory failure.

Assessment findings

Signs and symptoms vary in severity. The patient may complain of nasal congestion, coughing, wheezing, malaise, sore throat, earache, dyspnea, and fever. Although uncommon, signs of central nervous system infection, such as weakness, irritability, and nuchal rigidity, also may be observed.

Inspection usually reveals inflamed mucous membranes in the nose and throat. Other findings are variable. For example, with otitis media, you may see a hyperemic eardrum on otoscopic examination; with severe respiratory distress, you may note nasal flaring, retraction, cyanosis, and tachypnea. With a lower respiratory tract infection, you may hear or auscultate wheezes, rhonchi, and crackles.

Diagnostic tests

• Cultures of nasal and pharyngeal secretions may show respiratory syncytial virus; however, the virus is very labile, so cultures aren't always reliable.
• Serum antibody titers may be elevated, but in infants under age 6 months, maternal antibodies may impair test results.
• Two serologic techniques that give rapid results are indirect immunofluorescence and the enzyme-linked immunosorbent assay (ELISA). However, these tests are an impractical diagnostic tool because serum specimens aren't obtained until 4 weeks after onset of illness. They're mainly used for epidemiologic studies.

Treatment

Appropriate treatment aims to support respiratory function, maintain fluid balance, and relieve symptoms. Ribavirin, a broad-spectrum antiviral agent, is being used successfully to treat infants with severe lower respiratory tract infection caused by the respiratory syncytial virus. The aerosol form of the drug is given by way of tent, oxygen hood, mask, or ventilator for 2 to 5 days, 12 to 18 hours a day. With this drug therapy, patients show less severe symptoms and improvements in arterial oxygen saturation.

Nursing diagnoses

• Activity intolerance
• Altered family processes
• Altered nutrition: Less than body requirements
• Diversional activity deficit
• Fatigue

• Impaired gas exchange
• Impaired social interaction
• Ineffective airway clearance
• Ineffective family coping
• Risk for aspiration
• Risk for fluid volume deficit
• Risk for infection

Nursing interventions

• Monitor the patient's respiratory status. Observe the rate and pattern; watch for nasal flaring or retraction, cyanosis, pallor, and dyspnea; listen or auscultate for wheezes, rhonchi, or other signs of potential respiratory distress. Monitor arterial blood gases and arterial oxygen saturation.
• Maintain a patent airway, and be especially watchful during periods of acute dyspnea. Perform percussion, and provide drainage and suction, when necessary. Administer oxygen, as ordered. If appropriate, use a croup tent to provide a high-humidity atmosphere. Semi-Fowler's position may help prevent aspiration of secretions.
• Carefully monitor intake and output. Observe for signs of dehydration, such as decreased skin turgor. Encourage the intake of high-calorie fluids, and administer I.V. fluids, as needed.
• Promote bed rest. Plan your nursing care to allow uninterrupted rest.
• Hold, talk to, and play with infants and young children. Offer diversional activities suited to the child's condition and age. Encourage parents to visit often and to cuddle their child.
• To prevent nosocomial infection on pediatric units, don't care for infants with respiratory syncytial virus infection if you have a respiratory illness yourself. Place infants with this infection on contact isolation (those infected with the same organism can share a room). Enforce strict hand washing for staff members and visitors, and impose oral secretions precautions.

Patient teaching

• Describe respiratory syncytial virus infection transmission methods to parents, and caution against taking infants into crowds.
• Explain all procedures and treatments to parents and, when appropriate, to children.
• If the patient is being cared for at home, explain the need for adequate rest, fluids, and nourishment.
• Teach the parents about drugs the child is taking and about adverse effects that should be reported.

• Teach the parents what signs and symptoms of serious complications to watch for and report.

PARAINFLUENZA

Widespread in infants and children and rare in adults, parainfluenza resembles influenza but is milder and seldom fatal. This self-limiting disease causes both upper and lower respiratory tract illness and is more common in children in the winter and spring.

Causes

Parainfluenza refers to any of a group of respiratory illnesses caused by paramyxoviruses, a subgroup of the myxoviruses. It's transmitted by direct contact or by inhalation of contaminated airborne droplets, and it has an incubation period of about 3 to 6 days.

Paramyxoviruses occur in four forms—Para 1 to 4—that are linked to several diseases: croup (Para 1, 2, and 3), acute febrile respiratory illnesses (1, 2, and 3), the common cold (1, 3, and 4), pharyngitis (1, 3, and 4), bronchitis (1 and 3), and bronchopneumonia (1 and 3). Para 3 is the second most common infecting organism that causes lower respiratory tract infections in children (respiratory syncytial virus infection ranks first). Para 4 seldom causes symptomatic infections in humans.

By age 8, most children demonstrate antibodies to Para 1 and Para 3. Most adults have antibodies to all four types as a result of childhood infections and subsequent multiple exposures. Reinfection usually is less severe and affects only the upper respiratory tract.

Complications

Possible complications include croup, bronchiolitis, and pneumonia. Bacterial complications are uncommon.

Assessment findings

The patient may complain of signs and symptoms that are similar to those of other respiratory diseases: nasal discharge, cough, chills, and muscle pain. A temperature over 100° F (37.8° C) for 2 or 3 days is common.

Inspection may reveal pharyngeal erythema (with little or no exudate). Other findings depend on whether complications develop. For example, nasal flaring and sternal retractions indicate respiratory distress; listlessness may indicate hypoxemia.

Palpation may reveal the absence of cervical adenopathy. Chest auscultation usually detects rhonchi or, in croup, stridor of the upper airways.

Diagnostic tests

Parainfluenza usually is clinically indistinguishable from similar viral infections. Isolation of the virus and serum antibody titers differentiate parainfluenza from other respiratory illness, but they seldom are done.

Treatment

No antiviral therapy or vaccine has been developed for parainfluenza infections.

Parainfluenza may require no treatment, or it may require bed rest, antipyretics, analgesics, and antitussives, depending on the severity of symptoms. Hospitalization seldom is necessary unless complications, such as croup or pneumonia, develop.

Nursing diagnoses

• Activity intolerance
• Fatigue
• Hyperthermia
• Knowledge deficit
• Pain
• Risk for fluid volume deficit
• Risk for infection

Nursing interventions

• Administer analgesics, antipyretics, and antitussives, as ordered.
• Encourage adequate rest and fluid intake.
• Promote careful hand washing.

Patient teaching

• Instruct the patient or family about the need for bed rest, antipyretics, analgesics, and antitussives, as well as the need for adequate fluids and for performing careful hand washing.
• Teach the patient or parents about the various signs and symptoms of complications. Tell them to call the doctor if these occur because additional treatment will be needed.

ADENOVIRAL INFECTIONS

Adenoviruses cause acute, self-limiting, febrile infections, with inflammation of the respiratory or the ocular mucous membranes or both. There are 35 known serotypes. These viruses produce five major infections, all of which occur in epidemics. They are common in all age-groups and may remain latent for years.

Adenoviruses affect almost everyone early in life, although maternal antibodies offer some protection during the first 6 months.

COMPARING MAJOR ADENOVIRAL INFECTIONS

Use this chart to review major adenoviral infections, the age-group affected, and characteristic clinical features.

Infection	Age-group	Clinical features
Acute febrile respiratory illness	Children	Nonspecific coldlike signs, similar to those of other viral respiratory illnesses: fever, pharyngitis, tracheitis, bronchitis, pneumonitis
Acute respiratory disease	Adults (usually military recruits)	Malaise, fever, chills, headache, pharyngitis, hoarseness, and dry cough
Viral pneumonia	Children and adults	Sudden onset of high fever, rapid infection of upper and lower respiratory tracts, rash, diarrhea, intestinal intussusception
Acute pharyngoconjunctival fever	Children (particularly after swimming in pools or lakes)	Spiking fever lasting for several days, headache, pharyngitis, conjunctivitis, rhinitis, cervical adenitis
Acute follicular conjunctivitis	Adults	Unilateral tearing and mucoid discharge; later, milder symptoms in other eye
Epidemic keratoconjunctivitis	Adults	Unilateral or bilateral ocular redness and edema, periorbital swelling, local discomfort, superficial opacity of the cornea without ulceration

Causes

Transmission occurs by direct inoculation into the eye, by fecal-oral contamination (adenoviruses may persist in the GI tract for years after infection), or by inhalation of an infected droplet. The incubation period usually is less than 1 week. Although the acute illness lasts less than 5 days, it may be followed by prolonged asymptomatic reinfection.

Complications

Acute conjunctivitis, sinusitis, pharyngitis, and pneumonia are potential complications of adenoviral infections.

Assessment findings

Clinical features vary with the type of infection. (For more information, see *Comparing major adenoviral infections.*)

Diagnostic tests

Definitive diagnosis requires isolation of the virus from respiratory or ocular secretions or from fecal smears. During epidemics, typical symptoms alone allow the doctor to make a diagnosis. Because adenoviral illnesses resolve quickly, serum antibody titers aren't useful for diagnosis. Blood tests show lymphocytosis in children. A chest X-ray may show pneumonitis when a respiratory disease is present.

Treatment

No specific drugs are effective against adenoviruses, so treatment is mainly supportive. Ocular infections may require corticosteroids and direct supervision by an ophthalmologist. Infants with pneumonia should be hospitalized to monitor for and treat symptoms that can cause death; those with keratoconjunctivitis require hospitalization to treat symptoms that can cause blindness. An experimental treatment, enteric-coated oral vaccines, has been used successfully in military recruits. Parenteral vaccines, which were used previously, aren't recommended because they caused a hybrid virus.

Nursing diagnoses

• Altered nutrition: Less than body requirements
• Diarrhea
• Fatigue
• Hyperthermia

- Impaired gas exchange
- Impaired skin integrity
- Pain
- Risk for fluid volume deficit
- Risk for infection
- Sensory or perceptual alterations

Nursing interventions
- During the acute stage, monitor the patient's respiratory status and intake and output. Provide respiratory care measures for the infant hospitalized with pneumonia.
- Check the patient's eyes for redness, itching, and drainage.
- Plan care to provide rest periods.
- Ensure adequate fluid and nutritional intake.
- Administer ordered medications to relieve symptoms.

Patient teaching
- Explain supportive care measures, such as bed rest, adequate fluid intake, analgesics, and antipyretics.
- To help minimize the incidence of adenoviral disease, teach the patient proper hand-washing techniques to reduce fecal-oral transmission.
- Inform the patient, patient groups, and other health care workers that keratoconjunctivitis can be prevented by avoiding swimming pools during epidemics of keratoconjunctivitis, by adequately chlorinating swimming pools, and by sterilizing ophthalmic instruments.

INFLUENZA
Also called the grippe or the flu, influenza is an acute, highly contagious infection of the respiratory tract.

Although it affects all age-groups, the highest incidence occurs in schoolchildren. The greatest severity is in young children, elderly people, and those with chronic diseases. In these groups, influenza may even lead to death.

Influenza occurs sporadically or in epidemics (usually during the colder months). Epidemics usually peak within 2 to 3 weeks after initial cases and subside within a month. The catastrophic pandemic of 1918 was responsible for an estimated 20 million deaths. The most recent pandemics—in 1957, 1968, and 1977—began in mainland China.

Causes
Influenza results from three types of virus. Type A, the most prevalent, strikes every year, with new serotypes causing epidemics every 3 years. Type B also strikes annually but only causes epidemics every 4 to 6 years. Type C is endemic and causes only sporadic cases.

The infection is transmitted by inhaling a respiratory droplet from an infected person or by indirect contact, such as drinking from a contaminated glass. The virus then invades the epithelium of the respiratory tract, causing inflammation and desquamation. (See *How influenza viruses multiply,* page 160.)

One remarkable feature of the influenza virus is its capacity for antigenic variation—that is, its ability to mutate into different strains so that no immunologic resistance is present in those at risk. Antigenic variation is characterized as *antigenic drift* (minor changes that occur yearly or every few years) and *antigenic shift* (major changes that lead to pandemics).

Complications
The most common complication of influenza is pneumonia, which can be primary influenza viral pneumonia or secondary to bacterial infection. Influenza also may cause myositis, exacerbation of chronic obstructive pulmonary disease, Reye's syndrome and, rarely, myocarditis, pericarditis, transverse myelitis, and encephalitis.

Assessment findings
The patient's history usually reveals recent exposure to a person with influenza. Most patients say that they didn't receive the influenza vaccine during the past season.

After an incubation period of 24 to 48 hours, flu symptoms appear. The patient may report sudden onset of chills, fever (101° to 104° F [38.3° to 40° C]), headache, malaise, myalgia (particularly in the back and limbs), photophobia, a nonproductive cough and, occasionally, laryngitis, hoarseness, rhinitis, and rhinorrhea. Fever usually is higher in children, who also may show signs of croup. These signs usually subside in 3 to 5 days, but cough and weakness may persist. Some patients (especially elderly people) may feel tired and listless for several weeks.

Inspection initially may reveal red, watery eyes; erythema of the nose and throat without exudate; and clear nasal discharge.

As the disease progresses, respiratory findings become more apparent. The patient frequently coughs and looks tired. If pulmonary complications occur, tachypnea, cyanosis, and shortness of breath may be noted.

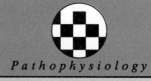

Pathophysiology

HOW INFLUENZA VIRUSES MULTIPLY

Classified as type A, B, or C, an influenza virus contains the genetic material ribonucleic acid (RNA) covered and protected by protein. The RNA is arranged in genes that carry the instruction for viral replication. This genetic material has an extraordinary ability to mutate, causing the generation of new serologically distinct strains of influenza virus. Being a virus, the pathogen cannot reproduce or carry out chemical reactions on its own. It needs a host cell.

Following attachment to the host cell, the viral

RNA enters the host cell and uses host components to replicate its genetic material and protein, which are then assembled into the new virus particles. These newly produced viruses can burst forth to invade other healthy cells.

The viral invasion destroys the host cells, impairing respiratory defenses, especially the mucociliary transport system, and predisposing the patient to secondary bacterial infection.

1. Virus attaches to host.

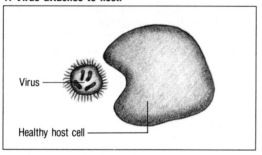

Virus

Healthy host cell

2. Viral RNA enters host cell.

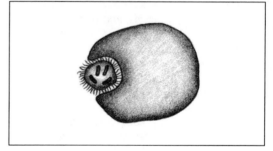

3. Viral RNA replicates within host cell.

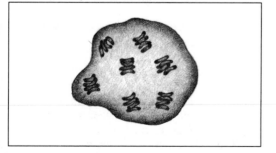

4. New virus particles are assembled and released.

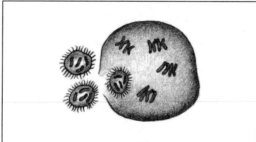

With bacterial pneumonia, you'll see purulent or bloody sputum.

Palpation may reveal cervical adenopathy and tenderness, especially in children. Auscultation may disclose transient gurgles or crackles. With pneumonia, breath sounds may be diminished in areas of consolidation.

Diagnostic tests

At the beginning of an influenza epidemic, many patients are misdiagnosed with other respiratory disorders. Because signs and symptoms of influenza aren't pathognomonic, isolation of the influenza virus through inoculation of chicken embryos (with nasal secretions from infected patients) is essential at the first sign of an epidemic. In addition, nose and throat cultures and increased serum antibody titers help confirm the diagnosis.

Once an epidemic is confirmed, diagnosis requires only observation of clinical signs and symptoms. Uncomplicated cases show decreased white blood cells with an increase in lymphocytes.

Treatment

The patient with uncomplicated influenza needs bed rest, adequate fluid intake, acetaminophen or aspirin to relieve fever and muscle pain (children should only receive acetaminophen), and guaifenesin or another expectorant to relieve nonproductive coughing. Prophylactic antibiotics aren't recommended; they have no effect on the influenza virus.

The antiviral agent amantadine has effectively reduced the duration of influenza A infection. In influenza complicated by pneumonia, the patient needs supportive care (fluid and electrolyte replacements, oxygen, and assisted ventilation) and treatment of bacterial superinfection with appropriate antibiotics. No specific therapy exists for cardiac, central nervous system, or other complications.

Nursing diagnoses

- Altered health maintenance
- Fatigue
- Hyperthermia
- Impaired skin integrity
- Ineffective breathing pattern
- Pain
- Risk for fluid volume deficit
- Risk for infection

Nursing interventions

- Administer analgesics, antipyretics, and decongestants, as ordered.
- Watch for signs and symptoms of developing pneumonia, such as crackles, increased fever, chest pain, dyspnea, and coughing accompanied by purulent or bloody sputum.
- Follow respiratory and blood and body fluid precautions.
- Provide cool, humidified air, but change the water daily to prevent *Pseudomonas* superinfection.
- Encourage the patient to rest in bed and drink plenty of fluids. Administer I.V. fluids, as ordered.
- Administer oxygen therapy, if warranted.
- Help the patient to gradually return to his normal activities.

Patient teaching

- Influenza usually doesn't require hospitalization. Teach the home patient about supportive care measures and signs and symptoms of serious complications.
- Advise the patient to use mouthwash or warm saline gargles to ease sore throat.
- Teach the patient the importance of increased fluids to prevent dehydration.
- Suggest a warm bath or a heating pad to relieve myalgia.
- Advise the patient to use a vaporizer to provide cool, moist air, but to clean the reservoir and change the water every 8 hours.
- Teach the patient how to dispose of tissues properly and proper hand-washing technique to prevent the virus from spreading.
- Discuss influenza immmunization. Suggest that high-risk patients and health care workers get an annual inoculation at the start of flu season (late autumn). Explain that each year's vaccine is based on the previous year's virus and usually is about 75% effective.

Tell a patient receiving the vaccine about possible adverse effects (discomfort at the vaccination site, fever, malaise and, rarely, Guillain-Barré syndrome).

Remember that the vaccine isn't recommended for pregnant women unless they have chronic diseases and are highly susceptible to influenza. The vaccine also shouldn't be given to anyone who's allergic to eggs, feathers, or chickens because it's made from chicken embryos. (Amantadine is an effective alternative for these people.)

HANTAVIRUS PULMONARY SYNDROME

Mainly occurring in the southwestern United States, hantavirus pulmonary syndrome is a new viral disease first reported in May 1993. The syndrome, which causes flulike symptoms and rapidly progresses to respiratory failure, is known for its high mortality. The hantavirus strain that causes disease in Asia and Europe — mainly hemorrhagic fever and renal disease — is distinctly different from the one currently found in North America. (See *Sin Nombre virus,* page 162.)

Causes

A member of the Bunyaviridae family, the genus *Hantavirus* (first isolated in 1977) is responsible for hantavirus pulmonary syndrome. Disease transmission is associated with exposure to infected rodents, which

SIN NOMBRE VIRUS

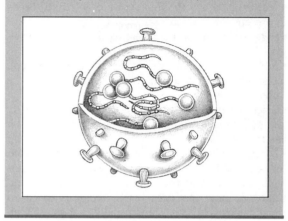

This illustration shows the Sin Nombre virus, the most common cause of hantavirus pulmonary syndrome in the United States and Canada. It exists primarily in western states and provinces.

are the primary reservoir for this virus. Data suggest that deer mice are the main source, but piñon mice, brush mice, and western chipmunks living in close proximity to humans in rural areas are also carriers. Hantavirus infections have been documented in people whose activities are associated with rodent contact, such as farming, hiking or camping in rodent-infested areas, and occupying rodent-infested dwellings.

Infected rodents manifest no apparent illness. However, they shed the virus in their feces, urine, and saliva. Human infection may occur from inhalation, ingestion (of contaminated food or water, for example), contact with rodent excrement, or rodent bites. Other means of transmission—from person to person or by mosquitos, fleas, or other arthropods—have not been reported.

Complications
Hantavirus pulmonary syndrome can very quickly progress to respiratory failure, possibly leading to death.

Assessment findings
Noncardiogenic pulmonary edema distinguishes this syndrome. Common chief complaints include myalgia, fever, headache, nausea, vomiting, and cough. Respiratory distress typically follows the onset of a cough. Fever, hypoxia and, in some patients, serious hypotension typify the hospital course.

Other signs and symptoms include a rising respiratory rate (28 breaths/minute or more) and an increased heart rate (120 beats/minute or more).

Diagnostic tests
Despite ongoing efforts to identify clinical and laboratory features that distinguish hantavirus pulmonary syndrome from other infections with similar features, diagnosis currently rests mainly on clinical suspicion in conjunction with a process of elimination developed by the Centers for Disease Control and Prevention (CDC) with the Council of State and Territorial Epidemiologists. (See *Screening for hantavirus pulmonary syndrome.*)

Note: The CDC and state health departments can perform definitive testing for hantavirus exposure and antibody formation.

Laboratory studies usually reveal an elevated white blood cell count with a predominance of neutrophils, myeloid precursors, and atypical lymphocytes. Tests also show an elevated hematocrit level, a decreased platelet count, an elevated partial thromboplastin time, and a normal fibrinogen level. Usually, laboratory findings demonstrate only minimal abnormalities in renal function, with serum creatinine levels no higher than 2.5 mg/dl.

Chest X-rays eventually show bilateral diffuse infiltrates in almost all patients (findings consistent with adult respiratory distress syndrome).

Treatment
Primarily supportive, treatment consists of maintaining adequate oxygenation, monitoring vital signs, and intervening to stabilize the patient's heart rate and blood pressure.

Drug therapy includes administration of vasopressors, such as dopamine or epinephrine, for hypotension. Fluid volume replacement may also be necessary, although precautions must be taken not to overhydrate the patient.

Recent investigational drug therapy involves ongoing clinical trials with ribavirin.

Nursing diagnoses
- Altered health maintenance
- Fatigue
- Hyperthermia
- Impaired gas exchange
- Ineffective breathing pattern
- Pain
- Risk for fluid volume deficit
- Risk for infection

SCREENING FOR HANTAVIRUS PULMONARY SYNDROME

The Centers for Disease Control and Prevention (CDC) has developed a screening procedure to track cases of hantavirus pulmonary syndrome. The screening criteria identify potential and actual cases.

Potential cases
For a diagnosis of possible hantavirus pulmonary syndrome, a patient must have one of the following:
• a febrile illness (temperature equal to or above 101° F [38.3° C]) occurring in a previously healthy person and characterized by unexplained adult respiratory distress syndrome
• bilateral interstitial pulmonary infiltrates that develop within 1 week of hospitalization and cause respiratory compromise that requires supplemental oxygen
• an unexplained respiratory illness that results in death and autopsy findings that demonstrate non-cardiogenic pulmonary edema without an identifiable specific cause of death.

Exclusions
Of the patients who meet the criteria for having potential hantavirus pulmonary syndrome, the CDC excludes those who have any of the following:

• a predisposing underlying medical condition (for example, severe underlying pulmonary disease, solid tumors or hematologic cancers, congenital or acquired immunodeficiency disorders) or a medical condition such as rheumatoid arthritis or organ transplantation that requires immunosuppressive drug therapy (for example, steroids or cytotoxic chemotherapy)
• an acute illness that provides a likely explanation for the respiratory illness—for example, a recent major trauma, burn, or surgery; a recent seizure disorder or history of aspiration; bacterial sepsis; another respiratory disorder such as respiratory syncytial virus in young children; influenza; or pneumonia caused by *Legionella*.

Confirmed cases
Cases of confirmed hantavirus pulmonary syndrome must include the following:
• at least one serum or tissue specimen that shows evidence of hantavirus infection
• in a patient with a compatible clinical illness, serologic evidence (presence of hantavirus-specific immunoglobulin M or rising titers of immunoglobulin G), polymerase chain reaction for hantavirus ribonucleic acid, or a positive immunohistochemistry test for the hantavirus antigen.

Nursing interventions
• Assess the patient's respiratory status and arterial blood gas values often.
• Monitor serum electrolyte levels and correct imbalances as appropriate.
• Maintain a patent airway by suctioning. Ensure adequate humidification, and check mechanical ventilator settings frequently.
• If the patient is hypoxic, assess his neurologic status frequently as well as his heart rate and blood pressure.
• Administer drug therapy and monitor the patient's response.
• Provide I.V. fluid therapy based on results of hemodynamic monitoring.
• Provide emotional support for the patient and his family.
• Report cases of hantavirus pulmonary syndrome to your state health department.
• Provide patients with prevention guidelines. (Until more is known about hantavirus pulmonary syndrome, preventive measures currently focus on rodent control.)

Patient teaching
• Teach the patient about his disorder, and answer any questions he might have.
• Fully discuss all treatments, procedures, and diagnostic tests with the patient, and explain why they have been ordered.

INFECTIOUS MONONUCLEOSIS
An acute infectious disease, mononucleosis causes fever, sore throat, and cervical lymphadenopathy, the hallmarks of the disease. It also causes hepatic dysfunction, increased lymphocytes and monocytes, and development and persistence of heterophil antibodies. The disease primarily affects young adults and children, although in children, it's usually so mild that it's often overlooked.

The disease is fairly prevalent in the United States, Canada, and Europe, and both sexes are affected equally. Incidence varies seasonally among college students but not among the general population.

The prognosis is excellent, and major complications are uncommon.

Causes

Infectious mononucleosis is caused by the Epstein-Barr virus (EBV), a member of the herpes group. Apparently, the reservoir of EBV is limited to humans.

The disease probably spreads by the oropharyngeal route. About 80% of patients carry EBV in the throat during the acute stage and for an indefinite time afterward. It also can be transmitted by blood transfusion and has been reported in cardiac surgery patients as the "post-pump perfusion" syndrome. The disease is probably contagious from before symptoms develop until the fever subsides and oropharyngeal lesions disappear.

Complications

Although major complications are rare, mononucleosis may cause splenic rupture, aseptic meningitis, encephalitis, hemolytic anemia, pericarditis, and Guillain-Barré syndrome.

Assessment findings

The patient's history may reveal contact with a person who has infectious mononucleosis.

After an incubation period of about 10 days in children and 30 to 50 days in adults, the patient may experience prodromal symptoms. He usually reports headache, malaise, profound fatigue, anorexia, myalgia, and, possibly, abdominal discomfort. After 3 to 5 days, he develops a sore throat, which he may describe as the worst he's ever had, and dysphagia related to adenopathy. He'll usually have a fever, typically with a late afternoon or evening peak of 101° to 102° F (38.3° to 38.9° C).

Your inspection commonly reveals exudative tonsillitis, pharyngitis, and, sometimes, palatal petechiae, periorbital edema, maculopapular rash that resembles rubella, and jaundice.

On palpation, you'll probably note that nodes are mildly tender. You'll usually find cervical adenopathy with slight tenderness, but the patient also may have inguinal and axillary adenopathy. You may detect splenomegaly and, less commonly, hepatomegaly.

Auscultation of the chest usually is normal.

Diagnostic tests

The following abnormal laboratory test results confirm infectious mononucleosis:
• An increase in white blood cell (WBC) count of 10,000 to 20,000/mm³ during the second and third weeks of illness. Lymphocytes and monocytes account for 50% to 70% of the total WBC count; 10% of the lymphocytes are atypical.
• A fourfold rise in heterophil antibodies (agglutinins for sheep red blood cells) in serum drawn during the acute phase and at 3- to 4-week intervals.
• Antibodies to EBV and cellular antigens shown on indirect immunofluorescence. Such testing usually is more definitive than heterophil antibodies but may not be necessary because the vast majority of patients are heterophil-positive.
• Abnormal liver function studies.

Treatment

Infectious mononucleosis isn't easily prevented, and it's resistant to standard antimicrobial treatment. Thus, therapy is essentially supportive: relief of symptoms, bed rest during the acute febrile period, and aspirin or another salicylate for headache and sore throat.

If severe throat inflammation causes airway obstruction, steroids can relieve swelling and prevent a tracheotomy. Splenic rupture, marked by sudden abdominal pain, requires splenectomy. About 20% of patients with infectious mononucleosis also have streptococcal pharyngotonsillitis and should receive antibiotic therapy for at least 10 days.

Nursing diagnoses

• Activity intolerance
• Altered nutrition: Less than body requirements
• Altered role performance
• Fatigue
• Hyperthermia
• Impaired skin integrity
• Impaired social interaction
• Knowledge deficit
• Pain
• Risk for fluid volume deficit
• Risk for injury

Nursing interventions

• Administer medications to treat symptoms, as needed.
• Provide warm saline gargles for symptomatic relief of sore throat.
• Provide adequate fluids and nutrition.
• Plan care to provide frequent rest periods.

Patient teaching

• Explain that convalescence may take several weeks, usually until the patient's WBC count returns to normal.

• Stress the need for bed rest during the acute illness. Warn the patient to avoid excessive activity, which could lead to splenic rupture.

• If the patient is a student, tell him that he can continue less demanding school assignments and see his friends but that he should avoid long, difficult projects until after recovery.

• To minimize throat discomfort, encourage the patient to drink milk shakes, fruit juices, and broths, and to eat cool, bland foods. Advise using warm saline gargles, analgesics, and antipyretics, as needed.

CYTOMEGALOVIRUS INFECTION

Also called generalized salivary gland disease and cytomegalic inclusion disease, cytomegalovirus (CMV) occurs worldwide. A herpesvirus, the disease is transmitted by human contact.

About four out of five persons over age 35 have been infected with CMV, usually during childhood or early adulthood. In most, the disease is so mild that it's overlooked. However, CMV can be devastating to a fetus or to an immunosuppressed patient.

Causes

The infection results from the cytomegalovirus, an ether-sensitive, DNA virus belonging to the herpes family. CMV has been found in the saliva, urine, semen, breast milk, feces, blood, and vaginal and cervical secretions of infected people.

Transmission occurs through direct contact with secretions and excretions, through blood transfusions, transplacentally, and through transplanted organs (patients who receive organs from a CMV-seropositive donor run a 90% chance of contracting the infection). CMV in cervical secretions can infect a sexual partner, or an infant during passage through the birth canal. CMV is present in the semen of homosexual men and may be transmitted through sexual activity; such transmission hasn't yet been proved in heterosexual men.

The disease probably spreads through the body in lymphocytes or mononuclear cells to the lungs, liver, GI tract, eyes, and central nervous system (CNS), where it often produces inflammatory reactions.

Complications

Immunosuppressed patients, such as those with acquired immunodeficiency syndrome, may develop opportunistic infections, such as pneumonia, hepatitis, ulceration of the GI tract, retinitis, and encephalopathy.

Congenital CMV can lead to stillbirth, neonatal retinitis, microcephaly, mental retardation, seizures and, later, hearing loss. The infant also can develop thrombocytopenia and hemolytic anemia.

Assessment findings

The adult patient's history may reveal an immunosuppressive condition. He may complain of mild, nonspecific clinical symptoms, such as fatigue, myalgia, and headache – or he may have no symptoms.

Other immunosuppressed patients may suffer extensive organ involvement. For example, a patient with CMV pneumonia may complain of a nonproductive cough and dyspnea with hypoxia. A patient with CMV colitis may report explosive watery diarrhea. A patient with CMV ulcerative disease may have GI bleeding. And a patient with CMV retinitis may complain of blurred vision and scotoma, which can progress to blindness in one or both eyes.

Fever is common. In an immunocompetent patient with CMV mononucleosis, 3 or more weeks of irregular high fever may be the only symptom.

Inspection findings vary in immunosuppressed patients. With respiratory involvement, you may note tachypnea, shortness of breath, cyanosis, and coughing, but seldom sputum production. With liver involvement, you may note jaundice and spider angiomas.

Inspection of an infant with congenital CMV infection may reveal signs of CNS damage, such as mental retardation and hearing loss, or jaundice, a petechial rash, seizures, and respiratory distress.

Palpation in all CMV patients may reveal splenomegaly and hepatomegaly.

Diagnostic tests

Isolating the virus or demonstrating rising serologic titers allows diagnosis of CMV. Complement fixation studies, hemagglutination inhibition antibody tests, and, in congenital infections, indirect immunofluorescent tests for CMV immunoglobulin M antibody may be performed. Chest X-ray typically shows bilateral, diffuse, white infiltrates.

The perfection of the CMV early antigen test has led to improved diagnosis and early treatment.

Treatment

Although antiviral therapy for herpesviruses has had encouraging results, CMV is more difficult to prevent and treat than other herpesviruses. Ganciclovir and, less frequently, high-dose acyclovir prove helpful for certain patients, although relapse may occur. Immunoglobulin G specific to CMV can also be given with ganciclovir. The second line of therapy is foscarnet.

Nursing diagnoses
• Activity intolerance
• Altered nutrition: Less than body requirements
• Altered parenting
• Diarrhea
• Fatigue
• Hyperthermia
• Impaired gas exchange
• Ineffective breathing pattern
• Ineffective family coping
• Pain
• Risk for infection
• Risk for injury
• Sensory or perceptual alterations

Nursing interventions
• Institute universal precautions before coming into contact with the patient's blood or other body fluids. Secretion precautions are especially important for infants known to be shedding CMV.
• Administer medications to treat symptoms as needed.
• Monitor intake and output. Offer nutritionally adequate meals. If the patient has diarrhea, replace fluids.
• Provide emotional support and counseling to the parents of a child with severe CMV infection. Help them find support systems, and coordinate referrals to other health care professionals.
• Monitor a patient with splenomegaly for signs of rupture, and protect him from excess activity and injury.
• For the patient with impaired vision, provide a safe environment and encourage optimal independence. Make referrals to community resources, as needed.
• For the patient with respiratory involvement, frequently assess ventilation status, and administer oxygen and assist ventilation, as needed. Position the patient in a semi-Fowler's or sitting position to facilitate ventilation.

Patient teaching
• Advise women health care workers trying to get pregnant to have CMV titers drawn to identify their risk of contracting the infection. A study done by the Centers for Disease Control showed that 50% of pregnant women exposed to CMV also had fetal exposure, with 20% of the fetuses contracting the infection.

• Urge the patient (especially if the patient is a child, who may be unconcerned with personal hygiene) to wash his hands thoroughly to help prevent contagion.
• Tell parents—especially the mother, if she's of child-bearing age—to wear gloves when coming into contact with secretions or changing diapers of a baby with congenital CMV. They should dispose of diapers and soiled articles properly and wash their hands thoroughly.
• Warn an immunosuppressed or pregnant patient to avoid contact with any person who has confirmed or suspected CMV infection.
• Tell an immunosuppressed patient who is CMV-seronegative to carry this information with him and to relay it to any caregiver. This way, he won't be given CMV-positive blood.

POLIOMYELITIS
Also called polio and infantile paralysis, poliomyelitis is an acute communicable disease caused by the poliovirus. It ranges in severity from inapparent infection to fatal paralytic illness.

First recognized in 1840, the disease became epidemic in Norway and Sweden in 1905. Outbreaks reached pandemic proportions in Europe, North America, Australia, and New Zealand during the first half of this century. Incidence peaked during the 1940s and early 1950s and led to the development of the Salk vaccine. (See *Polio protection*.)

Minor polio outbreaks still occasionally occur among nonimmunized groups, such as the Amish of Pennsylvania in 1979. Otherwise, only 5 to 10 cases (associated with the use of oral poliovirus vaccine) are reported in the United States annually.

Polio strikes most often during the summer and fall. Once mainly confined to infants and children, it's now more common in people over age 15. Among children, it most often paralyzes boys; girls and adults are at greater risk of infection but not of paralysis.

The prognosis largely depends on the site affected. If the central nervous system (CNS) is spared, the prognosis is excellent. However, CNS infection can cause paralysis and death. The mortality for all types of polio is 5% to 10%.

Causes
The poliovirus (an enterovirus) has three antigenically distinct serotypes—types 1, 2, and 3—that cause polio. These polioviruses are found worldwide and are transmitted from person to person by direct contact with infected oropharyngeal secretions or

POLIO PROTECTION

Dr. Jonas Salk's poliomyelitis vaccine, which became available in 1955, has been one of the miracle drugs of modern medicine. The vaccine contains dead (formalin-inactivated) polioviruses that stimulate production of circulating antibodies in the human body. It has effectively eliminated the once-feared disease.

The vaccine of choice

However, even miracle drugs can be improved. Today, the Sabin vaccine, which can be taken orally and is more than 90% effective, is the vaccine of choice in preventing poliomyelitis. This vaccine is available in trivalent and monovalent forms. Both forms contain live but weakened viruses. The trivalent form is the vaccine of choice because it contains all three poliovirus serotypes in one solution.

It's preferred to the monovalent form, which contains only one viral type and is useful only when the particular serotype is known.

Sabin vaccine risks

Because of the small risk of contracting polio from the vaccine, it's contraindicated in patients with immunodeficiency diseases, leukemia, or lymphoma, and in those receiving corticosteroids, antimetabolites, other immunosuppressants, or radiation therapy. These patients usually are immunized with the Salk vaccine, instead.

When possible, immunodeficient patients should avoid contact with family members who've received the Sabin vaccine for at least 2 weeks after vaccination.

The Sabin vaccine is no longer routinely advised for adults unless they're apt to be exposed to the disease or plan to travel to endemic areas.

---

feces. The incubation period ranges from 5 to 35 days (7 to 14 days is average).

The virus usually enters the body through the alimentary tract, multiplies in the oropharynx and lower intestinal tract, and then spreads to regional lymph nodes and blood. Factors that increase the probability of paralysis include pregnancy, old age, unusual physical exertion at or just before the clinical onset of poliomyelitis, and localized trauma, such as a recent tonsillectomy, tooth extraction, or inoculation.

Most major cases in the United States are related to the oral poliovirus vaccine (OPV) and occur in children under age 4. Infection occurs 7 to 21 days after administration of OPV and usually is associated with the first dose of the vaccine. OPV-related cases also occur in young adults, who show symptoms 20 to 29 days later.

Complications

Possible complications include respiratory failure, pulmonary edema, pulmonary embolism, hypertension, urinary tract infection, urolithiasis, atelectasis, pneumonia, myocarditis, cor pulmonale, soft-tissue and skeletal deformities, and paralytic ileus.

In polio survivors, latent poliomyelitis can lead to muscle spasticity and weakness 10 to 15 years after the initial infection. Delayed poliomyelitis also can affect respiratory muscles, leading to hypoxemia.

Assessment findings

Today, most cases of polio are so minor that the patient doesn't even visit the doctor. Inapparent, or subclinical, poliomyelitis (95% of all cases) has no symptoms. Abortive poliomyelitis (4% to 8% of all cases) is over in about 72 hours, with the patient experiencing only a slight fever, malaise, headache, sore throat, and vomiting.

The third type, major poliomyelitis, is most likely to be reported. It involves the CNS and takes two forms: nonparalytic and paralytic. In children, the course often is biphasic, with the onset of major illness occurring after recovery from the minor illness stage.

The most perilous paralytic form, bulbar paralytic poliomyelitis, occurs when the virus affects the medulla of the brain. This type usually weakens the muscles supplied by the cranial nerves (particularly the ninth and tenth).

A patient with nonparalytic poliomyelitis complains of moderate fever, headache, vomiting, lethargy, irritability, and pains in the neck, back, arms, legs, and abdomen.

Paralytic poliomyelitis usually develops within 5 to 7 days after the onset of fever. The patient complains of symptoms similar to those of nonparalytic poliomyelitis and then develops weakness and paralysis. The patient also may report related signs and symptoms, such as paresthesia, urine retention, constipation, and abdominal distention.

The patient with bulbar paralytic poliomyelitis may complain of facial weakness, dysphasia, difficulty in chewing, inability to swallow or expel saliva, regurgitation of food through the nasal passages, and dyspnea.

Your examination of the patient with nonparalytic poliomyelitis may reveal muscle tenderness and spasms in the extensors of the neck and back and sometimes in the hamstring and other muscles. (These spasms may be observed during maximum range-of-motion exercises.) This type of polio usually lasts about 1 week, with meningeal irritation persisting for about 2 weeks.

Examination of the patient with paralytic poliomyelitis may show asymmetrical weakness and flaccid paralysis of various muscles. He'll display Hoyne's sign — his head will fall back when he's supine and his shoulders are elevated. He also won't be able to raise his legs a full 90 degrees. The extent of paralysis depends on the level of the spinal cord lesions, which may be cervical, thoracic, or lumbar.

In both nonparalytic and paralytic polio, you may observe resistance to neck flexion — the patient will extend his arms behind him for support ("tripod") when he sits up.

Diagnostic tests

Isolation of the poliovirus from throat washings early in the disease and from stools throughout the disease confirms the diagnosis. If the patient has a CNS infection, cerebrospinal fluid cultures may aid diagnosis. Coxsackievirus and echovirus infections must be ruled out. Convalescent serum antibody titers four times greater than acute titers support a diagnosis of poliomyelitis.

Treatment

Poliomyelitis calls for supportive treatment, including analgesics to ease headache, back pain, and leg spasms. Morphine is contraindicated because of the danger of additional respiratory depression. Moist heat applications also may reduce muscle spasm and pain.

Bed rest is necessary until extreme discomfort subsides. It also helps prevent increased paralysis. Patients with paralytic polio may be bedridden for a long time and then require long-term rehabilitation, using physical therapy, braces, and corrective shoes. Orthopedic surgery also may be necessary.

Bladder involvement may require catheterization, and respiratory muscle involvement may require mechanical ventilation. Postural drainage and suction may be sufficient to manage pooling of secretions in patients with nonparalytic polio.

Nursing diagnoses

- Activity intolerance
- Altered family processes
- Altered growth and development
- Altered urinary elimination
- Constipation
- Impaired gas exchange
- Impaired physical mobility
- Impaired skin integrity
- Impaired social interaction
- Impaired swallowing
- Ineffective airway clearance
- Ineffective breathing pattern
- Ineffective family coping
- Ineffective individual coping
- Pain
- Powerlessness
- Risk for aspiration
- Risk for disuse syndrome
- Risk for infection
- Self-care deficit
- Sensory or perceptual alterations

Nursing interventions

- Observe for signs of paralysis and other neurologic damage, which can occur rapidly. Maintain a patent airway, and look for respiratory weakness and difficulty swallowing. Endotracheal intubation commonly is performed at the first sign of respiratory distress, and the patient is placed on a ventilator.
- Perform a brief neurologic assessment at least once a day, but don't demand any vigorous muscle activity. Encourage a return to mild activity as soon as possible.
- Frequently check blood pressure, especially if the patient has bulbar poliomyelitis. This form of the disease can cause hypertension or shock.
- Watch for signs of fecal impaction, caused by dehydration and intestinal inactivity. To prevent this, give enough fluids to ensure an adequate daily urine output of low specific gravity (1.5 to 2 liters/day for adults).
- Monitor the bedridden patient's food intake to make sure he's receiving an adequate, well-balanced diet. Provide tube feedings when needed.
- To prevent pressure ulcers, provide good skin care, reposition the patient often, and keep the bed linens dry.

• Assess bladder distention. Muscle paralysis may cause bladder weakness or transient bladder paralysis with urine retention.

• Have the patient wear high-top sneakers or use a footboard to prevent footdrop. To alleviate discomfort, use foam rubber pads and sandbags or light splints, as ordered.

• To control the spread of infection, wash your hands thoroughly after contact with the patient or any of his excretions.

• Provide emotional support to the patient and his family. Long-term support and encouragement are essential for maximum rehabilitation. Reassure the nonparalytic patient that his chances for recovery are good.

• When caring for a paralytic patient, help set up an interdisciplinary rehabilitation program with physical and occupational therapists and doctors. A psychiatrist also may help the patient and family accept the patient's physical disabilities.

• Report all polio cases to local public health authorities.

Patient teaching

• Inform the ambulatory patient about the need for careful hand washing.

• Warn any hospital worker who hasn't been vaccinated against polio to avoid contact with the patient.

• Instruct the patient or caregivers about measures needed to manage symptoms and prevent complications.

• Help the patient establish a support system of family, friends, or health care workers to assist him at home.

• Encourage parents to have children vaccinated against polio. Reassure them that the risk of vaccine-related disease is small.

VARICELLA

Chicken pox, the common name for varicella, is an acute, highly contagious infection that can occur at any age but is most common in children ages 2 to 8. Congenital varicella may affect infants whose mothers had acute infections in their first or early second trimester. Neonatal infection is rare, probably because of transient maternal immunity. Second attacks also are rare.

Chicken pox occurs worldwide and is endemic in large cities. Outbreaks occur sporadically and with varying severity, usually in areas with large groups of susceptible children. It affects all races and both sexes equally. Seasonal distribution varies; in temperate

Warning

CHICKEN POX AND REYE'S SYNDROME

If Reye's syndrome develops in a patient with chicken pox, signs and symptoms usually appear in the later stages of the disease. In the hospitalized patient, watch for such signs and symptoms as vomiting, restlessness, irritability, and a progressively decreased level of consciousness—all associated with progressive cerebral edema. The patient eventually develops encephalopathy, characterized by elevated serum ammonia and transaminase levels, bleeding diathesis, and hyperglycemia.

If the patient will be cared for at home, teach the signs and symptoms of Reye's syndrome to his parents. Also, because aspirin use has been linked to the development of Reye's syndrome, warn parents *not* to give aspirin to their child.

areas, incidence is higher during late autumn, winter, and spring.

Most children recover completely. However, potentially fatal complications may affect children receiving corticosteroids, antimetabolites, or other immunosuppressants, and those with leukemia, other malignant diseases, or immunodeficiency disorders. Congenital and adult varicella also may have severe effects.

Causes

Chicken pox is caused by the varicella-zoster herpesvirus—the same virus that, in its latent stage, causes herpes zoster (shingles). Transmission occurs through direct contact (primarily with respiratory secretions, less often with skin lesions) and indirect contact (through airwaves).

The incubation period lasts from 13 to 17 days. The disease probably is communicable from 1 day before lesions erupt to 6 days after vesicles form. It's most contagious in the early stages of lesion eruption.

Complications

Severe pruritus with this rash may provoke scratching, which can lead to infection, scarring, impetigo, furuncles, and cellulitis. Rare complications include Reye's syndrome (see *Chicken pox and Reye's syndrome*), pneumonia, myocarditis, bleeding disorders, arthritis, nephritis, hepatitis, and acute myositis.

Congenital varicella causes hypoplastic deformity and limb scarring, retarded growth, and central nervous system and eye problems.

Assessment findings

The patient's history reveals exposure within the past 2 to 3 weeks to someone with chicken pox.

During the prodromal phase, the patient complains of malaise, headache, and anorexia. When lesions develop, he also may report pruritus.

Your examination may reveal a temperature of 101° to 103° F (38.3° to 39.4° C), which usually persists for 3 to 5 days but, in the immunocompromised patient, may last for more than 7 days.

Within 24 hours of the prodromal phase onset, you may observe the rash, beginning as crops of small, erythematous macules on the trunk or scalp. The macules progress to papules and then clear vesicles on an erythematous base (the so-called dewdrop on a rose petal). The vesicles become cloudy and break easily; then scabs form. The rash spreads to the face and, rarely, to the extremities.

New vesicles continue to appear for 3 to 4 days, so the rash contains a combination of red papules, vesicles, and scabs in various stages. Shallow ulcers may develop on mucous membranes of the mouth, conjunctivae, and genitalia.

Inspection of an immunocompromised patient reveals more numerous lesions. These often are hemorrhagic and take longer to heal.

Diagnostic tests

Although diagnosis usually doesn't require laboratory tests, the virus can be isolated from vesicular fluid within the first 3 to 4 days of the rash. Giemsa stain distinguishes the varicella-zoster virus from the vaccinia-variola virus. Serum samples contain antibodies 7 days after onset of symptoms.

Treatment

Chicken pox calls for strict isolation until all the vesicles and most of the scabs disappear (usually for 1 week after the onset of the rash). Children can go back to school if just a few scabs remain; at this stage, chicken pox is no longer contagious. Congenital chicken pox requires no isolation.

Treatment consists of local or systemic antipruritics, such as calamine lotion, diphenhydramine or another antihistamine, or cool sponge baths with baking soda.

The patient doesn't need antibiotics unless bacterial infection develops. Salicylates are contraindicated because of their link with Reye's syndrome. Instead, the patient can receive acetaminophen as an analgesic and antipyretic. Antiviral drugs and corticosteroids aren't used to treat immunocompetent patients.

Immunosuppressed patients may need special treatment. When given up to 72 hours after exposure to chicken pox, varicella-zoster immune globulin may provide passive immunity. Vidarabine may slow vesicle formation, speed skin healing, and control the systemic spread of infection.

Nursing diagnoses

- Hyperthermia
- Impaired skin integrity
- Risk for infection
- Social isolation

Nursing interventions

- Observe an immunocompromised patient for manifestations of complications, such as pneumonitis and meningitis, and report them immediately.
- Provide skin care comfort measures. Use calamine lotion or cornstarch to relieve itching. Sponge baths or showers may increase comfort (tub baths may encourage the spread of the vesicles).
- If ordered, administer acetaminophen. Also administer varicella-zoster immune globulin, if ordered, to lessen the severity of the disease. Institute strict isolation measures until all skin lesions have crusted.
- To help prevent the spread of chicken pox, don't admit a child exposed to chicken pox to a unit that contains children who receive immunosuppressants or who have leukemia or immunodeficiency disorders.

Patient teaching

- Explain that the patient will probably receive treatment at home if he's immunocompetent.
- Teach the child and his family how to correctly apply topical antipruritic medications. Stress the importance of good hygiene.
- Tell the patient not to scratch the lesions. Because the need to scratch may be overwhelming, tell parents to trim their child's fingernails, tie mittens on his hands, or, possibly, use sedatives.
- Warn the parents to watch for and immediately report signs of complications. Severe skin pain, burning, or purulent discharge may indicate a serious secondary infection and require prompt medical attention.

• Caution the parents not to give the child aspirin because of its association with Reye's syndrome.
• To manage a fever, instruct the parents to give acetaminophen and tepid sponge baths, to dress the child in light clothing, and to maintain a cool environment.

RUBELLA

Commonly called German measles, rubella is an acute, mildly contagious viral disease that produces a distinctive 3-day rash and lymphadenopathy.

Worldwide in distribution, rubella flourishes during the spring (particularly in big cities), with epidemics occurring sporadically. It occurs most commonly among children ages 5 to 9, adolescents, and young adults.

The disease is self-limiting, and the prognosis is excellent—except for congenital rubella, which can have disastrous consequences.

Causes

The rubella virus is transmitted through contact with the blood, urine, stools, or nasopharyngeal secretions of infected people. It's communicable from about 10 days before until 5 days after the rash appears. Rubella can also be transmitted transplacentally. Humans are the only known hosts for the virus.

Complications

Rubella can cause arthritis, which usually is transient and mainly affects women; hemorrhagic problems, seen more often in children; and, less commonly, encephalitis, myocarditis, thrombocytopenia, and hepatitis. Complications associated with congenital rubella are serious and may be fatal.

Assessment findings

The patient's history may reveal inadequate immunization, exposure to someone with rubella infection within the past 2 to 3 weeks, or recent travel to an endemic area without reimmunization.

Children usually don't have prodromal symptoms, but adolescents and adults may report headache, malaise, anorexia, coryza, sore throat, and cough before the rash appears. Some adults also report symptoms of polyarthralgias and polyarthritis.

In all patients, the rash may be accompanied by a low-grade fever (99° to 101° F [37.2° to 38.3° C]), which usually disappears after the first day of the rash. In rare instances, a patient's temperature may reach 104° F (40° C).

Examination reveals an exanthematous, maculopapular, mildly pruritic rash that typically begins on the face and then spreads rapidly, often covering the trunk and extremities within hours. Small, red, petechial macules on the soft palate (Forschheimer spots) may precede or accompany the rash.

By the end of the second day, the rash begins to fade in the opposite order in which it appeared. The facial rash subsides, but the trunk rash may be confluent and hard to distinguish from a scarlet fever rash. It usually disappears on the third day but may persist for 4 to 5 days, sometimes accompanied by mild coryza and conjunctivitis. The rapid appearance and disappearance of the rubella rash distinguishes it from rubeola.

Palpation detects suboccipital, postauricular, and postcervical lymph node enlargement, a hallmark of rubella.

Diagnostic tests

Clinical signs and symptoms usually are sufficient to make a diagnosis, so laboratory tests seldom are done. Cell cultures of the throat, blood, urine, and cerebrospinal fluid, along with convalescent serum that shows a fourfold rise in antibody titers, confirm the diagnosis. Rubella-specific IgM antibody also can be determined by laboratory testing.

Congenital rubella can be diagnosed by determining the presence of rubella-specific IgM antibody in cord blood.

Treatment

Because the rubella rash is self-limiting and only mildly pruritic, it doesn't require topical or systemic medication. Treatment consists of antipyretics and analgesics for fever and joint pain. Bed rest isn't necessary, but the patient should be isolated until the rash disappears.

Immunization with the live rubella virus vaccine (RA 27/3), the only rubella vaccine available in the United States, is necessary for prevention. The vaccine should be given with measles and mumps vaccines at age 15 months to decrease the cost and number of injections needed. Repeat immunizations should be given to anyone immunized before 1960 and then every 10 years thereafter.

Nursing diagnoses

• Altered parenting
• Diversional activity deficit
• Fear
• Hyperthermia

• Impaired skin integrity
• Ineffective family coping (with congenital rubella)
• Pain

Nursing interventions
• Make the patient with active rubella as comfortable as possible. Keep the skin clean and dry.
• Administer antipyretics and analgesics, as ordered.
• If the patient is a child, give him books to read or games to play to keep him occupied.
• Institute isolation precautions until 5 days after the rash disappears. An infant with congenital rubella needs to be isolated for 3 months, until three throat cultures are negative.
• Ensure that only hospital workers who aren't at risk for rubella provide patient care. If ordered, administer immune globulin to anyone seeing the patient who hasn't been immunized.
• Report confirmed cases of rubella to local public health officials.
• Know how to manage rubella immunization before giving the vaccine. First, ask about allergies, especially to neomycin. If the patient has this allergy or if he's had a reaction to any immunization in the past, check with the doctor before giving the vaccine.

If the patient is a woman of childbearing age, ask her if she's pregnant. If she is or thinks she may be, *don't* give the vaccine.

Give the vaccine at least 3 months after any administration of immune globulin or blood. These substances may have antibodies that could neutralize the vaccine.

Don't vaccinate an immunocompromised patient, a patient with immunodeficiency diseases, or a patient receiving immunosuppressant, radiation, or corticosteroid therapy. Instead, administer immune serum globulin, as ordered, to prevent or reduce infection.

After giving the vaccine, observe for signs of anaphylaxis for at least 30 minutes. Keep epinephrine 1:1,000 nearby.
• Provide the parents of an infant with congenital rubella with support, counseling, and referrals, as needed.

Patient teaching
• Explain to the hospitalized patient or his family why respiratory isolation is necessary.
• Warn family members and visitors that rubella can be devastating to an unborn baby. Be sure the patient understands how important it is to avoid exposing pregnant women to this disease.

• Warn women who receive the rubella vaccine to use an effective means of birth control for at least 3 months after immunization.
• After giving the vaccine, warn about possible mild fever, slight rash, transient arthralgia (in adolescents), and arthritis (in elderly people). If the patient is an adult, suggest treating fever with aspirin or acetaminophen. Tell the parents of a child receiving the vaccine not to give him aspirin because of the danger of Reye's syndrome.
• Advise the patient to apply warmth to the injection site on and off for 24 hours after immunization to help the body absorb the vaccine. If swelling persists after 24 hours, suggest a cold compress to promote vasoconstriction and prevent antigenic cyst formation.
• Explain congenital rubella to the parents of an infant with that disease.

RUBEOLA
Also called morbilli and commonly called measles, rubeola is an acute, highly contagious infection that causes a characteristic rash. Measles is one of the most common and most serious communicable childhood diseases.

Although the measles vaccine has reduced the number of cases in children, the disease is becoming more prevalent in adolescents and adults, probably because of inadequate immunization. (See *Administering measles vaccine.*) In fact, a 300% increase in reported cases has occurred in the United States since 1986.

In temperate zones, incidence is highest in late winter and early spring. Before the measles vaccine, epidemics occurred every 2 to 5 years in large urban areas.

In the United States, the prognosis usually is excellent, but measles is a major cause of death in children in underdeveloped countries.

Causes
Measles is caused by the rubeola virus, a paramyxovirus. It's spread by direct contact or by contaminated airborne respiratory droplets. The portal of entry is the upper respiratory tract.

Complications
Severe infection may lead to secondary bacterial infection and to autoimmune reaction or organ invasion by the virus. This can result in otitis media, cervical adenitis, laryngitis, laryngotracheitis, pneumonia, and encephalitis.

ADMINISTERING MEASLES VACCINE

Follow these steps whenever you administer measles vaccine:
• Warn the patient or his parents that possible adverse effects of measles vaccine include anorexia, malaise, rash, mild thrombocytopenia or leukopenia, and fever. These reactions usually occur within 7 to 10 days.
• Ask about known allergies, especially to neomycin, because each dose contains a small amount of this drug. A patient who's allergic to eggs may receive the vaccine because it contains only minimal amounts of albumin and yolk components.
• Ask a woman patient of childbearing age if she's pregnant. If she is or thinks she might be, don't give the vaccine.
• Caution a woman patient to use reliable birth control methods for at least 3 months after vaccination.
• Don't vaccinate a child who has untreated tuberculosis, immunodeficiency, leukemia, or lymphoma, or a child who is receiving immunosuppressants. Instead, recommend that he receive gamma globulin if he's exposed to measles. (Gamma globulin won't prevent measles but will lessen its severity.)
   An older, nonimmunized child who has been exposed to measles for more than 5 days also may require gamma globulin, but be sure to immunize him 3 months later.
• Delay vaccination for 8 to 12 weeks after administration of whole blood, plasma, or gamma globulin;

measles antibodies in these components may neutralize the vaccine.
• Watch for signs of anaphylaxis for 30 minutes after vaccination. Keep epinephrine 1:1,000 handy.
• Advise the patient to apply a warm compress to the vaccination site to facilitate absorption of the vaccine. If swelling occurs within 24 hours after vaccination, tell the patient to apply cold compresses to promote vasoconstriction and prevent antigenic cyst formation.

Other considerations
One bout of measles usually renders immunity (a second infection is rare and may represent misdiagnosis). Infants under age 4 months may be immune because of circulating maternal antibodies.
   Under normal conditions, measles vaccine isn't administered to children younger than age 15 months. However, during an epidemic, infants as young as 6 months may receive the vaccine; then they will need reimmunization at age 15 months. An alternate approach calls for administration of gamma globulin to infants between ages 6 and 15 months who are likely to be exposed to measles. The risk of measles substantially increases after age 12 for people who received the vaccine at age 15 months. Because of this, the American Academy of Pediatrics recommends a second dose of measles vaccine before junior high school.

Subacute sclerosing panencephalitis, a rare and invariably fatal complication, may develop several years after measles. This complication is less common in patients who have received the measles vaccine.

Immunosuppressive measles encephalitis is an opportunistic infection that afflicts immunocompromised patients and occurs from 5 weeks to 6 months after measles. It causes progressive neurologic deterioration and can be fatal.

Assessment findings
The patient's history may reveal inadequate immunization and exposure to someone with measles within the past 10 to 14 days.

Symptoms begin and greatest communicability occurs during a 4- to 5-day prodromal phase about 11 days after exposure. The patient may complain of photophobia, malaise, anorexia, coryza, hoarseness, and a hacking cough. His temperature also may be elevated during this phase, peaking to 103° to 105° F (39.4° to 40.6° C).

Throughout the disease, symptoms vary in severity. They're usually mild in patients with partial immunity (conferred by administration of gamma globulin), in infants with transplacental antibodies, and in children. More severe symptoms and complications may develop in young infants, adolescents, adults, and immunocompromised patients.

During the prodromal phase, your examination may reveal periorbital edema and red, irritated conjunctiva. At the end of the prodromal phase, you may see Koplik's spots, the hallmark of the disease. These are tiny, bluish gray specks surrounded by a red halo that appear on the oral mucosa opposite the molars and occasionally bleed.

About 5 days after Koplik's spots appear, you may note that the patient's temperature rises sharply, spots slough off, and a slightly pruritic rash appears. This rash starts as faint macules behind the ears and on the neck and cheeks. The macules become papular and erythematous, rapidly spreading over the face, neck, eyelids, arms, chest, back, abdomen, and thighs. When the rash reaches the feet (2 to 3 days later), it begins to fade in the same sequence it appeared, leaving a brown discoloration that disappears in 7 to 10 days.

The disease climax occurs 2 to 3 days after the rash appears. At this time, your assessment may reveal a severe cough, puffy red eyes, and rhinorrhea. About 5 days after the rash appears, other symptoms disappear and communicability ends.

At any point in the disease, palpation may detect lymphadenopathy.

If the patient received the killed measles vaccine instead of the live, attenuated vaccine currently used, he may develop signs and symptoms of atypical measles. On examination, the patient appears acutely ill, with a fever and a maculopapular rash that's most obvious in the arms and legs. He may have pulmonary involvement and no skin lesions.

Diagnostic tests

Several tests may be ordered to differentiate measles from rubella, roseola infantum, enterovirus infection, toxoplasmosis, and drug eruptions. If necessary, measles virus may be isolated from the blood, nasopharyngeal secretions, and urine during the febrile period. Serum antibodies appear within 3 days after onset of the rash and reach peak titers 2 to 4 weeks later.

Treatment

The patient should receive antipyretics to control fever. Vaporizers and a warm environment help reduce respiratory irritation, but cough preparations and antibiotics are usually ineffective. Therapy also must combat complications.

Nursing diagnoses

- Altered nutrition: Less than body requirements
- Altered oral mucous membrane
- Fatigue
- Hyperthermia
- Impaired skin integrity
- Risk for infection
- Sensory or perceptual alterations (visual)

Nursing interventions

- Institute respiratory isolation measures for 4 days after the onset of the rash. Also follow universal blood and body fluid precautions.
- Encourage bed rest during the acute period.
- Administer saline eyedrops for irritation and antipyretics for fever.
- If you're using a vaporizer, clean it and change the water every 8 hours.
- If ordered, administer immune globulin to provide passive immunization to people at high risk who come in contact with the patient.
- To prevent the spread of disease, administer measles vaccine.
- Report measles cases to local health authorities.

Patient teaching

- Teach the patient or his parents supportive measures. Stress the need for isolation, bed rest, and increased fluids. The skin should be kept clean and dry. Eye irritation can be soothed by removing crusts and secretions with warm water. If photophobia occurs, advise darkening the room or using sunglasses. Fever can be reduced with antipyretics and tepid sponge baths.
- If a vaporizer is used, remind the patient or his parents to clean it and change the water every 8 hours.
- Warn parents to watch for and report the early signs and symptoms of complications.

MUMPS

An acute inflammation of one or both parotid glands, mumps (also called infectious or epidemic parotitis) is most prevalent in children older than age 5 and younger than age 9. The disease seldom occurs in infants under age 1 because of passive immunity from maternal antibodies.

Peak incidence takes place during late winter and early spring. The prognosis for complete recovery is good, although some patients, especially postpubertal males, have serious complications. One attack of mumps (even with only unilateral infection) usually confers lifelong immunity.

Causes

A paramyxovirus found in the saliva of an infected person causes mumps. Transmitted by droplets or by direct contact, the virus can be detected in the saliva 6 days before to 9 days after the parotid glands swell. The disease probably is most communicable in the 48 hours immediately before the onset of swelling. The incubation period ranges from 12 to 25 days (the average is 18 days).

Complications

Epididymo-orchitis occurs in about 25% of postpubertal males who contract mumps. This complication results in testicular swelling and tenderness, scrotal erythema, lower abdominal pain, nausea, vomiting, fever, and chills. Swelling and tenderness may last for several weeks. Epididymitis may precede or accompany orchitis. About 50% of men with mumps-induced orchitis exhibit testicular atrophy, with sterility occurring only when both testes are affected.

Mumps meningitis occurs in about 10% of mumps victims and affects male patients three to five times more often than female patients. Symptoms include fever, meningeal irritation (nuchal rigidity, headache, and irritability), vomiting, drowsiness, and a cerebrospinal fluid (CSF) lymphocyte count from 500 to 2,000/mm³.

Less common complications include pancreatitis, transient sensorineural hearing loss, transverse myelitis, arthritis, myocarditis, pericarditis, oophoritis, pancreatitis, diabetes mellitus, arthritis, thyroiditis, and nephritis.

Assessment findings

The typical patient history points to inadequate immunization and exposure to someone with mumps within the preceding 2 to 3 weeks. The clinical features of mumps vary widely. Up to 50% of susceptible people have subclinical illness without symptoms. In apparent disease, mumps usually begins with prodromal symptoms that last for 24 hours. Besides complaining of myalgia, anorexia, malaise, headache, an earache aggravated by chewing, and pain when drinking sour or acidic liquids, the patient may report a temperature of 101° to 104° F (38.3° to 40° C).

Inspection may reveal swelling and tenderness of the parotid glands and simultaneous (or a little later) swelling of one or more other salivary glands. (See *Parotid inflammation in mumps*.) Diagnosis usually is made after the characteristic signs and symptoms develop, especially parotid gland enlargement with a history of exposure to mumps.

Diagnostic tests

Glandular swelling confirms the diagnosis. Serologic testing to detect the mumps antibodies can verify the diagnosis if the patient's glands do not swell. If comparisons between a saliva, urine, or CSF specimen obtained during the acute phase of illness and another specimen obtained 3 weeks later show a fourfold rise in antibodies, the patient probably had mumps. Serum amylase levels also may be elevated.

PAROTID INFLAMMATION IN MUMPS

The mumps virus (paramyxovirus) attacks the parotid glands—the main salivary glands. Inflammation causes characteristic swelling and discomfort associated with eating, drinking, swallowing, and talking.

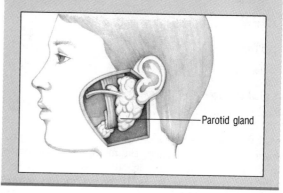

Parotid gland

Treatment

Appropriate treatment includes analgesics for pain, antipyretics for fever, and adequate fluid intake to prevent dehydration from fever and anorexia. If the patient can't swallow, treatment may include I.V. fluid replacement.

Nursing diagnoses

- Altered nutrition: Less than body requirements
- Altered thought processes
- Anxiety
- Body image disturbance
- Fluid volume deficit
- Hyperthermia
- Impaired swallowing
- Pain
- Risk for infection

Nursing interventions

- Give analgesics, and apply warm or cool compresses to the neck area to relieve pain. Give antipyretics and tepid sponge baths for fever. Increase fluids to prevent dehydration. Provide a high-calorie, nutritionally sound diet. Avoid spicy, irritating foods that trigger salivation or require a lot of chewing.
- Closely observe the patient for complications, especially for signs of central nervous system involvement, such as altered level of consciousness and nuchal rigidity.

COMPARING COMMON RASH-PRODUCING INFECTIONS

Infection	Incubation (days)	Duration (days)
Roseola	10 to 15	3 to 6
Varicella	10 to 14	7 to 14
Rubeola	13 to 17	5
Rubella	16 to 18	3
Herpes simplex	2 to 12	7 to 21

• Until symptoms subside, consider implementing respiratory isolation because the mumps virus remains in the patient's saliva throughout the disease course.
• Provide comfort measures. If the patient has scrotal swelling, support the scrotum with a small pillow. Or make an adhesive tape bridge to place between the thighs. Use a nonadhesive material for the portion that will elevate and support the scrotum.
• Report all cases of mumps to local public health authorities.

Patient teaching
• Encourage bed rest during the febrile period.
• To minimize pain and anorexia, recommend eating bland, nonirritating foods that require minimal chewing.
• Advise administering antipyretics and tepid sponge baths to reduce fever and increasing fluids to prevent dehydration.
• List complications to watch for and report to the doctor.
• Urge parents to have children immunized with live attenuated mumps vaccine at age 15 months—or older, if applicable. Among those susceptible to mumps and its complications are nonimmunized males who are approaching or past puberty. For these people, immunization within 24 hours of exposure may prevent or attenuate the actual disease. Explain that immunity to mumps lasts for at least 12 years after vaccination.
• Reassure the patient with epididymo-orchitis that even if testicular atrophy occurs, it won't cause impotence. Also inform him that sterility occurs only with bilateral orchitis.

ROSEOLA INFANTUM
An acute, benign infection, roseola infantum (exanthema subitum) affects infants and young children typically between ages 6 months and 3 years.

Roseola, which affects both sexes equally, occurs year-round, mostly in the spring and fall. Overt roseola, the most common exanthem in children under age 2, affects about 30% of all children; inapparent roseola (febrile illness without a rash) may affect the rest.

Causes
Human herpesvirus 6 is thought to cause roseola, although this is unconfirmed. The mode of transmission isn't known. Rarely does an infected child transmit roseola to a sibling. The incubation period lasts from 10 to 15 days.

Complications
Encephalopathy and thrombocytopenic purpura are rare complications.

Assessment findings
The patient history is unremarkable. The parents of a child with roseola usually report an abruptly rising, unexplainable fever that peaks between 103° and 105° F (39.4° and 40.6° C) for 3 to 5 days and then drops suddenly. Parents also report these symptoms: anorexia, irritability, and listlessness, although the child doesn't seem particularly ill. (Seizures may accompany a high fever.)

Accompanying the abrupt drop in temperature is a maculopapular, nonpruritic rash that blanches with pressure. This rash, which is profuse on the child's trunk, arms, and neck and mild on the face and legs, fades within 24 hours. (See *Comparing common rash-producing infections*.)

Diagnostic tests
Laboratory test results can't confirm roseola infantum because the causative organism remains unconfirmed.

Treatment
Because roseola is self-limiting, treatment is supportive and symptomatic: antipyretic medications to lower fever and, if necessary, anticonvulsants to relieve seizures.

Nursing diagnoses
• Altered nutrition: Less than body requirements
• Fluid volume deficit

- Hyperthermia
- Impaired skin integrity

Nursing interventions
- Give tepid sponge baths and administer antipyretics, as ordered, to reduce fever.
- Monitor fluid intake and output. Replace fluids and electrolytes as needed.
- Institute seizure precautions and monitor for seizures.

Patient teaching
- Teach parents how to lower the child's fever by giving tepid sponge baths, dressing the child in lightweight clothing, keeping the environment at a comfortable temperature, and administering antipyretics, as ordered.
- Stress the need for adequate fluid intake to promote hydration. Advise parents that strict bed rest isn't necessary.
- Tell parents to keep the child's skin clean and dry.
- Reassure parents that brief febrile seizures won't cause brain damage and will stop as the fever subsides. If the doctor prescribes phenobarbital to control seizures, explain that this medication may cause drowsiness. However, if it causes stupor, instruct the parents to call the doctor immediately.

HERPES SIMPLEX

A common infection, herpes simplex virus (HSV) occurs subclinically in about 85% of patients. In the rest, it causes localized lesions. HSV may be latent for years, but after the initial infection, the patient becomes a carrier susceptible to recurrent attacks. The outbreaks may be provoked by fever, menses, stress, heat, cold, lack of sleep, sun exposure, and contact with reactivated disease (for example, by kissing or by sharing cosmetics). In recurrent infections, the patient usually has no constitutional signs and symptoms. (See *Understanding the genital herpes cycle,* page 178.)

Generally not serious in an otherwise healthy adult, HSV infection in a neonate or an immunocompromised patient, such as one with acquired immunodeficiency syndrome (AIDS), can produce severe illness. In fact, serious HSV infections occur commonly in patients with AIDS.

HSV infection occurs worldwide and equally in males and females. Lower socioeconomic groups are infected more often, probably because of crowded living conditions.

Causes
Herpesvirus hominis, a widespread infectious agent, causes two serologically distinct HSV types. Seen most commonly in children, *type 1 (HSV-1)* is transmitted primarily by contact with oral secretions. It mainly affects oral, labial, ocular, or skin tissues. (See *Recognizing herpetic whitlow,* page 179.) *Type 2 (HSV-2),* transmitted primarily by contact with genital secretions, mainly affects genital structures, typically in adolescents and young adults.

In homosexual men, HSV-2 anal and perianal infection is common. However, with changing sexual practices, some studies report an increasing incidence of genital HSV-1 and oral HSV-2 infections. Although HSV most frequently occurs in the structures mentioned, it may infect any epithelial tissue. The incubation period varies, depending on the infection site. The average incubation for generalized infection is 2 to 12 days; for localized genital infection, 3 to 7 days.

Complications
Primary (or initial) HSV infection during pregnancy can lead to abortion, premature labor, microcephaly, and uterine growth retardation. Congenital herpes transmitted during vaginal birth may produce a subclinical neonatal infection or severe infection with seizures, chorioretinitis, skin vesicles, and hepatosplenomegaly.

In infants, HSV-1 can cause life-threatening nonepidemic encephalitis. And primary HSV infection is a leading cause of gingivostomatitis in children ages 1 to 3.

Blindness may result from ocular infection. Females with HSV may be at increased risk for cervical cancer. Urethral stricture may result from recurrent genital herpes.

Perianal ulcers, colitis, esophagitis, pneumonitis, and various neurologic disorders, resulting from HSV infection, are serious complications in patients with AIDS and other immunocompromised conditions.

Assessment findings
The patient's history may reveal oral, vaginal, or anal sexual contact with an infected person or other direct contact with lesions. With recurrent infection, the patient may identify various precipitating factors.

In *primary perioral HSV,* the patient may have generalized or localized infection. The patient with generalized infection usually reports a sore throat, fever, increased salivation, halitosis, anorexia, and severe mouth pain. If pain prevents adequate fluid intake, you

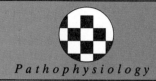

Pathophysiology

UNDERSTANDING THE GENITAL HERPES CYCLE

After a patient is infected with genital herpes, a latency period follows. The virus takes up permanent residence in the nerve cells surrounding the lesions, and intermittent viral shedding may take place.

Repeated outbreaks may develop at any time, again followed by a latent stage during which the lesions heal completely. Outbreaks may recur as often as three to eight times yearly.

Although the cycle continues indefinitely, some people remain symptom-free for years.

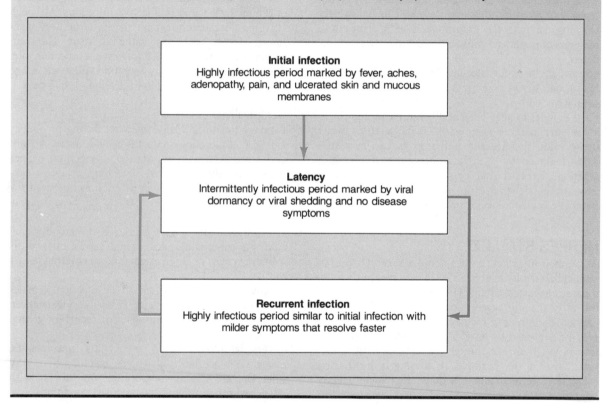

Initial infection
Highly infectious period marked by fever, aches, adenopathy, pain, and ulcerated skin and mucous membranes

Latency
Intermittently infectious period marked by viral dormancy or viral shedding and no disease symptoms

Recurrent infection
Highly infectious period similar to initial infection with milder symptoms that resolve faster

also may note such signs of dehydration as poor skin turgor. After a brief prodromal tingling and itching, typical primary lesions erupt.

Examination of the pharyngeal and oral mucosa may disclose edema and small vesicles on an erythematous base. These vesicles eventually rupture, leaving a painful ulcer that is followed by yellow crusting. Vesicles most commonly occur on the tongue, gingiva, and cheeks, but any part of the oral mucosa may be involved. Palpation reveals tender cervical adenopathy. A generalized infection usually runs its course in 4 to 10 days.

With *primary genital HSV,* the patient usually complains first of malaise, dysuria, dyspareunia, and, in females, leukorrhea. Then fluid-filled vesicles appear.

In examining a female patient, you may detect vesicles on the cervix (the primary infection site) and, possibly, on the labia, perianal skin, vulva, and vagina. In male patients, vesicles develop on the glans penis, foreskin, and penile shaft. Extragenital lesions may be seen on the mouth or anus. Ruptured vesicles appear as extensive, shallow, painful ulcers, with redness, marked edema, and characteristic oozing, yellow centers. Lesions may persist for several weeks. Palpation may reveal tender inguinal adenopathy.

The patient with *recurrent perioral or genital HSV* also may report prodromal symptoms (pain, tingling, or itching) at the site. Typically, the disease course is shorter than that of the primary infection. Recurrent perioral infection usually triggers no systemic symptoms, but the outer lip may be affected and painful. A male patient with recurrent genital herpes usually has less severe systemic symptoms and less local involvement. A female patient may have more symptoms and report severe discomfort. Palpation may reveal tender cervical adenopathy.

The patient with a *primary ocular infection* may report localized signs and symptoms, such as photophobia and excessive tearing. Follicular conjunctivitis or blepharitis with vesicles on the eyelid, eyelid edema, and chemosis also may occur. Systemic signs and symptoms may include lethargy and fever. The infection usually is unilateral, healing in 2 to 3 weeks. Recurrent ocular infections may cause decreased visual acuity and even permanent vision loss. Palpation may reveal regional adenopathy.

Diagnostic tests
Confirmation of HSV infection requires isolating the virus from local lesions and a histologic biopsy. In primary infection, a rise in antibodies and moderate leukocytosis may support the diagnosis.

Treatment
Symptomatic and supportive therapy is the rule. Generalized primary infection usually requires antipyretic and analgesic medications to reduce fever and pain. Anesthetic mouthwashes, such as viscous lidocaine, may reduce the pain of gingivostomatitis, enabling the patient to consume food and fluids and thus promote hydration. (Avoid offering alcohol-based mouthwashes, which can increase discomfort.) A bicarbonate-based mouth rinse may be used for oral care. Drying agents, such as calamine lotion, may soothe labial and skin lesions. Avoid using petrolatum-based salves or dressings because they promote viral spread and slow healing.

Refer patients with eye infections to an ophthalmologist. Topical corticosteroids are contraindicated in active infection, but ophthalmic medications, such as

RECOGNIZING HERPETIC WHITLOW

A finger infection caused by the microorganism that causes herpes simplex virus (HSV), herpetic whitlow commonly affects nurses—usually only in one finger. Typical signs and symptoms in the affected finger begin with tingling followed by:
• pain, redness, and swelling
• vesicular eruptions bordered by red halos
• vesicular ulceration or coalescence
• related effects, including satellite vesicles, fever, chills, malaise, and a red streak up the arm.

Healing occurs in 2 to 3 weeks. In health care workers, the infecting organism usually is HSV-1. In others, the infection usually is secondary to HSV-2 infection.

idoxuridine, trifluridine, and vidarabine, may be effective.

Acyclovir is a major agent for combating genital herpes, particularly primary infection. The drug may reduce symptoms, viral shedding, and healing time. And although it's mostly ineffective in treating recurrent attacks, it may be prescribed to treat and suppress HSV in immunocompromised patients and those with severe and frequent recurrences. Acyclovir therapy also may help treat perioral herpes, especially primary infection. The drug is available in topical, oral, and I.V. form (usually reserved for severe infection).

Nursing diagnoses
• Altered oral mucous membrane
• Altered sexuality patterns
• Altered thought processes
• Impaired skin integrity
• Impaired social interaction
• Knowledge deficit
• Pain
• Powerlessness
• Risk for infection
• Risk for injury
• Sensory or perceptual alterations
• Social isolation

Nursing interventions
• Observe universal precautions. For the patient with extensive cutaneous, oral, or genital lesions, institute drainage and secretion precautions.
• Instruct caregivers with active oral or cutaneous infections not to care for a patient in a high-risk group until the caregiver's lesions crust and dry. Also, insist

that the caregiver wear protective coverings, including a mask and gloves.
• Administer pain medications and prescribed antiviral agents, as ordered.
• As appropriate, refer the patient to a support group, such as the Herpes Resource Center.

Patient teaching
• Tell the patient with cold sores not to kiss infants or people with eczema. Tell the patient with genital herpes to wash his hands carefully after using the bathroom or touching his genitalia, to avoid spreading the infection to infants or other susceptible people.
• Instruct the patient with oral lesions to use lip balm with sunscreen to avoid reactivating lesions.
• Encourage the patient to get adequate rest and nutrition and to keep his lesions dry, except for applying prescribed medications.
• Teach the patient how to apply medications, using aseptic technique.
• Urge the patient with genital herpes to avoid sexual intercourse during the active disease stage before lesions completely heal.
• Instruct the patient with genital herpes to inform any sexual partner of his condition. Advise patients and partners to be screened for other sexually transmitted diseases, including human immunodeficiency virus infection.
• If the patient is pregnant, explain the potential risk to the infant during vaginal delivery. Answer her questions about cesarean delivery if she has an HSV outbreak when labor begins and if her membranes haven't ruptured.
• Advise the female patient with genital herpes to have a Papanicolaou test yearly if results have been normal. If results have been abnormal, advise her to be tested more frequently.
• Instruct the patient with herpetic whitlow not to share towels or eating utensils with uninfected people. Educate hospital staff members and other susceptible people about the risk of contracting the disease.
• Accept the patient's feelings of powerlessness as normal. Help him to identify and develop coping mechanisms, strengths, and resources for support.
• Provide a nonthreatening, nonjudgmental atmosphere to encourage the patient with genital herpes to voice his feelings about perceived changes in sexuality and behavior. Provide him and his partner with current information about the disease and treatment options. Offer to refer them for appropriate counseling, as needed.

HERPES ZOSTER
An acute unilateral and segmental inflammation of the dorsal root ganglia, herpes zoster (shingles) produces localized vesicular skin lesions confined to a dermatome. The patient with shingles may have severe neuralgic pain in the areas bordering the inflamed nerve root ganglia. (See *Tracking herpes zoster.*)

The infection, found primarily in adults over age 50, seldom recurs. The prognosis is good, and most patients recover completely unless the infection spreads to the brain. Herpes zoster is more severe in the immunocompromised patient but seldom is fatal.

Causes
The varicella-zoster virus, a herpesvirus, causes shingles. For unknown reasons and by an unidentified process, the disease erupts when the virus reactivates after dormancy in the cerebral ganglia (extramedullary ganglia of the cranial nerves) or the ganglia of posterior nerve roots. Although the process is unclear, the virus may multiply as it reactivates, and antibodies remaining from the initial infection may neutralize it. Without opposition from effective antibodies, the virus continues to multiply in the ganglia, destroys neurons, and spreads down the sensory nerves to the skin.

Herpes zoster may be more prevalent in people who had chicken pox at a very young age, especially before age 1 — but this is still a hypothesis.

Complications
Herpes zoster ophthalmicus may result in vision loss. Complications of generalized infection may involve acute urine retention and unilateral paralysis of the diaphragm. In postherpetic neuralgia (most common in elderly patients), intractable neurologic pain may persist for years, and scars may be permanent. In rare cases, herpes zoster may be complicated by generalized central nervous system (CNS) infection, muscle atrophy, motor paralysis (usually transient), acute transverse myelitis, and ascending myelitis.

Assessment findings
The typical patient reports no history of exposure to others with the varicella-zoster virus. He may complain of fever, malaise, pain that mimics appendicitis, pleurisy, musculoskeletal pain, or other conditions. In 2 to 4 days, he may report severe, deep pain; pruritus; and paresthesia or hyperesthesia (usually affecting the trunk and occasionally the arms and legs). Pain — described as intermittent, continuous, or debilitating — usually lasts from 1 to 4 weeks.

TRACKING HERPES ZOSTER

The herpes zoster virus infects the nerves that inner-vate the skin, the eyes, and the ears. Each nerve (tagged for its corresponding vertebral source) ema-nates from the spine, banding and branching around the body to innervate a skin area called a derma-tome. The herpes zoster rash erupts along the course of the affected nerve fibers, covering the skin in one or several of the dermatomes (as shown).

The thoracic (T) and lumbar (L) dermatomes are the most commonly affected, but others, such as those covering the cervical (C) and sacral (S) areas, can also be affected. Dermatome levels can vary and overlap.

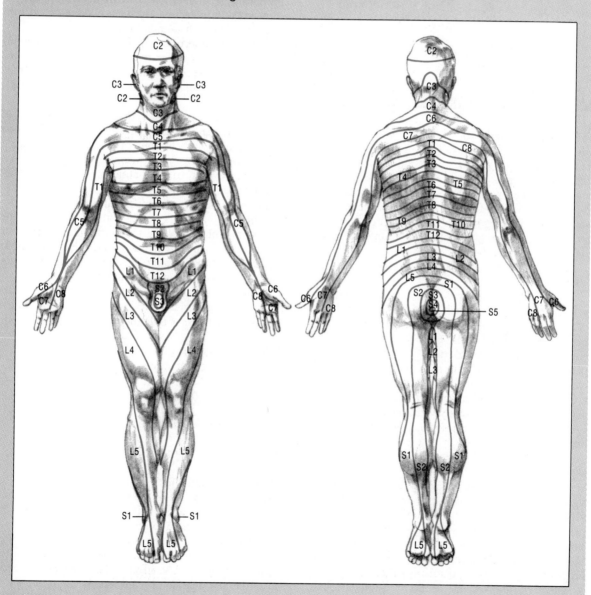

A LOOK AT HERPES ZOSTER

These characteristic herpes zoster lesions are fluid-filled vesicles that dry and form scabs after about 10 days.

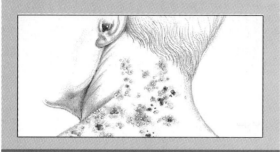

During examination of the patient within 2 weeks after his initial symptoms, you may observe small, red, nodular skin lesions spread unilaterally around the thorax or vertically over the arms or legs. Or instead of nodules, you may see vesicles filled with clear fluid or pus. About 10 days after they appear, these vesicles dry, forming scabs. (See *A look at herpes zoster.*) The lesions are most vulnerable to infection after rupture; some even become gangrenous.

During palpation, you may detect enlarged regional lymph nodes.

Herpes zoster may involve the cranial nerves (especially the trigeminal and geniculate ganglia or the oculomotor nerve). With geniculate involvement, you may observe vesicle formation in the external auditory canal and ipsilateral facial palsy. The patient may complain of hearing loss, dizziness, and loss of taste. With trigeminal involvement, the patient may complain of eye pain. He also may have corneal and scleral damage and impaired vision. Rarely, oculomotor involvement causes conjunctivitis, extraocular weakness, ptosis, and paralytic mydriasis.

Diagnostic tests

Vesicular fluid and infected tissue analyses typically show eosinophilic intranuclear inclusions and varicella virus. Differentiation of herpes zoster from localized herpes simplex requires staining antibodies from vesicular fluid and identification under fluorescent light. Usually, though, the locations of herpes simplex and herpes zoster lesions are distinctly different.

With CNS involvement, results of a lumbar puncture indicate increased pressure, and cerebrospinal fluid analysis demonstrates increased protein levels and, possibly, pleocytosis.

Treatment

Primary therapeutic goals include relief of itching with antipruritics (such as calamine lotion) and relief of neuralgic pain with analgesics (such as aspirin, acetaminophen or, possibly, codeine). Tricyclic antidepressants help relieve neuritic pain. A similar goal involves preventing secondary infection by applying a demulcent and skin protectant (such as collodion or tincture of benzoin) to unbroken lesions.

If bacteria infect ruptured vesicles, treatment includes an appropriate systemic antibiotic. Herpes zoster affecting trigeminal and corneal structures calls for instillation of idoxuridine ointment or another antiviral agent.

To help a patient cope with the intractable pain of postherpetic neuralgia, a systemic corticosteroid, such as cortisone or corticotropin, may be ordered to reduce inflammation. The doctor also may order tranquilizers, sedatives, or tricyclic antidepressants with phenothiazines.

In an immunocompromised patient at high risk for complications and in a patient with an infection of the ophthalmic branch of the trigeminal nerve, acyclovir may be prescribed. This drug halts the progressing rash, reduces the duration of viral shedding and acute pain, and prevents visceral complications.

As a last resort for pain relief, transcutaneous peripheral nerve stimulation, patient-controlled analgesia, or a small dose of radiotherapy may be considered.

Nursing diagnoses
• Altered thought processes
• Body image disturbance
• Diversional activity deficit
• Impaired skin integrity
• Impaired social interaction
• Pain
• Sensory or perceptual alterations

Nursing interventions
• Administer topical therapies as directed. If the doctor orders calamine, apply it liberally to the patient's lesions. Avoid blotting contaminated swabs on unaffected skin areas. Be prepared to administer drying therapies, such as oxygen, if the patient has severe disseminated lesions. Use silver sulfadiazine, as ordered, to soften and debride infected lesions.
• Give analgesics exactly as scheduled to minimize severe neuralgic pain. For a patient with postherpetic

neuralgia, consult with a pain specialist, and follow his recommendations to maximize pain relief without risking tolerance to the analgesic.
• Maintain meticulous hygiene to prevent spreading the infection to other parts of the patient's body.
• If the patient has open lesions, follow contact isolation precautions to prevent the spread of infection to immunocompromised patients.

Patient teaching
• To decrease discomfort from oral lesions, tell the patient to use a soft toothbrush, eat soft foods, and use a saline- or bicarbonate-based mouthwash and oral anesthetics.
• Stress the need for rest during the acute phase.
• Reassure the patient that herpes zoster isn't contagious (except to immunocompromised patients), but stress the need for meticulous hygiene to prevent spreading infection to other body parts.
• Reassure the patient that herpetic pain eventually will subside. Suggest diversionary or relaxation activities to take his mind off the pain and pruritus.

HERPANGINA
This infectious disease characteristically produces vesicular lesions on the mucous membranes of the soft palate, tonsillar pillars, and throat. Herpangina usually affects children under age 10 but seldom occurs in neonates (who are protected by maternal antibodies). It occurs slightly more often in late summer and fall and can be sporadic, endemic, or epidemic.

Causes
Group A coxsackieviruses and, less commonly, group B coxsackieviruses and echoviruses cause herpangina. Transmitted by fecal-oral transfer, herpangina has a 2- to 9-day incubation period. (For more information, see *Learning about enteroviruses.*)

Complications
Dehydration is possible.

Assessment findings
The patient history usually is unremarkable, although the patient may seek treatment during a known outbreak of herpangina, especially in warm months. After the incubation period, the patient or his parents may report the following signs and symptoms: a sore throat and pain on swallowing (the primary symptoms), transient headache, anorexia, vomiting, malaise, diar-

LEARNING ABOUT ENTEROVIRUSES

Enteroviruses inhabit the GI tract. Included among them are 3 known polioviruses, 23 group A coxsackieviruses, 6 group B coxsackieviruses, and 34 echoviruses.

They usually infect humans as a result of ingesting fecally contaminated material. They cause a wide range of diseases, such as aseptic meningitis, myocarditis, pericarditis, gastroenteritis, poliomyelitis, and hand-foot-and-mouth disease.

Enteroviruses can appear in the pharynx, feces, blood, cerebrospinal fluid, and central nervous system tissue. Infections from these microorganisms are more prevalent in the summer and fall.

rhea, and pain in the stomach, back of the neck, legs, and arms. A temperature of 100° to 104° F (37.8° to 40° C) occurs suddenly and persists for 1 to 4 days.

After initial symptoms, you may observe up to 12 grayish white papulovesicles on the soft palate. Less commonly, you may see lesions on the tonsils, uvula, tongue, and larynx. These lesions grow from about 1 to 2 mm in diameter to large, punched-out ulcers surrounded by small, inflamed margins. Usually all signs and symptoms subside in 4 to 7 days.

Diagnostic tests
The virus may be isolated from mouth washings or feces. Elevated specific antibody titers confirm herpangina, but these tests seldom are done. Other laboratory test findings are normal except for slight leukocytosis.

Treatment
Symptomatic treatment to relieve discomfort includes measures to reduce fever, prevent seizures, and promote hydration.

Nursing diagnoses
• Altered nutrition: Less than body requirements
• Altered oral mucous membrane
• Hyperthermia
• Impaired swallowing
• Pain
• Risk for fluid volume deficit

Nursing interventions
• Although herpangina doesn't require isolation precautions, practice careful hand washing and dispose of excretions properly.
• Provide adequate fluids, enforce bed rest, give tepid sponge baths, and administer prescribed antipyretic and analgesic medications, such as acetaminophen. Serve soft or pureed foods that minimize oral irritation.

Patient teaching
• Teach parents effective infection-control measures.
• Instruct caregivers in techniques to promote patient comfort and recovery.

GENITAL WARTS
A common sexually transmitted disease, genital warts are papillomas that consist of fibrous tissue overgrowth from the dermis and thickened epithelial coverings. Also known as venereal warts and condylomata acuminata, these growths are rare before puberty or after menopause. In people under age 25, genital warts are the fastest-growing sexually transmitted disease.

Causes
Genital warts result from infection with one of the more than 60 known strains of human papillomavirus. Transmitted by sexual contact, the virus incubates from 1 to 6 months (the average is 2 months) before warts erupt.

Complications
During pregnancy, genital warts in the vaginal and cervical walls may grow so large that they impede vaginal delivery. Other complications include possible genital tract dysplasia or cancer. (Studies show an association between human papillomavirus types 11, 16, and 18 and cervical dysplasia and cancer.)

Assessment findings
The patient's health history may include reported unprotected sexual contact with a partner with a known infection, a new partner, or many partners.

On examination, you'll observe warts growing on the moist genital surfaces, such as the subpreputial sac, the urethral meatus and, less commonly, on the penile shaft or scrotum in male patients and on the vulva and vaginal and cervical walls in female patients. In both sexes, papillomas spread to the peri-

neum and the perianal area. On inspection, you may find warts that begin as tiny red or pink swellings. These warts may grow as large as 4″ (10 cm) and may become pedunculated. Multiple swellings have a cauliflower-like appearance. Most patients report no symptoms; a few complain of itching or pain. Infected lesions become malodorous.

Diagnostic tests
Dark-field microscopy of wart-cell scrapings shows marked epidermal cell vascularization. This differentiates genital warts from condylomata lata associated with second-stage syphilis.

Another test involves applying 5% acetic acid (white vinegar) to the warts, which will turn white if they are papillomas.

Treatment
Genital warts occasionally resolve spontaneously. To remove small warts, the doctor usually recommends topical drug therapy. Medications of choice include 10% to 25% podophyllum resin in tincture of benzoin (contraindicated in pregnancy), trichloroacetic acid, and bichloroacetic acid. (Treatment aims to remove exophytic warts and ameliorate signs and symptoms, not to eradicate the human papillomavirus.)

Warts that grow larger than 1″ (2.5 cm) usually are removed by carbon dioxide laser, cryosurgery, electrocautery, or fluorouracil cream debridement. Conventional surgery may be recommended to remove perianal warts.

Rarely, immune therapy may be prescribed. This involves excising the warts and using them to prepare a vaccine to stimulate antibodies. Interferon therapy is under evaluation.

Nursing diagnoses
• Altered sexuality patterns
• Body image disturbance
• Knowledge deficit
• Risk for infection
• Risk for injury

Nursing interventions
• Use universal precautions when examining the patient, collecting a specimen, or performing associated procedures.
• Provide a nonthreatening, nonjudgmental atmosphere that encourages the patient to verbalize feelings about perceived changes in sexual identity and behavior.

Patient teaching
• Tell the patient to remove podophyllum resin with soap and water 4 to 6 hours after applying it to warts.
• Recommend sexual abstinence or condom use during intercourse until healing is complete.
• Advise the patient to inform his sexual partners about the risk of genital warts and of the need for evaluation.
• Urge the patient and his sexual partners to be tested for human immunodeficiency virus infection and other sexually transmitted diseases.
• Emphasize that genital warts can recur and that the virus can mutate, causing infection with warts of a different strain.
• Remind the patient to report for weekly treatments until all warts are removed. Then instruct him to schedule a checkup 3 months after all warts are gone.
• Encourage female patients to have a Papanicolaou test every 6 months.

RABIES

An acute central nervous system (CNS) infection, rabies (hydrophobia) usually is transmitted by an animal bite and is almost always fatal once symptoms occur. Fortunately, immunization that begins soon after infection may prevent fatal CNS invasion. (See *Schedules for rabies prophylaxis.*) Increased domestic animal control and vaccination in the United States have reduced cases of rabies in humans. Consequently, most human rabies can be traced to dog bites that occurred in other countries or bites from wild animals, such as raccoons.

Causes
Rabies is caused by the rabies virus, a rhabdovirus. The rabies virus is transmitted to a human from the bite of an infected animal through the skin or mucous membranes. The virus begins replicating in the striated muscle cells at the entry site and spreads along the nerve pathways to the spinal cord and brain, where it replicates. Finally, it moves through the nerves into other tissues, including the salivary glands. Airborne droplets and infected tissue transplants occasionally can transmit the virus. The incubation period is hours to weeks.

Complications
Untreated rabies can lead to life-threatening complications, including respiratory failure, peripheral vascular collapse, and central brain failure.

SCHEDULES FOR RABIES PROPHYLAXIS

The most important treatment consideration for the person exposed to rabies is immunization to prevent full-blown disease. If the patient never had a rabies immunization, he will need passive immunization with rabies immune globulin (RIG) and active immunization with human diploid cell vaccine (HDCV). Treatment with both should begin on the day of exposure.

If the patient received HDCV, and if he has an adequate rabies antibody titer, he won't need RIG vaccine. Nevertheless, he will need a booster dose of HDCV.

Review these schedules for people receiving rabies vaccine.

For passive immunization
The typical inoculation dose for the patient receiving RIG is 20 IU/kg (50% infiltrated around the wound and 50% injected I.M. in the buttock).

If RIG isn't available, the doctor may give antirabies serum (ARS) interferon. Of equine origin, this serum may produce severe adverse reactions. Administered like RIG, the typical ARS dose is 40 IU/kg.

For active immunization
The patient receiving HDCV will have five I.M. injections (1 ml each), usually in the deltoid muscle. Follow the first injection with doses at 3, 7, 14, and 28 days later.

An alternative to this schedule is four HDCV I.M. injections administered as follows: 2 ml on the day of exposure (given as two 1-ml injections), 1 ml administered in 7 days, and 1 ml administered in 21 days.

Nursing considerations
• Be sure to prepare RIG and HDCV in separate syringes.
• Never combine vaccines.
• Avoid injecting RIG and HDCV in the same site. Doing so will inactivate the vaccine.
• With active immunization, check the antibody titer after the last inoculation and at 2 to 3 weeks. Expect RFFIT findings to show an antibody titer of at least 1:5. This indicates growing immunity.

Assessment findings
The patient usually seeks treatment after an animal bite or after open wound contact with an infected animal's saliva. The patient initially complains of local or radiating pain or burning and a sensation of cold, pruritus, and tingling at the bite site. He also may report prodromal symptoms, such as malaise, headache, an-

FIRST AID FOR ANIMAL BITES

Follow these steps when caring for the patient bitten by an animal:
• Wash the bite vigorously with soap and water for at least 10 minutes to remove the animal's saliva. As soon as possible, flush the wound with a viricidal agent and then rinse with clear water.
• Apply a sterile dressing when you're sure the wound is clean. If possible, don't suture the wound, and don't immediately stop the bleeding (unless it's massive) because blood flow helps to clean the wound.
• Question the patient about the animal bite. Ask if he provoked the animal (if so, chances are it's not rabid). Also ask him to identify the animal or its owner (because the animal may need to be confined for observation).

orexia, nausea, sore throat, and a persistent loose cough.

In this patient, you may observe nervousness, anxiety, irritability, hyperesthesia, photophobia, sensitivity to loud noises, and excessive salivation, lacrimation, and perspiration. He also may have a slight fever, with his body temperature ranging from 100° to 102° F (37.8° to 38.9° C).

About 2 to 10 days after prodromal signs and symptoms begin, an excitation phase occurs, marked by intermittent hyperactivity, anxiety, apprehension, pupillary dilation, shallow respirations, and altered level of consciousness. With cranial nerve dysfunction, you may see ocular palsies, strabismus, asymmetrical pupillary dilation or constriction, absence of corneal reflexes, facial muscle weakness, and hoarseness. During this phase, the patient's temperature rises to about 103° F (39.4° C).

About 50% of patients exhibit hydrophobia during which forceful, painful pharyngeal muscle spasms expel fluids from the mouth, causing dehydration and, possibly, apnea, cyanosis, and death. Swallowing difficulty causes frothy drooling. Soon, the sight, sound, or thought of water triggers uncontrollable pharyngeal muscle spasms and excessive salivation. During this phase, you may observe nuchal rigidity and seizures (possibly accompanied by cardiac arrhythmias or arrest).

Between excitatory and hydrophobic episodes, the patient usually remains cooperative and lucid. After about 3 days, excitation and hydrophobia subside, and progressive paralysis, leading to coma, begins.

Palpating the peripheral pulses may detect tachycardia or bradycardia when the patient has signs of severe systemic disease. Hypotension usually accompanies coma.

Diagnostic tests

No tests can confirm the rabies diagnosis in humans before onset. In the United States, the rapid fluorescent focus inhibition test (RFFIT) is the standard measure for rabies neutrality antibody. The results of this in vitro cell culture neutralization test are available within 24 hours. The Centers for Disease Control considers complete neutralization at the 1:5 level by RFFIT an adequate antibody titer.

The rabies virus also may be isolated from certain infected tissue or secretions in animals or humans. Histologic examination of brain tissue from human rabies victims typically shows perivascular inflammation of the gray matter, neuronal degeneration, and characteristic cytoplasmic inclusion bodies (Negri bodies).

Treatment

Immunization as soon as possible after exposure and meticulous wound care are the treatments for rabies.

Before performing wound care, remember to put on gloves to avoid contact with infected blood. Thoroughly wash all wounds and abrasions with soap and water. (See First aid for animal bites.) Check the patient's immunization status, and administer tetanus-diphtheria prophylaxis, if needed. Take measures to control bacterial infection, as ordered. If the wound requires suturing, special techniques may be used to ensure proper wound drainage.

Although no specific drugs are available to treat rabies, postexposure prophylaxis usually is successful in preventing disease when used appropriately during the rabies incubation period. Treatment is mainly supportive, with special attention given to the cardiovascular and respiratory systems.

Nursing diagnoses

• Altered nutrition: Less than body requirements
• Anxiety
• Decreased cardiac output
• Hyperthermia
• Impaired swallowing
• Impaired tissue integrity
• Ineffective breathing pattern
• Risk for fluid volume deficit

- Risk for infection
- Sensory or perceptual alterations

Nursing interventions

- When injecting rabies vaccine, rotate injection sites on the upper arm or thigh. Don't use the buttocks. Watch for and symptomatically treat redness, itching, pain, and tenderness at the injection site.
- If rabies develops, begin aggressive supportive care. Monitor cardiac, neurologic, and pulmonary function. Administer I.V. fluids, as ordered.
- Isolate the patient, as needed. Wear a gown, gloves, mask, and protective eyeglasses when handling saliva and articles contaminated with saliva. Take precautions to avoid being bitten by the patient during the excitation phase.
- Keep the patient's room dark and quiet.
- Establish communication with the patient and his family. Provide psychological support to help them cope with the patient's symptoms and probable death.
- Assist in the prophylactic administration of rabies vaccine to high-risk people, such as farm workers, forest rangers, spelunkers (cave explorers), veterinarians, and other animal handlers.

Patient teaching

- Reassure the patient receiving prophylactic rabies vaccine that this will prevent rabies. Tell him how many times and on what dates he'll need to be vaccinated. Discuss possible adverse effects, such as redness and tenderness at the injection site.
- If the patient has rabies, explain the need for isolation precautions to him and his family. Also explain the probable course of the disease and any treatments.
- To help prevent this disease, urge any patient to have household pets immunized. Warn people not to try to touch wild animals, especially if they appear ill or docile (a possible sign of rabies).

COLORADO TICK FEVER

A benign infection, Colorado tick fever occurs in the Rocky Mountain region of the United States, mostly in April and May at lower altitudes and in June and July at higher altitudes. Because of occupational or recreational exposure, it's more common in men than in women. Colorado tick fever apparently confers long-lasting immunity against reinfection.

Causes

Colorado tick fever results from the Colorado tick fever virus, an arbovirus. A hard-shelled wood tick called *Dermacentor andersoni* transmits the disease to humans. After the adult tick acquires the virus from biting an infected rodent, the tick becomes permanently infected. The virus's incubation period is 3 to 6 days.

Complications

Rare complications of Colorado tick fever include pericarditis, myocarditis, epididymitis, orchitis, atypical pneumonia, and meningoencephalitis, a potentially fatal disorder.

Assessment findings

The patient's history may include a known tick bite or recent exposure to ticks or tick-infested areas. Soon after exposure, he may report the abrupt onset of chills; severe aching of the back, arms, and legs; lethargy; and headache with eye movement. He may experience photophobia, abdominal pain, nausea, and vomiting. He also may complain of a fever that begins abruptly, with his temperature increasing to 104° F (40° C). The fever may subside after 2 to 3 days and then recur for another 2 to 3 days.

Inspection may reveal conjunctival infection, altered level of consciousness (with central nervous system involvement), and a maculopapular or, less commonly, petechial rash.

Diagnostic tests

A complete blood count demonstrating leukopenia and serologic findings or viral isolation confirms the diagnosis.

Treatment

After correct removal of the tick, supportive treatment relieves symptoms, combats secondary infection, and maintains fluid balance.

Nursing diagnoses

- Altered thought processes
- Hyperthermia
- Knowledge deficit
- Pain
- Risk for fluid volume deficit
- Risk for injury
- Self-care deficit

Nursing interventions

- Carefully remove the tick by grasping it with forceps or gloved fingers and pulling gently. Be careful not to crush the tick's body. Keep it for identification. Thoroughly wash the wound with soap and water. If the

EBOLA ZAIRE

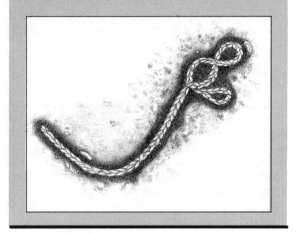

This illustration shows Ebola Zaire, one of three strains of the Ebola virus that cause hemorrhagic illness in humans.

tick's head remains embedded, surgical removal is necessary. Give a tetanus-diphtheria booster, as ordered.
• Be alert for secondary infection.
• Monitor the patient's intake, output, and body weight daily for evidence of fluid and electrolyte imbalance. Replace fluids and electrolytes as needed.
• Help the patient with personal hygiene and self-care during the acute stage of the illness.
• Relieve pain and reduce fever with antipyretic, analgesic medications, such as acetaminophen. Discourage using aspirin because of its bleeding potential. Also provide or suggest tepid sponge baths.

Patient teaching
• To prevent Colorado tick fever, educate patients to avoid tick-infested areas. If this isn't possible, recommend wearing protective clothing, using insect repellants, frequently checking for ticks, and removing them before they attach and feed.
• Teach patients and caregivers the correct technique for removing a tick. If the technique fails and the tick can't be removed, tell the patient to seek medical attention immediately.
• Alert patients and caregivers to the signs and symptoms of Colorado tick fever and the need for medical attention before symptoms advance and prostration and dehydration occur.

EBOLA VIRUS INFECTION

One of the most frightening viruses to come out of the African subcontinent, the Ebola virus first appeared in 1976. More than 400 people in Zaire and the neighboring Sudan were killed by the hemorrhagic fever that it caused. Ebola virus has been responsible for several outbreaks in the years since then, including one that occurred in Zaire in the summer of 1995.

An unclassified ribonucleic acid (RNA) virus, Ebola is morphologically similar to the Marburg virus. Both viruses cause headache, malaise, myalgia, and high fever, progressing to severe diarrhea, vomiting, and internal and external hemorrhage.

Four strains of the Ebola virus are know to exist: Ebola Zaire, Ebola Sudan, Ebola Tai, and Ebola Reston. (See *Ebola Zaire.*) All four types are structurally similar, although they have different antigenic properties. However, Ebola Reston causes illness only in monkeys, not in humans as do the other three.

The prognosis for Ebola virus infection is extremely poor, with a mortality as high as 90%. The incubation period ranges from 2 to 21 days.

Causes
Ebola virus infection is caused by an unclassified RNA virus that is passed from person to person by direct contact with infected blood, body secretions, or organs. Nosocomial and community-acquired transmission can occur. Contaminated needles can also cause the infection. Transmission through semen may occur up to 7 weeks after clinical recovery. The virus remains contagious even after the patient has died.

Complications
As the infection progresses, severe complications, including liver and kidney dysfunction, dehydration, and hemorrhage, may develop. In pregnant women, the Ebola virus leads to abortion and massive hemorrhage. Death usually results during the second week of illness from organ failure or hemorrhage.

Assessment findings
The patient's health history usually reveals contact with an infected person. However, no clear line of infection may be apparent at the beginning of an Ebola virus outbreak. The patient usually complains of flulike symptoms (such as headache, malaise, myalgia, fever, cough, and sore throat), which first appear within 3 days of infection.

As the virus spreads through the body, inspection reveals bruising as capillaries rupture and dead blood cells infiltrate the skin. A maculopapular eruption appears after the fifth day of infection. The patient may also display melena, hematemesis, epistaxis, and bleeding gums. In the final stages of the disease, the skin blisters and sloughs off, blood seeps from all body orifices, and the patient begins vomiting his liquefied internal organs.

Diagnostic tests

Specialized laboratory tests reveal specific antigens or antibodies and may show the isolated virus. As with other types of hemorrhagic fever, tests also demonstrate neutrophil leukocytosis, hypofibrinogenemia, thrombocytopenia, and microangiopathic hemolytic anemia.

Treatment

No cure exists for Ebola virus infection; treatment consists mainly of intensive supportive care. Administration of I.V. fluids helps offset the effects of severe dehydration. The patient may receive replacement of plasma heparin before the onset of clinical shock.

Experimental treatments include administration of plasma that contains Ebola virus–specific antibodies. Although this treatment has resulted in diminished levels of the Ebola virus in the body, further evaluation is needed.

Throughout treatment, the patient should remain in isolation. If diagnostic tests indicate that the patient is free of the virus—which typically occurs 21 days after onset in those few who survive—the patient can be released.

Nursing diagnoses

• Activity intolerance
• Altered nutrition: Less than body requirements
• Fatigue
• Fear
• Hyperthermia
• Impaired skin integrity
• Knowledge deficit
• Pain
• Risk for fluid volume deficit
• Risk for infection
• Risk for injury

Nursing interventions

• Follow the guidelines for universal precautions published by the Centers for Disease Control and Prevention when assessing a patient who may have Ebola virus

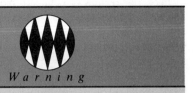
Warning

PREVENTING THE SPREAD OF EBOLA VIRUS

When caring for a patient in the early stages of Ebola virus infection, practicing universal precautions will generally prevent its transmission. As the disease progresses, however, the patient develops diarrhea and begins vomiting and hemorrhaging, greatly increasing the risk of the disease spreading through contact with infected blood and body fluids. The CDC recommends the following guidelines to help prevent the spread of this deadly disease:
• Keep the patient in isolation throughout the course of the disease.
• If possible, place the patient in a negative-pressure room at the beginning of hospitalization to avoid the need for transfer as the disease progresses.
• Restrict nonessential staff members from entering the patient's room.
• Make sure that anyone who enters the patient's room wears gloves and a gown to prevent contact with any surface in the room that may have been soiled.
• Use barrier precautions to prevent skin or mucous membrane exposure to blood or other body fluids, secretions, or excretions when caring for the patient.
• If you must come within 3′ (1 m) of the patient, also wear a face shield or surgical mask and goggles or eyeglasses with side shields.
• *Don't* reuse gloves or gowns unless they have been completely disinfected.
• Make sure any patient who dies of the disease is promptly buried or cremated: Precautions to prevent contact with the patient's body fluids and secretions should continue even after the patient's death.

infection. More extreme precautions are called for as the disease progresses. (See *Preventing the spread of Ebola virus.*)
• Watch for any changes in the rate and pattern of the patient's respirations.
• Closely monitor the patient's fluid and electrolyte balance.
• Monitor the patient's intake and output, looking for signs of dehydration.

- Check the results of complete blood count and co-agulation studies for signs of blood loss and coagulopathy.
- Assess the patient daily for petechiae, ecchymoses, and oozing blood. Note and document the size of ecchymoses at least every 24 hours.
- Test stools, urine, and vomitus for occult blood.
- Protect all areas of petechiae and ecchymoses from further injury.
- Watch for frank bleeding, including GI bleeding and, in women, menorrhagia. Note and document the amount of bleeding every 24 hours or more often.
- Monitor the patient's family and other close contacts for fever and other signs of infection.
- Provide emotional support for the patient and family during the course of this devastating disease. Encourage the patient and family to ask questions and discuss any concerns they have about the disease and its treatment.

Patient teaching
- Teach the patient's family about Ebola virus infection.
- Explain the importance of reporting any signs of bleeding.
- Explain the purpose of any diagnostic tests and procedures that the patient may undergo.

RICKETTSIA

Named for Howard Taylor Ricketts, who discovered them, rickettsiae are parasitic microorganisms that grow only inside living cells. These small, modified forms of bacteria cause Rocky Mountain spotted fever and other rickettsial diseases.

ROCKY MOUNTAIN SPOTTED FEVER
An acute infectious, febrile, and rash-producing illness, Rocky Mountain spotted fever is associated with outdoor activities, such as camping and hiking. Endemic throughout the continental United States, the disease is particularly prevalent in the southeastern, southwestern, southern, and eastern states. As outdoor activities increase in popularity, so does the risk for contracting Rocky Mountain spotted fever—especially in the spring and summer months. (See *Rocky Mountain spotted fever: Tracing its rise and fall.*)

Without early and appropriate treatment, the disease can be fatal (with mortality up to 40%). Appropriate treatment reduces the risk of death to less than 10%. The usual incubation period is 7 days, but it can range from 2 to 12 days. As a rule, the shorter the incubation time, the more severe the infection.

Causes
The *Rickettsia rickettsii* organism causes Rocky Mountain spotted fever. Transmitted by the wood tick (*Dermacentor andersoni*) in the western United States and by the dog tick (*D. variabilis*) in the eastern United States, the rickettsial organism enters humans or small animals with the prolonged bite (4 to 6 hours) of an adult tick. This disease occasionally is acquired through inhalation or through contact of abraded skin with tick excreta or tissue juices. (This explains why people shouldn't crush ticks between their fingers when removing them from others.) In most tick-infested areas, 1% to 5% of the ticks harbor *R. rickettsii*.

Complications
Although uncommon, complications can include lobar pneumonia, pneumonitis, otitis media, parotitis, disseminated intravascular coagulation (DIC), shock, and renal failure.

Assessment findings
The patient's history may show recent exposure to ticks or tick-infested areas, or a known tick bite, although about 25% of patients with the disease have no history of a tick bite.

The patient typically complains of symptoms that began abruptly, including a persistent fever with temperature ranging between 102° and 104° F (38.9° to 40° C); generalized, excruciating headache; and aching in the bones, muscles, joints, and back. He also may report anorexia, nausea, vomiting, constipation, and abdominal pain.

Inspection may disclose the tongue covered with a thick white coating that gradually turns brown as the fever persists and the patient's temperature rises. The skin initially may appear flushed, but in 2 to 5 days, eruptions begin at the wrists, ankles, or forehead and spread centrally. Within 2 days, the rash covers the entire body (including the scalp, palms, and soles). It consists of erythematous macules 1 to 5 mm in diameter that blanch on pressure. Untreated, the rash may become petechial and maculopapular. By the third week, the skin peels off; sometimes gangrene develops over the elbows, fingers, and toes.

ROCKY MOUNTAIN SPOTTED FEVER: TRACING ITS RISE AND FALL

According to the Centers for Disease Control, reported cases of Rocky Mountain spotted fever are either cyclical or declining—probably as a result of public health education efforts. The graph below plots the fever's incidence (per 10,000 population) in the United States over nearly 70 years.

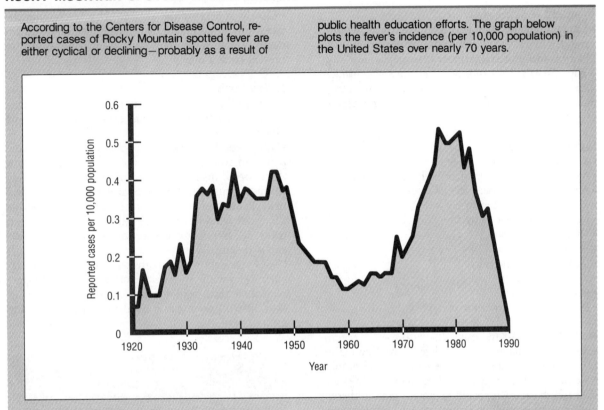

The patient may have a bronchial cough, a rapid respiratory rate (up to 60 breaths/minute), insomnia, restlessness, and, in extreme cases, delirium and circulatory collapse. Urine output decreases considerably, and the urine, which appears dark, contains albumin.

At disease onset, palpation may reveal a strong pulse, which gradually becomes rapid (possibly reaching 150 beats/minute) and thready. The rapid pulse rate and hypotension (less than 90 mm Hg systolic) herald imminent death from vascular collapse. Additionally, you may detect hepatomegaly, splenomegaly, and generalized pitting edema. Postauricular adenopathy may be palpated on one side if the tick bit the patient's head.

Diagnostic tests

Blood cultures to isolate the rickettsial organism can confirm the diagnosis. Some laboratories conduct direct immunofluorescence of cutaneous tissue to detect *R. rickettsii.*

Serologic tests performed during the patient's convalescence can confirm the diagnosis retrospectively. Four tests are performed together (separately, test findings are nonspecific). Diagnostically significant findings include:
- complement fixation titer—1:16 or more
- indirect hemagglutination titer—1:128 or more
- indirect immunofluorescence titer—1:64 or more
- latex agglutination titer—1:64 or more.

Other laboratory test findings may include a decreased platelet count, white blood cell count, and fibrinogen levels; prolonged prothrombin time and partial thromboplastin time; decreased serum protein levels, especially albumin; hyponatremia and hypochloremia associated with increased aldosterone excretion; and abnormal hepatic function.

Mild mononuclear pleocytosis with slightly elevated protein content in cerebrospinal fluid is common.

Treatment

In Rocky Mountain spotted fever, treatment requires careful removal of the tick and administration of antibiotics, such as tetracycline or chloramphenicol, until 3 days after the fever subsides. Treatment also includes measures to relieve symptoms. If DIC occurs, treatment includes heparin administration and platelet transfusion.

Nursing diagnoses

• Activity intolerance
• Altered nutrition: Less than body requirements
• Altered thought processes
• Altered tissue perfusion
• Decreased cardiac output
• Fluid volume deficit
• Hyperthermia
• Impaired skin integrity
• Pain
• Risk for infection
• Risk for injury

Nursing interventions

• Administer analgesics, as ordered. Avoid giving aspirin, which increases the patient's risk for bleeding.
• Monitor vital signs, and watch for profound hypotension and shock. Be prepared to provide oxygen therapy and assisted ventilation for pulmonary complications.
• Record intake and output. Watch closely for decreased urine output—a possible indicator of renal failure.
• Monitor the I.V. fluid infusion rate hourly. Deliver enough fluids to prevent dehydration, provided the patient has adequate urine output.
• Give antipyretic medications, as ordered, and tepid sponge baths to reduce fever.
• Administer antibiotics at ordered administration times.
• Provide meticulous mouth and skin care. Offer mentholated lotions to soothe itching resulting from the rash.
• Observe for petechiae.
• Frequently turn the patient to prevent pressure ulcers and pneumonia. Encourage incentive spirometry and deep breathing to reduce the patient's risk for atelectasis.
• Plan care to promote adequate rest periods.

• Provide the patient with frequent, small, high-protein, high-calorie meals, or administer tube feedings if necessary.
• Closely supervise the patient. Use restraining devices only if necessary. Administer sedatives, as ordered. Implement any safety measures needed to prevent patient injury.

Patient teaching

• Instruct the patient to report any recurrent symptoms to the doctor at once so that treatment can resume promptly.
• To prevent Rocky Mountain spotted fever, advise the patient to avoid tick-infested areas. If he does frequent these areas, instruct him to inspect his entire body (including his scalp) every 3 to 4 hours for attached ticks. Remind him to wear protective clothing, such as a long-sleeved shirt and slacks firmly tucked into laced boots. Tell him to apply insect repellant to clothes and exposed skin.
• Teach patients and caregivers how to correctly remove ticks with tweezers or forceps and steady traction. Show them how to avoid leaving mouth parts in skin. Instruct them not to handle the tick or tick fragments.

PROTOZOA

Such diseases as *Pneumocystis carinii* pneumonia, malaria, amebiasis, giardiasis, toxoplasmosis, and trichomoniasis result from minute but complex unicellular animals known as protozoa. These pathogens are known for their well-defined life cycles.

PNEUMOCYSTIS CARINII PNEUMONIA

Because of its association with human immunodeficiency virus (HIV) infection, *Pneumocystis carinii* pneumonia (PCP), an infectious, opportunistic infection, has increased in incidence since the 1980s. Before PCP prophylaxis, this disease was the first clue in about 60% of patients that an HIV infection was present.

PCP occurs in up to 90% of HIV-infected patients in the United States during their lifetime. It also is associated with other immunosuppressive conditions, including organ transplantation, leukemia, and lymphoma.

Causes

P. carinii, the cause of PCP, usually is classified as a protozoan, although some investigators consider it more closely related to fungi. The organism exists as a saprophyte in the lungs of humans and various animals. Part of the normal flora in most healthy people, *P. carinii* becomes an aggressive pathogen in the immunocompromised patient. Impaired cell-mediated (T-cell) immunity is thought to be more important than impaired humoral (B-cell) immunity in predisposing the patient to PCP, but the immune defects involved are poorly understood.

The organism invades the lungs bilaterally and multiplies extracellularly. As the infestation grows, alveoli fill with organisms and exudate, impairing gas exchange. The alveoli hypertrophy and thicken progressively, eventually leading to extensive consolidation.

The primary transmission route seems to be air, although the organism is already resident in most people. The incubation period probably lasts for 4 to 8 weeks.

Complications

PCP can progress to pulmonary insufficiency and, possibly, death. Disseminated infection doesn't occur.

Assessment findings

The patient typically has a history of an immunocompromising condition or procedure, such as HIV infection, leukemia, lymphoma, or organ transplantation.

PCP begins insidiously with increasing shortness of breath and a nonproductive cough. Anorexia, generalized fatigue, and weight loss may be reported. Although the patient may have hypoxemia and hypercapnea, he may not exhibit significant clinical symptoms. Throughout the illness, he may report a low-grade, intermittent fever.

Inspection may reveal tachypnea, dyspnea, and accessory muscle use when the patient breathes. With acute illness, he may appear cyanotic.

Late in the disease, when consolidation develops, chest percussion discloses dullness. Auscultation findings include crackles (in about one-third of patients) and decreased breath sounds (in patients with advanced pneumonia). (See *Planning care for the patient with PCP,* page 194.)

Diagnostic tests

Histologic studies can confirm *P. carinii.* In many patients with HIV, initial examination of a first-morning sputum specimen (induced by inhaling an ultrasoni-

cally dispersed saline mist) may be sufficient. This technique usually is ineffective in patients without HIV.

In all patients, fiber-optic bronchoscopy remains the most commonly used diagnostic tool to confirm PCP. Invasive procedures, such as transbronchial biopsy and open lung biopsy, are less commonly used.

In addition, a chest X-ray may show slowly progressing, fluffy infiltrates and occasional nodular lesions or a spontaneous pneumothorax. These findings must be differentiated from findings in other types of pneumonia or adult respiratory distress syndrome.

A gallium scan may show increased uptake over the lungs even when the chest X-ray appears relatively normal.

In PCP, arterial blood gas studies detect hypoxia and an increased A-a gradient.

Treatment

PCP may respond to drug therapy with co-trimoxazole or pentamidine isethionate. Because of immune system impairment, many patients with HIV experience severe adverse reactions to drug therapy. These reactions include bone marrow suppression, thrush, fever, hepatoxicity, and anaphylaxis. Nausea, vomiting, and rashes are common. To treat the latter effects, the doctor may prescribe diphenhydramine.

Leucovorin may reduce bone marrow suppression and may be used prophylactically in patients with HIV infection.

Pentamidine may be administered I.V. or in aerosol form. I.V. pentamidine is associated with severe toxic effects, whereas the inhaled form usually is well tolerated. However, inhaled pentamidine may not effectively reach the lung apices. Aerosolized pentamidine, co-trimoxazole, or dapsone may be given prophylactically to high-risk patients.

Supportive measures, such as oxygen therapy, mechanical ventilation, adequate nutrition, and fluid balance, are important adjunctive therapies. Oral morphine sulfate solution may reduce respiratory rate and anxiety, enhancing oxygenation.

Nursing diagnoses

- Activity intolerance
- Altered nutrition: Less than body requirements
- Diversional activity deficit
- Fear
- Fluid volume deficit
- Hyperthermia
- Impaired gas exchange

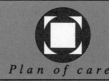

Plan of care

PLANNING CARE FOR THE PATIENT WITH P.C.P.

How can you best help a patient with PCP? Use your assessment findings to select nursing diagnoses and devise a care plan. For example, consider ways to care for Jack Taylor, a 30-year-old attorney.

Patient history

Mr. Taylor tells you that he has been short of breath, especially when he walks his dog. He has a dry cough and, in the past 6 weeks, he has lost about 20 lb (9 kg). He feels exhausted and has no appetite. He thinks his symptoms began about 2 months ago with the flu. He treated himself with rest, aspirin, and orange juice. As you talk, you learn that Mr. Taylor's family consists of an elderly father, a sister, and his longtime roommate, Tom Barnes. He explains that from what he has read and learned from his friends, he may be infected with human immunodeficiency virus (HIV). You offer reassurance as you proceed.

Assessment findings

Your baseline assessment begins with Mr. Taylor's vital signs. His temperature is 100.4° F (38° C); his respiratory rate, 30 breaths/minute. His pulse is shallow at 100 beats/minute, and his blood pressure registers 140/76 mm Hg.

On inspection, you see a pallid white man in moderate respiratory distress. He's dyspneic even when speaking. He uses accessory muscles when breathing. His lips and oral mucous membranes appear dry.

Palpation of Mr. Taylor's lymph nodes reveals enlarged cervical, axillary, and inguinal nodes. Chest auscultation discloses crackles.

Reviewing test results, you find that bilateral interstitial infiltrates were seen on chest X-ray. Arterial blood gas (ABG) analysis reveals:

- PaO_2: 70 mm Hg
- SaO_2: 92%
- $PaCO_2$: 30 mm Hg
- HCO_3: 24 mEq/liter
- pH: 7.40.
  The complete blood count shows:
- hemoglobin: 11 g/dl
- hematocrit: 32%
- platelet count: 173,000/mm³
- white blood cell count: 12,500/mm³.
  The suspected medical diagnosis is PCP. Mr. Taylor is scheduled for fiber-optic bronchoscopy today to obtain a tissue specimen for culture.

Nursing diagnoses

Based on your assessment findings, you devise a list of nursing diagnoses, including the following:
- Impaired gas exchange related to pulmonary infection
- Activity intolerance related to fatigue and shortness of breath
- Altered nutrition: Less than body requirements, related to infection and anorexia
- Anxiety related to hypoxemia and possible diagnosis of HIV infection
- Ineffective individual coping related to suspected diagnosis of HIV infection
- Risk for infection related to suspected immunodeficiency
- Risk for infection: Others, related to risk of transmissible organism.

Expected outcomes

You define the following goals for the patient. Mr. Taylor will:
- improve oxygenation to restore optimal respiratory performance
- modify activity levels to increase his comfort
- stabilize body weight
- prevent contagion.

Implementation

Which steps will you take to promote these outcomes for Mr. Taylor?

To improve oxygenation
- Reassess respiratory status and

monitor ABG levels every 4 hours. Alter care measures as needed.
- Administer oxygen therapy, encouraging deep-breathing exercises and incentive spirometry to promote gas exchange.
- Place the patient in semi-Fowler's or Fowler's position to assist lung expansion.
- Give ordered antimicrobial drugs to combat infection. Monitor for adverse reactions.

To modify activity levels
- Provide diversional activities.
- Coordinate activities of the health care team to allow Mr. Taylor adequate rest between procedures.
- Teach him energy conservation techniques.
- Encourage ambulation when his condition improves.

To stabilize weight
- Provide high-calorie, high-protein foods in small portions.
- Eliminate appetite-suppressing strong or offensive food odors by serving food that tastes best cold or at room temperature.
- Reduce anxiety by providing a relaxing environment, eliminating excessive environmental stimuli, and allowing ample time for meals.
- Provide nutritional supplements.

To prevent contagion
- Observe universal precautions.

Evaluation

Reassess Mr. Taylor's plan of care, altering it as needed. To evaluate it, answer such questions as these:

Have breathing exercises helped to improve oxygenation? Are ABG levels improved? Does Mr. Taylor exhibit less dyspnea with increased activity? Does he report increased energy with ambulation and rest periods? Has his appetite improved? Has he stopped losing weight?

- Impaired social interaction
- Impaired verbal communication
- Ineffective breathing pattern
- Powerlessness
- Self-care deficit

Nursing interventions

- Implement universal precautions.
- Frequently assess the patient's respiratory status, and monitor arterial blood gas levels. Administer oxygen therapy, as ordered.
- Encourage ambulation, deep-breathing exercises, and incentive spirometry to facilitate effective gas exchange.
- Administer antipyretics, as ordered, to relieve fever.
- Monitor intake and output and daily weight to evaluate fluid balance. Replace fluids as ordered.
- Give antimicrobial drugs, as ordered. Never give pentamidine I.M. because it can cause pain and sterile abscesses. Administer the I.V. drug form slowly over 60 minutes to reduce the risk of hypotension.
- Monitor for adverse effects of antimicrobial drugs. If the patient is receiving co-trimoxazole, watch for nausea, vomiting, rash, bone marrow suppression, thrush, fever, hepatoxicity, and anaphylaxis. If he's receiving pentamidine, watch for cardiac arrhythmias, hypotension, dizziness, azotemia, hypocalcemia, and hepatic disturbances.
- Provide diversional activities and adequate rest periods.
- Supply nutritional supplements as needed. Encourage the patient to eat a high-calorie, protein-rich diet. Offer small, frequent meals if the patient cannot tolerate large amounts of food.
- Give emotional support and help the patient identify and use meaningful support systems.

Patient teaching

- Instruct the patient about the medication regimen, especially about the adverse effects.
- Teach the patient energy conservation techniques.
- If the patient requires oxygen therapy at home, explain that an oxygen concentrator may be most effective.

MALARIA

An acute tropical, as well as a subtropical, infectious disease, malaria is most prevalent in Southeast Asia, the Middle East, Haiti, the Dominican Republic, India, Africa, Papua New Guinea, and Central and South America. Falciparum malaria is the most severe form of the disease. When treated, malaria seldom is fatal; untreated, it's fatal in 10% of victims, usually as a result of complications.

Untreated primary attacks last from a week to a month or longer. Relapses are common and can recur sporadically for several years. Susceptibility to the disease is universal.

Since 1940, only rarely have cases of malaria been contracted in the United States, and the incidence has markedly decreased since the end of the Vietnam war. But worldwide, nearly 270 million new cases are contracted each year, causing nearly 2 million deaths.

Causes

Malaria is caused by *Plasmodium vivax, P. malariae, P. falciparum,* and *P. ovale,* all of which are transmitted to humans by mosquito vectors.

Malaria literally means "bad air," and for centuries, it was thought to result from the inhalation of swamp vapors. It's now known that malaria is transmitted by the bite of female *Anopheles* mosquitoes, which abound in humid, swampy areas. When an infected mosquito bites, it injects *Plasmodium* sporozoites into the wound. The infective sporozoites migrate by blood circulation to parenchymal cells of the liver; there they form cystlike structures that contain thousands of merozoites.

On release, each merozoite invades an erythrocyte and feeds on hemoglobin. The erythrocyte eventually ruptures, releasing heme (malaria pigment), cell debris, and more merozoites that, unless destroyed by phagocytes, enter other erythrocytes. At this point, the infected person becomes a reservoir of malaria who infects any mosquito that feeds on him, thus beginning a new cycle of transmission.

As parasites, *P. vivax, P. ovale,* and *P. malariae* may persist for years in the liver and are responsible for the chronic carrier state. Because blood transfusions and street-drug paraphernalia also can spread malaria, drug addicts have a higher incidence of the disease.

Complications

Falciparum malaria can cause renal failure, liver failure, congestive heart failure, pulmonary edema, disseminated intravascular coagulation (DIC), circulatory collapse, severe normocytic anemia, seizures, hypoglycemia, splenic rupture, cerebral dysfunction, and death.

During pregnancy, malaria can lead to premature delivery, spontaneous abortion, stillbirth, and low-birth-weight infants.

Warning

PALPATION PRECAUTIONS IN MALARIA

To decrease the risk of splenic rupture in malaria, avoid vigorous palpation of the spleen. The patient's spleen is enlarged, so it may be extremely fragile. Nevertheless, spontaneous rupture may occur. The spleen is especially prone to rupture in *P. vivax* malaria.

Assessment findings

The patient's history may reveal travel to an endemic area, a recent blood transfusion, or I.V. drug use.

After an incubation period of 12 to 30 days, the patient may report malaria's prodromal signs and symptoms, such as chills, fever, headache, fatigue, and myalgia interspersed with periods of well-being (the hallmark of the benign form of malaria). Acute attacks (paroxysms) occur when erythrocytes rupture. These attacks have three stages:
• *cold stage,* lasting for 1 to 2 hours, ranging from chills to extreme shaking
• *hot stage,* lasting for 3 to 4 hours, characterized by a high fever (up to 107° F [41.7° C]) accompanied by cough, headache, backache, abdominal pain, nausea, vomiting, and delirium
• *wet stage,* lasting for 2 to 4 hours, characterized by profuse sweating.

Between paroxysms, the patient typically experiences a period of well-being, except in *P. falciparum* infection.

Inspection reveals pale skin. Rigors can be seen in the cold stage, and flushing, tachypnea, and mental confusion may accompany the hot stage.

Less frequently, inspection findings may include urticaria, jaundice, and petechial rash. Anemia and oliguria may be noted if acute renal failure occurs in the patient with *P. falciparum* infection. If cerebral complications develop, you may note hemiplegia, seizures, altered mental processes, and coma.

Palpation may reveal moderate splenomegaly and tender hepatomegaly. Lymphadenopathy usually is not present. Tachycardia accompanies paroxysms. Orthostatic hypotension commonly occurs in the hot stage of paroxysms. (See *Palpation precautions in malaria.*)

Chest auscultation may reveal scattered crackles.

Diagnostic tests

Unequivocal diagnosis depends on laboratory identification of the parasites in red blood cells of peripheral blood smears. The Centers for Disease Control can identify donors responsible for transmitting malaria through indirect fluorescent serum antibody tests. These tests are unreliable in the acute phase because antibodies can be undetectable for 2 weeks after onset.

Supplementary laboratory test values that support this diagnosis include decreased hemoglobin, a normal or decreased white blood cell (WBC) count (as low as 3,000/mm^3), and protein and WBCs in urine sediment. In falciparum malaria, serum values reflect DIC: a reduced platelet count (20,000 to 50,000/mm^3), prolonged prothrombin time (18 to 20 seconds), prolonged partial thromboplastin time (60 to 100 seconds), and decreased plasma fibrinogen levels.

Treatment

Malaria is best treated with oral chloroquine in all but chloroquine-resistant *P. falciparum* infection. Within 24 hours after such therapy begins, signs and symptoms and parasitosis decrease, and the patient usually recovers within 3 to 4 days. If the patient is comatose or vomiting frequently, chloroquine is given I.M. instead. Although rare, toxic reactions include GI upset, pruritus, headache, and visual disturbances.

Malaria caused by *P. falciparum,* which is resistant to chloroquine, requires treatment with oral quinine for 10 days, given concurrently with pyrimethamine with sulfadoxine and a sulfonamide, such as sulfadiazine. Relapses require the same treatment, or quinine alone, followed by tetracycline. Mefloquine also may be used for chloroquine-resistant malaria.

The only drug effective against the hepatic stage of the disease that is available in the United States is primaquine phosphate, given daily for 14 days. This drug can induce DIC from increased hemolysis of RBCs; consequently, it's contraindicated during an acute attack. (See *Nursing considerations for antimalarial drugs.*)

For travelers spending less than 3 weeks in areas where malaria exists, weekly prophylaxis includes oral chloroquine, beginning 2 weeks before and ending 6 weeks after the trip. Chloroquine and pyrimethamine with sulfadoxine may be ordered for those staying longer than 3 weeks, although combination treatment can cause severe adverse reactions. If the traveler isn't sensitive to either component of pyrimethamine with sulfadoxine, he may be given a single dose to take if he has a febrile episode. (See *How to prevent malaria*, page 198.)

Any traveler who develops an acute febrile illness should seek prompt medical attention, regardless of prophylaxis measures taken.

Nursing diagnoses
• Activity intolerance
• Altered thought processes
• Decreased cardiac output
• Diversional activity deficit
• Fatigue
• Fluid volume deficit
• Hyperthermia
• Impaired gas exchange
• Impaired physical mobility
• Impaired skin integrity
• Pain
• Risk for infection
• Risk for injury
• Self-care deficit

Nursing interventions
• Assess the patient on admission and daily thereafter for fatigue, fever, orthostatic hypotension, disorientation, myalgia, and arthralgia. Enforce bed rest during periods of acute illness.
• Institute universal precautions. Protect the patient from secondary bacterial infection by following proper hand washing and aseptic techniques. Double-bag all contaminated linens, and send them to the laundry as an isolation item.
• To reduce fever, administer antipyretics, as ordered. Document the onset and duration of fever as well as symptoms before, during, and after each episode. Administer analgesics, as ordered.
• Fluid balance is fragile, so keep a strict record of intake and output. Closely monitor I.V. fluids. Avoid fluid overload (especially in falciparum malaria) because it can lead to pulmonary edema and the aggravation of cerebral symptoms. Observe blood chemistry levels for hyponatremia and increased blood urea nitrogen, creatinine, and bilirubin levels. Monitor urine output hourly, and maintain it at 40 to 60 ml/hour for an adult and 15 to 30 ml/hour for a child. Immediately report any decrease in urine output or the onset of hematuria—a possible sign of renal failure.
• Slowly administer packed RBCs or whole blood while checking for crackles, tachycardia, and shortness of breath.

NURSING CONSIDERATIONS FOR ANTIMALARIAL DRUGS

Follow these guidelines for administering antimalarial drugs, such as chloroquine, primaquine, pyrimethamine, and quinine.

Chloroquine
• Perform baseline and periodic ophthalmic examinations, and report blurred vision, increased sensitivity to light, and muscle weakness to the doctor.
• Consult the doctor about altering therapy if muscle weakness appears.
• Suggest an audiometric examination before, during, and after therapy.
• Caution the patient to avoid excessive exposure to the sun to prevent exacerbating drug-induced dermatoses.

Primaquine
• Give with meals or antacids.
• Discontinue administration if you observe a sudden fall in hemoglobin concentration or in red blood cell or white blood cell count, or a marked darkening of urine, suggesting an impending hemolytic reaction.

Pyrimethamine
• Administer with meals to minimize GI distress.
• Check blood counts (including platelets) twice a week. If signs of folic or folinic acid deficiency develop, reduce the dosage or discontinue administration while the patient receives parenteral folinic acid until blood counts become normal.

Quinine
• Use with caution in the patient with a cardiovascular condition. Discontinue administration if you see any signs of idiosyncrasy or toxicity, such as headache, epigastric distress, diarrhea, rashes, or pruritus, in a mild reaction; or delirium, seizures, blindness, cardiovascular collapse, asthma, hemolytic anemia, or granulocytosis, in a severe reaction.
• Frequently monitor blood pressure while administering quinine I.V. Rapid administration causes marked hypotension.

• If humidified oxygen is ordered because of anemia, note the patient's response, particularly any changes in rate or character of respirations, or improvement in mucous membrane color.
• Watch for and immediately report signs of internal bleeding, such as tachycardia, hypotension, and pallor.

HOW TO PREVENT MALARIA

Follow these guidelines for preventing malaria, particularly if you practice or travel in mosquito-infested regions.
• Drain, fill, and eliminate breeding areas of the *Anopheles* mosquito.
• Install screens or mosquito netting in living and sleeping quarters in endemic areas.
• Use a residual insecticide on clothing and skin to discourage mosquito bites.
• Seek treatment for known cases of malaria.
• Question blood donors for a history of, or possible exposure to, malaria. They may give blood if they haven't taken any antimalarial drugs and are asymptomatic after 6 months outside an endemic area; if they were asymptomatic after treatment for malaria more than 3 years ago; or if they were asymptomatic after receiving malaria prophylaxis more than 3 years ago.
• Seek prophylactic drug therapy before traveling to an endemic area.

• Encourage frequent coughing and deep breathing, especially if the patient is on bed rest or has pulmonary complications. Record the amount and color of sputum.
• Watch for adverse effects of drug therapy, and take measures to relieve them.
• If the patient is comatose, change his position frequently and perform passive range-of-motion exercises every 3 to 4 hours. If the patient is unconscious or disoriented, provide proper supervision, use restraints only as needed, and keep an airway or padded tongue blade available.
• Provide emotional support and reassurance, especially in critical illness.
• Report all cases of malaria to local public health authorities.

Patient teaching
• Explain the procedures and treatment to the patient and his family. Listen sympathetically, and answer questions clearly. Suggest that family members be tested for malaria. Emphasize the need for follow-up care to check the effectiveness of treatment and to manage residual problems.

AMEBIASIS
Also called amebic dysentery, amebiasis can take the form of either an acute or a chronic protozoal infection. Extraintestinal amebiasis can induce hepatic abscess

and infection of the lungs, pleural cavity, pericardium, peritoneum and, rarely, the brain.

Amebiasis occurs worldwide, affecting about 10% of the population. It's most common in the tropics, subtropics, and other areas with poor sanitation and health practices.

Incidence in the United States averages between 2% and 5%. The disease most commonly occurs among migrant workers, homosexuals, institutionalized people, and patients with acquired immunodeficiency syndrome (AIDS), in whom fecal-oral contamination is common.

The prognosis is good, although complications increase the risk of death.

Causes
Amebiasis is caused by *Entamoeba histolytica*. This protozoan has two stages: during the cystic stage, it can survive outside the body; during the trophozoite stage, it can't.

Transmission occurs through ingesting feces-contaminated food or water or through oral-anal sexual practices. The ingested cysts pass through the intestine, where digestive secretions break them down, freeing the motile trophozoites within. The trophozoites then multiply, and either invade and ulcerate the mucosa of the large intestine or simply feed on intestinal bacteria. As the trophozoites are carried slowly toward the rectum, they are encysted and then excreted in feces. Humans are the principal carriers.

Complications
Amebiasis can cause chronic, recurrent episodes of diarrhea and abdominal pain, ameboma, megacolon, intussusception, extraintestinal abscesses, and intestinal stricture, hemorrhage, or perforation. Rarely, it causes a brain abscess, which usually is fatal.

Assessment findings
The patient may have a history of recent travel to an area with poor sanitation, sexual practices involving oral-anal contact, eating or drinking suspect food or water, or institutionalization.

The patient's signs and symptoms vary with the severity of the infestation, from no symptoms or only mild diarrhea to fulminating dysentery.

If the patient has *acute amebiasis,* he'll complain of chills and abdominal cramping; profuse, bloody diarrhea with tenesmus; and diffuse abdominal tenderness (caused by extensive rectosigmoid ulcers). He'll also have a sudden high fever, with a temperature of 104° to 105° F (40° to 40.6° C.)

A patient with *chronic amebiasis* may report intermittent diarrhea that lasts for 1 to 4 weeks and recurs several times a year. Such diarrhea produces 4 to 8 (or, in severe diarrhea, up to 18) foul-smelling mucus- and blood-tinged stools daily. The patient also may report vague abdominal cramps and, possibly, weight loss. Any fever he has is mild.

During inspection, you may note perianal ulceration and systemic signs of dehydration or anemia. Palpation may reveal diffuse abdominal tenderness and hepatomegaly. On auscultation of the abdomen, you may note hyperactive bowel sounds, particularly in the lower quadrants, when the patient has acute diarrhea.

Diagnostic tests
Isolating *E. histolytica* in fresh feces or in aspirates from abscesses, ulcers, or tissue confirms acute amebiasis. Endoscopy can aid in diagnosis, unless it's contraindicated by fulminant disease.

Other tests that support the diagnosis include:
• indirect hemagglutination test (positive with current or previous infection)
• complement fixation (usually positive only during active disease)
• a liver scan, which may reveal abscesses.

Treatment
The patient with amebiasis may receive metronidazole or emetine, both amebicides, for intestinal and extraintestinal infection. If he has just an intestinal infection, he'll receive either iodoquinol or paromomysin. For liver abscess without intestinal infections, he'll receive chloroquine.

The patient also may receive tetracycline along with metronidazole, emetine, iodoquinol, or paromomysin; the tetracycline supports the antiamoebic effect of these drugs by destroying the intestinal bacteria on which the amoebae normally feed.

Diloxanide furoate, an intestinal amebicide, and dehydroemetine, for intestinal and extraintestinal infections, also are useful in treating amebiasis. They're available through the Centers for Disease Control and Prevention.

Exploratory surgery is hazardous because it can lead to peritonitis, perforation, and pericecal abscess.

Nursing diagnoses
• Altered nutrition: Less than body requirements
• Altered sexuality patterns
• Diarrhea
• Fatigue
• Fluid volume deficit
• Impaired skin integrity
• Knowledge deficit
• Pain
• Risk for infection

Nursing interventions
• Institute enteric precautions.
• Obtain a stool specimen for examination. Don't give the patient a soap or hypotonic enema, bismuth, antacids, laxatives, barium preparations, or antibiotics (such as erythromycin or tetracycline) before collecting the sample because they interfere with the test. Send the specimen to the laboratory immediately.
• Monitor the frequency of the patient's bowel movements and the characteristics of his stools.
• Keep the patient's perianal area clean. Provide skin care after each bowel movement.
• Don't use fecal incontinence bags because they may spread disease.
• Administer amebicide medications, as ordered. Monitor the patient for toxic effects.
• Make sure the patient gets adequate rest, but provide him with diversional activities between rest periods.
• Assess the patient for signs of dehydration, and administer I.V. fluids, as ordered. Encourage him to drink fluids as soon as he can tolerate them.

Patient teaching
• Teach the patient about amebicide therapy, including precautions he should take and adverse effects of the medication. Explain to the patient taking metronidazole that he should avoid drinking alcohol while taking the drug and for 3 days after he has finished taking it; otherwise, a disulfiram-like reaction could result. Signs and symptoms include confusion, nausea, vomiting, headache, and seizures. Also warn him that the drug may turn his urine dark brown.
• Encourage the patient to return for follow-up appointments at scheduled intervals. If he's taking dehydroemetine, explain that he'll need routine electrocardiograms to monitor for cardiac arrhythmias, an adverse effect of the drug.
• Advise the patient's family and sexual partners to seek medical attention for amebiasis.
• Teach the patient and his family how to handle infectious material and about the need for careful hand washing. When warranted, teach the patient about safe sexual practices.

• Advise travelers to endemic areas and campers. to boil untreated or contaminated water to prevent the disease.

GIARDIASIS

Also called *Giardia* enteritis and lambliasis, giardiasis is a protozoal infection of the small bowel.

Giardiasis occurs worldwide but is most common in developing countries and other areas where sanitation and hygiene are poor.

In the United States, giardiasis most frequently occurs in travelers who have recently returned from endemic areas, campers who drink unpurified water from contaminated streams, male homosexuals, patients with congenital IgA deficiency, and children in day-care centers. Children in general are more likely to develop giardiasis than adults, probably because of frequent hand-to-mouth activity. Over the past 10 years, the parasite responsible for the disease has been found in municipal water sources, nursing homes, and day-care centers.

The prognosis is good; with treatment, the patient recovers completely. Without treatment, symptoms continue to wax and wane. Also, giardiasis doesn't confer immunity, so reinfections may occur.

Causes

Giardiasis is caused by the symmetrical flagellate protozoan *Giardia lamblia,* which has two stages: the cystic stage and the trophozoite stage. Ingestion of *G. lamblia* cysts in fecally contaminated water or the fecal-oral transfer of cysts by an infected person results in giardiasis.

When cysts enter the small bowel, they release trophozoites, which attach themselves with their sucking disks to the bowel's epithelial surface. This attachment causes superficial mucosal invasion and destruction, inflammation, and irritation. After that, the trophozoites encyst again, travel down the colon, and are excreted. Unformed feces that pass quickly through the intestine may contain trophozoites as well as cysts.

Complications

The mucosal destruction caused by the protozoa decreases food transit time through the small intestine and results in malabsorption. Other complications include dehydration and lactose intolerance.

Assessment findings

The patient's history may include recent travel to an area with poor sanitation, sexual practices that involve oral-anal contact, drinking suspect water, or institutionalization.

A patient with acute giardiasis may complain of abdominal cramps accompanied by explosive, pale, loose, greasy, malodorous, and frequent stools (from 2 to 10 daily). He will also report nausea. In chronic giardiasis, the patient also may complain of fatigue, weight loss, and flatulence. A mild infection may cause no intestinal symptoms.

Auscultation of the abdomen may reveal hyperactive bowel sounds in the right upper and left lower quadrants just before bowel movements, although you may not detect these sounds between episodes. You're most likely to notice alterations 30 minutes to 1 hour after the patient eats.

On palpation, you won't elicit localized tenderness, although you may note general upper and right lower quadrant discomfort and guarding.

Diagnostic tests

An accurate diagnosis depends on examination of a fresh stool specimen for cysts or examination of duodenal aspirate or biopsy for trophozoites.

Treatment

Giardiasis responds readily to oral quinacrine. Or the patient may instead be given metronidazole or furazolidone, although they're not as effective. If the patient has severe diarrhea and oral fluid intake is inadequate, he may need parenteral fluid replacement to prevent dehydration.

Nursing diagnoses

• Altered nutrition: Less than body requirements
• Diarrhea
• Fatigue
• Fluid volume deficit
• Impaired skin integrity
• Knowledge deficit
• Pain
• Risk for infection

Nursing interventions

• Institute enteric precautions, and quickly dispose of all fecal material. (Normal sewage systems adequately remove and process infected feces.) Pay strict attention to hand washing, particularly after handling feces. If

the patient is a child or an incontinent adult, he'll need a private room.
• Monitor the frequency of the patient's bowel movements and the characteristics of his stools. Keep his perianal area clean, making sure to clean his skin thoroughly after each bowel movement.
• Make sure the patient takes in adequate fluids. If necessary, administer I.V. fluid therapy. Provide nutritionally adequate foods, and monitor the patient's nutritional intake to prevent malnutrition.
• Administer medication, as ordered, carefully monitoring for adverse effects. If the patient is taking quinacrine, he may experience headache, diarrhea, nightmares, dizziness and, possibly, toxic psychosis. The patient taking metronidazole may have headache, GI upset, a metallic taste in his mouth, and a disulfiram-like reaction if alcohol is ingested. The patient taking furazolidone may experience headache, nausea, vomiting, an allergic reaction, and a disulfiram-like reaction when alcohol is ingested.
• Report epidemic situations to public health authorities.

Patient teaching
• Teach the patient about his medication, including precautions he should take and adverse effects. Caution the patient taking metronidazole or furazolidone not to drink alcohol while taking the drug and for 3 days after he has finished taking it. Otherwise, he may experience a disulfiram-like reaction (confusion, nausea, vomiting, headache, and seizures). Also warn him that his urine may turn dark brown.
• Encourage the patient to return for follow-up appointments because relapses can occur.
• Advise family members and others who may have been in contact with the patient to have their stools tested for *G. lamblia* cysts.
• Teach the patient and his family about the need for good personal hygiene, particularly proper hand-washing technique, and how to handle infectious material. When warranted, teach the patient about safe sexual practices.
• Teach travelers to endemic areas not to drink tap or suspect water or to eat uncooked and unpeeled fruits or vegetables, which may have been rinsed in contaminated water. Explain that prophylactic drug therapy isn't recommended.
• Advise campers to purify all stream and lake water before drinking it.

TOXOPLASMOSIS
Depending on their environment and eating habits, up to 70% of people in the United States are infected with *Toxoplasma gondii* — making toxoplasmosis one of the most common infectious diseases. Occurring worldwide, it's less common in cold or hot, arid climates and at high elevations.

The disease usually causes localized infection. However, it may produce significant generalized infection, especially in immunodeficient patients, such as neonates, acquired immunodeficiency syndrome (AIDS) patients, patients who've recently had an organ transplant, those with lymphoma, and those receiving immunosuppressant therapy.

Once infected, the patient may carry the organism for life. Reactivation of the acute infection can occur. Congenital toxoplasmosis, characterized by lesions in the central nervous system (CNS), may result in stillbirth or serious birth defects.

Causes
Toxoplasmosis is caused by the protozoan *T. gondii*, which exists in trophozoite forms in the acute stages of infection and in cystic forms (tissue cysts and oocysts) in the latent stages. The infection is transmitted by ingestion of tissue cysts in raw or undercooked meat (heating, drying, or freezing destroys these cysts) or by fecal-oral contamination from infected cats. Toxoplasmosis also occurs in vegetarians who aren't exposed to cats, so some other means of transmission may exist.

Congenital toxoplasmosis follows transplacental transmission from a mother who acquires primary toxoplasmosis shortly before or during pregnancy. Congenital infection is more severe when acquired early in the pregnancy.

Complications
Toxoplasmosis may cause encephalitis, myocarditis, pneumonitis, hepatitis, or polymyositis. If the disease is acquired in the first trimester of pregnancy, it commonly results in stillbirth. About one-third of infants who survive have congenital toxoplasmosis with CNS involvement and chorioretinitis (see also *Ocular toxoplasmosis*, page 202).

Assessment findings
The patient's history may reveal an immunocompromised state, exposure to cat feces, or frequent ingestion of poorly cooked meat.

OCULAR TOXOPLASMOSIS

Characterized by focal necrotizing retinitis, ocular toxoplasmosis (active chorioretinitis) accounts for about 25% of all cases of granulomatous uveitis. Although usually the result of a congenital infection, it may not appear until adolescence or young adulthood, when infection is reactivated.
    Symptoms include blurred vision, scotoma, pain, photophobia, and impairment or loss of central vision. Vision improves as inflammation subsides but usually without recovery of lost visual acuity. Ocular toxoplasmosis may subside after treatment with prednisone.

A patient with localized (mild, lymphatic) toxoplasmosis may complain of mononucleosis-like symptoms: malaise, myalgia, headache, fatigue, and sore throat. He'll also have a fever. A patient with generalized (fulminating, disseminated) infection may complain of headache, vomiting, cough, and dyspnea. His temperature may run as high as 106° F (41.1° C).

Inspection of the patient with generalized disease reveals delirium and seizures—signs of encephalitis. You also may note a diffuse maculopapular rash (except on the palms, soles, and scalp) and cyanosis.

Inspection of an infant with congenital toxoplasmosis may reveal hydrocephalus or microcephalus, seizures, jaundice, purpura, and rash. Other defects, which may not become apparent until months or years later, include strabismus, blindness, epilepsy, and mental retardation.

Palpation of the neonate reveals lymphadenopathy, splenomegaly, and hepatomegaly.

Auscultation of a patient with toxoplasmosis may reveal coarse crackles.

Diagnostic tests

Isolation of *T. gondii* in mice after their inoculation with specimens of body fluids, blood, and tissue, or *T. gondii* antibodies in such specimens, confirms toxoplasmosis.

Treatment

Most effective during the acute stage, treatment consists of drug therapy with sulfonamides and pyrimethamine for 4 to 6 weeks. The patient also may receive folinic acid to control pyrimethamine's adverse effects.

These drugs act synergistically against the trophozoites but don't eliminate already developed tissue cysts. For this reason, and because they don't alleviate the underlying immune system defect in AIDS, an AIDS patient needs toxoplasmosis treatment for life.

An AIDS patient who can't tolerate sulfonamides may receive clindamycin instead. This drug also is the primary treatment in ocular toxoplasmosis.

Nursing diagnoses

- Activity intolerance
- Fatigue
- Fluid volume deficit
- Hyperthermia
- Impaired skin integrity
- Ineffective breathing pattern
- Pain
- Risk for injury
- Sensory or perceptual alterations

Nursing interventions

- Give antipyretics and, possibly, tepid sponge baths to decrease fever.
- Make sure the patient with a high fever, vomiting, and sore throat receives sufficient fluid intake. Provide nutritionally adequate foods and, if needed, small, frequent feedings.
- Promote bed rest during the acute stage. Later, help the patient gradually increase his level of activity.
- Frequently assess respiratory status, especially in the immunocompromised patient. Provide chest physiotherapy and administer oxygen, as needed. Assist ventilation if needed.
- Assess the patient for signs of neurologic involvement and increased intracranial pressure.
- Don't palpate the patient's abdomen vigorously; this could lead to a ruptured spleen. For the same reason, discourage vigorous activity.
- Modify the environment, as needed, to protect a patient with neurologic manifestations or chorioretinitis. Refer him for rehabilitation or counseling, as needed.
- Carefully monitor the patient's drug therapy.
- Because sulfonamides cause blood dyscrasias and pyrimethamine depresses bone marrow, closely monitor the patient's hematologic values.
- Report all cases of toxoplasmosis to the local public health department.

Patient teaching

- Teach the patient about necessary medications, including the need for frequent blood tests.

• Emphasize the importance of regularly scheduled follow-up care.
• Advise all people to wash their hands after working with soil because it may be contaminated with cat oocysts; to cook meat thoroughly and to freeze it promptly if it's not for immediate use; to change cat litter daily (cat oocysts don't become infective until 1 to 4 days after excretion); to cover children's sand boxes; and to keep flies away from food because flies transport oocysts.

TRICHOMONIASIS

A protozoal infection of the lower genitourinary tract, trichomoniasis affects about 20% of sexually active women and 10% of sexually active men. The infection usually involves only the vagina or urethra.

The disease occurs worldwide. In women, the condition may be acute or chronic. The prognosis is good, especially if both sexual partners receive treatment concurrently; otherwise, the disease may recur. Symptoms may subside even if the disease isn't treated, although *Trichomonas vaginalis* infection will persist, possibly resulting in abnormal cytologic cervical smears.

Causes

A tetraflagellated, motile protozoan, *T. vaginalis* causes trichomoniasis in women by infecting the vagina, the urethra, and, possibly, the endocervix, Bartholin's glands, Skene's glands, and bladder. In men, it infects the lower urethra and, possibly, the prostate gland, seminal vesicles, and epididymis.

The organism grows best when the vaginal mucosa is more alkaline than normal (pH about 5.5 to 5.8). Factors that raise the vaginal pH—use of oral contraceptives, pregnancy, bacterial overgrowth, exudative cervical or vaginal lesions, and frequent douching, which disturbs lactobacilli that normally live in the vagina and maintain acidity—may predispose women to trichomoniasis.

Trichomoniasis usually is transmitted by intercourse; less often, by contaminated douche equipment and moist washcloths. An infected mother may transmit the infection to her newborn child through vaginal delivery.

Complications

Chronic trichomoniasis may lead to significant vaginal infection with mucosal irritation and erosion. Pelvic inflammatory disease also may occur.

Assessment findings

The patient's history may reveal unprotected sexual contact with an infected partner, a previous sexually transmitted disease, or a current sexually transmitted disease. About 70% of women—including those with chronic infections—and most men with trichomoniasis are asymptomatic.

A female patient with signs and symptoms may complain of vaginal discharge, severe itching, vulvovaginal irritation, dyspareunia, dysuria, urinary frequency and, occasionally, postcoital spotting, menorrhagia, and dysmenorrhea. These signs and symptoms may persist for a week to several months and may be more pronounced just after menstruation or during pregnancy. A male patient may complain of dysuria and urinary frequency.

In a female patient, your inspection may reveal vulvar and vaginal erythema and edema, frank excoriation, and a copious gray or greenish yellow, malodorous, and possibly profuse and frothy discharge that usually can be seen in the posterior vaginal fornix.

Diagnostic tests

Direct microscopic examination of vaginal or seminal discharge confirms the diagnosis when it reveals *T. vaginalis,* a motile, pear-shaped organism. Examination of urine specimens also may reveal *T. vaginalis.*

Cervical examination by colposcopy may demonstrate punctate cervical hemorrhages, giving the cervix a strawberry appearance that is almost pathognomonic for this disorder. Visual inspection seldom reveals this sign.

Treatment

Oral metronidazole given simultaneously to both sexual partners effectively cures trichomoniasis. The recommended dosage is 250 mg of oral metronidazole given three times a day for 7 days, or one 2-g oral dose.

Oral metronidazole hasn't been proven safe during the first trimester of pregnancy. A pregnant patient in the first trimester may insert a clotrimazole vaginal tablet at bedtime for 7 days for symptomatic relief. Sitz baths may help relieve symptoms.

Nursing diagnoses

• Altered sexuality patterns
• Altered urinary elimination
• Anxiety
• Impaired skin integrity
• Knowledge deficit

• Pain
• Sexual dysfunction

Nursing interventions
• Institute universal precautions when examining the patient or collecting specimens.
• Administer sitz baths to relieve discomfort.
• If the patient is pregnant, make sure she receives adequate treatment before delivery to prevent the neonate from contracting the infection.
• Encourage the patient to notify sexual partners so that they can be checked for the disease.

Patient teaching
• Instruct the patient not to douche before being examined for trichomoniasis.
• To help prevent reinfection during treatment, urge abstinence from intercourse and encourage the use of condoms. Refer sexual partners for treatment even if they're asymptomatic.
• If vaginal tablets are ordered, teach the patient the correct way to insert them.
• Warn the patient to abstain from alcoholic beverages while taking metronidazole and for at least 3 days after he has finished taking it. Alcohol consumption may provoke a disulfiram-like reaction (confusion, headache, cramps, vomiting, and seizures). Also, tell the patient this drug may turn his urine dark brown.
• Instruct the patient to notify the doctor if signs of candidal superinfection occur.
• Caution the patient to avoid douches and vaginal sprays because chronic use can alter vaginal pH.
• Tell the patient to scrub the bathtub with a disinfecting cleanser before and after sitz baths.
• Inform the patient that she can reduce the risk of genitourinary bacterial growth by wearing loose-fitting cotton underwear that allows ventilation. Bacteria flourish in a warm, dark, moist environment.

CRYPTOSPORIDIOSIS
This intestinal infection typically results in acute, self-limited diarrhea. However, in immunocompromised patients, cryptosporidiosis causes chronic, severe, and life-threatening symptoms.

The disease is prevalent in immunocompromised patients, such as malnourished children, patients with hypogammaglobulinemia, and those who receive immunosuppressants for cancer therapy or organ transplantation. It's especially prevalent in patients with acquired immunodeficiency syndrome (AIDS), in whom the incidence can run as high as 30%.

Cryptosporidiosis occurs worldwide. In addition to immunocompromised patients, travelers to foreign countries, medical personnel caring for patients with the disease, and children are at particular risk. Incidence in children with gastroenteritis in Western countries ranges from 1% to 4%; in developing countries, up to 11% of children with gastroenteritis have cryptosporidiosis.

Cryptosporidiosis is increasingly recognized as a major cause of diarrhea in the United States. An outbreak in Milwaukee in 1993, caused by contamination of the public water supply, resulted in an estimated 400,000 cases. Other outbreaks have been traced to contaminated swimming pools and fresh-pressed apple cider.

Causes
Cryptosporidiosis is caused by the protozoan *Cryptosporidium*. These small spherules inhabit the microvillus border of the intestinal epithelium. There, the protozoa shed infected oocysts into the intestinal lumen, where they pass into the feces. (See *Cryptosporidium oocyst*.)

These oocysts are particularly hardy, resisting destruction by routine water chlorination. This increases the risk of infection spreading through contact with contaminated water. The disease can also be transmitted via contaminated food and person-to-person contact.

Complications
Complications can be particularly severe in immunocompromised patients. In these patients, profuse, watery diarrhea can lead to severe fluid and electrolyte depletion and malnutrition. Rectal excoriation and breakdown can also result.

If the biliary tract becomes affected, papillary stenosis, sclerosing cholangitis, or cholecystitis can occur.

Assessment findings
Although asymptomatic infections can occur in both normal and immunocompromised patients, the typical patient with cryptosporidiosis develops symptoms after an incubation period of approximately 7 days. (The incubation period may be shorter in an immunocompromised patient.) The patient initially complains of watery, nonbloody diarrhea. He may also report abdominal pain, anorexia, nausea, fever, and weight loss. In the 10% of patients who develop biliary tract in-

volvement, right upper abdominal pain may be severe. Signs and symptoms usually subside within 2 weeks, but may recur sporadically for months to years.

The history of an immunocompromised patient typically reveals a more gradual onset of symptoms. Such a patient may also develop more severe diarrhea with daily fluid losses as high as 20 liters.

For all patients, auscultation of the abdomen may reveal hyperactive bowel sounds. Palpation may reveal abdominal tenderness.

Diagnostic tests

Cryptosporidiosis often goes undetected as the cause of profuse diarrhea because the acid-fast stain needed to detect the organism isn't routinely used. However, the acid-fast stain as well as microscopic examination of stool samples reveals the presence of oocysts. If too few oocysts are excreted to show up readily under microscopic examination, Sheather's cover-slip flotation method can make detection easier by concentrating the oocysts.

The infecting organisms can also be detected by light and electron microscopy at the apical surfaces of intestinal epithelium obtained through biopsies of the small bowel. Although serologic tests exist, their value in diagnosing acute or chronic infections in immunocompromised patients hasn't been determined.

With biliary tract involvement, studies may reveal an elevated alkaline phosphatase level, gallbladder wall thickening, and dilated bile ducts.

Treatment

Although no treatment currently exists that can eradicate the infecting organism, several medications are being investigated to control the disease in patients with AIDS. (See *Drug treatment for cryptosporidiosis,* page 206.)

Treatment of cryptosporidiosis consists mainly of supportive measures to control symptoms. Such measures include fluid replacement to prevent dehydration as well as administration of analgesics to relieve pain and antidiarrheal and antiperistaltic agents to control diarrhea. Occasionally, a patient—especially one who is immunocompromised—may require I.V. hyperalimentation therapy to maintain adequate nutrition.

Nursing diagnoses
• Altered nutrition: Less than body requirements
• Anxiety
• Diarrhea

CRYPTOSPORIDIUM OOCYST

This illustration shows the oocyst that causes cryptosporidiosis.

• Knowledge deficit
• Pain
• Risk for altered body temperature
• Risk for fluid volume deficit
• Risk for impaired tissue integrity
• Risk for infection

Nursing interventions
• Closely monitor the patient's fluid and electrolyte balance.
• Encourage an adequate intake of fluids, especially those rich in electrolytes.
• Monitor the patient's intake and output, and weigh him daily to evaluate the need for fluid replacement. Watch him closely for signs of dehydration, and provide fluid replacement as ordered.
• Administer analgesics, antidiarrheal and antiperistaltic agents, and antibiotics, as ordered. Observe the patient for signs of adverse reactions as well as therapeutic effects.
• If the patient is receiving I.V. hyperalimentation therapy, monitor him carefully. Provide meticulous skin care to maintain skin integrity at the I.V. site.
• Apply perirectal protective cream to prevent excoriation and skin breakdown.
• Encourage small, frequent meals to help prevent nausea.

DRUG TREATMENT FOR CRYPTOSPORIDIOSIS

Because cryptosporidiosis can cause life-threatening complications in patients with acquired immunodeficiency syndrome, several drugs are under investigation for treating the disease. However, no effective therapy yet exists to eradicate the organism.

Drugs under investigation include the antiviral agent zidovudine, which has proven somewhat effective in patients who haven't previously taken the drug. Cryptosporidiosis is the sole indication for the orphan drug spiramycin, an oral aminoglycoside. Unfortunately, this drug — along with diclazuril, the antidiarrheal agent somatostatin, and the antibacterial drug azithromycin — has yielded inconsistent results. The antiprotozoal agent albendazole, although not yet commercially available in the United States, is also undergoing clinical trials.

Patient teaching

• Teach the patient about his medications. Make sure he understands how to take the drugs and what adverse reactions to watch for. Stress the importance of calling his doctor immediately if he develops an adverse reaction.
• Teach the patient and his family to recognize the signs and symptoms of dehydration, including weight loss, poor skin turgor, oliguria, irritability, and dry flushed skin. Tell them to report such findings to the doctor.
• Teach the patient and family about good personal hygiene, especially proper hand-washing technique. Explain to them how to safely handle potentially infectious material, such as soiled bed sheets.
• Advise the patient's family members and close contacts to have their stools tested.

HELMINTHS

Helminthic disorders result from infection with parasitic worms, such as the fluke, tapeworm, and roundworm.

TRICHINOSIS

Also called trichiniasis and trichinellosis, trichinosis is a chronic infection that occurs worldwide. It's especially common in populations that eat pork or bear meat.

Trichinosis may produce multiple symptoms; respiratory, central nervous system (CNS), and cardiovascular complications; and, rarely, death. In the United States trichinosis usually is mild.

Causes

Trichinosis is caused by larvae of the intestinal roundworm *Trichinella spiralis*. Transmission occurs through ingestion of uncooked or undercooked meat that contains *T. spiralis* cysts. Such cysts are found primarily in swine and less often in dogs, cats, bears, horses, wild boars, foxes, wolves, and marine animals. These cysts result from the animals' ingestion of similarly contaminated flesh. In swine, such infection is caused by eating table scraps or raw garbage. Human-to-human transmission doesn't occur.

Once the cyst enters the body, gastric juices free the worm from the cyst capsule. It reaches sexual maturity in a few days. Then the female roundworm burrows into the intestinal mucosa and reproduces. The larvae are transported through the lymphatic system and the bloodstream. They become embedded as cysts in striated muscle, especially in the diaphragm, chest, arms, and legs.

Complications

Trichinosis can cause such complications as encephalitis, myocarditis, pneumonia, and respiratory failure.

Assessment findings

The patient's history may reveal ingestion of uncooked or undercooked meat, especially pork. Most patients are asymptomatic. Even when symptoms do occur, their frequency and severity vary.

During the first week, the patient may complain of intestinal symptoms, most commonly diarrhea. He also may report other symptoms, such as abdominal discomfort and vomiting.

During the second week, the patient may complain of systemic symptoms, most prominently muscle pain. He also may experience headache, weakness, fatigue, cough, shortness of breath, and dysphagia. His temperature usually will be elevated, ranging from 102° to 104° F (38.9° to 40° C).

With the appearance of systemic symptoms, inspection may reveal periorbital edema, possibly related to subconjunctival hemorrhages, and chemosis. You'll occasionally observe retinal hemorrhage. You may note a rash, along with edema in affected muscles (including the eye, masseter, neck and lumbrical muscles, as well as limb flexors).

Diagnostic tests
Infection may be difficult to prove. Stools may contain mature worms and larvae during the invasion stage. Skeletal muscle biopsies can show encysted larvae 10 days after ingestion. If a sample of the contaminated meat is available, analysis also shows larvae.

Skin testing done within 17 to 20 days of ingestion may show a positive histamine-like reaction 15 minutes after intradermal injection of the antigen. Such a result may remain positive for up to 5 years after exposure. Elevated acute and convalescent antibody titers (determined by flocculation tests 3 to 4 weeks after infection) confirm the diagnosis.

Other abnormal test results include elevated serum alanine aminotransferase (formerly SGPT), aspartate aminotransferase (formerly SGOT), creatine phosphokinase, and lactate dehydrogenase levels and an elevated eosinophil count (up to 15,000/mm³) during the acute stages. A normal or increased lymphocyte level (up to 300/mm³) and increased protein levels in cerebrospinal fluid indicate CNS involvement.

Treatment
Mebendazole may prevent symptomatic trichinosis when given in the first few days after ingestion of infected meat. This disease usually is self-limiting, and complete recovery occurs within a few months.

Supportive therapy, such as bed rest, administration of salicylates, and physical therapy to maintain and enhance muscle function, usually proves effective.

If symptoms persist for several years, the patient may need mebendazole therapy. He'll need corticosteroids only if he has a fever, allergic symptoms, leukocytosis, and eosinophilia.

Nursing diagnoses
• Activity intolerance
• Diarrhea
• Hyperthermia
• Impaired physical mobility
• Impaired skin integrity
• Impaired swallowing
• Ineffective breathing pattern
• Knowledge deficit
• Pain
• Risk for fluid volume deficit
• Sensory or perceptual alterations (visual)

Nursing interventions
• Reduce the patient's fever with tepid baths, cooling blankets, or antipyretics. Relieve muscle pain with analgesics, bed rest, and proper body alignment.
• If the patient has a fever, vomiting, and diarrhea, monitor his intake and output and daily weight. Replace fluids as needed.
• Provide skin care after bowel movements to prevent excoriation.
• To prevent pressure sores, frequently reposition the patient and gently massage bony prominences.
• Assess the patient's respiratory status. Administer oxygen and assist respiration, as needed.
• Encourage the patient to exercise to maintain muscle strength and function.
• Provide safety measures for the visually impaired patient, and assist with mobility during convalescence.
• Report all cases of trichinosis to local public health authorities.

Patient teaching
• Explain the importance of bed rest. Sudden death from cardiac involvement may occur in a patient with moderate to severe infection who has resumed activity too soon. Warn the patient to continue bed rest into the convalescent stage to avoid a serious relapse and, possibly, death.
• To help prevent trichinosis, teach patients about correct cooking and storing methods, not only for pork and pork products, but also for meat from carnivores. To kill trichinae, internal meat temperatures should reach 150° F (66° C), and meat color should change from pink to gray (unless the meat has been cured or frozen for at least 10 days at low temperatures).
• Warn travelers to other countries or to poor areas in the United States to avoid eating pork. Swine in these areas often are fed raw garbage.

HOOKWORM DISEASE
A helminthic infection of the upper intestine, hookworm disease (also called uncinariasis) is chronic and debilitating. The disease's major sign is anemia. Sandy soil, high humidity, a warm climate, and failure to wear shoes all favor its transmission.

In the United States, hookworm disease is most common in the Southeast. Although it can cause cardiopulmonary complications, it's seldom fatal, except in debilitated people and in infants.

Causes

Hookworm disease is caused by *Ancylostoma duodenale* in the eastern hemisphere and *Necator americanus* in the western hemisphere. Both forms of hookworm disease are transmitted to humans through direct skin penetration (usually in the foot) by hookworm larvae in soil contaminated with feces that contain hookworm ova. These ova develop into infectious larvae in 1 to 3 days.

Larvae travel through the lymphatic system to the pulmonary capillaries, where they penetrate alveoli and move up the bronchial tree to the trachea and epiglottis. There they are swallowed and enter the GI tract. When they reach the small intestine, they mature, attach to the jejunal mucosa, and suck blood, oxygen, and glucose from the intestinal wall. These mature worms then deposit ova, which are excreted in the stool, starting the cycle anew. Hookworm larvae mature in 5 to 6 weeks.

Complications

In severe and chronic infection, anemia from blood loss may lead to cardiomegaly (a result of increased oxygen demands), heart failure, and generalized, massive edema.

Assessment findings

The patient may report that he recently walked barefoot in an area with contaminated soil. He may have few symptoms, and the disease may be overlooked until the worms are passed in the stool. The earliest findings are irritation and pruritus at the entry site.

When the larvae reach the lungs, the patient may complain of sore throat and cough, possibly productive of bloody sputum. When intestinal infection occurs, he may report fatigue, nausea, weight loss, dizziness, uncontrolled diarrhea, and black, tarry stool. Fever occurs when larvae migrate through the lungs.

Inspection may reveal edema and an erythematous papulovesicular rash at the entry site. You also may observe irregular respirations during the migration of larvae through the lungs. Other possible signs include weight loss and growth retardation.

Auscultation of the chest may reveal crackles as larvae migrate through the lungs.

Diagnostic tests

Identification of hookworm ova in a fecal smear confirms the diagnosis. Anemia suggests severe chronic infection. In an infected patient, blood studies show:
• hemoglobin of 5 to 9 g/dl (in a severe case)

• white blood cell count as high as 47,000/mm³
• eosinophil count of 500 to 700/mm³.

Treatment

Mebendazole or pyrantel pamoate is prescribed for hookworm infection. The patient also needs an iron-rich diet or iron supplements to prevent or correct anemia.

Nursing diagnoses

• Altered growth and development
• Altered nutrition: Less than body requirements
• Diarrhea
• Fatigue
• Impaired gas exchange
• Ineffective breathing pattern
• Risk for infection

Nursing interventions

• If the patient has confirmed hookworm infestation, institute universal stool precautions, wear gloves, and wash your hands thoroughly after every patient contact. Promptly dispose of feces.
• If the patient has severe anemia, administer humidified oxygen, if ordered, at a low to moderate flow. (Humidification helps the patient with upper airway irritation from the parasites.) Encourage coughing and deep breathing to stimulate removal of blood or secretions from involved lung areas and to prevent secondary infection.
• Plan your care to allow frequent rest periods because the patient may tire easily. If anemia causes immobility, reposition him often to prevent skin breakdown.
• Closely monitor the patient's intake and output. Note the quantity and frequency of diarrheal stools.
• To help assess nutritional status, weigh the patient daily. To combat malnutrition, emphasize the importance of good nutrition, particularly foods high in iron and protein. If the patient receives iron supplements, explain that they'll darken his stools.
• Administer anthelmintics on an empty stomach.
• Interview the family and other close contacts to see if they have any symptoms.

Patient teaching

• To help prevent reinfection, teach the patient proper hand-washing technique and sanitary disposal of feces. Tell him to wear shoes in endemic areas.

ASCARIASIS

Also called roundworm infection, ascariasis is the most common helminthic infection. It occurs worldwide but is most common in tropical areas with poor sanitation and in the Orient, where farmers use human feces as fertilizer. In the United States, it's more prevalent in the South, particularly among children ages 4 to 12.

Causes

Ascariasis is caused by *Ascaris lumbricoides,* a large roundworm that resembles an earthworm. It's transmitted to humans by ingestion of soil contaminated with human feces that harbor *A. lumbricoides* ova. Ingestion may occur directly (by eating contaminated soil) or indirectly (by eating poorly washed raw vegetables grown in contaminated soil).

Ascariasis never passes directly from person to person. After ingestion, *A. lumbricoides* ova hatch and release larvae, which penetrate the intestinal wall and reach the lungs through the bloodstream. After about 10 days in pulmonary capillaries and alveoli, the larvae migrate to the bronchioles, bronchi, trachea, and epiglottis. There they are swallowed and returned to the intestine to mature into worms.

Complications

Ascariasis may lead to biliary or intestinal obstruction and pulmonary disease.

Assessment findings

The patient's history may reveal ingestion of poorly washed raw vegetables grown in contaminated soil. Most patients with ascariasis are asymptomatic. Some patients exhibit pulmonary symptoms, such as transitory coughing.

Mild intestinal infection may cause only vague stomach discomfort. The first clue may be vomiting a worm or passing a worm in the stool. Severe infection results in stomach pain, vomiting, restlessness, disturbed sleep, and, in extreme cases, intestinal obstruction. Fever may occur when larvae are migrating through the lungs.

Inspection eventually may reveal weight loss and impaired growth. Bowel sounds may be hyperactive above the obstruction and diminished or absent below the obstruction. Auscultation of the chest may detect wheezing.

Palpation of the abdomen may reveal distention.

Diagnostic tests

The key to diagnosis is identifying ova in the stools, or adult worms, which may be passed rectally or by mouth.

Treatment

Anthelmintic therapy, the primary treatment, uses pyrantel pamoate or piperazine to temporarily paralyze the worms, permitting peristalsis to expel them. Mebendazole also is used to block helminth nutrition. These drugs are up to 95% effective, even after a single dose.

In multiple helminthic infection, one of these drugs must be the first treatment; using some other anthelmintic first may stimulate *A. lumbricoides* perforation into other organs. No specific treatment exists for migratory infection because anthelmintics affect only mature worms.

In intestinal obstruction, nasogastric suctioning controls vomiting. When suctioning can be discontinued, instill piperazine and clamp the nasogastric tube. If vomiting does not occur, give a second dose of piperazine orally 24 hours later, as ordered. If this is ineffective, surgery probably will be required. Endoscopic retrograde cholangiopancreatography and papillotomy may be required for helminth removal.

Nursing diagnoses
- Altered growth and development
- Altered nutrition: Less than body requirements
- Altered thought processes
- Colonic constipation
- Hyperthermia
- Ineffective breathing pattern
- Knowledge deficit
- Pain
- Risk for fluid volume deficit
- Risk for infection

Nursing interventions
- Although isolation is unnecessary, properly dispose of feces and soiled linen, and carefully wash your hands after patient contact.
- If the patient is receiving nasogastric suction, be sure to provide mouth care.
- Maintain nasogastric tube patency and check for secretion returns every 4 hours.
- Administer antipyretics and give tepid sponge baths to reduce fever.
- Monitor respiratory status and administer oxygen or assist ventilation if pulmonary complications develop.

INCIDENCE OF TAPEWORM INFESTATION

The geographic areas and groups affected by tapeworm infestation vary as follows.

Taenia saginata
The beef tapeworm is found worldwide but is most prevalent in Europe and East Africa.

Taenia solium
The incidence of the pork tapeworm is highest in Mexico and Latin America; it's lowest among Muslims and Jews.

Diphyllobothrium latum
The fish tapeworm is endemic in Finland, northern Russia, Japan, Alaska, Australia, the Great Lakes region of the United States, Switzerland, Chile, and Argentina.

Hymenolepis nana
The most common tapeworm in humans, the dwarf tapeworm is particularly common among institutionalized mentally retarded children and in underdeveloped countries.

• Question family members and other contacts about symptoms.
• Weigh the patient daily and monitor intake and output. Replace fluids as needed. Provide a nutritionally adequate diet and administer nutritional supplements, as prescribed.
• Administer anthelmintic drug therapy, as ordered. Monitor nasogastric tube aspirate to ensure drug absorption.

Patient teaching
• Teach the patient to prevent reinfection by washing hands thoroughly, especially before eating and after defecating, and by bathing and changing underwear and bed linens daily.
• Inform the patient of drug adverse effects. Tell him that piperazine may cause stomach upset, dizziness, and urticaria. Remember, piperazine is contraindicated in patients with seizure disorders. Pyrantel produces red stools and vomitus and may cause stomach upset, headache, dizziness, and rash; mebendazole may cause abdominal pain and diarrhea.

TAENIASIS
Also called cestodiasis and commonly called tapeworm, taeniasis is a parasitic infection that can result from several types of parasites. The incidence of tapeworm infestation varies with the type. (See *Incidence of tapeworm infestation.*)

Tapeworm usually is a chronic but benign intestinal disease. However, infestation with *Taenia solium* may cause dangerous systemic and central nervous system (CNS) symptoms if larvae invade the brain and striated muscle of vital organs. Tapeworm seldom is fatal unless it's not treated.

Causes
Taeniasis is caused by *Taenia saginata* (beef tapeworm), *T. solium* (pork tapeworm), *Diphyllobothrium latum* (fish tapeworm), or *Hymenolepis nana*, (dwarf tapeworm).

T. saginata, T. solium, and *D. latum* are transmitted to humans by ingestion of uncooked or undercooked beef, pork, or fish (such as pike, trout, salmon, and turbot) that contains tapeworm cysts. Gastric acids break down these cysts in the stomach, freeing them to mature. The mature tapeworms then fasten to the intestinal wall and produce ova that pass from the body in feces.

H. nana is transmitted directly from person to person and requires no intermediate host. It completes its life cycle in the intestine. Its spread is facilitated by inadequate hand washing.

Complications
Severe tapeworm infection can lead to dehydration and malnutrition.

Assessment findings
Signs and symptoms vary with the type of infestation. A patient with beef tapeworm may complain of a crawling sensation in the perianal area (caused by worm segments that have been passed rectally) and intestinal obstruction (the result of long worm segments that have twisted in the intestinal lumen).

Pork tapeworm can cause seizures, headache, and personality changes. A patient with fish tapeworm may experience signs and symptoms of anemia (his hemoglobin may drop as low as 6 to 8 g/dl).

The signs and symptoms of a patient with dwarf tapeworm depend on his nutritional status and the number of parasites. A patient with a mild infestation commonly has no symptoms. If the infestation is severe, he may complain of anorexia, diarrhea, restlessness, dizziness, and apathy.

Diagnostic tests
Observation of tapeworm ova or body segments in feces allows diagnosis of a tapeworm infestation. Because ova aren't excreted continuously, confirmation may require multiple specimens.

Treatment
Administration of niclosamide or praziquantal cures up to 95% of patients. In beef, pork, and fish tapeworm infestation, the patient receives the drug once; in severe dwarf tapeworm infestation, twice (5 to 7 days each, spaced 2 weeks apart).

In beef tapeworm infestation, the absence of strobilae (multiple tapeworm segments) in feces within 2 to 3 hours of such treatment calls for administration of a laxative. During treatment for pork tapeworm, laxatives and induced vomiting are contraindicated because of the danger of autoinfection and systemic disease.

After drug treatment, all types of tapeworm infestation require follow-up stool specimens during the next 3 to 5 weeks to check for remaining ova or worm segments. Persistent infestation requires a second course of medication.

Nursing diagnoses
• Altered nutrition: Less than body requirements
• Altered thought processes
• Altered tissue perfusion
• Diarrhea
• Risk for fluid volume deficit
• Risk for infection

Nursing interventions
• Carefully dispose of the patient's excretions. Wear gloves when providing personal care and handling fecal excretions, bedpans, and bed linens. Afterward, wash your hands thoroughly and make sure the patient does the same.
• After administering niclosamide, document the passage of strobilae.
• Ask the patient for a list of people he has had contact with. If possible, advise them to seek medical attention to determine if they're infected.
• Document the patient's level of consciousness, and report any changes immediately. If he develops CNS symptoms, keep an artificial airway or padded tongue blade close at hand, raise side rails, keep the bed low, and help him with walking, as needed.
• Monitor intake and output and nutritional status. Replace fluids as needed. Offer a nutritionally adequate diet and administer supplements, as prescribed.
• Use enteric and secretion precautions for a patient with pork tapeworm. Avoid procedures and drugs that may cause vomiting or gagging. Make sure the patient has a private room if he is a child or is incontinent.

Patient teaching
• To prevent reinfection, teach the patient proper hand-washing technique and the need to cook meat and fish thoroughly. Stress the need for follow-up evaluations to monitor the success of therapy and to detect possible reinfection.
• If the patient needs niclosamide therapy, tell him not to consume anything after midnight on the day he starts taking the drug. He must take the drug on an empty stomach.

ENTEROBIASIS
A benign intestinal disease, enterobiasis has several other names, including oxyuriasis and pinworm and seatworm infection. Found worldwide, this disease is common even in temperate regions with good sanitation. It's the most prevalent helminthic infection in the United States.

Infection and reinfection most often occurs in children between ages 5 and 14 and in certain institutionalized groups because of poor hygiene and frequent hand-to-mouth activity. Crowded living conditions commonly enhance its spread to several members of a family.

Causes
Enterobiasis is caused by the nematode *Enterobius vermicularis*. Adult pinworms live in the intestine until the female worms migrate to the perianal region to deposit their ova.

Direct transmission occurs when the patient's hands transfer infective eggs from the anus to the mouth. *Indirect transmission* occurs when the patient comes in contact with contaminated articles, such as linens and clothing.

Complications
Although uncommon, complications may include salpingitis, appendicitis, bowel ulceration, and pelvic granuloma.

SCHISTOSOMAL DERMATITIS

Commonly called swimmers' itch or clam diggers' itch, schistosomal dermatitis affects those who bathe in and camp along freshwater lakes in the eastern and western United States. It's caused by schistosomal cercariae harbored by migratory birds.

The cercariae can penetrate the skin, causing a pruritic papular rash. Initially mild, the reaction grows more severe with repeated exposure. Treatment consists of 5% copper sulfate solution as an antipruritic and 2% methylene blue as an antibacterial agent.

Assessment findings

The patient's history may reveal contact with an infected person or infected articles.

Enterobiasis may be overlooked when it causes no symptoms. In symptomatic infection, the patient complains of intense perianal pruritus, especially at night, when the female worm crawls out of the anus to deposit ova. The pruritus causes the patient to wake up and scratch, disturbing his sleep and causing irritability. He usually doesn't have a fever.

Inspection may reveal perianal erythema and irritation.

Diagnostic tests

Identification of *Enterobius* ova recovered from the perianal area with a cellophane tape swab confirms the diagnosis. A stool sample usually is ova- and worm-free because these worms deposit the ova outside the intestine and die after migration to the anus.

Treatment

Drug therapy with pyrantel pamoate, piperazine, or mebendazole destroys these parasites. Effective eradication requires simultaneous treatment of family members and, in institutions, other patients.

Nursing diagnoses

• Impaired skin integrity
• Risk for infection
• Sleep pattern disturbance

Nursing interventions

• Obtain a specimen for evaluation. Place cellophane tape—sticky side out—on the base end of a test tube, and roll the tube around the perianal region. Make sure you collect the sample before the patient bathes and defecates in the morning. Then send the tape for examination under a microscope.
• Administer drugs, as ordered, to combat infection and relieve distressing symptoms.
• Before giving piperazine, obtain a history of seizure disorders. Because piperazine may aggravate these disorders, it is contraindicated in a patient with such a history.
• Before giving the tablet form of pyrantel, make sure the patient isn't sensitive to aspirin. The tablet has an aspirin coating.
• As warranted, follow up on others who have come in contact with the patient.
• Report all outbreaks of enterobiasis to school authorities.

Patient teaching

• To help prevent the spread of this disease, tell parents to bathe their children daily (showers are preferable to tub baths) and to change underwear and bed linens daily.
• Teach a child with the disease about proper personal hygiene, and stress the need for careful hand washing after defecation and before handling food. Discourage nail biting. If the child can't stop, suggest that he wear gloves until the infection clears.
• If the patient receives pyrantel, tell him and his family that this drug colors the stool bright red and may cause vomiting; the vomitus also will be red.

SCHISTOSOMIASIS

Also called bilharziasis, schistosomiasis is a slowly progressive disease whose incidence is increasing worldwide. It is most prevalent in agricultural areas in Asia, Africa, and South America.

The degree of infection determines the intensity of illness. If untreated, significant morbidity and even mortality can result.

Causes

Schistosomiasis is caused by blood flukes of the class Trematoda. Three major types of these parasites exist: *Schistosoma mansoni* and *S. japonicum* infect the intestinal tract; *S. haematobium* infects the urinary tract.

The parasite is transmitted through bathing, swimming, wading, or working in water contaminated with *Schistosoma* larvae, which are known as cercariae during their infective stage. (Also see *Schistosomal dermatitis*.)

ASSESSMENT FINDINGS IN SCHISTOSOMIASIS

Organism	Incidence	Assessment findings
S. japonicum	Affects men more than women; particularly prevalent among farmers in Japan, China, and the Philippines	May cause acute infection, with sudden onset of fever, chills, headache, and cough. Palpation may reveal such complications as hepatosplenomegaly and lymphadenopathy.
S. mansoni	Prevalent in Western hemisphere, particularly Puerto Rico, Lesser Antilles, Brazil, and Venezuela; also occurs in the Nile delta, Sudan, and central Africa	May cause chronic infection, with irregular fever, fatigue related to anemia, abdominal pain, intermittent diarrhea, and weight loss. If liver involvement develops, palpation reveals hepatomegaly followed by splenomegaly. Inspection may reveal hematemesis related to esophageal varices.
S. haematobium	Africa, Cyprus, Greece, India	Causes terminal hematuria, dysuria, and ureteral colic with secondary infection (symptoms include colicky pain, intermittent flank pain, and vague GI complaints); may culminate in total renal failure.

These cercariae penetrate the skin or mucous membranes and eventually work their way to the liver's venous portal circulation. There, they mature in 1 to 3 months. The adults then migrate to other parts of the body.

The female cercariae lay spiny eggs in blood vessels surrounding the large intestine or bladder. After penetrating the mucosa of these organs, the eggs are excreted in feces or urine. If the eggs hatch in fresh water, the first-stage larvae (miracidia) penetrate freshwater snails, which act as passive intermediate hosts. Cercariae produced in snails escape into water and begin a new life cycle.

Complications

Portal hypertension, hepatosplenomegaly, pulmonary hypertension, ascites, and hematemesis from ruptured esophageal varices can all result from schistosomiasis — as can heart and renal failure, possibly fatal complications.

Rarely, central nervous system complications occur. Granulomatous reactions to the eggs may lead to urinary obstruction or bladder irregularities. Hydronephrosis occurs late in the disease.

Assessment findings

The patient's history may reveal travel to an endemic area or swimming in contaminated water. Signs and symptoms of schistosomiasis depend on the specific causative parasite, the infection site, and the disease stage. (See *Assessment findings in schistosomiasis.*)

Diagnostic tests

The presence of ova in the urine or stool or a mucosal lesion biopsy confirms the diagnosis. A white blood cell count shows eosinophilia.

Treatment

The treatment of choice is the anthelmintic drug praziquantel. The patient needs to be examined again 3 to 6 months after treatment. If this checkup detects any living eggs, treatment may be resumed.

Nursing diagnoses

• Altered nutrition: Less than body requirements
• Diarrhea
• Fatigue
• Fluid volume deficit
• Hyperthermia
• Pain

Nursing interventions

• Plan your care to allow for sufficient rest periods. During the acute stage, the patient may need bed rest.
• Monitor the frequency of the patient's bowel movements and the characteristics of his stools, his intake and output, and his daily weight. If his urinary tract is involved, monitor his frequency of urination and the color and amount of urine.
• Replace fluids as needed, and provide adequate, nutritionally balanced meals. Administer nutritional supplements as needed.

Warning

SIGNS OF DISSEMINATED STRONGYLOIDIASIS

This potentially fatal disease occurs in immuno-compromised patients, such as those with lymphoma, leukemia, lepromatous leprosy, or human immunodeficiency virus infection, and those taking corticosteroids.

If your patient is at risk for this disorder, be alert for severe generalized abdominal pain, diffuse pulmonary infiltrates, pericarditis, myocarditis, hepatic granulomas, cholecystitis, ileus, shock, and signs of meningitis or sepsis from gram-negative bacilli. (Diagnostic tests may not show eosinophilia.)

• Assess the patient for bleeding and anemia. Also check his blood work.
• Administer anthelmintics, analgesics, and antipyretics, as ordered.

Patient teaching
• Explain the medication regimen to the patient.
• Inform the patient about the need for follow-up testing. He should have stool specimens examined 1 to 2 months after therapy ends.
• To help prevent the spread of schistosomiasis, teach the patient to avoid contaminated water.
• If the patient lives in an endemic area, explain the importance of working toward getting the local water supply purified. If he must enter this water, tell him to wear protective clothing and to dry himself afterward.

STRONGYLOIDIASIS

A parasitic intestinal infection, strongyloidiasis (threadworm infection) occurs worldwide. It's endemic in the tropics and subtropics as well as areas associated with poor hygiene. Outbreaks also occur in institutions. Its incidence in the United States is low.

Susceptibility to strongyloidiasis is universal; infection doesn't confer immunity. Because the reproductive cycle of the threadworm may continue in the untreated

host for as long as 45 years after the initial infection, autoinfection is highly probable.

Most patients with strongyloidiasis recover completely, but debilitation from protein loss occasionally is fatal. Massive autoinfection, especially in immunocompromised patients, also can be fatal.

Causes
Strongyloidiasis is caused by the helminth *Strongyloides stercoralis*. Transmission to humans usually occurs through contact with soil that contains infective *S. stercoralis* filariform larvae. Such larvae develop from noninfective rhabdoid (rod-shaped) larvae in human feces. The filariform larvae penetrate the human skin, usually at the feet, and then migrate by way of the lymphatic system to the bloodstream and the lungs.

Once they enter the pulmonary circulation, the filariform larvae break through the alveoli and migrate upward to the pharynx, where they are swallowed. Then they lodge in the small intestine, where they deposit eggs that mature into noninfective rhabdoid larvae. Next, these larvae migrate into the large intestine and are excreted in feces, starting the cycle again. The threadworm life cycle—which begins with penetration of the skin and ends with excretion of rhabdoid larvae—takes 17 days.

In autoinfection, rhabdoid larvae mature within the intestine to become infective filariform larvae.

Complications
If the infection is severe, malnutrition from substantial fat and protein loss, anemia, and lesions resembling ulcerative colitis may result in a secondary bacterial infection. Ulcerated intestinal mucosa may lead to perforation.

Possibly fatal septicemia and massive invasion of organs can occur. These effects of autoinfection are most likely to develop in immunocompromised patients. (See *Signs of disseminated strongyloidiasis*.)

Assessment findings
The patient's history may reveal an immunocompromised state or institutionalization. The patient may report walking in contaminated soil without shoes.

The patient may be asymptomatic, or he may complain of a cough during the stage of larval migration through the lungs. After that, he may complain of such intestinal symptoms as colicky abdominal pain and diarrhea. He also may develop fatigue, weakness, and weight loss. During the pulmonary stage, he may have a fever.

During inspection, you may note an erythematous, pruritic, papular rash at the entrance site, particularly the feet. The rash may become generalized.

Auscultation may reveal normal or hyperactive bowel sounds. You also may hear crackles during the pulmonary stage.

Diagnostic tests
Observation of *S. stercoralis* larvae in a fresh stool specimen allows diagnosis (2 hours after excretion, rhabdoid larvae look like hookworm larvae). Repeated testing may be needed. During the pulmonary phase, sputum may show many eosinophils and larvae.

Treatment
Because of the potential for autoinfection, the patient needs treatment with thiabendazole for 2 to 3 days. The total dose shouldn't exceed 3 g. He also may need protein replacement, blood transfusions, and I.V. fluids.

Retreatment is necessary if *S. stercoralis* remains in stools after therapy. Corticosteroids are contraindicated because they increase the risk of autoinfection and dissemination and also predispose the patient to GI ulceration.

Nursing diagnoses
• Altered nutrition: Less than body requirements
• Diarrhea
• Ineffective breathing pattern
• Pain
• Risk for fluid volume deficit
• Risk for infection

Nursing interventions
• Monitor the patient's intake and output and daily weight, especially if treatment includes blood transfusions and I.V. fluids. Ask the dietary department to provide a high-protein diet. The patient may need nutritional supplements or tube feedings to increase his caloric intake.
• Assess the frequency of the patient's bowel movements and the characteristics of his stools.
• Monitor serum protein levels.
• Wear gloves when handling bedpans or giving perineal care, and promptly dispose of feces.
• Because direct person-to-person transmission doesn't occur, the patient doesn't need isolation. However, label all stool specimens for the laboratory as contaminated.
• Check the patient's family and close contacts for signs of infection.
• If the patient has pulmonary infection, reposition him frequently; encourage incentive spirometry, coughing, and deep breathing; and administer oxygen, as ordered.
• Administer anthelmintic therapy, as ordered.

Patient teaching
• Teach the patient about anthelmintic drug therapy.
• Emphasize the need for follow-up stool examination, continuing several weeks after treatment.
• Warn the patient that thiabendazole may cause mild nausea, vomiting, drowsiness, and giddiness.
• To prevent reinfection, teach the patient proper handwashing technique. Stress the importance of washing his hands before eating and after defecating, and of wearing shoes when in endemic areas.

MISCELLANEOUS INFECTIONS

This category includes chlamydial infections and chronic fatigue and immune dysfunction syndrome.

CHLAMYDIAL INFECTIONS
Urethritis in men, cervicitis in women, and—much less commonly in the United States—lymphogranuloma venereum in both sexes all result from chlamydial infections. And all are linked to one organism: *Chlamydia trachomatis*. (See *Chlamydia trachomatis*, page 216.) These infections are the most common sexually transmitted diseases in the United States, afflicting an estimated 4 million Americans each year.

Children born of infected mothers may contract associated otitis media, pneumonia, and trachoma inclusion conjunctivitis during passage through the birth canal. Although trachoma inclusion conjunctivitis seldom occurs in the United States, it's a leading cause of blindness in Third World countries.

Causes
Transmission of *C. trachomatis*, an intracellular obligate bacterium, primarily follows vaginal or rectal intercourse or oral-genital contact with an infected person. Because signs and symptoms of chlamydial in-

CHLAMYDIA TRACHOMATIS

In chlamydial infections, microscopic examination reveals *Chlamydia trachomatis*, a unicellular parasite with a rigid cell wall.

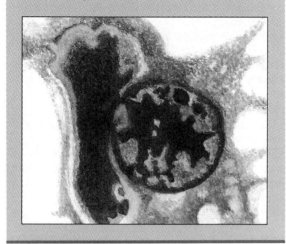

fections commonly appear late in the course of the disease, sexual transmission of the organism occurs unknowingly.

Complications

Untreated, chlamydial infections can lead to acute epididymitis, salpingitis, pelvic inflammatory disease (PID) and, eventually, sterility. In pregnant women, chlamydial infections are associated with spontaneous abortion, premature rupture of membranes, premature delivery, and neonatal death, although a direct link with *C. trachomatis* hasn't been established.

Complications of lymphogranuloma venereum include urethral and rectal strictures, perirectal abscesses, and rectovesical-rectovaginal and ischiorectal fistulas. Elephantiasis with enlargement of the penis or vulva occasionally occurs.

Assessment findings

The patient may have a history of unprotected sexual contact with an infected person, an unknown partner, or multiple sex partners. He also may have another sexually transmitted disease or have had one in the past.

Symptoms vary with the specific type of chlamydial infection; many patients have no symptoms. If the patient has cervicitis, she may complain of pelvic pain and dyspareunia. If PID develops, she may report se-

vere abdominal pain, nausea, vomiting, fever, chills, breakthrough bleeding, and bleeding after intercourse. A woman with urethral syndrome may experience dysuria and urinary frequency.

A male patient with urethritis may complain of dysuria, urinary frequency, and pruritus. If epididymitis develops, he may complain of severe scrotal pain. Prostatitis may cause lower back pain, urinary frequency, dysuria, nocturia, and painful ejaculation.

If the infection involves the rectum, the patient may complain of diarrhea, tenesmus, and pruritus.

A patient with lymphogranuloma venereum may have such systemic signs and symptoms as myalgia, headache, weight loss, backache, fever, and chills.

Inspection by speculum of the patient with cervicitis may reveal cervical erosion and mucopurulent discharge. Inspection of a male patient with urethritis may disclose urethral discharge, which may be copious and purulent, and meatal erythema. If he develops epididymitis, you'll note scrotal swelling and urethral discharge.

In a patient with proctitis, you may note mucopurulent discharge and diffuse or discrete ulceration in the rectosigmoid colon. Inspection of a patient with lymphogranuloma venereum may reveal a primary lesion—a painless vesicle or nonindurated ulcer. Such an ulcer usually is 2 to 3 mm in diameter and occurs on the glans or shaft of the penis; on the labia, vagina, or cervix; or in the rectum. It commonly goes unnoticed.

If a female patient with cervicitis develops PID, palpation reveals tenderness over the lower quadrant, abdominal distention and, sometimes, rigidity.

Palpation of a patient with lymphogranuloma venereum may reveal enlarged inguinal lymph nodes, especially in a male patient. These nodes may become fluctuant, tender masses. Regional nodes draining the initial lesion may enlarge and appear as a series of bilateral buboes. Untreated buboes may rupture and form sinus tracts that discharge a thick, yellow, granular secretion. The patient eventually may develop a scar or an indurated inguinal mass.

Diagnostic tests

Laboratory tests provide definitive diagnosis of chlamydial infection. A swab culture from the infection site (urethra, cervix, or rectum) usually establishes urethritis, cervicitis, salpingitis, endometritis, and proctitis. Culture of aspirated blood, pus, or cerebrospinal fluid establishes epididymitis, prostatitis, and lymphogranuloma venereum.

If the infection site is accessible, the doctor may first attempt direct visualization of cell scrapings or exudate with Giemsa stain or fluorescein-conjugated monoclonal antibodies. However, tissue cell cultures are more sensitive and specific.

Serologic studies to determine previous exposure to *C. trachomatis* include complement fixation tests and immunofluorescence microscopy. The enzyme-linked immunosorbent assay (ELISA) detects the *C. trachomatis* antibody as effectively as the immunofluorescence microscopy test and is useful as a screening test.

Treatment

The recommended first-line treatment for chlamydial infection consists of 100 mg of doxycycline four times a day for 7 to 21 days, or 500 mg of erythromycin four times a day for 7 days. Or the patient can receive 300 mg of ofloxacin every 12 hours for 7 days.

A patient with lymphogranuloma venereum needs extended treatment. A pregnant woman with a chlamydial infection should receive erythromycin stearate.

Nursing diagnoses
• Altered sexuality patterns
• Altered urinary elimination
• Impaired skin integrity
• Knowledge deficit
• Pain
• Risk for infection
• Sexual dysfunction

Nursing interventions
• Use universal precautions when examining the patient, giving patient care, and handling contaminated material. Properly dispose of all soiled dressings and contaminated instruments.
• Monitor the patient for complications.
• Examine and test the patient's sexual contacts for chlamydial infection.
• Check the newborn infant of an infected mother for signs of infection. Take specimens for culture from the infant's eyes, nasopharynx, and rectum. Positive rectal cultures will peak by 5 to 6 weeks postpartum.
• If required in your state, report all cases of chlamydial infection to local public health authorities for follow-up on sexual contacts. (The doctor or laboratory personnel may have done this already.)

Patient teaching
• Teach the patient the dosage requirements of his prescribed medication. Stress the importance of taking all of his medication, even after symptoms subside.
• Teach the patient to follow proper hygiene measures.
• To prevent eye contamination, tell the patient to avoid touching any discharge and to wash his hands before touching his eyes.
• To prevent reinfection during treatment, recommend that the patient abstain from intercourse, or encourage him to use condoms.
• Urge the patient to inform sexual partners of his infection so that they can seek treatment also. Explain that they should receive treatment regardless of their test results.
• Suggest that the patient and his sexual partners receive testing for the human immunodeficiency virus.
• Tell the patient to return for follow-up testing.

CHRONIC FATIGUE AND IMMUNE DYSFUNCTION SYNDROME

Also called chronic fatigue syndrome, chronic Epstein-Barr virus, myalgic encephalomyelitis, and Yuppie flu, this syndrome is characterized by incapacitating fatigue. The patient's symptoms may wax and wane, but they're often severely debilitating and may last for months or years.

Although most prevalent among professionals in their 20s and 30s, the syndrome affects people of all ages, occupations, and income levels. The diagnosis is more common in women than in men or children, especially women under age 45. Sporadic incidence as well as epidemic clusters have been observed.

Causes

The precise cause of chronic fatigue syndrome isn't known. Although the cause originally was attributed to the Epstein-Barr virus, that hypothesis has since been rejected on the basis of serologic and epidemiologic observation.

Several other causative viruses have been proposed and investigated, including cytomegalovirus, herpes simplex virus types 1 and 2, human herpesvirus 6, Inoue-Melnick virus, human adenovirus 2, enteroviruses, measles virus, and a retrovirus that resembles human T-cell lymphotropic virus type II. The onset in some patients suggests a viral illness, but whether the syndrome results from a new or a reactivated infection isn't known.

DIAGNOSTIC CRITERIA IN CHRONIC FATIGUE SYNDROME

The Centers for Disease Control uses two major and several minor criteria for diagnosing chronic fatigue and immune dysfunction syndrome. Keep in mind that they were developed for research purposes, not clinical use.

Major criteria

The patient has persistent or relapsing debilitating fatigue or must tire easily, with no previous history of similar symptoms. The fatigue doesn't resolve with bed rest and is severe enough so that the patient can maintain an average level of activity of less than 50% of normal for at least 6 months.

A thorough evaluation that includes a patient history, a physical examination, and appropriate laboratory findings has ruled out other clinical conditions that produce similar symptoms.

Minor criteria

In addition to the criteria above, the patient must exhibit at least eight of the following symptoms, or six symptoms plus at least two signs. He must have first experienced these at the same time or after the onset of fatigue, and they must have persisted or recurred for at least 6 months. The signs must be documented by a doctor on at least two occasions, at least 1 month apart.

Symptoms
• Reported mild fever (oral temperature of 99.5° to 101.5° F [37.5° to 38.6° C]), as measured by the patient) or chills
• Sore throat
• Painful anterior or posterior cervical or axillary lymph nodes
• Unexplained generalized muscle weakness
• Muscle discomfort or myalgia
• Generalized fatigue that persists for 24 hours or longer after levels of exercise that the patient could have tolerated easily when healthy
• Migratory arthralgia without joint swelling or redness
• One or more neuropsychiatric complaints (photophobia, transient visual scotomata, forgetfulness, excessive irritability, confusion, difficulty thinking, inability to concentrate, depression)
• Sleep disturbance (hypersomnia or insomnia)
• Description of the main symptom complex as first developing over a few hours to a few days (considered equivalent to the symptoms above in meeting the requirements of the case definition)

Signs
• Low-grade fever (oral temperature of 99.5° to 101.5° F [37.5° to 38.6° C] or rectal temperature of 100° to 103.8° F [37.8° to 39.9° C])
• Nonexudative pharyngitis
• Palpable or tender anterior or posterior cervical or axillary lymph nodes ¾" (2 cm) in diameter

---

Another theory holds that some symptoms may result from an overactive immune system. In addition, genetic predisposition, age, hormonal balance, neuropsychiatric factors, sex, previous illness, environment, and stress appear to have a role in the syndrome.

Complications

Chronic fatigue syndrome causes few complications. Its debilitating nature, however, greatly influences the patient's sense of well-being.

Assessment findings

The patient characteristically complains of prolonged, overwhelming fatigue, along with other signs and symptoms, including sore throat, myalgia, and cognitive dysfunction. The Centers for Disease Control uses a working case definition to group symptoms and severity. (See *Diagnostic criteria in chronic fatigue syndrome.*) When assessing the patient, keep in mind that this definition was developed for research purposes, not clinical use. Use the definition as a guide, not as the basis for determining the patient's need for care.

Diagnostic tests

No definitive test exists for this disorder. Diagnostic testing should include tests to rule out other illnesses, such as Epstein-Barr virus, leukemia, and lymphoma.

Some patients with chronic fatigue syndrome have reduced natural killer cell cytotoxicity, abnormal CD4:CD8 T-cell ratios, decreases in immunoglobulin subclasses, mild lymphocytosis, circulating immune complexes, and increased levels of antimicrosomal antibodies. But because these findings vary from patient to patient, they're of uncertain clinical significance.

A psychiatric screening may aid diagnosis because many patients have an underlying psychiatric disorder. Also, they commonly experience depression and anxiety after the syndrome's onset.

Treatment

Polyribonucleotide, an investigational antiviral agent and immunomodulator, is in clinical trials as a treatment for this disease.

Acyclovir, I.V. immune globulin, and I.M. magnesium sulfate also have been studied, but acyclovir has been found no better than a placebo. The role of immune globulin remains unclear after two clinical trials that provided contradictory results. I.M. magnesium sulfate can improve the patient's energy and emotional state and relieve pain.

Treatment focuses on supportive care. The patient with myalgia or arthralgia can benefit from nonsteroidal anti-inflammatory drugs. A patient who sleeps excessively can receive an antidepressant such as fluoxetine. A patient who has trouble sleeping or who experiences pain may benefit from amitriptyline.

Nursing diagnoses

• Activity intolerance
• Altered role performance
• Altered thought processes
• Fatigue
• Pain
• Powerlessness
• Self-esteem disturbance
• Sleep pattern disturbance

Nursing interventions

• Give the patient emotional support through the often long period of diagnostic testing and the protracted, often debilitating course of illness.
• Refer the patient for counseling as needed and to a local support group, if available. Make sure that the group advocates helping the patient lead as normal a life as possible. If necessary, refer him to a mental health center or a career counselor.

Patient teaching

• Suggest that the patient decrease activities when his fatigue is greatest. But advise him to avoid bed rest, which has no proven therapeutic value. A graded exercise program, although often difficult for the patient to accept, may help him feel better. Stress the importance of starting with a short exercise period and slowly increasing exercise time.
• If the patient needs medication, explain the medication regimen. If the doctor prescribes an antidepressant, explain how the medication can help relieve other signs and symptoms, such as sleep pattern disturbances and appetite changes.

• Help the patient return to a normal life-style. Begin by helping him plan a gradual return to work.

SELECTED REFERENCES

Avery, M.E., and First, L.R. *Pediatric Medicine*, 2nd ed. Baltimore: Williams & Wilkins Co., 1994.

Gubler, D.J., et al. "A Field Guide to Animal-Borne Infections," *Patient Care* 28(16):23-25, 29-32, 35-38, October 15, 1994.

Isselbacher, K., et al., eds. *Harrison's Principles of Internal Medicine*, 13th ed. New York: McGraw-Hill Book Co., 1995.

Long, B.C., and Phipps, W.J. *Medical-Surgical Nursing: A Nursing Process Approach*, 3rd ed. St. Louis: Mosby-Year Book, Inc., 1993.

Mandell, G.L., et al. *Principles and Practices of Infectious Diseases*, 4th ed. New York: Churchill Livingstone, 1994.

Nursing Timesavers: Immune and Infectious Disorders, Springhouse, Pa.: Springhouse Corp., 1994.

Tierney, L., et al. *Current Medical Diagnosis and Treatment 1995*. East Norwalk, Conn.: Appleton & Lange, 1995.

Winson, G. "Winning a Losing Battle: Wasting, Physiology, Nutrition — the Most Devastating Aspects of AIDS," *Nursing Times* 91(23):40-43, June 7-13, 1995.

3 TRAUMA

INTRODUCTION

Trauma is the third leading cause of death in the United States, outranked only by cardiovascular disease and cancer. In people under age 44, it's *the* leading cause of death.

Three types of trauma exist: blunt trauma, which leaves the body surface intact; penetrating trauma, which disrupts the body surface; and perforating trauma, which leaves entrance and exit wounds as an object passes through the body.

The basic elements of trauma care include triage, assessment and maintenance of ABCs (airway, breathing, and circulation), protection of the cervical spine, assessment of the patient's level of consciousness (LOC), and, as necessary, patient preparation for transport and, possibly, surgery.

Triage: First things first

Triage is the setting of emergency care priorities by making sound, rapid assessments. You'll base these assessments and subsequent interventions on the severity and number of injuries as well as on the available immediate and long-term resources. These resources include adequate personnel to provide care and facilities to save the patient's life.

Triage involves classifying patients by the urgency of their needs and by their likelihood of survival if treated. For instance, if mass casualties occur, some patients with massive injuries may not receive immediate care because the available personnel and facilities make survival unlikely.

The need for triage often arises at the scene of injury and continues in the emergency department. Following hospital protocol, you'll decide which patient to treat first, which of his injuries to treat first, how best to use other members of the medical team, and how to control patient and staff traffic.

Victims usually are assigned to one of the following categories:
• *Emergent.* A patient in this category has a life-threatening injury that requires treatment within a few minutes to prevent death or further injury. The category covers patients with respiratory distress or cardiopulmonary arrest and severe hemorrhage or shock.
• *Urgent.* A patient with a serious but not immediately life-threatening injury—a stable head, chest, or abdominal injury or a long-bone fracture—falls in this category. He should receive treatment within 1 hour.
• *Delayed.* Included in this category is a patient who has a minor injury, such as a laceration or an abrasion, and can wait 4 to 6 hours for treatment.

• *Indefinite.* A patient in this category can wait indefinitely for treatment or be referred to a clinic. In a disaster or military situation, this category also applies to any patient with massive injuries who has a marginal chance for recovery even with immediate, vigorous care.
• *Deceased.*

When caring for a trauma victim, talk to him while giving care. Explain what you're going to do before you touch him. Also, try to handle difficult situations diplomatically and intelligently, recognize your limitations, and ask for help when you need it.

Keep in mind that trauma care takes its toll on you, too. In many cases, you must deal with patients and families who are emotionally upset, angry, belligerent, intoxicated, or frightened; some may speak only a foreign language. So work calmly and rationally.

Begin with the ABCs

Always begin your care of an injured patient with a brief assessment of the ABCs: airway, breathing, and circulation. Obtain a brief history from the patient, family, friends, or medical personnel who saw the patient before he entered the hospital.

To assess airway patency, check for respiratory distress or signs of obstruction, such as stridor, choking, and cyanosis. Be especially alert for respiratory distress in a patient who inhaled chemicals or was in a fire, particularly if he has upper body burns. If his airway is obstructed, first check cervical alignment: He should have a secure cervical collar, towel rolls on both sides of his head, and tape across his forehead. Then, remove the obstruction, such as vomitus, dentures, blood clots, or foreign bodies, from his mouth.

To open the airway, use a jaw-thrust maneuver. (*Don't* use the head-tilt maneuver for a trauma patient. Suspect cervical spine injury until X-rays rule it out.) Then insert an oropharyngeal or nasopharyngeal airway (except in a patient with massive facial trauma or possible basal skull fracture). As necessary, assist with endotracheal tube insertion or cricothyroidotomy. If rescue personnel have inserted an esophageal obturator airway, leave it in place until the patient has been intubated. This will prevent him from aspirating if he vomits.

Next, make sure the patient's breathing is adequate. Look, listen, and feel for respirations: See if the patient's chest is rising and falling symmetrically, and check breath sounds. Note the rate and depth of respirations, use of accessory and abdominal muscles for breathing, and tracheal position. Also look for jugular vein distention and any open wounds. If the patient isn't breathing, call for help immediately and begin mouth-to-mouth, bag, valve, or mask resuscitation. Also administer supplemental oxygen.

To assess circulation, check for carotid and peripheral pulses. If he has neck injuries, palpate the femoral pulse instead. If circulation has stopped, start cardiopulmonary resuscitation at once.

If you see an external hemorrhage, apply direct pressure to the bleeding site; if the wound is on an extremity, elevate it above heart level, if possible. If this measure doesn't control the bleeding, apply direct pressure to the pressure point proximal to the site. Apply a tourniquet only if the hemorrhage is life-threatening. Because a tourniquet halts distal circulation, its use could cause the patient to lose an arm or a leg.

If the patient's head and neck aren't already immobilized, use an immobilization device, sandbags, a backboard, or tape to do so. Then obtain cervical spine X-rays to rule out spinal cord injury before moving the patient again.

Assess vital signs

Monitor the patient's vital signs, even if he appears stable, because changes can occur rapidly. Document the patient's baseline vital sign readings, and obtain new readings every 5 to 15 minutes until his condition stabilizes. Then place the patient on a cardiac monitor and pulse oximeter for continuous monitoring.

Check the patient's pupillary and motor responses to assess neurologic status. Report his LOC, using a stimulus-response method rather than categorizing; don't use words like "semiconscious" or "stuporous." Report decorticate (flexor) or decerebrate (extensor) postures immediately.

Remember, a patient without a head injury also can have an abnormal neurologic response. Any injury that impairs ventilation or perfusion can cause cerebral edema and raise intracranial pressure. If the patient has neurologic symptoms and is hypotensive, look for an extracranial cause because intracranial bleeding usually is not the cause of hypotension.

Next, perform a secondary survey of the patient by systematically assessing the entire body. Carefully log-roll the patient over, and assess for multiple injuries.

Give the patient oxygen. Then draw samples for arterial blood gas measurement, and calculate the effects of the supplemental oxygen. This lets you establish a baseline for oxygen and acid-base therapy. A patient with multiple injuries always needs supplemental oxygen because of blood loss and overwhelming physiologic stress. If he's conscious, he should show compensatory hyper-

ventilation. If he doesn't, suspect neurologic involvement or chest injury.

Draw blood for typing and cross matching, a complete blood count, prothrombin time, partial thromboplastin time, platelet levels, and routine blood studies, including amylase, electrolyte, and glucose levels. Then begin at least two I.V. lines with 14G or 16G catheters for fluid resuscitation with 0.9% sodium chloride or lactated Ringer's solution.

If the wound is tetanus-prone, ask the patient or a family member when he had his last tetanus immunization. Administer tetanus prophylaxis, as ordered. (See *Tetanus prophylaxis.*)

As indicated, insert an indwelling urinary catheter, unless you see blood at the meatus or in the scrotum, if you suspect an anterior pelvic fracture, or if the patient has a displaced prostate gland.

Then insert a nasogastric tube or, if the patient has facial fractures, an orogastric tube. During tube insertion, maintain cervical spine immobilization. Next, administer prophylactic antibiotics. As ordered, arrange for appropriate diagnostic studies, such as peritoneal lavage or excretory urography, and notify appropriate medical or surgical specialists.

Combat shock

Because severe injuries commonly lead to shock, inspect the patient's skin for color and feel it, noting temperature and moisture. Make sure he's receiving I.V. fluids (lactated Ringer's or 0.9% sodium chloride solution), followed by blood or blood products.

In all cases of massive external or suspected internal bleeding, watch for hypovolemia and estimate the amount of blood lost. Remember that a blood loss of 500 to 1,000 ml might not change systolic blood pressure, but it might elevate the patient's pulse rate.

Stay alert for signs of occult bleeding, common in the chest, abdomen, and thigh. Assess for occult bleeding by taking serial girth measurements at these sites. Use a tape measure and mark where you placed it on the body with a marking pen so that you measure in exactly the same place each time. This way you can accurately detect any enlargement. Increased diameter of the abdomen, chest, or thigh typically means leakage of blood into these tissues. Such blood loss will induce classic signs of hypovolemic shock (tachycardia, tachypnea, hypotension, restlessness, decreased urine output, delayed capillary refill, and cold, clammy skin).

Observe for faint, irregularly formed hemorrhagic patches on the skin around the umbilicus (Cullen's sign), which may signal retroperitoneal hematoma. Retroperi-

TETANUS PROPHYLAXIS

When administering tetanus prophylaxis to a trauma patient, the preferred agent for people ages 7 and older is adsorbed tetanus and diphtheria toxoid (Td).

When you're administering tetanus immune globulin (TIG) concurrently with Td, use separate syringes and administration sites. Give 0.5 ml of Td and 250 units of TIG to adults.

Remember, children under age 7 receive diphtheria and tetanus toxoids and pertussis vaccine (DTP) as part of a routine immunization program. If the child needs a booster dose, DTP is the preferred agent.

Use the following chart as a guide for giving tetanus prophylaxis to a trauma patient.

History of tetanus immunization (number of doses)	Tetanus-prone wounds		Non–tetanus-prone wounds	
	Td	TIG	Td	TIG
Uncertain	Yes	Yes	Yes	No
0 to 2	Yes	Yes	Yes	No
3 or more	No (*yes* if more than 5 years since last dose)	No	No (*yes* if more than 10 years since last dose)	No

toneal bleeding may not cause abdominal tenderness.

If the patient shows clinical signs of hypovolemia, begin I.V. therapy immediately with two or more large-bore catheters, and regulate fluids according to the severity of hypovolemia. Assist with the insertion of a central venous pressure or pulmonary artery catheter to monitor circulating blood volume.

Splinting for transport

Look for limb fractures and dislocations, and check the patient's circulation and neurovascular status distal to the injury. Do this by palpating pulses distal to the injury and looking for the classic signs and symptoms of arterial insufficiency—decreased or absent pulse, pallor, paresthesia, pain, and paralysis. Splint the injury and apply traction, as needed.

Next, prepare the victim for transport. Use special care in suspected cervical spine injury. Splint the areas above and below the injury site to prevent further soft-tissue and neurovascular damage and to minimize pain. For instance, if the forearm is injured, splint the wrist and elbow, too.

Types of splints include:
• *soft splint*—a nonrigid splint, such as a pillow or towels
• *hard splint*—a rigid splint with a firm surface, such as a long or short board, an aluminum ladder splint, or a cardboard splint
• *air splint*—an inflatable splint
• *traction splint*—a splint that uses traction to decrease

angulation and reduce pain, such as a Hare or Thomas splint.

Tips on applying a splint

When splinting a patient's injury, keep in mind the following guidelines:
• Splint most injuries "as they lie," except when neurovascular status is compromised.
• Have one person support the injured part while another applies padding and the splint.
• Secure the splint with straps or gauze—*not* with an elastic bandage.
• To apply an air splint, slide the splint backward over your arm and grasp the distal portion of the injured extremity. Then slip the splint from your arm onto the patient's extremity and inflate the splint.

HEAD INJURIES

Injuries to the head range from minor concussions to life-threatening hematomas and herniation. They also include injuries to structures of the head, such as the jaw.

CONCUSSION

By far the most common head injury, a concussion results from an acceleration-deceleration injury or a blow

WHAT YOUR PATIENT NEEDS TO KNOW AFTER A CONCUSSION

Before the patient's discharge, follow these teaching guidelines:
• Instruct the caregiver to awaken the patient every 2 hours through the night and to ask his name, where he is, and whether he can identify the caregiver.
• Advise the caregiver to return the patient to the hospital immediately if he is difficult to arouse, is disoriented, has seizures, or experiences a persistent or worsening headache, forceful or constant vomiting, blurred vision, any change in personality, abnormal eye movements, a staggering gait, or twitching.
• If the patient is a child, explain to the parents that some children have no apparent ill effects immediately after a concussion but may grow lethargic or somnolent a few hours later.
• Teach the patient the signs of postconcussion syndrome—headache, vertigo, anxiety, personality changes, memory loss, and fatigue. Explain that these signs may persist for several weeks.

to the head hard enough to jostle the brain and make it strike the skull, causing temporary neural dysfunction, but not hard enough to cause a cerebral contusion. Most concussion victims recover within 48 hours. Repeated concussions, however, exact a cumulative toll on the brain.

Causes
The blow that causes a concussion usually is sudden and forceful—a fall to the ground, a punch to the head, a motor vehicle crash. Sometimes, such a blow results from child, spouse, or elder abuse.

Complications
A concussion usually causes no significant anatomic brain injury. Seizures, persistent vomiting, or both may occur. Rarely, a concussion leads to intracranial hemorrhage.

Assessment findings
The patient's history may reveal a short-term loss of consciousness, vomiting, and anterograde and retrograde amnesia: He can't recall what happened immediately after

the injury and has difficulty recalling events that led up to it. Typically, he repeats the same questions. The presence of anterograde amnesia and the duration of retrograde amnesia reliably correlate with the injury's severity.

A family member or friend may report that the patient is behaving out of character. The patient usually complains of dizziness, nausea, and severe headache.

During inspection, you may note that an adult patient behaves irritably or lethargically. Skull palpation may reveal tenderness or hematomas caused by the injury. Neurologic assessment findings usually are normal.

Diagnostic tests
Computed tomography and magnetic resonance imaging help rule out fractures and more serious injuries.

Treatment
Most patients require no treatment except bed rest, observation, and nonnarcotic analgesics for headache.

Nursing diagnoses
• Anxiety
• Pain
• Risk for fluid volume deficit
• Risk for injury

Nursing interventions
• Initially, monitor vital signs continuously and check for additional injuries.
• Check vital signs, level of consciousness, and pupil size every 15 minutes. If the patient's condition worsens or fluctuates, he should be admitted for neurosurgical consultation. If he remains stable after 4 or more hours of observation, he may be discharged (with a head injury instruction sheet) in the care of a responsible adult.
• Observe the patient for headache, dizziness, irritability, and anxiety. If his condition worsens, perform a complete neurologic evaluation and notify the doctor.
• Observe seizure precautions if seizures have occurred.
• Monitor fluid and electrolyte levels and replace them as necessary.

Patient teaching
• Explain to the patient who is discharged from the emergency department that a responsible adult, such as a family member or friend, should continue to observe his condition at home. (See *What your patient needs to know after a concussion*.) If this isn't possible, the patient may be hospitalized for a brief time.
• Tell him not to take anything stronger than nonnarcotic analgesics for a headache. Warn him not to take aspirin

UNDERSTANDING INTRACRANIAL HEMORRHAGE, HEMATOMA, AND TENTORIAL HERNIATION

Left untreated, intracranial hemorrhage, hematoma, and tentorial herniation can be life-threatening. These conditions are among the most serious consequences of head injury.

Causes
A rapid accumulation of blood between the skull and the dura mater is an epidural hemorrhage or hematoma. A subdural hemorrhage or hematoma is a slow accumulation of blood between the dura mater and the subarachnoid membrane. An intracerebral hemorrhage or hematoma occurs within the cerebrum itself. Tentorial herniation results from injured brain tissue that swells and forces itself through the tentorial notch, constricting the brain stem.

Signs and symptoms
An epidural hemorrhage or hematoma can cause immediate loss of consciousness, followed by a lucid interval that lasts from minutes to hours. This eventually gives way to a rapidly progressive decrease in level of consciousness. Other effects include contralateral hemiparesis, progressively severe headache, ipsilateral pupillary dilation, and signs of increased intracranial pressure (ICP). These disorders also cause a decrease in pulse and respiratory rates and an increase in systolic blood pressure.

With a subacute or chronic subdural hemorrhage or hematoma, blood accumulates slowly, so symptoms may not occur until days after the injury. In an acute subdural hematoma, symptoms appear earlier because blood accumulates within 24 hours of the injury. Loss of consciousness occurs, typically with weakness or paralysis.

An intracerebral hemorrhage or hematoma usually causes nuchal rigidity, photophobia, nausea, vomiting, dizziness, seizures, decreased respiratory rate, and progressive obtundation.

Signs and symptoms of tentorial herniation include drowsiness, confusion, dilation of one or both pupils, hyperventilation, nuchal rigidity, bradycardia, and decorticate or decerebrate posturing. Irreversible brain damage or death can occur rapidly.

Treatment
An intracranial hemorrhage may require a craniotomy to locate and control bleeding and to aspirate blood. Epidural and subdural hematomas usually are drained by aspiration through burr holes in the skull. Increased ICP—which can occur in hemorrhage, hematoma, and tentorial herniation—may be controlled with mannitol I.V., steroids, or diuretics, but emergency surgery usually is required.

---

because it may heighten the risk of bleeding.
• If vomiting occurs, instruct the patient to eat lightly until it stops. (Occasional vomiting is normal after sustaining a concussion.)

CEREBRAL CONTUSION

More serious than a concussion, a cerebral contusion is an ecchymosis of brain tissue that results from a severe blow to the head. A contusion disrupts normal nerve functions in the bruised area and may cause loss of consciousness, hemorrhage, edema, and even death.

Causes

A cerebral contusion results from acceleration-deceleration or coup-contrecoup injuries. Such injuries can occur directly beneath the site of impact (coup) when the brain rebounds against the skull from the force of a blow (a beating with a blunt instrument, for example), when the force of the blow drives the brain against the opposite side of the skull (contrecoup), or when the head is hurled forward and stopped abruptly (as in a motor vehicle crash when the driver's head strikes the windshield). The brain

continues moving and slaps against the skull (acceleration) and then rebounds (deceleration).

This injury also is seen in child, spouse, and elder abuse.

Complications

When injuries cause the brain to strike against bony prominences inside the skull (especially the sphenoidal ridges), intracranial hemorrhage or hematoma can occur. The patient also may suffer tentorial herniation. (See *Understanding intracranial hemorrhage, hematoma, and tentorial herniation.*)

Residual headache and vertigo may complicate recovery. Secondary effects, such as brain swelling, may accompany serious contusions, resulting in increased intracranial pressure (ICP) and herniation.

Assessment findings

The patient's history (obtained from family, friends, and emergency personnel, if necessary) reveals a severe traumatic impact to the head, often against a blunt surface, such as a car dashboard. A period of unconsciousness, possibly lasting 6 hours or more, may follow the trauma.

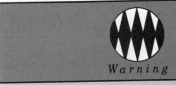

Warning

PREVENTING C.N.S. INFECTION

Avoid cleaning or suctioning the ears or nose of a patient with a head injury. Doing so could introduce microorganisms into the central nervous system (CNS).

Signs and symptoms vary, depending on the location of the contusion and the extent of damage. An unconscious patient may appear pale and motionless, whereas a conscious patient may appear drowsy or easily disturbed by any form of stimulation, such as noise or light. A conscious patient may become agitated, even violent.

Assessment of an unconscious patient may reveal below-normal blood pressure and temperature. His pulse rate may be within normal levels but feeble, and his respirations may be shallow. In a conscious patient, temperature, pulse rate, and respiratory status vary, depending on his physical and emotional status.

Inspection may reveal severe scalp wounds, labored respirations and, possibly, involuntary evacuation of the bowels and bladder. Palpation may disclose less obvious head injuries, such as hematoma. On palpation, the unconscious patient's skin will feel cold.

Neurologic findings may include hemiparesis, decorticate or decerebrate posturing, and unequal pupillary response. With effort, you may be able to rouse an unconscious patient temporarily. If you're performing a neurologic examination after the acute stage of the injury, you may find that the patient has returned to a relatively alert state, perhaps with temporary aphasia, slight hemiparesis, or unilateral numbness.

Diagnostic tests

Cerebral angiography outlines vasculature, and a computed tomography (CT) scan shows ischemic or necrotic tissue, cerebral edema, areas of petechial hemorrhage, and subdural, epidural, and intracerebral hematomas. A CT scan also may reveal a shift in brain tissue.

Treatment

Immediate treatment may include establishing a patent airway and, if necessary, a tracheotomy or endotracheal intubation. Treatment also may consist of I.V. fluids (lactated Ringer's or 0.9% sodium chloride solution), I.V. mannitol to reduce ICP, and restricted fluid intake to decrease intracerebral edema. Dexamethasone may be given I.M. or I.V. for several days to control cerebral edema.

The patient's ICP may be reduced by maintaining his partial pressure of arterial carbon dioxide ($PaCO_2$) between 30 and 35 mm Hg, which will constrict cerebral blood vessels. If necessary, additional treatments may include blood transfusion and craniotomy to control bleeding and aspirate blood.

Nursing diagnoses

- Altered thought processes
- Anxiety
- Impaired verbal communication
- Pain
- Risk for fluid volume deficit
- Risk for infection
- Risk for injury
- Sensory or perceptual alterations
- Sleep pattern disturbance

Nursing interventions

- Maintain a patent airway. Assist with endotracheal intubation or tracheotomy as necessary.
- If the patient is intubated, hyperventilate him to a $PaCO_2$ of 30 to 35 mm Hg. A decreased $PaCO_2$ constricts cerebral blood vessels and reduces cerebral blood flow, thus reducing ICP. Serial arterial blood gas studies allow monitoring of oxygenation.
- Monitor vital signs and respirations regularly (usually every 15 minutes). Abnormal respirations could indicate a breakdown in the respiratory center in the brain stem and possibly an impending tentorial herniation—a neurologic emergency.
- Frequently check the patient's neurologic status, including his level of consciousness. Assess him for restlessness, orientation, and pupillary response.
- Administer medications, as ordered.
- Protect the patient from injury according to his condition. Use side rails, assist the unsteady patient when walking, stay with the patient while he uses the bathroom, and place the confused patient where he can be easily observed.
- To decrease the patient's anxiety, speak calmly to him and explain your actions, even if he's unconscious.
- Insert an indwelling urinary catheter, as ordered. Monitor intake and output.
- If the patient is unconscious, insert a nasogastric tube to prevent aspiration—but only after a basilar skull frac-

ture has been ruled out. Otherwise, the tube may be inserted into the cranial vault.

• Carefully observe the patient for leakage of cerebrospinal fluid (CSF). Check the bed sheets for a blood-tinged spot surrounded by a lighter ring (halo sign). If CSF leakage develops and spinal injury is ruled out, raise the head of the bed 30 degrees. If you detect CSF leakage from the nose, place a gauze pad under the nostrils. If CSF leaks from the ear, position the patient so that his ear drains naturally; don't pack the ear or nose. (See *Preventing CNS infection.*)

• If the patient is unconscious and spinal injury is ruled out, elevate the head of the bed and maintain the patient's head in the midline position to decrease ICP. If his head is turned to the side, he may have poor jugular venous return, which can increase ICP.

• Restrict total fluid intake to reduce volume and intracerebral swelling.

• After the patient is stabilized, clean and dress any superficial scalp wounds. (If the skin has been broken, the patient may need tetanus prophylaxis.) Assist with suturing, if needed.

• If the patient develops temporary aphasia, provide an alternative means of communication.

Patient teaching

• Tell the patient not to cough, sneeze, or blow his nose because these activities may increase ICP.

• Instruct the patient to observe for CSF drainage and to be alert for signs of infection.

• Teach the patient and his family how to observe for mental status changes. Tell them to return to the hospital or to call the doctor if such changes occur.

SKULL FRACTURES

Because the first concern in a skull fracture is possible damage to the brain, rather than the fracture itself, the injury is considered a neurosurgical condition. Signs and symptoms reflect the severity and extent of the head injury.

Skull fractures may be simple (closed) or compound (open) and may or may not displace bone fragments. They're also described as linear, comminuted, or depressed. A linear, or hairline, fracture doesn't displace structures and seldom requires treatment. A comminuted fracture splinters or crushes the bone into several fragments. A depressed fracture pushes the bone toward the brain; it is considered serious only if it compresses or lacerates underlying structures. A child's thin, elastic skull allows a depression without a fracture.

Skull fractures also are classified according to location, such as cranial vault or basilar. A basilar fracture occurs at the base of the skull and involves the cribriform plate and the frontal sinuses. Because of the danger of cranial nerve complications, dural tears, and meningitis, basilar fractures usually are far more serious than vault fractures.

Causes

Like concussions and cerebral contusions or lacerations, skull fractures invariably result from a traumatic blow to the head. Motor vehicle crashes, bad falls, and severe beatings (especially in children and elderly people) top the list of causes.

Complications

Skull fractures can lead to infection, intracerebral hemorrhage and hematoma, brain abscess, and increased intracranial pressure (ICP) from edema. A linear fracture across a suture line in an infant increases the possibility of epidural hematoma.

Recovery from the injury also can be complicated by the residual effects of the injury, such as seizure disorders, hydrocephalus, and organic brain syndrome.

Assessment findings

The patient's history—obtained from the patient, his family, eyewitnesses, or emergency personnel—reveals a traumatic injury to the skull. The patient may or may not have lost consciousness and developed other neurologic changes. If conscious, he may complain of a persistent, localized headache.

Your assessment may reveal decreased pulse and respiratory rates as well as labored respirations. On inspection, a conscious patient with a linear fracture and a concussion may appear dazed. If he has another type of skull fracture, he may appear anxious and, depending on his neurologic status, may have normal responses or appear agitated and irritable.

Because scalp wounds commonly accompany skull fractures, inspection of the scalp may reveal abrasions, contusions, lacerations, or avulsions. If the scalp was lacerated or torn away, you may note profuse bleeding. The patient, however, may be in shock from other injuries or from medullary failure if the head injury is severe. You'll also note swelling and ecchymosis in the area of the injury, a sign that a fracture has occurred.

Other findings on inspection may include bleeding in the nose, pharynx, or ears; under the conjunctivae; under the periorbital skin (raccoon's eyes); and behind the eardrum. You may also observe Battle's sign.

Inspection of the ears and nose may reveal cerebrospinal fluid (CSF) and brain tissue leakage. The halo sign—a blood-tinged spot surrounded by a lighter ring caused by leakage of CSF—may also appear on the patient's pillowcase or bed linens.

Palpation of the head may reveal palpable fractures, areas of swelling and, possibly, hematoma. A vault fracture commonly causes soft-tissue swelling near the site, which makes the fracture difficult to detect without X-rays.

During your neurologic assessment, you may observe altered level of consciousness (LOC) along with other classic signs and symptoms of brain injury. These include agitation and irritability, abnormal deep tendon reflexes, altered pupillary and motor responses, hemiparesis, dizziness, seizures, and projectile vomiting. Loss of consciousness may last for hours, days, weeks, or indefinitely. Keep in mind that linear fractures associated only with concussion don't produce loss of consciousness.

Your neurologic assessment also may reveal vision loss in a patient with a sphenoidal fracture, and unilateral hearing loss or facial paralysis in a patient with a temporal fracture.

Diagnostic tests

Computed tomography may locate the fracture. (Cranial vault fractures aren't visible or palpable.) Reagent strips reveal the presence or absence of CSF in nasal or ear drainage. (*Note:* A positive result also will occur if the patient is hyperglycemic.)

Cerebral angiography locates vascular disruptions from internal pressure or injury. Magnetic resonance imaging, a computed tomography scan, and a radioisotope scan disclose intracranial hemorrhage from ruptured blood vessels.

Treatment

Although a simple linear skull fracture can tear an underlying blood vessel or cause a CSF leak, most linear fractures require only supportive treatment. Such treatment includes mild analgesics (acetaminophen) as well as cleaning, debriding, and suturing the wound after injection of a local anesthetic.

If the patient hasn't lost consciousness, he should be observed in the emergency department for at least 4 hours. After this period, a patient with stable vital signs can be discharged. He should receive an instruction sheet for 24 to 48 hours of observation at home.

More severe vault fractures, especially depressed fractures, usually require a craniotomy to elevate or remove fragments that have been driven into the brain and to extract foreign bodies and necrotic tissue. This reduces the risk of infection and further brain damage. Cranioplasty follows the use of tantalum mesh or acrylic plates to replace the removed skull section. The patient commonly requires antibiotics, tetanus prophylaxis, and (in profound hemorrhage) blood transfusions.

For status epilepticus, the patient may receive an anticonvulsant—usually 10 to 15 mg/kg of I.V. phenytoin sodium administered at a rate of not more than 50 mg/minute.

A basilar fracture calls for immediate prophylactic antibiotics to prevent meningitis from CSF leaks. The patient also needs close observation for secondary hematomas and hemorrhages; surgery may be necessary. Also, a patient with either a basilar or a vault fracture requires I.V. or I.M. dexamethasone to reduce cerebral edema and minimize brain tissue damage.

Nursing diagnoses

- Altered nutrition: Less than body requirements
- Altered thought processes
- Anxiety
- Impaired skin integrity
- Ineffective breathing pattern
- Ineffective family coping
- Pain
- Risk for infection
- Risk for injury
- Sensory or perceptual alterations

Nursing interventions

- Establish and maintain a patent airway; the patient may need intubation. Suction him through the mouth, not the nose, to avoid introducing bacteria into CSF if the patient has a CSF leak.
- If the patient's nose is draining CSF, wipe it—*don't* let him blow it. If an ear is draining, cover it lightly with sterile gauze—*don't* pack it or use a cotton-tipped applicator.
- Position a patient with a head injury so that secretions can drain properly. If he has a CSF leak, elevate the head of the bed 30 degrees; if he doesn't, leave the head of the bed flat, but position him on his side or abdomen. Remember that such a patient is at risk for jugular compression, leading to increased ICP, when he's not positioned on his back. So be sure to keep his head properly aligned. (See *Position to avoid for a head-injured patient*.)
- Carefully cover scalp wounds with a sterile dressing; control any bleeding, as necessary.

• Institute seizure precautions, but don't restrain the patient. Agitated behavior may be due to hypoxia or increased ICP, so be alert for these. Carefully monitor an elderly patient. He may have brain atrophy and therefore more space for cerebral edema under the cranium. He may have increased ICP but no signs. Speak in a calm, reassuring voice, and touch the patient gently. Don't make any sudden, unexpected moves.

• To help relieve the patient's anxiety, explain all procedures to him and tell him what to expect before performing the procedure.

• Don't administer narcotics or sedatives because they may depress respirations, increase carbon dioxide levels, and lead to increased ICP. They also can mask changes in neurologic status. Give acetaminophen for pain, as ordered.

• If the patient needs surgery for the skull fracture, obtain consent, as needed, to shave his head. Explain that you're doing this to provide a clean area for surgery. Then type and cross match his blood. Obtain orders for baseline laboratory studies, such as a complete blood count, electrolyte levels, and urinalysis.

• After surgery, monitor the patient's vital signs and neurologic status often (usually every 5 minutes until he's stable and then every 15 minutes for 1 hour). Report any changes in LOC. Because skull fractures and brain injuries heal slowly, don't expect dramatic postoperative improvement.

• During the patient's recovery from surgery, frequently monitor intake and output and maintain indwelling urinary catheter patency. Ensure adequate fluid intake. Because hypotonic fluids (even dextrose 5% in water) can increase cerebral edema, give them only as ordered.

• If the patient is unconscious, provide parenteral nutrition, as ordered, or use a nasoenteric feeding tube. The patient may regurgitate and aspirate food if you use a nasogastric tube.

• If the patient's fracture doesn't require surgery, wear sterile gloves and gently clean lacerations and the surrounding area. Assist with suturing if necessary. Cover the lacerations with sterile gauze.

• Provide emotional support for the patient and his family. Explain the need for procedures to reduce the risk of brain injury.

Patient teaching

• Before discharge, instruct the patient's family to watch closely for changes in mental status, LOC, and respirations. Tell them to return the patient to the hospital immediately if LOC decreases, if headache persists after

POSITION TO AVOID FOR A HEAD-INJURED PATIENT

If your patient has a head injury, don't place him in the low (Trendelenburg) position. Such a position increases intracranial pressure and produces cerebral venous stasis. The pressure of the abdomen on the diaphragm also causes respiratory distress.

several doses of acetaminophen, if he vomits more than once, or if weakness develops in arms or legs.

• Instruct the patient to take acetaminophen for his headache.

• Teach the patient and his family how to care for his scalp wound. Emphasize the need to return for suture removal and follow-up evaluation.

FRACTURED NOSE

The most common facial fracture, a fractured nose usually results from blunt injury and often is associated with other facial fractures. The severity of the fracture depends on the direction, force, and type of the blow. A severe comminuted fracture may cause extreme swelling or bleeding that may jeopardize the airway and require a tracheotomy during early treatment.

Causes

Fractures of the nasal bones usually result from direct trauma. The causative injury can be relatively minor, such as a fall, or more severe, such as a motor vehicle accident.

Complications

Nasal fractures may cause septal deviation and bone displacement, resulting in an airway obstruction. These complications can be permanent if treatment is inadequate or delayed. The patient also may develop septal hematoma, leading to abscess formation and avascular and septic necrosis. Other possible complications include cerebrospinal fluid (CSF) leakage and intracranial air penetration, which may lead to meningitis.

Assessment findings

The patient's history reveals a direct blow to the nose. He usually reports the immediate onset of pain, a nosebleed (ranging from minimal trickling to hemorrhage), and soft-tissue swelling. If his nasal passages are obstructed, he may breathe noisily.

If you perform inspection soon after the injury, you may note a swollen nose with bleeding, and deformity or displacement of the nose from the midline. A fracture may not be obvious, however, because swelling may have obscured the break.

Inspection performed several hours after the injury may reveal periorbital ecchymoses (raccoon's eyes), nasal displacement, and deformity.

You may be able to identify the fracture on palpation.

Diagnostic tests

X-rays help to confirm the diagnosis and determine the extent of injury.

Treatment

The patient may not need treatment unless he has suffered bone displacement, septal deviation, or a cosmetic deformity.

When necessary, prompt treatment restores normal facial appearance and reestablishes bilateral nasal passages after swelling subsides. Reduction of the fracture (restoring the displaced bone fragments to their normal positions) corrects alignment; immobilization (intranasal packing and an external splint shaped to the nose and taped) maintains it.

Nasal fractures should be reduced within the first 24 hours if possible, using local anesthesia for an adult and general anesthesia for a child. Severe swelling may delay treatment for several days to a week, making reduction more difficult. In this case, the patient may need general anesthesia.

If CSF leakage occurs, the patient needs close observation and antibiotic therapy. Septal hematoma requires incision and drainage to prevent necrosis.

Nursing diagnoses

• Body image disturbance
• Impaired tissue integrity
• Ineffective airway clearance
• Pain
• Risk for infection

Nursing interventions

• Start treatment immediately to reduce swelling, control bleeding, and relieve pain.

• While waiting for X-rays, apply ice packs to the nose to minimize swelling. Wrap the ice packs in a light towel to prevent ice from directly contacting the skin. To control anterior bleeding, gently apply local pressure. Posterior bleeding is rare and requires internal tamponade.
• After packing and splinting, apply ice in a plastic bag.
• Administer ordered pain medications as required.

Patient teaching

• The patient will find breathing more difficult as the swelling increases, so instruct him to breathe slowly through his mouth. To warm the inhaled air during cold weather, tell him to cover his mouth with a handkerchief or scarf. To prevent subcutaneous emphysema or intracranial air penetration (and potential meningitis), warn him not to blow his nose.
• Tell the patient to open his mouth when sneezing. Explain that this helps prevent infection and movement of bony fragments. Also advise him to avoid decongestant sprays, which can decrease the nasal blood supply needed for healing.

DISLOCATED OR FRACTURED JAW

A displacement of the temporomandibular joint results in a dislocated jaw. A break in one or both of the two maxillae (upper jawbones) or the mandible (lower jawbone) constitutes a fractured jaw. Treatment usually restores jaw alignment and function.

Causes

Simple fractures or dislocations usually are caused by a manual blow along the jawline as may occur in cases of child, spouse, or elder abuse; more serious compound fractures frequently result from motor vehicle crashes.

Complications

Infection can be a serious complication of a fractured jaw. A fracture can cause a large sublingual hematoma, which may compromise the airway. Injury also can traumatize the nerves that innervate the jaw and face.

Assessment findings

The patient's history reveals an injury to the jaw, and the patient reports mandibular pain beginning right after the injury.

Inspection reveals malocclusion (the most obvious sign of dislocation or fracture), swelling, ecchymosis, loss of function, and asymmetry.

Palpation of the injured area reveals pain and swelling. During palpation, note if the patient experiences any altered sensation. A mandibular fracture that damages the alveolar nerve produces paresthesia or anesthesia of the chin and lower lip.

Diagnostic tests
X-rays confirm the diagnosis.

Treatment
As in all traumatic injuries, treatment involves first checking for a patent airway, adequate breathing, and circulation. After that, treatment focuses on controlling hemorrhage and caring for any other injuries. The patient may need an oropharyngeal airway, nasotracheal intubation, or a tracheotomy to help maintain an adequate airway.

Treatment also includes:
• medications to relieve pain and anxiety, and to prevent infection before and after surgery, if indicated
• in dislocated jaw, manual reduction under anesthesia
• in fractured jaw, surgical reduction and fixation by wiring to restore mandibular and maxillary alignment (wiring usually is removed after 6 to 8 weeks)
• in maxillary fracture, reconstruction and repair of soft-tissue injuries, as necessary
• if possible, reimplantation of any lost teeth within 6 hours, while they're still viable. Teeth and bone fragments aren't removed during surgery unless they must be.

Nursing diagnoses
• Altered nutrition: Less than body requirements
• Anxiety
• Impaired verbal communication
• Ineffective airway clearance
• Pain
• Risk for aspiration
• Risk for fluid volume deficit
• Risk for infection
• Sensory or perceptual alterations

Nursing interventions
• Before and after surgery, administer medications for pain and anxiety, as needed.
• Before surgery, maintain the patient's airway and monitor vital signs. For a patient with a mandibular fracture and soft-tissue injuries, administer tetanus prophylaxis, as ordered.
• After surgery, position the patient on his side, with his head slightly elevated. A nasogastric tube usually is in place, with low suction to remove gastric contents and

GAINING ACCESS TO THE AIRWAY
If the patient's jaws are wired, keep a pair of wire clippers at the bedside to cut the wires in an emergency—for instance, to prevent aspiration if the patient vomits. When the patient becomes ambulatory, have him keep wire clippers available at all times, and make sure he knows which wires to cut if an emergency should occur.

prevent nausea, vomiting, and aspiration of vomitus. As necessary, suction the nasopharynx through the nose or by pulling the cheek away from the teeth and inserting a small suction catheter through any natural gap between the teeth.
• As soon as the patient awakes after surgery, remind him that he can't open his mouth if he has a fixation device in place.
• If the patient isn't intubated, provide nourishment through a straw. If a natural gap exists between his teeth, insert the straw there; if not, one or two teeth may have to be extracted. Such extraction should be avoided when possible. Start with clear liquids. After the patient can tolerate fluids, offer milk shakes, eggnog, broth, juices, pureed foods, and commercially prepared nutritional supplements. If possible, give soft foods with a straw. Give water after each liquid feeding, followed by mouthwash.
• If the patient can't tolerate oral fluids, administer I.V. fluids to maintain hydration.
• Record the patient's baseline weight, and perform a nutrition and hydration assessment.
• Administer antiemetics, as ordered, to minimize the patient's nausea and prevent aspiration of vomitus (a very real danger in a patient who has a wired jaw). Keep a pair of wire cutters at the patient's bedside to snip the wires if the patient should vomit. (See *Gaining access to the airway.*)
• An oral irrigating device may be used for mouth care while the wires are intact. Brush teeth and gums as soon as swelling subsides. Oral hygiene enhances comfort, aids healing of oral wounds, and prevents severe infections. You also can apply paraffin wax to wire ends to protect buccal surfaces.

• Because the patient will have difficulty talking while his jaw is wired, provide him with a toy slate or a pencil and paper. Also, suggest appropriate diversions.

Patient teaching
• Instruct family members to obtain help immediately if the patient appears to have trouble breathing.
• Explain to the patient and his family the importance of high-calorie food supplements, and teach them how to puree foods.
• Advise the patient to avoid alcohol. Explain that it may cause nausea, interact with medications, and dull reflexes necessary for airway clearance.
• Tell the patient to avoid carbonated beverages because the foaming action may cause airway problems.
• Teach the patient how to perform adequate mouth care. Stress the importance of oral hygiene, and suggest that he use a soft, child-sized toothbrush. Tell him to brush his teeth after each meal and at bedtime.
• Encourage the patient to keep follow-up appointments so that the doctor can make sure his fixation device is functioning properly.
• Tell the patient to avoid swimming and other water activities until the jaw wiring is removed; if he should accidentally get water in his lungs or start to drown, it would be difficult to clear the airway rapidly with the jaw wired shut.

PERFORATED EARDRUM
Resulting from a rupture of the tympanic membrane, a perforated eardrum may cause hearing loss.

Causes
The usual cause of a perforated eardrum is trauma: the deliberate or accidental insertion of a sharp object (such as a hair pin) or a sudden excessive change in pressure (from an explosion, a blow to the head, flying, or diving). The injury also may result from untreated otitis media and, in children, from acute otitis media.

Complications
Especially if untreated, a perforated eardrum can result in infection, such as mastoiditis and meningitis, and permanent hearing loss.

Assessment findings
The patient's history usually reveals some type of mild or severe trauma to the ear. The patient may report introducing a foreign object into the ear, or he may have a middle ear infection.

The patient may complain of the sudden onset of a severe earache and bleeding from the ear, usually the first indications of a perforated eardrum. He also may report hearing loss, tinnitus, and vertigo.

During your assessment, you may observe signs of hearing loss, such as the patient turning his unaffected ear toward you when you speak. If inspection of the outer ear reveals drainage, note its color and odor: Purulent otorrhea within 24 to 48 hours of injury signals infection.

An otoscopic examination reveals the perforated tympanic membrane and confirms the diagnosis.

A neurologic examination of the facial nerves should reveal normal voluntary facial movements if no facial nerve damage has occurred from the injury.

Diagnostic tests
Audiometric testing allows evaluation of middle ear function. Culture of the drainage can identify a causative organism, if infection caused the rupture.

Treatment
Most eardrum perforations heal spontaneously. If necessary, treatment includes local and systemic antibiotic therapy and analgesics for pain.

A large perforation with uncontrolled bleeding may require immediate surgery to approximate the ruptured edges. If the patient needs surgical closure, he may undergo a myringoplasty or tympanoplasty.

Nursing diagnoses
• Anxiety
• Knowledge deficit
• Pain
• Risk for infection
• Risk for injury
• Sensory or perceptual alterations (auditory)

Nursing interventions
• If the patient is bleeding from the ear, use a sterile, cotton-tipped applicator to absorb the blood, and check for purulent drainage or evidence of cerebrospinal fluid leakage (clear fluid).
• Apply a sterile dressing over the outer ear.
• Administer prescribed analgesics as necessary.
• Administer prescribed antibiotics.
• If the patient has difficulty hearing, face him, speak distinctly and slowly, and try to ensure quiet when talking with him.

Patient teaching
• Make sure the patient understands the ordered treatment. If he needs surgery, reinforce the doctor's explanation and answer any questions the patient may have.
• Warn against irrigating the ear.
• Caution the patient not to clean the middle ear canal with a cotton-tipped applicator. Explain that this may further injure the eardrum.
• Advise the patient and his family to exercise care when washing the patient's hair. Water may enter the middle ear and cause infection.
• Tell the patient to avoid swimming unless the doctor gives permission and then to use ear plugs to prevent water from entering the ears.
• Stress the importance of completing the course of antibiotic therapy as prescribed.

NECK AND SPINAL INJURIES

Because of the risk of paralysis, neck and spinal injuries call for especially careful treatment.

ACCELERATION-DECELERATION INJURIES

Also known as whiplash, acceleration-deceleration cervical injuries result from sharp hyperextension and flexion of the neck that damages muscles, ligaments, disks, and nerve tissue. The prognosis is excellent; symptoms usually subside with symptomatic treatment.

Causes
Any injury that forcibly causes hyperextension and flexion of the neck can result in whiplash. Common causes include motor vehicle crashes, sports accidents, and falls. For example, in a motor vehicle crash, a rear-end collision propels the patient's trunk forward on the pelvis, throwing the head into hyperextension and stretching the anterior structure of the neck; a head-on impact initially produces acute flexion and subsequently a reflex hyperextension.

Complications
Although rare, a possible complication of acceleration-deceleration injuries is nerve damage that results in numbness, tingling, or weakness.

Assessment findings
The patient's history reveals an acceleration-deceleration injury. He usually reports that symptoms first appeared 12 to 24 hours after the injury. If the injury is mild, symptoms may not appear until another 12 to 24 hours have passed.

The patient typically complains of moderate to severe pain in the anterior and posterior neck. Within several days, the anterior pain diminishes but posterior pain persists or even intensifies. (You may not see the patient until he has reached this point because many patients don't seek medical attention at first.) He also may report dizziness, headache, and vomiting.

During inspection of the neck, you may note neck muscle asymmetry. Neurologic examination may reveal gait disturbances, rigidity or numbness in the arms, and spacial instability that affects balance. Palpation reveals pain at the exact location of the injury.

Diagnostic tests
Full cervical spine X-rays rule out cervical fracture.

Treatment
Until X-rays rule out cervical fracture, treatment focuses on protecting the cervical spine. Initial treatment includes bed rest, the use of a soft cervical collar, and application of ice packs. Oral analgesics provide pain relief, and oral corticosteroids help reduce inflammation and relieve chronic discomfort. To restore flexibility, physical therapy, including mobilization exercises, is started at 72 hours after the injury. It is combined with application of moist heat and a gradually decreased use of the soft cervical collar.

If the patient experiences persistent ligamentous or articular pain, he may benefit from cervical traction and diathermy treatment.

Nursing diagnoses
• Altered role performance
• Anxiety
• Impaired physical mobility
• Knowledge deficit
• Pain

Nursing interventions
• As in all suspected spinal injuries, assume that the patient has an injured spine until proved otherwise. If you're at the scene of the accident, make sure a patient with suspected whiplash or other injuries receives careful transportation to the hospital. Immobilize his neck with tape and a hard cervical collar or sandbags.

• Until an X-ray rules out cervical fracture, move the patient as little as possible. Before X-rays are taken, carefully remove any neck jewelry the patient is wearing. Warn him against movements that could injure his spine.
• Administer medications for pain as ordered.
• Apply a soft cervical collar as directed.

Patient teaching

• The patient with whiplash is likely to be discharged immediately. To help decrease his anxiety, reassure him that uncomplicated whiplash has an excellent prognosis. Be sure he fully understands the treatment and why he must restrict his activity.
• Stress the importance of limiting activity during the first 72 hours after the injury. Tell the patient to rest for a few days and not to lift heavy objects.
• If the patient needs a soft cervical collar, teach him how to put it on.
• If a narcotic has been prescribed for pain relief, emphasize the need for safety in the home. Tell the patient not to drive and to avoid the use of alcohol while taking the medication.
• Warn the patient to return to the hospital or to call the doctor immediately if he develops persistent pain or numbness, tingling, or weakness on one side.

SPINAL INJURIES

Usually the result of trauma to the head or neck, spinal injuries (other than spinal cord damage) include fractures, contusions, and compressions of the vertebral column. Spinal injuries most commonly occur in the twelfth thoracic, first lumbar, and fifth, sixth, and seventh cervical areas. The real danger from such injuries lies in associated damage to the spinal cord.

Causes

Most serious spinal injuries result from motor vehicle crashes, falls, diving into shallow water, and gunshot and related wounds. Less serious spinal injuries typically are caused by improper lifting of heavy objects and by minor falls.

Complications

Spinal injury can be complicated by spinal cord damage, resulting in paralysis and even death. The extent of cord damage depends on the level of injury to the spinal column.

Assessment findings

The patient's history may reveal trauma, a neoplastic lesion, an infection that could produce a spinal abscess, or an endocrine disorder. The patient typically complains of muscle spasm and back or neck pain that worsens with movement. In cervical fractures, point tenderness may be present; in dorsal and lumbar fractures, pain may radiate to other body areas, such as the legs.

Physical assessment (including a neurologic assessment) helps locate the level of injury and detect any cord damage. General observation of the patient reveals that he limits movement and activities that cause pain. Inspection reveals any surface wounds that occurred with the spinal injury. Palpation can identify pain location, loss of sensation, deformity, and the presence of areflexia.

If the injury damages the spinal cord, you'll note clinical effects that range from mild paresthesia to quadriplegia and shock.

Diagnostic tests

Spinal X-rays, myelography, and computed tomography and magnetic resonance imaging scans are used to locate the fracture and site of the compression.

Treatment

The primary treatment after spinal injury is immediate immobilization to stabilize the spine and prevent cord damage; other treatment is supportive.

Cervical injuries require immobilization by application of a cervical collar, towel rolls or rigid foam blocks on both sides of the patient's head, or skeletal traction with skull tongs or a halo device.

Treatment of stable lumbar and dorsal fractures consists of bed rest on a firm surface (such as a bed board), analgesics, and muscle relaxants until the fracture stabilizes (usually in 10 to 12 weeks). Later treatment includes exercises to strengthen the back muscles and a back brace or corset to provide support while walking.

An unstable dorsal or lumbar fracture requires a plaster cast, a turning frame, and, in severe fracture, laminectomy and spinal fusion.

When the damage results in compression of the spinal column, neurosurgery may relieve the pressure. If the cause of compression is a neoplastic lesion, chemotherapy and radiation may relieve the compression by shrinking the lesion. Surface wounds that accompany the spinal injury require wound care and tetanus prophylaxis unless the patient has recently been immunized.

Nursing diagnoses
- Anxiety
- Diversional activity deficit
- Fluid volume deficit
- Impaired physical mobility
- Ineffective airway clearance
- Ineffective breathing pattern
- Pain
- Risk for aspiration
- Risk for disuse syndrome
- Risk for impaired skin integrity
- Risk for infection
- Sensory or perceptual alterations

Nursing interventions
- As in all spinal injuries, suspect cord damage until proved otherwise.
- During the initial assessment and X-rays, immobilize the patient on a firm surface with towel rolls or rigid foam blocks on both sides of his head. Tell him not to move. Avoid moving him because hyperflexion can damage the cord. If you must move him, get at least two other members of the staff to help you logroll him so that you don't disturb his body alignment.
- Offer comfort and reassurance to the patient, talking to him quietly and calmly. Remember, the fear of possible paralysis will be overwhelming. Allow a family member who isn't too distraught to stay with him.
- If the injury necessitates surgery, administer prophylactic antibiotics, as ordered. Catheterize the patient, as ordered, to avoid urine retention, and monitor defecation patterns to avoid impaction.
- If the patient has a halo or skull tong traction device, clean the pin sites daily, trim his hair short, and provide analgesics for headaches. During traction, turn the patient often to prevent pneumonia, embolism, and skin breakdown. Perform passive range-of-motion exercises to maintain muscle tone. If available, use a CircOlectric bed or Stryker frame to facilitate turning and to avoid spinal cord injury.
- To prevent aspiration, turn the patient on his side during feedings. Create a relaxed atmosphere at mealtimes.
- If necessary, insert a nasogastric tube to prevent gastric distention.
- Suggest appropriate diversionary activities to fill the hours of immobility. Offer prism glasses for reading.
- Watch closely for neurologic changes. Immediately report changes in skin sensation and loss of muscle strength. Either could point to pressure on the spinal cord, possibly as a result of edema or shifting bone fragments.

- Help the patient walk as soon as the doctor allows; he'll probably have to wear a back brace.

Patient teaching
- Explain traction methods to the patient and his family, and reassure them that halo or skull tong traction devices don't penetrate the brain.
- Tell the patient about the prescribed regimen for home care.
- Teach the patient exercises to maintain physical mobility.
- Instruct the patient about his medications, including adverse effects and the duration of treatment.
- Stress the importance of follow-up examinations.

THORACIC AND ABDOMINAL INJURIES

Blunt and penetrating chest and abdominal injuries often are life-threatening and require immediate treatment.

BLUNT CHEST INJURIES
Types of blunt chest injuries include myocardial and pulmonary contusions and rib and sternal fractures. Such fractures can be simple, multiple, displaced, or jagged. Chest injuries account for one-fourth of all trauma deaths in the United States.

Causes
Most blunt chest injuries result from motor vehicle crashes. Other causes include sports, fights, and blast injuries.

Complications
Potentially fatal complications, such as hemothorax, hemorrhagic shock, pneumothorax and tension pneumothorax, flail chest, and diaphragmatic rupture, can result from rib and sternal fractures that commonly occur with blunt chest trauma.

Hemothorax occurs when a rib lacerates lung tissue or an intercostal artery, causing blood to collect in the pleural cavity. This compresses the lung, limiting respiratory capacity.

Pneumothorax occurs when a fractured rib tears the pleura and punctures a lung, allowing air to fill the pleural cavity and possibly leading to tension pneumothorax. Multiple rib fractures may cause flail chest: A portion of the chest wall "caves in," resulting in a loss of chest wall integrity and inadequate lung inflation.

Diaphragmatic rupture (usually on the left side) causes severe respiratory distress. Unless treated early, abdominal viscera may herniate (with resulting bowel sounds in the chest) through the rupture into the thorax, compromising both circulation and the lungs' vital capacity.

Other complications of blunt chest trauma include rupture of the aorta, which is almost always immediately fatal; myocardial tears; cardiac tamponade; pulmonary artery tears; ventricular rupture; and bronchial, tracheal, or esophageal tears or rupture.

Assessment findings
The patient's history reveals a recent blunt injury to the chest, and the patient may complain of dyspnea and chest pain. Other clinical features vary with the complications caused by the chest injury.

A patient with a sternal fracture – usually a transverse fracture located in the middle or upper sternum – may complain of persistent chest pain, even at rest. A patient with a rib fracture may complain of tenderness over the fracture site and pain that worsens with deep breathing and movement. Inspection reveals shallow, splinted respirations (a result of the painful breathing). Palpation reveals slight edema over the fracture site. You may note hypoventilation on auscultation.

If the patient develops a hemothorax, he'll report chest pain after the injury along with some form of respiratory distress. Depending on the seriousness of the hemothorax, inspection may disclose no obvious respiratory distress, mild respiratory distress, or severe dyspnea with restlessness and pallor or cyanosis. The patient may have asymmetrical chest movements and flat neck veins. In a massive hemothorax, you may observe bloody sputum or hemoptysis.

Palpation of a hemothorax may reveal unilateral decreased fremitus and decreased chest expansion on inspiration. If the hemothorax is small, percussion won't detect any changes. If the hemothorax is moderate or massive, percussion reveals dullness over the area of fluid collection. Auscultation may reveal unilateral diminished breath sounds or, in a more severe hemothorax, unilateral absent breath sounds. The patient with moderate or massive hemothorax also has hypotension and tachycardia.

If the patient develops a pneumothorax, he'll usually complain of acute, sharp chest pain and shortness of breath. Inspection of this patient may disclose an obviously increased respiratory rate, cyanosis, agitation and, possibly, asymmetrical chest expansion.

Percussion reveals unilateral hyperresonance. On auscultation, breath sounds are diminished or absent on the affected side. You'll also note a crunching sound that occurs with each heartbeat – Hamman's sign, which indicates mediastinal air accumulation.

If a tension pneumothorax develops, the patient may complain of acute chest pain. Upon inspection, you may observe cyanosis, increasing dyspnea, tracheal deviation, distended neck veins, and asymmetrical or paradoxical neck movement. Palpation confirms the tracheal deviation and may disclose subcutaneous crepitus in the neck and upper chest area. Percussion usually reveals unilateral hyperresonance. On auscultation, you'll note unilateral absent breath sounds, muffled heart sounds, and hypotension.

A patient who develops flail chest may report severe pain (from the rib fractures) and extreme shortness of breath. On inspection, you may note that he appears restless. You also may see bruising and disfigurement in the chest area; rapid, shallow respirations; cyanosis; and paradoxical chest movements. (See *Paradoxical breathing in flail chest.*) Palpation may reveal tachycardia, bony crepitus at the fracture site, and subcutaneous crepitus. Auscultation may disclose hypotension and diminished breath sounds.

In a patient with pulmonary contusions, assessment findings include hemoptysis, pallor or cyanosis, dyspnea and, possibly, signs of airway obstruction. Myocardial contusions produce tachycardia, ecchymosis, chest pain, and ECG abnormalities. Diaphragmatic rupture causes severe respiratory distress. If the patient doesn't receive immediate treatment, assessment reveals a decrease in the vital capacity and serious circulatory changes – the result of herniation of the abdominal contents into the thorax.

Diagnostic tests
The following findings support a diagnosis of blunt chest injury, along with specific complications:
• Chest X-rays may confirm rib and sternal fractures, pneumothorax, flail chest, pulmonary contusions, lacerated or ruptured aorta, tension pneumothorax (mediastinal shift), diaphragmatic rupture, lung compression, or atelectasis with hemothorax.
• With cardiac damage, an electrocardiogram may show right bundle-branch block. In myocardial contusions, arrhythmias, conduction abnormalities, and ST-T wave changes may occur.
• Serum levels of aspartate aminotransferase (formerly SGOT), alanine aminotransferase (formerly SGPT), lac-

tate dehydrogenase, creatine phosphokinase (CPK), and the isoenzyme CPK-MB are elevated.

• Angiography reveals aortic laceration or rupture.
• Contrast studies and liver and spleen scans detect diaphragmatic rupture.
• Echocardiography, computed tomography, and nuclear heart and lung scans show the extent of injury.

Treatment

Blunt chest injuries call for controlling bleeding and maintaining a patent airway, adequate ventilation, and fluid and electrolyte balance. Further treatment depends on the specific injury and complications.

• Single fractured ribs are managed conservatively with mild analgesics and follow-up examinations to check for indications of a pneumothorax or hemothorax.
• Treatment for a pneumothorax involves inserting a spinal or 14G or 16G needle into the second intercostal space at the midclavicular line to release pressure. Then the doctor inserts a chest tube in the affected side to normalize pressure and reexpand the lung. The patient also receives oxygen and I.V. fluids.
• Shock related to hemothorax calls for I.V. infusion of lactated Ringer's or 0.9% sodium chloride solution. If the patient loses more than 1,500 ml of blood or more than 30% of circulating blood volume, he'll also need a transfusion of packed red blood cells or an autotransfusion. He'll also receive oxygen and will have chest tubes inserted into the fifth or sixth intercostal space at the midaxillary line to remove blood.
• Treatment of flail chest may include endotracheal intubation and mechanical ventilation. The patient also may receive I.V. muscle relaxants. If the patient requires controlled ventilation, he'll receive a neuromuscular blocking agent. If an air leak occurs, the patient may need operative fixation of the flail chest.
• Pulmonary contusions are managed with colloids to replace volume and maintain oncotic pressure. (Steroid use is controversial.) The patient also may need endotracheal intubation and mechanical ventilation as well as antibiotics and analgesics.
• Myocardial contusions call for intensive monitoring to detect arrhythmias and prevent cardiogenic shock. Drug therapy depends on the type of arrhythmia. Treatment is similar to that for myocardial infarction.
• For myocardial rupture, septal perforation, and other cardiac lacerations, immediate surgical repair is mandatory. Less severe ventricular wounds require use of a digital or balloon catheter. Atrial wounds require a clamp or balloon catheter.

PARADOXICAL BREATHING IN FLAIL CHEST

Flail chest causes a distinctive breathing pattern.

Inspiration
The chest wall normally expands during inspiration, drawing air into the lungs. But in flail chest, the injured free-floating section retracts as the patient inhales. Atelectasis can occur because lung tissue beneath the injury can't expand.

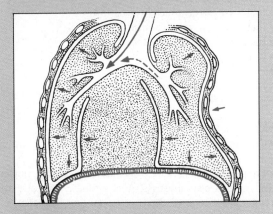

Expiration
During expiration, the flail section moves contrary to the rest of the chest wall, bulging outward. As a result, the patient can't expel air effectively.

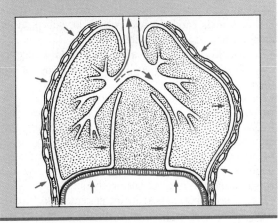

• The rare patient with an aortic rupture or laceration who reaches the hospital alive needs immediate surgery, using synthetic grafts or anastomosis to repair the damage. He requires a large volume of I.V. fluids (usually lactated Ringer's solution) and whole blood along with oxygen at a very high rate. A pneumatic antishock garment is applied, and the patient is promptly transported to the operating room.

• For a patient with a diaphragmatic rupture, a nasogastric tube is inserted to temporarily decompress the stomach, and the patient is prepared for surgical repair.

Nursing diagnoses

• Anxiety
• Decreased cardiac output
• Fluid volume deficit
• Impaired gas exchange
• Impaired physical mobility
• Ineffective airway clearance
• Ineffective breathing pattern
• Knowledge deficit
• Pain
• Risk for impaired skin integrity
• Risk for infection

Nursing interventions

• Continuously monitor any patient with a blunt chest injury.

• Frequently check pulses (including peripheral pulses) and level of consciousness. Also evaluate the color and temperature of skin, depth of respiration, use of accessory muscles, and length of inhalation compared with exhalation.

• Look for tracheal deviation, a sign of tension pneumothorax. Also look for distended jugular veins and paradoxical chest motion. Listen to the patient's heart and breath sounds carefully, and palpate for subcutaneous emphysema and fractured ribs.

• For simple rib fractures, administer mild analgesics, encourage bed rest, and apply heat. Don't strap or tape the chest.

• Anticipate the possible need to insert chest tubes, especially if bleeding is prolonged. To prevent atelectasis, frequently turn the patient, and encourage him to perform coughing and deep breathing.

• For more severe fractures, assist with administration of intercostal nerve blocks. (Obtain X-rays before and after this treatment to rule out pneumothorax.)

• For pneumothorax, assist during placement of the chest tube. Administer oxygen and I.V. fluids, as ordered.

• For flail chest, place the patient in semi-Fowler's position. To oxygenate the patient, intubate him, and provide controlled mechanical ventilation until paradoxical motion of the chest wall ceases. Observe for signs of tension pneumothorax. Suction the patient frequently and as completely as possible. Start I.V. therapy, and observe closely for signs of excessive or insufficient fluid resuscitation and of acid-base imbalance.

• For hemothorax, assist with chest tube insertion, observe the volume and consistency of chest drainage, and administer oxygen. Begin autotransfusion, if indicated. Monitor and document vital signs and blood loss. Immediately report falling blood pressure, rising pulse rate, and uncontrolled hemorrhage—all of which require a thoracotomy to stop bleeding.

• If the patient with a flail chest requires mechanical ventilation and paralyzing agents, also be sure to administer analgesics to control pain and decrease anxiety.

• For pulmonary contusions, monitor blood gas levels to ensure adequate ventilation. Provide oxygen therapy, mechanical ventilation, chest tube care, and I.V. therapy as needed. Administer ordered colloids, analgesics, and corticosteroids.

• For suspected cardiac damage, care is essentially the same as for a patient with a myocardial infarction. Close intensive care with cardiac monitoring or telemetry may detect arrhythmias and prevent cardiogenic shock. Impose bed rest in semi-Fowler's position (unless the patient requires the Trendelenburg position). As needed, administer oxygen, analgesics, and supportive drugs such as digitalis, as ordered, to control heart failure or supraventricular arrhythmia. Watch for cardiac tamponade, which calls for pericardiocentesis.

• If the patient has decreased mobility, reposition him at least every 2 hours to maintain skin integrity. Inspect his skin and keep it clean and dry.

Patient teaching

• Reinforce the doctor's explanation of the patient's condition and treatment plan. Make sure the patient and his family understand the care required.

• Teach the patient about the type of respiratory therapy he needs to have, such as incentive spirometry or postural drainage.

• Teach the patient breathing exercises to maintain effective pulmonary function. Explain the need for turning, coughing, and deep breathing.

• Discuss the medications prescribed for pain, including their adverse effects.

• Teach splinting techniques for turning, deep breathing, and ambulation.

• Encourage the patient not to smoke. Explain that smoking increases tracheobronchial secretions and decreases blood oxygen saturation.

• Teach the patient with rib or sternal fractures that pain will persist for several weeks. Tell him to take analgesics as prescribed.

• Advise the patient to notify the doctor if pain worsens or is accompanied by fever, a productive cough, and shortness of breath. These may indicate infection.
• Tell the patient to avoid contact sports until the pain is resolved and the doctor permits him to resume such activities.

PENETRATING CHEST WOUNDS

Depending on its size, a penetrating chest wound may cause varying degrees of damage to bones, soft tissue, blood vessels, and nerves.

The risk of death and disease from a chest wound depends on the size and severity of the wound. Gunshot wounds usually are more serious than stab wounds because they cause more severe lacerations and rapid blood loss and because ricochet often damages large areas and multiple organs. With prompt, aggressive treatment, up to 90% of patients with penetrating chest wounds recover.

Causes
Stab wounds from a knife or an ice pick and gunshot wounds are the most common penetrating chest wounds. Wartime explosions or firearms fired at close range are the usual source of large, gaping wounds.

Complications
Penetrating chest wounds may lead to arrhythmias; cardiac tamponade; mediastinitis; subcutaneous emphysema; bronchopleural fistula; myocardial rupture; shock, tears, and lacerations of the tracheobronchial tree; pneumothorax; and rib and sternal fractures.

Assessment findings
The patient's history reveals the cause of the chest wound. The patient may be groaning and crying with pain. The chest wound may be obvious, possibly accompanied by a sucking sound as the diaphragm contracts and air enters the chest cavity through the opening in the chest wall.

The patient's level of consciousness depends on the extent of the injury. If he's awake and alert, he may be in severe pain. This will cause him to splint his respirations, reducing his vital capacity.

Inspection reveals the location and type of chest wound. (If you observe the wound in the lower thoracic area, consider it a thoracoabdominal injury until proved otherwise.) If hemopneumothorax is present, the patient will appear dyspneic, tachypneic, anxious, and cyanotic.

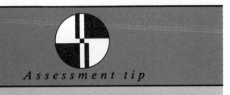

Assessment tip

HOW SEVERE IS THE WOUND?
Examining the wound site helps you to determine the severity of a penetrating wound. To help assess the severity of a stab wound, you'll also need to determine the type and size of the weapon used to inflict the wound and the location and angle of entry. For a gunshot wound, you'll need to determine the following:
• weapon and missile type
• missile velocity
• victim's distance from weapon
• location of entrance and exit wounds.

He may try to sit up to catch his breath. You may note tracheal deviation, depending on the severity.

On palpation, you'll note a weak, thready pulse, the result of massive blood loss and hypovolemic shock. Percussion reveals flatness over areas of blood collection in the pleural or pericardial sac. Auscultation reveals decreased blood pressure and tachycardia from anxiety and blood loss. It also reveals diminished breath sounds over the area of lung collapse in hemopneumothorax. (See *How severe is the wound?*)

Diagnostic tests
Chest X-rays allow evaluation of the injury and confirm chest tube placement. Arterial blood gas analysis helps evaluate the patient's respiratory status. A complete blood count may show low hemoglobin and hematocrit, reflecting severe blood loss. Additional tests may include arteriography, aortography, bronchoscopy, computed tomography, echocardiography, and esophagoscopy.

Treatment
In a penetrating chest wound, treatment involves maintaining a patent airway and providing ventilatory support as needed. Chest tube insertion allows the reestablishment of intrathoracic pressure and drainage of blood from a hemothorax.

The patient's wound will need surgical repair. The patient also may need analgesics, antibiotics, tetanus prophylaxis, and infusion of blood products and I.V. fluids.

Nursing diagnoses
- Altered tissue perfusion
- Anxiety
- Decreased cardiac output
- Fluid volume deficit
- Impaired gas exchange
- Impaired skin integrity
- Ineffective breathing pattern
- Pain
- Risk for infection

Nursing interventions
- Immediately evaluate the patient's ABCs—airway, breathing, and circulation. Establish a patent airway, and provide ventilatory support as needed. Monitor pulses frequently for rate and quality.
- Look for entrance and exit wounds, leaving them undisturbed for forensic evaluation.
- Apply wound dressings as needed, always using sterile technique.
- Place an occlusive dressing (for example, petroleum gauze) over a sucking wound. Monitor the patient for signs of tension pneumothorax. If such signs develop, temporarily remove the occlusive dressing to create a simple pneumothorax.
- Assist with insertion of central lines for monitoring and fluid replacement, if indicated.
- Monitor for signs of hemorrhagic shock.
- Ensure adequate I.V. access with at least two large-bore peripheral catheters.
- Obtain blood samples for type and cross matching.
- Estimate blood loss (also remember to look *under* the patient to estimate loss) and control bleeding. Replace blood and fluids as necessary.
- If warranted, obtain and set up equipment for autotransfusion, particularly when the patient has massive blood loss.
- Assist with chest X-ray and placement of chest tubes (using water-seal drainage) to reestablish intrathoracic pressure and to drain blood in a hemothorax. A second X-ray will evaluate the position of tubes and their function.
- After chest tubes are in place, be sure to watch for bleeding and substantial air leakage through chest tubes, a sign of lung lacerations. Also monitor closely for a blood loss of more than 200 ml/hour through chest tubes, the result of severe vascular injury. Report such findings to the doctor immediately.
- Provide ordered analgesics to relieve pain.
- Throughout treatment, monitor central venous pressure and vital signs to detect hypovolemia.

- Monitor pulse oximetry.
- Stabilize impaled objects.

Patient teaching
- Reassure the patient, especially if he's been the victim of a violent crime. Report the incident to the police in accordance with local laws. Help contact the patient's family, and offer them reassurance as well.
- Reinforce the doctor's explanation of the patient's condition and treatment plan. Make sure the patient and his family understand the care required.
- Teach the patient about the type of respiratory therapy he needs. Also teach him breathing exercises to maintain effective pulmonary function. Explain the need for turning, coughing, and deep breathing.
- Discuss the medications prescribed for pain, including adverse effects.
- Encourage the patient not to smoke. Explain that smoking increases tracheobronchial secretions and decreases blood oxygen saturation.
- Advise the patient to notify the doctor if pain worsens or is accompanied by fever, a productive cough, and shortness of breath. These may indicate infection.
- Tell the patient to avoid contact sports until the pain is resolved and the doctor lets him resume such activities.

BLUNT AND PENETRATING ABDOMINAL INJURIES

Potentially fatal, blunt and penetrating abdominal injuries may damage major blood vessels and internal organs. The prognosis depends on the extent of injury and the organs damaged but is improved by prompt diagnosis and surgical repair.

Causes
Blunt (nonpenetrating) abdominal injuries usually result from motor vehicle crashes, fights, falls from heights, and sports accidents; penetrating abdominal injuries, from stabbings and gunshots.

Complications
Immediate life-threatening complications include hemorrhage and hypovolemic shock. Later complications include infection and dysfunction of major organs, such as the liver, spleen, pancreas, and kidneys.

Assessment findings
The patient's history reveals an accidental or forcibly inflicted abdominal injury. Symptoms vary with the degree

of injury and the organs damaged. The patient with a blunt or penetrating abdominal injury typically is in obvious discomfort or pain.

A patient with a blunt abdominal injury may report severe pain that radiates beyond the abdomen to the shoulders, as well as nausea and vomiting. A penetrating abdominal wound may be obvious, especially if the patient is bleeding in the abdominal area. (If you observe the wound in the upper abdominal area, consider it a thoracoabdominal injury until proved otherwise.)

Inspection pinpoints the type of abdominal injury and helps determine its severity. Depending on the severity of the injury, the patient may be pale or cyanotic or dyspneic. Inspection of the patient with a blunt abdominal injury also reveals bruises, abrasions, contusions and, possibly, distention. (See *Effects of blunt abdominal trauma*.) For a patient with a penetrating abdominal injury, inspection reveals the type of wound and associated blood loss.

Palpation may reveal the extent of pain and tenderness and, in blunt abdominal injuries, abdominal splinting or rigidity. Rib fractures often accompany blunt abdominal injuries. Auscultation may disclose tachycardia, decreased breath sounds, absent or decreased bowel sounds, or bowel sounds in the chest. The patient also may have hypotension.

Diagnostic tests

Specific tests vary with the patient's condition but usually include abdominal films and examination of the stools and stomach contents for blood. Chest X-rays, preferably done with the patient upright, show free air.

Several blood studies usually are performed. Decreased hematocrit and hemoglobin levels point to blood loss. Coagulation studies evaluate clotting ability. White blood cell count normally is elevated but doesn't necessarily point to infection. Typing and cross matching precede blood transfusion.

Arterial blood gas analysis evaluates respiratory status. A pancreatic injury typically results in elevated serum amylase levels. Also, levels of aspartate aminotransferase (formerly SGOT) and alanine aminotransferase (formerly SGPT) increase with tissue injury and cell death.

Excretory urography and cystourethrography show renal and urinary tract damage. Radioisotope scanning and ultrasound examination detect liver, kidney, and spleen injuries. Angiography detects specific injuries, especially to the kidneys.

Peritoneal lavage is performed to check for blood, amylase, bile, food, fiber, and feces. Computed tomography scanning helps detect the extent of the injury and other

EFFECTS OF BLUNT ABDOMINAL TRAUMA

When a blunt object strikes a person's abdomen, it raises his intra-abdominal pressure. Depending on the force of the blow, the trauma can lacerate the liver and spleen, rupture the stomach, bruise the duodenum, and even damage the kidneys.

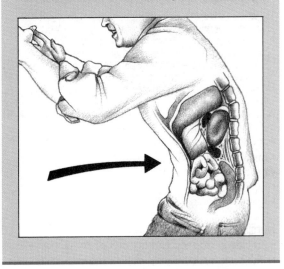

injuries that may have occurred. Exploratory laparotomy detects specific injuries when other clinical evidence is incomplete.

Treatment

The patient needs an immediate infusion of I.V. fluids and blood components to control hemorrhage and prevent hypovolemic shock. He also may require intubation and mechanical ventilation or supplemental oxygen, as well as insertion of a nasogastric (NG) tube and an indwelling urinary catheter. (See *Caring for a penetrating injury*, page 242.)

After stabilization, most abdominal injuries require surgical repair. Analgesics, withheld until after a definitive diagnosis, increase patient comfort, and antibiotics prevent infection.

The patient will probably require hospitalization; if he's asymptomatic, he may require observation for only 6 to 24 hours.

Nursing diagnoses
• Altered tissue perfusion
• Anxiety
• Decreased cardiac output

Warning

CARING FOR A PENETRATING INJURY

When administering emergency care to a patient with a penetrating abdominal injury, *don't* remove the penetrating object. Not only could that cause further damage, but it could also make determining the nature of the injury more difficult. Instead, secure the penetrating object and leave it in place until the surgical team is ready to remove it.

- Fluid volume deficit
- Impaired gas exchange
- Impaired skin integrity
- Pain
- Risk for infection

Nursing interventions

- Provide emergency care as needed to support the patient's vital functions.
- To maintain airway and breathing, intubate the patient and provide mechanical ventilation, as necessary. Otherwise, provide supplemental oxygen.
- When possible, explain each procedure to the patient before performing it to alleviate his anxiety.
- Using large-bore needles, start two I.V. lines for monitoring and rapid fluid infusion, using lactated Ringer's solution. Draw a blood sample for laboratory studies. Also, insert an NG tube and, if necessary, an indwelling urinary catheter; monitor stomach aspirate and urine for blood.
- Obtain vital signs for baseline data. Continue monitoring them every 15 minutes until the patient's condition stabilizes.
- Apply a sterile dressing to any open wounds. Splint a suspected pelvic injury on arrival by tying the patient's legs together with a pillow between them. Move such a patient as little as possible.
- If evisceration has occurred, minimize unnecessary movement of the patient. Apply a wet saline dressing to exposed abdominal contents.
- Administer analgesics, as ordered. Narcotics usually aren't recommended, but if the patient has severe pain,

they may be administered in small, titrated I.V. doses, as ordered.
- Give tetanus prophylaxis and prophylactic I.V. antibiotics, as ordered.
- Stabilize impaled objects and leave the wound uncleaned and intact for forensic evaluation.
- Prepare the patient for surgery. Obtain a consent form signed by the patient or a responsible relative.
- If the injury was caused by a motor vehicle crash, find out if the police were notified; if they weren't, notify them. If the patient suffered a gunshot or stab wound, also notify the police, place all his clothes in a bag, and retain them for the police. Document the number and sites of the wounds.

Patient teaching

- A patient with a blunt abdominal injury may be assessed and discharged from the emergency department. But some injuries, such as delayed rupture of the spleen, may not become apparent for several hours or days. Tell the patient to notify the doctor if he experiences any of the following: increased abdominal pain; shoulder pain that's not the result of shoulder trauma (Kehr's sign); malaise, lethargy, or dizziness (signs of slow blood loss); unexplained fever; nausea or vomiting, particularly if it's persistent; hematemesis or melena; or light-headedness, restlessness, diaphoresis, or hemoptysis.

INJURIES OF THE EXTREMITIES

These injuries can range from mild sprains or strains to traumatic amputation.

SPRAINS AND STRAINS

Usually a relatively minor injury, a sprain is a complete or incomplete tear in the supporting ligaments surrounding a joint. (A sprained ankle is a common joint injury.) A strain—which can be acute or chronic—is an injury to a muscle or tendinous attachment. Both injuries usually heal without surgical repair. (See *Classifying sprains and strains.*)

Causes

A sprain usually follows a sharp twisting motion of the affected joint. An acute strain usually results from vigorous muscle overuse, overstress, or overstretching of a single muscle or muscle group.

Complications

A sprain can result in an avulsion fracture, which occurs when a bone fragment is pulled out of place by a ligament. A chronic strain results from the accumulated effects of repeated muscle overuse.

Assessment findings

The patient's history reveals how the sprain or strain occurred.

If the patient has a sprain, his history also will reveal if he's physically active (which may have caused the injury) or sedentary (which puts him at increased risk for musculoskeletal injury) and if he's had similar injuries or a systemic disease that could cause musculoskeletal problems (for example, foot neuropathy in a diabetic patient could cause a sprain). He may report local pain that worsens during joint movement and loss of mobility. This loss of mobility may not occur until several hours after the injury.

The patient with an acute strain may report sharp, transient pain and rapid swelling. When the severe pain has subsided, he may complain of muscle tenderness. He may tell you he heard a snapping or popping noise at the time of the injury. The patient with a chronic strain reports stiffness, soreness, and generalized tenderness.

Inspection of a sprain reveals ecchymosis from blood extravasating into surrounding tissues and swelling, a key sign of a sprain. Palpation may reveal point tenderness in a moderate or severe sprain.

Inspection of a strain reveals swelling over the injury site and, if the injury is several days old, ecchymosis. Palpation reveals the degree of swelling and defines the area of tenderness.

Diagnostic tests

X-rays rule out fractures and confirm damage to ligaments. (See *Sprains and strains: An inside view,* page 244.)

Treatment

Ice should be applied to the injury site as soon as possible to control swelling. After 24 to 48 hours, treatment should switch to heat to encourage reabsorption of blood and to promote healing and comfort.

The patient may need the injury splinted or immobilized to promote comfort and aid healing. The patient may need surgery if the muscle, tendon, or ligament ruptured or if the ligaments torn by the sprain don't heal properly, causing recurrent dislocation. A rehabilitation or exercise program may help ensure a gradual progression of activity.

CLASSIFYING SPRAINS AND STRAINS

The guide below will help you classify the severity of sprains and strains.

Sprains
• Grade 1 (mild): minor or partial ligament tear with normal joint stability and function
• Grade 2 (moderate): partial tear with mild joint laxity and some function loss
• Grade 3 (severe): complete tear or incomplete separation of ligament from bone, causing total joint laxity and function loss

Strains
• Grade 1 (mild): microscopic muscle or tendon tear (or both) with no loss of strength
• Grade 2 (moderate): incomplete tear with bleeding into muscle tissue and some loss of strength
• Grade 3 (severe): complete rupture, usually resulting from separation of muscle from muscle, muscle from tendon, or tendon from bone. (This type of strain usually stems from sudden, violent movement or direct injury.)

Nursing diagnoses

• Impaired physical mobility
• Knowledge deficit
• Pain
• Risk for injury

Nursing interventions

• Immediately after the injury, control swelling by elevating the joint above the level of the patient's heart and by intermittently applying ice, as ordered, during the first 12 to 48 hours. To prevent a cold injury, place a towel between the ice pack and the skin.
• Immobilize a sprain with an elastic bandage. If the sprain is severe, use a soft cast. For a sprained ankle, apply the elastic bandage from the toes to midcalf.
• Depending on the severity of the injury, the patient may need codeine or another analgesic. If he has a sprained ankle, he may need crutches.
• Perform range-of-motion exercises, progressing from passive to active, to prevent joint contractures and muscle atrophy.

Patient teaching

• Make sure you provide comprehensive teaching because a patient with a sprain or strain seldom requires hospitalization.

SPRAINS AND STRAINS: AN INSIDE VIEW

Except for possible swelling and discoloration, you can't see a sprain or a strain. But the patient can surely feel one. In a *sprain,* he feels the stretching or tearing of a ligament—the fibrous tissue that binds joints together. He'll feel a partial muscle tear in an acute or chronic *strain.* A strain also may affect tendons—the fibrous tissue that connects muscle to bone. Here's what each type of injury looks like.

Knee sprain

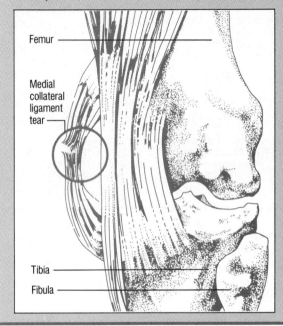

Femur

Medial collateral ligament tear

Tibia

Fibula

Calf strain

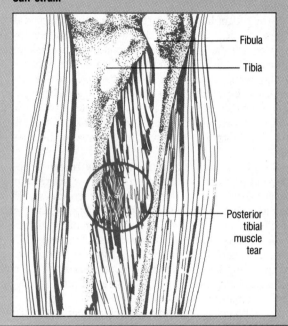

Fibula

Tibia

Posterior tibial muscle tear

• Instruct the patient to elevate the joint for 48 to 72 hours after the injury. (Explain that he can use pillows to elevate the joint while he's sleeping.) Also teach him to apply ice intermittently for the first 12 to 48 hours. Advise him to switch to intermittent applications of heat after that.

• If the joint has been wrapped in an elastic bandage, teach the patient how to reapply it by wrapping from below to above the injury, forming a figure eight. Tell him to remove the bandage before going to sleep and to loosen it if the leg becomes pale, numb, or painful.

• Stress the need for movement to alleviate the effects of immobility. Teach the patient how to perform range-of-motion exercises.

• Tell the patient to use aspirin, acetaminophen, or other prescribed analgesics for discomfort. Make sure he understands the purpose of the prescribed medication and any adverse reactions that could occur.

• Provide crutch-gait training for the patient with a sprained ankle.

• Instruct the patient to call the doctor if the pain worsens or persists. If so, an additional X-ray may detect a fracture that initially was missed.

• Warn the patient that he may further injure the joint if he overstresses it before healing is complete. This is especially true if he has an ankle or a knee injury.

DISLOCATIONS AND SUBLUXATIONS

Often causing extreme pain, dislocations are displacements of joint bones so that their articulating surfaces totally lose contact; subluxations are partial displacements of the articulating surfaces. Dislocations and subluxations occur at the joints of the shoulders, elbows, wrists, digits, hips, knees, ankles, and feet.

These injuries may accompany fractures of these joints or result in deposition of fracture fragments between joint surfaces. Even without a concomitant fracture, a displaced bone may damage surrounding muscles, ligaments, nerves, and blood vessels, especially if reduction is delayed.

Causes

A dislocation or subluxation may be caused by a congenital problem (such as congenital dislocation of the hip), or it may follow trauma or disease of surrounding joint tissues (for example, Paget's disease of the bone).

Complications

Nerve injury and vascular impairment, such as avascular necrosis, may complicate a dislocation or subluxation. Bone necrosis also may occur.

Assessment findings

The patient's history may reveal the direct cause of the injury. If trauma caused the injury, it may be accompanied by joint surface fractures. The patient may complain of extreme pain.

Inspection may reveal a deformity around the joint and a change in the length of the involved extremity. Palpation may detect impaired joint mobility and point tenderness.

Diagnostic tests

X-rays confirm the diagnosis and identify any associated fractures.

Treatment

Immediate reduction and immobilization can prevent additional tissue damage and vascular impairment. (See *Immobilizing a shoulder dislocation*.) Closed reduction consists of manual traction under general anesthesia or local anesthesia and sedatives. During reduction, meperidine I.V. controls pain; diazepam I.V. controls muscle spasm and facilitates muscle stretching during traction. Some injuries require open reduction under regional block or general anesthesia. Such surgery may include wire fixation of the joint, skeletal traction, and ligament repair.

After reduction, a splint, a cast, traction, or another device immobilizes the joint. In most cases, immobilizing the digits for 2 weeks, hips for 6 to 8 weeks, and other dislocated joints for 3 to 6 weeks allows surrounding ligaments to heal.

Nursing diagnoses
• Altered peripheral tissue perfusion
• Impaired physical mobility

IMMOBILIZING A SHOULDER DISLOCATION

Once a shoulder dislocation has been reduced, an external immobilization device, such as the elastic shoulder immobilizer or the stockinette Velpeau splint, can maintain the position until healing takes place. The device should remain on for about 3 weeks.

Elastic shoulder immobilizer

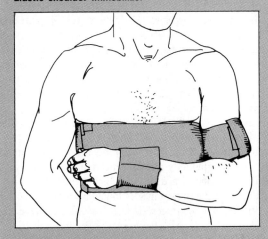

Stockinette Velpeau splint

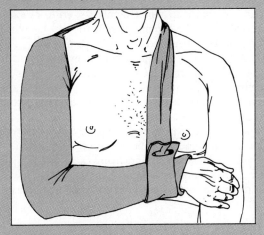

• Impaired skin integrity
• Knowledge deficit
• Pain
• Risk for disuse syndrome
• Self-care deficit

Nursing interventions

• Assess vascular condition to establish a baseline; reassess intermittently to detect vascular compromise.
• Report immediately signs of severe vascular compromise, such as pallor, pain, loss of pulses, paralysis, and paresthesia. If such signs develop, the patient will need an immediate orthopedic examination.
• Until reduction immobilizes the dislocated joint, do not attempt manipulation. Apply ice to ease pain and edema. Splint the extremity "as it lies," even if the angle is awkward.
• When a patient receives I.V. drugs to relieve pain and to relax him, he may develop respiratory depression or even respiratory arrest. So during and after reduction, keep an airway and a hand-held resuscitation bag nearby, and monitor pulse oximetry readings and vital signs.
• To avoid skin damage, watch for signs of pressure injury inside and outside the dressing.
• Encourage prescribed active range-of-motion exercises for adjacent nonimmobilized joints.
• After removal of the cast or splint, inform the patient that he may gradually return to normal joint activity.
• After reduction of a dislocated hip (required immediately), stress the importance of follow-up visits to detect aseptic femoral head necrosis from vascular damage.

Patient teaching

• To avoid injury from a dressing that is too tight, instruct the patient to report numbness, pain, cyanosis, and coldness of the extremity below the cast or splint.
• Explain prescribed medications for pain relief.
• Teach the patient and his family to evaluate skin integrity and neurovascular status while the joint is immobilized.
• Show the patient how to use assistive devices, such as crutches or a sling, as needed.
• As appropriate, explain that the patient may need help with self-care until the joint can be used again.
• Stress the importance of gradually exercising the joint after splint removal.
• At discharge, emphasize the need for follow-up visits.

ARM AND LEG FRACTURES

Usually caused by major trauma, an arm or a leg fracture is a break in the continuity of the bone. A fracture can result in substantial muscle, nerve, and other soft-tissue damage. The prognosis varies with the extent of disability or deformity, the amount of tissue and vascular damage, the adequacy of reduction and immobilization, and the patient's age, health, and nutrition. Children's bones usually heal rapidly and without deformity; the bones of adults in poor health or those with osteoporosis or impaired circulation may never heal properly.

Causes

Most arm and leg fractures result from major trauma, such as a fall on an outstretched arm, a skiing or motor vehicle crash, and child, spouse, or elder abuse (shown by multiple or repeated episodes of fractures). However, in a person with a pathologic bone-weakening condition, such as osteoporosis, bone tumor, or metabolic disease, a mere cough or sneeze can cause a fracture. Prolonged standing, walking, or running can cause stress fractures of the foot and ankle — usually in nurses, postal workers, soldiers, and joggers.

Complications

Possible complications of fractures include arterial damage, nonunion, fat embolism, infection, shock, avascular necrosis, and peripheral nerve damage. (See *Identifying peripheral nerve injuries.*)

Severe fractures, especially of the femoral shaft, may cause substantial blood loss and life-threatening hypovolemic shock.

Assessment findings

The patient's history usually reveals what caused the fracture. The patient typically reports pain that increases with movement and an inability to intentionally move the part of the arm or leg distal to the injury. The severity of the pain depends on the fracture type. (See *Classifying fractures,* pages 248 and 249.) The patient also may complain of a tingling sensation distal to the injury, possibly indicating nerve and vessel damage.

Inspection may disclose soft-tissue edema, an obvious deformity or shortening of the injured limb, and discoloration over the fracture site. Open fractures produce an obvious skin wound and bleeding. Gentle palpation usually reveals warmth, crepitus and, possibly, dislocation. Numbness distal to the injury and cool skin at the end of the extremity may indicate nerve and vessel damage.

Auscultation may reveal loss of pulses distal to the injury, an indication of possible arterial compromise or nerve damage.

Diagnostic tests

Anteroposterior and lateral X-rays of the suspected fracture, as well as X-rays of the joints above and below it, confirm the diagnosis. Angiography can help assess concurrent vascular injury.

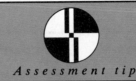

Assessment tip

IDENTIFYING PERIPHERAL NERVE INJURIES

The chart below lists signs and symptoms that can help you pinpoint where a patient has nerve damage. Keep in mind that you will not be able to rely on these signs and symptoms in a patient with severed extension tendons or severe muscle damage.

Nerve	Associated injury	Sign or symptom
Radial	Fracture of the humerus (especially the middle and distal thirds)	The patient can't extend his thumb.
Ulnar	Fracture of the medial humeral epicondyle	The patient can't perceive pain in the tip of his little finger.
Median	Elbow dislocation or wrist or forearm injury	The patient can't perceive pain in the tip of his index finger.
Peroneal	Tibia or fibula fracture or dislocation of knee	The patient can't extend his foot (this also may indicate sciatic nerve injury).
Sciatic and tibial	Rare with fractures or dislocations	The patient can't perceive pain in his sole.

Treatment

The primary goals of treatment are to return the injured limb to maximal function, to prevent complications, and to obtain the best possible cosmetic results.

Emergency treatment consists of splinting the limb above and below the suspected fracture, applying a cold pack, and elevating the limb — all of which reduce edema and pain. (See *Caring for an injured limb,* page 250.) A severe fracture that causes blood loss calls for direct pressure to control bleeding. The patient with a severe fracture also may need fluid replacement (including blood products) to prevent or treat hypovolemic shock.

After a fracture has been confirmed, treatment begins with reduction (restoring displaced bone segments to their normal position). This is followed by immobilization with a splint, a cast, or traction.

In closed reduction (manual manipulation), a local anesthetic — such as lidocaine — and an analgesic — such as morphine I.M. — minimize pain; a muscle relaxant — such as diazepam I.V. — or a sedative — such as midazolam — facilitates the muscle stretching necessary to realign the bone. (An X-ray confirms reduction and proper bone alignment.) General anesthesia may be needed for closed reduction.

When closed reduction is impossible, open reduction during surgery reduces and immobilizes the fracture by means of rods, plates, or screws. Afterward, the patient usually must wear a plaster cast.

When a splint or cast fails to maintain the reduction, immobilization requires skin or skeletal traction, using a series of weights and pulleys. In skin traction, elastic bandages and moleskin coverings attach the traction devices to the patient's skin. In skeletal traction, a pin or wire inserted through the bone distal to the fracture and attached to a weight allows more prolonged traction.

Treatment for an open fracture also requires careful wound cleaning, tetanus prophylaxis, prophylactic antibiotics and, possibly, additional surgery to repair soft-tissue damage.

Nursing diagnoses
• Altered tissue perfusion
• Anxiety
• Diversional activity deficit
• Fear
• Impaired physical mobility
• Impaired skin integrity
• Ineffective individual coping

CLASSIFYING FRACTURES

One of the best-known systems for classifying fractures uses a combination of general terms to describe the fracture—a simple, nondisplaced, oblique fracture, for example.

General classification of fractures
• *Simple (closed):* Bone fragments don't penetrate the skin.

• *Compound (open):* Bone fragments penetrate the skin.
• *Incomplete (partial):* Bone continuity isn't completely interrupted.
• *Complete:* Bone continuity is completely interrupted.
   Below you'll find definitions of the terms used to describe fractures along with illustrations of fragment positions and fracture lines.

Classification by fragment position

Comminuted
The bone breaks into small pieces.

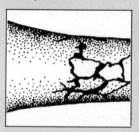

Impacted
One bone fragment is forced into another.

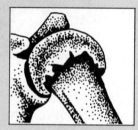

Angulated
Fragments lie at an angle to each other.

Displaced
Fracture fragments separate and are deformed.

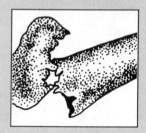

Nondisplaced
The two sections of bone maintain essentially normal alignment.

Overriding
Fragments overlap, shortening the total bone length.

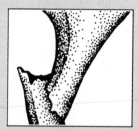

Segmental
Fractures occur in two adjacent areas with an isolated central segment.

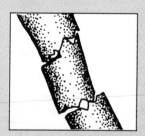

Avulsed
Fragments are pulled from normal position by muscle contractions or ligament resistance.

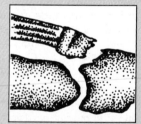
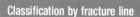

Classification by fracture line

Linear
The fracture line runs parallel to the bone's axis.

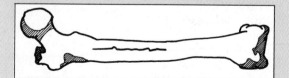

Longitudinal
The fracture line extends in a longitudinal (but not parallel) direction along the bone's axis.

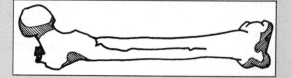

CLASSIFYING FRACTURES *(continued)*

Classification by fracture line *(continued)*

Oblique
The fracture line crosses the bone at roughly a 45-degree angle to the bone's axis.

Spiral
The fracture line crosses the bone at an oblique angle creating a spiral pattern.

Transverse
The fracture line forms a right angle with the bone's axis.

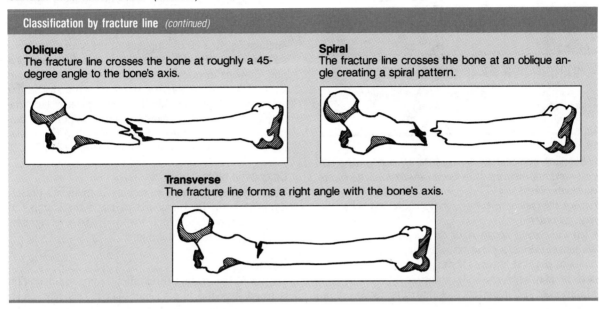

- Pain
- Risk for disuse syndrome
- Risk for fluid volume deficit
- Risk for infection
- Risk for injury
- Self-care deficit

Nursing interventions
- Reassure the patient with a fracture, who will probably be frightened and in pain. Ease pain with analgesics, as needed.
- If the patient has a severe open fracture of a large bone, such as the femur, watch for signs of shock. Monitor his vital signs; a rapid pulse, decreased blood pressure, pallor, and cool, clammy skin may indicate shock. Administer I.V. fluids, as ordered.
- If the fracture requires long-term immobilization with traction, reposition the patient often to increase comfort and prevent pressure ulcers. Assist with active range-of-motion exercises to prevent muscle atrophy. Encourage deep breathing and coughing to avoid hypostatic pneumonia.
- In long-term immobilization, urge adequate fluid in-take to prevent urinary stasis and constipation. Watch for signs of renal calculi (flank pain, nausea, and vomiting).
- Provide for diversional activity. Allow the patient to express his concerns over lengthy immobilization and the problems it creates.
- Provide good cast care. While the cast is wet, support it with pillows. Observe for skin irritation near cast edges, and check for foul odors or discharge, particularly after open reduction, compound fracture, or skin lacerations and wounds on the affected limb.
- Encourage the patient to start moving around as soon as he can, and help him with walking. (Remember, the patient who's been bedridden for some time may be dizzy at first.)
- After cast removal, refer the patient for physical therapy to restore limb mobility.

Patient teaching
- Help the patient set realistic goals for recovery.
- Show the patient how to use his crutches properly.
- Tell the patient with a cast to report signs of impaired circulation (skin coldness, numbness, tingling, or dis-

CARING FOR AN INJURED LIMB

When giving emergency care to a patient with an injured joint, *don't* attempt to straighten it. Instead, immobilize and splint the limb as it is.

coloration) immediately. Warn him against getting the cast wet, and instruct him not to insert foreign objects under the cast.

• Teach the patient to exercise joints above and below the cast, as ordered.

• Tell the patient not to walk on a leg cast or foot cast without the doctor's permission. Plaster casts require 48 hours to dry and harden. If the patient has a fiberglass cast, he may be able to walk immediately.

• Emphasize the importance of returning for follow-up care.

TRAUMATIC AMPUTATION

The accidental loss of a body part, traumatic amputation usually involves a finger, a toe, an arm, or a leg. In complete amputation, the member is totally severed; in partial amputation, some soft-tissue connection remains.

The prognosis has improved because of early, improved emergency and critical care management, new surgical techniques, early rehabilitation, prosthesis fitting, and new prosthesis designs. New limb reimplantation techniques have been moderately successful, but incomplete nerve regeneration remains a major limiting factor.

Causes

A traumatic amputation may result from a cutting, tearing, or crushing insult, involving the use of factory, farm, or power tools, or from a motor vehicle crash.

Complications

Hypovolemic shock and sepsis are possible complications in traumatic amputation. If reimplantation is attempted, residual paralysis may occur.

Assessment findings

The patient history reveals the type of accident that caused the amputation. Inspection typically reveals a partially or completely severed body part with hemorrhage and soft-tissue damage. Inspection also discloses the type of amputation. In a clean amputation, the wound has well-defined edges and damage is local. In a crush amputation, damage involves the tissue and arterial intima. In an avulsive amputation, the tissue is torn and vascular and neural structures may become separated near the damaged bone or cartilage. In a partial amputation, palpation detects the status of pulses distal to the amputation.

Diagnostic tests

Ultrasonography is used to monitor the patient's pulses. X-rays of both the amputated part and the stump can help determine the extent of fractures, and arteriography can help evaluate arterial injury.

Treatment

The greatest immediate threat after traumatic amputation is blood loss and hypovolemic shock. Therefore, emergency treatment consists of local measures to control bleeding, fluid replacement with sterile 0.9% sodium chloride or lactated Ringer's solution and colloids, and blood replacement as needed.

Reimplantation, especially for straight-edged amputation, is becoming more common and successful because of advances in microsurgery. If reconstruction or reimplantation is possible, surgery attempts to preserve the patient's usable joints. When arm or leg amputations are performed, the surgeon creates a stump to be fitted with a prosthesis. A rigid dressing permits early prosthesis fitting and rehabilitation.

Nursing diagnoses

• Altered peripheral tissue perfusion
• Altered role performance
• Body image disturbance
• Fear
• Fluid volume deficit
• Impaired skin integrity
• Ineffective individual coping
• Knowledge deficit
• Pain
• Risk for infection

Nursing interventions

• In emergency treatment, monitor vital signs (especially in hypovolemic shock). If amputation involved an extremity, ensure I.V. access with at least two large-bore catheters (probably unnecessary with single-digit involvement). Clean the wound and give tetanus prophylaxis, analgesics, and antibiotics, as ordered.

• After a complete amputation, wrap the amputated part in wet dressings moistened with sterile 0.9% sodium chloride solution (*don't* place the part directly in formalin, water, or sterile 0.9% sodium chloride solution, and *don't* put a tag on the part). Place the amputated part in a dry, clean plastic bag, seal the bag tightly, and label it. Then place the bag on ice (not dry ice). Flush the wound with sterile 0.9% sodium chloride solution, apply a sterile pressure dressing, and elevate the limb (don't use a tourniquet). Notify the reimplantation team.

• After a partial amputation, position the limb in normal alignment, and drape it with towels or dressings soaked in sterile 0.9% sodium chloride solution.

• Preoperative care includes thorough wound irrigation and debridement (using local anesthesia). Postoperative dressing changes require sterile technique to help prevent skin infection and ensure skin graft viability.

• Encourage the patient to verbalize his feelings about his altered body image.

• Allow the patient to verbalize his concerns and fear about his future after the amputation. If necessary, consult with a rehabilitation counselor to help the patient learn a new skill.

• If reimplantation is not viable, inform the patient about community support services and rehabilitation programs.

Patient teaching

• Reinforce the doctor's explanation of the surgery, as necessary, and clear up any misconceptions the patient or his family may have.

• After surgery, tell the patient to report any drainage through the cast and any warmth, tenderness, or foul odor. Teach him to immediately wrap the stump with an elastic bandage if the cast slips off. Or show him how to slip on a custom-fitted, elastic stump shrinker.

• Teach the patient how to care for his stump. Instruct him to call the doctor if the incision appears to be opening, looks red or swollen, feels warm, is painful to touch, or is seeping drainage.

• Reinforce the need to follow the prescribed exercise program to minimize complications, maintain muscle tone and strength, and prevent contractures. Also stress the importance of correct positioning to prevent contractures.

• Caution the patient to protect the stump from additional trauma.

WHOLE BODY INJURIES

Affecting the entire body, these injuries frequently are life-threatening.

BURNS

A major burn is a horrifying injury, requiring painful treatment and a long period of rehabilitation. It's often fatal or permanently disfiguring and incapacitating, both emotionally and physically.

In the United States, about 1.4 million people are burned annually. Of these, up to 100,000 are seriously burned, and more than 6,000 die of burn injuries, making burns the fourth largest cause of accidental death.

Causes

Thermal burns, the most common type, frequently result from residential fires, motor vehicle crashes, playing with matches, improperly stored gasoline, space heater or electrical malfunctions, and arson. Other causes include improper handling of firecrackers, scalding accidents, and kitchen accidents (such as a child climbing on top of a stove or grabbing a hot iron). Sometimes burns are traced to child or elder abuse.

Chemical burns result from the contact, ingestion, inhalation, or injection of acids, alkalies, or vesicants. Electrical burns commonly occur after contact with faulty electrical wiring or with high-voltage power lines, or when electric cords are chewed (by young children). Friction, or abrasion, burns happen when the skin is rubbed harshly against a coarse surface. Sunburn follows excessive exposure to sunlight.

Complications

The most common complications and leading causes of death are respiratory complications and sepsis. Other possible complications include hypovolemic shock, anemia, and malnutrition.

Assessment findings

The patient's history usually reveals the cause of the burn. It also may disclose preexisting medical conditions—such as a cardiac or pulmonary problem, diabetes mellitus, peripheral vascular disease, chronic alcohol or drug abuse, or a psychiatric disorder—that could complicate burn treatment and recovery.

As well, the history will reveal the patient's age. If he's under age 5 or over age 65, he'll have a higher incidence of complications and, consequently, a higher risk of death.

Obtain all this information as soon as possible because medications, confusion resulting from the injury, or the use of an endotracheal tube may prevent the patient from giving an accurate history later.

Your assessment provides a general idea of burn severity. First, determine the depth of tissue damage. A partial-thickness burn damages the epidermis and part of the dermis, whereas a full-thickness burn also affects the subcutaneous tissue. The more traditional method is to gauge burns by degree, although most burns are a combination of degrees and thicknesses.

The following can help you gauge a burn's severity:
• *First-degree (superficial)*. Erythema appears, and the patient will complain of pain. Damage is limited to the epidermis.
• *Second-degree (partial thickness)*. Blisters and mild to moderate edema develop, and the patient will report pain. Both the epidermis and the dermis are damaged.
• *Third-degree (full thickness)*. Tissue appears white, brown, pale yellow, cherry red, or black and leathery with thrombosed vessels; no blisters appear. Both epidermis and dermis are damaged. Damage may extend through deeply charred subcutaneous tissue to muscle and bone.

Next, assess the size of the burn. This usually is expressed as the percentage of the body surface area (BSA) covered by the burn. Determine this percentage with an assessment tool, such as the Rule of Nines or the Lund and Browder Chart. (See *Estimating the extent of a burn*.) You usually don't need to calculate the total BSA in a patient with a first-degree burn.

Then estimate the severity of the burn by correlating its depth and size, as follows:
• *Major*. This category includes third-degree burns on more than 10% of the patient's BSA; second-degree burns on more than 25% of an adult's BSA or more than 20% of a child's; burns of the hands, face, feet, or genitalia; burns complicated by fractures or respiratory damage; electrical burns; and all burns in poor-risk patients.
• *Moderate*. This category covers third-degree burns on 3% to 10% of a patient's BSA, or second-degree burns on 15% to 25% of an adult's BSA or 10% to 20% of a child's.
• *Minor*. Third-degree burns that appear on less than 3% of a patient's BSA, or second-degree burns on less than 15% of the BSA — 10% in a child — make up this category.

Inspection reveals other characteristics of the burn as well, including location and extent. Keep in mind that burns on the face, hands, feet, and genitalia are most serious because of a possible loss of function or severe impact on body image. Also note the burn's configuration. If the patient has a circumferential burn, he runs the risk of edema totally occluding circulation in his extremity. If he has burns on his neck, he may suffer airway obstruction; burns on the chest can lead to restricted respiratory excursion.

Inspect the patient for other injuries that may complicate his recovery. In particular, look for signs of pulmonary damage from smoke inhalation — singed nasal hairs, mucosal burns, voice changes, coughing, wheezing, soot in the mouth or nose, and darkened sputum. Also, look for respiratory distress and cyanosis — signs of systemic complications from noxious fumes such as cyanide from burning carpets.

Palpation reveals edema and pulse rate, strength, and regularity.

Lung auscultation may reveal respiratory distress, including stridor, wheezing, crackles, and rhonchi. Heart auscultation may detect an S_3 or S_4 gallop or murmur, a sign of myocardial injury or decompensation. The patient with severe burns may be hypotensive, indicating hypovolemia and, possibly, shock. (You can take the blood pressure even if all extremities are burned by placing a $4'' \times 4''$ sterile gauze pad or sterile towel on the extremity before applying the blood pressure cuff.)

Abdominal auscultation may disclose absent bowel sounds if the patient has an ileus, which usually accompanies a burn that covers more than 25% of total BSA.

Diagnostic tests

Routine blood work for a patient with a burn injury includes a complete blood count, platelet count, clotting studies, liver function studies, and carboxyhemoglobin, electrolyte, blood urea nitrogen, glucose, and creatinine levels. A urinalysis may reveal myoglobinuria and hemoglobinuria. If the patient is age 35 or over, he'll also need an electrocardiogram. Chest X-ray films and arterial blood gas levels allow the evaluation of alveolar function. Fiber-optic bronchoscopy shows the condition of the trachea and bronchi.

Treatment

For a patient with severe facial burns or suspected pulmonary injury, treatment to prevent hypoxia includes endotracheal intubation, administration of high concentrations of oxygen, and positive-pressure ventilation.

Treatment for moderate or severe burns includes administration of lactated Ringer's solution through a large-bore I.V. line to expand vascular volume. Central I.V. lines and arterial lines are inserted as necessary. An adult patient also needs I.V. fluids sufficient to maintain a urine output of 30 to 50 ml/hour; the output of a child under 66 lb (30 kg) should be maintained at 1 ml/kg/hour. An

ESTIMATING THE EXTENT OF A BURN

You can quickly estimate the extent of an adult patient's burns by using the Rule of Nines, shown below at left. This method divides an adult's body surface into percentages.

To use this method, mentally transfer your patient's burns to the body chart shown here. Then add up the corresponding percentages for each burned body section. The total—a rough estimate of the extent of your patient's burns—enters into

the formula to determine his initial fluid replacement needs.

You can't use this method with an infant or a child because his body section percentages differ from those of an adult. (For instance, an infant's head accounts for 17% of his total body surface, compared with 7% for an adult.) Instead, use the Lund and Browder chart (below right).

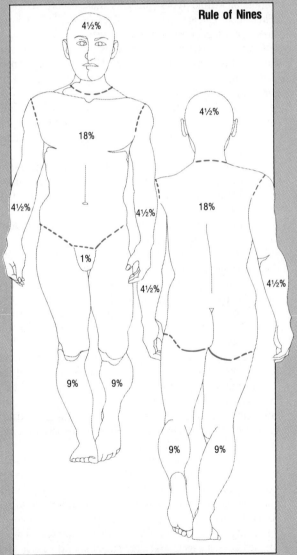

Rule of Nines

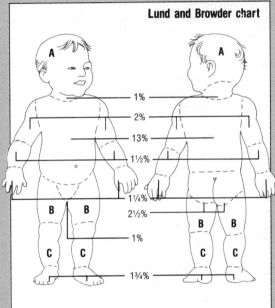

Lund and Browder chart

Relative percentages of areas affected by growth

At birth	0 to 1 yr	2 to 4 yr	5 to 9 yr	10 to 15 yr	Adult
A: Half of head					
9½%	8½%	6½%	5½%	4½%	3½%
B: Half of thigh					
2¾%	3¼%	4%	4¼%	4½%	4¾%
C: Half of leg					
2½%	2½%	2¾%	3%	3¼%	3½%

indwelling urinary catheter permits accurate monitoring of urine output. I.V. morphine (2 to 4 mg) alleviates pain and anxiety. The patient also will need a nasogastric (NG) tube to prevent gastric distention and accompanying ileus from hypovolemic shock.

All burn patients need a booster of 0.5 ml of tetanus toxoid administered I.M. Most burn centers don't recommend administering prophylactic antibiotics because overuse of antibiotics fosters the development of resistant bacteria.

Treatment of the burn wound itself includes:
• initial debriding by washing the surface of the wound area with mild soap
• sharp debridement of loose tissue and blisters (blister fluid contains agents that reduce bactericidal activity and increase inflammatory response)
• covering the wound with an antimicrobial agent and an occlusive cotton gauze dressing
• escharotomy, if the patient is at risk for vascular, circulatory, or respiratory compromise.

Nursing diagnoses
• Altered nutrition: Less than body requirements
• Altered peripheral tissue perfusion
• Altered protection
• Anxiety
• Body image disturbance
• Decreased cardiac output
• Fluid volume deficit
• Hypothermia
• Impaired gas exchange
• Impaired physical mobility
• Impaired skin integrity
• Ineffective airway clearance
• Ineffective individual coping
• Knowledge deficit
• Pain
• Risk for infection
• Sensory or perceptual alterations

Nursing interventions
• Provide immediate, aggressive burn treatment to increase the patient's chance for survival. Later, provide supportive measures and use strict aseptic technique to minimize the risk of infection. Keep in mind that good nursing care can make the difference between life and death in a burn patient. (See *Planning care for a patient with a major burn*.)
• Make sure the patient with major or moderate burns has adequate airway, breathing, and circulation. If needed, assist with endotracheal intubation. Administer 100% oxygen, as ordered, and adjust the flow to maintain adequate gas exchange. Also draw blood samples, as ordered.
• Take steps to control bleeding, and remove any clothing that's still smoldering. If it's stuck to the patient's skin, soak it first in saline solution. Also remove rings and other constricting items.
• Cover the burns with a clean, dry, sterile bed sheet. *Never* cover large burns with saline-soaked dressings, which can drastically lower body temperature.
• Start I.V. therapy at once to prevent hypovolemic shock and maintain cardiac output. Use lactated Ringer's solution or a fluid replacement formula, as ordered. (See *Fluid replacement: The first 24 hours,* page 257.) Closely monitor the patient's intake and output.
• Assist with the insertion of a central venous pressure line and additional arterial and I.V. lines (using venous cutdown, if necessary) as necessary. Insert an indwelling urinary catheter, as ordered.
• Continue fluid therapy, as ordered, to combat fluid evaporation through the burn and the release of fluid into interstitial spaces (possibly resulting in hypovolemic shock).
• Check the patient's vital signs every 15 minutes. Maintain his core body temperature by covering him with a sterile blanket and exposing only small areas of his body at a time.
• Insert an NG tube, as ordered, to decompress the stomach and avoid aspiration of stomach contents.
• Provide a diet high in potassium, protein, vitamins, fats, nitrogen, and calories to keep the patient's weight as close to his preburn weight as possible. If necessary, feed the patient through a small NG tube (as soon as bowel sounds return if he's had paralytic ileus) until he can tolerate oral feedings. Weigh him every day at the same time.
• If the patient will be transferred to a specialized burn care unit within 4 hours after the injury, don't treat the burn wound itself in the emergency department. Instead, prepare him for transport by wrapping him in a sterile sheet and a blanket for warmth and elevating the burned extremity to decrease edema. Then, transport him immediately.
• If the patient has only minor burns, immerse the burned area in cool saline solution (55° F [12.8° C]) or apply cool compresses, making sure he doesn't develop hypothermia. Next, soak the wound in a mild antiseptic solution to clean it, and give ordered pain medication.
• Debride the devitalized tissue. Cover the wound with an antibacterial agent and a nonstick bulky dressing, and administer tetanus prophylaxis, as ordered.

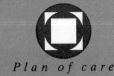

Plan of care

PLANNING CARE FOR A PATIENT WITH A MAJOR BURN

You need to develop a comprehensive care plan for the patient with a major burn to give him the best chance for survival and recovery. Here's one such plan, developed for Bill Tamel, age 56.

Patient history and emergency treatment

Mr. Tamel was working in a paper container factory when a flash fire broke out. Rescue workers didn't reach him until 11 minutes after his co-workers reported the blaze.

The paramedics report that Mr. Tamel was unconscious and had shallow respirations during transport to the hospital. They noted that his face, neck, hands, and arms appeared severely burned and that he was missing several digits. His blood pressure was barely palpable, and he had a rapid, thready, and irregular femoral pulse.

As he's wheeled into the trauma room, Mr. Tamel stops breathing. He receives an emergency tracheostomy (needed because of severe burns to his airway and edema) and is placed on a ventilator. He's given lactated Ringer's solution I.V. and has an indwelling urinary catheter inserted. To promote respiratory excursion during the emergent (shock or fluid accumulation) phase, emergency escharotomies are performed on both arms and over the chest.

When you talk with Mr. Tamel's co-workers, they tell you that he takes insulin every morning and that he carefully protects his feet and legs during the cooler weather. An examination of his medical records shows a 7-year history of insulin-dependent diabetes mellitus, peripheral vascular disease, and mild arteriosclerotic cerebrovascular disease. The records also reveal that Mr. Tamel quit smoking shortly after he was diagnosed with diabetes.

Assessment findings

Your initial assessment reveals that Mr. Tamel has a blood pressure of 50/0 mm Hg and a pulse rate of 122 beats/minute, with frequent premature atrial and ventricular contractions and short runs of ventricular tachycardia—all signs of shock. He's receiving 12 breaths/minute on the ventilator, with a tidal volume of 700 cc and an FIO_2 of 0.8. His level of consciousness is still fluctuating, but you can rouse him.

On inspection, you note that secretions suctioned from Mr. Tamel's endotracheal tube are frothy, blood-tinged, and full of charred particles. His nose, lips, and eyelids appear severely swollen, and his neck circumference is increasing. You estimate that partial- and full-thickness burns cover 45% of his body surface area.

Chest X-rays show diffuse infiltrates without atelectasis. Analysis of Mr. Tamel's arterial blood gas (ABG) levels reveals a pH of 7.22, a PaO_2 of 58 mm Hg, a $PaCO_2$ of 35 mm Hg, and an HCO_3 of 19 mEq/liter. He also has the following venous blood values:
• glucose—244 mg/dl
• potassium—6.2 mEq/liter
• sodium—121 mEq/liter
• hematocrit—54%.

Nursing diagnoses

Based on your assessment findings, you devise the following nursing diagnoses to cover the next 24 to 48 hours—the emergent phase of Mr. Tamel's burn injuries:
• Fluid volume deficit related to hypovolemia, hyperkalemia, hyponatremia, and metabolic acidosis
• Impaired gas exchange and ineffective airway clearance related to third-space shifts of fluid in the lungs
• Risk for infection related to loss of protective skin barrier, septic aerobic and anaerobic microorganisms, wound contamination, and altered nutrition
• Altered nutrition: Less than body requirements, related to increased metabolic demand and loss of protein and nutrients
• Pain related to exposed nerve endings and hypoxia
• Anxiety related to pain, sudden injury, mechanical ventilation, and fear of death
• Hypothermia related to skin and fluid loss.

Expected outcomes

Next, you set several immediate goals for Mr. Tamel. To increase his chances for survival and recovery, Mr. Tamel will have:
• a stable fluid volume and electrolyte balance
• improved oxygenation and perfusion to vital organs and tissues
• decreased risk of infection
• improved nutrition
• reduced pain and anxiety levels
• adequate body temperature.

Implementation

You'll need to take several steps to implement your care plan.

To correct Mr. Tamel's fluid volume and electrolyte imbalance
• Monitor his vital signs (possibly with a central venous line, or through pulmonary artery, arterial, or intracranial pressure monitoring) and intake and output.

(continued)

PLANNING CARE FOR A PATIENT WITH A MAJOR BURN (continued)

• Watch for signs of hypovolemia and hypervolemia.
• Observe the pattern of third-space shifting (generalized edema, ascites, and pulmonary and intracranial edema).
• Monitor Mr. Tamel's potassium levels and watch for signs of hyperkalemia (slowed, irregular heart rate; cardiac rhythm strip changes; weakness; and diarrhea).
• Monitor sodium levels and watch for signs of hyponatremia (increasing confusion, twitching, seizures, abdominal pain, nausea, and vomiting).
• Watch for signs of metabolic acidosis (headache, disorientation, drowsiness, nausea and vomiting, and rapid, shallow breathing), and monitor test results (for low pH and $PaCO_2$, negative base excess, and an anion gap greater than 15 mEq/liter).

To improve oxygenation and maintain perfusion to vital organs and tissues

• Maintain a patent airway, clear secretions, and deliver oxygen based on Mr. Tamel's ABG results.
• Assess lung sounds and patterns and chest expansion, and watch for signs of hypoxia.
• Perform an escharotomy, as ordered, to allow chest expansion.
• Monitor mechanical ventilation, making sure the equipment is working properly and checking the settings and Mr. Tamel's response.
• Maintain adequate pulmonary hygiene through turning and performing postural drainage.
• Watch for signs of decreased tissue perfusion, increased confusion, and agitation.

To reduce the risk of infection

• Use aseptic technique for all patient care, including maintenance of I.V. or other invasive tubing; this includes hand washing and wearing protective isolation clothing, masks, and gloves.
• Administer I.V. and topical antibiotics.
• Meticulously clean unburned skin daily.
• Assess Mr. Tamel daily for purulent drainage, redness, swelling, and fever.

To ensure adequate nutrition

• Provide a high-calorie, high-protein diet.
• Use a gastric or nasoenteric feeding tube for enteral feedings if the patient can't eat.
• Observe for diarrhea and notify the doctor if it occurs.
• Administer total parenteral nutrition if GI dysfunction exists.
• Maintain sterility at the insertion site to prevent infection.
• Monitor the patient for signs of infection at the insertion site.

To reduce pain and anxiety

• Ensure adequate I.V. analgesia, especially before extensive cleaning and debridement.
• Explain the purpose for all treatments and procedures to Mr. Tamel.
• Provide emotional support and reassurance.
• Teach Mr. Tamel relaxation techniques (such as imagery), and provide diversional activities (such as listening to music).

To maintain an adequate body temperature

• Use a heated mattress, blankets, or heat lamps.
• Cover Mr. Tamel's burns with dressings whenever possible.
• Clean and debride wounds as quickly as possible to prevent prolonged exposure.
• Monitor Mr. Tamel's rectal temperature.

Evaluation

You've met your goals if you've stabilized Mr. Tamel's fluid volume and electrolyte balance, improved his oxygenation, maintained perfusion to vital organs, prevented infection, improved his nutritional status, and maintained his body temperature. Mr. Tamel also should be in less pain and feel less anxious. By meeting these goals, you'll greatly improve Mr. Tamel's chances for survival—and put him on the road to recovery.

• Explain all procedures to the patient before performing them. Speak calmly and clearly to help alleviate his anxiety. Encourage him to actively participate in his care as much as possible.
• Give the patient opportunities to voice his concerns, especially about altered body image. If appropriate, arrange for him to meet a patient with similar injuries. When possible, show the patient how his bodily functions are improving. If necessary, refer him for mental health counseling.

For a patient with an electrical or a chemical burn:
• Keep in mind that tissue damage from an electrical burn is difficult to assess because internal destruction along the conduction pathway usually is greater than the surface burn would indicate. An electrical burn that ignites the patient's clothes may cause thermal burns as well.
• If the electric shock caused ventricular fibrillation and cardiac and respiratory arrest, begin cardiopulmonary resuscitation at once. Get an estimate of the voltage that caused the injury.
• If the patient has a chemical burn, irrigate the wound with copious amounts of water or 0.9% sodium chloride solution. Using a weak base (such as sodium bicarbonate) to neutralize hydrofluoric acid, hydrochloric acid, or sulfuric acid on skin or mucous membranes is controversial, particularly in the emergent phase, because the

neutralizing agent can produce more heat and tissue damage.

• If the chemical entered the patient's eyes, flush them with large amounts of water or 0.9% sodium chloride solution for at least 30 minutes. In an alkali burn, irrigate until the pH of the conjunctival cul-de-sacs returns to 7.0. Have the patient close his eyes, and cover them with a dry, sterile dressing. Note the type of chemical that caused the burn and any noxious fumes. The patient will need an ophthalmologic examination.

Patient teaching

• If the patient has only a minor burn, stress the importance of keeping his dressing dry and clean, elevating the burned extremity for the first 24 hours, taking analgesics as ordered, and returning for a wound check in 2 days.
• For a patient with a moderate or major burn, discharge teaching involves the entire burn team. Teaching topics include wound management; signs and symptoms of complications; use of pressure dressings, exercises, and splints; and resocialization. Make sure the patient understands the treatment plan, including why it's necessary and how it will help his recovery.
• Explain to the patient that a home health nurse can assist with wound care. Provide the patient with the phone numbers of a doctor or nurse who can answer questions.
• Give the patient written discharge instructions for later reference.

ELECTRIC SHOCK

When an electric current passes through the body, the damage it does depends on the intensity of the current (amperes, milliamperes, or microamperes), the resistance of the tissues it passes through, the kind of current (AC, DC, or mixed), and the frequency and duration of current flow.

Mild electric shock can cause a local, unpleasant tingling or a painful sensation. Severe electric shock can cause ventricular fibrillation, asystole, respiratory paralysis, burns, and even death. Even the smallest electric current—if it passes through the heart—may induce ventricular fibrillation or another arrhythmia that progresses to fibrillation or myocardial infarction.

In the United States, about 1,000 persons die of electric shock each year. Electric shock is a particular hazard in the hospital. (See *Preventing electric shock*, page 258.)

The greatest threats to life from electric shock include cardiac arrhythmias, renal failure secondary to the pre-

FLUID REPLACEMENT: THE FIRST 24 HOURS

Use one of these formulas as a general guideline for the amount of fluid replacement, according to hospital protocol. Vary the infusions according to the patient's response, especially urine output.

Baxter formula
Administer 4 ml of lactated Ringer's solution per kilogram of body weight per percentage of body surface area (BSA) over 24 hours. Give one-half of the total over the first 8 hours after the burn, one-fourth over the next 8 hours, and the remainder over the last 8 hours.

Modified Brooke formula
With this formula, you'll administer various fluids:
• 0.5 ml of a colloid (plasma, plasmanate, or dextran) per kilogram of body weight per percentage of BSA
• 1.5 ml lactated Ringer's solution per kilogram of body weight per percentage of BSA
• 2,000 ml dextrose 5% in water for adults (less for children).
   Give one-half of the total over the first 8 hours after the burn, one-fourth over the next 8 hours, and the remainder over the last 8 hours.

cipitation of myoglobin and hemoglobin in the kidneys, and electrolyte abnormalities, such as hyperkalemia and hypocalcemia from massive muscle breakdown.

The prognosis depends on the site and extent of damage, the patient's state of health, and the speed and adequacy of treatment. Dry, calloused, unbroken skin offers more resistance to electric current than mucous membrane, an open wound, or thin, moist skin.

Causes

Electric shock usually follows accidental contact with an exposed part of an electrical appliance or wiring. It also may result from lightning or the flash of electric arcs from high-voltage power lines or machines.

The current can cause a true electrical injury if it passes through the body. If it doesn't pass through the body, it can cause arc or flash burns. Thermal surface burns can result from associated heat and flames.

Complications

Although complications can occur in almost any part of the body, the most common include sepsis; neurologic, cardiac, or psychiatric dysfunction; renal failure; electrolyte abnormalities; peripheral nerve injuries; vascular disruption; and thrombi.

PREVENTING ELECTRIC SHOCK

Take the following steps to help prevent electric shock in the hospital:
• Check for cuts, cracks, or frayed insulation on electric cords, call buttons (also check for warm call buttons), and electrical devices attached to the patient's bed. Report any problems to maintenance personnel.
• Keep all electrical devices away from hot or wet surfaces and sharp corners. Also, don't set glasses of water, damp towels, or other wet items on electrical equipment. Wipe up accidental spills before they leak into electrical equipment.
• Avoid using extension cords because they may circumvent the ground; if they're necessary, don't place them under carpeting or where they'll be walked on.
• Make sure ground connections on electrical equipment are intact. Line cord plugs should have three prongs; the prongs should be straight and firmly fixed. Check that prongs fit wall outlets properly and that outlets aren't loose or broken. Don't use adapters on plugs.

• If a machine sparks, smokes, seems unusually hot, or gives you or your patient a slight shock, unplug it immediately, if doing so won't endanger the patient's life. Promptly report such equipment to maintenance personnel. Also, check inspection labels, and report equipment overdue for inspection.
• Be especially careful when using electrical equipment near a patient with a pacemaker or direct cardiac line because a cardiac catheter or pacemaker can create a direct, low-resistance path to the heart; even a small shock may cause ventricular fibrillation.
• Make sure defibrillator paddles are free of dry, caked gel before applying fresh gel. Otherwise, the patient may suffer burns from poor electrical contact. Also, don't apply too much gel. If the gel runs over the edge of the paddle and touches your hand, you'll receive some of the defibrillator shock, and the patient will lose some of the energy in the discharge.

Assessment findings

The patient's history reveals the source of the electric current and the approximate length of exposure. Varying signs and symptoms depend on the amount and type of current, the duration and area of exposure, and the pathway the current took through the body. If the shock was severe, the patient or an observer may report that the patient lost consciousness. After regaining consciousness, the patient may complain of muscle pain, fatigue, headache, and nervous irritability.

When electric shock results from a high-frequency current (which generates more heat in tissues than a low-frequency current), inspection usually reveals burns and local tissue coagulation and necrosis. Electric shock resulting from low-frequency current may produce serious burns if contact is concentrated in a small area (for example, when a toddler bites into an electric cord). When the electric current passes through the patient's body, inspection reveals entrance and exit injuries that appear as round or oval yellow-brown lesions.

Depending on the action of the current, inspection and palpation also may reveal contusions, evidence of fractures, and other injuries that can result from violent muscle contractions or falls during the shock. If ventricular fibrillation occurs, you won't be able to palpate the pulse or auscultate heart sounds, and the patient will be unconscious. Respirations may continue for a short time and then cease.

If respiratory failure occurs, inspection discloses cyanosis, absent respirations, markedly decreased blood pressure, cold skin, and unconsciousness; pulses, however, can still be palpated.

Neurologic examination may reveal numbness or tingling or sensorimotor deficits.

Diagnostic tests

An electrocardiogram (ECG), arterial blood gas analysis, urine myoglobin tests, and X-rays of injured areas are used to evaluate internal damage and guide treatment.

Treatment

The first step in treatment involves separating the victim from the current source by turning it off or unplugging it. If this isn't possible, the victim is pulled free with a nonconductive device, such as a loop of dry cloth or rubber, a dry rope, or a leather strap.

After interrupting the current source, perform emergency measures, including assessing vital functions and instituting cardiopulmonary resuscitation (CPR) if the patient has no respirations or pulse.

When the patient is revived, treatment includes:
• assessment for shock, acid-base imbalance, cardiac arrhythmias, hemorrhage, myoglobinuria, traumatic injury, and neurologic damage
• use of a cardiac monitor to permit rapid identification and treatment of arrhythmias

• use of a cervical collar and backboard until spinal injury has been ruled out
• vigorous fluid replacement using lactated Ringer's solution, along with central venous pressure and urine output monitoring
• administration of an osmotic diuretic (mannitol) for myoglobinuria once intravascular volume has been replaced
• administration of tetanus prophylaxis
• administration of sodium bicarbonate to prevent arrhythmias.

Nursing diagnoses
• Altered tissue perfusion
• Anxiety
• Decreased cardiac output
• Impaired skin integrity
• Ineffective breathing pattern
• Pain
• Risk for injury
• Sensory or perceptual alterations

Nursing interventions
• If it hasn't already been done, separate the victim from the current source and then begin emergency treatment. If necessary, start CPR at once. Continue until vital signs return or emergency help arrives with a defibrillator and other life-support equipment.
• After emergency treatment, monitor the patient's cardiac rhythm continuously and obtain a 12-lead ECG.
• Because internal tissue destruction may be much greater than skin damage suggests, give a rapid I.V. infusion of 1 to 2 liters of lactated Ringer's solution, as ordered, to maintain a urine output of 75 to 100 ml/hour. Insert an indwelling urinary catheter, and send the first specimen to the laboratory.

Measure intake and output hourly and watch for tea- or port wine–colored urine, which occurs when coagulation necrosis and tissue ischemia liberate myoglobin and hemoglobin. These proteins can precipitate in the renal tubules, causing tubular necrosis and renal shutdown. To promote diuresis and myoglobin excretion, give mannitol, as ordered.
• Frequently assess the patient's neurologic status because central nervous system damage may result from ischemia or demyelination. If necessary, institute seizure precautions according to hospital policy.

Because a spinal cord injury may follow cord ischemia or a compression fracture, continue to watch for sensorimotor deficits. Ensure proper spinal immobilization until

fractures have been ruled out.
• Check for neurovascular damage in the extremities by assessing peripheral pulses and capillary refill and by asking about numbness, tingling, and pain. Elevate any injured extremities.
• Care for the burned area as indicated. If ordered, apply a sterile dressing and administer topical and systemic antibiotics to help reduce the risk of infection.

Patient teaching
• Reinforce the doctor's explanation of all treatments and procedures. Allow the patient to discuss his experience with you to help decrease his anxiety.
• Tell the patient how to avoid electrical hazards at home and at work. Warn him not to use electrical appliances while showering or wet. Also warn him *never* to touch electrical appliances while touching faucets or cold water pipes in the kitchen; these pipes may provide the ground for all circuits in the house.
• If the patient is a young child, advise his parents to put safety guards on all electrical outlets and to keep him away from electrical devices.

COLD INJURIES
Caused by overexposure, cold injuries occur in two major forms: localized injuries (frostbite) and systemic injuries (hypothermia).

Frostbite may be superficial or deep. Superficial frostbite affects skin and subcutaneous tissue, especially of the face, ears, extremities, and other exposed body areas. Deep frostbite extends beyond the subcutaneous tissue and usually affects the hands and feet. Untreated or improperly treated frostbite can lead to gangrene, requiring amputation.

Hypothermia—core body temperature below 95° F (35° C)—effects chemical changes in the body. Severe hypothermia can be fatal.

The risk of serious cold injuries—especially hypothermia—is increased by youth, old age, lack of insulating body fat, wet or inadequate clothing, drug abuse, cardiac disease, smoking, fatigue, malnutrition and depletion of caloric reserves, and excessive alcohol intake.

Causes and pathophysiology
Frostbite results from prolonged exposure to freezing temperatures or to cold, wet environments. The cold causes ice crystals to form within and around tissue cells. This in turn causes cell membranes to rupture, interrupting enzymatic and metabolic activities. Increased capillary permeability accompanies the release of his-

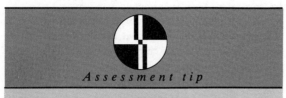

tamine, resulting in aggregation of red blood cells and microvascular occlusion.

Hypothermia results from cold-water near drowning and prolonged exposure to cold temperatures. It also can occur in normal temperatures if the patient's homeostasis is altered by disease or debility. Administration of large amounts of cold blood or blood products can cause hypothermia. In hypothermia, metabolic changes slow the functions of most major organ systems, resulting in decreased renal blood flow and decreased glomerular filtration, for example.

Complications

Tissue and muscle damage caused by frostbite may lead to renal failure and rhabdomyolysis. Avascular necrosis and gangrene also may result from frostbite.

Common complications associated with hypothermia include severe infection, aspiration pneumonia, cardiac arrhythmias, hypoglycemia or hyperglycemia, metabolic acidosis, pancreatitis, and renal failure.

Assessment findings

The history of a patient with a cold injury reveals the cause, the temperature to which the patient was exposed, and the length of exposure. A patient with superficial frostbite may report burning, numbness, tingling, and itching, although he may not notice symptoms until he returns to a warm place. A patient with deep frostbite reports paresthesia and stiffness while the part is still frozen, a burning pain when the part thaws, and then warmth and numbness.

On inspection, an area with superficial frostbite appears swollen, with a mottled, blue-gray skin color. An area affected by deep frostbite appears white or yellow until it's thawed; then it turns purplish blue. You also may note edema, skin blisters, and necrosis.

Palpation of superficial frostbite reveals the extent and severity of swelling. Palpation of deep frostbite may reveal skin immobility. In either type of frostbite, palpation also reveals the presence or absence of associated peripheral pulses.

Your assessment findings in a patient with hypothermia vary with the patient's body temperature. (See *Determining core body temperature.*) A patient with moderate hypothermia—a core body temperature of 86° to 89.6° F (30° to 32° C)—is unresponsive, with peripheral cyanosis and muscle rigidity. If the patient was improperly rewarmed, he may show signs of shock.

A patient with severe hypothermia—a core body temperature of 77° to 86° F (25° to 30° C)—appears dead, with no palpable pulse and no audible heart sounds. His pupils may be dilated, and he may appear to be in a state of rigor mortis. Ventricular fibrillation and a loss of deep tendon reflexes commonly occur.

A patient with a body temperature below 77° F (25° C) will suffer cardiopulmonary arrest.

Diagnostic tests

Technetium pertechnetate scanning shows perfusion defects and deep tissue damage and can identify nonviable bone. Doppler and plethysmographic studies help determine pulses and the extent of frostbite after thawing.

Essential laboratory tests during treatment of moderate or severe hypothermia include a complete blood count, coagulation profile, urinalysis, and serum amylase, electrolyte, hemoglobin, glucose, liver enzyme, blood urea nitrogen, creatinine, and arterial blood gas levels.

Treatment

For frostbite injuries, treatment consists of rapidly rewarming the injured part to slightly above ideal body temperature to preserve viable tissue. Slow rewarming may increase tissue damage. Treatment also includes administration of antibiotics and tetanus prophylaxis, as needed, and narcotic analgesics to relieve pain when the affected part begins to rewarm.

After rewarming, the affected part is kept elevated, uncovered, at room temperature. A regimen of whirlpool treatments for 3 or more weeks cleans the skin and debrides sloughing tissue. After the early stage, active range-of-motion exercises restore mobility. Surgery usually isn't required; however, if gangrene develops, amputation may be necessary.

Treatment for hypothermia consists of supportive measures and specific rewarming techniques, including:
• passive rewarming (the patient rewarms on his own)

• active external rewarming with heating blankets, warm water immersion, heated objects such as water bottles, and radiant heat
• active core rewarming with heated I.V. fluids; genitourinary tract irrigation; extracorporeal rewarming; hemodialysis; and peritoneal, gastric, and mediastinal lavage.

Any arrhythmias that may develop usually convert to normal sinus rhythm with rewarming. If the patient has no pulse or respirations, he'll need cardiopulmonary resuscitation (CPR) until he's been rewarmed to a core temperature of at least 89.6° F (32° C).

Administration of oxygen, endotracheal intubation, controlled ventilation, I.V. fluids, and treatment of metabolic acidosis depend on test results and careful patient monitoring.

Nursing diagnoses
• Altered health maintenance
• Altered tissue perfusion
• Anxiety
• Decreased cardiac output
• Hypothermia
• Impaired gas exchange
• Impaired physical mobility
• Impaired skin integrity
• Risk for disuse syndrome
• Risk for infection

Nursing interventions
• If the patient has a localized cold injury, remove all constrictive clothing and jewelry.
• When the affected part begins to rewarm, the patient will feel pain, so give analgesics, as ordered. Check for a pulse. Be careful not to rupture any blebs. If the injury is on the foot, place cotton or gauze sponges between the toes to prevent maceration. Instruct him not to walk.
• If the injury has caused an open skin wound, give antibiotics and tetanus prophylaxis, as ordered.
• Rewarm the affected part by immersing it in tepid water (about 100° F [37.8° C]). Give the patient warm fluids to drink. *Never* rub the injured area—this aggravates tissue damage.
• If the patient has systemic hypothermia, first check for a pulse and respirations. If you can't detect them, begin CPR immediately. Continue CPR until the patient's core body temperature rises to at least 89.6° F (32° C). (Keep in mind that hypothermia helps protect the brain from anoxia, which normally accompanies prolonged cardiopulmonary arrest. So even if the patient has been un-responsive for a long time, CPR may resuscitate him, especially after a cold-water near drowning.)
• Assist with rewarming techniques as necessary. In moderate to severe hypothermia, aggressive rewarming should be attempted only by experienced personnel.
• During rewarming, provide supportive measures as ordered. These include mechanical ventilation and heated, humidified therapy to maintain tissue oxygenation, and I.V. fluids that have been warmed with a warming coil to correct hypotension and maintain urine output.
• Insert an indwelling catheter to monitor urine output.
• Frequently monitor the patient's core body temperature and other vital signs during and after initial rewarming. Also, continuously monitor his cardiac status.

If the patient's core temperature is below 89.6° F, use internal and external warming methods to bring up his body core and surface temperatures 1° to 2° F (0.2° to 1.1° C) per hour. *Note:* Make sure you rewarm the patient internally and externally at the same time; rewarming the surface first could cause rewarming shock with potentially fatal ventricular fibrillation.

Patient teaching
• To prevent cold injuries, teach the patient that in cold weather, he should wear mittens—not gloves; windproof, water-resistant, many-layered clothing; two pairs of socks (cotton next to the skin and then wool); and a scarf and a hat that covers the ears (to avoid substantial heat loss through the head).
• Before anticipated prolonged exposure to cold, advise the patient not to drink alcohol or smoke, and to get adequate food and rest. If he gets caught in severe cold weather, he should find shelter early or increase physical activity to maintain body warmth.

HEAT SYNDROME
Humans normally adjust to excessive temperatures by complex cardiovascular and neurologic changes, which are coordinated by the hypothalamus. Heat loss offsets heat production to regulate the body temperature. It does this by evaporation (sweating) or vasodilation, which cools the body's surface by radiation, conduction, and convection.

Sometimes both environmental and internal factors can increase heat production or decrease heat loss beyond the body's ability to compensate. When this happens, heat syndrome results. This syndrome falls into three categories: heat cramps, heat exhaustion, and heatstroke.

Causes

Heat syndrome may result from conditions that increase heat production, such as excessive exercise, infection, and drugs (for example, amphetamines). It also can stem from factors that impair heat dissipation. These include high temperatures or humidity, lack of acclimatization, excess clothing, cardiovascular disease, obesity, dehydration, sweat gland dysfunction, and drugs, such as phenothiazines and anticholinergics.

Heatstroke often is seen in elderly people during excessively hot summer days, particularly when they are inside with windows and doors closed and have no air conditioning. They may not open windows and doors because they are afraid someone may break in and injure them.

Complications

Heatstroke, a medical emergency, can lead to hypovolemic or cardiogenic shock, cardiac arrhythmias, and renal failure caused by rhabdomyolysis, disseminated intravascular coagulation, and hepatic failure.

Assessment findings

Signs and symptoms vary with the type of heat syndrome.

The history of a patient with heat cramps almost always reveals vigorous activity immediately preceding onset. The patient typically appears alert and complains of pain.

On assessment, the patient usually has normal vital signs (except for tachycardia) with a normal or slightly elevated body temperature. Inspection reveals muscle twitching and spasm. Palpation reveals moist, cool skin and muscle tenderness. Involved muscle groups may feel hard and lumpy. The neurologic examination usually is normal, although the patient may appear agitated.

The history of a patient with heat exhaustion usually reveals prolonged activity in a very warm or hot environment, without adequate salt intake. He may complain of muscle cramps. More often, he reports nausea and vomiting, thirst, weakness, and oliguria. He also may complain of headache and fatigue and may be anxious.

Assessment reveals a rectal temperature over 100° F (37.8° C). On inspection, you may note pale skin. The patient's pulse feels thready and rapid, and his skin is cool and moist. Auscultation reveals decreased blood pressure. When heat exhaustion is mainly due to water depletion, examination may reveal mental confusion, giddiness, syncope, impaired judgment, and anxiety paresthesia. Assessment also may reveal hyperventilation, which can lead to respiratory alkalosis. If you note that

sweating ceases, the patient may be progressing from heat exhaustion to heatstroke.

The history of a patient with heatstroke may reveal the specific cause, such as exposure to high temperature and humidity without any wind. He may exhibit weakness, dizziness, nausea, vomiting, and blurred vision, confusion, hallucinations, and decreased muscle coordination.

Your assessment shows a rectal temperature of at least 106° F (41.1° C). On inspection and palpation, the patient's skin is red, diaphoretic, and hot in early stages; gray, dry, and hot in later stages. He may have a rapid pulse rate. On auscultation, his blood pressure is slightly elevated in early stages; decreased in later stages. The neurologic examination of the conscious patient may reveal dilated pupils, emotional lability, confusion, and—as heatstroke progresses—delirium, seizures, collapse and, finally, unconsciousness. You also may note hyperpnea at any time, which leads to respiratory alkalosis and compensatory metabolic acidosis. In late stages, you may note slow, deep respirations, which progress to Cheyne-Stokes respirations.

Diagnostic tests

Serum electrolyte and arterial blood gas levels may reveal respiratory alkalosis, hyponatremia, and hypokalemia in heat exhaustion and heatstroke. In heatstroke, blood studies reveal leukocytosis, elevated blood urea nitrogen levels, hemoconcentration, and decreased serum potassium, calcium, and phosphorus levels. Blood studies also may reveal thrombocytopenia, increased bleeding and clotting times, fibrinolysis, and consumption coagulopathy. Urinalysis results show concentrated urine, with elevated protein levels, tubular casts, and myoglobinuria.

Treatment

For heat cramps, treatment consists of moving the patient to a cool environment, providing rest, and administering oral or I.V. fluid and electrolyte replacement (for example, Lytren or Rehydralyte for adults and Pedialyte for children). Salt tablets aren't recommended because of their comparatively slow absorption.

Treatment for heat exhaustion involves moving the patient to a cool environment, providing rest, and administering oral fluid and electrolyte replacement. If I.V. replacement is necessary, laboratory test results determine the choice of I.V. solution—usually saline or isotonic glucose solution.

Heatstroke therapy focuses on lowering the body temperature as rapidly as possible. The patient's clothing is removed, and cool water is applied to the skin, followed by fanning with cool air. Shivering is controlled with diazepam or chlorpromazine. Application of hypothermia blankets and ice packs to the groin and axillae also helps lower body temperature. Treatment continues until the body temperature drops to 102.2° F (39° C). Supportive measures include oxygen therapy, central venous pressure and pulmonary artery wedge pressure monitoring, and, if necessary, endotracheal intubation. The patient is closely observed for complications.

Nursing diagnoses
• Altered thought processes
• Decreased cardiac output
• Fluid volume deficit
• Hyperthermia
• Impaired gas exchange
• Impaired home maintenance management
• Knowledge deficit
• Sensory or perceptual alterations

Nursing interventions
• Monitor the patient's vital signs and pulse oximetry readings. If he's unstable, use a rectal probe to assess his body temperature.
• Perform or assist with the cooling procedure as needed. If ordered, place the patient on a cooling mattress.

If the patient has heatstroke, remove his clothing and place him in the lateral recumbent position, or support him in the knee-chest position so that as much skin as possible is exposed to the air. Then spray his entire body with water as cool air is passed over the body. Use fans to provide air movement, which increases heat loss through convection and evaporation. Or cover the patient with a damp sheet, and fan him with cool air.
• Assist with supportive measures as necessary. These may include assisting with insertion of an endotracheal tube and caring for it to maintain an adequate airway. Provide supplemental oxygen, as ordered.
• Encourage adequate fluid intake as required. If necessary, ensure peripheral I.V. access, as ordered.
• Monitor the patient for complications. Note his level of consciousness, cardiac rhythm, and cardiac output. If a central line is in place, monitor central venous pressure and pulmonary artery wedge pressure.
• Administer medication as ordered to inhibit shivering.
• Monitor urine output. Insert an indwelling urinary catheter, as needed, and monitor myoglobin test results, as ordered.
• Referral to a social service agency may be necessary for an elderly patient who experiences heat syndrome because of a compromised home environment.

Patient teaching
• Advise the patient to avoid immediate reexposure to high temperatures. He may remain hypersensitive to heat for a while.
• Teach the patient the importance of maintaining an adequate fluid intake, wearing loose clothing, and limiting activity in hot weather.
• Advise athletes to monitor fluid losses, replace fluids, and use a gradual approach to physical conditioning.
• In hot weather, encourage elderly patients to spend time in air-conditioned areas, such as shopping malls and libraries.

ASPHYXIA
A condition of insufficient oxygen and accumulating carbon dioxide in the blood and tissues, asphyxia results from interference with respiration. It leads to cardiopulmonary arrest and is fatal without prompt treatment.

Causes
Asphyxia results from any internal or external condition or substance that inhibits respiration. Some examples include:
• hypoventilation, stemming from narcotic abuse, medullary disease or hemorrhage, respiratory muscle paralysis, or cardiopulmonary arrest
• intrapulmonary obstruction, associated with airway obstruction, pulmonary edema, pneumonia, and near drowning
• extrapulmonary obstruction, as in tracheal compression from a tumor, pneumothorax, strangulation, trauma, or suffocation
• inhalation of toxic agents, resulting from carbon monoxide poisoning, smoke inhalation, and excessive oxygen inhalation.

Complications
Without timely intervention, asphyxia can lead to neurologic damage and death.

Assessment findings
The patient's history (obtained from a family member, friend, or emergency personnel) reveals the cause of the asphyxia. Signs and symptoms depend on the duration and degree of asphyxia.

On general observation, the patient typically appears anxious, agitated or confused, and dyspneic, with prominent neck muscles. Other common signs and symptoms include wheezing, stridor, altered respiratory rate (apnea, bradypnea, occasional tachypnea), and a fast, slow, or absent pulse.

Inspection may reveal little or no air moving in or out of the nose and mouth. You may note intercostal rib retractions as the intercostal muscles pull against resistance. You also may note pale skin and, depending on the severity of the asphyxia, cyanosis in mucous membranes, lips, and nail beds. Trauma-induced asphyxia may cause erythema and petechiae on the upper chest, up to the neck and face. In late-stage carbon monoxide poisoning, mucous membranes appear cherry-red. Auscultation reveals decreased or absent breath sounds.

Diagnostic tests
Arterial blood gas (ABG) analysis, the most important test, indicates decreased PaO_2 (less than 60 mm Hg) and increased $PaCO_2$ (more than 50 mm Hg). Chest X-rays may detect a foreign body, pulmonary edema, or atelectasis. Toxicology tests may show drugs, chemicals, or abnormal hemoglobin. Pulmonary function tests may indicate respiratory muscle weakness.

Treatment
Asphyxia requires immediate respiratory support with cardiopulmonary resuscitation (CPR), endotracheal intubation, supplemental oxygen, mechanical ventilation, and pulse oximetry, as needed. It also calls for prompt treatment of the underlying cause: bronchoscopy for extraction of a foreign body; a narcotic antagonist, such as naloxone, for narcotic overdose; and gastric lavage for poisoning.

Nursing diagnoses
• Anxiety
• Decreased cardiac output
• Impaired gas exchange
• Ineffective airway clearance
• Ineffective breathing pattern
• Risk for aspiration
• Risk for suffocation

Nursing interventions
• If a foreign body is blocking the patient's airway, perform the abdominal thrust.
• In an unconscious patient, the tongue may obstruct the airway. You may be able to open the airway by simply repositioning the patient.
• If the patient has no spontaneous respirations and no pulse, begin CPR.
• If necessary, assist with endotracheal intubation to provide an airway, and give supplemental oxygen or provide mechanical ventilation, as ordered. Monitor ABG levels, the best indicator of oxygenation and acid-base status.
• Ensure I.V. access, monitor I.V. fluids, and obtain laboratory specimens, as ordered.
• If the patient ingested poison, insert a nasogastric tube or an Ewald tube for lavage.
• Administer medications, such as naloxone for narcotic overdose, as ordered.
• Monitor the patient's cardiac status, vital signs, and neurologic status throughout treatment.
• Continually reassure the patient throughout treatment. Respiratory distress is terrifying.
• If asphyxia was intentionally induced, such as carbon monoxide poisoning, refer the patient to a psychiatrist.

Patient teaching
• To prevent drug-induced asphyxia, warn the patient about the danger of taking alcohol with other central nervous system depressants.
• If the patient works with toxic chemicals, stress the importance of adequate ventilation in the workplace and the use of protective gear supplied by the employer.

NEAR DROWNING
In near drowning, the victim has survived (at least temporarily) the physiologic effects of submersion in fluid. Hypoxemia and acidosis are the primary problems in victims of near drowning.

Near drowning occurs in three forms. In "dry" near drowning, the victim doesn't aspirate fluid but suffers respiratory obstruction or asphyxia (10% to 15% of patients). In "wet" near drowning, the victim aspirates fluid and suffers from asphyxia or secondary changes from fluid aspiration (about 85% of patients). And in secondary near drowning, the victim suffers recurrence of respiratory distress (usually aspiration pneumonia or pulmonary edema) within minutes or 1 to 2 days after a near-drowning incident.

Causes
Near drowning typically results from an inability to swim. In swimmers, it can result from panic, a boating accident, sudden acute illness (seizure or myocardial infarction) or a blow to the head while in the water, venomous stings from aquatic animals, drinking heavily before swimming, a suicide attempt, or decompression sickness from deep-water diving.

Complications

Near drowning may result in neurologic impairment, seizure disorders, pulmonary edema, renal damage, bacterial aspiration, and pulmonary or cardiac complications, such as arrhythmias and decreased blood pressure.

Assessment findings

The patient's history (obtained from a family member, friend, or emergency personnel, if necessary) reveals the cause of the near drowning. The patient may display any of a host of signs and symptoms. If he's conscious, he may complain of a headache or substernal chest pain.

Your initial assessment of the patient's vital signs may detect fever; rapid, slow, or absent pulse; shallow, gasping, or absent respirations; confusion; and seizures. If the patient was exposed to cold temperatures, he may experience hypothermia.

On initial observation, the patient may be unconscious, semiconscious, or awake. If he's awake, he usually appears apprehensive, irritable, restless, or lethargic, and he may vomit. Inspection may reveal cyanosis or pink, frothy sputum (indicating pulmonary edema). Palpation of the abdomen may disclose abdominal distention.

Auscultation of the lungs may reveal crackles, rhonchi, wheezing, or apnea. You may note tachycardia, an irregular heartbeat (arrhythmias), or cardiac arrest when you auscultate the heart. The patient also may be hypotensive.

Diagnostic tests

Supportive tests include:
• arterial blood gas (ABG) analysis to show the degree of hypoxia, intrapulmonary shunt, and acid-base balance
• serum electrolyte levels to monitor electrolyte balance
• complete blood count to determine hemolysis
• blood urea nitrogen and creatinine levels and urinalysis to evaluate renal function
• cervical spine X-ray to rule out fracture
• serial chest X-rays to evaluate pulmonary changes
• electrocardiogram (ECG) to detect myocardial ischemia.

Treatment

Prehospital care includes spinal precautions, cardiopulmonary resuscitation (CPR) as needed, and supplemental oxygen.

After the patient reaches the hospital, resuscitation continues. His oxygenation and circulation are maintained. X-rays confirm cervical spine integrity, and the patient's blood pH and electrolyte imbalances are corrected. If he's hypothermic, steps are taken to rewarm him.

ABG results help guide pulmonary therapy and determine the need for sodium bicarbonate to treat metabolic acidosis.

If the patient can't maintain an open airway, has abnormal ABG levels and pH, or doesn't have spontaneous respirations, he may need endotracheal intubation and mechanical ventilation. If he develops bronchospasm, he may need bronchodilators. Central venous pressure or pulmonary artery wedge pressure determines the need for fluid replacement and cardiac drug therapy. The patient also may require standard treatment for pulmonary edema. Nasogastric (NG) tube drainage prevents vomiting, and an indwelling urinary catheter allows monitoring of urine output.

Nursing diagnoses

• Decreased cardiac output
• Hypothermia
• Impaired gas exchange
• Ineffective airway clearance
• Ineffective breathing pattern
• Risk for aspiration
• Risk for infection

Nursing interventions

• Continue CPR as indicated.
• If the patient has been submerged in cold water, use a rectal probe to determine the degree of hypothermia.
• If the patient is hypothermic, start rewarming procedures during resuscitation. Don't stop resuscitation until the patient's body temperature ranges between 86° and 90.5° F (30° to 32.5° C).
• Protect the cervical spine until fracture is ruled out.
• Ensure peripheral I.V. access and administer I.V. fluids as necessary.
• If ordered, insert an NG tube to remove swallowed water and reduce the risk of vomiting and aspiration.
• Insert an indwelling urinary catheter to monitor urine output. Metabolic acidosis may develop to compensate for impaired renal function.
• Assess ABG levels and obtain an ECG. The patient will probably need continuous cardiac monitoring.
• Continually monitor the patient's vital signs and neurologic status. He may have central nervous system damage despite treatment for hypoxia and shock.
• Obtain baseline serum electrolyte levels; continue monitoring these levels.
• If the patient has a central line in place, closely monitor all hemodynamic parameters: cardiac output, central venous pressure, pulmonary artery wedge pressure, heart

rate, and arterial blood pressure.
• Administer bronchodilator and antibiotic agents to the patient as ordered.

Patient teaching
• To prevent near drowning, advise the patient to avoid use of alcohol or drugs before swimming, to observe water safety measures (such as the "buddy system"), and to take a water safety course given by the Red Cross, YMCA, or YWCA.

DECOMPRESSION SICKNESS
Also known as caisson disease, diver's paralysis, or "the bends," decompression sickness is a painful condition that results from too rapid change from high- to low-pressure environments (decompression). The victims usually are scuba divers who ascend too quickly from water deeper than 33' (10 m). Signs and symptoms appear during or within 30 minutes of rapid decompression, although they may be delayed for as long as 24 hours.

Causes
The sickness results from an abrupt change in air or water pressure that causes nitrogen to spill out of tissues faster than it can be diffused through respiration. As a result, gas bubbles form in blood and body tissues. These bubbles can accumulate over several dives.

Complications
Massive venous air embolization, intravascular volume depletion, vascular occlusion, and avascular necrosis may complicate decompression sickness.

Assessment findings
Characteristic clinical features vary, depending on the number and location of gas bubbles. The patient's history (obtained, if necessary, from a family member or friend) reveals the cause of the disorder. The history and physical examination also may reveal predisposing factors, such as excessive use of alcohol or drugs, obesity, dehydration, recent injury, exposure to cold temperatures, and hypoxia.

The patient typically complains of "the bends," which is severe or incapacitating joint, muscle, and bone pain (Type I). He also may report urinary retention, fecal incontinence, and back pain, as well as neurologic disturbances, such as headache, confusion, dizziness, deafness, and visual disturbances (Type II). A detailed neurologic examination of the patient may demonstrate hemiplegia, paresthesia and hyperesthesia of the legs, and an unsteady gait.

As well, the patient may report respiratory distress, known as "the chokes," which includes chest pain, retrosternal burning, and a cough that may become paroxysmal and uncontrollable.

Diagnostic tests
The doctor may order laboratory studies, such as arterial blood gas analysis, to evaluate the patient's signs and symptoms.

Treatment
Consisting of supportive measures, treatment includes recompression and oxygen administration. Recompression takes place in a hyperbaric chamber (not available in all hospitals), in which air pressure is increased to 2.8 absolute atmospheric pressure over 1 to 2 minutes. This rapid rise in pressure reduces the size of the circulating nitrogen bubbles and relieves pain and other clinical effects. Analgesics, such as aspirin, also may be given for pain.

During recompression, intermittent oxygen administration, with periodic maximal exhalations, promotes gas bubble diffusion. Once signs and symptoms subside and diffusion of gas bubbles is complete, a slow air pressure decrease in the chamber allows for gradual, safe decompression.

Supportive measures may include fluid replacement in hypovolemic shock and sometimes corticosteroids to reduce the risk of spinal edema. Short-acting barbiturates may be given to treat seizures. Narcotics are contraindicated because they may further depress impaired respiration.

Nursing diagnoses
• Altered urinary elimination
• Anxiety
• Decreased cardiac output
• Fatigue
• Fluid volume deficit
• Hypothermia
• Impaired gas exchange
• Pain
• Sensory or perceptual alterations

Nursing interventions
• Administer supplemental 100% oxygen by mask at 6 to 8 liters/minute.

• Give emergency medications as ordered. Ensure I.V. access for drugs and parenteral fluids.
• Catheterize the patient with bladder paralysis, and accurately monitor intake and output.
• Continuously monitor neurologic status, cardiac output, and respiratory function to quickly identify changes in the patient's condition.

Patient teaching
• Explain procedures to the patient and listen to his concerns to help alleviate anxiety.
• To help prevent decompression sickness, advise divers and fliers to follow the U.S. Navy's ascent guidelines closely.

RADIATION EXPOSURE

Expanded use of ionized radiation has vastly increased the incidence of radiation exposure. Cancer patients who receive radiation therapy and nuclear power plant workers are among the most likely victims of radiation exposure.

The amount of radiation absorbed by a human body is measured in radiation absorbed doses (rad), not to be confused with roentgens, which are used to measure radiation emissions. A person can absorb up to 200 rad without fatal consequences. A dose of 450 rad is fatal in about half the cases; more than 600 rad is nearly always fatal. When radiation is focused on a small area, the body can absorb and survive many thousands of rads if they are administered in carefully controlled doses over a long period. This basic principle is the key to safe and successful radiation therapy.

Causes
Exposure to radiation can occur by inhalation, ingestion, or direct contact. The existence and severity of tissue damage depend on the amount of body area exposed (the smaller, the better), length of exposure, dosage absorbed, distance from the source, and presence of protective shielding. (For guidelines to help minimize radiation exposure, see *Preventing radiation exposure,* page 268.) Ionized radiation (X-rays, protons, neutrons, and alpha, beta, and gamma rays) may cause immediate cell necrosis or disturbed deoxyribonucleic acid synthesis, which impairs cell function and division.

Rapidly dividing cells—bone marrow, hair follicles, gonads, and lymph tissue—are the most susceptible to radiation damage; highly differentiated cells—nerve, bone, and muscle—can resist radiation more successfully.

Complications
Delayed complications include leukemia and thyroid carcinoma. For people in the childbearing years, long-term exposure may cause fetal growth retardation or genetic defects in offspring.

Assessment findings
The effects of ionized radiation can be immediate and acute or delayed and chronic. Acute effects may be hematopoietic (after 100 to 600 rad), GI (after 600 to 2,000 rad), cerebral (after 1,000 or more rad), or cardiovascular (after 5,000 rad). They depend strictly on the *amount* of radiation absorbed.

An accurate patient history should reveal the radiation exposure, its type, duration, and organs exposed.

A patient with *acute hematopoietic radiation toxicity* may report bleeding from the skin as well as from the GI and genitourinary tracts, the result of thrombocytopenia. During the latent period that follows, pancytopenia develops, and the patient may report no apparent signs or symptoms. As the latent period ends, the patient may report nosebleeds, hemorrhage, and increased susceptibility to infection (from an impaired immune response). Inspection may reveal petechiae, pallor, weakness, and oropharyngeal abscesses.

A patient with *radiation exposure that affects the GI system* may report intractable nausea, vomiting, and diarrhea. (This may result in severe fluid and electrolyte imbalance.) Inspection of the mouth and throat may reveal ulceration and infection. In later stages of exposure, the breakdown of intestinal villi will cause plasma loss that can lead to circulatory collapse and may end in death.

A patient with *cerebral radiation toxicity* may report nausea, vomiting, and diarrhea within hours after brief exposure to large amounts of radiation. Shortly after these signs develop, the patient may complain of lethargy. Inspection may disclose tremors, which may be followed by seizures, confusion, coma, and even death within hours or days.

A patient with *cardiovascular radiation toxicity* may experience hypotension, shock, and cardiac arrhythmias.

Delayed or chronic effects from repeated, prolonged exposure to small doses of radiation over a long time may seriously damage the skin, causing dryness, erythema, atrophy, and malignant lesions. (Such damage also can follow acute exposure.)

Other delayed effects may include alopecia, brittle nails, hypothyroidism, amenorrhea, cataracts, decreased fertility, anemia, leukopenia, thrombocytopenia, malignant

PREVENTING RADIATION EXPOSURE

Proper shielding and other safety precautions can help you minimize the risk of exposing yourself and your patients to radiation.

Protecting yourself
• When caring for a patient exposed to radiation, cover your entire body with disposable, protective clothing. Wear a surgical mask, cap, goggles, gown, pants, bootcaps, and double gloves. Tape all glove, gown, and boot connections.
• Double-bag all equipment and clothing that come in contact with a radiation-contaminated patient, and attach a label noting that the bag contains radioactive waste. Make sure the label includes the magenta-colored "radiation" insignia to avoid the danger of improper disposal.
• Wear proper shielding devices when performing X-ray or radiation treatments. If you work in areas where radiation is present, also wear a radiation detection badge and periodically have it read.

• If you are or may be pregnant, ask to be excused from caring for a patient with known or suspected radiation contamination.

Protecting your patient
• When performing diagnostic or treatment procedures that use radiation, shield the patient's reproductive organs from exposure, if feasible.
• Perform fluoroscopic examinations as quickly as possible.

Protecting your patient and yourself
• Ensure that areas housing X-ray and nuclear materials are properly shielded.
• Make sure that X-ray equipment is periodically checked for reliability of output and that filters are used properly.
• If accidental contamination occurs, immediately remove all clothing and wash the body vigorously with soap and water.

neoplasms, bone necrosis and fractures, and a shortened life span.

Diagnostic tests
Supportive laboratory findings show decreased hematocrit, hemoglobin, and platelets; thrombocytopenia, leukopenia, and lymphopenia; and decreased levels of serum electrolytes (potassium and chloride) from vomiting and diarrhea. Bone marrow studies show blood dyscrasia; X-rays may reveal bone necrosis. A Geiger counter may help determine the amount of radiation in open wounds.

Treatment
Initial treatment of a patient exposed to radiation involves managing any life-threatening injuries. After the patient's airway, breathing, and circulation are secure, a Geiger counter helps determine whether radioactive material was ingested or inhaled. Treatment of local radiation effects depends on the extent, degree, and location of tissue injury. Treatment of systemic effects is symptomatic and supportive.

Chelating agents are used to remove internal radioactive contamination. If contamination remains, the patient's wounds are cleaned, irrigated, debrided, and left open for 24 hours. With severe contamination, amputation, although rare, may be required.

Other treatments may include potassium iodide, which

blocks the uptake of radioactive iodine by the thyroid if given within a few hours of exposure; aluminum phosphate gel, which reduces the intestinal absorption of radioactive strontium (by 85%); and barium sulfate, which precipitates radium.

Nursing diagnoses
• Altered nutrition: Less than body requirements
• Altered oral mucous membrane
• Altered thought processes
• Anxiety
• Fluid volume deficit
• Impaired skin integrity
• Risk for infection

Nursing interventions
• Prepare to intervene as necessary to support respiratory and cardiac functions.
• To minimize radiation exposure, properly dispose of contaminated clothing. Wear protective clothing when handling contaminated clothing and body fluids. If the patient's skin is contaminated, wash his body thoroughly with mild soap and water. Debride and irrigate open wounds. If the patient recently ingested radioactive material, perform gastric lavage and whole bowel irrigation, and administer activated charcoal, as ordered. Check hospital policy to ensure proper disposal of contami-

nated excrement and body fluids.

• Monitor intake and output, and maintain fluid and electrolyte balance. Give I.V. fluids and electrolytes, as ordered. If the patient can take oral feedings, encourage a high-protein, high-calorie diet. Tell him to use a soft toothbrush to minimize gum bleeding. Offer lidocaine to soothe painful mouth ulcers.

• To prevent skin breakdown, make sure the patient avoids extreme temperatures, tight clothing, and drying soaps. Use rigid aseptic technique.

• Prevent complications. Monitor vital signs and watch for signs of hemorrhage.

• Provide emotional support for the patient and his family, especially after severe exposure. Suggest genetic counseling and screening, as needed.

• Encourage a patient who has been exposed to significant amounts of radiation to receive genetic counseling. Refer him to a genetic counselor.

Patient teaching
• Teach the patient how to deal with the effects of radiation exposure.

• If the patient recovers from exposure, teach him how to prevent a recurrence.

MISCELLANEOUS INJURIES

Common environmental injuries, such as poisoning, poisonous snakebites, and insect bites and stings, affect large numbers of patients. As well, home, work, or motor vehicle accidents commonly result in open trauma wounds. Finally, acts of violence, such as gunshot wounds, stabbings, and rape, account for such injuries as open trauma wounds and rape-trauma syndrome.

POISONING

Inhalation, ingestion, or injection of, or skin contamination from, any harmful substance is a common problem. In the United States, about 1 million people are poisoned annually, 800 of them fatally. The prognosis depends on the amount of poison absorbed, its toxicity, and the time interval between poisoning and treatment.

Causes
Because of their curiosity and ignorance, children are the most common poison victims. In fact, accidental poisoning—usually from the ingestion of salicylates (aspirin), cleaning agents, insecticides, paints, cosmetics, and plants—is the fourth leading cause of death in children.

In adults, poisoning is most common among chemical company employees, particularly those in companies that use chlorine, carbon dioxide, hydrogen sulfide, nitrogen dioxide, and ammonia, and in companies that ignore safety standards. Other causes of poisoning in adults include improper cooking, canning, and storage of food; ingestion of, or skin contamination from, plants (for example, dieffenbachia, mistletoe, azalea, and philodendron); and accidental or intentional drug overdose (usually barbiturates) or chemical ingestion.

Complications
Depending on the poison, possible complications vary widely but can include hypotension, cardiac arrhythmias, seizures, coma, and death.

Assessment findings
The patient's history should reveal the source of poison and the form of exposure (ingestion, inhalation, injection, or skin contact). Assessment findings vary with the poison. (See *Pinpointing poison's effects,* page 270.)

Diagnostic tests
Toxicologic studies (including drug screens) of poison levels in the mouth, vomitus, urine, feces, or blood or on the victim's hands or clothing confirm the diagnosis. If possible, have the family or patient bring the container holding the poison to the emergency department for comparable study. In inhalation poisoning, chest X-rays may show pulmonary infiltrates or edema; in petroleum distillate inhalation, X-rays may show aspiration pneumonia. Abdominal X-rays may reveal iron pills or other radiopaque substances.

Arterial blood gas and serum electrolyte levels and a complete blood count are used to evaluate oxygenation, ventilation, and the metabolic status of seriously poisoned patients.

Treatment
Initial treatment includes emergency resuscitation; support for the patient's airway, breathing, and circulation; and prevention of further absorption of poison. After this, treatment consists of continuing supportive or symptomatic care and, when possible, administration of a specific antidote.

A poisoning victim who exhibits an altered level of consciousness (LOC) routinely receives oxygen, glucose, and naloxone. Activated charcoal has proved effective in eliminating many toxic substances. The specific treatment depends on the poison.

PINPOINTING POISON'S EFFECTS

Review the assessment findings and possible toxins listed below to help you determine what type of poison is causing your patient's signs and symptoms.

Agitation, delirium
Alcohol, amphetamines, atropine, barbiturates, physostigmine, scopolamine

Coma
Atropine, barbiturates, bromide, carbon monoxide, chloral hydrate, ethanol, ethchlorvynol, paraldehyde, salicylates, scopolamine

Constricted pupils
Barbiturates, chloral hydrate, morphine, propoxyphene

Diaphoresis
Alcohol, fluoride, insulin, physostigmine

Diarrhea, nausea, vomiting
Alcohol (ethanol, methanol, ethylene glycol), digitalis, heavy metals (lead, arsenic), morphine and its analogues, salicylates

Dilated pupils
Alcohol, amphetamines, belladonna alkaloids (such as atropine and scopolamine), botulin toxin, cocaine, cyanide, ephedrine, glutethimide, meperidine, parasympatholytics, sympathomimetics

Dry mouth
Antihistamines, belladonna alkaloids, botulin toxin, morphine, phenothiazines, tricyclic antidepressants

Extrapyramidal tremor
Phenothiazines

Hematemesis
Fluoride, mercuric chloride, phosphorus, salicylates

Kussmaul's respirations
Ethanol, ethylene glycol, methanol, salicylates

Partial or total blindness
Methanol

Pink skin
Atropine (flushed and dry skin), carbon monoxide, cyanide, phenothiazines

Seizures
Alcohol (ethanol, methanol, ethylene glycol), amphetamines, carbon monoxide, cholinesterase inhibitors, hydrocarbons, phenothiazines, propoxyphene, salicylates, strychnine

Nursing diagnoses
• Altered thought processes
• Anxiety
• Diarrhea
• Fluid volume deficit
• Impaired skin integrity
• Ineffective breathing pattern
• Knowledge deficit
• Pain
• Risk for aspiration
• Risk for injury
• Sensory or perceptual alterations

Nursing interventions
• Carefully monitor the patient's vital signs and LOC. If necessary, begin cardiopulmonary resuscitation.
• Depending on the poison, prevent further absorption of ingested poison by inducing emesis, using syrup of ipecac, or by administering gastric lavage and cathartics (magnesium sulfate). The treatment's effectiveness depends on the speed of absorption and the time elapsed between ingestion and removal. With syrup of ipecac, give warm water (usually less than 1 qt [less than 1 liter]) until vomiting occurs, or give another dose of ipecac, as ordered.
• Never induce emesis if you suspect corrosive acid poisoning, if the patient is unconscious or has seizures, or if the gag reflex is impaired even in a conscious patient. Instead, neutralize the poison by instilling the appropriate antidote by nasogastric (NG) tube. Common antidotes include milk, magnesium salts (milk of magnesia), activated charcoal, or other chelating agents (such as deferoxamine or edetate disodium).

When possible, add the antidote to water or juice. (Note: Methods of removing a poisonous hydrocarbon are controversial. In the conscious patient, because there is a lower risk of aspiration with ipecac-induced emesis than with lavage, emesis may be the preferred treatment, but some doctors still use lavage. Moreover, some believe that because of poor absorption, kerosene [a hydrocarbon] doesn't require removal from the GI tract;

others believe that removal depends on the amount ingested.)

• When you do want to induce emesis and the patient has already taken syrup of ipecac, don't give activated charcoal to neutralize the poison until *after* emesis; activated charcoal absorbs ipecac.

• To perform gastric lavage, instill 30 ml of fluid by NG tube; then aspirate the liquid. Repeat until the aspirate is clear. Save vomitus and aspirate for analysis. (To prevent aspiration in the unconscious patient, an endotracheal tube should be in place before lavage.)

• If several hours have passed since the patient ingested the poison, use large quantities of I.V. fluids to diurese the patient. The kind of fluid you'll use depends on the patient's acid-base balance and cardiovascular status and on the flow rate necessary for effective diuresis of poison.

• If ingested poisoning is severe and peritoneal dialysis or hemodialysis is necessary, assist as necessary.

• To prevent further absorption of inhaled poison, remove the patient to fresh or uncontaminated air. Provide supplemental oxygen and, if needed, intubation. To prevent further absorption from skin contamination, remove the clothing covering the contaminated skin, and immediately flush the area with large amounts of water.

• If the patient is in severe pain, give analgesics, as ordered; frequently monitor fluid intake and output, vital signs, and LOC.

• Keep the patient warm, and provide support in a quiet environment.

• If the poison was ingested intentionally, refer the patient for counseling to help prevent future attempts at suicide.

• For more specific treatment, contact the local poison center or a national center.

Patient teaching

• To prevent accidental poisoning, instruct the patient to read the label before he takes medication. Tell him to store all medications and household chemicals properly, keep them out of reach of children, and discard old medications. Warn him not to take medications prescribed for someone else, not to transfer medications from their original containers to other containers without labeling them properly, and never to transfer poisons to food containers. Parents should avoid taking medication in front of their young children or calling medication "candy" to get children to take it.

• Tell the patient to keep syrup of ipecac available. Emphasize the importance of understanding the directions for proper use.

• Advise parents to use childproof caps on medication containers.

• Make sure the patient understands the importance of using toxic sprays only in well-ventilated areas and of following instructions carefully. Tell him to use pesticides carefully and to keep the number of his poison control center handy.

POISONOUS SNAKEBITES

Each year, poisonous snakes bite about 8,000 persons in the United States. Occurring most often during summer afternoons, in grassy or rocky habitats, poisonous snakebites are medical emergencies. With prompt, correct treatment, they need not be fatal. However, antivenin against an exotic venomous snake is not always readily available.

Causes

The only poisonous snakes found in nature in the United States are pit vipers (Crotalidae) and coral snakes (Elapidae). Pit vipers include rattlesnakes, water moccasins (cottonmouths), and copperheads. They have a pitted depression between their eyes and nostrils, and two fangs ¾" to 1¼" (1.9 to 3.2 cm) long. (See *Pit viper,* page 272.) Because a snake's fangs may break off or grow behind old ones, these snakes can have anywhere from one to four fangs.

Because coral snakes are nocturnal and placid, their bites are less common than pit viper bites; pit vipers also are nocturnal but are more active. Coral snake fangs are short but have teeth behind them. Coral snakes have distinctive red, black, and yellow bands (yellow bands always border red ones), tend to bite with a chewing motion, and may leave multiple fang marks, small lacerations, and extensive tissue destruction.

Many snakebites are associated with activities involving amateur snake keeping and handling and commonly result from carelessness or daring on the part of the snake handler. Handling snakes that appear to be dead may lead to a venomous snakebite secondary to postmortem reflex action of the snake's head, or a snakebite may occur even by inadvertently striking fingers against a fang of a preserved snake.

Complications

In a pit viper bite, delayed administration of specific antivenin may result in extensive vasculitis, necrosis, and sloughing of the skin and subcutaneous tissue. An untreated coral snake bite can result in respiratory arrest and, if shock develops, cardiovascular collapse and death.

PIT VIPER

A pitted depression between the eyes and nostrils and two long fangs are characteristic of a pit viper, the most common poisonous snake.

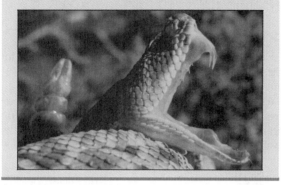

Assessment findings

Inspection usually reveals evidence of the bite on the arms and legs, below the elbow or knee. Bites to the head or trunk are most dangerous, but any bite into a blood vessel is dangerous.

Most pit viper bites that result in envenomation cause immediate and progressively severe pain and edema. In fact, the entire extremity may swell within a few hours. (See *Severe edema in snakebite.*) Additional assessment findings may include local elevation in skin temperature, fever, discoloration of the skin, petechiae, ecchymoses, blebs, blisters, and bloody wound discharge, as well as local necrosis.

The patient may have several complaints, including headache, a metallic or rubber taste in the mouth, nausea, vomiting, and diarrhea. Because pit viper venom is neurotoxic, he also may report local and facial numbness and tingling, fasciculation, and twitching of skeletal muscles.

You may note seizures (especially in children), extreme anxiety, difficulty in speaking, fainting, weakness, dizziness, excessive sweating, tachycardia, hypotension, occasional paralysis, mild to severe respiratory distress, blurred vision, and marked thirst. Severe envenomation may result in coma and death. Pit viper venom also may impair coagulation and cause hematemesis, hematuria, melena, bleeding gums, and internal bleeding. Palpation may reveal lymphadenopathy.

The patient's reaction to a coral snakebite usually is delayed — perhaps up to several hours. These snakebites cause little or no local tissue reaction, such as local pain, swelling, or necrosis. However, because a coral snake's venom is neurotoxic, the reaction can progress swiftly, producing such wide-ranging effects as local paresthesia, weakness, euphoria, drowsiness, nausea, vomiting, difficulty swallowing, marked salivation, dysphonia, ptosis, blurred vision, miosis, respiratory distress and possible respiratory failure, loss of muscle coordination, abnormal reflexes, peripheral paralysis and, possibly, shock with cardiovascular collapse and death. Coral snakebites also can cause coagulotoxicity. (See *Assessing snakebites,* page 274.)

Diagnostic tests

Laboratory test values can help to identify the extent of envenomation and to provide guidelines for supportive treatment. Abnormal test results may include prolonged bleeding time and partial thromboplastin time, decreased hemoglobin and hematocrit levels, sharply decreased platelet count (less than $200,000/mm^3$), urinalysis showing hematuria, and, in infection (snake mouths contain gram-negative bacteria), increased white blood cell count.

Chest X-rays may show pulmonary edema or emboli; an electrocardiogram may show tachycardia and ectopic beats; and severe envenomation may produce abnormal findings on an EEG.

Treatment

Prompt, appropriate first aid can reduce venom absorption and prevent severe symptoms. It should be followed by antivenin administration and other treatments.
• If possible, identify the snake, but don't waste time trying to find it.
• Immediately immobilize the patient's limb below heart level in a horizontal position, and instruct the victim to remain as quiet as possible.
• If indicated, apply a slightly constrictive band (one that obstructs only lymphatic and superficial venous blood flow) about 4″ (10 cm) above the fang marks or just above the first joint proximal to the bite. The band should be loose enough to allow a finger's width between the band and the skin. Don't apply a constrictive band if more than 30 minutes have elapsed since the bite. Also, total constrictive band time should not exceed 2 hours nor should it delay antivenin administration. Once the band is in place, don't remove it until the patient is examined by the doctor.
• Wash the skin over the fang marks.
• Never give the victim alcoholic drinks or stimulants; these speed venom absorption. Never apply ice to a

snakebite: It increases tissue damage. Don't incise and suction the affected area. The risk of trauma to underlying structures caused by unskilled performance of the technique is greater than the amount of venom that can be recovered.

• Transport the victim as quickly as possible, keeping him warm and quiet. Record the signs and symptoms of progressive envenomation and when they develop.

• Antivenin administration is required in life-threatening circumstances. Prepare and administer the antivenin according to the manufacturer's directions. Watch the patient closely for signs of sensitivity and anaphylaxis. Keep emergency epinephrine on hand in case the patient develops such problems.

Other treatments include tetanus toxoid or tetanus immune globulin (human); broad-spectrum antibiotics; and, depending on respiratory status, severity of pain, and type of snakebite (narcotics are contraindicated in coral snakebites), codeine, morphine, or meperidine.

All snakebites require administration of I.V. isotonic fluids. If bleeding is severe, blood transfusions also may be necessary. Antihistamines help relieve pruritus and urticaria.

Most necrotic tissue resulting from a snakebite needs surgical debridement after 3 or 4 days. Although controversial, fasciotomy may be required within 2 or 3 hours of the bite if intense, rapidly progressive edema develops. Extreme envenomation may require limb amputation and subsequent reconstructive surgery, rehabilitation, and physical therapy.

Nursing diagnoses
• Anxiety
• Decreased cardiac output
• Diarrhea
• Fear
• Fluid volume deficit
• Impaired skin integrity
• Ineffective breathing pattern
• Pain
• Risk for infection
• Risk for injury
• Sensory or perceptual alterations

Nursing interventions
• When the patient arrives at the hospital, immobilize the extremity if this hasn't already been done. If a tight tourniquet has been applied within the past hour, apply a loose tourniquet proximally and remove the first tourniquet. Release the second tourniquet gradually during

SEVERE EDEMA IN SNAKEBITE

After snakebite, the affected extremity develops severe edema within hours.

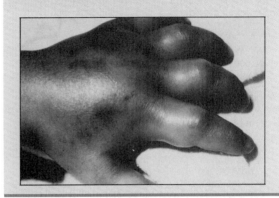

antivenin administration, as ordered. A sudden release of venom into the bloodstream can cause cardiopulmonary collapse, so keep emergency equipment handy.

• On a flow sheet, document vital signs, level of consciousness, skin color, swelling, respiratory status, description of the bite and surrounding area, and symptoms. Monitor vital signs every 15 minutes, and check for a pulse in the affected limb.

• Start an I.V. line with a large-bore needle for antivenin administration. Severe bites that result in coagulotoxic signs and symptoms may require two I.V. lines: one for antivenin, the second for blood products.

• Have blood samples drawn for clotting studies, platelet count, fibrinogen levels, fibrin split products, type and cross matching, and other ordered tests.

• Before antivenin administration, obtain a patient history of allergies (especially to horse serum) and other medical problems. Do hypersensitivity tests, as ordered, and assist with desensitization, as needed. During antivenin administration, keep epinephrine, oxygen, and vasopressors available to combat anaphylaxis from an allergic reaction to horse serum.

• If signs of hypersensitivity occur during antivenin administration, stop the infusion and administer diphenhydramine, cimetidine, or ranitidine, as ordered. Start the infusion at a slower rate and closely monitor the patient.

• Administer packed red blood cells, whole blood, I.V. fluids and, possibly, fresh frozen plasma or platelets, as ordered, to counteract any coagulotoxicity and maintain the patient's blood pressure. If he develops respiratory

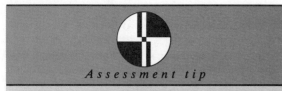

Assessment tip

ASSESSING SNAKEBITES

When examining a patient who has sustained a poisonous snakebite, keep in mind the following hints:
• Absence of fang marks precludes envenomation.
• Marks without bleeding or with clotted blood probably denote a lack of envenomation or an insect bite, or the marks are factitious.
• In the presence of venom injection, the fang marks continue oozing nonclotting blood.
• A pit viper bite produces immediate, severe, burning pain. Soon after the bite, mild ecchymoses appear around the fang marks.
• Absence of microhematuria after a pit viper bite indicates a lack of severe envenomation.

distress, assist with endotracheal intubation or tracheotomy, as ordered.
• Give analgesics, as needed. *Don't* give narcotics to victims of coral snakebites.
• Clean the snakebite using sterile technique. Open, debride, and drain any blebs and blisters because they may contain venom. Be sure to change dressings daily.
• If the patient requires hospitalization for longer than 24 to 48 hours, position him carefully to avoid contractures. Perform passive range-of-motion exercises until the fourth day after the bite and then active exercises and whirlpool treatments, as ordered.
• For information on the proper antivenin for exotic snakes, contact the Arizona Poison and Drug Information Center at (602) 626-6016.
• For those likely to encounter venomous snakes, additional protection is given by pretesting for sensitivity to horse serum.

Patient teaching
• Stress the importance of protecting extremities in snake-infested areas, as many venomous snakes have long, sharp fangs that can easily penetrate clothing.

INSECT BITES AND STINGS

Among the most common traumatic complaints are insect bites and stings. The more serious include those of a tick, brown recluse spider, black widow spider, scorpion, bee, wasp, yellow jacket, and fire ant. Emergencies develop when a number of stings occur at one time or when the patient develops an allergic response to the protein substances in the insect venom.

With a bee, wasp, or yellow jacket sting, the shorter the interval between the sting and systemic signs and symptoms, the worse the prognosis. Without prompt treatment, signs and symptoms may progress to cyanosis, coma, and death.

Causes
Reactions to insect bites and stings are caused by the toxic effects of the injected venom or a hypersensitivity response to it.

Complications
About 25% of people are hypersensitive to Hymenoptera venoms (bees, wasps, hornets, and yellow jackets) and may develop anaphylaxis.

Assessment findings
With a *tick* bite, the patient may complain of itching at the affected site. After several days, he may develop tick paralysis (acute flaccid paralysis, starting as paresthesia and pain in the legs and resulting in respiratory failure from bulbar paralysis). If the tick carried Rocky Mountain spotted fever or Lyme disease, the patient will develop signs and symptoms of the disease. (For more information, see "Rocky Mountain Spotted Fever" and "Lyme Disease" in Chapter 2.)

With a *brown recluse (violin) spider* bite, localized vasoconstriction begins within 2 to 8 hours after the bite and is the result of a coagulotoxic venom. The small, reddened puncture wound forms a bleb and then becomes ischemic, eventually leading to ischemic necrosis. In about 3 to 4 days, the center darkens and hardens. Within 1 to 2 weeks, an ulcer forms. Rarely, thrombocytopenia and hemolytic anemia develop and lead to death within the first 24 to 48 hours (usually in a child or in a patient with a history of cardiac disease). In some cases, the bite may result in renal failure, disseminated intravascular coagulation, and cardiogenic shock, which may lead to death.

The patient may complain of minimal initial pain that increases over time. He also may complain of fever, chills, malaise, weakness, nausea, vomiting, and joint pain. Inspection may reveal petechiae.

With a *black widow spider* bite, the patient may report feeling a pinprick sensation, followed by dull, numbing pain. Initially a tiny, edematous, red bite mark may be noted. The injected venom is neurotoxic, and the severity and progression of the signs and symptoms depend on the patient's age, size, and sensitivity.

If the bite is on a leg, the patient may have severe pain and large-muscle cramping. Palpation may reveal a rigid, painful abdomen. If the bite is on an arm, rigidity and pain in the chest, shoulders, and back may occur.

Systemic signs and symptoms may include extreme restlessness, vertigo, sweating, chills, pallor, seizures (especially in children), hyperactive reflexes, hypertension, tachycardia, thready pulse, circulatory collapse, nausea, vomiting, headache, ptosis, eyelid edema, urticaria, pruritus, fever, and urine retention.

With a *scorpion* sting, the patient may experience an anaphylactic or neurotoxic reaction. You may note local swelling and tenderness and skin discoloration at the bite site. The patient may complain of a sharp burning sensation and paresthesia. Palpation may reveal regional lymph gland swelling.

If the reaction is neurotoxic, the patient may experience immediate, sharp pain; hyperesthesia; drowsiness; itching of the nose, throat, and mouth; impaired speech; salivation; lacrimation; diarrhea and gastric cramping; sweating; jaw muscle spasms; laryngospasm; incontinence; seizures; and nausea and vomiting. Death may follow cardiovascular or respiratory failure. These signs and symptoms usually last from 24 to 78 hours. The bite site recovers last.

With a *bee, wasp,* or *yellow jacket* sting, the patient may have either a localized or a systemic reaction. In a local reaction, you'll observe a raised, reddened wheal, possibly with a protruding stinger from the bee. It's usually painful and pruritic.

In a systemic reaction, signs and symptoms of hypersensitivity usually appear within 20 minutes, including weakness, chest tightness, dizziness, nausea, vomiting, abdominal cramps, throat constriction, and wheezing and decreased blood pressure (signs of cardiovascular collapse).

With a *fire ant* sting, the patient will report immediate pain, itching, and burning. Within 4 to 8 hours, clear vesicles develop with surrounding erythema. After 24 hours, you'll note the characteristic pustule.

Diagnostic tests

Identification of the insect is difficult, unless the patient was stung by a honeybee or a bumblebee. These insects usually leave a stinger (with venom sac) in the lesion. Tests showing hemolytic anemia or thrombocytopenia may indicate a brown recluse spider bite; hematuria and an increased white blood cell count may point to a black widow spider bite.

Treatment

For a *tick* bite, treatment involves removing the tick, applying antipruritics for itching, and providing symptomatic therapy for severe symptoms, such as assisted ventilation for respiratory failure. Treatment for Rocky Mountain spotted fever and Lyme disease includes such antibiotics as tetracycline, erythromycin, and penicillin.

No known specific treatment exists for a *brown recluse spider* bite. Combination therapies including corticosteroids, antibiotics, antihistamines, tranquilizers, I.V. fluids, and tetanus prophylaxis reduce signs and symptoms and prevent complications. Lesion excision in the first 10 to 12 hours may relieve pain. A split-thickness skin graft closes the wound. Without grafting, healing may take 6 to 8 weeks. A large chronic ulcer may require skin grafting.

For a *black widow spider* bite, treatment consists of antivenin I.V. to neutralize the venom and ice packs applied to the bite area. When skin or eye tests show sensitivity to horse serum, desensitization precedes antivenin treatment.

Symptomatic treatment may include calcium gluconate I.V. to control muscle spasms, diazepam for severe muscle spasms, adrenalin or antihistamines for hypersensitivity symptoms, oxygen by nasal cannula or mask for respiratory difficulty, and tetanus immunization and antibiotics to prevent infection.

For a *scorpion* sting, antivenin (made from goat serum) may be used if available. (For information on how to obtain this agent, contact the Arizona Poison and Drug Information Center, [602] 626-6016.) Symptomatic treatment may include calcium gluconate I.V. for muscle spasm and phenobarbital I.M. for seizures.

For *bee, wasp, yellow jacket,* or *fire ant* stings, treatment of local reactions includes applying ice to the affected area. If the entire extremity shows signs, treatment involves elevating the affected extremity and administering 25 to 50 mg oral diphenhydramine every 4 hours. More severe reactions may require administration of prednisone for 5 to 7 days.

For patients who are extremely allergic to stings, self-treatment with injectable epinephrine as soon as possible after the sting may prevent anaphylaxis and respiratory obstruction. The patient should then seek immediate medical attention.

Supportive treatment includes airway management, I.V. fluids for volume expansion, vasopressors, theophylline for bronchospasm, and corticosteroids to reduce allergic response. Venom immunotherapy may be indicated for patients with a history of severe reactions who are at increased risk for repeated stings.

Nursing diagnoses
• Impaired skin integrity
• Knowledge deficit
• Pain
• Risk for poisoning
• Sensory or perceptual alterations

Nursing interventions
• Monitor the patient's vital signs, general appearance, and any changes at the bite or sting site.
• Keep the patient quiet and warm and the affected part immobile.
• Clean the bite or sting site with antiseptic, and apply ice to relieve pain, reduce swelling, and slow circulation.
• Have epinephrine and emergency resuscitation equipment on hand in case of anaphylactic reaction.
• When giving analgesics, monitor respiratory status.
• To remove a tick, cover it with mineral, salad, or machine oil, or alcohol on a gauze pad. This blocks the tick's breathing pores, causing it to withdraw from the skin. Don't squeeze or crush the tick when removing it. If it doesn't disengage after the pad has been in place for 30 minutes, carefully remove all parts of it with tweezers.
• For a brown recluse spider bite, clean the lesion with a 1:20 Burow's aluminum acetate solution and, as ordered, apply antibiotic ointment. Reassure the patient with a disfiguring ulcer that skin grafting can help.
• If a bee, wasp, or yellow jacket stinger is in place, scrape it off. Don't pull or squeeze it; squeezing releases more toxin. Clean the site and apply ice.

Patient teaching
• To reduce the risk of being bitten by a tick, tell the patient to keep away from wooded areas, to wear protective clothes, and to examine the body carefully for ticks after being outdoors.
• Teach the patient how to safely remove ticks.
• To prevent brown recluse and black widow spider bites, advise the patient to spray infested areas, to tuck pant legs into socks in such areas, to wear gloves and heavy clothes when working around woodpiles or sheds, to inspect outdoor work clothes for spiders before use, and to discourage children from playing near infested areas.
• Tell the patient who is allergic to bee stings to wear a medical identification bracelet or carry a card, and to carry an anaphylaxis kit. Explain how to use the kit, and refer him to an allergist for hyposensitization.
• To prevent bee stings, warn the patient to avoid using fragrant cosmetics during insect season, wearing bright colors or going barefoot, and touching flowers and fruits that attract bees. Advise using an insect repellent.

OPEN TRAUMA WOUNDS
Resulting from accidental injury or acts of violence, open trauma wounds include abrasions, lacerations, avulsions, crush wounds, puncture wounds, and missile injuries. (For more information, see *Types and causes of open trauma wounds.*)

Causes
Most commonly, open wounds result from an accidental injury at home or work or from a motor vehicle crash. Other open wounds, such as stab and gunshot wounds, may be intentionally inflicted by the victim or by someone else. Open wounds occasionally are self-inflicted by patients with psychiatric disorders or suicidal ideations.

Complications
Infection is the major complication. Organ tissue damage, scarring, and dysfunction also may occur.

Assessment findings
The patient's history (possibly obtained from witnesses) may include such details as the mechanism and time of injury and any treatment already provided. Inspection usually reveals the extent of injury, level of consciousness, obvious skeletal damage, local and generalized neurologic deficits, and the patient's general condition.

Inspection of an *abrasion* may reveal epidermal scrapes, reddish welts, embedded dirt and debris, and bruises in the affected area. The patient usually complains of pain at the site.

With a *laceration*, you'll note an open skin area, extending deep into the epithelium. The edges may be even (possibly indicating a knife wound) or torn and ragged.

With an *avulsion*, you'll note torn tissue or skin that appears peeled away. Bleeding usually is significant, depending on the location and size.

In a *crush wound*, you'll observe severe ecchymoses, hematomas, edema, hemorrhage and, possibly, split skin over the affected area. Damage to the underlying tissues may not be evident.

With a *puncture wound* or a *missile injury*, external damage may be minimal. The entrance site will be visible, and bleeding will vary. Sometimes, no bleeding is present. If the object causing the puncture is still in place, its presence may maintain hemostasis, preventing extensive external blood loss.

Depending on the injury's cause, the wound may contain foreign bodies, such as stones or dirt. You may detect peripheral nerve damage — a common complication in lacerations and other open trauma wounds — as well as fractures and dislocations. Signs of peripheral nerve damage vary with location:

- *radial nerve* — weak wrist extension, inability to extend thumb in a hitchhiker's sign, numbness in dorsum of thumb
- *median nerve* — numbness in index finger tip, finger abduction, and apposition of thumb and fingers
- *ulnar nerve* — numbness in little finger tip, finger fanning (abduction)
- *peroneal nerve* — inability to extend foot or big toe, footdrop, numbness in lateral dorsum and first-toe web space
- *sciatic and tibial nerves* — plantar flexion, weakness in leg, numbness in sole.

Diagnostic tests

X-rays, magnetic resonance imaging, and computed tomography scans help determine bone involvement and soft-tissue injury, particularly organ injury. A complete blood count helps evaluate blood loss. In patients with suspected nerve involvement, electromyography, nerve conduction, and electrical stimulation tests can provide more detailed information about possible peripheral nerve damage.

Treatment

For all types of traumatic wounds, treatment includes administration of a local anesthetic, if necessary; thorough cleaning and irrigation of the affected area; and administration of tetanus prophylaxis when indicated.

Small avulsions require a nonadhesive pressure dressing. Larger avulsed areas may be repaired by reattaching the avulsed tissue or by split-thickness grafting.

Grossly contaminated lacerations require treatment with a broad-spectrum antibiotic. Lacerations are closed by suture or Steri-Strips. Crush and puncture wounds may require surgery, debridement, and repair.

Missile injuries and some puncture wounds require stabilization of life-threatening insults. Endotracheal intubation, volume replacement (with lactated Ringer's solution), and surgery may be necessary.

Nursing diagnoses

- Anxiety
- Decreased cardiac output
- Impaired gas exchange
- Impaired physical mobility
- Impaired skin integrity
- Pain
- Risk for fluid volume deficit
- Risk for infection

TYPES AND CAUSES OF OPEN TRAUMA WOUNDS

Common open trauma wounds and their causes include the following:
- Abrasions — partial-thickness denudations of skin, resulting from falls, scrapes, and cycling accidents
- Lacerations — skin openings that penetrate deep into the epithelium, resulting from tearing, sharp cutting, or compression forces
- Avulsions — full-thickness tissue loss, usually seen in fingertip or nose injuries and caused by tearing of the tissue from its usual location
- Crush injuries — skin, epithelium, and underlying tissue injuries, resulting from injury sustained from a heavy falling object or being pulled into machinery
- Puncture wounds — penetrating skin, epithelium, and, possibly, tissue wounds, usually a result of stepping on broken glass, nails, tacks, or other sharp objects
- Missile injuries — high-pressure penetrating wounds, usually caused by stabbing or gunshots.

Nursing interventions

For all injuries:
- Check for bleeding tendencies and anticoagulant use.
- Administer analgesics and tetanus prophylaxis, if necessary.
- Thoroughly clean the injured area with soap and water. Irrigate all minor wounds with 0.9% sodium chloride solution after removing any foreign objects.
- Assess for neuromuscular, tendon, and circulatory damage.
- If injury resulted from foul play, notify the police.

For an abrasion:
- Clean the injured site gently with topical germicide and irrigate; too vigorous scrubbing of abrasions will increase tissue damage. Apply light, water-soluble antibiotic cream to prevent infection.
- If the wound is severe, apply a loose, protective dressing that allows air to circulate.

For a laceration less than 8 hours old or any affecting the face and areas of possible functional disability (such as the elbow):
- Apply pressure and elevate the injured extremity to control hemorrhage.
- As necessary, debride necrotic margins, and close the wound, using strips of tape or sutures.
- Severe laceration with underlying structural damage may require surgery.

For a grossly contaminated laceration or one more than 8 hours old (except on the face and areas of possible functional disability):
• Administer a broad-spectrum antibiotic, such as tetracycline, for at least a 5-day course, as ordered.
• *Don't* close the wound immediately.
• Instruct the patient to elevate the injured extremity for 24 hours after injury to reduce swelling.
• Tell him to keep the dressing clean and dry and to watch for signs of infection.
• After 5 to 7 days, close the wound with sutures or a butterfly dressing if it appears uninfected and contains healthy granulated tissue.
• Apply a sterile dressing and splint, as necessary.
For an avulsion:
• Record the time of injury to help determine if tissue is salvageable. Preserve tissue (if available) in cool saline solution for possible split-thickness graft or flap.
• Control hemorrhage with pressure, absorbable gelatin sponge, or topical thrombin.
• Clean the wound gently, irrigate with 0.9% sodium chloride solution, and debride, if necessary. Cover with a bulky dressing.
For a crush wound:
• Control hemorrhage by applying pressure and a cold pack. Apply a dry, sterile bulky dressing.
• Immobilize the injured extremity, and encourage the patient to rest. Monitor vital signs, and check peripheral pulses and circulation often.
• If the injury is severe, infuse lactated Ringer's or 0.9% sodium chloride solution with a large-bore catheter, as ordered. Assist with surgery, debridement, and repair, as ordered.
For a puncture wound:
• Don't remove impaling objects until the injury is completely evaluated. (If the eye is injured, call an ophthalmologist immediately.)
• Leave human bite wounds open. Apply a dry, sterile dressing to other minor puncture wounds.
• If the puncture wound resulted from a bite, determine the risk of rabies and, if needed, administer vaccine.
• Deep wounds that damage underlying tissues and retention of injuring object require surgery.
For a missile injury:
• Control hemorrhage with pressure, if possible. Use large-bore catheters to start two infusions, using lactated Ringer's or 0.9% sodium chloride solution for volume replacement, and prepare for possible surgery.
• Maintain a patent airway, and monitor for signs of hy-

povolemia, shock, and cardiac arrhythmias. Check the patient's vital signs and neurovascular response often.
• Cover a sucking chest wound during exhalation with petroleum gauze and an occlusive dressing.
• If damage is minor, apply a dry sterile dressing.
• Obtain X-rays to detect retained fragments.
• If possible, determine the caliber of the weapon.
• If the wound becomes infected, culture the wound and scrub with surgical soap preparation. Remove some or all sutures, and give a broad-spectrum antibiotic, as ordered.

Patient teaching
• Teach the patient how to care for the wound at home. Tell him to report any swelling, numbness, or tingling, which may indicate neurovascular compromise.
• Direct him to use an ice pack as indicated.
• Tell the patient to take analgesics, as prescribed, and to complete the course of prescribed antibiotics.
• Stress the need for follow-up care and suture removal.
• Point out the signs and symptoms of infection: redness, warmth, drainage, swelling, increased pain. If the patient suspects an infection, tell him to notify the doctor. If soaks are ordered, instruct the patient to soak the wound in warm, soapy water for 15 minutes, three times daily, and to return for follow-up care every 2 to 3 days, until the wound heals.

RAPE-TRAUMA SYNDROME
The term rape refers to illicit sexual intercourse without consent. In this violent assault, sexual intercourse is used as a weapon. Rape inflicts varying degrees of physical and psychological trauma. Rape-trauma syndrome occurs after the rape or attempted rape; it refers to the victim's early-stage (short-term) and later-stage (long-term) reactions and to the methods the victim uses to cope with this trauma.

In the United States, a rape is reported every 4.8 minutes (300 per day; 109,062 per year). The incidence of reported rape is highest in large cities and is rising. However, more than 90% of assaults may never be reported, making statistics inaccurate.

Known victims of rape range in age from 2 months to 97 years. (This covers all types of rape, including incest, child sexual abuse, and date rape.) The age-group most affected is the 10- to 19-year-olds; the average victim's age is 13½. About one out of seven reported rapes involves a prepubertal child.

In most cases, the rapist is a man and the victim is a woman. However, rapes do occur between people of the same sex, especially in prisons, schools, hospitals, and other institutions. Also, children often are the victims of rape; most of these cases involve manual, oral, or genital contact with the child's genitals. The rapist usually is a member of the child's family. A man or child can also be sexually abused by a woman.

The prognosis for rape-trauma syndrome is good if the rape victims receive physical and emotional support and counseling to help them deal with their feelings. Victims who articulate their feelings are able to cope with fears, interact with others, and return to normal routines faster than those who do not.

Causes
Rape-trauma syndrome results from rape or attempted rape.

Complications
As with other posttraumatic distress syndromes, possible complications of rape-trauma syndrome include lasting psychiatric problems (such as depression, guilt, and anxiety) and, in some cases, suicide.

Assessment findings
If the patient is in the early stage of rape-trauma syndrome, a complete history and physical examination usually are necessary. The patient's history may reveal information pertinent to physical assessment. (Furthermore, assessment notes may be used as evidence if the rapist is tried.)

The patient's history also may disclose information pertinent to treatment, such as allergies to penicillin and other drugs and any recent illnesses (especially a sexually transmitted disease [STD]). If the victim is a woman, her history should note whether she was pregnant at the time of the attack, the date of her last menstrual period, and details of her obstetric and gynecologic history.

Record the victim's statements in the first person, using quotation marks. Also document objective information provided by others. In your assessment notes, include the time the victim arrived at the hospital, the date and time of the alleged rape, and the time the victim was examined.

Depending on the specific body areas attacked, the patient may complain of a sore throat, difficulty swallowing, vaginal pain, rectal pain, or pain from other injuries incurred during the assault.

If the patient is in the early stage of rape-trauma syndrome, she may exhibit psychological signs and symptoms, such as disbelief, panic, severe anxiety, anger, self-blame, humiliation, and depression. Alternatively, she may appear outwardly calm, compliant, glib, and talkative.

Even if the victim wasn't beaten, physical examination will probably identify signs of physical trauma, especially if the assault was prolonged. General observation will reveal the patient's general physical appearance and demeanor. Inspection of clothing may detect signs of bleeding. General inspection of the victim's body may reveal signs of physical trauma, such as injuries and bleeding. Depending on the specific body areas attacked, inspection also may show a reddened (sore) throat, mouth irritation, ecchymoses, or rectal pain and bleeding.

If the victim is a female, a vaginal examination will determine injury. Inspection may reveal lacerations, contusions, and abrasions to the vulva, cervix, and the vaginal walls. A bimanual examination determines the size of the ovaries and the uterus. A speculum examination is performed when necessary. If the victim is a male, a full genital examination and anal examination may disclose lacerations, contusions, and abrasions.

If additional physical violence accompanied the rape, physical examination also may identify hematomas, lacerations, bleeding, fractures, severe internal injuries, and hemorrhage. If the rape occurred outdoors, examination may reveal that the patient is suffering from exposure.

If the assessment is performed several weeks after the rape, mental status findings may include a history of anxiety, nightmares, flashbacks, depression, anger, disinterest in sex, anorgasmy, and suicidal ideation.

Diagnostic tests
Victims should be examined as soon as possible after the rape. Evidence for deoxyribonucleic acid testing should be collected within 48 hours. Recent advances in laboratory evaluation include acid phosphatase detection in vaginal washings; the male-specific semen protein p30; and MHS-5, a sperm-coating antigen from human seminal vesicles. As appropriate, specimens are obtained from the cervical canal, throat, or rectum.

Routine laboratory tests include an STD screen and a rapid plasma reagin test. A pregnancy test, a drug screen, and an alcohol level determination also may be performed. Other tests are determined by patient injuries; for example, X-rays are performed if fractures are suspected.

Laboratory tests that detect consequences of sexual contact (such as STD or pregnancy) and provide evidence for possible assault charges often are processed by the police laboratory. If the rape occurred in the past 7 days, specimens obtained may include a blood sample; hair samples of a different color from that of the victim or that are obviously out of place; fiber samples, such as paint or wool; any soiled or torn material; and body fluids, such as blood or semen, not belonging to the victim.

Treatment

Abrasions, lacerations, and other physical injuries receive standardized care, as appropriate. Tetanus prophylaxis is given when indicated. In addition, all sexual assault victims receive STD prophylaxis, according to guidelines established by the Centers for Disease Control and Prevention. Women should receive information on pregnancy prevention.

Long-term treatment includes crisis intervention and counseling. Also, female patients should schedule a follow-up gynecologic examination after 7 to 14 days to ensure adequate pregnancy and STD prophylaxis; male patients should have a follow-up urologic examination.

Nursing diagnoses

- Altered oral mucous membrane
- Anxiety
- Ineffective individual coping
- Pain
- Powerlessness
- Rape-trauma syndrome
- Risk for infection
- Self-esteem disturbance
- Sleep pattern disturbance

Nursing interventions

- If the rape victim is not seriously injured, allow her to remain clothed, and take her to a private room, where she can talk with you or a counselor before the necessary physical examination. Remember, immediate reactions to rape differ and include crying, laughing, hostility, confusion, withdrawal, and outward calm. Often anger and rage don't surface until later. During the assault, the victim may have felt demeaned, helpless, and afraid for her life; afterward, she may feel ashamed, guilty, shocked, and vulnerable and experience a sense of disbelief and lowered self-esteem.
- Offer emotional support, reassurance, and acceptance. Help the patient explore her feelings; listen, convey trust and respect, and remain nonjudgmental. Don't leave the patient alone unless requested.
- Monitor the patient's mental status. Reorient her to her surroundings and help her interpret reality, as needed.

- Thoroughly explain the examination and why it's necessary (to rule out internal injuries, obtain a specimen for STD testing, and acquire evidence for possible prosecution). Obtain informed consent for treatment and for the police report. Allow the victim some control, if possible; for instance, ask if she's ready to be examined or if she'd rather wait.
- Before the examination, ask the victim whether she douched, bathed, or washed before coming to the hospital. Note this on her chart. Have her change into a hospital gown, and place her clothing in *paper bags*. (*Never* use plastic bags because secretions and seminal stains will mold, destroying valuable evidence.) Label each bag and its contents.
- Tell the victim she may urinate (preferably after the examination), but warn her not to wipe or otherwise clean the perineal area. Stay with her, or ask a counselor to stay with her, throughout the examination.
- Assist throughout the examination, providing support and reassurance, and carefully labeling all possible evidence. Before the victim's pelvic area is examined, take vital signs and, if the patient is wearing a tampon, remove it, wrap it, and label it as evidence. This examination often is distressing to the rape victim. Reassure her, and allow her as much control as possible.
- During the examination, assist in specimen collection, including those for semen and STD. Carefully label all specimens with the patient's name, the doctor's name, and the site from which the specimen was obtained. List all specimens in your notes. If the case comes to trial, specimens will be used for evidence, so accuracy is vital.
- Carefully collect and label fingernail scrapings and foreign material obtained by combing the victim's pubic hair; these also provide valuable evidence. Note to whom these specimens are given.
- For a male victim, be especially alert for injury to the mouth, perineum, and anus. As ordered, obtain a pharyngeal sample for a gonorrhea culture and rectal aspirate for acid phosphatase or sperm analysis.
- Assist in photographing the patient's injuries (this may be delayed for a day or repeated when bruises and ecchymoses are more apparent).
- Most states require hospitals to report all incidents of rape. The patient may elect not to press charges and not to assist the police investigation.
- If the police interview the patient in the hospital, stay with the patient, be supportive, and encourage her to recall details of the rape. Your kindness and empathy are invaluable.
- If requested, notify the patient's family. Help the patient verbalize anticipation of her family's response.

• If severe injuries require hospitalization, introduce the patient to her primary nurse, if possible.

• If the patient is having trouble sleeping, administer medications, as ordered, to promote sleep, educate the patient in relaxation techniques, create a quiet environment conducive to sleep, and discourage excessive napping.

Patient teaching

• Before discharge, provide clear verbal and written instructions. If antibiotics were prescribed to prevent STD, stress the importance of completing the course of medication.

• Explain to the patient the need for follow-up care to safeguard against acquired immunodeficiency syndrome, pregnancy, and STD.

• Encourage the patient not to stay alone. Inform her of self-help groups in the community, and refer her to an appropriate follow-up agency (medical clinic, rape counseling center, or psychiatric service). Also advise her how to contact a 24-hour crisis intervention service, if one is available.

SELECTED REFERENCES

Black, J., and Matassarin-Jacobs, E., eds. *Luckmann and Sorensen's Medical-Surgical Nursing: A Psychophysiologic Approach,* 4th ed. Philadelphia: W.B. Saunders Co., 1993.

Emergency Nurses Association. *Emergency Nursing Core Curriculum,* 4th ed. Philadelphia: W.B. Saunders Co., 1994.

Emergency Nurses Association. *Standards of Emergency Nursing Practice,* 3rd ed. Chicago: Emergency Nurses Association, 1995.

Gulanick, M., et al. *Nursing Care Plans: Nursing Diagnosis and Intervention,* 3rd ed. St. Louis: Mosby-Year Book, Inc., 1994.

Isselbacher, K., et al., eds. *Harrison's Principles of Internal Medicine,* 13th ed. New York: McGraw-Hill Book Co., 1995.

Kitt, S., et al. *Emergency Nursing: A Physiologic and Clinical Perspective,* 2nd ed. Philadelphia: W.B. Saunders Co., 1995.

Neff, J.A., and Kidd, P.S. *Trauma Nursing: The Art and Science.* St. Louis: Mosby-Year Book, Inc. 1993.

O'Brien, G.M., et al. "Chronic Pulmonary Disease in the Trauma Patient," *Critical Care Clinics* 10(3):507-22, July 1994.

Phipps, W.J., et al. *Medical-Surgical Nursing: Concepts and Clinical Practice,* 5th ed. St. Louis: Mosby-Year Book, Inc., 1995.

Rakel, R.E., ed. *Conn's Current Therapy 1996.* Philadelphia: W.B. Saunders Co., 1996.

Sheehy, S.B., and Lombardi, J.E. *Manual of Emergency Care,* 4th ed. St. Louis: Mosby-Year Book, Inc., 1994.

Smeltzer, S., and Bare, B. *Brunner and Suddarth's Textbook of Medical-Surgical Nursing,* 8th ed. Philadelphia: J.B. Lippincott Co., 1996.

Taylor, C.M., and Sparks, S.M. *Nursing Diagnosis Reference Manual,* 3rd ed. Springhouse, Pa.: Springhouse Corp., 1995.

Textbook of Advanced Cardiac Life Support. Dallas: American Heart Association, 1994.

Tierney, L., et al. *Current Medical Diagnosis and Treatment 1995.* East Norwalk, Conn.: Appleton & Lange, 1995.

Tintinalli, J., et al. *Emergency Medicine: A Comprehensive Study Guide,* 4th ed. New York: McGraw-Hill Book Co., 1995.

Wilson, R.F. "Trauma in Patients with Preexisting Cardiac Disease," *Critical Care Clinics* 10(3):461-506, July 1994.

4 NEOPLASMS

INTRODUCTION

Second only to cardiovascular disease as a cause of death in North America, cancer is predicted by some epidemiologists to be the leading cause of death by the year 2010. More than 1 million cancer cases are diagnosed each year. And the disease kills about 500,000 Americans annually. The incidence of cancer increases with age; however, only accidents exceed it as a cause of death in children.

Abnormal cell growth

Classified by histologic origin, malignant tumors derived from epithelial tissues are called carcinomas; from epithelial and glandular tissues, adenocarcinomas; from connective, muscle, and bone tissues, sarcomas; from glial cells, gliomas; from pigmented cells, melanomas; and from plasma cells, myelomas. When tumors are derived from erythrocytes, they are called erythroleukemia; from lymphocytes, leukemia; and from lymphatic tissue, lymphoma.

Cancer cells grow larger and divide more rapidly than normal cells, and serve no useful purpose. The most characteristic difference is the cancer cell's ability to grow and spread rapidly, uncontrollably, and independently from the primary site to other tissues where it establishes secondary foci called metastases. Cancer cells metastasize by way of the circulation through the blood or lymphatics, by accidental transplantation from one site to another during surgery, and by local extension.

What causes cancer?

Evidence suggests that carcinogenesis (a cell's transformation from normal to cancerous) results from complex interactions of viruses, physical and chemical carcinogens, diet, genetic predisposition, immunologic, and hormonal factors.

Viruses

In animal studies of viral ability to transform cells, some human viruses show carcinogenic potential. For example, researchers currently link the Epstein-Barr virus, which causes infectious mononucleosis, with lymphomas and nasopharyngeal cancer. They link some viruses from deoxyribonucleic acid (DNA), such as herpes simplex, type 2, with cancer of the cervix and some viruses from ribonucleic acid (RNA) with breast cancer. Hepatitis B virus causes hepatocellular carcinoma, and human T-cell leukemia virus (HTLV-1) probably causes adult T-cell leukemia.

Radiation

The relation between excessive radiation exposure and cancer is well established and supported by detailed studies of widespread exposures, such as those that occurred in nuclear explosions in Hiroshima and Nagasaki in 1945. In addition, the sun's ultraviolet rays can cause cancer on exposed skin. Although radiation can induce tumor development, other factors, such as the patient's tissue type, age, and hormonal status, interact to promote its carcinogenic effect.

Environment

Many substances commonly found in the environment may induce carcinogenesis by damaging cellular DNA. Some proven carcinogens in humans include:
• asbestos (mesothelioma of the lung)
• vinyl chloride (angiosarcoma of the liver)
• airborne aromatic hydrocarbons and benzpyrene (lung cancer)
• alkylating agents (leukemia)
• tobacco (lung, mouth and upper airways, esophagus, pancreas, kidneys, and bladder).

Diet

Especially in the development of GI cancer, diet has been implicated as a result of high-protein and high-fat diets. Food additives, such as nitrates, and certain food preparation methods, particularly charbroiling, may also induce carcinogenesis.

Genetic predisposition

Some cancers and some precancerous lesions result from genetic predisposition either directly (as in Wilms' tumor and retinoblastoma) or indirectly (as in Down's syndrome and inherited immunodeficiency diseases). Expressed as autosomal recessive, X-linked, or autosomal dominant disorders, their common characteristics include:
• early onset of malignant disease
• increased incidence of bilateral cancer in paired organs (breasts, adrenal glands, kidneys, and eighth cranial nerves—acoustic neuroma, for example)
• increased incidence of multiple primary cancers in nonpaired organs
• abnormal chromosome complement in tumor cells.

Ineffective immune response

Other factors that interact to increase susceptibility to cancer include immunologic competence, age, nutritional status, and response to stress. Theoretically, the body develops cancer cells continuously, but the immune system recognizes them as foreign cells and destroys them. This defense mechanism, *immunosurveillance,* has two major components: the humoral immune response and the cell-mediated immune response. Their interaction promotes antibody production, cellular immunity, and immunologic memory. Presumably, the intact human immune system is responsible for spontaneous regression of tumors.

Theoretically, the *cell-mediated immune response* begins when T lymphocytes, also known as T cells, become sensitized by contact with a specific antigen. After repeated contacts, the sensitized T cells release chemical factors called *lymphokines,* some of which begin to destroy the antigen. This reaction transforms the additional T cells into "killers" of antigen-specific cells—in this case, cancer cells.

Similarly, the *humoral immune response* reacts to an antigen by triggering the release of antibodies from plasma cells and activating the serum-complement system, which destroys the antigen-bearing cell. An opposing immune factor, a "blocking antibody," enhances tumor growth by protecting cancer cells from immune destruction. Theoretically, cancer arises when any one of several factors disrupts the immune system, for example:
• *Aging cells,* when reproducing their genetic material, may err, giving rise to mutations. The aging immune system may not recognize these mutations as foreign, thereby allowing them to proliferate and form a cancerous tumor.
• *Cytotoxic drugs* or *steroidal agents* decrease antibody production and destroy circulating lymphocytes.
• *Extreme stress* or *certain viral infections* can depress the immune system.
• *Increased susceptibility to infection* (resulting from radiation, cytotoxic drug therapy, or lymphoproliferative and myeloproliferative diseases, such as lymphatic and myelocytic leukemia) may cause bone marrow depression, which may impair leukocyte function.
• *Acquired immunodeficiency syndrome* (AIDS) weakens cell-mediated immunity.
• *Cancer* itself suppresses the immune system. Advanced cancer exhausts the immune response and leads to anergy, the absence of immune reactivity.

Hormones
The role of hormones in carcinogenesis remains controversial. However, evidence points to excessive hormone use—especially estrogen—as a cancer source in animals. Also, the synthetic estrogen diethylstilbestrol (DES) causes vaginal cancer in some daughters of women who were treated with DES during pregnancy. Whether hormonal changes retard or stimulate cancer development remains unclear.

Cancer assessment
Careful cancer assessment is crucial. In most cancers, the earlier the detection, the more effective the treatment and the better the prospect for cure. To perform the assessment, you'll need to learn about the patient's risk factors, such as cigarette smoking and hazardous working conditions. You'll also need to be alert for cancer's warning signs. Use *CAUTION,* the American Cancer Society's mnemonic device, to assess for the following cancer signs in your patients:
• *C* hange in bowel or bladder habits
• *A* sore that doesn't heal
• *U* nusual bleeding or discharge
• *T* hickening or lump in the breast or elsewhere
• *I* ndigestion or difficulty swallowing
• *O* bvious change in a wart or mole
• *N* agging cough or hoarseness.

Patient health history
Remember that the patient may be worried that he has cancer, so establish rapport and keep the interview as open as possible.

First, obtain biographical information, including the patient's current and previous occupations, his ethnic background, and his previous places of residence. These factors may inform you about the patient's exposure to possible carcinogens.

Investigate the patient's current complaints. What are his symptoms? How long has he had them? What precipitates, exacerbates, or relieves his symptoms? Typically, the chief complaint is one of the cancer warning signs set forth by the American Cancer Society.

Examine the patient's medical history for additional clues. Does he have allergies? Has he undergone medical treatments, been hospitalized, or had surgery? Because of a link with melanoma or other skin cancer, even the removal of a tiny mole may be important. Investigate also whether he's had chemotherapy or ionizing radiation, procedures associated with secondary cancers.

Ask the patient about previous drug therapy and any current drug regimen. Taken over prolonged periods, some medications, such as phenytoin (an anticonvulsant), azathiopine (an immunosuppressant), and estrogen (a hormone commonly used postmenopausally), may lead to cancer.

Question the patient about his family history. Have family members or other relatives had cancer, such as breast, colorectal, or lung cancer (suggesting a possible genetic susceptibility)? Ask about the incidence of specific inherited conditions, such as colonic polyposis, which almost always develops into cancer.

Review the patient's life-style for behaviors that predispose him to cancer. Discuss his food habits, for example. Diets high in fiber and vitamins A, C, and E and low in animal fats and proteins may support cancer prevention. Diets that feature heavy meat consumption may place the patient at added risk for breast, colon, and uterine cancer.

Physical examination

- Take the patient's vital signs. Note whether his temperature is above or below normal. Also note any hypertension, tachycardia or bradycardia, and tachypnea. Keep in mind that intermittent fever occurs in leukemia.
- Inspect the patient's skin for abnormal masses, lesions, or unusual pigmentation. Note any moles that show evidence of bleeding. Look for bruises, petechiae, or purpura, which may indicate bleeding tendencies. Observe the patient's color for pallor, cyanosis, jaundice, and redness. Check the patient's hair distribution; unusual patterns may suggest endocrine tumors. Palpate the skin and note its temperature; cool limbs may indicate a circulation problem caused by a tumor.
- Inspect the patient's face for signs of paralysis, which may result from a tumor with nerve involvement. Look at the patient's eyes. Observe conjunctival color for signs of anemia. Check the sclera for icterus. Jaundice may indicate cancer of the pancreas, liver, or biliary tract. Check the ears for drainage that may signal cancer.
- Observe the breasts for symmetry. Look for dimpling, flattening, puckering, erythema, edema, ulceration, and venous patterns. Check for nipple inversion, masses, discharge, and retraction. Note the color, consistency, and amount of any discharge. Palpate the breasts for a lump or thickening with the patient seated and again with the patient reclining.
- Inspect the patient's chest for respiratory fremitus. Weak or absent fremitus suggests fluid, a mass, or obstruction in the pleural space. Percuss the chest, checking for dullness over the lungs, which may indicate a mass. Auscultate the lungs. Decreased or absent breath sounds point to fluid or tissue obstruction.
- Inspect the abdomen. Consider shape, tone, and symmetry. A distorted contour may indicate tumor growth or organ enlargement. Palpate the abdomen for abnormal masses and the lymph nodes for enlargement that may indicate spreading cancer. (See *Evaluating the lymph nodes.*) Auscultate the abdomen for hyperactive, tinkling, or high-pitched rushes, which point to intestinal obstruc-

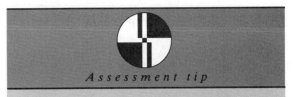

Assessment tip

EVALUATING THE LYMPH NODES

Cells from a primary tumor can spread, or metastasize, to other body areas through the lymphatic system. Lymph nodes normally aren't palpable. Those that are usually result from an inflammatory response to infection. However, superficial or gross adenopathy occurs in a high percentage of patients with lymphoma and metastatic disease.

To palpate lymph nodes, begin in the preauricular, or parotid gland, area (shown below). Proceed downward from the head and neck to the axillary and inguinal areas.

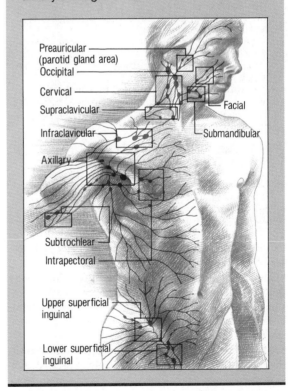

tion. A harsh bruit over the liver can signal a vascular tumor, such as a hepatoma. A friction rub may indicate surface tumor nodules. Percuss the abdomen for ascites; malignant ascites typically occurs with ovarian, endometrial, breast, and colon cancers. Next, percuss the liver. A span of dullness greater than 4¾" (12 cm) along

STAGING CANCER BY THE T.N.M. SYSTEM

Most diagnosticians stage cancer by the internationally recognized TNM (tumor, node, metastasis) system developed by the American Joint Committee on Cancer. This system offers a convenient structure to guide treatment, present a prognosis, and standardize research by ensuring reliable comparisons of patients in various institutions. Some differences in classification may occur, depending on the primary cancer site.

T for primary tumor
The anatomic extent of the primary tumor depends on its size, depth of invasion, and surface spread. Tumor stages progress from TX to T4 as follows:
TX—primary tumor can't be assessed
T0—no evidence of primary tumor
Tis—carcinoma in situ
T1, T2, T3, T4—increasing size or local extent or both of the primary tumor

N for nodal involvement
Nodal involvement reflects the tumor's spread to the lymph nodes, as follows:
NX—regional lymph nodes can't be assessed
N0—no evidence of regional lymph node metastasis
N1, N2, N3—increasing involvement of regional lymph nodes

M for distant metastasis
Metastasis denotes the extent (or spread) of disease. Levels range from MX to M1 as follows:
MX—distant metastasis can't be assessed
M0—no evidence of distant metastases
M1—distant metastasis

the midclavicular line indicates hepatomegaly and possibly cancer.

• Observe the extremities. Note any signs of immobility or fractures, which may indicate bone metastasis.

• Inspect female genitalia for growths, lesions, inflammation, and discharge. Inspect male genitalia, noting any ulcers, nodules, or discharge.

• Perform the neurologic assessment with the patient sitting upright. Cancer patients commonly experience various neurologic problems, such as spinal cord compression and peripheral neuropathies.

Diagnosing cancer

A thorough medical history and physical examination should precede sophisticated diagnostic procedures. Useful tests for detecting early cancerous lesions include X-rays, lymphangiography, mammography, endoscopy, barium studies, and isotope, computed tomography, and magnetic resonance imaging scans.

The single most important diagnostic tool is a biopsy for direct histologic study of tumor tissue. Biopsy tissue samples can be taken by curettage, fluid aspiration (pleural effusion), needle aspiration biopsy (breast), dermal punch (skin or mouth), endoscopy (rectal polyps), and surgical excision (visceral tumors and nodes).

Although it doesn't confirm a diagnosis by itself, a tumor marker—carcinoembryonic antigen (CEA)—can signal cancer that affects the large bowel, stomach, pancreas, lungs, or breasts, and sometimes sarcomas, such as leukemias and lymphomas, as well. CEA titers range from normal levels (less than 5 ng/ml) to suspicious levels (5 to 10 ng/ml) to very suspicious levels (more than 10 ng/ml). During chemotherapy, CEA values provide a valuable baseline for evaluating the tumor's spread, regulating drug dosage, predicting the effectiveness of surgery or radiation, and detecting tumor recurrence.

Although no more specific than CEA, alpha-fetoprotein, a fetal antigen rare in adults, can suggest testicular, ovarian, gastric, pancreatic, and primary lung cancers. Beta–human chorionic gonadotropin may point to testicular cancer or choriocarcinoma. The test for prostate-specific antigen helps detect and evaluate prostatic cancer, whereas CA125 is useful for monitoring ovarian cancer.

Staging and grading cancer
Choosing effective therapeutic options depends on correct *staging* of malignant tumors. Although cancer staging systems vary according to cancer site and pathologists' preferences, the widely used TNM (tumor, node, metastasis) staging system quantifies cancer and allows reliable comparison of cancer treatments and survival rates among large populations. The TNM system describes the tumor, lymph node involvement, and metastasis to other areas. (See *Staging cancer by the TNM system.*)

Grading, another objective way to define a tumor, takes into account the resemblance of tumor tissue to normal cells (differentiation) and the tumor's estimated growth rate. Grading has limitations, in that results reflect only a portion of the tumor. Most tumors have cells in various stages of development, so as a tumor develops, the grade may change.

Grading also names the lesion according to corresponding normal cells, such as lymphoid or mucinous lesions. (See *Differences between a benign and a malignant tumor.*)

DIFFERENCES BETWEEN A BENIGN AND A MALIGNANT TUMOR

Factor	Benign	Malignant
Growth	Expands slowly, pushing aside surrounding tissues but not infiltrating	Usually infiltrates surrounding tissues rapidly, expanding in all directions
Limitation	Typically encapsulated	Seldom encapsulated and commonly poorly delineated
Recurrence	Seldom recurs after surgical removal	Commonly recurs when removed surgically because of infiltration into surrounding tissues
Morphology	Closely resembles tissue of origin	Differs considerably from tissue of origin
Differentiation	Well-differentiated cells	Poorly differentiated or undifferentiated cells
Mitotic activity	Slight	Extensive
Tissue destruction	Usually slight	Extensive, owing to infiltration and metastatic lesion
Spread	No metastasis	Metastasis by way of blood or lymph system or both, with establishment of secondary tumors
Effect on body	Cachexia rare; usually not fatal but may obstruct vital organs, exert pressure, produce excess hormones; can become malignant	Cachexia typical—anemia, loss of weight, weakness, general ill health; fatal if untreated

Cancer treatments

Treatment options include surgery, radiation, chemotherapy, and immunotherapy (biotherapy), used independently or in combination. In each patient, treatment depends on the type, stage, localization, and responsiveness of the tumor, as well as the patient's limitations.

Surgery

Once the mainstay of cancer treatment, surgery is now regularly combined with radiation, chemotherapy, and immunotherapy. Surgery removes the bulk of the tumor, and the other treatments discourage residual cell proliferation. Surgery also can relieve pain, correct obstruction, and alleviate pressure. Less radical surgery (for example, a lumpectomy instead of a radical mastectomy) is more acceptable to patients.

Radiation therapy

This treatment aims to destroy the rapidly dividing cancer cells and, at the same time, damage normal cells as little as possible. Two types of radiation therapy are common: ionizing radiation and particle radiation. Both target cellular DNA, but particle radiation causes less skin damage.

Treatment approaches include external beam radiation and intracavitary and interstitial implants (requiring personal radiation protection for all staff members who come in contact with the patient). For more information, see *Preparing for external radiation therapy,* page 288.

Normal and malignant cells respond to radiation differently, depending on blood supply, oxygen saturation, previous irradiation, and immune status. In most instances, normal cells recover from radiation faster than malignant cells. The success of the treatment and damage to normal tissue vary with radiation's intensity. Although a large single dose of radiation has greater cellular effects than fractions of the same amount delivered sequentially, a protracted schedule allows time for normal tissue to recover in the intervals between individual sublethal doses.

Radiation may be chosen for palliative therapy to relieve pain, obstructions, malignant effusions, cough, dyspnea, ulcerative lesions, and hemorrhage. It also can promote the repair of pathologic fractures and delay tumor spread. Radiation can give a cancer patient an im-

PREPARING FOR EXTERNAL RADIATION THERAPY

Follow these guidelines to help relieve your patient's anxiety before he undergoes his first radiation treatment:
• Show the patient the radiation therapy department and introduce him to the staff.
• Before treatment, help him remove all metal objects (pens, buttons, jewelry) that may interfere with therapy. Explain that the areas to be treated will be marked with ink. Tell him not to wash these areas because the markings ensure that radiation reaches the same target at each treatment.
• Reinforce the doctor's explanation of the procedure, and answer questions as honestly as you can. Realistically explain the benefits and adverse effects of radiation therapy. If you don't know the answer to a question, refer the patient to the doctor.
• Discuss the adverse effects to watch for and report. Because radiation therapy may increase susceptibility to infection, warn the patient to avoid people with colds or other infections during therapy.
• Reassure the patient that the actual treatment is painless and won't make him radioactive. Stress that he'll be under constant surveillance during radiation administration and can call the therapist if he needs anything.

portant psychological lift just by shrinking a visible tumor.

Combining radiation and surgery can minimize radical surgery, prolong survival, and preserve physiologic function. For example, small preoperative doses of radiation can shrink a tumor, making it removable by surgery while preventing further spread of the disease during surgery. After the wound heals, larger postoperative doses of radiation prevent residual cancer cells from multiplying or metastasizing.

Systemic adverse effects of radiation include weakness, fatigue, and possibly anorexia, nausea, vomiting, anemia, and diarrhea. (See *Managing adverse effects of radiation.*) These adverse effects may subside after treatment with antiemetics, sedatives, corticosteroids, frequent small meals, fluid maintenance, medications to control diarrhea, and rest. Systemic effects are seldom severe enough to require discontinuation of treatment; however, they may require a readjustment of radiation dosage. Radiation therapy also requires frequent blood counts (with particular attention to white blood cells and platelets).

Chemotherapy

Treatment with antineoplastic drugs may induce tumor regression and prevent or delay metastasis. Useful for controlling residual disease or as an adjunct to surgery or radiation therapy, chemotherapy can induce long remissions and possibly cures, especially in patients with childhood leukemia, Hodgkin's disease, choriocarcinoma, and testicular cancer. As palliative treatment, chemotherapy aims to improve the patient's quality of life by relieving pain and other symptoms. The major cancer chemotherapeutic agents include the following:
• *Alkylating agents* and *nitrosoureas* inhibit cell growth and division by reacting with DNA. Nitrosoureas can cross the blood-brain barrier.
• *Antimetabolites* prevent cell growth by competing with metabolites in producing nucleic acid.
• *Antitumor antibiotics* block cell growth by binding with DNA and interfering with DNA-dependent RNA synthesis.
• *Plant alkaloids* prevent cellular reproduction by disrupting cell mitosis.
• *Steroidal hormones* inhibit hormone-susceptible tumor growth by changing the chemical environment.

Antineoplastic drugs that kill cancer cells can also kill cells in normal tissues, especially in tissues that contain rapidly proliferating cells. For example, antineoplastic drugs typically depress bone marrow function, causing anemia, leukopenia, and thrombocytopenia. They irritate GI epithelial cells, causing ulceration, bleeding, and vomiting. What's more, they destroy hair follicles and skin cells, causing alopecia and dermatitis. Many I.V. anticancer drugs may irritate the vein, causing venous sclerosis and, if extravasated, deep cutaneous necrosis that requires debridement and skin grafting. Only nurses with special preparation and certification in chemotherapy should administer chemotherapeutic drugs.

Besides encouragement and support, all patients who undergo chemotherapy need special nursing care to prevent infection, maintain hydration, promote safety, and help them cope with drug adverse effects.
• Watch for signs of infection, especially in the patient who is receiving simultaneous radiation treatment. Be alert for a low-grade fever when the granulocyte count falls below 500/mm^3. Take the patient's temperature frequently. Even a slight fever may indicate sepsis. At the same time, keep in mind that the patient's temperature may not rise significantly. This phenomenon may result from few or no granulocytes or from steroid therapy.
• Increase the patient's fluid intake before and throughout chemotherapy.

MANAGING ADVERSE EFFECTS OF RADIATION

Area treated	Effect	Management
Abdominopelvic	Cramps, diarrhea	Administer loperamide and diphenoxylate with atropine; provide a low-residue diet; maintain fluid and electrolyte balance.
Head	Alopecia	Protect the scalp with gentle combing and grooming; avoid frequent shampooing. Provide a soft head covering (scarf, hat, wig) to conserve body heat and protect scalp from sunburn and injuries.
	Mucositis	Provide mouthwash with viscous lidocaine; offer cool liquids, ice pops, and a soft, nonirritating diet. Avoid spicy food and alcohol.
	Monilia	Provide medicated mouthwash (avoid commercial mouthwash).
	Dental caries	Apply fluoride to teeth prophylactically; provide gingival care.
	Xerostomia	Encourage fluid intake, especially water; offer commercially available saliva substitutes.
Chest	Pulmonary irritation	Tell the patient to stop smoking and to avoid people with upper respiratory tract infections; administer steroid therapy, as ordered; provide humidifier, if necessary.
	Pericarditis, myocarditis	Control arrhythmias with appropriate agents (procainamide, disopyramide) as ordered; provide pain relief; monitor for heart failure.
	Esophagitis	Provide total parenteral nutrition; maintain fluid balance.
Kidneys	Nephritis, hypertensive nephropathy	Maintain fluid and electrolyte balance; watch for signs of renal failure.

• Inform the patient that he may have some hair loss if his drug regimen causes alopecia. Reassure him that his hair should grow back after therapy ends (although it may return in a different color and texture). If the patient expresses interest in a hairpiece or wig, encourage him to obtain one before therapy begins. In this way, he can match his current hair color and style.

• Check skin for petechiae, ecchymoses, and chemical cellulitis and for secondary infection during treatment.

• Minimize possible tissue irritation and damage by checking I.V. needle placement before and during drug infusion. Instruct the patient to report any discomfort, burning sensation, or pain during the infusion.

• Frequently check for blood return, and observe the I.V. site during the infusion for signs of infiltration. If you're infusing a vesicant and you suspect infiltration (extravasation), *stop the infusion*. Then aspirate the drug from the I.V. needle, and give the appropriate antidote according to established protocol. (These protocols must be established for each drug to allow for immediate treatment.)

• Administer chemotherapeutic drugs by the recommended route (orally, subcutaneously, intramuscularly, intravenously, intracavitarily, intrathecally, intraperitoneally, or intra-arterially), depending on the drug and its action. You'll usually follow procedures for intermittent administration to allow for bone marrow recovery between doses.

• Check the dosage, which usually is calculated according to the patient's body surface area, with adjustments for general condition and degree of myelosuppression. Be sure that dosage calculation is based on current information because the dosages may change as a consequence of research findings.

• Encourage apprehensive patients to express their concerns and fears. Provide simple, truthful information. Explain that not all patients who receive chemotherapy experience nausea and vomiting. For those who do, antiemetic drugs, relaxation therapy, and diet can minimize discomfort.

Immunotherapy

Usually combined with surgery, chemotherapy, or radiation, immunotherapy may be most effective in early cancer stages. Because much immunotherapy remains investigational, its availability may depend on the treatment facility. And adverse effects may be unpredictable. The following immunotherapies offer promise:

• *Nonspecific immunostimulation* uses biological agents, such as bacille Calmette-Guérin (BCG) vaccine or *Corynebacterium parvum,* to stimulate the reticuloendothelial system, thereby augmenting the patient's immune system and combating the immunosuppressive effects of cancer and treatment.

• *Intralesional stimulation* involves injecting a biological agent directly into the tumor. This initiates specific and nonspecific responses that trigger local cancer cell destruction.

• *Active specific immunostimulation* uses specific tumor antigen vaccines to stimulate the patient's immune system to control or reject malignant cells by producing antibodies and lymphocytes.

• *Adoptive transfer of immunity* involves transferring immunologically active cells from a donor with established immunity to stimulate active immunity in the patient.

Additional advances in three other areas of immunotherapy are promising. *Interferons,* once confined to antiviral applications, are now used to stimulate antibody production and cell-mediated immunity. Usually combined with other treatments, *bone marrow transplantation* restores hematologic and immunologic function in some cancer patients. A third treatment involves injecting *monoclonal antibodies* tagged with radioisotopes into the body. These agents help detect cancer by attaching to tumor cells. Some investigational findings indicate a link between monoclonal antibodies and certain toxins that destroy specific cancer cells without disturbing healthy cells.

Nursing interventions

Strive to provide adequate nutrition and maintain fluid balance. Keep in mind that tumors grow at the expense of normal tissue by competing for nutrients; this leaves some patients with a protein deficiency. And cancer treatments themselves may produce nutritional and fluid and electrolyte disturbances, resulting from vomiting, diarrhea, draining fistulas, altered taste sensations, and anorexia.

Also, implement measures to relieve pain and increase comfort. Help the patient with terminal cancer deal with his diagnosis and explore hospice care, if appropriate.

Maintaining nutrition and hydration

• Base nutritional planning on the patient's dietary history. Pinpoint possible nutritional problems and their causes (such as diabetes) before the patient selects a menu.

• Ask the dietitian to provide a liquid, high-protein, high-carbohydrate, high-calorie diet if the patient can't tolerate solid foods. If the patient has stomatitis, provide soft, bland foods.

• Encourage the patient's family to bring foods from home, if he requests them and if appropriate.

• Provide a relaxed, pleasant mealtime. Encourage visitors to eat with the patient or, if possible, encourage him to dine with other patients. Let him choose from a varied menu.

• If appropriate, suggest a glass of wine or a cocktail before dinner to promote relaxation and stimulate appetite. Urge the patient to drink juice and other calorie-rich beverages instead of water.

• If the patient is unable to eat a large meal, suggest small, frequent meals instead.

• Avoid highly aromatic foods. Therapy may alter the patient's sense of smell and inhibit appetite. On the other hand, if he complains that food tastes bland or metallic, try adding mild seasonings to food. Sugar counteracts some metallic flavors, as do sour candies.

• Experiment with foods. Because treatments may alter the chemical receptors on the tongue, foods that normally displease the patient may appeal to him.

• Deliver nourishment by nasogastric (NG) tube if the patient can't eat, can't accept table food (after head, neck, or GI surgery, for example), or can't swallow easily. If he needs the tube after discharge, teach him how to insert it, how to test its position in his stomach by aspirating stomach contents, and how to instill the nutritional supplement. Alternatives to NG tube feedings may involve gastrostomy, jejunostomy and, occasionally, esophagostomy tubes.

• Caution the patient that gastric or intestinal juices that spill on the skin will cause excoriation if not washed off immediately. Flush the tube well with water after each feeding.

• Provide adequate hydration by instilling up to 6 oz (177 ml) of water or another clear liquid between meals. After jejunostomy, begin with very small feedings, slowly and carefully increasing the amount of nutritional supplement. Provide additional fluids and calories during limited feeding periods by supplementing jejunostomy feedings with I.V. fat emulsions.

• Discuss advantages and disadvantages of parenteral feeding if your patient will need it, especially during aggressive chemotherapy or radiation therapy. Tell him that patients who receive parenteral nutrition during cancer therapy experience less nausea, vomiting, diarrhea, and weight loss than patients who don't. And because of their improved nutritional status, they may respond better to treatment. Explain also that parenteral nutrition can restore protein balance to help him better tolerate surgery, if indicated. Other advantages include a slight weight gain, better wound healing, and decreased risk for infection after radical surgery.

Controlling pain

Most cancer patients fear overwhelming pain, making pain control a major concern at every cancer stage — from localized cancer to advanced metastasis. Cancer pain may result from inflammation or from pressure of the tumor on pain-sensitive structures, tumor infiltration of nerves or blood vessels, or metastatic extension to bone. Chronic and unrelenting pain can undermine the patient's tolerance, interfere with eating and sleeping, and color his life with anger, despair, and anxiety.

Opioid analgesics (also called narcotic analgesics), either alone or combined with nonnarcotic analgesics or antianxiety agents, are the mainstay of pain relief in advanced cancer. In terminal illness, drug dosages may be high, especially for the patient who develops drug tolerance and whose addiction danger is unimportant.

Use the following guidelines for pain relief:

• Provide analgesics generously, as needed and as ordered. Anticipate the need for pain relief, and schedule it so that pain doesn't become unbearable. Make an agreement with the patient that you'll provide pain medication before pain becomes severe. This will decrease the patient's anxiety level and help in pain control. If

PATIENT-CONTROLLED ANALGESIA

Cancer care centers across the United States report encouraging results with the pain relief system known as patient-controlled analgesia (PCA).

How PCA works
This system permits the patient to self-administer an analgesic at the press of a button. The button, stationed at bedside, activates a pump fitted with a prefilled analgesic-containing syringe. Small, intermittent doses of the analgesic administered I.V., subcutaneously, or epidurally maintain medication levels in the bloodstream to ensure the patient's comfort and minimize sedation.

Locked safely inside the pump, the medication syringe or cassette dispenses only preset doses at preset intervals. This allows the patient to achieve his maximum comfort level but not to overdose. The computerized system usually includes a "breakthrough" option for additional doses that the nurse or patient can activate.

PCA advantages
Clinical studies show that patients who use a PCA system deliver analgesic drugs effectively and maintain comfort without oversedation. They use less of the drug than the amount normally given by I.M. injection.

PCA provides other significant advantages. Patients using this system:
• stay alert and active during daytime hours
• need not endure pain while waiting for an injection
• have reduced anxiety levels
• remain free from pain caused by injections
• need not call the nurse away from other essential clinical duties.

possible, use patient-controlled analgesia. (See *Patient-controlled analgesia*.)

• Initiate noninvasive pain-relief techniques, as needed. Tell the patient that these can be used alone or with drug therapy. Popular noninvasive techniques include cutaneous stimulation, relaxation, biofeedback, distraction, and guided imagery.

• Explain palliative treatments, if ordered. These measures can relieve pressure and discomfort caused by inflamed necrotic tissue. Radiation therapy can shrink metastatic tissue and control bone pain. When a tumor invades nervous system tissues, pain control may require anesthetics, destructive nerve blocks, electronic nerve stimulation with a dorsal column or transcutaneous electrical nerve stimulator, rhizotomy, or chordotomy.

Exploring hospice care

A holistic approach to patient care modeled after St. Christopher's Hospice in London, the hospice program provides comprehensive physical, psychological, social, and spiritual care for terminally ill patients. Many hospices are associated with hospitals, but some are independent or provide home care programs. As a variation of the hospice approach, several large cities in the United States have facilities that offer children with leukemia and their families a homelike environment during outpatient treatment at a nearby hospital.

When referring the patient to hospice care:
• Explain that the hospice care goal is to help each patient live his remaining life to the fullest, without pain, and surrounded by whom he chooses. Pain control, a priority, uses all possible avenues available to the patient. Morphine is still the drug of choice for pain control.
• Urge family members to assume an active role in patient care. Point out that hospice care relies on a coordinated team effort to overcome the anxiety, fear, and depression that typically affect the terminally ill patient.
• Provide a warm and secure setting to help family members work out their grief before the patient dies.
• Encourage everyone involved in hospice care (staff, patient, and family) to be committed to high-quality care, accept emotional involvement, and feel comfortable with personal feelings about death and dying.
• Foster open communication to evaluate patient care and to help staff members cope with their own feelings.

Cancer's emotional aspect

Few illnesses evoke as profound an emotional response as cancer. Patients express this response in several ways. A few face this difficult reality immediately. Many initially use denial as a coping mechanism and refuse to accept the diagnosis. As evidence of cancer becomes inescapable, the patient may plunge into depression. Family members may express denial by encouraging unproven treatments. This can delay effective care.

Some patients cope by intellectualizing their disease, enabling them to obscure its reality and to regard it as unrelated to themselves. For most patients, intellectualization is a more productive coping behavior than denial because the patient is receiving treatment.

Watch for these behavioral responses so you can identify them and offer support. For many cancers, you can offer realistic hope for long-term survival or remission. And even in advanced disease, you can offer short-term, achievable goals, such as a comfortable afternoon or a pleasant visit with a loved one.

To help a patient cope with cancer, first try to understand your own feelings about it. Then listen sensitively to the patient so that you can offer genuine understanding and comfort. When caring for a patient with terminal cancer, increase your own effectiveness by seeking others to help you through your grieving.

HEAD, NECK, AND SPINAL NEOPLASMS

Cancers in this region of the body are among the deadliest and most disfiguring. Involvement of speech and sense organs, as well as the central nervous system (CNS) itself, can have an enormous impact on the patient's quality of life.

MALIGNANT BRAIN TUMORS

Slightly more common in men than in women, malignant brain tumors (gliomas, meningiomas, and schwannomas) have an overall incidence of 5 per 100,000. They cause CNS changes by invading and destroying tissues and by secondary effect — mainly compression of the brain, cranial nerves, and cerebral vessels; cerebral edema; and increased intracranial pressure (ICP).

Tumors can occur at any age. In adults, incidence is highest between ages 40 and 60, and the most common tumor types are gliomas and meningiomas. They usually occur above the covering of the cerebellum (supratentorial tumors).

Most tumors in children occur before age 1 or between ages 2 and 12. The most common are astrocytomas, medulloblastomas, ependymomas, and brain stem gliomas. Brain tumors are one of the most common causes of cancer death in children.

Causes

The cause of brain tumors is unknown.

Complications

In malignant brain tumors, life-threatening complications from increasing ICP include coma, respiratory or cardiac arrest, and brain herniation.

Assessment findings

The patient's history usually reveals an insidious onset of signs and symptoms. If the brain tumor has already been diagnosed, his history may also show an early misdiagnosis—a common occurrence.

Signs and symptoms result from increased ICP. Specific assessment findings vary with the type of tumor, its location, and the degree of invasion. Neurologic assessment findings often help to pinpoint the location of the tumor. (See *Brain tumors: Site-specific signs and symptoms*, page 294, and *Assessment findings in malignant brain tumors*, pages 296 and 297.)

Diagnostic tests
Skull X-rays, brain scans, computed tomography and magnetic resonance imaging scans, and cerebral angiography help locate the tumor. Biopsy of the lesion allows identification of the histologic type and grading of the tumor. Grade 1 tumors are well differentiated; grade 2, moderately well differentiated; grade 3, poorly differentiated; and grade 4, extremely poorly differentiated. The higher the grade, the poorer the prognosis.

The patient may also receive a lumbar puncture, which shows increased cerebrospinal fluid (CSF) pressure, which reflects ICP; increased protein levels; decreased glucose levels; and, occasionally, tumor cells in CSF.

Treatment
Specific treatments vary with the tumor's histologic type, radiosensitivity, and location. Such treatments may include surgery, radiation therapy, chemotherapy, and decompression of increased ICP (with diuretics, corticosteroids or, possibly, ventriculoatrial or ventriculoperitoneal shunting of the CSF).

Treatment of a glioma usually consists of resection by craniotomy. Radiation therapy and chemotherapy follow resection. The combination of carmustine, lomustine, or procarbazine with radiation therapy is more effective than radiation alone.

For low-grade cystic cerebellar astrocytomas, surgical resection permits long-term survival. For other astrocytomas, treatment consists of repeated surgery, radiation therapy, and shunting of fluid from obstructed CSF pathways. Radiation therapy works best in radiosensitive astrocytomas; some astrocytomas are radioresistant.

Treatment for oligodendrogliomas and ependymomas includes surgical resection and radiation therapy. Medulloblastomas call for surgical resection and, possibly, intrathecal infusion of methotrexate or another antineoplastic drug. Meningiomas require surgical resection, including dura mater and bone. (Operative mortality may reach 10% because of large tumor size.)

For schwannomas, microsurgical technique allows complete resection of the tumor and preservation of the facial nerve. Although schwannomas are moderately radioresistant, treatment still calls for postoperative radiation therapy.

Treatment for malignant brain tumors also includes chemotherapy with nitrosoureas, which cross the blood-brain barrier and allow other chemotherapeutic drugs to go through as well. Intrathecal and intra-arterial administration maximizes drug action.

Palliative measures for gliomas, astrocytomas, oligodendrogliomas, and ependymomas include dexamethasone for cerebral edema and antacids and histamine receptor antagonists for stress ulcers. These tumors and schwannomas may also require anticonvulsants.

New treatments under investigation include bone marrow transplantation and hyperthermia.

Treatment of brain tumors can cause several complications. Surgery can result in immediate or delayed CNS infections, with symptoms that mimic tumor progression or recurrence. If fever or rapidly progressive neurologic symptoms develop, bacterial and fungal cultures will confirm the infection.

Early delayed radiation encephalopathy may stem from temporary demyelination. Anorexia, somnolence, lethargy, and headache occur 2 to 6 weeks after the therapy but resolve spontaneously in about 6 weeks.

Late delayed radiation encephalopathy stems from brain necrosis and small-vessel occlusion. Symptoms can mimic disease advancement and may include intracranial hypertension and focal neurologic dysfunction. Both are irreversible and potentially fatal complications.

Corticosteroid therapy predisposes the patient to cushingoid symptoms and GI ulceration.

Nursing diagnoses
• Activity intolerance
• Altered role performance
• Anxiety
• Body image disturbance
• Energy field disturbance
• Fear
• Hopelessness
• Impaired physical mobility
• Impaired skin integrity
• Ineffective breathing pattern
• Ineffective family coping
• Ineffective individual coping

BRAIN TUMORS: SITE-SPECIFIC SIGNS AND SYMPTOMS

A brain tumor usually produces signs and symptoms specific to its location. Recognizing these typical effects helps identify the tumor site and guide treatment before and after surgery. It can also help you spot life-threatening complications, such as increasing ICP and imminent brain herniation. A brain tumor may cause all, some, or none of the effects listed below.

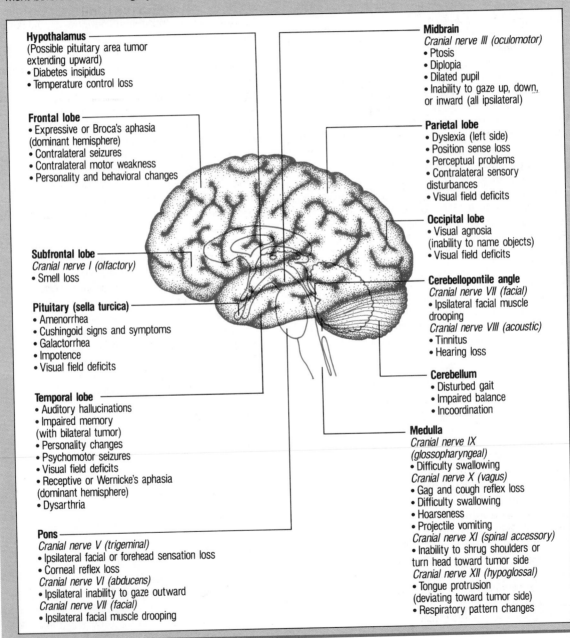

Hypothalamus
(Possible pituitary area tumor extending upward)
• Diabetes insipidus
• Temperature control loss

Frontal lobe
• Expressive or Broca's aphasia (dominant hemisphere)
• Contralateral seizures
• Contralateral motor weakness
• Personality and behavioral changes

Subfrontal lobe
Cranial nerve I (olfactory)
• Smell loss

Pituitary (sella turcica)
• Amenorrhea
• Cushingoid signs and symptoms
• Galactorrhea
• Impotence
• Visual field deficits

Temporal lobe
• Auditory hallucinations
• Impaired memory (with bilateral tumor)
• Personality changes
• Psychomotor seizures
• Visual field deficits
• Receptive or Wernicke's aphasia (dominant hemisphere)
• Dysarthria

Pons
Cranial nerve V (trigeminal)
• Ipsilateral facial or forehead sensation loss
• Corneal reflex loss
Cranial nerve VI (abducens)
• Ipsilateral inability to gaze outward
Cranial nerve VII (facial)
• Ipsilateral facial muscle drooping

Midbrain
Cranial nerve III (oculomotor)
• Ptosis
• Diplopia
• Dilated pupil
• Inability to gaze up, down, or inward (all ipsilateral)

Parietal lobe
• Dyslexia (left side)
• Position sense loss
• Perceptual problems
• Contralateral sensory disturbances
• Visual field deficits

Occipital lobe
• Visual agnosia (inability to name objects)
• Visual field deficits

Cerebellopontile angle
Cranial nerve VII (facial)
• Ipsilateral facial muscle drooping
Cranial nerve VIII (acoustic)
• Tinnitus
• Hearing loss

Cerebellum
• Disturbed gait
• Impaired balance
• Incoordination

Medulla
Cranial nerve IX (glossopharyngeal)
• Difficulty swallowing
Cranial nerve X (vagus)
• Gag and cough reflex loss
• Difficulty swallowing
• Hoarseness
• Projectile vomiting
Cranial nerve XI (spinal accessory)
• Inability to shrug shoulders or turn head toward tumor side
Cranial nerve XII (hypoglossal)
• Tongue protrusion (deviating toward tumor side)
• Respiratory pattern changes

• Ineffective thermoregulation
• Pain
• Powerlessness
• Self-care deficit
• Sensory or perceptual alterations

Nursing interventions

• Carefully document the occurrence, nature, and duration of seizure activity.
• Maintain a patent airway.
• Take steps to protect the patient's safety.
• Administer anticonvulsant drugs, as ordered.
• Monitor for changes in the patient's neurologic status, and watch for increased ICP. (See *Imminent transtentorial herniation.*)
• Monitor respiratory changes carefully. An abnormal respiratory rate and depth may point to rising ICP or herniation of the cerebellar tonsils from expanding infratentorial mass.
• Monitor the patient's temperature carefully. Fever commonly follows hypothalamic anoxia, but it can also indicate meningitis. Use hypothermia blankets before and after surgery to keep the patient's temperature down and minimize cerebral metabolic demands.
• As ordered, administer steroids and osmotic diuretics, such as mannitol, and restrict fluid intake to reduce cerebral edema. Monitor the patient's fluid and electrolyte balance to avoid dehydration.
• Observe and report signs of stress ulcers: abdominal distention, pain, vomiting, and tarry stools. Administer antacids, as ordered.
• If the patient requires surgery, he'll need special care. After a craniotomy, monitor the patient's general neurologic status, and watch for signs of increased ICP, such as an elevated bone flap and typical neurologic changes. To reduce the risk of increased ICP, restrict fluids to 1,500 ml/24 hours, as ordered.

   To promote venous drainage and reduce cerebral edema after supratentorial craniotomy, elevate the head of the bed about 30 degrees. Position the patient on his side to allow drainage of secretions and prevent aspiration. As appropriate, instruct him to avoid Valsalva's maneuver and isometric muscle contractions when moving or sitting up in bed; these can increase intrathoracic pressure and ICP. Withhold oral fluids, which may provoke vomiting and, consequently, raise ICP.

   After infratentorial craniotomy, keep the patient flat for 48 hours, but logroll him every 2 hours to minimize complications of immobilization. Prevent other complications by paying careful attention to ventilatory status and to cardiovascular, GI, and musculoskeletal functions.

Warning

IMMINENT TRANSTENTORIAL HERNIATION

If your patient develops sudden unilateral pupillary dilation with loss of light reflex, notify the doctor at once. This ominous change indicates imminent transtentorial herniation.

• The patient usually won't receive radiation therapy until after the surgical wound heals, but it can induce wound breakdown even then. So observe the wound carefully for signs of infection and sinus formation. Because radiation may cause brain inflammation, also watch for signs of rising ICP.
• Before chemotherapy, give prochlorperazine or another antiemetic, as ordered, to minimize nausea and vomiting.
• Because brain tumors may cause residual neurologic deficits that handicap the patient physically or mentally, begin rehabilitation early. Consult with occupational and physical therapists to encourage independence in daily activities. As necessary, provide aids for self-care and mobilization, such as bathroom rails for wheelchair patients. If the patient is aphasic, arrange for consultation with a speech pathologist.
• Throughout therapy, provide emotional support to help the patient and his family cope with the treatment, potential disabilities, and changes in life-style resulting from his tumor.

Patient teaching

• Because some of the antineoplastic agents (carmustine, lomustine, semustine, and procarbazine, for example) used as adjuncts to radiation therapy and surgery can cause delayed bone marrow depression, tell the patient to watch for and immediately report any signs of infection or bleeding that appear within 4 weeks after the start of chemotherapy.
• As appropriate, explain adverse effects from chemotherapy and other treatments. Explain what actions the patient can take to alleviate them.
• Teach the patient and his family the early signs of tumor recurrence, and encourage their compliance with the treatment regimen.

(Text continues on page 298.)

ASSESSMENT FINDINGS IN MALIGNANT BRAIN TUMORS

Tumor and characteristics	Assessment findings
Glioblastoma multiforme (spongioblastoma multiforme) • Most common glioma, accounting for 60% of all gliomas • Peak incidence between ages 50 and 60; more common in men than in women • Unencapsulated, highly malignant; grows rapidly and infiltrates the brain extensively; may become enormous before diagnosed • Occurs most often in cerebral hemispheres, especially frontal and temporal lobes (rarely in brain stem and cerebellum) • Occupies more than one lobe of affected hemisphere; may spread to opposite hemisphere by corpus callosum; may metastasize into CSF, producing tumors in distant parts of the nervous system	*General* • Increased ICP (nausea, vomiting, headache, papilledema) • Mental and behavioral changes • Altered vital signs (increased systolic pressure, widened pulse pressure, respiratory changes) • Speech and sensory disturbances • In children, irritability and projectile vomiting *Localizing* • Midline: headache (bifrontal or bioccipital) that's worse in morning; intensified by coughing, straining, or sudden head movements • Temporal lobe: psychomotor seizures • Central region: focal seizures • Optic and oculomotor nerves: visual defects • Frontal lobe: abnormal reflexes and motor responses
Astrocytoma • Second most common malignant glioma, accounting for 10% of all gliomas • Occurs at any age; incidence higher in males than in females • Occurs most often in central and subcortical white matter; may originate in any part of the CNS • Cerebellar astrocytomas usually confined to one hemisphere	*General* • Headache and mental activity changes • Decreased motor strength and coordination • Seizures and scanning speech • Altered vital signs *Localizing* • Third ventricle: changes in mental activity and level of consciousness, nausea, and pupillary dilation and sluggish light reflex; paresis or ataxia in later stages of the disease • Brain stem and pons: ipsilateral trigeminal, abducens, and facial nerve palsies in early stages; cerebellar ataxia, tremors, and other cranial nerve deficits as the disease progresses • Third or fourth ventricle or aqueduct of Sylvius: secondary hydrocephalus • Thalamus or hypothalamus: various endocrine, metabolic, autonomic, and behavioral changes
Oligodendroglioma • Third most common glioma that accounts for less than 5% of all gliomas • Occurs in middle adult years; more common in women than in men • Slow-growing	*General* • Mental and behavioral changes • Decreased visual acuity and other visual disturbances • Increased ICP *Localizing* • Temporal lobe: hallucinations and psychomotor seizures • Central region: seizures (confined to one muscle group or unilateral) • Midbrain or third ventricle: pyramidal tract symptoms (dizziness, ataxia, paresthesias of the face) • Brain stem and cerebrum: nystagmus, hearing loss, dizziness, ataxia, paresthesias of the face, cranial nerve palsies, hemiparesis, suboccipital tenderness, loss of balance

ASSESSMENT FINDINGS IN MALIGNANT BRAIN TUMORS *(continued)*

Tumor and characteristics	Assessment findings
Ependymoma • Rare glioma • Most common in children and young adults • Locates most often in fourth and lateral ventricles	*General* • Increased ICP and obstructive hydrocephalus, depending on tumor size • Other assessment findings similar to those of oligodendroglioma
Medulloblastoma • Rare glioma • Incidence highest in children ages 4 to 6 • Affects males more than females • Frequently metastasizes by way of CSF	*General* • Increased ICP *Localizing* • Brain stem and cerebrum: papilledema, nystagmus, hearing loss, perception of flashing lights, dizziness, ataxia, paresthesias of the face, cranial nerve palsies (V, VI, VII, IX, X, primarily sensory), hemiparesis, suboccipital tenderness; compression of supratentorial area produces other general and focal symptoms
Meningioma • Most common nongliomatous brain tumor, constituting 15% of primary brain tumors • Occurs most frequently among people in their 50s; rare in children; more common in females than in males (ratio 3:2) • Arises from the meninges • Common locations include parasagittal area, sphenoidal ridge, anterior part of the base of the skull, cerebellopontile angle, and spinal canal • Benign, well-circumscribed, highly vascular tumor that compresses underlying brain tissue by invading overlying skull	*General* • Headache • Seizures (in two-thirds of patients) • Vomiting • Changes in mental activity • Other assessment findings similar to those of schwannomas *Localizing* • Skull changes (bony bulge) over tumor • Sphenoidal ridge, indenting optic nerve: unilateral visual changes and papilledema • Prefrontal parasagittal: personality and behavioral changes • Motor cortex: contralateral motor changes • Anterior fossa compressing both optic nerves and frontal lobes: headaches and bilateral vision loss • Pressure on cranial nerves, causing varying symptoms
Schwannoma (acoustic neurinoma, neurilemoma, cerebellopontile angle tumor) • Accounts for about 10% of all intracranial tumors • Onset of symptoms between ages 30 and 60; higher incidence in women than in men • Affects the craniospinal nerve sheath, usually cranial nerve VIII; also, V and VII, and to a lesser extent, VI and X on the same side as the tumor • Benign, but often classified as malignant because of its growth patterns; slow-growing—may be present for years before symptoms occur	*General* • Unilateral hearing loss with or without tinnitus • Stiff neck and suboccipital discomfort • Secondary hydrocephalus • Ataxia and uncoordinated movements of one or both arms due to pressure on brain stem and cerebellum *Localizing* • V: early signs including facial hypoesthesia and paresthesia on the side of hearing loss; unilateral loss of corneal reflex • VI: diplopia • VII: paresis progressing to paralysis (Bell's palsy) • X: weakness of palate, tongue, and nerve muscles on same side as tumor

• Refer the patient to resource and support services, such as the social service department, home health care agencies, and the American Cancer Society.

PITUITARY TUMORS

Originating most often in the anterior pituitary (adenohypophysis), pituitary tumors constitute 10% to 15% of intracranial neoplasms. They occur in adults of both sexes, usually between ages 30 and 50.

The most common tumor tissue types include chromophobe adenoma (90%), basophil adenoma, and eosinophil adenoma. As pituitary adenomas grow, they replace normal glandular tissue and enlarge the sella turcica, which houses the pituitary gland. The prognosis is fair to good, depending on the extent to which the tumor spreads beyond the sella turcica.

Causes

The exact cause is unknown, but a predisposition to a pituitary tumor may be inherited through an autosomal dominant trait. A pituitary tumor isn't malignant in the strict sense; however, its invasive growth categorizes it as a neoplastic condition.

Chromophobe adenoma may be associated with production of corticotropin, melanocyte-stimulating hormone, growth hormone, and prolactin; basophil adenoma, with excess corticotropin production and, consequently, with Cushing's syndrome; and eosinophil adenoma, with excessive growth hormone.

Complications

The loss of pituitary hormone action results in endocrine abnormalities throughout the body if lost hormones are not replaced. Tumor compression of the hypothalamus may result in diabetes insipidus.

Assessment findings

The patient's history may reveal complaints related to neurologic and endocrine abnormalities. Typically, the patient complains of a frontal headache and visual disturbances (blurred vision progressing to field cuts and, eventually, blindness). The patient's family may describe personality changes or dementia. The patient may also report amenorrhea, decreased libido, impotence, lethargy, weakness, increased fatigability, sensitivity to cold, constipation (from decreased production of corticotropin and thyroid-stimulating hormone), and seizures.

Inspection may reveal rhinorrhea, a sign that the tumor has eroded the base of the skull. History and inspection may reveal cranial nerve (III, IV, VI) involvement from lateral extension of the tumor. With cranial nerve involvement, the patient typically reports diplopia and dizziness. You may observe head tilting to compensate for diplopia, conjugate deviation of gaze, nystagmus, eyelid ptosis, and limited eye movements.

Inspection may also disclose skin changes that indicate endocrine involvement. Examples include a waxy appearance, fewer wrinkles (which the patient may report during the history), and pubic and axillary hair loss.

Inspection of the eyes may reveal strabismus.

Diagnostic tests

• *Skull X-rays with tomography* may show an enlarged sella turcica or erosion of its floor. If growth hormone secretion predominates, X-ray findings show enlarged paranasal sinuses and mandible, thickened cranial bones, and separated teeth.
• *Carotid angiography* may identify displacement of the anterior cerebral and internal carotid arteries from tumor enlargement. This study can also rule out an intracerebral aneurysm.
• *Computed tomography scan* may confirm an adenoma and accurately depict its size.
• *Cerebrospinal fluid (CSF) analysis* may disclose increased protein levels.
• *Endocrine function tests* may or may not contribute helpful information. In many cases, results are ambiguous and inconclusive.
• *Magnetic resonance imaging scan* differentiates healthy, benign, and malignant tissues and blood vessels.

Treatment

Surgical options include transfrontal removal of large tumors impinging on the optic apparatus and transsphenoidal resection for smaller tumors confined to the pituitary fossa. Radiation therapy is the primary treatment for small, nonsecretory tumors confined to the sella turcica or for patients considered poor surgical risks. Otherwise, radiation is an adjunct to surgery, especially when only part of the tumor can be removed.

Postoperative measures include replacement therapy with corticosteroids or thyroid or sex hormones, correction of electrolyte imbalances and, as necessary, insulin therapy. Other drug therapy may include bromocriptine, an ergot derivative that shrinks prolactin-secreting and growth hormone–secreting tumors. Cyproheptadine, an antiserotonin drug, can reduce increased corticosteroid levels in Cushing's syndrome.

Cryohypophysectomy (freezing the area with a probe inserted transsphenoidally) is an alternative to surgical resection.

Nursing diagnoses
• Fatigue
• Impaired social interaction
• Ineffective family coping
• Ineffective individual coping
• Pain
• Risk for injury
• Sensory or perceptual alterations
• Sexual dysfunction

Nursing interventions
• Use the patient's comprehensive health history and physical assessment data as the baseline for later comparison.
• Establish a supportive, trusting relationship with the patient and family to help them cope with the diagnosis, treatment, and potential long-term consequences of this disease. Make sure they understand the need for lifelong health evaluations and, possibly, hormone replacement.
• Maintain a safe, clutter-free environment for the visually impaired or acromegalic patient. Reassure him that treatment will probably restore his eyesight.
• Provide for periods of rest to avoid undue fatigue.
• Administer analgesics, as ordered, to relieve headache.
   For a *supratentorial or transsphenoidal hypophysectomy:*
• Elevate the patient's head about 30 degrees to promote venous drainage from the head and reduce cerebral edema.
• Position the patient on his side to let secretions drain and to prevent aspiration.
• Withhold oral fluids, which may trigger vomiting and subsequently increase intracranial pressure (ICP). Don't allow a patient recovering from transsphenoidal surgery to blow his nose. Watch for CSF drainage from the nose, and monitor for signs of infection from the contaminated upper respiratory tract.
   For a *craniotomy:*
• Monitor vital signs.
• Perform a baseline neurologic assessment to use for planning further care and evaluating progress. Continuously assess level of consciousness.
• Maintain a patent airway, and suction as necessary.
• Give the patient nothing by mouth for 24 to 48 hours, to prevent aspiration or vomiting, which increases ICP.
• Observe for cerebral edema, bleeding, and CSF leakage.
• Provide a restful, quiet environment.

• Monitor intake and output to detect fluid and electrolyte imbalances.
• Reassure the patient that some symptoms caused by pituitary dysfunction, such as altered sex drive, impotence, infertility, hair loss, and emotional lability, will subside with treatment.

Patient teaching
• Provide necessary preoperative instruction, taking care that the patient understands the information and recognizes possible postoperative problems. Inform the patient having transsphenoidal surgery that he'll lose his sense of smell.
• If surgery (such as transsphenoidal hypophysectomy) will disrupt the patient's dura, caution him to avoid such activities as coughing, sneezing, and bending over. These may increase ICP or cause CSF leakage.
• Instruct the patient to immediately report a persistent postnasal drip or constant swallowing—signs of CSF drainage, not necessarily nasal drainage.
• Encourage the patient to wear a medical identification bracelet that identifies his hormonal condition and its proper treatment.

LARYNGEAL CANCER
Squamous cell carcinoma constitutes about 95% of laryngeal cancers. Rare laryngeal cancer forms—adenocarcinoma and sarcoma—account for the rest. The disease affects men about five times more often than women, and most victims are between ages 50 and 65.

   A tumor on the true vocal cord seldom spreads because underlying connective tissues lack lymph nodes. On the other hand, a tumor on another part of the larynx tends to spread early. Laryngeal cancer is classified by its location:
• supraglottis (false vocal cords)
• glottis (true vocal cords)
• subglottis (rare downward extension from vocal cords).

Causes
The cause of laryngeal cancer is unknown. Major risk factors include smoking and alcoholism. Minor risk factors include chronic inhalation of noxious fumes, familial disposition, and a history of frequent laryngitis and vocal straining.

Complications
Untreated, laryngeal cancer causes increasing swallowing difficulty and pain.

STAGING LARYNGEAL CANCER

Review the following classification developed by the American Joint Committee on Cancer. This TNM (tumor, node, metastasis) system helps define the advancement of your patient's laryngeal cancer and direct treatment. The T stages cover supraglottic, glottic, and subglottic tumors.

Primary tumor
TX—primary tumor can't be assessed
T0—no evidence of primary tumor
Tis—carcinoma in situ

Supraglottic tumor stages
T1—tumor confined to one subsite in supraglottis; vocal cords retain normal motion
T2—tumor extends to other sites in supraglottis, or to glottis; vocal cords retain motion
T3—tumor confined to larynx, but vocal cords lose motion; or tumor extends to the postcricoid area, the pyriform sinus, or the preepiglottic space, and vocal cords lose motion; or both
T4—tumor extends through thyroid cartilage, or extends to tissues beyond the larynx (such as the oropharynx or soft tissues of the neck), or both

Glottic tumor stages
T1—tumor confined to vocal cords, which retain normal motion; may involve anterior or posterior commissures
T2—tumor extends to supraglottis or subglottis or both; vocal cords may lose motion
T3—tumor confined to larynx, but vocal cords lose motion
T4—tumor extends through thyroid cartilage, or extends to tissue beyond the larynx (such as the oropharynx or soft tissues of the neck), or both

Subglottic tumor stages
T1—tumor confined to the subglottis
T2—tumor extends to vocal cords; vocal cords may lose motion
T3—tumor confined to larynx with vocal cord fixation
T4—tumor extends through cricoid or thyroid cartilage, or extends to tissues beyond the larynx (such as the oropharynx or soft tissues of the neck), or both

Regional lymph nodes
NX—regional lymph nodes can't be assessed
N0—no evidence of regional lymph node metastasis
N1—metastasis in a single ipsilateral lymph node, 3 cm or less in greatest dimension
N2—metastasis in one or more ipsilateral lymph nodes, or in bilateral or contralateral nodes, larger than 3 cm but less than 6 cm in greatest dimension
N3—metastasis in a node larger than 6 cm in greatest dimension

Distant metastasis
MX—distant metastasis can't be assessed
M0—no evidence of distant metastasis
M1—distant metastasis

Staging categories
Laryngeal cancer progresses from mild to severe as follows:
Stage 0—Tis, N0, M0
Stage I—T1, N0, M0
Stage II—T2, N0, M0
Stage III—T3, N0, M0; T1, N1, M0; T2, N1, M0; T3, N1, M0
Stage IV—T4, N0 or N1, M0; any T, N2 or N3, M0; any T, any N, M1

Assessment findings
Varied assessment findings in laryngeal cancer depend on the tumor's location and its stage. (See *Staging laryngeal cancer.*)

With Stage I disease, the patient may complain of local throat irritation or hoarseness that lasts about 2 weeks. In Stages II and III, he usually reports hoarseness. He may also have a sore throat, and his voice volume may be reduced to a stage whisper. In Stage IV, he typically reports pain radiating to his ear, dysphagia, and dyspnea. In advanced (Stage IV) disease, palpation may detect a neck mass or enlarged cervical lymph nodes.

Diagnostic tests
The usual workup includes laryngoscopy, xeroradiography, biopsy, laryngeal tomography and computed tomography scans, and laryngography to visualize and define the tumor and its borders. Chest X-ray findings can help detect metastases.

Treatment
Early lesions may respond to laser surgery or radiation therapy; advanced lesions to laser surgery, radiation therapy, and chemotherapy. Treatment aims to eliminate cancer and preserve speech. If speech preservation isn't possible, speech rehabilitation may include esophageal speech or prosthetic devices. (See *Reviewing alternative*

REVIEWING ALTERNATIVE SPEECH METHODS

During convalescence, your patient may work with a speech pathologist who can teach him new ways to speak, using various communication techniques, such as the following.

Esophageal speech

By drawing air in through the mouth, trapping it in the upper esophagus, and releasing it slowly while forming words, the patient can again communicate by voice. With training and practice, a highly motivated patient can master esophageal speech in about a month. Recognize that speech will sound choppy at first, but with increasing skill, words will flow more smoothly and understandably.

Because esophageal speech requires strength, an elderly patient or one with asthma or emphysema may find it too physically demanding to learn. And because it also requires frequent sessions with a speech pathologist, a chronically ill patient may find esophageal speech overwhelming.

Artificial larynges

The throat vibrator and the Cooper-Rand device are basic artificial larynges. Both types vibrate to produce speech that's easy to understand, although it sounds monotonous and mechanical.

Tell the patient to operate a throat vibrator by holding it in place against his neck. A pulsating disk in the device vibrates the throat tissue as the patient forms words with his mouth. The throat vibrator may be difficult to use immediately after surgery, when the patient's neck wounds are still sore.

The Cooper-Rand device vibrates sounds piped into the patient's mouth through a thin tube, which the patient positions in the corner of his mouth. Easy to use, this device may be preferred soon after surgery.

Surgically implanted prostheses

Most surgical implants generate speech by vibrating when the patient manually closes the tracheostomy, forcing air upward. One such device is the Blom-Singer voice prosthesis. Only hours after it's inserted through an incision in the stoma, the patient can speak in a normal voice. The surgeon may implant the device when radiation therapy ends or within a few days (or even years) after laryngectomy.

To speak, the patient covers his stoma while exhaling. Exhaled air travels through the trachea, passes through an airflow port on the bottom of the prosthesis, and exits through a slit at the esophageal end of the prosthesis. This creates the vibrations needed to produce sound.

Not all patients are eligible for tracheoesophageal puncture, the procedure needed to insert the prosthesis. Considerations include the extent of the laryngectomy; pharyngoesophageal muscle status; stomal size and location; and the patient's mental and emotional status, visual and auditory acuity, hand-eye coordination, bimanual dexterity, and self-care skills.

---

speech methods.) Surgical techniques to construct a new voice box are experimental.

In early disease, laser surgery destroys precancerous lesions; in advanced disease, it can help clear obstructions. Other surgical procedures vary with tumor size and include cordectomy, partial or total laryngectomy, supraglottic laryngectomy, and total laryngectomy with laryngoplasty.

Radiation therapy alone or combined with surgery can create complications, including airway obstruction, pain, and loss of taste (xerostomia).

Chemotherapy is minimally beneficial in treating laryngeal cancer.

Nursing diagnoses

- Anxiety
- Body image disturbance
- Energy field disturbance
- Impaired gas exchange
- Impaired skin integrity
- Impaired swallowing
- Impaired verbal communication
- Ineffective airway clearance
- Ineffective breathing pattern
- Ineffective individual coping
- Knowledge deficit
- Pain
- Risk for infection

Nursing interventions

- Provide supportive psychological, preoperative, and postoperative care to minimize complications and speed recovery.
- If the patient is scheduled to undergo chemotherapy, you'll need to assess his bone marrow and pulmonary function before treatment begins. Once chemotherapy is under way, reassess these important functions. If moderate impairment results from folate deficiency, reduce

RECOGNIZING AND MANAGING COMPLICATIONS OF LARYNGEAL SURGERY

Once your patient returns from surgery, you'll need to monitor his recovery, watching carefully for complications, such as fistula formation, a ruptured carotid artery, and stenosis of the tracheostomy site.

Fistula formation
Warning signs of fistula formation include redness, swelling, and secretions on the suture line. The fistula may form between the reconstructed hypopharynx and the skin. This eventually heals spontaneously, although the process may take weeks or months.

Feed the patient who has a fistula through a nasogastric tube. Otherwise, food will leak through the fistula and delay healing.

Ruptured carotid artery
Bleeding, a cardinal sign of a ruptured carotid artery, may occur in a patient who received preoperative radiation therapy or in a patient with a fistula that constantly bathes the carotid artery with oral secretions.

If rupture occurs, apply pressure to the site. Call for help immediately, and take the patient to the operating room for carotid ligation.

Tracheostomy stenosis
Constant shortness of breath alerts you to this complication, which may occur weeks to months after laryngectomy.

Management includes fitting the patient with successively larger tracheostomy tubes until he can tolerate insertion of a full-sized one.

the dose, as ordered. Also, monitor for renal toxicity related to chemotherapy.
• Encourage the patient to voice his concerns before surgery. Help him choose a temporary, alternative way to communicate, such as writing or using sign language or an alphabet board. If appropriate, arrange for a laryngectomee to visit him.

After *partial laryngectomy:*
• Give I.V. fluids and, usually, tube feedings for the first 2 days after surgery; then resume oral fluids. Keep the tracheostomy tube (inserted during surgery) in place until tissue edema subsides.
• Make sure the patient doesn't use his voice until the doctor gives permission (usually 2 to 3 days postoperatively). Then caution the patient to whisper until he heals completely.

After *total laryngectomy:*
• As soon as the patient returns to his room from surgery, position him on his side and elevate his head 30 to 45 degrees. When you move him, remember to support the back of his neck to prevent tension on sutures and, possibly, wound dehiscence.
• If the patient has a laryngectomy tube in place, care for it as you would a tracheostomy tube. Shorter and thicker than a tracheostomy tube, the laryngectomy tube stays in place until the stoma heals (about 7 to 10 days).
• Watch the stoma for crusting and secretions, which can cause skin breakdown. To prevent crusting, provide adequate room humidification. Remove crusts with petrolatum, antimicrobial ointment, and moist gauze.

• Monitor vital signs. Be especially alert for fever, which indicates infection. Record fluid intake and output, and watch for dehydration. Also, be alert for and report postoperative complications. (See *Recognizing and managing complications of laryngeal surgery.*)
• Provide frequent mouth care. Clean the patient's tongue and the sides of his mouth with a soft toothbrush or a terry washcloth, and rinse his mouth with a deodorizing mouthwash.
• Suction gently. Unless ordered otherwise, do not attempt deep suctioning, which could penetrate the suture line. Suction through both the tube and the patient's nose because the patient can no longer blow air through his nose. Suction his mouth gently.
• After inserting a drainage catheter (usually connected to a blood drainage system or a GI drainage system), don't stop suction without the doctor's consent. After removing the catheter, check the dressings for drainage.
• Give analgesics, as ordered. Keep in mind that opioid analgesics depress respiration and inhibit coughing.
• If the doctor orders nasogastric (NG) tube feeding, check tube placement, and elevate the patient's head to prevent aspiration. Be ready to perform suction after NG tube removal or oral fluid intake because the patient may have difficulty swallowing.
• Support the patient through inevitable grieving. If his depression becomes severe, consider referring him for appropriate counseling.

Patient teaching

• Before partial or total laryngectomy, instruct the patient in good oral hygiene practices. If appropriate, instruct a male patient to shave off his beard to facilitate postoperative care.

• Explain postoperative procedures, such as suctioning, NG tube feeding, and laryngectomy tube care. Carefully discuss the effects of these procedures (breathing through the neck and speech alteration, for example).

• Also, prepare the patient for other functional losses. Forewarn him that he won't be able to smell aromas, blow his nose, whistle, gargle, sip, or suck on a straw.

• Reassure the patient that speech rehabilitation measures (including laryngeal speech, esophageal speech, an artificial larynx, and various mechanical devices) may help him communicate again.

• Encourage the patient to take advantage of services and information offered by the American Speech-Learning-Hearing Association, the International Association of Laryngectomees, the American Cancer Society, or the local chapter of the Lost Chord Club.

THYROID CANCER

Although thyroid cancer occurs in all age-groups, patients who have had radiation therapy in the neck area are especially susceptible. Before the 1950s, radiation therapy was commonly given to children to shrink enlarged thymus glands, tonsils, or adenoids and to treat acne and other skin disorders. About 25% of those who had these treatments later developed thyroid nodules; 25% of those nodules became malignant.

The risk of developing a malignant tumor after radiation correlates with the dose (a threshold dose has not been defined) and the patient's age (a malignant tumor is rare in patients who begin radiation therapy after age 21). Papillary and follicular carcinomas are the most common forms of thyroid cancers and are usually associated with the longest survival times.

Papillary carcinoma accounts for about 60% of thyroid cancer in adults. It can occur at any age but is most common in women of childbearing age. Usually multifocal and bilateral, it metastasizes slowly into regional nodes of the neck, mediastinum, lungs, and other distant organs. It is the least virulent form of thyroid cancer.

Less common (about 20% of all cases), follicular carcinoma is more likely to recur and metastasize to the regional lymph nodes and spread through blood vessels into the bones, liver, and lungs.

Medullary (solid) carcinoma originates in the parafollicular cells derived from the last branchial pouch and contains amyloid and calcium deposits. It can produce calcitonin, histaminase, corticotropin (producing Cushing's syndrome), and prostaglandin E_2 and F_3 (producing diarrhea). This form of thyroid cancer is familial, possibly inherited as an autosomal dominant trait, and usually associated with pheochromocytoma. A rare (5%) form of thyroid cancer, it typically occurs in women over age 40. It is curable when detected before it causes symptoms. Untreated, it grows rapidly, frequently metastasizing to bones, liver, and kidneys.

Anaplastic carcinoma resists radiation and is almost never curable by resection. This cancer metastasizes rapidly, causing death by invading the trachea and compressing adjacent structures. It accounts for between 10% and 15% of thyroid cancers and occurs most often in patients over age 60.

Causes

Besides exposure to radiation, suspected causes of thyroid cancer include prolonged secretion of thyroid-stimulating hormone (TSH) (through radiation or heredity), familial predisposition, and chronic goiter.

Complications

Dysphagia and stridor are typical complications of thyroid cancer—especially in untreated disease. They usually result from pressure caused by a space-occupying lesion that extends into neck structures. Additional complications include hormone alterations and distant metastases.

Assessment findings

The first indication of disease may be a painless nodule discovered incidentally or detected during physical examination.

If the tumor grows large enough to destroy the thyroid gland, the patient's history may include sensitivity to cold and mental apathy (hypothyroidism). If the tumor triggers excess thyroid hormone production, the patient may report sensitivity to heat, restlessness, and overactivity (hyperthyroidism). The patient may also complain of diarrhea, dysphagia, anorexia, irritability, and ear pain. When speaking with the patient, you may hear hoarseness and vocal stridor.

On inspection, you may detect a disfiguring thyroid mass, especially if the patient is in the later stages of anaplastic thyroid cancer. (See *Anaplastic thyroid cancer,* page 304.)

Palpation may disclose a hard nodule in an enlarged thyroid gland or palpable lymph nodes with thyroid enlargement.

ANAPLASTIC THYROID CANCER

The most disfiguring, destructive, and deadly form of thyroid cancer, anaplastic carcinoma has the poorest prognosis. Although this tumor rarely metastasizes to distant organs, its rapid growth and size produce severe anatomic distortion of nearby structures. Treatment usually consists of total thyroidectomy, which seldom is successful.

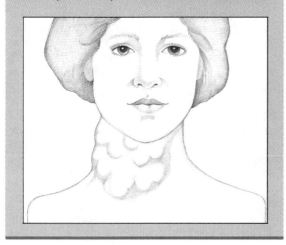

By auscultation, you may discover bruits if thyroid enlargement results from an increase in TSH, which increases thyroid vascularity.

Diagnostic tests
• *Fine-needle aspiration biopsy* may help to differentiate benign from malignant thyroid nodules. And histologic analysis will help to stage the disease and guide treatment. (See *Staging thyroid cancer.*)
• *Thyroid scan* may differentiate functional nodes (rarely malignant) from hypofunctional nodes (commonly malignant) by measuring how readily nodules trap isotopes compared with the rest of the thyroid gland. In thyroid cancer, scintigraphy findings may demonstrate a "cold," nonfunctioning nodule.
• *Ultrasonography* evaluates changes in the size of thyroid nodules after thyroxine suppression therapy, guides fine-needle aspiration, and detects recurrent disease.
• *Magnetic resonance imaging* and *computed tomography scans* provide information for treatment planning because they establish the extent of the disease within the thyroid and in surrounding structures.
• *Calcitonin assay* is a reliable clue to silent medullary carcinoma. The calcitonin level is measured during a

resting state and during a calcium infusion (15 mg/kg) over a 4-hour period. An elevated fasting calcitonin level and an abnormal response to calcium stimulation—a high release of calcitonin from the node in comparison with the rest of the gland—are indicative of medullary cancer.

Treatment
Surgery is recommended initially for all forms of thyroid cancer, but the extent of surgery and the postoperative treatments vary. Ideally before surgery, the patient should have normal thyroid function (euthyroid) as demonstrated by normal thyroid function tests, pulse rate, and electrocardiogram.

Treatment may include one or a combination of the following:
• total or subtotal thyroidectomy with modified node dissection (bilateral or homolateral) on the side of the primary cancer (for papillary or follicular cancer)
• total thyroidectomy and radical neck excision (for medullary or anaplastic cancer)
• radioisotope (iodine 131) therapy with external radiation (sometimes postoperatively in lieu of radical neck excision) or alone (for metastasis)
• adjunctive thyroid suppression (with exogenous thyroid hormones suppressing TSH production) and simultaneous administration of an adrenergic blocking agent, such as propranolol, to increase tolerance to surgery and radiation therapy
• chemotherapy limited to treating symptoms of widespread metastasis, as a palliative measure; doxorubicin has some antitumor activity in about 20% of cases.

Nursing diagnoses
• Altered nutrition: Less than body requirements
• Anxiety
• Body image disturbance
• Diarrhea
• Impaired gas exchange
• Impaired skin integrity
• Impaired swallowing
• Impaired verbal communication
• Pain

Nursing interventions
• Prepare the patient for scheduled surgery.
• Encourage the patient to voice his concerns, and offer reassurance.
• Before surgery, establish a way for the patient to communicate postoperatively (pad and pencil, head nodding for yes and no, or other ways).

STAGING THYROID CANCER

Thyroid cancer classifications signify the tumor's (T) size and extent at its origin, its invasion of regional (cervical and upper mediastinal) lymph nodes (N), and the disease's spread or metastasis (M) to other structures. After accumulating data about the tumor and its spread, staging further defines the disease process.

The following summarizes the classification and staging systems adopted by the American Joint Committee on Cancer.

Primary tumor
TX—primary tumor can't be assessed
T0—no evidence of primary tumor
T1—tumor 1 cm or less in greatest dimension and limited to the thyroid
T2—tumor more than 1 cm but less than 4 cm in greatest dimension and limited to the thyroid
T3—tumor more than 4 cm and limited to the thyroid
T4—tumor (any size) extends beyond the thyroid

Regional lymph nodes
NX—regional lymph nodes can't be assessed
N0—no evidence of regional lymph node metastasis
N1—regional lymph node metastasis
N1a—metastasis in ipsilateral cervical nodes
N1b—metastasis in bilateral, midline, or contralateral cervical or mediastinal lymph nodes

Distant metastasis
MX—distant metastasis can't be assessed
M0—no evidence of distant metastasis
M1—distant metastasis

Staging categories for papillary or follicular cancer
Papillary or follicular cancer progresses from mild to severe as follows:
Stage I—any T, any N, M0 (patient under age 45); T1, N0, M0 (patient age 45 or over)
Stage II—any T, any N, M1 (patient under age 45); T2, N0, M0; T3, N0, M0 (patient age 45 or over)
Stage III—T4, N0, M0; any T, N1, M0 (patient age 45 or over)
Stage IV—any T, any N, M1 (patient age 45 or over)

Staging categories for medullary cancer
Medullary cancer progresses from mild to severe as follows:
Stage I—T1, N0, M0
Stage II—T2, N0, M0; T3, N0, M0; T4, N0, M0
Stage III—any T, N1, M0
Stage IV—any T, any N, M1

Staging categories for undifferentiated cancer
All cases are Stage IV.
Stage IV—any T, any N, any M

Take the following steps postoperatively:
• When the patient regains consciousness, keep him in the semi-Fowler's position. To avoid pressure on the suture line, his head should be neither hyperextended nor flexed. Support his head and neck with sandbags and pillows. When you move him, continue this support with your hands.
• After monitoring vital signs, check the patient's dressing, neck, and back for blood. If he complains that the dressing feels tight, loosen it and call the doctor immediately.
• Check serum calcium levels daily because hypocalcemia may develop if the parathyroid glands were removed.
• Watch for and report other complications—for example, hemorrhage and shock (elevated pulse rate and hypotension), tetany (carpopedal spasm, twitching, seizures), thyroid storm (high fever, severe tachycardia, delirium, dehydration, and extreme irritability), and respiratory obstruction (dyspnea, crowing respirations, retraction of neck tissues).

• Keep a tracheotomy set and oxygen equipment handy for use if respiratory obstruction occurs. Use continuous steam inhalation in the patient's room until his chest sounds clear.
• Administer pain medications, as ordered, and make sure that the patient feels as comfortable as possible.
• Provide I.V. fluids or a soft diet, as needed. Many patients can tolerate a regular diet within 24 hours of surgery.
• Provide the same postsurgical care after extensive tumor and node excision as you would after radical neck surgery.

Patient teaching
• Preoperatively, advise the patient to expect temporary voice loss or hoarseness for several days after surgery. Also, explain the operation and postoperative procedures and positioning.
• Before discharge, ensure that the patient knows the date and time of his next appointment. Answer his questions about his treatment and home care. Be sure he un-

derstands the purpose of his medications, dosage, administration times, and possible adverse effects.
• Refer the patient to resource and support services, such as the social service department, home health care agencies, hospices, and the American Cancer Society.

SPINAL NEOPLASMS

Similar to intracranial tumors but involving the spinal cord or its roots, untreated spinal neoplasms can eventually cause paralysis. As primary tumors, they originate in the meningeal coverings, the parenchyma of the cord or its roots, the intraspinal vasculature, or the vertebrae. They can also occur as metastatic foci from primary tumors, but death usually results from the primary condition.

Primary tumors of the spinal cord may be extramedullary (occurring outside the spinal cord) or intramedullary (occurring within the cord). Extramedullary tumors may be intradural (meningiomas and schwannomas) and account for about 60% of all primary spinal cord neoplasms. Extramedullary tumors may also be extradural (metastatic tumors from breasts, lungs, prostate, leukemia, or lymphomas) and account for about 25% of these neoplasms.

Intramedullary tumors, or gliomas (astrocytomas or ependymomas), are comparatively rare and account for only about 10% of spinal neoplasms. In children, these lesions are low-grade astrocytomas.

Spinal cord tumors are rare compared with intracranial tumors (ratio of 1:4). They occur with equal frequency in men and women, except for meningiomas, which occur more often in women. Spinal cord tumors can grow anywhere along the cord or its roots.

The prognosis depends on tumor control and the extent of residual neurologic deficit.

Causes

Little is known about the cause of spinal cord tumors. They have been associated with central von Recklinghausen's disease, however, and research is ongoing.

Complications

Motor and sensory deficits range from weakness to paralysis as the disease progresses. They may lead to loss of sphincter control and subsequent bladder and bowel dysfunction.

In late stages of disease, especially with paralysis, the complications of immobility, such as skin breakdown, may occur. Other complications depend on the tumor's location. For example, respiratory problems occur in high cervical tumors, whereas chronic urinary tract problems are associated with tumors lower in the spine.

Assessment findings

Because the spinal cord adjusts to a slow-growing tumor, a tumor may grow for several years and produce minimal neurologic signs. The patient's history, however, may reveal pain described as most severe directly over the tumor and radiating around the trunk or down the limb on the affected side. The patient may report that few measures relieve the pain, not even bed rest. Some patients also complain of constipation.

In the early stages, the patient may express difficulty in emptying the bladder or notice changes in the urinary stream. If you suspect a spinal cord tumor, ask the patient about bladder emptying because many patients overlook or dismiss this sign.

In later stages, urine retention is an inevitable sign of spinal cord compression. If the patient has a cauda equina tumor, he may report bladder and bowel incontinence, usually resulting from flaccid paralysis.

On inspection and palpation, you may find symmetrical spastic weakness, decreased muscle tone, exaggerated reflexes, and a positive Babinski's sign. If the tumor is at the cauda equina level, you may notice muscle wasting. Palpation may reveal muscle flaccidity, wasting, weakness, and progressive diminution in tendon reflexes.

Neurologic examination may disclose contralateral loss of sensation to pain, temperature, and touch (Brown-Séquard syndrome). These losses are less obvious to the patient than functional motor changes. Caudal lesions invariably produce parasthesias in the nerve pathways of the involved roots.

Diagnostic tests

• *Lumbar puncture* reveals clear yellow cerebrospinal fluid (CSF), resulting from increased protein levels if the flow is completely blocked. If the flow is partially blocked, protein levels rise, but the fluid appears only slightly yellow in proportion to the CSF protein level. A Papanicolaou test of the CSF may show malignant cells of metastatic carcinoma.
• *X-rays* show distortions of the intervertebral foramina; changes in the vertebrae or collapsed areas in the vertebral body; and localized enlargement of the spinal canal, indicating an adjacent blockage.
• *Myelography* identifies the lesion's level by outlining the tumor if it causes a partial obstruction. The myelogram shows the anatomic relation to the cord and the dura. If the tumor causes a complete obstruction, the injected

contrast agent can't flow past the tumor. This study is dangerous in instances of nearly complete cord compression because withdrawn or escaping CSF will allow the tumor to exert greater pressure against the cord.
• *Radioisotope bone scan* demonstrates metastatic invasion of the vertebrae by detecting a characteristic increase in osteoblastic activity.
• *Computed tomography* and *magnetic resonance imaging scans* show cord compression and tumor location.
• *Frozen section biopsy* performed during surgery identifies the tissue type.

Treatment

Spinal cord tumors are treated with decompression or radiation therapy. Not usually indicated for metastatic tumors, laminectomy may be done for primary tumors that produce spinal cord or cauda equina compression. If the tumor progresses slowly or if it's treated before the cord degenerates from compression, signs and symptoms are likely to subside and function may be restored.

In a patient with metastatic carcinoma or lymphoma who suddenly experiences complete transverse myelitis with spinal shock, functional improvement is unlikely, even with treatment. This patient's prognosis is poor.

If the patient has incomplete paraplegia of rapid onset, emergency surgical decompression may save cord function. Steroid therapy may minimize cord edema until he undergoes surgery.

Partial removal of intramedullary gliomas, followed by radiation therapy, may temporarily ease signs and symptoms. Metastatic extradural tumors can be controlled with radiation therapy, analgesics and, in hormone-mediated tumors (breast and prostate), appropriate hormone therapy.

Transcutaneous electrical nerve stimulation (TENS) may relieve radicular pain from spinal cord tumors and is a useful alternative to opioid analgesics. TENS works by applying an electrical charge to the skin, thereby stimulating large-diameter nerve fibers and inhibiting the transmission of pain impulses along nerve fibers.

The risk of infection is increased by treatment in many cases, but the risk also increases as the patient's condition deteriorates.

Nursing diagnoses

• Altered urinary elimination
• Anxiety
• Constipation
• Impaired physical mobility
• Impaired skin integrity
• Ineffective breathing pattern
• Ineffective family coping
• Ineffective individual coping
• Knowledge deficit
• Pain
• Risk for infection
• Risk for injury
• Total incontinence

Nursing interventions

• Set up the patient's care plan to foster emotional support and skilled intervention during acute and chronic disease phases. Aim for early recognition of recurrence, prevention or treatment of complications, and maintenance of the quality of life.
• Use the baseline data from the initial neurologic evaluation to help plan future care and evaluate changes in the patient's clinical status.
• Encourage the patient to voice his concerns about his illness and treatment. Answer any questions. Provide brief, easy-to-understand explanations before performing procedures.
• Recognize that the patient needs emotional support, rehabilitation (including bowel and bladder retraining), and medications and other measures to relieve pain. Prevent infection and skin breakdown.
• If the patient experiences urine retention, provide necessary care, such as intermittent catheterization or indwelling urinary catheter care. Monitor intake and output as needed. If the patient has constipation, administer laxatives and enemas, as ordered.
• After laminectomy, perform neurologic checks frequently. Change the patient's position by logrolling. Administer analgesics, as ordered, monitor for signs of infection, and assist the patient in early walking.
• Institute safety precautions for the patient with impaired sensation and motor deficits. Use side rails if the patient is bedridden. If he's not, encourage him to wear flat shoes for walking. Remove scatter rugs and clutter to prevent falls.
• Encourage the patient to perform daily activities as independently as possible. To avoid aggravating pain, move the patient slowly, making sure his body is aligned properly when you give personal care.
• If the patient has respiratory problems, provide rest periods between activities. Provide oxygen, as ordered, and assist him into a position that allows maximal chest expansion.
• After radiation therapy, administer steroid and antacid medications, as ordered, for spinal cord edema. Monitor for sensory or motor dysfunction (which indicates the need for increased steroid therapy).

• Enforce bed rest for the patient who has vertebral body involvement until the doctor says he can safely walk. Body weight alone can cause vertebral column collapse and cord laceration from bone fragments.
• Logroll and position the patient on his side every 2 hours to prevent pressure ulcers and other complications of immobility.
• If the patient requires a back brace, make sure he wears it whenever he gets out of bed.
• Help the patient and his family to understand and cope with the spinal tumor diagnosis, treatment, potential disabilities, and necessary changes in life-style.

Patient teaching
• Refer the patient, family, and close friends to support groups, the social service department, and home health care agencies, as appropriate.
• Instruct the patient and family in the care the patient requires, including how to administer medications, maintain skin integrity, reduce discomfort (for example, by using TENS to block radicular pain), prevent infection and injury, and cope with incontinence.

THORACIC NEOPLASMS

The lung and breast are the most common sites for thoracic cancer. Although rare, soft-tissue sarcomas may also develop in the chest region.

LUNG CANCER
The most common forms of lung cancer are squamous cell (epidermoid) carcinoma, small-cell (oat cell) carcinoma, adenocarcinoma, and large-cell (anaplastic) carcinoma. The most common site is the wall or epithelium of the bronchial tree.

For most patients, the prognosis is poor, depending on the cancer's extent when diagnosed and the cells' growth rate. Only about 13% of patients with lung cancer survive 5 years after diagnosis. Although the disease is largely preventable, it's the most common cause of cancer death in men. In women, lung cancer ranks with breast cancer as a leading cause of death.

Causes
Lung cancer's exact cause remains unclear. Risk factors include tobacco smoking, exposure to carcinogenic and industrial air pollutants (asbestos, arsenic, chromium, coal dust, iron oxides, nickel, radioactive dust, and uranium), and genetic predisposition.

Complications
Disease progression and metastasis cause various complications. When the primary tumor spreads to intrathoracic structures, complications may include tracheal obstruction; esophageal compression with dysphagia; phrenic nerve paralysis with hemidiaphragm elevation and dyspnea; sympathetic nerve paralysis with Horner's syndrome; eighth cervical and first thoracic nerve compression with ulnar and Pancoast's syndrome (shoulder pain radiating to the ulnar nerve pathways); lymphatic obstruction with pleural effusion; and hypoxemia. Other complications are anorexia and weight loss, sometimes leading to cachexia, digital clubbing, and hypertrophic osteoarthropathy. Endocrine syndromes may involve production of hormones and hormone precursors.

Assessment findings
Because early lung cancer may cause no symptoms, the disease may be advanced when it's diagnosed. While taking the patient's history, be sure to assess his exposure to carcinogens. If he's a smoker, determine pack years. (See *Determining pack years.*)

The patient's chief complaints may include coughing (induced by tumor stimulation of nerve endings), hemoptysis, dyspnea (from the tumor occluding air flow) and, sometimes, hoarseness (from tumor or tumor-bearing lymph nodes pressing on the laryngeal nerve).

On inspection, you may notice the patient become short of breath when he walks or exerts himself. You may also observe finger clubbing; edema of the face, neck, and upper torso; dilated chest and abdominal veins (superior vena cava syndrome); weight loss; and fatigue.

Palpation may reveal enlarged lymph nodes and an enlarged liver. Percussion findings may include dullness over the lung fields in a patient with pleural effusion.

Auscultation may disclose decreased breath sounds, wheezing, and pleural friction rub (with pleural effusion).

Diagnostic tests
• *Chest X-rays* usually show an advanced lesion and can detect a lesion up to 2 years before signs and symptoms appear. Findings may indicate tumor size and location.
• *Cytologic sputum analysis,* which is 75% reliable, requires a sputum specimen expectorated from the lungs and tracheobronchial tree, *not* from postnasal secretions or saliva.

• *Bronchoscopy* can identify the tumor site. Bronchoscopic washings provide material for cytologic and histologic study. The flexible fiber-optic bronchoscope increases test effectiveness.
• *Needle biopsy* of the lungs relies on biplanar fluoroscopic visual control to locate peripheral tumors before withdrawing a tissue specimen for analysis. This procedure allows a firm diagnosis in 80% of patients.
• *Tissue biopsy* of metastatic sites (including supraclavicular and mediastinal nodes and pleura) helps to assess disease extent. Based on histologic findings, staging determines the disease's extent and prognosis and helps direct treatment. (See *Staging lung cancer,* page 310.)
• *Thoracentesis* allows chemical and cytologic examination of pleural fluid.

Additional studies include chest tomography, bronchography, esophagography, and angiocardiography (contrast studies of bronchial tree, esophagus, and cardiovascular tissues). Tests to detect metastasis include a bone scan (abnormal findings may lead to a bone marrow biopsy, which is typically recommended in patients with small-cell carcinoma); a computed tomography scan of the brain; liver function studies; and gallium scans of the liver and spleen.

Treatment

Various combinations of surgery, radiation therapy, and chemotherapy improve the prognosis and prolong patient survival. Because lung cancer is usually advanced at diagnosis, most treatment is palliative.

Surgery is the primary treatment for Stage I, Stage II, or selected Stage III squamous cell carcinoma, adenocarcinoma, and large-cell carcinoma, unless the tumor is inoperable or other conditions (such as cardiac disease) rule out surgery. Surgery may involve partial lung removal (wedge resection, segmental resection, lobectomy, radical lobectomy) or total removal (pneumonectomy, radical pneumonectomy).

Preoperative radiation therapy may reduce tumor bulk to allow for surgical resection and may also improve response rates. Radiation therapy is ordinarily recommended for Stage I and Stage II lesions if surgery is contraindicated, and for Stage III disease confined to the involved hemithorax and the ipsilateral supraclavicular lymph nodes. Radiation therapy usually begins about 1 month after surgery (to allow the wound to heal). It's directed to the chest area most likely to develop metastasis.

Chemotherapy drug combinations of fluorouracil, vincristine, mitomycin, cisplatin, and vindesine induce a response rate, ranging from 30% to 50%, yet have minimal

DETERMINING PACK YEARS

Patients who smoke cigarettes are at a higher risk for such respiratory diseases as lung cancer, emphysema, and bronchitis. Use the following formula to calculate pack years and assess a patient's risk for lung disease: pack years = number of packs smoked daily × number of years smoked.

For example, a patient who smokes two packs of cigarettes daily for 42 years has accumulated 84 pack years.

Normally, the more pack years, the greater the risk for lung disease.

effect on long-term survival. Promising combinations of drugs for treating small-cell carcinomas include cyclophosphamide, doxorubicin, and vincristine; cyclophosphamide, doxorubicin, vincristine, and etoposide; and etoposide, cisplatin, cyclophosphamide, and doxorubicin.

Immunotherapy is investigational. Nonspecific regimens using bacille Calmette-Guérin (BCG) vaccine or, possibly, *Corynebacterium parvum* offer the most promise.

In laser therapy, also largely investigational, a laser beam is directed through a bronchoscope to destroy local tumors.

Nursing diagnoses
• Altered nutrition: Less than body requirements
• Anxiety
• Fatigue
• Fluid volume deficit
• Impaired gas exchange
• Impaired physical mobility
• Impaired skin integrity
• Ineffective airway clearance
• Ineffective breathing pattern
• Knowledge deficit
• Pain
• Risk for infection
• Risk for injury

Nursing interventions
• Give comprehensive supportive care and provide patient teaching to minimize complications and speed the patient's recovery from surgery, radiation therapy, and chemotherapy.

STAGING LUNG CANCER

Using the TNM (tumor, node, metastasis) classification system, the American Joint Committee on Cancer stages lung cancer as follows.

Primary tumor
TX—primary tumor can't be assessed, or malignant tumor cells detected in sputum or bronchial washings but undetected by X-ray or bronchoscopy
T0—no evidence of primary tumor
Tis—carcinoma in situ
T1—tumor 3 cm or less in greatest dimension, surrounded by normal lung or visceral pleura; no bronchoscopic evidence of cancer closer to the center of the body than the lobar bronchus
T2—tumor larger than 3 cm; or one that involves the main bronchus and is 2 cm or more from the carina; or one that invades the visceral pleura; or one that's accompanied by atelectasis or obstructive pneumonitis that extends to the hilar region but doesn't involve the entire lung
T3—tumor of any size that extends into neighboring structures, such as the chest wall, diaphragm, or mediastinal pleura; or tumor in the main bronchus that doesn't involve but is less than 2 cm from the carina; or tumor that's accompanied by atelectasis or obstructive pneumonitis of the entire lung
T4—tumor of any size that invades the mediastinum, heart, great vessels, trachea, esophagus, vertebral body, or carina; or tumor with malignant pleural effusion

Regional lymph nodes
NX—regional lymph nodes can't be assessed
N0—no detectable metastasis to lymph nodes
N1—metastasis to the ipsilateral peribronchial or hilar lymph nodes or both
N2—metastasis to the ipsilateral mediastinal and the subcarinal lymph nodes or both
N3—metastasis to the contralateral mediastinal or hilar lymph nodes, the ipsilateral or the contralateral scalene, or the supraclavicular lymph nodes

Distant metastasis
MX—distant metastasis can't be assessed
M0—no evidence of distant metastasis
M1—distant metastasis

Staging categories
Lung cancer progresses from mild to severe as follows:
Occult carcinoma—TX, N0, M0
Stage 0—Tis, N0, M0
Stage I—T1, N0, M0; T2, N0, M0
Stage II—T1, N1, M0; T2, N1, M0
Stage IIIA—T1, N2, M0; T2, N2, M0; T3, N0, M0; T3, N1, M0; T3, N2, M0
Stage IIIB—any T, N3, M0; T4, any N, M0
Stage IV—any T, any N, M1

• Urge the patient to voice his concerns, and schedule time to answer his questions. Be sure to explain procedures before performing them. This will help reduce the patient's anxiety.
• Before and after surgery give ordered analgesics as necessary.

After *thoracic surgery:*
• Maintain a patent airway, and monitor chest tubes to reestablish normal intrathoracic pressure and prevent postoperative and pulmonary complications.
• Check vital signs and watch for and report abnormal respiration and other changes.
• Suction the patient often, and encourage him to begin deep breathing and coughing as soon as possible. Check secretions often. Initially, sputum will appear thick and dark with blood, but it should become thinner and grayish yellow within 1 day.
• Monitor and document amount and color of closed chest drainage. Keep chest tubes patent and draining effectively. Watch for fluctuation in the water seal chamber on inspiration and expiration, indicating that the chest tube remains patent. Watch for air leaks, and report them immediately. Position the patient on the surgical side to promote drainage and lung reexpansion.
• Watch for and report any foul-smelling discharge or excessive drainage on surgical dressings. Usually, you'll remove the dressing after 24 hours, unless the wound appears infected.
• Monitor intake and output. Maintain adequate hydration.
• Watch for and be prepared to treat infection, shock, hemorrhage, atelectasis, dyspnea, mediastinal shift, and pulmonary embolus.
• To help prevent pulmonary embolus, apply antiembolism stockings, and encourage the patient to perform range-of-motion exercises.

For *chemotherapy:*
• Ask the dietary department to provide soft, nonirritating, protein-rich foods. Encourage the patient to eat high-calorie, between-meal snacks.
• Give antiemetics and antidiarrheals, as needed.

• Schedule patient care to help the patient conserve his energy.
• Impose reverse isolation if bone marrow suppression develops during treatment.

For *radiation therapy:*
• Provide meticulous skin care to minimize skin breakdown.

Patient teaching

• Before surgery, supplement and reinforce what the doctor has told the patient about the disease and the operation itself.
• Teach the patient about postoperative procedures and equipment. Discuss urinary catheterization, chest tubes, endotracheal tubes, dressing changes, and I.V. therapy. Teach him how to cough and breathe deeply from the diaphragm and how to perform range-of-motion exercises. Reassure him that analgesics and proper positioning will help to control postoperative pain.
• Warn an outpatient to avoid tight clothing, sunburn, and harsh ointments on his chest. Teach him exercises to prevent shoulder stiffness.
• If the patient is receiving chemotherapy or radiation therapy, explain possible adverse effects of these treatments. Teach him ways to avoid complications, such as infection. Also review reportable adverse effects.
• Educate high-risk patients in ways to reduce their chances of developing lung cancer or recurrent cancer.
• Refer smokers to local branches of the American Cancer Society or Smokenders. Provide information about group therapy, individual counseling, and hypnosis.
• Urge all heavy smokers over age 40 to have a chest X-ray annually and cytologic sputum analysis every 6 months. Also encourage patients who have recurring or chronic respiratory tract infections, chronic lung disease, or a nagging or changing cough to seek prompt medical evaluation.

MESOTHELIOMA

Originating in the serosal lining of the pleural cavity, mesotheliomas account for less than 10% of all cancer-related deaths. Incidence is high, however, in asbestos workers and their immediate families and among people who live along major routes used for transporting large quantities of asbestos.

With a latency period ranging from 20 to 45 years from exposure to tumor discovery, a mesothelioma usually occurs in people over age 50 and is invariably fatal. Typically, less than 2 years pass between the onset of symptoms and death.

Causes and pathophysiology

The link between this tumor and asbestos exposure is well established. Only seldom does predisposition, chronic inflammation, radiation, or recurrent lung infections account for a mesothelioma. Smoking alone doesn't increase the risk for developing a mesothelioma; coupled with asbestos exposure, it increases the risk by about 50%.

Whether a mesothelioma begins in the visceral or parietal pleura is uncertain; in animals, tumor-causing asbestos fibers migrate to mesothelial cells, penetrating the pleura. From there, the pleural lymphatics carry them to the pleural surface. Signs and symptoms result from pleural effusion, restricted lung function, tumor mass, infection, and advanced disease.

Complications

Disease progression and metastasis can lead to severe dyspnea, infection, and complications of immobility, such as skin breakdown.

Assessment findings

The patient's history will probably reveal asbestos exposure at some time in the patient's life. His chief complaints may be chest pain and dyspnea. Other complaints include cough, hoarseness, anorexia, weight loss, weakness, and fatigue.

Vital signs may reflect an elevated temperature. Inspection reveals shortness of breath and, in some cases, finger clubbing. You may discover dullness over lung fields on chest percussion and diminished chest sounds on auscultation.

Diagnostic tests

• *Open pleural biopsy* is necessary to obtain a specimen. Then histologic study can confirm the diagnosis.
• *Chest X-rays* exhibit nodular, irregular, unilateral pleural thickening and varying degrees of unilateral pleural effusion.
• *Computed tomography scan* of the chest defines the tumor's extent.

Treatment

No standard treatment exists for a mesothelioma. Surgery, radiation therapy, chemotherapy, and a combination of treatments are usually tried, but they seldom control the disease in most patients.

If surgery is performed, a pleuropneumonectomy is the usual procedure. Cisplatin and mitomycin are the most successful chemotherapy drug combinations. Doxorubicin and methotrexate achieve less successful results.

Nursing diagnoses
- Anxiety
- Fatigue
- Fluid volume excess
- Hopelessness
- Impaired gas exchange
- Impaired physical mobility
- Impaired skin integrity
- Ineffective breathing pattern
- Risk for infection

Nursing interventions
- Listen to the patient's fears and concerns. Give him clear, concise explanations of all procedures and actions, and remain with him during periods of severe anxiety. Encourage him to identify those actions that promote comfort. Then be sure to perform them and to encourage the patient and his family to help. Include the patient in decisions related to his care whenever possible.
- Administer ordered pain medication as required. Monitor and document the medication's effectiveness.
- Perform comfort measures, such as repositioning and relaxation techniques.
- Monitor respiratory status. Provide oxygen as ordered, and assist the patient to a comfortable position (Fowler's position, for example) that allows for maximal chest expansion to relieve respiratory distress.
- If mobility decreases, turn the patient frequently. Provide skin care, particularly over bony prominences. Encourage him to be as active as possible.
- Prevent infection. Adhere to strict aseptic technique when suctioning the patient, changing dressings or I.V. tubing, and performing any type of invasive procedure. Monitor body temperature and white blood cell count closely.
- Monitor I.V. fluid intake to avoid circulatory overload and pulmonary congestion.
- Watch for treatment complications by observing and listening to the patient. Also monitor laboratory studies and vital signs. Perform appropriate nursing measures to prevent or alleviate complications. Report complications.

Patient teaching
- Show the patient how to perform relaxation techniques. Also demonstrate breathing and positioning variations to ease the dyspnea associated with progressive disease.
- Explain all procedures and treatments. Schedule time to answer the patient's questions.
- Teach the patient measures (such as increasing fluid intake) to minimize adverse effects of treatment.

- When appropriate, teach the patient and his family procedures to maximize breathing and prevent the complications of immobility.
- Explain how to practice meticulous hand washing and aseptic techniques to avoid infection.
- Refer the patient to the social services department, support groups, and community or professional mental health resources to help him and his family cope with terminal illness.

BREAST CANCER
Along with lung cancer, breast cancer is a leading killer of women ages 35 to 54. Breast cancer strikes about 10% of all women. The disease seldom occurs in men.

Although breast cancer may develop any time after puberty, about 70% of cases develop in women over age 50; about 20% in women under age 30. Five-year survival rates show increasing improvement: from 53% in the 1940s, to 70% in the 1980s, and 76% in the 1990s because of earlier diagnosis and better treatment. Mortality, however, hasn't changed in the past 50 years.

The most reliable breast cancer detection method is regular breast self-examination, followed by immediate professional evaluation of any abnormality. Another detection method, mammography, is probably responsible for an increase in reported cases.

Causes and pathophysiology
The causes of breast cancer remain elusive. Significant risk factors include a family history of breast cancer (mother, sister, grandmother, aunt) and being a woman over age 45 and premenopausal. Other risk factors may include a long menstrual cycle, early onset of menses, or late menopause; first pregnancy after age 35; a high-fat diet; endometrial or ovarian cancer; radiation exposure; estrogen therapy; antihypertensive therapy; alcohol and tobacco use; and preexisting fibrocystic disease. The recent discovery of the breast cancer gene BRCA 1 confirms the theory that the disease can be inherited from either the mother or the father.

About half of all breast cancers develop in the upper outer quadrant. (For more information, see *Breast tumor sources and sites.*) Growth rates vary. Theoretically, slow-growing breast cancer may take up to 8 years to become palpable at 3/8″ (1 cm). It spreads by way of the lymphatic system and the bloodstream through the right side of the heart to the lungs and to the other breast, chest wall, liver, bone, and brain.

The estimated breast cancer growth rate is called its *doubling time,* or the time it takes malignant cells to double in number. Survival time is based on tumor size and the number of involved lymph nodes.

Classified by histologic appearance and the lesion's location, breast cancer may be described as:
• *adenocarcinoma* (ductal) — arising from the epithelium
• *intraductal* — developing within the ducts (includes Paget's disease)
• *infiltrating* — occurring in the breast's parenchymal tissue
• *inflammatory (rare)* — growing rapidly and causing overlying skin to become edematous, inflamed, and indurated
• *lobular carcinoma in situ* — involving the lobes of glandular tissue
• *medullary or circumscribed* — enlarging tumor with rapid growth rate.

Coupled with a staging system, these classifications provide a clearer picture of the cancer's extent. The most common system for staging, both before and after surgery, is the TNM (tumor, node, metastasis) system. (See *Staging breast cancer,* page 314.)

Assessment findings

The patient most often reports that she detected a painless lump or mass in her breast or that she noticed a thickening of breast tissue. Otherwise, the disease most commonly appears on a mammogram before a lesion becomes palpable. The patient's history may indicate several risk factors for breast cancer. (See *Planning care for the patient with breast cancer,* pages 315 and 316.)

Inspection may reveal clear, milky, or bloody nipple discharge, nipple retraction, scaly skin around the nipple, and skin changes, such as dimpling, peau d'orange, or inflammation. Arm edema, also identified on inspection, may indicate advanced nodal involvement.

Palpation may identify a hard lump, mass, or thickening of breast tissue. Palpation of the cervical supraclavicular and axillary nodes may also disclose lumps or enlargement.

Complications

Disease progression and metastasis lead to site-specific complications, including infection, decreased mobility if the disease metastasizes to the bone, central nervous system effects if the tumor metastasizes to the brain, and respiratory problems if it spreads to the lung.

BREAST TUMOR SOURCES AND SITES

About 90% of all breast tumors arise from the epithelial cells lining the ducts. About half of all breast cancers develop in the breast's upper outer quadrant — the section containing the most glandular tissue.

The second most common cancer site is the nipple, where all the breast ducts converge.

The next most common site is the upper inner quadrant, followed by the lower outer quadrant and, finally, the lower inner quadrant.

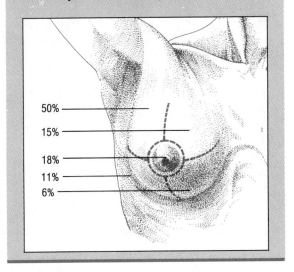

50%
15%
18%
11%
6%

Diagnostic tests

• *Mammography,* the essential test for breast cancer, can detect a tumor too small to palpate.
• *Fine-needle aspiration* and *excisional biopsy* provide cells for histologic examination to confirm the diagnosis.
• *Ultrasonography* can distinguish between a fluid-filled cyst and a solid mass.
• *Chest X-rays* can pinpoint metastases in the chest.
• *Scans* of the bone, brain, liver, and other organs can detect distant metastases.
• *Laboratory tests,* such as alkaline phosphatase levels and liver function, can uncover distant metastases.
• *Hormonal receptor assay* can determine whether the tumor is estrogen- or progesterone-dependent. This test guides decisions to use therapy that blocks the action of the estrogen hormone that supports tumor growth.

Treatment

Choice of treatment usually reflects the disease's stage and type, the woman's age and menopausal status, and

STAGING BREAST CANCER

Cancer staging helps form a prognosis and a treatment plan. For breast cancer, most clinicians use the TNM (tumor, node, metastasis) system developed by the American Joint Committee on Cancer.

Primary tumor

TX—primary tumor can't be assessed
T0—no evidence of primary tumor
Tis—carcinoma in situ: intraductal carcinoma, lobular carcinoma in situ, or Paget's disease of the nipple with no tumor
T1—tumor 2 cm or less in greatest dimension
T1a—tumor 0.5 cm or less in greatest dimension
T1b—tumor more than 0.5 cm but not more than 1 cm in greatest dimension
T1c—tumor more than 1 cm but not more than 2 cm in greatest dimension
T2—tumor more than 2 cm but not more than 5 cm in greatest dimension
T3—tumor more than 5 cm in greatest dimension
T4—tumor of any size that extends to the chest wall or skin
T4a—tumor extends to the chest wall
T4b—tumor accompanied by edema (including *peau d'orange*), ulcerated breast skin, or satellite skin nodules on the same breast
T4c—both T4a and T4b
T4d—inflammatory carcinoma

Regional lymph nodes

NX—regional lymph nodes can't be assessed
N0—no evidence of nodal involvement
N1—movable ipsilateral axillary nodal involvement
N2—ipsilateral axillary nodal involvement with nodes fixed to one another or to other structures
N3—ipsilateral internal mammary nodal involvement

Distant metastasis

MX—distant metastasis can't be assessed
M0—no evidence of distant metastasis
M1—distant metastasis (including metastasis to ipsilateral supraclavicular nodes)

Staging categories

Breast cancer progresses from mild to severe as follows:
Stage 0—Tis, N0, M0
Stage I—T1, N0, M0
Stage IIA—T0, N1, M0; T1, N1, M0; T2, N0, M0
Stage IIB—T2, N1, M0; T3, N0, M0
Stage IIIA—T0, N2, M0; T1, N2, M0; T2, N2, M0; T3, N1 or N2, M0
Stage IIIB—T4, any N, M0; any T, N3, M0
Stage IV—any T, any N, M1

---

the disfiguring effects of the surgery. Therapy may include any combination of surgery, radiation, chemotherapy, and hormonal therapy.

Surgery includes lumpectomy, partial mastectomy, total mastectomy, and modified radical mastectomy.

• *Lumpectomy.* Through a small incision near the nipple, the surgeon removes the tumor, surrounding tissue and, possibly, nearby lymph nodes. Typically, the patient will undergo radiation therapy after lumpectomy.

Lumpectomy is used for patients with small, well-defined lesions. Fewer than 20% of cancer patients undergo this operation. In some cases, the surgeon will perform a lumpectomy by freezing the tumor with a cryoprobe (which chills the tumor to −292° F [−180° C]), thawing the tumor, and then repeating the procedure four more times. Finally, he refreezes the tumor and then performs the surgery.

This cell-destroying technique, called *cryolumpectomy,* is recommended only for small, early, primary tumors. Radiation therapy may follow cryolumpectomy, which has few complications, and may prevent local recurrence.

• *Partial mastectomy.* The surgeon removes the tumor along with a wedge of normal tissue, skin, fascia and, possibly, axillary lymph nodes. Radiation therapy or chemotherapy usually follows in an effort to destroy undetected disease in other breast areas.

• *Total mastectomy.* Also called simple mastectomy, a total mastectomy is removal of the entire breast. The surgeon uses this procedure if the cancer appears confined to breast tissue and no lymph node involvement is detected. The operation may be followed by chemotherapy or radiation therapy.

After mastectomy, reconstructive surgery can create a breast mound if the patient desires it and if she doesn't have advanced disease.

• *Modified radical mastectomy.* The surgeon removes the entire breast, axillary lymph nodes, and the lining that covers the chest muscles. If the lymph nodes contain cancer cells, radiation therapy and chemotherapy follow the surgery. *Modified radical* mastectomy differs from *radical* mastectomy in that it preserves the patient's pectoral muscles. Modified radical mastectomy has replaced

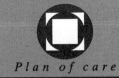

Plan of care

PLANNING CARE FOR THE PATIENT WITH BREAST CANCER

When caring for a patient with breast cancer, you need to address not only physical needs but also emotional ones. How, though, do you develop a plan of care that satisfies these needs? Well, you can begin this way: consider that you've just met Lilly Jennings, age 54. She is a sportswear buyer and has no children. Her friend brings her to the hospital.

Patient history
Ms. Jennings tells you her story calmly and with little emotion. She says that until recently she hadn't seen a gynecologist or had a mammogram for more than 5 years. She describes herself as healthy and active. In sporadic breast self-examinations, she never noticed anything extraordinary.

Three weeks ago, she saw her gynecologist and had a mammogram. Two days later, she had a needle biopsy. The results: a 5-cm, malignant Stage II tumor in the upper outer quadrant of her left breast. The gynecologist suspects axillary node involvement. Ms. Jennings expects to have a simple mastectomy tomorrow morning. She quietly states that she knows she should have gone to the doctor every year for a checkup. You reassure her that the records point to a localized tumor and that surgery and chemotherapy offer excellent possibilities for a cure.

As you inquire further, you learn that Ms. Jennings has an older sister who has "heart problems" and who lives with and cares for her 78-year-old parents on their farm 60 miles away. Both parents are in relatively good health.

Assessment findings
Your initial examination of Ms. Jennings reveals little that is abnormal or unusual. Her vital signs are stable. Her temperature is normal, and she reports no pain anywhere.

On inspection, you see a slightly obese, carefully groomed white woman. You defer breast palpation because test findings have localized the tumor. You observe no breast asymmetry and no discharge.

Lung auscultation reveals full expansion without wheezing or crackles. Heart sounds and rhythm are regular. Bowel sounds are present in all quadrants.

Nursing diagnoses
Based on your assessment findings, you select these nursing diagnoses:
• Fear, anxiety, and ineffective individual coping related to cancer treatment and related adverse effects, the possibility of premature death, lack of family support system, potential sexual rejection by her partner, and altered body image
• Impaired skin integrity related to tissue trauma from surgery, radiation therapy, or metastasis
• Body image disturbance related to surgery, radiation therapy, or chemotherapy
• Pain related to treatment
• Self-care deficit related to fatigue, weakness, and partial immobility of upper extremity after surgery

Expected outcomes
To provide effective care, you'll need to help Ms. Jennings:
• decrease fear, stress, and anxiety
• maintain skin and tissue integrity and pain-free status
• adapt to changes in body image
• return to self-care, increase activity tolerance, and avoid immobility.

Implementation
You next plan interventions to achieve expected outcomes.

To minimize fear and stress and promote coping
• Help Ms. Jennings express her feelings. Then provide information to help her understand her disease and its treatment. This will help to minimize her fear of the unknown. (It also will help establish a trusting relationship.)
• Help Ms. Jennings identify coping strategies that have worked for her in the past. Doing so will help the health care team use known coping strategies to offer comfort.
• Provide emotional support through all phases of care; encourage other health care team members, family, and friends to do the same.
• Encourage questions from Ms. Jennings and others. Set aside daily time to keep Ms. Jennings up-to-date on information, test results, and available ancillary services that promote recovery.
• Ensure adequate rest during the day and sleep at night without pain.

To maintain skin integrity and diminish pain
• Promote optimal nutrition. Increase protein, carbohydrate, and fat intake, as needed, to meet greater metabolic needs. During chemotherapy and radiation therapy, provide antiemetics and oral anesthetics, as ordered and needed.
• Give irradiated skin gentle cleaning, air exposure, and water-based lubricants. Advise Ms. Jennings to wear comfortable, loose, soft, cotton clothing. Encourage her to change position often to avoid prolonged pressure while at rest.

(continued)

PLANNING CARE FOR THE PATIENT WITH BREAST CANCER
(continued)

• Explain the need for and provide opioid analgesics to relieve pain caused by exposed, damaged, or irradiated nerve endings. Provide anti-inflammatory drugs to combat adverse effects of therapy.
• Encourage early mobility and range-of-motion exercises on the affected side to stimulate vascular and neurologic function.

To adapt to body changes
• Help Ms. Jennings confront obvious changes, such as breast tissue and hair losses. Reassure her that scars will heal, and hair will grow back. Discuss prostheses constructed with comfort and contour in mind.
• Help the patient recognize that it's normal to grieve over the loss of a body part. Then help her to accept

the loss, and to participate in care, dressing, and visiting with family and friends.
• Offer information and referral to local mastectomy support groups. Also offer a referral for appropriate psychological counseling.

To promote self-care and restore mobility
• Encourage early participation in all postoperative care and activities of daily living.
• Keep Ms. Jennings as comfortable as possible before starting activity.
• Assess her activity limits. Encourage her to exercise when her energy levels permit.
• Explain that energy levels and activity tolerance may diminish during therapy, but will improve after treatment.

Evaluation
During this hospitalization and

possible subsequent hospitalizations for chemotherapy or radiation therapy or both, reassess and alter your plan of care according to Ms. Jennings's needs. Is she coping well with each readmission?

To help you evaluate the success of your plan of care, ask: How is Ms. Jennings coping at home? Is she keeping follow-up medical appointments? Are her energy and mobility levels returning? Is her skin integrity restored? Has she returned to work? Is she adopting healthful behaviors to maintain or enrich her quality of life? Is her diet adequate to meet her increased metabolic needs? Is she exercising regularly? Have her social relationships resumed or changed? Does she attend a self-help group for mastectomy patients?

---

radical mastectomy as the most widely used surgical procedure for treating breast cancer.

Before or after tumor removal, primary radiation therapy may be effective for a patient who has a small tumor in early stages without distant metastases. Radiation therapy can also prevent or treat local recurrence. Furthermore, preoperative breast irradiation helps to "sterilize" the field, making the tumor more manageable surgically—especially in inflammatory breast cancer.

Various cytotoxic drug combinations may be administered either as adjuvant therapy or as primary therapy. The patient may base her decision to undergo chemotherapy on several factors, including the cancer's stage and hormonal receptor assay results.

Chemotherapy commonly relies on a combination of drugs, such as cyclophosphamide, fluorouracil, methotrexate, doxorubicin, vincristine, and prednisone. A typical regimen is cyclophosphamide, methotrexate, and fluorouracil; it's used in premenopausal and postmenopausal women.

Hormonal therapy lowers levels of estrogen and other hormones suspected of nourishing breast cancer cells. For example, antiestrogen therapy (specifically tamoxifen, which is most effective against tumors identified as estrogen-receptor–positive) is used in postmenopausal

women. Alternatively, the patient may receive antiandrogen therapy (aminoglutethimide) or androgen (fluoxymesterone), estrogen (diethylstilbestrol), or progestin (megestrol) therapy.

Nursing diagnoses
• Altered nutrition: Less than body requirements
• Anxiety
• Body image disturbance
• Decisional conflict
• Energy field disturbance
• Fear
• Impaired physical mobility
• Impaired skin integrity
• Ineffective individual coping
• Knowledge deficit
• Pain
• Risk for infection
• Self-care deficit

Nursing interventions
• Evaluate the patient's feelings about her illness, and determine her level of knowledge. Listen to her concerns, and stay with her during periods of severe anxiety.

• Administer ordered analgesics as required. Monitor and record their effectiveness.
• Perform comfort measures, such as repositioning, to promote relaxation and relieve anxiety.
• If immobility develops late in the disease, prevent complications by frequently repositioning the patient, using a convoluted foam mattress, and providing skin care (particularly over bony prominences).
• Watch for treatment complications, such as nausea, vomiting, anorexia, leukopenia, thrombocytopenia, GI ulceration, and bleeding. Provide comfort measures and prescribed treatments to relieve these complications.

After surgery:
• Inspect the dressing anteriorly and posteriorly. Report excessive bleeding promptly.
• Record the amount and color of drainage. Drainage appears bloody during the first 4 hours; then it becomes serous.
• Monitor vital signs. If a general anesthetic was given during surgery, monitor intake and output for at least 48 hours.
• Prevent lymphedema of the arm, which may be an early complication of lymph node dissection. Such prevention is crucial because lymphedema can't be treated effectively.
• Use strict aseptic technique when changing dressings or I.V. tubing or performing any invasive procedure. Monitor temperature and white blood cell count closely.
• Inspect the incision. Encourage the patient and her partner to look at her incision as soon as feasible—when the first dressing is removed, if possible.

Patient teaching
• Clearly explain all procedures and treatments.
• Besides the usual preoperative teaching, show the mastectomy patient how to ease postsurgical pain by lying on the affected side or by placing a hand or pillow on the incision. Point out where the incision will be. Inform the patient that after the operation, she'll receive analgesics because pain relief encourages coughing and turning and promotes well-being. Explain that a small pillow placed under the arm anteriorly may provide comfort.
• Tell her that she may move about and get out of bed as soon as possible—usually as soon as the effects of the anesthetic subside or the first evening after surgery.
• Explain that she may have an incisional drain or some type of suction to remove accumulated fluid, to relieve tension on the suture line, and to promote healing.
• Urge the patient to avoid activities that may injure her arm and hand on the side of her surgery. Caution her not to let blood be drawn from or allow injections into

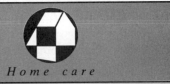

Home care

MANAGING MASTECTOMY AFTER DISCHARGE

Follow these guidelines when providing home care for the mastectomy patient:
• If the patient agrees, refer her to the American Cancer Society's Reach for Recovery program.
• Teach the patient how to examine her breasts, and observe as she performs a self-examination.
• Encourage the patient to talk about her feelings. Discuss such issues as grief over the loss of a body part, loss of "femininity," breast reconstruction, and the diagnosis of cancer.
• During each visit, look closely for signs of infection at the incision site.
• Make sure the amount of drainage continues to decrease. Report any increases, changes in color, or foul odor.
• Teach the patient to:
—wash her hands before touching the incision site
—empty the drainage device at least every 8 hours and record the amount
—notify you if the drainage suddenly increases, changes in color, or has a foul odor
—perform arm exercises at least four times a day, increasing them as tolerated and stopping at the point of pain
—avoid shaving and using depilatory creams and strong deodorants in the affected area
—avoid any constriction of the affected area (for example, from wearing tight clothing).

that arm. She should also refuse to have blood pressure taken or I.V. therapy administered on the affected arm.
• To help prevent lymphedema, instruct the patient to exercise her hand and arm on the affected side regularly and to avoid activities that might allow infection of this hand or arm. Tell her that infection increases the risk of lymphedema. (See *Managing mastectomy after discharge.*)
• Inform the patient that she may experience "phantom breast syndrome," a tingling or pins-and-needles sensation in the area where the breast was removed.
• Women who have had breast cancer in one breast are at higher risk for cancer in the other breast or for recurrent cancer in the chest wall. For this reason, urge the patient to continue examining the other breast and to comply with recommended follow-up treatment.

SITES OF GASTRIC CANCER

The illustration below shows how frequently gastric cancer occurs in different parts of the stomach.

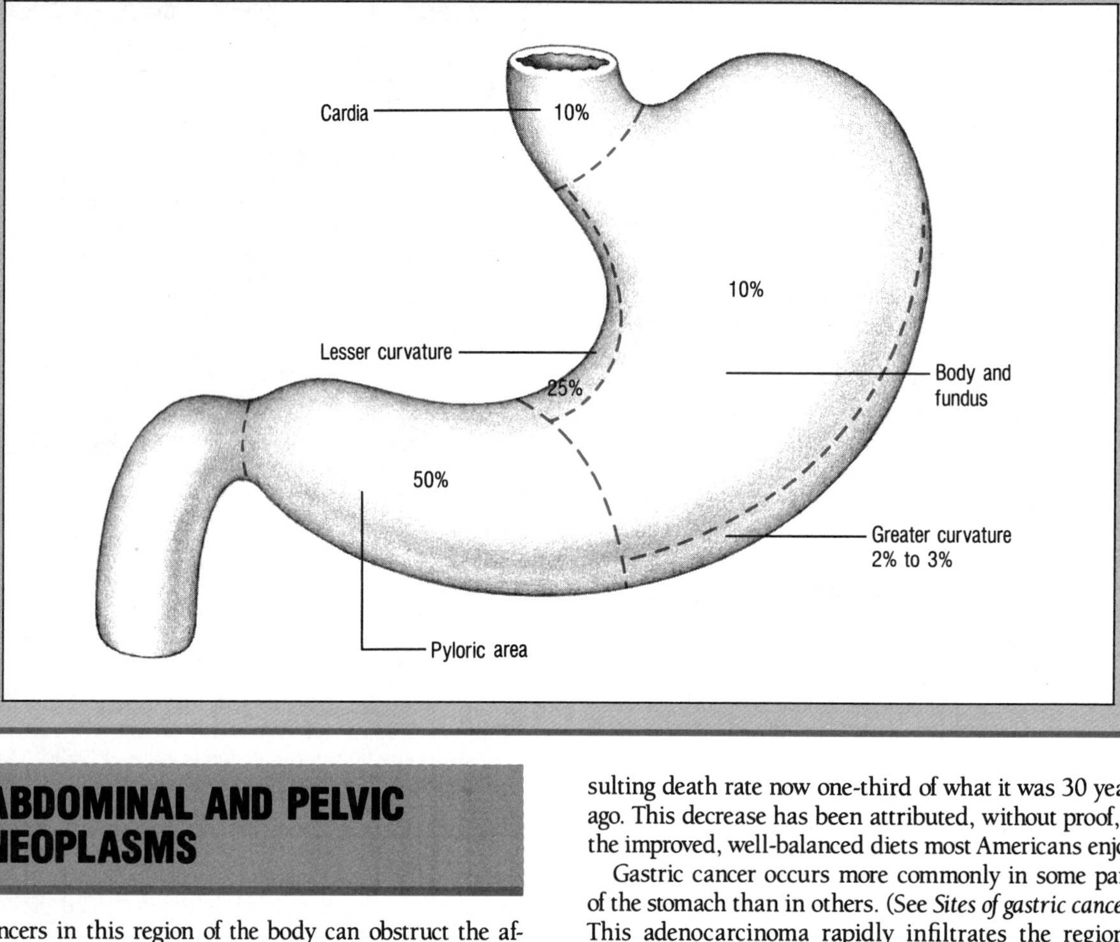

Cardia — 10%

10%

Lesser curvature —

25%

Body and fundus

50%

Greater curvature 2% to 3%

Pyloric area

ABDOMINAL AND PELVIC NEOPLASMS

Cancers in this region of the body can obstruct the affected organ or disrupt its secretory or absorptive functions and obstruct the flow of GI contents.

GASTRIC CANCER

Although gastric cancer is common throughout the world in people of all races, its incidence exhibits unexplained geographic, cultural, and gender differences. For example, mortality from this disorder is high in Japan, Iceland, Chile, and Austria. Incidence is also higher in men over age 40.

Over the past 25 years in the United States, the incidence of gastric cancer has fallen 50%, with the resulting death rate now one-third of what it was 30 years ago. This decrease has been attributed, without proof, to the improved, well-balanced diets most Americans enjoy.

Gastric cancer occurs more commonly in some parts of the stomach than in others. (See *Sites of gastric cancer.*) This adenocarcinoma rapidly infiltrates the regional lymph nodes, omentum, liver, and lungs by way of the walls of the stomach, duodenum, and esophagus; the lymphatic system; adjacent organs; the bloodstream; and the peritoneal cavity.

The patient's prognosis depends on the stage of the disease at the time of diagnosis. Overall, the 5-year survival rate is about 15%.

Causes

Although the cause of gastric cancer is unknown, predisposing factors, such as gastritis with gastric atrophy, increase the risk. Genetic factors have also been implicated. People with type A blood have a 10% increased risk, and the disease occurs more commonly in people with a family history of such cancer.

Dietary factors also seem to have an effect. For instance, certain types of food preparation and preservation (especially smoked foods, pickled vegetables, and salted fish and meat) and physical properties of some foods increase the risk. Furthermore, high alcohol consumption and smoking increase the chances of developing gastric cancer.

Complications
Malnutrition occurs when the stomach can't digest protein, and GI obstruction develops as the tumor enlarges. Iron deficiency anemia results as the tumor causes ulceration and bleeding. If the patient has pernicious anemia, the tumor can interfere with the production of intrinsic factor needed for vitamin B_{12} absorption. As the cancer metastasizes to other structures, related complications appear.

Assessment findings
In the early stages, the patient may complain of pain in his back or in the epigastric or retrosternal areas that is relieved with nonprescription medications. (He may not report this symptom because he doesn't realize its significance.) The patient typically reports a vague feeling of fullness, heaviness, and moderate abdominal distention after meals.

Depending on cancer progression, the patient may report weight loss, resulting from appetite disturbance, nausea, and vomiting. (He may report coffee-ground vomitus if the tumor is located in the cardia.) He may also complain of weakness and fatigue. If the tumor is located in the proximal area of the stomach, he may experience dysphagia.

Palpation of the abdomen may disclose a mass. You may also be able to palpate enlarged lymph nodes, especially the supraclavicular and axillary nodes. Other assessment findings depend on the extent of the disease and the location of metastasis.

Diagnostic tests
• *Barium X-rays of the GI tract with fluoroscopy* show changes that suggest gastric cancer. Changes include a tumor or filling defect in the outline of the stomach, loss of flexibility and distensibility, and abnormal gastric mucosa with or without ulceration.
• *Gastroscopy with fiber-optic endoscope* helps rule out other diffuse gastric mucosal abnormalities by allowing direct visualization. Gastroscopic biopsy permits evaluation of gastric mucosal lesions. Photography during gastroscopy provides a permanent record of gastric lesions that can later be used to judge disease progression and the effectiveness of treatment.
• *Gastric acid stimulation test* determines whether the stomach secretes acid properly.
• *Blood studies* monitor the course of the disease, complications, and the effectiveness of treatment. These studies include a complete blood count, chemistry profiles, arterial blood gas analysis, liver function studies, and a carcinoembryonic antigen radioimmunoassay.

Certain other studies may rule out specific organ metastases. These include computed tomography scans, chest X-rays, liver and bone scans, and liver biopsy. (See *Staging gastric cancer,* page 320.)

Treatment
Surgery to remove the tumor often is the treatment of choice. Excision of the lesion with appropriate margins is possible in more than one-third of patients. Even in a patient whose disease isn't considered surgically curable, resection eases symptoms and improves the potential benefits of the chemotherapy and radiation therapy that usually follow surgery.

The nature and extent of the lesion determine the type of surgery. Surgical procedures include gastroduodenostomy, gastrojejunostomy, partial gastric resection, and total gastrectomy. If metastasis has occurred, the omentum and spleen may have to be removed. (See *Understanding gastric surgery,* page 321.)

Chemotherapy for GI tumors may help control signs and symptoms and prolong survival. Gastric adenocarcinomas respond to several agents, including fluorouracil, carmustine, doxorubicin, and mitomycin. Antiemetics can control nausea, which intensifies as the tumor grows. In the more advanced stages, the patient may need sedatives and tranquilizers to control overwhelming anxiety. Opioid analgesics can relieve severe and unremitting pain.

If the patient has a nonresectable or partially resectable tumor, radiation therapy is effective if combined with chemotherapy. The patient should receive this therapy on an empty stomach but not preoperatively because it may damage viscera and impede healing.

Treatment with antispasmodics and antacids may help relieve GI distress.

Nursing diagnoses
• Altered nutrition: Less than body requirements
• Altered oral mucous membrane
• Anxiety
• Diarrhea

STAGING GASTRIC CANCER

Both prognosis and treatment of gastric cancer depend on its type and stage. Using the TNM (tumor, node, metastasis) system, the American Joint Committee on Cancer describes the following stages of gastric cancer.

Primary tumor
TX—primary tumor can't be assessed
T0—no evidence of primary tumor
Tis—carcinoma in situ: intraepithelial tumor doesn't penetrate the lamina propria
T1—tumor penetrates the lamina propria or submucosa
T2—tumor penetrates the muscularis propria or subserosa
T3—tumor penetrates the serosa (visceral peritoneum) without invading adjacent structures
T4—tumor invades adjacent structures

Regional lymph nodes
NX—regional lymph nodes can't be assessed
N0—no evidence of regional lymph node metastasis
N1—involvement of perigastric lymph nodes within 3 cm of the edge of the primary tumor
N2—involvement of the perigastric lymph nodes more than 3 cm from the edge of the primary tumor, or in lymph nodes along the left gastric, common hepatic, splenic, or celiac arteries

Distant metastasis
MX—distant metastasis can't be assessed
M0—no evidence of distant metastasis
M1—distant metastasis

Staging categories
Gastric cancer stages progress from mild to severe as follows:
Stage 0—Tis, N0, M0
Stage IA—T1, N0, M0
Stage IB—T1, N1, M0; T2, N0, M0
Stage II—T1, N2, M0; T3, N0, M0
Stage IIIA—T2, N2, M0; T3, N1, M0; T4, N0, M0
Stage IIIB—T3, N2, M0; T4, N1, N0
Stage IV—T4, N2, M0; any T, any N, M1

- Fatigue
- Fear
- Impaired gas exchange
- Impaired skin integrity
- Impaired swallowing
- Knowledge deficit
- Pain
- Risk for infection

Nursing interventions

- Provide a high-protein, high-calorie diet to help the patient avoid or recover from the weight loss, malnutrition, and anemia associated with gastric cancer. This diet also helps the patient tolerate surgery, radiotherapy, and chemotherapy; helps prevent wound dehiscence; and promotes wound healing. Plus, it provides enough protein, fluid, and potassium to aid glycogen and protein synthesis.
- Give the patient dietary supplements, such as vitamins and iron, and provide small, frequent meals. If the patient has an iron deficiency, give him iron-rich foods, such as spinach and dried fruit.
- To stimulate a poor appetite, administer steroids or antidepressants to the patient, as ordered. Wine or brandy may also help stimulate his appetite.
- If the patient can't tolerate oral foods, provide parenteral nutrition.

- Administer an antacid to relieve heartburn and acid stomach and a histamine$_2$-receptor antagonist, such as cimetidine or famotidine, to decrease gastric secretions. Give opioid analgesics, as ordered, to relieve pain.
- After surgery, provide meticulous supportive care to promote recovery and help prevent complications.
- After any type of gastrectomy, turn the patient hourly; administer opioid analgesics (which depress respiration), as ordered; and regularly assist the patient with coughing, deep breathing, and turning to help prevent respiratory problems. If respiratory complications develop, the patient may need oxygen.

If the patient can't breathe effectively on his own, use intermittent positive pressure breathing or incentive spirometry to completely expand his lungs. Also, make sure you position him properly—usually in semi-Fowler's position.

- After total gastrectomy, support the patient during episodes of dumping syndrome, which stems from the stomach's inability to store food. Keep an emesis basin at the bedside, and provide small meals six to eight times a day when the patient is allowed food by mouth.
- Monitor the patient's nasogastric (NG) tube for drainage. Expect little or no drainage from the tube because no secretions form after the stomach is removed.
- Watch for signs of vitamin B$_{12}$ malabsorption, the result of an absence of intrinsic factor from gastric secretions.

UNDERSTANDING GASTRIC SURGERY

What type of surgery is performed depends on where the tumor occurs and how far it has spread. The dotted lines below show the areas removed.

Gastroduodenostomy
Also called a Billroth I, gastroduodenostomy may be performed to remove a tumor in the pyloric region. The surgeon resects the distal one-third to one-half of the stomach and anastomoses the remaining stomach portion to the duodenum.

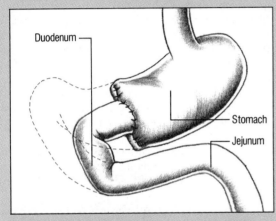

Gastrojejunostomy
Used for a stomach tumor located in the antrum, or pyloric region, this surgery is called a Billroth II. The surgeon removes the distal portion of the antrum, anastomoses the remaining stomach to the jejunum, and then closes the duodenal stump.

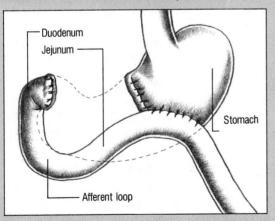

Partial gastric resection
If a tumor lies in a defined area of the stomach, the surgeon performs a gastric resection by removing the diseased stomach portion and attaching the remaining stomach to the jejunum.

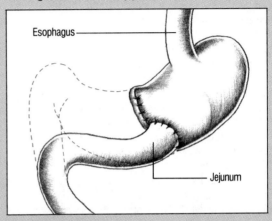

Total gastrectomy
If a tumor develops in the cardia or high in the fundus, the patient may require total gastrectomy. The surgeon removes the entire stomach and attaches the lower end of the esophagus to the jejunum (esophagojejunostomy) at the entrance to the small intestine.

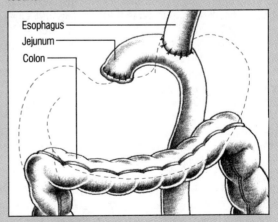

• If the patient has poor digestion and absorption after a gastrectomy, provide him with a special diet. He'll need frequent feedings of small amounts of clear liquids, increasing to small, frequent feedings of bland food. If necessary, administer pancreatin and sodium bicarbonate after meals to prevent or control steatorrhea and dyspepsia.

• Observe the surgical wound regularly for signs of infection (redness, swelling, warmth) and failure to heal. If needed, administer vitamin C to help improve wound healing.

• During radiation treatment, offer fluids, such as orange juice, grapefruit juice, or ginger ale, to minimize nausea and vomiting. Also watch for adverse effects, such as nausea, vomiting, alopecia, malaise, and diarrhea. Provide comfort measures and reassurance as needed.

• During chemotherapy, watch for complications, such as infection, and expected adverse effects, such as nausea, vomiting, mouth ulcers, and alopecia.

• Throughout treatment, listen to the patient's fears and concerns, and offer reassurance when appropriate. Stay with him during periods of severe anxiety.

• Encourage the patient to identify actions and care measures that will promote comfort and relaxation. Try to perform these measures, and encourage the patient and his family to do so, too.

• Whenever possible, include the patient and his family in decisions related to the patient's care.

• If all treatments fail, keep the patient comfortable and free from unnecessary pain, and provide psychological support. Encourage him to express his feelings and fears and to ask questions about his illness. Answer such questions honestly; evasive answers will make the patient retreat and feel isolated.

• Also talk with family members, and answer their questions. Advise them to let the patient talk about his future; encourage them to maintain a realistic outlook.

Patient teaching

• Before surgery, prepare the patient for its effects. Explain postsurgical procedures, such as insertion of an NG tube.

• If the patient is having a partial gastric resection, reassure him that he eventually may be able to eat normally. If he's having a total gastrectomy, prepare him for a slow recovery and only partial return to a normal diet. Explain that he'll have to eat small meals for the rest of his life.

• After surgery, emphasize the importance of deep breathing and changing position every 2 hours.

• Stress the importance of sound nutrition. Explain that the patient must take vitamins (to prevent B_{12} deficiency) and iron for the rest of his life.

• Teach the patient about dumping syndrome after gastric resection. Early dumping syndrome, which may be mild or severe, occurs a few minutes after eating and lasts up to 45 minutes. Onset is sudden, with nausea, weakness, sweating, palpitations, dizziness, flushing, borborygmi, explosive diarrhea, and increased blood pressure and pulse rate. Late dumping syndrome, which is less serious, occurs 2 to 3 hours after eating. The patient may experience profuse sweating, anxiety, and fine hand and leg tremors, along with vertigo, exhaustion, lassitude, palpitations, throbbing headache, faintness, sensation of hunger, glycosuria, and a marked decrease in blood pressure and in glucose levels. Tell him that these symptoms may persist from a year after surgery to the rest of his life.

• Explain the ordered treatments to the patient and his family. Describe the adverse effects the treatment may cause, and tell the patient to notify the doctor if these effects persist.

• Prepare the patient for chemotherapy's adverse effects, such as nausea and vomiting, and suggest measures, such as drinking plenty of fluids, that may help relieve these problems.

• Encourage the patient to follow his normal routine as much as possible after recovering from surgery and during radiation therapy and chemotherapy. Leading a near-normal life will help foster feelings of independence and control and will reduce complications of immobility.

• Caution the patient to avoid crowds and people with known infections because chemotherapy and radiation therapy diminish the body's natural resistance to infection.

• Encourage the patient to learn and practice relaxation and pain management techniques to help control anxiety and discomfort.

• If appropriate, direct the patient and his family to hospital and community support personnel and services. These include social workers, psychologists, cancer support groups, home health care agencies, and hospices.

ESOPHAGEAL CANCER

Most common in men over age 60, esophageal cancer is nearly always fatal. The disease occurs worldwide, but incidence varies geographically. It is most commonly found in Japan, Russia, China, the Middle East, and the Transkei region of South Africa, where esophageal cancer has reached almost epidemic proportions. In the United

States, more than 8,000 cases of esophageal cancer are reported annually.

Esophageal tumors are usually fungating and infiltrating. In most cases, the tumor partially constricts the lumen of the esophagus. Regional metastasis occurs early by way of submucosal lymphatics, often fatally invading adjacent vital intrathoracic organs. If the patient survives primary extension, the liver and lungs are the usual sites of distant metastases. Unusual metastasis sites include the bone, kidneys, and adrenal glands.

Most cases (98%) arise in squamous cell epithelium, although a few are adenocarcinomas and fewer still, melanomas and sarcomas. About half the squamous cell cancers occur in the lower portion of the esophagus, 40% in the midportion, and the remaining 10% in the upper or cervical esophagus. Regardless of cell type, the prognosis for esophageal cancer is grim: 5-year survival rates are less than 5%, and most patients die within 6 months of diagnosis.

Causes

Although the cause of esophageal cancer is unknown, several predisposing factors have been identified. These include chronic irritation from heavy smoking or excessive use of alcohol; stasis-induced inflammation, as in achalasia or stricture; previous head and neck tumors; and nutritional deficiency, as in untreated sprue and Plummer-Vinson syndrome.

Complications

Direct invasion of adjoining structures may lead to severe complications, such as mediastinitis, tracheoesophageal or bronchoesophageal fistula (causing an overwhelming cough when swallowing liquids), and aortic perforation with sudden exsanguination.

Other complications include an inability to control secretions, obstruction of the esophagus, and loss of lower esophageal sphincter control, which can result in aspiration pneumonia.

Assessment findings

Early in the disease, the patient may report a feeling of fullness, pressure, indigestion, or substernal burning. He may also tell you he uses antacids to relieve GI upset. Later, he may complain of dysphagia and weight loss. The degree of dysphagia varies, depending on the extent of disease. At first, the dysphagia is mild, occurring only after the patient eats solid foods, especially meat. Later, the patient has difficulty swallowing coarse foods and, in some cases, liquids.

The patient may complain of hoarseness (from laryngeal nerve involvement), a chronic cough (possibly from aspiration), anorexia, vomiting, and regurgitation of food. This results from the tumor size exceeding the limits of the esophagus. He may also complain of pain on swallowing or pain that radiates to his back.

If you observe the patient in the late stages of the disease, he appears very thin, cachexic, and dehydrated.

Diagnostic tests

• *X-rays of the esophagus, with barium swallow and motility studies,* delineate structural and filling defects and reduced peristalsis.
• *Chest X-rays* or *esophagography* may reveal pneumonitis.
• *Esophagoscopy, punch and brush biopsies,* and *exfoliative cytologic tests* confirm esophageal tumors.
• *Bronchoscopy* (usually performed after an esophagoscopy) may reveal tumor growth in the tracheobronchial tree.
• *Endoscopic ultrasonography* of the esophagus combines endoscopy and ultrasound technology to measure the depth of penetration of the tumor.
• *Computed tomography scan* may help diagnose and monitor esophageal lesions.
• *Magnetic resonance imaging scan* permits evaluation of the esophagus and adjacent structures.
• *Liver function studies* and other laboratory tests may reveal abnormalities. If so, a *liver scan* and *mediastinal tomography scan* can help reveal the extent of the disease. (See *Staging esophageal cancer,* page 324.)

Treatment

Esophageal cancer usually is advanced when diagnosed, so surgery and other treatments can only relieve disease effects.

Palliative therapy consists of treatment to keep the esophagus open, including dilation of the esophagus, laser therapy, radiation therapy, and installation of prosthetic tubes (such as the Celestin tube) to bridge the tumor. Radical surgery can excise the tumor and resect either the esophagus alone or the stomach and esophagus. Chemotherapy and radiation therapy can slow the growth of the tumor. Gastrostomy or jejunostomy can help provide adequate nutrition. A prosthesis can be used to seal any fistula that develops. Endoscopic laser treatment and bipolar electrocoagulation can help restore swallowing by vaporizing cancerous tissue. If the tumor is in the upper esophagus, however, the laser can't be positioned properly.

Analgesics are used for pain control.

STAGING ESOPHAGEAL CANCER

The prognosis and treatment of esophageal cancer depend on its type and stage. Using the TNM (tumor, node, metastasis) system, the American Joint Committee on Cancer has established the following stages for esophageal cancer.

Primary tumor
TX—primary tumor can't be assessed
T0—no evidence of primary tumor
Tis—carcinoma in situ
T1—tumor invades lamina propria or submucosa
T2—tumor invades muscularis propria
T3—tumor invades adventitia
T4—tumor invades adjacent structures

Regional lymph nodes
NX—regional lymph nodes can't be assessed
N0—no regional lymph node metastasis
N1—regional lymph node metastasis

Distant metastasis
MX—distant metastasis can't be assessed
M0—no known distant metastasis
M1—distant metastasis

Staging categories
Esophageal cancer progresses from mild to severe as follows:
Stage 0—Tis, N0, M0
Stage I—T1, N0, M0
Stage IIA—T2, N0, M0; T3, N0, M0
Stage IIB—T1, N1, M0; T2, N1, M0
Stage III—T3, N1, M0; T4, any N, M0
Stage IV—any T, any N, M1

Nursing diagnoses
• Altered nutrition: Less than body requirements
• Anxiety
• Fatigue
• Fear
• Fluid volume deficit
• Impaired swallowing
• Pain
• Risk for aspiration
• Risk for infection

Nursing interventions
• Monitor the patient's nutritional and fluid status, and provide him with high-calorie, high-protein foods. If he's having trouble swallowing solids, puree or liquefy his food, and offer a commercially available nutritional supplement. As ordered, provide tube feedings, and prepare him for supplementary parenteral nutrition.

• To prevent food aspiration, place the patient in Fowler's position for meals and allow plenty of time to eat. If he regurgitates food after eating, provide mouth care.
• If the patient has a gastrostomy tube, give food slowly—by gravity—in prescribed amounts (usually 200 to 500 ml). Offer him something to chew before each feeding. This promotes gastric secretions and provides some semblance of normal eating.
• Administer ordered analgesics for pain relief as necessary. Provide comfort measures, such as repositioning, and distractions to help decrease discomfort.
• After surgery, monitor the patient's vital signs, fluid and electrolyte balance, and intake and output. Immediately report any unexpected changes in the patient's condition. Monitor him for such complications as infection, fistula formation, pneumonia, empyema, and malnutrition.
• If an anastomosis to the esophagus was performed, position the patient flat on his back to prevent tension on the suture line. Watch for signs of an anastomotic leak.
• If the patient had a prosthetic tube inserted, make sure it doesn't become blocked or dislodged. This could cause a perforation of the mediastinum or precipitate tumor erosion.
• After radiation therapy, monitor the patient for such complications as esophageal perforation, pneumonitis and fibrosis of the lungs, and myelitis of the spinal cord.
• After chemotherapy, take steps to decrease adverse effects, such as providing normal saline mouthwash to help prevent mouth ulcers. Allow the patient plenty of rest, and administer medications, as ordered, to reduce adverse effects.
• Protect the patient from infection.
• Throughout therapy, answer the patient's questions, and tell him what to expect from surgery and other therapies. Listen to his fears and concerns, and stay with him during periods of severe anxiety.
• Encourage the patient to identify actions and care measures that will promote his comfort and relaxation. Try to perform these measures, and encourage the patient and his family to do so, too.
• Whenever possible, include the patient in care decisions.

Patient teaching
• Explain the procedures the patient will undergo after surgery—closed chest drainage, nasogastric suctioning, and placement of gastrostomy tubes.
• If appropriate, instruct the family in gastrostomy tube care. This includes checking tube patency before each feeding, providing skin care around the tube, and keeping the patient upright during and after feedings.

• Stress the need to maintain adequate nutrition. Ask a dietitian to instruct the patient and his family. If the patient has difficulty swallowing solids, instruct him to puree or liquefy his food and to follow a high-calorie, high-protein diet to minimize weight loss. Also, recommend that he add a commercially available, high-calorie supplement to his diet.

• Encourage the patient to follow as normal a routine as possible after recovery from surgery and during radiation therapy and chemotherapy. Tell him that this will help him maintain a sense of control and reduce the complications associated with immobility.

• Advise the patient to rest between activities and to stop any activity that tires him or causes pain.

• Refer the patient and his family to appropriate organizations, such as the American Cancer Society.

PANCREATIC CANCER

Pancreatic cancer is the fourth most lethal of all carcinomas. It occurs most often among blacks, particularly in men between ages 35 and 70. Incidence of pancreatic cancer is highest in Israel, the United States, Sweden, and Canada and lowest in Switzerland, Belgium, and Italy. The prognosis is poor: Most patients die within a year of diagnosis.

Causes and pathophysiology

Evidence suggests that pancreatic cancer is linked to inhalation or absorption of carcinogens that are then excreted by the pancreas. Examples of such carcinogens include:

• cigarette smoke (pancreatic cancer is three to four times more common among smokers)

• excessive fat and protein (a diet high in fat and protein induces chronic hyperplasia of the pancreas, with increased turnover of cells)

• food additives

• industrial chemicals, such as beta-naphthalene, benzidine, and urea.

Other possible predisposing factors include chronic pancreatitis, diabetes mellitus, and chronic alcohol abuse.

Tumors of the pancreas are almost always adenocarcinomas. They arise most frequently (67% of the time) in the head of the pancreas. Tumors in this location commonly obstruct the ampulla of Vater and common bile duct and metastasize directly to the duodenum. Adhesions anchor the tumor to the spine, stomach, and intestines.

ISLET CELL TUMORS

Relatively uncommon, islet cell tumors (insulinomas) may be benign or malignant. They produce symptoms in three stages, and despite treatment, the prognosis is unfavorable.

Slight hypoglycemia
Fatigue, restlessness, malaise, and excessive weight gain result from slight hypoglycemia.

Compensatory secretion of epinephrine
This stage is characterized by pallor, clamminess, perspiration, palpitations, finger tremors, hunger, decreased temperature, and increased pulse rate and blood pressure.

Severe hypoglycemia
Ataxia, clouded sensorium, diplopia, and episodes of violence and hysteria are the effects of severe hypoglycemia.

Therapy and prognosis
Treatment consists of enucleation of benign tumors, or chemotherapy with streptozocin or resection to include pancreatic tissue for malignant tumors. Most islet cell tumors metastasize to the liver only. Some metastasize to the bone, brain, and lungs. Death results from a combination of hypoglycemic reactions and widespread metastasis.

Less frequently, tumors arise in the body and tail of the pancreas. When this happens, large nodular masses become fixed to retropancreatic tissues and the spine. The spleen, left kidney, suprarenal gland, and diaphragm are directly invaded, and the celiac plexus becomes involved, resulting in splenic vein thrombosis and spleen infarction. Among the rarest of pancreatic tumors are islet cell tumors. (See *Islet cell tumors.*)

In pancreatic cancer, two main tissue types form fibrotic nodes: Cylinder cells arise in ducts and degenerate into cysts, and large, fatty, granular cells arise in parenchyma.

Complications

Related to the progression of the disease, complications may include malabsorption of nutrients, insulin-dependent diabetes, liver and GI problems, and mental status changes.

Assessment findings

A patient who seeks treatment early in the disease usually reports a dull, intermittent epigastric pain. Later, he

STAGING PANCREATIC CANCER

Using the TNM (tumor, node, metastasis) system, the American Joint Committee on Cancer has established the following stages for pancreatic cancer.

Primary tumor
TX—primary tumor can't be assessed
T0—no evidence of primary tumor
T1—tumor limited to the pancreas
T1a—tumor 2 cm or less in greatest dimension
T1b—tumor more than 2 cm in greatest dimension
T2—tumor penetrates the duodenum, bile duct, or peripancreatic tissues
T3—tumor penetrates the stomach, spleen, colon, or adjacent large vessels

Regional lymph nodes
NX—regional lymph nodes can't be assessed
N0—no evidence of regional lymph node metastasis
N1—regional lymph node metastasis

Distant metastasis
MX—distant metastasis can't be assessed
M0—no known distant metastasis
M1—distant metastasis

Staging categories
Pancreatic cancer progresses from mild to severe as follows:
Stage I—T1, N0, M0; T2, N0, M0
Stage II—T3, N0, M0
Stage III—any T, N1, M0
Stage IV—any T, any N, M1

---

may report continuous pain that radiates to the right upper quadrant or dorsolumbar area. He may describe it as colicky, dull, or vague and unrelated to posture or activity. Or he may state that meals seem to aggravate the epigastric pain. He also may report anorexia, nausea, vomiting, and a rapid, profound weight loss.

Inspection may reveal jaundice. On palpation, you may note a palpable, well-defined, large mass in the subumbilical or left hypochondrial region—an indication that the tail of the pancreas is involved. The mass may adhere to the large vessels or the vertebral column and may produce a pulsation. If the tumor has involved or compressed the splenic artery, auscultation of the left hypochondrium may reveal an abdominal bruit.

Diagnostic tests

Several tests may be ordered to help diagnose the disease and determine its extent. (See *Staging pancreatic cancer.*)

Percutaneous fine-needle aspiration biopsy of the pancreas may detect tumor cells, and laparotomy with a biopsy allows a definitive diagnosis. However, a biopsy may miss relatively small or deep-seated cancerous tissue or create a pancreatic fistula. Retroperitoneal insufflation, cholangiography, scintigraphy and, particularly, barium swallow (to locate the neoplasm and detect changes in the duodenum or stomach relating to carcinoma of the head of the pancreas) also can be performed to detect the disease.

Ultrasonography helps identify a mass but not its histology. A computed tomography scan shows greater detail of the mass than ultrasonography. A magnetic resonance imaging scan discloses the tumor's location and size in great detail.

Angiography reveals the tumor's vascular supply. Endoscopic retrograde cholangiopancreatography also allows visualization, instillation of contrast medium, and specimen biopsy.

A secretin test reveals the absence of pancreatic enzymes and suggests pancreatic duct obstruction and tumors of the body and tail.

Other laboratory tests that support the diagnosis include:
• serum bilirubin (increased)
• serum amylase-lipase (occasionally increased)
• prothrombin time (prolonged)
• aspartate aminotransferase (formerly SGOT) and alanine aminotransferase (formerly SGPT) (elevated enzyme levels when liver cell necrosis is present)
• alkaline phosphatase (markedly elevated with biliary obstruction)
• plasma insulin immunoassay (shows measurable serum insulin in the presence of islet cell tumors)
• hemoglobin and hematocrit (may show mild anemia)
• fasting blood glucose (may indicate hypoglycemia or hyperglycemia)
• stool studies (may show occult blood if ulceration in the GI tract or ampulla of Vater has occurred)
• specific tumor markers for pancreatic cancer, including carcinoembryonic antigen, pancreatic oncofetal antigen, alpha-fetoprotein, and serum immunoreactive elastase I (all levels elevated in the presence of cancer).

Treatment

Because pancreatic cancer may metastasize widely before it's diagnosed, treatment seldom succeeds in curing the disease. Treatment consists of surgery and, possibly, chemotherapy and radiation therapy.

Some surgical procedures help increase the survival rate slightly.

• Total pancreatectomy may increase survival time by resecting a localized tumor or by controlling postoperative gastric ulceration.

• Cholecystojejunostomy, choledochoduodenostomy, and choledochojejunostomy have partially replaced radical resection. They bypass the obstructing common bile duct extensions, easing jaundice and pruritus.

• If radical resection isn't indicated and duodenal obstruction is expected to develop later, a gastrojejunostomy is performed.

Whipple's operation, or radical pancreatoduodenectomy, has a high mortality but can obtain wide lymphatic clearance—except with tumors located near the portal vein, superior mesenteric vein and artery, and celiac axis. This seldom used procedure removes the head of the pancreas; the duodenum; portions of the body and tail of the pancreas, stomach, jejunum, and pancreatic duct; and the distal portion of the bile duct.

Although pancreatic cancer usually responds poorly to chemotherapy, recent studies using combinations of fluorouracil, streptomycin, mitomycin, and doxorubicin show a trend toward longer survival time.

Radiation therapy usually doesn't increase long-term survival, although it may prolong survival time from 6 to 11 months when used as an adjunct to fluorouracil chemotherapy. It also can ease the pain associated with nonresectable tumors.

Medications used in pancreatic cancer include:
• antibiotics to prevent infection and relieve symptoms
• anticholinergics, particularly propantheline, to decrease GI tract spasm and motility and reduce pain and secretions
• antacids to decrease secretion of pancreatic enzymes and suppress peptic activity, thus reducing stress-induced damage to gastric mucosa
• diuretics to mobilize extracellular fluid from ascites
• insulin to provide an adequate exogenous insulin supply after pancreatic resection
• opioid analgesics to relieve pain (used only after other analgesics fail because morphine, meperidine, and codeine can lead to biliary tract spasm and increase common bile duct pressure)
• pancreatic enzymes to assist with digestion of proteins, carbohydrates, and fats when pancreatic juices are insufficient because of surgery or obstruction.

Nursing diagnoses
• Altered nutrition: Less than body requirements
• Anxiety
• Constipation
• Fluid volume deficit
• Fluid volume excess
• Impaired skin integrity
• Ineffective family coping
• Ineffective individual coping
• Knowledge deficit
• Pain
• Risk for injury

Nursing interventions
• Monitor the patient's fluid balance, abdominal girth, metabolic state, and weight daily. If weight loss occurs, replace nutrients through an I.V. line, by mouth, or through a nasogastric (NG) tube. If the patient gains weight (from ascites), impose dietary restrictions, such as a low-sodium diet, as ordered. Maintain a 2,500-calorie diet.
• Serve small, frequent meals. Consult the dietitian to ensure proper nutrition, and make mealtimes as pleasant as possible. Administer an oral pancreatic enzyme at mealtimes, if needed. As ordered, give an antacid to prevent stress ulcers.
• Before surgery, make sure the patient is medically stable—particularly regarding nutrition. This may take 4 to 5 days. If he can't tolerate oral feedings, provide total parenteral nutrition and I.V. fat emulsions to correct deficiencies and maintain a positive nitrogen balance.

Administer blood transfusions (to combat anemia), vitamin K (to overcome prothrombin deficiency), antibiotics (to prevent postoperative complications), and gastric lavage (to maintain gastric decompression), as ordered.
• After surgery, watch for and report complications, such as fistula, pancreatitis, fluid and electrolyte imbalance, infection, hemorrhage, skin breakdown, nutritional deficiency, liver failure, renal insufficiency, and diabetes.
• If the patient is receiving chemotherapy, watch for and symptomatically treat its toxic effects.
• To prevent constipation, administer laxatives, stool softeners, and cathartics, as ordered. Also modify the patient's diet and increase his fluid intake. To increase GI motility, position him properly during and after meals, and assist him with walking.
• Ensure adequate rest and sleep (with a sedative, if necessary). Assist with range-of-motion and isometric exercises, as appropriate.

• Administer analgesics for pain, and antibiotics and antipyretics for fever, as ordered.
• Watch for signs of hypoglycemia or hyperglycemia, and give the patient glucose or an antidiabetic agent (such as tolbutamide), as ordered. Monitor the patient's blood glucose, urine glucose, and acetone levels and his response to treatment.
• Document the progression of jaundice.
• Provide scrupulous skin care to prevent pruritus and necrosis, and keep the patient's skin clean and dry. If he develops overwhelming pruritus, you can prevent excoriation by clipping his nails and having him wear light cotton gloves.
• Watch for signs of upper GI bleeding. Test stools and emesis for blood, and maintain a flow sheet of frequent hemoglobin and hematocrit determinations.

To control active bleeding, promote gastric vasoconstriction with medication and iced saline lavage through an NG or a duodenal tube. Replace any lost fluids.
• Ease discomfort from pyloric obstruction with an NG tube.
• To prevent thrombosis, apply antiembolism stockings and assist with range-of-motion exercises. If thrombosis occurs, elevate the patient's legs and apply moist heat to the thrombus site. Give an anticoagulant, such as aspirin, as ordered, to prevent further clot formation and pulmonary embolus.
• Throughout therapy, answer any questions the patient has, and tell him what to expect from surgery and other therapies. Listen to his fears and concerns, and stay with him during periods of severe stress and anxiety.
• Encourage the patient to identify actions and care measures that will promote his comfort and relaxation. Try to perform these measures, and encourage the patient and his family to do so, too.
• Whenever possible, include the patient and his family in care decisions.

Patient teaching
• Describe expected postoperative procedures and adverse effects of radiation therapy and chemotherapy.
• If appropriate, provide information on diabetes.
• Help the patient and his family cope with the impending reality of death.
• Refer the patient to resource and support services, such as the social service department, local home health care agencies, hospices, and the American Cancer Society.
• Encourage the patient to follow as normal a routine as possible. Explain that leading a near-normal life will help foster feelings of independence and control.

COLORECTAL CANCER
The second most common visceral neoplasm in the United States and Europe, colorectal cancer is equally distributed between men and women. It occurs more frequently in those over age 40.

Malignant tumors of the colon or rectum are almost always adenocarcinomas. About half of these are sessile lesions of the rectosigmoid area; the rest, polypoid lesions.

Colorectal cancer progresses slowly, remaining localized for a long time. Unless the tumor has metastasized, the 5-year survival rate is relatively high: about 80% for rectal cancer and more than 85% for colon cancer. If left untreated, the disease is invariably fatal.

Causes
Although the exact cause of colorectal cancer is unknown, studies show a greater incidence in areas of higher economic development, suggesting a relation to diet (excess animal fat, particularly beef, and low fiber).

Other factors that magnify the risk of developing colorectal cancer include diseases of the digestive tract, a history of ulcerative colitis (cancer usually starts in 11 to 17 years), and familial polyposis (cancer almost always develops by age 50).

Complications
As the tumor grows and encroaches on the abdominal organs, abdominal distention and intestinal obstruction occur. Anemia may develop if rectal bleeding isn't treated.

Assessment findings
Signs and symptoms depend on the tumor's location. If it develops on the colon's right side, the patient probably won't have signs and symptoms in the early stages because the stool is still in liquid form in that part of the colon. He may have a history of black, tarry stools, however, and report anemia, abdominal aching, pressure, and dull cramps. As the disease progresses, he may complain of weakness, diarrhea, obstipation, anorexia, weight loss, and vomiting.

A tumor on the left side of the colon causes symptoms of obstruction even in the early disease stages because stools are more completely formed when they reach this part of the colon. The patient may report rectal bleeding (often ascribed to hemorrhoids), intermittent abdominal fullness or cramping, and rectal pressure.

As the disease progresses, obstipation, diarrhea, or ribbon- or pencil-shaped stools may develop. The patient may note that the passage of flatus or stool relieves his pain. He may also report obvious bleeding during defecation and dark or bright red blood in the feces and mucus in or on the stools.

A patient with a rectal tumor may report a change in bowel habits, often beginning with an urgent need to defecate on arising ("morning diarrhea") or obstipation alternating with diarrhea. He also may notice blood or mucus in the stools and complain of a sense of incomplete evacuation. Late in the disease, he may complain of pain that begins as a feeling of rectal fullness and progresses to a dull, sometimes constant ache confined to the rectum or sacral region.

Inspection of the abdomen may reveal distention or visible masses. Abdominal veins may appear enlarged and visible from portal obstruction. The inguinal and supraclavicular nodes may also appear enlarged. You may note abnormal bowel sounds on abdominal auscultation. Palpation may reveal abdominal masses. Right side tumors usually feel bulky; tumors of the transverse portion are more easily detected. (See *Palpating a patient with colorectal cancer*.)

Diagnostic tests
Several tests support a diagnosis of colorectal cancer.
• *Digital rectal examination* can detect almost 15% of colorectal cancers. Specifically, it can detect suspicious rectal and perianal lesions.
• *Fecal occult blood test* can detect blood in stools, a warning sign of rectal cancer.
• *Proctoscopy* or *sigmoidoscopy* permits visualization of the lower GI tract. It can detect up to 66% of colorectal cancers.
• *Colonoscopy* permits visual inspection and photography of the colon up to the ileocecal valve and provides access for polypectomies and biopsies of suspected lesions.
• *Excretory urography* verifies bilateral renal function and allows inspection for displacement of the kidneys, ureters, or bladder by a tumor pressing against these structures.
• *Barium enema studies,* using a dual contrast of barium and air, allow the location of lesions that aren't detectable manually or visually. Barium examination shouldn't precede colonoscopy or excretory urography because barium sulfate interferes with these tests.
• *Computed tomography scan* allows better visualization if a barium enema yields inconclusive results or if metastasis to the pelvic lymph nodes is suspected.
• *Carcinoembryonic antigen,* although not specific or sensitive enough for early diagnosis of colorectal cancer, permits patient monitoring before and after treatment to

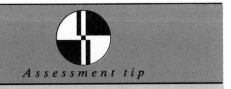

Assessment tip

PALPATING A PATIENT WITH COLORECTAL CANCER

A patient who complains of generalized tenderness may make accurate palpation difficult. To accurately assess tenderness in such a patient, place your stethoscope on his abdomen. But instead of auscultating, press into the abdomen with the stethoscope as you would with your hands and see if the patient still complains of pain.

detect metastasis or recurrence. (See *Staging colorectal cancer,* page 330.)

Treatment
The most effective treatment for colorectal cancer is surgery to remove the malignant tumor and adjacent tissues, along with any lymph nodes that may contain cancer cells. After surgery, treatment continues with chemotherapy, radiation therapy, or both.

The type of surgery depends on tumor location:
• *Cecum and ascending colon.* Tumors in these areas call for right hemicolectomy (for advanced disease). Surgery may include resection of the terminal segment of the ileum, cecum, ascending colon, and right half of the transverse colon with corresponding mesentery.
• *Proximal and middle transverse colon.* Surgery consists of right colectomy that includes the transverse colon and mesentery corresponding to midcolic vessels, or segmental resection of the transverse colon and associated midcolic vessels.
• *Sigmoid colon.* Surgery usually is limited to the sigmoid colon and mesentery.
• *Upper rectum.* A tumor in this area usually requires anterior or low anterior resection. A newer method, using a stapler, allows for much lower resections than previously possible.
• *Lower rectum.* Abdominoperineal resection and permanent sigmoid colostomy are required.

If metastasis has occurred, or if the patient has residual disease or a recurrent inoperable tumor, he needs chemotherapy. Drugs used in such treatment commonly include fluorouracil combined with levamisole or leuco-

STAGING COLORECTAL CANCER

Named for pathologist Cuthbert Dukes, the Dukes cancer classification assigns tumors to four stages. These stages (with substages) reflect the extent of bowel mucosa and bowel wall infiltration, lymph node involvement, and metastasis. Use this summary to clarify your patient's cancer stage and prognosis.

Stage A
Malignant cells are confined to the bowel mucosa, and the lymph nodes contain no cancer cells. Treated promptly, about 80% of these patients remain disease-free 5 years later.

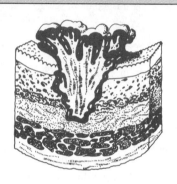

Stage B
Malignant cells extend through the bowel mucosa but remain within the bowel wall. The lymph nodes are normal. In substage B_2, all bowel wall layers and immediately adjacent structures contain malignant cells, but the lymph nodes remain normal. About 50% of patients with substage B_2 survive for 5 or more years.

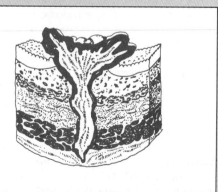

Stage C
Malignant cells extend into the bowel wall and the lymph nodes. In substage C_2, malignant cells extend through the entire thickness of the bowel wall. The lymph nodes also contain malignant cells. The 5-year survival rate for patients with stage C disease reaches about 25%.

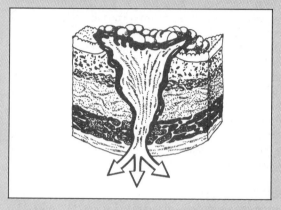

Stage D
Metastasized to distant organs by way of the lymph nodes and mesenteric vessels, malignant cells typically lodge in the lungs and liver. Only 5% of patients with stage D cancer survive 5 or more years.

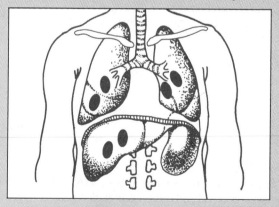

vorin. Researchers are evaluating the effectiveness of flu-orouracil with recombinant interferon alfa-2a.

Radiation therapy, used before or after surgery, induces tumor regression.

Nursing diagnoses
• Altered nutrition: Less than body requirements
• Altered oral mucous membrane
• Anxiety
• Body image disturbance
• Constipation
• Diarrhea
• Fear
• Fluid volume deficit
• Impaired skin integrity
• Ineffective family coping
• Ineffective individual coping
• Knowledge deficit
• Pain
• Risk for infection
• Sexual dysfunction

Nursing interventions
• Before colorectal surgery, monitor the patient's diet modifications, and administer laxatives, enemas, and antibiotics, as ordered. These measures help clean the bowel and decrease abdominal and peritoneal cavity contamination during surgery.
• After surgery, monitor the patient's vital signs, intake and output, and fluid and electrolyte balance. Also monitor him for complications, including anastomotic leaks, hemorrhage, irregular bowel function, phantom rectum, ruptured pelvic peritoneum, stricture, urinary dysfunction, and wound infection.
• Care for the patient's incision and, if appropriate, his stoma. To decrease discomfort, administer ordered analgesics as necessary, and perform comfort measures, such as positioning.
• Encourage the patient to look at the stoma and to participate in its care as soon as possible. Teach good hygiene and skin care. Allow him to shower or bathe as soon as the incision heals.
• Consult with an enterostomal therapist, if available, for questions on setting up a postoperative regimen for the patient.
• Watch for adverse effects of radiation therapy (nausea, vomiting, hair loss, malaise), and provide comfort measures and reassurance.
• During chemotherapy, watch for complications (such as infection) and expected adverse effects. Prepare the patient for these problems. Take steps to reduce these ef-

fects; for example, by rinsing the patient's mouth with normal saline mouthwash to deter ulcers.
• To help prevent infection, use strict aseptic technique when caring for I.V. catheters and providing wound care. Change I.V. tubing and sites as directed by hospital policy. Have the patient wash his hands before and after meals and after going to the bathroom.
• Listen to the patient's fears and concerns, and stay with him during periods of severe stress and anxiety.
• Encourage the patient to identify actions and care measures that will promote his comfort and relaxation. Try to perform these measures, and encourage the patient and his family to do so, too.
• Whenever possible, include the patient and his family in care decisions.

Patient teaching
• Throughout therapy, answer the patient's questions, and tell him what to expect from surgery and other therapy.
• If appropriate, explain that the stoma will be red, moist, and swollen; reassure the patient that postoperative swelling eventually will subside.
• Show the patient a diagram of the intestine before and after surgery, stressing how much of the bowel remains intact. Supplement your teaching with instruction booklets (available for a fee from the United Ostomy Association, and free from various companies that manufacture ostomy supplies). Arrange a postsurgical visit from a recovered ostomy patient.
• Prepare the patient for the I.V. lines, nasogastric tube, and indwelling urinary catheter he'll have postoperatively.
• Preoperatively, teach the patient the coughing and deep-breathing exercises he should use postoperatively.
• Explain to the patient's family that their positive reactions will foster the patient's adjustment.
• If appropriate, instruct the patient with a sigmoid colostomy to perform his own irrigation as soon as he's able after surgery. Advise him to schedule irrigation for the time of the day when he normally evacuates. Many patients find that irrigating every 1 to 3 days is necessary for regulation.
• Direct the patient to follow a high-fiber diet.
• If flatus, diarrhea, or constipation occurs, tell the patient to eliminate suspected causative foods from his diet. Explain that he may reintroduce them later. Teach him which foods may alleviate constipation, and encourage him to increase his fluid and fiber intake.
• If diarrhea is a problem, advise the patient to try eating applesauce, bananas, or rice. Caution him to take laxa-

UNILATERAL KIDNEY TUMOR

In kidney cancer, tumors—such as this one in the upper kidney pole—usually occur unilaterally.

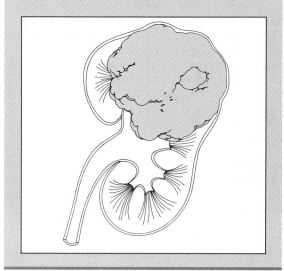

tives or antidiarrheal medications only as prescribed by his doctor.

• When appropriate, explain that after several months, many patients with an ostomy establish control with irrigation and no longer need to wear a pouch. A stoma cap or gauze sponge placed over the stoma protects it and absorbs mucoid secretions. Explain that before achieving such control, the patient can resume physical activities—including sports—provided he's not at risk of injuring the stoma or surrounding abdominal muscles.

• If the patient wants to swim, he can place a pouch or stoma cap (if regulated) over the stoma. He should avoid heavy lifting, which can cause herniation or prolapse through weakened muscles in the abdominal wall. Suggest that he consider a structured, gradually progressive exercise program to strengthen abdominal muscles. Such a program can be instituted under a doctor's supervision.

• Emphasize the need for keeping follow-up appointments. Anyone who has had colorectal cancer runs an increased risk of developing another primary cancer. The patient should have yearly screenings (sigmoidoscopy, digital rectal examination, stool test for blood) and follow-up testing.

• If the patient will undergo radiation therapy or chemotherapy, explain the treatment to him. Be sure he understands the adverse effects that usually occur and the measures he can take to decrease their severity or prevent their occurrence.

• Instruct the patient and his family about the American Cancer Society's guidelines for colorectal cancer screening: a digital rectal examination annually starting at age 40, periodic sigmoidoscopy and colonoscopy, and a stool test for occult blood annually starting at age 50.

• Refer the patient to a home health care agency that can check on his physical care at home.

• For male patients, suggest sexual counseling; most are impotent for a time after colostomy.

KIDNEY CANCER

About 85% of kidney cancers—also called nephrocarcinoma, renal cell carcinoma, hypernephroma, and Grawitz's tumor—originate in the kidneys. Others are metastases from various primary-site carcinomas.

Most kidney tumors are large, firm, nodular, encapsulated, unilateral, and solitary. (See *Unilateral kidney tumor.*) They may affect either kidney; occasionally they're bilateral or multifocal.

The incidence of kidney cancer is rising, possibly from exposure to environmental carcinogens and increased longevity. Even so, kidney cancer accounts for only about 2% of all adult cancers. Twice as common in men as in women, kidney cancer typically strikes after age 40, with peak incidence between ages 50 and 60. Renal pelvic tumors and Wilms' tumor occur most commonly in children.

Kidney cancer can be separated histologically into clear cell, granular cell, and spindle cell types. Sometimes the prognosis is considered better for the clear cell type than for the other types; in general, however, the prognosis depends more on the cancer's stage than on its type. (See *Staging kidney cancer.*)

Overall prognosis has improved considerably, with the 5-year survival rate about 50% and the 10-year survival rate at 18% to 23%. Left untreated, kidney cancer is fatal.

Causes
Although the cause of kidney cancer is unknown, some studies implicate particular factors, including heavy cigarette smoking. Patients who receive regular hemodialysis also may be at increased risk.

Complications
Complications include hemorrhage, respiratory problems from metastasis to the lungs, neurologic problems from

STAGING KIDNEY CANCER

Using the TNM (tumor, node, metastasis) system, the American Joint Committee on Cancer has established the following stages for kidney cancer.

Primary tumor

TX—primary tumor can't be assessed
T0—no evidence of primary tumor
T1—tumor 2.5 cm or less in greatest dimension and limited to the kidney
T2—tumor greater than 2.5 cm in greatest dimension and limited to the kidney
T3—tumor extends into major veins or invades adrenal gland or perinephric tissues, but not beyond Gerota's fascia
T3a—tumor extends into adrenal gland or perinephric tissues, but not beyond Gerota's fascia
T3b—tumor grossly extends into renal veins or vena cava
T4—tumor extends beyond Gerota's fascia

Regional lymph nodes

NX—regional lymph nodes can't be assessed
N0—no evidence of regional lymph node metastasis
N1—metastasis in a single lymph node, 2 cm or less in greatest dimension
N2—metastasis in a single lymph node, between 2 and 5 cm in greatest dimension, or metastases to several lymph nodes, none more than 5 cm in greatest dimension
N3—metastasis in a lymph node more than 5 cm in greatest dimension

Distant metastasis

MX—distant metastasis can't be assessed
M0—no known distant metastasis
M1—distant metastasis

Staging categories

Kidney cancer progresses from mild to severe as follows:
Stage I—T1, N0, M0
Stage II—T2, N0, M0
Stage III—T1, N1, M0; T2, N1, M0; T3a, N0, M0; T3a, N1, M0; T3b, N0, M0; T3b, N1, M0
Stage IV—T4, any N, M0; any T, N2, M0; any T, N3, M0; any T, any N, M1

---

brain metastasis, and GI problems from liver metastasis.

Assessment findings

The patient may complain of hematuria and often a dull, aching flank pain. He also may report weight loss, although this is uncommon. Rarely, his temperature may be elevated. Palpation may reveal a smooth, firm, nontender abdominal mass.

Diagnostic tests

Renal ultrasonography and a computed tomography scan can distinguish between simple cysts and renal cancer. In many cases, these tests eliminate the need for renal angiography. Other tests that aid diagnosis and help in staging include excretory urography, nephrotomography, and kidney-ureter-bladder radiography.

Additional relevant tests include liver function studies, which show increased alkaline phosphatase, bilirubin, and transaminase levels and prolonged prothrombin time. Such results may point to liver metastasis. If the tumor hasn't metastasized, these abnormal values reverse after tumor resection.

Treatment

Radical nephrectomy, with or without regional lymph node dissection, offers the only chance of cure. It's the treatment of choice in localized cancer or with tumor extension into the renal vein and vena cava. Nephrectomy won't help in disseminated disease.

Because this disease resists radiation, this treatment is used only when the cancer has spread into the perinephric region or the lymph nodes or when the primary tumor or metastatic sites can't be completely excised. Then the patient usually needs high radiation doses.

Chemotherapy and hormonal therapy have no effect on kidney cancer. Immunotherapy with lymphokine-activated killer cells plus recombinant interleukin-2 shows promise but is expensive and causes many adverse reactions. Interferon is somewhat effective in treating advanced disease.

Nursing diagnoses

• Altered tissue perfusion
• Anxiety
• Fear
• Impaired physical mobility
• Impaired tissue integrity
• Ineffective breathing pattern
• Pain
• Risk for injury

Nursing interventions

• Before surgery, assure the patient that his body will adequately adapt to the loss of a kidney.

• Administer prescribed analgesics as necessary. Provide comfort measures, such as positioning and distractions, to help the patient cope with his discomfort.
• After surgery, encourage diaphragmatic breathing and coughing.
• Assist the patient with leg exercises, and turn him every 2 hours to reduce the risk of phlebitis.
• Check dressings often for excessive bleeding. Watch for signs of internal bleeding, such as restlessness, sweating, and increased pulse rate.
• Position the patient on the operative side to allow the pressure of adjacent organs to fill the dead space at the operative site, improving dependent drainage.
• If possible, assist the patient with walking within 24 hours of surgery.
• Provide adequate fluid intake, and monitor intake and output.
• Monitor laboratory test results for anemia, polycythemia, and abnormal blood chemistry values that may point to bone or hepatic involvement or may result from radiation therapy or chemotherapy.
• Provide symptomatic treatment for adverse effects of chemotherapeutic drugs.
• Encourage the patient to express his anxieties and fears, and remain with him during periods of severe stress and anxiety.

Patient teaching
• Tell the patient what to expect from surgery and other treatments.
• Before surgery, teach him diaphragmatic breathing and effective coughing techniques, such as how to splint his incision.
• Explain the possible adverse effects of radiation and drug therapy. Advise the patient on how to prevent and minimize these problems.
• When preparing the patient for discharge, stress the importance of compliance with any prescribed outpatient treatment. This includes an annual follow-up chest X-ray to rule out lung metastasis and excretory urography every 6 to 12 months to check for contralateral tumors.
• If appropriate, refer the patient and his family to hospital and community services, such as cancer support groups and hospice care.

LIVER CANCER

Having a high mortality, primary liver cancer accounts for roughly 2% of all cancers in North America and for 10% to 50% of cancers in Africa and parts of Asia. It's most prevalent in men, particularly those over age 60, and the incidence increases with age.

Most primary liver tumors (90%) originate in the parenchymal cells and are hepatomas (also called hepatocellular carcinomas, or primary liver cell carcinomas). Some primary tumors originate in the intrahepatic bile ducts and are known as cholangiomas (also known as cholangiocarcinomas, or cholangiocellular carcinomas). Rarer tumors include a mixed-cell type, Kupffer cell sarcoma, and hepatoblastoma, which occurs almost exclusively in children. Roughly 30% to 70% of patients with hepatomas also have cirrhosis, and a person with cirrhosis is about 40 times more likely to develop hepatomas than someone with a normal liver.

The liver is one of the most common sites of metastasis from other primary cancers, particularly melanoma and cancers of the colon, rectum, stomach, pancreas, esophagus, lung, or breast. In North America, metastatic liver cancer is about 20 times more common than primary liver cancer and, after cirrhosis, is the leading cause of fatal hepatic disease. Liver metastasis may occur as a solitary lesion, the first sign of recurrence after a remission.

No particular staging system exists for liver cancer. Although most hepatoblastomas are resectable and curable, the prognosis is almost always poor. The disease is rapidly fatal—usually within 6 months—from GI hemorrhage, progressive cachexia, liver failure, or metastatic spread. When cirrhosis is present, the prognosis is especially grim, with death from liver failure usually occurring within 2 months of diagnosis.

Causes
The immediate cause is unknown, but in children, it's commonly attributed to congenital factors. Adult liver cancer may result from environmental exposure to carcinogens, including the chemical compound aflatoxin (a mold that grows on rice and peanuts), thorium dioxide (a contrast medium used for liver radiography in the past), *Senecio* alkaloids and, possibly, androgens and oral estrogens. Another high-risk factor is exposure to the hepatitis B virus.

Whether cirrhosis is a premalignant state or whether alcohol or malnutrition predisposes the liver to hepatomas is unclear.

Complications
Progression of this disease may cause GI hemorrhage, progressive cachexia, and liver failure.

Assessment findings

The patient's history may show weight loss, resulting from anorexia, as well as weakness, fatigue, and fever. The patient also may complain of severe pain in the epigastrium or the right upper quadrant.

On inspection, you may note jaundice (including scleral icterus) and dependent edema. Peripheral edema may suggest decreased plasma albumin levels related to liver dysfunction and malnutrition. Auscultation may reveal a bruit, hum, or rubbing sound if the tumor involves a large part of the liver. Percussing the abdomen may uncover an increased span of liver dullness, indicating an enlarged liver. Dull sounds on percussion indicate ascites. Palpation may disclose a mass in the right upper quadrant and a tender, nodular liver.

Diagnostic tests

These findings support a diagnosis of liver cancer:
• *Liver biopsy*, by needle or open biopsy, reveals cancerous cells.
• *Liver function studies* are abnormal.
• *Alpha-fetoprotein* levels rise above 500 mcg/ml.
• *Chest X-rays* may rule out metastasis to the lungs.
• A *liver scan* may show filling defects.
• *Arteriography* may define large tumors.
• *Electrolyte studies* may indicate increased sodium retention (resulting in functional renal failure), hypoglycemia, hypercalcemia, or hypocholesterolemia.

Treatment

Because liver cancer may reach an advanced stage before diagnosis, few hepatic tumors are resectable. A resectable tumor must be solitary and not accompanied by cirrhosis, jaundice, or ascites. Resection is performed by lobectomy or partial hepatectomy.

Radiation therapy may be used alone or with chemotherapy. Chemotherapeutic drugs include fluorouracil, doxorubicin, methotrexate, cyclophosphamide, and vincristine. Both therapies combined produce a better response rate than either therapy used alone.

Nursing diagnoses

• Altered nutrition: Less than body requirements
• Altered thought processes
• Altered tissue perfusion
• Anxiety
• Fatigue
• Fear
• Fluid volume excess
• Hyperthermia
• Impaired gas exchange
• Impaired skin integrity
• Ineffective family coping
• Ineffective individual coping
• Pain

Nursing interventions

• Give analgesics as ordered, and encourage the patient to identify care measures that promote comfort.
• Monitor the patient's diet throughout his illness. Most patients need a special diet that restricts sodium, fluids, and protein and prohibits alcohol. Weigh the patient daily, and note intake and output accurately.
• Control ascites. If signs develop—peripheral edema, orthopnea, and dyspnea on exertion—measure and record the patient's abdominal girth daily.
• To increase venous return and prevent edema, elevate the patient's legs whenever possible.
• Monitor respiratory function. Note any shortness of breath or increase in respiratory rate. Bilateral pleural effusion (evident on chest X-ray) and metastasis to the lungs are common. Watch carefully for signs of hypoxemia from intrapulmonary arteriovenous shunting.
• Keep the patient's fever down. Administer sponge baths and aspirin suppositories if the patient has no signs of GI bleeding. Avoid acetaminophen; the diseased liver can't metabolize it. If a high fever develops, the patient has an infection and needs antibiotics.
• Provide meticulous skin care. Turn the patient frequently, and keep his skin clean to prevent pressure ulcers. Apply lotion to prevent chafing, and administer an antipruritic for severe itching.
• Watch for encephalopathy. Many patients develop end-stage symptoms of ammonia intoxication, including confusion, restlessness, irritability, agitation, delirium, asterixis, lethargy and, finally, coma. Monitor the patient's serum ammonia level, vital signs, and neurologic status.
• As ordered, control ammonia accumulation with sorbitol (to induce osmotic diarrhea), neomycin (to reduce bacterial flora in the GI tract), lactulose (to control bacterial elaboration of ammonia), and sodium polystyrene sulfonate (to lower the potassium level).
• If the patient has a transhepatic catheter in place to relieve obstructive jaundice, irrigate it frequently with the prescribed solution (0.9% sodium chloride or, sometimes, 5,000 units of heparin in 500 ml dextrose 5% in water). Monitor his vital signs frequently for any indication of bleeding or infection.
• After surgery, watch for intraperitoneal bleeding and sepsis, which may precipitate coma. Monitor for renal failure by checking the patient's urine output, blood urea nitrogen, and serum creatinine levels hourly.

• Throughout therapy, provide comprehensive supportive care and emotional assistance. Remember that throughout this intractable illness, your primary concern is to keep the patient as comfortable as possible.
• At all times, listen to the concerns and fears of the patient and his family.

Patient teaching
• Explain the treatments to the patient and his family, including adverse effects the patient may experience.
• Explain the importance of restricting sodium and protein intake and eliminating alcohol from the diet.
• Encourage the patient to learn and practice relaxation techniques to promote comfort and ease anxiety.
• If appropriate, direct the patient and his family to local support groups and services.

BLADDER CANCER
Benign or malignant tumors may develop on the bladder wall surface or grow within the wall itself and quickly invade underlying muscles. About 90% of bladder cancers are transitional cell carcinomas, arising from the transitional epithelium of mucous membranes. They may result from malignant transformation of benign papillomas. Less common bladder tumors include adenocarcinomas, epidermoid carcinomas, squamous cell carcinomas, sarcomas, tumors in bladder diverticula, and carcinoma in situ.

Bladder tumors are most prevalent in people over age 50, are more common in men than in women, and occur more often in densely populated industrial areas. Bladder cancer accounts for about 2% to 4% of all cancers.

Despite treatment, the patient with superficial disease has up to an 80% chance for recurrence. Only about 10% of superficial bladder cancers develop into invasive disease; in invasive disease, however, the patient's chances for metastasis increase up to 90%. With treatment, about 50% of patients with invasive cancer experience complete remission; 20% have partial remission.

Causes
Certain environmental carcinogens, such as 2-naphthylamine, tobacco, nitrates, and coffee, are known to predispose a person to transitional cell tumors. This places certain industrial workers at high risk for developing such tumors, including rubber workers, weavers, aniline dye workers, hairdressers, petroleum workers, spray painters, and leather finishers. The latency period between exposure to the carcinogen and development of signs and symptoms is about 18 years.

Squamous cell carcinoma of the bladder is common in geographic areas where schistosomiasis is endemic, such as Egypt. What's more, it's also associated with chronic bladder irritation and infection in people with renal calculi, indwelling urinary catheters, chemical cystitis caused by cyclophosphamide, and pelvic irradiation.

Complications
If bladder cancer progresses, complications include bone metastases and problems resulting from tumor invasion of contiguous viscera.

Assessment findings
The patient typically reports gross, painless, intermittent hematuria (often with clots). He may complain of suprapubic pain after voiding (which suggests invasive lesions). He also may complain of bladder irritability, urinary frequency, nocturia, and dribbling. If he reports flank pain, he may have an obstructed ureter.

Diagnostic tests
• To confirm a bladder cancer diagnosis, the patient typically undergoes *cystoscopy* and *biopsy*. If the test results show cancer cells, further studies will determine the cancer stage and treatment. (See *Comparing staging systems for bladder cancer*.) Cystoscopy should be performed when hematuria first appears. If the patient receives an anesthetic during the procedure, he also may undergo a bimanual examination to detect whether the bladder is fixed to the pelvic wall.
• *Excretory urography* can identify a large, early-stage tumor or an infiltrating tumor; delineate functional problems in the upper urinary tract; assess hydronephrosis; and detect rigid deformity of the bladder wall.
• *Urinalysis* can detect blood and malignant cells in the urine.
• *Retrograde cystography* evaluates bladder structure and integrity. Test results also help confirm a bladder cancer diagnosis.
• *Bone scan* can detect metastases.
• *Computed tomography scan* can define the thickness of the involved bladder wall and disclose enlarged retroperitoneal lymph nodes.
• *Ultrasonography* can find metastases in tissues beyond the bladder and can distinguish a bladder cyst from a bladder tumor.
• *Laboratory tests,* such as a complete blood count and chemistry profile, may be ordered to evaluate conditions, such as anemia, associated with bladder cancer.

COMPARING STAGING SYSTEMS FOR BLADDER CANCER

Staging helps determine the most appropriate treatment for bladder cancer. One of two staging systems may be used: the TNM (tumor, node, metastasis) system or the JSM (Jewett-Strong-Marshall) system.

The JSM system grades cancers O and A through D. Both systems distinguish superficial bladder cancers from invasive bladder cancers, which penetrate bladder muscle and may spread to other sites.

TNM system	Stage	JSM system
Superficial tumor		
TX	Primary tumor can't be assessed	—
T0	No tumor	0
Tis	Carcinoma in situ	0
Ta	Noninvasive papillary tumor	0
Invasive tumor		
T1	Tumor invades subepithelial connective tissue	—
T2	Tumor invades superficial muscle (inner half)	B_1
T3a	Tumor invades deep muscle	B_2
T3b	Tumor invades perivesical fat	C
T4	Tumor invades prostate, uterus, vagina, pelvic wall, or abdominal wall	D_1
NX	Regional lymph nodes can't be assessed	—
N0	No evidence of lymph node involvement	—
N1	Metastasis in a single lymph node, 2 cm or less in greatest dimension	D_1
N2	Metastasis in a single lymph node, between 2 and 5 cm in greatest dimension, or metastases to several lymph nodes, none greater than 5 cm in greatest dimension	—
N3	Metastasis in a lymph node more than 5 cm in greatest dimension	—
MX	Distant metastasis can't be assessed	—
M0	No evidence of distant metastasis	—
M	Distant metastasis	D_2

Treatment

The cancer's stage and the patient's life-style, other health problems, and mental outlook will influence selection of therapy. Surgery, chemotherapy, radiation therapy, or one of several investigational treatments may be used. (For more information, see *Investigational bladder cancer treatments,* page 338.)

Superficial bladder tumors are removed cystoscopically by *transurethral resection* and electrically by *fulguration.* This usually is adequate treatment if the tumor hasn't

INVESTIGATIONAL BLADDER CANCER TREATMENTS

Current investigational therapies offer promise for bladder cancer patients. Treatments include immunotherapy, neoadjuvant radiation therapy and chemotherapy, and photodynamic therapy.

Immunotherapy
Also called biotherapy, this experimental treatment uses the intravesical route to instill interferon alfa and tumor necrosis factor. These agents are believed to stimulate the patient's immune system to produce natural substances that kill abnormal cells or delay their growth.

Adverse effects from interferon alfa include alopecia, leukopenia, and flulike symptoms. Adverse effects associated with tumor necrosis factor are being studied.

Neoadjuvant therapy
Patients with localized bladder tumors judged too extensive for surgical removal may benefit from an experimental combination of radiation therapy and chemotherapy. This treatment shrinks the tumors so that surgery can be more effective or the bladder can be retained.

The adverse effects are those associated with radiation therapy and the particular chemotherapeutic agents used.

Photodynamic therapy
This treatment requires I.V. injection of a photosensitizing agent called hematoporphyrin derivative (HPD). Malignant tissue appears to have an affinity for HPD, so superficial bladder cancer cells readily absorb the drug. A cystoscope is then used to introduce laser energy into the bladder; exposing the HPD-impregnated tumor cells to laser energy kills them.

However, HPD sensitizes not only tumor tissue but also normal tissue. So any patient who receives this therapy must avoid sunlight for about 30 days. Precautions involve wearing protective clothing (including gloves and a face mask), drawing heavy curtains at home during the day, scheduling outdoor travel for night, and conducting exercises inside or outdoors at night to promote circulation, joint mobility, and muscle activity. After 30 days, the patient can gradually return to normal daylight activities.

---

invaded the muscle. Additional tumors may develop, however, and fulguration may have to be repeated every 3 months for years. Once the tumors penetrate the muscle layer or recur frequently, cystoscopy with fulguration is no longer appropriate.

Intravesical chemotherapy is used for treating superficial tumors (especially tumors in many sites) and for preventing tumor recurrence. This therapy directly washes the bladder with anticancer drugs. Commonly used agents include thiotepa, doxorubicin, and mitomycin.

Intravesical administration of the live, attenuated *bacille Calmette-Guérin (BCG) vaccine* has proved successful in treating superficial bladder cancers, particularly primary and relapsed carcinoma in situ.

Tumors too large to be treated cystoscopically require *segmental bladder resection*. This surgery, which removes a full-thickness section of the bladder, is feasible only if the tumor isn't near the bladder neck or ureteral orifices. Bladder instillations of thiotepa after transurethral resection also may help.

For infiltrating bladder tumors, the treatment of choice is *radical cystectomy* with a pretreatment course of 2,000-rad external beam radiation therapy directed at the bladder. During the operation, the surgeon removes the bladder with perivesical fat, lymph nodes, urethra, and the

prostate and seminal vesicles (in men) or the uterus and adnexa uteri (in women). Next, he constructs a urinary diversion, usually an ileal conduit (ileal loop). After surgery, the patient will wear an external pouch continuously. Other diversions are *ureterostomy, nephrostomy, continent vesicostomy (Kock pouch), ileal bladder,* and *ureterosigmoidostomy.* (For more information, see *Common urinary diversions.*)

Note: A male patient may become impotent after radical cystectomy and urethrectomy because the operation damages the sympathetic and the parasympathetic nerves that control erection and ejaculation. At a later date, treatment may include a penile implant to make sexual intercourse (without ejaculation) possible.

Treatment for patients with advanced bladder cancer includes cystectomy to remove the tumor, radiation therapy, and combination systemic chemotherapy with cisplatin, the most active agent. Other agents include methotrexate, vinblastine, and doxorubicin. In some instances, this combined treatment successfully arrests the disease.

Nursing diagnoses
• Altered urinary elimination
• Anxiety
• Body image disturbance

COMMON URINARY DIVERSIONS

Various urinary diversions may be done for bladder cancer patients. Two of the most commonly performed types include the continent vesicostomy and the ileal conduit.

Continent vesicostomy
This alternative to the ileal conduit diverts urine to a reservoir reconstructed from part of the bladder wall. The reservoir empties through a stoma on the abdomen. Accumulated urine can be drained by inserting a catheter through the stoma.

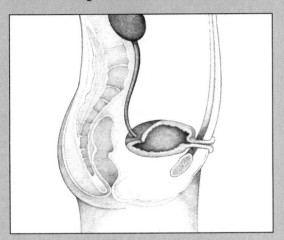

Ileal conduit
This preferred procedure diverts urine through a segment of the ileum to a stoma on the abdomen (as shown). Because urine empties continuously, the patient will need to wear a collecting device (or pouch).

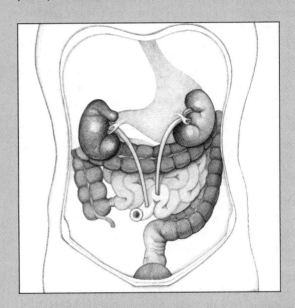

• Fear
• Impaired skin integrity
• Ineffective family coping
• Ineffective individual coping
• Pain
• Risk for infection
• Sexual dysfunction

Nursing interventions
• Listen to the patient's fears and concerns. Stay with him during periods of severe stress and anxiety, and provide psychological support. As appropriate, encourage him to express typical concerns about the cancer's extent, the surgical procedure, an altered body image (especially if he undergoes urinary diversion surgery), and sexual dysfunction.

• To relieve discomfort, provide ordered pain medications as necessary. Implement comfort measures and distractions that will help the patient relax.
• Before surgery, offer information and support when the patient and enterostomal therapist select a stoma site. The therapist assesses the patient's abdomen in various positions. The typical site—in the rectus muscle—minimizes the risk of subsequent herniation. Advise the patient to make sure that he can easily see the selected site.
• After surgery, encourage the patient to look at the stoma. If he has difficulty doing this, leave the room for a few minutes when the stoma is exposed. Offer him a mirror to make viewing easier.
• To obtain a specimen for culture and sensitivity tests after urinary diversion surgery, catheterize the patient,

using sterile technique. Insert a lubricated catheter tip into the stoma about 2″ (5 cm). Many hospitals use a double telescope-type catheter for ileal conduit catheterization.

• After ileal conduit surgery, watch for these complications: wound infection, enteric fistulas, urine leaks, ureteral obstruction, bowel obstruction, and pelvic abscesses. After radical cystectomy and construction of a urine reservoir, watch for these complications: incontinence, difficult catheterization, urine reflux, obstruction, bacteriuria, and electrolyte imbalances.

• If the patient is receiving chemotherapy, watch for complications resulting from the particular drug regimen.

• If the patient is having radiation therapy, watch for these complications: radiation enteritis, colitis, and skin reactions. Preoperative radiation therapy may produce radiation enteritis, requiring aggressive parenteral support postoperatively. Residual damage of the bowel and the skin resembles the damage that occurs after radiation therapy for prostate cancer. As appropriate, implement measures to prevent or alleviate complications.

Patient teaching

• Tell the patient what to expect from diagnostic tests. For example, be sure he understands that he may be anesthetized for cystoscopy. After the test results are known, explain the implications to the patient and his family.

• Provide complete preoperative teaching. Include an explanation of the operation the patient will undergo. Discuss equipment and procedures that the patient can expect postoperatively. Also demonstrate essential coughing and deep-breathing exercises. Encourage the patient to ask questions.

For the patient with a urinary stoma:

• Teach the patient how to care for his urinary stoma. Instruction usually begins 4 to 6 days after surgery. Encourage appropriate relatives or other caregivers to attend the teaching session. Advise them beforehand that a negative reaction to the stoma can impede the patient's adjustment.

• If the patient will wear a urine collection pouch, teach him how to prepare and apply it. First, find out whether he will wear a reusable pouch or a disposable pouch. If he chooses a reusable pouch, he'll need at least two to wear alternately.

• Teach the patient to select the right-sized pouch by measuring the stoma and choosing a pouch with an opening that leaves a ⅛″ (0.3 cm) margin of skin around the stoma.

• Instruct the patient to remeasure the stoma after he goes home, in case the size changes.

• Advise him to be sure the pouch has a push-button or twist-type valve at the bottom to allow for drainage.

• Tell him to empty the pouch when it's one-third full, or every 2 to 3 hours.

• Offer the patient tips on effective skin seal. Explain that urine tends to destroy skin barriers that contain mostly karaya (a natural skin barrier). Suggest that he select a barrier made of urine-resistant synthetics with little or no karaya. Advise him to check the pouch frequently to ensure that the skin seal remains intact. Explain that a good skin seal can last from 3 to 6 days, so he need only change the pouch that often. If desired, he can wear a loose-fitting elastic pouch belt for added security. Tell the patient that the ileal conduit stoma should reach its permanent size about 2 to 4 months after surgery.

• Explain that the surgeon constructs the ileal conduit from the intestine, which normally produces mucus. For this reason, the patient will see mucus in the drained urine. Assure him that this is normal.

• Teach the patient to provide stoma care. Show him how to keep the skin around the stoma clean and free of irritation. Instruct him to remove the pouch, wash the skin with water and mild soap, and rinse well with clear water to remove soapy residue. Tell him to gently pat the skin dry. Never rub.

• Demonstrate how to place a gauze sponge soaked in vinegar water (1 part vinegar to 3 parts water) over the stoma for a few minutes to prevent a buildup of uric acid crystals. When he cares for his skin, suggest that he place a rolled-up dry sponge over the stoma to collect (or wick) draining urine.

• Next, instruct him to coat his skin with a silicone skin protectant and then cover with the collection pouch. If skin irritation or breakdown occurs, he should apply a layer of antacid precipitate to the clean, dry skin before coating it with the silicone skin protectant.

• To ensure a better seal and minimize skin breakdown, teach the patient how to use various products to level uneven abdominal surfaces, such as gullies, scars, and wedges.

• If the patient with surgically induced impotence was sexually active before surgery, encourage the patient's partner to express support and understanding. Suggest alternative methods of sexual expression.

• Postoperatively, tell the patient with a urinary stoma to avoid heavy lifting and contact sports. Encourage him to participate in his usual athletic and physical activities.

• Refer the patient to the American Cancer Society or the United Ostomy Association, as appropriate.
• Before discharge, arrange for follow-up home nursing care. Also refer the patient for services provided by the enterostomal therapist.

GALLBLADDER AND BILE DUCT CANCERS

Usually discovered coincidentally in patients with cholecystitis (about 90% have gallstones), gallbladder and bile duct cancers account for less than 1% of all cancer cases. The predominant type is adenocarcinoma (responsible for 85% to 95% of cases). Squamous cell carcinoma accounts for between 5% and 15%. Mixed-tissue types are rare.

Gallbladder cancer is most prevalent in women over age 60. And because it's usually discovered after cholecystectomy and at an advanced stage, the prognosis is poor. If the cancer invades gallbladder musculature, the survival rate is less than 5% — even after extensive surgery. Although some long-term survivals (4 to 5 years) have been reported, few patients survive more than 6 months after surgery. In most patients — with or without surgery — the disease progresses rapidly. Patients seldom live a year after diagnosis.

Carcinoma of the extrahepatic bile duct causes less than 1% of all cancer deaths in the United States. This disease affects more men than women (ratio of 5:2) between ages 60 and 70. The usual site is the bifurcation in the common bile duct. About 50% of patients also have gallstones. And carcinoma at the distal end of the common duct is commonly confused with carcinoma of the pancreas. Metastasis affects local lymph nodes, the liver, the lungs, and the peritoneum. Patients typically die of hepatic failure. No staging protocol exists for this type of cancer.

Causes

Whereas tumors of the biliary system are usually related to cholelithiasis, bile duct cancer seems to accompany infestation by liver flukes or other parasites.

The cause of extrahepatic bile duct cancer isn't known; however, statistics show an unexplained increase of this cancer in patients with sclerosing cholangitis, portal bacteremia, viral infections, or ulcerative colitis. Suspected causes include failure of an immune mechanism or chronic use of certain drugs by the colitis patient.

Complications

Cholangitis from obstructed bile ducts may develop as disease progresses. Typically, lymph node metastases appear in up to 70% of patients at diagnosis. Direct extension to the liver is also common (affecting up to 90% of patients). Direct extension to the cystic and the common bile ducts, stomach, colon, duodenum, and jejunum also occurs, and produces obstructions. Metastases further spread by portal or hepatic veins to the peritoneum, ovaries, and lower lung lobes.

Assessment findings

The patient history may reveal pain centered in the epigastric area or in the right upper quadrant. The patient may describe the pain as sporadic rather than continuous. Like a patient with cholecystitis, she may report weight loss and fatigue, resulting from anorexia, nausea, and vomiting. She also may report pruritus.

Inspection may identify scleral or gingival jaundice (usually associated with advanced disease in gallbladder cancer patients).

Palpation in the right upper quadrant will reveal gallbladder enlargement.

Diagnostic tests

• *Liver function tests* — to evaluate bilirubin, urine bile and bilirubin, and urobilinogen balances — show elevated levels in more than half of gallbladder cancer patients. Serum alkaline phosphatase levels are consistently elevated.
• *Liver-spleen scan* detects abnormalities.
• *Cholecystography* may demonstrate stones or calcification (the "porcelain" gallbladder).
• *Magnetic resonance imaging* may show areas of tumor growth.
• *Cholangiography* may outline a common bile duct obstruction.

The following tests help to confirm extrahepatic bile duct carcinoma:
• *Liver function studies* indicate biliary obstruction; elevated bilirubin (5 to 30 mg/dl), alkaline phosphatase, and blood cholesterol levels; prolonged prothrombin time; and response to vitamin K.
• *Endoscopic retrograde cholangiopancreatography* identifies the tumor site and permits tissue specimen retrieval for biopsy.

Treatment

The treatment of choice for gallbladder cancer, surgery includes cholecystectomy, common bile duct exploration, T-tube drainage, and wedge excision of hepatic tissue.

As a rule, surgery can relieve obstruction and jaundice, resulting from extrahepatic bile duct cancer. The procedure depends on the cancer site and may include cholecystoduodenostomy or T-tube drainage of the common bile duct.

Radiation therapy may be palliative, and adjuvant chemotherapy (infrequently used) may produce some good results.

Nursing diagnoses
• Altered nutrition: Less than body requirements
• Altered tissue perfusion
• Anxiety
• Fear
• Impaired skin integrity
• Ineffective breathing pattern
• Ineffective family coping
• Ineffective individual coping
• Pain
• Risk for infection
• Risk for injury

Nursing interventions
• Listen to the patient's fears and concerns. Stay with her when her stress and anxiety levels increase. Encourage her to identify actions and care measures that promote comfort and relaxation.

After *biliary resection:*
• Provide meticulous skin care, using strict aseptic technique when caring for the incision and surrounding tissue.
• Give pain medications as ordered. Place the patient in low Fowler's position to promote comfort.
• Prevent respiratory problems by encouraging the patient to cough and breathe deeply despite the high incision, which will make her prefer taking shallow breaths. Provide analgesics. Also show the patient how to splint the abdomen with a pillow or an abdominal binder. This will ease discomfort and promote greater respiratory efforts.
• Check the patient's intake and output carefully. Watch for electrolyte imbalances. Monitor I.V. solutions to avoid overloading the cardiovascular system.
• If the patient has a nasogastric (NG) tube and a T tube in place after surgery, record the amount and color of drainage at each shift. These tubes may remain for 24 to 72 hours to relieve distention and to promote drainage of blood, bile, and serosanguineous fluid.
• Secure the T tube and the NG tube to minimize tension and to prevent them from being pulled out.
• Encourage deep-breathing and coughing exercises.

During *radiation therapy:*
• Encourage the patient to eat high-calorie, well-balanced meals.
• Offer fluids, such as ginger ale, to minimize nausea and vomiting.
• Watch for radiation's adverse effects, such as nausea, vomiting, hair loss, malaise, and diarrhea; promote comfort measures and offer reassurance as appropriate.

During *chemotherapy:*
• Watch for complications, such as infection. Prepare the patient to cope with expected adverse effects.

Patient teaching
• Offer information and support to help the patient and her family deal with their initial fears and reactions to the diagnosis.
• Explain postoperative procedures. Prepare the patient for intubation with an NG tube, a T tube, or I.V. tubes.
• Preoperatively, teach coughing and deep-breathing exercises that the patient should perform postoperatively.
• Discuss ordered treatments, such as radiation therapy and chemotherapy, with the patient and her family. Make sure the patient understands the implications of treatments. Describe potential adverse effects, and advise her to notify the doctor if they persist.
• If appropriate, direct the patient and her family to hospital and community services, such as cancer support groups and hospice care.

NEOPLASMS OF THE MALE AND FEMALE GENITALIA

Besides their impact on physiologic function, cancers of the reproductive system have profound implications for the patient's body image and self-esteem.

PROSTATIC CANCER
The most common neoplasm in men over age 50, prostatic cancer is a leading cause of male cancer death. Adenocarcinoma is the most common form; only seldom does prostatic cancer occur as a sarcoma. About 85% of prostatic cancers originate in the posterior prostate gland, with the rest growing near the urethra. Malignant prostatic tumors seldom result from the benign hyperplastic enlargement that commonly develops around the prostatic urethra in older men.

STAGING PROSTATIC CANCER

Developed by the American Joint Committee on Cancer, descriptive categories, known as the TNM (tumor, node, metastasis) cancer staging system, interpret prostatic cancer's progress.

Primary tumor
TX—primary tumor can't be assessed
T0—no evidence of primary tumor
T1—tumor an incidental histologic finding
T1a—three or fewer microscopic foci of cancer
T1b—more than three microscopic foci of cancer
T2—tumor limited to the prostate gland
T2a—tumor less than 1.5 cm in greatest dimension, with normal tissue on at least three sides
T2b—tumor larger than 1.5 cm in greatest dimension or present in more than one lobe
T3—unfixed tumor extends into the prostatic apex or into or beyond the prostatic capsule, bladder neck, or seminal vesicle
T4—tumor fixed or invades adjacent structures not listed in T3

Regional lymph nodes
NX—regional lymph nodes can't be assessed

N0—no evidence of regional lymph node metastasis
N1—metastasis in a single lymph node, 2 cm or less in greatest dimension
N2—metastasis in a single lymph node, between 2 and 5 cm in greatest dimension, or metastasis to several lymph nodes, none more than 5 cm in greatest dimension
N3—metastasis in a lymph node more than 5 cm in greatest dimension

Distant metastasis
MX—distant metastasis can't be assessed
M0—no known distant metastasis
M1—distant metastasis

Staging categories
Prostatic cancer progresses from mild to severe as follows:
Stage 0 or Stage I—T1a, N0, M0; T2a, N0, M0
Stage II—T1b, N0, M0; T2b, N0, M0
Stage III—T3, N0, M0
Stage IV—T4, N0, M0; any T, N1, M0; any T, N2, M0; any T, N3, M0; any T, any N, M1

Slow-growing prostatic cancer seldom produces signs and symptoms until it's well advanced. Typically, when primary prostatic lesions spread beyond the prostate gland, they invade the prostatic capsule and then spread along the ejaculatory ducts in the space between the seminal vesicles or perivesicular fascia. When prostatic cancer is treated in its localized form, the 5-year survival rate is 70%; after metastasis, it's under 35%. When prostatic cancer is fatal, death usually results from widespread bone metastases.

Prostatic cancer accounts for about 22% of all cancers, with highest incidence among blacks and lowest among Asians. It appears unaffected by socioeconomic status or fertility.

Causes
Risk factors for prostatic cancer include age (the cancer seldom develops in men under age 40) and infection. Endocrine factors may also have a role, leading researchers to suspect that androgens may speed tumor growth.

Complications
Progressive disease can lead to spinal cord compression, deep vein thrombosis, pulmonary emboli, and myelophthisis.

Assessment findings
The patient's history may reveal urinary problems, such as dysuria, frequency, retention, back or hip pain, and hematuria. The patient with these complaints may have advanced disease, with back or hip pain signaling bone metastasis. The patient usually has no signs or symptoms in early disease. Inspection may reveal edema of the scrotum or leg in advanced disease. During digital rectal examination (DRE), prostatic palpation may detect a nonraised, firm, nodular mass with a sharp edge (in early disease) or a hard lump (in advanced disease).

Diagnostic tests
• *DRE* (recommended yearly by the American Cancer Society for men over age 40) is the standard screening test.
• *Blood tests* may show elevated levels of prostate-specific antigen (PSA). Although most men with metastasized prostatic cancer will have an elevated PSA level, the finding also occurs with other prostatic disease. So the PSA level should be assessed in light of DRE findings.
• *Transrectal prostatic ultrasonography* may be used for patients with abnormal DRE and PSA test findings.
• *Bone scan* and *excretory urography* may determine the disease's extent. (See *Staging prostatic cancer.*)
• *Magnetic resonance imaging* and *computed tomography scans* can help define the tumor's extent.

Treatment

Therapy varies by cancer stage and may include radiation, prostatectomy, orchiectomy (removal of the testes) to reduce androgen production, and hormonal therapy with synthetic estrogen (diethylstilbestrol). Radical prostatectomy is usually effective for localized lesions without metastasis. A transurethral resection of the prostate may be performed to relieve an obstruction.

Radiation therapy may cure locally invasive lesions in early disease and may relieve bone pain from metastatic skeletal involvement. It also may be used prophylactically for patients with tumors in regional lymph nodes. Alternatively, internal beam radiation may be recommended because it permits increased radiation to reach the prostate but minimizes the surrounding tissues' exposure to radiation.

If hormonal therapy, surgery, and radiation therapy aren't feasible or successful, chemotherapy may be tried. Chemotherapy for prostatic cancer (combinations of cyclophosphamide, doxorubicin, fluorouracil, cisplatin, and vindesine) offers limited benefits. Research continues to seek the most effective chemotherapeutic regimen.

Nursing diagnoses
- Altered urinary elimination
- Anxiety
- Fear
- Ineffective family coping
- Ineffective individual coping
- Pain
- Risk for infection
- Sexual dysfunction
- Urinary retention

Nursing interventions
- At all times, encourage the patient to express his fears and concerns, including those about changes in his sexual identity, owing to surgery. Offer reassurance when possible.
- Administer ordered analgesics as necessary. Provide comfort measures to reduce pain. Encourage the patient to identify care measures that promote his comfort and relaxation.

After *prostatectomy*:
- Regularly check the dressing, incision, and drainage systems for excessive blood. Also watch for signs of bleeding (pallor, restlessness, falling blood pressure, and rising pulse rate).
- Be alert for signs of infection (fever, chills, inflamed incisional area). Maintain adequate fluid intake (at least 2,000 ml daily).

- Give antispasmodics, as ordered, to control postoperative bladder spasms. Also provide analgesics as needed.
- Because urinary incontinence commonly follows prostatectomy, keep the patient's skin clean and dry.

After *suprapubic prostatectomy*:
- Keep the skin around the suprapubic drain dry and free from drainage and urine leakage. Encourage the patient to begin perineal exercises between 24 and 48 hours after surgery.
- Allow the patient's family to assist in his care, and encourage them to provide psychological support.
- Give meticulous catheter care. After prostatectomy, a patient usually has a three-way catheter with a continuous irrigation system. Check the tubing for kinks, mucus plugs, and clots, especially if the patient complains of pain. Warn the patient not to pull on the tubes or the catheter.

After *transurethral resection*:
- Watch for signs of urethral stricture (dysuria, decreased force and caliber of urine stream, and straining to urinate). Also observe for abdominal distention (a result of urethral stricture or catheter blockage by a blood clot). Irrigate the catheter, as ordered.

After *perineal prostatectomy*:
- Avoid taking the patient's temperature rectally or inserting enema or other rectal tubes. Provide pads to absorb draining urine. Assist the patient with frequent sitz baths to relieve pain and inflammation.

After *perineal* or *retropubic prostatectomy*:
- Give reassurance that urine leakage after catheter removal is normal and will subside in time.

After *radiation therapy*:
- Watch for the common adverse effects of radiation to the prostate. These include proctitis, diarrhea, bladder spasms, and urinary frequency. Internal radiation of the prostate almost aways results in cystitis in the first 2 to 3 weeks of therapy. Encourage the patient to drink at least 2,000 ml of fluid daily. Administer analgesics and antispasmodics to decrease his discomfort.

After *hormonal therapy*:
- When a patient receives hormonal therapy with diethylstilbestrol, watch for adverse effects (gynecomastia, fluid retention, nausea, and vomiting). Be alert for thrombophlebitis (pain, tenderness, swelling, warmth, and redness in calf).

Patient teaching
- Before surgery, discuss the expected results. Explain that radical surgery always produces impotence. Up to 7% of patients experience urinary incontinence.

• To help minimize incontinence, teach the patient how to do perineal exercises while he sits or stands. To develop his perineal muscles, tell him to squeeze his buttocks together and hold this position for a few seconds; then relax. He should repeat this exercise 10 times as frequently as ordered by the doctor.
• Prepare the patient for postoperative procedures, such as dressing changes and intubation.
• If appropriate, discuss the adverse effects of radiation therapy. All patients who receive pelvic radiation therapy will develop such symptoms as diarrhea, urinary frequency, nocturia, bladder spasms, rectal irritation, and tenesmus.
• Encourage the patient to maintain as nearly normal a life-style as possible during recovery.
• When appropriate, refer the patient to the social service department, local home health care agencies, hospices, and other support organizations.

TESTICULAR CANCER

Malignant testicular tumors are the most prevalent solid tumors in men ages 20 to 40. Testicular cancer is rare in nonwhite men and accounts for less than 1% of all male cancer deaths. Rarely, when testicular cancer occurs in children, about 50% of tumors are detectable before age 5.

With few exceptions, testicular tumors originate from germinal cells. About 40% become *seminomas*. These tumors, which are characterized by uniform, undifferentiated cells, resemble primitive gonadal cells. Other tumors—*nonseminomas*—show various degrees of differentiation.

The prognosis depends on the cancer cell type and stage. When treated with surgery, chemotherapy, and radiation therapy, 100% of patients with Stage I or Stage II seminomas and 90% of those with Stage I nonseminomas survive beyond 5 years. The prognosis is poor, however, if the disease advances beyond Stage II. Typically, when testicular cancer extends beyond the testes, it spreads through the lymphatic system to the iliac, para-aortic, and mediastinal nodes. Metastases affect the lungs, liver, viscera, and bone.

Causes

Although researchers don't know the immediate cause of testicular cancer, they suspect that cryptorchidism (even when surgically corrected) plays a role in the developing disease. (See *Cryptorchidism and testicular cancer.*) A history of mumps orchitis, inguinal hernia in childhood, or maternal use of diethylstilbestrol (DES) or other estro-

CRYPTORCHIDISM AND TESTICULAR CANCER

In men with cryptorchidism (the failure of a testicle to descend into the scrotum), testicular tumors are about 50 times more common than in men with normal anatomic structure. However, a simple surgical procedure, called orchiopexy, can bring the testicle to its normal position in the scrotum and reduce the testicular cancer risk. Nevertheless, testicular tumors occur more commonly in a surgically descended testicle than in a naturally descended one.

What happens in orchiopexy
In this procedure, the surgeon incises the groin area and separates the testicle and its blood supply from surrounding abdominal structures. Then, he creates a "tunnel" into the scrotum to accommodate the descent of the testicle.

Reducing the risk further
After orchiopexy, urge the patient to examine himself monthly to detect a tumor at its earliest stage.

gen-progestin combinations during pregnancy also increases the risk for this disease.

Complications
Disease progression may induce back or abdominal pain from retroperitoneal adenopathy, dyspnea, cough, and hemoptysis from lung metastases, and ureteral obstruction.

Assessment findings
The patient history may disclose previous injuries to the scrotum, viral infections (such as mumps), or the use of DES or other estrogen-progestin drugs by the patient's mother during pregnancy. The patient may describe a feeling of heaviness or a dragging sensation in the scrotum. He may also report swollen testes or a painless lump found while performing testicular self-examination. In late disease stages, the patient may complain of weight loss, a cough, hemoptysis, shortness of breath, lethargy, and fatigue.

On inspection, you may notice that the patient has enlarged testes. Gynecomastia, a sign that the tumor produces chorionic gonadotropins or estrogen, may be obvious also. In later stages of testicular cancer, the patient may appear lethargic, thin, and pallid.

Palpation findings include a firm, smooth testicular mass and enlarged lymph nodes in surrounding areas.

STAGING TESTICULAR CANCER

Using the TNM (tumor, node, metastasis) system, the American Joint Committee on Cancer has established the following stages for testicular cancer.

Primary tumor
TX—primary tumor can't be assessed (this stage is used in the absence of radical orchiectomy)
T0—histologic scar or no evidence of primary tumor
Tis—intratubular tumor: preinvasive cancer
T1—tumor limited to testicles, including the rete testis
T2—tumor extends beyond tunica albuginea or into epididymis
T3—tumor extends into spermatic cord
T4—tumor invades scrotum

Regional lymph nodes
NX—regional lymph nodes can't be assessed
N0—no evidence of regional lymph node metastasis
N1—metastasis in a single lymph node, 2 cm or less in greatest dimension

N2—metastasis in a single lymph node, between 2 and 5 cm in greatest dimension, or metastases to several lymph nodes, none more than 5 cm in greatest dimension
N3—metastasis in a lymph node more than 5 cm in greatest dimension

Distant metastasis
MX—distant metastasis can't be assessed
M0—no known distant metastasis
M1—distant metastasis

Staging categories
Testicular cancer progresses from mild to severe as follows:
Stage 0—Tis, N0, M0
Stage I—T1, N0, M0; T2, N0, M0
Stage II—T3, N0, M0; T4, N0, M0
Stage III—any T, N1, M0
Stage IV—any T, N2, M0; any T, N3, M0; any T, any N, M1

In later disease stages, palpation may disclose an abdominal mass as well.

On auscultation you may hear decreased breath sounds.

Diagnostic tests
• *Serum analyses* may be done to evaluate beta-subunit human chorionic gonadotropin (HCG) and alpha-fetoprotein (AFP) levels. Elevated levels of these proteins (tumor markers) suggest testicular cancer and can differentiate a seminoma from a nonseminoma: elevated HCG and AFP levels point to a nonseminoma; elevated HCG and normal AFP levels indicate a seminoma.
• *Computed tomography scan* can detect metastases.
• *Excretory urography* may detect ureteral displacement, which is caused by metastasis to a para-aortic lymph node.
• *Chest X-rays* may demonstrate pulmonary metastases.
• *Lymphangiography, ultrasonography,* and *magnetic resonance imaging scan* may disclose additional metastases.
• *Biopsy* can confirm the diagnosis, help stage the disease, and plan treatment. (See *Staging testicular cancer.*)

Treatment
In testicular cancer, treatment includes surgery, radiation therapy, and chemotherapy. Treatment intensity varies with the tumor cell type and stage.

Surgical options include orchiectomy and retroperitoneal node dissection to prevent disease extension and assess its stage. Most surgeons remove just the testis, not the scrotum. The patient may need hormonal replacement therapy after bilateral orchiectomy.

Treatment of seminomas involves postoperative radiation to the retroperitoneal and homolateral iliac nodes. Patients whose disease extends to retroperitoneal structures may be given prophylactic radiation to the mediastinal and supraclavicular nodes. Treatment of nonseminomas includes radiation directed to all cancerous lymph nodes.

Chemotherapy is most effective for late-stage seminomas and most nonseminomas when used for recurrent cancer after orchiectomy and removal of the retroperitoneal lymph nodes.

Autologous bone marrow transplantation is usually reserved for patients who don't respond to standard therapy. It involves giving high-dose chemotherapy, removing and treating the patient's bone marrow to kill remaining cancer cells, and returning the processed bone marrow to the patient.

Nursing diagnoses
• Altered oral mucous membrane
• Anxiety
• Body image disturbance
• Fear

- Ineffective family coping
- Ineffective individual coping
- Pain
- Risk for infection
- Sexual dysfunction

Nursing interventions
- Focus on responding to the psychological impact of the disease, preventing postoperative complications, and minimizing and controlling the complications of radiation therapy and chemotherapy.
- Listen to the patient's fears and concerns. Remember that the patient with testicular cancer typically fears sexual impairment and disfigurement. (See *Sex after testicular cancer surgery.*) When possible, provide reassurance. Stay with the patient during periods of severe anxiety and stress.
- Encourage the patient to ask questions. Base your relationship on trust so that he feels comfortable expressing his concerns.

    After *orchiectomy:*
- For the first day after surgery, apply an ice pack to the scrotum and provide analgesics, as ordered.
- Check for excessive bleeding, swelling, and signs of infection, such as drainage from the incision, fever, pain, and redness.
- Supply an athletic supporter to minimize scrotal pain during ambulation.

    During *chemotherapy:*
- Know what problems to expect and how to prevent or ease them.
- Give antiemetics, as ordered, to prevent severe nausea and vomiting.
- Offer the patient small, frequent feedings to maintain oral intake despite anorexia. Devise a mouth care regimen, making sure to check regularly for stomatitis.
- Be alert for signs of myelosuppression. If the patient receives vinblastine, monitor for signs and symptoms of neurotoxicity (peripheral paresthesia, jaw pain, muscle cramps). If he receives cisplatin, check for ototoxicity. To prevent renal damage, encourage increased fluid intake. To maximize hydration, give I.V. fluids, as ordered, with a potassium supplement. Provide diuresis, as ordered, by administering furosemide or mannitol.

    During *radiation therapy:*
- Watch for and report adverse effects.
- Implement appropriate comfort and safety measures. For example, avoid rubbing the skin near radiation target sites. This helps to prevent or alleviate pain, skin breakdown, and infection.

SEX AFTER TESTICULAR CANCER SURGERY

Patients with testicular cancer typically are anxious about their future. Besides the usual apprehensions about living with cancer, these patients fear loss of sexual function after surgery (orchiectomy). To help patients face their fear, provide support and a clear explanation of how orchiectomy affects sexual activity.

After unilateral orchiectomy
Unilateral orchiectomy doesn't cause sterility or impotence. And because most surgeons remove only the diseased testicle and leave the scrotum, later reconstructive surgery can be done. This involves implanting a gel-filled testicular prosthesis, which weighs the same as and feels like a normal testicle. The patient can resume sexual activity after the incision heals.

After bilateral orchiectomy
Bilateral testicular cancer is uncommon. However, if the patient will lose both testes, he will be sterile. And if nerve or vascular damage (or both) occur with surgery, he will also be impotent.

Be as positive and supportive as possible. Clearly express that a loss of fertility doesn't mean a loss of masculinity. Typically, the patient will take synthetic hormones to replace or supplement depleted male hormone levels.

Patient teaching
- Provide reassurance that sterility and impotence usually don't follow unilateral orchiectomy. Explain that synthetic hormones can supplement depleted hormonal levels. Inform the patient that most surgeons don't remove the scrotum. Also explain that a testicular prosthetic implant can correct disfigurement.
- As suitable, review sperm banking procedures before the patient begins treatment, especially if infertility and impotence may result from surgery.
- Explain tests and treatments that the patient will undergo. Make sure he understands each treatment, its purpose, possible complications, and the care required during and after the treatment.
- Teach the patient how to perform testicular self-examination. Tell him that this is the best way to detect a new or recurrent tumor.
- Refer the patient to organizations, such as the American Cancer Society, that offer information and support during and after treatment.

CERVICAL CANCER

The third most common cancer of the female reproductive system, cervical cancer is classified as either preinvasive or invasive.

Preinvasive cancer ranges from minimal cervical dysplasia, in which the lower third of the epithelium contains abnormal cells, to carcinoma in situ, in which the full thickness of epithelium contains abnormally proliferating cells (also known as cervical intraepithelial neoplasia). Preinvasive cancer is curable in 75% to 90% of patients with early detection and proper treatment. If untreated, it may progress to invasive cervical cancer, depending on the form.

In invasive disease, cancer cells penetrate the basement membrane and can spread directly to contiguous pelvic structures or disseminate to distant sites by way of lymphatic routes. Invasive cancer of the uterine cervix accounts for 4,500 deaths annually in the United States. In 95% of cases, the histologic type is squamous cell carcinoma, which varies from well-differentiated cells to highly anaplastic spindle cells. Only 5% of cases are adenocarcinomas. Invasive cancer typically occurs between ages 30 and 50; rarely, under age 20. Women age 65 or older account for 24% of new cases and 40% of deaths.

Causes

Although the cause is unknown, several predisposing factors have been associated with cervical cancer: frequent intercourse at a young age (under 16), multiple sexual partners, multiple pregnancies, human papillomavirus (HPV), and other bacterial or viral venereal infections.

Complications

Disease progression can cause flank pain from sciatic nerve or pelvic wall invasion, and hematuria and renal failure associated with bladder involvement.

Assessment findings

Preinvasive cancer produces no symptoms or other clinical changes. In early invasive cervical cancer, the patient history will include abnormal vaginal bleeding, such as a persistent vaginal discharge that may be yellowish, blood-tinged, and foul-smelling; postcoital pain and bleeding; and bleeding between menstrual periods or unusually heavy menstrual periods. The patient history may suggest one or more of the predisposing factors for this disease.

If the cancer has advanced into the pelvic wall, the patient may report gradually increasing flank pain, which can indicate sciatic nerve involvement. Leakage of urine may point to metastasis into the bladder with formation of a fistula. Leakage of feces may indicate metastasis to the rectum with fistula development.

Inspection may disclose vaginal discharge or leakage of urine or feces.

Diagnostic tests

• *Papanicolaou (Pap) test* identifies abnormal cells, and *colposcopy* determines the source of the abnormal cells seen on the Pap test.
• *Cone biopsy* is performed if endocervical curettage is positive.
• *Vira pap test,* under investigation, permits examination of the specimen's deoxyribonucleic acid (DNA) structure to detect HPV.

Additional studies, such as lymphangiography, cystography, and major organ and bone scans, can detect metastasis. (See *Staging cervical cancer.*)

Treatment

Accurate clinical staging will determine the type of treatment. Preinvasive lesions may be treated with total excisional biopsy, cryosurgery, laser destruction, conization (followed by frequent Pap test follow-ups) or, rarely, hysterectomy. Therapy for invasive squamous cell carcinoma may include radical hysterectomy and radiation therapy (internal, external, or both). Rarely, pelvic exenteration may be performed for recurrent cervical cancer.

Complications of surgery include bladder dysfunction, formation of lymphocysts or seromas after lymphadenectomy, and pulmonary embolism. Complications of radiation therapy include diarrhea, abdominal cramping, dysuria, and leukopenia. Combined surgery and irradiation in the abdomen and pelvis may lead to small-bowel obstruction, stricture and fibrosis of the intestine or rectosigmoid, and rectovaginal or vesicovaginal fistula.

Nursing diagnoses

• Altered sexuality patterns
• Anxiety
• Diversional activity deficit
• Fear
• Impaired physical mobility
• Impaired skin integrity
• Ineffective individual coping
• Pain
• Risk for infection
• Sexual dysfunction

STAGING CERVICAL CANCER

Treatment decisions depend on accurate staging. The International Federation of Gynecology and Obstetrics defines cervical cancer stages as follows:

Stage 0
Carcinoma in situ, intraepithelial carcinoma

Stage I
Cancer confined to the cervix (extension to the corpus should be disregarded)

Stage IA
Preclinical malignant lesions of the cervix (diagnosed only microscopically)

Stage IA1
Minimal microscopically evident stromal invasion

Stage IA2
Lesions detected microscopically, measuring 5 mm or less from the base of the epithelium, either surface or glandular, from which it originates; lesion width shouldn't exceed 7 mm

Stage IB
Lesions measuring more than 5 mm deep and 7 mm wide, whether seen clinically or not (preformed space involvement shouldn't alter the staging but should be recorded for future treatment decisions)

Stage II
Extension beyond the cervix but not to the pelvic wall; the cancer involves the vagina but hasn't spread to the lower third

Stage IIA
No obvious parametrial involvement

Stage IIB
Obvious parametrial involvement

Stage III
Extension to the pelvic wall; on rectal examination, no cancer-free space exists between the tumor and the pelvic wall; the tumor involves the lower third of the vagina; this includes all cases with hydronephrosis or nonfunctioning kidney

Stage IIIA
No extension to the pelvic wall

Stage IIIB
Extension to the pelvic wall and hydronephrosis, or nonfunctioning kidney, or both

Stage IV
Extension beyond the true pelvis or involvement of the bladder or the rectal mucosa

Stage IVA
Spread to adjacent organs

Stage IVB
Spread to distant organs

Nursing interventions

• Listen to the patient's fears and concerns, and offer reassurance when appropriate. Encourage her to use relaxation techniques to promote her comfort during the diagnostic procedures.
• If you assist with a biopsy, drape and prepare the patient as for a routine Pap test and pelvic examination. Have a container of formaldehyde ready to preserve the specimen during transfer to the pathology laboratory. Assist the doctor as needed, and provide support for the patient throughout the procedure.
• If you assist with cryosurgery or laser therapy, drape and prepare the patient as for a routine Pap test and pelvic examination. Assist the doctor as necessary, and provide support for the patient throughout the procedure.
• After any surgery, monitor vital signs every 4 hours. Watch for and immediately report signs of complications, such as bleeding, abdominal distention, severe pain, and

wheezing or other breathing difficulties. Encourage deep breathing and coughing. Administer analgesics and prophylactic antibiotics, as ordered.

For *internal radiation therapy:*
• Check to see whether the radioactive source will be inserted while the patient is in the operating room (preloaded) or at bedside (afterloaded). If the source is preloaded, the patient will return to her room "hot," and safety precautions will begin immediately.
• Remember that safety precautions—time, distance, and shielding—begin as soon as the radioactive source is in place. Inform the patient that she'll require a private room.
• Encourage the patient to lie flat and to limit movement while the source is in place. If she prefers, elevate the head of the bed slightly.
• Check the patient's vital signs every 4 hours; watch for skin reactions, vaginal bleeding, abdominal discomfort,

GUIDELINES FOR USING A DILATOR

After undergoing intracavitary radiation, the patient may need to use a dilator to relieve vaginal narrowing, resulting from scar tissue. She should insert the dilator once or twice a day and leave it in her vagina for about 5 minutes. Also, note the following:
• The dilator should feel smooth; if it has flaws or rough spots, the patient should use another one.
• Before and after each insertion, the patient should wash the dilator with soap and water.
• The patient should apply a water-soluble lubricant (such as K-Y Jelly) to the tip of the dilator before insertion.
• To properly insert the dilator, the patient lies on her back with her knees slightly apart. Then she inserts it into the vagina as far as possible without causing pain.
• The dilator use may cause mild discomfort or a pink or slightly bloody discharge. Significant, menstrual-like bleeding should not occur.

and evidence of dehydration. Make sure the patient can reach everything she needs without stretching or straining.
• Assist the patient in range-of-motion arm exercises. Avoid leg exercises and other body movements that could dislodge the source. If ordered, administer a tranquilizer to help the patient relax and remain still. Organize your time with the patient to minimize your exposure to radiation.
• Provide diversional activities that require minimal movement.
• Inform visitors of safety precautions, and hang a sign listing these precautions on the patient's door.
• Watch for treatment complications by listening to and observing the patient and monitoring laboratory studies and vital signs. When appropriate, perform measures to prevent or alleviate complications.

Patient teaching

For a *biopsy:*
• Explain to the patient that she may feel pressure, minor abdominal cramps, or a pinch from the punch forceps. Reassure her that the pain will be minimal because the cervix has few nerve endings.

For *cryosurgery:*
• Explain to the patient that the procedure takes about 15 minutes, during which time the doctor will use refrigerant to freeze the cervix. Caution her that she may

experience abdominal cramps, headache, and sweating, but reassure her that she'll feel little, if any, pain.

For *laser surgery:*
• Explain that the procedure takes about 30 minutes and may cause abdominal cramps.
• After excisional biopsy, cryosurgery, or laser therapy, tell the patient to expect a discharge or spotting for about 1 week. Advise her not to douche, use tampons, or engage in sexual intercourse during this time. Caution her to report signs of infection. Stress the need for a follow-up Pap test and a pelvic examination in 3 to 4 months and periodically thereafter. Also, tell her what to expect postoperatively if a hysterectomy is necessary.
• Find out whether the patient will have internal or external therapy or both. Usually, internal radiation therapy is the first procedure.

For *preloaded internal radiation therapy:*
• Explain to the patient that the procedure requires a 2- to 3-day hospital stay, bowel preparation, a povidone-iodine vaginal douche, a clear liquid diet, and nothing by mouth the night before the implantation. It also requires an indwelling urinary catheter.
• Inform the patient that the procedure is performed in the operating room under general anesthesia. She will be placed in the lithotomy position, and an applicator will be inserted. The radioactive source, such as radium, will be implanted in the applicator by the doctor.

For *afterloaded internal radiation therapy:*
• Explain to the patient that a member of the radiation team will implant the source after the patient has returned to her room from surgery.
• If the patient will undergo outpatient external radiation therapy, explain that it continues for about 4 to 6 weeks. Describe the procedure and measures she can take at home to prevent complications, such as providing care around the radiation site to prevent skin breakdown.
• Review the possible complications of radiation therapy. Remind the patient to watch for and report uncomfortable adverse effects. Because radiation therapy may increase susceptibility to infection by lowering the white blood cell count, warn the patient to avoid people with obvious infections during therapy.
• Inform the patient that vaginal narrowing caused by scar tissue can occur after internal radiation. This condition can be managed by having regular sexual intercourse, by using a dilation procedure, or both. If appropriate, teach the patient how to use a dilator. (See *Guidelines for using a dilator.*)
• Describe the complications that can occur even years after high-dose radiation therapy. GI problems (usually within the first 2 years after radiation therapy) include

bowel obstruction, rectovaginal fistula, and small-bowel fistula. Urinary tract problems (usually 3 to 4 years after treatment) include urinary fistula and hematuria.

For *all patients with cervical cancer:*
• Reassure the patient that this disease and its treatment shouldn't radically alter her life-style or prohibit sexual intimacy.
• Explain the importance of complying with follow-up visits to the gynecologist and oncologist. Stress the value of follow-up visits in detecting disease progression or recurrence.

UTERINE CANCER

The most common gynecologic cancer, uterine cancer (cancer of the endometrium) typically afflicts postmenopausal women between ages 50 and 60. It's uncommon between ages 30 and 40 and rare before age 30. Most premenopausal women who develop uterine cancer have a history of anovulatory menstrual cycles or other hormonal imbalance. About 33,000 new cases of uterine cancer are reported annually; of these, roughly 5,500 are eventually fatal.

Causes and pathophysiology

Uterine cancer appears linked to several predisposing factors:
• low fertility index and anovulation
• history of infertility or failure of ovulation
• abnormal uterine bleeding
• obesity, hypertension, diabetes, or nulliparity
• familial tendency
• history of uterine polyps or endometrial hyperplasia
• prolonged estrogen therapy with exposure unopposed by progesterone.

In most patients, uterine cancer is an adenocarcinoma that metastasizes late, usually from the endometrium to the cervix, ovaries, fallopian tubes, and other peritoneal structures. It may spread to distant organs, such as the lungs and the brain, by way of the blood or the lymphatic system. Lymph node involvement can also occur. Less common uterine tumors include adenoacanthoma, endometrial stromal sarcoma, lymphosarcoma, mixed mesodermal tumors (including carcinosarcoma), and leiomyosarcoma.

Complications

Intestinal obstruction, ascites, increasing pain, and hemorrhage are complications related to disease progression.

Assessment findings

The patient history may reflect one or more predisposing factors. In the younger patient, it may also reveal spotting and protracted, heavy menstrual periods. The postmenopausal woman may report that bleeding began 12 or more months after menses had stopped. In either case, the patient may describe the discharge as watery at first, then blood-streaked, and gradually becoming bloodier.

In more advanced stages, palpation may disclose an enlarged uterus.

Diagnostic tests

• *Endometrial, cervical,* or *endocervical biopsy* confirms cancer cells.
• *Fractional dilatation and curettage* identifies the problem when the disease is suspected but the endometrial biopsy is negative.

Positive diagnosis requires the following tests to provide baseline data and permit staging:
• *multiple cervical biopsies* and *endocervical curettage* to pinpoint cervical involvement
• *Schiller's test,* the staining of the cervix and vagina with an iodine solution that turns healthy tissues brown (cancerous tissues resist the stain)
• *computed tomography scan* or *magnetic resonance imaging* to detect metastasis to the myometrium, cervix, lymph nodes, and other organs
• *excretory urography* and, possibly, *cystoscopy* to evaluate the urinary system
• *proctoscopy* or *barium enema studies,* which may be performed if bladder and rectal involvement are suspected
• *blood studies, urinalysis,* and *electrocardiography* may also help in staging the disease. (For more information, see *Staging uterine cancer,* page 352.)

Treatment

Depending on the extent of the disease, the treatment may include one or more of the following:
• *Surgery* usually involves total abdominal hysterectomy, bilateral salpingo-oophorectomy or, possibly, omentectomy with or without pelvic or para-aortic lymphadenectomy. Total pelvic exenteration removes all pelvic organs, including the rectum, bladder, and vagina, and is only performed when the disease is sufficiently contained to allow surgical removal of diseased parts. This surgery seldom is curative, especially in nodal involvement.
• *Radiation therapy* is used when the tumor isn't well differentiated. Intracavitary radiation, external radiation, or both may be given 6 weeks before surgery to inhibit recurrence and lengthen survival time.

STAGING UTERINE CANCER

The International Federation of Gynecology and Obstetrics defines uterine (endometrial) cancer stages as follows:

Stage 0
Carcinoma in situ

Stage I
Carcinoma confined to the corpus

Stage IA
Length of the uterine cavity 8 cm or less

Stage IB
Length of the uterine cavity more than 8 cm

Stage I cases are subgrouped by the following histologic grades of the adenocarcinoma:

G1 — Highly differentiated adenomatous carcinoma

G2 — Moderately differentiated adenomatous carcinoma with partly solid areas

G3 — Predominantly solid or entirely undifferentiated carcinoma

Stage II
Carcinoma has involved the corpus and the cervix but has not extended outside the uterus

Stage III
Carcinoma has extended outside the uterus but not outside the true pelvis

Stage IV
Carcinoma has extended outside the true pelvis or has obviously involved the mucosa of the bladder or rectum

Stage IVA
Spread of the growth to adjacent organs

Stage IVB
Spread to distant organs

• *Hormonal therapy,* using tamoxifen, shows a response rate of 20% to 40%.
• *Chemotherapy,* including both cisplatin and doxorubicin, is usually tried when other treatments have failed.

Nursing diagnoses
• Altered urinary elimination
• Anxiety
• Body image disturbance
• Diversional activity deficit
• Fear
• Impaired tissue integrity
• Ineffective individual coping
• Pain
• Risk for infection
• Sexual dysfunction
• Social isolation

Nursing interventions
• Listen to the patient's fears and concerns. She may be fearful for her survival and concerned that treatment will alter her life-style or prevent sexual intimacy. Remain with the patient during periods of severe stress and anxiety.
• Administer ordered pain medications as necessary. Patients who require pain medications for this disease are often in the later stages. Encourage the patient to identify actions that promote comfort and then be sure to perform them as often as possible. Provide distractions and help her perform relaxation techniques that may ease her discomfort.

After *surgery:*
• Measure fluid contents of the blood drainage system every shift. Notify the doctor immediately if drainage exceeds 400 ml.
• If the patient has received subcutaneous heparin, continue administration, as ordered, until she is fully ambulatory. Give prophylactic antibiotics as ordered, and provide good indwelling urinary catheter care.
• Check the patient's vital signs every 4 hours. Watch for and immediately report any sign of complications, such as bleeding, abdominal distention, severe pain, and wheezing or other breathing difficulties. Provide analgesics as ordered.
• Regularly encourage the patient to breathe deeply and cough. Promote the use of an incentive spirometer once every waking hour to help keep lungs expanded.
• Find out whether the patient will have internal or external radiation or both. Usually, internal radiation therapy is used first.

For *internal radiation therapy:*
• Check to see whether the radioactive source will be inserted while the patient is in the operating room (preloaded) or at the bedside (afterloaded). If the source is

preloaded, the patient will return to her room "hot," and safety precautions will begin immediately.

• Remember that safety precautions—time, distance, and shielding—must be imposed as soon as the radioactive source is in place. Inform the patient that she'll require a private room.

• Encourage the patient to limit movement while the source is in place. If she prefers, slightly elevate the head of the bed. Make sure the patient can reach everything she needs (the call bell, telephone, water) without stretching or straining. Assist her in range-of-motion arm exercises; leg exercises and other body movements could dislodge the source.

• If ordered, administer a tranquilizer to help the patient relax and remain still.

• Provide diversional activities that require minimal movement.

• Check the patient's vital signs every 4 hours; watch for skin reaction, vaginal bleeding, abdominal discomfort, and evidence of dehydration.

• Inform visitors of safety precautions, and hang a sign listing these precautions on the patient's door.

For *internal* and *external radiation therapy:*
• Be alert for the possible adverse effects of radiation. Perform measures that help prevent them.

• Organize the time you spend with the patient to minimize your exposure to radiation.

Patient teaching
• Emphasize that prompt treatment significantly improves a patient's likelihood of survival. Discuss tests to diagnose and stage the disease, and explain treatments, which may include radiation therapy, surgery, hormonal therapy, or chemotherapy, or a combination of these.

For *surgery:*
• Reinforce what the doctor told the patient about the surgery, and explain the routine tests (such as repeated blood tests the morning after surgery) and postoperative care. If the patient is to have a lymphadenectomy *and* a total hysterectomy, explain that she'll probably have a blood drainage system for about 5 days after surgery. Also explain indwelling catheter care. Fit the patient with antiembolism stockings for use during and after surgery. Make sure the patient's blood has been typed and cross-matched. If the patient is premenopausal, inform her that removal of her ovaries will induce menopause.

• As appropriate, explain that except in total pelvic exenteration, the vagina remains intact and that once she recovers, sexual intercourse is possible.

For *internal radiation therapy:*
• Describe the procedure for radiation therapy to the patient. Answer the patient's questions and counsel her about radiation's adverse effects. Advise her to rest frequently and to maintain a well-balanced diet.

• Explain that the *preloaded* internal radiation procedure requires a 2- to 3-day hospital stay, bowel preparation, a povidone-iodine vaginal douche, a clear liquid diet, and nothing taken by mouth the night before the implantation, as well as an indwelling catheter. Inform the patient that the procedure is performed in the operating room under general anesthesia. She will be placed in a dorsal position, with knees and hips flexed and heels resting in footrests. The doctor will implant the radiation source in the vagina.

• Explain that in *afterloaded* internal radiation therapy, a member of the radiation team will implant the source while the patient is in her room.

For *external radiation therapy:*
• Teach the patient and her family about the therapy before it begins. Tell the patient that treatment is usually given 5 days a week for 6 weeks. Warn her not to scrub body areas marked with indelible ink because these markings direct treatment to exactly the same area each time.

• Instruct the patient to maintain a high-protein, high-carbohydrate, low-residue diet to reduce bulk and yet maintain calories. Administer diphenoxylate with atropine, as ordered, to minimize diarrhea, a possible adverse effect of pelvic radiation.

• To minimize skin breakdown and reduce the risk of skin infection, tell the patient to keep the treatment area dry, to avoid wearing clothes that rub against the area, and to avoid using heating pads, alcohol rubs, or irritating skin creams. Because radiation therapy increases susceptibility to infection (possibly by lowering the white blood cell [WBC] count), encourage the patient to avoid people with colds or other infections.

For *chemotherapy* or *immunotherapy:*
• Explain the therapy and be sure the patient understands what adverse effects to expect and how to alleviate them. If the patient is receiving a synthetic form of progesterone, such as hydroxyprogesterone (Delalutin), medroxyprogesterone (Provera), or megestrol (Megace), tell her to watch for depression, dizziness, backache, swelling, breast tenderness, irritability, and abdominal cramps. Instruct her to report signs of thrombophlebitis, such as pain in the calves, numbness, tingling, or loss of leg function.

• Advise the patient receiving chemotherapy that WBC counts must be checked weekly, and reinforce the im-

STAGING VAGINAL CANCER

The International Federation of Gynecology and Obstetrics has established this staging system as a guide to the treatment and the prognosis of vaginal cancer.

Stage 0
Carcinoma in situ, intraepithelial carcinoma.

Stage I
The carcinoma is limited to the vaginal wall.

Stage II
The carcinoma has involved the subvaginal tissue but has not extended to the pelvic wall.

Stage III
The carcinoma has extended to the pelvic wall.

Stage IV
The carcinoma has extended beyond the true pelvis or has involved the mucosa of the bladder or rectum.

portance of preventing infection. Assure her that hair loss is temporary.
• If the patient works and is undergoing chemotherapy, point out that continuing to work during this period may offer an important diversion. Advise her to talk with her employer about a flexible work schedule.
• Refer the patient to the social service department and to community services that offer psychological support and information, such as the American Cancer Society.

VAGINAL CANCER

The rarest gynecologic cancer, vaginal cancer usually appears as squamous cell carcinoma, but occasionally as melanoma, sarcoma, or adenocarcinoma. Vaginal cancer usually occurs in women in their early to middle 50s, but some rarer types do appear in younger women, and rhabdomyosarcoma appears in children.

Causes and pathophysiology

Although the relation is unclear, certain factors predispose the patient to the development of squamous cell carcinoma of the vagina. These include trauma, chronic pessary use, and the use of chemical carcinogens, such as those in some sprays and douches.

The likeliest risk factor appears to be advanced age combined with any of the above. Cancer in this area may also be an extension of a previous cancer of the endometrium, vulva, or cervix. In addition, vaginal adenocarcinoma has been associated with the use of diethylstilbestrol (DES) by the patient's mother during pregnancy.

Because the vagina is a thin-walled structure with rich lymphatic drainage, cancer here varies in severity, depending on its exact location and effect on lymphatic drainage. Vaginal cancer resembles cervical cancer in that it may progress from an intraepithelial tumor to an invasive cancer. It spreads more slowly than cervical cancer, however.

A lesion in the upper third of the vagina, the most common site, usually metastasizes to the groin nodes; a lesion in the lower third, the second most common site, usually metastasizes to the hypogastric and iliac nodes. A lesion in the middle third metastasizes erratically. A posterior lesion displaces and distends the vaginal posterior wall before spreading to deep layers. By contrast, an anterior lesion spreads more rapidly into other structures and deep layers because unlike the posterior wall, the anterior vaginal wall is not flexible.

Complications

Metastasis may affect the cervix, uterus, and rectum.

Assessment findings

The history may reveal one or more risk factors and the most frequent presenting signs—bloody vaginal discharge and irregular or postmenopausal bleeding. The patient may also complain of urine retention or urinary frequency if the lesion is close to the neck of the bladder. Vaginal examination may reveal a small or large ulcerated lesion in any area of the vagina.

Diagnostic tests

Several tests help identify and stage vaginal cancer:
• *Papanicolaou (Pap) test* shows abnormal cells.
• *Biopsy of the lesion* is performed to identify cancerous cells. Biopsy of the cervix and vulva may also be performed to rule out these areas as primary cancer sites.
• *Colposcopy* may be used to locate lesions that may have been missed during the pelvic examination.
• *Lugol's solution* painted on the suspected area helps identify malignant areas by staining glycogen-containing normal tissue; abnormal tissue resists staining.
• *Barium enema* is performed to rule out rectal metastasis. (See *Staging vaginal cancer.*)

Treatment

Early-stage treatment aims to treat the malignant area and preserve the vagina. Topical chemotherapy with fluorouracil and laser surgery can be used for Stages 0 and I. Recommendations for radiation therapy and surgery vary with the size, depth, and location of the lesion, and the patient's desire to preserve a functional vagina. Such preservation is possible only in the early stages. Survival rates are the same for patients treated with radiation as for those who undergo surgery.

Surgery may be recommended only when the tumor is so extensive that exenteration is needed because the vagina's close proximity to the bladder and rectum allows only minimal tissue margins around resected vaginal tissue. Radiation therapy is the preferred treatment for all stages of vaginal cancer. Most patients need preliminary external radiation treatment to shrink the tumor before internal radiation can begin. Then, if the tumor is localized to the vault and the cervix is present, radiation (radium or cesium) can be given with an intrauterine tandem and colpostats (ovoids); if the cervix is absent, then a specially designed vaginal applicator is used instead. To minimize complications, radioactive sources and filters are carefully placed away from radiosensitive tissues, such as the bladder and rectum. Such treatment lasts 48 to 72 hours, depending on the dosage.

Nursing diagnoses

- Altered sexuality patterns
- Anxiety
- Diversional activity deficit
- Fear
- Impaired physical mobility
- Impaired tissue integrity
- Ineffective individual coping
- Pain
- Risk for infection
- Social isolation

Nursing interventions

- Listen to the patient's fears and concerns and offer psychological support. The patient may fear both the disease and its impact on her sexual behavior.
- When appropriate, administer ordered analgesics and provide comfort measures and distractions that help minimize pain.

  For *internal radiation therapy:*
- Before treatment, find out if the radiation source will be inserted in the operating room or the patient's room, so that you can minimize your radiation exposure.

- Because radiation effects are cumulative, wear a radiosensitive badge and a lead shield when you enter the patient's room. Check with the radiation therapist concerning the maximum recommended time that you can safely spend providing direct care. Organize care to minimize your exposure.
- While the radiation source is in place, the patient must lie flat on her back and limit movement. The head of the bed can be slightly elevated. Insert an indwelling urinary catheter if this wasn't done in the operating room, and don't change the patient's linens unless they are soiled. Give only partial bed baths, and make sure the patient has a call bell, telephone, water, and anything else she needs within easy reach. The doctor will order a clear liquid or low-residue diet and an antidiarrheal drug to prevent bowel movements.
- Provide diversional activities that require minimal movement.
- Inform visitors of safety precautions, and hang a sign listing these precautions on the patient's door.
- To compensate for immobility, encourage the patient to do active range-of-motion exercises with both arms.
- Watch for the complications of prescribed treatments. Perform measures that help prevent or alleviate complications of radiation therapy and chemotherapy.

Patient teaching

- Explain all treatments to the patient and, as appropriate, her family.
- Before external radiation therapy, stress the importance of providing good skin care to the target site after treatment to maintain skin integrity. Tell the patient to avoid constrictive clothing over the area, to avoid extremes of hot or cold, and to avoid vigorously rubbing the area. Also stress the need to take measures to prevent infection, such as avoiding crowds and washing her hands.
- Before internal radiation therapy, explain the necessity of immobilization during therapy, and tell the patient what this therapy entails (such as no linen changes and the use of an indwelling catheter).
- After internal radiation therapy, instruct the patient to use a stent or prescribed dilator exercises to prevent vaginal stenosis. Coitus also helps prevent such stenosis.
- Refer the patient for psychological counseling, if necessary, or to the social service department and support groups, such as the American Cancer Society.

OVARIAN CANCER

After cancers of the lung, breast, and colon, primary ovarian cancer ranks as the most common cause of cancer death among American women. In women with previously treated breast cancer, metastatic ovarian cancer is more common than cancer of any other organ.

Incidence is higher in women of upper socioeconomic status between the ages of 20 and 54. However, the disease may occur during childhood or even pregnancy.

The prognosis varies with the histologic type and staging of the disease, but it's often poor because ovarian tumors are difficult to diagnose and progress rapidly. Although about 40% of women with ovarian cancer survive for 5 years, no major improvement in the overall survival rate has been made in the past 30 years.

Causes and pathophysiology

Environmental and life-style factors seem to play a role in ovarian cancer. Women who live in industrialized nations are at greater risk, as are those whose diet is high in saturated fat. Other risk factors include infertility problems or nulliparity, celibacy, exposure to asbestos and talc, a history of breast or uterine cancer, and a family history of ovarian cancer.

Primary epithelial tumors arise in the müllerian epithelium; germ cell tumors, in the ovum itself; and sex cord tumors, in the ovarian stroma. Ovarian tumors spread rapidly intraperitoneally by local extension or surface seeding and, occasionally, through the lymphatics and the bloodstream. In most cases, extraperitoneal spread is through the diaphragm into the chest cavity, which may cause pleural effusions. Other metastasis is rare.

Three main types of ovarian cancer exist:
• *Primary epithelial tumors* account for 90% of all ovarian cancers and include serous cystadenocarcinoma, mucinous cystadenocarcinoma, and endometrioid and mesonephric malignant tumors.
• *Germ cell tumors* include endodermal sinus malignant tumors, embryonal carcinoma (a rare ovarian cancer that appears in children), immature teratomas, and dysgerminoma.
• *Sex cord (stromal) tumors* include granulosa cell tumors (which produce estrogen and may have feminizing effects), thecomas, and the rare arrhenoblastomas (which produce androgen and have virilizing effects).

Complications

Fluid and electrolyte imbalance, leg edema, ascites, and intestinal obstruction, causing nausea, malnutrition, and hunger, are common complications of progressive disease. Profound cachexia and recurrent malignant effusions, such as pleural effusions, may also occur.

Assessment findings

Because of ovarian cancer's lack of obvious signs, it's seldom diagnosed early. Usually, the cancer has metastasized before a diagnosis is made. Signs and symptoms vary with the tumor's size and the extent of metastasis.

In later stages, the history may disclose urinary frequency, constipation, pelvic discomfort, distention, and weight loss. The patient may complain of pain, possibly associated with tumor rupture, torsion, or infection. In a young patient, the pain may mimic that of appendicitis.

Inspection reveals a patient who is alert but gaunt. It often discloses a grossly distended abdomen accompanied by ascites—typically the sign that prompts the patient to seek treatment.

Palpation of the abdominal organs and peritoneum may disclose masses. On palpation, an ovarian tumor may vary from a rocky hardness to a rubbery or cyst-like quality. Postmenopausal women who have palpable, premenopausal-size ovaries require further evaluation for an ovarian tumor.

Diagnostic tests

Tests ordered to help assess the patient's condition may include a complete blood count, blood chemistries, electrocardiography (see *Staging ovarian cancer*), and the following:
• *Exploratory laparotomy,* including lymph node evaluation and tumor resection, is required for accurate diagnosis and staging.
• *Abdominal ultrasonography, computed tomography scan,* or *X-rays* delineate tumor size.
• *Excretory urography* provides information on renal function and possible urinary tract obstruction.
• *Chest X-rays* can help identify distant metastasis and pleural effusions.
• *Barium enema* (especially in patients with GI symptoms) may reveal obstruction and tumor size.
• *Lymphangiography* can show lymph node involvement.
• *Mammography* can rule out primary breast cancer.
• *Liver function studies* or a *liver scan* can help identify metastasis with ascites.
• *Aspiration of ascitic fluid* can reveal atypical cells.
• *Laboratory tumor marker studies,* such as ovarian carcinoma antigen, carcinoembryonic antigen, and human chorionic gonadotropin, are also evaluated.

Treatment

Depending on the cancer's stage and the patient's age, treatment requires varying combinations of surgery, chemotherapy and, possibly, radiation therapy.

STAGING OVARIAN CANCER

The International Federation of Gynecology and Obstetrics has established this staging system, which is based on findings at clinical examination, surgical exploration, or both. Histology is taken into consideration, as is cytology in effusions. Ideally, biopsies should be obtained from any suspicious areas outside of the pelvis.

To evaluate the impact on the prognosis of the different criteria for allotting cases to Stage IC or IIC, consider (1) if rupture of the capsule was (a) spontaneous or (b) caused by the surgeon, or (2) if the source of malignant cells detected was (a) peritoneal washings or (b) ascites.

Stage I
Growth limited to the ovaries.

Stage IA
Growth limited to one ovary; no ascites. No tumor on the external surface; capsule intact.

Stage IB
Growth limited to both ovaries; no ascites. No tumor on the external surfaces; capsules intact.

Stage IC
Tumor either Stage IA or IB but with tumor on surface of one or both ovaries; or with capsule ruptured; or with ascites present containing malignant cells or with positive peritoneal washings.

Stage II
Growth involving one or both ovaries with pelvic extension.

Stage IIA
Extension or metastasis, or both, to the uterus or tubes (or both).

Stage IIB
Extension to other pelvic tissues.

Stage IIC
Tumor either Stage IIA or IIB, but with tumor on surface of one or both ovaries; or with capsule (or capsules) ruptured; or with ascites present containing malignant cells or with positive peritoneal washings.

Stage III
Tumor involving one or both ovaries with peritoneal implants outside the pelvis or positive retroperitoneal or inguinal nodes. Superficial liver metastasis equals Stage III.

Tumor limited to the true pelvis but with histologically proved malignant extension to small bowel or omentum.

Stage IIIA
Tumor grossly limited to the true pelvis with negative nodes but with histologically confirmed microscopic seeding of abdominal peritoneal surfaces.

Stage IIIB
Tumor of one or both ovaries with histologically confirmed implants of abdominal peritoneal surfaces none exceeding 2 cm in greatest dimension. Nodes are negative.

Stage IIIC
Abdominal implants greater than 2 cm in greatest dimension or positive retroperitoneal or inguinal nodes or both.

Stage IV
Growth involving one or both ovaries with distant metastasis. If pleural effusion is present, there must be positive cytology to suggest Stage IV.

Parenchymal liver metastasis equals Stage IV.

Occasionally, in girls or young women with a unilateral encapsulated tumor who wish to maintain fertility, the following conservative approach may be appropriate:
• resection of the involved ovary
• biopsies of the omentum and the uninvolved ovary
• peritoneal washings for cytologic examination of pelvic fluid
• careful follow-up, including periodic X-rays, to rule out metastasis.

However, ovarian cancer usually requires more aggressive treatment, including total abdominal hysterectomy and bilateral salpingo-oophorectomy with tumor resection, omentectomy, appendectomy, lymph node palpation with probable lymphadenectomy, tissue biopsies,

and peritoneal washings. Complete tumor resection is impossible if the tumor has matted around other organs or if it involves organs that can't be resected. Bilateral salpingo-oophorectomy in a prepubertal girl necessitates hormonal replacement therapy, beginning at puberty, to induce the development of secondary sex characteristics.

Chemotherapy after surgery extends survival time in most patients but is largely palliative in advanced disease, although prolonged remissions are achieved in some patients. Drugs used include melphalan, chlorambucil, thiotepa, methotrexate, cyclophosphamide, doxorubicin, vincristine, vinblastine, dactinomycin, bleomycin, and cisplatin. These drugs are usually given in combination. Intraperitoneal administration of cisplatin or paclitaxel has slowed disease progression and increased survival.

Radiation therapy isn't commonly used because it causes myelosuppression, which limits the effectiveness of chemotherapy. Radioisotopes have been used as adjuvant therapy but cause small-bowel obstructions and stenosis.

Under investigation, immunotherapy consists of I.V. injection of *Corynebacterium parvum* or bacille Calmette-Guérin (BCG) vaccine, lymphokine-activated killer cells, and interleukin-2.

Nursing diagnoses

- Altered growth and development (in a child)
- Altered nutrition: Less than body requirements
- Anticipatory grieving
- Anxiety
- Fear
- Fluid volume excess
- Hopelessness
- Impaired skin integrity
- Ineffective family coping
- Ineffective individual coping
- Pain
- Risk for infection
- Sexual dysfunction

Nursing interventions

- Listen to the patient's concerns and fears. Answer her questions honestly. Provide support for the patient and her family. If the patient is a young woman who must undergo surgery and lose her childbearing ability, help her and her family overcome feelings of despair. If the patient is a child, find out whether or not her parents have told her she has cancer, and respond to her questions accordingly.
- After surgery, frequently monitor the patient's vital signs and check I.V. fluids. Monitor intake and output while maintaining good catheter care. Check the dressing regularly for excessive drainage or bleeding, and watch for signs of infection.
- Provide abdominal support and be alert for abdominal distention. Encourage coughing and deep breathing. Reposition the patient often, and encourage her to walk shortly after surgery.
- If the patient has pain, make her as comfortable as possible. Give analgesics as needed, provide distractions, and have the patient perform relaxation techniques.
- Monitor and treat adverse effects of therapy. If the patient is undergoing intraperitoneal chemotherapy, help alleviate her discomfort by infusing the fluid at a slower rate and repositioning her in an attempt to distribute the fluid evenly.
- If the patient is receiving immunotherapy, watch for flu-like symptoms that may last 12 to 24 hours after drug administration. Give aspirin or acetaminophen for fever. Keep the patient covered with blankets, and provide warm liquids to relieve chills. Administer an antiemetic, as needed.
- If the patient has effusions and must undergo paracentesis and thoracentesis, assist with the procedure as necessary. Be sure to help the patient find a comfortable position during the procedure and help her maintain it, using pillows. After the procedure, encourage fluids and monitor intake and output.
- For the malnourished patient, administer supplementary enteral or parenteral nutrition, as ordered. If the GI tract is intact, offer the patient frequent, small meals. If the GI tract is obstructed, discuss the possibility of a gastrostomy tube or a jejunostomy tube with the doctor and the patient.

Patient teaching

- Teach the patient relaxation techniques and other measures that may help ease her discomfort.
- Stress the importance of preventing infection, emphasizing good hand-washing technique.
- Explain measures that may help maintain adequate nutrition, such as eating small, frequent meals.
- If the patient will undergo drug therapy or radiation therapy, explain the adverse effects that she can expect and suggest ways to alleviate and prevent them.
- Before surgery, thoroughly explain all preoperative tests, the expected course of treatment, and surgical and postoperative procedures.
- In premenopausal women, explain that bilateral oophorectomy artificially induces early menopause. Such patients may experience hot flashes, headaches, palpitations, insomnia, depression, and excessive perspiration.
- As appropriate, refer the patient and her family to the social service department, home health care agencies, hospices, and support groups, such as the American Cancer Society.

BONE, SKIN, AND SOFT-TISSUE NEOPLASMS

Cancer in bone, skin, and soft tissue can be just as serious as cancer in some major organs. Both primary malignant tumors and metastatic lesions may afflict these structures.

PRIMARY MALIGNANT BONE TUMORS

Sarcomas of the bone, primary malignant bone tumors are rare, constituting less than 0.5% of all malignant tumors. Most bone tumors result from metastasis from another malignant tumor.

Primary bone tumors occur more commonly in males than in females, especially in children and adolescents, although some types occur in people between ages 35 and 60.

Causes and pathophysiology

Although the cause of primary malignant bone tumors remains unknown, some researchers hypothesize that primary malignant bone tumors arise in centers of rapid skeletal growth because children and young adults with these tumors seem to be much taller than average. Other theories point to heredity factors, trauma, and excessive radiotherapy as causes.

Prior exposure to carcinogens, an underlying condition, such as Paget's disease, or radiation exposure has been linked with the development of osteogenic sarcomas, chondrosarcomas, and fibrosarcomas.

Primary malignant bone tumors may originate in osseous or nonosseous tissue. (See *Types of primary malignant bone tumors,* page 360.) Osseous tumors arise from the bony structure itself as well as from cartilage, fibrous tissue, and bone marrow. They include osteogenic sarcoma (the most common), parosteal osteogenic sarcoma, chondrosarcoma (malignant cartilage tumor), and malignant giant cell tumor. Together, these make up about 60% of all malignant bone tumors.

Nonosseous tumors arise from hematopoietic, vascular, and neural tissues. They include Ewing's sarcoma, fibrosarcoma, and chordoma. Osteogenic and Ewing's sarcomas are the most common bone tumors of children.

Complications

A life-threatening complication, hypercalcemia commonly occurs from excessive calcium release associated with tumor destruction of bone. When the calcium reaches a level that exceeds the renal and GI capacity to excrete it, the calcium blood level rises above normal. (See *Counteracting hypercalcemia,* page 361.)

Assessment findings

The patient may complain of bone pain and describe it as a dull ache. The pain is usually localized, although it may be referred from the hip or spine. The patient may describe the pain as more intense at night and note that movement doesn't aggravate the pain.

Inspection may reveal weakness in the affected limb; you may also note that the patient walks with a limp. In late stages, the patient may appear cachectic, with fever and impaired mobility.

Palpation may disclose a mass or tumor, possibly accompanied by swelling. You may also find a pathologic fracture.

Diagnostic tests

A biopsy (by incision or aspiration) confirms primary malignant bone tumors. Bone X-rays and radioisotope bone and computed tomography scans delineate the tumor size. A patient with sarcoma also usually has elevated serum alkaline phosphatase levels.

Treatment

Treatment focuses on preserving the limb as well as controlling the cancer. Surgical resection of the tumor (often with preoperative radiation *and* postoperative chemotherapy) saves many limbs from amputation. Some hospitals may perform both preoperative and postoperative radiation therapy and chemotherapy, or various other combinations.

Sometimes treatment calls for radical surgery, such as hemipelvectomy. When any type of surgical amputation is indicated, a 3″ to 4″ (8- to 10-cm) margin of healthy tissue should be left.

Intensive chemotherapy combines cyclophosphamide, vincristine, doxorubicin, and dacarbazine. Adjuvant therapies include immunotherapy with interferon and hyperthermia, which is still under investigation.

Nursing diagnoses

• Altered nutrition: Less than body requirements
• Altered tissue perfusion
• Anxiety
• Body image disturbance
• Fear
• Impaired physical mobility
• Impaired tissue integrity
• Ineffective family coping
• Ineffective individual coping
• Pain
• Risk for infection

TYPES OF PRIMARY MALIGNANT BONE TUMORS

Type	Clinical features	Treatment
Osseous origin		
Osteogenic sarcoma	• Osteoid tumor present in specimen • Arises from bone-forming osteoblast and bone-digesting osteoclast • Occurs most commonly in femur, but also in tibia and humerus; occasionally, in fibula, ileum, vertebra, or mandible • Usually develops in males ages 10 to 30	• Surgery (tumor resection, high thigh amputation, hemipelvectomy) • Radiation therapy • Chemotherapy • Combination of above
Parosteal osteogenic sarcoma	• Develops on surface of bone instead of interior • Progresses slowly • Occurs most commonly in distal femur, but also in tibia, humerus, and ulna • Usually develops in women ages 30 to 40	• Surgery (tumor resection, possible amputation, hemipelvectomy) • Chemotherapy • Combination of above
Chondrosarcoma	• Develops from cartilage • Doesn't cause pain; grows slowly, but is locally recurrent and invasive • Occurs most commonly in pelvis, proximal femur, ribs, and shoulder girdle • Usually develops in men ages 30 to 50	• Hemipelvectomy, surgical resection (ribs) • Radiation therapy (palliative) • Chemotherapy
Malignant giant cell tumor	• Arises from benign giant cell tumor • Found most commonly in long bones, especially in knee area • Usually develops in women ages 18 to 50	• Curettage • Total excision • Radiation therapy
Nonosseous origin		
Ewing's sarcoma	• Originates in bone marrow and invades shafts of long and flat bones • Usually affects lower extremities, most commonly in femur, innominate bones, ribs, tibia, humerus, vertebra, and fibula; may metastasize to lungs • Causes increasingly severe and persistent pain • Usually develops in males ages 10 to 20 • Has poor prognosis	• High-voltage radiation therapy (tumor is very radiosensitive) • Chemotherapy to slow growth • Amputation (only if no evidence of metastases)
Fibrosarcoma	• Occurs relatively rarely • Originates in fibrous tissue of bone • Invades long or flat bones (femur, tibia, mandible) but also involves periosteum and overlying muscle • Usually develops in men ages 30 to 40	• Amputation • Radiation therapy • Chemotherapy • Bone grafts (with low-grade fibrosarcoma)
Chordoma	• Derived from embryonic remnants of notochord • Progresses slowly • Usually found at end of vertebral column and in spheno-occipital, sacrococcygeal, and vertebral areas • Characterized by constipation and visual disturbances • Usually develops in men ages 50 to 60	• Surgical resection (often resulting in neural defects) • Radiation therapy (palliative, or when surgery not applicable, as in occipital area)

Warning

COUNTERACTING HYPERCALCEMIA

When hypercalcemia first develops, it causes lethargy, anorexia, nausea, vomiting, constipation, and dehydration. The patient may also develop pathologic fractures from weakening of involved bone and kidney stones from excessive glomerular filtration of calcium. If the condition continues uninterrupted, the patient's serum calcium levels will become markedly elevated (above 15 mg/dl) and interfere with normal conduction and muscle contraction. This can result in life-threatening cardiac arrhythmias, coma and, eventually, cardiac arrest.

If the patient develops any of these signs, take the following steps:
• To reduce the risk of renal damage and help decrease the patient's serum calcium level, immediately start a 1,000-ml infusion of 0.9% sodium chloride solution. Repeat this infusion every 4 to 6 hours to promote diuresis. Monitor the patient's urine output and adjust the infusion accordingly.

• If the sodium chloride solution doesn't promote adequate diuresis, give furosemide, as ordered. *Don't* give thiazide diuretics, which inhibit calcium excretion.
• Administer drugs, such as calcitonin, mithramycin, corticosteroids and, possibly, sodium bicarbonate, as ordered, to decrease serum calcium levels. Watch for adverse drug effects and for rebound hypocalcemic tetany. If the patient isn't responsive to conventional drug therapy, give gallium nitrate (Ganite) I.V., as ordered.
• Obtain an electrocardiogram (ECG) to check for cardiac arrhythmias. Carefully monitor the patient's vital signs and watch for signs of impending cardiac arrest.
• Repeat the ECG and serum calcium determination, as ordered, and continue to monitor the patient.

Nursing interventions
• Before surgery, start I.V. infusions to maintain the patient's fluid and electrolyte balance and to keep a vein open if he needs blood or plasma during surgery.
• Administer analgesics as necessary.
• After surgery, check the patient's vital signs every hour for the first 4 hours, every 2 hours for the next 4 hours, and then every 4 hours if the patient is stable.
• Check the dressing for oozing often, and tape a tourniquet to the bed in case of hemorrhage. Elevate the foot of the bed or the stump on a pillow for the first 24 hours (but not more than 48 hours; contractures are possible).
• Make sure the patient has received his analgesic before morning care. If necessary, brace him with pillows, keeping the affected part at rest.
• Provide foods high in protein, vitamins, and folic acid. Administer laxatives, if necessary. Encourage fluids to prevent dehydration, and record intake and output.
• A nasogastric (NG) tube and an indwelling urinary catheter usually are inserted during hemipelvectomy surgery to prevent abdominal distention. Continue low gastric suction for 2 days after surgery or until the patient can tolerate a soft diet. Administer antibiotics, as ordered, to prevent infection. Give transfusions if necessary. Keep drains in place to facilitate wound drainage

and prevent infection. Keep the indwelling urinary catheter in place until the patient can void voluntarily.
• Because the patient may have thrombocytopenia, make sure he uses a soft toothbrush and an electric razor to avoid bleeding. Don't give I.M. injections or take rectal temperatures. Be careful not to bump the patient's arms or legs; low platelet count causes bruising.
• To encourage rehabilitation, start physical therapy 24 hours postoperatively. The patient usually won't have severe pain after amputation. If he does, check for such wound complications as hematoma, excessive stump edema, and infection.
• Wash the stump, massage it gently, and keep it dry until it heals. Make sure the bandage is firm and stays on day and night. When you reapply the bandage, make sure you wrap the stump so that you shape it for a prosthesis.
• During radiation therapy, watch for such adverse effects as nausea, vomiting, and dry skin with excoriation.
• During chemotherapy, watch for such complications as infection and for expected adverse effects, including nausea, vomiting, mouth ulcers, and alopecia. Take measures to reduce these effects, such as providing the patient with plenty of fluids to drink and normal saline mouthwash for gargling.

• Throughout treatment, be sensitive to the enormous emotional strain of amputation. Encourage communication, and help the patient set realistic goals.
• Listen to the patient's fears and concerns, and offer reassurance when appropriate. Stay with the patient during periods of severe stress and anxiety.
• Whenever possible, include the patient and the family in care decisions.

Patient teaching
• Help the patient and his family understand the disease. Reinforce the doctor's explanations and provide information that will help the patient and his family make informed decisions about treatment.
• Prepare the patient for the effects of surgery.
• Explain the procedures the patient will undergo, such as insertion of I.V. lines, NG tubes, and indwelling urinary catheters.
• If amputation is inevitable, teach the patient how to readjust his body weight so that he can get in and out of his bed and wheelchair. Teach exercises that will help him do this even before surgery. If appropriate, have an amputee visit the patient.
• Emphasize the importance of deep breathing and turning every 2 hours immediately after surgery.
• Stress the importance of getting plenty of rest and sleep to promote recovery, but encourage some physical exercise.
• Teach the patient about phantom limb syndrome. Explain that he may sense an itch or tingling in the amputated extremity. Reassure him this sensation is normal after amputation and usually subsides within several hours. Explain, however, that the sensation may recur off and on for years.
• To avoid contractures and ensure the best conditions for wound healing, teach the patient *not* to hang the stump over the edge of the bed; sit in a wheelchair with the stump flexed; place a pillow under his hip, knee, or back, or between his thighs; lie with knees flexed; rest an above-the-knee stump on the crutch handle; or abduct an above-the-knee stump.
• Help the patient select a prosthesis. Explain the needs he must consider and the types of prostheses available. The rehabilitation staff will make the final decision, but most patients know nothing about choosing a prosthesis and appreciate some basic guidelines.
• When discussing prostheses, keep in mind the patient's age. Children need relatively simple devices, whereas elderly patients may require prostheses that provide more stability. Consider personal and family finances as well.

Children outgrow prostheses, so parents may need to select inexpensive ones.
• Teach the patient and a family member how to care for the stump. Stress the need for following aseptic technique to prevent infection.
• Emphasize the importance of sound nutrition. Ask the dietitian to provide instruction for the patient and his family.
• Teach the patient and his family about the complications of any postoperative treatments. Explain actions that he can take to alleviate and prevent them.
• Refer the patient and his family to the social service department, home health care agencies, and support groups, such as the American Cancer Society, as appropriate.
• Try to help the patient develop a positive attitude toward recovery, and urge him to resume an independent life-style. If he's elderly, refer him to community health services as necessary. Suggest tutoring for a child to help him keep up with his schoolwork.

MULTIPLE MYELOMA
Also called malignant plasmacytoma, plasma cell myeloma, and myelomatosis, multiple myeloma is a disseminated neoplasm of marrow plasma cells. The disease infiltrates bone to produce osteolytic lesions throughout the skeleton (flat bones, vertebrae, skull, pelvis, and ribs). In late stages, it infiltrates the body organs as well (liver, spleen, lymph nodes, lungs, adrenal glands, kidneys, skin, and GI tract).

Multiple myeloma strikes about 12,300 persons yearly—mostly men over age 68. It usually carries a poor prognosis because, by the time it's diagnosed, it has already infiltrated the vertebrae, pelvis, skull, ribs, clavicles, and sternum. By then, skeletal destruction is widespread and, without treatment, leads to vertebral collapse. Within 3 months of diagnosis, 52% of patients die; within 2 years, 90% die. If the disease is diagnosed early, treatment can often prolong life by 3 to 5 years.

Causes
Although the cause of multiple myeloma isn't known, genetic factors and occupational exposure to radiation have been linked to the disease.

Complications
Multiple myeloma can cause infections, such as pneumonia, pyelonephritis (caused by tubular damage from large amounts of Bence Jones protein, hypercalcemia, and hyperuricemia), renal calculi, renal failure, hema-

tologic imbalance, fractures, hypercalcemia, hyperuricemia, and dehydration. Patients may also develop a predisposition toward bleeding—the result of M protein coating the platelets. This bleeding usually occurs in the GI tract or the nose.

Assessment findings

The patient may have a history of neoplastic fractures. He usually complains of severe, constant back pain, which may increase with exercise. He may also report other symptoms similiar to those of arthritis, such as aches, joint swelling, and tenderness, probably from vertebral compression. Other complaints include numbness, prickling, and tingling of the extremities (peripheral paresthesia).

Inspection may reveal that the patient has pain on movement or weight bearing, especially in the thoracic and lumbar vertebrae.

As the disease advances, the patient will become progressively weaker because of veterbral compression, anemia, and weight loss. As the nerves associated with respiratory function are affected, he may develop pneumonia as well as noticeable thoracic deformities and a reduction in body height of 5″ (13 cm) or more as vertebral collapse occurs.

Diagnostic tests

• *Complete blood count* shows moderate or severe anemia. The differential may show 40% to 50% lymphocytes but seldom more than 3% plasma cells. Rouleaux formation, often the first clue, is seen on differential smear and results from elevation of the erythrocyte sedimentation rate.
• *Urine studies* may show protein urea, Bence Jones protein, and hypercalciuria. Absence of Bence Jones protein doesn't rule out multiple myeloma, but its presence almost invariably confirms the disease. (See *Bence Jones protein.*)
• *Bone marrow aspiration* detects myelomatous cells (abnormal number of immature plasma cells); 10% to 95% instead of the normal 3% to 5%.
• *Serum electrophoresis* shows an elevated globulin spike that is electrophoretically and immunologically abnormal.
• *X-rays* during the early stages may reveal only diffuse osteoporosis. Eventually, they show multiple, sharply circumscribed osteolytic (punched out) lesions, particularly on the skull, pelvis, and spine—the characteristic lesions of multiple myeloma.
• *Excretory urography* can assess renal involvement. To avoid precipitation of Bence Jones protein, iothalamate or

BENCE JONES PROTEIN

The hallmark of multiple myeloma, this protein—a light chain of gamma globulin—was named for Henry Bence Jones, an English doctor. In 1848, he noticed that patients with a certain bone disease excreted a unique protein—unique in that it coagulated at 113° to 131° F (45° to 55° C), then redissolved when heated to boiling.

It remained for Otto Kahler, an Austrian, to demonstrate in 1889 that Bence Jones protein was related to myeloma. Bence Jones protein isn't found in the urine of all multiple myeloma patients, but it's almost never found in patients without this disease.

diatrizoate is used instead of the usual contrast medium.

Treatment

Long-term treatment of multiple myeloma consists mainly of chemotherapy to suppress plasma cell growth and control pain. Combinations of melphalan and prednisone or of cyclophosphamide and prednisone are used. Adjuvant local radiation reduces acute lesions and relieves the pain of collapsed vertebrae.

Other treatment usually includes administration of analgesics for pain. If the patient develops vertebral compression, he may require a laminectomy; if he has renal complications, he may need dialysis. Maintenance therapy with interferon may prolong the plateau phase once the initial chemotherapy is complete.

Because the patient may have bone demineralization and may lose large amounts of calcium into blood and urine, he's a prime candidate for renal calculi, nephrocalcinosis and, eventually, renal failure from hypercalcemia. Hydration, diuretics, corticosteroids, oral phosphate, and gallium I.V. to decrease serum calcium levels control the hypercalcemia. Plasmapheresis removes the M protein from the blood and returns the cells to the patient, although this effect is only temporary.

Nursing diagnoses

• Altered nutrition: Less than body requirements
• Altered protection
• Anxiety
• Energy field disturbance
• Fear
• Hopelessness
• Impaired physical mobility
• Ineffective breathing pattern
• Ineffective family coping

- Ineffective individual coping
- Pain
- Sensory alteration

Nursing interventions
• Encourage the patient to drink 3,000 to 4,000 ml of fluids daily, particularly before excretory urography. Monitor fluid intake and output, which shouldn't fall below 1,500 ml.
• Administer ordered analgesics for pain as necessary. Provide comfort measures, such as repositioning and relaxation techniques.
• During chemotherapy, watch for complications, such as fever and malaise, which may signal the onset of infection. Also watch for signs of other problems, such as severe anemia and fractures.
• If the patient is taking melphalan, a phenylalanine derivative of nitrogen mustard that depresses bone marrow, obtain a platelet and white blood cell count before each treatment. If he's taking prednisone, closely watch for signs of infection, which this drug masks.
• After laminectomy, try to get the patient out of bed within 24 hours, if possible, and encourage him to walk. This helps prevent pneumonia and diminish the bone demineralization that immobilization can cause. But never allow the patient to walk unaccompanied, and make sure he uses a walker or other supportive aid to prevent falls. Reassure him if he's fearful, and allow him to move at his own pace; these patients are particularly vulnerable to pathologic fractures.
• If the patient is bedridden, change his position every 2 hours. Provide passive range-of-motion and deep-breathing exercises; promote active exercises when he can tolerate them.
• Check for hemorrhage, motor or sensory deficits, and loss of bowel or bladder function. Position the patient as ordered, maintain alignment, and logroll him when turning.
• Throughout therapy, listen to the patient's fears and concerns. Offer reassurance when appropriate, and stay with him if he experiences periods of severe stress and anxiety.
• Encourage the patient to identify actions and measures that promote comfort and relaxation. Try to perform these measures, and encourage the patient and his family to do so, too.
• Involve the patient and his family in decisions about his care whenever possible.
• Help relieve the patient's and his family's anxiety by answering their questions.

Patient teaching
• Reinforce the doctor's explanation of the disease, diagnostic tests, treatment options, and prognosis. Make sure the patient understands what to expect from the treatment and diagnostic tests (including painful procedures, such as bone marrow aspiration and biopsy). Tell him to notify the doctor if the adverse effects of treatment persist.
• Prepare the patient for the effects of surgery.
• Explain the procedures the patient will undergo, such as insertion of an I.V. line and an indwelling urinary catheter.
• Emphasize the importance of deep breathing and changing position every 2 hours after surgery.
• Tell the patient to dress appropriately because multiple myeloma may make him particularly sensitive to cold.
• Caution the patient to avoid crowds and people with known infections because chemotherapy diminishes the body's natural resistance to infection.
• If appropriate, direct the patient and his family to community resources, such as the American Cancer Society, for support.

MULTIPLE ENDOCRINE NEOPLASIA
In this hereditary disorder, two or more endocrine glands develop hyperplasia, adenoma, or carcinoma—either concurrently or consecutively. Two well-documented types of multiple endocrine neoplasia (MEN) occur: MEN I (Werner's syndrome), involving hyperplasia and adenomatosis of the parathyroid glands, pancreatic islet cells, pituitary and, rarely, adrenal glands and thyroid gland; and MEN II (Sipple's syndrome), involving medullary thyroid carcinoma, with hyperplasia and adenomatosis of the adrenal medulla (pheochromocytoma) and parathyroid glands. MEN I is more common.

This disorder affects both males and females and may appear at any time from adolescence to old age.

Causes
Multiple endocrine neoplasia usually results from autosomal dominant inheritance.

Complications
Depending on the gland affected, MEN I can cause GI bleeding, perforation, and obstruction from peptic ulceration; rarely, it causes renal and skeletal complications. MEN II commonly causes renal calculus formation.

Assessment findings

Signs and symptoms of MEN vary, depending on the type and the glands involved. With MEN I, the history usually reveals peptic ulcers, perhaps associated with Zollinger-Ellison syndrome. The patient may complain of sharp, gnawing, or burning epigastric pain that occurs when he takes antacids or eats. If hypoglycemia develops (caused by increased insulin production from pancreatic islet cell tumors), he may report periods of dizziness, headache, and clouded vision. Palpation may reveal epigastric tenderness. Auscultation, if performed early in ulcer development, may disclose hyperactive bowel sounds. These sounds may disappear as the ulcer develops.

When MEN I affects the parathyroid glands, the patient is usually asymptomatic. If he does have symptoms, they result from the hypercalcemia caused by hyperparathyroidism. He may complain that he tires quickly or has weakness; he also may have vague abdominal discomfort.

When MEN I causes a pituitary tumor, it usually triggers pituitary hypofunction, but it can also cause hyperfunction. Signs and symptoms include amenorrhea and infertility, decreased beard and body hair, cold intolerance, fatigue, recent weight loss, and anorexia.

If MEN II causes medullary carcinoma of the thyroid, the patient may have a history of fractures and may complain of weakness, fatigue, and emotional changes—all signs of Cushing's syndrome. Inspection may reveal the characteristic moon face and buffalo hump. If the patient has an enlarged thyroid, palpation may disclose the mass.

If MEN II causes a tumor in the adrenal medulla, the patient may complain of a headache. You may detect an irregular, rapid pulse rate (possibly caused by a tachyarrhythmia) and hypertension. If MEN II causes adenomatosis or hyperplasia of the parathyroid glands, the patient history may disclose previous problems with renal calculi or urinary tract infection.

Diagnostic tests

Investigating the causes of pituitary tumor, hypoglycemia, hypercalcemia, or GI hemorrhage may lead to a diagnosis of MEN. Diagnostic tests must carefully evaluate each affected endocrine gland.

For example, a radioimmunoassay showing increased levels of gastrin in a patient with peptic ulcers and Zollinger-Ellison syndrome suggests the need for follow-up studies for MEN I because 50% of patients with the syndrome have MEN. After confirmation of MEN, family members must also be tested for this syndrome.

Treatment

The immediate goal is eradicating the tumor; subsequent therapy controls residual symptoms. Primary treatment of peptic ulcers emphasizes control of bleeding or resection of necrotic tissue. Appropriate treatment of hypoglycemia caused by insulinoma consists of oral administration of diazoxide or glucose to keep blood glucose levels within acceptable limits. However, the patient commonly needs subtotal (partial) pancreatectomy. Because all parathyroid glands have the potential for neoplastic enlargement, the patient may also need subtotal parathyroidectomy, along with transsphenoidal hypophysectomy.

In MEN II, treatment for adrenal medullary tumor includes antihypertensive drugs and tumor resection.

Nursing diagnoses

• Anxiety
• Fatigue
• Fear
• Impaired skin integrity
• Impaired tissue integrity
• Ineffective family coping
• Ineffective individual coping
• Pain
• Risk for infection
• Sensory or perceptual alterations

Nursing interventions

• Provide supportive care. Manage peptic ulcers, hypoglycemia, and other complications, as needed.
• Administer ordered analgesics as necessary, and monitor their effectiveness. Provide comfort measures, such as position changes. Also, encourage the patient to practice relaxation techniques to promote comfort. Provide periods of rest if the patient tires easily.
• If the disease involves the pancreas, monitor blood glucose levels frequently. If it affects the adrenal glands, monitor blood pressure closely, especially during drug therapy.
• If the patient may have a pituitary tumor, watch for signs of pituitary trophic hormone dysfunction, which may affect any of the endocrine glands. Also watch for signs of pituitary apoplexy—sudden severe headache, altered level of consciousness, and visual disturbances.
• After surgery, monitor intake and output, I.V. fluids, and vital signs. Watch for and report complications. Provide aseptic wound care to prevent infection. Ask the patient to cough and breathe deeply.
• Throughout therapy, listen to the patient's fears and concerns and provide psychological support.

IDENTIFYING BASAL CELL CARCINOMA

This photograph shows an enlarged nasal nodule in basal cell carcinoma. Note its depressed center and firm, elevated border.

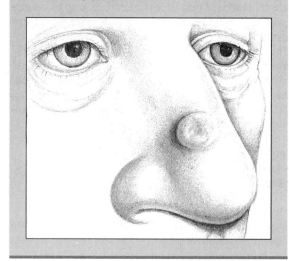

Patient teaching
• Teach the patient about his illness. Make sure he understands what symptoms to expect and the treatment required. Answer his questions honestly.
• If the patient needs surgery, reinforce the doctor's explanation of the procedure, and be sure the patient understands the possible complications. Provide preoperative teaching, including coughing and deep-breathing exercises, and explain what to expect postoperatively.
• As appropriate, refer the patient to the social service department, home health care agencies, and support groups such as the American Cancer Society.

BASAL CELL EPITHELIOMA

This slow-growing, destructive skin tumor usually occurs in people over age 40. Basal cell epithelioma is most prevalent in blond, fair-skinned men, and it's the most common malignant tumor that affects whites. The two major types of basal cell epithelioma are noduloulcerative and superficial.

Causes and pathophysiology
Prolonged sun exposure is the most common cause of basal cell epithelioma — 90% of tumors occur on sun-exposed areas of the body — but arsenic ingestion, radia-

tion exposure, burns, immunosuppression and, rarely, vaccinations are other possible causes.

Although the pathogenesis is uncertain, some experts hypothesize that basal cell epithelioma originates when undifferentiated basal cells become carcinomatous instead of differentiating into sweat glands, sebum, and hair.

Complications
Disease progression can lead to disfiguring lesions of the eyes, nose, and cheeks.

Assessment findings
The patient history may reveal that the patient became aware of an odd-looking skin lesion, which prompted him to seek medical examination. The history may also disclose prolonged exposure to the sun sometime in the patient's life or other risk factors for this disease.

Inspection of the face, particularly the forehead, eyelid margins, and nasolabial folds, may reveal lesions characterized as small, smooth, pinkish, and translucent papules (early-stage noduloulcerative). Telangiectatic vessels cross the surface, and the lesions may be pigmented. As the lesions enlarge, their centers become depressed and their borders become firm and elevated. These ulcerated tumors are called rodent ulcers.

Inspection of the chest and back may disclose multiple oval or irregularly shaped, lightly pigmented plaques. These may have sharply defined, slightly elevated, threadlike borders (superficial basal cell epitheliomas).

Inspection of the head and neck may show waxy, sclerotic, yellow to white plaques without distinct borders. These plaques may resemble small patches of scleroderma and may suggest sclerosing basal cell epitheliomas (morphea-like epitheliomas). (See *Identifying basal cell carcinoma*.)

Diagnostic tests
All types of basal cell epitheliomas are diagnosed by clinical appearance. Incisional or excisional biopsy and histologic study may help to determine the tumor type and histologic subtype.

Treatment
Depending on the size, location, and depth of the lesion, treatment may include curettage and electrodesiccation, chemotherapy, surgical excision, irradiation, or chemosurgery.
• *Curettage and electrodesiccation* offer good cosmetic results for small lesions.

• *Topical fluorouracil* is often used for superficial lesions. This medication produces marked local irritation or inflammation in the involved tissue but no systemic effects.

• Microscopically controlled *surgical excision* carefully removes recurrent lesions until a tumor-free plane is achieved. After removal of large lesions, skin grafting may be required.

• *Irradiation* is used if the tumor location requires it. It's also preferred for elderly or debilitated patients who might not tolerate surgery.

• *Chemosurgery* may be necessary for persistent or recurrent lesions. It consists of periodic applications of a fixative paste (such as zinc chloride) and subsequent removal of fixed pathologic tissue. Treatment continues until tumor removal is complete.

• *Cryotherapy,* using liquid nitrogen, freezes the cells and kills them.

Nursing diagnoses
• Altered nutrition: Less than body requirements
• Anxiety
• Body image disturbance
• Fear
• Impaired skin integrity
• Ineffective family coping
• Ineffective individual coping
• Risk for infection
• Self-esteem disturbance

Nursing interventions
• Listen to the patient's fears and concerns. Offer reassurance when appropriate. Remain with the patient during periods of severe stress and anxiety. Provide positive reinforcement for the patient's efforts to adapt.

• Arrange for the patient to interact with others who have a similar problem.

• Assess the patient's readiness for decision making; then involve him and his family in decisions related to his care whenever possible.

• Watch for complications of treatment, including local skin irritation from chemotherapeutic agents applied topically and infection.

• Watch for radiation's adverse effects, such as nausea, vomiting, hair loss, malaise, and diarrhea. Provide reassurance and comfort measures when appropriate.

Patient teaching
• Instruct the patient to eat frequent, small, high-protein meals. Advise him to include egg nogs, blenderized foods, and liquid protein supplements if the lesion has invaded the oral cavity and is causing eating difficulty.

• To prevent disease recurrence, tell the patient to avoid excessive sun exposure and to use a strong sunscreen or sunshade to protect his skin from damage by ultraviolet rays.

• Advise the patient to relieve local inflammation from topical fluorouracil with cool compresses or with corticosteroid ointment.

• Instruct the patient with noduloulcerative basal cell epithelioma to wash his face gently when ulcerations and crusting occur; scrubbing too vigorously may cause bleeding.

• As appropriate, direct the patient and his family to hospital and community support services — for example, social workers, psychologists, and cancer support groups.

SQUAMOUS CELL CARCINOMA
Arising from keratinizing epidermal cells, squamous cell carcinoma of the skin is an invasive tumor with potential for metastasis. It occurs most commonly in fair-skinned white men over age 60. Outdoor employment and residence in a sunny, warm climate (southern United States and Australia, for example) greatly increase the risk for squamous cell carcinoma.

Lesions on sun-damaged skin tend to be less invasive with less tendency to metastasize than lesions on unexposed skin. (See *Squamous cell carcinoma nodule,* page 368.) Notable exceptions are squamous cell lesions on the lower lip and the ears; almost invariably, these are markedly invasive metastastic lesions with a poor prognosis.

Causes and pathophysiology
Predisposing factors associated with squamous cell carcinoma include overexposure to the sun's ultraviolet rays, radiation therapy, ingestion of herbicides containing arsenic, chronic skin irritation and inflammation, exposure to local carcinogens (such as tar and oil), hereditary diseases (such as xeroderma pigmentosum and albinism), and the presence of premalignant lesions (such as actinic keratosis or Bowen's disease). See *Comparing premalignant skin lesions,* page 369.

Rarely, squamous cell carcinoma may develop on the site of smallpox vaccination, psoriasis, or chronic discoid lupus erythematosus.

Transformation from a premalignant lesion to squamous cell carcinoma may begin with induration and inflammation of the preexisting lesion. When squamous cell carcinoma arises from normal skin, the nodule grows slowly on a firm, indurated base. If untreated, this

SQUAMOUS CELL CARCINOMA NODULE

This ulcerated nodule with an indurated base and a raised, irregular border is a typical lesion in squamous cell carcinoma.

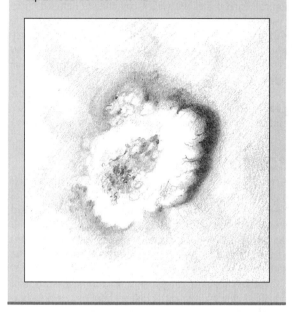

nodule eventually ulcerates and invades underlying tissues.

Complications

Lymph node involvement and visceral metastasis, resulting in respiratory problems, are possible complications from disease progression.

Assessment findings

The patient history may disclose areas of chronic ulceration, especially on sun-damaged skin.

Inspection may reveal lesions on the face, ears, and dorsa of the hands and forearms and on other sun-damaged skin areas. The lesions may appear scaly and keratotic with raised, irregular borders. In late disease, the lesions grow outward (exophytic), are friable, and tend toward chronic crusting.

As the disease progresses and metastasizes to the regional lymph nodes, the patient may complain of pain and malaise. He may also complain of anorexia and resulting fatigue and weakness.

Diagnostic tests

An excisional biopsy provides a definitive diagnosis of squamous cell carcinoma. Appropriate laboratory tests depend on systemic symptoms. (See *Staging squamous cell carcinoma,* page 370.)

Treatment

The size, shape, location, and invasiveness of a squamous cell tumor and the condition of the underlying tissue determine the treatment method; a deeply invasive tumor may require a combination of techniques. All the major treatment methods have excellent cure rates. In most cases, the prognosis is better with a well-differentiated lesion than with a poorly differentiated one in an unusual location. Depending on the lesion, treatment may consist of wide surgical excision; curettage and electrodesiccation, which offer good cosmetic results for smaller lesions; radiation therapy, which is generally for older or debilitated patients; chemotherapy; and chemosurgery, which is reserved for resistant or recurrent lesions.

The chemotherapeutic agent fluorouracil is available in various strengths (1%, 2%, and 5%) as a cream or solution. Local application causes immediate stinging and burning. Later effects include erythema, vesiculation, erosion, superficial ulceration, necrosis, and reepithelialization. The 5% solution induces the most severe inflammatory response but provides complete involution of the lesions with little recurrence.

Fluorouracil treatment is continued until the lesions reach the ulcerative and necrotic stages (usually 2 to 4 weeks). Then a corticosteroid preparation as an anti-inflammatory agent may be applied. Complete healing occurs within 1 to 2 months, with excellent results.

Be careful to keep fluorouracil away from the eyes, scrotum, or mucous membranes. Warn the patient to avoid excessive exposure to the sun during the course of treatment because it intensifies the inflammatory reaction. Possible adverse effects of treatment include post-inflammatory hyperpigmentation.

Nursing diagnoses

• Altered nutrition: Less than body requirements
• Anxiety
• Body image disturbance
• Fatigue
• Fear
• Impaired skin integrity
• Ineffective family coping

COMPARING PREMALIGNANT SKIN LESIONS

Review the chart below to help you differentiate among diseases associated with premalignant skin lesions, including their causes, the people at risk, lesion descriptions, and treatment.

Disease	Cause	People at risk	Lesion description	Treatment
Actinic keratosis	Solar radiation	White men with fair skin (middle-aged to elderly)	Reddish brown lesions 1 mm to 1 cm in size (may enlarge if untreated) on face, ears, lower lip, bald scalp, dorsa of hands and forearms	Topical fluorouracil, cryosurgery using liquid nitrogen, or curettage and electrodesiccation
Bowen's disease	Unknown	White men with fair skin (middle-aged to elderly)	Brown to reddish brown lesions, with scaly surface on exposed and unexposed areas	Surgical excision, topical fluorouracil
Erythroplasia of Queyrat	Bowen's disease of the mucous membranes	Men (middle-aged to elderly)	Red lesions, with a glistening or granular appearance on mucous membranes, particularly the glans penis in uncircumcised men	Surgical excision
Leukoplakia	Smoking, alcohol, chronic cheek-biting, ill-fitting dentures, misaligned teeth	Men (middle-aged to elderly)	Lesions on oral, anal, and genital mucous membranes, varying in appearance from smooth and white to rough and gray	Elimination of irritating factors, surgical excision, or curettage and electrodesiccation (if lesion is still premalignant)

• Ineffective individual coping
• Knowledge deficit

Nursing interventions
• Although disfiguring lesions are distressing, try to accept the patient as he is to increase his self-esteem and to strengthen a caring relationship.
• Listen to the patient's fears and concerns. Offer reassurance when appropriate. Remain with the patient during periods of severe stress and anxiety.
• Accept the patient's perception of himself. Help the patient and his family set realistic goals and expectations.
• Assess the patient's readiness for decision making; then involve him in making choices and decisions related to his care. Provide positive reinforcement for the patient's efforts to adapt.
• Coordinate a consistent care plan for changing the patient's dressings. A standard routine helps the patient

and his family learn how to care for the wound.
• To promote healing and prevent infection, keep the wound dry and clean.
• Try to control odor with balsam of Peru, yogurt flakes, oil of cloves, or other odor-masking substances, even though they may be ineffective for long-term use. Topical or systemic antibiotics also temporarily control odor and eventually alter the lesion's bacterial flora.
• Provide periods of rest between procedures if the patient fatigues easily.
• Be prepared for the adverse effects of radiation therapy, such as nausea, vomiting, hair loss, malaise, and diarrhea.
• Provide small, frequent meals of a high-protein, high-calorie diet if the patient is anorexic. Consult with the dietitian to incorporate foods that the patient enjoys into his diet.

STAGING SQUAMOUS CELL CARCINOMA

Using the TNM (tumor, node, metastasis) system, the American Joint Committee on Cancer has established the following staging system for squamous cell carcinoma.

Primary tumor
TX—primary tumor can't be assessed
T0—no evidence of primary tumor
Tis—carcinoma in situ
T1—tumor 2 cm or less in greatest dimension
T2—tumor between 2 and 5 cm in greatest dimension
T3—tumor more than 5 cm in greatest dimension
T4—tumor invades deep extradermal structures (such as cartilage, skeletal muscle, or bone)

Regional lymph nodes
NX—regional lymph nodes can't be assessed
N0—no evidence of regional lymph node involvement
N1—regional lymph node involvement

Distant metastasis
MX—distant metastasis can't be assessed
M0—no known distant metastasis
M1—distant metastasis

Staging categories
Squamous cell carcinoma progresses from mild to severe as follows:
Stage 0—Tis, N0, M0
Stage I—T1, N0, M0
Stage II—T2, N0, M0; T3, N0, M0
Stage III—T4, N0, M0; any T, N1, M0
Stage IV—any T, any N, M1

Patient teaching
• Explain all procedures and treatments to the patient and his family. Encourage the patient to ask questions, and then answer them honestly.
• Instruct the patient to avoid excessive sun exposure to prevent recurrence. Direct him to wear protective clothing (hats, long sleeves) whenever he is outdoors.
• Urge the use of a strong sunscreen or sunshade to protect the skin from ultraviolet rays. Strong sunscreening agents containing para-aminobenzoic acid, benzophenone, and zinc oxide are most effective. Apply these agents 30 to 60 minutes before sun exposure, as well as lipscreens to protect the lips from sun damage.
• Advise the patient to relieve local inflammation from topical fluorouracil with cool compresses or with corticosteroid ointment.
• Teach the patient to periodically examine the skin for precancerous lesions and to have any removed promptly.
• If appropriate, direct the patient and his family to hospital and community support services, such as social workers, psychologists, and cancer support groups.

MALIGNANT MELANOMA

A neoplasm that arises from melanocytes, malignant melanoma is potentially the most lethal of the skin cancers. It's also relatively rare, accounting for only 1% to 2% of all malignant tumors. Melanoma is slightly more common in women than in men and is unusual in children. Peak incidence occurs between ages 50 and 70, although the incidence in younger age-groups is increasing.

Melanoma spreads through the lymphatic and vascular systems and metastasizes to the regional lymph nodes, skin, liver, lungs, and central nervous system. Its course is unpredictable, however, and recurrence and metastases may not appear for more than 5 years after resection of the primary lesion. The prognosis varies with the tumor thickness. In most patients, superficial lesions are curable, whereas deeper lesions tend to metastasize.

Common sites for melanoma are the head and neck in men, the legs in women, and the backs of people exposed to excessive sunlight. Up to 70% of malignant melanomas arise from a preexisting nevus. (See *Recognizing potentially malignant nevi.*) It seldom appears in the conjunctiva, choroid, pharynx, mouth, vagina, or anus.

The four types of melanomas are as follows:
• *Superficial spreading melanoma*, the most common type (accounting for 50% to 70% of cases), usually develops between ages 40 and 50.
• *Nodular melanoma* usually develops between ages 40 and 50 (accounting for 12% to 30% of cases). It grows vertically, invades the dermis, and metastasizes early.
• *Acral-lentiginous melanoma* is the most common melanoma among Hispanics, Asians, and Blacks. It occurs on palms and soles and in sublingual locations.
• *Lentigo maligna melanoma* is relatively rare (accounting for 10% to 15% of cases). This is the most benign, the slowest growing, and the least aggressive of the four

RECOGNIZING POTENTIALLY MALIGNANT NEVI

Often pigmented, nevi (moles) are skin lesions that may be hereditary. They begin to grow in childhood (occasionally, they're congenital) and become more numerous in young adulthood. Up to 70% of patients with melanoma have a history of a preexisting nevus at the tumor site. Of these, about one-third are reported to be congenital; the remainder develop later in life.

Changes in nevi (color, size, shape, texture, ulceration, bleeding, or itching) suggest possible malignant transformation. The presence or absence of hair within a nevus has no significance.

Types of nevi
Junctional nevi are flat or slightly raised and light to dark brown, with melanocytes confined to the epidermis. Usually, they appear before age 40. These nevi may change into compound nevi if junctional nevus cells proliferate and penetrate into the dermis.

Compound nevi are usually tan to dark brown and slightly raised, although size and color vary. They contain melanocytes in both the dermis and epidermis and seldom undergo malignant transformation. Excision is necessary only to rule out malignant transformation or for cosmetic reasons.

Dermal nevi are elevated lesions from 2 to 10 mm in diameter. They vary in color from flesh to brown.

They usually develop in people over age 40, typically on the upper body. Excision is necessary only to rule out malignant transformation.

Blue nevi are flat or slightly elevated lesions from 0.5 to 1 cm in diameter. Twice as common in women as in men, they appear on the head, neck, arms, and dorsa of the hands. Their blue color results from pigment and collagen in the dermis, which reflect blue light but absorb other wavelengths. Excision is necessary to rule out pigmented basal cell epithelioma or melanoma, or for cosmetic reasons.

Dysplastic nevi are generally greater than 5 mm in diameter, with irregularly notched or indistinct borders. Coloration is a mixture of tan and brown, sometimes with red, pink, and black pigmentation. No two lesions are alike. They occur in great numbers (typically more than 100 at a time), never singly, usually appearing on the back, scalp, chest, and buttocks. Dysplastic nevi are potentially malignant, especially in patients with a personal or family history of melanoma. Skin biopsy confirms diagnosis; treatment is by surgical excision, followed by regular physical examinations (every 6 months) to detect any new lesions or changes in existing lesions.

---

types. It most commonly occurs in areas heavily exposed to the sun. It arises from a lentigo maligna on an exposed skin surface and usually occurs between ages 60 and 70.

Causes
Several factors may influence the development of melanoma:
- *Excessive exposure to sunlight.* Melanoma occurs most commonly in sunny, warm areas and often develops on body parts that are exposed to the sun.
- *Skin type.* Most people who develop melanoma have blond or red hair, fair skin, and blue eyes; are prone to sunburn; and are of Celtic or Scandinavian ancestry. Melanoma is rare among Blacks; when it does develop, it usually arises in lightly pigmented areas (the palms, plantar surface of the feet, or mucous membranes).
- *Hormonal factors.* Pregnancy may increase the risk of melanoma and exacerbate growth.
- *Family history.* Melanoma occurs slightly more often within families.
- *Past history of melanoma.* A person who has had one melanoma is at greater risk of developing a second.

Complications
This cancer has a strong tendency to metastasize, and complications result from disease progression to the lungs, liver, or brain.

Assessment findings
A sore that doesn't heal, a persistent lump or swelling, and changes in preexisting skin markings, such as moles, birthmarks, scars, freckles, or warts, may be part of the patient history. Suspect melanoma when any preexisting skin lesion or nevus enlarges, changes color, becomes inflamed or sore, itches, ulcerates, bleeds, changes texture, or shows signs of surrounding pigment regression.

In superficial spreading melanoma, inspection may reveal lesions on the ankles or the inside surfaces of the knees. These lesions may appear red, white, or blue over a brown or black background. They may have an irregular, notched margin. Palpation may reveal small, elevated tumor nodules that may ulcerate and bleed. These tumors may grow horizontally for years, but when vertical growth occurs, the prognosis worsens.

In nodular malignant melanoma, inspection of the knees and ankles may reveal a uniformly discolored nodule. It may appear grayish and resemble a blackberry. Occasionally, this melanoma is flesh-colored, with flecks of pigment around its base, which may be inflamed. Palpation may disclose polypoidal nodules that resemble the surface of a blackberry.

In acral-lentiginous melanoma, inspection may show pigmented lesions on the palms and soles and under the nails. The color may resemble a mosaic of rich browns, tans, and black. Inspection of the nail beds may reveal a streak in the nail associated with an irregular tan or brown stain that diffuses from the nail bed.

In lentigo maligna melanoma, the patient history may reveal a long-standing lesion that has now ulcerated. Inspection may disclose a large lesion (3 to 6 cm) that appears as a freckle of tan, brown, black, whitish, or slate color on the face, back of the hand, or under the fingernails. There may be irregular scattered black nodules on the surface. Palpation may reveal a flat nodule with smaller nodules scattered over the surface.

Diagnostic tests
• *Excisional biopsy* and *full-depth punch biopsy* with histologic examination can distinguish malignant melanoma from a benign nevus, seborrheic keratosis, or pigmented basal cell epithelioma and can also determine tumor thickness and disease stage. (See *Staging malignant melanoma.*)
• *Baseline laboratory studies* may include complete blood count with differential, erythrocyte sedimentation rate, platelet count, and liver function studies, in addition to urinalysis.

Depending on the depth of tumor invasion and any metastatic spread, baseline diagnostic studies may also include such tests as chest X-rays, computed tomography (CT) scans of the chest and abdomen, and a gallium scan. Signs of bone metastasis may require a bone scan; central nervous system metastasis, a CT scan of the brain. Magnetic resonance imaging may be used to assess metastasis.

Treatment
A patient with malignant melanoma always requires surgical resection to remove the tumor (a 3- to 5-cm margin is desired). The extent of resection depends on the size and location of the primary lesion. Closure of a wide resection may necessitate a skin graft. If so, plastic surgery techniques provide excellent cosmetic repair. Surgical treatment may also include regional lymphadenectomy.

Deep primary lesions may merit adjuvant chemotherapy. The most consistently used drugs have been dacarbazine and carmustine. After surgical removal of a mass, intra-arterial isolation perfusions are performed to prevent recurrence and metastatic spread.

Although still experimental, immunotherapy, consisting of treatment with bacille Calmette-Guérin (BCG) vaccine, offers hope to patients with advanced melanoma. In theory, immunotherapy combats cancer by boosting the body's disease-fighting systems.

Chemotherapy is useful only in metastatic disease. Dacarbazine and the nitrosoureas have generated some response. Similarly, radiation therapy is usually reserved for metastatic disease. It doesn't prolong survival but may reduce tumor size and relieve pain.

Regardless of treatment, melanomas require close long-term follow-up care to detect metastases and recurrences. Statistics show that about 13% of recurrences develop more than 5 years after primary surgery.

Nursing diagnoses
• Altered nutrition: Less than body requirements
• Anticipatory grieving
• Anxiety
• Body image disturbance
• Fear
• Impaired skin integrity
• Ineffective family coping
• Ineffective individual coping
• Knowledge deficit
• Pain
• Risk for infection

Nursing interventions
• Listen to the patient's fears and concerns. Stay with him during episodes of stress and anxiety. Include the patient and family in care decisions.
• Provide positive reinforcement as the patient attempts to adapt to his disease.
• Watch for complications associated with chemotherapy, such as mouth sores, hair loss, weakness, fatigue, and anorexia. Offer orange and grapefruit juices and ginger ale to help with nausea and vomiting.
• Provide an adequate diet for the patient, one that is high in protein and calories. If the patient is anorexic, provide small, frequent meals. Consult with the dietitian to incorporate foods that the patient enjoys into his diet.
• After surgery, take precautions to prevent infection. Check dressings often for excessive drainage, foul odor, redness, and swelling. If surgery included lymphadenectomy, apply a compression stocking, and instruct the pa-

STAGING MALIGNANT MELANOMA

Several systems exist for staging malignant melanoma, including the TNM (tumor, node, metastasis) system, developed by the American Joint Committee on Cancer, and Clark's system, which classifies tumor progression according to skin layer penetration.

Primary tumor

TX—primary tumor can't be assessed
T0—no evidence of primary tumor
Tis—melanoma in situ (atypical melanotic hyperplasia, severe melanotic dysplasia), not an invasive lesion (Clark's Level I)
T1—tumor 0.75 mm in thickness or less invades the papillary dermis (Clark's Level II)
T2—tumor between 0.75 and 1.5 mm thick, or tumor invades the interface between the papillary and reticular dermis (Clark's Level III), or both
T3—tumor between 1.5 and 4 mm thick, or tumor invades the reticular dermis (Clark's Level IV), or both
T3a—tumor between 1.5 and 3 mm thick
T3b—tumor between 3 and 4 mm thick
T4—tumor more than 4 mm thick, or tumor invades subcutaneous tissue (Clark's Level V), or tumor has one or more satellites within 2 cm of the primary tumor
T4a—tumor more than 4 mm thick, or invades subcutaneous tissue, or both
T4b—one or more satellites exist within 2 cm of the primary tumor

Regional lymph nodes

NX—regional lymph nodes can't be assessed
N0—no evidence of regional lymph node involvement
N1—metastasis 3 cm or less in greatest dimension in any regional lymph node
N2—metastasis greater than 3 cm in greatest dimension in any regional lymph node, or in-transit metastasis, or both

Distant metastasis

MX—distant metastasis can't be assessed
M0—no evidence of distant metastasis
M1—distant metastasis
M1a—metastasis in skin, subcutaneous tissue, or lymph nodes beyond the regional nodes
M1b—visceral metastasis

Staging categories

Malignant melanoma progresses from mild to severe as follows:
Stage I—T1, N0, M0; T2, N0, M0
Stage II—T3, N0, M0
Stage III—T4, N0, M0; any T, N1, M0; any T, N2, M0
Stage IV—any T, any N, M1

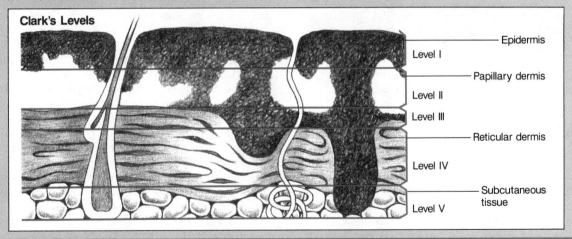

Clark's Levels

- Epidermis
- Level I
- Papillary dermis
- Level II
- Level III
- Reticular dermis
- Level IV
- Subcutaneous tissue
- Level V

tient to keep the extremity elevated to minimize lymphedema.

In advanced metastatic disease:
• Control and prevent pain with regularly scheduled administration of analgesics.

• If the patient is dying, identify the needs of patient, family, and friends, and provide appropriate support and care.

Patient teaching

• Make sure the patient understands the procedures and treatments associated with his diagnosis. Review the doctor's explanation of treatment alternatives. Honestly answer any questions he may have about surgery, chemotherapy, and radiation therapy.

• Tell the patient what to expect before and after surgery, what the wound will look like, and what type of dressing he'll have. Warn him that the donor site for a skin graft may be as painful, if not more so, than the tumor excision site.

• Teach the patient and his family relaxation techniques to help relieve anxiety. Encourage the patient to continue these after he is discharged.

• Emphasize the need for close follow-up care to detect recurrences early. Explain that recurrences and metastases, if they occur, are often delayed, so follow-up must continue for years. Teach the patient how to recognize the signs of recurrence.

• To help prevent malignant melanoma, stress the detrimental effects of overexposure to solar radiation, especially to fair-skinned, blue-eyed patients. Recommend that they use a sunblock or a sunscreen.

• When appropriate, refer the patient and his family to community support services, such as the American Cancer Society or a hospice.

BLOOD AND LYMPH NEOPLASMS

When cancer affects the circulatory systems, the entire body may become rapidly involved in the disease.

HODGKIN'S DISEASE

A neoplastic disorder, Hodgkin's disease is characterized by painless, progressive enlargement of the lymph nodes, spleen, and other lymphoid tissue. This enlargement results from proliferation of lymphocytes, histiocytes, eosinophils, and Reed-Sternberg cells. The latter cells are the special histologic feature of Hodgkin's disease.

Hodgkin's disease occurs in all races but is slightly more common in whites. Its incidence peaks in two age-groups—15 to 38 and after age 50. It occurs most commonly in young adults—except in Japan, where it occurs exclusively among people over age 50. It has a higher incidence in men than in women. A family history of Hodgkin's disease increases the likelihood of acquiring the disorder.

Untreated, Hodgkin's disease follows a variable but relentlessly progressive and ultimately fatal course. However, recent advances in therapy make Hodgkin's disease potentially curable, even in advanced stages. Appropriate treatment yields a 5-year survival rate of about 90%.

Causes

Although the cause of Hodgkin's disease is unknown, some studies point to genetic, viral, or environmental factors.

Complications

Hodgkin's disease can cause multiple organ failure.

Assessment findings

Most commonly, the patient's history will reveal painless swelling of one of the cervical lymph nodes or sometimes the axillary or inguinal lymph nodes. The history may also reveal a persistent fever and night sweats. The patient may complain of weight loss despite an adequate diet, with resulting fatigue and malaise. As the disease advances, the patient may become increasingly susceptible to infection.

Inspection during the advanced stages of the disease may reveal edema of the face and neck, and jaundice.

Palpation may identify enlarged, rubbery lymph nodes in the neck. These nodes enlarge during periods of fever and then revert to normal size.

Diagnostic tests

Tests must first rule out other disorders that enlarge the lymph nodes.

Lymph node biopsy confirms the presence of Reed-Sternberg cells, abnormal histiocyte proliferation, and nodular fibrosis and necrosis. (See *Spotting Reed-Sternberg cells.*)

Lymph node biopsy also helps determine lymph node and organ involvement, as do bone marrow, liver, mediastinal, and spleen biopsies; routine chest X-rays; abdominal computed tomography, lung, and bone scans; lymphangiography; and laparoscopy.

Hematologic tests show mild to severe normocytic anemia; normochromic anemia (in 50% of patients); and elevated, normal, or reduced white blood cell count and differential, showing any combination of neutrophilia, lymphocytopenia, monocytosis, and eosinophilia. Elevated serum alkaline phosphatase levels indicate liver or bone involvement.

A staging laparotomy is necessary for patients under age 55 and for those without obvious Stage III or Stage IV disease, lymphocyte predominance subtype histology, or medical contraindications. (See *Staging Hodgkin's disease,* page 376.)

Treatment

Depending on the stage of the disease, the patient may receive chemotherapy, radiation therapy, or both. Correct treatment allows longer survival and may even induce a cure in many patients.

A patient with Stage I or Stage II disease receives radiation therapy alone; a patient with Stage III disease receives radiation therapy and chemotherapy. For Stage IV, the patient receives chemotherapy alone, sometimes inducing a complete remission. As an alternative, he may receive chemotherapy and radiation therapy to involved sites.

Chemotherapy consists of various combinations of drugs. The well-known MOPP protocol (mechlorethamine, vincristine [Oncovin], procarbazine, and prednisone) was the first to provide significant cures for generalized Hodgkin's disease. Another useful combination is ABVD (doxorubicin [Adriamycin], bleomycin, vinblastine, and dacarbazine). Treatment with these drugs may require concomitant administration of antiemetics, sedatives, and antidiarrheals to combat GI adverse effects.

Other treatments include autologous bone marrow transplantation and immunotherapy, which by itself hasn't proved effective.

Nursing diagnoses

• Altered nutrition: Less than body requirements
• Altered oral mucous membrane
• Anxiety
• Fatigue
• Fear
• Impaired skin integrity
• Ineffective family coping
• Ineffective individual coping
• Knowledge deficit
• Pain
• Risk for infection

Nursing interventions

• Watch for complications during chemotherapy, including anorexia, nausea, vomiting, alopecia, and mouth ulcers.
• Provide a well-balanced, high-calorie, high-protein diet. If the patient is anorexic, provide frequent, small

SPOTTING REED-STERNBERG CELLS

The illustration below shows Reed-Sternberg cells. Note the large, distinct nucleoli.

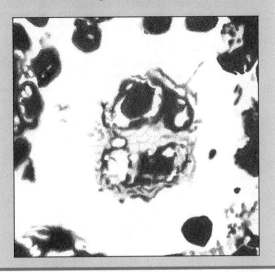

meals. Consult with the dietitian to incorporate foods the patient enjoys into his diet.
• Be alert for adverse effects of radiation therapy, such as hair loss, nausea, vomiting, and anorexia.
• Offer the patient grapefruit juice, orange juice, or ginger ale to alleviate nausea and vomiting.
• Perform comfort measures that promote relaxation. Provide for periods of rest if the patient tires easily. Administer pain medication, as ordered, and monitor its effectiveness.
• Watch for the development of hypothyroidism, sterility, and a second neoplastic disease, including late-onset leukemia and non-Hodgkin's lymphoma. Although these are complications of the treatments, they also indicate the success of treatment.
• Throughout therapy, listen to the patient's fears and concerns. Encourage him to express his feelings, and stay with him during periods of extreme stress and anxiety. Provide emotional support to the patient and his family.
• Involve the patient and his family in all aspects of his care.

Patient teaching

• Explain all procedures and treatments associated with the plan of care.

STAGING HODGKIN'S DISEASE

Treatment of Hodgkin's disease depends on the stage it has reached—that is, the number, location, and degree of involved lymph nodes. The Ann Arbor classification system, adopted in 1971, divides Hodgkin's disease into four stages.

Stage I
Hodgkin's disease appears in a single lymph node region (I) or a single extralymphatic organ (IE).

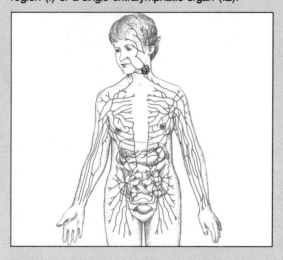

Stage II
The disease appears in two or more nodes on the same side of the diaphragm (II) and in an extralymphatic organ (IIE).

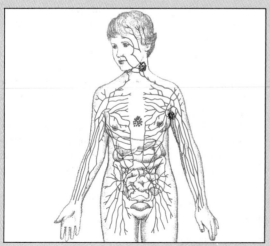

Stage III
Hodgkin's disease spreads to both sides of the diaphragm (III) and perhaps to an extralymphatic organ (IIIE), the spleen (IIIS), or both (IIIES).

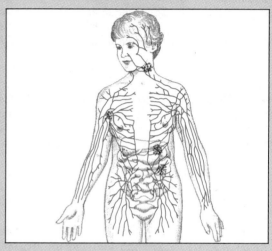

Stage IV
The disease disseminates, involving one or more extralymphatic organs or tissues, with or without lymph node involvement.

Doctors subdivide each stage into categories. Category A includes patients without defined signs and symptoms, and category B includes patients who experience such defined signs as recent unexplained weight loss, fever, and night sweats.

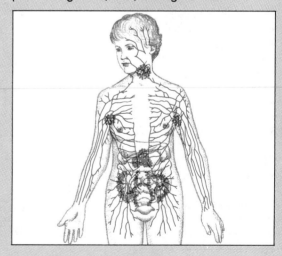

• Because sudden withdrawal of prednisone is life-threatening, advise the patient taking this medication not to change his drug dosage or discontinue the drug without contacting his doctor.

• If the patient is a woman of childbearing age, advise her to delay pregnancy until long-term remission occurs. Radiation therapy and chemotherapy can cause genetic mutations and spontaneous abortions.

• Stress the importance of maintaining good nutrition (aided by eating small, frequent meals of the patient's favorite foods) and drinking plenty of fluids.

• Instruct the patient to pace his activities to counteract therapy-induced fatigue. Teach him how to use relaxation techniques to promote comfort and reduce anxiety.

• Stress the importance of good oral hygiene to prevent stomatitis. To control pain and bleeding, teach the patient to use a soft toothbrush, a cotton swab, or an anesthetic mouthwash, such as viscous lidocaine (as prescribed); to apply petroleum jelly to his lips; and to avoid astringent mouthwashes.

• Advise the patient to avoid crowds and any person with a known infection. Emphasize that he should notify the doctor if he develops any infections.

• Because enlarged lymph nodes may indicate disease recurrence, teach the patient the importance of checking his lymph nodes.

• Make sure the patient understands the possible adverse effects of his treatments. Tell him to notify the doctor if these signs and symptoms persist.

• When appropriate, refer the patient and his family to community organizations, such as psychological counseling services, support groups, and hospices.

• Advise the patient to seek follow-up care after he has completed the initial treatment.

MALIGNANT LYMPHOMAS

Also called non-Hodgkin's lymphomas and lymphosarcomas, malignant lymphomas are a heterogeneous group of malignant diseases that originate in lymph glands and other lymphoid tissue. Lymphomas are usually classified according to histologic, anatomic, and immunomorphic characteristics developed by the National Cancer Institute. However, the Rappaport histologic and Lukes classifications also are used in some settings (see *Classifying malignant lymphomas,* page 378).

Malignant lymphomas occur three times more commonly than Hodgkin's disease—and the incidence is increasing, especially in patients with autoimmune disorders and those receiving immunosuppressant treatment. Nodular lymphomas yield a better prognosis than the diffuse form of the disease, but in both, the prognosis is less hopeful than in Hodgkin's disease.

Causes
Although some theories point to a viral source, the cause of malignant lymphomas is unknown.

Complications
Malignant lymphomas can lead to hypercalcemia, hyperuricemia, lymphomatosis, meningitis, and anemia from bone marrow involvement. As tumors grow, they may produce liver, kidney, and lung problems. Central nervous system involvement can lead to increased intracranial pressure.

Assessment findings
The symptoms of malignant lymphomas may mimic those of Hodgkin's disease. Most commonly, the patient history reveals painless, swollen lymph glands. The swelling may have appeared and disappeared over several months.

As the lymphoma progresses, the patient may complain of fatigue, malaise, weight loss, and night sweats. If the patient is a child, he may have trouble breathing and have a cough, probably the result of enlarged lymph nodes.

Inspection may reveal enlarged tonsils and adenoids, and palpation may disclose rubbery nodes in the cervical and supraclavicular areas.

Diagnostic tests
Biopsies—of lymph nodes; of tonsils, bone marrow, liver, bowel, or skin; or, as needed, of tissue removed during exploratory laparotomy—differentiate a malignant lymphoma from Hodgkin's disease. Chest X-rays; lymphangiography; liver, bone, and spleen scans; a computed tomography scan of the abdomen; and excretory urography indicate disease progression.

A complete blood count may show anemia. The patient may have a normal or elevated uric acid level and an elevated serum calcium level, resulting from bone lesions.

The same staging system used for Hodgkin's disease is used for malignant lymphomas.

Treatment
Radiation and chemotherapy serve as the main treatments for lymphomas. Radiation therapy is used mainly during the localized stage of the disease. Total nodal irradiation often effectively treats both nodular and diffuse lymphomas.

CLASSIFYING MALIGNANT LYMPHOMAS

Several classification and staging systems are in current use for evaluating the extent of malignant lymphoma. Among the most common are the National Cancer Institute's (NCI) system (named the "Working formulation for classification of non-Hodgkin's lymphomas for clinical usage"), the Rappaport histologic classification, and Lukes classification. The three systems appear below.

NCI working formulation	Rappaport histologic classification	Lukes classification
Low grade		
• Small lymphocytic	• Diffuse well-differentiated lymphocytic	• Small lymphocytic and plasmacytoid lymphocytic
• Follicular, predominantly small cleaved cell	• Nodular poorly differentiated lymphocytic	• Small cleaved follicular center cell, follicular only or follicular and diffuse
• Follicular mixed, small and large cell	• Nodular mixed lymphoma	• Small cleaved follicular center cell, follicular; large cleaved follicular center cell, follicular
Intermediate grade		
• Follicular, predominantly large cell	• Nodular histiocytic lymphoma	• Large cleaved or noncleaved follicular center cell, or both, follicular
• Diffuse, small cleaved cell	• Diffuse poorly differentiated lymphoma	• Small cleaved follicular center cell, diffuse
• Diffuse mixed, small and large cell	• Diffuse mixed lymphocytic-histiocytic	• Small cleaved, large cleaved, or large noncleaved follicular center cell, diffuse
• Diffuse large cell, cleaved or non-cleaved	• Diffuse histiocytic lymphoma	• Large cleaved or noncleaved follicular center cell, diffuse
High grade		
• Diffuse large cell immunoblastic	• Diffuse histiocytic lymphoma	• Immunoblastic sarcoma, T-cell or B-cell type
• Large cell, lymphoblastic	• Lymphoblastic, convoluted or nonconvoluted	• Convoluted T cell
• Small noncleaved cell	• Undifferentiated, Burkitt's and non-Burkitt's diffuse undifferentiated lymphoma	• Small noncleaved follicular center cell
Miscellaneous		
• Composite • Mycosis fungoides • Histiocytic • Extramedullary plasmacytoma • Unclassifiable		

Chemotherapy is most effective with combinations of antineoplastic agents. For example, the CHOP protocol (cyclophosphamide, doxorubicin, vincristine [Oncovin], and prednisone) can induce a complete remission in 70% to 80% of those with nodular lymphoma and in 20% to 55% of those with diffuse lymphoma. Other combinations—such as MACOP-B (methotrexate, leucovorin, doxorubicin [Adriamycin], cyclophosphamide, vincristine [Oncovin], prednisone, and bleomycin)—can induce a prolonged remission and possibly a cure for diffuse lymphoma.

Recent studies show that lower intensity and shorter duration of chemotherapy can produce the same response rate as high-intensity and long-term chemotherapy in children with a localized malignant lymphoma.

Because perforation commonly occurs in patients with gastric lymphomas, these patients usually undergo a debulking procedure before chemotherapy, such as a sub-total or—in some cases—a total gastrectomy.

Nursing diagnoses
• Altered nutrition: Less than body requirements
• Altered protection
• Anxiety
• Fatigue
• Fear
• Ineffective family coping
• Ineffective individual coping
• Pain
• Risk for infection

Nursing interventions
• Administer ordered pain medication and monitor its ef-fectiveness.
• Provide for rest periods if patient tires easily.
• Watch for complications of chemotherapy, such as nau-sea and vomiting, anorexia, hair loss, mouth ulcers, and infection.
• Offer the patient fluids, such as grapefruit juice, orange juice, or ginger ale, to counteract nausea.
• Because this disease causes large numbers of tumors, provide the patient with lots of fluids to help flush out the cells that are destroyed during treatment. This helps prevent tumor lysis syndrome.
• Provide a well-balanced, high-calorie, high-protein diet. Consult with the dietitian and plan small, frequent meals that include the patient's favorite foods. Schedule meals around the patient's treatment.
• If the patient can't tolerate oral feedings, administer I.V. fluids. If necessary, give antiemetics and sedatives, as ordered.
• Throughout therapy, listen to the patient's fears and concerns. Stay with him during periods of severe stress or anxiety. Encourage him to express his anger and con-cerns, and offer reassurance when appropriate.
• Involve the patient and his family in his care whenever possible.

Patient teaching
• Make sure the patient receives thorough explanations about all forms of his treatment.
• Instruct the patient to keep irradiated skin dry.
• Before surgery, explain preoperative and postoperative procedures thoroughly to the patient. Tell him that he may have a nasogastric tube or an indwelling urinary catheter inserted postoperatively.
• After chemotherapy and radiation therapy, advise the patient to avoid crowds and anyone who has an infection.

Urge him to report any infection he develops to his doc-tor.
• Stress the importance of maintaining a well-balanced, high-calorie, high-protein diet.
• Emphasize the importance of maintaining good oral hy-giene during treatment to prevent stomatitis. Instruct the patient to clean his teeth with a soft-bristled toothbrush and to avoid commercial mouthwashes.
• Teach the patient relaxation and comfort measures and encourage him to use them.
• If appropriate, refer the patient to the social service de-partment, home health care agencies, hospices, and sup-port groups such as the American Cancer Society.

MYCOSIS FUNGOIDES
Also called malignant cutaneous reticulosis and granu-loma fungoides, mycosis fungoides is a rare, chronic form of T-cell lymphoma. It originates in the reticuloendothe-lial system of the skin and eventually affects lymph nodes and internal organs. Three clinical stages have been identified: premycotic (or erythematous), plaque, and tumor.

In the United States, this disease strikes more than 1,000 patients of all races annually. Most are between 40 and 60 years old.

Unlike other lymphomas, mycosis fungoides has an average life expectancy of 8 to 9 years after diagnosis. If correctly treated—particularly before it has spread past the skin—the disease may go into remission for many years. After it reaches the tumor stage, however, progression to severe disability and death is rapid.

Causes
Although its cause is unknown, mycosis fungoides has been associated with exposure to certain chemicals, a family history of Hodgkin's disease or lymphoma, and defects in host immunosurveillance.

Complications
Fissures on the palms and soles, alopecia, and infection can develop during the course of the disease.

Assessment findings
In the premycotic stage of mycosis fungoides, the patient may complain of general itching and superficial skin eruptions that he may describe as appearing and dis-appearing spontaneously. Inspection may disclose le-sions of varying sizes that appear as scaling, macular, erythematous patches. The lesions may be localized or scattered over the entire skin surface. In this early stage,

mycosis fungoides is commonly mistaken for psoriasis or dermatitis.

In the plaque stage, the patient may complain of great discomfort and itching in the lesion areas. Inspection may disclose an irregular thickening of the skin with raised and irregularly shaped plaques. You may also note lesions on the palms and soles, which the patient describes as painful, and alopecia.

In the tumor stage, inspection reveals mass lesions that may appear anywhere—in previously normal skin, in plaques, and in previous mycotic lesions. Although these lesions can develop anywhere on the body, they most commonly appear on the face and body folds, such as the axilla, groin, cubital folds, neck, and breasts. You may also be able to palpate the patient's lymph nodes.

Diagnostic tests
A complete blood count and differential and a fingerstick smear for Sézary cells (abnormal circulating lymphocytes) aid diagnosis of this disease. Blood chemistry studies allow screening for visceral dysfunction. Chest X-rays, liver-spleen isotopic scanning, lymphangiography, and lymph node biopsy help to assess histologic involvement and to stage the disease.

Treatment
In mycosis fungoides, the type of treatment is based on the patient's age and clinical status, the treatment facilities available, the stage of the disease, its rate of progression, and past treatments and their effects.

Treatment may include phototherapy, methoxsalen photochemotherapy, radiation therapy, or topical, intralesional, or systemic corticosteroids or mechlorethamine (nitrogen mustard). Topical mechlorethamine is the preferred treatment for inducing remission in the pretumorous stage. Total-body electron beam radiation, which is less toxic to internal organs than standard photon beam radiation, has induced remission in some patients with early-stage disease.

Other kinds of systemic chemotherapy can help patients with tumor-stage (advanced) disease. Such agents include cyclophosphamide, methotrexate, doxorubicin, and bleomycin.

Nursing diagnoses
• Anxiety
• Body image disturbance
• Fear
• Impaired skin integrity
• Ineffective family coping
• Ineffective individual coping
• Pain
• Risk for infection

Nursing interventions
• Administer ordered pain medications and antipruritics as necessary. Help make the patient comfortable by providing distractions and having him perform relaxation techniques. Also, help him identify care measures that will promote his comfort and relaxation, and try to perform these measures whenever possible.
• If the patient has difficulty applying the mechlorethamine to all involved skin surfaces, help him do so. But be sure to wear gloves to prevent contact sensitization.
• Watch for and immediately report any complications of treatment, particularly infection. During drug therapy, provide measures that prevent or alleviate anticipated problems with the prescribed drugs.
• If the patient is receiving systemic cytotoxic therapy, watch for such complications as transient leukopenia and thrombocytopenia and ulcerations at active disease sites.
• If the patient is receiving electron beam radiation therapy, monitor him for acute and long-term effects. Acute toxicity results in radiation dermatitis, hyperpigmentation, blistering, and temporary hair loss. Long-term effects include weight loss, increased skin pigmentation, permanent hair loss, and wrinkled, dry skin.
• Provide positive reinforcement if radiation therapy or the disease's scalp involvement results in alopecia. Suggest a head covering to protect the scalp.
• Remember that the patient with pruritus has an overwhelming desire to scratch—often to the point of removing skin and replacing itching with pain, which he may find easier to endure. You can't keep such a patient from scratching, but you can help minimize the damage. Make sure he keeps his fingernails short and clean, and provide him with a pair of soft, white cotton gloves when itching becomes unbearable.
• Because pruritus typically intensifies at night, provide the patient with larger bedtime doses of antipruritics or sedatives, as ordered, to ensure adequate sleep. When pruritus has interrupted his sleep, postpone early-morning care to allow him more sleep.
• Throughout therapy, listen to the patient's fears and concerns. Remain with him during periods of severe stress and anxiety. Provide reassurance and support by demonstrating a positive but realistic attitude. Reinforce your verbal support by touching the patient without any hint of anxiety or distaste.
• Include the patient and his family in care decisions whenever possible.

Patient teaching
• The patient with malignant skin lesions is likely to be depressed, fearful, and self-conscious. So fully explain the disease and its stages to help him and his family understand and accept the disease.
• Teach the patient the importance of preventing infection by careful hand washing and maintaining good hygiene.
• Refer the patient to support groups, such as the American Cancer Society, as appropriate.

ACUTE LEUKEMIA
Beginning as a malignant proliferation of white blood cell (WBC) precursors, or blasts, in bone marrow or lymph tissue, acute leukemia results in an accumulation of these cells in peripheral blood, bone marrow, and body tissues.

The most common forms of acute leukemia include acute lymphoblastic (lymphocytic) leukemia (ALL), characterized by abnormal growth of lymphocyte precursors (lymphoblasts); acute myeloblastic (myelogenous) leukemia (AML), which causes rapid accumulation of myeloid precursors (myeloblasts); and acute monoblastic (monocytic) leukemia, or Schilling's type, which results in a marked increase in monocyte precursors (monoblasts). Other variants include acute myelomonocytic leukemia and acute erythroleukemia.

Acute leukemia ranks 20th among causes of cancer-related death among people of all ages. In the United States, an estimated 11,000 persons develop acute leukemia annually. The disease is more common in males than in females, in whites (especially those of Jewish ancestry), in children between ages 2 and 5 (80% of all leukemias in this age-group are ALL), and in those who live in urban and industrialized areas. Among children, acute leukemia is the most common form of cancer.

Untreated, acute leukemia is invariably fatal, usually because of complications resulting from leukemic cell infiltration of bone marrow or vital organs. With treatment, the prognosis varies.

In ALL, treatment induces remissions in 90% of children (average survival time: 5 years) and in 65% of adults (average survival time: 1 to 2 years). Children between ages 2 and 8 have the best survival rate—about 50%—with intensive therapy.

In AML, the average survival time is only 1 year after diagnosis, even with aggressive treatment. Remissions lasting 2 to 10 months occur in 50% of children; adults survive only about 1 year after diagnosis, even with treatment.

Causes and pathophysiology
The exact cause of acute leukemia is unknown; however, radiation (especially prolonged exposure), certain chemicals and drugs, viruses, genetic abnormalities, and chronic exposure to benzene are likely contributing factors.

In children, Down's syndrome, ataxia, and telangiectasia may increase the risk, as may such congenital disorders as albinism and congenital immunodeficiency syndrome.

Although the pathogenesis isn't clearly understood, immature, nonfunctioning WBCs appear to accumulate first in the tissue where they originate (lymphocytes in lymph tissue, granulocytes in bone marrow). These immature WBCs then spill into the bloodstream. From there, they infiltrate other tissues.

Complications
Acute leukemia increases the risk of infection and, eventually, organ malfunction through encroachment or hemorrhage.

Assessment findings
The patient's history usually shows a sudden onset of high fever and abnormal bleeding, such as bruising after minor trauma, nosebleeds, gingival bleeding, purpura, ecchymoses, petechiae, and prolonged menses. He may also report fatigue and night sweats. More insidious symptoms include weakness, lassitude, recurrent infections, and chills.

The patient with ALL, AML, or acute monoblastic leukemia may also complain of abdominal or bone pain. When assessing this patient, you may note tachycardia and, during auscultation, decreased ventilation, palpitations, and a systolic ejection murmur.

Inspection of any patient with acute leukemia may reveal pallor. On palpation, you may note lymph node enlargement as well as liver or spleen enlargement.

Diagnostic tests
Bone marrow aspiration showing a proliferation of immature WBCs confirms acute leukemia. If the aspirate is dry or free of leukemic cells but the patient has other typical signs of leukemia, a bone marrow biopsy—usually of the posterior superior iliac spine—must be performed.

Blood counts show thrombocytopenia and neutropenia, and a WBC differential determines the cell type. Lumbar puncture detects meningeal involvement. A computed tomography scan shows the affected organs, and cerebrospinal fluid analysis detects abnormal WBC invasion of the central nervous system.

Treatment

Systemic chemotherapy aims to eradicate leukemic cells and induce remission. It's used when fewer than 5% of blast cells in the marrow and peripheral blood are normal. The specific chemotherapeutic and radiation treatment varies with the diagnosis:

• For meningeal infiltration, the patient receives an intrathecal instillation of methotrexate or cytarabine with cranial radiation.

• For ALL, the treatment is vincristine, prednisone, high-dose cytarabine, and daunorubicin. Because ALL carries a 40% risk of meningeal infiltration, the patient also receives intrathecal methotrexate or cytarabine. If brain or testicular infiltration has occurred, the patient also needs radiation therapy.

• For AML, treatment consists of a combination of I.V. daunorubicin and cytarabine. If these fail to induce remission, treatment involves some or all of the following: a combination of cyclophosphamide, vincristine, prednisone, or methotrexate; high-dose cytarabine alone or with other drugs; amsacrine; etoposide; and azacytidine and mitoxantrone.

• For acute monoblastic leukemia, the patient receives cytarabine and thioguanine with daunorubicin or doxorubicin.

Treatment may also include antibiotic, antifungal, and antiviral drugs and granulocyte injections to control infection, as well as transfusions of platelets to prevent bleeding and of red blood cells to prevent anemia. Bone marrow transplantation is performed in some patients.

Nursing diagnoses

• Altered nutrition: Less than body requirements
• Altered oral mucous membrane
• Altered parenting
• Altered protection
• Anticipatory grieving
• Anxiety
• Fatigue
• Fear
• Impaired tissue integrity
• Ineffective family coping
• Ineffective individual coping
• Pain
• Risk for altered body temperature
• Risk for infection
• Risk for injury

Nursing interventions

• Develop a plan of care for the leukemic patient that emphasizes comfort, minimizes the adverse effects of chemotherapy, promotes preservation of veins, manages complications, and provides teaching and psychological support. Because so many of these patients are children, be especially sensitive to their emotional needs and to those of their families when developing your plan.

• Before treatment begins, help establish an appropriate rehabilitation program for the patient during remission.

• Watch for signs of meningeal infiltration (confusion, lethargy, and headache). If it develops, the patient will need intrathecal chemotherapy.

• After drug instillation, place the patient in Trendelenburg's position for 30 minutes. Make sure he receives enough fluids, and keep him supine for 4 to 6 hours. Check the lumbar puncture site often for bleeding.

• Take steps to prevent hyperuricemia, a possible result of rapid, chemotherapy-induced leukemic cell lysis. Make sure the patient receives about 2 liters of fluid daily, and give acetazolamide, sodium bicarbonate tablets, and allopurinol, as ordered. Check the patient's urine pH often; it should be above 7.5. Watch for a rash or other hypersensitivity reactions to allopurinol.

• If the patient receives daunorubicin or doxorubicin, watch for early indications of cardiotoxicity, such as arrhythmias and signs of heart failure.

• To control infection, place the patient in a private room and impose reverse isolation if necessary (although the benefits of reverse isolation are controversial). Coordinate care so that the patient doesn't come into contact with staff members who also care for patients with infections or infectious diseases. Screen staff members and visitors for contagious diseases, and watch for and report any signs of infection. Don't use an indwelling urinary catheter or give I.M. injections; they provide an avenue for infection.

• Keep the patient's skin and perianal area clean, apply mild lotions or creams to keep the skin from drying and cracking, and thoroughly clean the skin before all invasive skin procedures. Change I.V. tubing according to your hospital's policy. Use strict aseptic technique and a metal scalp vein needle (metal butterfly needle) when starting an I.V. line. If the patient is receiving total parenteral nutrition, provide scrupulous subclavian catheter care.

• Monitor the patient's temperature every 4 hours. If his temperature rises over 101° F (38.3° C) and his WBC count decreases, he will need prompt antibiotic therapy.

• Watch for bleeding. If it occurs, apply ice compresses and pressure, and elevate the extremity. Avoid giving the patient aspirin or aspirin-containing drugs or rectal suppositories, taking a rectal temperature, or performing a digital rectal examination.

• After bone marrow transplantation, keep the patient in a sterile room, administer antibiotics, and transfuse packed red blood cells as necessary.

• Administer prescribed pain medications as needed, and monitor their effectiveness. Provide comfort measures, such as position changes and distractions, to alleviate the patient's discomfort.

• Control mouth ulceration by checking often for obvious ulcers and gum swelling and by providing frequent mouth care and saline rinses.

• Check the rectal area daily for induration, swelling, erythema, skin discoloration, and drainage.

• Minimize stress by providing a calm, quiet atmosphere that's conducive to rest and relaxation. Especially if the patient is a child, be flexible with patient care and visiting hours so that he has time to be with his family and friends and to play and do schoolwork.

• Establish a trusting relationship to promote communication. Allow the patient and his family to express their anger, anxiety, and depression.

• Let the patient and his family participate in his care as much as possible.

• If the patient doesn't respond to treatment and has reached the terminal phase of the disease, he'll need supportive nursing care. Take steps to manage pain, fever, and bleeding; make sure the patient is comfortable; and provide emotional support for him and his family. If the patient wishes, provide for religious counseling. Discuss the option of home or hospice care.

Patient teaching

• Explain the course of the disease to the patient.

• Teach the patient and his family how to recognize signs and symptoms of infection (fever, chills, cough, sore throat). Tell them to report an infection to the doctor.

• Explain to the patient that his blood may not have enough platelets for proper clotting, and teach him the signs of abnormal bleeding (bruising, petechiae). Explain that he can apply pressure and ice to the area to stop such bleeding. Also, teach him steps he can take to prevent bleeding. Urge him to report excessive bleeding or bruising to the doctor.

• Inform the patient that drug therapy is tailored to his type of leukemia. Explain that he'll probably need a combination of drugs; teach him about the ones he'll receive. Make sure he understands their adverse effects and the measures he can take to prevent or alleviate them.

• Explain that if the chemotherapy causes weight loss and anorexia, the patient will need to eat and drink high-calorie, high-protein foods and beverages. If he loses his appetite, advise him to eat small, frequent meals. If the chemotherapy and adjunctive prednisone instead cause weight gain, he'll need dietary counseling.

• Instruct the patient to use a soft toothbrush and to avoid hot, spicy foods and commercial mouthwashes, which can irritate the mouth ulcers that result from chemotherapy.

• If the patient receives cranial radiation, explain what the treatment is and how it will help him. Be sure to discuss potential adverse effects and the steps he can take to minimize them.

• If the patient needs a bone marrow transplant, reinforce the doctor's explanation of the treatment, its possible benefits, and the potential adverse effects. Teach him about total-body irradiation and the chemotherapy that he'll undergo before transplantation. Tell the patient what to expect after the transplantation.

• Advise the patient to limit his activities and to plan rest periods during the day.

• Refer the patient to the social service department, home health care agencies, and support groups such as the American Cancer Society.

CHRONIC GRANULOCYTIC LEUKEMIA

Also called chronic myelogenous (or myelocytic) leukemia, chronic granulocytic leukemia is characterized by the abnormal overgrowth of granulocytic precursors (myeloblasts, promyelocytes, metamyelocytes, and myelocytes) in bone marrow, peripheral blood, and body tissues.

The disease is most common in young and middle-aged adults, slightly more common in men than in women, and rare in children. In the United States, between 3,000 and 4,000 cases of chronic granulocytic leukemia develop annually, accounting for about 20% of all leukemias.

The clinical course of chronic granulocytic leukemia proceeds in two distinct phases: the insidious *chronic phase,* characterized by anemia and bleeding abnormalities, and eventually the *acute phase (blast crisis),* in which myeloblasts, the most primitive granulocytic precursors, proliferate rapidly.

The disease is always deadly. Average survival time is 3 to 4 years after onset of the chronic phase and 3 to 6 months after onset of the acute phase.

Causes

Although the exact causes remain unknown, almost 90% of patients with this leukemia have the Philadelphia chromosome, an abnormality in which the long arm of chromosome 22 translocates to chromosome 9. Radiation and carcinogenic chemicals may induce this abnormality.

Myeloproliferative diseases also may increase the incidence of chronic granulocytic leukemia. Some researchers suspect that an unidentified virus causes this leukemia.

Complications

Complications include infection, hemorrhage, and pain.

Assessment findings

The patient history may reveal renal calculi or gouty arthritis (from increased uric acid excretion). The patient may relate symptoms of anemia: fatigue, weakness, dyspnea, decreased exercise tolerance, and headache. Evidence of bleeding and clotting disorders may include bleeding gums, nosebleeds, easy bruising, and hematuria. Additionally, the patient may report recent weight loss and anorexia.

The patient's vital signs may include a low-grade fever and tachycardia. Inspection may reveal pallor and difficulty breathing, and ophthalmoscopic examination may disclose retinal hemorrhage.

Palpation may uncover hepatosplenomegaly with abdominal discomfort and pain (in splenic infarction from leukemic cell infiltration) and sternal and rib tenderness (from leukemic infiltration of the periosteum).

Auscultation may disclose hypoventilation, especially if the patient has dyspnea.

Diagnostic tests

• *Chromosomal studies* of peripheral blood or bone marrow showing the Philadelphia chromosome and low leukocyte alkaline phosphatase levels confirm chronic granulocytic leukemia.
• *Serum analysis* shows white blood cell (WBC) abnormalities: leukocytosis (WBC count over 50,000/mm³, rising as high as 250,000/mm³); occasionally leukopenia (WBC count under 5,000/mm³); neutropenia (neutrophil count under 1,500/mm³) despite high WBC count; and increased circulating myeloblasts.

Additional findings may include a decreased hemoglobin level (below 10 g/dl), low hematocrit (less than 30%), and thrombocytosis (more than 1 million thrombocytes/mm³). The serum uric acid level may exceed 8 mg/dl.
• *Bone marrow aspirate* — or *biopsy* (performed only if the aspirate is dry) — may be hypercellular, characteristically showing bone marrow infiltration by a significantly increased number of myeloid elements; in the acute phase, myeloblasts predominate.
• *Computed tomography scan* may identify the organs affected by this leukemia.

Treatment

In the chronic phase, treatment strives to control leukocytosis and thrombocytosis. Commonly used drugs include busulfan and hydroxyurea. Aspirin may be given to prevent a cerebrovascular accident if the patient's platelet count exceeds 1 million/mm³.

Bone marrow transplantation may be tried. During the chronic phase, more than 60% of patients who receive a transplant achieve remission.

Ancillary treatments may include the following:
• local splenic radiation or splenectomy to increase the platelet count and to decrease adverse effects associated with splenomegaly
• leukapheresis (selective leukocyte removal) to reduce the WBC count
• allopurinol to prevent secondary hyperuricemia or colchicine to relieve gouty attacks caused by elevated serum levels of uric acid
• prompt antibiotic treatment of infections that may result from chemotherapy-induced bone marrow suppression.

During the acute phase of this leukemia, either lymphoblastic or myeloblastic disease may develop. Treatment is similar to that for acute lymphoblastic leukemia. Remission, if achieved, is commonly short-lived.

Despite vigorous treatment, chronic granulocytic leukemia rapidly advances after onset of the acute phase.

Nursing diagnoses

• Altered nutrition: Less than body requirements
• Altered oral mucous membrane
• Altered protection
• Anticipatory grieving
• Anxiety
• Constipation
• Fatigue
• Fear
• Impaired tissue integrity
• Ineffective family coping
• Ineffective individual coping
• Pain
• Risk for altered body temperature
• Risk for infection
• Risk for injury

Nursing interventions

Take the following steps during the chronic phase of chronic granulocytic leukemia when the patient is hospitalized:

• If the patient has persistent anemia, plan your care to minimize his fatigue. Schedule laboratory tests and physical care with frequent rest periods in between. Assist the patient with walking if necessary. Regularly check the patient's skin and mucous membranes for pallor, petechiae, and bruising.

• To minimize bleeding and infection risks, provide the patient with a soft-bristled toothbrush, an electric razor, and other safety devices.

• To minimize the abdominal discomfort of splenomegaly, provide small, frequent meals. For the same reason, prevent constipation with a stool softener or laxative, as needed. Maintain adequate fluid intake, and ask the dietary department to provide a high-bulk diet.

• To prevent atelectasis, help the patient perform coughing and deep-breathing exercises.

• Listen to the patient's fears and concerns, and provide emotional support. Stay with the patient during periods of severe stress, and answer his questions honestly. Encourage his participation in care decisions whenever possible.

• Administer ordered pain medications as necessary, and monitor their effectiveness. Provide comfort measures and distractions to help the patient cope with his discomfort. Instruct the patient in appropriate relaxation techniques.

• Watch for adverse effects of treatment, and take measures that will reduce or prevent them. For example, the patient who is undergoing chemotherapy should rinse his mouth with normal saline mouthwash to reduce the severity of ulcers.

• After bone marrow transplantation, keep the patient in a sterile room, and administer antibiotics and packed red blood cells as ordered. Watch for signs of infection.

For more information about nursing interventions during the acute phase, see "Acute Leukemia" in this chapter.

Patient teaching

• At the time of diagnosis, repeat and reinforce the doctor's explanation of the disease and its treatment to the patient and his family.

• Take extra care to provide sound patient teaching because the patient with chronic granulocytic leukemia typically receives outpatient chemotherapy throughout the chronic phase.

• Explain diagnostic test procedures to the patient. Be sure he understands why the tests are necessary.

• Explain expected adverse effects of chemotherapy, especially bone marrow suppression (bleeding, infection). Inform the patient that he'll receive a combination of drugs tailored to his leukemia type.

• Teach the patient the signs and symptoms of infection to watch for and report: any temperature over 100° F (37.8° C), chills, redness or swelling anywhere on the skin, sore throat, or cough.

• Instruct the patient to watch for signs of thrombocytopenia and to apply ice and pressure immediately to any external bleeding site. Unless his doctor tells him to do otherwise, advise him to avoid using aspirin and aspirin-containing compounds, which may increase his bleeding risk.

• Urge the patient to obtain adequate rest to minimize fatigue from anemia.

• To minimize the toxic effects of chemotherapy, encourage the patient to eat foods high in calories and protein. Explain that these foods will help him maintain his strength and prevent body tissues from breaking down. Suggest that he eat small, frequent meals throughout the day, especially if he has little appetite.

• If the patient will undergo bone marrow transplantation, reinforce the doctor's explanation of the procedure, its possible outcome, and potential adverse effects. Be sure the patient fully understands the therapy. Teach him about total body irradiation, which usually takes place before the procedure, and discuss any chemotherapy that he will undergo.

• As appropriate, refer the patient and his family to the social service department, home health care agencies, hospices, and support groups such as the American Cancer Society.

CHRONIC LYMPHOCYTIC LEUKEMIA

A generalized, progressive disease, chronic lymphocytic leukemia is marked by an uncontrollable spread of abnormal, small lymphocytes in lymphoid tissue, blood, and bone marrow. Once these cells infiltrate bone marrow, lymphoid tissue, and organ systems, clinical signs begin to appear.

This disease occurs most commonly in elderly people; nearly all those afflicted are men over age 50. According to the American Cancer Society, chronic lymphocytic leukemia accounts for almost one-third of new leukemia cases annually.

Chronic lymphocytic leukemia is the most benign and the most slowly progressive form of leukemia. However, the prognosis is poor if anemia, thrombocytopenia, neutropenia, bulky lymphadenopathy, and severe lymphocytosis develop. Gross bone marrow replacement by abnormal lymphocytes is the most common cause of death, usually within 4 to 5 years of diagnosis.

Causes
Although the cause of the disease is unknown, researchers suspect hereditary factors because a higher incidence has been recorded within families. Undefined chromosomal abnormalities and certain immunologic defects, such as ataxia-telangiectasia or acquired agammaglobulinemia, are also suspected. The disease doesn't seem to result from radiation exposure.

Complications
The most common complication is infection, which can be fatal. In the end stage of the disease, possible complications include anemia, progressive splenomegaly, leukemic cell replacement of the bone marrow, and profound hypogammaglobulinemia, which usually terminates with fatal septicemia.

Assessment findings
In the early stages of the disease, the patient usually complains of fatigue, malaise, fever, weight loss, and frequent infections.

Inspection may reveal macular or nodular eruptions, evidence of skin infiltration. On palpation, you may note enlarged lymph nodes, liver, and spleen, along with bone tenderness and edema from lymph node obstruction.

As the disease progresses, you may note anemia, pallor, weakness, dyspnea, tachycardia, palpitations, bleeding, and infection from bone marrow involvement. You may also see signs of opportunistic fungal, viral, or bacterial infections, which commonly occur in late stages.

Diagnostic tests
Typically, chronic lymphocytic leukemia is an incidental finding during a routine blood test that reveals numerous abnormal lymphocytes. In the early stages, the patient has a mildly but persistently elevated white blood cell (WBC) count. Granulocytopenia is the rule, although the WBC count climbs as the disease progresses.

Blood studies also reveal a hemoglobin count under 11 g/dl, hypogammaglobulinemia, and depressed serum globulin levels. Other common developments include neutropenia (less than 1,500/mm³), lymphocytosis (more than 10,000/mm³), and thrombocytopenia (less than 150,000/mm³).

Bone marrow aspiration and biopsy show lymphocytic invasion. A computed tomography scan identifies affected organs.

Treatment
Systemic chemotherapy includes alkylating agents, usually chlorambucil or cyclophosphamide, and sometimes corticosteroids (prednisone) when autoimmune hemolytic anemia or thrombocytopenia occurs.

When chronic lymphocytic leukemia causes obstruction or organ impairment or enlargement, local radiation therapy can reduce organ size, and splenectomy can help relieve the symptoms. Allopurinol can prevent hyperuricemia, a relatively uncommon finding.

Radiation therapy can help relieve symptoms. It's generally used to treat enlarged lymph nodes, painful bony lesions, or massive splenomegaly.

Nursing diagnoses
• Altered nutrition: Less than body requirements
• Altered protection
• Anticipatory grieving
• Anxiety
• Fatigue
• Fear
• Impaired tissue integrity
• Ineffective family coping
• Ineffective individual coping
• Pain
• Risk for infection
• Risk for injury

Nursing interventions
• Help establish an appropriate rehabilitation program for the patient during remission.
• To control infection, place the patient in a private room and impose reverse isolation if necessary (although the benefits of reverse isolation are controversial). Coordinate care so that the patient doesn't come into contact with staff members who also care for patients with infections or infectious diseases. Screen staff members and visitors for contagious diseases. Don't use an indwelling urinary catheter or give I.M. injections; they provide an avenue for infection. If the patient does develop signs of infection—a temperature over 100° F (37.8° C), chills, or redness or swelling of any body part—report them at once.
• Clean the patient's skin daily with mild soap and water, and provide frequent soaks if ordered. Keep the patient's perianal area clean, apply mild lotions or creams to keep the skin from drying and cracking, and thoroughly clean

the skin before all invasive skin procedures. Change I.V. tubing according to your hospital's policy. Use strict aseptic technique and a metal scalp vein needle (metal butterfly needle) when starting an I.V. line. If the patient is receiving total parenteral nutrition, provide scrupulous subclavian catheter care.
• Watch for bleeding. If it occurs, apply ice compresses and pressure, and elevate the extremity. Don't give the patient aspirin or aspirin-containing drugs, and don't administer rectal suppositories, take a rectal temperature, or perform a digital rectal examination.
• Watch for signs of thrombocytopenia (easy bruising and nosebleeds, bleeding gums, black, tarry stools) and anemia (pale skin, weakness, fatigue, dizziness, palpitations).
• Be alert for adverse effects of treatment, and take measures to prevent or alleviate them. For instance, you can control mouth ulceration by checking often for obvious ulcers and gum swelling and by providing frequent mouth care and saline rinses.
• Check the rectal area daily for induration, swelling, erythema, skin discoloration, and drainage.
• Administer blood component therapy as necessary.
• Establish a trusting relationship to promote communication. Allow the patient and his family to express their anger, anxiety, and depression. Let the family participate in the patient's care as much as possible.
• The patient with chronic lymphocytic leukemia is likely to be elderly and may feel frightened, so take time to listen to his fears. Try to keep his spirits up by concentrating on little things, such as improving his personal appearance, providing a pleasant environment, and asking questions about his family. If possible, provide opportunities for his favorite activities.
• Minimize stress by maintaining a calm, quiet atmosphere that's conducive to rest and relaxation.
• Administer prescribed pain medications as appropriate, and monitor their effectiveness. Provide comfort measures, such as position changes and distractions, to help alleviate the patient's discomfort.
• If the patient doesn't respond to treatment and has reached the terminal phase of the disease, he'll need supportive nursing care. Take steps to manage pain, fever, and bleeding; make sure the patient is comfortable; and provide emotional support for him and his family. If the patient wishes, provide for religious counseling. Discuss the option of home or hospice care.

Patient teaching
• Describe the disease course, diagnostic tests, and treatments and their adverse effects.

• Teach the patient and his family how to recognize signs and symptoms of infection (fever, chills, cough, sore throat).
• Warn the patient about to be discharged to avoid coming into contact with obviously ill people, especially children with common contagious childhood diseases.
• Explain that if the chemotherapy causes weight loss and anorexia, the patient will need to eat and drink high-calorie, high-protein foods and beverages. If he loses his appetite, advise him to eat small, frequent meals. If the chemotherapy and adjunctive prednisone instead cause weight gain, he'll need dietary counseling.
• Instruct the patient to use a soft toothbrush and to avoid hot, spicy foods and commercial mouthwashes to prevent irritating the mouth ulcers that result from chemotherapy.
• Warn the patient to take care to prevent bleeding because his blood may not have enough platelets for proper clotting. Tell him to avoid aspirin and aspirin-containing drugs, and teach him how to recognize drugs that contain aspirin. Teach him the signs of abnormal bleeding (bruising, petechiae) and how to apply pressure and ice to the area to stop such bleeding. Urge him to report excessive bleeding or bruising to his doctor.
• Advise the patient to limit his activities and to plan rest periods during the day.
• Stress the importance of follow-up care, frequent blood tests, and taking all medications exactly as prescribed. Teach the patient the signs of recurrence (swollen lymph nodes in the neck, axilla, and groin; increased abdominal size or discomfort), and tell him to notify his doctor immediately if these signs occur.
• As appropriate, refer the patient and his family to the social service department, home health care agencies, hospices, and support groups such as the American Cancer Society.

KAPOSI'S SARCOMA
Initially, this cancer of the lymphatic cell wall was described as a rare blood vessel sarcoma, occurring mostly in elderly Italian and Jewish men. In recent years, the incidence of Kaposi's sarcoma has risen dramatically along with the incidence of acquired immunodeficiency syndrome (AIDS). Currently, it's the most common AIDS-related cancer.

Characterized by obvious, colorful lesions, Kaposi's sarcoma causes structural and functional damage. When associated with AIDS, it progresses aggressively, involving the lymph nodes, the viscera, and possibly GI structures.

LAUBENSTEIN'S STAGES IN KAPOSI'S SARCOMA

The following staging system was proposed by L.J. Laubenstein for use in evaluating and treating patients who have AIDS and Kaposi's sarcoma:
Stage I — locally indolent cutaneous lesions
Stage II — locally aggressive cutaneous lesions
Stage III — mucocutaneous and lymph node involvement
Stage IV — visceral involvement.

Within each stage, a patient may have different symptoms classified as a stage subtype — A or B, as follows:
• Subtype A — no systemic signs or symptoms
• Subtype B — one or more systemic signs and symptoms, including 10% weight loss, fever of unknown origin that exceeds 100° F (37.8° C) for more than 2 weeks, chills, lethargy, night sweats, anorexia, and diarrhea.

Causes

The exact cause of Kaposi's sarcoma is unknown, but the disease may be related to immunosuppression. Genetic or hereditary predisposition is also suspected.

Complications

Disease progression can cause severe pulmonary involvement, resulting in respiratory distress, and GI involvement, leading to digestive problems.

Assessment findings

The health history typically reveals that the patient has AIDS. If the sarcoma advances beyond the early stages or if a lesion breaks down, the patient may report pain. Usually, however, the lesions remain pain-free unless they impinge on nerves or organs.

On inspection, you may observe several lesions in various shapes, sizes, and colors (ranging from red-brown to dark purple) on the skin, buccal mucosa, hard and soft palates, lips, gums, tongue, tonsils, conjunctiva, and sclera (the most common sites). In advanced disease, the lesions may join, becoming one large plaque. Untreated lesions may appear as large, ulcerative masses. You may notice that the patient has dyspnea, especially if pulmonary involvement occurs.

Palpation and inspection may also disclose edema from lymphatic obstruction.

Auscultation may uncover wheezing and hypoventilation. Respiratory distress usually results from bronchial blockage. The most common extracutaneous sites are the lungs and GI tract (esophagus, oropharynx, and epiglottis).

Diagnostic tests

Usually, the patient will undergo a tissue biopsy to determine the lesion's type and stage. Then, a computed tomography scan may be performed to evaluate metastasis. (See *Laubenstein's stages in Kaposi's sarcoma*.)

Treatment

Radiation therapy, chemotherapy, and drug therapy with biological response modifiers are treatment options. Radiation therapy offers palliation of symptoms, including pain from obstructing lesions in the oral cavity or extremities and edema caused by lymphatic blockage. It may also be used for cosmetic improvement.

Chemotherapy includes combinations of doxorubicin, vinblastine, vincristine, and etoposide (VP-16). The biological response modifier interferon alfa-2b may be prescribed in AIDS-related Kaposi's sarcoma. It reduces the number of skin lesions but is ineffective in advanced disease.

Nursing diagnoses

• Altered nutrition: Less than body requirements
• Anticipatory grieving
• Anxiety
• Body image disturbance
• Fatigue
• Fear
• Impaired gas exchange
• Impaired skin integrity
• Ineffective breathing pattern
• Ineffective family coping
• Ineffective individual coping
• Pain
• Risk for infection

Nursing interventions

• Listen to the patient's fears and concerns and answer his questions honestly. Stay with him during periods of severe stress and anxiety. Allow him to participate in care decisions whenever possible, and encourage him to participate in self-care measures as much as he can.
• Inspect the patient's skin every shift. Look for new lesions and skin breakdown. If the patient has painful lesions, help him into a more comfortable position.
• Administer pain medications. Suggest distractions, and help the patient with relaxation techniques.
• To help the patient adjust to changes in his appearance, urge him to share his feelings. Give encouragement.

• Supply the patient with high-calorie, high-protein meals. If he can't tolerate regular meals, provide him with frequent, smaller meals. Consult with the dietitian, and plan meals around the patient's treatment. If the patient can't take food by mouth, administer I.V. fluids. Give antiemetics and sedatives, as ordered.
• Provide rest periods if the patient tires easily.
• Be alert for adverse effects of radiation therapy or chemotherapy—such as anorexia, nausea, vomiting, and diarrhea—and take steps to prevent or alleviate them.

Patient teaching
• Offer emotional support to help the patient and family cope with the diagnosis and prognosis. Provide opportunities for them to discuss their concerns.
• Reinforce the doctor's explanation of treatments. Be sure the patient understands which adverse effects to expect and how to manage them. For example, during radiation therapy, instruct the patient to keep irradiated skin dry to avoid possible breakdown and subsequent infection.
• Explain infection prevention techniques and, if necessary, demonstrate basic hygiene measures to prevent infection. These measures are especially important if the patient also has AIDS.
• Stress the need for ongoing treatment and care.
• As appropriate, refer the patient to the social service department support groups.

SELECTED REFERENCES

American Joint Committee on Cancer. *Manual for Staging of Cancer,* 4th ed. Philadelphia: J.B. Lippincott Co., 1992.

Beutler, E., et al. *Williams' Hematology,* 5th ed. New York: McGraw-Hill Book Co., 1995.

Friedman, L. "Commentary on Kaposi's Sarcoma as a Sexually Transmissible Infection: An Analysis of Australian AIDS Surveillance Data," *ONS Nursing Scan in Oncology* 3(3):15, May-June 1994.

Illustrated Manual of Nursing Practice, 2nd ed. Springhouse, Pa.: Springhouse Corp., 1994.

Isselbacher, K., et al., eds. *Harrison's Principles of Internal Medicine,* 13th ed. New York: McGraw-Hill Book Co., 1995.

Macdonald, J., et al. *Manual of Oncologic Therapeutics,* 3rd ed. Philadelphia: J.B. Lippincott Co., 1995.

Purandare, L. "Caring for Patients with Chronic Leukaemia," *Nursing Times* 91(31):27-28, August 2, 1995.

Rakel, R.E., ed. *Conn's Current Therapy 1996.* Philadelphia: W.B. Saunders Co., 1996.

5   IMMUNE DISORDERS

INTRODUCTION

The human body protects itself from disease caused by microorganisms through an elaborate network of safeguards — the immune system.

The immune system: Structures and strategies

Also known as the host defense system, the immune system consists of physical and chemical barriers to infection, the inflammatory response, and the immune response.

Physical barriers, such as the skin and mucous membranes, bar invasion by most organisms. Harmful organisms that do penetrate these barriers simultaneously trigger a second line of defense: the inflammatory and immune responses. Both responses call on cells derived from a hematopoietic stem cell in the bone marrow.

The inflammatory response mobilizes polymorphonuclear leukocytes, basophils, mast cells, and platelets. The immune response primarily involves forces of T lymphocytes (popularly called T cells) and B lymphocytes (often called B cells), macrophages, and macrophage-like cells and their products. Some of these cells circulate continuously, whereas others stand guard in the tissues and organs of the immune system, including the thymus, lymph nodes, Peyer's patches of the intestines, spleen, and tonsils.

The thymus contributes to the maturation of T cells (the blood cells associated with *cell-mediated immunity*). Here, these cells are "educated" to differentiate self from nonself. In contrast, the bone marrow serves as the site of B lymphocyte maturation. The B cells provide *humoral immunity*. The key humoral effector mechanism is the complement cascade. The lymph nodes, spleen, and intestinal lymphoid tissue then help to destroy and remove any antigens circulating in the blood and lymph.

Antigens

To understand the immune response, you need to know about antigens and the concepts of specificity and memory. An antigen is any substance that can induce an immune response. T and B cells have specific receptors that respond to specific antigen molecular shapes (epitopes). In B cells, this receptor is an immunoglobulin (Ig) or antibody molecule known as IgD or IgM. This molecule also is called a surface immunoglobulin. The T-cell antigen receptor recognizes an antigen only in association with specific cell surface antigen determinants called the major histocompatibility complex (MHC). (See *Major histocompatibility complex,* page 392.) Slightly different antigen receptors can recognize many distinct antigens coded for distinct, variable (V)-region genes.

Groups, or clones, of lymphocytes exist with identical receptors for a specific antigen. The lymphocytic clones rapidly proliferate after exposure to a specific antigen. Some lymphocytes, however, further differentiate, and others become memory cells, allowing a faster response — the memory or *anamnestic response* — to a subsequent challenge by the antigen.

Many factors influence antigenicity (the ability to produce an immune response). Among them are the physical and chemical characteristics of the antigen, its relative foreignness, and a person's genetic makeup. Most antigens are large molecules, such as proteins or polysaccharides. (Smaller molecules, such as drugs, that aren't antigenic by themselves are known as haptens. These haptens can bind with larger molecules, or carriers, and become antigenic or immunogenic.)

The relative foreignness of the antigen influences the intensity of the immune response. For example, little or no immune response may follow transfusion of serum proteins between humans; however, a vigorous immune response (serum sickness) commonly follows transfusion of horse serum proteins to a human.

Genetic makeup may also determine why some people respond to certain antigens, whereas others do not. The genes responsible for this phenomenon — the immune response genes — are located within the MHC.

T cells

T cells and macrophages are the chief participants in cell-mediated immunity. Immature T cells derive from the bone marrow and migrate to the thymus, where they mature in a process that appears linked to products of the MHC: human leukocyte antigen (HLA) genes.

Mature T cells can distinguish self from nonself. T cells acquire certain surface molecules, or markers. These markers combined with the T-cell antigen receptor promote a particular activation of each type of T cell. They can become CD4 T cells with helper-cell potential or CD8 T cells with cytotoxic potential.

T-cell activation requires presentation of antigen as a specific HLA. Helper T cells require class II HLA; cytotoxic T cells require class I HLA. T-cell activation also involves interleukin-1, produced by macrophages, and interleukin-2, produced by T cells. (Interleukins are growth factors that stimulate the production of other immune cells.)

B cells

B cells and their product, immunoglobulins, are responsible for humoral immunity. The binding of a soluble antigen with B-cell antigen receptors initiates the humoral

MAJOR HISTOCOMPATIBILITY COMPLEX

Playing a pivotal role in the immune response is the major histocompatibility complex (MHC), a cluster of genes located on human chromosome 6. Also known as human leukocyte antigen (HLA) genes, these structures are inherited in an autosomal codominant manner.

Each person receives a set of MHC genes (haplotype) from each parent. And both gene sets are expressed on the person's cells. These genes play an essential role in the recognition of self versus nonself, and by coding for cell surface proteins, they participate in the interaction of immunologically active cells.

Classifications

HLAs are grouped into three classes. *Class I antigens* appear on nearly all body cells. They include HLA-A, HLA-B, and HLA-C. During tissue graft rejection, they are the chief antigens recognized by the host. When cytotoxic T cells lyse a virally infected antigen, they recognize it as a Class I antigen.

Class II antigens only appear on B cells, macrophages, and activated T cells. They include HLA-D and HLA-DR. Class II antigens promote efficient collaboration between immunocompetent cells. To become activated, T cells must be presented with a Class II antigen. Because Class II antigens determine whether a person responds to a particular antigen, they're also known as immune response genes.

Class III antigens include certain complement proteins (C2, C4, and factor B).

immune response. The activated B cells differentiate into plasma cells that secrete immunoglobulins—or antibodies. This response is regulated by T cells and their products—for example, B-cell growth factor and B-cell differentiating factor.

The immunoglobulin molecules secreted by plasma cells have four chains—two heavy and two light. Any B-cell clone has one antigen specificity determined by the V regions of its light and heavy chains. However, the clone can change the class of immunoglobulin that it makes by altering the association between its V-region genes and its heavy-chain, constant (C)-region genes (a process known as isotype switching). For example, a B-cell clone genetically directed to recognize tetanus toxoid will first make an IgM antibody against tetanus toxoid and later an IgG or other antibody against the toxoid.

Natural killer cells

A discrete population of large lymphocytes, natural killer (NK) cells resemble T cells. NK cells recognize surface changes on body cells infected with a virus; they then bind to and usually kill the infected cells.

Macrophages: Key antigen-presenting cells

Important cells of the reticuloendothelial system, macrophages influence both the inflammatory and immune responses. Macrophage precursors (monocytes) circulate in the blood. When they collect in various tissues and organs, such as the liver, spleen, lungs, and connective tissue, they develop into macrophages with varying characteristics, depending on the receptor tissue. Unlike B and T cells, macrophages lack surface receptors for specific antigens. Instead, they have receptors for the C region of the heavy chain (fragment, crystallizable [Fc] region) of immunoglobulin, for fragments of the third component of complement (C3), and for other factors, such as carbohydrate molecules.

A primary function of macrophages is the presentation of an antigen to T cells. Macrophages ingest and process an antigen and then deposit it on their own surfaces with HLA. T cells become activated when they recognize this complex. Macrophages also function in the inflammatory response by producing interleukin-1, which generates fever, and by synthesizing complement proteins and other mediators, which produce phagocytic, microbicidal, and tumoricidal effects.

Complement system

The chief humoral effector of the inflammatory response, the complement system consists of more than 20 serum proteins. When activated, these proteins interact in a cascadelike process that has profound biological effects. Complement activation occurs along one of two pathways. In the classical pathway, an immunoglobulin (IgM or IgG) and an antigen bind to form antigen-antibody complexes that activate the first complement component (C1). This, in turn, activates C4, C2, and C3. In the alternate pathway, activating surfaces, such as bacterial membranes, directly amplify spontaneous cleavage of C3. Once C3 is activated in either pathway, activation of the terminal components—C5 to C9—follows.

The major biological effects of complement activation include phagocyte attraction (chemotaxis) and activation, histamine release, viral neutralization, promotion of phagocytosis by opsonization, and lysis of cells and bacteria. Other mediators of inflammation derived from the kinin and coagulation pathways interact with the complement system.

Polymorphonuclear leukocytes

Besides macrophages and complement, other key participants in the inflammatory response are the polymorphonuclear leukocytes—neutrophils, eosinophils, and basophils. Neutrophils, the most numerous of these cells, derive from bone marrow and proliferate dramatically in response to infection and inflammation. Highly mobile cells, neutrophils are attracted to areas of inflammation; in fact, they're the primary constituent of pus. Neutrophils have surface receptors for immunoglobulins and complement fragments. And they avidly ingest opsonized particles, such as bacteria. Ingested organisms are then promptly killed by toxic oxygen metabolites and enzymes, such as lysozymes. The neutrophils are so effective that they may damage host tissues even as they act to protect them by killing invading organisms.

Also derived from bone marrow, eosinophils multiply in allergic disorders and parasitic infestations. Although their phagocytic function isn't clearly understood, evidence suggests that they participate in host defense against parasites. Their products may also dampen the inflammatory response in allergic disorders.

Two other cells that function in allergic disorders are basophils and mast cells. Basophils circulate in peripheral blood, whereas mast cells accumulate in connective tissue, particularly in the lungs, intestines, and skin. Both cells have surface receptors for IgE. When crosslinked by an IgE-antigen complex, they release substances (mediators) characteristic of the allergic response.

Immune disorders

For various reasons, the complex processes involved in the host defense and immune response may malfunction. When the body's defenses are exaggerated, misdirected, or absent or depressed, the result may be a hypersensitivity, autoimmune, or immunodeficiency disorder, respectively.

Hypersensitivity disorders

An exaggerated or inappropriate immune response may lead to various hypersensitivity disorders. Such disorders are classified as Type I through Type IV, although some overlap exists. (See *Classifying hypersensitivity reactions*, pages 386 and 387.)
• *Type I hypersensitivity (allergic disorders)*. In some people, certain antigens (allergens) induce B-cell production of IgE, which binds to the Fc receptors on mast cell surfaces. When these cells are reexposed to the same antigen, the antigen binds with the surface IgE, cross-links the Fc receptors, and causes mast cell degranulation

with release of various mediators. (Degranulation may also be triggered by complement-derived anaphylatoxins—C3a and C5a—or by certain drugs, such as morphine.) Some of these mediators are preformed, whereas others are synthesized with mast cell activation. Preformed mediators include heparin, histamine, proteolytic and other enzymes, and chemotactic factors for eosinophils and neutrophils. Newly synthesized mediators include prostaglandins and leukotrienes.

These mediators cause vasodilation, smooth-muscle contraction, bronchospasm, increased vascular permeability, edema, mucus secretion, and cellular infiltration by eosinophils and neutrophils. Classic associated signs and symptoms include hypotension, wheezing, swelling, urticaria, and rhinorrhea.

Examples of Type I hypersensitivity disorders are anaphylaxis, hay fever (allergic rhinitis) and, in some cases, asthma.
• *Type II hypersensitivity (antibody-dependent cytotoxicity)*. In this form of hypersensitivity, antibody is directed against cell surface antigens. (Alternately, though, antibody may be directed against small molecules adsorbed to cells or against cell surface receptors, rather than against cell constituents themselves.) Type II hypersensitivity then causes tissue damage through several mechanisms. Antigen-antibody binding activates complement, which ultimately disrupts cellular membranes. Another mechanism is mediated by various phagocytic cells with receptors for immunoglobulin (Fc region) and complement fragments.

In a process called phagocytosis, these cells envelop and destroy opsonized targets, such as red blood cells, leukocytes, and platelets. Antibodies to these cells may be visualized by immunofluorescence. Cytotoxic T cells and NK cells contribute to tissue damage in Type II hypersensitivity.

Examples of Type II hypersensitivity include transfusion reactions and Goodpasture's syndrome.
• *Type III hypersensitivity (immune complex disease)*. In this disorder, excessive circulating antigen results in the deposition of immune complexes in tissue—most commonly in the kidneys, joints, skin, and blood vessels. (Normally, immune complexes are effectively cleared by the reticuloendothelial system.) These deposited immune complexes activate the complement cascade, resulting in local inflammation. They also trigger platelet release of vasoactive amines that increase vascular permeability, augmenting deposition of immune complexes in vessel walls.

Type III hypersensitivity may be associated with infections, such as hepatitis B and bacterial endocarditis;
(Text continues on page 396.)

CLASSIFYING HYPERSENSITIVITY REACTIONS

In 1962, British immunologists P.G.H. Gell and R.R.A. Coombs classified four ways in which immune system activity causes tissue damage. With some modifications, the system remains applicable today.

Type I

In Type I hypersensitivity, when IgE antibodies bind antigens to the mast cell surface, allergy mediators are released, causing vasodilation, increased capillary permeability, smooth-muscle contraction, and eosinophilia.

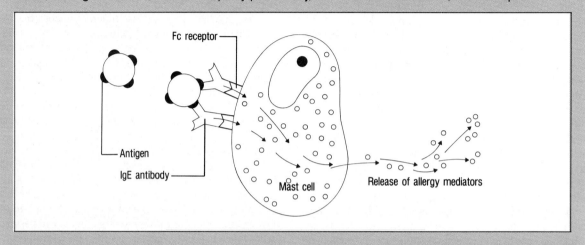

Type II

In Type II hypersensitivity, binding of IgG or IgM antibodies to cellular or exogenous antigens activates the complement cascade, resulting in phagocytosis or cytolysis.

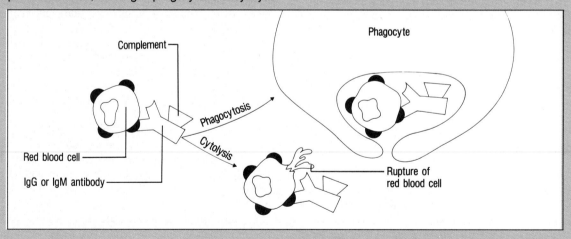

CLASSIFYING HYPERSENSITIVITY REACTIONS *(continued)*

Type III
In Type III hypersensitivity, activation of complement by immune complexes causes infiltration of polymorphonuclear leukocytes and release of lysosomal enzymes and permeability factors. This produces an inflammatory reaction.

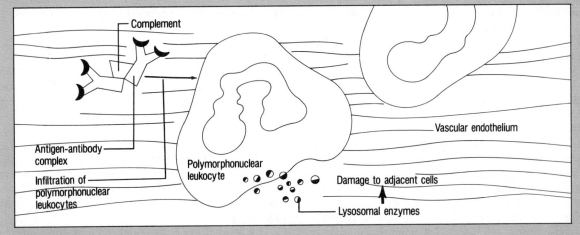

Type IV
In Type IV hypersensitivity, an antigen-presenting cell presents an antigen to T cells in association with the major histocompatibility complex (MHC). The sensitized T cells release lymphokines, which stimulate macrophages. Then lysozymes are released, and surrounding tissue sustains damage.

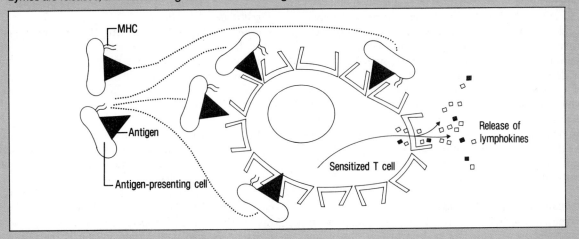

malignant diseases, in which a serum sickness–like syndrome may occur; and autoimmune disorders, such as systemic lupus erythematosus (SLE). This type of hypersensitivity reaction may also follow drug or serum therapy.

• *Type IV hypersensitivity (delayed hypersensitivity)*. In this form of hypersensitivity, the macrophages process the antigens and present the result to the T cells. The sensitized T cells then release lymphokines, which recruit and activate other lymphocytes, monocytes, macrophages, and polymorphonuclear leukocytes. The coagulation, kinin, and complement pathways contribute to tissue damage in this type of reaction.

Examples of Type IV hypersensitivity include tuberculin reactions and contact hypersensitivity.

Autoimmune disorders
Characterized by a misdirected immune response, autoimmunity results when the immune system becomes self-destructive. What causes this abnormal response puzzles researchers. Although they do know that recognition of self through the MHC is a key to the effective immune response, they do not know how to prevent a response against self. Nor do they know which cells are primarily responsible. Autoimmunity may result from a combination of factors.

Characteristic of many autoimmune disorders is B-cell hyperactivity, which is marked by proliferation of B cells and autoantibodies and by hypergammaglobulinemia. T-cell abnormalities—especially suppressor T-cell deficiency—are also common. Viruses may contribute to autoimmunity by causing proliferation (Epstein-Barr virus) or destruction (human immunodeficiency virus [HIV]) of lymphocytes; so may macrophage abnormalities, which interfere with antigen processing and presentation. Hormonal and genetic factors strongly influence the incidence of autoimmune disorders; for example, SLE predominantly affects women of childbearing age, and certain HLA haplotypes are associated with increased risk of specific autoimmune disorders.

Immunodeficiency disorders
Increased susceptibility to infection is a hallmark of immunodeficiency. Caused by a depressed or absent immune response, the disorder may be classified as primary or secondary. Primary immunodeficiency denotes a defect involving T cells, B cells, or lymphoid tissues, such as the thymus. Secondary immunodeficiency results from an underlying disease or factor that depresses or blocks the immune response.

Iatrogenic immunodeficiency may result from drug treatments or from treatments to prevent the body from rejecting a donor organ. (See *Understanding iatrogenic immunodeficiency.*)

Assessing the immune system
Performing an accurate assessment of the immune system can challenge your skills. Immune disorders may cause vague symptoms, which initially seem related to other body systems.

Patient history
Begin by reviewing the patient's chief complaint. With an immune disorder, he may complain of vague symptoms, such as lack of energy, light-headedness, frequent infections or bruising, and slow wound healing.

Ask about changes in the patient's overall health because the immune system affects all body functions. Has he developed unexplained rashes, visual disturbances, fever, or changes in elimination patterns? If the patient is a woman, find out if she has noted changes in her menstrual pattern—commonly an early sign of platelet dysfunction.

Ask about the patient's social and work environments to detect exposure to chemicals or pathogens that may affect immune function. Finally, investigate the family history for immune disorders or cancer.

Physical examination
• *Inspection.* Begin by observing the patient's appearance. Does he show signs of acute illness? Does he grimace with pain or seem extremely tired? Does he show signs of chronic illness, such as emaciation or pronounced listlessness? Does he look older than his stated age, possibly from malnutrition related to chronic illness?

Watch the patient's movements, posture, and gait for signs that may indicate joint, spinal, and neurologic changes caused by an immune disorder. Find out whether the patient has pain when he moves.

Inspect the patient's skin. Note any pallor, cyanosis, or jaundice. Note the character and distribution of any rashes. Does the rash appear red and raised, as in urticaria associated with an allergy? Or is the rash distributed across the nose like the butterfly rash associated with SLE? Does the rash itch?

Check the nose for pale, boggy turbinates (associated with chronic allergy) or the ulcerated mucous membranes associated with SLE. Look inside the patient's mouth. White patches may indicate candidiasis associated with immunosuppression. Lacy white plaques on

UNDERSTANDING IATROGENIC IMMUNODEFICIENCY

Although immunodeficiency or immunosuppression may occur as a complication of chemotherapy or other treatment, it may be the therapeutic goal itself. For instance, in an autoimmune disorder such as SLE, treatment aims to suppress immune-mediated tissue damage. Immunosuppression is also desirable to prevent a rejection reaction — after organ transplantation, for example.

Iatrogenic immunodeficiency may be induced by drugs, radiation therapy, or surgery.

Drug-induced immunodeficiency

Immunosuppressants include cytotoxic drugs and corticosteroids. Cytotoxic drugs kill immunocompetent cells while they're replicating. However, most cytotoxic drugs aren't selective so they interfere with all rapidly proliferating cells, reducing lymphocytes and phagocytes as well. Besides depleting lymphocyte populations, cytotoxic drugs interfere with lymphocyte synthesis and the release of immunoglobulins and lymphokines.

Cyclophosphamide, a potent and frequently used immunosuppressant, initially depletes B cells, thereby suppressing humoral immunity. Long-term cyclophosphamide therapy also depletes T cells, suppressing cell-mediated immunity as well. Cyclophosphamide may be given for SLE, Wegener's granulomatosis and other systemic vasculitides, and certain autoimmune disorders.

Other cytotoxic drugs used for immunosuppression are *azathioprine* (after kidney transplantation) and *methotrexate* (in rheumatoid arthritis, psoriasis, mycosis fungoides, and cancer).

Corticosteroids possess potent anti-inflammatory and immunosuppressive effects. As a result, they're widely used to treat immune-mediated disorders. They act to stabilize the vascular membrane and block tissue infiltration by neutrophils and monocytes. This inhibits inflammation. Corticosteroids also "kidnap" T cells in the bone marrow, causing lymphopenia. However, because these drugs aren't cytotoxic, lymphocyte concentrations can quickly return to normal levels 24 hours after therapy stops.

Corticosteroids also appear to inhibit immunoglobulin synthesis and to interfere with the binding of immunoglobulin to antigen or to cells with Fc receptors. The most commonly used oral corticosteroid is *prednisone.* Other corticosteroids used for immunosuppression include *hydrocortisone, methylprednisolone,* and *dexamethasone.*

Some relatively new immunosuppressants, such as *cyclosporine* and *antithymocyte globulin (ATG),* selectively suppress the proliferation and development of helper T cells. This results in depressed cell-mediated immunity. Typical uses for cyclosporine include prevention of kidney, liver, and heart transplant rejection. Its use in other disorders is investigational.

ATG also has been used effectively to prevent cell-mediated rejection of tissue grafts and transplants.

Radiation-induced immunodeficiency

Because radioactive energy kills proliferating and intermitotic cells, including most lymphocytes, radiation therapy may induce profound lymphopenia, resulting in immunosuppression. Irradiation of all major lymph node areas — a procedure known as total nodal irradiation — is used to treat certain disorders, such as Hodgkin's disease. Its effectiveness in treating severe rheumatoid arthritis and lupus nephritis and in preventing kidney transplant rejection is investigational.

Surgery-induced immunodeficiency

Splenectomy may be performed to manage various disorders, including splenic injury or trauma, tumor, Hodgkin's disease, hairy-cell leukemia, Felty's syndrome, Gaucher's disease, idiopathic thrombocytopenic purpura, hereditary spherocytosis and hereditary elliptocytosis, thalassemia major, and chronic lymphocytic leukemia.

---

the buccal mucosa may be the hairy leukoplakia associated with acquired immunodeficiency syndrome (AIDS).

Observe the eyes for redness and infection. Do the eyes tear sufficiently, or does the patient complain of burning, dry eyes? Assess the fundus with an ophthalmoscope. Do you see areas that suggest hemorrhage, aneurysm, or infiltration? These may indicate vasculitis.

Evaluate skin integrity. Does the skin appear inflamed or infected? Particularly, check for infection in areas of recent invasive procedures (such as venipunctures).

Inspect the arms, hands, legs, and feet for signs of peripheral vascular insufficiency associated with vasculitis, systemic sclerosis, and SLE. Observe for blanching and cyanosis, pallor, and reddening.

Assess the patient's level of consciousness (LOC) and mental status. Altered blood flow and inflammation of the central nervous system (CNS) may affect LOC. CNS changes may affect patients with SLE or AIDS.

Assess other body systems, as appropriate, to determine immune-related effects.

• *Palpation and percussion.* Take the patient's vital signs. Are they within normal limits and stable? Fever, with or without chills, may signal infection. Assess pulse and respiratory rates and depth. Percussion that discloses lobar dullness may point to lung consolidation associated with pneumonia. Measure the patient's blood pressure while he lies down, sits, and stands.

Feel the lymph nodes, noting any enlargement. This may indicate inflammation. Tender nodes may indicate acute infection. Generalized lymphadenopathy (involving three or more node groups) can indicate an autoimmune disorder, such as SLE, or an infectious or neoplastic disorder.

Palpate and percuss various organs. Be alert for tenderness associated with enlargement, inflammation, or masses. If findings suggest splenic enlargement, suspect an infection, typical in patients with immunodeficiency.

Assess musculoskeletal integrity and range of motion, particularly in the hands, wrists, and knees. Palpate the joints to detect swelling, tenderness, and pain. Autoimmune disorders, such as SLE and rheumatoid arthritis, limit range of motion and cause joint enlargement.

• *Auscultation.* To detect abnormal breath sounds, auscultate the lungs. Pneumonia associated with immunodeficiency may cause crackles and decreased breath sounds.

Identify heart sounds. Listen for abnormal rate, rhythm, and sounds. Particularly note pericardial friction rub, which occurs in about 50% of SLE patients.

Listen for bowel sounds in all abdominal quadrants. Increased sounds may occur in autoimmune disorders that cause diarrhea. Decreased sounds may occur in disorders that cause constipation.

Diagnostic tests
• *General cellular and humoral studies.* These include such tests as T- and B-cell assays to help diagnose primary and secondary immunodeficiencies and complement assays to help detect immunomediated disease.
• *Protein electrophoresis.* By measuring various proteins in serum or urine, this test helps detect diseases associated with excess or deficient gamma globulin.
• *Immunoelectrophoresis.* This test aims to differentiate monoclonal from polyclonal increases in immunoglobulins, to identify IgA, IgG, and IgM, and to help identify abnormal immunoglobulins and an allergic response.
• *Immunofixation electrophoresis.* This electrophoresis provides results more rapidly and shows higher resolution of low levels of monoclonal immunoglobulin chains.
• *Erythrocyte sedimentation rate.* A sensitive but nonspecific indicator of inflammatory disorders, this test helps detect rheumatoid arthritis and systemic sclerosis.

• *Delayed hypersensitivity skin tests.* Patch and scratch allergy tests and intradermal skin tests help evaluate cell-mediated immunity. Viral, bacterial, and fungal tests help diagnose specific infections, such as candidiasis.
• Another disorder-specific test is the *enzyme-linked immunosorbent assay* (ELISA). Test results can show exposure to HIV, to rheumatoid factor (to confirm rheumatoid arthritis), and to lupus erythematosus cell (to confirm SLE).

ALLERGIC DISORDERS

Characterized by a harmful reaction to extrinsic materials or allergens, allergic disorders include allergic rhinitis, atopic dermatitis, anaphylaxis, urticaria and angioedema, and blood transfusion reactions.

ALLERGIC RHINITIS
Inhaled, airborne allergens may trigger an immune response in the upper airway in susceptible people. Depending on the allergen, the resulting rhinitis and conjunctivitis may occur seasonally (hay fever) or year-round (perennial allergic rhinitis). The term "hay fever" is a misnomer because hay doesn't cause allergic rhinitis nor is fever associated with it. Nonetheless, by affecting more than 20 million Americans, allergic rhinitis ranks as the most common atopic allergic reaction. Although the disorder can affect anyone at any age, it's most prevalent in young children and adolescents.

Causes
Hay fever is an IgE-mediated Type I hypersensitivity response to an environmental antigen (allergen) in a genetically susceptible person. It's usually induced by airborne pollens: in spring by tree pollens (oak, elm, maple, alder, birch, cottonwood); in summer by grass and weed pollens (fescue, bluegrass, English plantain, sheep sorrel); and in the fall by weed pollens (ragweed). Occasionally, in summer and fall, it's induced by mold spores.

In perennial allergic rhinitis, inhaled allergens provoke antigen responses that produce signs and symptoms year-round. Major perennial allergens and irritants include house dust and dust mites that feed on the dust, feathers (in pillows and quilts), molds, tobacco smoke, processed materials or industrial chemicals, and animal danders. In many patients, the offending allergens can't be identified. Seasonal pollen allergy may exacerbate symptoms of perennial rhinitis.

Complications
Swelling of the turbinates and mucous membranes may trigger secondary sinus and middle ear infections, especially in perennial allergic rhinitis. Nasal polyps, which may result from edema and infection, may increase nasal obstruction.

Assessment findings
In seasonal allergic rhinitis, the patient typically complains of paroxysmal sneezing, profuse watery rhinorrhea, nasal obstruction or congestion, pruritus of the nose and eyes, and headache or sinus pain. Some patients also complain of an itchy throat, malaise, and fever. Inspection may reveal pale, cyanotic, edematous nasal mucosa; red and edematous eyelids and conjunctivae; and excessive lacrimation.

In perennial allergic rhinitis, the patient seldom reports conjunctivitis and other extranasal effects. He commonly complains of chronic and extensive nasal obstruction or stuffiness, which can obstruct the eustachian tube, particularly in children. Inspection may reveal nasal polyps.

In both conditions, dark circles may appear under the patient's eyes (allergic shiners), a result of venous congestion in the maxillary sinuses. The severity of signs and symptoms may vary from year to year.

To distinguish between allergic rhinitis and other disorders of the nasal mucosa, remember these differences:
• In chronic vasomotor rhinitis, signs and symptoms don't affect the eyes, rhinorrhea is mucoid, and seasonal variation is absent.
• In infectious rhinitis (the common cold), the nasal mucosa appears beet red; nasal secretions contain polymorphonuclear (not eosinophilic) exudate; and signs and symptoms include fever and sore throat.
• In rhinitis medicamentosa, which results from excessive use of nasal sprays or drops, nasal drainage and mucosal redness and swelling subside when medication is discontinued.

Diagnostic tests
Microscopic examination of sputum and nasal secretions shows a high number of eosinophils. IgE levels may be normal or elevated. The patient's history and skin test results (including documented responses to various environmental stimuli) can help pinpoint the responsible allergens.

In children, the differential diagnosis should rule out a foreign body (such as a bean or a pea) lodged in the nose.

Treatment
Appropriate therapy aims to control signs and symptoms by eliminating the environmental antigen, if possible, and by drug therapy and immunotherapy in ongoing allergic rhinitis.

Antihistamines effectively block histamine effects (such as a runny nose and watery eyes) but commonly produce unpleasant effects, such as sedation, dry mouth, nausea, dizziness, blurred vision, and nervousness. Nonsedating antihistamines, such as terfenadine and astemizole, produce fewer annoying effects and are less likely to cause drowsiness.

Taken as prescribed, topical intranasal corticosteroids may reduce local inflammation with minimal systemic adverse effects. Commonly used drugs are flunisolide and beclomethasone. Usually, these drugs aren't effective for acute exacerbations; nasal decongestants and oral antihistamines may be used instead. Cromolyn sodium may help prevent allergic rhinitis. However, this drug may take up to 4 weeks to produce a satisfactory effect and must be taken regularly during allergy season. Drug therapy for seasonal allergies requires particularly close dosage regulation.

Long-term management includes immunotherapy or desensitization with injections of allergen extracts administered preseasonally, coseasonally, or perennially.

Nursing diagnoses
• Altered health maintenance
• Impaired skin integrity
• Knowledge deficit
• Pain

Nursing interventions
• Implement measures to relieve signs and symptoms and increase the patient's comfort.
• Increase the patient's fluid intake to loosen secretions.
• Monitor the patient's compliance with the prescribed drug regimen. Note any changes in control of signs and symptoms or any indications of drug misuse.
• Before desensitization injections, assess the patient's current symptoms. After giving the injection, observe him for 30 minutes to detect adverse reactions, including anaphylaxis and severe localized erythema. Be sure epinephrine and emergency resuscitation equipment are ready to use. Instruct him to call the doctor if he experiences a delayed reaction.

Patient teaching

• Instruct the patient to reduce environmental exposure to airborne allergens by sleeping with the windows closed; avoiding the countryside during pollination season; using air conditioning, if possible, to filter allergens and to minimize humidity and dust; keeping pets outside; and removing dust-collecting items, such as wool blankets, deep-pile carpets, and heavy draperies, from the home.

• Tell him to apply a skin protectant on and below the nose to help prevent excoriation from constant nose blowing.

• In severe and resistant allergic rhinitis, discuss possible life-style changes, such as relocation to a pollen-free area either seasonally or year-round.

ATOPIC DERMATITIS

Marked by superficial skin inflammation and intense itching, this chronic skin disorder may appear at any age. Typically, atopic dermatitis begins during infancy or early childhood. It may then subside spontaneously, followed by exacerbations in late childhood, adolescence, or early adulthood. Atopic dermatitis affects less than 1% of the population.

Causes

Several theories attempt to explain the causes of atopic dermatitis. One theory suggests an underlying metabolically or biochemically induced skin disorder, genetically linked to elevated serum IgE levels and possibly causing IgE-dependent recognition of otherwise nontoxic substances. Another theory suggests defective T-cell function.

Atopic dermatitis is exacerbated by certain irritants, infections (commonly *Staphylococcus aureus*), and some allergens. The disorder has not been definitely linked to exposure to inhalant allergens, such as house dust and animal dander. However, exposure to food allergens, such as soybeans, fish, or nuts, may coincide with flare-ups.

Complications

Excoriation from scratching may lead to a bacterial skin infection.

Assessment findings

The patient with atopic dermatitis typically complains of intense pruritus. On inspection, the skin appears erythematous. You also may see weeping lesions caused by scratching. The lesions usually appear in areas of flexion and extension, such as the neck, antecubital fossa, popliteal folds, and behind the ears. They may appear scaly and lichenified. The patient's history may disclose unusually severe viral infections, bacterial and fungal skin infections, ocular complications, and allergic contact dermatitis.

Depending on the extent and appearance of the skin lesions, the patient may show signs of social withdrawal. This may result from his perception of his appearance and others' response to it, leaving him less willing to associate with others.

Diagnostic tests

During an episode of atopic dermatitis, serum analysis may reveal eosinophilia and elevated IgE levels. Additional allergy testing may identify the causative allergen.

Treatment

Drug therapy typically consists of corticosteroids and antipruritics. Active dermatitis usually responds to topical corticosteroids, such as fluocinolone acetonide and flurandrenolide. These drugs should be applied immediately after bathing for optimal skin penetration. Oral antihistamines, especially hydroxyzine, and phenothiazine derivatives, such as methdilazine and trimeprazine, are commonly recommended to control itching. A bedtime dose of antihistamines may reduce involuntary scratching during sleep. If secondary infection develops, antibiotics may be prescribed.

Nursing diagnoses

• Body image disturbance
• Impaired skin integrity
• Impaired social interaction
• Knowledge deficit
• Risk for infection

Nursing interventions

• Provide meticulous skin care. Because dry skin aggravates itching, frequently apply nonirritating, water-based topical lubricants, especially after bathing or showering. Moisturizing lotions may be better tolerated than creams or ointments because the creams and ointments tend to seal in body heat, which may aggravate the dermatitis.
• Inspect the skin for signs of secondary infection in areas that have been scratched.
• Reduce or minimize environmental exposure to offending allergens and irritants, such as wools and harsh detergent residues. If the offending substance remains unknown, gradually eliminate suspected substances.

Keep a record showing whether symptoms subside or continue.
• Monitor the patient's compliance with drug therapy.

Patient teaching
• Emphasize the importance of performing a regular personal hygiene regimen, using only water. Or suggest bathing with hypoallergenic soap.
• Advise the patient to use bath soap and laundry detergents sparingly. Tell him to avoid additives, such as bleach and fabric softeners. Suggest rinsing clothes twice during the laundering to remove the maximum amount of detergent from the clothing.
• Identify reportable signs of secondary infection.
• If the patient modifies his diet to exclude food allergens, teach him how to monitor his nutritional status. Provide a list of foods to replace nutrients lost by avoiding the offending foods.
• Demonstrate how to apply topical corticosteroids. Then review the patient's application schedule.
• If the patient's disorder poses a severe strain on family and social relationships, refer him for appropriate counseling. Offer encouragement and support as the patient learns to cope.

ANAPHYLAXIS
A dramatic, acute atopic reaction, anaphylaxis is marked by the sudden onset of rapidly progressive urticaria and respiratory distress. A severe reaction may initiate vascular collapse, leading to systemic shock and, possibly, death.

Causes
Anaphylactic reactions result from systemic exposure to sensitizing drugs or other specific antigens. Such substances may be serums (usually horse serum), vaccines, allergen extracts (such as pollen), enzymes (L-asparaginase), hormones, penicillin and other antibiotics, sulfonamides, local anesthetics, salicylates, polysaccharides (such as iron dextran), diagnostic chemicals (sodium dehydrocholate, radiographic contrast media), foods (legumes, nuts, berries, seafood, egg albumin) and sulfite-containing food additives, insect venom (honeybees, wasps, hornets, yellow jackets, fire ants, and certain spiders) and, rarely, a ruptured hydatid cyst.

The most common anaphylaxis-causing antigen is penicillin. This drug induces a reaction in 1 to 4 of every 10,000 patients treated with it. Penicillin is most likely to induce anaphylaxis after parenteral administration or prolonged therapy.

After initial exposure to an antigen, the immune system responds by producing specific immunoglobulin (Ig) antibodies in the lymph nodes. Helper T cells enhance the process. These antibodies (IgE) then bind to membrane receptors located on mast cells (found throughout connective tissue) and basophils.

Once the body reencounters the antigen, the IgE antibodies, or cross-linked IgE receptors, recognize the antigen as foreign. This activates a series of cellular reactions. (See *What happens in anaphylaxis*, pages 402 and 403.)

Complications
Untreated anaphylaxis causes respiratory obstruction, systemic vascular collapse, and death—in minutes to hours after the first symptoms (although a delayed or persistent reaction may occur for up to 24 hours).

Assessment findings
The patient, a relative, or another responsible person will report the patient's exposure to an antigen. Immediately after exposure, the patient may complain of a feeling of impending doom or fright, weakness, sweating, sneezing, dyspnea, nasal pruritus, and urticaria. He may impress you as extremely anxious. Keep in mind that the sooner signs and symptoms begin after exposure to the antigen, the more severe the anaphylaxis.

On inspection, the patient's skin may display well-circumscribed, discrete cutaneous wheals with erythematous, raised serpiginous borders, and blanched centers. They may coalesce to form giant hives.

Angioedema may cause the patient to complain of a "lump" in his throat, or you may hear hoarseness or stridor. Wheezing, dyspnea, and complaints of chest tightness suggest bronchial obstruction. These are early signs of impending, potentially fatal respiratory failure.

Other effects may follow rapidly. The patient may report GI and genitourinary effects, including severe stomach cramps, nausea, diarrhea, and urinary urgency and incontinence. Neurologic effects may include dizziness, drowsiness, headache, restlessness, and seizures. Cardiovascular effects include hypotension, shock and, sometimes, cardiac arrhythmias, which, if untreated, may precipitate vascular collapse.

Diagnostic tests
No tests are required to identify anaphylaxis. The patient's history and signs and symptoms establish the diagnosis. If signs and symptoms occur without a known allergic stimulus, other possible causes of shock, such as

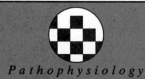

Pathophysiology

WHAT HAPPENS IN ANAPHYLAXIS

An anaphylactic reaction requires previous sensitization or exposure to the specific antigen. The following illustrates the anaphylactic process.

1. Response to the antigen

IgM and IgG recognize the antigen as a foreign substance and attach themselves to it.

The antigen destruction process (known as the complement cascade) begins but can't finish—either because of insufficient amounts of the protein catalyst A or because the antigen inhibits certain complement enzymes. The patient has no signs and symptoms at this stage.

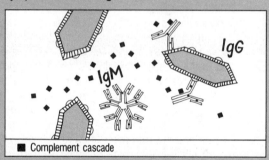

■ Complement cascade

2. Released chemical mediators

The antigen's continued presence activates IgE (attached to basophils). The activated IgE promotes the release of mediators, including histamine, serotonin, and slow-reacting substance of anaphylaxis (SRS-A).

The sudden release of histamine causes vasodilation and increases capillary permeability. The patient begins to have signs and symptoms, including sudden nasal congestion; itchy, watery eyes; flushing; sweating; weakness; and anxiety.

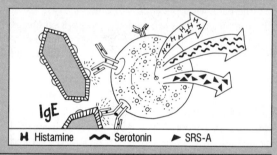

H Histamine   ∿ Serotonin   ▶ SRS-A

3. Intensified response

The activated IgE also stimulates mast cells located in connective tissue along the venule walls. These mast cells release more histamine (H) and eosinophil chemotactic factor of anaphylaxis (ECF-A). These substances produce disruptive lesions, which weaken the venules.

Now, itchy red skin, wheals, and swelling appear. Signs and symptoms worsen.

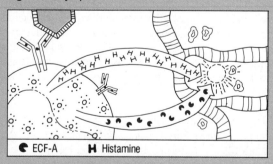

❤ ECF-A   H Histamine

4. Distress

In the lungs, the histamine causes endothelial cells to burst and endothelial tissue to tear away from surrounding tissue. Fluids leak into the alveoli, and SRS-A prevents alveoli from expanding, thereby reducing pulmonary compliance.

Tachypnea, crowing, use of accessory muscles for breathing, and cyanosis signal respiratory distress. Resulting neurologic signs and symptoms include changes in level of consciousness, severe anxiety and, possibly, seizures.

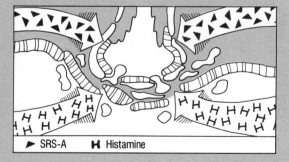

▶ SRS-A   H Histamine

WHAT HAPPENS IN ANAPHYLAXIS *(continued)*

5. Deterioration

Meanwhile, basophils and mast cells begin to release prostaglandins and bradykinin, along with histamine and serotonin. These substances increase vascular permeability, causing fluids to leak from the vessels.

Shock and confusion; cool, pale skin; generalized edema; tachycardia; and hypotension signal rapid vascular collapse.

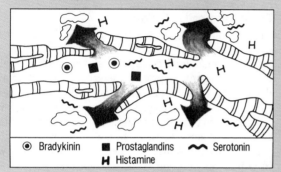

◉ Bradykinin   ■ Prostaglandins   ∿ Serotonin
Ħ Histamine

6. Failed compensatory mechanisms

Damage to endothelial cells causes basophils and mast cells to release heparin. Eosinophils release arylsulfatase B (to neutralize SRS-A), phospholipase D (to neutralize heparin), and cyclic adenosine monophosphate and the prostaglandins E_1 and E_2 (to increase the metabolic rate). But this response can't reverse anaphylaxis.

Hemorrhage, disseminated intravascular coagulation, and cardiopulmonary arrest result.

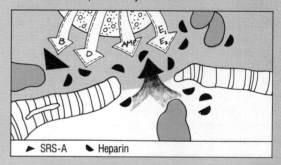

➤ SRS-A   🌢 Heparin

---

acute myocardial infarction, status asthmaticus, or congestive heart failure, must be ruled out.

Skin testing may help to identify a specific allergen. However, because skin tests can cause serious reactions, a scratch test should be done first in high-risk situations.

Treatment

Always an emergency, anaphylaxis requires an *immediate* injection of epinephrine 1:1,000 aqueous solution, 0.1 to 0.5 ml for mild signs and symptoms. If signs and symptoms are severe, repeat the dose every 5 to 20 minutes, as directed.

In the early stages of anaphylaxis, when the patient remains conscious and normotensive, give epinephrine intramuscularly or subcutaneously. Speed it into circulation by massaging the injection site. In severe reactions, when the patient is unconscious and hypotensive, give the drug intravenously, as ordered.

Establish and maintain a patent airway. Watch for early signs of laryngeal edema (stridor, hoarseness, and dyspnea), which will probably require endotracheal tube insertion or a tracheotomy and oxygen therapy.

If cardiac arrest occurs, begin cardiopulmonary resuscitation. Assist with ventilation, closed-chest cardiac massage, and sodium bicarbonate administration as ordered.

Watch for hypotension and shock. As ordered, maintain circulatory volume with volume expanders (plasma, plasma expanders, 0.9% sodium chloride solution, and albumin) as needed. As prescribed, administer I.V. vasopressors, norepinephrine, and dopamine to stabilize blood pressure. Monitor blood pressure, central venous pressure, and urine output.

Nursing diagnoses

- Altered thought processes
- Anxiety
- Decreased cardiac output
- Fear
- Impaired gas exchange
- Impaired skin integrity
- Ineffective breathing pattern
- Knowledge deficit
- Pain
- Risk for suffocation

Nursing interventions

- Provide supplemental oxygen and observe the patient's response. If hypoxia continues, prepare to help insert an artificial airway.
- Insert a peripheral I.V. line for administering emergency drugs and volume expanders, as needed.

• After the initial emergency, administer other medications, as ordered: subcutaneous epinephrine, longer-acting epinephrine, corticosteroids, and diphenhydramine I.V. for urticaria; and aminophylline I.V. for bronchospasm. (*Caution:* Rapid infusion of aminophylline may cause or aggravate severe hypotension.)

• Continually reassure the patient, and explain all tests and treatments to reduce fear and anxiety. If necessary, reorient the patient to the situation and surroundings.

• If the patient undergoes skin or scratch testing, monitor for signs of a serious allergic response. Keep emergency resuscitation equipment nearby during and after the test.

• If the patient must receive a drug to which he's allergic, prevent a severe reaction by making sure he receives careful desensitization with gradually increasing doses of the antigen or with advance administration of corticosteroids. Of course, a person with a history of allergies should receive a drug with high anaphylactic potential only after cautious pretesting for sensitivity. Closely monitor the patient during testing. Be sure you have resuscitation equipment and epinephrine at hand. When any patient takes a drug with high anaphylactic potential (particularly parenteral drugs), make sure he receives close medical observation.

• Monitor the patient undergoing diagnostic procedures, such as excretory urography, cardiac catheterization, and angiography, that use radiographic contrast media.

Patient teaching

• Teach the patient to avoid exposure to known allergens. If he has a food or drug allergy, instruct him not to consume the offending food or drug in any of its combinations and forms. If he's allergic to insect stings, he should avoid open fields and wooded areas during the insect season.

• Advise the patient to carry an anaphylaxis kit whenever he's outdoors. Urge him to familiarize himself with the kit and the directions before he needs them.

• Tell the patient to wear medical identification naming his allergy or allergies.

URTICARIA AND ANGIOEDEMA

Also known as hives, urticaria and angioedema are common allergic reactions. Urticaria is an episodic, rapidly occurring, usually self-limiting skin reaction. It involves only the superficial portion of the dermis, which erupts with local wheals surrounded by an erythematous flare. Angioedema, another dermal eruption, involves additional skin layers (including the subcutaneous tissue) and produces deeper, larger wheals (usually on the hands, feet, lips, genitalia, and eyelids). Angioedema causes diffuse swelling of loose subcutaneous tissue and also may affect the upper respiratory and GI tracts.

Urticaria and angioedema can occur separately or simultaneously, but angioedema may persist longer. Urticaria and angioedema affect about 20% of the general population at some time. Episodes tend to occur more often after adolescence with the highest incidence in people in their 30s. Recurrent acute episodes last less than 6 weeks; episodes that persist longer than 6 weeks are considered chronic.

Causes and pathophysiology

Urticaria and angioedema may result from allergy to drugs, foods, insect stings and, occasionally, inhalant allergens (animal danders, cosmetics) that provoke an IgE-mediated response to protein allergens. However, certain drugs may cause urticaria without an IgE response. When urticaria and angioedema are part of an anaphylactic reaction, they almost always persist long after the systemic response subsides because circulation to the skin is restored last after an allergic reaction. This slows histamine reabsorption at the reaction site.

Urticaria and angioedema not triggered by an allergen are probably also related to histamine release. External physical stimuli, such as cold (usually in young adults), heat, water, and sunlight, may also provoke urticaria and angioedema. Dermatographism, which develops after stroking or scratching the skin, may affect as much as 20% of the population. Such urticaria develops with varying pressure, most often under tight clothing, and is aggravated by scratching.

Several mechanisms and disorders may provoke urticaria and angioedema: These include IgE-induced release of mediators from cutaneous mast cells; binding of IgG or IgM to antigen, resulting in complement activation; and disorders such as localized or secondary infection (respiratory infection), neoplastic disease (Hodgkin's disease), connective tissue diseases (systemic lupus erythematosus), collagen vascular disease, and psychogenic disease.

Angioedema without urticaria occurs with C1 inhibitor deficiency, which can occur as an autosomal dominant characteristic (hereditary angioedema) or be acquired with lymphoproliferative disorders.

Complications

Skin abrasion and secondary infection may result from scratching. Angioedema that involves the upper respiratory tract may cause life-threatening laryngeal edema.

GI involvement may cause severe abdominal colic that may lead to unnecessary surgery.

Assessment findings

The patient's history may or may not reveal the source of the offending substance. Check the drug history, including nonprescription preparations, such as vitamins, aspirin, and antacids.

Investigate frequently troublesome foods, such as strawberries, milk products, and seafood. Environmental allergens may include pets, clothing (wool or down), soap, inhalants (hair sprays), cosmetics, hair dyes, and insect bites or stings. Remember to inquire about exposure to physical factors, such as cold, sunlight, exercise, and trauma (dermatographism).

Skin inspection typically discloses distinct, raised, evanescent dermal wheals surrounded by a reddened flare (urticaria). Varied in size, these lesions typically erupt on the extremities, external genitalia, and face, particularly around the eyes and lips. In cholinergic urticaria, the wheals may appear tiny and blanched with an erythematous rim.

Angioedema characteristically produces nonpitted swelling of deep subcutaneous tissue on the eyelids, lips, genitalia, and mucous membranes. Usually, these swellings don't itch but may burn and tingle.

With upper respiratory tract involvement, auscultation may detect respiratory stridor caused by laryngeal obstruction. The patient may appear anxious and gasping for breath. With GI involvement, he may complain of abdominal colic with or without nausea and vomiting.

Diagnostic tests

Careful skin testing with the suspected offending substance to see if a local wheal and flare result can confirm diagnosis. Diagnosis may also be confirmed by injecting the patient's serum into a skin site of a normal recipient, resulting in a wheal and flare reaction to the antigen (Prausnitz-Küstner reaction). Total IgE elevation or peripheral eosinophilia may be present.

An elimination diet and a food diary documenting foods eaten and times, amounts, and circumstances may help to pinpoint provoking allergens. Or the food diary may suggest other allergies. For instance, a patient allergic to fish may also be allergic to an iodine-based radiographic contrast medium.

Laboratory tests (complete blood count, urinalysis, and erythrocyte sedimentation rate) and chest X-rays may be done to rule out infections.

Recurrent angioedema without urticaria, along with a family history of angioedema, points to hereditary angioedema. Decreased serum levels of C1, C4, and C2 inhibitors confirm the diagnosis.

Treatment

Appropriate treatment aims to prevent or limit the patient's contact with triggering factors. Once the triggering stimulus has been removed, urticaria usually subsides in a few days—unless it results from a drug reaction. Then it may persist for as long as the drug remains in the tissues.

Treatment may involve desensitization to the triggering antigen. During desensitization, progressively larger doses of specific antigens (identified by skin testing) are injected intradermally. Diphenhydramine or another antihistamine can ease itching and swelling.

Nursing diagnoses
- Altered oral mucous membrane
- Impaired skin integrity
- Knowledge deficit
- Risk for infection
- Risk for suffocation

Nursing interventions
- Reduce or minimize environmental exposure to offending allergens and irritants, such as wools and harsh detergents. This may be easier if the offending substance is known. If it isn't, gradually eliminate suspected substances, and monitor the patient's condition to document improvement.
- If food is a suspected cause, gradually eliminate foods from the diet, and watch for improvement of signs and symptoms.
- Inspect the skin for signs of secondary infection caused by scratching.

Patient teaching
- To help identify the cause of urticaria and angioedema, teach the patient how to keep a diary. Elements to record include exposure to suspected offending substances and signs and symptoms that appear after exposure.
- If the patient modifies his diet to exclude food allergens, teach him to monitor his nutritional status. Provide him with a list of food replacements for nutrients lost by excluding allergy-provoking foods and beverages.
- Instruct him to keep his fingernails short to avoid abrading the skin when scratching.
- Review signs and symptoms that indicate a skin infection. Explain hygiene measures for managing minor infection, and direct the patient to seek medical attention as needed.

UNDERSTANDING THE Rh SYSTEM

The Rh system contains more than 30 antibodies and antigens. Of the world's population, about 85% are Rh-positive, which means that their RBCs carry the D or Rh antigen. The rest of the population are Rh-negative and don't have this antigen.

Effects of sensitization
When an Rh-negative person receives Rh-positive blood for the first time, he becomes sensitized to the D antigen but shows no immediate reaction to it. If he receives Rh-positive blood a second time, he develops a massive hemolytic reaction.

For example, an Rh-negative mother who delivers an Rh-positive baby is sensitized by the baby's Rh-positive blood. During her next Rh-positive pregnancy, her sensitized blood will cause a hemolytic reaction in fetal circulation.

Preventing sensitization
To prevent the formation of antibodies against Rh-positive blood, an Rh-negative mother should receive $Rh_o(D)$ immune globulin (human) (RhoGAM) I.M. within 72 hours after delivering an Rh-positive baby.

BLOOD TRANSFUSION REACTION

Mediated by immune or nonimmune factors, a transfusion reaction accompanies or follows I.V. administration of blood components. Its severity varies from mild (fever and chills) to severe (acute renal failure or complete vascular collapse and death), depending on the amount of blood transfused, the type of reaction, and the patient's general health.

Causes and pathophysiology
The immune response to blood can be directed against red or white blood cells, platelets, or one or more of the immunoglobulins.

A hemolytic reaction follows the transfusion of mismatched blood. Transfusion with serologically incompatible blood triggers the most serious reaction, marked by intravascular agglutination of red blood cells (RBCs). The recipient's antibodies (IgG or IgM) attach to the donor RBCs, leading to widespread clumping and destruction of the recipient's RBCs.

Transfusion with Rh-incompatible blood triggers a less serious reaction, known as Rh isoimmunization, within several days to 2 weeks. Rh reactions are most likely to occur in women sensitized to RBC antigens by prior

pregnancy or unknown factors, such as bacterial or viral infection, and in people who have received more than five transfusions. (See *Understanding the Rh system.*)

A febrile nonhemolytic reaction, the most common type of reaction, apparently develops when cytotoxic or agglutinating antibodies in the recipient's plasma attack antigens on transfused lymphocytes, granulocytes, or plasma cells.

Although fairly common, allergic reactions are only occasionally serious. In this type of reaction, transfused soluble antigens react with surface IgE molecules on mast cells and basophils, causing degranulation and release of allergic mediators. Antibodies against IgA in an IgA-deficient recipient can also trigger a severe allergic reaction (anaphylaxis).

Complications
The patient may develop bronchospasm (possibly leading to acute respiratory failure), acute tubular necrosis leading to acute renal failure, anaphylactic shock, vascular collapse, or disseminated intravascular coagulation (DIC).

Assessment findings
The immediate effects of a hemolytic transfusion reaction develop within a few minutes or hours after transfusion begins. The patient may complain of chills, nausea, vomiting, chest tightness, and chest and back pain.

Vital signs may show fever, tachycardia, and hypotension. The patient may appear dyspneic and apprehensive. Skin inspection may reveal urticaria and angioedema. Auscultation may reveal wheezing if bronchospasm occurs. The patient may also show signs of anaphylaxis, shock, congestive heart failure, and pulmonary edema. In a surgical patient, anesthesia masks these signs, but you'll note blood oozing from mucous membranes or the incision site.

A hemolytic reaction that occurs several weeks after the transfusion can produce fever, an unexpected fall in serum hemoglobin level, and jaundice.

The patient with an allergic reaction has similar signs and symptoms except no fever. However, mild to severe fever is the hallmark of a febrile nonhemolytic reaction that begins at the start of transfusion or within 2 hours after its completion.

Diagnostic tests
Confirming a hemolytic transfusion reaction requires proof of blood incompatibility and evidence of hemolysis, such as hemoglobinuria, anti-A or anti-B antibodies in

the serum, and low serum hemoglobin and elevated bilirubin levels. The patient suspected of having such a reaction should have his blood retyped and crossmatched with the donor's blood.

After a hemolytic transfusion reaction, laboratory tests show increased indirect bilirubin and serum hemoglobin levels, decreased haptoglobin levels, and hemoglobin in urine. As the reaction progresses, tests may show signs of DIC, such as thrombocytopenia, increased prothrombin time, and decreased fibrinogen level, and signs of acute tubular necrosis, such as increased serum blood urea nitrogen and creatinine levels.

Treatment
If a hemolytic reaction occurs, the transfusion should be stopped immediately. Osmotic or loop diuretics can prevent acute tubular necrosis. Other symptomatic treatment includes I.V. vasopressors and 0.9% sodium chloride solution to combat shock, epinephrine to treat dyspnea and wheezing, diphenhydramine to combat cellular histamine released from mast cells, corticosteroids to reduce inflammation, and mannitol or furosemide to maintain urinary tract function.

Treatment for a nonhemolytic febrile reaction calls for antipyretics.

Nursing diagnoses
• Anxiety
• Decreased cardiac output
• Impaired gas exchange
• Impaired tissue integrity
• Pain
• Risk for altered body temperature
• Risk for injury

Nursing interventions
• Monitor the patient's vital signs every 15 to 30 minutes, watching for signs of shock.
• Maintain a patent I.V. line with 0.9% sodium chloride solution, and insert an indwelling urinary catheter. Monitor intake and output.
• Cover the patient with blankets to ease chills.
• In the surgical or semicomatose patient, deliver supplemental oxygen at a low flow rate through a nasal cannula or hand-held resuscitation bag.
• Afterward, fully document the transfusion reaction on the patient's chart, noting the duration of the transfusion and the amount of blood absorbed. Provide a complete description of the reaction and any interventions.
• To prevent a hemolytic transfusion reaction, first make sure you know your hospital's policy about giving blood before giving a blood transfusion. Then make sure you have the right blood and the right patient. Check and double-check the patient's name, hospital number, ABO group, and Rh status. If you find even a small discrepancy, don't give the blood. Notify the blood bank immediately and return the unopened unit.

Patient teaching
• During the transfusion reaction, explain what's happening. After recovery, tell the patient what kind of transfusion reaction he had, and answer his questions.

AUTOIMMUNE DISORDERS

Marked by an abnormal immune response to oneself, autoimmunity leads to a sequence of tissue reactions and damage that may produce diffuse, systemic signs and symptoms. Among the autoimmune disorders are rheumatoid arthritis, juvenile rheumatoid arthritis, psoriatic arthritis, ankylosing spondylitis, Sjögren's syndrome, lupus erythematosus, Goodpasture's syndrome, Reiter's syndrome, systemic sclerosis, polymyositis and dermatomyositis, and vasculitis.

RHEUMATOID ARTHRITIS
A chronic, systemic, symmetrical inflammatory disease, rheumatoid arthritis primarily attacks peripheral joints and surrounding muscles, tendons, ligaments, and blood vessels. Spontaneous remissions and unpredictable exacerbations mark the course of this potentially crippling disease.

Rheumatoid arthritis occurs worldwide, affecting more than 6.5 million people in the United States alone. The disease strikes women three times more often than men. Although it can occur at any age, the peak onset period for women is between ages 35 and 50.

Rheumatoid arthritis usually requires lifelong treatment and, sometimes, surgery. In most patients, the disease follows an intermittent course and allows normal activity, although 10% suffer total disability from severe articular deformity or associated extra-articular symptoms, or both. The prognosis worsens with the development of nodules, vasculitis, and high titers of rheumatoid factor.

Causes and pathophysiology
What causes the chronic inflammation characteristic of rheumatoid arthritis isn't known, but various theories

JOINT DEFORMITY

In advanced rheumatoid arthritis, marked edema and congestion cause spindle-shaped interphalangeal joints and severe flexion deformities.

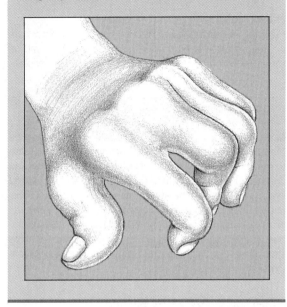

point to infectious, genetic, and endocrine factors. A genetically susceptible person may develop abnormal or altered IgG antibodies when exposed to an antigen. The body doesn't recognize these altered IgG antibodies as "self," and the person forms an antibody known as rheumatoid factor against them. By aggregating into complexes, rheumatoid factor generates inflammation.

Eventually, the cartilage damage that results from the inflammation triggers further immune responses, including complement activation. Complement, in turn, attracts polymorphonuclear leukocytes and stimulates the release of inflammatory mediators, which exacerbates joint destruction.

Much more is known about the pathophysiology of rheumatoid arthritis than about its causes. If unarrested, joint inflammation occurs in four stages. First, synovitis develops from congestion and edema of the synovial membrane and joint capsule. Formation of pannus — thickened layers of granulation tissue — marks the onset of the second stage. Pannus covers and invades cartilage and eventually destroys the joint capsule and bone.

Progression to the third stage is characterized by fibrous ankylosis — fibrous invasion of the pannus and scar formation that occludes the joint space. Bone atrophy and misalignment cause visible deformities and disrupt the articulation of opposing bones, causing muscle atrophy and imbalance and, possibly, partial dislocations or subluxations. In the fourth stage, fibrous tissue calcifies, resulting in bony ankylosis and total immobility.

Complications

Pain associated with movement may restrict active joint use and cause fibrous or bony ankylosis, soft-tissue contractures, and joint deformities. (See *Joint deformity*.)

Between 15% and 20% of patients develop Sjögren's syndrome with keratoconjunctivitis sicca. Rheumatoid arthritis can also destroy the odontoid process, part of the second cervical vertebra. Rarely, spinal cord compression may occur, particularly in patients with longstanding deforming rheumatoid arthritis.

Assessment findings

The patient's history may reveal an insidious onset of nonspecific symptoms, including fatigue, malaise, anorexia, persistent low-grade fever, weight loss, and vague articular symptoms.

Later, more specific localized articular symptoms develop, frequently in the fingers at the proximal interphalangeal, metacarpophalangeal, and metatarsophalangeal joints. These symptoms usually occur bilaterally and symmetrically and may extend to the wrists, elbows, knees, and ankles.

The patient may report that affected joints stiffen after inactivity, especially on rising in the morning. She may complain that joints are tender and painful, at first only when she moves them, but eventually even at rest. Ultimately, joint function is diminished. She may also experience tingling paresthesia in the fingers, the result of synovial pressure on the median nerve from carpal tunnel syndrome.

Other complaints include stiff, weak, or painful muscles. If the patient has peripheral neuropathy, she may report numbness or tingling in the feet or weakness or loss of sensation in the fingers. If pleuritis develops, she may complain of pain on inspiration (although pleuritis often causes no symptoms). The patient with pulmonary nodules or fibrosis may complain of shortness of breath.

Inspection of the patient's joints may show deformities and contractures, especially if active disease continues. The fingers may appear spindle-shaped from marked edema and congestion in the joints. Proximal interphalangeal joints may develop flexion deformities or become hyperextended. Metacarpophalangeal joints may swell dorsally, and volar subluxation and stretching of tendons may pull the fingers to the ulnar side (ulnar drift). The fingers may become fixed in a characteristic swan-neck deformity or in a boutonnière deformity. The hands appear foreshortened, and the wrists boggy. Inspection of pressure areas, such as the elbows, may reveal rheumatoid nodules—subcutaneous, round or oval, nontender masses—the most common extra-articular finding.

If the patient has vasculitis, you may observe such extra-articular signs as lesions, leg ulcers, and multiple systemic complications. If she has scleritis or episcleritis, you may observe redness of the eye.

Palpation may reveal joints that are hot to the touch. If the patient has pericarditis, auscultation may reveal pericardial friction rub (although pericarditis may cause no signs).

If spinal cord compression occurs, your assessment may also reveal signs of upper motor neuron disorder, such as a positive Babinski's sign and weakness. You may also detect signs of other extra-articular findings, including temporomandibular joint disease, infection, osteoporosis, myositis, cardiopulmonary lesions, lymphadenopathy, and peripheral neuritis.

Diagnostic tests

Although no test definitively diagnoses rheumatoid arthritis, the following are useful:

• *X-rays.* In early stages, X-rays show bone demineralization and soft-tissue swelling. Later, they help determine the extent of cartilage and bone destruction, erosion, subluxations, and deformities. They also show the characteristic pattern of these abnormalities, particularly symmetrical involvement, although no particular pattern is conclusive for rheumatoid arthritis.

• *Rheumatoid factor test.* This test is positive in 75% to 80% of patients, as indicated by a titer of 1:160 or higher. Although the presence of rheumatoid factor doesn't confirm rheumatoid arthritis, it does help determine the prognosis; a patient with a high titer usually has more severe and progressive disease with extra-articular manifestations.

• *Synovial fluid analysis.* Analysis shows increased volume and turbidity, but decreased viscosity and complement (C3 and C4) levels. The white blood cell count often exceeds 10,000/mm³.

• *Serum protein electrophoresis.* This test may show elevated serum globulin levels.

• *Erythrocyte sedimentation rate.* The rate is elevated in 85% to 90% of patients. Because an elevated sedimentation rate frequently parallels disease activity, this test may help monitor the patient's response to therapy (as may a C-reactive protein test).

• *Complete blood count.* This test usually shows moderate anemia and slight leukocytosis.

The criteria for classifying rheumatoid arthritis developed by the American Rheumatism Association can also serve as guidelines for establishing a diagnosis. But keep in mind that failure to meet these criteria—particularly early in the disease—doesn't exclude the diagnosis. (See *Classifying rheumatoid arthritis,* page 410.)

Treatment

Treatment requires a multidisciplinary health care team to reduce the patient's pain and inflammation, preserve functional capacity, resolve pathologic processes, and bring about improvement.

Salicylates, particularly aspirin, are the mainstay of therapy because they decrease inflammation and relieve joint pain. The patient may also receive other nonsteroidal anti-inflammatory drugs (such as indomethacin, fenoprofen, and ibuprofen), antimalarials (hydroxychloroquine), gold salts, penicillamine, and corticosteroids (prednisone)—although corticosteroid therapy can cause osteoporosis. Other therapeutic drugs include such immunosuppressants as cyclophosphamide, methotrexate, and azathioprine, which are used in the early stages of the disease. (See *Drug therapy for rheumatoid arthritis,* page 411.)

Supportive measures include increased sleep—8 to 10 hours every night—frequent rest periods between daily activities, and splinting to rest inflamed joints (although, like corticosteroid therapy, immobilization can cause osteoporosis).

A physical therapy program that includes range-of-motion exercises and carefully individualized therapeutic exercises forestalls the loss of joint function; application of heat relaxes muscles and relieves pain. Moist heat (hot soaks, paraffin baths, whirlpools) usually works best for patients with chronic disease. Ice packs help during acute episodes.

Useful surgical procedures include metatarsal head and distal ulnar resectional arthroplasty, and insertion of a Silastic prosthesis between the metacarpophalangeal and proximal interphalangeal joints. Arthrodesis (joint fusion) may bring about stability and relieve pain, but only at the price of decreased joint mobility. Synovectomy (removal of destructive, proliferating synovium, usually in the wrists, fingers, and knees) may halt or delay the course of the disease. Osteotomy (the cutting of bone or excision of a wedge of bone) can realign joint surfaces and redistribute stresses. Tendons that rupture spontaneously need surgical repair. Tendon transfers may prevent deformities or relieve contractures. The patient may

CLASSIFYING RHEUMATOID ARTHRITIS

Revised in 1987, the criteria of the American Rheumatism Association allow the classification of rheumatoid arthritis.

Guidelines
A patient who meets four of seven criteria is classified as having rheumatoid arthritis. She must experience the first four criteria for at least 6 weeks, and a doctor must observe the second through fifth criteria.

A patient with two or more other clinical diagnoses can also be diagnosed with rheumatoid arthritis.

Criteria
• Morning stiffness in and around the joints that lasts 1 hour before full improvement
• Arthritis in three or more joint areas, with at least three joint areas (as observed by a doctor) exhibiting soft-tissue swelling or joint effusions, not just bony overgrowth (the 14 possible areas involved include the right and left proximal interphalangeal, metacarpophalangeal, wrist, elbow, knee, ankle, and metatarsophalangeal joints)
• Arthritis of hand joints, including the wrist, the metacarpophalangeal joint, or the proximal interphalangeal joint
• Arthritis that involves the same joint areas on both sides of the body
• Subcutaneous rheumatoid nodules over bony prominences
• Demonstration of abnormal amounts of serum rheumatoid factor by any method that produces a positive result in less than 5% of patients without rheumatoid arthritis
• Radiographic changes, which usually are seen on posteroanterior hand and wrist radiographs; these must show erosions or unequivocal bony decalcification localized in or most noticeable adjacent to the involved joints.

---

need joint reconstruction or total joint arthroplasty in advanced disease.

Nursing diagnoses
• Activity intolerance
• Altered health maintenance
• Altered peripheral tissue perfusion
• Altered protection
• Altered role performance
• Anticipatory grieving
• Energy field disturbance
• Fatigue
• Fear
• Hopelessness
• Impaired physical mobility
• Knowledge deficit
• Pain
• Powerlessness
• Risk for impaired skin integrity
• Risk for infection
• Self-care deficit
• Sexual dysfunction

Nursing interventions
• Monitor the patient's vital signs, and note weight changes, sensory disturbances, and level of pain. Administer analgesics, as ordered, and watch for adverse reactions.

• Give meticulous skin care. Check for rheumatoid nodules. Also monitor for pressure ulcers and skin breakdown, especially if the patient is in traction or wearing splints. These can result from immobility, vascular impairment, corticosteroid treatment, and improper splinting. Use lotion or cleansing oil—not soap—on dry skin.
• Monitor the duration of morning stiffness. Duration more accurately reflects the severity of the disease than the intensity.
• Supply a zipper-pull, easy-to-open beverage cartons, lightweight cups, and unpackaged silverware to make it easier for the patient to perform activities of daily living, such as dressing and feeding herself. Allow the patient enough time to calmly perform these tasks.
• Provide emotional support. Remember that the patient can easily become depressed, discouraged, and irritable. Encourage discussion of her fears concerning dependency, disability, sexuality, body image, and self-esteem. Refer her to appropriate counseling, as needed.

After total knee or hip arthroplasty:
• Monitor and record vital signs. Watch for complications, such as steroid crisis and shock in a patient receiving corticosteroids. Monitor the patient's distal leg pulses often, marking them with a waterproof marker to make them easier to find.
• As soon as the patient awakens, have her perform active dorsiflexion; if she can't, report this immediately. Supervise isometric exercises every 2 hours. After total hip arthroplasty, check traction for pressure areas, and keep

DRUG THERAPY FOR RHEUMATOID ARTHRITIS

Drug and adverse effects	Nursing interventions
aspirin Prolonged bleeding time; GI disturbances, including nausea, dyspepsia, anorexia, ulcers, and hemorrhage; hypersensitivity reactions ranging from urticaria to anaphylaxis; salicylism (mild toxicity: tinnitus, dizziness; moderate toxicity: restlessness, hyperpnea, delirium, marked lethargy; and severe toxicity: coma, seizures, severe hyperpnea)	• Don't use in neonates and in patients with GI ulcers, bleeding, or hypersensitivity. • Give with food, milk, an antacid, or a large glass of water to reduce adverse GI effects. • Remember that toxicity can develop rapidly in febrile, dehydrated children. • Monitor salicylate levels. • Teach the patient to reduce the dose, one tablet at a time, if tinnitus occurs. • Teach the patient to watch for signs of bleeding, such as bruising, melena, and petechiae.
fenoprofen, ibuprofen, naproxen, piroxicam, sulindac, and tolmetin Prolonged bleeding time; central nervous system abnormalities (headache, drowsiness, restlessness, dizziness, tremors); GI disturbances, including hemorrhage and peptic ulcer; increased blood urea nitrogen (BUN) and liver enzyme levels	• Don't use in patients with renal disease, in asthmatics with nasal polyps, or in children. • Use cautiously in patients with GI disorders or cardiac disease and in patients allergic to other nonsteroidal anti-inflammatory drugs. • Give with milk or food to reduce adverse GI effects. • Tell the patient that the therapeutic effect may be delayed for 2 to 3 weeks. • Monitor renal, hepatic, and auditory functions in long-term therapy. Stop the drug if abnormalities develop.
gold (oral and parenteral) Dermatitis, pruritus, rash, stomatitis, nephrotoxicity, blood dyscrasias, nitritoid crisis, and, with the oral form, GI distress and diarrhea	• Observe for nitritoid crisis (flushing, fainting, sweating). • Check the patient's urine for blood and albumin before each dose. If you get a positive result, withhold the drug and notify the doctor. • Stress the need for regular follow-up examinations, including blood and urine testing. • To avoid local nerve irritation, mix the drug well and give an I.M. injection deep in the buttock. • Advise the patient not to expect an improvement for 3 to 6 months. • Instruct the patient to report rash, bruising, bleeding, hematuria, and oral ulcers.
indomethacin Blood dyscrasias; hemolytic, aplastic, and iron deficiency anemias; headache; blurred vision; corneal and retinal damage; hearing loss; tinnitus; GI disturbances, including GI ulcer and hematuria	• Don't use in children under age 14 or in patients with aspirin intolerance or GI disorders. • Severe headache may occur within 1 hour. Stop the drug if headache persists. • Tell the patient to report any visual changes. Stress the need for regular eye examinations during long-term therapy. • Always give with food or milk. • Administer a single dose at bedtime to alleviate morning stiffness.
methotrexate Bone marrow depression; stomatitis, nausea, and vomiting; alopecia; tubular necrosis, cirrhosis, hepatic fibrosis, and hyperuricemia; pulmonary infiltrates; diarrhea, possibly leading to hemorrhagic enteritis and intestinal perforation	• If adverse GI reactions occur, you may need to stop the drug as ordered. Administer antiemetics, as ordered, to control nausea and vomiting. • Report rash, redness, or ulcerations in mouth and pulmonary adverse reactions, which may signal serious complications. • Monitor the patient's serum uric acid, serum creatinine, and BUN levels during therapy. As ordered, reduce the dose if the patient's BUN level reaches 20 to 30 mg/dl or her serum creatinine level reaches 1.2 to 2 mg/dl. Stop the drug, as ordered, if her BUN level rises above 30 mg/dl or her serum creatinine level reaches more than 2 mg/dl.
penicillamine Blood dyscrasias, glomerulonephropathy	• Give on an empty stomach, before meals, and separately from other drugs or milk. • Monitor the patient's urine for protein and blood. Also monitor liver function studies and complete blood count. • Tell the patient to report fever, sore throat, chills, bruising, and bleeding.

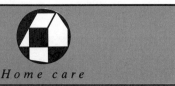

Home care

LIVING WITH RHEUMATOID ARTHRITIS

Follow these guidelines to help your patient learn to live with rheumatoid arthritis:
• Teach the patient how to use correct posture when standing, sitting, and walking.
• Recommend using chairs with high seats and armrests. If that's not possible, suggest putting blocks of wood under the legs of a favorite chair.
• Recommend using a raised toilet seat.
• Teach the patient proper body mechanics—avoiding flexion, keeping her hands close to the center of the body, and sliding rather than lifting objects.
• Suggest that the patient take a hot shower or bath just before bed or in the morning to help relieve pain.
• Refer the patient for physical and occupational therapy to help increase her mobility, strength, and ability to perform activities of daily living.
• Reinforce instructions about the need for adaptive devices, such as dressing aids (long-handled shoehorn, reacher, elastic shoelaces, zipper pull, and button hook) and eating utensils.
• Inspect the patient's home for possible safety hazards, and work with the patient and family to remove them. Encourage the use of grab bars and safety mats or strips in the tub or shower.
• Advise the patient to save her strength by pacing her activities and dressing in a sitting position whenever possible.
• Refer the patient to the Arthritis Foundation.

the head of the bed raised between 30 and 45 degrees.
• Change or reinforce dressings, as needed, using aseptic technique. Check wounds for hematoma, excessive drainage, color changes, and foul odor—all possible signs of hemorrhage or infection. (The rheumatoid arthritis patient's wounds may heal slowly.) Make sure you don't contaminate dressings when helping the patient use the urinal or bedpan.
• Administer blood replacement products, antibiotics, and pain medication, as ordered. Monitor serum electrolyte and hemoglobin levels and hematocrit.
• Have the patient turn, cough, and breathe deeply every 2 hours; then percuss her chest.
• After total knee arthroplasty, keep the patient's leg extended and slightly elevated.

• After total hip arthroplasty, keep the patient's hip in abduction to prevent dislocation. Watch for and immediately report any inability to rotate the hip or bear weight on it, increased pain, or a leg that appears shorter. All may indicate dislocation.
• As soon as possible, help the patient get out of bed and sit in a chair, keeping her weight on the unaffected side. When she's ready to walk, consult with the physical therapist for walking instruction and aids.

Patient teaching
• Explain the nature of rheumatoid arthritis. Make sure the patient and her family understand that rheumatoid arthritis is a chronic disease that may require major changes in life-style and that so-called miracle cures don't work.
• Explain all diagnostic tests and procedures.
• Encourage a balanced diet, but make sure the patient understands that special diets won't cure rheumatoid arthritis. Stress the need for weight control because obesity further stresses the joints.
• Discuss the patient's sexual concerns. If pain creates problems during intercourse, discuss trying alternative positions, taking analgesics beforehand, and using moist heat to increase mobility.
• Before discharge, make sure the patient knows how and when to take prescribed medications and how to recognize possible adverse effects. (See *Living with rheumatoid arthritis*.)

If the patient requires total knee or hip arthroplasty, she'll need special preoperative teaching:
• Explain all preoperative and surgical procedures. If possible, show the patient the prosthesis that will be used.
• Teach postoperative exercises (such as isometrics) and supervise her practice. Also, teach the deep-breathing and coughing exercises she must perform after surgery.
• Explain that total hip or knee arthroplasty requires frequent range-of-motion exercises of the leg after surgery; total knee arthroplasty also requires frequent leg-lift exercises.
• Show the patient how to use a trapeze to move herself about in bed after surgery, and make sure she has a fracture bedpan handy.
• Tell her what kind of dressings to expect after surgery. After total knee arthroplasty, the patient's knee may be placed in a constant-passive-motion device to increase mobility and prevent emboli. After total hip arthroplasty, she'll have an abduction pillow between her legs to help keep the hip prosthesis in place.

JUVENILE RHEUMATOID ARTHRITIS TYPES

Signs and symptoms of JRA vary according to type. The types include systemic, polyarticular, and pauciarticular JRA.

Systemic JRA
• Accounts for 20% to 30% of JRA cases
• Can affect any joint and either sex
• Causes a "sawtooth" fever pattern—an intermittent fever that begins suddenly, spikes to 103° F (39.4° C) or more once or twice daily (usually in late afternoon), and rapidly returns to normal or subnormal
• Can't be easily detected by laboratory tests because serum findings are negative for rheumatoid factor (RF) and antinuclear antibodies (ANAs)
• Develops into severe arthritis in about 20% of patients

Polyarticular JRA
This type of arthritis may be mild (RF-negative) or severe (RF-positive).

RF-negative polyarticular JRA
• Affects girls eight times more often than boys
• Involves five or more joints
• Usually develops insidiously
• Mostly affects the wrists, elbows, knees, ankles, and small joints of the hands and feet, but can also affect larger joints, including the temporomandibular and those of the cervical spine, hips, and shoulders
• Results in negative findings for RF; however, in about 25% of patients, test findings disclose ANAs
• Develops into severe arthritis in about 10% of patients

RF-positive polyarticular JRA
• Affects girls six times more often than boys
• Usually occurs late in childhood

• Can affect any joint
• Is marked by positive RF findings in serum tests; in about 75% of patients, test findings disclose ANAs
• Mimics adult rheumatoid arthritis in about 50% of patients who have severe, destructive disease

Pauciarticular JRA
Some subtypes of this arthritis include pauciarticular JRA with iridocyclitis and pauciarticular JRA with sacroiliitis. Pauciarticular JRA involves four or fewer joints.

Pauciarticular JRA with iridocyclitis
• Accounts for about 45% of pauciarticular JRA cases
• Strikes girls under age 6 about seven times more often than boys
• Affects mostly knee, elbow, and ankle joints, and the iris
• Involves chronic iridocyclitis in about 40% of patients
• Develops into polyarthritis in about 20% of patients
• Is marked by negative RF findings in serum tests; about 60% of patients have positive ANA test findings

Pauciarticular JRA with sacroiliitis
• Strikes boys over age 8 nine times more often than girls
• Is marked by positive HLA-B27 findings in serum tests
• Involves the hip, sacroiliac, heel, and foot
• Shows no RF or ANAs on test findings
• May later develop into the sacrolumbar arthritis characteristic of ankylosing spondylitis
• May occur with acute iritis

JUVENILE RHEUMATOID ARTHRITIS

Affecting children under age 17, juvenile rheumatoid arthritis (JRA) consists of several conditions characterized by chronic synovitis, joint swelling, pain, and tenderness. The disease may also produce extra-articular signs and symptoms, involving organs such as the skin, heart, lungs, liver, spleen, and eyes. Major types of JRA include *systemic* (Still's disease or acute febrile type), *polyarticular*, and *pauciarticular*. (See *Juvenile rheumatoid arthritis types*.)

Depending on the type, JRA may occur as early as age 6 weeks—though seldom before age 6 months—with peak onset between ages 1 and 3, and 8 and 12. Considered the major chronic rheumatic disorder of childhood, JRA occurs in an estimated 150,000 to 250,000 children in the United States, affecting twice as many girls as boys.

Causes
Studies continue to probe for the causes of JRA. Various findings suggest links to genetic factors or to an abnormal immune response. Viral or bacterial (particularly streptococcal) infection, trauma, and emotional stress may be precipitating factors, but their exact relation to the disease remains unclear.

Complications
JRA may involve structures besides the joints, including the skin, heart, lungs, liver, spleen, lymph nodes, and eyes. Unheralded by obvious early signs or symptoms,

chronic iridocyclitis (insidious inflammation of the iris and ciliary body) may lead to such complications as ocular damage and loss of vision. Growth disturbances, such as overgrowth or undergrowth adjacent to inflamed joints, are also complications of JRA.

Assessment findings

Almost all patients complain of joint stiffness in the morning or after periods of inactivity. Young children with JRA are typically irritable and listless. Other signs and symptoms vary with the type of JRA.

With *systemic JRA,* the child may experience mild, transient arthritis or frank polyarthritis associated with fever and rash. Joint involvement may not be evident at first, but the child's behavior may clearly suggest joint pain. For example, she may always favor sitting in a flexed position. She may walk very little or refuse to walk at all.

An intermittent, spiking (sawtooth) fever is common. (In fact, this sign helps to differentiate the disease from other inflammatory disorders.) When fever spikes, inspect the skin for a characteristic evanescent rheumatoid rash. Small, pale or salmon-pink macules most commonly appear on the trunk and proximal extremities and, occasionally, on the face, palms, and soles. Massaging or applying heat intensifies this rash, which usually is most conspicuous in areas subjected to rubbing or pressure (for example, from underclothing).

The child may complain of painful breathing (if she has pleuritis with systemic JRA) and nonspecific abdominal pain.

If the child has myocarditis, she may also report or you may note fatigue, shortness of breath, palpitations, and fever. Assessment may also disclose resting or exertional tachycardia; arrhythmias; neck vein distention; increased amplitude of S_1, S_2, and S_4 gallops; and systolic ejection murmurs—all suggesting heart failure.

Palpation and percussion may reveal hepatic, splenic, and lymph node enlargement. Auscultation findings may include a friction rub associated with pericarditis.

With *polyarticular JRA,* the child may complain mostly of pain in the wrists, elbows, knees, ankles, and small joints of the hands and feet. However, she may also complain of pain in larger joints, including the temporomandibular and those of the cervical spine, hips, and shoulders.

On inspection, you may notice joint swelling. Tenderness and stiffness are also typical. Usually the arthritis occurs symmetrically. It may be remittent or indolent. The child may have a low-grade fever with daily peaks. Parents may report weight loss in the child and describe her as listless. You may also observe noticeable developmental retardation.

Palpation and percussion may disclose hepatic, splenic, and lymph node enlargement. You may also find subcutaneous nodules on the elbows or heels.

With *pauciarticular JRA,* the child typically complains of pain in the hip, knees, heels, feet, ankles, and elbows. With inflammation of the iris and ciliary body, she may complain of pain, redness, blurred vision, and photophobia. With sacroiliitis, she typically reports lower back pain.

Diagnostic tests

• *Complete blood count* usually shows decreased hemoglobin levels and increased neutrophil (neutrophilia) and platelet (thrombocytosis) levels. Other findings include an elevated erythrocyte sedimentation rate and elevated C-reactive protein, serum haptoglobin, immunoglobulin, and C3 complement levels.

• *Antinuclear antibody* test results may be positive in patients with polyarticular JRA and in patients with pauciarticular JRA with chronic iridocyclitis.

• *Rheumatoid factor* (RF) appears in about 15% of patients with JRA. In contrast, about 85% of patients with rheumatoid arthritis test positive for RF. Patients with polyarticular JRA may or may not test positive for RF.

• *Human leukocyte antigen (HLA)-B27* appearing in blood tests may forecast later development of ankylosing spondylitis.

• *X-ray studies* demonstrate early structural changes associated with JRA. These include soft-tissue swelling, effusion, and periostitis in affected joints. Later evidence includes osteoporosis and accelerated bone growth followed by subchondral erosions, joint space narrowing, bone destruction, and fusion.

Treatment

Successful JRA management usually calls for anti-inflammatory drugs, physical therapy, carefully planned nutrition and exercise, and regular eye examinations. Both the child and the parents must be involved in therapy.

Aspirin is the initial drug of choice. Dosages are based on the child's weight. Additional nonsteroidal anti-inflammatory drugs (NSAIDs) may be used. If these prove ineffective, gold salts, hydroxychloroquine, and penicillamine may be tried. Because of adverse effects, corticosteroids are reserved for treating systemic disorders (such as pericarditis or iritis) that resist treatment with NSAIDs. Corticosteroids and mydriatic drugs are commonly prescribed for iridocyclitis. Investigational drug therapy includes low-dose cytotoxic agents, such as methotrexate.

Physical therapy promotes regular exercise to maintain joint mobility and muscle strength, thereby preventing contractures, deformity, and disability. Good posture, gait training, and joint protection are also beneficial. Splints help reduce pain, prevent contractures, and maintain correct joint alignment.

Surgery is usually limited to soft-tissue releases to improve mobility. Joint replacement is delayed until the child has matured physically and can tolerate vigorous rehabilitation.

Nursing diagnoses
• Activity intolerance
• Altered role performance
• Fatigue
• Impaired physical mobility
• Ineffective family coping
• Knowledge deficit
• Pain
• Risk for injury
• Self-care deficit
• Sensory or perceptual alterations

Nursing interventions
• Focus nursing care on reducing the patient's pain and promoting mobility.
• During inflammatory exacerbations, be sure to administer NSAIDs or prescribed medication on a regular schedule. The patient will be more likely to participate in physical therapy exercises if she has minimal pain before beginning.
• Consult an occupational therapist to assess the patient's home care needs. Provide specialized eating utensils, a high commode or toilet seat, a lowered sink, and a tub or shower chair as needed.
• Allow the patient to rest frequently throughout the day to conserve energy for times when she must be mobile.
• Arrange the patient's environment for participation in activities of daily living so that she feels capable of accomplishing tasks.

Patient teaching
• Advise parents and health care professionals to encourage the child to be as independent as possible and to develop a positive attitude toward school, social development, and vocational planning.
• Encourage regular slit-lamp examinations to help ensure early diagnosis and treatment of iridocyclitis. Children with pauciarticular JRA with chronic iridocyclitis

should be checked every 3 months during periods of active disease and every 6 months during remissions.
• Teach parents about reportable signs of bleeding secondary to aspirin or NSAID therapy.

PSORIATIC ARTHRITIS
Marked by rheumatoid-like joint disease and psoriasis of the skin and nails, psoriatic arthritis usually occurs in a mild form with intermittent flare-ups. Rarely, the disease progresses to crippling arthritis mutilans.

Although the arthritis component of this syndrome usually appears clinically indistinguishable from rheumatoid arthritis, rheumatoid nodules do not develop, and serologic test results for rheumatoid factor (RF) are negative. Psoriatic arthritis affects men and women equally. Usually, onset occurs between ages 30 and 35. Nearly 20% of patients with psoriasis have coexisting arthritic disease.

Causes
Evidence suggests that predisposition to psoriatic arthritis is hereditary. Blood test results show about 45% of patients with human leukocyte antigen (HLA)-B27. A streptococcal infection or trauma usually precedes onset.

Complications
Severe complications are rare with psoriatic arthritis. About 75% of patients with a hereditary predisposition to psoriatic arthritis develop the disease; in about half of these, crippling arthritis and inflammatory ocular complications (conjunctivitis, acute anterior uveitis, and episcleritis) occur.

Assessment findings
About 25% of patients have a history of psoriatic lesions before arthritis signs and symptoms occur. Sometimes a patient may have only one skin lesion. This patient may be unaware that the lesion constitutes psoriasis.

The patient with severe psoriatic arthritis may report arthritis symptoms and skin lesions occurring simultaneously. He may also complain of malaise and fever.

Inspection of an affected joint typically reveals swelling, tenderness, warmth, and restricted movement. One or several joints may be involved. Arthritis may be distributed symmetrically or asymmetrically. It can develop in any peripheral joint but most commonly occurs in the distal interphalangeal joints of the hands. Affected fingers may appear sausagelike. Characteristic nail changes include pitting, transverse ridging, onycholysis, keratosis, and yellowing. In some patients, the disease may destroy the entire nail.

Carefully inspect the skin for psoriatic lesions. Remember that psoriatic arthritis can occur even if only one lesion exists, although it is most common in patients with severe skin disease.

Diagnostic tests

X-ray studies can confirm joint involvement. They may show eroded terminal phalangeal tufts, "whittling" of the distal terminal phalanges, "pencil-in-cup" distal interphalangeal joint deformities, sacroiliitis, and relative absence of osteoporosis. X-rays may also demonstrate atypical spondylitis with syndesmophyte formation, resulting in hyperostosis and paravertebral ossification, which may lead to vertebral fusion.

Blood test findings typically include no RF, an elevated erythrocyte sedimentation rate, and an increased uric acid level.

Diagnostic tests also aim to rule out disorders that mimic psoriatic arthritis—fungal infections, Reiter's disease, gout, and rheumatoid arthritis, for example.

Treatment

For mild psoriatic arthritis, treatment is supportive and consists of immobilizing the affected joints with bed rest or splints, isometric exercises, paraffin baths, heat therapy, and aspirin and other nonsteroidal anti-inflammatory drugs (NSAIDs). Some patients respond well to low-dose systemic corticosteroids and topical corticosteroids to help control skin lesions.

In resistant cases, gold salts and methotrexate therapy may help to relieve both the articular and the cutaneous effects of psoriatic arthritis. Antimalarial agents are contraindicated because they can provoke exfoliative dermatitis.

Nursing diagnoses

- Altered protection
- Altered role performance
- Body image disturbance
- Fatigue
- Impaired physical mobility
- Impaired skin integrity
- Ineffective individual coping
- Pain

Nursing interventions

- Plan nursing care to relieve the patient's pain, preserve his skin integrity and joint mobility, and restore his body image and self-confidence.

- Provide active range-of-motion exercises during exacerbations.
- As ordered, administer NSAIDs and corticosteroids.
- Reassure the patient that psoriatic lesions aren't contagious. Avoid showing revulsion to unsightly psoriatic patches. Doing so will only reinforce the patient's altered self-image and fear of rejection.
- Encourage the patient to express his anxieties and concerns about restricted mobility and his physical appearance.
- Provide alternating activity and rest periods to help the patient avoid fatigue.

Patient teaching

- Explain the disease and treatment to the patient and his family.
- Encourage low-stress exercise—particularly swimming—to maintain the patient's strength and range of motion.
- Teach the patient how to apply skin care products and medications correctly; discuss possible adverse effects.
- Stress the importance of adequate rest and protection for affected joints.
- Encourage regular, moderate exposure to the sun.
- As needed, refer the patient to the local chapter of the Arthritis Foundation for self-help and support groups.

ANKYLOSING SPONDYLITIS

Also called rheumatoid spondylitis or Marie-Strümpell disease, ankylosing spondylitis primarily affects the sacroiliac, the axial spine, and the adjacent ligamentous or tendinous attachments to the bone.

Typically beginning in adults before age 40, this inflammatory disease progressively restricts spinal movement. It begins in the sacroiliac and gradually progresses to the lumbar, thoracic, and cervical spine. Bone and cartilage deterioration leads to fibrous tissue formation and eventual fusion of the spine or the peripheral joints. Symptoms progress unpredictably into remission, exacerbation, or arrest at any stage.

Usually ankylosing spondylitis occurs as a primary disorder, but it also may occur secondary to various GI, genitourinary, and cutaneous disorders. For example, with GI disease, ankylosing spondylitis may occur in association with ulcerative colitis, regional enteritis, Whipple's disease, gram-negative dysentery, and yersiniosis. With genitourinary disease, it's associated with chlamydial or mycoplasmic infections, and with cutaneous disease, it's associated with psoriasis, acne conglobata, and hidradenitis suppurativa.

In primary disease, sacroiliitis is usually bilateral and symmetrical; in secondary disease, it's usually unilateral and asymmetrical. The patient may also have extra-articular disease, such as acute anterior iritis (in about 25% of patients), proximal root aortitis and heart block, and apical pulmonary fibrosis. Rarely, extra-articular disease appears as caudal adhesive leptomeningitis and IgA nephropathy.

Ankylosing spondylitis affects men three to four times more often than women. Progressive disease is well recognized in men but often overlooked or missed in women, who tend to have more peripheral joint involvement.

Causes
Studies suggest a familial tendency for ankylosing spondylitis; however, the exact cause of the disease is unknown. In more than 90% of patients with this disease, circulating immune complexes and human leukocyte antigen (HLA)-B27 (the histocompatibility antigen) suggest immune system activity.

Complications
Rarely, disease progression can impose severe physical restrictions on activities of daily living and occupational functions. Atlantoaxial subluxation is a rare complication of primary ankylosing spondylitis.

Assessment findings
Varying assessment findings depend on the disease stage. The patient may first complain of intermittent low back pain that's most severe in the morning or after inactivity and relieved by exercise. He may also report mild fatigue, fever, anorexia, and weight loss. If he has symmetrical or asymmetrical peripheral arthritis, he may describe pain in his shoulders, hips, knees, and ankles.

The patient may also complain of pain over the symphysis pubis, which may lead to its mistaken identity as pelvic inflammatory disease. (See *Detecting spondylitis in women.*)

Observe the patient's movements. Note stiffness or limited motion of the lumbar spine; pain and limited expansion of the chest, resulting from costovertebral and sternomanubrial joint involvement; and limited range of motion, resulting from hip deformity.

Inspect the spine. In advanced disease, you'll see kyphosis (caused by chronic stooping to relieve discomfort). Inspect the eyes for redness and inflammation resulting from iritis.

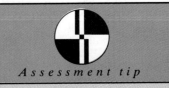

Assessment tip

DETECTING SPONDYLITIS IN WOMEN
Because ankylosing spondylitis seldom occurs in women, the disorder may be easily overlooked. Typically, if a woman's symptoms include pelvic pain, diagnosticians suspect pelvic inflammatory disease rather than ankylosing spondylitis. That's one reason to assess carefully if your female patient has apparent pelvic inflammatory disease but culture results identify no apparent cause. In compiling a thorough health and social history, investigate any possible family history of ankylosing spondylitis.

Otherwise, misdiagnosis may lead to unwarranted invasive tests and treatments and cause the patient needless anxiety related to contracting a sexually transmitted disease.

Palpate affected joints. Note any warmth, swelling, or tenderness.

Auscultate the heart and listen for an aortic murmur caused by regurgitation and cardiomegaly. Also auscultate the lungs. When present, upper lobe pulmonary fibrosis, which mimics tuberculosis, may reduce vital capacity to 70% or less of predicted volume.

Diagnostic tests
Diagnosis of primary ankylosing spondylitis requires meeting established criteria. (See *Diagnosing primary ankylosing spondylitis,* page 418.) Laboratory tests never confirm the diagnosis; however, the following findings may support the diagnosis:
• *Serum findings* include HLA-B27 in about 95% of patients with primary ankylosing spondylitis and up to 80% of patients with secondary disease. The absence of rheumatoid factor helps to rule out rheumatoid arthritis, which produces similar symptoms.
• *Erythrocyte sedimentation rate* and *alkaline phosphatase* and *creatine phosphokinase levels* may be slightly elevated in active disease.
• *Serum IgA levels* may be elevated.
• *X-ray studies* define characteristic changes in ankylosing spondylitis. However, these changes may not appear for up to 3 years after the disease's onset. They include bilateral sacroiliac involvement (the hallmark of the disease); blurring of the joints' bony margins in early dis-

DIAGNOSING PRIMARY ANKYLOSING SPONDYLITIS

The following are the diagnostic criteria for primary ankylosing spondylitis. For a reliable diagnosis, the patient must meet the following:
• criterion 7 and any one of criteria 1 through 5 *or*
• any five of criteria 1 through 6 if he doesn't have criterion 7.

Seven criteria
1. Axial skeleton stiffness of at least 3 months' duration relieved by exercise
2. Lumbar pain that persists at rest
3. Thoracic cage pain of at least 3 months' duration that persists at rest
4. Past or current iritis
5. Decreased lumbar range of motion
6. Decreased chest expansion (age-related)
7. Bilateral, symmetrical sacroiliitis demonstrated by radiographic studies

ease; patchy sclerosis with superficial bony erosions; eventual squaring of vertebral bodies; and "bamboo spine" with complete ankylosis.

Treatment
Because no treatment reliably stops disease progression, management aims to delay further deformity by good posture, stretching and deep-breathing exercises and, if appropriate, braces and lightweight supports. Heat, ice, and nerve stimulation measures may relieve symptoms in some patients. Nonsteroidal anti-inflammatory drugs, such as aspirin, indomethacin, and sulindac, control pain and inflammation.

Severe hip involvement, which affects about 15% of patients, usually necessitates hip replacement surgery. Severe spinal involvement may require a spinal wedge osteotomy to separate and reposition the vertebrae. Usually, this surgery is reserved for selected patients because of possible spinal cord damage and a lengthy convalescence.

Nursing diagnoses
• Activity intolerance
• Altered protection
• Fatigue
• Impaired gas exchange
• Impaired physical mobility
• Knowledge deficit
• Pain

Nursing interventions
• Keep in mind the patient's limited range of motion when planning self-care tasks and activities.
• Offer support and reassurance.
• Give analgesics, as ordered.
• Apply heat locally and massage as indicated. Assess mobility and comfort levels frequently.
• Have the patient perform active range-of-motion exercises to prevent restricted, painful movement.
• Pace periods of exercise and rest to help the patient achieve comfortable energy levels and oxygenation of lungs.
• If treatment includes surgery, ensure proper body alignment and positioning.
• Because ankylosing spondylitis is a chronic, progressively crippling condition, you'll need to involve other caregivers, such as a social worker, visiting nurse, and dietitian.

Patient teaching
• To minimize deformities, advise the patient to avoid any physical activity that places stress on the back, such as lifting heavy objects.
• Teach the patient to stand upright, to sit upright in a high, straight-backed chair, and to avoid leaning over a desk.
• Instruct him to sleep in a prone position on a hard mattress and to avoid using pillows under the neck or knees.
• Advise the patient to avoid prolonged walking, standing, sitting, or driving; to perform regular stretching and deep-breathing exercises; and to swim regularly, if possible.
• Instruct him to have his height measured every 3 to 4 months to detect kyphosis.
• Suggest that he seek vocational counseling if work requires standing or prolonged sitting at a desk.
• Tell him to contact the local arthritis agency or the Ankylosing Spondylitis Association for additional information and support.

SJÖGREN'S SYNDROME
The next most common autoimmune disorder after rheumatoid arthritis, Sjögren's syndrome results from a chronic exocrine gland dysfunction. Marked by diminished lacrimal and salivary gland secretion (sicca complex), the syndrome affects more women (about 90%) than men. The mean age of occurrence is 50.

Sjögren's syndrome may be a primary disorder, or it may be associated with inflammatory connective tissue disorders, such as rheumatoid arthritis (about 50% of patients), scleroderma, systemic lupus erythematosus, primary biliary cirrhosis, Hashimoto's thyroiditis, polyarteritis, and interstitial pulmonary fibrosis.

Nephritis (seldom leading to chronic renal failure) may affect up to 40% of patients with primary Sjögren's syndrome and may result in renal tubular acidosis in about 25% of patients.

Patients with Sjögren's syndrome may also have Raynaud's phenomenon (about 20%) and vasculitis (usually limited to the skin and may be systemic or localized in the legs). Sensory polyneuropathy and biochemical hypothyroidism (resembling Hashimoto's thyroiditis) occur in up to 50% of patients. Rarely, systemic necrotizing vasculitis develops and involves the skin, peripheral nerves, and GI tract.

Overall, the prognosis for a patient with Sjögren's syndrome is good.

Causes and pathophysiology

No one knows what causes Sjögren's syndrome. However, researchers think that genetic and environmental factors may contribute to its development. Viral or bacterial infection—or possibly exposure to pollen—may trigger this disease in a genetically susceptible person. Tissue damage results from infiltration by lymphocytes or deposition of immune complexes. Lymphocytic infiltration may be classified as benign lymphoma, malignant lymphoma, or pseudolymphoma (nonmalignant, but tumorlike, aggregates of lymphoid cells).

Complications

The disease seldom produces significant complications.

Assessment findings

The patient typically reports slowly developing dryness affecting the eyes (xerophthalmia), the mouth (xerostomia), and other organs. Initially, she may describe a foreign body sensation in the eye (gritty, sandy eye) along with redness, burning, photosensitivity, eye fatigue, itching, and mucoid discharge. She may also complain of a film across her eyes.

With oral dryness, the patient may report difficulty swallowing and talking; an abnormal taste or smell sensation (or both); thirst; ulcers of the tongue, mouth, and lips (especially at the corners of the mouth); and severe dental caries. (See *Dry mouth: Sign of Sjögren's syndrome?*)

With other dryness—of the respiratory tract, for example—the patient may report epistaxis, hoarseness, chronic nonproductive cough, recurrent otitis media, and

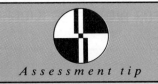

DRY MOUTH: SIGN OF SJÖGREN'S SYNDROME?

If the patient's history suggests Sjögren's syndrome, be sure to find out which prescription and nonprescription drugs she takes. Keep in mind that more than 200 commonly used drugs produce dry mouth.

frequent respiratory tract infections. With vaginal dryness, the patient may report dyspareunia and pruritus.

Additional complaints include generalized itching, fatigue, recurrent low-grade fever, and arthralgia or myalgia.

Inspection may disclose mouth ulcers, dental caries and, possibly, enlarged salivary glands.

Palpable purpura may be evident if the patient also has vasculitis. Palpable lymph node enlargement may be the first sign of malignant lymphoma or pseudolymphoma.

Diagnostic tests

For a diagnosis of Sjögren's syndrome, symptoms must meet specific criteria. (See *Criteria for diagnosing Sjögren's syndrome,* page 420.)

Laboratory test values in patients with Sjögren's syndrome include:
• elevated erythrocyte sedimentation rate in more than 90% of patients
• mild anemia and leukopenia in about 30% of patients
• hypergammaglobulinemia in about 50% of patients.

Various autoantibodies are also common, including antisalivary duct antibodies. Typically, 75% to 90% of patients test positive for rheumatoid factor, and between 50% and 80% of patients test positive for antinuclear antibodies.

Other test findings help support the diagnosis. To measure eye involvement, the patient may undergo Schirmer's test and a slit-lamp examination with rose bengal dye. Labial biopsy (to detect lymphoid foci) is a simple procedure with minimal risk—and the only specific diagnostic technique.

Salivary gland involvement may be evaluated by measuring the volume of parotid saliva, by secretory sialog-

CRITERIA FOR DIAGNOSING SJÖGREN'S SYNDROME

For a diagnosis of Sjögren's syndrome, the patient must have the following:
• keratoconjunctivitis sicca
• diminished salivary gland flow
• a positive salivary gland biopsy, showing mononuclear cell infiltration
• the presence of autoantibodies in a serum sample, indicating a systemic autoimmune process.

raphy, and by salivary scintigraphy. Salivary gland biopsy results typically show lymphocytic infiltration in Sjögren's syndrome; lower lip biopsy findings show salivary gland infiltration by lymphocytes.

Diagnosis must rule out other causes of ocular and oral dryness, including sarcoidosis, endocrine disorders, anxiety or depression, and effects of certain therapies, such as radiation to the head and neck. In patients with salivary gland and lymph node enlargement, diagnosis also must rule out cancer.

Treatment

Aimed at relieving symptoms, treatment includes conservative measures to moisten the eyes and mouth. Artificial tears and sustained-release cellulose capsules help to relieve ocular dryness. If an eye infection develops, the patient receives antibiotics; topical steroids should be avoided.

Mouth dryness can be relieved by using a methylcellulose swab or spray and by drinking plenty of fluids, especially at mealtime. Meticulous oral hygiene includes regular flossing, brushing, and fluoride treatments at home and frequent dental checkups.

Other treatment measures vary according to extraglandular effects. For parotid gland enlargement, treatment involves local heat and analgesia. For interstitial pulmonary and renal disease, treatment relies on corticosteroids. For cutaneous vasculitis, however, corticosteroids work less effectively.

If the patient has lymphoma, treatment includes a combination of chemotherapy, surgery, and radiation therapy.

Nursing diagnoses

• Altered oral mucous membrane
• Altered sexuality patterns
• Fatigue
• Impaired skin integrity
• Impaired swallowing
• Impaired tissue integrity
• Pain
• Risk for infection
• Risk for injury
• Sensory or perceptual alterations
• Sexual dysfunction

Nursing interventions

• Instill artificial tears as often as every 30 minutes to prevent eye damage (corneal ulcerations, corneal opacifications) from insufficient tear secretions. The patient may also benefit from instilling an eye ointment at bedtime or from using sustained-release cellulose capsules twice daily.
• Provide plenty of fluids—especially water—for the patient to drink and sugarless chewing gum or candies to promote oral moisture without promoting tooth decay.

Patient teaching

• Teach the patient how to instill eyedrops, ointments, or sustained-release capsules.
• Recommend that she wear sunglasses to protect her eyes from dust, wind, and strong light. Because dry eyes are more susceptible to infection, direct the patient to keep her face clean and to avoid rubbing her eyes.
• Instruct the patient to perform meticulous oral hygiene, including rinsing her mouth with a sodium bicarbonate solution (1 tsp [5 ml] per 8 oz [240 ml] water) to slow bacterial growth.
• Advise the patient to avoid saliva-decreasing drugs, such as atropine derivatives, antihistamines, anticholinergics, and antidepressants. Many nonprescription drugs contain these compounds.
• If mouth lesions make eating painful, suggest high-calorie, protein-rich liquid supplements to prevent malnutrition.
• Instruct the patient to avoid sugar, which contributes to dental caries, and tobacco, alcohol, and spicy, salty, or highly acidic foods, which cause mouth irritation.
• Urge the patient to humidify her home and work environments to help relieve respiratory tract dryness. Suggest using normal saline solution (in drop or spray form) to relieve nasal dryness.
• Advise the patient to avoid prolonged hot showers and baths and to use moisturizing lotions on dry skin. Suggest using a water-soluble gel as a vaginal lubricant.
• As appropriate, refer the patient to the Sjögren's Syndrome Foundation for further information and support.

DISCOID LUPUS ERYTHEMATOSUS

A form of lupus erythematosus marked by chronic skin eruptions, DLE can cause scarring and permanent disfigurement if untreated. About 5% of patients with DLE later develop SLE. An estimated 60% of patients with DLE are women in their late 20s or older. The disease seldom occurs in children. Its exact cause isn't known, although evidence suggests an autoimmune process.

Assessment findings
The patient with DLE has lesions that appear as raised, red, scaling plaques with follicular plugging and central atrophy. The raised edges and sunken centers give the lesions a coinlike appearance. Although these lesions can appear anywhere on the body, they usually erupt on the face, scalp, ears, neck, and arms or on any part of the body that is exposed to sunlight. Such lesions can resolve completely or may cause hypopigmentation or hyperpigmentation, atrophy, and scarring. Facial plaques sometimes assume the butterfly pattern characteristic of SLE. Hair becomes brittle and may fall out in patches.

Diagnostic tests
As a rule, the patient's history and the rash are enough to form the diagnosis. Positive findings in the LE cell test (in which polymorphonuclear leukocytes engulf cell nuclei to form so-called LE cells) occur in less than 10% of patients. Positive lesional skin biopsy results typically disclose immunoglobulins or complement components. SLE must be ruled out.

Treatment
Patients with DLE must avoid prolonged exposure to the sun, fluorescent lighting, and reflected sunlight. They should wear protective clothing, use sunscreens, avoid outdoor activity during peak sunlight periods (between 10 a.m. and 2 p.m.), and report any changes in the lesions.

As in SLE, drug treatment consists of topical, intralesional, and systemic medications.

LUPUS ERYTHEMATOSUS

A chronic inflammatory autoimmune disorder affecting the connective tissues, lupus erythematosus takes two forms: discoid lupus erythematosus (DLE) and systemic lupus erythematosus (SLE). DLE affects only the skin (see *Discoid lupus erythematosus*), whereas SLE affects multiple organs (including the skin) and can be fatal.

Researchers think that clinical signs and symptoms result from antibody-antigen trapping in specific organ capillaries. Like rheumatoid arthritis, SLE is characterized by recurrent seasonal remissions and exacerbations, especially during the spring and summer.

The annual incidence of SLE in urban populations varies from 15 to 50 per 100,000 persons. It strikes women 8 times more often than men (15 times more often during childbearing years). SLE occurs worldwide but is most prevalent among Asians and blacks.

The prognosis improves with early detection and treatment but remains poor for patients who have cardiovascular, renal, or neurologic complications or severe bacterial infections. The disease is incurable.

Causes and pathophysiology
The exact cause of SLE remains a mystery, but available evidence points to interrelated immune, environmental, hormonal, and genetic factors. Scientists think that autoimmunity is the primary cause. In autoimmunity, the body produces antibodies, such as antinuclear antibodies (ANAs), against its own cells. The formed antigen-antibody complexes then suppress the body's normal immunity and damage tissues. A significant feature in patients with SLE is their ability to produce antibodies against many different tissue components, such as red blood cells (RBCs), neutrophils, platelets, lymphocytes, or almost any organ or tissue in the body.

Certain predisposing factors may make a person susceptible to SLE. These include stress, streptococcal or viral infections, exposure to sunlight or ultraviolet light, immunization, pregnancy, and abnormal estrogen metabolism.

Complications
Concomitant infections, particularly urinary tract infections, and renal failure represent the leading causes of death for SLE patients.

Assessment findings
The onset of SLE, which may be acute or insidious, produces no characteristic clinical pattern. However, the patient may complain of fever, anorexia, weight loss, malaise, fatigue, abdominal pain, nausea, vomiting, diarrhea, constipation, rashes, and polyarthralgia. When taking the patient history, be sure to check the medication history. (See *Drug effects or SLE?* page 422.)

SLE can involve every organ system. Women may report irregular menstruation or amenorrhea, particularly

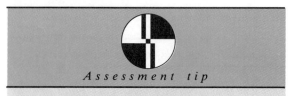

during flareups. In about 90% of patients, joint involvement resembles that of rheumatoid arthritis. Raynaud's phenomenon affects about 20% of patients. The patient may complain that sunlight (or ultraviolet light) provokes or aggravates skin eruptions. She may report chest pain (indicating pleuritis) and dyspnea (suggesting parenchymal infiltrates and pneumonitis).

Cardiopulmonary signs and symptoms occur in about 50% of patients. Watch for repeated arterial clotting to manifest itself in dyspnea, tachycardia, central cyanosis, and hypotension. These signs and symptoms may herald pulmonary emboli. Also be alert for altered level of consciousness, weakness of the extremities, and speech disturbances that point to cerebrovascular accident.

Seizure disorders and mental dysfunction may indicate neurologic damage. And some signs and symptoms signal added central nervous system (CNS) involvement. They include emotional instability, psychosis, organic brain syndrome, headaches, irritability, and depression.

If the patient reports oliguria, be alert for possible renal failure. If she complains of urinary frequency, dysuria, and bladder spasms, watch for other signs of urinary tract infection.

During inspection, observe for skin lesions. Ordinarily, these eruptions appear as an erythematous rash in areas exposed to light. The classic butterfly rash over the nose and cheeks appears in less than 50% of patients. The rash may vary in severity from malar erythema to discoid lesions (plaque). Also watch for patchy alopecia, which is common.

Check the patient's vital signs, intake and output, and weight. Inspect the mucous membranes, noting any painless ulcers. Look at the patient's hands and feet. Vasculitis may develop, especially in the digits. Inspect the skin of the arms and legs for infarctive lesions, necrotic leg ulcers, and digital gangrene.

With palpation, you may detect lymph node enlargement (diffuse or local and nontender). During auscultation, note any signs of cardiopulmonary abnormalities, such as pericardial friction rub (signaling pericarditis). Also note tachycardia and other signs of myocarditis and endocarditis.

Diagnostic tests

Laboratory tests include a complete blood count with differential (which may show anemia and a reduced white blood cell [WBC] count); platelet count (which may be decreased); erythrocyte sedimentation rate (usually elevated); and serum electrophoresis (which may detect hypergammaglobulinemia).

Difficult to detect, CNS involvement may account for abnormal EEG results in about 70% of patients. But brain and magnetic resonance imaging scans may be normal in patients with SLE despite CNS disease. (For more information, see *Diagnostic signs of SLE.*) Specific tests for SLE include the following studies:

• *ANA, anti-DNA,* and *lupus erythematosus (LE) cell tests* produce positive findings in most patients with active SLE, but they're only marginally useful in diagnosing the disease. The ANA test is sensitive but not specific for SLE, the anti-DNA test is specific but not sensitive, and the LE cell test is neither sensitive nor specific for SLE.

• *Urine studies* may detect RBCs, WBCs, urine casts and sediment, and significant protein loss (more than 3.5 g in 24 hours).

• *Blood studies* may demonstrate decreased serum complement (C3 and C4) levels, indicating active disease. Leukopenia, mild thrombocytopenia, and anemia also are seen during active disease.

• *Chest X-rays* may disclose pleurisy or lupus pneumonitis.

• *Electrocardiography* may show a conduction defect with cardiac involvement or pericarditis.

• *Renal biopsy* can show progression of SLE and the extent of renal involvement.

Treatment

The mainstay of SLE treatment is drug therapy. The patient with mild disease requires little or no medication. Nonsteroidal anti-inflammatory drugs, including aspirin, usually control arthritis and arthralgia symptoms. Skin lesions need topical medications and protection from exposure to the sun. Recommend that the patient use sunscreening agents with a sun protection factor of at least 15. Topical corticosteroid creams, such as triamcinolone and hydrocortisone, may be administered for mild disease.

Fluorinated steroids may control acute or discoid lesions. And refractory skin lesions may respond to intralesional or systemic corticosteroids or antimalarials, such as hydroxychloroquine and chloroquine. Because hydroxychloroquine and chloroquine can cause retinal damage, such treatment requires ophthalmologic examination every 6 months. Dapsone helps many patients.

Corticosteroids remain the treatment of choice for systemic symptoms of SLE, for acute generalized exacerbations, and for serious disease-related injury to vital organ systems from pleuritis, pericarditis, nephritis related to SLE, vasculitis, and CNS involvement. With initial prednisone doses (equivalent to 60 mg or more), the patient's condition usually improves noticeably within 48 hours. Then with symptoms under control, the patient discontinues, or tapers, prednisone's use slowly. (*Note:* Rising serum complement levels and decreasing anti-DNA titers indicate patient response.)

If the patient has glomerulonephritis, she'll need treatment with large doses of corticosteroids. Then, if renal failure occurs despite treatment, dialysis or kidney transplantation may be necessary.

In some patients, cytotoxic drugs, such as azathioprine, cyclophosphamide, and methotrexate, may delay or prevent renal deterioration. Antihypertensive drugs and dietary changes may also be effective. Additionally, warfarin is indicated for antiphospholipid antibodies, which can cause clotting in vascular structures.

Nursing diagnoses
- Altered nutrition: Less than body requirements
- Altered oral mucous membrane
- Altered protection
- Altered urinary elimination
- Body image disturbance
- Constipation
- Decreased cardiac output
- Diarrhea
- Fatigue
- Impaired physical mobility
- Impaired skin integrity
- Impaired tissue integrity
- Impaired verbal communication
- Ineffective breathing pattern
- Knowledge deficit
- Pain
- Risk for infection
- Sensory or perceptual alterations

DIAGNOSTIC SIGNS OF S.L.E.

Diagnosing SLE is far from easy because the disease so often mimics other disorders. Signs may be vague and may vary from patient to patient. For these reasons, the American Rheumatism Association has devised criteria for identifying SLE. Usually, four or more of the following signs must appear at some time in the disease course:
- discoid rash
- facial erythema (butterfly rash)
- hematologic abnormality (hemolytic anemia, leukopenia, lymphopenia, or thrombocytopenia)
- immune dysfunction (identified by positive LE cell, anti-DNA, or anti-Sm tests; or false-positive test results for syphilis for more than 6 months)
- neurologic disorder
- nonerosive arthritis
- oral ulcers
- photosensitivity
- positive ANA test results
- renal disorder
- serositis.

Nursing interventions
- Continually assess for signs and symptoms of organ involvement while offering the patient encouragement, emotional support, and thorough patient teaching.
- Monitor especially for hypertension, weight gain, and other signs of renal involvement.
- Evaluate possible neurologic damage signaled by personality changes, paranoid or psychotic behavior, depression, ptosis, and diplopia.
- Check urine, stools, and GI secretions for blood. Check the scalp for hair loss, and skin and mucous membranes for petechiae, bleeding, ulceration, pallor, and bruising.
- Provide a balanced diet. Foods high in protein, vitamins, and iron help maintain optimum nutrition and prevent anemia. However, renal involvement may mandate a low-sodium, low-protein diet. Provide bland, cool foods if the patient has a sore mouth.
- Urge the patient to get plenty of rest. Schedule diagnostic tests and procedures to allow adequate rest.
- Explain all tests and procedures. Tell the patient that several blood samples are needed initially, then periodically, to monitor progress.
- Apply heat packs to relieve joint pain and stiffness. Encourage regular exercise to maintain full range of motion and to prevent contractures.
- Explain the expected benefit of prescribed medications, and watch for adverse effects, especially when ad-

ministering high doses of corticosteroids or nonsteroidal anti-inflammatory drugs.

• Institute seizure precautions if you suspect CNS involvement.

• Warm and protect the patient's hands and feet if she has Raynaud's phenomenon.

• Arrange a physical therapy and occupational therapy consultation if musculoskeletal involvement compromises the patient's mobility.

• Support the patient's self-image. Offer female patients helpful tips. Suggest hypoallergenic cosmetics. As needed, refer her to a hairdresser who specializes in scalp disorders. Offer male patients similar advice, suggesting hypoallergenic hair care and shaving products.

Patient teaching

• Teach range-of-motion exercises and body alignment and postural techniques.

• Be sure the patient understands ways to avoid infection. Direct her to avoid crowds and people with known infections.

• Advise the patient to notify the doctor if fever, cough, or rash occurs or if chest, abdominal, muscle, or joint pain worsens.

• Instruct the photosensitive patient to wear protective clothing (hat, sunglasses, long-sleeved shirts or sweaters, and slacks) and to use a sunscreen when outdoors.

• Teach the patient to perform meticulous mouth care to relieve discomfort and prevent infection.

• Because SLE usually strikes women of childbearing age, questions associated with pregnancy commonly arise. The best evidence available indicates that a woman with SLE can have a safe, successful pregnancy if she sustains no serious renal or neurologic impairment. Advise her to seek additional medical care from a rheumatologist during her pregnancy. As indicated, explain that her doctors may order low-dose aspirin to reduce the risk of thrombosis during pregnancy.

• Warn the patient against trying unproven "miracle" drugs to relieve arthritis symptoms.

• Refer the patient to the Lupus Foundation of America and the Arthritis Foundation, as necessary.

GOODPASTURE'S SYNDROME

In this disorder, hemoptysis and rapidly progressive glomerulonephritis result from the deposition of antibodies against the alveolar and glomerular basement membranes. Goodpasture's syndrome may occur at any age but most commonly strikes men between ages 20 and 30. The prognosis improves with aggressive immuno-suppressant and antibiotic therapy and with dialysis or kidney transplantation.

Causes and pathophysiology

The cause of Goodpasture's syndrome is unknown. Although some cases have been associated with exposure to hydrocarbons or type 2 influenza, many have no precipitating events. The high incidence of human leukocyte antigen DR2 in patients with this disorder suggests a genetic predisposition.

Abnormal production and deposition of antibodies against glomerular basement membrane (GBM) and alveolar basement membrane activate the complement and inflammatory responses, resulting in glomerular and alveolar tissue damage.

Complications

Renal failure, requiring dialysis or transplantation, and severe pulmonary complications, such as pulmonary edema and hemorrhage, may occur.

Assessment findings

Initially, the patient with Goodpasture's syndrome may complain of malaise, fatigue, and pallor — signs and symptoms associated with severe iron deficiency anemia.

Your assessment may reveal hematuria and signs of peripheral edema associated with renal involvement. You may also note signs of pulmonary involvement, such as dyspnea and hemoptysis, ranging from a cough with blood-tinged sputum to frank pulmonary hemorrhage. The patient may have had subclinical pulmonary bleeding for months or years before developing overt hemorrhage and signs of renal disease.

Diagnostic tests

Measurement of circulating anti-GBM antibodies by radioimmunoassay, as well as linear staining of GBM and alveolar basement membrane by immunofluorescence, confirm the diagnosis.

Immunofluorescence of alveolar basement membrane shows linear deposition of immunoglobulins, as well as C3 and fibrinogen. Immunofluorescence of GBM also shows linear deposition of immunoglobulins. This finding, along with circulating anti-GBM antibodies, distinguishes Goodpasture's from other pulmonary-renal syndromes, such as Wegener's granulomatosis, polyarteritis, and systemic lupus erythematosus.

Lung biopsy shows interstitial and intra-alveolar hemorrhage with hemosiderin-laden macrophages. Chest X-rays reveal pulmonary infiltrates in a diffuse, nodular pattern, and renal biopsy frequently shows focal necrotic lesions and cellular crescents.

Serum creatinine and blood urea nitrogen (BUN) levels typically increase to two to three times normal. Urinalysis may reveal red blood cells and cellular casts, which typify glomerular inflammation. Tests may also show granular casts and proteinuria.

Treatment
Plasmapheresis may be used to remove antibodies, and immunosuppressants to suppress antibody production. Patients with renal failure may benefit from dialysis or kidney transplantation. Aggressive ultrafiltration helps relieve pulmonary edema that may aggravate pulmonary hemorrhage. High-dose I.V. corticosteroids also help control pulmonary hemorrhage.

Nursing diagnoses
• Activity intolerance
• Altered oral mucous membrane
• Altered urinary elimination
• Fatigue
• Fluid volume excess
• Impaired gas exchange
• Ineffective breathing pattern

Nursing interventions
• Elevate the head of the bed and administer humidified oxygen to promote adequate oxygenation. Assess respiratory rate and breath sounds regularly, and note the quantity and quality of the patient's sputum.
• Encourage the patient to conserve his energy. If he's bedridden, provide range-of-motion exercises. Assist with activities of daily living, and provide frequent rest periods.
• Monitor the patient's vital signs, arterial blood gas levels, hematocrit, and coagulation studies.
• Monitor the patient's daily intake and output, daily weight, creatinine clearance, and BUN and creatinine levels, and observe his signs and symptoms to determine his renal function.
• Transfuse blood and administer corticosteroids, as ordered. Watch the patient closely for signs of a transfusion reaction or an adverse reaction to the corticosteroids.

Patient teaching
• Stress the importance of conserving energy, especially if the patient develops iron deficiency anemia.
• Teach the patient to follow an appropriate diet—usually a low-protein diet if renal disease is significant. Explain that his fluid intake may also be restricted. Stress the

importance of complying with these measures to prevent further deterioration of renal tissue.
• If the patient has a sore, dry mouth, advise him to suck on sugarless hard candy.
• Teach the patient and his family the signs of respiratory or genitourinary bleeding. Tell them to report any such signs to the doctor at once.
• If the patient needs dialysis or kidney transplantation, refer him to a renal support group.

REITER'S SYNDROME
The dominant feature of this self-limiting syndrome is polyarthritis. Reiter's syndrome also causes urethritis, mucocutaneous lesions, and conjunctivitis or, less commonly, uveitis.

Reiter's syndrome usually affects young men ages 20 to 40; it seldom occurs in women and children. Most patients recover in 2 to 16 weeks. About 50% of patients have recurring acute attacks, whereas the rest follow a chronic course, experiencing continued synovitis and sacroiliitis.

Causes
Although the exact cause of Reiter's syndrome is unknown, most cases follow venereal or enteric infection. The high incidence of human leukocyte antigen (HLA)-B27 in patients with Reiter's syndrome (between 75% and 85% of patients) suggests a genetic susceptibility. The disease has also followed infections caused by *Mycoplasma, Shigella, Campylobacter, Salmonella, Yersinia,* and *Chlamydia* organisms. It's common in patients infected with the human immunodeficiency virus and usually precedes or follows the onset of acquired immunodeficiency syndrome.

Complications
Chronic heel pain, ankylosing spondylitis, and persistent joint pain and swelling commonly result from Reiter's syndrome. Up to 25% of patients have such crippling effects that they must change occupations. If anterior uveitis doesn't respond to treatment, ocular disease may progress to blindness. Reiter's syndrome may also cause such genitourinary complications as prostatitis and hemorrhagic cystitis.

Assessment findings
The patient may initially complain of dysuria, hematuria, urgent and frequent urination, and mucopurulent penile discharge, with swelling and reddening of the urethral meatus. He may also report suprapubic pain,

fever, and anorexia with weight loss. Inspection of the penis may reveal small, painless ulcers on the glans penis (balanitis); these ulcers may coalesce to form irregular patches covering the penis and scrotum.

Arthritic symptoms usually follow genitourinary or enteric signs and symptoms and often last from 2 to 4 months. The patient is most likely to complain of asymmetrical and extremely variable polyarticular arthritis, usually in weight-bearing joints of the legs and sometimes in the low back or sacroiliac joints. If arthritis has developed, the patient may report warm, erythematous, and painful joints, or he may have only mild symptoms, with minimal synovitis.

On inspection, you may note muscle wasting near affected joints. The patient's fingers and toes may appear swollen and sausagelike.

Ocular signs and symptoms include mild bilateral conjunctivitis, possibly complicated by uveitis, keratitis, iritis, retinitis, or optic neuritis. In severe cases, the patient may complain of burning, itching, and profuse mucopurulent discharge. Inspection of the eyes may reveal redness and swelling.

In 30% of patients, you may observe skin lesions (keratoderma blennorrhagicum), which resemble pustular psoriasis with involvement of the skin and nails. These lesions develop 4 to 6 weeks after the onset of other signs and symptoms and may last for several weeks. They occur most commonly on the palms and soles but can develop anywhere on the trunk, extremities, or scalp.

You may also note that the patient's nails become thick, opaque, and brittle, with an accumulation of keratic debris under the nails. In many patients, painless, transient ulcerations erupt on the buccal mucosa, palate, and tongue.

Diagnostic tests

Most patients with Reiter's syndrome test positive for HLA-B27. Tests also show an elevated white blood cell (WBC) count and erythrocyte sedimentation rate and may show mild anemia. Examination of urethral discharge and synovial fluid reveals many WBCs, mostly polymorphonuclear leukocytes; synovial fluid is also grossly purulent and high in complement and protein. Cultures of urethral discharge and synovial fluid rule out other causes, such as disseminated gonococcal disease.

During the first few weeks of the syndrome, X-rays are normal. They may remain so, but in some patients, they may show osteoporosis in inflamed areas. If inflammation persists, X-rays may show erosions of the small joints, periosteal proliferation (new bone formation) of involved joints, and calcaneal spurs. Late findings include asymmetrical sacroiliitis.

Treatment

No specific treatment exists for Reiter's syndrome. During acute stages, the patient may be restricted to limited weight bearing or may need complete bed rest.

Nonsteroidal anti-inflammatory drugs (NSAIDs), such as indomethacin, can help relieve discomfort and fever. If the patient doesn't respond to NSAIDs, the doctor may prescribe such cytotoxic agents as azathioprine or methotrexate to alleviate debilitating signs and symptoms. Corticosteroids may help control persistent skin lesions; gold therapy may have limited value for bony erosion.

Physical therapy includes range-of-motion and strengthening exercises and the use of padded or supportive shoes to prevent contractures and deformities of the feet.

Nursing diagnoses
• Altered nutrition: Less than body requirements
• Altered oral mucous membrane
• Altered role performance
• Altered sexuality patterns
• Altered urinary elimination
• Fatigue
• Impaired physical mobility
• Impaired skin integrity
• Impaired tissue integrity
• Pain
• Risk for infection
• Sensory or perceptual alterations

Nursing interventions
• Maintain an accepting, nonjudgmental attitude to relieve any embarrassment the patient may feel if the disorder is associated with sexual activity.
• Follow universal precautions. Be particularly careful when handling linens, dressings, or clothing that touches the patient's genitalia.
• Provide rest and analgesia as needed.
• Provide a high-calorie, high-protein diet to ensure adequate nutrition.
• Develop an exercise regimen with the physical therapist and patient. Make sure it helps the patient maintain flexion, good body alignment, and posture.
• If the patient has severe or chronic joint impairment, arrange for occupational counseling.

Patient teaching
• Explain Reiter's syndrome to the patient. Counsel him to use condoms and to avoid multiple sex partners, and teach him steps he can take to avoid exposure to enteric pathogens, such as avoiding anal intercourse.
• Explain the recommended medications and their possible adverse effects. Warn the patient to take NSAIDs with meals or milk to prevent GI bleeding.
• Encourage normal daily activity and moderate exercise, as well as good posture and body mechanics. Suggest the patient use a firm mattress.

SYSTEMIC SCLEROSIS
Also called scleroderma, systemic sclerosis is a diffuse connective tissue disease. It's characterized by fibrotic, degenerative and, occasionally, inflammatory changes in skin, blood vessels, synovial membranes, skeletal muscles, and internal organs (especially the esophagus, intestinal tract, thyroid, heart, lungs, and kidneys).

Systemic sclerosis occurs in two distinct forms: localized (CREST syndrome) and diffuse. CREST syndrome, the more benign form, accounts for 80% of cases. It causes calcinosis cutis, Raynaud's phenomenon, esophageal dysfunction, sclerodactyly, and telangiectasia. Diffuse systemic sclerosis, which accounts for 20% of cases, is marked by generalized skin thickening and invasion of internal organ systems.

Eosinophilic fasciculitis, a rare variant of systemic sclerosis, causes skin changes similar to those of diffuse systemic sclerosis but limited to the fascia. Other differences from systemic sclerosis include eosinophilia, an absence of Raynaud's phenomenon, a good response to prednisone, and an increased risk of aplastic anemia.

Systemic sclerosis is twice as common in women as in men. It usually occurs between ages 30 and 50.

Causes
The cause of systemic sclerosis is unknown.

Complications
In advanced disease, cardiac and pulmonary fibrosis produce arrhythmias and dyspnea. Renal involvement usually causes malignant hypertension, the major cause of death from this disease.

Assessment findings
Ninety percent of patients complain of symptoms of Raynaud's phenomenon—blanching, cyanosis, and erythema of the fingers and toes in response to stress or exposure to cold. These symptoms may precede diagnosis of systemic sclerosis by months or even years. As the disease progresses, the patient may complain of pain, stiffness, and swelling of fingers and joints.

Eventually, the patient may complain of frequent reflux, heartburn, dysphagia (in 90% of patients), and bloating after meals, all stemming from motility abnormalities, GI fibrosis, and malabsorption. These symptoms may cause her to eat less and lose weight. Other common GI complaints include abdominal distention, diarrhea, constipation, and malodorous floating stools.

In the early stages, inspection may reveal thickened, hidelike skin with loss of normal skin folds. You may also note telangiectasia and areas of pigmentation and depigmentation. The patient's fingers may have shortened because of progressive phalangeal resorption. You may observe slowly healing ulcers on the tips of the fingers or toes—the result of compromised circulation. These ulcers may lead to gangrene.

Later, inspection may disclose taut, shiny skin over the entire hand and forearm from skin thickening. Facial skin may also appear tight and inelastic, causing a wrinkle-free, masklike appearance and a pinched mouth. As tightening progresses, contractures may develop.

With pulmonary involvement, you may observe dyspnea and auscultate decreased breath sounds. With cardiac involvement, you may auscultate an irregular cardiac rhythm, pericardial friction rub, and an atrial gallop. Your assessment may also reveal hypertension if renal involvement occurs.

Diagnostic tests
Typical cutaneous changes provide the first clue to diagnosis. Results of diagnostic tests include the following:
• *Blood studies* show mild anemia, slightly elevated erythrocyte sedimentation rate, hypergammaglobulinemia, positive rheumatoid factor (in 25% to 35% of patients), positive lupus erythematosus preparation, positive antinuclear antibody (low titer, speckled or nucleolar pattern) and, with diffuse systemic sclerosis, scleroderma antibody (in about 35% of patients).
• *Urinalysis* reveals proteinuria, microscopic hematuria, and casts (with renal involvement).
• *Hand X-rays* show terminal phalangeal tuft resorption, subcutaneous calcification, and joint space narrowing and erosion.
• *Chest X-rays* demonstrate bilateral basilar pulmonary fibrosis.
• *GI X-rays* disclose distal esophageal hypomotility and stricture, duodenal loop dilation, small-bowel malabsorption pattern, and large diverticula.

• *Pulmonary function studies* reveal decreased diffusion, vital capacity, and lung compliance.
• *ECG* detects possible nonspecific abnormalities related to myocardial fibrosis.
• *Skin biopsy* shows possible changes consistent with the progress of the disease, such as marked thickening of the dermis and occlusive vessel changes.

Treatment

No cure exists for systemic sclerosis. Treatment aims to preserve normal body functions and minimize complications. Immunosuppressants, such as chlorambucil, can help relieve symptoms. Used experimentally, corticosteroids and colchicine seem to stabilize symptoms; D-penicillamine may also be helpful. The patient should have her blood platelet levels monitored throughout immunosuppressant therapy.

Other treatment varies according to symptoms:
• *Raynaud's phenomenon.* Treatment consists of various vasodilators, calcium channel blockers, and antihypertensive agents (such as methyldopa), along with intermittent cervical sympathetic blockade or, rarely, thoracic sympathectomy.
• *Chronic digital ulcerations.* A digital plaster cast immobilizes the affected area, minimizes trauma, and maintains cleanliness; the patient may also need surgical debridement.
• *Esophagitis with stricture.* The patient receives antacids, a histamine₂ antagonist (such as omeprazole, cimetidine, or ranitidine), a soft bland diet, and periodic esophageal dilation.
• *Small-bowel involvement.* The patient receives broad-spectrum antibiotics, such as erythromycin or tetracycline, to counteract bacterial overgrowth in the duodenum and jejunum related to hypomotility.
• *Scleroderma kidney (with malignant hypertension and impending renal failure).* The patient needs dialysis, antihypertensives, and calcium channel blockers; if hypertensive crisis develops, she may receive an angiotensin-converting enzyme inhibitor.
• *Hand debilitation.* Treatment consists of physical therapy to maintain function and promote muscle strength, heat therapy to relieve joint stiffness, and patient teaching to help the patient perform activities of daily living.
• *Pulmonary manifestations.* The patient receives oral or parenteral cyclophosphamide to relieve symptoms of dyspnea, crackles, and constrictive pulmonary function.

Nursing diagnoses

• Activity intolerance
• Altered body image
• Altered family processes
• Altered nutrition: Less than body requirements
• Altered tissue perfusion
• Constipation
• Decreased cardiac output
• Diarrhea
• Fatigue
• Fear
• Impaired gas exchange
• Impaired physical mobility
• Impaired skin integrity
• Ineffective family coping
• Ineffective individual coping
• Pain
• Risk for infection

Nursing interventions

• Regularly assess mobility restrictions, vital signs, level of pain, intake and output, respiratory function, and daily weight.
• Because of compromised digital circulation, don't perform any finger-stick blood tests. Provide gloves or sock mittens after warming therapy.
• Use plaster wraps or topical ointments to lessen the painful effects of digital ulcerations.
• If the patient has cardiac and pulmonary fibrosis, provide rest and pulmonary exercises. Coughing, deep breathing, and chest physiotherapy will help keep her lungs clear.
• Provide a high-calorie diet that's smooth, cool, and palatable. Consult the dietitian to ensure the patient has a nutritious, appealing diet. Treat GI disturbances as necessary with antacids and antidiarrheals.
• If the patient suffers from delayed gastric emptying, offer her small, frequent meals and have her remain upright for at least 2 hours after eating. This should help improve her digestion and maintain weight.
• Whenever possible, let the patient participate in treatment by measuring her own intake and output, planning her own diet, assisting in dialysis, giving herself heat therapy, and performing prescribed exercises.
• Help the patient and her family accept the fact that this condition is incurable. Encourage them to express their feelings, and help them cope with their fears and frustrations.

Patient teaching

• Teach the patient and her family about the disease, its treatment, and relevant diagnostic tests.
• Warn the patient to avoid air conditioning, cool showers and baths, and preparing food under cold running water,

which may aggravate Raynaud's phenomenon. Also, advise her to wear gloves or mittens outside, even in mild weather; she may want to wear them indoors, too.

• Help the patient and her family adjust to her new body image and to the limitations and dependence that these changes cause. To reduce fatigue, teach the patient to pace her activities and organize schedules to include necessary rest and exercise.

• Advise the patient to avoid contact with people who have active infections (especially of the upper respiratory tract).

• Urge the patient to maintain a high-calorie diet. Warn her that supplements may not help her overall condition because they often contribute to diarrhea.

• Advise the patient with GI involvement to avoid late-night meals, to elevate the head of the bed, and to use prescribed antacids and histamine₂ antagonists to reduce the incidence of reflux and resulting scarring.

• If the patient needs dialysis, refer her to the National Kidney Foundation's local support group. Explain that she may have to limit certain foods and liquids for the rest of her life. Reassure her that dialysis can be done close to or in her home.

POLYMYOSITIS AND DERMATOMYOSITIS

Diffuse, inflammatory myopathies, polymyositis and dermatomyositis produce symmetrical weakness of striated muscle—primarily proximal muscles of the shoulder and pelvic girdle, neck, and pharynx. In dermatomyositis, such weakness is accompanied by cutaneous involvement. These diseases usually progress slowly, with frequent exacerbations and remissions.

Polymyositis and dermatomyositis are twice as common in women as in men (with the exception of dermatomyositis with cancer, which is most common in men over age 40). Generally, the prognosis worsens with age. Although 80% to 90% of affected children regain normal function if properly treated, untreated childhood dermatomyositis may rapidly progress to disabling contractures and muscle atrophy.

Causes and pathophysiology

Although the cause of polymyositis and dermatomyositis is unknown, the diseases may result from autoimmunity, perhaps combined with defective T-cell function. Presumably, the patient's T cells inappropriately recognize muscle fiber antigens as foreign, and release lymphotoxins that cause diffuse or focal muscle fiber degeneration.

Regeneration of new muscle cells then follows, producing remission.

These diseases may be associated with allergic reactions, systemic lupus erythematosus (SLE), scleroderma, rheumatoid arthritis, Sjögren's syndrome, penicillamine administration, systemic viral infection, and carcinomas of the lung, breast, and other organs.

Complications

Associated cancer, respiratory disease, and heart failure can cause death.

Assessment findings

Onset of polymyositis can be acute or insidious with weakness, tenderness, and discomfort. The patient may complain of these symptoms in such proximal muscles as the shoulder and pelvic girdle more commonly than in distal muscles; she may also complain of aching pain in the buttocks. She may report weakness that impairs ordinary activities. For instance, she may have trouble getting up from a chair or a kneeling position, combing her hair, reaching into a high cupboard, climbing stairs, or even raising her head from a pillow.

Other musculoskeletal signs and symptoms include an inability to move against resistance, proximal dysphagia (regurgitation of fluid through the nose), and dysphonia (nasal voice). The patient may also report signs of Raynaud's phenomenon. Palpation may reveal tenderness in the buttocks area.

A patient with dermatomyositis may report a rash over much of her upper body and swelling around her eyes. Inspection may reveal a dusky red rash, usually located on the butterfly area of the face, neck, upper back, chest, shoulders, and arms and around the nail beds. A characteristic heliotropic (purplish) rash may appear on the eyelids, accompanied by periorbital edema. Inspection of the fingers may disclose subungual erythema, cuticular telangiectasis, and scaly, violet, flat-topped patches over the dorsum of the proximal interphalangeal and metacarpophalangeal joints (Gottron's papules).

Diagnostic tests

Muscle biopsy that shows necrosis, degeneration, regeneration, and interstitial chronic lymphocytic infiltration allows diagnosis.

Appropriate laboratory tests differentiate polymyositis from diseases that cause similar muscular or cutaneous symptoms, such as muscular dystrophy, advanced trichinosis, psoriasis, seborrheic dermatitis, and SLE. Typical results in polymyositis include the following:

• mildly elevated erythrocyte sedimentation rate

• elevated white blood cell count
• elevated muscle enzyme levels (creatine phosphokinase, aldolase, aspartate aminotransferase [formerly SGOT]) not attributable to hemolysis of red blood cells or hepatic or other diseases
• increased urine creatine levels (more than 150 mg/24 hours)
• decreased creatinine levels
• electromyography showing polyphasic, short-duration potentials; fibrillation (positive spikes); and bizarre, high-frequency, repetitive changes
• positive antinuclear antibodies.

Treatment

High-dose corticosteroid therapy (40 to 60 mg/day) relieves inflammation and lowers muscle enzyme levels. Within 2 to 6 weeks after treatment, serum muscle enzyme levels usually return to normal and muscle strength improves, permitting a gradual titration of corticosteroid dosage. If the patient responds poorly to corticosteroids, treatment may include cytotoxic or immunosuppressant drugs, such as cyclophosphamide, azathioprine, and methotrexate given intermittently I.V. or daily by mouth.

Supportive therapy includes bed rest during the acute phase, range-of-motion exercises to prevent contractures, analgesics and application of heat to relieve painful muscle spasms, and diphenhydramine to relieve itching. Patients over age 40 need thorough assessment for coexisting cancer.

Nursing diagnoses

• Activity intolerance
• Altered urinary elimination
• Fatigue
• Fear
• Impaired physical mobility
• Impaired skin integrity
• Pain
• Risk for infection
• Self-care deficit

Nursing interventions

• Assess the patient's level of pain, weakness, and range of motion daily. Administer analgesics as needed.
• If the patient is confined to bed, prevent pressure ulcers by giving good skin care. To prevent footdrop and contractures, make sure the patient wears high-topped sneakers, and assist with passive range-of-motion exercises at least four times daily. Begin exercise therapy as soon as possible to prevent deterioration and contrac-

tures. Allow the patient's family to assist in performing these exercises.
• If 24-hour urine collection for creatine and creatinine tests are necessary, make sure the staff, patient, and family understand the collection procedure.
• When you assist with muscle biopsy, make sure the biopsy specimen isn't taken from an area of recent needle insertion, such as an injection or electromyography site.
• If the patient has a rash, warn her against scratching, which may cause infection. If antipruritic drugs don't relieve severe itching, apply tepid sponges or compresses. If the patient is young or scratches during her sleep, provide lightweight cotton gloves to protect the skin.
• Alternate activities with rest periods to prevent excessive fatigue.

Patient teaching

• Explain the disease and its complications to the patient and encourage her to express her anxiety. Ease her fear of dependence by reassuring her that weakness will probably pass.
• Prepare the patient and her family for diagnostic procedures and possible adverse effects of corticosteroid therapy, such as hirsutism and edema.
• Reassure the patient that corticosteroid-induced weight gain will diminish when therapy ends, but warn her not to discontinue the drug abruptly.
• Advise the patient to follow a low-sodium diet to prevent fluid retention.
• Teach the family how to help the patient with range-of-motion exercises. Involve the family in the prescribed home exercise program.
• Encourage the patient to feed and dress herself to the best of her ability but to ask for help when needed. Advise her to pace her activities to combat weakness.

VASCULITIS

An autoimmune condition, vasculitis includes a broad spectrum of disorders characterized by blood vessel inflammation and necrosis. Clinical effects depend on the vessels involved and reflect tissue ischemia caused by blood flow obstruction.

The prognosis varies with the disease form. For example, hypersensitivity vasculitis is usually benign and limited to the skin, whereas the more extensive polyarteritis nodosa can be rapidly fatal.

Except for the mucocutaneous lymph node syndrome, which affects only children, vasculitis can affect a person at any age. Vasculitis may be a primary disorder or secondary to other disorders, such as rheumatoid arthritis and systemic lupus erythematosus.

Causes and pathophysiology

Exactly how vascular damage develops in vasculitis isn't well understood. Some think that vasculitis may follow serious infectious disease, such as hepatitis B and bacterial endocarditis, and may be related to high doses of antibiotics.

Current theory holds that vasculitis is initiated by excessive circulating antigen, which triggers the formation of soluble antigen-antibody complexes. Then, because the reticuloendothelial system cannot effectively clear these complexes, they're deposited in blood vessel walls (Type III hypersensitivity). Theorists think that increased vascular permeability (associated with release of vasoactive amines by platelets and basophils) enhances this deposition. The deposited complexes activate the complement cascade. The result: chemotaxis of neutrophils, which release lysosomal enzymes, which in turn, cause vessel damage and necrosis. These effects may precipitate thrombosis, occlusion, hemorrhage, and tissue ischemia.

Another mechanism that may contribute to vascular damage is the cell-mediated (T-cell) immune response, whereby circulating antigen triggers sensitized lymphocytes to release soluble mediators. This attracts macrophages, which release intracellular enzymes, causing vascular damage. They can also transform into the epithelioid and multinucleated giant cells that typify the granulomatous vasculitides. Macrophagic phagocytosis of immune complexes enhances granuloma formation.

Complications

Renal, cardiac, and hepatic involvement can be fatal if vasculitis isn't treated. Renal failure, renal hypertension, glomerulitis, fibrous scarring of the lung tissue, cerebrovascular accident, and GI bleeding are a few of the severe complications associated with vasculitis.

Assessment findings

Patient history and physical assessment findings will vary, depending on the blood vessels involved. (See *Types of vasculitis*, pages 432 to 434.)

Diagnostic tests

Not all vasculitis disorders can be diagnosed definitively by specific tests. The most useful general diagnostic procedure is biopsy of the affected vessel. In some disorders, arteriography may be informative.

Treatment

Appropriate treatment aims to minimize irreversible tissue damage associated with ischemia. In primary vasculitis, treatment may involve removal of an offending antigen or use of anti-inflammatory or immunosuppressant drugs. Antigenic drugs, food, and other offending environmental substances should be identified and eliminated, if possible.

Drug therapy in primary vasculitis typically involves daily administration of low-dose oral cyclophosphamide and corticosteroids.

In rapidly fulminant vasculitis, the daily cyclophosphamide dose may be increased significantly for the first 2 to 3 days and then returned to the regular dose. In addition, the patient usually receives prednisone in daily divided doses for 7 to 10 days, with consolidation to a single morning dose by 2 to 3 weeks. When the vasculitis appears to be in remission, or when prescribed cytotoxic drugs take full effect, corticosteroid therapy is tapered to a single daily dose and then to an alternate-day schedule that may continue for 3 to 6 months.

In secondary vasculitis, treatment focuses on the underlying disorder.

Nursing diagnoses

- Activity intolerance
- Altered nutrition: Less than body requirements
- Altered oral mucous membrane
- Altered tissue perfusion
- Body image disturbance
- Decreased cardiac output
- Hyperthermia
- Impaired gas exchange
- Impaired physical mobility
- Impaired skin integrity
- Ineffective breathing pattern
- Pain
- Risk for infection
- Risk for injury
- Sensory or perceptual alterations

Nursing interventions

- Assess for dry nasal mucosa in patients with Wegener's granulomatosis. Instill nose drops to lubricate the mucosa and to minimize crusting. Or irrigate the nasal passages with warm 0.9% sodium chloride solution.
- Monitor vital signs. Use a Doppler ultrasonic flowmeter, if available, to auscultate blood pressure in patients who have Takayasu's arteritis and whose peripheral pulses are difficult to palpate.

(Text continues on page 434.)

TYPES OF VASCULITIS

Vasculitis is a diverse group of inflammatory conditions, all of which cause vascular necrosis. Notable types are listed here, together with typical assessment and diagnostic findings.

Type	Assessment findings	Diagnostic test findings
Polyarteritis nodosa		
• This disorder affects small to medium-size arteries throughout the body. Lesions, which tend to be segmental and located at arterial bifurcations and branchings, spread distally to arterioles. In patients with severe disease, lesions circumferentially involve adjacent veins. • Aneurysms, hemorrhage, thrombosis, and fibrosis occur. Although any vessel can be affected, commonly involved ones are in the kidneys, heart, liver, GI tract, muscle, and testes. • The disorder affects males twice as frequently as females. Average onset is at age 45.	• Abdominal pain, myalgia, headache, hypertension, joint pain, weakness, weight loss, and malaise may occur. • The patient may also report signs and symptoms of specific organ dysfunction, such as chest pain, seizures, altered mental status, and edema.	• Laboratory findings include elevated erythrocyte sedimentation rate (ESR); leukocytosis; anemia; thrombocytosis; hypergammaglobulinemia; depressed C3 complement levels; rheumatoid factor (RF) titer greater than 1:60; and circulating immune complexes. • Tissue biopsy reveals the disease's hallmark: acute necrotizing inflammation of the arterial media with fibrinoid necrosis and extensive inflammatory cell infiltration of all coats of the vessel and surrounding tissue. • Arteriography demonstrates characteristic abnormalities, such as aneurysms in the small and medium-size arteries of the kidneys and abdominal viscera.
Allergic angiitis and granulomatosis (Churg-Strauss syndrome)		
• These disorders affect small to medium-size arteries and arterioles, capillaries, and venules, mainly in the lungs but also in other organs. The disorders resemble polyarteritis nodosa but include intravascular and extravascular granuloma formation, eosinophilic tissue infiltration, and associated severe asthma and peripheral eosinophilia. • The disorders strike men more commonly than women. Average age at onset is 44, but the disorders can occur at any age.	• The patient usually reports symptoms similar to those of polyarteritis nodosa and severe pulmonary involvement (asthma).	• Typical laboratory results are similar to those in polyarteritis nodosa. Eosinophilia (greater than 1,000 cells/ml) may also be seen. • Tissue biopsy shows granulomatous inflammation with eosinophilic infiltration. • X-ray studies show pulmonary infiltrates.
Polyangiitis overlap syndrome		
• This syndrome affects small to medium-size arteries and other vessels in the lungs and other organs.	• The patient usually complains of symptoms of polyarteritis nodosa and allergic angiitis and granulomatosis.	• Laboratory findings are the same as those in polyarteritis nodosa and allergic angiitis and granulomatosis. • Tissue biopsy shows granulomatous inflammation with eosinophilic infiltration. • X-rays show pulmonary infiltrates.

TYPES OF VASCULITIS *(continued)*

Type	Assessment findings	Diagnostic test findings
Wegener's granulomatosis		
• This type of vasculitis involves small to medium-size vessels of the respiratory tract and the kidneys (causing glomerulonephritis). • The patient may be any age, but the average age at onset is 40. • The incidence is only slightly higher in men than in women.	• The patient usually reports fever, paranasal sinus pain and drainage, pulmonary congestion, cough, dyspnea, malaise, anorexia, and weight loss. Serous otitis media may occur. • Inspection may reveal saddle nose deformity, skin lesions, and purulent or bloody nasal discharge with or without nasal mucosal ulceration. You may also detect eye involvement, such as conjunctivitis, episcleritis, scleritis, granulomatous sclerouveitis, ciliary vessel vasculitis, and proptosis (bulging) from lesions of the retro-orbital mass. • Clinical findings may include pericarditis and, rarely, cardiomyopathy. Renal involvement may cause glomerulitis, possibly leading to renal failure.	• Laboratory tests may detect anemia and leukocytosis; mild hypergammaglobulinemia (particularly IgA); elevated ESR; mildly elevated RF levels; circulating immune complexes; and antineutrophil cytoplasmic autoantibodies. • Tissue biopsy may demonstrate necrotizing vasculitis with granulomatous inflammation.
Temporal arteritis (giant cell arteritis)		
• This disorder occurs in medium-size to large arteries, usually the branches of the carotid artery and particularly the temporal artery. • The typical patient is a woman over age 55. (The disorder seldom occurs in blacks.)	• The patient may complain of fever, myalgia, malaise, fatigue, anorexia, weight loss, sweats, arthralgia, jaw and tongue claudication, headache, and stiffness, aching, and pain in the muscles of the neck, shoulders, lower back, hips, and thighs associated with polymyalgia rheumatica. • The patient may also report sudden blindness (caused by ischemic optic neuritis).	• Laboratory results include monochromic or slightly hypochromic anemia, elevated ESR, and increased levels of alkaline phosphatase, IgG, complement, and circulating immune complexes. • Tissue biopsy shows panarteritis with infiltration of mononuclear cells, giant cells within the vessel wall, fragmentation of internal elastic lamina, and proliferation of intima.
Takayasu's arteritis (aortic arch syndrome)		
• This syndrome affects medium-size to large arteries, particularly the aortic arch and its branches and, possibly, the pulmonary artery. There, inflammatory mononuclear cell infiltrates and giant cells appear in the vessel wall, resulting in marked proliferation and fibrosis, scarring and vascularization of the media, and disruption and degeneration of the elastic lamina. Cardiomegaly and cardiac failure secondary to aortic or pulmonary hypertension commonly occur and may progress to cerebrovascular accident. • Most patients are adolescent and young women.	• The patient may report malaise, fever, nausea, night sweats, arthralgia, anorexia, weight loss, pain or paresthesia distal to affected areas, syncope, and—if the carotid artery is involved—diplopia and transient blindness. • On inspection, you may notice pallor. On palpation, you may not find a distal pulse. Auscultation may disclose bruits and aortic regurgitation.	• Laboratory reports may indicate anemia, leukocytosis, positive lupus erythematosus cell findings, elevated immunoglobulin levels, and elevated ESR. • Tissue biopsy findings include inflammation of vascular adventitia and intima and thickening of vessel walls. • Arteriography may disclose irregular vessel walls, stenosis, poststenotic dilation, aneurysms, and calcified, obstructed vessels.

(continued)

TYPES OF VASCULITIS *(continued)*

Type	Assessment findings	Diagnostic test findings
Hypersensitivity vasculitis		
• A heterogenous group of disorders thought to be caused by a hypersensitivity reaction, this vasculitis type involves small vessels, especially those of the skin. • The disorders affect both sexes and all age-groups.	• The patient typically reports such symptoms as fever, malaise, myalgia, and anorexia. • Inspection may reveal palpable purpura, papules, nodules, vesicles, bullae, ulcers, or chronic or recurrent urticaria.	• Laboratory findings usually include mild leukocytosis with or without eosinophilia and elevated ESR. • Tissue biopsy shows leukocytoblastic angiitis, usually in postcapillary venules, with infiltration of polymorphonuclear leukocytes, fibrinoid necrosis, and extravasation of erythrocytes.
Mucocutaneous lymph node syndrome (Kawasaki disease)		
• In this syndrome, small to medium-size vessels, primarily of the lymph nodes, are affected. Lesions may progress to involve coronary arteries. Other effects include intimal proliferation and infiltration of the vessel wall with mononuclear cells. Beadlike aneurysms and thromboses may occur along the artery. • The syndrome may progress to myocarditis, pericarditis, myocardial infarction, and cardiomegaly. Although usually benign and self-limiting, it can be fatal if coronary artery aneurysms develop.	• The patient usually reports fever and other signs, such as inflamed neck glands (nonsuppurative cervical adenitis), edema, and conjunctival congestion. • Inspection findings may include erythema of the mouth, lips, and palms and desquamation of the fingertips.	• Tissue biopsy shows intimal proliferation and vessel walls infiltrated with mononuclear cells.
Behçet's syndrome		
• This syndrome involves small vessels, primarily of the mouth and genitalia but also of the eyes, skin, joints, GI tract, and central nervous system. The underlying cause is leukocytoblastic venulitis. • The syndrome most commonly strikes young adults and proves more severe in men than women.	• The patient commonly reports recurrent aphthous ulcers and eye pain (from lesions caused by iritis, posterior uveitis, retinal vessel occlusions, and optic neuritis). • Inspection findings may include genital lesions and cutaneous lesions (folliculitis, erythema nodosum, and an acnelike exanthem). Nonspecific inflammatory skin reactions may also be seen.	• Laboratory tests may reveal leukocytosis, elevated ESR and C-reactive protein levels, and antibodies to human oral mucosa.

• Measure intake and output. Check daily for edema. Keep the patient well hydrated (about 3 liters of fluid daily) to reduce the risk of hemorrhagic cystitis associated with cyclophosphamide therapy.

• Monitor the patient's white blood cell and platelet count during cyclophosphamide therapy to avoid severe leukopenia and thrombocytopenia. Also assess for GI disturbances.

• Watch for signs and symptoms of organ involvement and treat accordingly.

• To prevent falls, ensure that the patient with decreased visual acuity has a safe environment.

• Regulate environmental temperature to prevent additional vasoconstriction caused by cold.

• Provide emotional support to help the patient and his family cope with an altered body image — the result of the disorder or its therapy. (For example, with Wegener's granulomatosis, saddle nose may develop. Corticosteroid therapy may cause weight gain, and cyclophosphamide therapy may cause alopecia.)

Patient teaching

• Teach the patient and his family to recognize adverse effects of drug therapy (for example, with corticosteroids) and to watch for signs of bleeding: black tarry stools, hemoptysis, epistaxis, and multiple ecchymoses. Instruct them to report any of these findings to the doctor.

• Advise the patient to wear warm clothes and gloves when going outside in cold weather.

IMMUNODEFICIENCY DISORDERS

Caused by an absent or a depressed immune response and manifested in various forms, immunodeficiency disorders include X-linked infantile agammaglobulinemia, common variable immunodeficiency, selective IgA deficiency, DiGeorge's syndrome, acquired immunodeficiency syndrome, chronic mucocutaneous candidiasis, immunodeficiency with eczema and thrombocytopenia, ataxia-telangiectasia, severe combined immunodeficiency disease, and complement deficiencies.

X-LINKED INFANTILE AGAMMAGLOBULINEMIA

Also known as Bruton's agammaglobulinemia, X-linked infantile agammaglobulinemia is a congenital disorder in which all five immunoglobulins (IgM, IgG, IgA, IgD, IgE) and circulating B cells and plasma cells in all lymphoid tissues are missing or deficient. (However, T cells are left intact.)

Affecting males almost exclusively, this disorder, which occurs in 1 in 50,000 to 100,000 births, causes recurrent infections during infancy. The prognosis is good with early treatment unless the infant contracts vaccine-induced polio or a persistent viral infection.

Causes

The disease is transmitted genetically in an X-linked recessive pattern. B cells and B-cell precursors may be in the bone marrow and peripheral blood, but for unknown reasons, they fail to mature and to secrete immunoglobulins. Researchers suspect that the disease results from a dysfunction in gene-chain linkages.

Complications

Infections are common because of increased susceptibility. Common complications include hepatitis and enteroviral infections caused by echovirus and poliovirus. Infections usually leave some permanent damage, especially in the nervous or respiratory system. Mycoplasmic infection can cause a form of arthritis, and viral infections can lead to fatal encephalitis. In some patients, a dermatomyositis-like syndrome may develop in conjunction with disseminated echovirus infection. This is usually fatal despite appropriate treatment.

Assessment findings

As you review the patient's history, you'll typically find that the infant with X-linked agammaglobulinemia stays symptom-free until age 6 months. At this age, he's no longer protected by the transplacental maternal immunoglobulins that provided immune response. Typical beginning infections include recurrent bacterial otitis media, pneumonia, dermatitis, bronchitis, and meningitis — usually caused by pneumococci, streptococci, *Haemophilus influenzae,* or other gram-negative organisms.

On inspection, observe the infant's eyes for purulent conjunctivitis, the mouth for dental caries (if the infant has teeth), and the joints for signs of polyarthritis, resembling rheumatoid arthritis. Also note any signs of malnutrition or failure to thrive because severe malabsorption associated with infestation by *Giardia lamblia* may result in retarded development.

Despite recurrent infections, lymphadenopathy and splenomegaly are usually absent.

Diagnostic tests

Reliably diagnosing X-linked agammaglobulinemia is difficult because recurrent infections are common even in normal infants (many of whom don't start producing their own antibodies until ages 18 to 20 months).

The diagnosis rests on detecting missing or decreased IgM, IgA, and IgG in the serum by a process such as immunoelectrophoresis (although this diagnostic method is usually not possible until the infant reaches age 9 months). Another diagnostic technique, antigenic stimulation, confirms the infant's inability to produce specific antibodies (although cell-mediated immunity remains intact).

Treatment

Infection prevention or control and immune globulin replacement therapy to boost the patient's immune response are the main treatments. Judicious antibiotic use helps to combat infection. Some patients need long-term administration of broad-spectrum antibiotics. Injection of immune globulin helps maintain immune response.

Other treatments include corticosteroid and antimetabolite therapy for dermatomyositis with echovirus. However, this treatment may be ineffective.

Nursing diagnoses
- Altered growth and development
- Altered protection
- Fluid volume deficit
- Impaired tissue integrity
- Pain
- Risk for infection

Nursing interventions
- Because immune globulin administration causes significant pain, administer the injection deeply into a large muscle mass, such as the gluteal or thigh muscle. Massage well. If the dose contains more than 1.5 ml, divide it and inject it into more than one site. For frequent injections, rotate the injection sites.
- Because immune globulin is composed primarily of IgG, the patient may also need fresh-frozen plasma infusions to provide IgA and IgM. (Mucosal secretory IgA cannot be replaced by therapy. This may result in crippling pulmonary disease.)
- Take vital signs frequently during infusion therapy. Immediately report fever, tachycardia, or tachypnea.
- During acute infection, monitor the patient closely. Maintain adequate nutrition and hydration, and perform chest physiotherapy if necessary.

Patient teaching
- Carefully explain all treatment measures and make sure the patient's family understands the disease. Suggest genetic counseling if the parents have questions about the vulnerability of future offspring.
- To help prevent severe infection, teach the family how to recognize early signs and symptoms and to report them promptly. Advise them to clean the patient's cuts and scrapes immediately and meticulously. Warn them to keep the patient out of crowds and away from people with known and active infections.

COMMON VARIABLE IMMUNODEFICIENCY

This immunodeficiency disorder is marked by progressive deterioration of humoral (B-cell) immunity, which results in increased susceptibility to infection. Unlike X-linked agammaglobulinemia, this disorder usually produces symptoms after infancy and childhood, manifesting itself between ages 25 and 40. It affects men and women equally and usually doesn't interfere with a normal life span or with normal pregnancy and offspring.

Common variable immunodeficiency (also known as acquired agammaglobulinemia or common variable agammaglobulinemia) may be associated with autoimmune diseases, such as systemic lupus erythematosus, rheumatoid arthritis, hemolytic anemia, and pernicious anemia, and with cancers, such as leukemia and lymphoma.

Causes
No one knows what causes common variable immunodeficiency. Most patients have a normal circulating B-cell count but defective synthesis or release of immunoglobulins. Many also exhibit progressive deterioration of cell-mediated (T-cell) immunity (detected by delayed hypersensitivity in skin testing).

Although no clear proof of genetic influence on disease occurrence exists, the disease does occur in siblings. Additionally, family members have a higher incidence of hypogammaglobulinemia, selective IgA deficiency, and autoimmune disease.

Complications
A spruelike syndrome with diarrhea, malabsorption, steatorrhea, and a protein-losing enteropathy (like inflammatory bowel disease) typically complicates common variable immunodeficiency. *Giardia lamblia* GI infection and upper and lower respiratory tract infections are also typical complications.

Assessment findings
Review the patient's history. Investigate disorders, such as pyogenic bacterial infections, which are characteristic of common variable immunodeficiency. Be alert also for a history of chronic rather than acute infections. Recurrent sinopulmonary infections, chronic bacterial conjunctivitis, atrophic gastritis with pernicious anemia, and malabsorption (often associated with infestation by *G. lamblia*) are usually the first clues to common variable immunodeficiency. Also, suspect the disorder in an adult patient with unexplained bronchiectasis. Other initial signs and symptoms include fever, weight loss, and a palpable spleen and lymph nodes.

Diagnostic tests
Characteristic diagnostic markers in this disorder are decreased serum IgM, IgA, and IgG levels detected by immunoelectrophoresis and a normal circulating B-cell

count. Plasma cells seldom appear in the lymph nodes, bone marrow, and spleen but may be found in intestinal lamina propria. Rheumatoid factor and positive Coombs' test findings may be present. Antigenic stimulation confirms an inability to produce specific antibodies; cell-mediated immunity may be intact or delayed.

X-rays usually show signs of chronic lung disease or sinusitis. Regular X-ray and pulmonary function studies monitor infection in the lungs.

Treatment

Care and treatment measures for patients with common variable immunodeficiency are essentially the same as for X-linked agammaglobulinemia. Antibiotics are preferred for combating infection. And weekly or monthly injections of immune globulin help to maintain the immune response.

Nursing diagnoses

- Altered health maintenance
- Altered nutrition: Less than body requirements
- Altered protection
- Diarrhea
- Fluid volume deficit
- Ineffective airway clearance
- Knowledge deficit
- Pain
- Risk for infection

Nursing interventions

- Because immune globulin administration causes significant pain, administer injections deep into a large muscle mass, such as the gluteal or thigh muscle. Massage well. If the dose is more than 1.5 ml, divide it. Then inject the divided doses into more than one site. For frequent injections, rotate the injection sites. Because immune globulin is composed primarily of IgG, the patient may also need fresh-frozen plasma infusions to provide IgA and IgM.
- As ordered, administer antibiotics and chest physiotherapy, including additional hydration and mucolytics, to forestall or treat infection.
- Institute diet therapy, as recommended, to counteract the depleting effects of malabsorption syndrome and anemias. Be sure to involve the dietitian and doctor in devising an optimal nutrition plan.

Patient teaching

- To help avoid severe infection, teach the patient and his family how to recognize its early signs and symptoms.

Warn him to avoid crowds and people who have active infections.
- Stress the importance of good nutrition and regular follow-up care. A cooked-food diet (one that contains no raw foods) may help reduce bacteria in foods and beverages.
- Explain to the patient that secondary conditions may coexist with the immunodeficiency. Advise him that these may require additional or specialized treatment.

SELECTIVE IgA DEFICIENCY

The most common immunoglobulin deficiency, selective IgA deficiency affects as many as 1 in 500 to 700 persons. IgA (the major immunoglobulin in human saliva, in nasal and bronchial fluids, and in intestinal secretions) guards against bacterial and viral infections. Consequently, selective IgA deficiency usually leads to chronic sinopulmonary infections, GI diseases, and other disorders.

Some patients, however, remain healthy throughout their lives; a few survive to age 70. These patients may have no signs or symptoms because they have extra amounts of low-molecular-weight IgM, which takes over IgA function and helps maintain immunity.

The age of onset varies. The prognosis is good for patients who receive correct treatment, especially if they have no associated disorders. Some IgA-deficient children with recurrent respiratory disease and middle ear inflammation may begin to synthesize IgA spontaneously as recurrent infections subside and their condition improves.

Causes

The exact cause of IgA deficiency is unknown. It may be linked with autosomal dominant or recessive inheritance, although the patterns aren't clearly established. An increased incidence is found in families with hypogammaglobulinemia.

Several other theories about the cause of IgA deficiency exist. Patients with IgA deficiency have a normal number of peripheral blood lymphocytes carrying IgA receptors and a normal amount of other immunoglobulins, which suggests that their B cells may not be secreting IgA. In an occasional patient, suppressor T cells appear to inhibit IgA. Patients with rheumatoid arthritis or systemic lupus erythematosus (SLE) are also IgA-deficient, pointing to a link between IgA deficiency and autoimmune disorders. A transient form of the deficiency seems to result from certain drugs, such as anticonvulsants. And toxoplasmosis, rubella, and cytomegalovirus have produced IgA deficiency through congenital intrauterine infections.

Complications
Mild to severe chronic pulmonary disease (such as asthma) and chronic diarrheal diseases commonly result from IgA deficiency. A patient who develops significant levels of antibodies to IgA may have a severe anaphylactic reaction if he receives a transfusion of normal blood or blood products.

Assessment findings
Some IgA-deficient patients have no signs or symptoms. Among those who do develop symptoms, the most common complaint is chronic sinopulmonary infection. The patient may also complain of symptoms of other disorders. These include respiratory allergy, often triggered by infection; GI tract diseases, such as spruelike disease, ulcerative colitis, and regional enteritis; autoimmune diseases, such as rheumatoid arthritis, SLE, chronic hepatitis, and immunohemolytic anemia; and malignant tumors, such as squamous cell carcinoma of the lungs, reticulum cell sarcoma, and thymoma.

Diagnostic tests
Hematologic analyses of the IgA-deficient patient show serum IgA levels below 5 mg/dl. Although the patient usually has no IgA in his secretions, such levels are occasionally normal. The patient has normal IgE levels; his IgM levels may be normal or elevated in serum and secretions. Normally absent low-molecular-weight IgM may be present.

Tests may also detect autoantibodies and antibodies against IgG (rheumatoid factor), IgM, and cow's milk. Cell-mediated immunity and secretory component (the glycopeptide that transports IgA) are usually normal, and most circulating B cells appear normal.

Treatment
Selective IgA deficiency has no known cure. Treatment aims to control symptoms of associated diseases, such as respiratory tract and GI infections, and is the same as for a patient with normal IgA. In severe recurrent infection, the patient may receive IgA-free gamma globulin preparation.

Nursing diagnoses
• Altered health maintenance
• Altered nutrition: Less than body requirements
• Altered protection
• Diarrhea

• Risk for infection

Nursing interventions
• Consult the dietitian to develop a nutritious diet that minimizes adverse effects from GI tract diseases, diarrhea, anemias, and autoimmune diseases.
• If the patient needs a transfusion with blood products, minimize the risk of an adverse reaction by using washed red blood cells. Or avoid the reaction completely by cross matching the patient's blood with that of an IgA-deficient donor.

Patient teaching
• Because IgA deficiency is lifelong, teach the patient steps he can take to prevent infection. Also teach him to recognize early signs of infection; tell him to seek treatment immediately if such signs occur.
• Advise the patient to use acetaminophen instead of aspirin and other nonsteroidal anti-inflammatory drugs for mild pain relief.

DiGEORGE'S SYNDROME
Also known as congenital thymic hypoplasia or aplasia, DiGeorge's syndrome is marked by a partial or total absence of cell-mediated immunity that results from a deficiency of T cells. It characteristically produces life-threatening hypocalcemia and is associated with abnormalities of the great vessels, atrial and ventricular septal defects, esophageal atresia, bifid uvula, short philtrum, mandibular hypoplasia, hypertelorism, and low-set notched ears. Also, the thymus may be absent or underdeveloped and abnormally located.

An infant with thymic hypoplasia (rather than aplasia) may experience a spontaneous return of cell-mediated immunity but can develop severe T-cell deficiencies later in life. This results in an exaggerated susceptibility to viral, fungal, and bacterial infections, which may be overwhelming.

Few patients live beyond age 2 without fetal thymic transplantation. If transplantation, correction of hypocalcemia, and repair of cardiac anomalies can take place, the prognosis improves.

Causes
DiGeorge's syndrome may result from abnormal fetal development of the third and fourth pharyngeal pouches (during the 12th week of gestation) that interferes with the formation of the thymus and parathyroid glands. As a result, the thymus is completely or partially absent and abnormally located, causing deficient cell-mediated im-

munity. (See *The thymus and immune response.*) This syndrome has been linked to maternal alcoholism and resultant fetal alcohol syndrome.

Complications
Failed parathyroid development results in life-threatening hypocalcemia that's unusually resistant to treatment. This can lead to seizures and central nervous system damage. Death commonly results from cardiac defects.

Assessment findings
The parents of an older infant may report a history of repeated infections. Usually, however, signs are obvious at birth or shortly thereafter. The child also commonly has signs of tetany, hyperphosphoremia, and hypocalcemia—the result of hypoparathyroidism, which is associated with DiGeorge's syndrome.

Inspection of an infant with DiGeorge's syndrome may reveal low-set ears, notched ear pinnae, a fish-shaped mouth, an undersized jaw, and abnormally wide-set eyes (hypertelorism) with antimongoloid eyelid formation (downward slant). Your assessment may also reveal signs of cardiovascular abnormalities, such as oxygen therapy–resistant cyanosis, tachypnea, and a palpable systolic bruit at the left sternal border.

Diagnostic tests
The sheep cell agglutination test reveals decreased or absent T cells. A chest X-ray shows that the thymus is absent. Immunoglobulin assays don't help in diagnosis because the infant's antibodies usually come from maternal circulation. Low serum calcium, elevated serum phosphorus, and absent parathyroid hormone levels confirm hypoparathyroidism.

Treatment
Life-threatening hypocalcemia needs immediate, aggressive treatment—for example, with a rapid I.V. infusion of 10% calcium gluconate. Transplantation of thymic tissue can help the patient develop immunocompetent T cells of host origin.

When possible, congenital cardiac deformities require surgical repair.

Nursing diagnoses
• Activity intolerance
• Altered growth and development
• Altered protection
• Knowledge deficit
• Risk for infection
• Risk for injury

THE THYMUS AND IMMUNE RESPONSE

Although the exact relation between the thymus and the immune system remains unclear, possible thymic functions include:
• destruction of T cells that would have mistaken components of the human organism as foreign during the fetal stage. This allows the fetus's immune system to establish the difference between self and nonself.
• maturation of T cells in the thymic epithelium or mesenchymal cells. These mature cells help regulate the humoral immune response.

Nursing interventions
• During calcium infusion, monitor the patient's heart rate and take steps to avoid infiltration. Remember that the patient *must* receive vitamin D, and sometimes also parathyroid hormone, with the calcium supplements to ensure effective use of calcium.
• Provide a low-phosphorus diet.
• Take steps to prevent infection.

Patient teaching
• Teach the infant's parents to watch for signs of infection and to seek immediate treatment if such signs occur. Also teach them to keep the infant away from crowds or any other potential sources of infection.
• Teach the parents to provide good hygiene, adequate nutrition, and hydration.

ACQUIRED IMMUNODEFICIENCY SYNDROME

A widely publicized disease, acquired immunodeficiency syndrome (AIDS) is a progressive impairment of the immune response marked by the gradual destruction of CD4+ T lymphocytes (T cells) by the human immunodeficiency virus (HIV). The resulting immunodeficiency predisposes the patient to opportunistic infections, unusual cancers, and other characteristic abnormalities.

Virtually any cell that has the CD4+ molecule on its surface may be infected by the virus. These include monocytes, macrophages, bone marrow progenitors, and glial, gut, and epithelial cells. Such infections can cause dementia, wasting syndrome, and hematologic abnormalities.

This syndrome was first described by the Centers for Disease Control (CDC) in 1981. Since then, the CDC

CLASSIFYING H.I.V. INFECTION

The current CDC classification system for human immunodeficiency virus (HIV) infection groups HIV infection into three categories reflecting CD4+ T-lymphocyte (T-cell) counts and three categories reflecting clinical disease. These groups form a matrix of nine mutually exclusive categories.

T-cell categories
The CD4+ T-cell ranges below are positive markers for HIV infection (along with various test results identifying HIV or the HIV antibody). The categories are:
1. ≥500 CD4+ T cells/µL of blood
2. 200 to 499 CD4+ T cells/µL of blood
3. <200 CD4+ T cells/µL of blood

Clinical categories
A. The patient has asymptomatic HIV infection, acute HIV infection or persistent generalized lymphadenopathy (PGL)
B. The patient does not have conditions in categories A or C but does have symptoms (for example, cervical dysplasia, herpes zoster, peripheral neuropathy)
C. The patient has what the CDC defines as AIDS-indicator conditions.

	Clinical conditions		
	A: Asymptomatic, acute (primary) HIV, or PGL	**B:** Symptomatic not A or C conditions	**C:** AIDS-indicator conditions
1: ≥500/µL	A1	B1	C1
2: 200-499/µL	A2	B2	C2
3: <200/µL AIDS-indicator T-cell count	A3	B3	C3

has issued a case surveillance definition for AIDS and has modified it several times, most recently in 1993. (See *Classifying HIV infection.*)

AIDS occurs most commonly in homosexual and bisexual men, I.V. drug users, neonates of HIV-infected women, recipients of contaminated blood or blood products (although the risk of receiving contaminated blood has been drastically reduced since 1985), and heterosexual partners of those in high-risk groups. Because of similar routes of transmission, AIDS shares epidemiologic patterns with other sexually transmitted diseases and hepatitis B.

Although the prevalence of HIV infection isn't known, estimates suggest that 1 to 1.5 million people in the United States alone have the infection, and more than 100,000 Americans had developed AIDS by 1989. The average duration between HIV exposure and diagnosis is 8 to 10 years, although the incubation period can vary.

The course of AIDS can vary, but the syndrome usually results in death from opportunistic infections. Antiretroviral therapy—with zidovudine, for instance—and prophylaxis and treatment of common opportunistic infections can delay but not stop the progression. Most experts believe that virtually everyone infected with HIV will develop AIDS.

Causes and pathophysiology
AIDS results from a retrovirus—HIV type I. This virus destroys CD4+ T cells, the essential regulators and effectors of the normal immune response. HIV is transmitted by contact with infected blood or body fluids. Transmission results from such high-risk behaviors as sharing a contaminated needle or having unprotected sexual contact, especially rectal intercourse, which results in mucosal trauma. Transmission may also occur through transfusion of contaminated blood or blood products. What's more, it can pass from an infected mother to the fetus through cervical or blood contact at delivery or through breast milk. The virus isn't transmitted by everyday household or social contact.

Complications
Repeated opportunistic infections eventually overwhelm the body's compromised immune defenses. These infections invade every body system, including the lungs, bone marrow, and brain. Neuropathy (HIV encephalopathy) occurs in 40% to 60% of infected patients.

Assessment findings
After initial exposure, the infected person may have no recognizable signs or symptoms, or he may experience a mononucleosis-like syndrome for 3 to 6 weeks and then remain asymptomatic for years. His history usually suggests exposure to HIV—most often through unprotected sexual relations with an infected partner or sharing of I.V. needles.

The patient's initial complaints include fever, rigors, arthralgia, myalgia, maculopapular rash, urticaria, abdominal cramps, and diarrhea. Symptoms of aseptic meningitis, such as severe headache and stiff neck, may also occur. As the syndrome progresses, the patient may experience neurologic symptoms from HIV encephalopathy or symptoms of an opportunistic infection or cancer.

Your assessment may disclose palpable lymph nodes in two or more extrainguinal sites, a sign of lymphade-

DIAGNOSTIC CRITERIA FOR A.I.D.S.

The CDC diagnoses a patient as having acquired immunodeficiency disease syndrome (AIDS) if he has HIV infection, a certain CD4 + T-lymphocyte count (specified by the CDC), and one or more of the following conditions (from the CDC's clinical HIV classification categories):

Category A conditions
Persistent generalized lymphadenopathy or acute (primary) HIV infection with accompanying illness or history of acute HIV infection

Category B conditions
Symptoms or diseases not included in category C, such as bacillary angiomatosis, oropharyngeal or persistent vulvovaginal candidiasis, fever or diarrhea lasting over 1 month, idiopathic thrombocytopenic purpura, pelvic inflammatory disease (particularly if complicated by tubo-ovarian abscess), and peripheral neuropathy

Category C conditions
The following disorders defined by the CDC as

AIDS-indicator conditions: Candidiasis of the bronchi, trachea, or lungs or esophagus; cervical cancer (invasive); coccidioidomycosis (disseminated or extrapulmonary); cryptococcosis (extrapulmonary); cryptosporidiosis (chronic intestinal); cytomegalovirus (CMV) disease affecting organs other than the liver, spleen, or lymph nodes; CMV retinitis with vision loss; encephalopathy related to HIV; herpes simplex involving chronic ulcers or herpetic bronchitis, pneumonitis, or esophagitis; histoplasmosis, disseminated or extrapulmonary; isosporiasis (chronic intestinal); Kaposi's sarcoma; lymphoma (Burkitt's or its equivalent); lymphoma (immunoblastic or its equivalent); lymphoma of the brain (primary); *Mycobacterium avium* complex or *M. kansasii,* (disseminated or extrapulmonary); *M. tuberculosis* at any site (pulmonary or extrapulmonary); *Mycobacterium* (any other species, disseminated or extrapulmonary); *Pneumocystis carinii* pneumonia; pneumonia (recurrent); progressive multifocal leukoencephalopathy; *Salmonella* septicemia (recurrent); toxoplasmosis of the brain; wasting syndrome caused by HIV.

nopathy. You may also observe behavioral, cognitive, and motor changes associated with progressive dementia, which occurs in about 30% of patients.

In children, the incubation time averages 17 months. A child's signs and symptoms resemble those of an adult, except that he's more likely to have a history of bacterial infections, such as otitis media, pneumonias other than those caused by *Pneumocystis carinii*, sepsis, chronic salivary gland enlargement, and lymphoid interstitial pneumonia.

Diagnostic tests
The CDC defines AIDS as an illness characterized by laboratory evidence of HIV infection coexisting with one or more indicator diseases. (See *Diagnostic criteria for AIDS.*) Most patients are diagnosed by these criteria. However, AIDS can also be diagnosed without laboratory evidence of HIV infection, or even with laboratory evidence against HIV infections.

Laboratory evidence of seroconversion occurs 8 to 12 weeks after HIV exposure. Antibody tests, the most commonly performed studies, indirectly indicate infection by revealing HIV antibodies. The recommended protocol calls for initial screening with an enzyme-linked immunosorbent assay (ELISA). If results are positive, the ELISA test is repeated. If still positive, the findings are confirmed by an alternate method, usually the Western blot or an immunofluorescence assay.

Antibody testing, however, isn't always reliable. That's because the duration needed to produce a detectable HIV antibody level varies from one patient to another. In fact, an infected patient can test negative anywhere from a few weeks to (in one documented case) as long as 35 months. Transferred maternal antibodies, which persist for up to 10 months, also make antibody tests unreliable in neonates.

Direct testing, though more involved, overcomes these problems by detecting HIV itself. Such testing includes antigen tests (p24 antigen), HIV cultures, nucleic acid probes of peripheral blood lymphocytes, and the polymerase chain reaction.

Further blood tests support the diagnosis and help evaluate the severity of immunosuppression. Such tests include CD4 + and CD8 + T-cell subset counts, erythrocyte sedimentation rate, complete blood count, serum beta (sub 2) microglobulin, p24 antigen, neopterin levels, and anergy testing.

Because many opportunistic infections in AIDS patients are reactivations of previous infections, patients also commonly receive testing for syphilis, hepatitis B, tuberculosis, toxoplasmosis and, in some geographic areas, histoplasmosis.

AIDS dementia requires a three-step diagnosis: Western blot confirmation of HIV infection, identification of signs of dementia, and exclusion of other conditions that may cause dementia, such as hypoxia, hypoglycemia, central nervous system tumors, and brain atrophy.

Treatment

No cure has yet been found for AIDS. However, several antiretroviral treatments can inhibit or temporarily inactivate HIV. Also, immunomodulatory drugs strengthen the immune system, and anti-infective and antineoplastic drugs combat opportunistic infections and associated cancers. Some anti-infectives also serve as prophylaxis against opportunistic infections. New protocols combine two or more of these drugs to produce the maximum benefit with the fewest adverse reactions. Combination therapy also helps inhibit the production of mutant HIV strains resistant to a particular drug.

Although many opportunistic infections respond to anti-infective drugs, they tend to recur after treatment. Because of this, the patient usually requires continued prophylaxis until the drug loses its effectiveness or can no longer be tolerated.

Zidovudine, the most commonly used antiretroviral, effectively slows the progression of HIV infection, decreasing the number of opportunistic infections, prolonging survival, and slowing the progress of associated dementia. However, the drug often produces severe adverse reactions and toxicities.

Initially, the zidovudine regimen consisted of 200 mg every 4 hours, for a total daily dose of 1,200 mg (or 1,000 mg if the patient didn't want to interrupt his sleep to take the sixth dose). Now, however, this regimen is giving way to a lower-dose one that calls for 100 mg every 4 hours, for a total daily dose of 600 mg (or 500 mg, if the patient doesn't want to interrupt his sleep). The lower-dose regimen appears to be just as effective, and reports indicate that it causes fewer adverse reactions and less toxicity.

Didanosine (DDI), a newly approved antiretroviral drug, is prescribed only for patients who cannot tolerate, or who no longer respond to, drug therapy with zidovudine.

Zalcitabine (DDC) is used in combination with zidovudine; in advanced HIV infection to boost—or enhance—the return of CD4+ T-cell counts. Additional treatment measures involve implementing supportive care, such as maintaining adequate nutrition and hydration and relieving pain and other distressing symptoms.

Nursing diagnoses

• Activity intolerance
• Altered family processes
• Altered health maintenance
• Altered nutrition: Less than body requirements
• Altered oral mucous membrane
• Altered protection
• Altered sexuality patterns
• Altered thought processes
• Anticipatory grieving
• Body image disturbance
• Defensive coping
• Denial
• Fatigue
• Hopelessness
• Hyperthermia
• Impaired skin integrity
• Impaired tissue integrity
• Ineffective individual coping
• Knowledge deficit
• Parental role conflict
• Powerlessness
• Risk for fluid volume deficit
• Risk for infection
• Social isolation

Nursing interventions

• To help prevent transmission of AIDS, follow universal precautions whenever a risk of exposure to blood, body fluids, or secretions exists.
• Monitor the patient for fever, noting any pattern, and for such signs of infection as skin breakdown, cough, sore throat, and diarrhea. Also, assess for swollen, tender lymph nodes, and check laboratory values regularly.
• Provide the patient with normal saline or bicarbonate mouthwash for daily oral rinsing. Avoid glycerin swabs, which dry the mucous membranes.
• Record the patient's caloric intake. He may need total parenteral nutrition, although this creates a potential route for infection.
• Ensure adequate fluids during episodes of diarrhea.
• Provide meticulous skin care, especially in the debilitated patient.
• Encourage the patient to maintain as much physical activity as he can tolerate. Make sure his schedule includes time for both exercise and rest.
• If the patient develops Kaposi's sarcoma, monitor the progression of the lesions.

• Monitor opportunistic infections or signs of disease progression, and treat infections as ordered.

• Recognize that a diagnosis of AIDS has a devastating impact on the patient, his socioeconomic status, and his family relationships. Help him cope with an altered body image and the emotional burden of serious illness and the threat of death.

Patient teaching

• Teach the patient and his family members, sexual partners, and friends about the syndrome and its transmission. Tell the patient not to donate blood, blood products, organs, tissue, or sperm.

• Urge him to inform potential sexual partners and health care workers that he has HIV infection.

• If the patient uses I.V. drugs, caution him not to share needles.

• Inform the patient that high-risk sexual practices for AIDS transmission are those that exchange body fluids, such as vaginal or anal intercourse without a condom. Discuss safe sexual practices, such as hugging, petting, mutual masturbation, and protected sexual intercourse.

• Advise the female patient of childbearing age to avoid pregnancy. Explain that an infant may become infected before birth, during delivery, or during breast-feeding.

• Identify the signs of impending infection, and stress the importance of seeking immediate medical attention.

• Involve the patient with hospice care early in treatment so he can establish a relationship. If he develops AIDS dementia in stages, help him understand the progression of this symptom.

CHRONIC MUCOCUTANEOUS CANDIDIASIS

Also called moniliasis, this form of candidiasis, which affects males and females alike, usually develops during the first year of life but occasionally occurs as late as age 20. Chronic mucocutaneous candidiasis is characterized by repeated infection with Candida albicans.

In some patients with chronic mucocutaneous candidiasis, an autoimmune response affects the endocrine system, inducing various endocrinopathies. In these patients, the prognosis depends on the severity of the associated endocrinopathy.

Causes

Although no characteristic immune system defects are known to cause this infection, anergy may play a role. Many patients have a diminished response to various an-

tigens or to Candida organisms alone. In some patients, anergy may result from deficient migration inhibiting factor, a mediator normally produced by the lymphocytes. This leads researchers to think that the disease may result from an inherited defect in cell-mediated (T-cell) immunity. (Humoral immunity, mediated by B cells, remains intact and produces a normal antibody response to C. albicans.)

Complications

Patients with chronic mucocutaneous candidiasis seldom develop systemic infection. However, hepatic and endocrine failure associated with this disorder can be fatal. Patients with associated endocrinopathy seldom live to age 40.

Other complications include psychiatric disorders associated with physical disfigurement and multiple endocrine aberrations.

Assessment findings

The patient may report speech and eating problems because of lesions of the mouth, nose, and palate. On inspection, you may see large, circular lesions on the skin, mucous membranes, nails, and vagina. The lesions may be beefy red and denuded.

The infection seldom produces systemic signs or symptoms, but in late stages, it may be associated with recurrent respiratory tract infections. Other associated conditions include severe viral infections that may precede the onset of endocrinopathy and, sometimes, hepatitis. If endocrinopathy develops as the disease progresses, the patient may complain of signs and symptoms related to the organs involved. For example, tetany commonly occurs as a result of hypoparathyroidism. You may also recognize symptoms of Addison's disease, hypothyroidism, diabetes mellitus, and pernicious anemia.

Diagnostic tests

Laboratory findings usually show a normal or decreased circulating T-cell count. In most patients, skin testing fails to detect delayed hypersensitivity to Candida even during the infectious stage (probably because migration-inhibiting factor, which appears when T cells are activated, may not respond to Candida).

Abnormalities not related to immune dysfunction result from endocrinopathy. Laboratory findings may point to hypocalcemia, abnormal hepatic function, hyperglycemia, iron deficiency, and abnormal vitamin B_{12} absorption (pernicious anemia).

Before diagnosing the patient's disease as chronic mucocutaneous candidiasis, diagnosis must rule out other immunodeficiency disorders associated with chronic candidal infection, especially DiGeorge's syndrome, ataxia-telangiectasia, and severe combined immunodeficiency disease. All of these diseases produce severe immunologic defects.

After diagnosis, typical studies include evaluation of adrenal, pituitary, thyroid, gonadal, pancreatic, and parathyroid functions, and other careful diagnostic follow-up.

Treatment
Infection control is the main aim of treatment. Although miconazole and nystatin may produce sustained improvement, these topical antifungal agents ultimately fail to control infection.

Systemic infections warrant vigorous treatment. Oral ketoconazole and injections of thymosin and levamisole may have a positive effect. Iron replacement therapy (administered orally or intramuscularly) may also be necessary.

Nursing diagnoses
• Body image disturbance
• Impaired skin integrity
• Impaired tissue integrity
• Pain
• Risk for infection
• Sexual dysfunction

Nursing interventions
• Because candidal infections can be painful, provide meticulous skin and mucous membrane care to help prevent infection.
• Supply bland, cool foods along with topical anesthetics for the patient with a sore mouth and tongue.
• Give calcium infusions, as ordered, when endocrinopathy produces hypocalcemia. Monitor vital signs and cardiac rhythm during infusion therapy.
• Refer the patient for appropriate counseling; for example, if he needs help coping with disfigurement or experiences sexual dysfunction.

Patient teaching
• Teach the patient to recognize and report progressive manifestations of the disease.
• Emphasize the importance of taking ordered medications properly and for the prescribed length of time.
• Instruct him to schedule and keep appointments with an endocrinologist for regular medical checkups.

IMMUNODEFICIENCY WITH ECZEMA AND THROMBOCYTOPENIA

Also known as Wiskott-Aldrich syndrome, this disorder arises from defective B-cell and T-cell function, which impairs cell-mediated immunity.

The disease affects only males, and the prognosis is poor. The average life span approaches 4 years; only seldom does a child with the disease live past age 10. The patient with the disease also has an increased risk for leukemia and lymphoma.

Causes
Wiskott-Aldrich syndrome results from an X-linked recessive trait. Boys with this genetic defect are born with a normal thymus gland and normal plasma cells and lymphoid tissues. However, an inherited defect in both B-cell and T-cell function compromises the immune system response, which increases vulnerability to infection. A boy with Wiskott-Aldrich syndrome also has a metabolic defect in platelet synthesis. The body produces only small, short-lived platelets. This results in thrombocytopenia.

Complications
Death usually follows massive bleeding (in infancy), cancer, or severe infection (in early childhood).

Assessment findings
In an infant, you'll observe characteristic signs of thrombocytopenia, such as bloody stools, a bleeding circumcisional site, petechiae, and purpura. As the infant ages, thrombocytopenia subsides. Beginning at about age 6 months, however, recurrent systemic infections develop, including chronic pneumonia, sinusitis, otitis media, and herpes simplex of the skin and eyes (which may cause keratitis and vision loss) with hepatosplenomegaly.

When the patient is about age 1, eczema develops and progressively worsens. Infection typically follows persistent scratching.

Diagnostic tests
The most important clues to diagnosing immunodeficiency with thrombocytopenia and eczema are bleeding disorders at birth and thrombocytopenia (coagulation test results show a platelet count below 100,000/mm³ and prolonged bleeding time). Laboratory test findings may detect normal or elevated IgE levels, decreased IgM levels, normal IgG and IgA levels, and low (or no) isohemagglutinin levels. In neonates, findings may point to

normal cell-mediated immunity initially. This immunity diminishes with age.

Sputum and throat cultures commonly identify *Streptococcus pneumoniae*, meningococci, and *Haemophilus influenzae* as infecting organisms.

Treatment

The main treatment goals include limiting bleeding by transfusing fresh, crossmatched platelets; preventing or controlling infection with prophylactic or early and aggressive antibiotic therapy; supplying passive immunity by infusing immune globulins; and controlling eczema with topical corticosteroids. (Systemic corticosteroids are contraindicated because they further compromise immunity.)

Additional therapy includes antipruritic agents to relieve itching. Although treatment with transfer factor achieves limited success, bone marrow transplantation has helped some patients. Splenectomy may reduce the patient's risk for serious hemorrhage by raising the platelet count.

Nursing diagnoses

• Altered parenting
• Altered protection
• Fatigue
• Fluid volume deficit
• Impaired tissue integrity
• Ineffective family coping
• Risk for infection

Nursing interventions

• Check the child's baseline platelet count before giving ordered platelet transfusions. Be sure to check the platelet count often during therapy; each transfused platelet unit should raise the count by 10,000/mm³.
• Give the patient cool baths, use garments and bed linens made only of natural fibers, and apply topical and systemic antipruritics to decrease the itching and provide comfort.
• Monitor vital signs. Report fever, tachycardia, or tachypnea immediately—especially if the patient is scheduled for bone marrow transplantation, which can't proceed if the child has an infection.
• Arrange genetic consultation, as appropriate, for the parents. Explain that the genetic counselor can answer questions about the vulnerability of future offspring.

Patient teaching

• Instruct the parents to watch for signs and symptoms of infection, such as fever, coldlike symptoms, and drainage and redness around any superficial wound. Direct them to report such signs promptly.
• Show the parents and the patient (if appropriate) how to perform meticulous mouth and skin care (including careful cleaning of all skin wounds, no matter how superficial). Also teach them ways to ensure optimal nutrition and adequate hydration.
• Urge the patient and his parents to prevent infections by avoiding crowds and people known to have active infections.
• Provide physical and emotional support along with careful teaching to help the patient and his family cope with this disease. When the patient is old enough, begin teaching him about the disease and his limitations.
• Instruct parents to watch the patient for such signs of bleeding as easy bruising, bloody stools, swollen joints, and tenderness in the trunk area. Assist them to plan activities to promote their child's safe but normal development. For example, the child may swim or ride a bike (if he wears protective headgear), although he must avoid contact sports, such as boxing, and roughhousing.

ATAXIA-TELANGIECTASIA

An autosomal recessive disorder, ataxia-telangiectasia is characterized by progressively severe ataxia, telangiectasia (particularly of the face, earlobes, and conjunctivae), and chronic, recurrent sinopulmonary infections that may reflect both humoral (B-cell) and cell-mediated (T-cell) immunodeficiencies. At one time, the disorder was considered a neurologic disease because its dominant sign is cerebellar ataxia. It's now known to have associated endocrine and vascular components.

Ataxia usually appears within 2 years of birth but may develop as late as age 9. The degree of immunodeficiency determines the rate of deterioration. Some patients die within several years; others survive into their 30s.

Causes

Immunodeficiency may result from defective embryonic development of the mesoderm, hormonal deficiency, or defective deoxyribonucleic acid repair.

Complications

Children with ataxia-telangiectasia are unusually vulnerable to lymphomas, particularly lymphosarcomas and lymphoreticular cancers. They may also develop leukemia, adenocarcinoma, dysgerminoma, or medulloblastoma. Severe abnormalities cause rapid deterioration and premature death from overwhelming sinopulmonary infection or cancer.

Assessment findings

Although some patients remain symptom-free for 10 or more years, about 80% have a history of recurrent or chronic respiratory tract infections because of IgA deficiency early in life. But the earliest and most dominant signs of cerebellar ataxia usually develop by the time the infant begins to use his motor skills.

Assessment usually discloses continual and involuntary jerky (choreoathetoid) movements, nystagmus, extrapyramidal signs (pseudoparkinsonism, dystonias, and motor restlessness), and posterior column signs (unsteady gait with forward leaning to maintain balance, decreased arm movements, and purposeless tremors).

Associated signs of telangiectasia usually appear later, sometimes not until age 9. At first, a vascular lesion appears on the sclera. Later, inspection may disclose lesions that appear on the bridge or side of the nose, the ear, or the antecubital or popliteal areas.

When you inspect an adolescent patient, you may detect a lack of secondary sex characteristics during puberty. Rarely, you may observe signs of progeria: premature graying, senile keratoses, and vitiligo. Eventually, the patient may develop signs of mental retardation.

Diagnostic tests

Diagnosis usually depends on immunologic tests. A patient with ataxia-telangiectasia may show:
• selective absence of IgA (in 60% to 80% of patients) or deficient IgA and IgE
• normal B-cell count but diminished antibody responses
• absence of Hassall's corpuscles on examination of thymic tissue
• high serum levels of oncofetal proteins
• decreased T cells.

Computed tomography and magnetic resonance imaging scans and pneumoencephalography show degenerative neurologic changes.

Treatment

No treatment exists to stop progression of ataxia-telangiectasia. But the patient must receive prophylactic or early and aggressive therapy with broad-spectrum antibiotics to prevent or control recurrent infections.

Immune globulin infusion or injection can passively replace missing antibodies in an IgG-deficient patient and may also help prevent infection, although this treatment may not help an IgA-deficient patient. The effec-tiveness of other forms of immunotherapy — such as fetal thymus transplantation and histocompatible bone marrow transplantation — is unproven.

Nursing diagnoses
• Activity intolerance
• Altered growth and development
• Altered health maintenance
• Altered parenting
• Altered protection
• Impaired physical mobility
• Ineffective family coping
• Knowledge deficit
• Risk for infection
• Self-care deficit

Nursing interventions
• Treat chronic respiratory tract infections with antibiotics, as ordered.
• Give immune globulin injections deep into the gluteal or femoral muscle. These injections are painful; massage the area well after the injection to help distribute the medication.
• Offer emotional support to the parents in distress. Allow them to verbalize their fears and frustrations. Help them identify and use effective coping strategies.
• The parents of a child with ataxia-telangiectasia may need genetic counseling to resolve questions about the vulnerability of future offspring. They may also need psychotherapy to help them cope with their child's long-term illness and inevitable early death, and to help them develop effective parenting skills.

Patient teaching
• To help parents protect their child from infections, advise them to avoid crowds and people who have infections, and teach them to recognize early signs of infection.
• If the patient has chronic bronchial infections, teach his parents chest physical therapy and postural drainage techniques.
• Stress the importance of proper nutrition and adequate hydration.

SEVERE COMBINED IMMUNODEFICIENCY DISEASE

Cell-mediated (T-cell) and humoral (B-cell) immunity are either deficient or absent in severe combined immunodeficiency disease (SCID). This deficiency predisposes the patient to infection from all classes of microorganisms during infancy. SCID affects seven times as many males as females.

Causes and pathophysiology

SCID is usually transmitted as an autosomal recessive trait, although it may be X-linked. In most cases, the genetic defect seems associated with failure of the stem cell to differentiate into T and B cells. Less commonly, SCID results from enzyme deficiency.

Complications

Without treatment, patients typically die of infection within 2 years of birth. Such infections usually result from *Salmonella*, *Escherichia coli*, *Pseudomonas*, cytomegalovirus, *Pneumocystis carinii*, or *Candida*. Common viral infections, such as chicken pox, are also usually fatal.

Assessment findings

An infant with SCID has a history of extreme susceptibility to infection in the first few months of life. But he probably won't show signs of any gram-negative infections until about age 6 months because of protection by maternal IgG.

On assessment, you may commonly observe that the infant appears emaciated and fails to thrive, and you may note signs of chronic otitis media and sepsis. You may also find signs of the usual childhood diseases, such as chicken pox. Other assessment findings depend on the type and site of infection. For instance, an infant with severe watery diarrhea may have a GI infection from *Salmonella* or *Escherichia coli*.

Diagnostic tests

Defective humoral immunity is hard to detect before an infant reaches age 5 months. Before that age, even normal infants have only small amounts of serum IgM and IgA, and normal IgG levels merely reflect maternal IgG. However, tests that show a severely diminished or absent T-cell number and function and a lymph node biopsy that shows an absence of lymphocytes can confirm a diagnosis of SCID.

A chest X-ray characteristically shows bilateral pulmonary infiltrates.

Treatment

Treatment aims to restore immune response and prevent infection. The patient needs histocompatible bone marrow transplantation to correct immunodeficiency. Bone marrow cells must be matched for histocompatibility—

using both human leukocyte antigen and mixed leukocyte culture—so siblings usually serve as donors. But parental marrow can now be used successfully—after it's depleted of T cells, which could cause fatal acute graft-versus-host disease. T cells are removed with monoclonal antibodies or lectin columns.

Fetal thymus and liver transplantation have met with limited success. Immune globulin may also play a role in treatment. Some SCID infants have received long-term protection by being isolated in a completely sterile environment. However, this approach doesn't work for the infant who already has had recurring infections.

Nursing diagnoses

- Altered growth and development
- Altered parenting
- Altered protection
- Anxiety
- Impaired gas exchange
- Ineffective family coping
- Pain
- Risk for infection
- Social isolation

Nursing interventions

- Constantly monitor the infant for early signs of infection. If infection develops, provide prompt and aggressive drug therapy and supportive care, as ordered.
- Watch for adverse effects of any medications given. Avoid vaccinations, and give only irradiated blood products if a transfusion is ordered.
- Although SCID infants must remain in strict protective isolation, try to provide a stimulating atmosphere to promote growth and development.
- Encourage parents to visit their child often, to hold him, and to bring him toys that can be easily sterilized.
- Maintain a normal day and night routine, and talk to the child as much as possible. If parents can't visit, call them often to report on the infant's condition.
- Provide emotional support for the family and encourage the parents to have genetic counseling.

Patient teaching

- Ensure that the parents understand the need and proper technique for strict protective isolation.

COMPLEMENT DEFICIENCIES

Complement is a series of circulating enzymatic serum proteins with nine functional components, labeled C1 through C9. Complement deficiency or dysfunction may

MAJOR DISORDERS ASSOCIATED WITH COMPLEMENT DEFICIENCIES

Deficiency	Associated clinical conditions
C1q	Glomerulonephritis, systemic lupus erythematosus (SLE)
C1r	SLE-like syndrome
C2	SLE, discoid lupus erythematosus, juvenile rheumatoid arthritis, glomerulonephritis
C3	Recurrent pyogenic infections, glomerulonephritis
C4	SLE-like syndrome
C5	Recurrent disseminated neisserial infections, SLE
C6	Recurrent disseminated neisserial infections
C7	Recurrent disseminated neisserial infections, Raynaud's phenomenon
C8	Recurrent disseminated neisserial infections
C9	None identified
Properdin	Recurrent pyogenic infections, fulminant meningococcemia
C1 esterase inhibitor	Hereditary angioedema, increased incidence of several autoimmune diseases

increase susceptibility to infection and seems to be related to certain autoimmune disorders.

Theoretically, any complement component may be deficient or dysfunctional, and many such disorders are under investigation. However, primary complement deficiencies are rare. The most common include C2, C6, and C8 deficiencies, and C5 familial dysfunction. (See *Major disorders associated with complement deficiencies*.) More common secondary complement abnormalities have been confirmed in patients with lupus erythematosus, in some with dermatomyositis, in one with scleroderma (and in his family), and in a few patients with gonococcal and meningococcal infections.

The prognosis varies with the abnormality and the severity of associated diseases.

Causes

Primary complement deficiencies are inherited as autosomal recessive traits, except for deficiency of C1 esterase inhibitor, which is autosomal dominant. Secondary deficiencies may follow complement-fixing (complement-consuming) immunologic reactions, such as drug-induced serum sickness, acute streptococcal glomerulonephritis, and acute active systemic lupus erythematosus.

Normally, IgG or IgM reacts with antigens as part of an immune response, activating C1, which then combines with C4, initiating the classical complement pathway, or cascade. (An alternative complement pathway involves the direct activation of C3 by the serum protein properdin, bypassing the initial components [C1, C4, and C2] of the classical pathway.) Complement then combines with the antigen-antibody complex and undergoes a sequence of complicated reactions that amplify the immune response against the antigen. This complex process is called complement fixation. Any deficiency in complement interferes with this system.

Complications

C1 esterase inhibitor deficiency may lead to severe or even fatal swelling of the larynx.

Assessment findings

Signs and symptoms vary with the specific deficiency.

A patient with C2 or C3 deficiency or C5 familial dysfunction is likely to have signs and symptoms of a bacterial infection, which may involve several body systems simultaneously. Your assessment may also show signs of such collagen vascular diseases as lupus erythematosus and chronic renal failure in a patient with C2 deficiency.

In an infant with familial C5 dysfunction, assessment may uncover a failure to thrive, diarrhea, and seborrheic dermatitis. You may observe periodic swelling in the face, hands, abdomen, or throat that may lead to airway obstruction in a patient with C1 esterase inhibitor deficiency.

Diagnostic tests

Diagnosis of a complement deficiency is difficult and requires careful interpretation of both clinical features and laboratory results. Various complement deficiencies cause a low total serum complement level. Specific assays may help confirm deficiency of specific complement components. For example, immunofluorescence of glomerular tissues in glomerulonephritis that reveals complement components and IgG strongly suggests complement deficiency.

Treatment

Although primary complement deficiencies have no known cure, the associated infections, collagen vascular disease, and renal disease require prompt treatment. Transfusion of fresh-frozen plasma replaces complement components, but this treatment is controversial because it doesn't cure complement deficiencies and provides only transient beneficial effects. Although helpful, bone marrow transplantation can cause potentially fatal graft-versus-host disease (GVHD). Anabolic steroids and antifibrinolytic agents reduce acute swelling in patients with C1 esterase inhibitor deficiency.

Nursing diagnoses

- Altered growth and development
- Altered protection
- Body image disturbance
- Impaired skin integrity
- Ineffective airway clearance
- Ineffective family coping
- Risk for fluid volume deficit
- Risk for infection
- Risk for injury
- Risk for suffocation
- Social isolation

Nursing interventions

- Closely monitor the intake and output, serum electrolyte levels, and acid-base balance of a patient with renal infection. Also, watch for signs of renal failure.
- To maintain adequate ventilation, provide chest physiotherapy as needed to the patient with a respiratory tract infection.
- After bone marrow transplantation, monitor the patient closely for signs of transfusion reaction and GVHD.
- When caring for a patient with C1 esterase inhibitor deficiency, be prepared for emergency management of laryngeal edema that may result from angioedema. Keep airway equipment on hand.
- Provide support to the parents in distress. Help them identify and use effective coping strategies. Refer them to a counselor, if needed.

Patient teaching

- Teach the patient (or his family, if he's a child) the importance of avoiding infection, how to recognize its early signs and symptoms, and the need for prompt treatment if it occurs.

SELECTED REFERENCES

Avery, M.E., and First, L.R. *Pediatric Medicine,* 2nd ed. Baltimore: Williams & Wilkins Co., 1994.

"Consult Stat: Research Finds an ERT/Lupus Connection," *RN* 58(7):60, July 1995.

Immune and Infectious Disorders. Nursing TimeSavers Series. Springhouse, Pa.: Springhouse Corp., 1994.

Isselbacher, K., et al., eds. *Harrison's Principles of Internal Medicine,* 13th ed. New York: McGraw-Hill Book Co., 1995.

Long, B.C., and Phipps, W.J. *Medical-Surgical Nursing: A Nursing Process Approach,* 3rd ed. St. Louis: Mosby-Year Book, Inc., 1993.

Moncur, C., et al. "Rheumatoid Arthritis: Status of Drug Therapies," *Physical Therapy* 75(6):511-25, June 1995.

Spraul, G., et al. "A Descriptive Study of Foot Problems in Children with Juvenile Rheumatoid Arthritis," *Arthritis Care and Research* 7(3):144-50, September 1994.

Stites, D.P., et al. *Basic and Clinical Immunology,* 8th ed. East Norwalk, Conn.: Appleton & Lange, 1994.

Taylor, C.M., and Sparks, S.M. *Nursing Diagnosis Reference Manual,* 3rd ed. Springhouse, Pa.: Springhouse Corp., 1995.

Tierney, L., et al. *Current Medical Diagnosis and Treatment 1995.* East Norwalk, Conn.: Appleton & Lange, 1995.

6 HEMATOLOGIC DISORDERS

INTRODUCTION

Blood, one of the body's major fluid tissues, continuously circulates through the heart and blood vessels, carrying vital elements to every part of the body.

Reviewing blood basics

Blood performs several physiologically vital functions through its special components: the liquid portion (plasma) and the formed constituents (erythrocytes, leukocytes, platelets) that are suspended in it. Erythrocytes, or red blood cells (RBCs), carry oxygen to the tissues and remove carbon dioxide from them. Leukocytes, or white blood cells (WBCs), participate in inflammatory and immune responses. Plasma carries antibodies and nutrients to tissues and carries waste away; coagulation factors in plasma, with platelets (thrombocytes), control clotting. (See *Coagulation factors,* page 452.)

The average person has 5 to 6 liters of circulating blood, which constitutes 5% to 7% of body weight (as much as 10% in premature neonates). Blood is three to five times more viscous than water, with an alkaline pH of 7.35 to 7.45, and is either bright red (arterial blood) or dark red (venous blood), depending on the degree of oxygen saturation and the hemoglobin level.

Formation and characteristics

Hematopoiesis occurs primarily in the red bone marrow of the long bones and axial skeleton where primitive blood cells (stem cells) produce the precursors of erythrocytes (normoblasts), leukocytes, and thrombocytes (megakaryocytes). During embryonic development, blood cells are derived from mesenchyma and form in the yolk sac. As the fetus matures, blood cells are produced in the liver, the spleen, and the thymus; by the fifth month of gestation, blood cells also begin to form in the bone marrow. After birth, blood cells are usually produced only in the marrow.

Blood's functions

The most important function of blood is to *transport oxygen* (bound to RBCs inside hemoglobin) from the lungs to the body tissues and to *return carbon dioxide* from these tissues to the lungs. Blood also performs the following vital defensive and protective functions:
• provision of complement, a group of immunologically important protein substances in plasma
• transportation of granulocytes and monocytes to defend the body against pathogens by phagocytosis
• production and delivery of antibodies (by way of WBCs) formed by plasma cells and lymphocytes

• provision of specific immunity against viruses and cancer cells through sensitized lymphocytes.

Blood's other functions include control of hemostasis by platelets, plasma, and coagulation factors that repair tissue injuries and prevent or halt bleeding; regulation of acid-base and fluid balance; regulation of body temperature by carrying off excess heat generated by the internal organs for dissipation through the skin; and transportation of nutrients and regulatory hormones to body tissues, and of metabolic wastes to the organs of excretion (kidneys, lungs, and skin).

Blood dysfunction

Because of the rapid reproduction of bone marrow cells and the short life span and minimal storage in the bone marrow of circulating cells, bone marrow cells and their precursors are particularly vulnerable to physiologic changes that can affect cell production. Resulting blood disorders may be primary or secondary, quantitative or qualitative, or both; they may involve some or all blood components.

Quantitative blood disorders result from increased or decreased cell production or cell destruction; qualitative blood disorders stem from intrinsic cell abnormalities or plasma component dysfunction. Specific causes of blood disorders include trauma, chronic disease, surgery, malnutrition, drugs, exposure to toxins and radiation, and genetic and congenital defects that disrupt production and function. For example, depressed bone marrow production or mechanical destruction of mature blood cells can reduce the number of RBCs, platelets, and granulocytes, resulting in pancytopenia (anemia, thrombocytopenia, granulocytopenia). Increased production of multiple bone marrow components can follow myeloproliferative disorders.

RBC development

The tissues' demand for oxygen and the blood cells' ability to deliver it regulate RBC production. Consequently, hypoxia (or tissue anoxia) stimulates RBC production by triggering the formation and release of erythropoietin, a hormone that activates bone marrow to produce RBCs. Erythropoiesis may also be stimulated by androgens.

The actual formation of an erythrocyte begins with an uncommitted stem cell that eventually may develop into an RBC. Such formation requires certain vitamins—B_{12} and folic acid—and minerals, such as copper, cobalt, and especially iron, which is vital to hemoglobin's oxygen-carrying capacity. Iron is obtained from various foods and is absorbed in the duodenum and upper jejunum, leaving any excess for temporary storage in reticuloen-

COAGULATION FACTORS

The following lists coagulation factors and their synonyms. All coagulation factors are located in plasma except for Factor III, which is found in tissue cells.

Factor	Synonym
Factor I	Fibrinogen
Factor II	Prothrombin
Factor III	Tissue thromboplastin
Factor IV	Calcium ion
Factor V	Labile factor
Factor VII	Conversion accelerator
Factor VIII	Antihemophilic factor
Factor IX	Plasma thromboplastin component
Factor X	Stuart-Prower factor
Factor XI	Plasma thromboplastin antecedent
Factor XII	Hageman factor
Factor XIII	Fibrin stabilizing factor

dothelial cells, especially those in the liver. Iron excess is stored as ferritin and hemosiderin until it's released for use in the bone marrow to form new RBCs.

RBC disorders

Both quantitative and qualitative abnormalities constitute RBC disorders. Deficiency of RBCs (anemia) can follow any condition that destroys or inhibits the formation of these cells. Common factors leading to this deficiency include:
• congenital or acquired defects that cause bone marrow aplasia and suppress general hematopoiesis (aplastic anemias) or erythropoiesis
• drugs, toxins, and ionizing radiation
• metabolic abnormalities (sideroblastic anemias)
• deficiencies of vitamins (vitamin B_{12} deficiency or pernicious anemia), iron, or minerals (iron, folic acid, copper, and cobalt deficiency anemias) that cause inadequate RBC production
• excessive chronic or acute blood loss (posthemorrhagic anemia)
• chronic illnesses, such as renal disease and cancer
• intrinsically or extrinsically defective RBCs (sickle cell anemia).

Comparatively few conditions lead to an increased RBC count. Such conditions include:
• abnormal proliferation of all bone marrow elements (polycythemia vera)

• a single-element abnormality (for instance, an increase in the RBC count that results from erythropoietin excess, which is the result of hypoxemia or pulmonary disease)
• reduced plasma cell volume, which causes an apparent corresponding rise—relative, not absolute—in RBC concentration
• chronic hypoxic lung disease.

WBC development and function

WBCs protect the body against harmful bacteria and infection. They are classified as granular leukocytes—basophils, neutrophils, and eosinophils—or as nongranular leukocytes—lymphocytes, monocytes, and plasma cells. (See *Two types of leukocytes.*) Most WBCs are produced in bone marrow; however, lymphocytes and plasma cells complete their maturation in the lymph nodes. Although WBCs have a poorly defined tissue life span, some granular leukocytes (granulocytes) have a circulating half-life of less than 6 hours, some monocytes may survive for weeks or months, and certain lymphocytes last for years.

Normally, WBCs range from 5,000 to 10,000/mm³ and comprise the following elements:
• *Neutrophils,* the predominant form of granulocyte, make up about 60% of WBCs; they help devour invading organisms by phagocytosis.
• *Eosinophils,* minor granulocytes, may defend against parasites and participate in allergic reactions, pulmonary infections, and dermatologic infections.
• *Basophils,* minor granulocytes, may release heparin and histamine into the blood and also participate in delayed hypersensitivity reactions.
• *Monocytes,* along with neutrophils, help devour invading organisms by phagocytosis. They also help process antigens for lymphocytes and form macrophages in the tissues.
• *Lymphocytes* primarily occur in two forms: B cells and T cells. B cells aid antibody synthesis and T cells regulate cell-mediated immunity.
• *Plasma cells* develop from lymphocytes that reside in the tissues and produce antibodies. A recently identified large granular lymphocyte is thought to become the important antitumor cell called a natural killer cell.

WBC disorders

A temporary increase in the production and release of mature WBCs is a normal response to infection. However, an abnormal increase in immature WBC precursors and their accumulation in bone marrow or lymphoid tissue are characteristic of leukemia. These nonfunctioning WBCs (blasts) provide no protection against infection, crowd out other vital components—RBCs, platelets, mature WBCs—and spill into the bloodstream, sometimes infiltrating organs and impairing their functions.

WBC deficiencies may result from inadequate cell production, drug reactions, ionizing radiation, infiltrated bone marrow (cancer), congenital defects, aplastic anemias, folic acid deficiency, and hypersplenism. The most common types of WBC deficiencies are granulocytopenia and lymphocytopenia; monocytopenia occurs less frequently.

Platelets and platelet disorders

Small (2 to 4 microns in diameter) and colorless, platelets are disk-shaped cytoplasmic cells split from cells in bone marrow called megakaryocytes. Platelets have a life span of 7 to 10 days and perform three vital functions:
• initiating contraction of damaged blood vessels to minimize blood loss
• forming hemostatic plugs in injured blood vessels
• with plasma, providing materials that accelerate blood coagulation—notably platelet Factor III.

Platelet disorders include thrombocytopenia (platelet decrease), thrombocytosis (platelet excess), and thrombocytopathy (platelet dysfunction). Thrombocytopenia may result from congenital deficiency or acquired deficiency (exposure to drugs and ionizing radiation, cancerous infiltration of the bone marrow, abnormal sequestration in the spleen, abnormal mechanical destruction, or infection).

Thrombocytosis occurs with certain diseases, such as cancer. Thrombocytopathy usually results from disease (such as uremia and liver failure) or medication (such as salicylates and nonsteroidal anti-inflammatory agents).

Plasma

A clear, straw-colored fluid, plasma consists mainly of proteins (chiefly albumin, globulin, and fibrinogen) held in aqueous suspension. Other components of plasma include glucose, lipids, amino acids, electrolytes, pigments, hormones, respiratory gases (oxygen and carbon dioxide), and products of metabolism, such as urea, uric acid, creatinine, and lactic acid. Plasma's fluid characteristics—including osmotic pressure, viscosity, and suspension qualities—depend on its protein content. Plasma components regulate acid-base balance and immune responses and mediate coagulation and nutrition.

Hemostasis and clotting

In a complex process called hemostasis, platelets, plasma, and coagulation factors interact to control bleeding. When tissue injury occurs, local vasoconstriction and platelet

TWO TYPES OF LEUKOCYTES

Leukocytes vary in size, shape, and number. They are classified as granular or nongranular.

Granulocytes
The most numerous leukocytes, granulocytes include basophils, containing cytoplasmic granules that stain readily with alkaline dyes; neutrophils, which are finely granular and recognizable by their multinucleated appearance; and eosinophils, which stain with acidic dyes.

Nongranulocytes
Nongranular leukocytes include lymphocytes, monocytes and plasma cells. They have few, if any, granulated particles in the cytoplasm.

clumping (aggregation) at the injury site initially help prevent hemorrhage.

The extrinsic pathway (stimulated by tissue injury) or intrinsic pathway (stimulated by vessel injury or a foreign body in the bloodstream) activates the clotting process. A stabler clot is formed when each pathway merges with the final common pathway. In the final common pathway, prothrombin is converted to thrombin, and fibrinogen is converted to fibrin, which creates a fibrin clot that lasts for 2 to 3 days.

Assessment

Because many signs and symptoms of hematologic disorders are nonspecific and systemic, such as malaise and light-headedness, assessment can be difficult. However, certain key findings may alert you to the possibility of a hematologic disorder. These include abnormal bleeding, petechiae, ecchymoses, fatigue, weakness, dyspnea with or without exertion, fever, lymphadenopathy, and joint and bone pain.

History

Biographic data, including the patient's ethnic background and current and previous occupations, can provide important clues in identifying disorders associated with toxin exposure and hereditary disorders, such as sickle cell anemia and pernicious anemia.

Exploring the patient's complaints may reveal useful information about his symptoms, including onset, duration, precipitating or exacerbating factors, and relief measures. His health history may yield additional clues, such as allergies, immunizations, previously diagnosed illnesses, past hospitalizations and surgeries, past blood product transfusions, and current medications. Note any past illnesses that required immunosuppressive therapy, such as cancer; any immunosuppressive treatments, such as splenectomy or certain drugs; and any disorders that affect bone marrow function, such as hepatitis.

A review of the patient's life-style may reveal behaviors that can adversely affect hematologic function (for instance, poor dietary habits causing malnutrition or increased alcohol intake causing folic acid deficiency).

Physical examination

The patient with a hematologic disorder may have above- or below-normal temperature, tachycardia, hypotension, and tachypnea. His skin color may appear pale (possibly indicating decreased hemoglobin content), cyanotic (possibly indicating excessive deoxygenated hemoglobin), ruddy (possibly indicating polycythemia), or erythematous (possibly accompanying inflammation and fever).

Red-streaked areas over the lymph nodes may indicate an acute lymphatic disorder, such as acute lymphadenitis. Inspection of the skin and mucous membranes may reveal jaundice and purpuric lesions, petechiae, ecchymoses, and telangiectases. Dry, coarse skin may indicate iron deficiency anemia; itchy skin may result from polycythemia vera; red palms may indicate iron deficiency anemia.

The patient's mucous membranes may reveal bleeding, swelling, redness, and ulcerations. A smooth tongue can indicate vitamin B_{12} deficiency or iron deficiency anemia.

Inspection of the patient's fingernails may reveal longitudinal striations, a sign of anemia; koilonychia (spoon nail), characteristic of iron deficiency anemia; or nail clubbing from chronic tissue hypoxia.

The patient's eyes may appear jaundiced and the conjunctivae may appear pale. Retinal hemorrhages and exudates suggest severe anemia and thrombocytopenia. On inspection, the patient's abdomen may appear enlarged, distended, or asymmetrical.

Auscultation over the liver and spleen may reveal rubbing sounds that fluctuate with respirations, possibly indicating peritoneal inflammation or infarction. Percussion over all four quadrants helps to determine liver and spleen size. Palpation of the lymph nodes, liver, and spleen may detect enlargement. Congestion caused by cell overproduction, as in polycythemia, or excessive cell destruction, as in hemolytic anemia, can cause hepatomegaly or splenomegaly. Tenderness of sternal nodes may indicate anemia.

Diagnosing hematologic disorders

Laboratory studies that help determine blood composition, production, and function are vital in diagnosing he-

matologic disorders. Other common studies include tests to evaluate the coagulation and agglutination properties of the blood, and biopsies to evaluate the blood's formed elements.

Overall composition

Commonly performed tests include the following:
• *Peripheral blood smear* shows maturity and morphologic characteristics of blood elements and determines qualitative abnormalities.
• *Complete blood count (CBC)* determines the actual number of blood elements in relation to volume and quantifies abnormalities (RBCs, WBCs, and platelets).

RBC function

Various tests evaluate RBC function, including the following:
• *Hematocrit (HCT),* or packed cell volume (PCV), measures the percentage of RBCs per fluid volume of whole blood.
• *Hemoglobin (Hb)* measures the amount (grams) of hemoglobin per 100 ml of whole blood, to determine oxygen-carrying capacity.
• *Reticulocyte count* assesses RBC production by determining concentration of this erythrocyte precursor.
• *Schilling test* determines absorption of vitamin B_{12} (necessary for erythropoesis) by measuring excretion of radioactive B_{12} in the urine.
• *Mean corpuscular volume (MCV)* describes the RBC in terms of size. Immature or iron-deficient cells have increased MCV.
• *Mean corpuscular hemoglobin (MCH)* determines average amount of hemoglobin per RBC. The MCH is decreased in iron deficiency anemia.
• *Mean corpuscular hemoglobin concentration (MCHC)* determines the average hemoglobin concentration of 100 ml of packed RBCs.
• *Sucrose hemolysis test* assesses the susceptibility of RBCs to hemolyze with complement.
• *Sideroblast test* detects stainable iron (available for hemoglobin synthesis) in normoblastic RBCs.
• *Hemoglobin electrophoresis* demonstrates abnormal hemoglobin such as sickle cell anemia.

Coagulation tests

Commonly performed tests include the following:
• *Platelet count* determines the number of platelets.
• *Bleeding time (Ivy bleeding time)* assesses the platelets' capacity to stop bleeding in capillaries and small vessels by measuring the duration of bleeding after a standard skin incision. Used along with the platelet count, it can

help detect the presence of such disorders as von Willebrand's disease, disseminated intravascular coagulation (DIC), severe hepatic or renal disease, and hemolytic disease of the newborn.

• *Capillary fragility test* measures the capillaries' ability to remain intact under increasing intracapillary pressure. It can help detect thrombocytopenia, DIC, polycythemia vera, and von Willebrand's disease.

• *Activated partial thromboplastin time (APTT)* evaluates intrinsic pathway clotting factors. It helps in preoperative screening for bleeding tendencies and aids in monitoring heparin therapy.

• *Partial thromboplastin time (PTT)* also aids in evaluating intrinsic pathway clotting factors. However, it is less sensitive and less frequently performed than APTT.

• *Prothrombin time (PT, Quick's test, or pro time)* indirectly measures prothrombin and helps evaluate prothrombin, fibrinogen, and extrinsic coagulation Factors V, VII, and X. It's used to monitor oral anticoagulant therapy.

• *Plasma thrombin time (thrombin clotting time),* which measures how quickly a clot forms, detects abnormalities in thrombin fibrinogen reaction. It helps identify a fibrinogen deficiency or defect, diagnose DIC and hepatic disease, and monitor heparin, streptokinase, and urokinase therapy.

• *Plasma fibrinogen* test determines the amount of fibrinogen (Factor I) available in plasma to help form fibrin clots. Fibrinogen levels are decreased in hepatic failure and DIC, but increased in hepatic cirrhosis and some lymphoproliferative disorders, such as lymphoma.

• *Fibrin degradation products (FDPs or fibrin split products)* show the amount of clot breakdown products in serum. Normally cleared rapidly, FDPs are elevated in such clotting disorders as DIC.

• *Antithrombin III test* helps determine the cause of impaired coagulation, especially hypercoagulation. Antithrombin III levels are decreased in clotting disorders, such as DIC, and may be increased during therapy with oral anticoagulants.

• *D-dimer test* measures a specific fibrin monomer fragment of FDPs to determine if FDPs are caused by normal mechanisms or by excessive fibrinolysis. The fibrin monomer fragments are present in severe clotting disorders, such as DIC.

• *Factor VIII assay* identifies the quantity of this factor, which commonly is reduced in hemophilia.

• *One-stage factor assays: Extrinsic coagulation system* helps detect a deficiency of Factor II, V, or X when PT and APTT are prolonged. The *intrinsic coagulation system* helps identify a deficiency of Factor VIII, IX, or XII when PT is normal and the APTT is abnormal.

WBC function
The following laboratory studies evaluate WBC function:
• *WBC count* and *differential* establishes the quantity and maturity of polymorphonuclear granulocytes or bands, basophils, eosinophils, lymphocytes, and monocytes.

• *Quantified T4/T8 lymphocyte test* determines helper and suppressor agents important to immune function in human immunodeficiency virus (HIV) infection; may also be reported as a T4/T8 ratio.

• *Complement fixation ratio* detects the quantity of complement and antibody complexes indicative of infection.

• *Absolute T4 helper count* provides the CD4$^+$ T-cell count, which is used to monitor patients with HIV infection.

• *Immunoglubulin test* measures the levels of immunoglobulins G, A, and M to detect immune incompetence caused by low antibody levels.

Plasma
The following laboratory studies assess aspects of plasma:
• *Erythrocyte sedimentation rate (ESR)* measures the rate of RBC settling out of plasma. It may detect infection or inflammation.

• *Electrophoresis of serum proteins* determines the amount of various serum proteins, which are classified by mobility in response to an electrical field.

• *Immunoelectrophoresis of serum proteins* separates and classifies serum antibodies (immunoglobulins), using specific antisera.

Agglutination tests
These tests evaluate the ability of the blood's formed elements to react to foreign substances by clumping together:
• *ABO blood typing* helps prevent lethal transfusion reactions. It types blood into A, B, AB, and O groups, according to the presence of major antigens A and B on RBC surfaces and according to serum antibodies anti-A and anti-B.

• *Rh typing* classifies blood by the presence or absence of the Rh$_o$(D) antigen on the surface of RBCs to ensure compatibility of transfused blood.

• *Cross matching* establishes the compatibility or incompatibility of donor and recipient blood before transfusion.

• *Direct antiglobulin test (direct Coombs' test)* demonstrates the presence of immunoglobulin G (IgG) antibodies (such as antibodies to Rh factor), complement, or both on the surface of circulating RBCs. It is used to diagnose hemolytic disease of the newborn and aid in differential diagnosis of hemolytic anemias.

• *Antibody screening test (indirect Coombs' test),* a two-step test, detects the presence of IgG antibodies on RBCs in recipient or donor serum before transfusion.

• *Leukoagglutinin test* differentiates between transfusion reactions by detecting antibodies that react with WBCs.

Bone marrow biopsy

Because most hematopoiesis occurs in bone marrow, histologic and hematologic bone marrow examination helps diagnose thrombocytopenia, anemias, polycythemia, and DIC.

ANEMIAS

Characterized by reduced hemoglobin levels, the anemias include pernicious anemia, folic acid deficiency anemia, aplastic or hypoplastic anemias, sideroblastic anemias, iron deficiency anemia, and sickle cell anemia. They may result from one or more of these pathophysiologic processes: diminished hemoglobin or red cell production, increased red cell destruction, or blood loss.

PERNICIOUS ANEMIA

Also known as Addison's anemia, pernicious anemia is a megaloblastic anemia characterized by decreased gastric production of hydrochloric acid and deficiency of intrinsic factor, a substance normally secreted by the parietal cells of the gastric mucosa that is essential for vitamin B_{12} absorption. The resulting deficiency of vitamin B_{12} causes serious neurologic, psychological, gastric, and intestinal abnormalities. Increasingly fragile cell membranes induce widespread destruction of red blood cells (RBCs), resulting in low hemoglobin levels.

In the United States, pernicious anemia is most common in New England and the Great Lakes region. It's rare in children, Blacks, and Asians. Onset typically is between ages 50 and 60; incidence rises with increasing age.

Causes and pathophysiology

Familial incidence of pernicious anemia suggests a genetic predisposition. This disorder is significantly more common in patients with immunologically related diseases, such as thyroiditis, myxedema, and Graves' disease.

These facts seem to support a widely held theory that an inherited autoimmune response causes gastric mucosal atrophy and, consequently, decreases hydrochloric acid and intrinsic factor production. Intrinsic factor deficiency impairs vitamin B_{12} absorption. The resultant vitamin B_{12} deficiency inhibits the growth of all cells, particularly RBCs, leading to insufficient and deformed RBCs with poor oxygen-carrying capacity.

Pernicious anemia also impairs myelin formation. Initially, it affects the peripheral nerves but gradually it extends to the spinal cord, causing neurologic dysfunction.

Secondary pernicious anemia can result from partial removal of the stomach, which limits the amount of productive mucosa.

Complications

Patients treated with vitamin B_{12} injections have few permanent complications. Those who go untreated may experience permanent neurologic disability (including paralysis) and psychotic behavior; they also may lose sphincter control of bowel and bladder, and some eventually may die of the disorder. Although the reason is unclear, the incidence of peptic ulcer disease is four to five times greater in patients with pernicious anemia than in the general population.

Assessment findings

Although pernicious anemia usually has an insidious onset, the patient's history may reveal the characteristic triad of symptoms: weakness, a beefy red sore tongue, and numbness and tingling in the extremities. The patient may also complain of nausea, vomiting, anorexia, weight loss, flatulence, diarrhea, and constipation. (See *Planning care for the patient with pernicious anemia.*)

On inspection, the lips, gums, and tongue appear markedly bloodless. Slightly jaundiced sclera and pale to bright yellow skin may be present with hemolysis-induced hyperbilirubinemia.

The pulse rate is rapid, and auscultation may reveal a systolic murmur. Percussion or palpation may reveal an enlarged liver and spleen.

When neurologic involvement occurs, the patient may complain of weakness in the extremities; peripheral numbness and paresthesias; disturbed position sense; lack of coordination; impaired fine finger movement; light-headedness; headache; altered vision (diplopia, blurred vision), taste, and hearing (tinnitus); loss of bowel and bladder control; and, in males, impotence.

You may observe that the patient is irritable, depressed, delirious, and ataxic, and has poor memory. You also may note positive Babinski's and Romberg's signs and optic muscle atrophy. Although some of these symptoms are temporary, irreversible central nervous system changes may have occurred before treatment is initiated.

Complaints of weakness, fatigue, and light-headedness stem from the impaired oxygen-carrying capacity of the blood owing to lowered hemoglobin levels. Compensatory increased cardiac output may cause palpita-

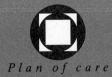

Plan of care

PLANNING CARE FOR THE PATIENT WITH PERNICIOUS ANEMIA

To help you develop an effective plan of care, suppose that you're caring for Frank Peterson, a 53-year-old apartment building janitor and handyman. Mr. Peterson was brought to the hospital last evening after losing his balance on a stepladder.

Patient history

Mr. Peterson complains of extreme tiredness despite sleeping more, plus anorexia, dyspepsia, and a sore mouth and tongue, progressively worsening over the past several months. If he walks up more than one flight of steps, he becomes winded. Many small jobs, requiring minor lifting or pushing, make him short of breath. He describes himself as a moderate drinker, consuming 1 pint of whiskey and one case of beer each week, usually in the evening. He also has smoked one to two packs of cigarettes each day for 35 years.

Mr. Peterson's family history is unremarkable. He can't remember much about his father and hasn't seen his two brothers for many years; he does remember that his mother had diabetes and had to give herself insulin every day. He describes his family as being poor and remembers many meals of soup and bread.

Assessment findings

Your initial assessment of Mr. Peterson begins with his vital signs, height, and weight. His oral temperature is 99.2° F (37.3° C). His pulse rate is irregular, rapid, and bounding at 98 beats/minute. His respiratory rate is 28 breaths/minute and shallow. His blood pressure is elevated at 158/96 mm Hg.

He weighs 151 lb (68.5 kg) and is 6′ (1.8 m) tall.

Inspection reveals a thin black man with pale pink gums, beefy red tongue, oral ulcerations, mildly jaundiced sclera, distended neck veins, and dry skin. He appears anxious and has difficulty with fine tremors when asked to close his eyes and hold his hands outstretched. Both hands and feet are cool with capillary refill greater than 4 seconds. Palpation of the abdomen reveals an enlarged, tender liver. Auscultation identifies diffuse crackles and diminished breath sounds. His heart sounds are distant, but an S_3 is audible.

Initial diagnostic tests showed:
• decreased RBC count, hematocrit, hemoglobin level, and platelet count
• decreased folate, ferritin, transferrin, iron-binding capacity, and vitamin B_{12} levels
• abnormal blood urea nitrogen and decreased serum albumin levels
• peripheral oximetry of 91%.

Because test findings suggest pernicious anemia, a Schilling test is scheduled to detect the absence of intrinsic factor. Bone marrow and gastric analyses are indicated, and stool tests to detect occult blood are ordered.

Nursing diagnoses

Based on your assessment, you select these nursing diagnoses:
• Activity intolerance and altered tissue perfusion related to lack of hemoglobin and oxygen delivery, manifested by fatigue and weakness
• Altered nutrition: Less than body requirements, related to inadequate intake of essential nutrients, oral pain, and anorexia
• Decreased cardiac output related to increased cardiac work load and reduced oxygenation
• Risk for injury related to falls and hand injuries associated with cerebral hypoxia, impaired proprioception, and paresthesias.

Expected outcomes

You plan the following goals for Mr. Peterson. He will:
• improve oxygenation and tissue perfusion
• supplement and stabilize his dietary intake of essential nutrients and decrease mouth pain
• improve proprioception, walking, and hand coordination, and decrease paresthesia
• decrease the heart's work load.

Implementation

You'll need to take the following steps to promote optimal outcomes for Mr. Peterson.

To improve tissue perfusion
• Administer oxygen as needed.
• Administer blood products to correct deficiencies in RBCs, WBCs, hemoglobin, and platelets; administer slowly because of cardiac compromise.
• Allow for bed rest with a gradual increase in activity according to the patient's tolerance level.
• Decrease anxiety by explaining the need for all tests, medications, transfusions, and rest. Assure Mr. Peterson that most of his symptoms will diminish with proper therapy.
• Instruct him to stop smoking. Refer him for counseling, as needed.

To supplement and stabilize nutrition and decrease mouth pain
• Consult the dietitian and provide frequent, small, attractive meals high in iron, folate, and vitamin B_{12}. Ensure that meals are neither too hot nor too cold, easy to chew, and composed of foods that appeal to Mr. Peterson.
• Add vitamin C to his diet and medications to promote iron absorption.
• Provide oral care with salt water

(continued)

PLANNING CARE FOR THE PATIENT WITH PERNICIOUS ANEMIA *(continued)*

before each meal and at bedtime. If glossitis increases, provide an oral anesthetic, such as viscous lidocaine (Xylocaine), as a swish up to 5 minutes before eating and as needed.
• Provide chemical agents (such as histamine₂-receptor antagonists) to protect the gastric mucosa from further irritation.
• Weigh Mr. Peterson three times per week to chart progression of weight gain and acceptance of new eating habits.

To reduce the risk of injury related to neurologic effects
• Administer oxygen, as needed.
• Provide assistance for walking, daily activities, and transferring by one-person assist or devices such as a walker.
• Clear the room of excess furnish-

ings. Provide good lighting while Mr. Peterson is moving about in the room.
• Keep his hands and feet covered and warm. Provide warm baths or showers to increase circulation.
• Assess for confusion, changes in mentation or level of consciousness, shortened attention span, and irritability.

To decrease cardiac work load
• Promote rest.
• Monitor Mr. Peterson's vital signs every 4 hours while he is awake. Before getting him out of bed, test for orthostatic hypotension.
• Monitor fluid intake and adjust it according to symptoms of pulmonary or venous congestion.
• Provide for optimal intake of oxygen by elevating the head of the bed, administering oxygen as ordered, providing small meals, and decreasing anxiety.
• Deliver and monitor for the effectiveness of medications that decrease cardiac work load (antiar-

rhythmics, cardiotonics, diuretics, vasodilators).
• Provide stool softeners to decrease the urge to use Valsalva's maneuver.

Evaluation
While Mr. Peterson remains in the hospital, his condition will change. Reevaluate his condition and alter your plans and goals as he progresses with therapy. Does he have sufficient information about diet, diet supplements, and ordered medications? Will he be able to afford his ordered medications and diet, and can he prepare foods well enough so that he will stay on his new diet? Does he understand the signs and symptoms associated with his anemia, and know when to notify the doctor if problems occur? Can he identify ways to reduce his risk for injury while performing his job? Will he comply with quarterly doctor's visits and laboratory tests?

---

tions, dyspnea, orthopnea, tachycardia, premature beats and, eventually, congestive heart failure.

Diagnostic tests
The results of blood studies, bone marrow examination, gastric analysis, and the Schilling test establish the diagnosis. Laboratory screening must rule out other anemias with similar symptoms, such as folic acid deficiency anemia, because treatment differs. Diagnosis must also rule out vitamin B₁₂ deficiency, resulting from malabsorption due to GI disorders, gastric surgery, radiation therapy, or drug therapy.

Blood study results that suggest pernicious anemia include:
• decreased hemoglobin levels (4 to 5 g/dl) and decreased RBC count
• increased mean corpuscular volume (under 120 mm³); because larger-than-normal RBCs *each* contain increased amounts of hemoglobin, mean corpuscular hemoglobin concentration is also increased
• possible low white blood cell (WBC) and platelet counts and large, malformed platelets
• serum vitamin B₁₂ levels less than 0.1 mcg/ml
• elevated serum lactate dehydrogenase levels.

Bone marrow studies reveal erythroid hyperplasia (crowded red bone marrow) with increased numbers of megaloblasts but few normally developing RBCs. Gastric analysis shows absence of free hydrochloric acid after histamine or pentagastrin injection.

The Schilling test is the definitive test for pernicious anemia. In this test, the patient receives a small (0.5 to 2 mcg) oral dose of radioactive vitamin B₁₂ after fasting for 12 hours. A larger (1 mg) dose of nonradioactive vitamin B₁₂ is given I.M. 2 hours later, as a parenteral flush, and the radioactivity of a 24-hour urine specimen is measured. About 7% of the radioactive B₁₂ dose is excreted in the first 24 hours; people with pernicious anemia excrete less than 3%. (Normally, vitamin B₁₂ is absorbed, and excess amounts are excreted in the urine; in pernicious anemia, the vitamin remains unabsorbed and is passed in the stool.) When the Schilling test is repeated with intrinsic factor added, the test shows normal excretion of vitamin B₁₂.

Treatment
Early I.M. vitamin B₁₂ replacement can reverse pernicious anemia and may prevent permanent neurologic damage. An initial high dose of parenteral vitamin B₁₂

causes rapid RBC regeneration. Within 2 weeks, hemoglobin should rise to normal, and the patient's condition should markedly improve. Because rapid cell regeneration increases the patient's iron requirements, concomitant iron replacement is necessary to prevent iron deficiency anemia. After the patient's condition improves, vitamin B_{12} doses can be decreased to maintenance levels and given monthly. Because such injections must be continued for life, patients should learn self-administration.

If anemia causes extreme fatigue, the patient may require bed rest until hemoglobin rises. If he is critically ill, with severe anemia and cardiopulmonary distress, he may need blood transfusions, digitalis, a diuretic, and a low-sodium diet for congestive heart failure. Most important is the replacement of vitamin B_{12} to control the condition that led to this failure. Antibiotics help combat accompanying infections, and topical anesthetics may relieve mouth pain.

Nursing diagnoses
• Activity intolerance
• Altered nutrition: Less than body requirements
• Altered oral mucous membrane
• Altered tissue perfusion
• Fatigue
• Impaired gas exchange
• Impaired physical mobility
• Impaired swallowing
• Knowledge deficit
• Pain
• Risk for infection
• Risk for injury
• Self-care deficit
• Sensory or perceptual alteration

Nursing interventions
• If the patient has severe anemia, plan activities, rest periods, and necessary diagnostic tests to conserve his energy. Monitor pulse rate often; tachycardia means his activities are too strenuous.
• Advise the patient to report signs and symptoms of decreased perfusion to vital organs--dyspnea, chest pain, dizziness--and symptoms of neuropathy, such as tingling in the periphery.
• To ensure accurate Schilling test results, make sure that all urine over a 24-hour period is collected and that the specimens remain uncontaminated by bacteria.
• Provide a well-balanced diet, including foods high in vitamin B_{12} (meat, liver, fish, eggs, and milk). Offer be-tween-meal snacks, and encourage the family to bring favorite foods from home.
• Because a sore mouth and tongue make eating painful, ask the dietitian to avoid giving the patient irritating foods. If these symptoms make talking difficult, supply a pad and pencil or some other aid to facilitate nonverbal communication; explain this problem to the family. Provide diluted mouthwash or, with severe conditions, swab the patient's mouth with tap water or warm saline solution. Oral anesthetics diluted in 0.9% sodium chloride solution also may be used.
• If the patient is incontinent, establish a regular bowel and bladder routine. After the patient is discharged, a visiting nurse should follow up on this schedule and make adjustments, as needed.
• If neurologic damage causes behavioral problems, assess mental and neurologic status often; if necessary, give tranquilizers, as ordered, and, if needed, apply a soft restraint at night.
• Institute safety precautions to prevent falls.

Patient teaching
• Warn the patient to guard against infections, and tell him to report signs of infection promptly, especially pulmonary and urinary tract infections, because the patient's weakened condition may increase susceptibility.
• Caution the patient with a sensory deficit to avoid exposure to extreme heat or cold on the extremities.
• If neurologic involvement is present, advise the patient to avoid clothing with small buttons and activities of daily living that require fine motor skills.
• Stress that vitamin B_{12} replacement isn't a permanent cure and that these injections *must* be continued for life, even after symptoms subside.
• If possible, teach the patient or his caregiver proper injection techniques.
• Teach family members to observe for confusion or irritability and to report these findings to the doctor.
• To prevent pernicious anemia, emphasize the importance of vitamin B_{12} supplements for patients who have had extensive gastric resections or who follow strict vegetarian diets.

FOLIC ACID DEFICIENCY ANEMIA
A common, slowly progressive megaloblastic anemia, folic acid deficiency anemia is most prevalent in infants, adolescents, pregnant and lactating females, alcoholics, elderly people, and in people with malignant or intestinal diseases.

FOODS HIGH IN FOLIC ACID CONTENT

Folic acid (pteroylglutamic acid, folacin) is found in most body tissues, where it acts as a coenzyme in metabolic processes involving 1-carbon transfer. It is essential for formation and maturation of RBCs and for synthesis of deoxyribonucleic acid. Although its body stores are comparatively small (about 70 mg), this vitamin is plentiful in most well-balanced diets.

However, because folic acid is water-soluble and heat-labile, it's easily destroyed by cooking. Also, about 20% of folic acid intake is excreted unabsorbed. Insufficient daily folic acid intake (less than 50 mcg/day) usually induces folic acid deficiency within 4 months. Below is a list of foods high in folic acid content.

Food	mcg/100 g
Asparagus spears	109
Beef liver	294
Broccoli spears	54
Collards (cooked)	102
Mushrooms	24
Oatmeal	33
Peanut butter	57
Red beans	180
Wheat germ	305

Causes
Alcohol abuse suppressing the metabolic effects of folate is probably the most common cause of folic acid deficiency anemia. Additional causes include:
• poor diet (common in alcoholics, narcotic addicts, elderly people who live alone, and infants, especially those with infections or diarrhea). Some adolescents whose diet mainly consists of nonnutritional food develop folate deficiency.
• impaired absorption (due to intestinal dysfunction from such disorders as celiac disease, tropical sprue, regional jejunitis, and bowel resection)
• bacteria competing for available folic acid
• excessive cooking of foods, which destroys the available nutrient

• limited storage capacity in infants
• prolonged drug therapy with such drugs as anticonvulsants, estrogens, and methotrexate
• increased folic acid requirements during pregnancy, during rapid growth periods in infancy (especially in surviving premature infants); during childhood and adolescence due to consumption of folate-poor cow's milk; and in patients with neoplastic diseases and some skin diseases, such as exfoliative dermatitis.

Complications
Folic acid deficiency anemia produces no complications.

Assessment findings
The patient's history may reveal severe, progressive fatigue, the hallmark of folic acid deficiency. Associated findings include shortness of breath, palpitations, diarrhea, nausea, anorexia, headaches, forgetfulness, and irritability. The impaired oxygen-carrying capacity of the blood from lowered hemoglobin levels may produce complaints of weakness and light-headedness.

Inspection may reveal generalized pallor and jaundice. The patient may appear wasted. Cheilosis and glossitis may be present. Folic acid deficiency anemia doesn't cause neurologic impairment unless it's associated with vitamin B_{12} deficiency.

Diagnostic tests
The Schilling test and a therapeutic trial of vitamin B_{12} injections distinguish between folic acid deficiency anemia and pernicious anemia. Significant findings on blood studies include macrocytosis, decreased reticulocyte count, increased mean corpuscular volume, abnormal platelets, and serum folate levels less than 4 mg/ml.

Treatment
Medical treatment consists primarily of folic acid supplements and elimination of contributing causes. Supplements may be given orally (1 to 5 mg/day) or parenterally (to patients who are severely ill, have malabsorption, or are unable to take oral medication). Many patients respond favorably to a well-balanced diet. (See *Foods high in folic acid content.*)

Nursing diagnoses
• Activity intolerance
• Altered growth and development
• Altered nutrition: Less than body requirements
• Altered oral mucous membrane
• Altered thought processes
• Altered tissue perfusion

- Diarrhea
- Fluid volume deficit
- Impaired gas exchange

Nursing interventions

- If the patient has severe anemia, plan activities, rest periods, and necessary diagnostic tests to conserve his energy. Monitor his pulse rate often; tachycardia means his activities are too strenuous.
- Advise the patient to report signs and symptoms of decreased perfusion to vital organs: dyspnea, chest pain, dizziness.
- If the patient has glossitis, emphasize the importance of good oral hygiene. Suggest regular use of a mild or diluted mouthwash and a soft toothbrush. Oral anesthetics may be used to allay discomfort.
- Because a sore mouth and tongue make eating painful, ask the dietitian to give the patient only nonirritating foods. If these symptoms make talking difficult, supply a pad and pencil or some other aid to facilitate nonverbal communication; explain this problem to the family.
- To ensure accurate Schilling test results, make sure that all urine over a 24-hour period is collected and that the specimens remain uncontaminated by bacteria.
- Provide a well-balanced diet, including foods high in folate, such as dark green leafy vegetables, organ meats, eggs, milk, oranges, bananas, dry beans, and whole-grain breads. Offer between-meal snacks, and encourage the family to bring favorite foods from home.
- Monitor fluid and electrolyte balance, particularly in the patient who has severe diarrhea and is receiving parenteral fluid replacement therapy.

Patient teaching

- To prevent folic acid deficiency anemia, emphasize the importance of a well-balanced diet high in folic acid. Identify alcoholics or other high-risk people with poor dietary habits, and try to arrange for appropriate counseling. Tell mothers who are not breast-feeding to use commercially prepared formulas.
- Teach the patient to meet daily folic acid requirements by including a food from each food group in every meal. If the patient has a severe deficiency, explain that diet only reinforces folic acid supplementation and isn't therapeutic by itself. Urge compliance with the prescribed course of therapy. Advise the patient not to stop taking the supplements when he begins to feel better.
- Warn the patient to guard against infections, and tell him to report signs of infection promptly, especially pulmonary and urinary tract infections, because the patient's weakened condition may increase susceptibility.

APLASTIC OR HYPOPLASTIC ANEMIAS

Potentially fatal, aplastic or hypoplastic anemias result from injury to or destruction of stem cells in bone marrow or the bone marrow matrix, causing pancytopenia (anemia, leukopenia, thrombocytopenia) and bone marrow hypoplasia.

Although often used interchangeably with other terms for bone marrow failure, aplastic anemias correctly refer to pancytopenia resulting from the decreased functional capacity of a hypoplastic, fatty bone marrow. These disorders usually produce fatal bleeding or infection, particularly when they're idiopathic or stem from chloramphenicol use or infectious hepatitis. Mortality for aplastic anemias with severe pancytopenia is 80% to 90%.

Causes

Aplastic anemias usually develop when damaged or destroyed stem cells inhibit red blood cell (RBC) production. Less commonly, they develop when damaged bone marrow microvasculature creates an unfavorable environment for cell growth and maturation. About half of such anemias result from drugs (such as chloramphenicol), toxic agents (such as benzene), or radiation. (See *Causes of acquired aplastic anemias*, page 462.) The rest may result from immunologic factors (suspected but unconfirmed), severe disease (especially hepatitis), viral infection (especially in children), or preleukemic and neoplastic infiltration of bone marrow.

Idiopathic anemias may be congenital. Two such forms of aplastic anemia have been identified: Congenital hypoplastic anemia (anemia of Blackfan and Diamond) develops between ages 2 months and 3 months; Fanconi's syndrome, between birth and age 10. In the absence of a consistent familial or genetic history of aplastic anemia, researchers suspect that these congenital abnormalities result from an induced change in fetal development, such as in maternal rubella or cytomegalovirus infection.

Complications

Life-threatening hemorrhage from the mucous membranes is the most common complication of aplastic or hypoplastic anemias because affected patients develop alloimmunization, which can make platelet transfusions ineffective. Immunosuppression can lead to secondary opportunistic infections.

CAUSES OF ACQUIRED APLASTIC ANEMIAS

Drugs, toxic agents, and radiation cause about half of all cases of acquired aplastic anemias. Examples and other causes are listed below.

Drugs
Antibiotics (chloramphenicol, cephalosporins, sulfonamides and, rarely, penicillins), anti-inflammatory drugs (phenylbutazone, indomethacin, gold, and penicillamine), anticonvulsants (especially phenytoin, ethosuximide, and carbamazepine), antineoplastics, diuretics (including hydrochlorothiazide), phenothiazines, antidiabetic drugs, antithyroid drugs, antimalarials, zidovudine, antiarrhythmics (procainamide)

Chemicals and toxins
Pesticides, aromatic hydrocarbons (benzene), heavy metals

Infections
Hepatitis C (non-A, non-B), Epstein-Barr virus, Venezuelan equine encephalitis, cytomegalovirus, miliary tuberculosis

Rheumatoid and autoimmune diseases
Systemic lupus erythematosus, rheumatoid arthritis, graft-versus-host disease

Other causes
Paroxysmal nocturnal hemoglobulinuria, radiation, thymoma, pregnancy, idiopathic causes

Assessment findings

The patient's history may not help establish the disease onset because the symptoms often develop insidiously. The patient may report signs and symptoms of anemia (progressive weakness and fatigue, shortness of breath, and headache) or signs of thrombocytopenia (easy bruising and bleeding, especially from the mucous membranes [nose, gums, rectum, vagina]).

Inspection may reveal pallor if the patient is anemic, and ecchymosis, petechiae, or retinal bleeding if thrombocytopenia is present. You may note alterations in the level of consciousness and weakness if bleeding into the central nervous system has occurred.

Auscultation may reveal bibasilar crackles, tachycardia, and a gallop murmur if severe anemia results in congestive heart failure.

The patient may also have signs and symptoms of an opportunistic infection (most commonly, a bacterial infection). Fever, oral and rectal ulcers, and sore throat may indicate the presence of an infection but without characteristic inflammation.

Diagnostic tests

Confirmation of aplastic anemia requires a series of laboratory tests. Characteristic blood study results include:
• RBC count of 1 million/mm^3 or less, usually with normochromic and normocytic cells (although macrocytosis [larger-than-normal erythrocytes] and anisocytosis [excessive variation in erythrocyte size] may exist); very low absolute reticulocyte count
• elevated serum iron levels (unless bleeding occurs), but normal or slightly reduced total iron-binding capacity; hemosiderin is present, and tissue iron storage is visible microscopically
• decreased platelet and white blood cell (WBC) counts.

Bone marrow biopsies performed at several sites may yield a dry tap or show severely hypocellular or aplastic marrow, with a varying amount of fat, fibrous tissue, or gelatinous replacement; absence of tagged iron (because the iron is deposited in the liver rather than in bone marrow) and megakaryocytes; and depression of erythroid elements.

Differential diagnosis must rule out paroxysmal nocturnal hemoglobinuria and other diseases in which pancytopenia is common.

Treatment

Effective treatment must eliminate any identifiable cause and provide vigorous supportive measures, such as packed RBC, platelet, and experimental histocompatibility antigen (HLA)-matched leukocyte transfusions. Even after elimination of the cause, recovery can take months or may never occur. Bone marrow transplantation is the treatment of choice for anemia due to severe aplasia and for patients who need constant RBC transfusions. (See *Nursing interventions in bone marrow transplantation.*)

The patient with low leukocyte counts is at risk for infection. Prevention of infection may range from frequent hand washing to filtered air flow. The infection itself may require specific antibiotics; however, these are not given prophylactically because they tend to encourage resistant strains of organisms. Patients with low hemoglobin counts may need respiratory support with oxygen, in addition to blood transfusions.

Other appropriate forms of treatment include corticosteroids to stimulate erythroid production (successful in children, unsuccessful in adults); marrow-stimulating agents, such as androgens (which are controversial); antilymphocyte globulin (experimental); and immunosup-

NURSING INTERVENTIONS IN BONE MARROW TRANSPLANTATION

In bone marrow transplantation, 500 to 700 ml of marrow usually are aspirated from the pelvic bones of an HLA-compatible (allogeneic) donor. In certain malignant disorders, autologous (self-donor) and peripheral stem cell transplants are performed. In such cases, stem cells are harvested and stored before the patient undergoes chemotherapy, which suppresses bone marrow. After chemotherapy, the stored cells are infused to repopulate the bone marrow and rescue the patient from aplasia. This procedure has effected long-term healthy survival in about half the patients with severe aplastic anemia. Bone marrow transplantation may also be effective in treating patients with hematologic malignancies (leukemia, lymphoma, and multiple myeloma), certain immunodeficiency diseases, and solid-tumor cancers.

Because bone marrow transplantation carries serious risks, it requires infection prevention techniques, such as good hand washing, particulate filter air flow, a primary nurse, and strict aseptic technique.

Before marrow infusion
• Assess the patient's understanding of bone marrow transplantation. If necessary, correct any misconceptions, and provide additional information, as appropriate. Explain that success rate depends on the disease stage and an HLA-identical sibling match.
• Explain that chemotherapy and, possibly, radiation therapy are necessary to remove existing cells that may cause resistance to transplantation.
• To suppress the patient's immune system, various preparatory regimens may be used, including parenteral cyclophosphamide. This treatment requires aggressive hydration to prevent hemorrhagic cystitis. In conjunction with cyclophosphamide, the patient may receive additional chemotherapy or total-body irradiation. To control nausea and vomiting, give the patient an antiemetic such as ondansetron, granisetron or, occasionally, lorazepam, as needed.
• Because alopecia is a common adverse effect of high-dose cyclophosphamide therapy, urge the patient to choose a wig or scarf before treatment begins.
• Total-body irradiation given in one dose or daily for several consecutive days follows chemotherapy, inducing total marrow aplasia. Inform the patient that cataracts, GI disturbances, and sterility are possible

adverse effects.
• Assess venous access. If necessary, the patient may have an indwelling central venous catheter inserted.

During marrow infusion
• Monitor the patient's vital signs to detect hypersensitivity reactions.
• Watch for complications of marrow infusion, such as pulmonary embolus and volume overload.
• Reassure the patient throughout the procedure.

After marrow infusion
• Continue to monitor vital signs every 4 hours. Watch for fever and chills, which may be the only signs of infection.
• Be alert for bradycardia, nausea, garlic taste in the mouth, and hypocalcemia, which can be caused by marrow preservatives.
• Give prophylactic antibiotics, as ordered.
• To reduce the possibility of bleeding, don't administer medication rectally or intramuscularly.
• Administer methotrexate, corticosteroids, or cyclosporine, as ordered, to prevent graft-versus-host (GVH) disease, a potentially fatal complication of transplantation. Watch for signs and symptoms of GVH disease, such as maculopapular rash, jaundice, joint pain, and diarrhea, and for signs of failure to engraft, such as pancytopenia.
• Administer vitamins, steroids, and iron and folic acid supplements, as ordered. Blood products, such as platelets and packed RBCs, may also be indicated, depending on the results of daily blood studies.
• Give good mouth care every 2 hours. Use chlorhexidine or other bactericidal mouthwash to prevent candidiasis and other mouth infections.
• Provide meticulous skin care, paying close attention to pressure points and open sites, such as I.V. sites.
• Teach the patient measures to prevent infection, such as avoiding crowds and people with known infections.
• Instruct the patient to avoid activities with an increased risk of injury or bleeding, such as playing contact sports or using a razor blade. Suggest that the patient shave with an electric razor.
• For more information, refer the patient to the Aplastic Anemia Foundation of America.

---

pressant agents (if the patient doesn't respond to other therapy).

A new group of agents called colony-stimulating factors encourage the growth of specific cellular components and show some promise in trials of patients who have received chemotherapy or radiation therapy. These agents include granulocyte colony-stimulating factor,

granulocyte-macrophage colony-stimulating factor, and erythropoietic stimulating factor.

Nursing diagnoses
• Activity intolerance
• Altered oral mucous membrane
• Altered thought processes
• Altered tissue perfusion

- Decreased cardiac output
- Fatigue
- Impaired gas exchange
- Impaired physical mobility
- Ineffective thermoregulation
- Pain
- Risk for infection

Nursing interventions

- Focus your efforts on helping to prevent or manage hemorrhage, infection, adverse effects of drug therapy, and blood transfusion reaction.
- If the patient's platelet count is low (less than 20,000/mm³), prevent hemorrhage by avoiding I.M. injections, suggesting the use of an electric razor and a soft toothbrush, humidifying oxygen to prevent drying of mucous membranes (dry mucosa may bleed), and promoting regular bowel movements through the use of a stool softener and a diet to prevent constipation (which can cause rectal mucosal bleeding). Also, apply pressure to venipuncture sites until bleeding stops. Detect bleeding early by checking for blood in urine and stool and assessing skin for petechiae.
- Help prevent infection by washing your hands thoroughly before entering the patient's room, by making sure the patient is receiving a nutritious diet (high in vitamins and proteins) to improve his resistance, and by encouraging meticulous mouth and perianal care.
- Make sure throat, urine, nasal, stool, and blood cultures are done regularly and correctly to check for infection.
- If the patient has a low hemoglobin level, which causes fatigue, schedule frequent rest periods. Administer oxygen therapy, as needed.
- Ensure a comfortable environmental temperature for a patient experiencing hypothermia or hyperthermia.
- If blood transfusions are necessary, assess for a transfusion reaction by checking the patient's temperature and watching for the development of other signs and symptoms, such as rash, urticaria, pruritus, back pain, restlessness, and shaking chills.
- To prevent aplastic anemia, monitor blood studies carefully in the patient receiving anemia-inducing drugs.

Patient teaching

- Teach the patient to avoid contact with potential sources of infection, such as crowds, soil, and standing water that can harbor organisms.
- Reassure and support the patient and his family by explaining the disease and its treatment, particularly if the patient has recurring acute episodes. Explain the purpose of all prescribed drugs, and discuss possible adverse reactions, including which ones he should report promptly.
- Tell the patient who doesn't require hospitalization that he can continue his normal life-style, with appropriate restrictions (such as regular rest periods), until remission occurs.
- Support efforts to educate the public about the hazards of toxic agents. Tell parents to keep toxic agents out of their children's reach. Encourage people who work with radiation to wear protective clothing and a radiation-detecting badge and to observe plant safety precautions. Those who work with benzene (solvent) should know that 10 parts per million is the highest safe environmental level and that a delayed reaction to benzene may develop.
- Refer the patient to the Aplastic Anemia Foundation of America for additional information and assistance.

SIDEROBLASTIC ANEMIAS

An umbrella term, sideroblastic anemias comprise a group of heterogenous disorders with a common defect—failure to use iron in hemoglobin synthesis despite the availability of adequate iron stores. As a result, iron is deposited in the mitochondria of normoblasts, and characteristic rings surround the nucleus of this cell.

Sideroblastic anemias may be hereditary or acquired; the acquired form, in turn, can be primary or secondary. Hereditary sideroblastic anemia often responds to treatment with pyridoxine (vitamin B₆). Correction of the secondary acquired form depends on the causative disorder; the primary acquired (idiopathic) form, however, resists treatment and usually proves fatal within 10 years after onset of complications or a concomitant disease.

Causes

Most prevalent in young males, hereditary sideroblastic anemia appears to be transmitted by X-linked inheritance; females are carriers and usually show no signs of this disorder.

The acquired form may be secondary to ingestion of or exposure to toxins, such as alcohol and lead, or to drugs, such as isoniazid and chloramphenicol. It can also occur as a complication of neoplastic and inflammatory diseases, such as lymphoma, rheumatoid arthritis, lupus erythematosus, multiple myeloma, tuberculosis, and severe infections.

The primary acquired form, whose cause is unknown, is most common in elderly people but occasionally develops in young people. It's often associated with thrombocytopenia or leukopenia.

Complications
Increased total body iron (hemochromatosis) can result in severe heart, liver, and pancreatic disease. Respiratory complications also can occur. These complications are most common in elderly patients who have primary acquired sideroblastic anemia. About 10% of patients with this disorder develop acute myelogenous leukemia.

Assessment findings
Sideroblastic anemias usually produce nonspecific clinical effects, which may exist for several years before being identified. The patient's history may reveal anorexia, fatigue, weakness, and dizziness. The patient may also have a history of dyspnea.

On inspection, you may observe pale skin and oral mucous membranes. You may also note slight jaundice, caused by excessive iron accumulation in the liver, and petechiae or bruises, caused by thrombocytopenia.

Palpation may reveal enlarged lymph nodes. If iron accumulates in the liver and the patient has jaundice, palpation also may disclose hepatosplenomegaly.

Hereditary sideroblastic anemia is associated with increased GI absorption of iron, causing signs of hemosiderosis (eventually, hepatomegaly, cardiomyopathy and, possibly, endocrine problems). Additional symptoms in secondary sideroblastic anemia depend on the underlying cause.

Diagnostic tests
Ringed sideroblasts on microscopic examination of bone marrow aspirate, stained with Prussian blue dye, confirm this diagnosis.

Microscopic examination of blood shows erythrocytes to be hypochromic or normochromic and slightly macrocytic. Red cell precursors may be megaloblastic, with anisocytosis (abnormal variation in red blood cell [RBC] size) and poikilocytosis (abnormal variation in RBC shape).

Vitamin B_{12} and folic acid levels are normal unless combined anemias are present. The reticulocyte count is low because young cells die in the marrow. Unlike iron deficiency anemia, sideroblastic anemia lowers hemoglobin levels and raises serum iron and transferrin levels. In turn, faulty hemoglobin production raises urobilinogen and bilirubin levels. Platelets and leukocytes remain normal, but occasionally, thrombocytopenia or leukopenia occurs.

Treatment
The underlying cause determines the course of treatment. Hereditary sideroblastic anemia usually responds to several weeks of treatment with high doses of pyridoxine.

The acquired secondary form subsides after the causative drug or toxin is removed or the underlying condition is adequately treated. Folic acid supplements may be beneficial when concomitant megaloblastic nuclear changes in RBC precursors are present. Deferoxamine may be used to treat chronic iron overload in selected patients.

Carefully crossmatched transfusions (providing needed hemoglobin) or high doses of androgens are effective palliative measures for some patients with the primary acquired form of sideroblastic anemia. However, this form is essentially refractory to treatment and usually leads to death from acute leukemia or from respiratory or cardiac complications.

Some patients with sideroblastic anemias may benefit from phlebotomy to prevent hemochromatosis. Phlebotomy increases the rate of erythropoiesis and uses up excess iron stores; thus, it reduces serum and total-body iron levels.

Clinical trials are being conducted to determine the effectiveness of recombinant cytokines, such as erythropoietin, granulocyte-macrophage colony-stimulating factor, and interleukin-3, in the treatment of sideroblastic anemias.

Nursing diagnoses
• Altered oral mucous membrane
• Decreased cardiac output
• Fatigue
• Impaired skin integrity
• Knowledge deficit
• Pain
• Risk for infection
• Risk for injury

Nursing interventions
• Provide frequent rest periods if the patient becomes easily fatigued. Plan activities and diagnostic tests so the patient can rest in between. Monitor his pulse rate often; tachycardia indicates that his activities are too strenuous.
• Because sideroblastic anemias often produce weakness, institute safety measures to prevent falls.
• Administer medications, as ordered. If the patient has pain from complications of the disorder, such as pancreatitis, give analgesics, as ordered, and monitor their ef-

IRON ABSORPTION AND STORAGE

Essential to erythropoiesis, iron is abundant throughout the body. Two-thirds of total-body iron is found in hemoglobin; the other third, mostly in the reticuloendothelial system (liver, spleen, and bone marrow), with small amounts in muscle, serum, and body cells.

Adequate dietary ingestion of iron and recirculation of iron released from disintegrating red cells maintain iron supplies. The duodenum and upper part of the small intestine absorb dietary iron. Such absorption depends on gastric acid content, the amount of reducing substances (ascorbic acid, for example) present in the alimentary canal, and dietary iron intake. If iron intake is deficient, the body gradually depletes its iron stores, causing decreased hemoglobin and, eventually, signs and symptoms of iron deficiency anemia.

fectiveness. Also provide comfort measures, and have the patient perform relaxation techniques to help him cope with associated pain.
• Administer ordered blood transfusions, and monitor the patient's tolerance of the treatment. Notify the doctor if signs of a transfusion reaction occur.
• If the patient has jaundice or pruritus, provide good skin care to prevent skin breakdown.
• Watch for the complications of therapy. Note any signs or symptoms of decreased perfusion to vital organs (dyspnea, chest pain, dizziness) or of neuropathy (peripheral tingling).
• Inquire about possible exposure to lead in the home (especially for children) or on the job.
• Identify patients who abuse alcohol; refer them for appropriate therapy.

Patient teaching
• Reinforce the doctor's explanation of the disorder and answer any questions. Be sure that the patient fully understands prescribed treatments and possible complications of organ involvement or preleukemia.
• Teach the patient the importance of continuing prescribed therapy, even after he begins to feel better.
• Advise parents to have all house paint checked for lead and not to allow children to eat paint chips.
• Provide instructions for a high-protein diet at home, especially if phlebotomy is used as a treatment.
• If androgens are used as part of the treatment, teach the patient to recognize and report adrenergic adverse effects.

• If phlebotomy is scheduled, explain the procedure to the patient to help reduce his anxiety. If this procedure must be repeated frequently, provide a high-protein diet to help replace the protein lost during phlebotomy.
• Teach the patient to recognize and report signs and symptoms of heart failure.
• Emphasize the need for proper hygiene and other measures to guard against infections because the patient's weakened condition may increase his susceptibility. Tell the patient to report signs and symptoms of infection promptly, especially urinary tract and pulmonary infections.

IRON DEFICIENCY ANEMIA

A common disease worldwide, iron deficiency anemia affects 10% to 30% of the adult population of the United States. It's most prevalent among premenopausal women, infants (particularly premature or low-birthweight infants), children, adolescents (especially girls), alcoholics, and elderly people (especially those unable to cook). The prognosis after replacement therapy is favorable.

Causes and pathophysiology
Iron deficiency anemia stems from an inadequate supply of iron for optimal formation of red blood cells (RBCs), which produces smaller (microcytic) cells with less color on staining. Body stores of iron, including plasma iron, decrease, as does transferrin, which binds with and transports iron. Insufficient body stores of iron lead to a depleted RBC mass and, in turn, to a decreased hemoglobin concentration (hypochromia) and decreased oxygen-carrying capacity of the blood. (See *Iron absorption and storage.*)

Iron deficiency can result from any of the following:
• inadequate dietary intake of iron, as in prolonged unsupplemented breast- or bottle-feeding of infants; during periods of stress, such as rapid growth in children and adolescents; and in elderly patients existing on a poorly balanced diet
• iron malabsorption, as in chronic diarrhea, partial or total gastrectomy, and malabsorption syndromes, such as celiac disease
• blood loss secondary to drug-induced GI bleeding (from anticoagulants, aspirin, steroids) or due to heavy menses, hemorrhage from trauma, GI ulcers, malignant tumors, and varices
• pregnancy, in which the mother's iron supply is diverted to the fetus for erythropoiesis
• intravascular hemolysis-induced hemoglobinuria or paroxysmal nocturnal hemoglobinuria

• mechanical erythrocyte trauma caused by a prosthetic heart valve or vena cava filter.

Complications

Possible complications of this disorder include infection and pneumonia. In a child, iron deficiency anemia can cause pica, which may lead to eating more lead-based paint and can result in lead poisoning. Another complication is bleeding, which may be identified by ecchymotic areas on the skin, hematuria, and gingival bleeding.

The most significant complication of iron deficiency anemia stems from overreplacement of oral or intramuscular iron supplements. Hemochromatosis (excessive iron deposits in tissue) can result, affecting the liver, heart, pituitary gland, and joints. Iron poisoning can occur in children when toxic levels are allowed to build up during therapy.

Assessment findings

Iron deficiency anemia may persist for years without signs and symptoms. The characteristic history of fatigue, inability to concentrate, headache, and shortness of breath (especially on exertion) may not develop until long after iron stores and circulating iron become low. The patient may report increased frequency of infections and pica, an uncontrollable urge to eat strange things, such as clay, starch, ice and, in children, lead. A female patient may give a history of menorrhagia.

In chronic iron deficiency anemia, the patient history may include complaints of dysphagia and neuromuscular effects, such as vasomotor disturbances, numbness and tingling of the extremities, and neuralgic pain. Inspection may reveal a red, swollen, smooth, shiny, and tender tongue (glossitis). The corners of the mouth may be eroded, tender, and swollen (angular stomatitis). Inspection may also reveal spoon-shaped, brittle nails.

A patient with advanced iron deficiency anemia may develop tachycardia because decreased oxygen perfusion causes the heart to compensate with increased cardiac output. In such a patient, the oxygen saturation level may be below 90%.

Diagnostic tests

Blood studies and stores in bone marrow may confirm iron deficiency anemia. However, the results of these tests can be misleading because of complicating factors, such as infection, pneumonia, blood transfusion, and iron supplements. Characteristic blood study results include:
• low hemoglobin levels (males, less than 12 g/dl; females, less than 10 g/dl)

• low hematocrit (males, less than 47 ml/dl; females, less than 42 ml/dl)
• low serum iron levels, with high binding capacity
• low serum ferritin levels
• low RBC count, with microcytic and hypochromic cells (in early stages, RBC count may be normal, except in infants and children)
• decreased mean corpuscular hemoglobin in severe anemia.

Bone marrow studies reveal depleted or absent iron stores (done by staining) as well as normoblastic hyperplasia.

GI studies, such as guaiac stool tests, barium swallow and enema, endoscopy, and sigmoidoscopy, rule out or confirm the diagnosis of bleeding causing the iron deficiency.

Diagnosis must rule out other forms of anemia, such as those that result from thalassemia minor, cancer, and chronic inflammatory, hepatic, and renal disease.

Treatment

First, the underlying cause of anemia must be determined. Then, iron replacement therapy can begin. The treatment of choice is an oral preparation of iron or a combination of iron and ascorbic acid (which enhances iron absorption). In rare cases, iron may have to be administered I.M. — for instance, if the patient is noncompliant with the oral preparation, if he needs more iron than he can take orally, if malabsorption prevents adequate iron absorption, or if a maximum rate of hemoglobin regeneration is desired. (See *Injecting iron solutions*, page 468.)

Total-dose I.V. infusions of supplemental iron can be administered to pregnant and elderly patients with severe iron deficiency anemia. The patient should receive this painless infusion of iron dextran in 0.9% sodium chloride solution over 8 hours. To minimize the risk of an allergic reaction to iron, an I.V. test dose of 0.5 ml should be given first.

Nursing diagnoses
• Activity intolerance
• Altered growth and development
• Altered nutrition: Less than body requirements
• Altered oral mucous membrane
• Altered thought processes
• Altered tissue perfusion
• Fatigue
• Impaired gas exchange

INJECTING IRON SOLUTIONS

For deep I.M. injections of iron solutions, use the Z-track technique to avoid subcutaneous irritation and discoloration from leaking medication.

Choose an injection site
Rotate the injection sites in the upper outer quadrant of the buttocks.

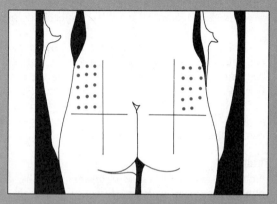

Displace tissues
Choose a 19- to 20-gauge, 2″ to 3″ (5- to 7.5-cm) needle. After drawing up the solution, change to a fresh needle to avoid tracking the solution through to subcutaneous tissue. Draw 0.5 cc of air into the syringe as an air-lock.

Displace the skin and fat at the injection site firmly to one side.

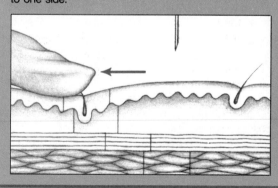

Inject the solution
Clean the area, and insert the needle. Aspirate to check for entry into a blood vessel. Inject the solution slowly, followed by the 0.5 cc of air in the syringe.

After injecting the solution, wait 10 seconds.

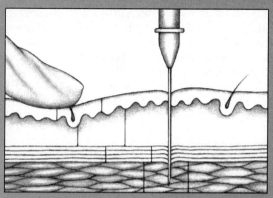

Release the tissues
Pull the needle straight out, and release the tissues.

Apply direct pressure to the site, but don't massage it. Caution the patient not to exercise vigorously for at least 15 minutes after the injection.

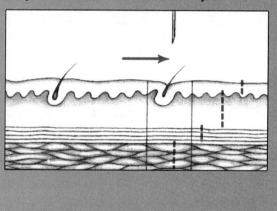

• Knowledge deficit
• Pain

Nursing interventions
• Note signs or symptoms of decreased perfusion to vital organs: dyspnea, chest pain, dizziness, and signs of neuropathy, such as tingling in the periphery. Provide oxygen therapy as necessary to help prevent and reduce hypoxia.
• Assess the family's dietary habits for iron intake, noting the influence of childhood eating patterns, cultural food preferences, and family income on adequate nutrition.

• Because a sore mouth and tongue make eating painful, ask the dietitian to give the patient nonirritating foods. If these symptoms make talking difficult, supply a pad and pencil or some other communication aid. Provide diluted mouthwash or, in especially severe conditions, swab the patient's mouth with tap water or warm saline solution. Oral anesthetic diluted in saline solution may also be used.

• As ordered, administer analgesics for headache and other discomfort, and monitor their effectiveness.

• Evaluate the patient's drug history. Certain drugs, such as pancreatic enzymes and vitamin E, may interfere with iron metabolism and absorption; aspirin, steroids, and other drugs may cause GI bleeding.

• Provide frequent rest periods to decrease physical exhaustion. Plan activities so that the patient has sufficient rest between them. Monitor the patient's pulse rate often; tachycardia indicates that his activities are too strenuous.

• If the patient receives iron I.V., monitor the infusion rate carefully, and observe for an allergic reaction. Stop the infusion and begin supportive treatment immediately if the patient shows signs of an adverse reaction. Also, watch for dizziness and headache and for thrombophlebitis around the I.V. site.

• Use the Z-track injection method when administering iron I.M. to prevent skin discoloration, scarring, and irritating iron deposits in the skin.

• Monitor the patient for iron replacement overdose. (See *Recognizing iron overdose*.)

• Provide good nutrition and meticulous care of I.V. sites, such as those used for blood transfusions, to help prevent infection.

• Monitor the patient's compliance with the prescribed iron supplement therapy.

Patient teaching

• Reinforce the doctor's explanation of the disorder, and answer any questions. Be sure the patient fully understands the prescribed treatments and possible complications.

• Ask about possible exposure to lead in the home (especially for children) or on the job. Teach the patient and his family about the dangers of lead poisoning, especially if the patient reports pica.

• Advise the patient not to stop therapy even if he feels better because replacement of iron stores takes time.

• Inform the patient that milk or an antacid interferes with absorption but that vitamin C can increase absorption. Instruct the patient to drink liquid supplemental iron through a straw to prevent staining his teeth.

Warning

RECOGNIZING IRON OVERDOSE

Excessive iron replacement is demonstrated when signs and symptoms, such as diarrhea, fever, severe stomach pain, nausea, and vomiting, occur.

Notify the doctor promptly when these signs and symptoms occur, and administer prescribed treatments. For this acute condition, treatment includes giving iron-binding agents (deferoxamine), inducing vomiting that produces systemic alkalinization, and giving anticonvulsants.

• Tell the patient to report any adverse effects of iron therapy, such as nausea, vomiting, diarrhea, and constipation, which may require a dosage adjustment or supplemental stool softeners.

• Teach the basics of a nutritionally balanced diet—red meats, green vegetables, eggs, whole wheat, iron-fortified bread, and milk. However, explain that no food in itself contains enough iron to *treat* iron deficiency anemia; an average-sized person with anemia would have to eat at least 10 lb (4.5 kg) of steak daily to receive therapeutic amounts of iron.

• Warn the patient to guard against infections because his weakened condition may increase his susceptibility. Stress the importance of meticulous wound care, periodic dental checkups, good hand-washing techniques, and other measures to prevent infection. Also tell the patient to report any signs of infection, including temperature elevation and chills.

• Because an iron deficiency may recur, explain the need for regular checkups and to comply with prescribed treatments.

SICKLE CELL ANEMIA

A congenital hemolytic disease, sickle cell anemia results from a defective hemoglobin molecule (hemoglobin S) that causes red blood cells (RBCs) to become sickle-shaped. Such cells impair circulation, resulting in chronic ill health (fatigue, dyspnea on exertion, swollen joints), periodic crises, long-term complications, and premature death.

COMPARING NORMAL AND SICKLED RED BLOOD CELLS

As you can see, the properties of normal round and sickled RBCs vary in more ways than shape.

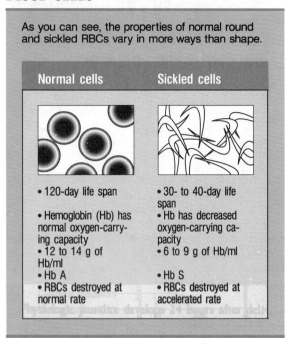

Normal cells	Sickled cells
• 120-day life span	• 30- to 40-day life span
• Hemoglobin (Hb) has normal oxygen-carrying capacity	• Hb has decreased oxygen-carrying capacity
• 12 to 14 g of Hb/ml	• 6 to 9 g of Hb/ml
• Hb A	• Hb S
• RBCs destroyed at normal rate	• RBCs destroyed at accelerated rate

Sickle cell anemia is most common in tropical Africans and in people of African descent; about 1 in 10 African-Americans carries the abnormal gene. If two such carriers have offspring, each child has a 1 in 4 chance of developing the disease. Overall, 1 in every 400 to 600 black children has sickle cell anemia. This disease also occurs in Puerto Rico, Turkey, India, the Middle East, and the Mediterranean area. Possibly, the defective hemoglobin S–producing gene has persisted because in areas where malaria is endemic, the heterozygous sickle cell trait provides resistance to malaria and is actually beneficial.

Penicillin prophylaxis can decrease morbidity and mortality from bacterial infections. Once, many patients with sickle cell anemia died in their early 20s, but now 50% to 70% live into their 40s and 50s.

Causes and pathophysiology

Sickle cell anemia results from homozygous inheritance of the hemoglobin S–producing gene, which causes substitution of the amino acid valine for glutamic acid in the beta hemoglobin chain. Heterozygous inheritance of this gene results in sickle cell trait, a condition with minimal or no symptoms. The patient with sickle cell trait is a carrier; he can pass the sickle cell gene to his offspring.

In sickle cell anemia, the abnormal hemoglobin S found in the patient's RBCs becomes insoluble whenever hypoxia occurs. As a result, these RBCs become rigid, rough, and elongated, forming a crescent or sickle shape. Such sickling can produce hemolysis (cell destruction). (See *Comparing normal and sickled red blood cells*.)

Each person with sickle cell anemia has a different hypoxic threshold and different factors that precipitate a sickle cell crisis. Illness, cold exposure, and stress are known to precipitate sickling crises in most people. (See *What happens in sickle cell crisis*.)

In addition, these altered cells accumulate in capillaries and smaller blood vessels, making the blood more viscous. Normal circulation is impaired, causing pain, tissue infarctions, and swelling. Such blockage causes anoxic changes that lead to further sickling and obstruction.

Complications

Sickle cell anemia causes long-term complications. An adult with this disease may develop chronic obstructive pulmonary disease, congestive heart failure (CHF), or organ infarction, such as retinopathy and nephropathy. Splenic infarctions are common and often cause significant necrosis early in life, so that splenomegaly leads to a small, nodular, and malfunctioning spleen. Infection or repeated occlusion of small blood vessels and consequent infarction or necrosis of major organs commonly cause premature death. For example, cerebral blood vessel occlusion causes cerebrovascular accident and is the most common cause of death in severe sickle cell disease. Frequent sickling and hyperviscosity can lead to heart murmurs and CHF.

Assessment findings

Signs and symptoms usually don't develop until after 6 months of age because large amounts of fetal hemoglobin protect infants for the first few months after birth.

Characteristically, the patient history in sickle cell anemia includes chronic fatigue, unexplained dyspnea or dyspnea on exertion, joint swelling, aching bones, chest pain, ischemic leg ulcers (especially around the ankles), and an increased susceptibility to infection. The patient's medical history may include pulmonary infarctions and cardiomegaly.

Inspection may reveal jaundice or pallor. A young child may appear small for his age, whereas an older child may experience delayed growth and puberty. Inspection of an adult usually reveals a spiderlike body build (narrow shoulders and hips, long extremities, curved spine, and barrel chest).

Typically, assessment of the patient's vital signs reveals tachycardia. Palpation may disclose hepatomegaly and, in children, splenomegaly. (Splenomegaly usually is absent in adulthood because the spleen shrinks over time.) Auscultation may detect systolic and diastolic murmurs.

In sickle cell crisis, assessment findings may include the following:
• history of recent infection, stress, dehydration, or other conditions that provoke hypoxia, such as strenuous exercise, high altitude, unpressurized aircraft, cold, and vasoconstrictive drugs
• complaints of sleepiness with difficulty awakening, severe pain and, sometimes, hematuria
• pale lips, tongue, palms, and nail beds; lethargy; listlessness; and often irritability
• body temperature over 104° F (40° C) or a temperature of 100° F (37.8° C) that persists for 2 or more days.

The following characteristic signs and symptoms help determine the type of crisis the patient is experiencing:
• A *painful crisis* (vaso-occlusive crisis, infarctive crisis), the most common crisis and the hallmark of this disease, usually appears periodically after age 5. It results from blood vessel obstruction by rigid, tangled sickle cells, which causes tissue anoxia and, possibly, necrosis.

Vaso-occlusive crisis is characterized by severe abdominal, thoracic, muscle, or bone pain and, possibly, increased jaundice, dark urine, or a low-grade fever. Patients with long-term disease may experience autosplenectomy, in which splenic damage and scarring is so extensive that the spleen shrinks and becomes impalpable. This can lead to increased susceptibility to *Streptococcus pneumoniae* sepsis, which can be fatal without prompt treatment. After the crisis subsides (in 4 days to several weeks), infection may develop, producing lethargy, sleepiness, fever, and apathy.
• An *aplastic crisis* (megaloblastic crisis) results from bone marrow depression and is associated with infection (usually viral). It's characterized by pallor, lethargy, sleepiness, dyspnea, possible coma, markedly decreased bone marrow activity, and RBC hemolysis.
• An *acute sequestration crisis* occurs in infants between ages 8 months and 2 years and may cause sudden, massive entrapment of RBCs in the spleen and liver. This rare crisis causes lethargy and pallor and, if untreated, commonly progresses to hypovolemic shock and death.
• A *hemolytic crisis* is rare and usually affects patients who have glucose-6-phosphate dehydrogenase (G6PD) deficiency with sickle cell anemia. It probably results

Pathophysiology

WHAT HAPPENS IN SICKLE CELL CRISIS

Sickle cell crisis occurs when a patient with sickle cell anemia experiences cellular oxygen deprivation—for example, from an infection, from exposure to cold or to high altitude, or from overexertion.

Sickle cell anemia results from an alteration in the molecular structure of hemoglobin: One amino acid is substituted for another. This deprives the RBCs of needed oxygen. In response, their altered hemoglobin molecules aggregate, sickling cells and causing cellular, vascular, and tissue damage. The result is disabling pain and, ultimately, tissue necrosis.

from complications of sickle cell anemia, such as infection, rather than from the disorder itself. In hemolytic crisis, degenerative changes cause liver congestion and hepatomegaly. Chronic jaundice worsens, although increased jaundice doesn't always indicate a hemolytic crisis.

Diagnostic tests

A positive family history and typical clinical features suggest sickle cell anemia; a stained blood smear showing sickle cells and hemoglobin electrophoresis showing hemoglobin S confirm it. Electrophoresis should be done on umbilical cord blood samples at birth to provide sickle cell disease screening for all neonates at risk. Additional laboratory studies show low RBC counts, elevated white blood cell (WBC) and platelet counts, decreased erythrocyte sedimentation rate, increased serum iron levels, decreased RBC survival, and reticulocytosis. Hemoglobin levels may be low or normal.

A lateral chest X-ray may be performed to detect the characteristic "Lincoln log" deformity. This spinal abnormality develops in many adults and some adolescents with sickle cell anemia, leaving the vertebrae resembling logs that form the corner of a cabin.

An ophthalmoscopic examination to detect corkscrew or comma-shaped vessels in the conjunctivae, another sign of this disease, may also be performed.

Treatment

Although sickle cell anemia can't be cured, treatments can alleviate symptoms and prevent painful crises. Certain vaccines, such as polyvalent pneumoccocal vaccine and Haemophilus influenzae B vaccine; anti-infectives, such as low-dose oral penicillin; and chelating agents, such as deferoxamine, can minimize complications resulting from the disease and from transfusion therapy.

Other medications, such as analgesics, may help to relieve the pain of vaso-occlusive crisis. Iron supplements may be given if folic acid levels are low. A good antisickling agent isn't yet available; the most commonly used drug, sodium cyanate, has many adverse effects.

Treatment begins before age 4 months with prophylactic penicillin. If the patient's hemoglobin level drops suddenly or if his condition deteriorates rapidly, hospitalization will be needed for transfusion of packed RBCs.

In an acute sequestration crisis, treatment may include sedation and administration of analgesics, blood transfusion, oxygen therapy, and large amounts of oral or I.V. fluids. Despite the effectiveness of transfusions, some clinicians limit them because they increase blood viscosity and the risk of vascular occlusion.

Nursing diagnoses

• Altered growth and development
• Altered tissue perfusion
• Body image disturbance
• Fatigue
• Hyperthermia
• Impaired gas exchange
• Impaired tissue integrity
• Knowledge deficit
• Pain
• Risk for fluid volume deficit

Nursing interventions

• Encourage the patient to talk about his fears and concerns. Try to stay with him during periods of severe crisis and anxiety. Provide reassurance, when possible, but always answer his questions honestly.
• If a male patient develops sudden, painful priapism, reassure him that such episodes are common and have no permanent harmful effects.
• Ensure that the patient receives adequate amounts of folic acid–rich foods, such as leafy green vegetables. Encourage adequate fluid intake to hydrate the patient; give parenteral fluids, if necessary. Provide eggnog, ice pops, and milkshakes to meet fluid requirements.

• Apply warm compresses, warmed thermal blankets, and warming pads or mattresses to painful areas of the patient's body. Consider the weight of the warming appliance, to avoid aggravating pain. Never apply cold to a painful area.
• Administer analgesics and antipyretics as necessary. Each patient's level of pain is different; some may require acetaminophen to control the pain; others may have continuous pain during crisis while receiving morphine.
• When cultures demonstrate the presence of infection, administer antibiotics, as ordered. Also administer prophylactic antibiotics, as ordered. Use strict aseptic technique when performing treatments.
• Encourage bed rest with the head elevated to decrease tissue oxygen demand. Administer oxygen only if the patient is experiencing severe dyspnea.
• Administer blood transfusions as ordered. Use strict aseptic technique.
• If the patient requires general anesthesia for surgery, help ensure that he receives adequate ventilation to prevent hypoxic crisis. Make sure the surgeon and the anesthesiologist are aware that the patient has sickle cell anemia, and provide a preoperative transfusion of packed RBCs, as needed.

Patient teaching

• To help prevent exacerbation of sickle cell anemia, advise the patient to avoid tight clothing that restricts circulation.
• Warn against strenuous exercise, vasoconstricting medications, cold temperatures (including drinking large amounts of ice water and swimming), unpressurized aircraft, high altitude, and other conditions that provoke hypoxia.
• Stress the importance of normal childhood immunizations, meticulous wound care, good oral hygiene, regular dental checkups, and a balanced diet as safeguards against infection.
• Emphasize the need for prompt treatment of infection.
• Explain the need to increase fluid intake to prevent dehydration that results from impaired ability to properly concentrate urine. Tell parents to encourage a child with sickle cell anemia to drink more fluids, especially in the summer, by offering milkshakes, ice pops, and eggnog.
• To encourage normal mental and social development, warn parents against being overprotective. Although the child must avoid strenuous exercise, he can enjoy most everyday activities.
• Refer parents of children with sickle cell anemia for genetic counseling to answer their questions about the risk to future offspring. Recommend screening of other

• Because delayed growth and late puberty are common, reassure an adolescent patient that he will grow and mature.

• Review the symptoms of vaso-occlusive crisis so that the patient and his family will recognize and treat it early. As appropriate, explain how to care for this condition at home. Prepare parents for an infant's first vaso-occlusive crisis (called "hand-foot crisis"), during which the infant's hands, feet, or both swell and become painful.

• Inform the patient and his parents that if he must be hospitalized for a vaso-occlusive crisis, I.V. fluids and parenteral analgesics may be administered. He also may receive oxygen therapy and blood transfusions.

• If appropriate, discuss how special conditions, such as surgery and pregnancy, may affect the patient.

• Stress to the patient the need to inform all health care providers that he has this disease before he undergoes any treatment—especially major surgery. Explain that any procedure that involves general anesthesia will require that the patient has adequate ventilation to prevent hypoxic crisis. Urge him to wear medical identification stating that he has sickle cell anemia.

• Warn women with sickle cell anemia that they're poor obstetric risks. However, their use of oral contraceptives is also risky; refer them for birth control counseling. If such women *do* become pregnant, they should maintain a balanced diet during pregnancy and may benefit from a folic acid supplement.

• If necessary, arrange for psychological counseling to help the patient cope. Suggest that he join an appropriate support group, such as the National Association for Sickle Cell Disease.

THALASSEMIA

Thalassemia, a group of hereditary hemolytic anemias, is characterized by defective synthesis in one or more of the polypeptide chains necessary for hemoglobin production. Because thalessemia affects hemoglobin production, it also impairs red blood cell (RBC) synthesis. This disorder is most common in individuals of Mediterranean ancestry (especially Italians and Greeks), but it also occurs in Blacks and people from southern China, southeast Asia, and India.

Two pairs of polypeptide chains—alpha chains and beta chains—make up hemoglobin. In thalassemia, diminished synthesis can affect either pair. Structurally, the chains are normal, but the genetic defect decreases their number. In alpha-thalassemia, alpha chain synthesis slows; in beta-thalassemia, beta chain synthesis slows. Some patients with beta-thalassemia have no normal hemoglobin, only hemoglobin S and the minor hemoglobins.

In the most severe form of alpha-thalassemia—hydrops fetalis—severe anemia and congestive heart failure render fetuses hydropic. These fetuses are stillborn or die shortly after birth. Prenatal testing can detect the condition.

Beta-thalassemia (by far, the most common form of this disorder) occurs in three clinical forms: thalassemia major, intermedia, and minor. The severity of the resulting anemia depends on whether the patient is homozygous or heterozygous for the thalassemic trait. The prognosis for beta-thalassemia varies. Patients with thalassemia major seldom survive to adulthood; children with thalassemia intermedia develop normally into adulthood, although puberty is usually delayed; patients with thalassemia minor can expect a normal life span.

Causes
Thalassemia major and thalassemia intermedia result from homozygous inheritance of the partially dominant autosomal gene responsible for this trait. Thalassemia minor is caused by heterozygous inheritance of the same gene. In all of three types of thalassemia, total or partial deficiency of beta polypeptide chain production impairs hemoglobin synthesis and results in continual production of fetal hemoglobin, even after the neonatal period has passed.

Complications
As children with thalassemia major grow older, they become susceptible to pathologic fractures. This occurs because the bone marrow cavities expand as the long bones thin. These patients are also subject to cardiac arrhythmias, heart failure, and other complications that result from iron deposits in the heart and other tissues caused by repeated blood transfusions.

Assessment findings
In thalassemia major (also known as Cooley's anemia, Mediterranean disease, and erythroblastic anemia), the infant is well at birth but develops severe anemia, bone abnormalities, failure to thrive, and life-threatening complications. Often, the first signs are pallor and yellow skin and scleras in infants between ages 3 and 6 months. Later signs and symptoms include severe anemia, splenomegaly or hepatomegaly with abdominal enlargement, frequent infections, bleeding tendencies (especially to-

ward epistaxis), and anorexia.

Children with thalassemia major commonly have small bodies and large heads and may also be mentally retarded. Infants may have mongoloid features because bone marrow hyperactivity has thickened the bone at the base of the nose.

Thalassemia intermedia comprises moderate thalassemic disorders in homozygotes. Patients with this condition show some degree of anemia, jaundice, and splenomegaly, and may exhibit signs of hemosiderosis caused by increased intestinal absorption of iron.

Thalassemia minor may cause mild anemia but usually produces no signs or symptoms and is often overlooked.

Diagnostic tests

In thalassemia major, laboratory test results show a decreased RBC count and hemoglobin (Hb) level, microcytosis, and increased reticulocyte, bilirubin, and urinary and fecal urobilinogen levels. A low serum folate level indicates increased folate use by hypertrophied bone marrow. A peripheral blood smear reveals target cells, microcytes, pale nucleated RBCs, and marked anisocytosis. X-rays of the skull and long bones show thinning and widening of the marrow space because of overactive bone marrow. The bones of the skull and vertebrae may appear granular. (See *Skull changes in thalassemia major.*) Long bones may show areas of osteoporosis. The phalanges may also be deformed (rectangular or biconvex). Quantitative Hb studies show a significant rise in Hb F and a slight increase in Hb A_2. Diagnosis must rule out iron deficiency anemia, which also produces hypochromia (slightly lower Hb level) and microcytic (notably small) RBCs.

In thalassemia intermedia, laboratory test results show hypochromia and microcytic RBCs, but the anemia is less severe than that in thalassemia major. In thalassemia minor, test results also show hypochromia and microcytic RBCs. Quantitative Hb studies show a significant increase in Hb A_2 levels and a moderate rise in Hb F levels.

Treatment

Treatment of thalassemia major is essentially supportive. For example, infections require prompt treatment with appropriate antibiotics. Folic acid supplements help maintain folic acid levels despite increased requirements. Transfusions of packed RBCs raise Hb levels but must be used judiciously to minimize iron overload. Splenectomy and bone marrow transplantation have been tried, but their effectiveness has not been confirmed.

SKULL CHANGES IN THALASSEMIA MAJOR

This illustration of an X-ray shows a characteristic skull abnormality in thalassemia major: diploetic fibers extending from internal lamina, resembling hair standing on end.

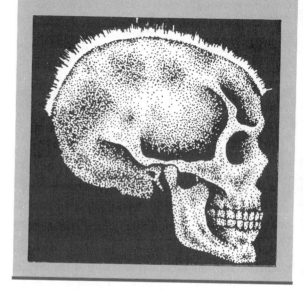

Thalassemia intermedia and thalassemia minor generally don't require treatment.

Iron supplements are contraindicated in all forms of thalassemia.

Treatment of children proves more difficult. Regular blood transfusions may minimize physical and mental retardation, but transfusions increase the risk of deadly hemosiderosis and iron overload. Continuous subcutaneous infusion of iron-chelating agents may help produce a negative overall iron balance. If rapid splenic sequestration of transfused RBCs necessitates more transfusions, a splenectomy may be performed.

Nursing diagnoses
• Altered growth and development
• Altered parenting
• Body image disturbance
• Knowledge deficit
• Risk for infection

Nursing interventions
• Watch for adverse reactions—shaking chills, fever, rash, itching, and hives—during and after RBC transfusions

for thalassemia major.
• Administer antibiotics as ordered. Observe the patient for signs of adverse reactions to them.
• Provide an adequate diet, and encourage increased consumption of fluids.
• Provide emotional support to help the patient and his family cope with the chronic nature of the illness and the need for lifelong transfusions.

Patient teaching
• Stress the importance of good nutrition, meticulous wound care, periodic dental checkups, and other measures to prevent infection.
• Discuss with the parents of a young patient various options for healthy physical and creative outlets. Such a child must avoid strenuous athletic activity because of the resulting increased oxygen demand and the inherent tendency toward pathologic fractures. Reassure the parents that the child may be allowed to participate in less stressful activities.
• Teach the parents to watch for signs of hepatitis and iron overload—always possible with frequent transfusions.
• Refer the parents of a child with thalassemia for genetic counseling if they have concerns or questions about the vulnerability of future offspring to this disorder. Also, refer adult patients with thalassemia minor and thalassemia intermedia for genetic counseling; they need to recognize the risk of transmitting thalassemia major to their children if they marry another person who has thalassemia. If such persons choose to marry and have children, all their children should be evaluated for thalassemia by age 1.
• Be sure to tell patients with thalassemia minor that their condition is benign.

POLYCYTHEMIAS

Characterized by an abnormal increase in the number of erythrocytes in the blood, polycythemias may be secondary to pulmonary or cardiac disease or to prolonged exposure to high altitudes. In the absence of a demonstrable cause, polycythemia is considered idiopathic.

POLYCYTHEMIA VERA
A chronic, myeloproliferative disorder, polycythemia vera is characterized by increased red blood cell (RBC) mass, leukocytosis, thrombocytosis, and increased hemoglobin concentration, with normal or decreased plasma volume. It usually occurs between ages 40 and 60, most commonly among men of Jewish ancestry; it seldom affects children or blacks and doesn't appear to be familial.

The onset of polycythemia is gradual, and the disease runs a chronic but slowly progressive course. The prognosis depends on age at diagnosis, treatment used, and complications. Mortality is high if polycythemia is untreated or is associated with leukemia or myeloid metaplasia. (Polycythemia vera is also known as primary polycythemia, erythremia, polycythemia rubra vera, splenomegalic polycythemia, and Vaquez-Osler disease.)

Cause and pathophysiology
In polycythemia vera, uncontrolled and rapid cellular reproduction and maturation cause proliferation or hyperplasia of all bone marrow cells (panmyelosis). The cause of such uncontrolled cellular activity is unknown, but it is probably the result of a multipotential stem cell defect.

Complications
Hyperviscosity may lead to thrombosis of small vessels with ruddy cyanosis of the nose and clubbing (stunting) of the digits. Further thromboembolic involvement can lead to splenomegaly, renal calculus formation, and abdominal organ thrombosis.

Paradoxically, hemorrhage is a complication of polycythemia vera. It may be due to defective platelet function or to hyperviscosity and the local effects from excess RBCs exerting pressure on distended venous and capillary walls.

Cerebrovascular accident (CVA) may also complicate the disease. As well, incidence of peptic ulcer disease is four to five times greater in patients with polycythemia vera than in the general population.

Assessment findings
In its early stages, polycythemia vera may produce no signs or symptoms. However, as altered circulation (secondary to increased RBC mass) produces hypervolemia and hyperviscosity, the patient may report a vague feeling of fullness in the head, rushing in the ears, tinnitus, headache, dizziness, vertigo, epistaxis, night sweats, epigastric and joint pain, and visual alterations, such as scotomas, double vision, and blurred vision. He may also report a decrease in urine output, possibly due to increased uric acid production.

Late in the disease, the patient may report pruritus (which worsens after bathing and may be disabling), a sense of abdominal fullness, and pain, such as pleuritic chest pain or left upper quadrant pain. (See *Common clin-*

COMMON CLINICAL FEATURES OF POLYCYTHEMIA VERA

Signs and symptoms	Causes
Eye and ear • Visual disturbances (blurring, diplopia, scotoma, engorged veins of fundus and retina) and congestion of conjunctiva, retina, and retinal veins	• Hypervolemia and hyperviscosity • Engorgement of capillary beds
Nose and mouth • Epistaxis or gingival bleeding • Oral mucous membrane congestion	• Hypervolemia and hyperviscosity • Engorgement of capillary beds
Central nervous system • Headache or fullness in the head, lethargy, weakness, fatigue, syncope, dizziness, vertigo, tinnitus, paresthesia of digits, and impaired mentation	• Hypervolemia and hyperviscosity
Cardiovascular system • Hypertension • Intermittent claudication, thrombosis and emboli, angina, thrombophlebitis • Hemorrhage	• Hypervolemia and hyperviscosity • Hypervolemia, thrombocytosis, and vascular disease • Engorgement of capillary beds
Skin • Pruritus (especially after hot bath) • Urticaria • Ruddy cyanosis • Night sweats • Ecchymosis	• Basophilia (secondary histamine release) • Altered histamine metabolism • Hypervolemia and hyperviscosity due to congested vessels, increased oxyhemoglobin and reduced hemoglobin levels • Hypermetabolism • Hemorrhage
GI system • Epigastric distress • Early abdominal fullness • Peptic ulcer pain • Hepatosplenomegaly • Weight loss	• Hypervolemia and hyperviscosity • Hepatosplenomegaly • Gastric thrombosis and hemorrhage • Congestion, extramedullary hemopoiesis, and myeloid metaplasia • Hypermetabolism
Respiratory system • Dyspnea	• Hypervolemia and hyperviscosity
Musculoskeletal system • Joint pain	• Increased urate production secondary to nucleoprotein turnover

ical features of polycythemia vera for a systematic listing of signs and symptoms.)

Diagnostic tests

Laboratory studies confirm polycythemia vera by showing increased RBC mass and normal arterial oxygen saturation in association with splenomegaly or two of the following:
• platelet count above 400,000/mm³ (thrombocytosis)

• white blood cell (WBC) count above 10,000/mm³ in adults (leukocytosis)
• elevated leukocyte alkaline phosphatase level
• elevated serum vitamin B_{12} levels or unbound B_{12}–binding capacity.

Another common finding is increased uric acid production, leading to hyperuricemia and hyperuricuria. Other laboratory results include increased blood histamine, decreased serum iron concentration, and decreased or absent urinary erythropoietin. Bone marrow biopsy reveals panmyelosis.

Treatment

Phlebotomy, the primary treatment, can be performed repeatedly and can reduce RBC mass promptly. It's best used for patients with mild disease or for young patients. The frequency of phlebotomy and the amount of blood removed each time depends on the patient's condition. Typically, 350 to 500 ml of blood can be removed every other day until the patient's hematocrit is reduced to the low-normal range. After repeated phlebotomies, the patient will develop iron deficiency, which stabilizes RBC production and reduces the need for phlebotomy. However, phlebotomy doesn't reduce the WBC or platelet count and won't control the hyperuricemia associated with marrow cell proliferation.

Myelosuppressive therapy may be used for patients with severe symptoms, such as extreme thrombocytosis, a rapidly enlarging spleen, and hypermetabolism. It's also used for elderly patients who have difficulty tolerating the phlebotomy procedure. Radioactive phosphorus (^{32}P) or chemotherapeutic agents, such as melphalan, busulfan, and chlorambucil, can satisfactorily control the disease in most cases. However, these agents may cause leukemia, and should be reserved for older patients and those with serious problems not controlled by phlebotomy. Patients of any age who have had previous thrombotic problems should be considered for myelosuppressive therapy.

Pheresis technology allows removal of RBCs, WBCs, and platelets individually or collectively (and provides these cellular components for blood banks). Pheresis also permits the return of plasma to the patient, thereby diluting the blood and reducing hypovolemic symptoms.

As appropriate, additional treatments include administration of cyproheptadine (12 to 16 mg/day) and allopurinol (300 mg/day) to reduce serum uric acid levels. Treatment usually improves symptomatic splenomegaly; rarely, splenectomy may be performed.

Nursing diagnoses
• Activity intolerance
• Altered nutrition: Less than body requirements
• Altered tissue perfusion
• Anxiety
• Fatigue
• Knowledge deficit
• Pain
• Risk for impaired skin integrity
• Risk for infection
• Risk for injury
• Sensory or perceptual alterations

Nursing interventions
• Encourage the patient to express any concerns about the disease, its treatment, and the effect that it may have on his life. Answer questions appropriately and provide emotional support. If possible, stay with him during periods of acute stress and anxiety.
• Keep the patient active and ambulatory to prevent thrombosis. If bed rest is necessary, prescribe a daily program of both active and passive range-of-motion exercises.
• Watch for complications, such as hypervolemia, thrombocytosis, signs of impending CVA (decreased sensation, numbness, transitory paralysis, fleeting blindness, headache, and epistaxis), and hypertension and congestive heart failure (caused by prolonged hyperviscosity).
• Regularly examine the patient for bleeding.
• To compensate for increased uric acid production, give the patient additional fluids, administer allopurinol, as ordered, and alkalinize the urine to prevent uric acid calculus formation.
• If the patient has symptomatic splenomegaly, suggest or provide small, frequent meals, followed by a rest period, to prevent nausea and vomiting.
• If the patient has pruritus, give medications, as ordered, and provide distractions to help him cope.
• Report acute abdominal pain immediately; it may signal splenic infarction, renal calculus formation, or abdominal organ thrombosis.
• Before phlebotomy, check the patient's blood pressure and pulse and respiratory rates. During phlebotomy, make sure the patient is lying down comfortably, to prevent vertigo and syncope. Stay alert for tachycardia, clamminess, and complaints of vertigo. If these effects occur, the procedure should be stopped.
• Immediately after phlebotomy, check the patient's blood pressure and pulse rate. Have the patient sit up for about 5 minutes before allowing him to walk; this prevents vasovagal attack and orthostatic hypotension. Also, administer 24 oz (710 ml) of juice or water to replenish fluid volume.

During myelosuppressive chemotherapy:
• Monitor complete blood count (CBC) and platelet count before and during therapy.
• Watch for and report all adverse effects that occur after administration of an alkylating agent.
• If nausea and vomiting occur, begin antiemetic therapy, and adjust the patient's diet.

During treatment with ³²P:

• Make sure you have a blood sample for CBC and platelet count before beginning treatment. (*Note:* The health care professional who administers ³²P should take radiation precautions to prevent contamination.)

• Have the patient lie down during I.V. administration (to facilitate the procedure and prevent extravasation) and for 15 to 20 minutes afterward.

Patient teaching

• Determine what the patient knows about the disease, especially if he has been diagnosed for some time. As necessary, reinforce the doctor's explanation of the disease process, signs and symptoms, and prescribed treatment.

• Tell the patient to remain as active as possible, to help maintain his self-esteem.

• Instruct the patient to use an electric razor to prevent accidental cuts, and to keep his environment free of clutter to minimize falls and contusions.

• Advise the patient to avoid high altitudes, which may exacerabate polycythemia.

• If the patient develops thrombocytopenia, tell him which are the most common bleeding sites (such as the nose, gingiva, and skin), so he can check for bleeding. Advise him to report any abnormal bleeding promptly.

• If the patient requires phlebotomy, describe the procedure and explain that it will relieve distressing symptoms. Tell the patient to watch for and report any symptoms of iron deficiency (pallor, weight loss, asthenia, glossitis).

• If the patient requires myelosuppressive therapy, tell him about possible adverse effects (nausea, vomiting, and susceptibility to infection) that may follow administration of an alkylating agent. As appropriate, mention that alopecia may follow the use of busulfan, cyclophosphamide, and uracil mustard and that sterile hemorrhagic cystitis may follow the use of cyclophosphamide (forcing fluids can prevent this adverse effect).

• If an outpatient develops leukopenia, reinforce instructions about preventing infection. Warn the patient that his resistance to infection is low; advise him to avoid crowds, and make sure he knows the symptoms of infection.

• If the patient requires treatment with ³²P, explain the procedure. Tell him that he may require repeated phlebotomies until ³²P takes effect.

• Refer the patient to the social service department and local home health care agencies, as appropriate.

SPURIOUS POLYCYTHEMIA

Characterized by increased hematocrit and normal or decreased red blood cell (RBC) total mass, spurious polycythemia results from decreasing plasma volume and subsequent hemoconcentration. This disease is also known as relative polycythemia, stress erythrocytosis, stress polycythemia, benign polycythemia, Gaisböck's syndrome, and pseudopolycythemia.

Causes and pathophysiology

Possible causes of spurious polycythemia include the following:

• *Dehydration.* Conditions that promote severe fluid loss decrease plasma levels and lead to hemoconcentration. Such conditions include persistent vomiting or diarrhea, burns, adrenocortical insufficiency, aggressive diuretic therapy, decreased fluid intake, diabetic ketoacidosis, and renal disease.

• *Hemoconcentration due to stress.* Nervous stress leads to hemoconcentration by some unknown mechanism, possibly by temporarily decreasing circulating plasma volume or by vascular redistribution of erythrocytes.

• *High normal RBC mass and low normal plasma volume.* In many patients, an increased hematocrit merely reflects a normally high RBC mass and low plasma volume.

Other factors that may be associated with spurious polycythemia include hypertension, thromboembolic disease, pregnancy, elevated serum cholesterol and uric acid levels, and familial tendency.

Complications

Spurious polycythemia can be complicated by hypercholesterolemia, hyperlipidemia, and hyperuricemia. Thromboembolic complications may result if the condition goes untreated.

Assessment findings

The patient with spurious polycythemia usually has no specific signs or symptoms but may have vague complaints, such as headache, dizziness, and fatigue. Less commonly, the patient may report diaphoresis, dyspnea, and claudication. The patient's history may reveal existing cardiac or pulmonary disease.

Inspection typically reveals a patient with a ruddy appearance and a short neck. Palpation usually discloses associated hepatosplenomegaly. Auscultation may detect slight hypertension and hypoventilation when the patient is recumbent.

Diagnostic tests

Spurious polycythemia is distinguishable from true polycythemia vera by its characteristic normal or decreased RBC mass, elevated hematocrit, and the absence of leukocytosis.

The results of other commonly performed laboratory tests include:
• elevated hemoglobin levels and hematocrit
• elevated RBC count
• normal arterial oxygen saturation and bone marrow studies
• normal or decreased plasma volume.

Treatment

The principal goals of treatment are to correct dehydration and to prevent life-threatening thromboembolism. Rehydration with appropriate fluids and electrolytes is the primary therapy for spurious polycythemia secondary to dehydration. Therapy must also include appropriate measures to prevent continuing fluid loss.

Nursing diagnoses

• Activity intolerance
• Altered tissue perfusion
• Anxiety
• Fatigue
• Fluid volume deficit
• Ineffective breathing pattern
• Pain

Nursing interventions

• Focus your care on rehydration, a cardiovascular diet and exercise regimen, and patient teaching about the condition and related stress factors.
• Encourage the patient to discuss his concerns about the disease, its treatments, and the effect it may have on his life. Answer questions appropriately and provide emotional support. If possible, stay with the patient during periods of severe stress and anxiety.
• Keep the patient active and ambulatory to prevent thrombosis. If he complains of fatigue, alternate periods of rest and activity.
• Auscultate breath sounds every 4 hours. If the patient hypoventilates when recumbent, assist him to a comfortable position by elevating the head of the bed.
• During rehydration, monitor intake and output to maintain fluid balance. Also monitor laboratory studies to maintain electrolyte balance.
• To prevent thromboemboli in predisposed patients, initiate a cardiovascular exercise program coupled with a reduced dietary cholesterol plan. (Studies show that hypertension and hypercholesterolemia can be reduced by the combination of regular exercise and a diet low in fat and cholesterol.) Antilipemics, such as cholestyramine or gemfibrozil, may be added to the treatment plan when exercise and dietary control are unsuccessful.

Patient teaching

• Thoroughly explain the disease, including its diagnosis and treatment. The hard-driving person who is predisposed to spurious polycythemia is likely to be more inquisitive and anxious than the average patient. Answer his questions honestly, and reassure him that he can effectively control symptoms by complying with the prescribed treatment.
• Emphasize the need for follow-up examinations every 3 to 4 months after leaving the hospital.
• Caution the patient to follow a doctor-prescribed exercise program and diet. Results should be checked during follow-up examinations.
• When appropriate, suggest counseling about the patient's work habits and lack of relaxation. If the patient is a smoker, emphasize the importance of stopping. Then refer him to an antismoking program, if necessary.
• Teach the patient to recognize and report signs and symptoms of increasing polycythemia and thromboembolism.
• Instruct the patient to use an electric razor and to maintain a clutter-free environment to minimize falls and contusions.
• Refer the patient to the social service department and local home health care agencies, as appropriate.

SECONDARY POLYCYTHEMIA

Also called reactive polycythemia, secondary polycythemia is characterized by excessive production of circulating red blood cells (RBCs) due to hypoxia, tumor, or disease. It occurs in about 2 out of every 100,000 people who live at or near sea level; incidence rises among people who live at high altitudes.

Causes and pathophysiology

Secondary polycythemia may result from increased production of erythropoietin. This hormone, which is possibly produced and secreted in the kidneys, stimulates bone marrow production of RBCs. This increased production may be an appropriate (compensatory) physiologic response to hypoxemia, which may result from:
• chronic obstructive pulmonary disease
• hemoglobin abnormalities (such as carboxyhemoglobinemia, which occurs in heavy smokers)

• congestive heart failure (causing a decreased ventilation-perfusion ratio)
• right-to-left shunting of blood in the heart (as in transposition of the great vessels)
• central or peripheral alveolar hypoventilation (as in barbiturate intoxication or pickwickian syndrome)
• low oxygen content of air at high altitudes.

Increased production of erythropoietin may also be an inappropriate (pathologic) response to renal disease (such as renovascular impairment, renal cysts, and hydronephrosis), to central nervous system disease (such as encephalitis and parkinsonism), to neoplasms (such as renal tumors, uterine myomas, and cerebellar hemangiomas), and to endocrine disorders (such as Cushing's syndrome and pheochromocytomas). Rarely, secondary polycythemia results from a recessive genetic trait.

Complications
A patient with secondary polycythemia has an increased risk of hemorrhage due to problems with platelet quality, especially during surgery. Thromboemboli secondary to hemoconcentration may occur spontaneously; after prolonged immobility, as may occur with arthritic conditions or decreased mobility; or after surgery.

Assessment findings
The patient's history usually reveals shortness of breath (associated with emphysema). Inspection reveals a ruddy cyanosis of the skin and, possibly, clubbing of the fingers (in underlying cardiac or pulmonary disease). Hypoxemia is found without hepatosplenomegaly or hypertension, which constitutes a major difference between primary (vera) and secondary polycythemia.

Secondary polycythemia that isn't caused by hypoxemia is usually an incidental finding during treatment for an underlying disease.

Diagnostic tests
Laboratory results for secondary polycythemia include:
• increased RBC mass, with increased hematocrit, hemoglobin levels, mean corpuscular volume, and mean corpuscular hemoglobin
• elevated urinary erythropoietin levels
• increased blood histamine levels
• decreased or normal arterial oxygen saturation.

Bone marrow biopsies reveal hyperplasia confined to the erythroid series. Unlike polycythemia vera, secondary polycythemia isn't associated with leukocytosis or thrombocytosis.

Treatment
The goal of treatment is correction of the underlying disease or environmental condition. In severe secondary polycythemia when altitude is a contributing factor, relocation may be advisable. If secondary polycythemia has produced hazardous hyperviscosity, or if the patient doesn't respond to treatment for the primary disease, reduction of blood volume by phlebotomy or pheresis may be effective.

Emergency phlebotomy is indicated for prevention of impending vascular occlusion and before emergency surgery. In the latter case, removal of excess RBCs and reinfusion of the patient's plasma is usually advisable.

Nursing diagnoses
• Activity intolerance
• Altered protection
• Anxiety
• Fatigue
• Fear
• Impaired gas exchange
• Knowledge deficit
• Risk for fluid volume deficit
• Risk for infection
• Risk for injury

Nursing interventions
• Encourage the patient to express any concerns about the disease, its treatments, and the effect that it may have on his life. Answer questions and provide emotional support. If possible, stay with him during periods of severe stress and anxiety.
• Before phlebotomy or pheresis, check the patient's blood pressure while he's lying down. Also note pulse and respiratory rates. During phlebotomy, make sure the patient is lying down comfortably to prevent vertigo and syncope. Stay alert for tachycardia, clamminess, and complaints of vertigo. If these effects occur, the procedure should be stopped.
• Immediately after phlebotomy, check the patient's blood pressure and pulse rate while he's lying down. Have the patient sit up for about 5 minutes before allowing him to walk; this prevents vasovagal stimulation and orthostatic hypotension. Also, administer 24 oz (710 ml) of juice or water to replenish fluid volume.
• Support the patient's efforts to perform activities.
• Keep the patient as active as possible to decrease the risk of thrombosis due to increased blood viscosity. Provide rest periods between activities, as needed; the well-rested patient may be more active. If bed rest is neces-

sary, prescribe a daily program of active and passive range-of-motion exercises.

• Reduce caloric and sodium intake to counteract the tendency to hypertension. Provide meals that meet these requirements.

• Administer ordered medications, such as analgesics for headaches, as appropriate. Administer oxygen, as ordered, to maintain adequate tissue perfusion.

Patient teaching

• Teach the patient and his family about the underlying disorder. Help them understand its relation to polycythemia and the measures to control both. Explain the disease process, its signs and symptoms, prescribed treatments, and any complications that may occur.

• Emphasize the importance of regular blood studies (every 2 to 3 months), even after the disease is controlled.

• Help the patient overcome potential noncompliance with a low-sodium, reduced-calorie diet. Suggest using herbs and spices to add flavor and removing fat and skin from meat before cooking. Refer the patient to the dietitian for additional teaching, if necessary.

• Instruct the patient to use an electric razor and to maintain a clutter-free environment to minimize falls and contusions.

• Caution the patient to avoid high altitudes, which may exacerabate polycythemia.

• Explain that alternating periods of rest and activity will reduce the body's demand for oxygen and prevent fatigue.

• Describe the advantages of following a cardiovascular fitness program (affirmed by the doctor), and encourage the patient to participate. If appropriate, suggest walking at a pace of at least 4 mph for 20 to 30 minutes four times per week.

• Refer the patient to the social service department and local home health care agencies, as appropriate.

HEMORRHAGIC DISORDERS

Characterized by uncontrolled bleeding, hemorrhagic disorders involve a rapid loss of a large amount of blood, either internally or externally. Hemorrhage may be arterial, venous, or capillary. Common hemorrhagic disorders include allergic purpuras, hereditary hemorrhagic telangiectasia, thrombocytopenia, idiopathic thrombocytopenic purpura, platelet function disorders, hemophilia, von Willebrand's disease, and disseminated intravascular coagulation.

ALLERGIC PURPURAS

A nonthrombocytopenic purpura, allergic purpura is an acute or chronic vascular inflammation that affects the skin, joints, and GI and genitourinary (GU) tracts in association with allergy symptoms. When allergic purpura primarily affects the GI tract, with accompanying joint pain, it is called Henoch-Schönlein syndrome or anaphylactoid purpura. However, the term allergic purpura applies to purpura associated with many other conditions, such as erythema nodosum. An acute attack of allergic purpura can last for several weeks.

Fully developed allergic purpura is persistent and debilitating. This disorder affects males more commonly than females and is most prevalent in children ages 3 to 7 years. The prognosis is more favorable for children than for adults. The course of Henoch-Schönlein syndrome is usually benign and self-limiting, lasting 1 to 6 weeks if renal involvement is not severe.

Causes

The most common identifiable cause of allergic purpura is probably an autoimmune reaction directed against vascular walls and triggered by a bacterial infection (particularly a streptococcal infection, such as scarlet fever). Typically, upper respiratory tract infection occurs 1 to 3 weeks before the onset of signs and symptoms. Other possible causes include allergic reactions to some drugs and vaccines; allergic reactions to insect bites; and allergic reactions to some foods (such as wheat, eggs, milk, and chocolate).

Complications

Renal disease (renal failure and acute glomerulonephritis) can be fatal. Hypertension and resulting blood loss from renal damage can further complicate the patient's condition.

Assessment findings

An accurate patient allergy history may yield information that helps ensure a positive outcome. The patient history may include pain and bleeding due to bleeding from the mucosal surfaces of the ureters, bladder, and urethra. In 25% to 50% of patients, allergic purpura is associated with GU symptoms. Other patient complaints include moderate, transient headaches; fever; anorexia; edema of the hands, feet, or scalp; and skin lesions, accompanied by pruritus, paresthesia and, occasionally, angioneurotic edema.

The patient with Henoch-Schönlein purpura may report a hypersensitivity to aspirin and food and drug additives. Typically, the patient complains of transient or severe colic, tenesmus, constipation, vomiting, and edema. He also may report hematuria and joint pain, mostly affecting the knees and ankles. Other symptoms include bleeding or hemorrhage of the mucous membranes of the bowel, resulting in GI bleeding, occult blood in the stool and, possibly, intussusception. Such GI abnormalities may precede overt, cutaneous signs of purpura.

Inspection findings in allergic purpuras include the characteristic skin lesions. Purple, macular, ecchymotic, and of varying sizes, these lesions result from vascular leakage into the skin and mucous membranes. The lesions usually appear in symmetrical patterns on the arms and legs. In children, skin lesions are generally urticarial; they expand and become hemorrhagic.

In Henoch-Schönlein purpura, inspection and palpation may disclose localized areas of edema, especially on the dorsal surfaces of the hands.

Diagnostic tests

No laboratory test clearly identifies allergic purpura (although white blood cell count and erythrocyte sedimentation rate are elevated). Diagnosis necessitates careful clinical observation, often during the second or third attack. The following laboratory test results may aid diagnosis:
• guaiac-positive stools
• hematuria identified on urinalysis
• elevated blood urea nitrogen and creatinine levels and proteinuria, indicating glomerular involvement
• normal coagulation and platelet function (with the exception of a positive tourniquet test).

Small-bowel X-rays may reveal areas of transient edema. Diagnosis must rule out other forms of nonthrombocytopenic purpura.

Treatment

In allergic purpura, treatment is usually based on symptoms; for example, severe allergic purpura may require corticosteroids to relieve edema and analgesics to alleviate joint and abdominal pain. Some patients with chronic renal disease may benefit from immunosuppression with azathioprine or corticosteroids, along with identification of the provocative allergen.

Nursing diagnoses

• Altered renal or GI tissue perfusion
• Anxiety
• Body image disturbance
• Impaired skin integrity
• Knowledge deficit

• Pain
• Risk for fluid volume deficit
• Risk for infection

Nursing interventions

For allergic purpuras:
• Monitor skin lesions and level of pain. Provide analgesics, as needed.
• Watch carefully for complications, including GI and GU tract bleeding, edema, nausea, vomiting, headache, hypertension (with nephritis), abdominal rigidity and tenderness, and absence of stool (with intussusception).
• To prevent muscle atrophy in the bedridden patient, provide passive or active range-of-motion exercises.
• Provide emotional support and reassurance, especially if the patient is temporarily disfigured by florid skin lesions.
• Administer fluids if required to maintain fluid level. Encourage fluid intake, as appropriate.
   For immunosuppressive therapy:
• Provide an environment free from the possibility of secondary infection.
• If corticosteroid therapy is added, watch for signs of Cushing's syndrome and labile emotional involvement.

Patient teaching

• Teach the patient about the disease, its symptoms, and treatment.
• Explain the need to protect against infection. Advise the patient to wash his hands frequently to avoid infecting his skin lesions. Teach him to protect edematous areas because the skin over these areas breaks down easily.
• After the acute stage, direct the patient to report immediately any recurrence of symptoms (most common about 6 weeks after initial onset). Tell him to return for follow-up urinalysis as scheduled.
• Encourage maintenance of an elimination diet to help identify specific allergenic foods so that these foods can be eliminated from the patient's diet.

HEREDITARY HEMORRHAGIC TELANGIECTASIA

Also called Osler-Rendu-Weber disease, hereditary hemorrhagic telangiectasia is an inherited vascular disorder in which venules and capillaries dilate to form fragile masses of thin convoluted vessels (telangiectases), resulting in an abnormal tendency to hemorrhage. This disorder affects both sexes but may cause less severe bleeding in females.

Causes

Hereditary hemorrhagic telangiectasia is transmitted by autosomal dominant inheritance. The disorder seldom skips generations. In its homozygous state, it may be fatal.

Complications

Secondary iron deficiency anemia from chronic bleeding is the most common complication. Rarely, vascular malformation may cause pulmonary arteriovenous fistulas; then, shunting of blood through the fistulas may lead to hypoxemia. Recurring cerebral embolism and brain abscess may also occur. Hemorrhagic shock, although rare, may occur in severe cases or in undiagnosed patients undergoing surgery or in victims of trauma.

Assessment findings

Although signs of hereditary hemorrhagic telangiectasia may be present in childhood, they increase in severity with age.

The history of a patient with this disorder reveals an established familial pattern of bleeding disorders. The patient may complain of epistaxis, hemoptysis, or tarry stools, indicating fragile mucous membranes in the nose, mouth, or stomach.

Inspection reveals localized aggregations of dilated capillaries on the skin of the face, ears, scalp, hands, arms, and feet, and under the nails. Characteristic telangiectases are violet, bleed spontaneously, may be flat or raised, blanch on pressure, and are nonpulsatile. They may be associated with vascular malformations, such as arteriovenous fistulas. Although they can't be seen on inspection, visceral telangiectases are common in the liver, bladder, respiratory tract, and stomach. The type and distribution of these lesions are usually similar among family members.

Inspection may also reveal generalized capillary fragility, evidenced by spontaneous bleeding, petechiae, ecchymoses, and spider hemangiomas of varying sizes. These signs of capillary fragility may exist without overt telangiectasia. (See *Typical lesions of hereditary hemorrhagic telangiectasia*.) A lesser form of this syndrome leads to clubbing of the digits.

An established familial pattern of bleeding disorders and clinical evidence of telangiectasia and hemorrhage establish the diagnosis.

TYPICAL LESIONS OF HEREDITARY HEMORRHAGIC TELANGIECTASIA

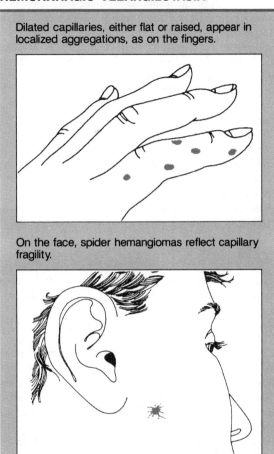

Dilated capillaries, either flat or raised, appear in localized aggregations, as on the fingers.

On the face, spider hemangiomas reflect capillary fragility.

Diagnostic tests

Bone marrow aspiration showing depleted iron stores confirms secondary iron deficiency anemia. Hypochromic, microcytic anemia is common; abnormal platelet function may also be found. Coagulation tests are essentially irrelevant because hemorrhage in telangiectasia results from vascular wall weakness.

Treatment

Supportive therapy includes blood transfusions and the administration of supplemental iron. Ancillary treatment may consist of applying pressure and topical hemostatic agents to bleeding sites; cauterizing bleeding sites not readily accessible; and protecting the patient from trauma and unnecessary bleeding.

Parenteral administration of supplemental iron enhances absorption to maintain adequate iron stores and prevents gastric irritation. Administering antipyretics or antihistamines before blood transfusion and using saline-washed cells, frozen blood, or other types of leukocyte-poor blood instead of whole blood transfusion may prevent febrile transfusion reactions.

Nursing diagnoses
• Activity intolerance
• Altered tissue perfusion
• Anxiety
• Body image disturbance
• Impaired skin integrity
• Knowledge deficit
• Risk for fluid volume deficit
• Risk for infection

Nursing interventions
• Provide emotional and psychological support. Encourage the patient to express his concerns about his disease and its treatment. If possible, stay with the patient during periods of severe stress and anxiety. As much as possible, include the patient in care decisions.
• Administer ordered blood transfusions. Set the flow rate, and observe the patient for tolerance of the infusion and possible adverse reactions. Take the patient's vital signs, and monitor the patient frequently according to hospital policy. Check for signs of febrile or allergic transfusion reaction (flushing, shaking chills, fever, headache, rash, tachycardia, hypertension).
• Encourage fluid intake if the patient is bleeding or is hypovolemic. Monitor intake and output.
• Provide good skin care and hygiene, and use aseptic techniques when caring for the patient. Lesions bleed easily, which may result in infection and skin breakdown.
• Throughout the patient's hospitalization, observe him for indications of GI bleeding, such as hematemesis and melena.
• Monitor organ function through routine physical examination and comparison with laboratory evaluations to detect possible renal, hepatic, or respiratory failure.

Patient teaching
• Teach the patient about the disease, its signs and symptoms, and treatment, reinforcing the doctor's explanation as necessary. Also teach the patient and his family about the hereditary nature of this disorder. Refer the patient for genetic counseling, as appropriate.
• If the patient requires an iron supplement, stress the importance of following dosage instructions and of taking oral iron with meals to minimize GI irritation. Warn that iron turns stools dark green or black and may cause constipation.
• Teach the patient and family how to manage minor bleeding episodes, especially recurrent epistaxis, and to recognize major ones that necessitate emergency intervention.
• Encourage routine medical care to monitor for visceral hemorrhage and organ failure.

THROMBOCYTOPENIA
The most common cause of hemorrhagic disorders, thrombocytopenia is characterized by a deficient number of circulating platelets. Because platelets play a vital role in coagulation, this disease poses a serious threat to hemostasis. The prognosis is excellent in drug-induced thrombocytopenia if the offending drug is withdrawn; in such cases, recovery may be immediate. Otherwise, the prognosis depends on the patient's response to treatment of the underlying cause.

Causes and pathophysiology
Thrombocytopenia may be congenital or acquired; the acquired form is more common. In either case, it usually results from decreased or defective production of platelets in the marrow (for example, in leukemia, aplastic anemia, and toxicity with certain drugs) or from increased destruction outside the marrow caused by an underlying disorder (such as cirrhosis of the liver, disseminated intravascular coagulation, and severe infection).

Less commonly, thrombocytopenia results from sequestration (hypersplenism, hypothermia) or platelet loss. Acquired thrombocytopenia may result from the use of certain drugs, such as quinine, quinidine, rifampin, heparin, nonsteroidal anti-inflammatory agents, histamine blockers, most chemotherapeutic agents, allopurinol, and alcohol.

Thrombocytopenia may also occur transiently after a viral infection (such as Epstein-Barr) or infectious mononucleosis. (See *Causes of decreased circulating platelets*.) An idiopathic form of thrombocytopenia also occurs. (For more information, refer to "Idiopathic Thrombocytopenic Purpura" in this chapter.)

Complications

Complications of thrombocytopenia are usually related to bleeding. Severe thrombocytopenia can cause acute hemorrhage, which may be fatal without immediate therapy. The most common sites of severe bleeding include the brain and the GI tract, although intrapulmonary bleeding and cardiac tamponade can also occur.

Assessment findings

Typically, a patient with thrombocytopenia reports sudden onset of petechiae and ecchymoses from bleeding into mucous membranes (GI, urinary, vaginal, or respiratory). He may also complain of malaise, fatigue, and general weakness (with or without accompanying blood loss). In acquired thrombocytopenia, the patient's history may include the use of one or several offending drugs.

Inspection typically reveals evidence of bleeding (petechiae, ecchymoses), along with slow, continuous bleeding from any injuries or wounds. Painless, round, and as tiny as pinpoints (1 to 3 mm in diameter), petechiae usually occur on dependent portions of the body, appearing and fading in crops and sometimes grouping to form ecchymoses. Another form of blood leakage and larger than petechiae, ecchymoses are purple, blue, or yellow-green bruises that vary in size and shape. They can occur anywhere on the body from traumatic injury. In patients with bleeding disorders, they usually appear on the arms and legs. In adults, inspection may reveal large, blood-filled bullae in the mouth. Gentle palpation of edematous ecchymotic areas may cause pain, indicating that these areas are actually hematomas. Superficial hematomas are red; deep hematomas are blue. They typically exceed 1 cm in diameter.

If the patient's platelet count is between 30,000 and 50,000/mm³, expect bruising with minor trauma; if it's between 15,000 and 30,000/mm³, expect spontaneous bruising and petechiae, mostly on the arms and legs. With a platelet count below 15,000/mm³, expect spontaneous bruising or, after minor trauma, mucosal bleeding, generalized purpura, epistaxis, hematuria, and GI or intracranial bleeding. Female patients may report menorrhagia.

Diagnostic tests

The following laboratory findings help establish a diagnosis of thrombocytopenia:
• diminished platelet count (in adults, less than 100,000/mm³)
• prolonged bleeding time (although this doesn't always indicate platelet quality)

CAUSES OF DECREASED CIRCULATING PLATELETS

Thrombocytopenia usually results from insufficient production or increased peripheral destruction of platelets. Less commonly, it results from sequestration or platelet loss.

Diminished or defective platelet production
Congenital
• Wiskott-Aldrich syndrome
• Maternal ingestion of thiazides
• Neonatal rubella
• Polycythemia
Acquired
• Aplastic anemia
• Marrow infiltration (acute and chronic leukemias, tumor)
• Nutritional deficiency (vitamin B₁₂, folic acid)
• Myelosuppressive agents
• Drugs that directly influence platelet production (thiazides, alcohol, hormones)
• Radiation
• Viral infections (measles, dengue)

Increased peripheral destruction (outside marrow)
Congenital
• Nonimmune (prematurity, erythroblastosis fetalis, infection)
• Immune (drug sensitivity, maternal idiopathic thrombocytopenic purpura [ITP])
Acquired
• Nonimmune (infection, disseminated intramuscular coagulation, thrombotic thrombocytopenic purpura)
• Immune (drug-induced, especially with quinine and quinidine; post-transfusion purpura; acute and chronic ITP; sepsis; alcohol)
• Invasive lines or devices (intra-aortic balloon pump, prosthetic cardiac valves)

Sequestration of platelets
• Hypersplenism
• Hypothermia

Platelet loss
• Hemorrhage
• Extracorporeal perfusion

• normal prothrombin and partial thromboplastin times.

Platelet antibody studies can help determine why the platelet count is low and help direct treatment. Platelet survival studies help differentiate between ineffective platelet production and inappropriate platelet destruction. (Platelet production disorders may occur after radiation exposure, medication ingestion, or an infectious disease. They may also occur idiopathically. Inappropriate platelet destruction may occur with splenic disease and platelet antibody disorders.)

In severe thrombocytopenia, a bone marrow study determines the number, size, and cytoplasmic maturity of the megakaryocytes (the bone marrow cells that release mature platelets). This information may identify ineffective platelet production as the cause of thrombocytopenia and rule out a malignant disease process at the same time.

Treatment

Removal of the offending agents in drug-induced thrombocytopenia or proper treatment of the underlying cause, when possible, is essential. Corticosteroids may be used to increase platelet production. Lithium carbonate or folate may also be used to stimulate bone marrow production of platelets. In cases of severe or refractory thrombocytopenia, I.V. gamma globulin has been used experimentally with moderate success.

Platelet transfusions may be used to stop episodic abnormal bleeding caused by a low platelet count. However, if platelet destruction results from an immune disorder, platelet infusions may have only a minimal effect and may be reserved for life-threatening bleeding.

Splenectomy may be necessary to correct thrombocytopenia caused by platelet destruction. A splenectomy should significantly reduce platelet destruction because the spleen acts as the primary site of platelet removal and antibody production.

Nursing diagnoses
• Activity intolerance
• Altered protection
• Anxiety
• Body image disturbance
• Fatigue
• Impaired skin integrity
• Knowledge deficit
• Risk for infection
• Risk for injury

Nursing interventions
• Provide emotional support as necessary. Encourage the patient to discuss his concerns about his condition. Reassure him that the ecchymoses and petechiae will heal as the disease resolves.
• Provide rest periods between activities if the patient tires easily.

• If the patient has painful hematomas, handle the area gently. Protect all areas of ecchymosis and petechiae from further injury.
• Take every possible precaution against bleeding. Protect the patient from trauma. Keep the bed's side rails raised, and pad them, if possible. Promote the use of an electric razor and a soft toothbrush. Avoid invasive procedures, such as venipuncture or urinary catheterization, if possible. When venipuncture is unavoidable, exert pressure on the puncture site for at least 20 minutes or until the bleeding stops.
• Monitor platelet count daily.
• Watch for bleeding (petechiae, ecchymoses, surgical or GI bleeding, menorrhagia). Identify the amount of bleeding or the size of ecchymoses at least every 24 hours. Test stool, urine, and emesis for blood.
• During active bleeding, maintain the patient on strict bed rest. Keep the head of the bed elevated to prevent gravity-related pressure increases, possibly leading to intracranial bleeding.
• When administering platelet concentrate, remember that platelets are extremely fragile, so infuse them quickly, using the administration set recommended by the blood bank.
• During platelet transfusion, monitor for a febrile reaction (flushing, chills, fever, headache, tachycardia, hypertension). Such reactions are common and a fever will destroy the blood products. HLA-typed platelets may be ordered to prevent febrile reaction. If the patient has a history of minor reactions, he may benefit from acetaminophen and diphenhydramine before the transfusion.
• One to 2 hours after administering platelet concentrate, monitor the patient's platelet count to assess his response to the infusion. A lack of platelet level increase indicates that the patient is making platelet antibodies and should receive HLA-matched platelets.

Patient teaching
• Teach the patient about his disorder and its cause, if known. If appropriate, reassure the patient that thrombocytopenia often resolves spontaneously.
• Teach the patient to recognize and report signs of intracranial bleeding (persistent headache, mood change, nausea, vomiting, and drowsiness) and other signs of bleeding (tarry stools, coffee-ground vomitus, epistaxis, menorrhagia, and gingival or urinary tract bleeding).
• Advise the patient to avoid straining at stool or coughing: Both can lead to increased intracranial pressure, possibly causing cerebral hemorrhage. Provide a stool softener, if necessary, because constipation and passage

CONTROLLING LOCAL BLEEDING

The following agents may be used at home and in the hospital to control local bleeding and capillary oozing.

Agents for home use

Let your patient know about preparations that may be used at home, such as absorbable gelatin sponges (Gelfoam), ice packs, and dicresulene polymer (Negatan).

If the doctor recommends Gelfoam to stop the bleeding—from a puncture wound (venipuncture) or tooth extraction, for example—tell the patient to saturate this foam-like wafer with an isotonic saline or a thrombin solution. Instruct him to place the sponge on the bleeding site and apply pressure for 10 to 15 seconds. Advise him to keep the sponge in place after the bleeding stops. Explain that this agent, which holds many times its weight in blood, can be systemically absorbed.

If the patient bleeds from a blood vessel or into a joint (hemarthrosis), instruct him to elevate the bleeding part and apply an ice pack to the site until the bleeding subsides.

Inform the patient that Negatan—an astringent and protein denaturant—may be applied to oral ulcers. Tell him first to clean and dry the ulcer and then to apply the preparation for 1 minute. Next, he should neutralize the area with large amounts of water. Because the agent may burn or sting, a topical anesthetic may be applied first.

Agents for hospital use

Inform the surgical patient that bleeding can be controlled with such agents as oxidized cellulose (Surgicel), microfibrillar collagen hemostat (Avitene), or thrombin (Thrombinar).

Surgicel, for instance, helps to control surgical bleeding or external bleeding at open wounds. This agent may remain in place until hemostasis occurs. The caregiver then irrigates it (to prevent fresh bleeding) and removes it with sterile forceps.

Another agent, Thrombinar, may be used during surgery or for GI bleeding. The caregiver mixes Thrombinar with sterile isotonic saline solution or sterile distilled water and applies it to the wound. Or she mixes the agent with milk, which the patient drinks to control GI bleeding. Some patients react to Thrombinar with hypersensitivity and fever.

---

of hard stools are likely to tear the rectal mucosa and cause bleeding.

• Discuss the diagnostic tests that may be performed throughout the course of the disease.

• Explain the function of platelets. Warn the patient that the lower his platelet count falls, the more cautious he'll have to be in his activities. Be sure he understands that in severe thrombocytopenia, even minor bumps or scrapes may result in bleeding.

• Teach the patient how to control local bleeding. (See *Controlling local bleeding.*)

• If thrombocytopenia is drug-induced, stress the importance of avoiding the offending drug.

• If the patient must receive long-term steroid therapy, teach him to watch for and report cushingoid symptoms. Emphasize that corticosteroids must be discontinued gradually. While the patient is receiving corticosteroid therapy, monitor his fluid and electrolyte balance, and watch for infection, pathologic fractures, and mood changes.

• Warn the patient to avoid taking aspirin in any form, as well as other drugs that impair coagulation. Teach him how to recognize aspirin compounds and nonsteroidal anti-inflammatory drugs listed on labels of over-the-counter remedies.

• If the patient experiences frequent nosebleeds, recommend that he use a humidifier at night. Also suggest that he moisten his inner nostrils twice a day with an anti-infective ointment.

• Teach the patient to monitor his condition by examining his skin for ecchymoses and petechiae. Instruct him how to test his stools for occult blood.

• Advise the patient to carry medical identification to alert others that he has thrombocytopenia.

IDIOPATHIC THROMBOCYTOPENIC PURPURA

Thrombocytopenia that results from immunologic platelet destruction is known as idiopathic thrombocytopenic purpura (ITP). This form of thrombocytopenia may be acute (postviral thrombocytopenia) or chronic (Werlhof's disease, purpura hemorrhagica, essential thrombocytopenia, or autoimmune thrombocytopenia). The acute form usually affects children between ages 2 and 6; the chronic form mainly affects adults under age 50, especially women between ages 20 and 40. The prognosis for the acute form is excellent: Nearly four out of five patients recover completely without specific treatment. The prognosis for the chronic form is good: Transient remissions lasting weeks or even years are common, especially among women.

Causes

ITP is an autoimmune disorder. Antibodies that reduce the life span of platelets have been found in nearly all patients. The spleen probably helps to remove platelets modified by the antibody. The acute form usually follows a viral infection, such as rubella or chicken pox, and can result from immunization with a live vaccine. The chronic form seldom follows infection and is often linked with other immunologic disorders, such as systemic lupus erythematosus.

Human immunodeficiency virus (HIV) infection has become a common cause of ITP and should be considered in the differential diagnosis. ITP can be the initial symptom of HIV infection—a symptom indicating AIDS-related complex or a complication of fully developed AIDS. It is also often a precursor to lymphoma.

Complications

As with other purpuric conditions, hemorrhage can severely complicate ITP. A major complication during the initial phase of the disease, cerebral hemorrhage is most likely to occur if the patient's platelet count falls below $500/mm^3$. As well, potentially fatal purpuric lesions may occur in vital organs, such as the brain and kidneys.

Assessment findings

The patient's history usually reveals clinical features common to all forms of thrombocytopenia: epistaxis, oral bleeding, and the development of purpura and petechiae. A female patient may complain of menorrhagia. In the acute form, the sudden onset of bleeding usually follows a recent viral illness, although bleeding can occur up to 21 days after the virus strikes. In the chronic form, the onset of bleeding is insidious.

Inspection typically reveals petechiae or ecchymoses in the skin or bleeding into mucous membranes (GI, urinary, vaginal, or respiratory). Palpation may reveal splenomegaly.

The patient's platelet count determines the type of abnormal bleeding he experiences. For example, a platelet count between 30,000 and $50,000/mm^3$ causes bruising with minor trauma. A platelet count between 15,000 and $30,000/mm^3$ produces spontaneous bruising and petechiae, mostly on the arms and legs. A platelet count below $15,000/mm^3$ triggers spontaneous bruising, or, after minor trauma, mucosal bleeding, generalized purpura, epistaxis, hematuria, and GI or intracranial bleeding.

Diagnostic tests

A platelet count less than $20,000/mm^3$ and prolonged bleeding time suggest ITP. Platelet size and morphologic appearance may be abnormal; anemia may be present if bleeding has occurred.

As in thrombocytopenia, bone marrow studies show an abundance of megakaryocytes (platelet precursors) and a shortened circulating platelet survival time (several hours or days rather than the usual 7 to 10 days).

Highly sensitive tests that quantitate platelet-associated immunoglobulin G (IgG) may help to establish the diagnosis; however, because these tests are nonspecific, their usefulness is limited. Half of all patients with thrombocytopenia show an increased IgG level on the platelet.

Treatment

Acute ITP may be allowed to run its course without intervention, or it may be treated with glucocorticoids or immune globulin. Treatment with plasmapheresis or plateletpheresis with transfusion has been attempted with limited success.

For chronic ITP, corticosteroids are the treatment of choice to suppress phagocytic activity, promote capillary integrity, and enhance platelet production. Patients who fail to respond spontaneously within 1 to 4 months, or who require high doses of corticosteroids to maintain platelet counts, require splenectomy.

Splenectomy may be up to 85% successful in adults when splenomegaly accompanies the initial thrombocytopenia. Before splenectomy, the patient may require blood, blood components, and vitamin K to correct anemia and coagulation defects. After splenectomy, he may need blood and component replacement and platelet concentrate. Normally, however, platelets multiply spontaneously after splenectomy.

Alternative treatments include immunosuppressants (cytoxan or vincristine sulfate, for example) and high-dose I.V. immune globulin in adults (85% effective).

The use of immunosuppressants requires weighing the risks against the benefits. Immune globulin treatment has a rapid effect, raising platelet counts within 1 to 5 days, but the beneficial effect lasts only about 1 to 2 weeks. Immune globulin is usually administered to prepare severely thrombocytic patients for emergency surgery.

Nursing diagnoses

- Activity intolerance
- Altered protection
- Anxiety

- Body image disturbance
- Fatigue
- Impaired skin integrity
- Knowledge deficit
- Risk for fluid volume deficit

Nursing interventions

- Patient care for ITP is essentially the same as for thrombocytopenia, but a key difference is the use of platelet support. Thrombocytopenia responds well to treatment with platelet replacement. But ITP is not usually treated with platelets because the body often rejects them.
- Provide emotional support and encourage the patient to discuss any concerns. Reassure him that any petechiae and ecchymoses will heal as the disease resolves.
- Protect all areas of petechiae and ecchymoses from further injury.
- Watch for signs of bleeding. Identify the amount of bleeding or the size of ecchymoses at least every 24 hours. Test stool, urine, and vomitus for blood.
- Provide rest periods between activities if needed.
- Guard against bleeding by protecting the patient from trauma. Keep the bed's side rails raised, and pad them, if possible. Promote the use of an electric razor and a soft toothbrush. Avoid invasive procedures, such as venipuncture or catheterization, if possible. When venipuncture is unavoidable, exert pressure on the puncture site for at least 20 minutes or until the bleeding stops.
- Monitor the patient's platelet count daily, and check for adverse reactions to platelet transfusions, such as fever, allergic responses, and alloimmunization.
- During active bleeding, maintain strict bed rest. Elevate the head of the bed to prevent gravity-related pressure increases, possibly leading to intracranial bleeding.
- If the patient is receiving corticosteroid therapy, monitor his fluid and electrolyte balance, and watch for infection, pathologic fractures, and mood changes.
- Before splenectomy, administer transfusions as ordered and according to hospital protocol. Take the patient's vital signs immediately before the transfusion; then monitor them closely after the transfusion has begun.
- After splenectomy, monitor the patient's vital signs and intake and output. Administer analgesics, I.V. infusions, and transfusions, as necessary.
- Closely monitor the patient receiving immunosuppressants (commonly given before splenectomy) for signs of bone marrow depression, infection, mucositis, GI tract ulceration, and severe diarrhea or vomiting.

Patient teaching

- Teach the patient about ITP. For a home care patient,

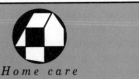

Home care

LIVING WITH I.T.P.

When teaching a patient how to live safely at home with ITP, include the following points:
- Caution the patient to avoid aspirin and other drugs that impair coagulation. Teach him how to recognize aspirin compounds and nonsteroidal anti-inflammatory drugs listed on labels of over-the-counter drugs.
- Instruct the patient to use a humidifier at night if he experiences frequent nosebleeds. Also suggest that he moisten his inner nostrils twice a day with an anti-infective ointment.
- Teach the patient how to examine his skin for ecchymoses and petechiae and how to test his stools for occult blood.
- Explain the importance of reporting signs of bleeding, such as tarry stools, coffee-ground vomitus, epistaxis, and gum or urinary tract bleeding.

explain how to cope with it. (See *Living with ITP*.)
- Warn the patient not to strain during defecation or coughing; both can lead to increased intracranial pressure, possibly causing cerebral hemorrhage. Provide a stool softener, if needed, because constipation and passage of hard stools can tear the rectal mucosa, causing bleeding.
- Explain the purpose of diagnostic tests and the function of platelets. Tell the patient how the results of platelet counts can help identify abnormal bleeding.
- Warn the patient that the lower his platelet count falls, the more precautions he'll need to take. In severe ITP, even minor bumps or scrapes can result in bleeding.
- Advise the patient to carry medical identification to alert others that he has ITP.

PLATELET FUNCTION DISORDERS

These hemorrhagic disorders resemble thrombocytopenia but stem from platelet dysfunction rather than platelet deficiency. They characteristically cause defects in platelet adhesion or procoagulation activity (ability to bind coagulation factors to their surface to form a stable fibrin clot). Such disorders may also create defects in platelet aggregation and thromboxane A_2 and may produce abnormalities by preventing the release of adenosine diphosphate (defective platelet release reaction). The prognosis varies widely.

Causes

Platelet function disorders may be inherited (autosomal recessive) or acquired. Inherited disorders cause the bone marrow to produce platelets that are ineffective in the clotting mechanism. Acquired disorders result from the effects of drugs, such as aspirin and carbenicillin; from systemic diseases, such as uremia; and from other hematologic disorders.

Complications

Hemorrhage is the most serious complication of platelet function disorders.

Assessment findings

The patient history discloses the sudden occurrence of excessive bruising and both nasal and gingival bleeding. It may also reveal the use of drugs (especially aspirin) that might be the cause of the problem or a family history of bleeding disorders that cause platelet dysfunction.

Skin inspection reveals petechiae and purpura. External hemorrhage may also be present. The patient's vital signs are usually normal. However, with hemorrhage, the patient's pulse and respiratory rates will rise and his blood pressure will decrease.

Another serious sign—internal hemorrhage into the muscles and visceral organs—may not be immediately obvious. Occasionally, this disorder is first identified by excessive bleeding during surgery.

Diagnostic tests

Prolonged bleeding time in a patient with both a normal platelet count and normal clotting factors suggests this diagnosis. Determination of the defective mechanism requires a blood film and a platelet function test to measure platelet release reaction and aggregation. Depending on the type of platelet dysfunction, some or all test results may be abnormal.

Other typical laboratory findings include poor clot retraction, decreased prothrombin conversion, and normal prothrombin, activated partial thromboplastin, and thrombin times. Baseline testing includes a complete blood count (CBC) and differential and appropriate tests to determine hemorrhage sites.

Treatment

Platelet replacement is the only satisfactory treatment for inherited platelet dysfunction. However, platelets may need to be HLA-matched to ensure that the body doesn't reject them. Cryoprecipitate infusions are used to treat uremia-induced platelet dysfunction.

Acquired platelet function disorders respond to adequate treatment of the underlying disease or discontinuation of damaging drug therapy.

Plasmapheresis effectively controls bleeding caused by a plasma element that's inhibiting platelet function. During this procedure, one or more units of whole blood are removed from the patient, the plasma is removed from the whole blood, and the remaining packed red blood cells are reinfused.

Nursing diagnoses

- Activity intolerance
- Altered protection
- Altered tissue perfusion
- Anxiety
- Body image disturbance
- Fatigue
- Impaired skin integrity
- Knowledge deficit
- Risk for fluid volume deficit
- Risk for impaired skin integrity
- Risk for infection
- Risk for injury

Nursing interventions

- Provide emotional support as necessary. Listen to the patient's fears and concerns. Reassure him when possible. If the patient is distressed by the appearance of the ecchymoses and petechiae, reassure him that they will heal as the disease resolves.
- Watch for bleeding (petechiae, ecchymoses, surgical or GI bleeding, menorrhagia, and bleeding from the skin, nose, gums, or an injury site). Identify the amount of bleeding or size of the ecchymoses at least every 24 hours. Test stools, urine, and vomitus for blood.
- Protect all areas of ecchymoses and petechiae from further injury and discomfort for the patient.
- Alert other care team members to the patient's hemorrhagic potential, especially before he undergoes diagnostic tests that may cause trauma and bleeding.
- Keep the bed's side rails raised, and pad them, if possible. Avoid invasive procedures, such as venipuncture and urinary catheterization, if possible. When venipuncture is unavoidable, exert pressure on the puncture site for at least 20 minutes or until the bleeding stops.
- Monitor the patient's platelet count daily.
- During active bleeding, maintain the patient on strict bed rest, if necessary, with the head of the bed elevated to prevent gravity-related pressure increases, possibly leading to intracranial bleeding.

• When administering platelet concentrate, remember that platelets are extremely fragile, so infuse them quickly, using the administration set recommended by the blood bank.

• During platelet transfusion, monitor for febrile reaction (flushing, chills, fever, headache, tachycardia, hypertension). Such reactions are common, and a fever will destroy the blood products. HLA-typed platelets may be ordered to prevent febrile reaction. If the patient has a history of minor reactions, he may benefit from acetaminophen and diphenhydramine before the transfusion.

• Perform a platelet count 1 to 2 hours after the platelet transfusion to evaluate the patient's response.

• Observe the patient undergoing plasmapheresis for hypovolemia, hypotension, tachycardia, vasoconstriction, and other signs of volume depletion.

Patient teaching

• Teach the patient about the disease, its signs and symptoms, and treatment.

• If platelet dysfunction is inherited, help the patient and his family understand and accept the disorder. Teach them how to manage potential bleeding episodes. Warn them that petechiae, ecchymoses, and bleeding from the nose, gums, and GI tract signal abnormal bleeding and should be reported immediately. Be sure that the patient knows the significance of tarry stools and coffee-ground vomitus. Advise the patient to use an electric razor to avoid skin injury.

• Teach the patient to avoid unnecessary trauma. Advise him to tell his dentist about this condition before undergoing oral surgery. Also, stress the need for good oral hygiene, using a soft toothbrush.

• Advise the patient to avoid straining at stool or coughing; both can lead to increased intracranial pressure, possibly causing cerebral hemorrhage in the patient with thrombocytopenia. Provide a stool softener, if necessary, because constipation and passage of hard stools are likely to tear the rectal mucosa and cause bleeding.

• Teach the patient to monitor his condition by examining his skin for ecchymoses and petechiae. Teach him how to test his stools for occult blood.

• Tell the patient with a known coagulopathy to avoid aspirin, aspirin compounds, and other agents that impair coagulation. Teach him how to recognize aspirin compounds and nonsteroidal anti-inflammatory drugs listed on the labels of over-the-counter remedies.

• Advise the patient to carry medical identification to alert others that he is a potential bleeder.

HEMOPHILIA

A hereditary bleeding disorder, hemophilia results from deficiency of specific clotting factors. Hemophilia A (classic hemophilia), which affects more than 80% of all hemophiliacs, results from deficiency of Factor VIII; hemophilia B (Christmas disease), which affects 15% of hemophiliacs, results from deficiency of Factor IX. However, other evidence suggests that hemophilia may actually result from nonfunctioning Factors VIII and IX, rather than from their deficiency.

Hemophilia is the most common X-linked genetic disease and occurs in about 1.25 in 10,000 live male births.

The severity and prognosis of bleeding disorders vary with the degree of deficiency and the site of bleeding. The overall prognosis is best in mild hemophilia, which doesn't cause spontaneous bleeding and joint deformities. Advances in treatment have greatly improved the prognosis, and many hemophiliacs live normal life spans.

Causes and pathophysiology

Hemophilia A and B are inherited as X-linked recessive traits. Therefore, female carriers have a 50% chance of transmitting the gene to each daughter, who would then be a carrier, and a 50% chance of transmitting the gene to each son, who would be born with hemophilia.

Hemophilia produces abnormal bleeding, which may be mild, moderate, or severe, depending on the degree of factor deficiency. After a person with hemophilia forms a platelet plug at a bleeding site, the lack of clotting factors impairs formation of a stable fibrin clot. Immediate hemorrhage is not prevalent, but delayed bleeding is common.

Complications

Bleeding into joints and muscles causes pain, swelling, extreme tenderness and, possibly, permanent deformity. Bleeding near peripheral nerves may cause peripheral neuropathies, pain, paresthesias, and muscle atrophy. If bleeding impairs blood flow through a major vessel, it can cause ischemia and gangrene. Pharyngeal, lingual, intracardial, intracerebral, and intracranial bleeding may all lead to shock and death.

Assessment findings

Varying assessment findings depend on the severity of the patient's condition. A patient with undiagnosed hemophilia typically presents with pain and swelling in a weight-bearing joint, such as the hip, knee, and ankle.

Mild hemophilia frequently goes undiagnosed until adulthood because the patient with a mild deficiency does not bleed spontaneously or after minor trauma but has prolonged bleeding if challenged by major trauma or surgery. Postoperative bleeding continues as a slow ooze or ceases and starts again, up to 8 days after surgery.

Moderate hemophilia causes symptoms similar to those of severe hemophilia but produces only occasional spontaneous bleeding episodes.

Severe hemophilia causes spontaneous bleeding. Often, the first sign of severe hemophilia is excessive bleeding after circumcision. Later, spontaneous bleeding or severe bleeding after minor trauma may produce large subcutaneous and deep I.M. hematomas.

The patient history may reveal prolonged bleeding after surgery (including dental extractions) or trauma or joint pain if episodes of spontaneous bleeding into muscles or joints have occurred. The history may disclose signs of internal bleeding, such as abdominal, chest, or flank pain, episodes of hematuria or hematemesis, and tarry stools. It should also reveal any activity or movement limitations that the patient has experienced in the past and any need he has for assistive devices, such as splints, canes, or crutches.

Inspection may reveal hematomas on the extremities or the torso or both and, if bleeding has occurred in joints, joint swelling. Joint range of motion may be limited, and the patient may complain of pain when this assessment is done if bleeding has occurred into the joints.

Diagnostic tests
Specific coagulation factor assays can diagnose the type and severity of hemophilia. A positive family history can also help diagnose hemophilia.

Characteristic findings in hemophilia A are:
• Factor VIII assay 0% to 25% of normal
• prolonged activated partial thromboplastin time (APTT)
• normal platelet count and function, bleeding time, and prothrombin time.

Characteristic findings in hemophilia B are:
• deficient Factor IX assay
• baseline coagulation results similar to those of hemophilia A, with normal Factor VIII.

In hemophilia A or B, the degree of factor deficiency determines severity:
• mild hemophilia—factor levels 5% to 25% of normal
• moderate hemophilia—factor levels 1% to 5% of normal
• severe hemophilia—factor levels less than 1% of normal.

Blood studies are the key diagnostic tool for assessing hemophilia, but additional tests may be ordered periodically to evaluate complications caused by bleeding.

For example, a computed tomography scan would be used for suspected intracranial bleeding, arthroscopy or arthrography for certain joint problems, and endoscopy for GI bleeding.

Treatment
Hemophilia is not curable, but treatment can prevent crippling deformities and prolong life. Correct treatment quickly stops bleeding by increasing plasma levels of deficient clotting factors to help prevent disabling deformities that result from repeated bleeding into muscles, joints, and organs.

In hemophilia A, cryoprecipitated antihemophilic factor (AHF), lyophilized AHF, or both, given in doses large enough to raise clotting factor levels above 25% of normal can permit normal hemostasis. Before surgery, AHF is administered to raise clotting factors to hemostatic levels. Levels are then kept within a normal range until the wound has healed. Fresh-frozen plasma can also be given, but it does have some drawbacks. (See *Using factor replacement products.*)

Inhibitors to Factor VIII develop after multiple transfusions in 10% to 20% of patients with severe hemophilia. This renders the patient resistant to Factor VIII infusions. Desmopressin may be given to stimulate the release of stored Factor VIII, raising the level in the blood.

In hemophilia B, administration of Factor IX concentrate during bleeding episodes increases Factor IX levels.

A person with hemophilia who undergoes surgery needs careful management by a hematologist with expertise in hemophilia care. The patient will require deficient factor replacement before and after surgery. Such replacement may be necessary even for minor surgery, such as a dental extraction. In addition, aminocaproic acid is frequently used for oral bleeding to inhibit the active fibrinolytic system present in the oral mucosa.

Nursing diagnoses
• Activity intolerance
• Altered tissue perfusion
• Anxiety
• Impaired adjustment
• Impaired physical mobility
• Ineffective individual coping
• Knowledge deficit
• Pain
• Powerlessness
• Risk for fluid volume deficit
• Risk for injury
• Social isolation

Nursing interventions

• Provide emotional support, and listen to the patient's fears and concerns. Reassure him when possible. Remember that people who may have been exposed to the human immunodeficiency virus (HIV) through contaminated blood products need special support and infection control.

• If the newly diagnosed patient has difficulty adjusting to his diagnosis, reassure him that his feelings are normal. Point out areas of his life where he can maintain control. Arrange for others with the same problem to speak with the patient and his family.

• Allow the patient private time with his family and friends to help overcome feelings of social isolation.

• Watch for signs and symptoms of decreased tissue perfusion, such as restlessness, anxiety, confusion, pallor, cool and clammy skin, chest pain, decreased urine output, hypotension, and tachycardia. Monitor the patient's blood pressure and pulse and respiratory rates. Observe him frequently for bleeding from the skin, mucous membranes, and wounds.

During bleeding episodes:

• If the patient has surface cuts or epistaxis, apply pressure—often the only treatment needed. With deeper cuts, pressure may stop the bleeding temporarily. Cuts deep enough to require suturing may also require factor infusions to prevent further bleeding. (See *Recognizing and managing bleeding,* page 494.)

• Give the deficient clotting factor or plasma, as ordered. The body uses up AHF in 48 to 72 hours, so repeat infusions, as ordered, until the bleeding stops.

• Watch for adverse reactions to blood products, such as flushing, headache, tingling, fever, chills, urticaria, and anaphylaxis.

• Apply cold compresses or ice bags and raise the injured part.

• To prevent recurrence of bleeding, restrict activity for 48 hours after bleeding is under control.

• Control pain with an analgesic, such as acetaminophen, propoxyphene, codeine, or meperidine, as ordered. Avoid I.M. injections because they may cause hematoma formation at the injection site. Aspirin and aspirin-containing medications are contraindicated because they decrease platelet adherence and may increase the bleeding.

• If the patient cannot tolerate activities because of blood loss, provide rest periods between activities.

If the patient has bled into a joint:

• Immediately elevate the joint.

• To restore joint mobility, if ordered, begin range-of-motion exercises at least 48 hours after the bleeding is con-

USING FACTOR REPLACEMENT PRODUCTS

Each of these agents replaces a specific clotting factor.

Cryoprecipitate
• Factor VIII (70 to 100 units/bag); does not contain Factor IX
• Can be stored frozen for up to 12 months, but must be used within 6 hours after it thaws
• Given through a blood filter; compatible only with 0.9% sodium chloride solution

Lyophilized Factor VIII or IX
• Derived from monoclonal antibodies
• May be freeze-dried and labeled with exact units of Factor VIII or IX contained in the vial (vials range from 200 to 1,500 units of Factor VIII or IX each and contain 20 to 40 ml after reconstitution with diluent); can be stored for 2 years at temperatures ranging from 36° to 46° F (2° to 8° C), or for 6 months at room temperature not exceeding 88° F (31° C)
• No blood filter needed; usually given by slow I.V. push through a butterfly infusion set

Fresh-frozen plasma
• Factor VIII (about 0.75 unit/ml) and Factor IX (about 1 unit/ml); impractical for most hemophiliacs because a large volume is needed to raise factors to hemostatic levels; a poor source of Factor VIII because freezing the plasma destroys the factor (in contrast, fresh plasma [not frozen] is a good source of Factor VIII)
• Can be stored frozen for up to 12 months, but must be used within 2 hours after it thaws
• Given through a blood filter; compatible only with 0.9% sodium chloride solution

trolled. Tell the patient to avoid weight bearing until bleeding stops and swelling subsides.

• Administer analgesics for the pain associated with hemarthrosis. Also, apply ice packs and elastic bandages to alleviate the pain.

After bleeding episodes and surgery:

• Watch closely for signs of further bleeding, such as increased pain and swelling, fever, and symptoms of shock.

• Closely monitor APTT.

Patient teaching

• Teach the patient the benefits of regular exercise. Explain that strong muscles help protect the joints and that this, in turn, reduces the incidence of hemarthrosis. Instruct him to perform isometric exercises. Explain that

RECOGNIZING AND MANAGING BLEEDING

Bleeding in hemophilia may occur spontaneously or stem from an injury. Inform your patient and his family about possible types of bleeding and their associ- ated signs and symptoms. Accordingly, advise them what actions to take and when to call for medical help.

Bleeding site	Signs and symptoms	Interventions
Intracranial	Change in personality or wakefulness (level of consciousness), headache, nausea	Instruct the patient or his family to notify the doctor immediately and treat symptoms as an emergency.
Joints (hemarthroses) Most often affects the knees, followed by elbows, ankles, shoulders, hips, and wrists	Joint pain and swelling, joint tingling and warmth (at onset of hemorrhage)	Tell the patient to begin antihemophilic factor (AHF) infusions and then to notify the doctor.
Muscles	Pain and reduced function of affected muscle; tingling, numbness, or pain in a large area away from the affected site (referred pain)	Urge the patient to notify the doctor and to start an AHF infusion if the patient is reasonably certain that bleeding results from recent injury (otherwise, call the doctor for instructions).
Subcutaneous tissue or skin	Pain, bruising, and swelling at the site (delayed oozing may also occur after an injury)	Show the patient how to apply appropriate topical agents, such as ice packs or absorbable gelatin sponges (Gelfoam), to stop bleeding.
Kidney	Pain in the lower back near the waist, decreased urine output	Instruct the patient to notify the doctor and to start AHF infusion if bleeding results from a known recent injury.
Heart (cardiac tamponade)	Chest tightness, shortness of breath, swelling (usually occurs in hemophiliacs who are very young or who have severe disease)	Instruct the patient to contact the doctor or to go to the nearest emergency department at once.

they can also help prevent muscle weakness and recurrent joint bleeding.
• Advise parents to protect their child from injury while avoiding unnecessary restrictions that impair his normal development. For example, for a toddler, padded patches can be sewn into the knees and elbows of clothing to protect these joints during frequent falls. An older child must be prevented from joining in contact sports, such as football, but he can be encouraged to swim or to play golf.
• Tell the patient to avoid such activities as heavy lifting and using power tools because they increase the risk of injury that can result in serious bleeding problems.
• If an injury occurs, direct the parents to apply cold compresses or ice bags and elevate the injured part, or to apply light pressure to the bleeding. To prevent recurrence of bleeding after treatment, instruct the parents to restrict the child's activity for 48 hours after bleeding is under control.
• Advise the parents to notify the doctor immediately after even a minor injury, especially to the head, neck or abdomen. Such injuries may require special blood factor replacement.
• Instruct parents to watch for signs of internal bleeding, such as severe pain or swelling in a joint or muscles, stiffness, decreased joint movement, severe abdominal pain, blood in urine, tarry stools, and severe headache.
• Explain to the patient and, if appropriate, his parents the importance of avoiding aspirin, combination medications that contain aspirin, and over-the-counter anti-inflammatory agents, such as ibuprofen compounds. Teach the patient and his parents how to recognize over-the-counter medications that contain aspirin. Tell them to use acetaminophen instead.

• Stress the importance of good dental care, including regular, careful toothbrushing to prevent the need for dental surgery. Have the child use a soft toothbrush to avoid gum injury. Emphasize that poor dental hygiene can lead to bleeding from inflamed gums.

• Tell the parents to check with the doctor before allowing dental extractions or any other surgery. Advise them to get the names of other doctors they can contact in case their regular doctor isn't available.

• Teach the patient the importance of protecting his veins for lifelong therapy.

• As necessary, encourage these patients to remain independent and be self-sufficient. Refer them for counseling as necessary.

• Tell the parents to make sure the child wears a medical identification bracelet at all times.

• Refer new patients to a hemophilia treatment center for evaluation. The center will devise a treatment plan for such patients' primary doctors and is a resource for other medical and school personnel, dentists, or others involved in their care. Explain that these centers also offer carrier testing, prenatal diagnosis, and other genetic counseling services.

For patients receiving blood components:

• Train the parents to administer blood factor components at home to avoid frequent hospitalization. Teach them proper venipuncture and infusion techniques, and urge them not to delay treatment during bleeding episodes. Tell parents to keep blood factor concentrate and infusion equipment available at all times, even on vacation.

• Review possible adverse reactions, such as blood-borne infection and factor inhibitor development, that can result from replacement factor procedures.

• If the patient develops flushing, headache, or tingling from replacement factors, inform him or his parents that these reactions occur most often with freeze-dried concentrate. Slowing the infusion rate may cause symptoms to abate.

• If fever and chills occur, indicating an allergy to white blood cell antigens, instruct the patient or his parents that this reaction occurs most often with plasma infusions. Acetaminophen may relieve the patient's discomfort.

• Tell the patient that urticaria is the most common reaction to cryoprecipitate or plasma. This hypersensitivity sign results from an allergy to a plasma protein. The wheals usually subside after administration of diphenhydramine or another antihistamine. Ideally, the patient who develops urticaria frequently should receive an an-

tihistamine about 45 minutes before a clotting factor infusion.

• Review the signs and symptoms of anaphylaxis: rapid or difficult breathing, wheezing, hoarseness, stridor, and chest tightness. (The same plasma proteins that cause urticaria may cause anaphylaxis.) Teach the patient to administer epinephrine and then to contact the doctor at once.

• Tell the patient or the parents to watch for early signs of hepatitis: headache, fever, decreased appetite, nausea, vomiting, abdominal tenderness, and pain over the liver. Explain that the patient who receives blood components risks hepatitis, which may appear 3 weeks to 6 months after treatment with blood components.

• Inform the patient that all donated blood and plasma are screened for antibodies to HIV, which causes acquired immunodeficiency syndrome. Also, all freeze-dried products are heat-treated to kill HIV.

• For more information, refer the patient's family to the National Hemophilia Foundation.

VON WILLEBRAND'S DISEASE

Also known as angiohemophilia, pseudohemophilia, or vascular hemophilia, this hereditary bleeding disorder is characterized by prolonged bleeding time, moderate deficiency of clotting Factor VIII (antihemophilic factor [AHF]), and impaired platelet function.

Von Willebrand's disease commonly causes bleeding from the skin or mucosal surfaces and, in females, excessive uterine bleeding. Bleeding may range from mild and asymptomatic to severe hemorrhage. The prognosis, however, is usually good because most cases are mild. Severe forms may cause hemorrhage after laceration or surgery, and GI bleeding. Excessive postpartum bleeding is uncommon because Factor VIII levels and bleeding time abnormalities become less pronounced during pregnancy. Massive soft-tissue hemorrhage and bleeding into joints seldom occur. Bleeding episodes occur sporadically—a patient may bleed excessively after one dental extraction but not after another. The severity of bleeding may lessen with age.

Causes and pathophysiology

Unlike hemophilia, von Willebrand's disease is inherited as an autosomal dominant trait, affecting both males and females. Scientists have identified an acquired form of this disease in patients with cancer and immune disorders.

One theory holds that mild to moderate deficiency of Factor VIII and defective platelet adhesion prolong co-

agulation time. More specifically, this results from a deficiency of von Willebrand's factor (Factor VIII$_{VWF}$), which appears to occupy the Factor VIII molecule and may be necessary for the production of Factor VIII and proper platelet function. Defective platelet function is characterized by:
• decreased agglutination and adhesion at the bleeding site
• reduced platelet retention when filtered through a column of packed glass beads
• diminished ristocetin-induced platelet aggregation.

Complications
Severe, potentially life-threatening hemorrhage is the major complication associated with von Willebrand's disease.

Assessment findings
The patient history may reveal a positive family history of the disease. Typically, the patient complains of easy bruising and frequent bleeding from the nose or gums. A female patient may report menorrhagia. If a patient has a severe form of the disease, he may report hemorrhage after a laceration or surgery, and he may have experienced episodes of GI bleeding. Inspection may reveal bruises.

Diagnostic tests
Because symptoms are usually mild, laboratory values are borderline, and Factor VIII levels fluctuate, diagnosis is difficult. Typical laboratory findings include:
• prolonged bleeding time (more than 6 minutes)
• slightly prolonged partial thromboplastin time (more than 45 seconds)
• absent or reduced levels of Factor VIII–related antigens and low Factor VIII activity level
• defective in vitro platelet aggregation (using the ristocetin coagulation factor assay test)
• normal platelet count and normal clot retraction.

Treatment
The aims of treatment are to shorten bleeding time by local measures and to replace Factor VIII (and, consequently, Factor VIII$_{VWF}$) by infusion of cryoprecipitate or blood fractions that are rich in Factor VIII.

In many cases, the disorder is so mild that no treatment may be required other than having the patient avoid taking aspirin unless surgical or dental procedures are required. However, preparation is necessary for these procedures even for patients with mild forms of the disease.

During bleeding episodes and before even minor surgery, I.V. infusion of cryoprecipitate or fresh plasma (in quantities sufficient to raise Factor VIII levels to 50% of normal) shortens bleeding time. Desmopressin may be effective in mild disease because it enhances cellular release of stored Factor VIII.

Nursing diagnoses
• Activity intolerance
• Altered tissue perfusion
• Anxiety
• Fatigue
• Ineffective family coping
• Ineffective individual coping
• Knowledge deficit
• Risk for fluid volume deficit
• Risk for injury

Nursing interventions
• Focus on measures to control bleeding and on patient teaching to prevent bleeding, unnecessary trauma, and complications.
• Provide emotional support as necessary. Listen to the patient's fears and concerns. If the newly diagnosed patient has difficulty adjusting to his diagnosis, reassure him that his feelings are normal. Arrange for others with the same problem to speak with the patient and his family.
• Watch for signs and symptoms of decreased tissue perfusion, such as restlessness, anxiety, confusion, pallor, cool and clammy skin, chest pain, decreased urine output, hypotension, and tachycardia. Monitor the patient's blood pressure and pulse and respiratory rates. Observe the patient frequently for bleeding from the skin, mucous membranes, and wounds.
• After surgery, monitor bleeding time or other identified clotting procedure for 24 to 48 hours, and watch for signs of new bleeding.
• During a bleeding episode, elevate the area, if possible, and apply cold compresses and gentle pressure to the bleeding site. (Pressure is often the only treatment necessary.) Monitor the patient's vital signs for tachypnea, tachycardia, and hypotensive changes.
• Give AHF or plasma, as ordered. The body uses up AHF in 48 to 72 hours, so repeat infusions, as ordered, until bleeding stops.
• Watch for adverse reactions to blood products, such as flushing, headache, tingling, fever, chills, urticaria, and anaphylaxis.

• After bleeding episodes and surgery, be alert for signs of further bleeding, such as increased pain and swelling, fever, and signs of shock.
• If the patient is fatigued after a bleeding episode, alternate activities and rest periods.
• Prevent potential injury by using an electric razor, keeping the room free from clutter, and providing a cushioned sitting and sleeping surface (such as a convoluted foam mattress).

Patient teaching
• Advise the patient to notify the doctor after even minor trauma and before all surgery, including dental procedures, to determine if replacement of blood components is necessary.
• Warn against using aspirin and other drugs that impair platelet function. Explain to the patient and, if appropriate, his parents the importance of not taking aspirin, combination medications that contain aspirin, and over-the-counter anti-inflammatory agents, such as ibuprofen compounds. Teach the patient and his parents how to recognize over-the-counter medications that contain aspirin.
• If the patient has a severe form of this disease, teach the patient and his parents special precautions to prevent bleeding episodes. Explain to them that all contact sports and activities must be avoided because they increase the risk of bleeding. Tell the patient to avoid such activities as heavy lifting and using power tools because they increase the risk of injury that can result in serious bleeding problems.
• Urge the patient to wear a medical identification bracelet.
• Refer parents of affected children for genetic counseling.

DISSEMINATED INTRAVASCULAR COAGULATION

Also known as consumption coagulopathy and defibrination syndrome, disseminated intravascular coagulation (DIC) complicates diseases and conditions that accelerate clotting, causing small–blood vessel occlusion, organ necrosis, depletion of circulating clotting factors and platelets, and activation of the fibrinolytic system. This, in turn, can provoke severe hemorrhage.

Clotting in the microcirculation usually affects the kidneys and extremities but may occur in the brain, lungs, pituitary and adrenal glands, and GI mucosa. Other conditions, such as vitamin K deficiency, hepatic

disease, and anticoagulant therapy, may cause a similar hemorrhage.

DIC is usually acute but may be chronic in cancer patients. The prognosis depends on early detection and treatment, the severity of the hemorrhage, and treatment of the underlying disease or condition.

Causes and pathophysiology
DIC may result from:
• infection—gram-negative or gram-positive septicemia; viral, fungal, or rickettsial infection; protozoal infection
• obstetric complications—abruptio placentae, amniotic fluid embolism, retained dead fetus, eclampsia, septic abortion, postpartum hemorrhage
• neoplastic disease—acute leukemia, metastatic carcinoma, lymphomas
• disorders that produce necrosis—extensive burns and trauma, brain tissue destruction, transplant rejection, hepatic necrosis, anorexia
• other disorders and conditions—heatstroke, shock, poisonous snakebite, cirrhosis, fat embolism, incompatible blood transfusion, drug reactions, cardiac arrest, surgery necessitating cardiopulmonary bypass, giant hemangioma, severe venous thrombosis, purpura fulminans, adrenal disease, adult respiratory distress syndrome, diabetic ketoacidosis, pulmonary embolism, and sickle cell anemia.

Why such conditions and disorders lead to DIC is unclear; furthermore, whether they lead to it through a common mechanism is uncertain. In many patients, the triggering mechanisms may be the entrance of foreign protein into the circulation and vascular endothelial injury.

Regardless of how DIC begins, the typical accelerated clotting results in generalized activation of prothrombin and a consequent excess of thrombin. Excess thrombin converts fibrinogen to fibrin, producing fibrin clots in the microcirculation. This process consumes exorbitant amounts of coagulation factors (especially platelets, Factor V, prothrombin, fibrinogen, and Factor VIII), causing thrombocytopenia, deficiencies in Factors V and VIII, hypoprothrombinemia, and hypofibrinogenemia.

Circulating thrombin activates the fibrinolytic system, which lyses fibrin clots into fibrinogen degradation products (FDPs). The hemorrhage that occurs may be due largely to the anticoagulant activity of FDPs, as well as to depletion of plasma coagulation factors.

Complications
DIC may be complicated by renal failure, hepatic damage, cerebrovascular accident, ischemic bowel, or respi-

ratory distress. Hypoxia and anoxia can occur and can lead to severe muscle pain. Shock and coma can also complicate care. Small vessel occlusion can cause necrosis and gangrene in fingers and toes. After fibrinolysis, severe to fatal hemorrhaging of vital organs can occur suddenly.

Assessment findings

The most significant clinical feature of DIC is abnormal bleeding *without* a history of a serious hemorrhagic disorder. Signs and symptoms are related to bleeding and thrombosis. Bleeding problems are usually more common than thrombotic problems unless coagulation occurs to a greater extent than fibrinolysis.

The patient history may reveal the presence of one of the causes of DIC. Although bleeding may occur from any site, the patient history may include signs of bleeding into the skin, such as cutaneous oozing, petechiae, ecchymoses, and hematomas. If the patient is receiving treatment for another disorder when this problem occurs, the history may also reveal bleeding from surgical or invasive procedure sites, such as incisions or venipuncture sites.

Other reported signs and symptoms may include nausea; vomiting; severe muscle, back, and abdominal pain; chest pain; hemoptysis; epistaxis; seizures; and oliguria.

Inspection may reveal petechiae and other signs of bleeding into the skin, acrocyanosis, and dyspnea.

On palpation, you may detect reduced peripheral pulses. Auscultation may disclose decreased blood pressure, and neurologic assessment may reveal mental status changes, including confusion.

Diagnostic tests

Abnormal bleeding in the absence of a known hematologic disorder suggests DIC. The following initial laboratory findings reflect coagulation deficiencies related to their utilization for clotting.
• decreased platelet count—less than 100,000/mm³
• decreased fibrinogen levels—less than 150 mg/dl
• prolonged prothrombin time—more than 15 seconds
• prolonged partial thromboplastin time—more than 60 to 80 seconds
• increased FDPs—often greater than 45 mcg/ml, or positive at less than 1:100 dilution
• positive D-dimer test (specific fibrinogen test for DIC)—positive at less than 1:8 dilution.

Other supportive data include prolonged thrombin time, positive fibrin monomers, diminished levels of Factors V and VIII, fragmentation of red blood cells (RBCs), and decreased hemoglobin levels (less than 10 g/dl). As-

sessment of renal status demonstrates reduction in urine output (less than 30 ml/hour), and elevated blood urea nitrogen levels (greater than 25 mg/dl) and serum creatinine levels (greater than 1.3 mg/dl).

Final confirmation of the diagnosis may be difficult because many of these test results also occur in other disorders (primary fibrinolysis, for example). However, the FDP and D-dimer tests are considered specific and diagnostic of DIC. Additional diagnostic measures determine the underlying disorder.

Treatment

Successful management of DIC requires prompt recognition and adequate treatment of the underlying disorder. Treatment may be supportive (when the underlying disorder is self-limiting, for example) or highly specific. If the patient isn't actively bleeding, supportive care alone may reverse DIC. Active bleeding may require administration of blood, fresh-frozen plasma, platelets, or packed RBCs to support hemostasis.

Heparin therapy is controversial. It may be used early in the disease to prevent microclotting but may be considered a last resort in the patient who is actively bleeding. If thrombosis does occur, heparin therapy is usually mandatory. In most cases, it's administered in combination with transfusion therapy.

Nursing diagnoses

• Altered tissue perfusion
• Anxiety
• Fatigue
• Fear
• Impaired gas exchange
• Impaired physical mobility
• Impaired tissue integrity
• Pain
• Risk for fluid volume deficit
• Risk for injury

Nursing interventions

• Focus on early recognition of signs of abnormal bleeding, prompt treatment of the underlying disorders, and prevention of further bleeding.
• Keep the family informed of the patient's progress. Prepare them for his appearance (I.V. lines, nasogastric tubes, bruises, dried blood). Provide emotional support. Listen to the patient's and his family's concerns. When possible, encourage the patient. As needed, enlist the aid of a social worker, chaplain, and other members of the health care team in providing such support.

• If the patient is unable to tolerate activities because of blood loss, provide rest periods.

• Administer prescribed analgesics for pain as necessary.

• Reposition the patient every 2 hours and provide meticulous skin care to prevent skin breakdown.

• Administer oxygen therapy as ordered.

• Test all stools and urine for occult blood.

• To prevent clots from dislodging and causing fresh bleeding, do not vigorously rub these areas when washing. Use a 1:1 solution of hydrogen peroxide and water to help remove crusted blood.

• Protect the patient from injury. Enforce complete bed rest during bleeding episodes. If the patient is very agitated, pad the side rails.

• If bleeding occurs, use pressure and topical hemostatic agents to control bleeding; for example, absorbable gelatin sponges (Gelfoam), microfibrillar collagen hemostat (Avitene Hemostat), or thrombin (Thrombinar).

• Check all venipuncture sites frequently for bleeding. After injection or removal of I.V. catheters or needles, apply pressure to injection sites for at least 10 minutes. Alert other personnel to the patient's tendency to hemorrhage. Limit venipunctures whenever possible.

• Monitor intake and output hourly in acute DIC, especially when administering blood products. Watch for transfusion reactions and signs of fluid overload.

• To measure the amount of blood lost, weigh dressings and linen and record drainage. Weigh the patient daily, particularly in renal involvement.

• Watch for bleeding from the GI and genitourinary (GU) tracts. If you suspect intra-abdominal bleeding, measure the patient's abdominal girth at least every 4 hours, and monitor closely for signs of shock. Perform bladder irrigations as ordered for GU bleeding.

• Monitor the results of serial blood studies (particularly hematocrit, hemoglobin levels, and coagulation times).

Patient teaching

• Explain the disorder to the patient and his family. Teach them about the signs and symptoms of the problem, the diagnostic tests required, and the treatment that the patient will receive.

MISCELLANEOUS DISORDERS

These disorders include hypersplenism, hyperbilirubinemia, and hemolytic disease of the newborn (erythroblastosis fetalis).

HYPERSPLENISM

A syndrome marked by exaggerated splenic activity and, possibly, splenomegaly, hypersplenism causes peripheral blood cell deficiency as the spleen traps and destroys these cells.

In this disorder, the spleen's normal filtering and phagocytic functions accelerate indiscriminately, automatically removing antibody-coated, aging, and abnormal cells, even though some cells may be functionally normal. The spleen may also temporarily sequester normal platelets and red blood cells (RBCs), withholding them from circulation. In this manner, the enlarged spleen may trap as much as 90% of the body's platelets and up to 45% of its RBC mass.

Causes

Hypersplenism may be idiopathic (primary) or secondary to an extrasplenic disorder, such as malaria, sickle cell anemia, or polycythemia vera. (See *Causes of splenomegaly,* page 500.)

Complications

Infection, anemia, and hemorrhage can complicate hypersplenism.

Assessment findings

Typically, the patient with hypersplenism has a history of frequent infections. He may also complain of weakness, easy bruising, a sore mouth and, rarely, abdominal pain. The patient history may reveal disorders, such as rheumatoid arthritis, in which hypersplenism occurs as a secondary disorder. Vital signs may disclose fever and a rapid pulse rate, and inspection of the oral mucosa may reveal lacerations. Palpation may reveal a tender and enlarged spleen. Auscultation may detect palpitations.

Other assessment findings include the signs and symptoms of the underlying problem when hypersplenism is a secondary disorder.

Diagnostic tests

Diagnosis requires evidence of abnormal splenic destruction or sequestration of RBCs or platelets and splenomegaly. The most definitive test measures the accumulation of erythrocytes in the spleen and liver after I.V. infusion of chromium-labeled RBCs or platelets. A high spleen-liver ratio of radioactivity indicates splenic destruction or sequestration.

The complete blood count (CBC) shows decreased hemoglobin levels (as low as 4 g/dl), white blood cell count

CAUSES OF SPLENOMEGALY

An enlarged spleen may develop in any of the disorders listed below.

Infectious disorders
Acute (abscesses, subacute bacterial endocarditis), chronic (tuberculosis, malaria, Felty's syndrome)

Congestive disorders
Cirrhosis, thrombosis

Hyperplastic disorders
Hemolytic anemia, polycythemia vera

Infiltrative disorders
Gaucher's disease, Niemann-Pick disease

Cystic or neoplastic disorders
Cysts, leukemia, lymphoma, myelofibrosis, Hodgkin's disease, multiple myeloma

(less than 4,000/mm³), and platelet count (less than 125,000/mm³) and an elevated reticulocyte count.

Splenic biopsy, scan, and angiography may be useful; biopsy is risky, however, and should be avoided if possible.

Treatment
Appropriate treatment depends on the problem's cause. Secondary hypersplenism necessitates treatment of the underlying disease. Splenectomy is indicated in a transfusion-dependent patient who fails to respond to other therapy. Splenectomy seldom cures the patient, but it does correct the effects of cytopenia. Occasionally, splenectomy may hasten blood cell destruction in the bone marrow and liver.

Nursing diagnoses
• Altered oral mucous membrane
• Altered tissue perfusion
• Anxiety
• Fatigue
• Pain
• Risk for altered body temperature
• Risk for fluid volume deficit
• Risk for infection

Nursing interventions
• Provide emotional support as necessary. Listen to the patient's fears and concerns. Reassure him when possible.
• If the patient has pain, administer analgesics as ordered, and provide distractions to help him cope with discomfort.
• Watch for signs and symptoms of decreased tissue perfusion, such as restlessness, anxiety, confusion, pallor, cool and clammy skin, chest pain, decreased urine output, hypotension, and tachycardia. Monitor the patient's vital signs at least every 4 hours. Observe him frequently for bleeding.
• If the patient tolerates activities poorly because of decreased tissue perfusion, provide rest periods between activities.
• Perform all procedures, using aseptic technique, to help prevent infection.
• If splenectomy is scheduled, administer preoperative transfusions of blood or blood products (fresh-frozen plasma, platelets), as ordered, to replace deficient blood elements. Treat symptoms or complications of any underlying disorder as ordered.
• Watch for adverse reactions to blood products, such as flushing, headache, tingling, fever, chills, urticaria, and anaphylaxis.
• Postoperatively, monitor intake and output, weight, central venous or pulmonary artery pressure, and fluid volume. Note hypovolemia that may be caused by intraperitoneal fluid shifts. Evaluate abdominal girth if intraperitoneal fluid shifts are suspected. Also, monitor vital signs. Keep the nasogastric (NG) tube patent. Listen for bowel sounds. Provide stool softeners. Check for excessive drainage or apparent bleeding.
• Watch for possible complications of surgery, such as infection, thromboembolism, paralytic ileus, and abdominal distention.

Patient teaching
Before surgery:
• Reinforce the doctor's explanation of the disease as necessary. Be sure the patient understands the problem and the care required.
• If splenectomy will be performed, teach the patient about the surgery. Also, inform him about postoperative care, such as insertion of I.V. and arterial lines. Provide preoperative teaching, including such topics as coughing and deep breathing.
• Explain the need to prevent infection, and teach the patient the value of good hand-washing technique.

• Explain the laboratory tests that will be performed repeatedly to monitor his status. These include serial CBCs, platelet counts, and chemistries performed to assess blood counts and help identify fluid shifts into the abdomen.

After surgery:
• Reinforce preoperative teaching as necessary. Instruct the patient to perform deep-breathing exercises, and encourage early ambulation to prevent respiratory complications and venous stasis. Explain the need to do range-of-motion exercises in bed.
• While the NG tube is in place and after its removal, instruct the patient to rinse his mouth with cool, soothing solutions to combat irritation.

Before discharge:
• Teach the patient the signs of infection (elevated temperature, weakness). Urge him to report all signs of infection after surgery, even if they seem minor.
• Explain the need to maintain a quiet, safe home environment, free of potentially infectious visitors.

HYPERBILIRUBINEMIA

Elevated serum bilirubin levels and mild jaundice are hallmarks of hyperbilirubinemia, also known as neonatal jaundice. The disorder can be physiologic (with jaundice the only symptom) or pathologic (resulting from an underlying disease). Physiologic jaundice is widespread and tends to be more common and severe in certain ethnic groups (Chinese, Japanese, Koreans, Native Americans) whose mean peak of unconjugated bilirubin is about twice that of the rest of the population.

Physiologic jaundice is self-limiting; the prognosis for pathologic jaundice varies, depending on the cause. Untreated, severe hyperbilirubinemia may cause kernicterus, a neurologic syndrome resulting from deposition of unconjugated bilirubin in the brain cells and characterized by severe neural symptoms.

Causes and pathophysiology

Hyperbilirubinemia stems from hemolytic processes in the neonate. As erythrocytes break down at the end of their neonatal life cycle, the hemoglobin separates into globin (protein) and heme (iron) fragments. Heme fragments form unconjugated (indirect) bilirubin, which binds with albumin for transport to liver cells to conjugate with glucuronide, forming direct bilirubin. Because unconjugated bilirubin is fat-soluble and cannot be excreted in the urine or bile, it may escape to extravascular tissue, especially fatty tissue and the brain, resulting in hyperbilirubinemia.

This pathophysiologic process may develop when:
• factors that disrupt conjugation and usurp albumin-binding sites are present, including drugs such as aspirin, tranquilizers, and sulfonamides, and conditions such as hypothermia, anoxia, hypoglycemia, and hypoalbuminemia
• decreased hepatic function results in reduced bilirubin conjugation
• increased erythrocyte production or breakdown results from hemolytic disorders or from Rh or ABO incompatibility
• biliary obstruction or hepatitis results in blockage of normal bile flow
• maternal enzymes present in breast milk inhibit the infant's glucuronyl-transferase conjugating activity. (See *Causes of hyperbilirubinemia*, page 502.)

Complications

Kernicterus (bilirubin encephalopathy) is the most dangerous complication of hyperbilirubinemia. It can be fatal, or it can cause profound neurologic disorders. Survivors may develop cerebral palsy, epilepsy, or mental retardation or have only minor sequelae, such as perceptual-motor handicaps and learning disorders.

Assessment findings

Identifying the underlying cause of hyperbilirubinemia requires a detailed patient history, including prenatal history and family history for paternal Rh factor and red blood cell defects.

Inspection of the face and sclera in fair-skinned infants in a well-lit room (without yellow or gold lighting) reveals a yellowish skin coloration (jaundice), particularly in the sclera. In dark-skinned infants, inspection of the oral mucosa and sclera reveals jaundice. Begin inspection with the head and face because jaundice first appears over the head and face area and then spreads, occurring in the lower extremities last. Jaundice can be verified by pressing the skin on the cheek or abdomen lightly with one finger and then releasing pressure and observing the skin color immediately. Keep in mind that jaundice does not become clinically apparent until serum bilirubin levels reach about 7 mg/dl.

Diagnostic tests

Jaundice and elevated levels of serum bilirubin confirm hyperbilirubinemia.

Signs of jaundice necessitate measuring and charting serum bilirubin levels every 4 hours. Testing may include direct and indirect bilirubin levels, particularly for pathologic jaundice.

CAUSES OF HYPERBILIRUBINEMIA

The infant's age at onset of hyperbilirubinemia may provide clues to the sources of this jaundice-causing disorder.

Day 1
• Blood type incompatibility (Rh, ABO, other minor blood groups)
• Intrauterine infection (rubella, cytomegalic inclusion body disease, toxoplasmosis, syphilis and, occasionally, bacteria such as *Escherichia coli,* staphylococci, *Pseudomonas, Klebsiella, Proteus,* and streptococci)

Day 2 or 3
• Infection (usually from gram-negative bacteria)
• Polycythemia
• Enclosed hemorrhage (skin bruises, subdural hematoma)
• Respiratory distress syndrome (hyaline membrane disease)
• Heinz-body anemia from drugs and toxins (vitamin K_3, sodium nitrate)
• Abnormal red blood cell (RBC) morphology

• RBC enzyme deficiencies (glucose-6-phosphate dehydrogenase [G6PD], hexokinase)
• Physiologic jaundice
• Blood group incompatibilities

Days 4 and 5
• Breast-feeding, maternal diabetes
• Respiratory distress syndrome
• Crigler-Najjar syndrome (congenital nonhemolytic icterus)
• Gilbert's syndrome

Day 7 and later
• Herpes simplex
• Pyloric stenosis
• Hypothyroidism
• Neonatal giant cell hepatitis
• Infection (usually acquired in neonatal period)
• Bile duct atresia
• Galactosemia
• Choledochal cyst

Physiologic jaundice develops 24 hours after delivery in 50% of term infants (usually day 2 to day 3) and 48 hours after delivery in 80% of premature infants (usually day 3 to day 5). It usually disappears by day 7 in term infants and by day 9 or day 10 in premature infants. Throughout physiologic jaundice, serum unconjugated bilirubin levels do not exceed 12 mg/dl.

Pathologic jaundice may appear anytime after the first day of life and may persist beyond 7 days with serum bilirubin levels greater than 12 mg/dl in a term infant, greater than 15 mg/dl in a premature infant, or increasing more than 5 mg/dl in 24 hours. Bilirubin levels that are excessively elevated or that vary daily suggest a pathologic process.

Both mother and infant should be tested for blood group incompatibilities, and their hematocrit and hemoglobin levels should be measured. The direct Coombs' test also should be performed on both mother and infant.

Treatment
Depending on the underlying cause, treatment may include phototherapy, exchange transfusions, albumin infusion and, possibly, drug therapy. Phototherapy is the treatment of choice for physiologic jaundice and pathologic jaundice due to hemolytic disease of the newborn (after the initial exchange transfusion). Phototherapy uses fluorescent light to decompose bilirubin in the skin

by oxidation. It usually is discontinued after bilirubin levels fall below 10 mg/dl and continue to decrease for 24 hours. However, phototherapy seldom is the only treatment for jaundice due to a pathologic cause.

An exchange transfusion, replacing the infant's blood with fresh blood (less than 48 hours old), thus removing some of the unconjugated bilirubin in serum, may be performed for severe hyperbilirubinemia.

Other therapy for excessive bilirubin levels includes albumin administration (1 g/kg of 25% salt-poor albumin), which provides additional albumin for binding unconjugated bilirubin. This may be done 1 to 2 hours before exchange or as a substitute for a portion of the plasma in the transfused blood.

Drug therapy, which is rare, usually consists of phenobarbital administered to the mother before delivery and to the infant several days after delivery. This drug stimulates the hepatic glucuronide-conjugating system.

Nursing diagnoses
• Altered parenting
• Knowledge deficit
• Risk for altered body temperature
• Risk for fluid volume deficit
• Risk for impaired skin integrity

Nursing interventions

• Observe the infant for jaundice. Identify the body areas affected, and note the time that you first noticed jaundice. Also, immediately note and report the jaundice and serum bilirubin levels.

• Provide emotional support and, as appropriate, reassurance to the infant's parents.

• Observe the infant's eye color every 4 to 8 hours, and also check the infant for lethargy, a sign of neurologic complications.

For the infant receiving phototherapy:

• Keep a record of how long each bilirubin light bulb is in use because these bulbs require frequent changing for optimum effectiveness.

• Undress the infant so that his entire body surface is exposed to the light rays. Keep him about 18″ to 30″ (about 46 to 76 cm) from the light source. Protect his eyes with shields that filter the light to prevent retinal damage. Remove the eye patches at least every 8 hours to provide visual stimulation.

• Monitor and maintain the infant's body temperature; high and low temperatures predispose him to kernicterus. Remove the infant from the light source every 3 to 4 hours, and take off the eye shields. Turn the infant every 2 hours to provide maximum skin exposure for photodecomposition.

• Encourage the parents to visit the nursery and sit by the infant as often as they desire. Allow the parents to feed him.

• Provide the infant with 2 oz of dextrose 5% in water or sterile water between feedings to help avoid fluid volume deficit, resulting from insensible fluid loss from the heat of the phototherapy lamp.

• The infant usually shows a decrease in serum bilirubin level 1 to 12 hours after the start of phototherapy. When the infant's bilirubin level is less than 10 mg/dl and has been decreasing for 24 hours, discontinue phototherapy, as ordered. Resume therapy, as ordered, if the serum bilirubin level increases several milligrams per 100 ml, as it often does, due to a rebound effect.

For the infant receiving exchange transfusions:

• Prepare the infant warmer and tray before the transfusion. Try to keep the infant quiet. Give him nothing by mouth for 3 to 4 hours before the procedure to reduce the risk of aspiration.

• Check the blood to be used for the exchange — type, Rh, age. Keep emergency equipment (resuscitation and intubation equipment, and oxygen) available.

• During the procedure, monitor respiratory and heart rates every 15 minutes; check the infant's temperature

PREVENTING HYPERBILIRUBINEMIA

Here are some steps to take to prevent hyperbilirubinemia:

• Maintain oral intake. Stress the importance of this to the infant's mother. Tell her not to skip any feedings because fasting stimulates the conversion of heme to bilirubin.

• Supplement breast-feeding with the administration of glucose water.

• If indicated, administer $Rh_o(D)$ immune globulin (human), as ordered:

—to an Rh-negative patient after amniocentesis
—to an Rh-negative patient during the third trimester of pregnancy (if she previously gave birth to an Rh-positive infant)
—to an Rh-negative patient after spontaneous or elective abortion.

every 30 minutes. Continue to monitor vital signs every 15 to 30 minutes for 2 hours.

• Measure intake and output. Observe for umbilical cord bleeding and complications, such as hemorrhage at the cannulization site, hypokalemia, hypoglycemia, infection at the cannulization site, thrombosis, and cardiac failure from fluid volume excess, sepsis, and shock. Report serum bilirubin and hemoglobin levels. Bilirubin levels may rise, due to a rebound effect, within 30 minutes after transfusion, necessitating repeat transfusions.

Patient teaching

• Teach parents to prevent hyperbilirubinemia. (See *Preventing hyperbilirubinemia.*)

• Reassure parents that most infants experience some degree of jaundice. Explain hyperbilirubinemia, its causes, diagnostic tests, and treatment. If possible, provide them with printed information about hyperbilirubinemia.

• Explain the prescribed treatment to the parents and the care that their infant will receive during the prescribed therapy.

• Inform the parents that their infant's stool contains some bile and may be greenish.

• Emphasize the importance of follow-up doctor visits.

HEMOLYTIC DISEASE OF THE NEWBORN

This disorder, formerly known as erythroblastosis fetalis, affects the fetus and neonate. It stems from an incompatibility of fetal and maternal blood, resulting in ma-

UNDERSTANDING A.B.O. INCOMPATIBILITY

A form of fetomaternal incompatibility, ABO incompatibility occurs between mother and fetus in about 25% of all pregnancies, with highest incidence among blacks. In about 1% of this number, it leads to hemolytic disease of the newborn. Although ABO incompatibility is more common than Rh isoimmunization, it is less severe. Low antigenicity of fetal or neonatal ABO factors may account for the milder clinical effects.

Each blood group has specific antigens on RBCs and specific antibodies in serum. Maternal antibodies form against fetal cells when blood groups differ. Infants with group A blood, born of group O mothers, account for about 50% of all ABO incompatibilities. Unlike Rh isoimmunization, which always follows sensitization during a previous pregnancy, ABO incompatibility is likely to develop in a firstborn infant.

Clinical effects of ABO incompatibility include jaundice (which usually appears in the neonate in 24 to 48 hours), mild anemia, and mild hepatosplenomegaly.

Diagnosis is based on clinical signs in the neonate, the presence of ABO incompatibility, a weak to moderate positive Coombs' test, and elevated serum bilirubin levels. Cord hemoglobin and indirect bilirubin levels indicate the need for exchange transfusion. An exchange transfusion is done with blood of the same group and Rh type as those of the mother. Because infants with ABO incompatibility respond so well to phototherapy, exchange transfusion is seldom necessary.

Blood group	Antigens on RBCs	Antibodies in serum	Most common incompatible groups
A	A	Anti-B	Mother A, infant B or AB
B	B	Anti-A	Mother B, infant A or AB
AB	A and B	No antibodies	Mother AB, infant (no incompatibility)
O	No antigens	Anti-A and anti-B	Mother O, infant A or B

ternal antibody activity against fetal red blood cells (RBCs).

Intrauterine transfusions can save 40% of fetuses with this problem. However, in severe, untreated hemolytic disease of the newborn, the prognosis is poor, especially if kernicterus develops. About 70% of these infants die, usually within the first week of life; survivors inevitably develop pronounced neurologic damage.

ABO incompatibility, another form of fetomaternal incompatibility, can also occur and can lead to hemolytic disease of the newborn. (See *Understanding ABO incompatibility*.)

Causes and pathophysiology

Although more than 60 RBC antigens can stimulate antibody formation, hemolytic disease of the newborn usually results from Rh isoimmunization—a condition that develops in about 7% of all pregnancies in the United States.

During her first pregnancy (whether it ends in delivery or abortion), an Rh-negative female becomes sensitized by exposure to Rh-positive fetal blood antigens inherited from the father. A female may also become sensitized by receiving blood transfusions with alien Rh antigens, causing agglutins to develop. This sensitization is the result of inadequate doses of $Rh_o(D)$ immune globulin (human) or from failure to receive $Rh_o(D)$ immune globulin after significant fetal-maternal leakage from abruptio placentae.

Subsequent pregnancy with an Rh-positive fetus causes increasing amounts of maternal agglutinating antibodies to cross the placental barrier, attach to Rh-positive cells in the fetus, and cause hemolysis and anemia in the fetus. To compensate for this, the fetus produces more RBCs, and erythroblasts (immature RBCs) appear in the fetal circulation. Extensive hemolysis results in the release of large amounts of unconjugated bilirubin, which the liver is unable to conjugate and excrete, causing hyperbilirubinemia and hemolytic anemia in the fetus. Before the development of $Rh_o(D)$ immune globulin, this condition was a major cause of kernicterus and neonatal death.

Complications

Untreated hemolytic disease of the newborn can lead to kernicterus, which produces pronounced neurologic defects, such as cerebral palsy, sensory impairment, and mental deficiencies.

Severely affected fetuses who develop hydrops fetalis—the most severe form of this disorder, associated with profound anemia and edema—are commonly stillborn; even if they're delivered alive, they seldom survive longer than a few hours.

Assessment findings

The mother's history may reveal that the infant's father is Rh-positive and the mother Rh-negative or that the mother has had a previous pregnancy in which she developed the antigen-antibody response. Previous pregnancies include stillbirths and abortions as well as any live births. The maternal history may also reveal previous blood transfusions.

Inspection of the mildly affected neonate reveals pallor and, 30 minutes to 24 hours after birth, jaundice. Palpation may uncover mild to moderate hepatosplenomegaly.

In severely affected neonates who survive birth, inspection usually reveals pallor, edema, petechiae, a bile-stained umbilical cord, and yellow or meconium-stained amniotic fluid. Grunting respirations are obvious. Palpation reveals hepatosplenomegaly. Auscultation discloses pulmonary crackles and, possibly, heart murmurs. On neurologic examination, you'll note poor muscle tone and, in some cases, unresponsiveness.

In the 10% of untreated neonates who develop kernicterus, neurologic assessment may reveal lethargy, poor sucking ability, retracted head, stiff extremities, squinting, a high-pitched cry, and seizures. Infants with kernicterus also commonly have anemia.

If the neonate with hydrops fetalis is born alive, inspection reveals signs of extreme hemolysis: marked pallor, edema (ranging from mild peripheral edema to anasarca), petechiae, and widespread ecchymosis in severe cases (indicating the presence of disseminated intravascular coagulation). Inspection also discloses smaller body size than that of infants of comparable gestational age and an enlarged placenta. (This disorder retards intrauterine growth. The neonate's lungs, kidneys, brain, and thymus are also small.)

Palpation and percussion may reveal hepatosplenomegaly, cardiomegaly, and ascites. Auscultation may reveal dyspnea and pulmonary crackles (signs of peritoneal and pleural effusions). In addition, the neonate may have fetal hypoxia and heart failure (with possible pericardial effusion and circulatory collapse).

Note: Identification of green or brown-tinged amniotic fluid before birth usually indicates that the infant will be stillborn.

Diagnostic tests

Diagnostic tests are performed on the mother and the neonate. The father may also be tested for blood group, Rh factor, and Rh zygosity.

Diagnostic tests performed on the mother to help identify hemolytic disease of the newborn and help determine treatment include:
• *Blood typing and screening*
• *Rh antibody titer tests* to determine changes in the degree of maternal immunization
• *Amniotic fluid analysis,* which may show increased bilirubin levels (indicating possible hemolysis) and elevations in Rh titers
• *Radiologic studies,* which may show edema and, in hydrops fetalis, the halo sign (edematous, elevated subcutaneous fat layers) and the Buddha position (fetus's legs are crossed).

Diagnostic tests performed on the neonate to help identify hemolytic disease of the newborn include:
• *Direct Coombs' test* of umbilical cord blood to measure RBC (Rh-positive) antibodies in the neonate (positive only when the mother is Rh-negative and the fetus is Rh-positive)
• *Cord hemoglobin count,* which signals severe disease if hemoglobin levels are low (less than 10 g/dl)
• *Stained RBC examination* (many nucleated peripheral RBCs).

Treatment

The choice of treatment depends on the degree of maternal sensitization and hemolytic effects on the fetus or neonate.
• Intrauterine transfusion is performed on a fetus when amniotic fluid analysis suggests that the fetus is severely affected and delivery is inappropriate because of fetal immaturity. The mother is admitted to the labor and delivery area and monitored closely. She is given a tocolytic agent I.V. to inhibit contractions, and ultrasonography is performed to locate the umbilical vein of the fetus. Then, using a procedure called percutaneous umbilical blood sampling, a needle is inserted into the umbilical vein, and a blood sample is taken to identify the fetal blood type, measure hemoglobin levels and hematocrit, and obtain other pertinent information. If the fetal blood sample verifies anemia, a blood transfusion of O-negative

blood in utero can take place through the sampling needle. This procedure may be repeated periodically (about every 2 weeks) until the fetus is mature enough for delivery.

• Planned delivery usually is done 2 to 4 weeks before term date, depending on maternal history, serologic tests, and amniocentesis; labor may be induced from the 34th to 38th week of gestation. During labor, the fetus should be monitored electronically; capillary blood sampling (from the scalp) determines acid-base balance. Any indication of fetal distress necessitates immediate cesarean delivery.

• Phenobarbital administered during the last 5 to 6 weeks of gestation may lower serum bilirubin levels in the neonate.

• An exchange transfusion removes antibody-coated RBCs and prevents hyperbilirubinemia through removal of the infant's blood and replacement with fresh group O, Rh-negative blood.

• Albumin infusion binds bilirubin, reducing the risk of hyperbilirubinemia.

• Phototherapy by exposure to ultraviolet light reduces bilirubin levels.

• Administration of gamma globulin that contains anti-Rh-positive antibody ($Rh_o[D]$) can provide passive immunization, which prevents maternal Rh isoimmunization in Rh-negative females. However, it's ineffective if sensitization has already resulted from a previous pregnancy, abortion, or transfusion.

Neonatal therapy for hydrops fetalis consists of maintaining ventilation by intubation, oxygenation, and mechanical assistance, when necessary, and removing excess fluid to relieve ascites and respiratory distress. Other appropriate measures include an exchange transfusion and maintenance of the neonate's body temperature.

Administration of $Rh_o(D)$ immune globulin (human) to an unsensitized Rh-negative mother as soon as possible after the birth of an Rh-positive infant, or after a spontaneous or elective abortion, prevents complications in subsequent pregnancies.

The following patients should be screened for Rh isoimmunization or irregular antibodies:

• all Rh-negative mothers during their first prenatal visit and at 24, 28, 32, and 36 weeks' gestation

• all Rh-positive mothers with histories of transfusion, a jaundiced baby, stillbirth, cesarean birth, induced abortion, placenta previa, or abruptio placentae.

Nursing diagnoses
• Altered parenting
• Altered tissue perfusion
• Impaired gas exchange
• Impaired tissue integrity
• Ineffective breathing pattern
• Knowledge deficit
• Risk for altered body temperature
• Risk for fluid volume deficit
• Risk for impaired skin integrity

Nursing interventions
• Administer $Rh_o(D)$ immune globulin I.M., as ordered, to all Rh-negative, antibody-negative females after transfusion reaction or ectopic pregnancy, or during the second and third trimesters to patients with abruptio placentae, placenta previa, or amniocentesis.

For intrauterine transfusion:
• Before intrauterine transfusion, obtain a baseline fetal heart rate through electronic monitoring. Afterward, carefully observe the mother for uterine contractions and fluid leakage from the puncture site. Monitor fetal heart rate for tachycardia or bradycardia.

For exchange transfusions:
• Prepare the infant warmer and tray before the transfusion. Try to keep the infant quiet. Obtain a baseline fetal heart rate.

• Check the blood to be used for the exchange—type, Rh, age. Keep emergency equipment (resuscitative and intubation equipment, and oxygen) available.

• During an exchange transfusion, maintain the infant's body temperature by placing him under a heat lamp or overhead radiant warmer. Monitor his respiratory and heart rates every 15 minutes; check his temperature every 30 minutes. Keep resuscitative and monitoring equipment handy, and warm blood before transfusion.

• Watch for complications of transfusion, such as lethargy, muscle twitching, seizures, dark urine, edema, and change in vital signs. Watch for postexchange serum bilirubin levels that are usually 50% of preexchange levels (although these levels may rise to 70% to 80% of preexchange levels due to rebound effect). Within 30 minutes of transfusion, bilirubin may rebound, requiring repeated exchange transfusions.

• After the exchange transfusion, continue to monitor the infant's vital signs every 15 to 30 minutes for 2 hours. Measure intake and output. Observe for umbilical cord bleeding and complications, such as hemorrhage, hypocalcemia, sepsis, and shock. Report serum bilirubin and hemoglobin levels.

For phototherapy:

• Keep a record of how long each bilirubin light bulb is in use because these bulbs require frequent changing for optimum effectiveness.

• Undress the infant, so that his entire body surface is exposed to the light rays. Keep him 18″ to 30″ (46 to 76 cm) from the light source. Protect his eyes with shields that filter the light to prevent retinal damage. Remove the eye patches at least every 8 hours to provide visual stimulation.

• Monitor and maintain the infant's body temperature; high and low temperatures predispose him to kernicterus. Remove the infant from the light source every 3 to 4 hours, and take off the eye shields. Turn the infant every 2 hours to provide maximum skin exposure for photodecomposition.

• To promote normal parental bonding, encourage the parents to visit the nursery and help care for their infant as often as possible.

• Provide the infant with 2 oz (57 g) of dextrose 5% in water or sterile water between feedings to help avoid a fluid volume deficit resulting from insensible fluid loss from the heat of the phototherapy lamp.

For all infants:

• Provide emotional support to the infant's parents, as appropriate. Reassure them that they're not at fault for having a child with this disorder. Encourage them to express their fears concerning possible complications of treatment.

• Organize nursing care to allow for extended periods of rest for the infant who is hemolyzing RBCs and is anemic and jaundiced.

• Keep the infant in an incubator to help reduce his energy expenditures until his condition stabilizes.

• Monitor vital signs frequently. Remember that tachycardia may occur in severe anemia.

• If the infant has hydrops fetalis, also administer oxygen as ordered, maintain the airway and mechanical ventilation as required, and assist in the removal of excess fluids to relieve ascites and respiratory distress.

Patient teaching

• Reinforce the doctor's explanation of the disease and its complications as necessary. Explain diagnostic tests and the prescribed treatment to the parents. Be sure they understand the care that the infant will receive.

GRANULOCYTOPENIA AND LYMPHOCYTOPENIA

Granulocytopenia is characterized by a marked reduction in the number of circulating granulocytes. Although this implies that all granulocytes (neutrophils, basophils, and eosinophils) are reduced, granulocytopenia usually refers to decreased neutrophils—a condition known as neutropenia. (See *Understanding neutropenia*, page 508.) This disorder, which can occur at any age, is associated with infections and ulcerative lesions of the throat, GI tract, other mucous membranes, and skin. Its severest form is known as agranulocytosis.

A rare disorder, lymphocytopenia (lymphopenia) is a deficiency of circulating lymphocytes (leukocytes produced mainly in lymph nodes).

In granulocytopenia and lymphocytopenia, the white blood cell (WBC) count may reach dangerously low levels, leaving the body unprotected against infection. Prognosis in both disorders depends on the underlying cause and whether it can be treated. Untreated, severe granulocytopenia can be fatal in 3 to 6 days.

Causes

Granulocytopenia may result from diminished production of granulocytes in bone marrow, increased peripheral destruction of granulocytes, or greater use of granulocytes. Diminished production of granulocytes in bone marrow generally stems from radiation therapy or drug therapy; it's a common adverse effect of antimetabolites and alkylating agents and may occur in the patient who is hypersensitive to phenothiazines, sulfonamides (and some sulfonamide derivatives, such as chlorothiazide), antibiotics, or antiarrhythmics. Drug-induced granulocytopenia usually develops slowly and typically correlates with the dosage and duration of therapy. Granulocyte production also decreases in such conditions as aplastic anemia and malignant bone marrow diseases and in some hereditary disorders (infantile genetic agranulocytosis).

The growing loss of peripheral granulocytes results from increased splenic sequestration, diseases that destroy peripheral blood cells (viral and bacterial infections), and drugs that act as haptens (carriers of antigens that attack blood cells, causing acute idiosyncratic or non–dose-related drug reactions). Infections such as mononucleosis may cause granulocytopenia because of increased use of granulocytes.

Similarly, lymphocytopenia may result from decreased production, increased destruction, or loss of lymphocytes. Decreased lymphocyte production may result from

UNDERSTANDING NEUTROPENIA

Neutropenia, a deficiency in the number of mature neutrophils, is the most common immune system deficiency. Common infections that occur secondary to neutropenia include aerobic gram-negative bacilli and *Staphylococcus aureus* and certain fungal infections, such as candidiasis and aspergillosis.

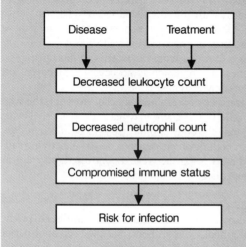

Assessment findings

Typically, patients with granulocytopenia experience slowly progressive fatigue and weakness. However, if they develop an infection, they can exhibit sudden onset of fever and chills and mental status changes. Overt signs of infection (pus formation) are usually absent. If granulocytopenia results from an idiosyncratic drug reaction, signs of infection develop abruptly, without causing slowly progressive fatigue and weakness.

In a patient with lymphocytopenia, palpation may reveal enlarged lymph nodes, spleen, and tonsils and signs of an associated disease.

Diagnostic tests

Diagnosis of granulocytopenia necessitates a thorough patient history to check for precipitating factors. Physical examination for clinical effects of underlying disorders is also essential.

Marked reduction in neutrophils (less than 500/mm³ leads to severe bacterial infections) and a WBC count below 2,000/mm³, with few observable granulocytes on the complete blood count (CBC), confirm granulocytopenia.

Bone marrow examination shows a scarcity of granulocytic precursor cells beyond the most immature forms, but this may vary, depending on the cause.

A lymphocyte count below 1,500/mm³ in adults or below 3,000/mm³ in children indicates lymphocytopenia. Evaluation of the patient's clinical status, bone marrow and lymph node biopsies, or other appropriate diagnostic tests can help identify the cause and establish the diagnosis.

Treatment

Effective management of granulocytopenia must identify and eliminate the cause and control infection until the bone marrow can generate more leukocytes. This often means drug or radiation therapy must be stopped and antibiotic treatment begun immediately, even before test results are known. Treatment may also include antifungal preparations. Administration of granulocyte- or granulocyte-macrophage colony-stimulating factor (G-CSF or GM-CSF) is a newer treatment used to stimulate bone marrow production of neutrophils. Spontaneous restoration of leukocyte production in bone marrow generally occurs within 1 to 3 weeks.

Treatment of lymphocytopenia includes eliminating the cause and managing the underlying disorder. For an infant with SCID, therapy may include bone marrow transplantation.

a genetic or thymic abnormality or from an immunodeficiency disorder, such as thymic dysplasia or ataxia-telangiectasia. Increased lymphocyte destruction may be caused by radiation therapy, chemotherapy, or human immunodeficiency virus (HIV) infection. Loss of lymphocytes may follow postoperative thoracic duct drainage, intestinal lymphangiectasia, or impaired intestinal lymphatic drainage (as in Whipple's disease). Lymphocyte depletion can also result from elevated plasma corticoid levels (due to stress, corticotropin or steroid therapy, or congestive heart failure). Other disorders associated with lymphocyte depletion include Hodgkin's disease, leukemia, aplastic anemia, sarcoidosis, myasthenia gravis, lupus erythematosus, protein-calorie malnutrition, renal failure, terminal cancer, tuberculosis and, in infants, severe combined immunodeficiency disease (SCID).

Complications

Localized infection can quickly become systemic (as in bacteremia) or can spread throughout an organ (as in pneumonia). All patients should be evaluated carefully to detect even subtle signs of infection because untreated infection can lead to septic shock in 8 to 24 hours.

Nursing diagnoses
- Altered parenting
- Altered tissue perfusion
- Fatigue
- Impaired tissue integrity
- Knowledge deficit
- Risk for infection
- Risk for fluid volume deficit

Nursing interventions
- Monitor vital signs frequently. Obtain cultures from blood, throat, urine, mouth, nose, rectum, vagina, and sputum, as ordered. Give antibiotics, as scheduled.
- Explain the necessity of infection-prevention procedures to the patient and his caregivers. Teach proper hand-washing technique and correct use of gowns and masks. Prevent patient contact with staff or visitors with respiratory infections.
- Maintain adequate nutrition and hydration because malnutrition aggravates immunosuppression. Make sure the patient with mouth ulcerations receives a high-calorie liquid diet. Offer a straw to make drinking less painful.
- Provide warm saline water gargles and rinses as well as analgesics and anesthetic lozenges. Good oral hygiene promotes comfort and healing.
- Ensure adequate rest, which helps mobilize the body's defenses against infection. Provide good skin and perineal care.
- Monitor the CBC and differential count, blood culture results, serum electrolyte levels, fluid intake and output, and daily weight.
- To help detect granulocytopenia and lymphocytopenia in the early, most treatable stages, monitor the WBC count of any patient receiving radiation or chemotherapy. After the patient has developed bone marrow depression, he must zealously avoid exposure to infection.
- Advise a patient with known or suspected sensitivity to a drug that can cause granulocytopenia or lymphocytopenia to alert medical personnel to this sensitivity in the future.

Patient teaching
- Reinforce the doctor's explanation of the disease. Answer any questions the patient may have.
- Teach effective personal hygiene and the importance of proper hand washing.
- Teach the patient to use a soft toothbrush and to maintain good oral hygiene.
- Teach the patient and family members how to institute and maintain infection precautions.

SELECTED REFERENCES

Betz, C., et al. *Family-Centered Nursing Care of Children,* 2nd ed. Philadelphia: W.B. Saunders Co., 1994.

Clinical Laboratory Tests: Values and Implications, 2nd ed. Springhouse, Pa.: Springhouse Corp., 1995.

Cunningham, F.G., et al. *Williams Obstetrics,* 19th ed. East Norwalk, Conn.: Appleton & Lange, 1993.

Fischbach, F. *A Manual of Laboratory and Diagnostic Tests,* 4th ed. Philadelphia: J.B. Lippincott Co., 1992.

Illustrated Manual of Nursing Practice, 2nd ed. Springhouse, Pa.: Springhouse Corp., 1994.

Isselbacher, K., et al. *Harrison's Principles of Internal Medicine,* 13th ed. New York: McGraw-Hill Book Co., 1995.

Mennell, J.S., et al. "Antenatal Management of the Thrombocytopenias," *Clinics in Perinatology* 21(3):591-614, September 1994.

Rakel, R.E., ed. *Conn's Current Therapy 1996.* Philadelphia: W.B. Saunders Co., 1996.

Rintels, P.B., et al. "Therapeutic Support of the Patient with Thrombocytopenia," *Hematology/Oncology Clinics of North America* 8(6):1131-1157, December 1994.

Smeltzer, S., and Bare, B. *Brunner and Suddarth's Textbook of Medical-Surgical Nursing,* 8th ed. Philadelphia: J.B. Lippincott Co., 1996.

Sparks, S.M., and Taylor, C.M. *Nursing Diagnosis Reference Manual,* 3rd ed. Springhouse, Pa.: Springhouse Corp., 1995.

Sutherland, M.A. "Wound Healing Problems in Haemophilia," *Journal of Wound Care* 4(4):166-168, April 1995.

Tierney, L., et al. *Current Medical Diagnosis and Treatment 1995.* East Norwalk, Conn.: Appleton & Lange, 1995.

Williams, W.J. *Williams Hematology,* 5th ed. New York: McGraw-Hill Book Co., 1995.

7 CARDIOVASCULAR DISORDERS

INTRODUCTION

The cardiovascular system begins its activity when the fetus is barely 4 weeks old and is the last system to cease activity at the end of life. This system is so vital that its activity helps define the presence of life.

Life-giving transport system

The heart, arteries, veins, and lymphatics form the cardiovascular network that serves as the body's transport system. This system brings life-supporting oxygen and nutrients to cells, removes metabolic waste products, and carries hormones from one part of the body to another.

The cardiovascular system, often called the circulatory system, may be divided into two branches: pulmonary circulation and systemic circulation. In *pulmonary circulation,* blood picks up oxygen and liberates the waste product carbon dioxide. In *systemic circulation* (which includes coronary circulation), blood carries oxygen and nutrients to all active cells while transporting waste products to the kidneys, liver, and skin for excretion.

Circulation requires normal function of the heart, which propels blood through the system by continuous rhythmic contractions. Located behind the sternum, the heart is a muscular organ the size of a man's fist. It has three layers: the *endocardium* — the smooth inner layer; the *myocardium* — the thick, muscular middle layer that contracts in rhythmic beats; and the *epicardium* — the thin, serous membrane, or outer surface of the heart. Covering the entire heart is a saclike membrane called the *pericardium.* This membrane has two layers: a *visceral* layer that's in contact with the heart and a *parietal,* or outer, layer. The pericardial space between these two layers contains a small amount of fluid, which is secreted by the serous membrane. This pericardial fluid lubricates the parietal pericardium when the heart moves against this layer during contraction, preventing irritation.

The heart has four chambers: two thin-walled chambers called *atria* and two thick-walled chambers called *ventricles.* The atria serve as reservoirs during ventricular contraction (systole) and as booster pumps during ventricular relaxation (diastole). The left ventricle propels blood through the systemic circulation. The right ventricle, which forces blood through the pulmonary circulation, is much thinner than the left ventricle because it meets only one-sixth the resistance.

Heart valves

Two kinds of valves work inside the heart: *atrioventricular* and *semilunar.* The atrioventricular valve between the right atrium and the right ventricle has three leaflets, or cusps, and three papillary muscles; hence, it's called the tricuspid valve. The atrioventricular valve between the left atrium and the left ventricle consists of two cusps shaped like a bishop's miter and two papillary muscles and is called the mitral valve. The tricuspid and mitral valves prevent blood backflow from the ventricles to the atria during ventricular contraction.

The leaflets of both valves are attached to the papillary muscles of the ventricle by thin, fibrous bands called chordae tendineae. These leaflets separate and descend funnel-like into the ventricles during diastole and are pushed upward and together during systole, to occlude the tricuspid and mitral orifices. The valves' action isn't entirely passive because papillary muscles contract during systole and prevent the leaflets from prolapsing into the atria during ventricular contraction.

The two semilunar valves, which resemble half moons, prevent blood backflow from the aorta and the pulmonary artery into the ventricles when those chambers relax and fill with blood from the atria. These semilunar valves are referred to as aortic and pulmonary for their respective arteries.

Cardiac cycle

Diastole is the phase of ventricular relaxation and filling. As diastole begins, ventricular pressure falls below atrial pressure, and the aortic and pulmonary valves close. As ventricular pressure continues to fall below atrial pressure, the mitral and tricuspid valves open, and blood flows rapidly into the ventricles. Atrial contraction then increases the volume of ventricular filling by pumping up to 20% more blood into the ventricles.

When systole begins, the ventricles contract, raising ventricular pressure above atrial pressure and closing the mitral and tricuspid valves. When ventricular pressure finally becomes greater than that in the aorta and the pulmonary artery, the aortic and pulmonary valves open, and the ventricles eject blood. Ventricular pressure continues to rise as blood is expelled from the heart. As systole ends, the ventricles relax and stop ejecting blood, and ventricular pressure falls, closing the aortic and pulmonary valves.

S_1 (the first heart sound) is heard as the ventricles contract and the atrioventricular valves close. S_1 is loudest at the apex of the heart, over the mitral area. S_2 (the second heart sound), which is normally rapid and sharp, occurs when the aortic and pulmonary valves close. S_2 is loudest at the base of the heart (second intercostal space on both sides of the sternum).

INTERPRETING PULSE CHARACTER

Peripheral pulse rhythm should correspond exactly to the auscultatory heart rhythm. You can palpate it most easily where the artery crosses a bone or other firm surface (at the wrist, for example).

The character of the pulse may offer useful information. For example, *pulsus alternans* is a strong beat followed by a weak one and can mean left ventricular failure. A *water-hammer* (or Corrigan's) *pulse* is forceful and bounding. It's best felt in the carotid arteries or in the forearm and accompanies increased pulse pressure—often with capillary pulsations of the fingernails (Quincke's sign). This pulse usually indicates patent ductus arteriosus or aortic regurgitation.

Pulsus biferiens, a double peripheral pulse for every apical beat, can signal aortic stenosis, hyperthyroidism, or another disease. *Pulsus bigeminus* is a coupled rhythm; you feel its beat in pairs. The second beat, indicating a premature ventricular contraction after each regular beat, sometimes occurs after myocardial infarction.

Pulsus paradoxus is exaggerated waxing and waning of the arterial pressure (a 15 mm Hg or greater decrease in systolic blood pressure during inspiration), seen in cardiac tamponade.

Normally, the right heart valves close a fraction of a second later than the left valves because of lower pressures in the right ventricle and pulmonary artery. Identifying these components during auscultation is usually difficult, except when inspiration coincides with the end of systole or when a right bundle-branch block exists. Either will cause a slightly prolonged right ventricular ejection time, when the delayed closing of the pulmonary valve is heard as a split S_2.

Ventricular distention during diastole, which can occur in heart failure, creates low-frequency vibrations that may be heard in early diastole as a third heart sound (S_3), or ventricular gallop. An atrial gallop (S_4) may appear at the end of diastole, just before S_1, if atrial filling is forced into a ventricle that has become less compliant or overdistended, or has a decreased ability to contract. A ventricular pressure rise and ventricular vibrations cause this sound.

Cardiac conduction

The heart's conduction system consists of specialized cells that are capable of generating and conducting rhythmic electrical impulses to stimulate heart contraction. This system includes the sinoatrial (SA) node, the atrioventricular (AV) junction, the bundle of His and its bundle branches, and the ventricular conduction tissue and Purkinje's fibers.

Normally, the SA node controls the heart rate and rhythm at 60 to 100 beats/minute. Because the SA node has the lowest resting potential, it's the heart's pacemaker. If it defaults, another part of the system takes over. The AV junction may emerge at 40 to 60 beats/minute; the bundle of His and its bundle branches at 30 to 40 beats/minute; and ventricular conduction tissue and Purkinje's fibers at 20 to 30 beats/minute.

Cardiac output

The amount of blood pumped by the left ventricle into the aorta each minute (cardiac output) is calculated by multiplying the stroke volume (the amount of blood the left ventricle ejects during each contraction) by the heart rate (number of beats per minute). When cellular demands increase, the stroke volume or heart rate must increase.

Stroke volume depends on the ventricle's blood volume and pressure at the end of diastole (preload), resistance to ejection (afterload), and the myocardium's contractile strength. Changes in preload, afterload, or contractile strength can alter the stroke volume.

Many factors affect the heart rate, such as exercise, pregnancy, and stress. When the sympathetic nervous system releases norepinephrine, the heart rate increases; when the parasympathetic system releases acetylcholine, the heart rate slows.

Circulation and pulses

Blood circulates through three types of vessels: *arteries, veins,* and *capillaries.* The sturdy, pliable walls of the arteries adjust to the volume of blood leaving the heart. The major artery arching out of the left ventricle is the aorta. Its segments and subbranches ultimately divide into minute, thin-walled (one-cell thick) capillaries. Capillaries pass the blood to the veins, which return it to the heart. In the veins, valves prevent blood backflow.

Pulses are best felt wherever an artery runs near the skin's surface and over a hard structure. (See *Interpreting pulse character.*) Easily found pulses are:
• the *radial artery,* at the anterolateral aspect of the wrist
• the *temporal artery,* in front of the ear, above and lateral to the eye
• the *common carotid artery,* at the side of the neck
• the *femoral artery,* in the groin.

The lymphatic system also plays a role in the cardiovascular network. Originating in tissue spaces, the lymphatic system drains fluid and other plasma components

CHARACTERIZING CHEST PAIN

Pericarditis	Angina	Myocardial infarction
Onset and duration		
Sudden onset, continuous pain lasting for days, residual soreness	Gradual or sudden onset, pain usually lasting less than 15 minutes and not more than 30 minutes (average: 3 minutes)	Sudden onset, pain lasting 30 minutes to 2 hours, residual soreness for 1 to 3 days
Location and radiation		
Substernal pain to left of midline, radiation to back or subclavicular area	Substernal or anterior chest pain or pressure, not sharply localized; radiation to back, neck, arms, jaws, even upper abdomen or fingers	Substernal, midline, or anterior chest pain; radiation to jaws, neck, back, shoulders, and one or both arms
Quality and intensity		
Mild ache to severe pain, deep or superficial; "stabbing," "knifelike"	Mild to moderate pressure; deep sensation; varied pattern of attacks; "tightness," "squeezing," "crushing"	Persistent, severe pressure; deep sensation; "crushing," "squeezing," "heavy," "oppressive"; sudden death
Signs and symptoms		
Precordial friction rub; increased pain with movement, inspiration, laughing, coughing; decreased pain with sitting or leaning forward (sitting up pulls the heart away from the diaphragm)	Dyspnea, diaphoresis, nausea, desire to void, belching, apprehension	Nausea, vomiting, apprehension, dyspnea, diaphoresis, increased or decreased blood pressure; gallop heart sound, "sensation of impending doom"; chest pressure may fluctuate initially and then become persistent
Precipitating factors		
Myocardial infarction or upper respiratory tract infection; no relation to effort; cardiac surgery, cardiac tumor, or penetrating chest wound	Exertion, stress, eating, cold or hot and humid weather	Physical exertion or emotional stress; may also occur when person is at rest

that build up in extravascular spaces and reroutes them back to the circulatory system as lymph, a plasmalike fluid. Lymphatics also extract bacteria and foreign bodies.

Cardiovascular assessment

The patient history and physical assessment provide vital information about cardiovascular status. (See *Characterizing chest pain.*) When performing the assessment:
• First, observe for general signs of cardiovascular disorders, such as central cyanosis (disturbance in gas exchange), edema (congestive heart failure or valvular disease), and clubbing (congenital cardiovascular disease).
• Next, palpate the peripheral pulses bilaterally, and evaluate their rate, equality, and quality on a scale from

0 (absent) to +4 (bounding). (See *Determining pulse amplitude,* page 514.)
• Inspect the carotid arteries for distention. Palpate them individually for thrills (fine vibrations due to irregular blood flow), and listen for bruits.
• Check for pulsations in the jugular veins (more easily seen than felt with tangential light). Watch for jugular venous distention—a possible sign of right ventricular failure, valvular stenosis, cardiac tamponade, or pulmonary embolism. Take blood pressure readings in both arms while the patient is lying, sitting, and standing.
• Systematically auscultate the anterior chest wall for each of the four heart sounds in the aortic area (second intercostal space at the right sternal border), pulmonary area (second intercostal space at the left sternal border), right ventricular area (lower half of the left sternal bor-

DETERMINING PULSE AMPLITUDE

To record your patient's pulse amplitude, use this standard scale.

0: Pulse is not palpable.

+1: Pulse is thready, weak, difficult to find, may fade in and out, and disappears easily with pressure.

+2: Pulse is constant but not strong; light pressure must be applied or pulse will disappear.

+3: Pulse considered normal. It is easily palpable and does not disappear with pressure.

+4: Pulse is strong, bounding, and does not disappear with pressure.

der), and mitral area (fifth intercostal space at the midclavicular line). For low-pitched sounds, use the bell of the stethoscope; for high-pitched sounds, the diaphragm. Inspect for pulsations, and palpate for thrills. Check the location of apical pulsation for deviations in normal size (⅜″ to ¾″ [1 to 2 cm]) and position (in the mitral area) — possible signs of left ventricular hypertrophy, left-sided valvular disease, or right ventricular disease.

• Auscultate for murmurs, the vibrating sound of turbulent blood flow through a stenotic or incompetent valve. Time the murmur to determine where it occurs in the cardiac cycle — between S_1 and S_2 (systolic), between S_2 and the next S_1 (diastolic), or throughout systole (holosystolic). Finally, listen for the scratching or squeaking of a pericardial friction rub.

If you hear a rub, determine if it is a pericardial or a pleural friction rub. Have the patient hold his breath while auscultating the anterior chest. If a rub persists while he is holding his breath, the rub is pericardial.

Special cardiovascular tests

After a thorough history, physical examination, and clinical observation, special tests provide valuable diagnostic information.

Electrocardiography (ECG) is a primary tool for evaluating cardiac status. Through electrodes placed on the patient's limbs and over the precordium (see *ECG lead placement*), an ECG measures electrical activity by recording currents transmitted by the heart. It can detect ischemia, conduction delay, chamber enlargement, injury, necrosis, bundle-branch blocks, fascicular blocks, and arrhythmias. In ambulatory ECG, or Holter monitoring, a tape recording tracks as many as 100,000 cardiac cycles over a 12- or 24-hour period. Sometimes this test is used to determine cardiac status after myocardial

infarction (MI), to assess the effectiveness of antiarrhythmic drugs, and to determine if arrhythmias are the cause of particular symptoms.

Chest X-rays may reveal an enlarged heart and aortic dilation. They also assess pulmonary circulation. When pulmonary venous and arterial pressures rise, characteristic changes appear, such as dilation of the pulmonary venous shadows. When pulmonary venous pressure exceeds oncotic pressure of the blood, capillary fluid leaks into lung tissues, causing pulmonary edema. This fluid may settle in the alveoli, producing a butterfly pattern, or the lungs may appear cloudy or hazy; in the interlobular septa, sharp linear densities (Kerley's lines) may appear.

Exercise testing using a bicycle ergometer, treadmill, or short flight of stairs can determine cardiac response to physical stress. This type of test measures blood pressure and ECG changes during increasingly rigorous exercises. Myocardial ischemia, abnormal blood pressure response, or arrhythmias indicate failure of the circulatory system to adapt to exercise.

Cardiac catheterization evaluates chest pain, the need for coronary artery surgery or angioplasty, congenital heart defects, and valvular heart disease, and determines the extent of heart failure.

Right ventricular catheterization involves threading a catheter through a vein into the right ventricle, pulmonary artery, and its branches in the lungs to measure right atrial, right ventricular, pulmonary artery, and pulmonary capillary wedge pressures. A pulmonary arterial thermodilution catheter can measure cardiac output.

Left ventricular catheterization entails inserting a catheter into an artery and threading it retrogradely through the aorta into the left ventricle. *Ventriculography* during left ventricular catheterization involves injecting radiopaque dye into the left ventricle to measure ejection fraction (portion of ventricular volume ejected per beat) and to disclose abnormal heart wall motion or mitral valve incompetence.

In *coronary arteriography*, radiopaque material injected into coronary arteries allows cineangiographic visualization of coronary arterial narrowing or occlusion.

Digital subtraction angiography evaluates the coronary arteries, using X-ray images that are digitally subtracted by computer. Time-based color enhancement shows blood flow in nearby areas.

Echocardiography uses echoes from pulsed high-frequency sound waves (ultrasound) to evaluate structures of the heart. A small transducer placed on the chest wall in various positions and angles acts as both transmitter and receiver. It provides information about valve leaflets, sizes and dimensions of heart chambers, and thicknesses and motions of the septum and the ventricular walls.

Echocardiography can also show intracardiac masses (atrial tumors and thrombi, for example), detect pericardial effusion, diagnose idiopathic hypertrophic subaortic stenosis, and estimate cardiac output and ejection fraction. Echocardiography can also evaluate possible aortic dissection when it involves the ascending aorta. Both M-mode and two-dimensional echocardiography exist, but the latter has greater diagnostic abilities.

In *multiple-gated acquisition scanning,* a radioactive isotope remains in the intravascular compartment, allowing measurement of stroke volume, ventricular ejection fraction, and wall motion. *Myocardial imaging* uses radioactive agents (most often thallium-201) to detect abnormalities in coronary artery perfusion. These agents concentrate in normally perfused myocardium but not in ischemic areas. Nonperfused areas, or "cold spots," may be permanent (scar tissue after MI) or temporary (induced by transient ischemia). Thallium scanning with exercise tests identifies exercise-induced ischemia and evaluates abnormal findings on a stress ECG.

Technetium pyrophosphate scanning documents muscle viability (not perfusion). Unlike thallium, technetium accumulates only in irreversibly damaged myocardial tissue. Areas of necrosis appear as "hot spots" and can be detected only with acute infarction. This test determines the size and location of infarction but can produce false results.

Cardiac enzyme assays confirm acute MI or severe cardiac trauma because these cellular proteins are released into the blood as a result of cell membrane injury. All cardiac enzymes—creatine phosphokinase (CPK), lactate dehydrogenase, and aspartate aminotransferase (formerly SGOT), for example—are also found in other cells, but their numbers peak in the presence of transmural MI. Total CPK levels peak 6 to 30 hours after the onset of symptoms. Fractionation of enzymes can determine the source of damaged cells. For example, three fractions of CPK are isolated, one of which (an isoenzyme called CPK-MB) is found only in myocardial cells. CPK-MB in the blood indicates injury to these cells and generally peaks 21 hours after insult.

Peripheral arteriography consists of fluoroscopic imaging after arterial injection of contrast media. Similarly, *phlebography* defines the venous system after injection of contrast media into a vein. *Impedance plethysmography* evaluates the venous system to detect pressure changes transmitted to lower leg veins.

E.C.G. LEAD PLACEMENT

The 12-lead ECG provides a three-dimensional view of cardiac activity through three sets of leads:
• Standard limb leads (I, II, III) record electrical activity from the heart to the limbs.
• Augmented leads (aV$_R$, aV$_L$, aV$_F$) measure activity from the heart to the limbs.
• Precordial or chest leads (V$_1$ to V$_6$) show ventricular electrical activity.

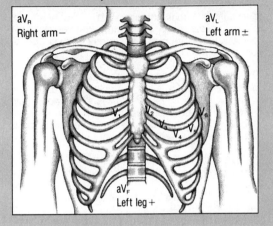

Doppler ultrasonography evaluates the peripheral vascular system and assesses arterial occlusive disease.

Endomyocardial biopsy can detect cardiomyopathy, infiltrative myocardial diseases, and rejection of transplants. Under fluoroscopic control, a right ventricular biopsy is done by way of the right internal jugular vein. Less commonly, a left ventricular biopsy is done by retrograde arterial catheterization.

Electrophysiologic studies help diagnose conduction system disease and serious arrhythmias. Electronic induction and termination of arrhythmias aid drug selection. *Endocardial mapping* detects an arrhythmia's focus, using a finger electrode. *Epicardial mapping* uses a computer and a fabric sock with electrodes that's slipped over the heart.

CONGENITAL DEFECTS

Abnormalities during fetal development may cause structural defects of the heart and great arteries. These defects may be acyanotic or cyanotic. Acyanotic defects include

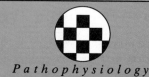

Pathophysiology

TYPES OF VENTRICULAR SEPTAL DEFECTS

The names for ventricular septal defects correspond to their anatomic locations, as shown. Defects of different types may appear together or converge.

Subpulmonary defects
These defects are located in the right ventricular outflow. Viewed from the left ventricle, they appear just below the aortic valve.

Membranous or perimembranous defects
When viewed from either ventricle, these defects involve the subaortic region of the membranous septum. Some experts use the term perimembranous because this type of defect may not be confined to the membranous septum.

Atrioventricular (AV) canal defects
These defects appear in the inflow of the right ventricle.

Muscular defects
Defects in the lower trabecular septum are known as muscular defects and more specifically as apical, midmuscular, anterior, and posterior defects. A large apical muscular defect may look like a single hole

when viewed from the left ventricle but have a "swiss cheese" appearance when viewed from the right ventricle. Right ventricular trabeculations cause this effect by partially covering the defect.

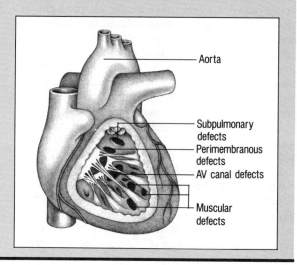

ventricular and atrial septal defects, coarctation of the aorta, and patent ductus arteriosus. Cyanotic defects include tetralogy of Fallot and transposition of the great arteries.

VENTRICULAR SEPTAL DEFECT

The most common congenital heart disorder, a ventricular septal defect is an abnormal opening in the ventricular septum that allows blood to escape from the left ventricle into the right. The result is that oxygenated blood returns to the lungs instead of proceeding into the aortic arch as it should.

A ventricular septal defect may be large or small and may involve one hole or several holes in any part of the septum. (See *Types of ventricular septal defects.*) Sometimes, the entire septum may be missing, which creates a single chamber. The amount of blood shunted between ventricles depends on the size of the defect and the amount of pulmonary and systemic resistance.

Up to 30% of smaller defects and 12% of larger ones close without treatment within a year after birth. Those that do—or those that are corrected surgically—have a good prognosis. Untreated defects that don't close on their own can be fatal during the first year after birth, usually due to secondary complications.

Causes and pathophysiology
Normally, the ventricular septum closes by the 6th week of gestation. But in about 200 of 100,000 neonates, the septum fails to close, resulting in a ventricular septal defect. The condition may not be obvious right away because right and left ventricular pressures are nearly equal at birth (so blood doesn't shunt through the defect). However, 4 to 8 weeks after birth, pulmonary vessels gradually relax and right ventricular pressure decreases. Blood begins to shunt and symptoms arise.

Although no one knows what causes a ventricular septal defect, genetic and environmental factors may influence its development. Fetal alcohol syndrome may play a role. And although most children with congenital heart defects are otherwise normal, those with a ventricular septal defect may have other birth defects. These include Down's syndrome and other autosomal trisomies, renal anomalies, and such cardiac defects as patent ductus arteriosus and coarctation of the aorta.

Complications
Pulmonary resistance rises because of the increased volume of blood being pumped to the lungs. Left-to-right shunting and increased pressure in the right ventricle cause hypertrophy, which causes the right atrium to enlarge as it works against the right ventricular resistance. The patient may develop heart failure and pulmonary hypertension.

Assessment findings
The clinical features of a ventricular septal defect vary with the defect's size, the effect of shunting on pulmonary vasculature, and the patient's age.

An infant with a small defect usually appears normal and has no sternal or costal retractions because a small defect allows little shunting, so pulmonary artery pressure and heart size remain normal. Auscultation reveals a loud murmur, usually loudest at the lower left sternal border and occurring within the first week after birth. Tachypnea of more than 60 breaths/minute may indicate mild heart failure.

An infant with a large defect typically will appear thin, small, restless, and irritable. He'll gain weight slowly and may have a history of feeding problems. With a moderate or large defect, auscultation typically reveals a pansystolic murmur—loudest at the lower left sternal border, fourth intercostal space—and usually produces a thrill. Also, the pulmonary component of S_2 sounds loud and is widely split.

An untreated ventricular septal defect that has progressed to heart failure will reveal tachycardia and an S_3 gallop rhythm that can be heard at the apex. An infant with heart failure will appear dusky and diaphoretic. You may see sternal and costal retractions during inspiration (particularly if the infant has pneumonia or atelectasis, or if he's aspirated something). The respiratory rate will be rapid, and the infant will have grunting respirations. Auscultation of the lung fields reveals crackles and gurgles. Palpation reveals that the point of maximal impulse has been displaced to the left. The liver, heart, and spleen enlarge as a result of systemic venous congestion.

With advanced heart failure and cardiac hypertrophy, you'll see cyanosis and, possibly, anterior chest wall prominence.

The older patient may display signs of fixed pulmonary hypertension, which can occur much later in life with right-to-left shunt (a condition called Eisenmenger complex). These signs include cyanosis and clubbing of the nail beds. Auscultation may reveal a diastolic murmur, a quieter systolic murmur, and a greatly accentuated S_2.

Diagnostic tests
• *Chest X-ray* results are normal if the patient has a small defect; for a large defect, chest X-rays reveal cardiomegaly, left atrial and left ventricular enlargement, and prominent pulmonary vascular markings.
• *Electrocardiography* results are normal for a small defect but show left and right ventricular hypertrophy (which suggests pulmonary hypertension) for a large defect. Large defects generate a right axis shift.
• *Echocardiography* may reveal a large defect and its location in the septum, estimate the degree of a left-to-right shunt, suggest pulmonary hypertension, and identify associated lesions and complications.
• *Cardiac catheterization* may be used to determine the size and location of the defect, to calculate the degree of shunting by comparing blood oxygen saturation between ventricles, to determine the extent of pulmonary hypertension, and to detect associated defects.

Treatment
Only about 15% of small defects in infants require surgical correction. Infants who don't require surgery may receive an antibiotic to prevent bacterial endocarditis.

For an infant with a large defect, treatment focuses on managing heart failure and improving growth. Specifically, the infant may receive digoxin, diuretics, a sodium-restricted diet, and nutritional supplements. If this regimen is effective, surgery may be delayed to give the defect time to shrink or close on its own. Surgery for large defects usually requires insertion of a patch graft, usually through the tricuspid valve, with the patient on cardiopulmonary bypass. If the child has other defects and will benefit from delaying surgery, the doctor may band the pulmonary artery. This procedure normalizes pressures and blood flow distal to the band and prevents pulmonary vascular disease.

Usually, postoperative treatment includes mechanical ventilation, analgesics, diuretics to increase urine output, continuous infusion of nitroprusside or adrenergic agents to regulate blood pressure and cardiac output and, in rare cases, a temporary pacemaker.

Nursing diagnoses
- Activity intolerance
- Altered growth and development
- Altered nutrition: Less than body requirements
- Altered parenting
- Decreased cardiac output
- Impaired gas exchange
- Ineffective family coping
- Risk for infection

Nursing interventions
- Administer ordered medications to the infant and monitor for adverse effects.
- Provide adequate nutrition. If the infant tires easily during feeding, he may need to be fed through a nasogastric tube.
- Monitor for signs of heart failure and administer symptomatic treatment as ordered.
- Encourage activity as tolerated.
- Recognize that the parents may have difficulty coping with the child's illness because of anxiety or economic problems. Assist the parents in identifying areas of concern and refer them to social service agencies as needed.

 After surgery:
- Monitor vital signs and intake and output. Maintain the infant's body temperature with an overbed warmer. Give catecholamines, nitroprusside, and diuretics, as ordered. Give analgesics as needed. Record the effectiveness of all medications given.
- Monitor central venous pressure, intra-arterial blood pressure, and left atrial or pulmonary artery pressure readings. Check heart rate and rhythm for signs of conduction block.
- Assess oxygenation, particularly in a child who requires mechanical ventilation. Suction as needed to maintain a patent airway and to prevent atelectasis and pneumonia.
- Monitor pacemaker effectiveness, if needed. Watch for signs of failure, such as bradycardia and hypotension.

Patient teaching
- Explain all tests thoroughly.
- Instruct the parents to watch for signs of heart failure, such as poor feeding, sweating, and heavy breathing.
- If the child is receiving digoxin or other medications, tell the parents how to give them and how to recognize adverse reactions. Caution them to keep medications out of the reach of all children.

- Teach the parents to recognize and report early signs of infection and to avoid exposing the child to people with obvious infections.
- Encourage the parents to let the child engage in normal activities as much as possible.
- Stress the importance of prophylactic antibiotics before and after surgery.
- Reassure the parents, and allow them to participate in their child's care.

ATRIAL SEPTAL DEFECT
In an atrial septal defect, an opening between the left atrium and the right atrium allows blood to shunt between the chambers. (See *Types of atrial septal defects.*) Because atrial pressure normally is slightly higher in the left atrium than in the right, blood typically shunts from left to right. The pressure difference may force large amounts of blood through the defect during diastole. If the hole is more than 1 cm in diameter, the atria act as a single chamber.

Most infants with an atrial septal defect have no significant left-to-right shunt and no symptoms because during diastole, blood flows toward the ventricular chamber (usually the right), which has thinner, more compliant walls.

Symptoms of left-to-right shunt typically develop in adolescents and young adults because the left ventricle becomes thicker over the years from increased left ventricular end-diastolic pressure. This increased ventricular resistance forces blood through the defect rather than into the ventricles.

An atrial septal defect is found in about 10% of children who have congenital heart disease and who have survived past their first birthday. The disorder is almost twice as common in females as in males and has a strong familial tendency.

Although an atrial septal defect is benign during infancy and childhood, delayed development of signs and symptoms and complications makes it one of the most common congenital heart defects diagnosed in adolescence and adulthood. The prognosis is excellent in asymptomatic people, but poor in those with cyanosis caused by large, untreated defects.

Causes and pathophysiology
The cause of an atrial septal defect is unknown. In this disorder, left-to-right shunt results in right ventricular volume overload, which affects the right atrium, right ventricle, and pulmonary arteries. Eventually, the right

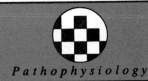

Pathophysiology

TYPES OF ATRIAL SEPTAL DEFECTS

Experts recognize three types of atrial septal defects, as shown. These defects can vary in size, but sinus venosus defects tend to be smaller than the others.

Sinus venosus
Usually located in the superior-posterior portion of the atrial septum, this defect sometimes extends into the superior vena cava and almost always is associated with abnormalities of the pulmonary veins as they enter the superior vena cava and the right atrium.

Ostium secundum
This defect, which may be single or multiple, occurs around the fossa ovalis and occasionally extends down close to the superior vena cava.

Ostium primum
A defect of the primitive septum, ostium primum occurs in the inferior portion of the septum primum and usually is associated with atrioventricular valve abnormalities (cleft mitral valve) and conduction defects.

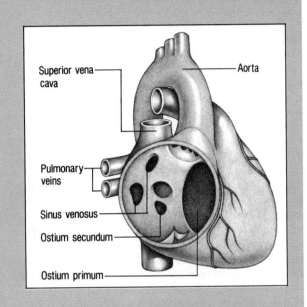

atrium enlarges and the right ventricle dilates to accommodate the increased blood volume.

Complications
In some adult patients, fixed (irreversible) pulmonary hypertension causes the shunt to reverse direction. Then, unoxygenated blood enters the systemic circulation, causing cyanosis. Right and left ventricular hypertrophy become significant. Atrial arrhythmias, heart failure, and emboli may occur.

Children with an atrial septal defect seldom develop heart failure, pulmonary hypertension, infective endocarditis, or other complications.

Assessment findings
Small defects typically go undetected in a preschooler, although the child may have a history of fatigue, shortness of breath after extreme exertion, and frequent respiratory tract infections.

A large defect may retard a child's growth. Cyanosis may develop, especially if right ventricular outflow is ob-

structed. Inspection of the jugular vein may reveal a strong pulse preceded by a systolic collapse. Inspection of the chest wall may reveal left chest prominence. An impulse may be palpable in that area.

In children, auscultation may reveal an early to midsystolic murmur, superficial in quality, heard at the second or third left intercostal space. If the patient has a large shunt—the result of increased tricuspid valve flow—you'll hear a low-pitched diastolic murmur at the lower left sternal border. The murmur will become more pronounced on inspiration. Although the murmur's intensity is a rough indicator of left-to-right shunt size, its low pitch may make it difficult to hear.

The most diagnostic sounds are a fixed, widely split S_2 (caused by delayed closure of the pulmonary valve) and a systolic click or late systolic murmur at the apex (resulting from mitral valve prolapse, which occasionally affects older children with an atrial septal defect).

As adults, many patients with an atrial septal defect complain of more pronounced symptoms, such as fatigue and dyspnea on exertion. Symptoms may become severe enough to sharply limit the patient's activities, especially after age 40.

If the patient has a large, uncorrected defect and fixed pulmonary hypertension, auscultation will reveal an accentuated S_2 and, possibly, a pulmonary ejection click and an audible S_4. The patient will become cyanotic and develop clubbed nails; severe pulmonary vascular disease may lead to syncope and hemoptysis.

Diagnostic tests

• *Chest X-rays* show an enlarged right atrium and right ventricle, a prominent pulmonary artery, and increased pulmonary vascular markings. The sinus venosus defect is characterized by an absent right superior vena cava shadow and entrance of the horizontal pulmonary vein into the upper right cardiac shadow.
• *Electrocardiography* results may be normal but usually show right axis deviation, a prolonged PR interval, varying degrees of right bundle-branch block, right ventricular hypertrophy, atrial fibrillation (particularly in severe cases after age 30) and, in ostium primum, left axis deviation.
• *Echocardiography* shows a volume overload on the right side of the heart and measures the right ventricular enlargement. It also may locate the defect and it estimates the size and direction of the shunt. (Other causes of right ventricular enlargement must be ruled out.)
• *Cardiac catheterization* confirms an atrial septal defect by demonstrating that right atrial blood is more oxygenated than superior vena cava blood, which indicates a left-to-right shunt. Catheterization also determines the degree of shunting and pulmonary vascular disease. Pulmonary artery systolic pressures are usually positive. Dye injection shows the defect's size and location, the location of pulmonary venous drainage, and atrioventricular valve competence. Cardiac catheterization is performed only when the patient's doctor strongly suspects an atrial septal defect but the patient has unusual symptoms.

Treatment

Because an atrial septal defect seldom produces complications in infants and toddlers, surgery may be delayed until they reach preschool or early school age. A large defect may need immediate surgical closure with sutures or a patch graft.

Nursing diagnoses

• Activity intolerance
• Decreased cardiac output
• Fatigue
• Impaired gas exchange
• Knowledge deficit
• Risk for infection

Nursing interventions

• Encourage the child to engage in any activity he can tolerate. Living as normally as possible is important to avoid illness-dependent behavior patterns.
  After surgery:
• Closely monitor vital signs, central venous and intra-arterial pressures, and intake and output.
• Watch for atrial arrhythmias.
• Give antibiotics and analgesics, as ordered.
• Provide range-of-motion exercises and coughing and deep-breathing exercises.

Patient teaching

• Before cardiac catheterization, explain pretest and posttest procedures to the patient (and parents, if the patient is a child). If possible, use drawings or other visual aids to help a child understand.
• If surgery is scheduled, teach the child and his parents about the intensive care unit, and introduce them to the staff. Show parents where they can wait during the operation. Explain postoperative procedures, tubes, dressings, and monitoring equipment.
• As needed, teach the patient or his family about the importance of antibiotic prophylaxis—especially before routine dental procedures—to prevent infective endocarditis.

COARCTATION OF THE AORTA

This disorder involves a narrowing (coarctation) of the aorta, usually just below the left subclavian artery and near the site where the ligamentum arteriosum joins the pulmonary artery to the aorta. (See *Understanding coarctation of the aorta.*) The ligamentum arteriosum is a remnant of a fetal blood vessel called the ductus arteriosus.

Coarctation may be associated with mitral or aortic valve lesions (usually the bicuspid aortic valve) and with severe cases of hypoplasia of the aortic arch, patent ductus arteriosus, or a ventricular septal defect.

This disorder accounts for about 8% of all congenital heart defects in children and is more common in males than in females. When it occurs in females, it commonly is associated with Turner's syndrome, a chromosomal disorder that causes ovarian dysgenesis.

The prognosis for coarctation of the aorta depends on the severity of associated cardiac anomalies. The prognosis is good if the condition can be surgically corrected before it induces severe systemic hypertension or degenerative changes in the aorta.

Causes

Coarctation of the aorta may develop as a result of smooth-muscle spasm and constriction as the ductus arteriosus closes. Contractile tissue may reach into the aortic wall, causing it to narrow.

Complications

Infective endocarditis represents the most common complication. Rarely, patients may develop such vascular complications as cerebrovascular accident, ruptured aorta, and cerebral thrombosis. Untreated, coarctation may lead to left ventricular failure.

If the patient has a ventricular septal defect and coarctation, blood shunts left to right, straining the right ventricle. This leads to pulmonary hypertension and, eventually, right ventricular hypertrophy and failure.

Assessment findings

An infant with coarctation may appear normal for up to 3 weeks after birth before signs and symptoms of left ventricular failure begin to surface. The infant may develop tachypnea, dyspnea, tachycardia, and pallor tinged with cyanosis. He also may exhibit signs of failure to thrive, such as inadequate weight gain.

Palpation may reveal an enlarged heart and liver, and absent or diminished femoral pulses.

Auscultation may disclose normal heart sounds or a narrowly split second sound with a loud pulmonary component. You may hear a third heart sound at the apex, possibly prolonged into a diastolic rumble. You may also hear an apical systolic blowing murmur that results from mitral incompetence. And you may hear a loud stenotic murmur over the spine (from the coarctation) or at the second right intercostal space or suprasternal notch (from associated aortic valve disease).

Patients with coarctation may remain asymptomatic until adolescence because collateral circulation develops to bypass the narrowed segment. During adolescence, however, the defect may cause signs and symptoms despite the collateral circulation. Signs and symptoms include dyspnea, muscle cramps after exercise, coolness in the lower extremities, headaches, epistaxis, and hypertension in the upper extremities.

These patients typically have resting systolic hypertension and wide pulse pressure. You'll find high diastolic pressure readings that are the same in both the arms and the legs.

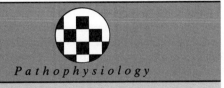

Pathophysiology

UNDERSTANDING COARCTATION OF THE AORTA

Normal fetal circulation includes three shunts that operate to bypass the fetus's liver and lungs. One of these shunts is called the ductus arteriosus; it connects the pulmonary artery with the aorta.

Most of the blood entering the main pulmonary artery bypasses the lungs and flows directly into the aorta through the ductus arteriosus.

After birth, when the neonate's lungs must function on their own, the ductus arteriosus closes, and the right ventricular output enters the left ventricle through the pulmonary capillaries, as it does in normal adult circulation.

If the ductus arteriosus closes improperly, coarctation may be the result.

By restricting blood flow, this abnormal constriction increases pressure on the left ventricle so much that it may fail, causing increased end-diastolic and pulmonary capillary pressures, pulmonary edema, a low output state and, possibly, sudden circulatory collapse. Restricted flow also increases the pressure load on the left ventricle, dilates the proximal aorta, and causes ventricular hypertrophy.

To compensate for the increased pressure, collateral circulation may develop to circumvent the narrowed aorta.

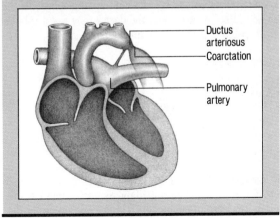

Coarctation may also produce a visible aortic pulsation in the suprasternal notch, a continuous systolic murmur, an accentuated S_2, and an S_4.

Diagnostic tests
• *Chest X-rays* may demonstrate left ventricular hypertrophy, left ventricular failure, a wide ascending and descending aorta, and notching of the undersurfaces of the ribs, caused by extensive collateral circulation.
• *Magnetic resonance imaging* or *digital angiography* allows visualization of the length and severity of the obstruction and the extent of collateral circulation.
• *Electrocardiography* may initially show right ventricular hypertrophy and left ventricular failure. If the coarctation isn't repaired, this test will eventually show left ventricular hypertrophy and a right axis deviation.
• *Echocardiography* may disclose increased left ventricular muscle thickness, coexisting abnormalities, and the coarctation site.
• *Cardiac catheterization* allows evaluation of collateral circulation and measurement of pressure in the right and left ventricles and the ascending and descending aortas (on both sides of the obstruction). When combined with *aortography,* catheterization locates the site and extent of coarctation. This procedure is performed only to identify associated abnormalities in infants with left ventricular failure.

Treatment
For an infant with left ventricular failure caused by coarctation of the aorta, treatment consists of medical management with prostaglandins, diuretics, and digoxin. Although most patients require surgery, the timing may be debatable. Most doctors recommend that surgery be done early. The procedure may involve end-to-end anastomosis or subclavian flap angioplasty. If the narrowed segment is long, the doctor may use a tubular graft, patch, or bypass conduit.

Nursing diagnoses
• Activity intolerance
• Altered parenting
• Decreased cardiac output
• Fatigue
• Knowledge deficit
• Risk for infection

Nursing interventions
• When coarctation in an infant requires rapid digitalization, monitor his vital signs closely, and watch for digitalis toxicity (poor feeding, vomiting).
• Balance intake and output carefully, especially if the infant is receiving diuretics and restricted fluids.

• If the infant can't maintain the proper body temperature, regulate environmental temperature with an overbed warmer.
• Monitor blood glucose levels to detect possible hypoglycemia, which may develop as glycogen stores decline.
   After corrective surgery:
• Monitor blood pressure closely, using an intra-arterial line. Take pressures on all extremities.
• Monitor fluid intake and output.
• If the patient develops hypertension and requires nitroprusside or trimethaphan, administer it as ordered, by continuous I.V. infusion. Use an infusion pump. Watch for severe hypotension, and regulate the dosage carefully.
• Check blood cyanide levels if the patient requires sustained nitroprusside therapy.
• Provide pain relief, and encourage a gradual increase in activity.
• Offer the parents emotional support.

Patient teaching
• Explain the disorder and appropriate diagnostic procedures and treatments. Tell parents what to expect after the surgery.
• For an older child, assess blood pressure in his extremities regularly, explain any exercise restrictions, and teach the family how to use blood pressure equipment for home monitoring.
• If an older child needs to continue antihypertensives after surgery, teach him and his parents about them; stress the need to take medications properly and to watch for adverse reactions.
• Stress the importance of continued endocarditis prophylaxis.

PATENT DUCTUS ARTERIOSUS
The ductus arteriosus is a blood vessel that connects the pulmonary artery to the descending aorta during fetal development. Normally, the ductus closes within days or weeks after birth. Its closure routes oxygenated blood to the body and unoxygenated blood to the lungs.

In patent ductus arteriosus, the lumen of the ductus remains open after birth. (See *A look at patent ductus arteriosus.*) This abnormal opening allows blood to shunt left to right from the aorta to the pulmonary artery. The result is recirculation of oxygenated arterial blood through the lungs.

The amount of blood shunted through the ductus depends on the relative resistances of pulmonary and systemic vasculature, and on the size of the ductus itself. The left atrium and left ventricle must accommodate increased pulmonary venous return, which raises left ventricular filling pressure and work load and could lead to left ventricular failure.

Patent ductus arteriosus typically affects twice as many females as males. When it occurs with rubella, however, it affects both sexes in equal numbers. It's the most common congenital heart defect found in adults; symptoms of pulmonary vascular disease appear by age 40. The prognosis is good if the shunt is small or can be surgically repaired.

Causes
Failure of the ductus to close—most prevalent in premature infants and those born at high altitudes—probably stems from abnormal oxygenation or from the relaxant action of prostaglandin E, which prevents the ductal spasm and contracture needed for closure. Patent ductus arteriosus may be familial, or it may have no known cause. It commonly accompanies rubella syndrome and may be associated with other congenital defects, such as coarctation of the aorta, a ventricular septal defect, and pulmonary and aortic stenoses.

Complications
In its final stages, untreated patent ductus arteriosus may advance to intractable—possibly fatal—left ventricular failure. The left-to-right shunt leads to chronic pulmonary artery hypertension that becomes fixed and unreactive. Children typically experience respiratory distress.

Assessment findings
Inspection may reveal a very slender infant, possibly with signs of failure to thrive, slow motor development, and a left chest deformity. An infant with a large shunt (especially a premature infant) may have dyspnea, tachycardia, edema, and other signs of left ventricular failure from the large volume of blood shunted to the lungs and the increased left ventricular work load.

Most children with patent ductus arteriosus have only cardiac signs and symptoms. But some may be physically underdeveloped, tire easily, and have a history of frequent respiratory tract infections.

An adult with undetected patent ductus arteriosus typically will present with signs and symptoms of pulmonary vascular disease and, by age 40, may tire easily and complain of dyspnea on exertion. About 1 in 10 adults may have signs of infective endocarditis.

In nearly all children with this anomaly, auscultation reveals the classic machinery murmur (Gibson murmur), best heard at the base of the heart, second left

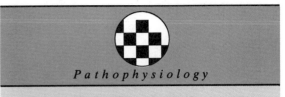

Pathophysiology

A LOOK AT PATENT DUCTUS ARTERIOSUS

This anomaly occurs when the ductus arteriosus—a tubular connection that shunts blood away from the fetus's pulmonary circulation—fails to close after birth. Blood then shunts from the aorta to the pulmonary artery.

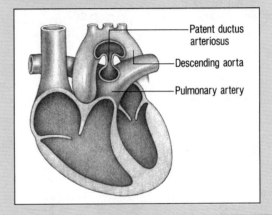

Patent ductus arteriosus

Descending aorta

Pulmonary artery

intercostal space under the left clavicle. (See *Auscultating for patent ductus arteriosus,* page 524.)

Palpation may reveal a thrill at the left sternal border and a prominent left ventricular impulse. Peripheral arterial pulses will be bounding (Corrigan's pulse). Pulse pressure will widen from a rise in systolic blood pressure and also from a drop in diastolic pressure.

Diagnostic tests
• *Chest X-rays* show increased pulmonary vascular markings, prominent pulmonary arteries, and enlargement of the left ventricle and the aorta. Results vary with the size of the shunt.
• *Electrocardiography (ECG)* results may be normal or may indicate left ventricular hypertrophy, left atrial enlargement and, in pulmonary vascular disease, biventricular hypertrophy.
• *Echocardiography* detects and helps estimate the size of a shunt. It also reveals an enlarged left atrium and left ventricle, or right ventricular hypertrophy from pulmonary vascular disease.

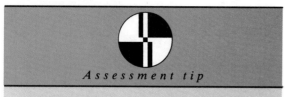

Assessment tip

AUSCULTATING FOR PATENT DUCTUS ARTERIOSUS

To detect patent ductus arteriosus, auscultate the base of the heart at the second left intercostal space under the left clavicle. You'll hear systolic clicks (C) and a continuous murmur during systole and diastole, not necessarily through the entire cycle but through the second sound in a crescendo-decrescendo manner, as shown below.

Normal

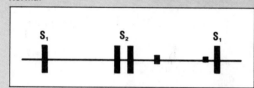

Patent ductus arteriosus

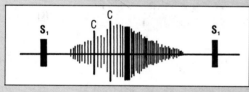

• *Cardiac catheterization* shows a pulmonary arterial oxygen content higher than the right ventricular content because of the influx of aortic blood. Increased pulmonary artery pressure indicates a large shunt or, if it exceeds systemic arterial pressure, severe pulmonary vascular disease. Catheterization allows calculation of the blood volume crossing the ductus and can rule out associated cardiac defects. Dye injection definitively demonstrates patent ductus arteriosus. This test is not used routinely to diagnose this disorder because of the risk involved.

Treatment

Asymptomatic infants require no immediate treatment. Those with left ventricular failure require fluid restriction, diuretics, and digitalis until surgery can be performed. If signs and symptoms are mild, surgical correction is usually delayed until the infant is 1 year old. Before surgery, the child requires antibiotics to protect against infective endocarditis. Experimental treatments include cardiac catheterization to deposit a plug or umbrella in the ductus, or administration of indomethacin I.V. to induce the ductus to spasm and close.

Nursing diagnoses
• Activity intolerance
• Altered growth and development
• Altered parenting
• Altered tissue perfusion
• Decreased cardiac output
• Fatigue
• Impaired gas exchange
• Ineffective breathing pattern
• Knowledge deficit
• Risk for infection

Nursing interventions

• Watch carefully for signs of patent ductus arteriosus in all premature infants. Be alert for respiratory distress symptoms that stem from left ventricular failure; they may develop rapidly in a premature infant. Frequently assess vital signs, ECG tracings, serum electrolyte levels, and fluid intake and output. Record the infant's response to diuretics and other therapy. Watch for signs of digitalis toxicity (such as poor feeding and vomiting).
• Ensure that the infant receives adequate nutrition to optimize growth and development.
• If the infant receives indomethacin to help close the ductus, watch for possible adverse reactions to the drug, such as diarrhea, jaundice, bleeding, and renal dysfunction.
• Before surgery, carefully explain all treatments and tests to the parents. Include the child in your explanations, if possible. Arrange for the child and the parents to meet the intensive care unit staff. Tell them about expected I.V. lines, monitoring equipment, and postoperative procedures.
• Immediately after surgery, the child may have a central venous pressure catheter and an arterial line in place. Carefully assess vital signs, fluid intake and output, and arterial and venous pressures. Provide pain relief as needed.

Patient teaching

• Before discharge, review what you've told the parents about activity restrictions based on the child's tolerance and energy levels. Advise parents not to become overprotective as their child's tolerance for physical activity increases.

• Stress the need for regular medical follow-up examinations. Tell the parents to inform any doctor who treats their child about his history of surgery for patent ductus arteriosus—even if the child is being treated for an unrelated medical problem.
• Teach the parents the importance of prophylactic antibiotics to reduce the child's risk of bacterial endocarditis.
• Urge the parents to seek medical attention whenever their child develops signs of infection, such as a sore throat, a cold, the flu, or an earache.

TETRALOGY OF FALLOT

This cardiac defect is really four defects that occur together: a ventricular septal defect, infundibular stenosis (possibly with pulmonary valve stenosis), right ventricular hypertrophy, and dextroposition of the aorta, which overrides the ventricular septal defect. (See *Defects in tetralogy of Fallot.*)

The degree of pulmonary stenosis, interacting with the ventricular septal defect's size and location, determines the clinical and hemodynamic effects of this complex anomaly. Blood may shunt left to right or right to left, depending on the defect's configuration.

Usually, the ventricular septal defect lies in the outflow tract of the right ventricle and is large enough to equalize right and left ventricular pressures. However, the ratio of systemic vascular resistance to pulmonary stenosis affects how much blood flows across the defect and the direction in which it flows.

When blood shunts right to left through the ventricular septal defect, unoxygenated blood mixes with oxygenated blood, which leads to cyanosis.

When right ventricular outflow is severely obstructed, blood flows right to left, which decreases arterial oxygen saturation and leads to cyanosis, reduced pulmonary blood flow, and hypoplasia of all the pulmonary vessels. Increased right ventricular pressure causes right ventricular hypertrophy.

Milder forms of pulmonary stenosis result in a left-to-right shunt or no shunt at all.

About 15% of infants born with a congenital heart defect have tetralogy of Fallot. It's equally common in males and females. Sometimes it coexists with other congenital heart defects, such as patent ductus arteriosus or an atrial septal defect. Before surgical techniques were available to correct this defect, about one-third of affected children died in infancy.

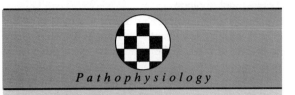

Pathophysiology

DEFECTS IN TETRALOGY OF FALLOT

This four-part complex includes a ventricular septal defect, an overriding (dextroposition of) aorta, infundibular pulmonary stenosis, and right ventricular hypertrophy. The severity of these defects influences hemodynamic changes. Milder defects may produce a left-to-right shunt. More severe defects produce a right-to-left shunt, through which unoxygenated blood directly enters the aorta.

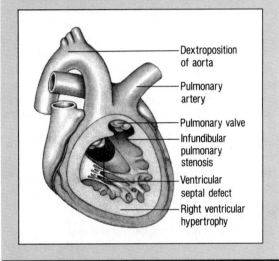

- Dextroposition of aorta
- Pulmonary artery
- Pulmonary valve
- Infundibular pulmonary stenosis
- Ventricular septal defect
- Right ventricular hypertrophy

Causes
Tetralogy of Fallot stems from embryonic hypoplasia of the right ventricle's outflow tract. No one knows what causes that hypoplasia. However, the defect has been associated with fetal alcohol syndrome and maternal ingestion of thalidomide during pregnancy.

Complications
Patients with tetralogy of Fallot risk developing cerebral abscess, pulmonary thrombosis, venous thrombosis or cerebral embolism, and infective endocarditis.

Affected females who live to childbearing age face an increased incidence of spontaneous abortion and premature birth and are more likely to have infants of low birth weight.

Assessment findings

Cyanosis is a hallmark of this defect. It usually becomes evident within a few months after birth; however, it may be present at birth if the infant has severe pulmonary stenosis.

Infants who normally appear pink may have hypercyanotic spells when they cry. They also may have tachycardia, tachypnea, dyspnea and, possibly, a period of unconsciousness or seizures.

After about age 3 months, inspection may reveal clubbing of the fingers and toes.

Older children may experience varying degrees of exercise intolerance and cyanosis, dyspnea on exertion, growth retardation, and eating difficulties. They commonly assume a squatting position after such exercise as walking or running. Signs and symptoms probably result from increased right-to-left shunting caused by spasm of the right ventricular outflow tract, increased systemic venous return, or decreased systemic arterial resistance.

Auscultation may detect an apical click, a loud (Grade 4 to 6) systolic murmur (best heard along the left sternal border), which may diminish or obscure the pulmonary component of S_2. In a patient who also has a large patent ductus, the continuous murmur of the ductus obscures the systolic murmur.

Palpation may reveal an obvious right ventricular impulse and a systolic thrill at the left sternal border that transmits to the suprasternal notch but not usually to the carotids. The inferior sternum appears prominent.

Diagnostic tests

• *Chest X-rays* may demonstrate normal or decreased pulmonary vascular markings, depending on the severity of the pulmonary obstruction. It also may reveal a large aorta and a normal-size heart with right ventricular enlargement in the lateral view. This configuration gives the cardiac silhouette a boot-shaped appearance. The main pulmonary artery segment on the left border of the heart may be diminished or have a concave appearance.
• *Electrocardiography* shows right ventricular hypertrophy with upright T waves in the right chest leads. These results are often associated with peaked P waves, right axis deviation and, possibly, right atrial hypertrophy.
• *Echocardiography* identifies a septal override of the aorta, the ventricular septal defect, and infundibular pulmonary stenosis. It also reveals the right ventricle's hypertrophied walls.
• *Laboratory tests* reveal diminished arterial oxygen saturation and polycythemia (hematocrit may be more than 60%) if the cyanosis is severe and long-standing. This condition predisposes the patient to thrombosis.

• *Cardiac catheterization* confirms the diagnosis by displaying pulmonary stenosis, the ventricular septal defect, and the overriding aorta. It also rules out other cyanotic heart defects and measures the degree of oxygen saturation in aortic blood.

Treatment

During cyanotic spells, oxygenation will improve if the patient assumes the knee-chest position and receives oxygen and morphine. Propranolol may prevent cyanotic episodes. Surgery that joins the subclavian artery to the pulmonary artery (Blalock-Taussig operation) may enhance blood flow to the lungs, reducing hypoxia.

Supportive measures include antibiotics administered before, during, and after dental treatments or surgery. Phlebotomy may also be needed in children with polycythemia.

Surgery to relieve pulmonary stenosis and close the ventricular septal defect requires cardiopulmonary bypass with hypothermia (to decrease oxygen utilization during surgery, especially in young children). Surgery is necessary when progressive hypoxia and polycythemia impair the patient's quality of life, usually before age 2.

Nursing diagnoses

• Altered growth and development
• Altered parenting
• Decreased cardiac output
• Impaired gas exchange
• Ineffective family coping
• Risk for injury

Nursing interventions

• Because of the right-to-left shunt through the ventricular septal defect, treat I.V. lines like arterial lines. A clot dislodged from a catheter tip in a vein can cross the shunt and cause cerebral embolism. The same thing can happen if air enters the venous lines.
• Allow parents time to grieve when they learn of their child's diagnosis. Encourage them to discuss their concerns and their feelings. Help them to deal with guilt if they experience it.
• Encourage parent-child bonding as much as possible.
  After surgery:
• If the child has undergone the Blalock-Taussig operation, don't use the arm on the operative side for measuring blood pressure, inserting I.V. lines, or drawing blood samples. Blood perfusion on that side diminishes greatly until collateral circulation develops. Note this restriction on the child's chart and at his bedside.

• Watch for right bundle-branch block or more serious disturbances of atrioventricular (AV) conduction and for ventricular ectopic beats.

• Be alert for other postoperative complications, such as bleeding, left ventricular failure, and respiratory failure. Transient left ventricular failure is common and may require treatment with digoxin and diuretics.

• Monitor left atrial pressure directly. A pulmonary artery catheter may be used to check central venous and pulmonary artery pressures.

• Check color and vital signs frequently. Obtain arterial blood gas measurements regularly to assess oxygenation. Suction as needed to prevent atelectasis and pneumonia. Monitor mechanical ventilation.

• Monitor and record intake and output accurately.

• If AV block develops with a low heart rate, a temporary external pacemaker may be necessary.

• For inadequate blood pressure or cardiac output, administer catecholamines as ordered by continuous I.V. infusion.

• To decrease left ventricular work load, administer nitroprusside, as ordered.

• Provide analgesics as needed.

• Keep the parents informed about their child's progress.

Patient teaching

• Explain tetralogy of Fallot to the parents. Inform them that their child will set his own exercise limits and will know when to rest. Make sure they understand that their child can engage in physical activity. Advise them not to be overprotective.

• Repeat your teaching information, if necessary, because learning is difficult in times of great stress.

• Teach the parents to recognize serious hypoxic spells, which can cause dramatically increased cyanosis; deep, sighing respirations; and loss of consciousness. Tell them to report such spells immediately. Emergency treatment may be necessary.

• After discharge, the child may require digoxin, diuretics, and other drugs. Stress the importance of complying with the prescribed regimen, and make sure the parents know how and when to administer the medications.

• Teach the parents to watch for signs of digitalis toxicity (anorexia, nausea, vomiting).

• To prevent infective endocarditis and other infections, warn the parents to keep their child away from people with known infections. Urge them to encourage good dental hygiene, and tell them to watch for ear, nose, and throat infections and dental caries, all of which necessitate immediate treatment. The child will still require

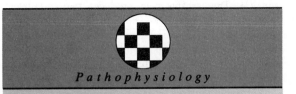

Pathophysiology

A LOOK AT TRANSPOSITION OF THE GREAT ARTERIES

In this anomaly, the aorta arises from the right ventricle and the pulmonary artery from the left ventricle, preventing the pulmonary and systemic circulations from mixing. Without associated defects that allow these circulatory systems to mix—such as patent ductus arteriosus or a septal defect—the neonate will die.

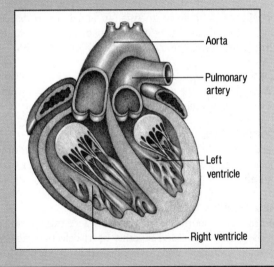

prophylactic antibiotics; tell parents to be sure the child completes the prescribed regimen.

• If the child requires medical attention for an unrelated problem, tell parents to inform the doctor immediately of the child's history of tetralogy of Fallot. Any treatment must take this defect into consideration.

TRANSPOSITION OF THE GREAT ARTERIES

In this congenital heart defect, the aorta and the pulmonary artery—known as the great vessels—are reversed from their normal positions. (See *A look at transposition of the great arteries.*) The aorta arises from the right ventricle, and the pulmonary artery from the left ventricle. This arrangement produces two circulatory systems (pulmonary and systemic). Oxygenated blood entering the left side of the heart returns to the lungs by the transposed pulmonary artery. Unoxygenated blood entering the right side of the heart returns to systemic circulation by the transposed aorta.

The two circulatory systems communicate somewhat only because of additional cardiac defects. In infants who have a condition called isolated transposition, oxygenated and unoxygenated blood mix slightly at the patent foramen ovale and the patent ductus arteriosus. In infants with other cardiac defects, blood may mix to a greater degree.

Transposition accounts for up to 5% of all congenital heart defects and commonly coexists with other congenital heart defects, such as a ventricular septal defect with or without pulmonary stenosis, an atrial septal defect, and patent ductus arteriosus. Transposition is two to three times more common in males than in females.

Causes
Transposition of the great arteries results from faulty embryonic development, but the cause is unknown.

Complications
Serious complications may include chronic heart failure, poor oxygenation, arrhythmias, and right ventricular failure.

Assessment findings
Within a few hours of birth, neonates with transposition of the great arteries and no other heart defects typically develop cyanosis and tachypnea that worsen with crying. After several days or weeks, such infants usually develop signs of heart failure (gallop rhythm, tachycardia, dyspnea, hepatomegaly, and cardiomegaly).

S_2 will be louder than normal because the aorta is transposed in an anterior direction and lies just behind the sternum; usually, however, no murmur can be heard during the first few days after birth. Associated defects (a ventricular septal defect, an atrial septal defect, or patent ductus arteriosus) cause their typical murmurs and may reduce cyanosis. However, they may cause other complications (especially severe heart failure). A ventricular septal defect with pulmonary stenosis produces a characteristic murmur and severe cyanosis.

As infants with this defect mature, cyanosis becomes their most prominent abnormality. However, they also develop exercise intolerance, fatigue, coughing, clubbing of the fingers, and — if they have a septal defect, patent ductus arteriosus, or pulmonary stenosis — more pronounced murmurs.

Diagnostic tests
• *Chest X-rays* are normal in the first days after birth. Within days or weeks, however, right atrial and right ventricular enlargement cause the heart to take on a characteristic egg shape. X-rays also reveal a narrow mediastinum and increased pulmonary vascular markings except when the infant also has pulmonary stenosis.
• *Electrocardiography* typically reveals right axis deviation and right ventricular hypertrophy, but results may be normal in a neonate.
• *Echocardiography* displays the reversed positions of the aorta and the pulmonary artery. Because of aortic valve displacement, it also records simultaneous echoes from the semilunar valves. It may also reveal other cardiac defects.
• *Cardiac catheterization* reveals decreased oxygen saturation in left ventricular blood and aortic blood; increased right atrial, right ventricular, and pulmonary artery oxygen saturation; and right ventricular systolic pressure equal to systemic pressure. Dye injection shows the transposed arteries and any other cardiac defects.
• *Arterial blood gas (ABG) measurements* indicate hypoxia and secondary metabolic acidosis.

Treatment
An infant with transposition of the great arteries may undergo atrial balloon septostomy (Rashkind procedure) during cardiac catheterization. This procedure enlarges the patent foramen ovale, which improves oxygenation by allowing more of the pulmonary and systemic blood to mix. Afterward, digoxin and diuretics can lessen heart failure until the infant can withstand corrective surgery (usually before age 1).

One of three surgical procedures can correct transposition. The *Mustard procedure* replaces the atrial septum with a Dacron or pericardial partition or baffle that channels systemic venous blood to the pulmonary artery. The pulmonary artery then carries the blood to the lungs for oxygenation. Oxygenated blood returning to the heart is channeled into the aorta. The *Senning procedure* accomplishes the same result by using the atrial septum to create partitions that redirect blood flow. In the arterial switch, or *Jantene procedure,* the transposed arteries are anastomosed to the correct ventricles.

Nursing diagnoses
• Activity intolerance
• Altered tissue perfusion

- Decreased cardiac output
- Fatigue
- Fluid volume excess
- Impaired gas exchange
- Risk for infection

Nursing interventions
- Explain cardiac catheterization and all necessary procedures to the parents. Offer them emotional support.
- Monitor the patient's vital signs, ABG measurements, urine output, and central venous pressure. Watch for signs of heart failure. Give digoxin and I.V. fluids as ordered, being careful to avoid fluid overload.
- Before corrective surgery, monitor ABG measurements, acid-base balance, intake and output, and vital signs.

  After corrective surgery:
- Monitor cardiac output by checking blood pressure, skin color, heart rate, urine output, central venous and left atrial pressures, and level of consciousness. Notify the doctor of abnormalities or changes.
- Monitor ABG measurements.
- Monitor the patient closely for supraventricular conduction blocks and arrhythmias. Watch for signs of atrioventricular blocks, atrial arrhythmias, and faulty sinoatrial function.
- After the Mustard or Senning procedure, watch for signs of baffle obstruction, such as marked facial edema.

Patient teaching
- Teach the parents to recognize signs of heart failure and digoxin toxicity (poor feeding, vomiting). Stress the importance of regular checkups to monitor cardiovascular status.
- Teach the parents to protect their infant from infection and to give prophylactic antibiotics.
- Tell the parents to let their child develop normally. They need not restrict activities; he'll set his own limits.
- If the patient is scheduled for surgery, explain the procedure to the parents (and the child, if he is old enough). Teach them about the intensive care unit, and introduce them to the staff. Also explain postoperative care.
- Encourage the parents to help their child assume new activity levels and become independent. Teach them about postoperative antibiotic prophylaxis for infective endocarditis.

CARDIAC DISORDERS

These disorders include inflammatory, valvular, and degenerative conditions, and cardiac complications. In inflammatory conditions (myocarditis, endocarditis, pericarditis, and rheumatic heart disease), scar formation and otherwise normal healing processes can cause debilitating structural damage. Valvular disorders result in stenosis (tissue thickening that narrows the valvular opening) or insufficiency (incomplete valve closure). Degenerative disorders (hypertension, coronary artery disease, myocardial infarction, heart failure, cardiomyopathies, and idiopathic hypertrophic subaortic stenosis) are the most common cardiovascular ailments. Cardiac complications include shock, ventricular aneurysm, cardiac tamponade, and arrhythmias.

MYOCARDITIS
A focal or diffuse inflammation of the myocardium, myocarditis typically is uncomplicated and self-limiting. It may be acute or chronic and can occur at any age. In many patients, myocarditis fails to produce specific cardiovascular symptoms or electrocardiogram (ECG) abnormalities. Recovery usually is spontaneous and without residual defects.

Occasionally, myocarditis may become serious and induce myofibril degeneration, right and left ventricular failure with cardiomegaly, and arrhythmias.

Causes
Myocarditis may result from any of the following:
- viruses—the most common causes in the United States and western Europe—including coxsackievirus A and B and, possibly, poliomyelitis, influenza, rubeola, rubella, human immunodeficiency virus, adenoviruses, and echoviruses
- bacteria, including diphtheria, tuberculosis, typhoid fever, tetanus, Lyme disease, and staphylococcal, pneumococcal, and gonococcal bacteria
- hypersensitive immune reactions, such as acute rheumatic fever and postcardiotomy syndrome
- radiation therapy, especially large doses to the chest during treatment of lung or breast cancer
- chemical poisons, such as chronic alcoholism
- parasitic infections, especially toxoplasmosis and South American trypanosomiasis (Chagas' disease) in infants and immunosuppressed adults
- helminthic infections, such as trichinosis.

The cause of giant cell myocarditis, a rare type of myocarditis, is unknown.

Complications

Occasionally, myocarditis is complicated by left ventricular failure. Rarely, it leads to cardiomyopathy. Sometimes myocarditis recurs or produces chronic valvulitis (when it results from rheumatic fever), cardiomyopathy, arrhythmias, or thromboembolism.

Assessment findings

The history commonly reveals a recent upper respiratory tract infection with fever, viral pharyngitis, or tonsillitis. The patient may complain of nonspecific symptoms, such as fatigue, dyspnea, palpitations, persistent tachycardia, and persistent fever, all of which reflect the accompanying systemic infection. Occasionally, the patient may complain of a mild, continuous pressure or soreness in the chest. This pain is unlike the recurring, stress-related pain of angina pectoris.

Auscultation usually reveals S_3 and S_4 gallops, a muffled S_1, possibly a murmur of mitral regurgitation (from papillary muscle dysfunction) and, if the patient has pericarditis, a pericardial friction rub. If the patient has left ventricular failure, you may notice pulmonary congestion, dyspnea, and resting or exertional tachycardia disproportionate to the degree of fever.

Diagnostic tests

Endomyocardial biopsy confirms a myocarditis diagnosis. The following test results can support the diagnosis:
• *Cardiac enzyme levels,* including creatine phosphokinase (CPK), CPK-MB, serum aspartate aminotransferase (formerly SGOT), and lactate dehydrogenase, are elevated.
• *White blood cell count* and *erythrocyte sedimentation rate* are elevated.
• *Antibody titers* are elevated, such as antistreptolysin-O titer in rheumatic fever.
• *Electrocardiography* typically shows diffuse ST-segment and T-wave abnormalities as in pericarditis, conduction defects (prolonged PR interval), and other ventricular and supraventricular ectopic arrhythmias.
• *Cultures* of stool, throat, pharyngeal washings, or other body fluids may identify the causative bacteria or virus.

Treatment

For most patients, treatment includes anti-infectives for the underlying causative infection, modified bed rest to decrease the heart's work load, and careful management of complications. Left ventricular failure requires activity restriction to minimize myocardial oxygen consumption, supplemental oxygen therapy, sodium restriction, diuretics to decrease fluid retention, and digitalis compounds to increase myocardial contractility. However, these compounds must be administered carefully because some patients with myocarditis may show a paradoxical sensitivity even to small doses.

Arrhythmias necessitate prompt but cautious administration of antiarrhythmics, such as quinidine or procainamide, to depress myocardial irritability. Thromboembolism requires anticoagulant therapy.

Treatment with corticosteroids or other immunosuppressants is controversial and therefore limited to combating life-threatening complications, such as intractable heart failure.

Nursing diagnoses

• Activity intolerance
• Altered role performance
• Anxiety
• Decreased cardiac output
• Diversional activity deficit
• Impaired gas exchange

Nursing interventions

• Stress the importance of bed rest. Assist the patient with bathing, if necessary. Provide a bedside commode because this method puts less stress on the heart than using a bedpan. Offer diversional activities that are physically undemanding.
• To reduce anxiety, allow the patient to express his concerns about the effects of activity restrictions on his responsibilities and routines. Reassure him that the restrictions are temporary.
• Assess cardiovascular status frequently, watching for signs of left ventricular failure (dyspnea, hypotension, and tachycardia). Check for changes in cardiac rhythm or conduction.
• Administer oxygen and evaluate arterial blood gas levels, as needed, to ensure adequate oxygenation.
• Observe for signs of digitalis toxicity (anorexia, nausea, vomiting, blurred vision, cardiac arrhythmias) and for complicating factors that may potentiate toxicity, such as electrolyte imbalance and hypoxia.
• Administer parenteral anti-infectives, as ordered.

Patient teaching

• Teach the patient about anti-infective drugs. Stress the importance of taking the drug and restricting his activities for as long as the doctor orders.

• If the patient will be taking digitalis at home, teach him to check his pulse for 1 full minute before taking the dose. Direct him to withhold the dose and notify the doctor if his heart rate falls below the predetermined rate (usually 60 beats/minute).

• During recovery, recommend that the patient resume normal activities slowly and avoid competitive sports.

ENDOCARDITIS

An infection of the endocardium, heart valves, or cardiac prosthesis, endocarditis results from bacterial or fungal invasion.

In infective endocarditis, fibrin and platelets cluster on valve tissue and engulf circulating bacteria or fungi. This produces vegetation, which, in turn, may cover the valve surfaces, causing deformities and destruction of valvular tissue. It may also extend to the chordae tendineae, causing them to rupture and leading to valvular insufficiency.

Sometimes vegetation forms on the endocardium, usually in areas altered by rheumatic, congenital, or syphilitic heart disease. It also may form on normal surfaces. Vegetative growth on the heart valves, endocardial lining of a heart chamber, or the endothelium of a blood vessel may embolize to the spleen, kidneys, central nervous system, and lungs.

Endocarditis can be classified as native valve endocarditis, endocarditis in I.V. drug users, and prosthetic valve endocarditis. It can be acute or subacute. Untreated, endocarditis is usually fatal. With proper treatment, however, about 70% of patients recover. The prognosis is worst when endocarditis causes severe valvular damage — leading to insufficiency and left ventricular failure — or when it involves a prosthetic valve.

Causes

Acute infective endocarditis usually results from bacteremia that follows septic thrombophlebitis, open-heart surgery involving prosthetic valves, or skin, bone, and pulmonary infections.

The most common causative organisms are group A nonhemolytic streptococci, staphylococci, and enterococci. However, almost any organism can cause endocarditis, including *Neisseria gonorrhoeae, Pseudomonas, Salmonella, Streptobacillus, Serratia marcescens,* bacteroids, *Haemophilus, Brucella, Mycobacterium,* N. *meningitidis, Listeria, Legionella,* diphtheroids, enteric gramnegative bacilli, spirochetes, rickettsiae, chlamydiae, and the fungi *Candida* and *Aspergillus.*

Subacute infective endocarditis typically occurs in people with acquired valvular or congenital cardiac lesions. It can also follow dental, genitourinary, gynecologic, and GI procedures. The most common infecting organisms are *Streptococcus viridans,* which normally inhabits the upper respiratory tract, and *Streptococcus faecalis* (enterococcus), typically found in GI and perineal flora.

Preexisting conditions can predispose a person to endocarditis (including rheumatic valvular disease), congenital heart disease, mitral valve prolapse, degenerative heart disease, calcific aortic stenosis (in elderly people), asymmetrical septal hypertrophy, Marfan syndrome, syphilitic aortic valve, I.V. drug abuse, and long-term hemodialysis with an arteriovenous shunt or fistula. However, up to 40% of affected patients have no underlying heart disease.

Complications

Typically, the heart compensates for the malfunctioning valves for years until left ventricular failure, valve stenosis or regurgitation, or myocardial erosion sets in. Also, vegetation on the valves can cause embolic debris to lodge in the small vasculature of the visceral tissue.

Assessment findings

The patient may report a predisposing condition and complain of nonspecific symptoms, such as weakness, fatigue, weight loss, anorexia, arthralgia, night sweats, and an intermittent fever that may recur for weeks.

Inspection may reveal petechiae of the skin (especially common on the upper anterior trunk) and the buccal, pharyngeal, or conjunctival mucosa, and splinter hemorrhages under the nails. Rarely, you may see Osler's nodes (tender, raised, subcutaneous lesions on the fingers or toes), Roth's spots (hemorrhagic areas with white centers on the retina), and Janeway lesions (purplish macules on the palms or soles). Clubbing of the fingers may be present in patients with long-standing disease.

Auscultation may reveal a murmur in all patients except those with early acute endocarditis and I.V. drug users with tricuspid valve infection. The murmur is usually loud and regurgitant, which is typical of the underlying rheumatic or congenital heart disease. A murmur that changes suddenly or a new murmur that develops in the presence of fever is a classic physical sign of endocarditis.

Percussion and palpation may reveal splenomegaly in long-standing disease.

In patients who have developed left ventricular failure, your assessment may reveal dyspnea, tachycardia, and bibasilar crackles.

In 12% to 35% of patients with subacute endocarditis, embolization from vegetating lesions or diseased valve tissue may produce typical characteristics of splenic, renal, cerebral, or pulmonary infarction, or peripheral vascular occlusion.

• Splenic infarction causes pain in the upper left quadrant, radiating to the left shoulder, and abdominal rigidity.
• Renal infarction causes hematuria, pyuria, flank pain, and decreased urine output.
• Cerebral infarction causes hemiparesis, aphasia, and other neurologic deficits.
• Pulmonary infarction causes cough, pleuritic pain, pleural friction rub, dyspnea, and hemoptysis. These signs are most common in right-sided endocarditis, which typically occurs among I.V. drug abusers and after cardiac surgery.
• Peripheral vascular occlusion causes numbness and tingling in an arm, leg, finger, or toe, or signs of impending peripheral gangrene.

Diagnostic tests
Three or more blood cultures during a 24- to 48-hour period identify the causative organism in up to 90% of patients. The remaining 10% may have negative blood cultures, possibly suggesting fungal or difficult-to-diagnose infections, such as *Haemophilus parainfluenzae*. Other abnormal but nonspecific laboratory results include:
• normal or elevated white blood cell count and differential
• abnormal histiocytes (macrophages)
• normocytic, normochromic anemia (in subacute infective endocarditis)
• elevated erythrocyte sedimentation rate and serum creatinine levels
• positive serum rheumatoid factor in about half of all patients with endocarditis after the disease is present for 6 weeks
• proteinuria and microscopic hematuria.

Echocardiography may identify valvular damage in up to 80% of patients with native valve disease. An electrocardiogram reading may show atrial fibrillation and other arrhythmias that accompany valvular disease.

Treatment
The goal of treatment is to eradicate all of the infecting organisms from the vegetation. Therapy should start promptly and continue over several weeks. Selection of an anti-infective drug is based on the infecting organism and sensitivity studies. Although blood cultures are negative in 10% to 20% of the subacute cases, the doctor may want to determine the *probable* infecting organism. I.V. antibiotic therapy usually lasts about 4 to 6 weeks.

Supportive treatment includes bed rest, aspirin for fever and aches, and sufficient fluid intake. Severe valvular damage, especially aortic regurgitation or infection of a cardiac prosthesis, may require corrective surgery if refractory heart failure develops or if an infected prosthetic valve must be replaced.

Nursing diagnoses
• Activity intolerance
• Altered role performance
• Decreased cardiac output
• Diversional activity deficit
• Impaired gas exchange
• Risk for injury

Nursing interventions
• Stress the importance of bed rest. Assist the patient with bathing, if necessary. Provide a bedside commode because this method puts less stress on the heart than using a bedpan. Offer diversional activities that are physically undemanding.
• To reduce anxiety, allow the patient to express his concerns about the effects of activity restrictions on his responsibilities and routines. Reassure him that the restrictions are temporary.
• Before giving antibiotics, obtain a patient history of allergies. Administer antibiotics on time to maintain consistent drug levels in the blood.
• Observe for signs of infiltration or inflammation at the venipuncture site, a possible complication of long-term I.V. administration. To reduce the risk of this complication, rotate venous access sites.
• Assess cardiovascular status frequently, and watch for signs of left ventricular failure, such as dyspnea, hypotension, tachycardia, tachypnea, crackles, and weight gain. Check for changes in cardiac rhythm or conduction.
• Administer oxygen and evaluate arterial blood gas values, as needed, to ensure adequate oxygenation.
• Watch for signs of embolization (hematuria, pleuritic chest pain, upper left quadrant pain, or paresis), a common occurrence during the first 3 months of treatment. Tell the patient to watch for and report these signs, which may indicate impending peripheral vascular occlusion or splenic, renal, cerebral, or pulmonary infarction.

• Monitor the patient's renal status (including blood urea nitrogen levels, creatinine clearance, and urine output) to check for signs of renal emboli and drug toxicity.

Patient teaching
• Teach the patient about the anti-infectives he'll continue to take. Stress the importance of taking the medication and restricting his activities for as long as the doctor orders.
• Tell the patient to watch closely for fever, anorexia, and other signs of relapse about 2 weeks after treatment stops.
• Make sure the susceptible patient understands the need for prophylactic antibiotics before, during, and after dental work, childbirth, and genitourinary, GI, or gynecologic procedures.
• Teach the patient how to recognize symptoms of endocarditis, and tell him to notify the doctor immediately if such symptoms occur.

PERICARDITIS
The pericardium is the fibroserous sac that envelops, supports, and protects the heart. Inflammation of this sac is called pericarditis.

This condition occurs in acute and chronic forms. The acute form can be fibrinous or effusive, with serous, purulent, or hemorrhagic exudate. The chronic form (called constrictive pericarditis) is characterized by dense fibrous pericardial thickening. (See *Understanding pericarditis*, page 534.)

The prognosis depends on the underlying cause but typically is good in acute pericarditis unless constriction occurs.

Causes
Common causes of this disorder include:
• bacterial, fungal, or viral infection (infectious pericarditis)
• neoplasms (primary or metastatic from lungs, breasts, or other organs)
• high-dose radiation to the chest
• uremia
• hypersensitivity or autoimmune disease, such as acute rheumatic fever (the most common cause of pericarditis in children), systemic lupus erythematosus, and rheumatoid arthritis
• drugs, such as hydralazine or procainamide
• idiopathic factors (most common in acute pericarditis)
• postcardiac injury, such as myocardial infarction (which later causes an autoimmune reaction known as

Dressler's syndrome in the pericardium). Other types of postcardiac injury include trauma and surgery that leaves the pericardium intact but allows blood to leak into the pericardial cavity.

Less common causes of pericarditis include aortic aneurysm with pericardial leakage, and myxedema with cholesterol deposits in the pericardium.

Complications
Pericardial effusion is the major complication of acute pericarditis. If fluid accumulates rapidly, cardiac tamponade may occur, resulting in shock, cardiovascular collapse and, eventually, death.

Assessment findings
The patient's history may include an event or disease that can cause pericarditis, such as chest trauma, myocardial infarction, or recent bacterial infection.

The patient with acute pericarditis typically complains of sharp, sudden pain, usually starting over the sternum and radiating to the neck, shoulders, back, and arms. The pain is usually pleuritic, increasing with deep inspiration and decreasing when the patient sits up and leans forward. This decrease occurs because leaning forward pulls the heart away from the diaphragmatic pleurae of the lungs. The patient may complain of dyspnea.

Pericarditis can mimic the pain of myocardial infarction. However, the patient may have no pain if he has slowly developing tuberculous pericarditis or postirradiation, neoplastic, or uremic pericarditis.

Auscultation almost always reveals a pericardial friction rub, which is a grating sound heard as the heart moves. You can hear it best during forced expiration, while the patient leans forward or is on his hands and knees in bed. The rub may have up to three components that correspond to atrial systole, ventricular systole, and the rapid-filling phase of ventricular diastole.

Occasionally, the friction rub is heard only briefly or not at all. If acute pericarditis has caused very large pericardial effusions, heart sounds may be distant.

Palpation may reveal a diminished or an absent apical impulse.

Constrictive pericarditis causes the membrane to calcify and become rigid. It also causes a gradual increase in systemic venous pressure and symptoms similar to those of chronic right ventricular failure (fluid retention, ascites, hepatomegaly).

Tachycardia, an ill-defined substernal chest pain, and a feeling of fullness in the chest may indicate pericardial effusion.

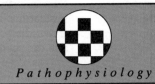

Pathophysiology

UNDERSTANDING PERICARDITIS

Pericarditis occurs when a pathogen or other substance attacks the pericardium, leading to the following events.

Inflammation

Pericardial tissue damaged by bacteria or other substances releases chemical mediators of inflammation (such as prostaglandins, histamines, bradykinins, and serotonins) into the surrounding tissue, starting the inflammatory process. Friction occurs as the inflamed pericardial layers rub against each other.

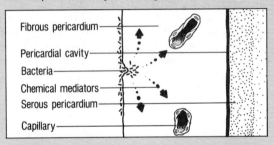

Vasodilation and clotting

Histamines and other chemical mediators cause vasodilation and increased vessel permeability. Local blood flow (hyperemia) increases. Vessel walls leak fluids and proteins (including fibrinogen) into tissues, causing extracellular edema. Clots of fibrinogen and tissue fluid form a wall, blocking tissue spaces and lymph vessels in the injured area. This wall prevents the spread of bacteria and toxins to adjoining healthy tissues.

Initial phagocytosis

Macrophages already present in the tissues begin to phagocytize the invading bacteria but usually fail to stop the infection.

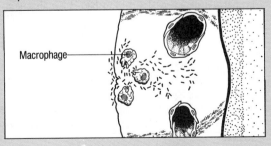

Enhanced phagocytosis

Substances released by the injured tissue stimulate neutrophil production in the bone marrow. Neutrophils then travel to the injury site through the bloodstream and join macrophages in destroying pathogens. Meanwhile, additional macrophages and monocytes migrate to the injured area and continue phagocytosis.

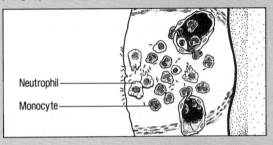

Exudation

After several days, the infected area fills with an exudate composed of necrotic tissue and dead and dying bacteria, neutrophils, and macrophages. Thinner than pus, this exudate forms until all infection ceases, creating a cavity that remains until tissue destruction stops. The contents of the cavity autolyze and are gradually reabsorbed into healthy tissue.

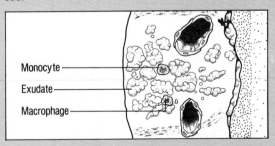

Fibrosis and scarring

As the end products of the infection slowly disappear, fibrosis and scar tissue may form. Scarring, which can be extensive, may ultimately cause heart failure if it restricts movement.

Pallor, clammy skin, hypotension, pulsus paradoxus (drop in systolic blood pressure of 15 mm Hg or greater during slow inspiration), neck vein distention, and dyspnea indicate cardiac tamponade.

Diagnostic tests

Laboratory results reflect inflammation and may identify the disorder's cause. They include the following:
• normal or elevated white blood cell count, especially in infectious pericarditis
• elevated erythrocyte sedimentation rate
• slightly elevated serum creatine phosphokinase-MB levels with associated myocarditis
• culture of pericardial fluid obtained by open surgical drainage or pericardiocentesis (which sometimes identifies a causative organism in bacterial or fungal pericarditis).

Other pertinent laboratory data include blood urea nitrogen levels to check for uremia, antistreptolysin-O titers to detect rheumatic fever, and a purified protein derivative skin test to check for tuberculosis.

Electrocardiography shows characteristic changes in acute pericarditis. They include elevated ST segments in the limb leads and most precordial leads. The QRS segments may be diminished when pericardial effusion is present. Rhythm changes may also occur, including atrial ectopic rhythms (such as atrial fibrillation) or sinus arrhythmias.

Echocardiography diagnoses pericardial effusion when it shows an echo-free space between the ventricular wall and the pericardium.

Treatment

Appropriate treatment aims to relieve symptoms, manage underlying systemic disease, and prevent or treat pericardial effusion and cardiac tamponade.

In idiopathic pericarditis, postmyocardial infarction pericarditis, and postthoracotomy pericarditis, treatment consists of bed rest as long as fever and pain persist and the administration of nonsteroidal drugs, such as aspirin and indomethacin, to relieve pain and reduce inflammation. If symptoms continue, the doctor may prescribe corticosteroids. Although they provide rapid and effective relief, corticosteroids must be used cautiously because the disorder may recur when drug therapy stops.

When infectious pericarditis results from disease of the left pleural space, mediastinal abscesses, or septicemia, the patient will require antibiotics, surgical drainage, or both. If cardiac tamponade develops, the doctor may perform emergency pericardiocentesis and may inject antibiotics directly into the pericardial sac.

Recurrent pericarditis may require partial pericardectomy, which creates a window that allows fluid to drain into the pleural space. In constrictive pericarditis, total pericardectomy may be necessary to permit the heart to fill and contract adequately. Treatment must also include management of rheumatic fever, uremia, tuberculosis, and other underlying disorders.

Nursing diagnoses
• Altered role performance
• Anxiety
• Decreased cardiac output
• Diversional activity deficit
• Ineffective breathing pattern
• Pain
• Risk for injury

Nursing interventions
• Stress the importance of bed rest. Assist the patient with bathing, if necessary. Provide a bedside commode because this method puts less stress on the heart than using a bedpan. Offer diversional activities that are physically undemanding.
• Place the patient in an upright position to relieve dyspnea and chest pain.
• Provide analgesics to relieve pain and oxygen to prevent tissue hypoxia.
• Because cardiac tamponade requires immediate treatment, keep a pericardiocentesis set handy whenever you suspect pericardial effusion.
• Assess cardiovascular status frequently, watching for signs of cardiac tamponade.
• To reduce anxiety, allow the patient to express his concerns about the effects of activity restrictions on his responsibilities and routines. Reassure him that the restrictions are temporary.
• Before giving antibiotics, obtain a patient history of allergies. Administer antibiotics on time to maintain consistent drug levels in the blood.
• Observe for signs of infiltration or inflammation at the venipuncture site, a possible complication of long-term I.V. administration. To reduce the risk of this complication, rotate venous access sites.
• Provide appropriate postoperative care, similar to that given after cardiothoracic surgery.

Patient teaching
• Explain all tests and treatments to the patient.
• If surgery will be necessary, teach the patient how to perform deep-breathing and coughing exercises before he undergoes the procedure.

• Tell the patient to resume his daily activities slowly and to schedule rest periods into his daily routine for a while.

RHEUMATIC FEVER AND RHEUMATIC HEART DISEASE

A systemic inflammatory disease of childhood, acute rheumatic fever develops after infection of the upper respiratory tract with group A beta-hemolytic streptococci.

Rheumatic fever principally involves the heart, joints, central nervous system, skin, and subcutaneous tissues. It commonly recurs.

The term rheumatic heart disease refers to the cardiac involvement of rheumatic fever—its most destructive effect. Cardiac involvement develops in up to 50% of patients and may affect the endocardium, myocardium, or pericardium during the early acute phase. It may later affect the heart valves, causing chronic valvular disease.

The extent of damage to the heart depends on where the disorder strikes. Myocarditis produces characteristic lesions called Aschoff's bodies in the acute stages, and cellular swelling and fragmentation of interstitial collagen, leading to formation of a progressively fibrotic nodule and interstitial scars. Endocarditis causes valve leaflet swelling; erosion along the lines of leaflet closure; and blood, platelet, and fibrin deposits, which form beadlike vegetation. It strikes the mitral valve most commonly in females and the aortic valve in males. In both, it affects the tricuspid valves occasionally and the pulmonary valve only rarely.

Long-term antibiotic therapy can minimize the recurrence of rheumatic fever, reducing the risks of permanent cardiac damage and valvular deformity.

Worldwide, 15 to 20 million new cases are reported each year. Although rheumatic fever tends to be familial, this tendency may merely reflect contributing environmental factors. For example, in lower socioeconomic groups, incidence is highest in children between ages 5 and 15, probably resulting from malnutrition and crowded living conditions. This disease strikes most often during cool, damp weather in the winter and early spring. In the United States, it's most common in the northern states.

Causes

Rheumatic fever appears to be a hypersensitivity reaction in which antibodies produced to combat streptococci react and produce characteristic lesions at specific tissue sites. How and why group A streptococcal infection initiates the process are unknown. Because few people infected with *Streptococcus* ever contract rheumatic fever (about 0.3%), altered host resistance probably is involved in its development or recurrence.

Complications

The mitral and aortic valves are often destroyed by rheumatic fever's long-term effects. Their malfunction leads to severe pancarditis and occasionally produces pericardial effusion and fatal heart failure. Of the patients who survive this complication, about 20% die within 10 years.

Assessment findings

Nearly all affected patients will report having a streptococcal infection a few days to 6 weeks earlier. They usually have a recent history of low-grade fever that spikes to at least 100.4° F (38° C) late in the afternoon, unexplained epistaxis, and abdominal pain.

Most patients complain of migratory joint pain (polyarthritis). Swelling, redness, and signs of effusion usually accompany such pain, which most commonly affects the knees, ankles, elbows, and hips.

If the patient has pericarditis, he may complain of sharp, sudden pain that usually starts over the sternum and radiates to the neck, shoulders, back, and arms. The pain commonly is pleuritic, increasing with deep inspiration and decreasing when the patient sits up and leans forward. (This position pulls the heart away from the diaphragmatic pleurae of the lungs.) The pain may mimic that of myocardial infarction.

A patient with heart failure caused by severe rheumatic carditis may complain of dyspnea, right upper quadrant pain, and a hacking, nonproductive cough.

Inspection may reveal skin lesions such as erythema marginatum, a nonpruritic, macular, transient rash. The lesions are red with blanched centers and well-demarcated borders. They typically appear on the trunk and extremities.

Near tendons or the bony prominences of joints, you may notice subcutaneous nodules that are firm, movable, nontender, and about 3 mm to 2 cm in diameter. They occur especially around the elbows, knuckles, wrists, and knees, and less often on the scalp and backs of the hands. These nodules persist for a few days to several weeks and, like erythema marginatum, often accompany carditis.

You may notice edema and tachypnea if the patient has left ventricular failure.

Up to 6 months after the original streptococcal infection, you may note transient chorea. Mild chorea may produce hyperirritability, a deterioration in handwriting, or inability to concentrate. Severe chorea causes purposeless, nonrepetitive, involuntary muscle spasms and speech disturbances; poor muscle coordination; and weakness. Chorea resolves with rest and causes no residual neurologic damage.

Auscultation may reveal a pericardial friction rub (a grating sound heard as the heart moves) if the patient has pericarditis. You can hear it best during forced expiration, with the patient leaning forward or on his hands and knees. Murmurs and gallops may also occur. With left ventricular failure, you may hear bibasilar crackles and a ventricular or an atrial gallop. The most common murmurs include the following:
• a systolic murmur of mitral insufficiency (high-pitched, blowing, holosystolic, loudest at apex, possibly radiating to the anterior axillary line)
• a midsystolic murmur caused by stiffening and swelling of the mitral leaflet
• occasionally, a diastolic murmur of aortic insufficiency (low-pitched, rumbling, almost inaudible). Valvular disease may eventually cause chronic valvular stenosis and insufficiency, including mitral stenosis and insufficiency and aortic insufficiency. In children, mitral insufficiency remains the major sequela of rheumatic heart disease.

Palpation may reveal a rapid pulse rate.

Diagnostic tests
No specific laboratory tests can determine the presence of rheumatic fever, but the following test results support the diagnosis:
• *White blood cell count* and *erythrocyte sedimentation rate* may be elevated (during the acute phase); blood studies show slight anemia caused by suppressed erythropoiesis during inflammation.
• *C-reactive protein* is positive (especially during acute phase).
• *Cardiac enzyme levels* may be increased in severe carditis.
• *Antistreptolysin-O titer* is elevated in 95% of patients within 2 months of onset.
• *Throat cultures* may continue to show the presence of group A streptococci; however, they usually occur in small numbers. Isolating them is difficult.
• *Electrocardiography* reveals no diagnostic changes, but 20% of patients show a prolonged PR interval.
• *Chest X-rays* show normal heart size (except with myocarditis, heart failure, and pericardial effusion).
• *Echocardiography* helps evaluate valvular damage, chamber size, ventricular function, and the presence of a pericardial effusion.

• *Cardiac catheterization* evaluates valvular damage and left ventricular function in severe cardiac dysfunction.

Treatment
Effective management eradicates the streptococcal infection, relieves symptoms, and prevents recurrence, thus reducing the chance of permanent cardiac damage. During the acute phase, treatment includes penicillin or (for patients with penicillin hypersensitivity) erythromycin. Salicylates, such as aspirin, relieve fever and minimize joint swelling and pain; if the patient has carditis or if salicylates fail to relieve pain and inflammation, the doctor may prescribe corticosteroids.

Supportive treatment requires strict bed rest for about 5 weeks during the acute phase with active carditis, followed by a progressive increase in physical activity. The increase depends on clinical and laboratory findings and the patient's response to treatment.

After the acute phase subsides, a monthly I.M. injection of penicillin G benzathine or daily doses of oral sulfadiazine or penicillin G may be used to prevent recurrence. Such preventive treatment usually continues for at least 5 years or until age 25.

Heart failure requires continued bed rest and diuretics. Severe mitral or aortic valvular dysfunction that causes persistent heart failure will require corrective surgery, such as commissurotomy (separation of the adherent, thickened leaflets of the mitral valve), valvuloplasty (inflation of a balloon within a valve), or valve replacement (with prosthetic valve). Corrective valvular surgery seldom is necessary before late adolescence.

Nursing diagnoses
• Activity intolerance
• Altered role performance
• Anxiety
• Decreased cardiac output
• Diversional activity deficit
• Fatigue
• Impaired gas exchange
• Knowledge deficit
• Pain
• Risk for infection
• Risk for injury

Nursing interventions
• Before giving penicillin, ask the patient (or, if the patient is a child, his parents) if he's ever had a hypersensitivity reaction to it. Even if he hasn't, warn him that such a reaction is possible.

• Administer antibiotics on time to maintain consistent antibiotic blood levels.

• Stress the importance of bed rest. Assist with bathing, as necessary. Provide a bedside commode because it puts less stress on the heart than using a bedpan. Offer diversional activities that are physically undemanding.

• Place the patient in an upright position to relieve dyspnea and chest pain, if needed.

• Provide analgesics to relieve pain and oxygen to prevent tissue hypoxia, as needed.

• To reduce anxiety, allow the patient to express his concerns about the effects of activity restrictions on his responsibilities and routines. Reassure him that the restrictions are temporary.

• If the patient is unstable because of chorea, clear his environment of objects that could make him fall.

• After the acute phase, encourage the patient's family and friends to spend as much time as possible with the patient to minimize his boredom. Advise the parents to secure a tutor to help their child keep up with schoolwork during the long convalescence.

• Help the parents overcome any guilt feelings they may have about their child's illness. Failure to seek treatment for streptococcal infection is common because the illness may seem no worse than a cold.

• Encourage the parents and the child to vent their frustrations during the long, tedious recovery. If the child has severe carditis, help them prepare for permanent changes in the child's life-style.

Patient teaching

• Explain all tests and treatments to the patient.

• Tell the patient to resume activities of daily living slowly and to schedule rest periods into his routine for a while.

• Tell the parents or patient to stop penicillin therapy and call the doctor immediately if the patient develops a rash, fever, chills, or other signs of allergy.

• Instruct the patient and his family to watch for and report early signs of left ventricular failure, such as dyspnea and a hacking, nonproductive cough.

• Teach the patient and his family about this disease and its treatment. Warn the parents to watch for and immediately report signs of recurrent streptococcal infection: sudden sore throat, diffuse throat redness and oropharyngeal exudate, swollen and tender cervical lymph glands, pain on swallowing, temperature of 101° to 104° F (38.3° to 40° C), headache, and nausea. Urge them to keep the child away from people with respiratory tract infections.

• Help the patient's family understand the frustrations associated with chorea (nervousness, restlessness, poor coordination, weakness, and inattentiveness). Emphasize that these effects are transient.

• Make sure the patient and his family understand the need to comply with prolonged antibiotic therapy and follow-up care, and the need for additional antibiotics during dental surgery. Arrange for a visiting nurse to oversee home care, if necessary.

MITRAL STENOSIS

In this disorder, valve leaflets become diffusely thickened by fibrosis and calcification. The mitral commissures fuse, the chordae tendineae fuse and shorten, the valvular cusps become rigid, and the apex of the valve becomes narrowed, obstructing blood flow from the left atrium to the left ventricle.

As a result of these changes, left atrial volume and pressure rise and the atrial chamber dilates. The increased resistance to blood flow causes pulmonary hypertension, right ventricular hypertrophy and, eventually, right ventricular failure. What's more, inadequate filling of the left ventricle reduces cardiac output.

Two-thirds of all patients with mitral stenosis are female.

Causes

Mitral stenosis most commonly results from rheumatic fever. It may also be associated with congenital anomalies.

Complications

Pulmonary hypertension caused by mitral stenosis can rupture pulmonary-bronchial venous connections, which results in hemorrhage. Pulmonary hypertension also increases transudation of fluid from pulmonary capillaries, which can cause fibrosis in the alveoli and pulmonary capillaries. This action reduces vital capacity, total lung capacity, maximal breathing capacity, and oxygen uptake per unit of ventilation.

Thrombi may form in the left atrium and, if they embolize, travel to the brain, kidneys, spleen, and extremities—possibly causing infarction. Embolization occurs most commonly in patients with arrhythmias.

Assessment findings

In mild mitral stenosis, the patient may have no symptoms. In moderate to severe mitral stenosis, you may find a history of dyspnea on exertion, paroxysmal nocturnal dyspnea, orthopnea, weakness, fatigue, and palpitations.

The presence of hemoptysis suggests rupture of pulmonary-bronchial venous connections.

Inspection may reveal peripheral and facial cyanosis, particularly in severe cases. The patient's face may appear pinched and blue, and she may have a malar rash. You may note jugular vein distention and ascites in the patient with severe pulmonary hypertension or associated tricuspid stenosis.

Palpation may reveal peripheral edema, hepatomegaly, and a diastolic thrill at the cardiac apex.

Auscultation may reveal a loud S_1 or opening snap and a diastolic murmur at the apex, along the left sternal border or at the base of the heart. (See *Identifying the murmur of mitral stenosis.*) In patients with pulmonary hypertension, the second heart sound is often accentuated, and the two components of the second heart sound are closely split. A pulmonary systolic ejection click may be heard in patients with severe pulmonary hypertension. Crackles may be heard when the lungs are auscultated.

Diagnostic tests
• *Cardiac catheterization* shows a diastolic pressure gradient across the valve. It also shows elevated pulmonary capillary wedge pressure (greater than 15 mm Hg) and pulmonary artery pressure in the left atrium with severe pulmonary hypertension. It detects elevated right ventricular pressure, decreased cardiac output, and abnormal contraction of the left ventricle. However, this test may not be indicated in patients who have isolated mitral stenosis with mild symptoms.
• *Chest X-rays* show left atrial and ventricular enlargement (in severe mitral stenosis), straightening of the left border of the cardiac silhouette, enlarged pulmonary arteries, dilation of the upper lobe pulmonary veins, and mitral valve calcification.
• *Echocardiography* discloses thickened mitral valve leaflets and left atrial enlargement.
• *Electrocardiography* reveals left atrial enlargement, right ventricular hypertrophy, right axis deviation, and (in 40% to 50% of cases) atrial fibrillation.

Treatment
In valvular heart disease, treatment depends on the nature and severity of associated symptoms. In asymptomatic mitral stenosis in a young patient, penicillin is an important prophylactic.

If the patient is symptomatic, treatment varies. Heart failure requires bed rest, digoxin, diuretics, a sodium-restricted diet and, in acute cases, oxygen. Small doses of beta blockers may also be used to slow the ventricular

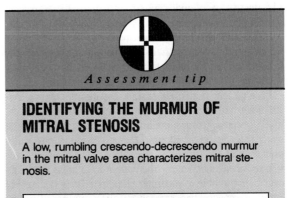

Assessment tip

IDENTIFYING THE MURMUR OF MITRAL STENOSIS
A low, rumbling crescendo-decrescendo murmur in the mitral valve area characterizes mitral stenosis.

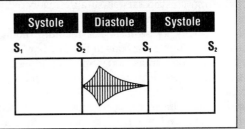

rate when cardiac glycosides fail to control atrial fibrillation or flutter. Synchronized cardioversion may be used to correct atrial fibrillation in an unstable patient.

If hemoptysis develops, the patient requires bed rest, salt restriction, and diuretics to decrease pulmonary venous pressure. Embolization mandates anticoagulants along with symptomatic treatments.

A patient with severe, medically uncontrollable symptoms may need open-heart surgery with cardiopulmonary bypass for commissurotomy or valve replacement.

Percutaneous balloon valvuloplasty may be used in young patients who have no calcification or subvalvular deformity, in symptomatic pregnant women, and in elderly patients with end-stage disease who couldn't withstand general anesthesia. This procedure is performed in the cardiac catheterization laboratory.

Nursing diagnoses
• Activity intolerance
• Altered role performance
• Altered tissue perfusion
• Decreased cardiac output
• Fatigue
• Fluid volume excess
• Impaired gas exchange
• Impaired physical mobility

• Ineffective individual coping

Nursing interventions

• Before giving penicillin, ask the patient if she's ever had a hypersensitivity reaction to it. Even if she never has, warn her that such a reaction is possible.
• If the patient needs bed rest, stress its importance. Assist with bathing, as necessary. Provide a bedside commode because using a commode puts less stress on the heart than using a bedpan. Offer diversional, physically undemanding activities.
• To reduce anxiety, allow the patient to express concerns over being unable to meet her responsibilities because of activity restrictions. Give reassurance that activity limitations are temporary.
• Watch closely for signs of heart failure, pulmonary edema, and adverse reactions to drug therapy.
• Place the patient in an upright position to relieve dyspnea, if needed. Administer oxygen to prevent tissue hypoxia, as needed.
• If the patient has had surgery, watch for hypotension, arrhythmias, and thrombus formation. Monitor vital signs, arterial blood gas levels, intake and output, daily weights, blood chemistry studies, chest X-rays, and pulmonary artery catheter readings.
• Keep the patient on a low-sodium diet; provide as many favorite foods as possible.

Patient teaching

• Explain all tests and treatments to the patient.
• Advise the patient to plan for periodic rest in her daily routine to prevent undue fatigue.
• Teach the patient about diet restrictions, medications, symptoms that should be reported, and the importance of consistent follow-up care.

MITRAL INSUFFICIENCY

Also known as mitral regurgitation, mitral insufficiency occurs when a damaged mitral valve allows blood from the left ventricle to flow back into the left atrium during systole. As a result, the atrium enlarges to accommodate the backflow. The left ventricle also dilates to accommodate the increased volume of blood from the atrium and to compensate for diminishing cardiac output.

Mitral insufficiency tends to be progressive because left ventricular dilation increases the insufficiency, which further enlarges the left atrium and ventricle, which further increases the insufficiency.

Causes

Damage to the mitral valve can result from rheumatic fever, idiopathic hypertrophic subaortic stenosis, mitral valve prolapse, myocardial infarction, severe left ventricular failure, or ruptured chordae tendineae.

In older patients, mitral insufficiency may occur because the mitral annulus has become calcified. The cause is unknown, but it may be linked to a degenerative process. Mitral insufficiency is sometimes associated with congenital anomalies, such as transposition of the great arteries.

Complications

Ventricular hypertrophy and increased end-diastolic pressure result in increased pulmonary artery pressure, eventually leading to left and right ventricular failure with pulmonary edema and cardiovascular collapse.

Assessment findings

Depending on the disorder's severity, the patient may be asymptomatic or complain of orthopnea, exertional dyspnea, fatigue, weakness, weight loss, chest pain, and palpitations.

Inspection may reveal jugular vein distention with an abnormally prominent *a* wave. You may also note peripheral edema.

Auscultation may detect a soft S_1 that may be buried in the systolic murmur. A Grade 3 to 6 or louder holosystolic murmur, most characteristic of mitral insufficiency, is best heard at the apex. You'll also hear a split S_2 and a low-pitched S_3. The S_3 may be followed by a short, rumbling diastolic murmur. A fourth heart sound may be evident in patients with a recent onset of severe mitral insufficiency and who are in normal sinus rhythm. (See *Identifying the murmur of mitral insufficiency.*)

Auscultation of the lungs may reveal crackles if the patient has pulmonary edema.

Palpation of the chest may disclose a regular pulse rate with a sharp upstroke. You can probably palpate a systolic thrill at the apex. In patients with marked pulmonary hypertension, you may be able to palpate a right ventricular tap and the shock of the pulmonary valve closing. When the left atrium is markedly enlarged, it may be palpable along the sternal border late during ventricular systole. It resembles a right ventricular lift. Abdominal palpation may reveal hepatomegaly if the patient has right ventricular failure.

Diagnostic tests

• *Cardiac catheterization* detects mitral insufficiency, with increased left ventricular end-diastolic volume and pressure, increased left atrial and pulmonary capillary wedge pressures, and decreased cardiac output.

• *Chest X-rays* demonstrate left atrial and ventricular enlargement, pulmonary venous congestion, and calcification of the mitral leaflets in long-standing mitral insufficiency and stenosis.

• *Echocardiography* reveals abnormal motion of the valve leaflets, left atrial enlargement, and a hyperdynamic left ventricle.

• *Electrocardiography* may show left atrial and ventricular hypertrophy, sinus tachycardia, and atrial fibrillation.

Treatment

The nature and severity of associated symptoms determine treatment in valvular heart disease. The patient may need to restrict activities to avoid extreme fatigue and dyspnea.

Heart failure requires digoxin, diuretics, a sodium-restricted diet and, in acute cases, oxygen. Other appropriate measures include anticoagulant therapy to prevent thrombus formation around diseased or replaced valves, and prophylactic antibiotics before and after surgery or dental care.

If the patient has severe signs and symptoms that can't be managed medically, he may need open-heart surgery with cardiopulmonary bypass for valve replacement.

Valvuloplasty may be used in elderly patients who have end-stage disease and who cannot tolerate general anesthesia.

Nursing diagnoses

• Activity intolerance
• Altered tissue perfusion
• Decreased cardiac output
• Fatigue
• Fluid volume excess
• Impaired gas exchange
• Impaired physical mobility
• Ineffective individual coping
• Risk for infection

Nursing interventions

• Provide periods of rest between periods of activity to prevent excessive fatigue.

• To reduce anxiety, allow the patient to express his concerns about the effects of activity restrictions on his responsibilities and routines. Reassure him that the restrictions are temporary.

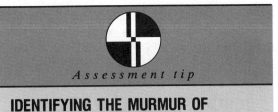

Assessment tip

IDENTIFYING THE MURMUR OF MITRAL INSUFFICIENCY

A high-pitched, rumbling pansystolic murmur that radiates from the mitral area to the left axillary line characterizes mitral insufficiency.

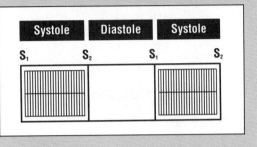

Systole	Diastole	Systole
S_1 S_2		S_1 S_2

• Keep the patient on a low-sodium diet; consult with the dietitian to ensure that the patient receives as many favorite foods as possible during the restriction.

• Monitor for left ventricular failure, pulmonary edema, and adverse reactions to drug therapy. Provide oxygen to prevent tissue hypoxia, as needed.

• If the patient has surgery, monitor postoperatively for hypotension, arrhythmias, and thrombus formation.

• Monitor the patient's vital signs, arterial blood gas levels, intake and output, daily weights, blood chemistry studies, chest X-rays, and pulmonary artery catheter readings.

• Before giving penicillin, ask the patient or his parents (if he's a child) if he's ever had a hypersensitivity reaction to it. Even if he hasn't, warn that such a reaction is possible. Administer antibiotics on time to maintain consistent drug levels in the blood.

Patient teaching

• Teach the patient about diet restrictions, medications, signs and symptoms that should be reported, and the importance of consistent follow-up care.

• Explain all tests and treatments.

• Make sure the patient and his family understand the need to comply with prolonged antibiotic therapy and follow-up care, and the need for additional antibiotics during dental surgery.

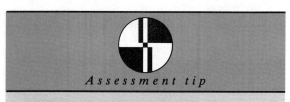

Assessment tip

IDENTIFYING THE MURMUR OF TRICUSPID STENOSIS

A low, rumbling crescendo-decrescendo murmur in the tricuspid area characterizes tricuspid stenosis.

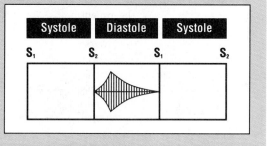

• Tell the parents or patient to stop the drug and call the doctor immediately if the patient develops a rash, fever, chills, or other signs of allergy *at any time* during penicillin therapy.
• Instruct the patient and his family to watch for and report early signs of heart failure, such as dyspnea and a hacking, nonproductive cough.

TRICUSPID STENOSIS

This relatively uncommon disorder obstructs blood flow from the right atrium to the right ventricle, which causes the right atrium to dilate and hypertrophy. Eventually, this leads to right ventricular failure and increases pressure in the vena cava.

Tricuspid stenosis seldom occurs alone and most often is associated with mitral stenosis. It's most common in women.

Causes

Although this disorder is caused most commonly by rheumatic fever, it also may be congenital.

Complications

Patients with untreated tricuspid stenosis may develop right ventricular failure.

Assessment findings

The patient with tricuspid stenosis may complain of dyspnea, fatigue, weakness, and syncope. Peripheral edema may cause her discomfort.

Inspection may reveal jugular vein distention with giant *a* waves in a patient who has normal sinus rhythm. The patient with severe tricuspid stenosis that has progressed to right ventricular failure may appear jaundiced, with severe peripheral edema and ascites. She also may appear malnourished.

Auscultation may reveal a diastolic murmur at the lower left sternal border and over the xiphoid process. It's most prominent during presystole in sinus rhythm. The murmur increases with inspiration and decreases with expiration and during Valsalva's maneuver. (See *Identifying the murmur of tricuspid stenosis*.)

Palpation may discover hepatomegaly when the patient has right ventricular failure.

Diagnostic tests

• *Cardiac catheterization* shows an increased pressure gradient across the valve, increased right atrial pressure, and decreased cardiac output.
• *Chest X-rays* demonstrate right atrial and superior vena cava enlargement.
• *Echocardiography* indicates thick tricuspid valve and right atrial enlargement.
• *Electrocardiography* reveals right atrial hypertrophy, right or left ventricular hypertrophy, and atrial fibrillation. Tall, peaked P waves appear in lead II and prominent, upright P waves appear in lead V_1.

Treatment

In tricuspid stenosis, treatment is based on the patient's symptoms. A sodium-restricted diet and diuretics can help to reduce hepatic congestion before surgery.

A patient with moderate to severe stenosis probably will require open-heart surgery for valvulotomy or valve replacement. Valvuloplasty may be performed on elderly patients with end-stage disease in the cardiac catheterization laboratory.

Nursing diagnoses
• Activity intolerance
• Altered tissue perfusion
• Decreased cardiac output
• Fatigue
• Fear
• Fluid volume excess
• Impaired gas exchange
• Impaired physical mobility

• Ineffective individual coping

Nursing interventions
• Alternate periods of activity and rest to prevent extreme fatigue and dyspnea.
• When the patient sits in a chair, elevate her legs to improve venous return to the heart.
• Elevate the head of the bed to improve ventilation.
• Keep the patient on a low-sodium diet. Consult with a dietitian to ensure that the patient receives foods that she likes while adhering to the diet restrictions.
• Monitor for signs of heart failure, pulmonary edema, and adverse reactions to the drug therapy.
• Allow the patient to express her fears and concerns about the disorder, its impact on her life, and any impending surgery. Reassure her as needed.
• If the patient has surgery, watch for hypotension, arrhythmias, and thrombus formation. Monitor her vital signs, arterial blood gas levels, intake and output, daily weights, blood chemistry studies, chest X-rays, and pulmonary artery catheter readings.

Patient teaching
• Teach the patient about diet restrictions, medications, signs and symptoms that should be reported, and the importance of consistent follow-up care.
• Urge the patient to elevate her legs whenever she sits down.

TRICUSPID INSUFFICIENCY
In this disorder, also known as tricuspid regurgitation, an incompetent tricuspid valve allows blood to flow back into the right atrium during systole, decreasing blood flow to the lungs and the left side of the heart. Cardiac output also decreases.

Causes
Tricuspid insufficiency results from marked dilation of the right ventricle and tricuspid valve ring. It most commonly occurs in the late stages of heart failure because of rheumatic or congenital heart disease.

Less commonly, it results from congenitally deformed tricuspid valves, atrioventricular canal defects, or Ebstein's malformation of the tricuspid valve. Other causes include infarction of the right ventricular papillary muscles, tricuspid valve prolapse, carcinoid heart disease, endomyocardial fibrosis, infective endocarditis, and trauma.

Complications
Fluid overload in the right side of the heart can lead to right ventricular failure.

Assessment findings
The patient may have a history of a disorder that can cause tricuspid insufficiency.

The patient may complain of dyspnea, fatigue, weakness, and syncope. Peripheral edema may cause him discomfort.

Inspection may reveal jugular vein distention with prominent v waves in a patient with normal sinus rhythm. In severe tricuspid insufficiency that has progressed to right ventricular failure, the patient may appear jaundiced, with severe peripheral edema and ascites.

Auscultation may disclose a blowing holosystolic murmur at the lower left sternal border that increases with inspiration and decreases with expiration and Valsalva's maneuver. (See *Identifying the murmur of tricuspid insufficiency,* page 544.)

Palpation may reveal hepatomegaly when the patient has right ventricular failure, systolic pulsations of the liver, and a positive hepatojugular reflex. You also may feel a prominent right ventricular pulsation along the left parasternal region.

Diagnostic tests
• *Cardiac catheterization* demonstrates markedly decreased cardiac output. The right atrial pressure pulse may exhibit no x descent during early systole, but instead a prominent c-v wave with a rapid y descent. The mean right atrial and right ventricular end-diastolic pressures typically are elevated.
• *Chest X-rays* show right atrial and ventricular enlargement.
• *Echocardiography* reveals right ventricular dilation and prolapse or flailing of the tricuspid leaflets.
• *Electrocardiography* discloses right atrial hypertrophy, right or left ventricular hypertrophy, atrial fibrillation, and incomplete right bundle-branch block.

Treatment
A sodium-restricted diet and diuretics help reduce hepatic congestion before surgery. When rheumatic fever has deformed the tricuspid valve and resulted in severe insufficiency, the patient usually will need open-heart surgery for tricuspid annuloplasty or tricuspid valve replacement.

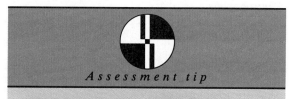

Assessment tip

IDENTIFYING THE MURMUR OF TRICUSPID INSUFFICIENCY

A high-pitched, blowing pansystolic murmur in the tricuspid area characterizes tricuspid insufficiency.

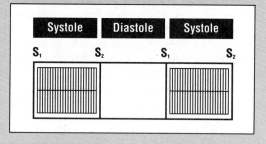

Nursing diagnoses
• Activity intolerance
• Altered tissue perfusion
• Decreased cardiac output
• Fatigue
• Fluid volume excess
• Impaired gas exchange
• Impaired physical mobility
• Ineffective individual coping
• Risk for infection

Nursing interventions
• Alternate periods of activity and rest to prevent extreme fatigue and dyspnea.
• Keep the patient's legs elevated while he's sitting in a chair to improve venous return to his heart.
• Elevate the head of his bed to improve ventilation.
• Maintain a low-sodium diet. Consult with a dietitian to ensure that the patient receives foods that he likes while adhering to the diet restrictions.
• Monitor for signs of heart failure, pulmonary edema, and adverse reactions to drug therapy.
• To reduce anxiety, allow the patient to express his concerns about the effects of activity restrictions on his responsibilities and routines. Reassure him that the restrictions are temporary.
• If the patient has surgery, watch for hypotension, arrhythmias, and thrombus formation. Monitor his vital signs, arterial blood gas levels, intake and output, daily weights, blood chemistry studies, chest X-rays, and pulmonary artery catheter readings.

Patient teaching
• Teach the patient about diet restrictions, medications, signs and symptoms that should be reported, and the importance of consistent follow-up care.
• Tell the patient to elevate his legs whenever he's sitting.

PULMONIC STENOSIS
In this disorder, obstructed right ventricular outflow causes right ventricular hypertrophy as the right ventricle attempts to overcome resistance to the narrow valvular opening.

A congenital defect, pulmonic stenosis is associated with other congenital heart defects, such as tetralogy of Fallot. It's rare among elderly people.

Causes
Pulmonic stenosis results from congenital stenosis of the pulmonary valve cusp or (infrequently) from rheumatic heart disease.

Complications
Right ventricular failure is the ultimate result of untreated pulmonic stenosis.

Assessment findings
Depending on the severity of the obstruction, the patient with mild stenosis may be asymptomatic. A patient with moderate to severe stenosis may complain of dyspnea on exertion, fatigue, chest pain, and syncope. Accompanying peripheral edema may cause him discomfort.

Inspection may reveal a prominent *a* wave in the jugular venous pulse. If severe stenosis has progressed to right ventricular failure, the patient may appear jaundiced, with severe peripheral edema and ascites. He may also appear malnourished.

Auscultation may reveal a fourth heart sound, a thrill at the upper left sternal border, a harsh systolic ejection murmur, and a holosystolic decrescendo murmur of tricuspid insufficiency, particularly if the patient has heart failure. (See *Identifying the murmur of pulmonic stenosis.*)

Palpation may detect hepatomegaly when the patient has right ventricular failure, presystolic pulsations of the liver, and a right parasternal lift.

Diagnostic tests
• *Chest X-rays* usually show normal heart size and normal lung vascularity, although the pulmonary arteries may be evident. With severe obstruction and right ventricular failure, the right atrium and ventricle typically appear enlarged.
• *Echocardiography* visualizes the pulmonary valve abnormality.
• *Electrocardiography* results may be normal in mild cases, or they may show right axis deviation and right ventricular hypertrophy. High-amplitude P waves in leads II and V_1 indicate right atrial enlargement.

Treatment
A low-sodium diet and diuretics help reduce hepatic congestion before surgery. Additionally, cardiac catheter balloon valvuloplasty is usually effective even with moderate to severe obstruction.

Nursing diagnoses
• Activity intolerance
• Altered tissue perfusion
• Decreased cardiac output
• Fatigue
• Fluid volume excess
• Impaired gas exchange
• Impaired physical mobility
• Ineffective individual coping
• Risk for infection

Nursing interventions
• Alternate periods of activity and rest to prevent extreme fatigue and dyspnea.
• Keep the patient's legs elevated while he sits in a chair to improve venous return to the heart.
• Elevate the head of the bed to improve ventilation.
• Keep the patient on a low-sodium diet. Consult with a dietitian to ensure that the patient receives foods that he likes while adhering to the diet restrictions.
• Monitor for signs of heart failure, pulmonary edema, and adverse reactions to drug therapy.
• To reduce anxiety, allow the patient to express his concerns about the effects of activity restrictions on his responsibilities and routines. Reassure him that the restrictions are temporary.
• After cardiac catheterization, apply firm pressure to the catheter insertion site, usually in the groin. Monitor the site for signs of bleeding every 15 minutes for at least 6 hours. If the site bleeds, remove the pressure dressing and manually apply firm pressure to the site.

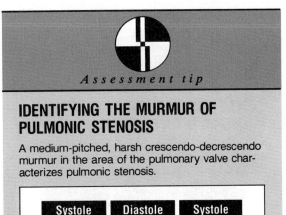

Assessment tip

IDENTIFYING THE MURMUR OF PULMONIC STENOSIS
A medium-pitched, harsh crescendo-decrescendo murmur in the area of the pulmonary valve characterizes pulmonic stenosis.

Systole	Diastole	Systole
S_1 S_2		S_1 S_2

• Notify the doctor of any changes in peripheral pulses distal to the insertion site, changes in cardiac rhythm and vital signs, and complaints of chest pain.

Patient teaching
• Teach the patient about diet restrictions, medications, signs and symptoms that should be reported, and the importance of consistent follow-up care.
• Teach the patient to elevate his legs whenever he sits.

PULMONIC INSUFFICIENCY
In this disorder, blood ejected into the pulmonary artery during systole flows back into the right ventricle during diastole, causing fluid overload in the ventricle, ventricular hypertrophy, and eventual right ventricular failure.

Causes
Pulmonic insufficiency may be congenital or may result from pulmonary hypertension. The most common acquired cause is dilation of the pulmonary valve ring from severe pulmonary hypertension.

Rarely, pulmonic insufficiency may result from prolonged use of a pressure monitoring catheter in the pulmonary artery.

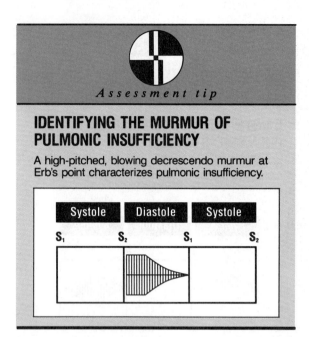

Assessment tip

IDENTIFYING THE MURMUR OF PULMONIC INSUFFICIENCY

A high-pitched, blowing decrescendo murmur at Erb's point characterizes pulmonic insufficiency.

Systole	Diastole	Systole	
S_1	S_2	S_1	S_2

Complications

If the patient has pulmonary hypertension, right ventricular failure may develop.

Assessment findings

The patient may complain of dyspnea on exertion, fatigue, chest pain, and syncope. Peripheral edema may cause him discomfort.

A patient with severe insufficiency that has progressed to right ventricular failure may appear jaundiced, with severe peripheral edema and ascites. He may also appear malnourished.

Auscultation may reveal a high-pitched, decrescendo, diastolic blowing murmur along the left sternal border (Graham Steell's murmur). This murmur may be difficult to distinguish from the murmur of aortic insufficiency. (See *Identifying the murmur of pulmonic insufficiency.*)

Palpation may disclose hepatomegaly when the patient has right ventricular failure.

Diagnostic tests

• *Cardiac catheterization* shows pulmonic insufficiency, increased right ventricular pressure, and associated cardiac defects.
• *Chest X-rays* show right ventricular and pulmonary arterial enlargement.
• *Echocardiography* visualizes the pulmonary valve abnormality.

• *Electrocardiography* findings may be normal in mild cases or reveal right ventricular hypertrophy.

Treatment

In pulmonic insufficiency, treatment is based on the patient's symptoms. A low-sodium diet and diuretics help to reduce hepatic congestion before surgery. Valvulotomy or valve replacement may be required in severe cases.

Nursing diagnoses

• Activity intolerance
• Altered tissue perfusion
• Decreased cardiac output
• Fatigue
• Fluid volume excess
• Impaired gas exchange
• Impaired physical mobility
• Ineffective individual coping
• Risk for infection

Nursing interventions

• Alternate periods of activity and rest to prevent extreme fatigue and dyspnea.
• Keep the patient's legs elevated while he sits in a chair to improve venous return to the heart.
• Elevate the head of the bed to improve ventilation.
• Keep the patient on a low-sodium diet. Consult with a dietitian to ensure that the patient receives foods that he likes while adhering to the diet restrictions.
• Monitor for signs of heart failure, pulmonary edema, and adverse reactions to drug therapy.
• To reduce anxiety, allow the patient to express his concerns about the effects of activity restrictions on his responsibilities and routines. Reassure him that the restrictions are temporary.
• If the patient has surgery, watch for hypotension, arrhythmias, and thrombus formation. Monitor his vital signs, arterial blood gas levels, intake and output, daily weights, blood chemistry studies, chest X-rays, and pulmonary artery catheter readings.

Patient teaching

• Teach the patient about diet restrictions, medications, symptoms that should be reported, and the importance of consistent follow-up care.
• Tell the patient to elevate his legs whenever he sits.

AORTIC STENOSIS

In this disorder, the opening of the aortic valve becomes narrowed, and the left ventricle exerts increased pressure to drive blood through the opening. The added work load increases the demand for oxygen, while diminished cardiac output reduces coronary artery perfusion, causes ischemia of the left ventricle, and leads to heart failure.

Sign and symptoms of aortic stenosis may not appear until the patient reaches ages 50 to 70, even though the lesion has been present since childhood. Incidence increases with age. Aortic stenosis is the most significant valvular lesion seen among elderly people. About 80% of patients with aortic stenosis are male.

Causes

Aortic stenosis may result from congenital aortic bicuspid valve (associated with coarctation of the aorta), congenital stenosis of pulmonary valve cusps, rheumatic fever or, in elderly patients, atherosclerosis.

Complications

Aortic stenosis leads to left ventricular failure, usually after age 70. It typically occurs within 4 years after the onset of signs and symptoms and is fatal in up to two-thirds of patients.

Sudden death, possibly caused by an arrhythmia, occurs in up to 20% of patients, usually around age 60.

Assessment findings

Even with severe aortic stenosis (narrowing to about one-third of the normal opening), the patient may be asymptomatic. Eventually, the patient will complain of dyspnea on exertion, fatigue, exertional syncope, angina, and palpitations. If left ventricular failure develops, the patient may complain of orthopnea and paroxysmal nocturnal dyspnea.

Inspection may reveal peripheral edema if the patient has left ventricular failure.

Palpation may detect diminished carotid pulses and pulsus alternans. If the patient has left ventricular failure, the apex of the heart may be displaced inferiorly and laterally. If the patient has pulmonary hypertension, you may be able to palpate a systolic thrill at the base of the heart, at the jugular notch, and along the carotid arteries. Occasionally, it may be palpable only during expiration and when the patient leans forward.

Auscultation may uncover an early systolic ejection murmur in children and adolescents who have noncalcified valves. The murmur begins shortly after S_1 and increases in intensity to reach a peak toward the middle of the ejection period. It diminishes just before the aortic

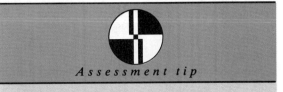

Assessment tip

IDENTIFYING THE MURMUR OF AORTIC STENOSIS

A low-pitched, harsh crescendo-decrescendo murmur that radiates from the aortic valve area to the carotid artery characterizes aortic stenosis.

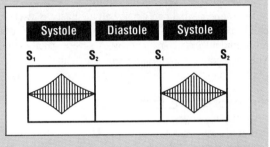

valve closes. (See *Identifying the murmur of aortic stenosis.*)

The murmur is low-pitched, rough, and rasping and is loudest at the base in the second intercostal space. In stenosis, the murmur is at least Grade 3 or 4. It disappears when the valve calcifies. A split S_2 (second heart sound) develops as aortic stenosis becomes more severe. An S_4 reflects left ventricular hypertrophy and may be heard at the apex in many patients with severe aortic stenosis.

Diagnostic tests

• *Cardiac catheterization* reveals the pressure gradient across the valve (indicating the obstruction's severity), increased left ventricular end-diastolic pressures (indicating left ventricular function), and the location of the left ventricular outflow obstruction.
• *Chest X-rays* show valvular calcification; left ventricular enlargement; pulmonary vein congestion; and, in later stages, left atrial, pulmonary artery, right atrial, and right ventricular enlargement.
• *Echocardiography* demonstrates a thickened aortic valve and left ventricular wall and, possibly, coexistent mitral valve stenosis.
• *Electrocardiography* reveals left ventricular hypertrophy. In advanced stages, the patient will exhibit ST-segment depression and T-wave inversion in standard leads I and

aV$_L$ and in the left precordial leads. Up to 10% of patients have atrioventricular and intraventricular conduction defects.

Treatment
Digitalis glycosides, a low-sodium diet, diuretics and, in acute cases, oxygen are used to treat heart failure. Nitroglycerin helps relieve angina.

In children who don't have calcified valves, simple commissurotomy under direct visualization is usually effective. Adults with calcified valves will need valve replacement once they become symptomatic or are at risk for developing left ventricular failure.

Percutaneous balloon aortic valvuloplasty is useful in children and young adults who have congenital aortic stenosis and in elderly patients with severe calcifications. This procedure may improve left ventricular function so that the patient can tolerate valve replacement surgery.

Nursing diagnoses
- Activity intolerance
- Altered role performance
- Altered tissue perfusion
- Decreased cardiac output
- Diversional activity deficit
- Fatigue
- Fluid volume excess
- Impaired gas exchange
- Impaired physical mobility
- Ineffective individual coping

Nursing interventions
- If the patient needs bed rest, stress its importance. Assist the patient with bathing if necessary; provide a bedside commode because using a commode puts less stress on the heart than using a bedpan. Offer diversional activities that are physically undemanding.
- Alternate periods of activity and rest to prevent extreme fatigue and dyspnea.
- To reduce anxiety, allow the patient to express his concerns about the effects of activity restrictions on his responsibilities and routines. Reassure him that the restrictions are temporary.
- Keep the patient's legs elevated while he sits in a chair to improve venous return to the heart.
- Place the patient in an upright position to relieve dyspnea, if needed. Administer oxygen to prevent tissue hypoxia, as needed.
- Keep the patient on a low-sodium diet. Consult with a dietitian to ensure that the patient receives foods that he likes while adhering to the diet restrictions.

- Monitor for signs of heart failure, pulmonary edema, and adverse reactions to drug therapy.
- Allow the patient to express his fears and concerns about the disorder, its impact on his life, and any impending surgery. Reassure him as needed.
- After cardiac catheterization, apply firm pressure to the catheter insertion site, usually in the groin. Monitor the site every 15 minutes for at least 6 hours for signs of bleeding. If the site bleeds, remove the pressure dressing and apply firm pressure.
- Notify the doctor of any changes in peripheral pulses distal to the insertion site, changes in cardiac rhythm and vital signs, and complaints of chest pain.
- If the patient has surgery, watch for hypotension, arrhythmias, and thrombus formation. Monitor his vital signs, arterial blood gas levels, intake and output, daily weights, blood chemistry studies, chest X-rays, and pulmonary artery catheter readings.

Patient teaching
- Advise the patient to plan for periodic rest in his daily routine to prevent undue fatigue.
- Teach the patient about diet restrictions, medications, symptoms that should be reported, and the importance of consistent follow-up care.
- Tell the patient to elevate his legs whenever he sits.

AORTIC INSUFFICIENCY
In this disorder (also called aortic regurgitation), blood flows back into the left ventricle during diastole. The ventricle becomes overloaded, dilated, and eventually hypertrophies. The excess fluid volume also overloads the left atrium and, eventually, the pulmonary system.

Aortic insufficiency by itself occurs most commonly among males. When associated with mitral valve disease, however, it's more common among females. This disorder also may be associated with Marfan syndrome, ankylosing spondylitis, syphilis, essential hypertension, and a ventricular septal defect, even after surgical closure.

Causes
Aortic insufficiency results from rheumatic fever, syphilis, hypertension, endocarditis, or trauma. In some patients, it may be idiopathic.

Complications
Left ventricular failure usually occurs. The patient may develop fatal pulmonary edema if a fever, an infection, or a cardiac arrhythmia develops. The patient also risks

myocardial ischemia because left ventricular dilation and elevated left ventricular systolic pressure alter myocardial oxygen requirements.

Assessment findings

In chronic severe aortic insufficiency, the patient may complain that he has an uncomfortable awareness of his heartbeat, especially when lying down. He may report palpitations along with a pounding head.

Dyspnea may occur with exertion, and the patient may experience paroxysmal nocturnal dyspnea with diaphoresis, orthopnea, and cough. He may become fatigued and syncopal with exertion or emotion. He may also have a history of anginal chest pain unrelieved by sublingual nitroglycerin.

On inspection, you may note that each heartbeat seems to jar the patient's entire body and that his head bobs with each systole. Inspection of arterial pulsations shows a rapidly rising pulse that collapses suddenly as arterial pressure falls late in systole. This is called a water-hammer pulse.

The patient's nail beds may appear to be pulsating. If you apply pressure at the nail tip, the root will alternately flush and pale (called Quincke's sign). Inspection of the chest may reveal a visible apical impulse. In left ventricular failure, the patient may have ankle edema and ascites.

In palpating the peripheral pulses, you may note rapidly rising and collapsing pulses (pulsus biferiens). If the patient has cardiac arrhythmias, pulses may be irregular. You'll be able to feel the apical impulse. (The apex will be displaced laterally and inferiorly.) A diastolic thrill probably will be palpable along the left sternal border, and you may be able to feel a prominent systolic thrill in the jugular notch and along the carotid arteries.

Auscultation may reveal an S_3, occasionally an S_4, and a loud systolic ejection sound. A high-pitched, blowing, decrescendo diastolic murmur is best heard at the left sternal border, third intercostal space. Use the diaphragm of the stethoscope to hear it, and have the patient sit up, lean forward, and hold his breath in forced expiration. (See *Identifying the murmur of aortic insufficiency.*)

You also may hear a midsystolic ejection murmur at the base of the heart. It may be a Grade 5 or 6 and typically is higher pitched, shorter, and less rasping than the murmur heard in aortic stenosis. Another murmur that may occur is a soft, low-pitched, rumbling, middiastolic or presystolic bruit (Austin Flint murmur). This murmur is best heard at the base of the heart.

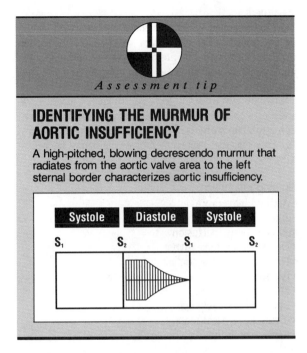

Assessment tip

IDENTIFYING THE MURMUR OF AORTIC INSUFFICIENCY

A high-pitched, blowing decrescendo murmur that radiates from the aortic valve area to the left sternal border characterizes aortic insufficiency.

Systole	Diastole	Systole	
S_1	S_2	S_1	S_2

Place the stethoscope lightly over the femoral artery, and you'll notice a booming pistol-shot sound and a to-and-fro murmur (Duroziez's sign). Arterial pulse pressure is widened. Auscultating blood pressure may be difficult because you can auscultate the patient's pulse without inflating the cuff. To determine systolic pressure, note when Korotkoff's sounds begin to muffle.

Diagnostic tests

• *Cardiac catheterization* shows reduction in arterial diastolic pressures, aortic insufficiency, other valvular abnormalities, and increased left ventricular end-diastolic pressure.

• *Chest X-rays* display left ventricular enlargement and pulmonary vein congestion.

• *Echocardiography* reveals left ventricular enlargement, dilation of the aortic annulus and left atrium, and thickening of the aortic valve. It also shows a rapid, high-frequency fluttering of the anterior mitral leaflet that results from the impact of aortic regurgitation.

• *Electrocardiography* shows sinus tachycardia, left ventricular hypertrophy, and left atrial hypertrophy in severe disease. ST-segment depressions and T-wave inversions appear in leads I, aV_L, V_5, and V_6 and indicate left ventricular strain.

Treatment

Valve replacement is the treatment of choice and should be performed before significant ventricular dysfunction occurs. This may not be possible, however, because signs and symptoms seldom occur until after myocardial dysfunction develops.

Digitalis glycosides, a low-sodium diet, diuretics, vasodilators, and especially angiotensin-converting enzyme inhibitors are used to treat left ventricular failure. In acute episodes, supplemental oxygen may be necessary.

Nursing diagnoses

• Activity intolerance
• Altered role performance
• Altered tissue perfusion
• Decreased cardiac output
• Diversional activity deficit
• Fatigue
• Fluid volume excess
• Impaired gas exchange
• Impaired physical mobility
• Ineffective individual coping

Nursing interventions

• If the patient needs bed rest, stress its importance. Assist with bathing if necessary. Provide a bedside commode because using a commode puts less stress on the heart than using a bedpan. Offer diversional activities that are physically undemanding.
• Alternate periods of activity and rest to prevent extreme fatigue and dyspnea.
• To reduce anxiety, allow the patient to express his concerns about the effects of activity restrictions on his responsibilities and routines. Reassure him that the restrictions are temporary.
• Keep the patient's legs elevated while he sits in a chair to improve venous return to the heart.
• Place the patient in an upright position to relieve dyspnea, if necessary, and administer oxygen to prevent tissue hypoxia.
• Keep the patient on a low-sodium diet. Consult a dietitian to ensure that the patient receives foods that he likes while adhering to the diet restrictions.
• Monitor for signs of heart failure, pulmonary edema, and adverse reactions to drug therapy.
• If the patient undergoes surgery, watch for hypotension, arrhythmias, and thrombus formation. Monitor his vital signs, arterial blood gas levels, intake and output, daily weights, blood chemistry studies, chest X-rays, and pulmonary artery catheter readings.

Patient teaching

• Advise the patient to plan for periodic rest in his daily routine to prevent undue fatigue.
• Teach the patient about diet restrictions, medications, symptoms that should be reported, and the importance of consistent follow-up care.
• Tell the patient to elevate his legs whenever he sits.

HYPERTENSION

This disorder is marked by an intermittent or sustained elevation of diastolic or systolic blood pressure. Generally, a sustained systolic pressure of 140 mm Hg or more or a diastolic pressure of 90 mm Hg or more qualifies as hypertension.

Aside from characteristic high blood pressure, hypertension is classified according to its cause, severity, and type. The two major types are *essential* (also called primary or idiopathic) *hypertension,* the most common (90% to 95% of cases), and *secondary hypertension,* which results from renal disease or another identifiable cause. *Malignant hypertension* is a severe, fulminant form of hypertension that commonly arises from both types. (See *Malignant hypertension.*) Hypertension affects more than 60 million adults in the United States. Blacks are twice as likely as whites to be affected, and they're four times as likely to die of the disorder.

Essential hypertension usually begins insidiously as a benign disease, slowly progressing to an accelerated or malignant state. If untreated, even mild hypertension can cause significant complications and a high mortality rate. (See *How hypertension develops,* page 552.) In many cases, however, treatment with stepped care offers patients an improved prognosis. (See *Stepped-care approach to antihypertensive therapy,* page 553.)

Causes

The cause of essential hypertension is unknown. Family history, race, stress, obesity, a diet high in sodium or saturated fat, use of tobacco or oral contraceptives, sedentary life-style, and aging have all been studied to determine their role in the development of hypertension.

Secondary hypertension may result from renovascular disease; renal parenchymal disease; pheochromocytoma; primary hyperaldosteronism; Cushing's syndrome; diabetes mellitus; dysfunction of the thyroid, pituitary, or parathyroid gland; coarctation of the aorta; pregnancy; and neurologic disorders. Use of oral contraceptives may be the most common cause of secondary hypertension, probably because these drugs activate the renin-angiotensin-aldosterone system.

Complications

Hypertension is a major cause of cerebrovascular accident, cardiac disease, and renal failure. Complications occur late in the disease and can attack any organ system. Cardiac complications may include coronary artery disease, angina, myocardial infarction, heart failure, arrhythmias, and sudden death. Neurologic complications include cerebral infarctions and hypertensive encephalopathy. Hypertensive retinopathy can cause blindness. Renovascular hypertension can lead to renal failure.

Assessment findings

In many cases, the hypertensive patient has no symptoms, and the disorder is revealed incidentally during evaluation for another disorder or during a routine blood pressure screening program. When symptoms do occur, they reflect the effect of hypertension on the organ systems.

The patient may report awakening with a headache in the occipital region, which subsides spontaneously after a few hours. This symptom usually is associated with severe hypertension. He may also complain of dizziness, palpitations, fatigue, and impotence.

With vascular involvement, the patient may complain of nosebleeds, bloody urine, weakness, and blurred vision. Complaints of chest pain and dyspnea may indicate cardiac involvement.

Inspection may reveal peripheral edema in late stages when heart failure is present. Ophthalmoscopic evaluation may reveal hemorrhages, exudates, and papilledema in late stages if hypertensive retinopathy is present.

Palpation of the carotid artery may disclose stenosis or occlusion. Palpation of the abdomen may reveal a pulsating mass, suggesting an abdominal aneurysm. Enlarged kidneys may point to polycystic disease, a cause of secondary hypertension.

Systolic or diastolic pressure, or both, may be elevated. A rise in diastolic blood pressure from a sitting to a standing position suggests essential hypertension, whereas a fall in blood pressure from the sitting to the standing position indicates secondary hypertension.

An abdominal bruit may be heard just to the right or left of the umbilicus midline, or in the flanks if renal artery stenosis is present. Bruits may also be heard over the abdominal aorta and femoral arteries.

Diagnostic tests

The following tests may elicit predisposing factors and help identify the cause of hypertension:
• *Urinalysis* may show protein, red blood cells, or white

Warning

MALIGNANT HYPERTENSION

Malignant hypertension is a medical emergency characterized by marked blood pressure elevation; papilledema; retinal hemorrhages and exudates; and manifestations of hypertensive encephalopathy, such as severe headache, vomiting, visual disturbances, transient paralysis, seizures, stupor, and coma. Cardiac decompensation and acute renal failure may also develop in this disorder.

The average age at diagnosis is 40, and the disorder affects more men than women. Before the availability of effective antihypertensives, most patients died within 2 years. Even with effective treatment, however, at least half the patients die within 5 years.

Causes
The cause of malignant hypertension isn't known. However, studies do show that dilation of cerebral arteries and generalized arteriolar fibrinoid necrosis contribute to the disorder. The cerebral arteries dilate because normal regulation of cerebral blood flow doesn't take place because of markedly high arterial pressure. The resulting excess in cerebral blood flow produces encephalopathy.

Treatment
Emergency treatment aims to quickly reduce blood pressure and identify the underlying cause.
• Diazoxide given rapidly I.V. can begin to reduce blood pressure in 1 to 3 minutes. Nitroprusside and trimethaphan, given by continuous infusion, may be tried. Other drugs for maintaining long-term control of blood pressure include hydralazine and methyldopa.
• With suspected pheochromocytoma, drugs that release additional catecholamines—such as methyldopa, reserpine, and guanethidine—are contraindicated.
• Furosemide and digitalis glycosides may be used to treat associated heart failure.

blood cells, suggesting renal disease; or glucose, suggesting diabetes mellitus.
• *Excretory urography* may reveal renal atrophy, indicating chronic renal disease; one kidney that is more than ⅝" (1.6 cm) shorter than the other suggests unilateral renal disease.

(Text continues on page 554.)

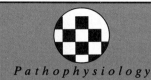

Pathophysiology

HOW HYPERTENSION DEVELOPS

Increased blood volume, cardiac rate, and stroke volume, or arteriolar vasoconstriction that increases peripheral resistance causes blood pressure to rise. Hypertension may also result from the breakdown or inappropriate response of the following intrinsic regulatory mechanisms.

Renin-angiotensin system
Renal hypoperfusion causes the release of renin. Angiotensinogen, a liver enzyme, converts the renin to angiotensin I, which increases preload and afterload. Angiotensin I then converts to angiotensin II in the lungs. A powerful vasoconstrictor, angiotensin II also helps increase preload and afterload by stimulating the adrenal cortex to secrete aldosterone. This serves to increase sodium reabsorption. Next comes hypertonic-stimulated release of antidiuretic hormone from the pituitary gland. This, in turn, increases water absorption, plasma volume, cardiac output, and blood pressure.

Autoregulation
Several intrinsic mechanisms work to change an artery's diameter to maintain tissue and organ perfusion despite fluctuations in systemic blood pressure. These mechanisms include stress relaxation and capillary fluid shift. In stress relaxation, blood vessels gradually dilate when blood pressure rises to reduce peripheral resistance. In capillary fluid shift, plasma moves between vessels and extravascular spaces to maintain intravascular volume.

When blood pressure drops, baroreceptors in the aortic arch and carotid sinuses decrease their inhibition of the medulla's vasomotor center. This action increases sympathetic stimulation of the heart by norepinephrine. And this increases cardiac output by strengthening the contractile force, raising the heart rate, and augmenting peripheral resistance by vasoconstriction. Stress can also stimulate the sympathetic nervous system to increase cardiac output and peripheral vascular resistance.

Blood vessel damage
Sustained hypertension damages blood vessels (as pictured below). Vascular injury begins with alternating areas of dilation and constriction in the arterioles. Increased intra-arterial pressure damages the endothelium (see left illustration). Independently, angiotensin induces endothelial wall contraction (see middle illustration), allowing plasma to leak through interendothelial spaces. Eventually, plasma constituents deposited in the vessel wall cause medial necrosis (see right illustration).

Vascular damage

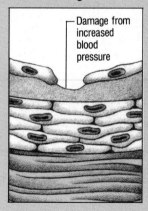

Damage from increased blood pressure

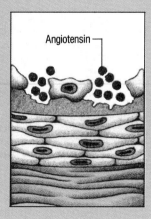

Angiotensin

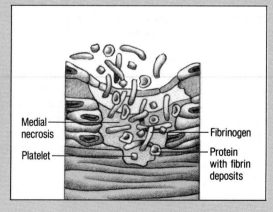

Medial necrosis

Platelet

Fibrinogen

Protein with fibrin deposits

STEPPED-CARE APPROACH TO ANTIHYPERTENSIVE THERAPY

The diagram below illustrates the four-step approach to antihypertensive therapy that is endorsed by the Joint National Committee on Detection, Evaluation, and Treatment of High Blood Pressure. The progression of therapy is based on the patient's response, which is defined in two ways: the patient has achieved the target blood pressure set by the doctor, or the patient is making considerable progress toward this goal.

STEP 1

Begin life-style modifications
- Weight reduction
- Moderation of alcohol intake
- Regular physical activity
- Reduction of sodium intake
- Smoking cessation

Inadequate response

STEP 2

Continue life-style modifications and begin drug regimen
- Beta blocker or diuretic drug of choice
- Angiotensin-converting enzyme inhibitor, calcium channel blocker, alpha-adrenergic blocker, or mixed alpha- and beta-adrenergic blocker (if a beta blocker or diuretic is not appropriate)

Inadequate response

STEP 3

Increase drug dosage
OR
Substitute another drug
OR
Add a second antihypertensive agent from a different class

Inadequate response

STEP 4

Add a second or third antihypertensive agent
Add a diuretic if not already prescribed

Source: U.S. Department of Health and Human Services. National Institutes of Health. National Heart, Lung, and Blood Institute. *The Fifth Report of the Joint National Committee on Detection, Evaluation, and Treatment of High Blood Pressure (JNC V)*. Washington, D.C.: Government Printing Office, 1992.

• *Serum potassium* levels less than 3.5 mEq/liter may indicate adrenal dysfunction (primary hyperaldosteronism).

• *Blood urea nitrogen* levels that are normal or elevated to more than 20 mg/dl and *serum creatinine* levels that are normal or elevated to more than 1.5 mg/dl suggest renal disease.

Other tests that help detect cardiovascular damage and other complications include electrocardiography, which may show left ventricular hypertrophy or ischemia, and chest X-rays, which may demonstrate cardiomegaly.

Treatment

Although essential hypertension has no cure, drugs and modifications in diet and life-style can control it. Generally, nondrug treatment, such as life-style modification, is tried first, especially in early, mild cases. If this is ineffective, treatment progresses in a stepwise manner to include various types of antihypertensives. This stepped-care approach may need modification. For instance, most blacks respond poorly to beta-adrenergic blocking agents; however, for unclear reasons, they respond well to a combination of a diuretic and an angiotensin-converting enzyme inhibitor. Many elderly patients can be treated with diuretics alone.

Treatment of secondary hypertension includes correcting the underlying cause and controlling hypertensive effects.

Severely elevated blood pressure (hypertensive crisis) may be refractory to medications and may be fatal.

Nursing diagnoses

• Altered tissue perfusion
• Fatigue
• Ineffective individual coping
• Knowledge deficit
• Noncompliance
• Risk for injury

Nursing interventions

• If a patient is hospitalized with hypertension, find out if he was taking prescribed antihypertensive medication. If he wasn't, ask why. If he can't afford the medication, refer him to the appropriate social service department.

• When routine blood pressure screening reveals elevated pressure, make sure the sphygmomanometer cuff size is appropriate for the patient's upper arm circumference. Take the pressure in both arms in lying, sitting, and standing positions. Ask the patient if he smoked, drank a beverage containing caffeine, or was emotionally upset before the test. Advise him to return for blood pressure testing at frequent and regular intervals.

• To help identify hypertension and prevent untreated hypertension, participate in public education programs dealing with hypertension and ways to reduce risk factors. Encourage public participation in blood pressure screening programs. Routinely screen all patients, especially those at risk (blacks and people with family histories of hypertension, cerebrovascular accident, or heart attack).

Patient teaching

• Teach the patient to use a self-monitoring blood pressure cuff and to record the reading at least twice weekly in a journal for review by the doctor at every office appointment. Tell the patient to take his blood pressure at the same hour each time with relatively the same type of activity preceding the measurement.

• Tell the patient and family to keep a record of drugs used in the past, noting especially which ones were or weren't effective. Suggest recording this information on a card so the patient can show it to his doctor.

• To encourage compliance with antihypertensive therapy, suggest establishing a daily routine for taking medication. Warn him that uncontrolled hypertension may cause stroke and heart attack. Tell him to report adverse effects of drugs. Advise him to avoid high-sodium antacids and over-the-counter cold and sinus medications containing harmful vasoconstrictors.

• Help the patient examine and modify his life-style. Suggest stress-reduction groups, dietary changes, and an exercise program, particularly aerobic walking, to improve cardiac status and reduce obesity and serum cholesterol levels.

• Encourage a change in dietary habits. Help the obese patient plan a reducing diet. Tell him to avoid high-sodium foods (pickles, potato chips, canned soups, cold cuts), table salt, and foods high in cholesterol and saturated fat.

CORONARY ARTERY DISEASE

The dominant effect of coronary artery disease is the loss of oxygen and nutrients to myocardial tissue because of diminished coronary blood flow. Fatty fibrous plaques or calcium-plaque deposits, or combinations of both, narrow the lumens of coronary arteries, reducing the volume of blood that can flow through them.

This disease is nearly epidemic in the Western world. Coronary artery disease is more prevalent in men, whites, and middle-aged and elderly people than in women or in people of other races and ages. More than 50% of men age 60 or older show signs of coronary artery disease on autopsy.

Causes

Atherosclerosis, the most common cause of coronary artery disease, has been linked to many risk factors. Some risk factors, such as the following, can't be controlled:
- *Age.* Atherosclerosis usually occurs after age 40.
- *Sex.* Men are eight times more susceptible than premenopausal women.
- *Heredity.* A positive family history of coronary artery disease increases the risk.
- *Race.* White men are more susceptible than nonwhite men; nonwhite women are more susceptible than white women.

However, the patient can modify other risk factors, such as the following, with good medical care and appropriate life-style changes:
- *Blood pressure.* Systolic blood pressure that is greater than 160 mm Hg or diastolic blood pressure that is greater than 95 mm Hg increases the risk.
- *Serum cholesterol levels.* Increased low-density lipoprotein and decreased high-density lipoprotein levels substantially heighten the risk.
- *Smoking.* Cigarette smokers are twice as likely to have a myocardial infarction and four times as likely to experience sudden death. The risk dramatically drops within 1 year after smoking ceases.
- *Obesity.* Added weight augments the risk of diabetes mellitus, hypertension, and elevated serum cholesterol levels.
- *Physical activity.* Regular exercise reduces the risk.
- *Stress.* Added stress or type A personality increases the risk.
- *Diabetes mellitus.* This disorder raises the risk, especially in women.
- *Other modifiable factors.* Increased levels of serum fibrinogen and uric acid; elevated hematocrit; reduced vital capacity; high resting heart rate; thyrotoxicosis; and use of oral contraceptives heighten the risk.

Uncommon causes of reduced coronary artery blood flow include dissecting aneurysms, infectious vasculitis, syphilis, and congenital defects in the coronary vascular system. Coronary artery spasms may also impede blood flow. (See *Understanding coronary artery spasm,* page 556.)

Complications

When a coronary artery goes into spasm or is occluded by plaques, blood flow to the myocardium supplied by that vessel decreases, causing angina pectoris. Failure to remedy the occlusion causes ischemia and, eventually, myocardial tissue infarction.

Assessment findings

The classic symptom of coronary artery disease is angina, the direct result of inadequate flow of oxygen to the myocardium. The patient usually describes it as a burning, squeezing, or crushing tightness in the substernal or precordial chest that may radiate to the left arm, neck, jaw, or shoulder blade. Typically, the patient clenches his fist over his chest or rubs his left arm when describing the pain. Nausea, vomiting, fainting, sweating, and cool extremities may accompany the tightness.

Angina commonly occurs after physical exertion but may also follow emotional excitement, exposure to cold, or a large meal. Angina may also develop during sleep from which symptoms awaken the patient.

The patient's history will suggest any pattern to the type and onset of pain. If the pain is predictable and relieved by rest or nitrates, it's called *stable angina.* If it increases in frequency and duration and is more easily induced, it's referred to as *unstable* or *unpredictable angina.* Unstable angina generally indicates extensive or worsening disease and, untreated, may progress to myocardial infarction. An effort-induced pain that occurs with increasing frequency and with decreasing provocation is referred to as *crescendo angina.* If severe non-effort-produced pain occurs at rest without provocation, it's called *variant* or *Prinzmetal's angina.*

Inspection may reveal evidence of atherosclerotic disease, such as xanthelasma and xanthoma. Ophthalmoscopic inspection may show increased light reflexes and arteriovenous nicking, suggesting hypertension, an important risk factor for coronary artery disease.

Palpation can uncover thickened or absent peripheral arteries, signs of cardiac enlargement, and abnormal contraction of the cardiac impulse, such as left ventricular akinesia or dyskinesia.

Auscultation may detect bruits, an S_3, an S_4, or a late systolic murmur (if mitral insufficiency is present).

Diagnostic tests

Diagnostic measures include the following:
- *Electrocardiography (ECG)* during angina shows ischemia as demonstrated by T-wave inversion or ST-segment depression and, possibly, arrhythmias, such as premature ventricular contractions. ECG results may or may not be normal during pain-free periods. Arrhythmias may occur without infarction, secondary to ischemia.

UNDERSTANDING CORONARY ARTERY SPASM

In coronary artery spasm, a spontaneous, sustained contraction of one or more coronary arteries causes ischemia and dysfunction of the heart muscle. This disorder may also cause Prinzmetal's angina and even myocardial infarction in patients with unoccluded coronary arteries.

Causes
The direct cause of coronary artery spasm is unknown, but possible contributing factors include:
• altered influx of calcium across the cell membrane
• intimal hemorrhage into the medial layer of the blood vessel
• hyperventilation
• elevated catecholamine levels
• fatty buildup in the lumen.

Signs and symptoms
The major symptom of coronary artery spasm is angina. But unlike classic angina, this pain commonly occurs spontaneously and may be unrelated to physical exertion or emotional stress; it may, however, follow cocaine use. It is usually more severe than classic angina, lasts longer, and may be cyclic—recurring every day at the same time. Ischemic episodes may cause arrhythmias, altered heart rate, lower blood pressure and, occasionally, fainting caused by decreased cardiac output. Spasm in the left coronary artery may result in mitral valve prolapse, producing a loud systolic murmur and, possibly, pulmonary edema, with dyspnea, crackles, and hemoptysis. Myocardial infarction and sudden death may occur.

Treatment
After diagnosis by coronary angiography and 12-lead electrocardiography, the patient may receive calcium channel blockers (verapamil, nifedipine, or diltiazem) to reduce coronary artery spasm and to decrease vascular resistance, and nitrates (nitroglycerin or isosorbide dinitrate) to relieve chest pain. During cardiac catheterization, the patient with clean arteries may receive ergotamine to induce the spasm and aid in the diagnosis.

Nursing interventions
When caring for a patient with coronary artery spasm, explain all necessary procedures and teach him how to take his medications safely. For calcium antagonist therapy, monitor the patient's blood pressure, pulse rate, and cardiac rhythm strips to detect arrhythmias.

For nifedipine and verapamil therapy, monitor digoxin levels, and check for signs of digitalis toxicity. Because nifedipine may cause peripheral and periorbital edema, watch for fluid retention.

Because coronary artery spasm is sometimes associated with atherosclerotic disease, advise the patient to stop smoking, avoid overeating, use alcohol sparingly, and maintain a balance between exercise and rest.

• *Treadmill* or *bicycle exercise test* may provoke chest pain and ECG signs of myocardial ischemia in response to physical exertion. Monitoring of electrical rhythm may demonstrate T-wave inversion or ST-segment depression in the ischemic areas.
• *Coronary angiography* reveals coronary artery stenosis or obstruction, collateral circulation, and the arteries' condition beyond the narrowing.
• *Myocardial perfusion imaging* with thallium-201 during treadmill exercise detects ischemic areas of the myocardium, visualized as "cold spots."

Treatment
The goal of treatment in patients with angina is to reduce myocardial oxygen demand or increase the oxygen supply and reduce pain. Activity restrictions may be required to prevent onset of pain. Rather than eliminating activities, performing them more slowly often averts pain. Stress reduction techniques are also essential, especially if known stressors precipitate pain.

Pharmacologic therapy consists primarily of nitrates, such as nitroglycerin, isosorbide dinitrate, or beta-adrenergic blockers.

Obstructive lesions may necessitate atherectomy or coronary artery bypass graft surgery, using vein grafts. Percutaneous transluminal coronary angioplasty (PTCA) may be performed during cardiac catheterization to compress fatty deposits and relieve occlusion. In patients with calcification, PTCA may reduce the obstruction by fracturing the plaque.

PTCA carries certain risks but causes fewer complications than surgery. Complications after PTCA can include circulatory insufficiency, death (rarely), myocardial infarction, restenosis of the vessels, retroperitoneal bleeding, sudden coronary occlusions, or vasovagal response and arrhythmias.

PTCA is a viable alternative to grafting in elderly patients or in those who otherwise cannot tolerate cardiac surgery. However, patients with a left main coronary artery occlusion, lesions in extremely tortuous vessels, or occlusions older than 3 months are not candidates for PTCA.

Laser angioplasty corrects occlusion by vaporizing fatty deposits with the excimer or hot-tip laser device.

Rotational ablation (or rotational atherectomy) removes atheromatous plaque with a high-speed, rotating burr covered with diamond crystals.

Because coronary artery disease is so widespread, prevention is important. Dietary restrictions aimed at reducing intake of calories (in obesity) and of salt, fats, and cholesterol minimize the risk, especially when supplemented with regular exercise. Abstention from smoking and reduction of stress are also essential.

Other preventive actions include control of hypertension (with diuretics or beta blockers), control of elevated serum cholesterol or triglyceride levels (with antilipemics), and measures to minimize platelet aggregation and the danger of blood clots (with aspirin, for example).

Nursing diagnoses
- Activity intolerance
- Altered nutrition: More than body requirements
- Altered role performance
- Altered sexuality patterns
- Altered tissue perfusion
- Anxiety
- Decreased cardiac output
- Denial
- Fluid volume deficit
- Fluid volume excess
- Health-seeking behaviors
- Impaired gas exchange
- Knowledge deficit
- Pain
- Risk for injury

Nursing interventions
- During anginal episodes, monitor blood pressure and heart rate. Take a 12-lead ECG during anginal episodes before administering nitroglycerin or other nitrates. Record duration of pain, amount of medication required to relieve it, and accompanying symptoms.
- Ask the patient to grade the severity of his pain on a scale of 1 to 10. This allows him to give his individual assessment of pain as well as of the effectiveness of pain-relieving medications.
- Keep nitroglycerin available for immediate use. Instruct the patient to call immediately whenever he feels chest, arm, or neck pain and before taking nitroglycerin.
- After catheterization, review the expected course of treatment with the patient and his family. Monitor the catheter site for bleeding. Also check for distal pulses. To counter the diuretic effect of the dye, increase I.V. fluids and make sure the patient drinks plenty of fluids. Assess potassium levels, and add potassium to the I.V. fluid, if necessary.
- During catheterization, monitor for dye reactions. If symptoms such as falling blood pressure, bradycardia, diaphoresis, and light-headedness appear, increase parenteral fluids as ordered, administer nasal oxygen, place the patient in Trendelenburg's position, and administer I.V. atropine if necessary.
- After PTCA, maintain heparinization, observe for bleeding systemically and at the site, and keep the affected leg immobile.
- After rotational ablation, monitor the patient for chest pain, hypotension, coronary artery spasm, and bleeding from the catheter site. Provide heparin and antibiotic therapy for 24 to 48 hours, as ordered.
- After bypass surgery, provide care for the I.V. set, pulmonary artery catheter, and endotracheal tube. Monitor blood pressure, intake and output, breath sounds, chest tube drainage, and cardiac rhythm, watching for signs of ischemia and arrhythmias. I.V. epinephrine, nitroprusside, dopamine, albumin, potassium, and blood products may be necessary. The patient may also need temporary epicardial pacing, especially if the surgery included replacement of the aortic valve.

Intra-aortic balloon pump insertion may be necessary until the patient stabilizes. Also observe for and treat chest pain. Perform vigorous chest physiotherapy and guide the patient in pulmonary toilet.

Patient teaching
- Before cardiac catheterization, explain the procedure to the patient. Make sure he knows why it's necessary, understands the risks, and realizes that it may indicate a need for interventional therapies such as PTCA, bypass surgery, atherectomy, and laser angioplasty.
- If the patient is scheduled for surgery, explain the procedure, provide a tour of the intensive care unit, introduce him to the staff, and discuss postoperative care.
- Help the patient determine which activities precipitate episodes of pain. Help him identify and select more effective coping mechanisms to deal with stress. Occupational change may be needed to prevent symptoms, but many patients reject this alternative.
- Stress the need to follow the prescribed drug regimen.
- Encourage the patient to maintain the prescribed low-sodium diet and start a low-calorie diet as well.
- Explain that recurrent angina symptoms after PTCA or rotational ablation may signal reobstruction.

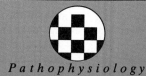

Pathophysiology

WHAT HAPPENS IN M.I.

When blood supply to the myocardium is interrupted, the following events occur:

1. Injury to the endothelial lining of the coronary arteries causes platelets, white blood cells, fibrin, and lipids to converge at the injured site. Foam cells, or resident macrophages, congregate under the damaged lining and absorb oxidized cholesterol, forming a fatty streak that narrows the arterial lumen.

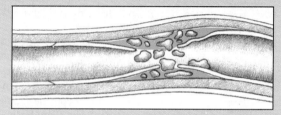

2. Because the arterial lumen narrows gradually, collateral circulation develops and helps maintain myocardial perfusion distal to the obstruction. During this stage, the patient may have chest pain when myocardial oxygen demand increases.

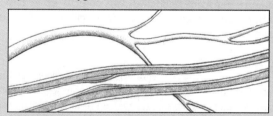

3. When myocardial demand for oxygen is more than the collateral circulation can supply, myocardial metabolism shifts from aerobic to anaerobic, producing lactic acid, which stimulates pain nerve endings. The patient experiences worsening angina that requires rest and medication for relief.

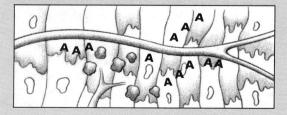

4. Lacking oxygen, the myocardial cells die. This decreases contractility, stroke volume, and blood pressure. Then the patient experiences tachycardia, hypotension, diminished heart sounds, cyanosis, tachypnea, and poor perfusion to vital organs.

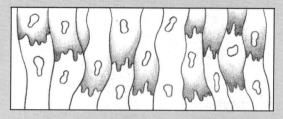

5. Hypoperfusion stimulates baroreceptors, which in turn stimulate the adrenal glands to release epinephrine and norepinephrine. These catecholamines increase heart rate and cause peripheral vasoconstriction, further increasing myocardial oxygen demand. The patient may experience tachyarrhythmias, changes in pulses, decreased level of consciousness, and cold, clammy skin.

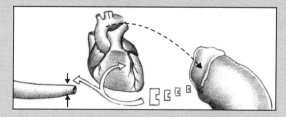

6. Damaged cell membranes in the infarcted area allow intracellular contents into the vascular circulation. Ventricular arrhythmias then develop with elevated serum levels of potassium, creatine phosphokinase (CPK), CPK-MB, aspartate aminotransferase (formerly SGOT), and lactate dehydrogenase.

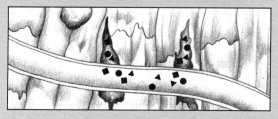

WHAT HAPPENS IN M.I. *(continued)*

7. All myocardial cells are capable of spontaneous depolarization and repolarization, so the electrical conduction system may be affected by infarct, injury, and ischemia. The patient may have a fever, leukocytosis, tachycardia, and ECG signs of tissue ischemia (altered T waves), injured tissue (altered ST segment), and infarcted tissue (deep Q waves).

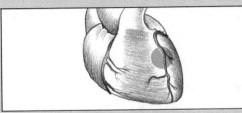

8. Extensive damage to the left ventricle may impair the ventricle's ability to pump, allowing blood to back up into the left atrium and, eventually, into the pulmonary veins and capillaries. When this occurs, the patient may be dyspneic, orthopneic, tachypneic, and cyanotic. Crackles may be heard in the lungs on auscultation. Pulmonary artery and capillary wedge pressures are increased.

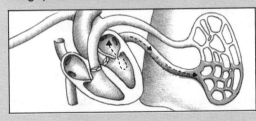

9. As back pressure rises, fluid crosses the alveolar-capillary membrane, impeding diffusion of oxygen (O_2) and carbon dioxide (CO_2). The patient experiences increasing respiratory distress, and arterial blood gases may show decreased partial pressure of oxygen (PaO_2) and arterial pH and increased partial pressure of carbon dioxide ($PaCO_2$).

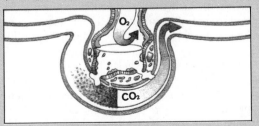

• Encourage regular, moderate exercise. Refer the patient to a cardiac rehabilitation center or cardiovascular fitness program near his home or workplace. The staff can set up a program of exercise that best meets the patient's needs and limitations. Encourage other family members or a friend to join in the physical activity to encourage the patient's commitment to the exercise program.
• Reassure the patient that he can resume sexual activity and that modifications can allow for sexual fulfillment without fear of overexertion, pain, or reocclusion.
• Refer the patient to a program to stop smoking. Acknowledge that this will be difficult but that he should make every attempt to stop smoking immediately and never restart.

MYOCARDIAL INFARCTION

Myocardial infarction (MI) results from reduced blood flow through one of the coronary arteries, which causes myocardial ischemia and necrosis. The infarction site depends on the vessels involved. For instance, occlusion of the circumflex coronary artery causes a lateral wall infarction; occlusion of the left anterior coronary artery causes an anterior wall infarction. True posterior and inferior wall infarctions result from occlusion of the right coronary artery or one of its branches. Right ventricular infarctions can also result from right coronary artery occlusion, can accompany inferior infarctions, and may cause right ventricular failure. In transmural (Q wave) MI, tissue damage extends through all myocardial layers; in subendocardial (non–Q wave) MI, usually only the innermost layer is damaged. (See *What happens in MI.*)

Men are more susceptible to MI than premenopausal women, although incidence is rising among women who smoke and take oral contraceptives. The incidence in postmenopausal women resembles that in men.

In North America and Western Europe, MI is one of the most common causes of death, which usually results from cardiac damage or complications. Mortality is about 25%. However, more than 50% of sudden deaths occur within 1 hour after onset of signs and symptoms, before the patient reaches the hospital. Of those who recover, up to 10% die within the first year.

Causes

MI results from occlusion of one of the coronary arteries. Such occlusion can stem from atherosclerosis, thrombosis, platelet aggregation, or coronary artery stenosis or spasm. Predisposing factors include:
• aging

- diabetes mellitus
- elevated serum triglyceride, low-density lipoprotein, and cholesterol levels, and decreased serum high-density lipoprotein levels
- excessive intake of saturated fats, carbohydrates, or salt
- hypertension
- obesity
- positive family history of coronary artery disease
- sedentary life-style
- smoking
- stress or a type A personality (aggressive, competitive attitude, addiction to work, chronic impatience).

In addition, use of drugs, such as amphetamines or cocaine, can cause an MI.

Complications

Cardiac complications of acute MI include arrhythmias, cardiogenic shock, heart failure causing pulmonary edema, and pericarditis. Other complications include rupture of the atrial or ventricular septum, ventricular wall, or valves; ventricular aneurysms; mural thrombi causing cerebral or pulmonary emboli; and extensions of the original infarction. Dressler's syndrome (post-MI pericarditis) can occur days to weeks after an MI and cause residual pain, malaise, and fever. (See *Complications of MI.*)

Typically, elderly patients are more prone to complications and death. Psychological problems can also occur, either from the patient's fear of another MI or from an organic brain disorder caused by tissue hypoxia. Occasionally, a patient may have a personality change.

Assessment findings

Typically, the patient reports the cardinal symptom of MI—persistent, crushing substernal pain that may radiate to the left arm, jaw, neck, and shoulder blades. He commonly describes the pain as heavy, squeezing, or crushing, and it may persist for 12 or more hours. However, in some patients—particularly elderly patients or those with diabetes—pain may not occur; in others, it may be mild and confused with indigestion.

Patients with coronary artery disease may report increasing anginal frequency, severity, or duration (especially when not precipitated by exertion, a heavy meal, or cold and wind). The patient may also report a feeling of impending doom, fatigue, nausea, vomiting, and shortness of breath. Sudden death, however, may be the first and only indication of MI.

Inspection may reveal an extremely anxious and restless patient with dyspnea and diaphoresis. If right ventricular failure is present, you may note jugular venous distention. Within the first hour after an anterior MI, about 25% of patients exhibit sympathetic nervous system hyperactivity, such as tachycardia and hypertension. Up to 50% of patients with an inferior MI exhibit parasympathetic nervous system hyperactivity, such as bradycardia and hypotension.

In patients who develop ventricular dysfunction, auscultation may disclose an S_4, an S_3, paradoxical splitting of S_2, and decreased heart sounds. A systolic murmur of mitral insufficiency may be heard with papillary muscle dysfunction secondary to infarction. A pericardial friction rub may also be heard, especially in patients who have a transmural MI or have developed pericarditis.

Fever is unusual at the onset of an MI. However, a low-grade fever may develop during the next few days.

Diagnostic tests

In MI, diagnostic tests may provide the following results:
- *Serial 12-lead electrocardiography (ECG)* readings may be normal or inconclusive during the first few hours after an MI. Characteristic abnormalities include serial ST-segment depression in subendocardial MI and ST-segment elevation and Q waves, representing scarring and necrosis, in transmural MI.
- *Serum creatine phosphokinase (CPK)* level is elevated, especially the CPK-MB isoenzyme, the cardiac muscle fraction of CPK.
- *Echocardiography* shows ventricular wall dyskinesia with a transmural MI and helps evaluate the ejection fraction.
- *Scans,* using I.V. technetium-99m pertechnetate, can identify acutely damaged muscle by picking up accumulations of radioactive nucleotide, which appears as a "hot spot" on the film. Myocardial perfusion imaging with thallium-201 reveals a "cold spot" in most patients during the first few hours after a transmural MI.

Treatment

The goals of treatment are to relieve chest pain, to stabilize heart rhythm, and to reduce cardiac work load. Treatment includes revascularization to preserve myocardial tissue. Arrhythmias, the most common problem during the first 48 hours after MI, may require antiarrhythmics, possibly a pacemaker and, rarely, cardioversion.

Drug therapy usually includes:
- lidocaine for ventricular arrhythmias; if lidocaine is ineffective, procainamide, quinidine sulfate, bretylium, or disopyramide
- atropine I.V. or a temporary pacemaker for heart block or bradycardia

COMPLICATIONS OF M.I.

Complication	Assessment	Treatment
Arrhythmias	• ECG shows premature ventricular contractions, ventricular tachycardia, or ventricular fibrillation; in inferior wall MI, bradycardia and junctional rhythms or atrioventricular (AV) block; in anterior wall MI, tachycardia or heart block.	• Antiarrhythmics, atropine, cardioversion, defibrillation, and pacemaker
Heart failure	• In left ventricular failure, chest X-rays show venous congestion and cardiomegaly. • Catheterization shows increases in pulmonary artery systolic and diastolic pressures, pulmonary capillary wedge pressure (PCWP), central venous pressure, and systemic vascular resistance (SVR).	• Diuretics, vasodilators, inotropics, and cardiac glycosides
Cardiogenic shock	• Catheterization shows decreased cardiac output, increased pulmonary artery systolic and diastolic pressures, decreased cardiac index, increased SVR, and increased PCWP. • Signs are hypotension, tachycardia, decreased level of consciousness, decreased urine output, neck vein distention, S_3 and S_4, and cool, pale skin.	• I.V. fluids, vasodilators, cardiotonics, cardiac glycosides, intra-aortic balloon pump (IABP), vasopressors, and beta-adrenergic stimulants
Mitral insufficiency	• Auscultation reveals apical holosystolic murmur. • Dyspnea is prominent. • Catheterization shows increased pulmonary artery pressure (PAP) and PCWP. • Echocardiogram shows valve dysfunction.	• Nitroglycerin, nitroprusside, IABP, and surgical replacement of the mitral valve and possible concomitant myocardial revascularization with significant coronary artery disease
Ventricular septal rupture	• In left-to-right shunt, auscultation reveals a harsh holosystolic murmur and thrill. • Catheterization shows increased PAP and PCWP. • Increased oxygen saturation of right ventricle and pulmonary artery confirms the diagnosis.	• Surgical correction (may be postponed, but more patients have surgery immediately or up to 7 days after septal rupture), IABP, nitroglycerin, nitroprusside, low-dose inotropics (dopamine), and cardiac pacing when high-grade AV blocks occur
Pericarditis or Dressler's syndrome	• Auscultation reveals a pericardial friction rub. • Chest pain is relieved in sitting position. • Sharp pain unlike previously experienced anginal pain.	• Anti-inflammatory agents, such as aspirin or other nonsteroidal anti-inflammatory drugs or corticosteroids
Ventricular aneurysm	• Chest X-rays may show cardiomegaly. • ECG may show arrhythmias and persistent ST-segment elevation. • Left ventriculography shows altered or paradoxical left ventricular motion.	• Cardioversion, defibrillation (if ventricular tachycardia or fibrillation occurs), antiarrhythmics, vasodilators, anticoagulants, cardiac glycosides, diuretics and, possibly, surgery
Cerebral or pulmonary embolism	• Dyspnea and chest pain or neurologic changes occur. • Nuclear scan shows ventilation-perfusion mismatch in pulmonary embolism. • Angiography shows arterial blockage.	• Oxygen and heparin • Cardiopulmonary resuscitation (CPR), epinephrine, or cardiac pacing
Ventricular rupture	• Cardiac tamponade occurs. • Arrhythmias, such as ventricular tachycardia and ventricular fibrillation, or sudden death results.	• Resuscitation for advanced cardiac life support protocol • Possible emergency surgical repair if CPR is successful

TREATING ACUTE M.I. WITH STREPTOKINASE

In the early stages of acute MI, therapy with the thrombolytic drug streptokinase, a first-generation thrombolytic, can dissolve the clot in an occluded artery. This action restores perfusion and limits the size of an infarction.

How streptokinase works
Streptokinase hastens fibrinolysis. It joins plasminogen to form a complex that then reacts with additional plasminogen to form plasmin. This proteolytic enzyme dissolves the clot and relieves the occlusion.

Because streptokinase causes antibodies to it to form, an allergic response may occur with subsequent administration. The antibodies usually last up to 6 months but can remain even longer. So a patient can't receive repeat streptokinase therapy for at least 6 months.

Procedure
Streptokinase may be given I.V. through central venous or intracoronary access following cardiac catheterization. However, during the treatment of acute MI, the I.V. route is most common.

To prevent potential allergic reaction, steroids and antihistamines are often administered. Streptokinase is then administered, usually over 30 to 60 minutes. Other protocols and regimens are continuously being investigated to achieve the highest and quickest rate of reperfusion.

Nursing considerations
During infusion:
• Monitor the patient's blood pressure for hypotension, an adverse reaction to streptokinase. If hypotension occurs, stop the drug until the blood pressure returns to a safe level and then restart the infusion.
After streptokinase therapy:
• Be alert for signs of bleeding. Because streptokinase alters the natural clotting mechanisms, it can produce hemorrhage, especially at the site of recent surgery, needle puncture, or trauma.
• Avoid giving the patient I.M. or I.V. injections for 24 hours.
• Check the infusion site for bleeding every 15 minutes for 1 hour, every 30 minutes for the next 2 hours, and then once every hour until the catheter is removed.
• Watch for signs and symptoms of GI bleeding.
• If a peripheral intracoronary catheter was used:
– Maintain alignment and immobility of the affected extremity if a peripheral artery was used. Don't raise the head of the bed more than 15 degrees.
– Document the patient's pulse rate, color, temperature, and sensitivity of both extremities when checking the site for bleeding.
– Apply direct pressure to the infusion site for at least 30 minutes after catheter removal. Assess the affected extremity distal to the pressure point, and keep the patient on bed rest for at least 6 hours with his leg straight and the head of the bed no higher than 15 degrees.

• nitroglycerin (sublingual, topical, transdermal, or I.V.); calcium channel blockers, such as nifedipine, verapamil, and diltiazem (sublingual, P.O., or I.V.); or isosorbide dinitrate (sublingual, P.O., or I.V.) to relieve pain by redistributing blood to ischemic area of the myocardium, increasing cardiac output, and reducing myocardial work load
• morphine I.V., the drug of choice for pain and sedation and, possibly, meperidine or hydromorphone
• drugs that increase contractility or blood pressure
• inotropic drugs, such as dobutamine and amrinone, to treat reduced myocardial contractility
• beta-adrenergic blockers, such as propranolol and timolol, after acute MI to help prevent reinfarction.

Other therapies may be used, as follows:
• Oxygen is usually administered (by face mask or nasal cannula) at a modest flow rate for 24 to 48 hours; a lower concentration is necessary if the patient has chronic obstructive pulmonary disease.
• Bed rest with bedside commode is enforced to decrease cardiac work load.

• Pulmonary artery catheterization may be performed to detect left or right ventricular failure and to monitor response to treatment, but it's not routinely done.
• Intra-aortic balloon pump may be used for cardiogenic shock.
• Revascularization therapy can be used if the patient is less than age 70 and doesn't have a history of cerebrovascular accident, bleeding, GI ulcers, marked hypertension, recent surgery, or chest pain lasting longer than 6 hours. Thrombolytic therapy must begin within 6 hours of the onset of symptoms, using intracoronary or systemic streptokinase (I.V.) or tissue plasminogen activator (t-PA). The best response occurs when treatment begins within the first hour after onset of symptoms. (See *Treating acute MI with streptokinase.*)
• Cardiac catheterization, percutaneous transluminal coronary angioplasty (PTCA), and coronary artery bypass grafting may also be performed.

Nursing diagnoses

- Activity intolerance
- Altered nutrition: Less than body requirements
- Altered sexuality patterns
- Altered tissue perfusion
- Anxiety
- Constipation
- Decreased cardiac output
- Denial
- Fatigue
- Fluid volume excess
- Ineffective individual coping
- Pain
- Risk for injury

Nursing interventions

- On admission to the intensive care unit (ICU), monitor and record the patient's ECG readings, blood pressure, temperature, and heart and breath sounds.
- Assess pain, and give analgesics, as ordered. Record the severity, location, type, and duration of pain. Don't give I.M. injections because absorption from the muscle is unpredictable, CPK may be falsely elevated, and I.V. administration gives more rapid relief of signs and symptoms.
- Check the patient's blood pressure after giving nitroglycerin, especially the first dose.
- Frequently monitor ECG rhythm strips to detect rate changes and arrhythmias. Analyze rhythm strips and place a representative strip in the patient's chart if any new arrhythmias are documented, if chest pain occurs, or at least every shift or according to institution protocol.
- During episodes of chest pain, obtain ECG readings and blood pressure and pulmonary artery catheter measurements (if applicable) to determine changes.
- Watch for crackles, cough, tachypnea, and edema, which may indicate impending left ventricular failure. Carefully monitor daily weight, intake and output, respiratory rate, serum enzyme levels, ECG readings, and blood pressure. Auscultate for adventitious breath sounds periodically (patients on bed rest frequently have atelectatic crackles, which may disappear after coughing) and for S_3 or S_4 gallops.
- Organize patient care and activities to maximize periods of uninterrupted rest.
- Ask the dietary department to provide a clear liquid diet until nausea subsides. A low-cholesterol, low-sodium diet, without caffeine-containing beverages, may be ordered.
- Provide a stool softener to prevent straining at stool, which causes vagal stimulation and may slow heart rate.

Allow the patient to use a bedside commode, and provide as much privacy as possible.
- Assist with range-of-motion exercises. If the patient is immobilized by a severe MI, turn him often. Antiembolism stockings help prevent venostasis and thrombophlebitis.
- Provide emotional support, and help reduce stress and anxiety; administer tranquilizers, as needed.
- If the patient has undergone PTCA, sheath care is necessary. Keep the sheath line open with a heparin drip. Observe for generalized and site bleeding. Keep the leg with the sheath insertion site immobile. Maintain strict bed rest. Check peripheral pulses in the affected leg frequently. Provide analgesics for back pain, if needed.
- After thrombolytic therapy, administer continuous heparin as ordered. Monitor the partial thromboplastin time every 6 hours, and monitor the patient for evidence of bleeding.
- Monitor ECG rhythm strips for reperfusion arrhythmias and treat them according to hospital protocol. If the artery reoccludes, the patient will experience the same symptoms as before. If this occurs, prepare the patient for return to the cardiac catheterization laboratory.

Patient teaching

- Explain procedures and answer questions for both the patient and his family. Explain the ICU environment and routine. Remember that you may need to repeat explanations once the emergency situation has resolved.
- To promote compliance with the prescribed medication regimen and other treatment measures, thoroughly explain dosages and therapy. Inform the patient of the drug's adverse reactions, and advise him to watch for and report signs of toxicity (for example, anorexia, nausea, vomiting, mental depression, vertigo, blurred vision, and yellow vision, if the patient is receiving digitalis).
- Review dietary restrictions with the patient. If he must follow a low-sodium or low-fat and low-cholesterol diet, provide a list of foods to avoid. Ask the dietitian to speak to the patient and his family.
- Encourage the patient to participate in a cardiac rehabilitation exercise program. The doctor and the exercise physiologist should determine the level of exercise and then discuss it with the patient and secure his agreement to a stepped-care program.
- Counsel the patient to resume sexual activity progressively. He may need to take nitroglycerin before sexual intercourse to prevent chest pain from the increased activity.
- Advise the patient about appropriate responses to new or recurrent symptoms.

CLASSIFYING HEART FAILURE

Although heart failure is usually classified by the site of heart failure (left ventricle, right ventricle, or both), it may also be classified by level of cardiac output, stage, and direction (high-output or low-output, acute or chronic, or forward or backward). These classifications represent different clinical aspects of heart failure, not distinct diseases.

Left-sided failure
Failure of the left ventricle to pump blood to the vital organs and periphery is usually caused by myocardial infarction (MI). Decreased left ventricular output causes fluid to accumulate in the lungs, precipitating dyspnea, orthopnea, and paroxysmal nocturnal dyspnea.

Right-sided failure
Resulting from failure of the right ventricle to pump sufficient blood to the lungs, this type usually is caused by disorders that increase pulmonary vascular resistance, such as pulmonary embolism, pulmonary stenosis, and pulmonary hypertension. Right ventricular failure produces congestive hepatomegaly, ascites, and edema.

High-output failure
Failure with an elevated cardiac output occurs when tissue demands for oxygenated blood exceed the heart's ability to supply it. High-output failure occurs in arteriovenous fistula, hyperthyroidism, anemia, sickle cell anemia, beriberi, Paget's disease of the bone, and thyrotoxicosis.

Low-output failure
Failure with decreased cardiac output is caused by decreased pumping ability of the myocardium. Low-output failure occurs in coronary artery disease, hy-

pertension, primary myocardial disease, and valvular disease.

Acute failure
This failure occurs suddenly, as in MI or ruptured cardiac valve. The sudden reduction in cardiac output results in systemic hypotension without peripheral edema. Acute failure may occur in a chronic condition, such as when a patient with chronic heart failure experiences acute heart failure with MI. It may also occur in any condition that stresses an already diseased heart.

Chronic failure
This type of heart failure occurs gradually and is sustained for long periods. The arterial blood pressure doesn't drop, but peripheral edema is present. Chronic failure may occur in cardiomyopathy or multivalvular disease, or in a healed, extensive MI.

Forward failure
The heart fails to expel enough blood into the arterial system. Sodium and water retention results from decreased renal perfusion and excessive proximal tubular sodium reabsorption or excessive distal tubular reabsorption, through activation of the renin-angiotensin-aldosterone system.

Backward failure
When backward heart failure occurs, one ventricle fails to empty its contents normally, and end-diastolic ventricular pressures rise. The pressures and volume in the atrium and venous system behind the failing ventricle also rise, and sodium and water retention occurs because of the elevated systemic venous and capillary pressures and the resulting transudation of fluid into the interstitial space.

• Advise the patient to report typical or atypical chest pain. Post-MI syndrome may develop, producing chest pain that must be differentiated from recurrent MI, pulmonary infarction, and heart failure.
• Stress the need to stop smoking. If necessary, refer the patient to a support group.

HEART FAILURE

When the myocardium cannot pump effectively enough to meet the body's metabolic needs, heart failure occurs. Pump failure usually occurs in a damaged left ventricle (left ventricular failure), but it may happen in the right ventricle (right ventricular failure) primarily, or secondary to left ventricular failure. Usually, however, left and

right ventricular failure develop simultaneously. Heart failure is classified as *high-output* or *low-output, acute* or *chronic, left-sided* or *right-sided,* and *forward* or *backward.* (See *Classifying heart failure.*)

For many patients, the symptoms of heart failure restrict the ability to perform activities of daily living, severely affecting quality of life. Advances in diagnostic and therapeutic techniques have greatly improved the outlook for these patients, but the prognosis still depends on the underlying cause and its response to treatment.

Causes and pathophysiology
Heart failure frequently results from a primary abnormality of the heart muscle (such as an infarction) that impairs ventricular function to the point that the heart

can no longer pump sufficient blood. (See *What happens in heart failure,* pages 566 and 567.) Heart failure can also result from causes not related to myocardial function. These include:

• mechanical disturbances in ventricular filling during diastole, which result from blood volume that's insufficient for the ventricle to pump. This occurs in mitral stenosis secondary to rheumatic heart disease or constrictive pericarditis and atrial fibrillation.

• systolic hemodynamic disturbances—such as excessive cardiac work load caused by volume overloading or pressure overload—that limit the heart's pumping ability. These disturbances can result from mitral or aortic insufficiency, which causes volume overloading, and aortic stenosis or systemic hypertension, which results in increased resistance to ventricular emptying.

In addition, certain conditions can predispose the patient to heart failure, particularly if he has some form of underlying heart disease. These include:

• arrhythmias—such as tachyarrhythmias, which can reduce ventricular filling time; bradycardia, which can reduce cardiac output; and arrhythmias that disrupt the normal atrial and ventricular filling synchrony

• pregnancy and thyrotoxicosis because of the increased demand for cardiac output

• pulmonary embolism because it elevates pulmonary arterial pressures that can cause right ventricular failure

• infections because increased metabolic demands further burden the heart

• anemia because to meet the oxygen needs of the tissues, cardiac output must increase

• increased physical activity, emotional stress, increased salt or water intake, or failure to comply with the prescribed treatment regimen for the underlying heart disease.

Complications

Pulmonary congestion can lead to pulmonary edema, a life-threatening condition. Decreased perfusion to major organs, especially the brain and kidneys, can cause these organs to fail. Myocardial infarction can occur because the oxygen demands of the overworked heart cannot be sufficiently met.

Assessment findings

The patient's history reveals a disorder or condition that can precipitate heart failure. The patient often complains of shortness of breath, which occurs in early stages during activity, and, in late stages, also at rest. He may report that dyspnea worsens at night when he lies down. He may use two or three pillows to elevate his head to sleep or have to sleep sitting up in a chair. He may relate that his shortness of breath wakes him up shortly after he falls asleep, causing him to sit bolt upright to catch his breath. Often he may remain dyspneic, coughing, and wheezing even when he sits up. This is referred to as paroxysmal nocturnal dyspnea.

The patient may report that his shoes or rings have become too tight, a result of peripheral edema. He may also report increasing fatigue, weakness, insomnia, anorexia, nausea, and a sense of abdominal fullness (particularly in right ventricular failure).

Inspection may reveal a dyspneic, anxious patient in respiratory distress. In mild cases, dyspnea may occur while the patient is lying down or active; in severe cases, it is not related to position. The patient may have a cough that produces pink, frothy sputum. You may note cyanosis of the lips and nail beds, pale skin, diaphoresis, dependent peripheral and sacral edema, and jugular venous distention. Ascites may also be present, especially in patients with right ventricular failure. If heart failure is chronic, the patient may appear cachectic.

When palpating the pulse, you may note that the skin feels cool and clammy. The pulse rate will be rapid, and a pulsus alternans may be present. Hepatomegaly and, possibly, splenomegaly also may be present.

Percussion reveals dullness over lung bases that are fluid-filled.

Auscultation of the blood pressure may detect decreased pulse pressure, reflecting reduced stroke volume. Heart auscultation may disclose an S_3 and S_4. Lung auscultation reveals moist, bibasilar crackles. If pulmonary edema is present, you'll hear crackles throughout the lung, accompanied by rhonchi and expiratory wheezing.

Diagnostic tests

• *Electrocardiography* reflects heart strain or enlargement, or ischemia. It may also reveal atrial enlargement, tachycardia, and extrasystoles.

• *Chest X-rays* show increased pulmonary vascular markings, interstitial edema, or pleural effusion and cardiomegaly.

• *Pulmonary artery pressure monitoring* typically demonstrates elevated pulmonary artery and capillary wedge pressures, left ventricular end-diastolic pressure in left ventricular failure, and elevated right atrial or central venous pressure in right ventricular failure.

Treatment

The aim of therapy is to improve pump function by reversing the compensatory mechanisms producing the

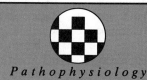

Pathophysiology

WHAT HAPPENS IN HEART FAILURE

These illustrations show, step-by-step, what happens when myocardial damage leads to heart failure.

Left ventricular failure
Increased work load and end-diastolic volume enlarge the left ventricle. Because of the lack of oxygen, however, the ventricle enlarges with stretched tissue rather than functional tissue. The patient may experience increased heart rate, pale and cool skin, tingling in the extremities, decreased cardiac output, and arrhythmias.

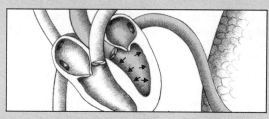

Diminished left ventricular function allows blood to pool in the ventricle and the atrium and eventually back up into the pulmonary veins and capillaries. At this stage, the patient may experience dyspnea on exertion, confusion, dizziness, postural hypotension, decreased peripheral pulses and pulse pressure, cyanosis, and an S_3 gallop.

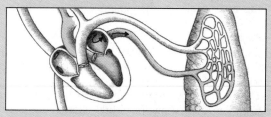

As the pulmonary circulation becomes engorged, rising capillary pressure pushes sodium and water into the interstitial space, causing pulmonary edema. You'll note coughing, subclavian retractions, crackles, tachypnea, elevated pulmonary artery pressure, diminished pulmonary compliance, and increased partial pressure of carbon dioxide.

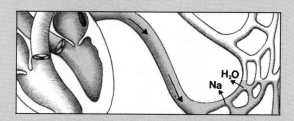

When the patient lies down, fluid in the extremities moves into systemic circulation. Because the left ventricle can't handle the increased venous return, fluid pools in the pulmonary circulation, worsening pulmonary edema. You may note decreased breath sounds, dullness on percussion, crackles, and orthopnea.

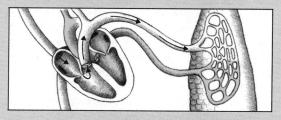

The right ventricle may now become stressed because it's pumping against greater pulmonary vascular resistance and left ventricular pressure. When this occurs, the patient's symptoms worsen.

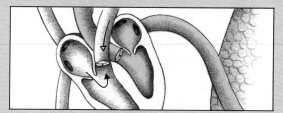

WHAT HAPPENS IN HEART FAILURE *(continued)*

Right ventricular failure
The stressed right ventricle hypertrophies with the formation of stretched tissue. Increasing conduction time and deviation of the heart from its normal axis can cause arrhythmias. If the patient doesn't already have left ventricular failure, he may experience increased heart rate, cool skin, cyanosis, decreased cardiac output, palpitations, and dyspnea.

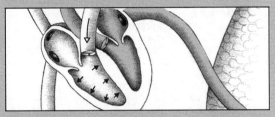

Blood pools in the right ventricle and right atrium. The backed-up blood causes pressure and congestion in the vena cava and systemic circulation. The patient will have elevated central venous pressure, jugular venous distention, and hepatojugular reflux.

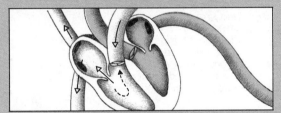

Backed-up blood also distends the visceral veins, especially the hepatic vein. As the liver and spleen become engorged, their function is impaired. The patient may develop anorexia, nausea, abdominal pain, palpable liver and spleen, weakness, and dyspnea secondary to abdominal distention.

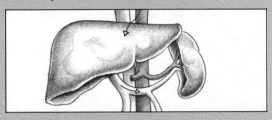

Rising capillary pressure forces excess fluid from the capillaries into the interstitial space. This causes tissue edema, especially in the lower extremities and abdomen. The patient may experience weight gain, pitting edema, and nocturia.

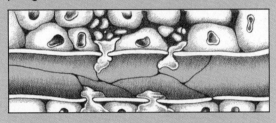

clinical effects. Heart failure can usually be controlled quickly by treatment consisting of:
• diuresis (with diuretics, such as furosemide, hydrochlorothiazide, ethacrynic acid, bumetanide, spironolactone, or triamterene) to reduce total blood volume and circulatory congestion
• prolonged bed rest
• oxygen administration to increase oxygen delivery to the myocardium and other vital organ tissues
• inotropic drugs, such as digoxin, to strengthen myocardial contractility; sympathomimetics, such as dopamine and dobutamine, in acute situations; or amrinone, to increase contractility and cause arterial vasodilation
• vasodilators to increase cardiac output or angiotensin-converting enzyme inhibitors to decrease afterload
• antiembolism stockings to prevent venostasis and possible thromboembolism formation.

Treatment of acute pulmonary edema requires morphine; nitroglycerin or nitroprusside as a vasodilator to diminish blood return to the heart; dobutamine, dopamine, or amrinone to increase myocardial contractility and cardiac output; diuretics to reduce fluid volume; supplemental oxygen; and high Fowler's position. (See *Managing pulmonary edema*, page 568.)

After recovery, the patient usually must continue taking digitalis, diuretics, and potassium supplements, and must remain under medical supervision. If the patient with valve dysfunction has recurrent acute heart failure, surgical replacement may be necessary.

Nursing diagnoses
• Activity intolerance
• Altered nutrition: Less than body requirements
• Altered tissue perfusion
• Decreased cardiac output

MANAGING PULMONARY EDEMA

Because of heart failure, fluid may accumulate in the extravascular spaces of the lungs. To intervene appropriately, you must accurately assess the severity of the patient's edema.

Initial stage
Signs and symptoms
- Persistent cough, which resembles throat-clearing when it begins
- Slight dyspnea and exercise intolerance
- Restlessness and anxiety
- Crackles at lung bases
- Diastolic gallop and S_3

Special considerations
- Check color and amount of expectoration.
- Start and maintain a keep-vein-open I.V. line.
- Position the patient for comfort and elevate the head of the bed.
- Auscultate the chest for crackles and S_3.
- Administer medications as ordered; morphine is the drug of choice.
- Administer diuretics and potassium replacement, if necessary.
- Monitor arterial blood gas (ABG) and electrolyte levels.
- Calculate intake and output accurately.
- Monitor apical and radial pulses.
- Help the patient conserve strength.
- Provide emotional support.

Acute stage
Signs and symptoms
- Acute dyspnea

- Rapid, noisy respirations (audible wheeze, crackles) in all lung fields
- More intense cough with frothy, blood-tinged sputum
- Cyanosis; cold, clammy skin
- Tachycardia; arrhythmias
- Hypotension
- Restlessness

Special considerations
- Administer supplemental oxygen, as necessary (preferably by high concentration mask or intermittent positive-pressure breathing apparatus).
- Aspirate the nasopharynx, as needed.
- Give inotropic drugs, such as digoxin, as ordered.
- Give nitrates, morphine, and potent diuretics, such as furosemide, as ordered.
- Insert an indwelling urinary catheter.
- Monitor and record intake and output.
- Monitor ABG levels.
- Attach cardiac monitor leads, and monitor heart rate and for arrhythmias. Keep resuscitation equipment available. Prepare for intubation and mechanical ventilation in case it's needed.
- Provide emotional support for the patient and family.

Advanced stage
Signs and symptoms
- Decreased level of consciousness
- Ventricular arrhythmias, bradycardia; shock
- Diminished breath sounds

Special considerations
- Assist with intubation and mechanical ventilation.
- Resuscitate the patient, if necessary.

- Fatigue
- Fluid volume excess
- Ineffective airway clearance
- Ineffective breathing pattern
- Knowledge deficit
- Risk for infection

Nursing interventions
- Place the patient in Fowler's position and give him supplemental oxygen to help him breathe more easily. Organize all activity to provide maximum rest periods.
- Weigh the patient daily (this is the best index of fluid retention), and check for peripheral edema. Also, monitor I.V. intake and urine output (especially in the patient receiving diuretics).
- Assess vital signs (for increased respiratory and heart rates and for narrowing pulse pressure) and mental status. Auscultate for abnormal heart and breath sounds.

Report any changes immediately.
- Frequently monitor blood urea nitrogen and serum creatinine, potassium, sodium, chloride, and magnesium levels.
- Provide continuous cardiac monitoring during acute and advanced stages to identify and treat arrhythmias promptly.
- To prevent deep vein thrombosis due to vascular congestion, assist the patient with range-of-motion exercises. Enforce bed rest, and apply antiembolism stockings. Watch for calf pain and tenderness.

Patient teaching
- Advise the patient to avoid foods high in sodium content, such as canned or commercially prepared foods and dairy products, to curb fluid overload.
- Prepare the patient to manage the disorder at home. (See *Dealing with heart failure.*)

DILATED CARDIOMYOPATHY

Also called congestive cardiomyopathy, this disorder results from extensively damaged myocardial muscle fibers. It interferes with myocardial metabolism and grossly dilates every heart chamber, giving the heart a globular shape. When hypertrophy coexists with dilated cardiomyopathy, the heart ejects blood less efficiently than normal, and a large volume of blood remains in the left ventricle after systole, causing signs of heart failure.

Dilated cardiomyopathy most commonly affects middle-aged men but can occur in any age-group. Because it isn't usually diagnosed until the advanced stages, the prognosis is generally poor. Most patients, especially those over age 55, die within 2 years of symptom onset.

Causes

The cause of most cardiomyopathies is unknown. Dilated cardiomyopathy can result from myocardial destruction by toxic, infectious, or metabolic agents; endocrine and electrolyte disorders; nutritional deficiencies; muscle disorders (myasthenia gravis, muscular dystrophy, myotonic dystrophy); infiltrative disorders (hemochromatosis, amyloidosis); and sarcoidosis.

Cardiomyopathy may be associated with alcoholism, viral myocarditis (especially after infection with coxsackievirus B, poliovirus, and influenza virus), and acquired immunodeficiency syndrome.

Metabolic cardiomyopathies are related to endocrine and electrolyte disorders and nutritional deficiencies. Dilated cardiomyopathy may develop in patients with hyperthyroidism, pheochromocytoma, beriberi, and kwashiorkor. Cardiomyopathy may also result from rheumatic fever, especially among children with myocarditis.

Cardiomyopathy may develop during the last trimester of pregnancy or within months after delivery. Its cause is unknown, but it occurs most frequently in multiparous women over age 30, particularly those with malnutrition or preeclampsia. In these patients, cardiomegaly and congestive heart failure may reverse with treatment, allowing a subsequent normal pregnancy. If cardiomegaly persists despite treatment, the prognosis is poor.

Dilated cardiomyopathy has been linked to the use of doxorubicin, cyclophosphamide, cocaine, and fluorouracil. Also, familial forms of this disorder may exist, possibly with an X-linked inheritance pattern.

Complications

Dilated cardiomyopathy can lead to intractable heart failure, arrhythmias, and emboli. Ventricular arrhythmias may lead to syncope and sudden death.

Home care

DEALING WITH HEART FAILURE

To help a patient with heart failure deal with the disorder at home, use the following interventions:
• Advise the patient to follow a low-sodium diet, if ordered. Identify low-sodium food substitutes and foods to avoid, and show how to read labels to assess sodium content. To evaluate compliance, analyze the patient's 24-hour dietary recall.
• Show the patient how to take a pulse by placing a finger on the radial artery and counting for 1 minute. Then have him demonstrate the procedure.
• Tell the patient to take digoxin at the same time each day, to check the pulse rate and rhythm before taking it, and to call the doctor if the rate is under 60 beats/minute or the rhythm is irregular.
• Teach the patient to report important signs and symptoms, such as dizziness, blurred vision, shortness of breath, persistent dry cough, palpitations, increased fatigue, paroxysmal nocturnal dyspnea, swollen ankles, and decreased urine output.
• Advise the patient to weigh himself at least three times per week and to report an increase of 3 to 5 pounds in 1 week.
• Instruct the patient taking a potassium-depleting diuretic to eat high-potassium foods, such as bananas and orange juice.

Assessment findings

The patient may have a history of a disorder that can cause cardiomyopathy. He often complains of a gradual onset of shortness of breath, orthopnea, dyspnea on exertion, paroxysmal nocturnal dyspnea, fatigue, a dry cough at night, palpitations, and vague chest pain.

Inspection may reveal peripheral edema, jugular venous distention, ascites, and peripheral cyanosis.

Palpation of peripheral pulses may disclose tachycardia even at rest and pulsus alternans in late stages. Palpation may also reveal hepatomegaly and splenomegaly.

Percussion may detect hepatomegaly. Dullness will be heard over lung areas that are fluid-filled.

Blood pressure auscultation may show a narrow pulse pressure. Cardiac auscultation reveals irregular rhythms, diffuse apical impulses, pansystolic murmur (mitral and tricuspid insufficiency caused by cardiomegaly and weak papillary muscles), and S_3 and S_4 gallop rhythms. Lung auscultation may reveal crackles and gurgles.

Diagnostic tests

No single test confirms dilated cardiomyopathy. Diagnosis requires elimination of other possible causes of heart failure and arrhythmias.

• *Electrocardiography (ECG)* and *angiography* rule out ischemic heart disease. The ECG may also show biventricular hypertrophy; sinus tachycardia; atrial enlargement; ST-segment and T-wave abnormalities; and, in 20% of patients, atrial fibrillation or left bundle-branch block. QRS complexes are decreased in amplitude.

• *Chest X-rays* demonstrate moderate to marked cardiomegaly, usually affecting all heart chambers, along with pulmonary congestion, pulmonary venous hypertension, and pleural effusion. Pericardial effusion may appear as a water bottle shape.

• *Echocardiography* may identify ventricular thrombi, global hypokinesis, and the degrees of left ventricular dilation and dysfunction.

• *Cardiac catheterization* can show left ventricular dilation and dysfunction, elevated left ventricular and often right ventricular filling pressures, and diminished cardiac output.

• *Gallium scans* may identify patients with dilated cardiomyopathy and myocarditis.

• *Transvenous endomyocardial biopsy* may be useful in some patients to determine the underlying disorder, such as amyloidosis or myocarditis.

Treatment

In dilated cardiomyopathy, the goal of treatment is to correct the underlying causes and to improve the heart's pumping ability with digitalis, diuretics, oxygen, anticoagulants, vasodilators, and a low-sodium diet supplemented by vitamin therapy. Antiarrhythmics may be used to treat arrhythmias. If cardiomyopathy is due to alcoholism, ingestion of alcohol must be stopped. A woman of childbearing age should avoid pregnancy.

Therapy may also include prolonged bed rest and selective use of corticosteroids, particularly when myocardial inflammation is present. Vasodilators reduce preload and afterload, thereby decreasing congestion and increasing cardiac output.

Acute heart failure necessitates vasodilation with nitroprusside I.V. or nitroglycerin I.V. Long-term treatment may include prazosin, hydralazine, isosorbide dinitrate and, if the patient is on prolonged bed rest, anticoagulants. Dopamine, dobutamine, and amrinone may be useful during the acute stage.

When these treatments fail, therapy may require heart transplantation for carefully selected patients.

Nursing diagnoses

• Activity intolerance
• Altered family processes
• Altered tissue perfusion
• Anxiety
• Decreased cardiac output
• Fatigue
• Fluid volume excess
• Hopelessness
• Impaired gas exchange
• Impaired physical mobility
• Ineffective breathing pattern
• Knowledge deficit

Nursing interventions

• Alternate periods of rest with required activities of daily living and treatments. Provide personal care as needed to prevent fatigue.

• Provide active or passive range-of-motion exercises to prevent muscle atrophy while the patient is on bed rest.

• Consult with the dietitian to provide a low-sodium diet that the patient can accept.

• Monitor for signs of progressive failure (decreased arterial pulses, increased neck vein distention) and compromised renal perfusion (oliguria, increased blood urea nitrogen and serum creatinine levels, and electrolyte imbalances). Weigh the patient daily.

• Administer oxygen as needed.

• If the patient is receiving vasodilators, check his blood pressure and heart rate frequently. If he becomes hypotensive, stop the infusion and place him supine with legs elevated to increase venous return and ensure cerebral blood flow.

• If the patient is receiving diuretics, monitor for signs of resolving congestion (decreased crackles and dyspnea) or too vigorous diuresis. Check serum potassium levels for hypokalemia, especially if therapy includes digitalis.

• Therapeutic restrictions and an uncertain prognosis usually cause profound anxiety and depression, so offer support and let the patient express his feelings. Be flexible with visiting hours. If hospitalization is prolonged, try to obtain permission for the patient to spend occasional weekends away from the hospital.

• Allow the patient and his family to express their fears and concerns. As needed, help them identify effective coping strategies.

Patient teaching

• Before discharge, teach the patient about his illness and its treatment.

• Emphasize the need to restrict sodium intake, to watch for weight gain, and to take digitalis as prescribed and watch for its toxic effects (anorexia, nausea, vomiting).
• Encourage family members to learn cardiopulmonary resuscitation because sudden cardiac arrest is possible.

HYPERTROPHIC CARDIOMYOPATHY

Also known as idiopathic hypertrophic subaortic stenosis, hypertrophic obstructive cardiomyopathy, and muscular aortic stenosis, this primary disease of cardiac muscle is characterized by left ventricular hypertrophy and disproportionate, asymmetrical thickening of the intraventricular septum and free wall of the left ventricle. It's also distinguished by a dynamic left ventricular outflow tract pressure gradient related to subaortic narrowing caused by septal hypertrophy in the mitral valve area. The obstruction produced may change between examinations and even from beat to beat.

In hypertrophic cardiomyopathy (HC), cardiac output may be low, normal, or high, depending on whether the stenosis is obstructive or nonobstructive. Eventually, left ventricular dysfunction—a result of rigidity and decreased compliance—causes pump failure. If cardiac output is normal or high, the stenosis may go undetected for years, but low cardiac output may lead to potentially fatal congestive heart failure.

The course of this disorder varies. Some patients demonstrate progressive deterioration, whereas others remain stable for several years.

Causes
About half of all cases of HC are transmitted as an autosomal dominant trait. Other causes aren't known.

Complications
Pulmonary hypertension and heart failure may occur secondary to left ventricular stiffness. Sudden death is also possible and usually results from ventricular arrhythmias, such as ventricular tachycardia and premature ventricular contractions.

Assessment findings
Generally, clinical features don't appear until the disease is well advanced. Then atrial dilation and, sometimes, atrial fibrillation abruptly reduce blood flow to the left ventricle. Most patients are asymptomatic but have a family history of HC. In some cases, death occurs suddenly, particularly in children and young adults. Patients who have symptoms complain of orthopnea and dyspnea on exertion. They often have anginal pain, fatigue, and syncope even at rest. Inspection of the carotid artery may show a rapidly rising carotid arterial pulse. Palpation of peripheral arteries reveals a characteristic double impulse (pulsus biferiens). Palpation of the chest reveals a double or triple apical impulse, which may be displaced laterally. Percussion may reveal bibasilar crackles if heart failure is present. Auscultation reveals a harsh systolic murmur, heard after S_1 at the apex near the left sternal border. The murmur is intensified by standing and with Valsalva's maneuver. An S_4 may also be audible.

Diagnostic tests
• *Echocardiography* shows left ventricular hypertrophy and a thick, asymmetrical intraventricular septum in obstructive HC, whereas hypertrophy affects various ventricular areas in nonobstructive HC. The septum may have a ground-glass appearance. Poor septal contraction, abnormal motion of the anterior mitral leaflet during systole, and narrowing or occlusion of the left ventricular outflow tract may also be seen in obstructive HC. The left ventricular cavity appears small, with vigorous posterior wall motion but reduced septal excursion.
• *Cardiac catheterization* reveals elevated left ventricular end-diastolic pressure and, possibly, mitral insufficiency. In a rare form of the disease, the left atrium will have a slipper-foot shape, and the left ventricle, a spade shape.
• *Electrocardiography* usually shows left ventricular hypertrophy, ST-segment and T-wave abnormalities, Q waves in leads II, III, aV_F, and in V_4 to V_6 (due to hypertrophy, not infarction), left anterior hemiblock, left axis deviation, and ventricular and atrial arrhythmias.
• *Chest X-rays* may show a mild to moderate increase in heart size.
• *Thallium scan* usually reveals myocardial perfusion defects.

Treatment
The goals of treatment are to relax the ventricle and to relieve outflow tract obstruction. Propranolol, a beta-adrenergic blocking agent, is the drug of choice. It slows the heart rate and increases ventricular filling by relaxing the obstructing muscle, thereby reducing angina, syncope, dyspnea, and arrhythmias. However, propranolol may aggravate symptoms of cardiac decompensation.

Calcium channel blockers may reduce elevated diastolic pressures and severity of outflow tract gradients and increase exercise tolerance. Disopyramide can be used to reduce left ventricular contractility and the outflow gradient.

Atrial fibrillation, a medical emergency with HC, necessitates cardioversion. It also calls for heparin administration before cardioversion and continuing until fibrillation subsides because of the high risk of systemic embolism.

If heart failure occurs, amiodarone may be used, unless an atrioventricular block exists. This drug seems to be effective in reducing ventricular and supraventricular arrhythmias, as well. Vasodilators (such as nitroglycerin), diuretics, and sympathetic stimulators (such as isoproterenol) are contraindicated.

If drug therapy fails, surgery is indicated. Ventricular myotomy (resection of the hypertrophied septum) alone or combined with mitral valve replacement may ease outflow tract obstruction and relieve symptoms. However, ventricular myotomy may cause complications, such as complete heart block and a ventricular septal defect, and is experimental.

Nursing diagnoses
• Activity intolerance
• Decreased cardiac output
• Fatigue
• Fluid volume excess
• Ineffective individual coping
• Knowledge deficit
• Pain
• Risk for infection

Nursing interventions
• Alternate periods of rest with required activities of daily living and treatments. Provide personal care as needed to prevent fatigue.
• Provide active or passive range-of-motion exercises to prevent muscle atrophy if the patient is on bed rest.
• If propranolol is to be discontinued, don't stop the drug abruptly; doing so may cause rebound effects, resulting in myocardial infarction or sudden death. To determine the patient's tolerance for an increased dose of propranolol, take his pulse to check for bradycardia, and have him stand and walk around slowly to check for orthostatic hypotension.
• Therapeutic restrictions and an uncertain prognosis usually cause profound anxiety and depression, so offer support and let the patient express his feelings. Be flexible with visiting hours. If hospitalization is prolonged, try to obtain permission for the patient to spend occasional weekends away from the hospital.
• Allow the patient and his family to express their fears and concerns. As needed, help them identify effective coping strategies.

Patient teaching
• Remind the patient and his family that propranolol may cause depression. Notify the doctor if symptoms occur.
• Instruct the patient to take his medication, as ordered. Tell him to notify any doctor caring for him that he shouldn't be given nitroglycerin, digitalis, or diuretics because they can worsen obstruction.
• Inform the patient that before dental work or surgery, he'll need antibiotic prophylaxis to prevent subacute bacterial endocarditis.
• Warn the patient against strenuous activity, which may precipitate syncope or sudden death. Also advise him to avoid Valsalva's maneuver or sudden position changes; both may worsen an obstruction. Urge his family to learn cardiopulmonary resuscitation.

HYPOVOLEMIC SHOCK
In this potentially life-threatening syndrome, reduced intravascular blood volume causes circulatory dysfunction and inadequate tissue perfusion. Tissue anoxia prompts a shift in cellular metabolism from aerobic to anaerobic pathways. This produces an accumulation of lactic acid, resulting in metabolic acidosis.

Without sufficient blood or fluid replacement, hypovolemic shock may lead to irreversible cerebral and renal damage, cardiac arrest and, ultimately, death. (See *How hypovolemic shock progresses.*) Hypovolemic shock syndrome necessitates early recognition of signs and symptoms and prompt, aggressive treatment to improve the prognosis.

Causes
Hypovolemic shock most often results from acute blood loss — about one-fifth of total volume. Massive blood loss may result from GI bleeding, internal hemorrhage (hemothorax, hemoperitoneum), external hemorrhage (accidental or surgical trauma) or any condition that reduces circulating intravascular plasma volume or other body fluids, such as in severe burns.

Other causes of hypovolemic shock include intestinal obstruction, peritonitis, acute pancreatitis, ascites and dehydration from excessive perspiration, severe diarrhea or protracted vomiting, diabetes insipidus, diuresis, and inadequate fluid intake.

Complications
Without immediate treatment, hypovolemic shock can cause adult respiratory distress syndrome, acute tubular necrosis and renal failure, disseminated intravascular coagulation, and multisystem organ failure.

Assessment findings

The patient's history will include disorders or conditions that reduce blood volume, such as GI hemorrhage, trauma, and severe diarrhea and vomiting. A patient with cardiac disease may complain of anginal pain because of decreased myocardial perfusion and oxygenation.

Inspection may reveal pale skin, decreased sensorium, and rapid, shallow respirations. Urine output is usually less than 20 ml/hour.

Palpation of peripheral pulses may disclose a rapid, thready pulse; the skin feels cold and clammy.

Auscultation of blood pressure usually detects a mean arterial pressure of less than 60 mm Hg in adults, and a narrowing pulse pressure. In patients with chronic hypotension, the mean pressure may fall below 50 mm Hg before any signs of shock appear.

Orthostatic vital signs and the tilt test may help determine the presence of hypovolemic shock. (See *Checking for early hypovolemic shock,* page 574.)

Central venous pressure, right atrial pressure, pulmonary artery pressures, pulmonary artery wedge pressure, and cardiac output are all reduced.

Diagnostic tests

Characteristic laboratory findings include:
• low hematocrit and decreased hemoglobin levels and red blood cell and platelet counts
• elevated serum potassium, sodium, lactate dehydrogenase, creatinine, and blood urea nitrogen levels
• increased urine specific gravity (greater than 1.020) and urine osmolality
• decreased urine creatinine levels
• decreased pH and partial pressure of oxygen in arterial blood and increased partial pressure of carbon dioxide in arterial blood.

In addition, X-rays, gastroscopy, aspiration of gastric contents through a nasogastric tube, and tests for occult blood identify internal bleeding sites. Coagulation studies may detect coagulopathy from disseminated intravascular coagulation.

Treatment

Emergency treatment measures must include prompt and adequate blood and fluid replacement to restore intravascular volume and to raise blood pressure and maintain it above 60 mm Hg. Infusion of 0.9% sodium chloride or lactated Ringer's solution and then possibly plasma proteins (albumin) or other plasma expanders may produce adequate volume expansion until packed cells can

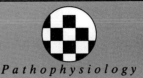

Pathophysiology

HOW HYPOVOLEMIC SHOCK PROGRESSES

Vascular fluid volume loss causes the extreme tissue hypoperfusion that characterizes hypovolemic shock. *Internal fluid loss* results from internal hemorrhage (such as GI bleeding) and third-space fluid shifting (such as in diabetic ketoacidosis). *External fluid loss* results from severe bleeding or from severe diarrhea, diuresis, or vomiting.

Inadequate vascular volume leads to decreased venous return and cardiac output. The resulting drop in arterial blood pressure activates the body's compensatory mechanisms in an attempt to increase vascular volume. If compensation is unsuccessful, decompensation and death may rapidly ensue.

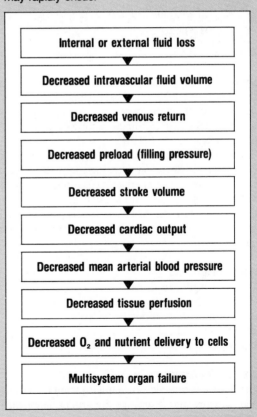

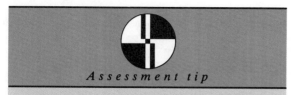

Assessment tip

CHECKING FOR EARLY HYPOVOLEMIC SHOCK

Orthostatic vital signs and tilt test results can help assess for the possibility of impending hypovolemic shock.

Orthostatic vital signs
Measure the patient's blood pressure and pulse rate while he's lying supine, sitting, and standing. Wait at least 1 minute between each position
• change. Consider a systolic blood pressure decrease of 10 mm Hg or more between positions or a pulse rate increase of 10 beats/minute or more a sign of volume depletion and impending hypovolemic shock.

Tilt test
With the patient lying supine, raise his legs above heart level. If his blood pressure rises significantly, the test is positive, indicating volume depletion and impending hypovolemic shock.

be matched. A rapid solution infusion system can provide these crystalloids or colloids at high flow rates.

In severe cases, an intra-aortic balloon pump, ventricular assist device, or pneumatic antishock garment may be helpful.

Treatment may also include oxygen administration, bleeding site identification, bleeding control by direct application of pressure and related measures, dopamine or another inotropic agent, and possibly surgery to correct the underlying problem. To be effective, dopamine or other inotropic agents must be used with vigorous fluid resuscitation.

Nursing diagnoses
• Altered thought processes
• Altered tissue perfusion
• Decreased cardiac output
• Fluid volume deficit
• Sensory or perceptual alterations

Nursing interventions
• Check for a patent airway and adequate circulation. If blood pressure and heart rate are absent, start cardiopulmonary resuscitation.

• Record the patient's blood pressure, pulse and respiratory rates, and peripheral pulses every 15 minutes until he is stabilized. Monitor cardiac rhythm continuously.
• When systolic blood pressure drops below 80 mm Hg, increase the oxygen flow rate, and notify the doctor immediately because systolic blood pressure less than 80 mm Hg usually results in inadequate coronary artery blood flow, cardiac ischemia, arrhythmias, and further complications of low cardiac output.
• Also, notify the doctor, and increase the infusion rate if the patient has a progressive drop in blood pressure accompanied by a thready pulse. This generally signals inadequate cardiac output from reduced intravascular volume.
• Start an I.V. infusion with 0.9% sodium chloride or lactated Ringer's solution, using a large-bore (14G to 18G) catheter, which allows easier administration of later blood transfusions. (*Caution:* Don't start an I.V. infusion in the legs of a shock patient who has suffered abdominal trauma because infused fluid may escape through the ruptured vessel into the abdomen.)
• Insert an indwelling urinary catheter if necessary to measure hourly urine output. If output is less than 30 ml/hour in adults, increase the fluid infusion rate, but watch for signs of fluid overload, such as an increase in pulmonary capillary wedge pressure (PCWP). Notify the doctor if urine output doesn't improve.
• An osmotic diuretic, such as mannitol, may be ordered to increase renal blood flow and urine output. Determine how much fluid to give by checking blood pressure, urine output, central venous pressure (CVP), or PCWP. (To increase accuracy, CVP should be measured at the level of the right atrium, using the same reference point on the chest each time.)
• Draw an arterial blood sample to measure blood gas levels. Administer oxygen by face mask or endotracheal tube to ensure adequate tissue oxygenation. Adjust the oxygen flow rate to a higher or lower level, as blood gas measurements indicate.
• Draw venous blood for a complete blood count, electrolyte measurements, type and cross matching, and coagulation studies.
• During therapy, assess skin color and temperature, and note any changes. Cold, clammy skin may be a sign of continuing peripheral vascular constriction, indicating progressive shock.
• Watch for signs of impending coagulopathy (petechiae, bruising, bleeding or oozing from gums or venipuncture sites).
• Provide emotional support to the patient and family.

Patient teaching

• Explain all procedures and their purpose to ease the patient's anxiety.
• Explain the risks associated with blood transfusions to the patient and his family.

CARDIOGENIC SHOCK

Sometimes called pump failure, cardiogenic shock is a condition of diminished cardiac output that severely impairs tissue perfusion. Cardiogenic shock occurs as a serious complication in nearly 15% of all patients who are hospitalized with acute myocardial infarction (MI). It typically affects patients whose area of infarction involves 40% or more of left ventricular muscle mass; in such patients, mortality may exceed 85%. Most patients with cardiogenic shock die within 24 hours of onset. The prognosis for those who survive is poor.

Causes and pathophysiology

Cardiogenic shock can result from any condition that causes significant left ventricular dysfunction with reduced cardiac output, such as MI (most common), myocardial ischemia, papillary muscle dysfunction, and end-stage cardiomyopathy.

Other causes include myocarditis and depression of myocardial contractility after cardiac arrest and prolonged cardiac surgery. Mechanical abnormalities of the ventricle, such as acute mitral or aortic insufficiency or an acutely acquired ventricular septal defect or ventricular aneurysm, may also result in cardiogenic shock.

Regardless of the cause, left ventricular dysfunction initiates a series of compensatory mechanisms that attempt to increase cardiac output and, in turn, maintain vital organ function. As cardiac output falls, aortic and carotid baroreceptors activate sympathetic nervous responses. These compensatory responses increase heart rate, left ventricular filling pressure, and peripheral resistance to flow to enhance venous return to the heart. The action initially stabilizes the patient but later causes deterioration with rising oxygen demands on the already compromised myocardium. These events constitute a vicious circle of low cardiac output, sympathetic compensation, myocardial ischemia, and even lower cardiac output.

Complications

Death usually ensues because the vital organs can't overcome the deleterious effects of extended hypoperfusion.

Assessment findings

Typically, the patient's history includes a disorder, such as MI or cardiomyopathy, that severely decreases left ventricular function. Patients with underlying cardiac disease may complain of anginal pain because of decreased myocardial perfusion and oxygenation. Urine output is usually less than 20 ml/hour.

Inspection usually reveals pale skin, decreased sensorium, and rapid, shallow respirations. Palpation of peripheral pulses may detect a rapid, thready pulse. The skin feels cold and clammy.

Auscultation of blood pressure usually discloses a mean arterial pressure of less than 60 mm Hg in adults, and a narrowing pulse pressure. In a patient with chronic hypotension, the mean pressure may fall below 50 mm Hg before he exhibits any signs of shock. Auscultation of the heart detects gallop rhythm, faint heart sounds and, possibly (if shock results from rupture of the ventricular septum or papillary muscles), a holosystolic murmur.

Although many of these clinical features also occur in heart failure and other shock syndromes, they are usually more profound in cardiogenic shock. Patients with pericardial tamponade may have distant heart sounds.

Diagnostic tests

• *Pulmonary artery pressure monitoring* reveals increased pulmonary artery pressure (PAP) and pulmonary capillary wedge pressure (PCWP), reflecting a rise in left ventricular end-diastolic pressure (preload) and heightened resistance to left ventricular emptying (afterload) caused by ineffective pumping and increased peripheral vascular resistance. Thermodilution catheterization reveals a reduced cardiac index (less than 1.8 liters/minute/m^2).
• *Invasive arterial pressure monitoring* shows systolic arterial pressure less than 80 mm Hg caused by impaired ventricular ejection.
• *Arterial blood gas analysis* may show metabolic and respiratory acidosis and hypoxia.
• *Electrocardiography* demonstrates possible evidence of acute MI, ischemia, or ventricular aneurysm.
• *Serum enzyme measurements* display elevated levels of creatine phosphokinase (CPK), lactate dehydrogenase (LDH), aspartate aminotransferase (formerly SGOT), and alanine aminotransferase (formerly SGPT), which point to MI or ischemia and suggest heart failure or shock. CPK and LDH isoenzyme levels may confirm acute MI.
• *Cardiac catheterization* and *echocardiography* reveal other conditions that can lead to pump dysfunction and

failure, such as cardiac tamponade, papillary muscle infarct or rupture, ventricular septal rupture, pulmonary emboli, venous pooling (associated with venodilators and continuous intermittent positive-pressure breathing), and hypovolemia.

Treatment

Treatment aims to enhance cardiovascular status by increasing cardiac output, improving myocardial perfusion, and decreasing cardiac work load with combinations of cardiovascular drugs and mechanical-assist techniques.

I.V. drugs may include dopamine, a vasopressor that increases cardiac output, blood pressure, and renal blood flow; amrinone or dobutamine, inotropic agents that increase myocardial contractility; and norepinephrine, when a more potent vasoconstrictor is necessary. Nitroprusside, a vasodilator, may be used with a vasopressor to further improve cardiac output by decreasing peripheral vascular resistance (afterload) and reducing left ventricular end-diastolic pressure (preload). However, the patient's blood pressure must be adequate to support nitroprusside therapy and must be monitored closely.

Treatment may also include the intra-aortic balloon pump (IABP), a mechanical-assist device that attempts to improve coronary artery perfusion and decrease cardiac work load. The inflatable balloon pump is inserted through the femoral artery into the descending thoracic aorta. The balloon inflates during diastole to increase coronary artery perfusion pressure and deflates before systole (before the aortic valve opens) to reduce resistance to ejection (afterload) and, therefore, lessen cardiac work load. Improved ventricular ejection, which significantly improves cardiac output, and a subsequent vasodilation in the peripheral vessels lead to lower preload volume.

When drug therapy and IABP insertion fail, a ventricular assist device may be used.

Nursing diagnoses

• Altered thought processes
• Altered tissue perfusion
• Anxiety
• Decisional conflict
• Decreased cardiac output
• Dysfunctional grieving
• Fear
• Fluid volume excess
• Hopelessness
• Impaired gas exchange

• Impaired physical mobility
• Risk for injury

Nursing interventions

• In the intensive care unit (ICU), start I.V. infusions with 0.9% sodium chloride or lactated Ringer's solution, using a large-bore (14G to 18G) catheter, which allows easier administration of later blood transfusions. (*Caution:* Don't start I.V. infusions in the legs of a shock patient who has suffered abdominal trauma because infused fluid may escape through the ruptured vessel into the abdomen.)
• Monitor and record blood pressure, pulse and respiratory rates, and peripheral pulses every 1 to 5 minutes until the patient is stabilized. Record hemodynamic pressure readings every 15 minutes. Monitor cardiac rhythm continuously. Systolic blood pressure less than 80 mm Hg usually results in inadequate coronary artery blood flow, cardiac ischemia, arrhythmias, and further complications of low cardiac output. When blood pressure drops below 80 mm Hg, increase the oxygen flow rate and notify the doctor immediately.

A progressive drop in blood pressure accompanied by a thready pulse generally signals inadequate cardiac output from reduced intravascular volume. Notify the doctor and increase the infusion rate.
• Using a pulmonary artery catheter, closely monitor PAP, PCWP, and cardiac output. A high PCWP indicates heart failure, increased systemic vascular resistance, decreased cardiac output, and decreased cardiac index, and should be reported immediately.
• Insert an indwelling urinary catheter if necessary to measure hourly urine output. If the output is less than 30 ml/hour in an adult, increase the fluid infusion rate, but watch for signs of fluid overload, such as an increase in PCWP. Notify the doctor if the patient's urine output doesn't improve.
• Administer an osmotic diuretic, such as mannitol, if ordered to increase renal blood flow and urine output. Determine how much fluid to give by checking blood pressure, urine output, central venous pressure (CVP), or PCWP. (To increase accuracy, measure CVP at the level of the right atrium, using the same reference point on the chest each time.)
• Draw an arterial blood sample to measure blood gas levels. Administer oxygen by face mask or airway to ensure adequate oxygenation of tissues. Adjust the oxygen flow rate to a higher or lower level, as blood gas measurements indicate. Many patients will need 100% oxygen and some will require 5 to 15 cm H_2O of positive

end-expiratory or continuous positive airway pressure ventilation.

• Monitor complete blood count and electrolyte levels.

• During therapy, assess skin color and temperature, and note any changes. Cold, clammy skin may be a sign of continuing peripheral vascular constriction, indicating progressive shock.

• When a patient is on the IABP, move him as little as possible. Never flex the patient's "ballooned" leg at the hip because this may displace or fracture the catheter. Never place the patient in a sitting position for any reason (including chest X-rays) while the balloon is inflated; the balloon will tear through the aorta and result in immediate death. Assess pedal pulses and skin temperature and color to make sure circulation to the leg is adequate. Check the dressing on the insertion site frequently for bleeding, and change it according to hospital protocol. Also check the site for hematoma or signs of infection, and culture any drainage.

• If the patient becomes hemodynamically stable, gradually reduce the frequency of balloon inflation to wean him from the IABP. During weaning, carefully watch for monitor changes, chest pain, and other signs of recurring cardiac ischemia and shock.

• To ease emotional stress, plan your care to allow frequent rest periods, and provide for as much privacy as possible. Allow family members to visit and comfort the patient as much as possible.

• Allow the family to express their anger, anxiety, and fear.

Patient teaching

• Because the patient and his family may be anxious about the ICU and about the IABP and other tubes and devices, offer explanations and reassurance.

• Prepare the patient and his family for a probable fatal outcome, and help them find effective coping strategies.

SEPTIC SHOCK

Low systemic vascular resistance and an elevated cardiac output characterize septic shock. The disorder is thought to occur in response to infections that release microbes or one of the immune mediators.

Septic shock is usually a complication of another disorder or invasive procedure and has a mortality as high as 25%. The incidence of septic shock approaches 500,000 cases annually.

Causes and pathophysiology

Any pathogenic organism can cause septic shock. Gram-negative bacteria, such as *Escherichia coli, Klebsiella pneumoniae, Serratia, Enterobacter,* and *Pseudomonas,* rank as the most common causes and account for up to 70% of all cases. Opportunistic fungi cause about 3% of cases. Rare causative organisms include mycobacteria and some viruses and protozoa.

Many organisms that are normal flora on the skin and in the intestines are beneficial and pose no threat. But when they spread throughout the body by way of the bloodstream (gaining entry through any alteration in the body's normal defenses or through artificial devices that penetrate the body, such as I.V., intra-arterial, and urinary catheters, and knife or bullet wounds), they can progress to overwhelming infection unless body defenses destroy them. Initially, these defenses activate chemical mediators in response to the invading organisms. The release of these mediators results in low systemic vascular resistance and increased cardiac output. Blood flow is unevenly distributed in the microcirculation, and plasma leaking from capillaries causes functional hypovolemia. Eventually, cardiac output falls, and poor tissue perfusion and hypotension cause multisystem organ failure and death.

Septic shock can occur in any person with impaired immunity, but neonates and elderly people are at greatest risk. About two-thirds of septic shock cases occur in hospitalized patients, most of whom have underlying diseases. Those at high risk include patients with burns; chronic cardiac, hepatic, or renal disorders; diabetes mellitus; immunosuppression; malnutrition; stress; and excessive antibiotic use. Also at risk are patients who have had invasive diagnostic or therapeutic procedures, surgery, or traumatic wounds.

Complications

In septic shock, complications include disseminated intravascular coagulation, renal failure, heart failure, GI ulcers, and abnormal liver function.

Assessment findings

The patient's history may include a disorder or treatment that can cause immunosuppression. Or it may include a history of invasive tests or treatments, surgery, or trauma. At onset, the patient may have fever and chills, although 20% of patients may be hypothermic.

The patient's signs and symptoms will reflect either the *hyperdynamic* or *warm phase* of septic shock (increased cardiac output, peripheral vasodilation, and decreased systemic vascular resistance) or the *hypodynamic* or *cold phase* (decreased cardiac output, peripheral vasoconstriction, increased systemic vascular resistance, and inadequate tissue perfusion).

In the hyperdynamic phase, the patient's skin may appear pink and flushed. His altered level of consciousness is reflected in agitation, anxiety, irritability, and shortened attention span. Respirations will be rapid and shallow. Urine output is below normal.

Palpation of peripheral pulses may detect a rapid, full, bounding pulse. The skin may feel warm and dry. Blood pressure may be normal or slightly elevated.

In the hypodynamic phase, the patient's skin may appear pale and, possibly, cyanotic. Peripheral areas may be mottled. His level of consciousness may be decreased; obtundation and coma may be present. Respirations may be rapid and shallow, and urine output may be less than 25 ml/hour or absent.

Palpation of peripheral pulses may reveal a rapid pulse that is weak, thready, or absent. It may also be irregular if arrhythmias are present. The skin may feel cold and clammy.

Auscultation of blood pressure may reveal hypotension, usually with a systolic pressure below 90 mm Hg or 50 to 80 mm Hg below the patient's previous level. Auscultation of the lungs may reveal crackles or rhonchi if pulmonary congestion is present.

If central pressures are being monitored, the pulmonary artery wedge pressure will be reduced or normal, and cardiac output will be moderately to severely increased or normal. Rarely, cardiac output will be decreased.

Diagnostic tests
The following are characteristic laboratory findings:
• *Blood cultures* are positive for the offending organism.
• *Complete blood count* shows the presence or absence of anemia and leukopenia, severe or absent neutropenia, and usually the presence of thrombocytopenia.
• *Serum lactate dehydrogenase* levels are elevated with metabolic acidosis.
• *Urine studies* show increased specific gravity (more than 1.020) and osmolality and decreased sodium.
• *Arterial blood gas analysis* demonstrates elevated blood pH and partial pressure of oxygen and decreased partial pressure of carbon dioxide with respiratory alkalosis in early stages.

Treatment
Location and treatment of the underlying sepsis is essential to treating septic shock. If any I.V., intra-arterial, or urinary drainage catheters are in place, they should be removed. Aggressive antimicrobial therapy appropriate for the causative organism must be initiated immediately. Culture and sensitivity tests help determine the most effective antimicrobial drug.

In patients who are immunosuppressed because of drug therapy, drugs should be discontinued or reduced. Granulocyte transfusions may be used in patients with severe neutropenia.

Oxygen therapy should be initiated to maintain arterial oxygen saturation greater than 95%. Mechanical ventilation may be required if respiratory failure occurs.

Colloid or crystalloid infusions are given to increase intravascular volume and raise blood pressure. After sufficient fluid volume has been replaced, diuretics, such as furosemide, can be given to maintain urine output above 20 ml/hour. If fluid resuscitation fails to increase blood pressure, a vasopressor, such as dopamine, can be started. Blood transfusion may be needed if anemia is present.

Nursing diagnoses
• Altered thought processes
• Altered tissue perfusion
• Anxiety
• Decreased cardiac output
• Fluid volume deficit
• Impaired gas exchange
• Risk for injury
• Sensory or perceptual alterations

Nursing interventions
• Remove any I.V., intra-arterial, or urinary drainage catheters and send to the laboratory to culture for the presence of the causative organism. New catheters can be reinserted in the intensive care unit.
• Start an I.V. infusion with 0.9% sodium chloride or lactated Ringer's solution, using a large-bore (14G to 18G) catheter, which allows easier administration of later blood transfusions. (*Caution:* Don't start I.V. infusions in the legs of a shock patient who has suffered abdominal trauma because infused fluid may escape through the ruptured vessel into the abdomen.)
• Record the patient's blood pressure, pulse and respiratory rates, and peripheral pulses every 1 to 5 minutes until he is stabilized. Record hemodynamic pressure readings every 15 minutes. Monitor cardiac rhythm continuously. Systolic blood pressure less than 80 mm Hg usually results in inadequate coronary artery blood flow, cardiac ischemia, arrhythmias, and further complications of low cardiac output. When blood pressure drops

below 80 mm Hg, increase the oxygen flow rate and notify the doctor immediately.

A progressive drop in blood pressure accompanied by a thready pulse generally signals inadequate cardiac output from reduced intravascular volume. Notify the doctor and increase the infusion rate.

• Administer appropriate antimicrobial drugs I.V. to achieve effective blood levels rapidly.

• Measure hourly urine output. If output is less than 30 ml/hour in adults, increase the fluid infusion rate, but watch for signs of fluid overload, such as an increase in pulmonary capillary wedge pressure. Notify the doctor if urine output doesn't improve. A diuretic may be ordered to increase renal blood flow and urine output.

• Draw an arterial blood sample to measure blood gas levels. Administer oxygen by face mask or airway to ensure adequate tissue oxygenation. Adjust the oxygen flow rate to a higher or lower level, as blood gas measurements indicate.

• Provide emotional support to the patient and his family.

• Document the occurrence of a nosocomial infection and report it to the infection-control nurse. Investigation of all hospital-acquired infections can help identify their sources and prevent future infections.

Patient teaching

• Explain all procedures and their purpose to ease the patient's anxiety.

• Explain the risks associated with blood transfusions to the patient and his family, and answer their questions as completely as possible.

VENTRICULAR ANEURYSM

This potentially life-threatening condition involves an outpouching—almost always of the left ventricle—that produces ventricular wall dysfunction in about 20% of patients after myocardial infarction (MI). Ventricular aneurysm may develop within days to weeks after MI or may be delayed for years. Resection improves the prognosis in patients with ventricular failure or ventricular arrhythmias.

Causes and pathophysiology

MI causes ventricular aneurysm. When MI destroys a large muscular section of the left ventricle, necrosis reduces the ventricular wall to a thin sheath of fibrous tissue. Under intracardiac pressure, this thin layer stretches and forms a separate noncontractile sac (aneurysm). Abnormal muscle wall movement accompanies ventricular

aneurysm. (See *Understanding ventricular aneurysm*, page 580.)

During systolic ejection, the abnormal muscle wall movements associated with the aneurysm cause the remaining normally functioning myocardial fibers to increase the force of contraction to maintain stroke volume and cardiac output. At the same time, a portion of the stroke volume is lost to passive distention of the noncontractile sac.

Complications

Ventricular aneurysms enlarge but seldom rupture. However, an untreated ventricular aneurysm can lead to ventricular arrhythmias, cerebral embolization, or heart failure and is potentially fatal.

Assessment findings

The patient may have a history of a previous MI. However, sometimes MI is silent, and the patient may be unaware of having had one. He may complain of palpitations and anginal pain.

If the patient has developed heart failure as a result of the aneurysm, he may complain of dyspnea, fatigue, and edema.

Inspection of the chest may reveal a visible or palpable systolic precordial bulge. Distended neck veins may appear if heart failure is present.

Palpation of peripheral pulses may reveal an irregular rhythm caused by arrhythmias (such as premature ventricular contractions). A pulsus alternans may be felt. Palpation of the chest usually detects a double, diffuse, or displaced apical impulse.

Auscultation of the heart may detect an irregular rhythm and a gallop rhythm. Crackles and rhonchi may be present in the lung if heart failure is present.

Diagnostic tests

The following tests may determine the presence of a ventricular aneurysm:

• *Two-dimensional echocardiography* demonstrates abnormal motion in the left ventricular wall.

• *Left ventriculography* reveals left ventricular enlargement, with an area of akinesia or dyskinesia (during cineangiography) and diminished cardiac function.

• *Electrocardiography* may show persistent ST-T wave elevations at rest. ST-segment elevation over the aneurysm creates an elevated rounded appearance.

• *Chest X-rays* may disclose an abnormal bulge distorting the heart's contour if the aneurysm is large; X-rays may be normal if the aneurysm is small.

UNDERSTANDING VENTRICULAR ANEURYSM

A ventricular aneurysm can cause the ventricular wall to contract in abnormal ways. In the sketches below, the arrows represent motion from end diastole to end systole.

Normal contraction
Change of 25% to 30% in outside wall diameter

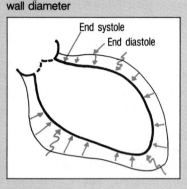

Hypokinesia
Decreased mobility

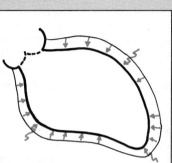

Asynergia
Decreased, inadequate movement

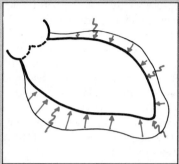

Akinesia
Lack of movement

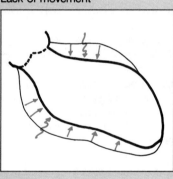

Dyskinesia
Paradoxical systolic expansion

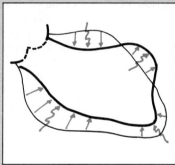

Asynchrony
Uncoordinated movement

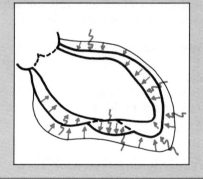

• *Noninvasive nuclear cardiology scan* may indicate the site of infarction and suggest the area of aneurysm.

Treatment
Depending on the size of the aneurysm and the presence of complications, treatment may require only routine medical examination to follow the patient's condition, or aggressive measures for intractable ventricular arrhythmias, heart failure, and emboli.

Emergency treatment of ventricular arrhythmia includes I.V. antiarrhythmics, cardioversion, and defibrillation. Preventive treatment continues with oral antiarrhythmics, such as procainamide, quinidine, or disopyramide.

Emergency treatment for heart failure with pulmonary edema includes oxygen, digitalis I.V., furosemide I.V., potassium replacement, morphine sulfate I.V. and, when necessary, nitroprusside I.V. and endotracheal intubation. Maintenance therapy may include oral nitrates, prazosin, and hydralazine.

Systemic embolization requires anticoagulation therapy or embolectomy. Refractory ventricular tachycardia, heart failure, recurrent arterial embolization, and persistent angina with coronary artery occlusion may require surgery. The most effective surgery is aneurysmectomy with myocardial revascularization.

Nursing diagnoses
- Altered tissue perfusion
- Anxiety
- Decreased cardiac output
- Fluid volume excess
- Impaired gas exchange
- Ineffective breathing pattern

Nursing interventions
- In a patient with heart failure, closely monitor vital signs, heart sounds, intake and output, fluid and electrolyte balance, and blood urea nitrogen and serum creatinine levels.
- Be alert for sudden changes in sensorium that indicate cerebral embolization and for any signs that suggest renal failure or MI.
- Arrhythmias require elective cardioversion. If the patient is conscious, give diazepam I.V., as ordered, before cardioversion.
- If the patient is receiving antiarrhythmics, check appropriate laboratory tests. For instance, if the patient takes procainamide, check antinuclear antibodies because the drug may induce signs and symptoms that mimic lupus erythematosus.
- Provide psychological support for the patient and his family to reduce anxiety.
- If the patient is scheduled to undergo resection, explain expected postoperative care in the intensive care unit (such as an endotracheal tube, a ventilator, hemodynamic monitoring, and chest tubes).
- After surgery, monitor vital signs, intake and output, heart sounds, and pulmonary artery catheter. Watch for signs of infection, such as fever and drainage.

Patient teaching
- Teach the patient how to check for pulse irregularity and rate changes. Encourage him to follow his prescribed medication regimen—even during the night—and to watch for adverse reactions.
- Because arrhythmias can cause sudden death, refer the family to a community-based cardiopulmonary resuscitation training program.

CARDIAC TAMPONADE
A rapid rise in intrapericardial pressure impairs diastolic filling of the heart in cardiac tamponade. The rise in pressure usually results from blood or fluid accumulation in the pericardial sac. If fluid accumulates rapidly, as little as 250 ml can create an emergency situation. Slow accumulation and rise in pressure, as in pericardial effusion associated with cancer, may not produce immediate signs and symptoms because the fibrous wall of the pericardial sac can gradually stretch to accommodate as much as 1 to 2 liters of fluid.

Causes
Cardiac tamponade may be idiopathic (Dressler's syndrome) or may result from:
- effusion (in cancer, bacterial infections, tuberculosis and, rarely, acute rheumatic fever)
- hemorrhage from trauma (such as gunshot or stab wounds of the chest, and perforation by catheter during cardiac or central venous catheterization, or after cardiac surgery)
- hemorrhage from nontraumatic causes (such as rupture of the heart or great vessels or anticoagulant therapy in a patient with pericarditis)
- viral, postirradiation, or idiopathic pericarditis
- acute myocardial infarction
- chronic renal failure during dialysis
- drug reaction (procainamide, hydralazine, minoxidil, isoniazid, penicillin, methysergide, and daunorubicin)
- connective tissue disorders (such as rheumatoid arthritis, systemic lupus erythematosus, rheumatic fever, vasculitis, and scleroderma).

Complications
Pressure resulting from fluid accumulation in the pericardium decreases ventricular filling and cardiac output, resulting in cardiogenic shock and death if untreated.

Assessment findings
The patient's history may show a disorder that can cause cardiac tamponade. He may report acute pain and dyspnea, sitting upright and leaning forward to facilitate breathing and lessen the pain. He may be orthopneic, diaphoretic, anxious, and restless, and appear pale or cyanotic. You may note neck vein distention produced by increased venous pressure, although this may not be present if the patient is hypovolemic.

Palpation of the peripheral pulses may disclose rapid, weak pulses. Palpation of the upper quadrant may reveal hepatomegaly.

Percussion may detect a widening area of flatness across the anterior chest wall, indicating a large effusion. Hepatomegaly may also be noted.

Auscultation of the blood pressure may demonstrate a decreased arterial blood pressure, pulsus paradoxus (an abnormal inspiratory drop in systemic blood pressure greater than 15 mm Hg), and narrow pulse pressure.

Heart sounds may be muffled. A quiet heart with faint sounds usually accompanies only severe tamponade and occurs within minutes of the tamponade, as happens with cardiac rupture or trauma. The lungs are clear.

Diagnostic tests
The following test results are characteristic:
• *Chest X-rays* show slightly widened mediastinum and enlargement of the cardiac silhouette.
• *Electrocardiography (ECG)* is useful to rule out other cardiac disorders. The QRS amplitude may be reduced, and electrical alternans of the P wave, QRS complex, and T wave may be present. Generalized ST-segment elevation is noted in all leads.
• *Pulmonary artery pressure monitoring* detects increased right atrial pressure, right ventricular diastolic pressure, and central venous pressure.
• *Echocardiography* records pericardial effusion with signs of right ventricular and atrial compression.

Treatment
The goal of treatment is to relieve intrapericardial pressure and cardiac compression by removing accumulated blood or fluid. Pericardiocentesis (needle aspiration of the pericardial cavity) or surgical creation of an opening dramatically improves systemic arterial pressure and cardiac output with aspiration of as little as 25 ml of fluid. A drain may be inserted into the pericardial sac to drain the effusion. This may be left in until the effusion process stops or the corrective action (pericardial window) is performed. In the case of infection, antibiotics can be instilled through the drain, clamped, and later drained off.

In the hypotensive patient, trial volume loading with I.V. 0.9% sodium chloride solution with albumin, and perhaps an inotropic drug, such as dopamine, is necessary to maintain cardiac output.

Depending on the cause of tamponade, additional treatment may include:
• in traumatic injury, blood transfusion or a thoracotomy to drain reaccumulating fluid or to repair bleeding sites
• in heparin-induced tamponade, the heparin antagonist protamine
• in warfarin-induced tamponade, vitamin K.

Nursing diagnoses
• Activity intolerance
• Altered tissue perfusion
• Anxiety
• Decreased cardiac output
• Impaired gas exchange
• Pain

Nursing interventions
• Monitor the patient with cardiac tamponade in the intensive care unit. Check for signs of increasing tamponade, increasing dyspnea, and arrhythmias.
   For pericardiocentesis:
• Reassure the patient to reduce anxiety.
• Gather a pericardiocentesis tray, an ECG machine, and an emergency cart with a defibrillator at the bedside. Make sure the equipment is turned on and ready for immediate use. Position the patient at a 45- to 60-degree angle. Connect the precordial ECG lead to the hub of the aspiration needle with an alligator clamp and connecting wire, and assist with fluid aspiration. When the needle touches the myocardium, you'll see an ST-segment elevation or premature ventricular contractions.
• Monitor blood pressure and central venous pressure (CVP) during and after pericardiocentesis. Infuse I.V. solutions, as ordered, to maintain blood pressure. Watch for a decrease in CVP and a concomitant rise in blood pressure, which indicate relief of cardiac compression.
• Administer oxygen therapy as needed.
• Watch for complications of pericardiocentesis, such as ventricular fibrillation, vagovagal arrest, and coronary artery or cardiac chamber puncture. Closely monitor cardiac rhythm strip changes, blood pressure, pulse rate, level of consciousness, and urine output.
   For thoracotomy:
• Give antibiotics, protamine, or vitamin K, as ordered.
• Postoperatively, monitor critical parameters, such as vital signs and arterial blood gas levels, and assess heart and breath sounds. Give pain medication, as ordered. Maintain the chest drainage system, and be alert for complications, such as hemorrhage and arrhythmias.

Patient teaching
• Explain the procedure (pericardiocentesis or thoracotomy) to the patient. Tell him what to expect postoperatively (chest tubes, drainage bottles, and administration of oxygen). Teach him how to turn, deep-breathe, and cough. If the patient is not in an acute situation preoperatively, teach these techniques then.

CARDIAC ARRHYTHMIAS
Arrhythmias result from abnormal electrical conduction or automaticity that changes heart rate and rhythm. They vary in severity, from those that are mild, asymptomatic,

and require no treatment (such as sinus arrhythmia, in which heart rate increases and decreases with respiration) to catastrophic ventricular fibrillation, which requires immediate resuscitation.

Arrhythmias are classified according to their origin as ventricular, atrial (supraventricular), or junctional. Their effect on cardiac output and blood pressure, partially influenced by the site of origin, determines their clinical significance.

Causes

Arrhythmias may be congenital or may result from myocardial ischemia or infarction, organic heart disease, drug toxicity, or degeneration of conductive tissue necessary to maintain normal heart rhythm (sick sinus syndrome).

Complications

In a patient with a normal heart, arrhythmias typically produce few symptoms. But even in a normal heart, persistently rapid or highly irregular rhythms can strain the myocardium and impair cardiac output.

Assessment findings

Depending on the arrhythmia, the patient may exhibit symptoms ranging from pallor, cold and clammy extremities, reduced urine output, palpitations, and weakness to chest pains, dizziness and, if cerebral circulation is severely impaired, syncope.

Diagnostic tests

Electrocardiography (ECG) allows detection and identification of arrhythmias. (See *Types of cardiac arrhythmias,* pages 584 to 588.)

Treatment

Effective treatment aims to return pacer function to the sinus node, increase or decrease ventricular rate to normal, regain atrioventricular synchrony, and maintain normal sinus rhythm. Such treatment corrects abnormal rhythms through therapy with antiarrhythmic drugs; electrical conversion with precordial shock (defibrillation and cardioversion); physical maneuvers, such as carotid massage and Valsalva's maneuver; temporary or permanent placement of a pacemaker to maintain heart rate; and surgical removal or cryotherapy of an irritable ectopic focus to prevent recurring arrhythmias.

Arrhythmias may respond to treatment of the underlying disorder, such as correction of hypoxia. However, arrhythmias associated with heart disease may require continuing and complex treatment.

Nursing diagnoses

• Activity intolerance
• Altered tissue perfusion
• Anxiety
• Decreased cardiac output
• Impaired gas exchange

Nursing interventions

• Carefully assess the patient's cardiac, electrolyte, and overall clinical status to determine the effect on cardiac output and whether the arrhythmia is life-threatening.
• Assess an unmonitored patient for rhythm disturbances. If the patient's pulse rate is abnormally rapid, slow, or irregular, watch for signs of hypoperfusion, such as hypotension and diminished urine output.
• Document any arrhythmias in a monitored patient, and assess for possible causes and effects.
• When life-threatening arrhythmias develop, rapidly assess the patient's level of consciousness and pulse and respiratory rates and initiate cardiopulmonary resuscitation, if indicated.
• Evaluate for altered cardiac output resulting from arrhythmias. Administer medications, as ordered, and prepare to assist with medical procedures, if indicated (for example, cardioversion).
• Monitor for predisposing factors, such as fluid and electrolyte imbalance, and signs of drug toxicity, especially with digoxin. If you suspect drug toxicity, report it to the doctor immediately and withhold the next dose.
• To prevent arrhythmias postoperatively, provide adequate oxygen and reduce heart work load, while carefully maintaining metabolic, neurologic, respiratory, and hemodynamic status.
• To avoid temporary pacemaker malfunction, install a fresh battery before each insertion. Carefully secure the external catheter wires and the pacemaker box. Assess the threshold daily. Watch closely for premature contractions, a sign of myocardial irritation.
• After pacemaker insertion, monitor the patient's pulse rate regularly, and watch for signs of pacemaker failure and decreased cardiac output.

Patient teaching

• Explain to the patient the importance of taking all ordered medications at the proper time intervals. Teach him how to take his pulse and recognize an irregular rhythm, and instruct him to report alterations from his baseline to the doctor.
• If the patient has a permanent pacemaker, warn him about environmental and electrical hazards, as indicated by the pacemaker manufacturer. Although hazards may

(Text continues on page 588.)

TYPES OF CARDIAC ARRHYTHMIAS

This chart reviews many common cardiac arrhythmias and outlines their causes, characteristics, and treatments. Use a normal ECG strip, if available, to compare normal cardiac rhythm configurations with the rhythm strips below. Characteristics of normal rhythm include:
• ventricular and atrial rates of 60 to 100 beats/minute
• regular and uniform QRS complexes and P waves
• PR interval of 0.12 to 0.2 second
• QRS duration <0.12 second
• identical atrial and ventricular rates, with constant PR interval.

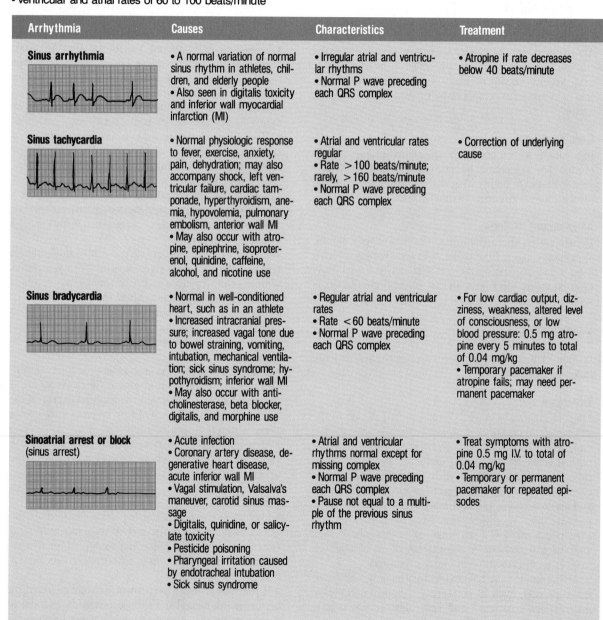

Arrhythmia	Causes	Characteristics	Treatment
Sinus arrhythmia	• A normal variation of normal sinus rhythm in athletes, children, and elderly people • Also seen in digitalis toxicity and inferior wall myocardial infarction (MI)	• Irregular atrial and ventricular rhythms • Normal P wave preceding each QRS complex	• Atropine if rate decreases below 40 beats/minute
Sinus tachycardia	• Normal physiologic response to fever, exercise, anxiety, pain, dehydration; may also accompany shock, left ventricular failure, cardiac tamponade, hyperthyroidism, anemia, hypovolemia, pulmonary embolism, anterior wall MI • May also occur with atropine, epinephrine, isoproterenol, quinidine, caffeine, alcohol, and nicotine use	• Atrial and ventricular rates regular • Rate >100 beats/minute; rarely, >160 beats/minute • Normal P wave preceding each QRS complex	• Correction of underlying cause
Sinus bradycardia	• Normal in well-conditioned heart, such as in an athlete • Increased intracranial pressure; increased vagal tone due to bowel straining, vomiting, intubation, mechanical ventilation; sick sinus syndrome; hypothyroidism; inferior wall MI • May also occur with anticholinesterase, beta blocker, digitalis, and morphine use	• Regular atrial and ventricular rates • Rate <60 beats/minute • Normal P wave preceding each QRS complex	• For low cardiac output, dizziness, weakness, altered level of consciousness, or low blood pressure: 0.5 mg atropine every 5 minutes to total of 0.04 mg/kg • Temporary pacemaker if atropine fails; may need permanent pacemaker
Sinoatrial arrest or block (sinus arrest)	• Acute infection • Coronary artery disease, degenerative heart disease, acute inferior wall MI • Vagal stimulation, Valsalva's maneuver, carotid sinus massage • Digitalis, quinidine, or salicylate toxicity • Pesticide poisoning • Pharyngeal irritation caused by endotracheal intubation • Sick sinus syndrome	• Atrial and ventricular rhythms normal except for missing complex • Normal P wave preceding each QRS complex • Pause not equal to a multiple of the previous sinus rhythm	• Treat symptoms with atropine 0.5 mg I.V. to total of 0.04 mg/kg • Temporary or permanent pacemaker for repeated episodes

TYPES OF CARDIAC ARRHYTHMIAS *(continued)*

Arrhythmia	Causes	Characteristics	Treatment
Wandering atrial pacemaker	• Rheumatic carditis as a result of inflammation involving the sinoatrial (SA) node • Digitalis toxicity • Sick sinus syndrome	• Atrial and ventricular rates vary slightly • Irregular PR interval • P waves irregular with changing configuration, indicating they're not all from SA node or single atrial focus; may appear after the QRS complex • QRS complexes uniform in shape but irregular in rhythm	• No treatment if asymptomatic • Treatment of underlying cause if symptomatic
Premature atrial contraction (PAC)	• Coronary or valvular heart disease, atrial ischemia, coronary atherosclerosis, heart failure, acute respiratory failure, chronic obstructive pulmonary disease (COPD), electrolyte imbalance, and hypoxia • Digitalis toxicity and aminophylline, adrenergics, or caffeine use • Anxiety	• Premature, abnormal-looking P waves, differing in configuration from normal P waves • QRS complexes after P waves, except in very early or blocked PACs • P wave often buried in the preceding T wave or identified in the preceding T wave	• No treatment usually
Paroxysmal atrial tachycardia (paroxysmal supraventricular tachycardia)	• Intrinsic abnormality of atrioventricular (AV) conduction system • Physical or psychological stress, hypoxia, hypokalemia, cardiomyopathy, congenital heart disease, MI, valvular disease, Wolff-Parkinson-White syndrome, cor pulmonale, hyperthyroidism, systemic hypertension • Digitalis toxicity; caffeine, marijuana, central nervous system stimulant use	• Atrial and ventricular rates regular • Heart rate >160 beats/minute; rarely exceeds 250 beats/minute • P waves regular but aberrant; difficult to differentiate from preceding T wave • P wave preceding each QRS complex • Sudden onset and termination of arrhythmia	• Vagal stimulation, Valsalva's maneuver, carotid sinus massage • Adenosine by rapid I.V. bolus injection to rapidly convert arrhythmia • Propranolol, quinidine, digoxin, verapamil, edrophonium to alter AV node conduction and maintain normal rhythm • Elective cardioversion, if patient is symptomatic and unresponsive to drugs
Atrial flutter	• Heart failure, tricuspid or mitral valve disease, pulmonary embolism, cor pulmonale, inferior wall MI, carditis • Digitalis toxicity	• Atrial rhythm regular; 250 to 400 beats/minute • Ventricular rate variable, depending on degree of AV block • Ventricular rhythm regular or irregular, depending on AV conduction • Sawtooth P-wave configuration possible (F waves) • QRS complexes uniform in shape, but irregular in rate	• Digitalis (unless arrhythmia is due to digitalis toxicity), verapamil, propranolol, or quinidine • May require synchronized cardioversion or atrial pacemaker

(continued)

TYPES OF CARDIAC ARRHYTHMIAS *(continued)*

Arrhythmia	Causes	Characteristics	Treatment
Atrial fibrillation	• Heart failure, COPD, thyrotoxicosis, constrictive pericarditis, ischemic heart disease, sepsis, pulmonary embolus, rheumatic heart disease, hypertension, mitral stenosis, digitalis toxicity (rarely), atrial irritation, complication of coronary bypass or valve replacement surgery • Nifedipine and digitalis use	• Atrial rhythm grossly irregular; rate >400 beats/minute • Ventricular rhythm grossly irregular • Ventricular rate normal, fast, or slow • QRS complexes of uniform configuration and duration • PR interval indiscernible • No P waves or erratic, irregular, baseline fibrillatory P waves	• Digitalis, propranolol, verapamil, and quinidine to slow ventricular rate, and quinidine to convert rhythm to normal sinus rhythm • May require elective cardioversion for rapid ventricular rate • Treatment of underlying cause
Junctional rhythm	• Inferior wall MI or ischemia, hypoxia, vagal stimulation, sick sinus syndrome • Acute rheumatic fever • Valve surgery • Digitalis toxicity	• Atrial and ventricular rhythms regular • Atrial rate 40 to 60 beats/minute • Ventricular rate usually 40 to 60 beats/minute (60 to 100 beats/minute is accelerated junctional rhythm) • P waves inverted and preceding, hidden within (absent), or after QRS complex • PR interval (when present) <0.12 second • QRS complex configuration and duration normal, except in aberrant conduction	• Atropine for symptomatic slow rate • Pacemaker insertion, if refractory to drugs • Discontinuation of digitalis, if appropriate
Premature junctional contractions (junctional premature beats)	• MI or ischemia • Digitalis toxicity and excessive caffeine or amphetamine use	• Atrial and ventricular rhythms irregular • P waves inverted; may precede, be hidden within, or follow QRS complex • PR interval <0.12 second, if P wave precedes QRS complex • QRS complex configuration and duration normal	• Correction of underlying cause • No treatment usually
First-degree AV block	• May be seen in a healthy person • Inferior wall myocardial ischemia or infarction, hypothyroidism, hypokalemia, hyperkalemia • Digitalis toxicity; quinidine, procainamide, or propranolol use	• Atrial and ventricular rhythms regular • PR interval >0.20 second • P wave preceding each QRS complex • QRS complex normal	• Cautious use of digitalis • Correction of underlying cause • Atropine may be used if PR interval exceeds 0.26 second or bradycardia develops

TYPES OF CARDIAC ARRHYTHMIAS *(continued)*

Arrhythmia	Causes	Characteristics	Treatment
Second-degree AV block Mobitz I (Wenckebach)	• Inferior wall MI, cardiac surgery, acute rheumatic fever, and vagal stimulation • Digitalis toxicity; propranolol, quinidine, or procainamide use	• Atrial rhythm regular • Ventricular rhythm irregular • Atrial rate exceeds ventricular rate • PR interval progressively, but only slightly, longer with each cycle until QRS complex disappears (dropped beat); PR interval shorter after dropped beat	• Treatment of underlying cause • Atropine or temporary pacemaker, for symptomatic bradycardia • Discontinuation of digitalis, if appropriate
Second-degree AV block Mobitz II	• Severe coronary artery disease, anterior MI, acute myocarditis • Digitalis toxicity	• Atrial rate regular • Ventricular rhythm regular or irregular, with varying degree of block • P-P interval constant • QRS complexes periodically absent	• Isoproterenol for symptomatic bradycardia • Temporary or permanent pacemaker • Discontinuation of digitalis, if appropriate
Third-degree AV block (complete heart block)	• Inferior or anterior wall MI, congenital abnormality, rheumatic fever, hypoxia, postoperative complications of mitral valve replacement, Lev's disease (fibrosis and calcification that spreads from cardiac structures to the conductive tissue) and Lenegre's disease (conductive tissue fibrosis) • Digitalis toxicity	• Atrial rate regular • Ventricular rate slow and regular • No relation between P waves and QRS complexes • No constant PR interval • QRS interval normal (nodal pacemaker), or wide and bizarre (ventricular pacemaker)	• Atropine for symptomatic bradycardia • Temporary or permanent pacemaker
Junctional tachycardia	• Myocarditis, cardiomyopathy, inferior wall MI or ischemia, acute rheumatic fever, valve replacement surgery • Digitalis toxicity	• Atrial rate > 100 beats/minute; however, P wave may be absent, hidden in QRS complex, or preceding T wave • Ventricular rate > 100 beats/minute • P wave inverted • QRS complex configuration and duration normal • Onset of rhythm often sudden, occurring in bursts	• Carotid sinus massage, elective cardioversion • Propranolol, verapamil, or edrophonium • Discontinuation of digitalis, if appropriate • Temporary atrial pacemaker to override the rhythm
Premature ventricular contraction (PVC)	• Heart failure; old or acute myocardial ischemia, infarction, or contusion; myocardial irritation by ventricular catheter, such as a pacemaker; hypercapnia; hypokalemia, hypocalcemia	• Atrial rate regular • Ventricular rate irregular • QRS complex premature, usually followed by a complete compensatory pause • QRS complex wide and distorted, usually > 0.14 second	• Treatment of underlying cause • No treatment if asymptomatic • Lidocaine or procainamide I.V. infusions, if symptomatic

(continued)

TYPES OF CARDIAC ARRHYTHMIAS *(continued)*

Arrhythmia	Causes	Characteristics	Treatment
Premature ventricular contraction (PVC) *(continued)*	• Drug toxicity (digitalis, aminophylline, tricyclic antidepressants, beta-adrenergics [isoproterenol or dopamine]) • Caffeine, tobacco, or alcohol use • Psychological stress; anxiety, pain, exercise	• Premature QRS complexes occurring singly, in pairs, or in threes; alternating with normal beats; focus from one or more sites • Most ominous when clustered, multifocal, with R wave on T pattern	• Potassium chloride I.V. if induced by hypokalemia
Ventricular tachycardia	• Myocardial ischemia, infarction, or aneurysm; coronary artery disease; rheumatic heart disease; mitral valve prolapse; heart failure; cardiomyopathy; ventricular catheters; hypokalemia; hypercalcemia; pulmonary embolism • Digitalis, procainamide, epinephrine, or quinidine toxicity • Anxiety	• Ventricular rate 140 to 220 beats/minute, regular or irregular • QRS complexes wide, bizarre, and independent of P waves • P waves not discernible • May start and stop suddenly	• Lidocaine, procainamide, or bretylium I.V. • Cardiopulmonary resuscitation (CPR) if pulses are absent, following advanced cardiac life support (ACLS) protocol • Synchronous cardioversion (emergency treatment), if pulses are present • Immediate defibrillation, if pulses are not present
Ventricular fibrillation	• Myocardial ischemia or infarction, untreated ventricular tachycardia, R-on-T phenomenon, hypokalemia, alkalosis, hyperkalemia, hypercalcemia, electric shock, hypothermia • Digitalis, epinephrine, or quinidine toxicity	• Ventricular rhythm rapid and chaotic • QRS complexes wide and irregular; no visible P waves	• CPR • Defibrillation • Epinephrine and lidocaine, procainamide, or bretylium I.V. • Treatment of underlying cause
Ventricular standstill (asystole)	• Myocardial ischemia or infarction, aortic valve disease, heart failure, hypoxemia, hypokalemia, severe acidosis, electric shock, ventricular arrhythmias, atrioventricular block, pulmonary embolism, heart rupture, cardiac tamponade, hyperkalemia, electromechanical dissociation • Cocaine overdose	• No atrial or ventricular rate or rhythm • No discernible P waves, QRS complexes, or T waves	• CPR, following ACLS protocol • Endotracheal intubation • Pacemaker • Treatment of underlying cause

not present a problem, in doubtful situations, a 24-hour ambulatory ECG (Holter monitoring) may be helpful. Tell the patient to report any light-headedness or syncope. Stress the importance of scheduling and keeping appointments for regular checkups.

VASCULAR DISORDERS

Vascular disorders can affect the arteries, the veins, or both types of vessels. Arterial disorders include aneurysms, which result from a weakening of the arterial wall; arterial occlusive disease, which commonly results from atherosclerotic narrowing of the artery's lumen; and Raynaud's disease, which may be linked to immunologic dysfunction. Thrombophlebitis, a venous disorder, results from inflammation or occlusion of the affected vessel.

THORACIC AORTIC ANEURYSM

Characterized by abnormal widening of the ascending, transverse, or descending part of the aorta, thoracic aortic aneurysm is a potentially life-threatening disorder. This aneurysm may be *saccular,* an outpouching of the arterial wall, with a narrow neck, involving only a portion of the vessel circumference; or *fusiform,* a spindle-shaped enlargement, encompassing the entire aortic circumference.

Dissection of the aneurysm is the circumferential or transverse tear of the aortic wall intima, usually within the medial layer. It occurs in about 60% of patients, is usually an emergency, and has a poor prognosis. (See *Classifying aortic dissection,* page 590.)

The ascending thoracic aorta is the most common site for the aneurysm, which occurs predominantly in men under age 60 who have coexisting hypertension. Descending thoracic aortic aneurysms are most common in younger patients who have had chest trauma.

Causes

Commonly, ascending thoracic aortic aneurysm results from atherosclerosis, which weakens the aortic wall and gradually distends the lumen in this area.

Descending thoracic aortic aneurysm usually occurs after blunt chest trauma that shears the aorta transversely (acceleration-deceleration injury), such as in a motor vehicle accident, or a penetrating chest injury, such as a knife wound. It also may be caused by hypertension.

Mycotic aneurysm develops from staphylococcal, streptococcal, or salmonella infections, usually at an atherosclerotic plaque.

Cystic medial necrosis caused by degeneration of the collagen and elastic fibers in the media of the aorta causes aneurysms during pregnancy and in patients with hypertension and Marfan syndrome. However, it can also be the cause without any underlying condition.

Other causes include congenital disorders, such as coarctation of the aorta, syphilis infection, and rheumatic vasculitis.

Complications

Some aneurysms progress to serious and, eventually, lethal complications, such as rupture of untreated thoracic dissecting aneurysm into the pericardium, with resulting cardiac tamponade.

Assessment findings

Thoracic aortic aneurysms fail to produce signs and symptoms until they expand and begin to dissect. Pain and other symptoms result from compression of the surrounding structures or from dissection of the aneurysm.

The patient may complain of hoarseness, dyspnea, throat pain, dysphagia, and a dry cough when a transverse aneurysm compresses the surrounding structures. Dissection of the aneurysm causes sudden pain and possibly syncope.

In *dissecting ascending aneurysm,* the patient may complain of pain with a boring, tearing, or ripping sensation in the thorax or the right anterior chest. It may extend to the neck, shoulders, lower back, and abdomen but seldom radiates to the jaw and arms. The pain is most intense at its onset and is often misdiagnosed as a transmural myocardial infarction (MI).

In *dissecting descending aneurysm,* the pain is sharp, tearing, and located between the shoulder blades, and often radiates to the chest. In *dissecting transverse aneurysm,* the pain is sharp, boring, and tearing and radiates to the shoulders.

In a patient with a thoracic aortic aneurysm, you may find pallor, diaphoresis, dyspnea, cyanosis, leg weakness or transient paralysis, and an abrupt onset of intermittent neurologic deficits. Palpation of peripheral pulses in dissecting ascending aneurysm may disclose abrupt loss of radial and femoral pulses and right and left carotid pulses. In dissecting descending aneurysm, carotid and radial pulses may be present and equal bilaterally.

Percussion of the chest may reveal an increasing area of flatness over the heart, suggesting cardiac tamponade and hemopericardium. Auscultation of the heart in dissecting ascending aneurysm may disclose a murmur of aortic insufficiency, a diastolic murmur, and (if hemopericardium is present) a pericardial friction rub. The blood pressure may be normal or significantly elevated, with a large difference in systolic blood pressure between the right and left arms.

In dissecting descending aneurysm, systolic blood pressure will be equal bilaterally, and you'll hear no murmur of aortic insufficiency or pericardial friction rub. You may detect bilateral crackles and rhonchi if pulmonary edema is present.

Diagnostic tests

In an asymptomatic patient, the diagnosis commonly occurs accidentally, through posteroanterior and oblique

CLASSIFYING AORTIC DISSECTION

These drawings illustrate the DeBakey classification of aortic dissections (shaded areas) according to location. Dissections can also be classified by their location in relation to the aortic valve. Thus, Types I and II are proximal; Type III, distal.

Type I
In this, the most common and lethal type of dissection, intimal tearing occurs in the ascending aorta, and the dissection extends into the descending aorta.

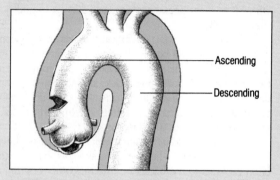

— Ascending

— Descending

Type II
In this type of dissection, which appears most commonly with Marfan syndrome, dissection is limited to the ascending or the transverse aorta.

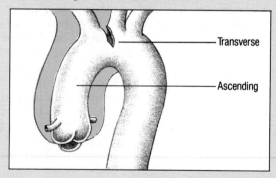

— Transverse

— Ascending

Type III
This form of dissection includes two formations. In the first, Type IIIa, the intimal tear is located in the descending aorta with distal propagation of the dissection. The second, Type IIIb, which has the same origin site, may extend to the aortic bifurcation.

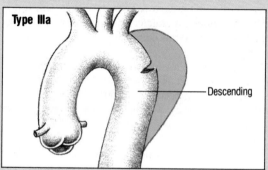

Type IIIa

— Descending

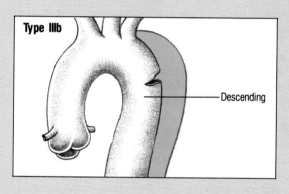

Type IIIb

— Descending

chest X-rays, showing widening of the aorta and mediastinum. The following tests help confirm the aneurysm:
• *Aortography,* the most definitive test, shows the lumen of the aneurysm, its size, and its location.

• *Magnetic resonance imaging* and a *computed tomography scan* help confirm and locate the presence of aortic dissection.
• *Electrocardiography* helps rule out the presence of MI as the cause of the symptoms.

• *Echocardiography* may help identify dissecting aneurysm of the aortic root.
• *Hemoglobin* levels may be normal or decreased, resulting from blood loss from a leaking aneurysm.

Treatment

For long-term treatment, beta-adrenergic blockers and other agents can control hypertension and cardiac output. In an emergency, antihypertensives, such as nitroprusside; negative inotropic agents, such as labetalol; oxygen for respiratory distress; narcotics for pain; I.V. fluids; and if needed, whole blood transfusions may be used.

In dissecting ascending aortic aneurysm—an extreme emergency—surgical resection of the aneurysm can restore normal blood flow through a Dacron or Teflon graft replacement. With aortic valve insufficiency, surgery consists of replacing the aortic valve.

Postoperative measures include careful monitoring and continuous assessment in the intensive care unit, antibiotics, insertion of endotracheal and chest tubes, ECG monitoring and, often, pulmonary artery catheterization and monitoring.

Nursing diagnoses

• Anxiety
• Decreased cardiac output
• Hopelessness
• Ineffective breathing pattern
• Knowledge deficit
• Pain

Nursing interventions

• In a nonemergency situation when a patient is diagnosed with a thoracic aneurysm, allow him to express his fears and concerns. Help him identify and use effective coping strategies.
• Offer the patient and family psychological support. Answer all questions honestly, and provide reassurance.
• In an acute situation, monitor blood pressure, pulmonary capillary wedge pressure (PCWP), and central venous pressure. Assess pain, breathing, and carotid, radial, and femoral pulses.
• Give analgesics to relieve pain, as ordered.
• Make sure laboratory tests include a complete blood count with differential, electrolyte measurements, typing and cross matching for whole blood, arterial blood gas analyses, and urinalysis.
• Insert an indwelling urinary catheter to monitor hourly outputs. Administer dextrose 5% in water or lactated Ringer's solution, and antibiotics, as ordered. Carefully monitor nitroprusside I.V.; use a separate I.V. line for infusion. Adjust the dose by slowly increasing the infusion rate. Meanwhile, check blood pressure every 5 minutes until it stabilizes. With suspected bleeding from an aneurysm, give whole blood transfusions, as ordered.

After repair of thoracic aneurysm:
• Carefully assess the patient's level of consciousness. Monitor vital signs, pulmonary artery and central venous pressures, PCWP, pulse rate, urine output, and pain.
• Check respiratory function. Carefully observe and record type and amount of chest tube drainage, and frequently assess heart and lung sounds.
• Monitor I.V. therapy and intake and output to determine the adequacy of renal function.
• Administer analgesics as ordered, especially before the patient performs breathing exercises or is moved.
• After stabilization of vital signs, encourage and assist the patient in turning, coughing, and deep breathing. If necessary, provide intermittent positive-pressure breathing to promote lung expansion. Help the patient walk as soon as he's able.
• Watch for signs of infection, especially fever, and excessive drainage on the dressing. Monitor for signs that resemble those of the initial dissecting aneurysm, suggesting a tear at the graft site.
• Assist with range-of-motion exercises of legs to prevent thromboemboli from venostasis during prolonged bed rest.

Patient teaching

• Explain any diagnostic tests. If surgery is scheduled, explain the procedure and expected postoperative care (I.V. lines, endotracheal and drainage tubes, cardiac monitoring, ventilation).
• Before discharge, ensure compliance with antihypertensive therapy by explaining the need for such drugs and the expected adverse effects. Teach the patient how to monitor his blood pressure. Refer him to community agencies for continued support and assistance, as needed.
• Direct the patient to call the doctor immediately if he has any sharp pain in the chest or back of the neck.

ABDOMINAL ANEURYSM

An abnormal dilation in the arterial wall, an abdominal aneurysm generally occurs in the aorta between the renal arteries and the iliac branches. Nearly 98% of all abdominal aneurysms are located in the infrarenal aorta. These aneurysms can be fusiform (spindle-shaped) or saccular (pouchlike) and develop slowly.

First, a focal weakness in the muscular layer of the aorta (tunica media), due to degenerative changes, allows the inner layer (tunica intima) and outer layer (tunica adventitia) to stretch outward. Blood pressure within the aorta progressively weakens the vessel walls and enlarges the aneurysm.

Abdominal aneurysms are seven times more common in hypertensive men than in women and are most common in whites ages 50 to 80.

Causes
About 95% of abdominal aortic aneurysms result from arteriosclerosis or atherosclerosis; the rest, from cystic medial necrosis, trauma, syphilis, and other infections.

Complications
More than 50% of all people with untreated abdominal aneurysms die of hemorrhage and shock from aneurysmal rupture within 2 years of diagnosis; more than 85%, within 5 years.

Assessment findings
Most patients with abdominal aneurysms are asymptomatic until the aneurysm enlarges and compresses surrounding tissue. A large aneurysm may produce signs and symptoms that mimic renal calculi, lumbar disk disease, and duodenal compression.

The patient may complain of gnawing, generalized, steady abdominal pain or low back pain that is unaffected by movement. He may have a sensation of gastric or abdominal fullness caused by pressure on the GI structures.

Sudden onset of severe abdominal pain or lumbar pain that radiates to the flank and groin from pressure on lumbar nerves may signify enlargement and imminent rupture. If the aneurysm ruptures into the peritoneal cavity, severe and persistent abdominal and back pain, mimicking renal or ureteral colic, occurs. If it ruptures into the duodenum, GI bleeding occurs with massive hematemesis and melena.

The patient may have a history of a syncopal episode that occurs when an aneurysm ruptures, causing hypovolemia and a subsequent drop in blood pressure. Once a clot forms and the bleeding stops, he may again be asymptomatic or have abdominal pain because of bleeding into the peritoneum.

Inspection of the patient with an intact abdominal aneurysm usually reveals no significant findings. However, if the person is not obese, you may note a pulsating mass in the periumbilical area. If the aneurysm has ruptured, you may note signs of hypovolemic shock, such as skin mottling, decreased level of consciousness (LOC), diaphoresis, and oliguria. The abdomen may appear distended and an ecchymosis or hematoma may be present in the abdominal, flank, or groin area.

Paraplegia may occur if aneurysm rupture reduces blood flow to the spine.

Auscultation of the abdomen may reveal a systolic bruit over the aorta caused by turbulent blood flow in the widened arterial segment. Hypotension occurs with aneurysm rupture.

Palpation of the abdomen may disclose some tenderness over the affected area. A pulsatile mass may be felt; however, avoid deep palpation to locate the mass because this may cause the aneurysm to rupture. Palpation of the peripheral pulses may reveal absent pulses distal to a ruptured aneurysm.

Diagnostic tests
Because an abdominal aneurysm seldom produces symptoms, it's typically detected accidentally on an X-ray or during a routine physical examination.

Several tests can confirm suspected abdominal aneurysm:
• *Abdominal ultrasonography* or *echocardiography* can determine the size, shape, and location of the aneurysm.
• *Anteroposterior* and *lateral X-rays* of the abdomen can detect aortic calcification, which outlines the mass, at least 75% of the time.
• *Computed tomography scan* can visualize the aneurysm's effect on nearby organs, particularly the position of the renal arteries in relation to the aneurysm.
• *Aortography* shows the condition of vessels proximal and distal to the aneurysm and the extent of the aneurysm but may underestimate aneurysm diameter because it visualizes only the flow channel and not the surrounding clot.

Treatment
Usually, abdominal aneurysm requires resection of the aneurysm and Dacron graft replacement of the aortic section. If the aneurysm is small and produces no symptoms, surgery may be delayed, and regular physical examination and ultrasound checks monitor progression of the aneurysm. Large aneurysms or those that produce symptoms risk rupture and require immediate repair. In patients with poor perfusion distal to the aneurysm, external grafting may be done.

In acute dissection, emergency treatment before surgery includes resuscitation with fluid and blood replacement, I.V. propranolol to reduce myocardial contractility, I.V. nitroprusside to reduce and maintain blood pressure to 100 to 120 mm Hg systolic, and analgesics to relieve pain. An arterial line and indwelling urinary catheter are inserted to monitor the patient's condition.

Nursing diagnoses
- Altered tissue perfusion
- Anxiety
- Decreased cardiac output
- Fluid volume deficit
- Impaired gas exchange
- Impaired physical mobility
- Impaired skin integrity
- Knowledge deficit
- Pain

Nursing interventions
In a nonacute situation:
- Allow the patient to express his fears and concerns. Help him identify effective coping strategies as he attempts to deal with his diagnosis.
- Offer the patient and his family psychological support. Answer all questions honestly, and provide reassurance.
- Before elective surgery, weigh the patient, insert an indwelling urinary catheter and an I.V. line, and assist with insertion of the arterial line and pulmonary artery catheter to monitor hemodynamic balance. Give prophylactic antibiotics, as ordered.

In an acute situation:
- Monitor the patient's vital signs on his admission to the intensive care unit (ICU).
- Insert an I.V. line with at least a 14G needle to facilitate blood replacement.
- As ordered, obtain blood samples for kidney function tests (blood urea nitrogen, creatinine, and electrolyte levels), a complete blood count with differential, blood typing and cross matching, and arterial blood gas (ABG) levels.
- Monitor the patient's cardiac rhythm strip. Insert an arterial line to allow for continuous blood pressure monitoring. Assist with insertion of a pulmonary artery line to monitor for hemodynamic balance.
- Administer ordered medications, such as antihypertensives and beta blockers to control aneurysm progression and analgesics to relieve pain.
- Be alert for signs of rupture, which may be immediately fatal. Watch closely for any signs of acute blood loss (decreasing blood pressure; increasing pulse and respiratory rates; cool, clammy skin; restlessness; and decreased sensorium).

- If rupture does occur, get the patient to surgery *immediately*. Medical antishock trousers may be used while transporting him to surgery.

After surgery:
- With the patient in the ICU, closely monitor vital signs, intake and hourly output, neurologic status (LOC, pupil size, sensation in arms and legs), and ABG levels.
- Assess fluid status and replace fluids as needed to ensure adequate hydration.
- Watch for signs of bleeding (increased pulse and respiratory rates, hypotension), which may occur retroperitoneally from the graft site.
- Check abdominal dressings for excessive bleeding or drainage. Assess the wound site for evidence of infection. Be alert for temperature elevations and other signs of infection. Use aseptic technique to change dressings.
- After nasogastric (NG) intubation for intestinal decompression, irrigate the tube frequently to ensure patency. Record the amount and type of drainage.
- Large amounts of blood may be needed during the resuscitative period to replace blood loss. Thus, renal failure due to ischemia is a major postoperative complication, possibly requiring hemodialysis.
- Assess for return of severe back pain, which can indicate that the graft is tearing.
- Mechanical ventilation is required after surgery. Assess the depth, rate, and character of respirations and breath sounds at least every hour. Have the patient cough, or suction the endotracheal tube as needed to maintain a clear airway. If the patient can breathe unassisted and has good breath sounds and adequate ABG levels, tidal volume, and vital capacity 24 hours after surgery, he will be extubated and will require oxygen by mask. Weigh the patient daily to evaluate fluid balance.
- Provide frequent turning, and help the patient walk as soon as he's able (generally the second day after surgery).

Patient teaching
- Provide psychological support for the patient and his family. Help ease their fears about the ICU, the threat of impending rupture, and surgery by providing appropriate explanations and answering all questions.
- Explain the surgical procedure and the expected postoperative care in the ICU for patients undergoing complex abdominal surgery (I.V. lines, endotracheal and NG intubation, mechanical ventilation).
- Instruct the patient to take all medications as prescribed and to carry a list of medications at all times, in case of an emergency.

• Tell the patient not to push, pull, or lift heavy objects until medically cleared by the doctor.

FEMORAL AND POPLITEAL ANEURYSMS

Because these aneurysms occur in the two major peripheral arteries, they're also known as peripheral arterial aneurysms. They may be *fusiform* (spindle-shaped) or *saccular* (pouchlike). Fusiform types are three times more common. They may be singular or multiple segmental lesions, often affecting both legs, and may accompany other arterial aneurysms located in the abdominal aorta or iliac arteries.

This condition is most common in men over age 50. Elective surgery before complications arise greatly improves the prognosis.

Causes

Femoral and popliteal aneurysms usually result from progressive atherosclerotic changes in the arterial walls (medial layer). Rarely, they result from congenital weakness in the arterial wall. They may also result from trauma (blunt or penetrating), bacterial infection, or peripheral vascular reconstructive surgery (which causes "suture line" aneurysms, also called false aneurysms, whereby a blood clot forms a second lumen).

Complications

If thrombosis, emboli, or gangrene occurs, poor tissue perfusion to areas distal to the aneurysm may require amputation.

Assessment findings

The patient may complain of pain in the popliteal space when a popliteal aneurysm is large enough to compress the medial popliteal nerve. Inspection may reveal edema and venous distention if the vein is compressed.

Femoral and popliteal aneurysms can produce signs and symptoms of severe ischemia in the leg or foot resulting from acute thrombosis within the aneurysmal sac, embolization of mural thrombus fragments and, rarely, rupture.

In acute aneurysmal thrombosis, the patient may complain of severe pain. Inspection may reveal distal petechial hemorrhages from aneurysmal emboli. The affected leg or foot may show loss of color. Palpation of the affected leg or foot may indicate coldness and a loss of pulse. Gangrene may develop.

Bilateral palpation that reveals a pulsating mass above or below the inguinal ligament in femoral aneurysm and behind the knee in popliteal aneurysm usually confirms the diagnosis. When thrombosis has occurred, palpation detects a firm, nonpulsating mass.

Diagnostic tests

Arteriography or ultrasonography may help resolve doubtful situations. Arteriography may also detect associated aneurysms, especially those in the abdominal aorta and the iliac arteries. Ultrasonography may also help determine the size of the femoral or popliteal artery.

Treatment

Femoral and popliteal aneurysms require surgical bypass and reconstruction of the artery, usually with an autogenous saphenous vein graft replacement. Arterial occlusion that causes severe ischemia and gangrene may require leg amputation.

Nursing diagnoses

• Activity intolerance
• Altered tissue perfusion
• Defensive coping
• Denial
• Diversional activity deficit
• Impaired physical mobility
• Impaired skin integrity
• Pain
• Risk for infection

Nursing interventions

Before arterial surgery:
• Assess and record the patient's circulatory status, noting location and quality of peripheral pulses in the affected leg.
• Administer prophylactic antibiotics or anticoagulants, as ordered.
   After arterial surgery:
• Monitor carefully for early signs of thrombosis or graft occlusion (loss of pulse, decreased skin temperature and sensation, severe pain) and infection (fever).
• Palpate distal pulses at least every hour for the first 24 hours and then as often as ordered. Correlate these findings with the preoperative circulatory assessment. Mark the sites on the patient's skin where pulses are palpable to facilitate repeated checks.
• Help the patient walk soon after surgery to prevent venous stasis and, possibly, thrombus formation.

Patient teaching

• Discuss expected postoperative procedures, review the explanation of the surgery, and answer the patient's questions.

• Tell the patient to immediately report any recurrence of symptoms because the saphenous vein graft replacement can fail or another aneurysm may develop.

• Explain to the patient with popliteal artery resection that swelling may persist for some time. If antiembolism stockings are ordered, make sure they fit properly, and teach the patient how to apply them. Warn against wearing constrictive apparel.

• If the patient is receiving anticoagulants, suggest measures to prevent accidental bleeding, such as using an electric razor. Tell the patient to report any signs of bleeding immediately (bleeding gums, tarry stools, easy bruising). Explain the importance of follow-up blood studies to monitor anticoagulant therapy. Warn the patient to avoid trauma, tobacco, and aspirin.

THROMBOPHLEBITIS

An acute condition characterized by inflammation and thrombus formation, thrombophlebitis may occur in deep or superficial veins. It typically occurs at the valve cusps because venous stasis encourages accumulation and adherence of platelet and fibrin. Thrombophlebitis usually begins with localized inflammation alone (phlebitis), but such inflammation rapidly provokes thrombus formation. Rarely, venous thrombosis develops without associated inflammation of the vein (phlebothrombosis).

Deep vein thrombophlebitis affects small veins, such as the lesser saphenous vein, or large veins, such as the vena cava, and the iliac, femoral, and popliteal veins. (See *Major venous pathways of the leg.*) It is more serious than superficial vein thrombophlebitis because it affects the veins deep in the leg musculature that carry 90% of the venous outflow from the leg. The incidence of deep vein thrombophlebitis involving the subclavian vein is rising with the increased use of subclavian vein catheters.

Some studies indicate that up to 35% of hospitalized patients develop deep vein thrombophlebitis. Some hospitalized patients are more at risk than others, however; the risk of developing deep vein thrombophlebitis increases dramatically after age 40 and triples with each additional 20 years.

Superficial vein thrombophlebitis is usually self-limiting and, because these veins have fewer valves than the deep veins, is less likely to cause complications.

MAJOR VENOUS PATHWAYS OF THE LEG

Thrombophlebitis can occur in any leg vein. It most commonly occurs at valve sites.

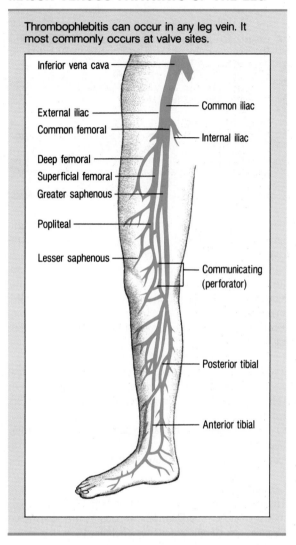

Inferior vena cava
External iliac
Common femoral
Deep femoral
Superficial femoral
Greater saphenous
Popliteal
Lesser saphenous
Common iliac
Internal iliac
Communicating (perforator)
Posterior tibial
Anterior tibial

Causes

Virchow, in 1846, identified three major factors that promote development of venous thrombosis. Known as Virchow's triad, they are hypercoagulability, venous stasis, and intimal damage.

Deep vein thrombophlebitis may be idiopathic, but it is more likely to occur in the presence of certain diseases, treatments, injuries, or other factors, such as the following:

• hypercoagulable states—cigarette smoking; circulating lupus anticoagulant; deficiencies of antithrombin III, pro-

DEALING WITH CHRONIC VENOUS INSUFFICIENCY

Chronic venous insufficiency results from the valvular destruction of deep vein thrombophlebitis, usually in the iliac and femoral veins and occasionally in the saphenous veins. It's often accompanied by incompetence of the communicating veins of the ankle, causing increased venous pressure and fluid migration into the interstitial tissue.

Signs and symptoms
Chronic venous insufficiency causes chronic swelling of the affected leg from edema, leading to tissue fibrosis and induration; skin discoloration from extravasation of blood in subcutaneous tissue; and stasis ulcers around the ankle.

Treatment
Appropriate treatment for small stasis ulcers consists of bed rest, elevation of the legs, warm soaks, and antimicrobial therapy for infection.

Treatment to counteract increased venous pressure, the result of reflux from the deep venous system to superficial veins, may include compression dressings, such as a sponge rubber pressure dressing or a zinc gelatin boot (Unna's boot). This therapy begins after massive swelling subsides.

Large stasis ulcers unresponsive to conservative treatment may require excision and skin grafting. Care includes daily inspection to assess healing and measures similar to those for varicose veins.

tein C, or protein S; disseminated intravascular coagulation; estrogen use; dysfibrinogenemia; myeloproliferative diseases; systemic infection
• intimal damage — infection, infusion of irritating I.V. solutions, trauma, venipuncture
• neoplasms — lung, ovary, pancreas, stomach, testicles, urinary tract
• surgery — abdominal, genitourinary, orthopedic, thoracic
• fracture of the spine, pelvis, femur, or tibia
• venous stasis — acute myocardial infarction, congestive heart failure, dehydration, immobility, incompetent vein valves, postoperative convalescence, cerebrovascular accident
• venulitis — Behçet's disease, homocystinuria, thromboangiitis obliterans
• other — pregnancy, previous deep vein thrombosis.

Complications
The major complications of thrombophlebitis are pulmonary embolism and chronic venous insufficiency. (See *Dealing with chronic venous insufficiency.*)

Assessment findings
In both deep vein and superficial vein thrombophlebitis, clinical features vary with the site of inflammation and length of the affected vein. Up to 50% of patients with deep vein thrombophlebitis may be asymptomatic, but others may complain of some tenderness, aching, or severe pain in the affected leg or arm, fever, chills, and malaise. Complete your physical examination carefully because much of the patient's subsequent care will depend on your findings. (See *Planning effective care for the patient with thrombophlebitis.*) Inspection may reveal

redness, swelling, and cyanosis of the affected leg or arm. Some patients with deep vein thrombophlebitis of a leg vein may have a positive Homans' sign (pain on dorsiflexion of the foot), but this is considered an unreliable sign. A positive cuff sign (elicited by inflating a blood pressure cuff until pain occurs) may be present in deep vein thrombophlebitis of either the arm or leg. When palpated, the affected leg or arm may feel warm.

Patients with superficial vein thrombophlebitis may also be asymptomatic, or they may complain of pain localized to the thrombus site. Inspection may disclose redness and swelling at the site and surrounding area. When palpated, the area feels warm, and a tender, hard cord extends over the affected vein's length.

Extensive vein involvement may cause lymphadenitis.

Diagnostic tests
Diagnosis must rule out arterial occlusive disease, lymphangitis, cellulitis, and myositis. Diagnosis of superficial vein thrombophlebitis is based on physical findings, whereas diagnosis of deep vein thrombophlebitis is based on the following characteristic test findings:
• *Doppler ultrasonography* identifies reduced blood flow to a specific area and any obstruction to venous flow, particularly in iliofemoral deep vein thrombophlebitis.
• *Plethysmography* shows decreased circulation distal to the affected area; it's more sensitive than ultrasonography in detecting deep vein thrombophlebitis.
• *Phlebography* usually confirms the diagnosis and shows filling defects and diverted blood flow.

Treatment
In deep vein thrombophlebitis, treatment includes bed rest, with elevation of the affected arm or leg; application

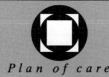

Plan of care

PLANNING EFFECTIVE CARE FOR THE PATIENT WITH THROMBOPHLEBITIS

To help you identify nursing diagnoses, using your assessment findings, and to help you plan, implement, and evaluate care, consider the case of Sarah Harris, a 42-year-old salesclerk. She came to the hospital this morning with severe pain and tenderness in her left calf.

Patient history
Mrs. Harris tells you that she has been experiencing increased fatigue in her calves and feet during a period of inventory taking and sales promotions. She has been on her feet constantly while working 9 to 10 hours a day for the past 3 weeks. The calf pain, which began about 3 days before admission, would subside after a hot bath and a night's sleep. But last night and this morning the pain was unrelieved, and now her left calf feels warm over a "lump." She denies smoking and alcohol use and has no known food or drug allergies. She takes oral contraceptives.

Mrs. Harris's medical history includes coronary artery disease, arteriosclerotic cerebrovascular disease, peripheral vascular disease, hyperlipoproteinemia, hypertension, and diabetes mellitus. In the past, her doctor has warned her to reduce dairy food consumption because her fasting cholesterol levels continually exceed 260 mg/dl.

Assessment findings
A mildly obese, fair-skinned woman, Mrs. Harris displays normal vital signs, has no elevated blood pressure, and is afebrile.

On inspection, her only apparent discomfort comes from the hot, tender calf of her left leg. Both feet are pale, but the right foot feels much warmer than the left foot. No pedal pulses can be palpated on the left foot, but right pedal pulses are strong, regular, and not easily occluded by touch. Capillary refill of the left toes is more than 5 seconds; of the right toes, less than 3 seconds.

Both legs appear to be equal in circumference, but a tape measure discloses a 1" (2.5 cm) increase around the widest part of the left calf. When her left foot is dorsiflexed, she complains of a sharp, shooting pain originating in that calf (positive Homans' sign).

Chest X-ray and auscultation reveal clear lungs bilaterally and slight cardiomegaly. The chest film is otherwise unremarkable. Mrs. Harris denies shortness of breath.

Her electrolyte levels, complete blood count, and arterial blood gas analysis are within normal ranges. The first of three consecutive stool samples is negative for occult blood.

Mrs. Harris is scheduled for two tests: Doppler ultrasonography and ^{125}I-fibrinogen venography.

Nursing diagnoses
Based on your assessment findings, you formulate relevant nursing diagnoses that include:
• Altered peripheral tissue perfusion related to vein inflammation and obstructed blood flow
• Pain related to swelling, inflammation, and obstructed blood flow to the left calf
• Self-care deficit related to lack of complete bed rest and need for left leg elevation
• Anxiety related to treatment, bed rest, and seriousness of possible embolus development.

Expected outcomes
Based on your careful assessment, you'll set care goals for Mrs. Harris. For example, she will:
• wear thigh-high antiembolism stockings to improve blood flow to her lower leg and decrease pain
• understand the importance of remaining on bed rest to decrease pain and swelling
• perform self-care activities while maintaining physical limitations and activity restrictions
• be less fearful and anxious once she understands her treatments, knows how to prevent thrombophlebitis, and recognizes when to contact the doctor.

Implementation
You realize that Mrs. Harris has come to the hospital during a time when preventive treatment will be beneficial. What can you do to prevent the clot in her leg from dislodging?

To reperfuse the left lower leg
• Administer and monitor heparin I.V. (or S.C.), as ordered; check partial thromboplastin time daily and watch for levels greater than 2½ times the normal level.
• Check Mrs. Harris's left leg for circulation, pain, tenderness, swelling, and heat every 4 hours; don't test for Homans' sign once thrombus formation has been documented.
• Apply thigh-high antiembolism stockings to both legs each day; remove them at least once per shift for 30 minutes, inspect the skin, note any abnormalities, and then reapply.
• Maintain a fluid intake of 2,500 to 3,000 ml daily.
• Place a cradle over the foot of the bed to keep the weight of the linens off the legs.

(continued)

PLANNING EFFECTIVE CARE FOR THE PATIENT WITH THROMBOPHLEBITIS *(continued)*

To reduce pain and swelling
• Establish a baseline for pain perception with Mrs. Harris; note irritability, facial grimaces, and other nonverbal expressions of pain.
• Provide analgesics, as ordered; increase or decrease dose, depending on her levels of pain expression.
• Change her position, and provide diversionary activities and rest.
• Keep Mrs. Harris on complete bed rest with her left leg elevated 30 degrees; provide a reduced-pressure mattress for the duration of bed rest.
• If heat therapy is ordered, apply warm compresses or an aquamatic K pad to the left calf.
• Remind Mrs. Harris not to rub or massage her calf.

To encourage limited self-care activities
• Establish a baseline of activities that Mrs. Harris can do while maintaining bed rest, such as washing her face, applying makeup, combing her hair, and performing mouth care.
• Keep bedside items (such as a call bell, water pitcher and cup, reading or diversionary material, telephone, notepaper and pen) within reach at all times.
• Start Mrs. Harris on an exercise regimen as soon as possible after the acute phase of thrombophlebitis to decrease problems associated with immobility.
• Allow Mrs. Harris to participate in treatment, such as having her keep a diary of fluid intake or levels of discomfort.

To reduce anxiety
• Explain all treatments and procedures, and allow Mrs. Harris to ask questions throughout the course of treatment. Involve her husband in patient-teaching sessions, and discuss signs and symptoms requiring medical attention.
• Reassure her that bed rest, heparin therapy, and adherence to limited mobility policies can help prevent recurrent thrombophlebitis, and that she's expected to do well.
• Assure her that any bruising noted over pressure points or at injection sites will dissipate.

Evaluation
You'll know Mrs. Harris has met her goals when her leg appears pink and feels warm, her pedal pulses are palpable on the affected leg, no edema is present, and her pain is relieved.

Mrs. Harris demonstrates the exercises she was taught to decrease the problems of immobility. She also shows no evidence of adverse drug reactions, including excessive bleeding.

Finally, Mrs. Harris discusses the importance of bed rest, explains ways to prevent thrombophlebitis, and lists the signs and symptoms that require her to contact the doctor.

---

of warm, moist compresses to the affected area; and analgesics. After the acute episode subsides, the patient may begin to ambulate while wearing antiembolism stockings (applied before he gets out of bed).

Treatment may include anticoagulants (initially, heparin; later, warfarin) to prolong clotting time. However, the full anticoagulant dose must be discontinued during any surgery to avoid the risk of hemorrhage. After some types of surgery, especially major abdominal or pelvic operations, prophylactic doses of anticoagulants may reduce the risk of deep vein thrombophlebitis.

For lysis of acute, extensive deep vein thrombophlebitis, treatment should include streptokinase or urokinase, if the risk of bleeding doesn't outweigh the potential benefits of thrombolytic treatment.

Rarely, deep vein thrombophlebitis may cause complete venous occlusion, which necessitates venous interruption through simple ligation to vein plication, or clipping. Embolectomy may be done if clots are being shed to the pulmonary and systemic vasculature and other treatment is unsuccessful. Caval interruption with transvenous placement of an umbrella filter can trap emboli, preventing them from traveling to the pulmonary vasculature.

Therapy for severe superficial vein thrombophlebitis may include an anti-inflammatory drug, such as indomethacin, along with antiembolism stockings, warm compresses, and elevation of the patient's leg.

Nursing diagnoses
• Activity intolerance
• Altered tissue perfusion
• Impaired skin integrity
• Pain
• Risk for infection
• Risk for injury

Nursing interventions
• Enforce bed rest, as ordered, and elevate the patient's affected arm or leg. If you plan to use pillows for elevating the leg, place them so they support its entire length to avoid compressing the popliteal space.
• Apply warm compresses or a covered aquamatic K pad to increase circulation to the affected area and to relieve

pain and inflammation. Give analgesics to relieve pain, as ordered.

• Mark, measure, and record the circumference of the affected arm or leg daily, and compare this measurement with that of the other arm or leg. To ensure accuracy and consistency of serial measurements, mark the skin over the area, and measure at the same spot daily.

• Administer heparin I.V., as ordered, with an infusion monitor or pump to control the flow rate, if necessary.

• Measure partial thromboplastin time regularly for the patient on heparin therapy. Measure prothrombin time for the patient on warfarin (therapeutic anticoagulation values for both are 1½ to 2 times control values).

• Watch for signs and symptoms of bleeding, such as tarry stools, coffee-ground vomitus, and ecchymoses. Watch for oozing of blood at I.V. sites, and assess gums for excessive bleeding.

• Be alert for signs of pulmonary emboli (crackles, dyspnea, hemoptysis, sudden changes in mental status, restlessness, and hypotension).

• To prevent thrombophlebitis in high-risk patients, perform range-of-motion exercises while the patient is on bed rest, use intermittent pneumatic calf massage during lengthy surgical or diagnostic procedures, apply antiembolism stockings postoperatively, and encourage early ambulation.

Patient teaching

• Before discharge, emphasize the importance of follow-up blood studies to monitor anticoagulant therapy.

• If the patient is being discharged on heparin therapy, teach him or his family how to give subcutaneous injections. If he requires further assistance, arrange for a home health care nurse.

• Tell the patient to avoid prolonged sitting or standing to help prevent a recurrence.

• Teach the patient how to properly apply and use antiembolism stockings. Tell him to report any complications, such as cold, blue toes.

• To prevent bleeding, encourage the patient to use an electric razor and to avoid medications that contain aspirin.

VARICOSE VEINS

Resulting from improper venous valve function, varicose veins are dilated, tortuous veins, engorged with blood. They can be either primary or secondary. Primary varicose veins originate in the superficial veins—the saphenous veins and their branches—whereas secondary varicose veins occur in the deep and perforating veins. (See *How varicose veins develop,* page 600.)

Primary varicose veins tend to run in families, affect both legs, and are twice as common in women as in men. Usually, secondary varicose veins only occur in one leg. Both types are more common in middle adulthood.

Causes

Primary varicose veins can result from congenital weakness of the valves or venous wall; from conditions that produce prolonged venous stasis, such as pregnancy or wearing tight clothing; or from occupations that necessitate standing for an extended period.

Secondary varicose veins result from disorders of the venous system, such as deep vein thrombophlebitis, trauma, and occlusion.

Complications

Long-standing varicose veins produce venous insufficiency and venous stasis ulcers, particularly around the ankles.

Assessment findings

The patient with varicose veins may be asymptomatic or complain of mild to severe leg symptoms, including a feeling of heaviness that worsens in the evening and in warm weather; cramps at night; diffuse, dull aching after prolonged standing or walking; aching during menses; and fatigue. Exercise may relieve symptoms because venous return improves.

Inspection of the affected leg reveals dilated, purplish, ropelike veins, particularly in the calf. Deep vein incompetence causes orthostatic edema and stasis of the calves and ankles. Palpation may reveal nodules along affected veins and valve incompetence, which can be checked by the manual compression test and Trendelenburg's test.

To do the *manual compression test,* palpate the dilated vein with the fingertips of one hand. With the other hand, firmly compress the vein at a point at least 8″ (20 cm) higher. Feel for an impulse transmitted to your lower hand. With competent saphenous valves, you won't detect any impulse. A palpable impulse indicates incompetent valves in a vein segment between your hands.

To do *Trendelenburg's test (retrograde filling test),* mark the distended veins with a pen while the patient stands. Then have him lie on the examination table and elevate his leg for about a minute to drain the veins. Next, have him stand while you measure venous filling time. Competent valves take at least 30 seconds to fill. If the veins fill in less than 30 seconds, have the patient lie on the examination table again and elevate his leg for 1 minute.

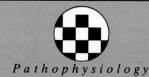

Pathophysiology

HOW VARICOSE VEINS DEVELOP

Varicose veins result when incompetent venous valves allow blood backflow and pooling. Normally, venous valves open and close smoothly and completely. This helps the blood along as it returns from the periphery to the heart.

Normal venous valves (open left, closed right)

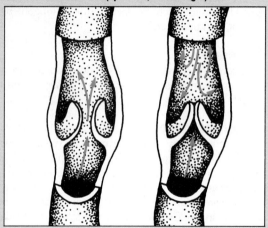

In varicose veins, injury to the valves, defective valvular structure or function, or venous occlusion leads to improper valve closure, resulting in venous blood backflow. As pressure builds, valves become incompetent, causing still more backflow. Progressive blood pooling produces the characteristic leg-vein dilation and leads to disturbed tissue oxygen and nutrient exchange.

Incompetent venous valve

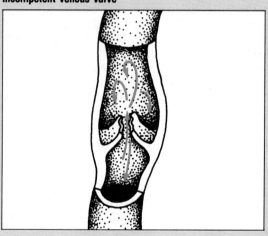

Then apply a tourniquet around his upper thigh. Next, have him stand. If leg veins still fill in less than 30 seconds, suspect incompetent perforating vein and deep vein valves (functioning valves block retrograde flow).

Now remove the tourniquet. If the veins fill again in less than 30 seconds, suspect incompetent superficial vein valves that allow backward blood flow.

To pinpoint incompetent valve location, repeat this procedure by applying the tourniquet just below the knee and then around the upper calf.

Diagnostic tests

• *Photoplethysmography,* a noninvasive test, characterizes venous blood flow by noting changes in the skin's circulation.

• *Doppler ultrasonography* quickly and accurately detects the presence or absence of venous backflow in deep or superficial veins.

• *Venous outflow* and *reflux plethysmography* can detect deep venous occlusion.

• *Ascending* and *descending venography* can demonstrate venous occlusion and patterns of collateral flow. It's an invasive test and not routinely used.

Treatment

In mild varicose veins, treatment involves wearing elastic stockings, avoiding tight clothing and prolonged standing, exercising, and elevating the legs. Treatment in moderate varicose veins consists of wearing antiembolism stockings or elastic bandages. Severe varicose veins may require custom-fitted, surgical-weight stockings with graduated pressure (highest at the ankle, lowest at the top). An exercise program, such as walking, promotes muscle contraction and forces blood through the veins, thereby minimizing venous pooling.

Severe varicose veins may require stripping and ligation or, in patients who are poor surgical risks, injection of a sclerosing agent into small segments of affected veins.

Nursing diagnoses
• Activity intolerance
• Altered tissue perfusion
• Fatigue
• Impaired skin integrity
• Impaired tissue integrity
• Pain

Nursing interventions
• After stripping and ligation or after injection of a sclerosing agent, administer analgesics, as ordered, to relieve pain.
• Frequently check circulation in toes (color and temperature), and observe elastic bandages for bleeding. When ordered, rewrap bandages at least once a shift, wrapping from toe to thigh, with the leg elevated.
• Watch for signs and symptoms of complications, such as sensory loss in the leg (which could indicate saphenous nerve damage), calf pain (thrombophlebitis), and fever (infection).

Patient teaching
• To promote comfort and minimize worsening of varicose veins, tell the patient to avoid wearing constrictive clothing.
• Tell the patient to elevate his legs above heart level when possible and to avoid prolonged standing or sitting.
• Teach the patient to put on the elastic, antiembolism, or compression stockings before getting out of bed in the morning. If he can't do that, tell him to lie with his legs raised for 1 minute and then to put on the stockings.
• Teach the patient to avoid injury to the lower legs, ankles, and feet and to observe for altered skin integrity of those areas. Have him report any problems to the doctor as soon as possible. Impaired tissue perfusion will reduce the leg's healing ability and predispose it to infection and further tissue damage.

RAYNAUD'S DISEASE
Also known as vasospastic arterial disease, Raynaud's disease is one of several primary arteriospastic disorders. These disorders are characterized by episodic vasospasm in the small peripheral arteries and arterioles precipitated by exposure to cold or stress.

Raynaud's disease occurs bilaterally and usually affects the hands or, less often, the feet and, rarely, the earlobes and the tip of the nose. The disease is five times more common in females than in males, particularly between late adolescence and age 40. The disorder is benign, requiring no specific treatment and with no serious sequelae.

Raynaud's phenomenon, however, is a condition often associated with several connective tissue disorders, such as scleroderma, systemic lupus erythematosus, and polymyositis. (For other disorders and conditions associated with Raynaud's phenomenon, see *Causes of Raynaud's phenomenon,* page 602.) Both disorders have a progressive course, leading to ischemia, gangrene, and amputation.

Causes
Although the cause is unknown, several conditions account for the reduced digital blood flow: intrinsic vascular wall hyperactivity to cold, ineffective basal heat production, increased vasomotor tone from sympathetic stimulation, stress, and an antigen-antibody immune response (the most probable theory because abnormal immunologic test results accompany Raynaud's phenomenon).

Complications
Severe, persistent vasoconstriction can lead to ischemia, gangrene, and amputation. Although extremely uncommon, full-thickness tissue necrosis and gangrene necessitate amputation of one or more phalanges.

Assessment findings
The patient with Raynaud's disease may complain of skin color changes induced by cold or stress.

The response to cold and stress is typically triphasic. Initially, the skin of affected areas appears markedly pale from severe vasoconstriction. During this phase, the patient may complain of numbness and tingling.

In the second phase, the skin appears cyanotic, resulting from dilation of cutaneous arterioles and venules.

Because vasoconstriction is diminished, reactive hyperemia results, so the skin in the third phase appears red and feels warm. During this phase, the patient may complain of a throbbing, burning, painful sensation.

Between attacks, the affected areas usually appear normal, although they may feel cool and perspire excessively. In long-standing disease, you may note trophic changes, such as sclerodactyly and ulcerations.

CAUSES OF RAYNAUD'S PHENOMENON

In primary or idiopathic Raynaud's phenomenon, more than 50% of patients have Raynaud's disease. Raynaud's phenomenon may also occur secondary to the following diseases and conditions as well as with the use of certain drugs.

Collagen vascular disease
- Dermatomyositis
- Polymyositis
- Rheumatoid arthritis
- Scleroderma
- Systemic lupus erythematosus

Arterial occlusive disease
- Acute arterial occlusion
- Atherosclerosis of the extremities
- Thoracic outlet syndrome
- Thromboangiitis obliterans

Neurologic disorders
- Carpal tunnel syndrome
- Cerebrovascular accident
- Invertebral disk disease
- Poliomyelitis
- Spinal cord tumors
- Syringomyelia

Blood dyscrasias
- Cold agglutinins
- Cryofibrinogenemia
- Cryoglobulinemia
- Myeloproliferative disorders
- Waldenström's disease

Trauma
- Cold injury
- Electric shock
- Hammer hand syndrome
- Keyboarding
- Piano playing
- Vibration injury

Drugs
- Beta-adrenergic blocking agents
- Bleomycin
- Cisplatin
- Ergot derivatives, such as ergotamine
- Methysergide
- Vinblastine

Other
- Pulmonary hypertension

Diagnostic tests

The ice water immersion test can help diagnose the disorder. In this test, the patient immerses his hand in ice water for 30 seconds after digital pulp temperature measurement with a thermistor probe. The hand is dried, and repeat pulp temperatures are taken every 5 minutes for 45 minutes until the temperature returns to normal. Ordinarily, this takes 10 minutes or less; in a patient with Raynaud's phenomenon, it takes much longer. Before Raynaud's phenomenon can be diagnosed as Raynaud's disease, however, secondary disease processes, such as chronic arterial occlusive disease and connective tissue disease, must be ruled out.

Arteriography and digital photoplethysmography may also help diagnose the presence of Raynaud's phenomenon.

Treatment

Initially, treatment consists of avoidance of cold, mechanical, or chemical injury; cessation of smoking; and reassurance that symptoms are benign. Because adverse reactions to drugs, especially vasodilators, may be more bothersome than the disease itself, drug therapy is reserved for unusually severe signs and symptoms. Such therapy may include phenoxybenzamine, nifedipine, reserpine, or guanethidine combined with prazosin. Biofeedback therapy may be useful if signs and symptoms are caused by stress.

Sympathectomy may be helpful when conservative treatment fails to prevent ischemic ulcers (occurring in less than 25% of patients).

Nursing diagnoses
- Altered role performance
- Altered tissue perfusion
- Impaired skin integrity
- Impaired tissue integrity
- Ineffective individual coping
- Ineffective thermoregulation
- Knowledge deficit
- Pain

Nursing interventions
- If signs and symptoms are caused by stress, help the patient identify stress-producing areas of her life, and help her identify and use effective coping strategies. If appropriate, refer her to a biofeedback program to help control signs and symptoms related to stress.
- Provide psychological support and reassurance to allay the patient's fear of amputation and disfigurement.
- Evaluate the patient's occupation and its effect on symptom occurrence. If needed, refer the patient to occupational rehabilitation to prevent progression to untreatable complications.

Patient teaching
• Warn against exposure to the cold. Tell the patient to wear mittens or gloves in cold weather or when handling cold items or defrosting the freezer.
• Advise the patient to avoid stress and to stop smoking. Refer her to a stop-smoking program, if needed.
• Instruct the patient to inspect her skin frequently and to seek immediate care for signs of skin breakdown or infection.
• Teach the patient about prescribed drugs, their proper use, and their adverse effects. Tell her to report any adverse effects to the doctor.

BUERGER'S DISEASE
An inflammatory, nonatheromatous occlusive condition, Buerger's disease causes segmental lesions and subsequent thrombus formation in the small and medium-size arteries (and sometimes the veins), resulting in decreased blood flow to the legs and feet.

Also called thromboangiitis obliterans, the disease affects the legs more commonly than the arms. Cerebral, visceral, and coronary vessels may also be affected. Incidence is highest among men of Asian and Jewish ancestry, ages 20 to 40, who smoke heavily.

Causes and pathophysiology
Although the cause of Buerger's disease is unknown, a definite link exists to smoking and an increased incidence of human leukocyte antigen (HLA)-B5 and HLA-A9, suggesting a hypersensitivity reaction to nicotine.

In the initial stages of the disease, polymorphonuclear leukocytes infiltrate the walls of the small and medium-size arteries and veins. The internal elastic lamina is preserved, and a thrombus may develop in the vascular lumen. As the disease progresses, mononuclear cells, fibroblasts, and giant cells replace the neutrophils. In later stages, perivascular fibrosis and recanalization occur.

Complications
Impaired tissue perfusion can cause ulcerations and poor wound healing, possibly leading to amputation if gangrene and systemic infection occur.

Assessment findings
The patient with Buerger's disease typically complains of painful, intermittent claudication of the instep, which is aggravated by exercise and relieved by rest.

During exposure to low temperature, the feet initially become cold and numb and appear cyanotic; later, they redden, become hot, and tingle. Occasionally, Buerger's disease also affects the hands, possibly resulting in severe digital ischemia, trophic nail changes, painful fingertip ulcerations, and gangrene.

Palpation of peripheral pulses reveals normal brachial and popliteal pulses but absent or diminished radial, ulnar, or tibial pulses.

Late in the disease, the patient may experience migratory superficial vein thrombophlebitis, peripheral ulceration, muscle atrophy, and gangrene.

Diagnostic tests
• *Doppler ultrasonography* may show diminished circulation in the peripheral vessels.
• *Plethysmography* helps to detect decreased circulation in the peripheral vessels.
• *Arteriography* helps locate lesions and rules out atherosclerosis. Smooth tapering segmental lesions in the distal vessels and collateral vessels at the site of vascular occlusion are characteristic findings.
• *Biopsy* of the affected vessel can confirm the diagnosis.

Treatment
Abstention from smoking tobacco is essential. An exercise program that uses gravity to fill and drain the blood vessels may also help in mild to moderate disease. Severe disease may require a lumbar sympathectomy or arterial bypass to increase blood supply to the skin. Parenteral or oral antibiotics may be used to treat secondary infections. Amputation may be necessary for non-healing ulcers, intractable pain, or gangrene.

Nursing diagnoses
• Activity intolerance
• Altered role performance
• Altered tissue perfusion
• Anxiety
• Impaired tissue integrity
• Ineffective individual coping
• Ineffective thermoregulation
• Risk for infection

Nursing interventions
• If the patient has ulcers and gangrene, enforce bed rest, and use a padded footboard or bed cradle to prevent pressure from bed linens. Protect the feet with soft padding. Wash them gently with a mild soap and tepid water, rinse thoroughly, and pat dry with a soft towel.
• Administer antibiotics, as ordered, and document the condition of ulceration daily.

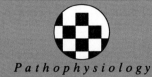

WHAT CAUSES ACUTE ARTERIAL OCCLUSION?

The most common cause of acute arterial occlusion is obstruction of a major artery by a clot. The occlusive mechanism may be endogenous, resulting from emboli formation, thrombosis, or plaques, or exogenous, resulting from trauma or fracture.

Embolism
Often the obstruction results from an embolus originating in the heart. Emboli typically lodge in the arms and legs, where blood vessels narrow or branch. In the arms, emboli usually lodge in the brachial artery but may occlude the subclavian or axillary arteries. Common leg sites include the iliac, femoral, and popliteal arteries. Emboli originating in the heart can cause neurologic damage if they enter the cerebral circulation.

Thrombosis
In a patient with atherosclerosis and marked arterial narrowing, thrombosis may cause acute intrinsic arterial occlusion. This complication typically arises in areas with severely stenotic vessels, especially in a patient who also has congestive heart failure, hypovolemia, polycythemia, or traumatic injury.

Plaques
Atheromatous debris (plaques) from proximal arterial lesions also may intermittently obstruct small vessels (usually in the hands or feet). These plaques also may develop in the brachiocephalic vessels and travel to the cerebral circulation, where they may lead to transient cerebral ischemia or infarction.

Exogenous causes
Acute arterial occlusion may stem from insertion of an indwelling arterial catheter, intra-arterial drug abuse, or peripheral arterial injection of foreign material.

In addition, extrinsic arterial occlusion can result from direct blunt or penetrating trauma to the artery.

• Provide emotional support. If necessary, refer the patient for psychological counseling to help him cope with restrictions imposed by this chronic disease.
• If the patient has undergone amputation, assess rehabilitative needs, especially regarding changes in body image. Refer him to a physical therapist, an occupational therapist, and the social service department, as needed.

Patient teaching
• Strongly urge the patient to quit smoking to enhance the effectiveness of treatment. If necessary, refer him to a self-help group or a psychologist.
• Warn the patient to avoid precipitating factors, such as stress, exposure to extreme temperatures, and trauma.
• Teach proper foot care, especially the importance of wearing well-fitting shoes and cotton or wool socks. Show the patient how to inspect his feet daily for cuts, abrasions, and signs of skin breakdown, such as redness and soreness. Remind him to seek medical attention immediately after any trauma.

ARTERIAL OCCLUSIVE DISEASE

An obstruction or narrowing of the lumen of the aorta and its major branches, arterial occlusive disease interrupts blood flow, usually to the legs and feet. This disorder may affect the carotid, vertebral, innominate, subclavian, mesenteric, and celiac arteries.

Arterial occlusive disease is more common in males than in females. The prognosis depends on the location of the occlusion, the development of collateral circulation to counteract reduced blood flow and, in acute disease, the time elapsed between the development of the occlusion and its removal.

Causes

Arterial occlusive disease is a common complication of atherosclerosis. (For more information, see *What causes acute arterial occlusion?*)

Predisposing factors include smoking; aging; conditions such as hypertension, hyperlipidemia, and diabetes mellitus; and family history of vascular disorders, myocardial infarction, or cerebrovascular accident.

SIGNS AND SYMPTOMS OF ARTERIAL OCCLUSIVE DISEASE

A patient with arterial occlusive disease may have a wide variety of signs and symptoms, depending on which portion of the vasculature is affected by the disorder.

Site of occlusion	Signs and symptoms
Internal and external carotid arteries	Transient ischemic attacks (TIAs) due to reduced cerebral circulation produce unilateral sensory or motor dysfunction (transient monocular blindness, hemiparesis), possible aphasia or dysarthria, confusion, decreased mentation, and headache. These recurrent clinical features usually last for 5 to 10 minutes but may persist for up to 24 hours and may herald a cerebrovascular accident. Absent or decreased pulsation with an auscultatory bruit over the affected vessels.
Vertebral and basilar arteries	TIAs of brain stem and cerebellum produce binocular visual disturbances, vertigo, dysarthria, and "drop attacks" (falling down without loss of consciousness). Less common than carotid TIA.
Innominate (brachiocephalic) artery	Signs and symptoms of vertebrobasilar occlusion. Indications of ischemia (claudication) of right arm; possible bruit over right side of neck.
Subclavian artery	Subclavian steal syndrome characterized by the backflow of blood from the brain through the vertebral artery on the same side as the occlusion, into the subclavian artery distal to the occlusion; clinical effects of vertebrobasilar occlusion and exercise-induced arm claudication. Possible gangrene, usually limited to the digits.
Mesenteric artery	Bowel ischemia, infarct necrosis, and gangrene; sudden, acute abdominal pain; nausea and vomiting; diarrhea; leukocytosis; and shock due to massive intraluminal fluid and plasma loss.
Aortic bifurcation (saddle block occlusion, a medical emergency associated with cardiac embolization)	Sensory and motor deficits (muscle weakness, numbness, paresthesia, paralysis), and signs of ischemia (sudden pain; cold, pale legs with decreased or absent peripheral pulses) in both legs.
Iliac artery (Leriche's syndrome)	Intermittent claudication of lower back, buttocks, and thighs, relieved by rest; absent or reduced femoral or distal pulses; shiny, scaly skin, subcutaneous tissue loss, and no body hair on affected limb; nail deformities; increased capillary refill time; blanching of feet on elevation; possible bruit over femoral arteries; impotence in males.
Femoral and popliteal arteries (associated with aneurysm formation)	Intermittent claudication of the calves on exertion; ischemic pain in feet; pretrophic pain (heralds necrosis and ulceration); leg pallor and coolness; shiny, scaly skin, subcutaneous tissue loss, and no body hair on affected limb; nail deformities; increased capillary refill time; blanching of feet on elevation; gangrene; no palpable pulses distal to occlusion. Auscultation over affected area may reveal a bruit.

Complications
Occlusions may be acute or chronic and often cause severe ischemia, skin ulceration, and gangrene.

Assessment findings
Varied assessment findings depend on the vessel involved. (For more information, see *Signs and symptoms of arterial occlusive disease*.)

Acute arterial occlusion occurs suddenly, often without warning. However, peripheral occlusion can often be recognized by the five *P*s:
• *Pain*, the most common symptom, occurs suddenly and is localized to the affected arm or leg.
• *Pallor* results from vasoconstriction distal to the occlusion.
• *Pulselessness* occurs distal to the occlusion.

• *Paralysis and paresthesia* occur in the affected arm or leg from disturbed nerve endings or skeletal muscles.
A sixth P, known as *poikilothermy,* refers to temperature changes that occur distal to the occlusion, making the skin feel cool.

Diagnostic tests

• *Arteriography* demonstrates the type, location, and degree of obstruction, and the establishment of collateral circulation. It is particularly useful in chronic disease or for evaluating candidates for reconstructive surgery.
• *Ultrasonography* and *plethysmography* are noninvasive tests that, in acute disease, show decreased blood flow distal to the occlusion.
• *Doppler ultrasonography* typically reveals a relatively low-pitched sound and a monophasic waveform.
• *Segmental limb pressures* and *pulse volume measurements* help evaluate the location and extent of the occlusion.
• *Ophthalmodynamometry* helps determine the degree of obstruction in the internal carotid artery by comparing ophthalmic artery pressure with brachial artery pressure on the affected side. More than a 20% difference between pressures suggests arterial insufficiency.
• *Electroencephalography* and a *computed tomography scan* may be necessary to rule out brain lesions.

Treatment

In mild chronic disease, treatment usually consists of supportive measures: elimination of smoking, hypertension control, walking exercise, and foot and leg care. In carotid artery occlusion, antiplatelet therapy may begin with dipyridamole and aspirin. For those patients with intermittent claudication caused by chronic arterial occlusive disease, pentoxifylline may improve blood flow through the capillaries. This drug is particularly useful for poor surgical candidates.

Thrombolytics, such as urokinase, streptokinase, and activase, can dissolve clots and relieve the obstruction caused by a thrombus.

Acute arterial occlusive disease usually requires surgery, such as the following:
• *Embolectomy.* A balloon-tipped Fogarty catheter is used to remove thrombotic material from the artery. Embolectomy is used mainly for mesenteric, femoral, or popliteal artery occlusion.
• *Thromboendarterectomy.* This involves the opening of the artery and removal of the obstructing thrombus and the medial layer of the arterial wall. Plaque deposits will remain intact. Thromboendarterectomy is usually performed after angiography and is often used in conjunc-

tion with autogenous vein or Dacron bypass surgery (femoropopliteal or aortofemoral).
• *Percutaneous transluminal coronary angioplasty (PTCA).* Using fluoroscopy and a special balloon catheter, PTCA dilates the stenosis or occluded artery to a predetermined diameter without overdistending it.
• *Laser surgery.* An excimer or a hot-tip laser obliterates the clot and plaque by vaporizing it.
• *Patch grafting.* This involves removal of the thrombosed arterial segment and replacement with an autogenous vein or Dacron graft.
• *Bypass graft.* Blood flow is diverted through an anastomosed autogenous or woven Dacron graft to bypass the thrombosed arterial segment.
• *Lumbar sympathectomy.* Depending on the condition of the sympathetic nervous system, this procedure may be an adjunct to reconstructive surgery.

Amputation may be necessary if arterial reconstructive surgery fails or if gangrene, uncontrollable infection, or intractable pain develops.

Other therapy includes heparin to prevent emboli (for embolic occlusion) and bowel resection after restoration of blood flow (for mesenteric artery occlusion).

Nursing diagnoses
• Activity intolerance
• Altered tissue perfusion
• Diversional activity deficit
• Impaired physical mobility
• Impaired skin integrity
• Ineffective individual coping
• Knowledge deficit
• Pain
• Risk for disuse syndrome
• Risk for infection

Nursing interventions
For chronic arterial occlusive disease:
• Prevent trauma to the affected extremity. Use minimal-pressure mattresses, heel protectors, a foot cradle, or a footboard to reduce pressure that could lead to skin breakdown. Keep the arm or leg warm but never use heating pads. If the patient is wearing socks, remove them frequently to check the skin.
• Avoid using restrictive clothing, such as antiembolism stockings.
• Administer analgesics, as ordered, to relieve pain.
• Allow the patient to express fears and concerns, and help him identify and use effective coping strategies.

For preoperative care during an acute episode:
• Assess the patient's circulatory status by checking for the most distal pulses and by inspecting his skin color and temperature.
• Administer analgesics for pain, as needed.
• Administer heparin or thrombolytics by continuous I.V. drip, as ordered. Use an infusion monitor or pump to ensure the proper flow rate.
• Wrap the patient's affected foot in soft cotton batting, and reposition it frequently to prevent pressure on any one area. Strictly avoid elevating or applying heat to the affected leg.
• Watch for signs of fluid and electrolyte imbalance, and monitor intake and output for signs of renal failure (urine output of less than 30 ml/hour).
• If the patient has carotid, innominate, vertebral, or subclavian artery occlusion, monitor him for signs of cerebrovascular accident, such as numbness in an arm or a leg and intermittent blindness.

For postoperative care:
• Monitor the patient's vital signs. Continuously assess his circulatory function by assessing skin color and temperature and by checking for distal pulses. In charting, compare earlier assessments and observations. Watch closely for signs of hemorrhage (tachycardia, hypotension), and check dressings for excessive bleeding.
• In carotid, innominate, vertebral, or subclavian artery occlusion, assess the patient's neurologic status frequently for changes in level of consciousness, pupil size, and muscle strength.
• In mesenteric artery occlusion, connect a nasogastric tube to low intermittent suction. Monitor intake and output (low urine output may indicate damage to renal arteries during surgery). Check bowel sounds for the return of peristalsis. Increasing abdominal distention and tenderness may indicate extension of bowel ischemia with resulting gangrene, necessitating further excision, or it may indicate peritonitis.
• In saddle block occlusion, check distal pulses for adequate circulation. Watch for signs of renal failure and mesenteric artery occlusion (severe abdominal pain), and for cardiac arrhythmias, which may precipitate embolus formation.
• If PTCA was performed, sheath (catheter) care must be done. The line must be kept open with a heparin infusion, so monitor the insertion site for bleeding. Keep the catheterized leg immobile, and keep the patient on strict bed rest. Monitor and record pulses in the catheterized leg. Provide analgesics for back pain associated with catheter placement.

• In iliac artery occlusion, monitor urine output for signs of renal failure from decreased perfusion to the kidneys as a result of surgery. Provide meticulous catheter care.
• In both femoral and popliteal artery occlusion, assist with early ambulation, but don't allow the patient to sit for an extended period.
• When caring for a patient who has undergone amputation, check the stump carefully for drainage. If drainage occurs, note and record its color and amount, and the time. Elevate the stump, as ordered, and administer adequate analgesics. Because phantom limb pain is common, explain this phenomenon to the patient.

Patient teaching
• When preparing the patient for discharge, instruct him to watch for signs of recurrence (pain, pallor, numbness, paralysis, absence of pulse) that can result from graft occlusion or occlusion at another site. Caution against wearing constrictive clothing, crossing his legs, or wearing garters. Tell him to avoid "bumping" injuries to affected limbs.
• Warn the patient to avoid all tobacco products.
• Tell the patient to avoid temperature extremes. If he must go outside in the cold, remind him to dress warmly and take special care to keep his feet warm.
• Instruct the patient to wash his feet daily and inspect them for signs of injury or infection. Remind him to report any abnormalities to the doctor.
• Advise the patient to wear sturdy, properly fitting shoes. Refer him to a podiatrist for any foot problems.

SELECTED REFERENCES

Braunwald, E. *Heart Disease: A Textbook of Cardiovascular Medicine,* 4th ed. Philadelphia: W.B. Saunders Co., 1992.

Illustrated Manual of Nursing Practice, 2nd ed. Springhouse, Pa.: Springhouse Corp., 1994.

Isselbacher, K., et al., eds. *Harrison's Principles of Internal Medicine,* 13th ed. New York: McGraw-Hill Book Co., 1995.

Kinney, M.R., et al. *AACN's Clinical Reference for Critical-Care Nursing,* 3rd ed. St. Louis: Mosby-Year Book, Inc., 1993.

Lieberman, K.S. "Markers of Reperfusion after Thrombolytic Therapy for Acute Myocardial Infarction," *Journal of Emergency Nursing* 21(2):112-15, April 1995.

Perra, B.M. "Managing Coronary Atherectomy Patients in a Special Procedure Unit," *Critical Care Nurse* 15(3):57-59, 63-68, June 1995.

Taylor, C.M., and Sparks, S.M. *Nursing Diagnosis Reference Manual,* 3rd ed. Springhouse, Pa.: Springhouse Corp., 1995.

8 RESPIRATORY DISORDERS

INTRODUCTION

The respiratory system provides vital gas exchange by distributing air to the alveoli. Here, pulmonary capillary blood takes on oxygen (O_2) and gives off carbon dioxide (CO_2). Various specialized structures within the respiratory system prepare air for the body to use.

The nose, for example, contains vestibular hairs that filter impurities from the air and an extensive vascular network to warm it. The nose also contains a layer of goblet cells and a moist mucosal surface. From this surface, water vapor enters the airstream to saturate the inspired air as it's warmed in the upper airways.

Ciliated mucosae in the posterior nose and the nasopharynx (and in major portions of the tracheobronchial tree) propel particles deposited by impaction or gravity to the oropharynx, where the particles are swallowed. Besides CO_2, other gases, such as carbon monoxide, may diffuse from pulmonary capillary blood to the alveoli, where they're excreted by the lungs.

External respiration

The external component of respiration—ventilation, or breathing—delivers inspired air (or gas) to the lower respiratory tract and alveoli. Expansion and contraction of the respiratory muscles move air into and out of the lungs. Ventilation begins with the contraction of the inspiratory muscles: The diaphragm, the major muscle of respiration, descends, while external intercostal muscles move the rib cage upward and outward. The accessory muscles of inspiration (which include the scalene and sternocleidomastoid muscles) raise the clavicles, upper ribs, and sternum. The accessory muscles aren't used in normal inspiration but are used in certain disease states.

An adult lung contains about 300 million alveoli, with many capillaries supplying each alveolus. To reach the capillary lumen, O_2 must cross the alveolocapillary membrane, which consists of an alveolar epithelial cell, a narrow interstitial space, the capillary basement membrane, and the capillary endothelial cell membrane. The tension created by O_2 entering the respiratory tract is about 160 mm Hg. In the alveoli, this inspired air mixes with CO_2 and water vapor, lowering pressure to about 100 mm Hg. Because the partial pressure of O_2 in alveolar blood (PAO_2) exceeds that in the mixed venous blood entering the pulmonary capillaries (about 40 mm Hg), O_2 diffuses across the alveolocapillary membrane into the blood.

Internal respiration and gas transport

Circulating blood delivers O_2 to the body's cells for metabolism and transports metabolic wastes and CO_2 from the tissues back to the lungs. When oxygenated arterial blood reaches tissue capillaries, O_2 diffuses from the blood into the cells again because of an oxygen tension gradient. The amount of O_2 available is determined by the level of hemoglobin (the principal carrier of O_2), regional blood flow, arterial oxygen tension, and carboxyhemoglobin tension.

Internal, or cellular, respiration occurs during cellular metabolism, which can occur with O_2 (aerobic) or without O_2 (anaerobic). The most efficient method of providing fuel (compounds such as adenosine triphosphate [ATP]) for cellular reactions is aerobic metabolism, which produces CO_2 and water besides ATP. Anaerobic metabolism is less efficient because a cell produces only a limited amount of ATP and releases both lactic acid and CO_2 as metabolic by-products.

Because circulation is continuous, CO_2 doesn't normally accumulate in tissues. CO_2 produced during cellular respiration diffuses from tissues to regional capillaries and is transported by systemic venous circulation. When CO_2 reaches the alveolar capillaries, it diffuses into the alveoli, where the partial pressure of CO_2 ($PACO_2$) is lower. During exhalation, CO_2 exits the alveoli.

Mechanisms of control

The central nervous system (CNS) controls respiration from the respiratory control center in the lateral medulla oblongata of the brain stem. Impulses travel along the phrenic nerves to the diaphragm and then along the intercostal nerves to the intercostal muscles, where the impulses control the rate and depth of respiration. The inspiratory and expiratory centers, located in the posterior medulla, establish the involuntary rhythm of the breathing pattern.

Apneustic and pneumotaxic centers in the pons influence the breathing pattern also. Stimulation of the lower pontine apneustic center (by trauma, tumor, or cerebrovascular accident, for example) produces forceful inspiratory gasps alternating with weak expiration. This pattern does not occur if the vagus nerve is intact. The apneustic center continuously excites the medullary inspiratory center and thereby facilitates inspiration. Signals from the pneumotaxic center and afferent impulses from the vagus nerve inhibit the apneustic center and "turn off" inspiration.

Arterial partial pressure of oxygen (PaO_2) and pH balances, as well as the pH of cerebrospinal fluid (CSF), influence output from the respiratory control center. CO_2 entering the CSF lowers the pH of CSF. This stimulates central chemoreceptors and increases ventilation.

The respiratory center also receives information from peripheral chemoreceptors in the carotid and aortic bodies. Although these chemoreceptors respond primarily to a decreased PaO_2 level, they also respond to reduced pH. Either change spurs respiratory drive within minutes.

Several other factors can alter the respiratory pattern. During exercise, stretch receptors in lung tissue and the diaphragm prevent the lungs from overdistending. During eating and drinking, the cortex can interrupt automatic control of ventilation. During sleep, the respiratory drive fluctuates, producing hypoventilation and periods of apnea. External sensations, drugs, chronic hypercapnia, and increased or decreased body heat can also alter the respiratory pattern.

Assessment

A complete respiratory assessment will help you identify existing and potential respiratory problems. It begins with a patient history followed by a physical examination.

Obtain the history

Ask the patient to describe his respiratory problem. How long has he had it? How long does each attack last? Does one attack differ from another? Does any activity in particular bring on an attack or make it worse? What relieves the symptoms?

Always ask about previous and current smoking habits: what the patient smokes, his daily use, and the number of years as a smoker. Record this information in pack years — the number of packs of cigarettes smoked daily multiplied by the number of years he has smoked. Remember also to ask about the patient's occupation, hobbies, and travel. Some activities may expose him to toxic or allergenic substances.

If the patient has dyspnea, find out whether it occurs during activity or rest. Does any specific position cause or worsen his dyspnea? How far can he walk? How many stairs can he climb? Can he relate dyspnea to allergies or environmental conditions?

If the patient has a cough, ask about its severity, persistence, and duration. If the cough produces sputum, ask the patient to describe its color, amount, and character. Also ask whether his cough and sputum have changed recently.

Observe the patient

Look for telltale signs of respiratory disease. The patient's appearance may provide clues. If he's frail or cachectic, he may have a chronic disease that impairs appetite. If he's diaphoretic, restless, irritable, or protective of a painful body part, he may be in acute distress. Also, assess behavior changes that may indicate hypoxia or hypercapnia. Confusion, lethargy, bizarre behavior, or quiet sleep from which he can't be aroused may signal hypercapnia. Restlessness, anxiety, or interrupted speech may indicate hypoxia. Watch for marked cyanosis, indicated by bluish or ashen skin (usually best seen on the lips, tongue, earlobes, and nail beds), which may result from hypoxemia or poor tissue perfusion.

Check chest configuration at rest and during ventilation. You may notice the following deviations:
• pigeon chest — anteriorly displaced sternum
• barrel chest — increased anteroposterior diameter
• funnel chest — depressed lower sternum
• kyphoscoliosis — raised shoulder and scapula, thoracic convexity, flared interspaces, and altered chest configuration (which, in turn, restricts breathing).

Assess the muscles used during inspiration with the patient in a semi-Fowler or flat position. Then note which muscles he uses when he breathes. If the epigastric area rises during inspiration, he's using his diaphragm. Use of the upper chest and neck muscles is normal only during physical stress.

Observe the patient's breathing rate and pattern. Certain disorders produce characteristic changes in breathing patterns. An acute respiratory disorder, for example, can produce tachypnea (rapid breathing), hypopnea (shallow breathing), or hyperpnea (deep breathing); intracranial lesions can produce Cheyne-Stokes or Biot's respirations; increased intracranial pressure can produce central hyperventilation and apneustic or ataxic breathing; metabolic disorders can produce Kussmaul's respirations; and airway obstruction can produce prolonged forceful expiration and pursed-lip breathing.

Observe posture and carriage. A patient with chronic obstructive pulmonary disease, for example, usually supports rib cage movement by placing his arms on the sides of a chair to increase expansion and leans forward during exhalation to help expel air. (See *Recognizing common respiratory patterns*.)

Perform a physical examination

You'll use such techniques as palpation, percussion, and auscultation to assess the respiratory system.

Palpation of the chest wall can help you detect masses, tender areas, and changes in fremitus (palpable vocal vibrations) or crepitus (air in subcutaneous tissues). To assess chest excursion and symmetry, place your hands bilaterally and horizontally on the posterior chest. Be sure your thumbs press lightly against the spine (as if to squeeze the skin over the spine into a fold or a pleat). As

RECOGNIZING COMMON RESPIRATORY PATTERNS

Use this chart as a visual guide to respiratory rate, rhythm, and depth patterns.

Pattern		Characteristics
Eupnea	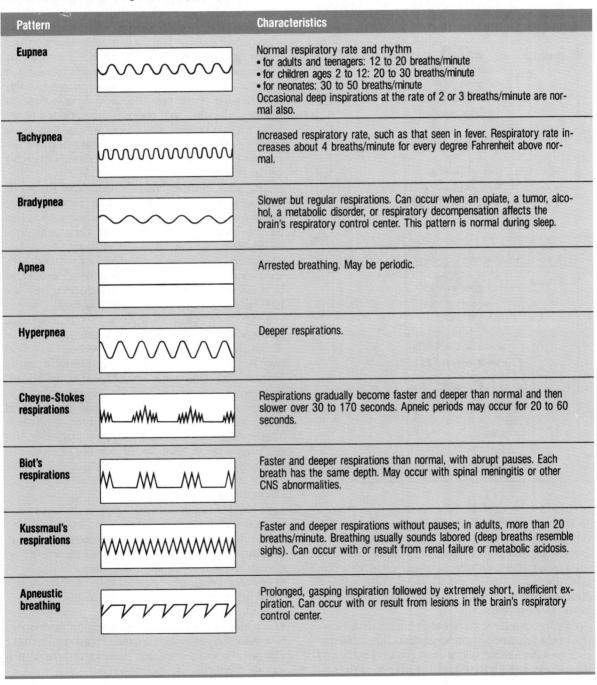	Normal respiratory rate and rhythm • for adults and teenagers: 12 to 20 breaths/minute • for children ages 2 to 12: 20 to 30 breaths/minute • for neonates: 30 to 50 breaths/minute Occasional deep inspirations at the rate of 2 or 3 breaths/minute are normal also.
Tachypnea		Increased respiratory rate, such as that seen in fever. Respiratory rate increases about 4 breaths/minute for every degree Fahrenheit above normal.
Bradypnea		Slower but regular respirations. Can occur when an opiate, a tumor, alcohol, a metabolic disorder, or respiratory decompensation affects the brain's respiratory control center. This pattern is normal during sleep.
Apnea		Arrested breathing. May be periodic.
Hyperpnea		Deeper respirations.
Cheyne-Stokes respirations		Respirations gradually become faster and deeper than normal and then slower over 30 to 170 seconds. Apneic periods may occur for 20 to 60 seconds.
Biot's respirations		Faster and deeper respirations than normal, with abrupt pauses. Each breath has the same depth. May occur with spinal meningitis or other CNS abnormalities.
Kussmaul's respirations		Faster and deeper respirations without pauses; in adults, more than 20 breaths/minute. Breathing usually sounds labored (deep breaths resemble sighs). Can occur with or result from renal failure or metabolic acidosis.
Apneustic breathing		Prolonged, gasping inspiration followed by extremely short, inefficient expiration. Can occur with or result from lesions in the brain's respiratory control center.

SEQUENCES FOR CHEST PALPATION

Follow this guide to conduct a thorough chest palpation. The numerical sequence ensures that all areas are examined and that bilateral findings can be easily compared.

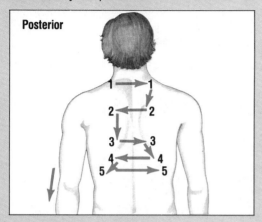

Posterior

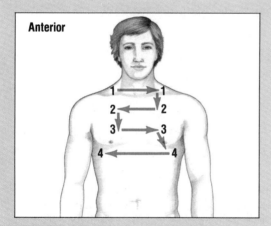

Anterior

the patient takes a deep breath, move your thumbs quickly and equally away from the spine. Repeat this with your hands placed anteriorly, at the costal margins (lower lobes) and clavicles (apices). Unequal movement indicates expansion differences, which occur in atelectasis, diaphragm or chest-wall muscle disease, and splinting with pain. (For more information, see *Sequences for chest palpation.*)

Percussion detects resonance over lung fields not covered by the heart or by bony structures. This technique relies on vibrations (resulting from precise finger taps) that strike underlying structures and rebound to the sur-

face, where you can feel and hear them. The quality of the vibration demarcates underlying chest structures. Dull percussion sounds typically signal consolidation or pleural disease. (See *Ensuring orderly percussion and auscultation,* opposite, and *Characterizing and interpreting percussion sounds,* page 614.)

Auscultation normally detects soft, vesicular breath sounds throughout most of the lung fields. When you auscultate your patient's lungs for normal and abnormal breath sounds, compare both lungs as you proceed from the apices to the bases. Note the pitch, intensity, quality, and duration of the breath sounds. Also evaluate for crackles, rhonchi, and wheezes. Adventitious breath sounds (or no breath sounds) may indicate fluid in the small airways or interstitial lung disease (crackles), secretions in the medium-size and large airways (rhonchi), and airflow obstruction (wheezes).

After characterizing breath sounds, have the patient whisper words while you auscultate peripheral lung fields. Whispering produces vibrations that you can hear on the chest's surface. Categorize these whispered sounds as:

• *bronchophony* — normally a low-pitched sound that intensifies as the patient talks louder, although words can't be deciphered. If you *can* hear words distinctly over the lung periphery, suspect consolidation or fluid.

• *egophony* — ordinarily a low-pitched sound that should clearly sound like "eee" when the patient says the letter "E." If the sound resembles a high-pitched "ate," fluid may be compressing the lung (as in pleural effusion). Normal egophonous sound intensifies over the affected lung area.

• *whispered pectoriloquy* — normally a high-pitched sound that renders the patient's words indistinct. If you hear clearly whispered words over peripheral lung fields, suspect consolidation. Again, sound intensity increases over the affected area.

Diagnostic tests

Once physical assessments are complete, the patient may undergo various respiratory tests.

• *Chest X-rays* identify lesions or such conditions as atelectasis, pleural effusion, infiltrates, pneumothorax, mediastinal shifts, and pulmonary edema.

• *Computed tomography scan* provides a three-dimensional picture that is 100 times more sensitive than chest X-ray films.

• *Lung scan,* ordered primarily to detect pulmonary emboli, demonstrates ventilation and perfusion patterns.

• *Magnetic resonance imaging* identifies obstructed vessels and highlights tissue perfusion.

ENSURING ORDERLY PERCUSSION AND AUSCULTATION

Percussion and auscultation can help you identify various lung abnormalities. To conduct a complete examination, percuss and auscultate along the points shown on the posterior shoulders. Then follow the sequence shown here. Remember to compare findings from one side of the body with those from the other side.

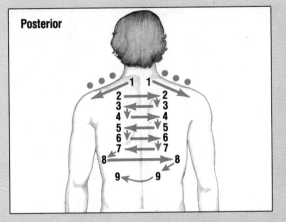

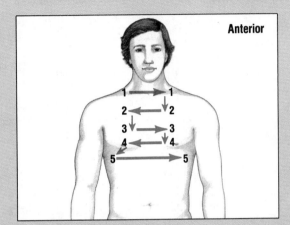

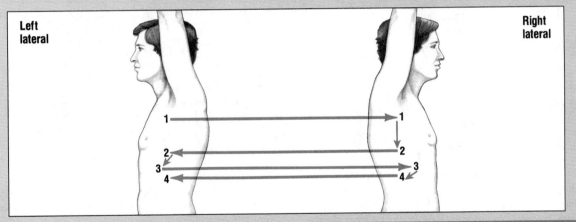

• *Sputum analysis* evaluates sputum quantity, color, viscosity, and odor. Stains and cultures can identify infectious organisms, whereas cytologic studies can detect abnormal respiratory cells.

• *Pulmonary function tests* measure lung volumes, flow rates, and compliance. Determined by body stature and age, normal values are reported as a percentage of the normal predicted value. (See *Defining static and dynamic values,* page 615.)

• *Pulse oximetry* continuously monitors arterial oxygen saturation (SaO_2).

• *Exercise stress tests* evaluate the lungs' ability to transport O_2 and remove CO_2 as metabolic demand increases.

• *Polysomnography* can detect sleep disorders.

• *Bronchoscopy* permits direct visualization of the trachea and the mainstem, lobar, segmental, and subsegmental bronchi. This procedure may help localize the site of lung hemorrhage, visualize masses in the airways, and collect respiratory tract secretions. This procedure allows biopsy.

• *Thoracentesis* permits removal of pleural fluid for analysis.

CHARACTERIZING AND INTERPRETING PERCUSSION SOUNDS

Several kinds of sounds may emanate from percussion. Known as flat, dull, resonant, hyperresonant, or tympanic, these sounds determine the location and density of various structures. During percussion, determining other tonal characteristics, such as pitch, intensity, and quality, will also help you identify respiratory structures. Use this chart as a guide to interpreting percussion sounds.

Character				Implications
Sound	Pitch	Intensity	Quality	
Flatness	High	Soft	Extremely dull	These sounds are normal over the sternum. Over the lung, they may indicate atelectasis or pleural effusion.
Dullness	Medium	Medium	Thudlike	Normal over the liver, heart, and diaphragm, these sounds over the lung may point to pneumonia, tumor, atelectasis, or pleural effusion.
Resonance	Low	Moderate to loud	Hollow	When percussed over the lung, these sounds are normal.
Hyperresonance	Lower than resonance	Very loud	Booming	These are normal findings with percussion over a child's lung. Over an adult lung, these findings may indicate emphysema, chronic bronchitis, asthma, or pneumothorax.
Tympany	High	Loud	Musical, drumlike	Over the stomach, these are normal findings; over the lung, they suggest tension pneumothorax.

• *Pleural biopsy* allows removal of pleural tissue for histologic examination and culture. This test can detect pleural neoplasms or granulomatous infections.

• *Transtracheal aspiration* obtains secretions from the trachea and proximal bronchi for microbiological analysis.

• *Arterial blood gas (ABG) analysis* evaluates gas exchange in the lungs by measuring the PaO_2, partial pressure of carbon dioxide ($PaCO_2$), SaO_2, bicarbonate (HCO_3) level, and the pH of an arterial blood sample. PaO_2 and SaO_2 indicate how much oxygen the lungs are delivering to the blood; $PaCO_2$ indicates how efficiently the lungs are eliminating CO_2. The pH reflects the blood's acid-base level. By evaluating pH, $PaCO_2$, and HCO_3 in a patient's arterial blood, you can determine his acid-base balance.

Respiratory care

The patient hospitalized with respiratory disease may require an artificial upper airway, chest tubes, mechanical ventilation, and chest physiotherapy.

Establishing an airway

In cardiopulmonary arrest, establishing an airway always takes precedence. Airway obstruction usually results when the tongue slides back and blocks the posterior pharynx. The head-tilt maneuver or—in suspected or confirmed cervical fracture or arthritis—the jaw-thrust maneuver can immediately move the tongue forward and relieve such obstruction. In some patients, endotracheal intubation and, sometimes, a tracheotomy may be needed.

Using chest tubes

To remove air or drain fluid from the pleural space, the patient may need a chest tube. This device allows a collapsed lung to reexpand to fill the evacuated pleural space. It also allows removal of pleural fluid for culture and analysis. Conditions that necessitate a chest tube include thoracic surgery, penetrating chest wounds, pleural effusion, and empyema. A chest tube facilitates evacuation of pneumothorax, hydrothorax, or hemothorax. Sometimes it's used to instill sclerosing drugs into the pleural space to prevent recurrent malignant pleural effusions.

The chest tube usually is placed in the sixth or seventh intercostal space, in the axillary region. Occasionally, in pneumothorax, the tube is placed in the second or third intercostal space, in the midclavicular region.

At times, the patient may have two chest tubes inserted, depending on the type of drainage required. One tube enters the chest anteriorly near the lung apex to drain air; the other tube is placed near the lung base to drain fluid.

The chest tube always connects to a system that provides a one-way valve mechanism to prevent outside air from entering the pleural space. Typically, this is a water seal, although waterless variations and flutter-valve styles are also available. Common plastic molded systems provide a water seal, a collection chamber for pleural fluid, and a suction chamber for medically ordered suction.

When caring for a patient with chest tubes, follow these guidelines:
• Monitor changes in suction pressure.
• Maintain tube patency by draining the tubes every 1 to 2 hours.
• Fasten tubing to the bed in a way that prevents dependent loops of tubing. To accommodate position changes, be sure to allow slack in the tube.
• Ensure that all system connections are tightly joined and secured with tape over the insertion sites.
• Check for air leaks, and add water to the suction system as needed. Don't clamp the tube if an air leak occurs.
• Record the amount, color, and consistency of drainage. When drainage appears to be excessive, be alert for signs of shock, such as tachycardia and hypotension.
• Always keep two hemostats at the bedside in case of chest tube disconnection. But keep in mind the risk related to using the hemostats: Tension pneumothorax may develop.
• If chest drainage proceeds by gravity rather than by suction, keep the collection chamber below chest level.

DEFINING STATIC AND DYNAMIC VALUES

The results of your patient's pulmonary function tests reflect static and dynamic values.

Static values
Test findings related to pulmonary volume are known as static values. They include:
• *tidal volume (VT)* — volume of air contained in a normal breath
• *functional residual capacity (FRC)* — volume of air remaining in the lungs after normal expiration
• *vital capacity (VC)* — volume of air that can be exhaled after maximal inspiration
• *residual volume (RV)* — amount of air remaining in the lungs after maximal expiration
• *total lung capacity (TLC)* — volume of air in the lungs after maximal inspiration.

Dynamic values
These findings characterize the movement of air into and out of the lungs and show changes in lung mechanics. They include:
• *forced expiratory volume in 1 second (FEV₁)* — maximum volume of air that can be expired in 1 second from TLC
• *maximal voluntary ventilation (MVV)* — volume of air that can be expired in 1 minute with the patient's maximum voluntary effort
• *forced vital capacity (FVC)* — maximum volume of air that the patient can exhale from TLC.

• Change the chest tube dressing if necessary and according to hospital policy, assessing the site for signs and symptoms of infection each time. Be sure to apply an occlusive dressing at each change.
• Tell the patient to cough once every hour, and have him take several deep breaths to enhance drainage and lung function.
• When the chest tube connects to a suction system, continuous bubbling in the water-seal chamber warns you that the system has an air leak. Locate the leak's source, and correct it or report it.
• If a chest tube dislodges from the patient's chest, apply petroleum gauze to the insertion site and notify the doctor.

Providing mechanical ventilation

When the patient has respiratory problems related to the CNS, hypoxemia, or failure of the normal bellows action provided by the diaphragm and rib cage, he may need breathing help from a mechanical ventilator.

Volume-cycled ventilators deliver a preset volume of gas. The tidal volume is set at 10 to 15 cc/kg of ideal body weight. You can use positive end-expiratory pressure (PEEP) to retain a certain amount of pressure in the lungs at the end of expiration, increasing functional residual capacity and improving gas exchange. PEEP is especially beneficial for patients with adult respiratory distress syndrome.

The primary hazards of PEEP include the increased incidence of pneumothorax and reduced venous return related to elevated intrathoracic pressure. High-frequency jet ventilation delivers small tidal volumes at high rates, resulting in low airway and intrathoracic pressures.

You can use several methods to wean a patient from a ventilator. Weaning begins when the patient meets specific criteria, which include stable ABG levels, tidal volume greater than 10 cc/kg, and a vital capacity greater than 15 cc/kg.

One weaning method calls for disconnecting the patient from the ventilator and using a T-piece (endotracheal tube oxygen adapter) that provides supplemental O_2 and humidification. The device allows the patient to breathe spontaneously without the ventilator for gradually increasing periods.

With another weaning method—intermittent mandatory ventilation—the ventilator supplies only a certain number of breaths while the patient breathes spontaneously between ventilator breaths. The frequency of ventilator breaths gradually decreases until the patient breathes entirely on his own.

Throughout weaning, assess the patient's status by monitoring vital signs, ABG levels, pulse oximetry values, symptoms, and other physical findings.

Performing chest physiotherapy

In respiratory conditions marked by excessive accumulation of lung secretions, chest physiotherapy can help remove the secretions. Chest physiotherapy includes chest assessment, effective breathing and coughing exercises, postural drainage, percussion, vibration, and evaluation of the therapy's effectiveness. Before beginning, review X-ray and assessment findings to locate the exact areas of secretions.
• *Deep breathing* maintains diaphragmatic tone, increases negative intrathoracic pressure, and promotes venous return. It's especially important when pain or dressings restrict chest movement. An incentive spirometer can provide positive visual reinforcement and further promote deep breathing.
• *Pursed-lip breathing* is used primarily in obstructive disease to slow expiration and prevent small-airway collapse. Such breathing funnels air through a narrow open-

ing, creating a positive back pressure that keeps the airways open.
• *Segmental breathing* (or *lateral costal breathing*) is used after lung resection or for a localized disorder. Place your hand over the affected lung area. Have the patient take a deep breath—deep enough to push that portion of his chest against your hand. If he's successful, you should feel the effort with your hand.
• *Coughing* that's controlled and staged gradually increases intrathoracic pressure, reducing the pain and bronchospasm of explosive coughing. When wound pain prevents effective coughing, splint the wound with a pillow, a towel, or your hand during coughing exercises.
• *Postural drainage* uses gravity to drain secretions into larger airways, from which they can be expectorated. This technique is used in patients with copious or tenacious secretions. Before postural drainage, auscultate the chest and review chest X-rays to determine the best position for maximum drainage. To reduce the patient's risk of vomiting, schedule postural drainage before or at least 1 hour after his meals.
• *Percussion* moves air against the chest wall to loosen lung secretions. It's contraindicated in severe pain, extreme obesity (which prevents effective contact with the chest wall), cancer that has metastasized to the ribs, crushing chest injuries, bleeding disorders, spontaneous pneumothorax, spinal compression fractures, osteoporosis, and pulmonary embolism.
• *Vibration* can be used with percussion or alone when percussion is contraindicated.

To evaluate therapy, auscultate the lung fields before and after therapy, and compare sputum findings.

PEDIATRIC DISORDERS

These disorders include respiratory distress syndrome, which is marked by widespread alveolar collapse and occurs mainly in premature infants, and sudden infant death syndrome, which strikes apparently healthy infants. They also include croup, a severe inflammation of the upper airway, and epiglottitis, an acute inflammation of the epiglottis that affects mainly young children.

RESPIRATORY DISTRESS SYNDROME

The most common cause of neonatal death, respiratory distress syndrome (also called hyaline membrane disease and RDS) causes 40,000 deaths every year. The syndrome occurs almost exclusively in infants born before the 37th gestational week (and in about 60% of those born before the 28th week). It's most common in infants of diabetic mothers, those delivered by cesarean section, and those delivered suddenly after antepartum hemorrhage.

In RDS, the premature infant develops widespread alveolar collapse from a deficiency of surfactant. Untreated, the syndrome causes death within 72 hours of birth in up to 14% of infants weighing less than 5½ lb (2,500 g). Aggressive management assisted by mechanical ventilation can improve the prognosis. A few patients who survive are left with bronchopulmonary dysplasia. Mild cases of the syndrome slowly subside after about 3 days.

Causes and pathophysiology

The immediate cause of RDS is lack of surfactant, a lipoprotein present in alveoli and respiratory bronchioles. In these structures, surfactant helps to lower surface tension, maintain alveolar patency, and prevent collapse, particularly at end expiration.

Although neonatal airways are developed by the 27th gestational week, the intercostal muscles are weak, and the alveoli and the capillary blood supplies are immature. Surfactant deficiency then leads to widespread atelectasis, which leads, in turn, to inadequate alveolar ventilation and shunting of blood through collapsed lung areas. The results are hypoxia and acidosis.

Complications

Respiratory insufficiency and shock may occur.

Assessment findings

The history typically indicates preterm birth (before 28 gestational weeks) or cesarean delivery. The maternal history may include diabetes or antepartal hemorrhage.

Although the neonate with RDS may breathe normally at first, within minutes to hours after birth, inspection may reveal rapid, shallow respirations with intercostal, subcostal, or sternal retractions, nasal flaring, and audible expiratory grunting. The grunting is a natural compensatory mechanism that produces positive end-expiratory pressure (PEEP) to prevent further alveolar collapse.

Additional findings may include hypotension, peripheral edema, and oliguria. In severe disease, the patient may display apnea, bradycardia, and cyanosis (from hypoxemia, left-to-right shunting through the foramen ovale, or right-to-left shunting through atelectatic lung areas). Other clinical features are pallor, frothy sputum, and low body temperature (resulting from an immature nervous system and inadequate subcutaneous fat).

Auscultation typically discloses diminished air entry and crackles, although crackles are rare early in the syndrome.

Diagnostic tests

Despite warning signs suggesting RDS, the diagnosis must be confirmed by chest X-rays and arterial blood gas (ABG) analysis.

• *Chest X-ray findings* may be normal for the first 6 to 12 hours in 50% of patients. However, later films show a fine reticulonodular pattern and dark streaks, indicating air-filled, dilated bronchioles.

• *ABG values* show a diminished PaO_2 level; normal, decreased, or increased $PaCO_2$ level; and reduced pH (a combination of respiratory and metabolic acidosis).

• The *lecithin-sphingomyelin ratio* helps to assess prenatal lung development and RDS risk. The test is usually ordered if a cesarean section will be performed before the 36th gestational week.

Treatment

The neonate with RDS requires vigorous respiratory support. Warm, humidified, oxygen-enriched gases are administered by oxygen hood or, if such treatment fails, by mechanical ventilation. The neonate with severe RDS may require mechanical ventilation with PEEP or continuous positive airway pressure (CPAP) administered by a tight-fitting face mask or, when necessary, endotracheal tube.

If the neonate can't maintain adequate gas exchange, high-frequency oscillation ventilation may be initiated to provide satisfactory minute volume (the total air breathed in 1 minute) with lower airway pressures.

Treatment also may include:

• a radiant warmer or an Isolette for thermoregulation

• I.V. fluids and sodium bicarbonate to control acidosis and maintain fluid and electrolyte balance

• tube feedings or total parenteral nutrition to maintain adequate nutrition if the neonate is too weak to eat

• drug therapy with pancuronium bromide (which paralyzes muscles to prevent spontaneous respirations during mechanical ventilation), prophylactic antibiotics, diuretics (to reduce pulmonary edema), and synthetic surfactant (to prevent atelectasis)

• investigational drug therapy—for example, with vitamin E to prevent complications associated with oxygen therapy, and corticosteroids administered maternally to stimulate surfactant production in fetuses at high risk for preterm birth.

Nursing diagnoses
- Impaired gas exchange
- Impaired skin integrity
- Ineffective airway clearance
- Risk for infection
- Risk for injury

Nursing interventions
- Continually assess the neonate. Monitor ABG levels and fluid intake and output.
- Check for arterial or venous hypotension, as appropriate, if the neonate has an umbilical catheter. Also watch for abnormal central venous pressure and for such complications as infection, thrombosis, and decreased circulation to the legs.
- If the neonate has a transcutaneous PO_2 monitor (an accurate method for determining PaO_2), change the site of the lead placement every 2 to 4 hours to avoid burning the skin.
- Use pulse oximetry to monitor SaO_2 levels.
- Weigh the infant once or twice daily.
- Regularly assess skin color, rate and depth of respirations, severity of retractions, nostril flaring, frequency of expiratory grunting, frothing at the lips, and restlessness.
- Regularly assess the effectiveness of oxygen or ventilator therapy. Evaluate every fraction of inspired oxygen (FIO_2) and PEEP or CPAP change by drawing arterial blood for analysis 20 minutes after each change. Be sure to adjust PEEP or CPAP as indicated by ABG levels.
- When the neonate receives mechanical ventilation, watch carefully for signs of barotrauma (increase in respiratory distress, subcutaneous emphysema) and accidental disconnection from the ventilator. Check ventilator settings frequently. Be alert for signals of complications of PEEP or CPAP therapy, such as decreased cardiac output, pneumothorax, and pneumomediastinum.
- Institute infection prevention measures if the infant receives mechanical ventilation.
- Provide suction, as necessary. Observe the oxygenation monitor or pulse oximeter before, during, and after suctioning to evaluate the patient's response to this therapy.
- Inspect the skin frequently for signs of breakdown.
- Provide mouth care every 2 hours. Lubricate the infant's nostrils and lips with water-soluble ointment.
- Observe for signs and symptoms of infection, resulting from invasive therapies and a weakened immune system.
- As needed, arrange for follow-up care with a neonatal ophthalmologist to detect possible retinal damage from oxygen therapy.

- Watch for additional complications of oxygen therapy, such as lung capillary damage, decreased mucus flow, impaired ciliary functioning, and widespread atelectasis. Additional problems include patent ductus arteriosus, congestive heart failure, retinopathy, pulmonary hypertension, necrotizing enterocolitis, and neurologic abnormalities.
- Help reduce mortality by detecting RDS early. Recognize intercostal retractions and grunting, especially in a premature infant, as signs of RDS. Make sure the patient receives immediate treatment.

Patient teaching
- Explain RDS to the parents. If possible, let them participate in care (using aseptic technique) to promote normal bonding.
- Explain the function of respiratory devices and equipment. Discuss alarm sounds and mechanical noise, and solicit the parents' feedback. Encourage them to ask questions and to express their fears and concerns.
- Advise parents that full recovery may take up to 12 months. When the prognosis is poor, prepare the parents for the neonate's possible death and offer emotional support. When appropriate, refer parents and family to professional staff, such as pastoral counselors and social workers.

SUDDEN INFANT DEATH SYNDROME
A medical mystery of early infancy, sudden infant death syndrome (SIDS) is the leading cause of death among apparently healthy infants ages 1 month to 1 year. The syndrome, also called crib death, occurs at the rate of 2 in every 1,000 live births. Each year in the United States, about 7,000 infants die of SIDS. Although the syndrome was known in ancient times, its cause remains obscure.

The peak incidence of SIDS occurs between ages 2 and 4 months; incidence declines rapidly between ages 4 and 12 months. About 60% of victims are male infants who die in their sleep, without warning, sound, or struggle. The incidence is slightly higher in preterm infants, Inuit infants, disadvantaged Black infants, infants of mothers under age 20, and infants of multiple births. Incidence is 10 times higher in SIDS siblings, slightly higher in infants whose mothers smoke, and up to 10 times higher in infants whose mothers are drug addicts.

Infants most commonly succumb to SIDS in the fall and winter. Many have a history of respiratory tract infections, suggesting viral infection as a cause. Studies show conflicting data about abnormal hepatic or pancreatic function. Although the link between apneic episodes and SIDS remains unclear, about 60% of infants with near-miss respiratory events have second episodes of apnea. Some succumb to apnea.

Causes
At one time, SIDS was attributed to abuse or to accidental suffocation during sleep. On postmortem examination, some SIDS-diagnosed infants show changes indicating chronic hypoxia, hypoxemia, and large-airway obstruction, leading researchers to suspect more than one cause.

Two leading hypotheses are the hypoxemia theory and the apnea theory. The hypoxemia theory suggests that SIDS occurs because of damage to the respiratory control center in the brain from chronic hypoxemia. The apnea theory holds that the SIDS victim experiences prolonged periods of sleep apnea and eventually dies during an episode.

Another proposed cause involves *Clostridium botulinum* toxin, which has been linked to a few SIDS deaths. A disproven theory is an association between SIDS and diphtheria, tetanus, and pertussis vaccines. Bottle-feeding and advanced parental age don't cause the syndrome, although breast-fed infants are at decreased risk for SIDS.

Complications
Because the syndrome is always fatal, it has no complications.

Assessment findings
The patient history supplied by the parents may reveal that they found the infant wedged in a crib corner or with blankets wrapped around his head. Despite such findings, autopsy results rule out suffocation as the cause of death. The history may also note frothy, blood-tinged sputum found around the infant's mouth or on the crib sheets. However, autopsy findings show a patent airway, ruling out aspiration of vomitus as the cause of death.

Typically, the parents report that the infant didn't cry and showed no signs of disturbed sleep. Reports of the infant found in a peculiar position or tangled in his blankets suggest movement before death, possibly from terminal spasm. Occasionally, the history may reveal a respiratory tract infection.

Documentation of events before discovery of the infant's death should be part of the history. Often, the bruising, possible fractured ribs, and the appearance of blood in the infant's mouth, nose, or ears from internal bleeding may be confused with abuse. Although this possibility shouldn't be dismissed, never assume that abuse caused the infant's death without obtaining further information. Also avoid assessment questions that may suggest parental responsibility for the death.

Depending on how long the infant has been dead, inspection may reveal an infant with mottled complexion and extremely cyanotic lips and fingertips. You may also see pooled blood in the legs and feet. These markings may be mistaken for bruises. The infant's diaper may be wet and full of stools.

Diagnostic tests
Diagnosis of SIDS requires an autopsy to rule out other causes of death. Characteristic histologic findings on autopsy include small or normal adrenal glands and petechiae over the visceral surfaces of the pleura, within the thymus (which is enlarged), and in the epicardium. Autopsy also reveals well-preserved lymphoid structures; signs of chronic hypoxemia, such as increased pulmonary artery smooth muscle; edematous, congestive lungs fully expanded; liquid (not clotted) blood in the heart; and stomach curd inside the trachea.

Treatment
Because most infants can't be resuscitated, treatment focuses on emotional support for the family. Any infant found apneic and successfully resuscitated, as well as any infant who has a sibling with apnea, may be at risk for SIDS. In such instances, a home apnea monitor may be recommended until the at-risk infant passes the age of vulnerability.

Nursing diagnoses
• Altered family processes
• Fear
• Hopelessness
• Knowledge deficit
• Spiritual distress

Nursing interventions
• Be sure both parents are present when the child's death is confirmed. The parents may lash out at emergency department personnel, the babysitter, or anyone else involved in the child's care—even at each other. Stay calm and let them express their feelings. Reassure them that they were not to blame.
• Let the parents see the infant in a private room. Allow them to express their grief. Stay in the room with them, if appropriate. Offer to call clergy, friends, or relatives. Return the infant's belongings to the parents.
• If your hospital's policy is to assign a home health nurse to the family, she will provide the continuing reassurance and assistance the parents will need. Assist her in

gathering the information necessary to implement appropriate follow-up care.

Patient teaching

• After the parents and other family members recover from the initial shock, explain the need for an autopsy to confirm the diagnosis. In some states, this is legally mandatory. At this time, provide the family with basic facts about SIDS, and encourage them to consent to the autopsy. Be sure they receive the autopsy report promptly.

• Refer the parents and family to community and hospital support services. Participants in such a program will contact the parents, ensure that they receive the autopsy report promptly, introduce them to a professional counselor, and maintain supportive telephone contact. Refer the parents to a local SIDS parents' group if one is available. Advise parents to contact the SIDS hot line (1-800-221-SIDS).

• If the parents decide to have another child, provide appropriate information to help them cope with the pregnancy and the first year of the new infant's life.

• Teach family members how to operate home apnea and cardiac monitors, if appropriate. If parents of healthy infants inquire about monitors for home use, explain that monitoring is recommended only for siblings of SIDS victims because of its high cost and sometimes disruptive effects on family dynamics.

• Teach family members and care givers how to perform one-person cardiopulmonary resuscitation or refer them to classes conducted by the American Red Cross if appropriate.

CROUP

A childhood disease that affects boys more often than girls (typically between ages 3 months and 3 years), croup is a severe inflammation and obstruction of the upper airway.

Croup usually occurs in the winter as acute laryngotracheobronchitis (the most common form), laryngitis, or acute spasmodic laryngitis and must be distinguished from epiglottitis. Usually mild and self-limiting, acute laryngotracheobronchitis appears mostly in children ages 3 months to 3 years. Acute spasmodic laryngitis affects children between ages 1 and 3, particularly those with allergies and a family history of croup. Overall, up to 15% of patients have a family history of croup. Recovery is usually complete.

Causes

Croup usually results from a viral infection. Parainfluenza viruses cause about two-thirds of such infections; adenoviruses, respiratory syncytial virus, influenza viruses, measles viruses, and bacteria (pertussis and diphtheria) account for the rest.

Complications

Airway obstruction, respiratory failure, and dehydration are complications of croup. Latent complications are ear infection and pneumonia.

Assessment findings

Typically, the child or his parents report a recent upper respiratory tract infection preceding croup.

On inspection, you may observe the use of accessory muscles with nasal flaring during breathing. You'll typically hear the child's sharp, barklike cough and hoarse or muffled vocal sounds. As croup progresses, the patient may display further upper airway obstruction with severely compromised ventilation. (See *How croup affects the upper airways.*)

Auscultation may disclose inspiratory stridor and diminished breath sounds. These signs and symptoms may last for only a few hours, or they may persist for 1 to 2 days.

Each form of croup has additional characteristics.

• In *laryngotracheobronchitis,* the patient may complain of fever and breathing problems that occur more often at night. Typically, the child becomes frightened because he can't breathe out (because inflammation causes edema in the bronchi and bronchioles).

During auscultation, you may hear diffusely decreased breath sounds, expiratory rhonchi, and scattered crackles.

• In *laryngitis,* which results from vocal cord edema, the patient usually reports mild signs and symptoms and no respiratory distress. If the patient is an infant, however, some respiratory distress may occur. In children, the history may include such signs and symptoms as a sore throat and cough that, rarely, may progress to marked hoarseness.

Inspection may disclose suprasternal and intercostal retractions, inspiratory stridor, dyspnea, diminished breath sounds, restlessness and, in later stages, severe dyspnea and exhaustion.

• In *acute spasmodic laryngitis,* the patient history may reveal mild to moderate hoarseness and nasal discharge, followed by the characteristic cough and noisy inspiration that often awaken the child at night. As the child understandably becomes anxious, this leads to increasing dyspnea and transient cyanosis.

Inspection may disclose labored breathing with retractions and clammy skin. Palpation may reveal a rapid pulse rate. These severe signs diminish after several hours but reappear in a milder form on the next one or two nights.

Diagnostic tests

• *Throat cultures* can identify infecting organisms—and their sensitivity to antibiotics when bacterial infection is the cause. Throat cultures can also rule out diphtheria.
• *Blood cultures* can distinguish between bacterial and viral infections.
• *X-ray studies* of the neck may show upper airway narrowing and edema in subglottic folds.
• *Laryngoscopy* may reveal inflammation and obstruction in epiglottal and laryngeal areas.

In evaluating the patient with croup, diagnosis should rule out the possibility of masses, cysts, and foreign body obstruction—a common cause of croupy cough in young children.

Treatment

For most children with croup, home care with rest, cool humidification during sleep, and antipyretic drugs, such as acetaminophen, relieve signs and symptoms. However, respiratory distress that interferes with oral hydration usually requires hospitalization and parenteral fluid replacement to prevent dehydration. If the patient has croup from a bacterial infection, he'll need antibiotic therapy. Oxygen therapy may also be required.

For moderately severe croup, aerosolized racemic epinephrine may temporarily reduce airway swelling. Intubation is performed only if other means of preventing respiratory failure are unsuccessful.

Several studies support the practice of prescribing corticosteroids for acute laryngotracheobronchitis.

Nursing diagnoses

• Anxiety
• Fear
• Hyperthermia
• Impaired gas exchange
• Ineffective airway clearance
• Knowledge deficit

Nursing interventions

• Monitor cough and breath sounds, hoarseness, severity of retractions, inspiratory stridor, cyanosis, respiratory

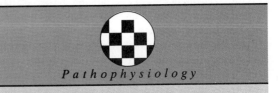

Pathophysiology

HOW CROUP AFFECTS THE UPPER AIRWAYS

In croup, inflammatory swelling and spasms constrict the larynx, thereby reducing airflow. This cross-sectional drawing (from chin to chest) shows the upper airway changes caused by croup. Inflammatory changes almost completely obstruct the larynx (which includes the epiglottis) and significantly narrow the trachea.

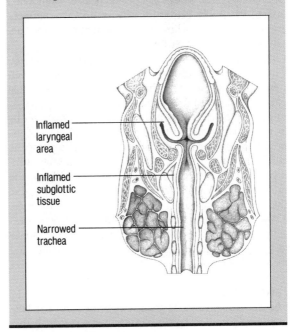

Inflamed laryngeal area

Inflamed subglottic tissue

Narrowed trachea

rate and character (especially prolonged and labored respirations), restlessness, fever, and heart rate.
• Keep the child as quiet as possible, but avoid sedation, which may depress respiration. If the patient is an infant, position him in an infant seat or prop him up with a pillow; place an older child in Fowler's position. If an older child requires a cool-mist tent to help him breathe, describe it to him and his parents and explain why it's needed.
• Change bed linens as necessary to keep the patient dry.

• Control the patient's energy output and oxygen demand by providing age-appropriate diversional activities to keep him quietly occupied.

• If possible, isolate patients suspected of having respiratory syncytial virus and parainfluenza infections. Wash your hands carefully before leaving the room, to avoid transmitting germs to other patients, particularly infants.

• Control fever with sponge baths and antipyretics. Keep a hypothermia blanket on hand if the patient's temperature rises above 102° F (38.9° C). Watch for seizures in infants and young children with high fevers. Give I.V. antibiotics, as ordered.

• Relieve sore throat with soothing, water-based ices, such as fruit sherbet and ice pops. Avoid thicker, milk-based fluids if the patient has thick mucus or swallowing difficulties. Apply petroleum jelly or another ointment around the nose and lips to decrease irritation from nasal discharge and mouth breathing.

• Institute measures to prevent the patient's crying, which increases respiratory distress. As necessary, adapt treatment to conserve the patient's energy and to include parents, who can provide reassurance.

• Reassure parents that they made the right decision by bringing their child to the emergency department — especially at night when the evening air may improve the child's breathing significantly, leaving the parents wondering if they overreacted. (Some doctors will ask the nurse to take the child outside for a few minutes to relieve the patient's croupiness.)

• Watch for signs of complete airway obstruction, such as increased heart and respiratory rates, use of respiratory accessory muscles in breathing, nasal flaring, and increased restlessness.

Patient teaching

• Because croup may be treated at home or in the hospital, you'll need to tailor your teaching accordingly. Because this disease primarily affects young children, patient teaching usually centers on the parents.

• Suggest using a cool-mist humidifier (vaporizer) in the home, then teach the parents how to use one, if necessary. If the patient is hospitalized, advise the parents that he may be placed in a cool-mist tent (with or without oxygen) to provide high humidity. To relieve acute croupy spells at home, instruct the parents to carry the child to the bathroom, shut the door, turn on the hot water, and allow steam to fill the air. Breathing warm, moist air should quickly ease an acute croup spell.

• Warn parents that ear infections and pneumonia may complicate croup. These disorders may follow croup about 5 days after recovery. Urge the parents to seek immediate medical attention if the patient has an earache, productive cough, high fever, or increased shortness of breath.

• If the patient has croup at home, tell the parents that bed rest is essential to conserve energy and limit oxygen needs. To ease the patient's breathing, advise the parents to use pillows to prop him into a sitting or semisitting (semi-Fowler's) position. Warn the parents never to rest a child or an infant with croup flat on his back. Advise them that keeping him quiet and comfortable will reduce his oxygen needs. Holding him as often as possible will soothe and comfort him. If the patient is hospitalized, explain that the same measures apply.

• If the parents are caring for the patient at home, urge them to ensure adequate hydration by giving him plenty of fluids. Suggest fluid electrolyte replacement (such as Gatorade), flavored gelatin dissolved in water, or ginger ale with the bubbles stirred out. Fluids should be at room temperature. Instruct them to avoid thicker, milk-based fluids. To relieve sore throat, suggest fruit sorbet or ice pops. Instruct the parents to withhold solid food until the child can breathe and swallow more easily. The child may have little or no appetite until he feels better.

• Explain that the hospitalized child may require hydration with I.V. fluids if he can't be hydrated orally.

• Warn parents not to give aspirin to reduce fever because of its link to Reye's syndrome.

EPIGLOTTITIS

A life-threatening emergency, this acute inflammation of the epiglottis and surrounding area rapidly causes edema and induration. Untreated, the disease results in complete airway obstruction. Epiglottitis proves fatal in 8% to 12% of patients, who are typically children between ages 2 and 8. However, the disease can occur from infancy to adulthood in any season.

Causes

Epiglottitis usually results from infection with the bacteria *Haemophilus influenzae* type B and, occasionally, pneumococci or group A streptococci.

Complications

Airway obstruction and death may occur within 2 hours of onset.

Assessment findings

The patient or his parents may report an earlier upper respiratory tract infection. Additional complaints include a sore throat and dysphagia and the sudden onset of a high fever.

On inspection, the patient may be febrile, drooling, pale or cyanotic, restless, apprehensive, and irritable. You may also observe nasal flaring. The patient may sit in a tripod position: upright, leaning forward with the chin thrust out, mouth open, and tongue protruding. This position helps relieve severe respiratory distress. The patient's voice usually sounds thick and muffled.

Because manipulation may trigger sudden airway obstruction, attempt throat inspection only when immediate intubation can be performed if necessary. (See *Airway crisis.*) The patient's throat will appear red and inflamed.

Auscultation of the lung fields may reveal rhonchi and diminished breath sounds, usually transmitted from the upper airway.

Diagnostic tests
• *Lateral neck X-rays* show an enlarged epiglottis and distended hypopharynx.
• *Direct laryngoscopy* reveals the hallmark of acute epiglottitis: a swollen, beefy-red epiglottis. The throat examination should follow X-ray studies and, in most cases, should *not* be performed if significant obstruction is suspected or if immediate intubation isn't possible.

Additional X-rays of the chest and cervical trachea help to confirm the diagnosis.

Treatment
A patient with acute epiglottitis and airway obstruction requires emergency hospitalization. He should be placed in a cool-mist tent with added oxygen. If complete or near-complete airway obstruction occurs, he may also need emergency endotracheal intubation or a tracheotomy. Arterial blood gas (ABG) monitoring or pulse oximetry may be used to assess his progress.

Treatment may also include parenteral fluids to prevent dehydration when the disease interferes with swallowing, and a 10-day course of parenteral antibiotics—usually ampicillin. If the patient is allergic to penicillin or could have ampicillin-resistant endemic *H. influenzae,* chloramphenicol or another antibiotic may be prescribed.

Although controversial, corticosteroids may be prescribed to reduce edema during early treatment. Oxygen therapy may also be used.

Keep in mind that preventive measures should be taken. In 1990, the American Academy of Pediatrics recommended that all children receive the haemophilus b conjugate vaccine, preferably at age 2 months. As more

Warning

AIRWAY CRISIS
Epiglottitis can progress to complete airway obstruction within minutes. To prepare for this medical emergency, keep the following tips in mind:
• Watch for increasing restlessness, tachycardia, fever, dyspnea, and intercostal and substernal retractions. These are warning signs of total airway obstruction and the need for an emergency tracheotomy.
• Keep the following equipment available at the patient's bedside in case of sudden, complete airway obstruction: a tracheotomy tray, endotracheal tubes, manual resuscitation bag, oxygen equipment, and a laryngoscope with blades of various sizes.
• Remember that using a tongue blade or throat culture swab can initiate sudden, complete airway obstruction.
• Before examining the patient's throat, request trained personnel (such as an anesthesiologist) to stand by if emergency airway insertion should be needed.

children become immunized, epiglottitis rates should decline.

Nursing diagnoses
• Anxiety
• Fear
• Fluid volume deficit
• Impaired gas exchange
• Impaired verbal communication
• Ineffective airway clearance
• Risk for suffocation

Nursing interventions
• Place the patient in a sitting position to ease his respiratory difficulty unless he finds another position more comfortable.
• Place the patient in a cool-mist tent. Change the sheets frequently because they quickly become saturated.
• Encourage the parents to remain with their child. Offer reassurance and support to relieve family anxiety and fear.
• Monitor the patient's temperature, vital signs, and respiration rate and pattern frequently. Also monitor ABG

levels (to detect hypoxia and hypercapnia) and pulse oximetry values (to detect decreasing oxygen saturation). Report any changes.

• Observe the patient continuously for signs of impending airway closure, which may develop at any time.

• Calm the patient during X-ray studies of his chest and cervical trachea.

• Minimize external stimuli.

• Start an I.V. line for antibiotic therapy and fluid replacement if the patient can't maintain adequate fluid intake. Draw blood for laboratory analysis, as ordered.

• Record intake and output precisely to monitor and prevent dehydration.

• If the patient has a tracheostomy, anticipate his needs because he'll be unable to cry or call out. Provide emotional support. Reassure him and his family that a tracheostomy is a short-term intervention (usually from 4 to 7 days). Monitor the patient for rising temperature, increasing pulse rate, and hypotension – signs of secondary infection.

Patient teaching

• Inform the patient and family that epiglottal swelling usually subsides after 24 hours of antibiotic therapy. The epiglottis usually returns to normal size within 72 hours.

• If the patient's home care regimen includes oral antibiotic therapy, emphasize the need for completing the entire prescription. Explain proper administration. Discuss drug storage, dosage, adverse effects, and whether or not the medication can be taken with food or milk.

• If the patient should require the haemophilus b conjugate vaccine, discuss the rationale for immunization, and help the family obtain the vaccine.

ACUTE DISORDERS

Acute respiratory disorders require prompt treatment and nursing care. They range from acute respiratory failure in chronic obstructive pulmonary disease to pleurisy.

ACUTE RESPIRATORY FAILURE IN C.O.P.D.

When the lungs can't adequately maintain arterial oxygenation or eliminate CO_2, acute respiratory failure results. Unchecked and untreated, the condition leads to tissue hypoxia. In patients with essentially normal lung tissue, acute respiratory failure usually produces a $PaCO_2$ above 50 mm Hg and a PaO_2 below 50 mm Hg.

These limits, however, don't apply to patients with chronic obstructive pulmonary disease (COPD). These patients consistently have a high $PaCO_2$ (hypercapnia) and a low PaO_2 (hypoxemia) level. So for them, only acute deterioration in arterial blood gas (ABG) values – and corresponding clinical deterioration – signals acute respiratory failure.

Causes

Acute respiratory failure may develop in COPD patients from any condition that increases the work of breathing and decreases the respiratory drive. These conditions may result from respiratory tract infection (such as bronchitis or pneumonia), bronchospasm, or accumulated secretions secondary to cough suppression. Other common causes are related to ventilatory failure, in which the brain fails to direct respiration, and gas exchange failure, in which respiratory structures fail to function properly. (See *Mechanics of acute respiratory failure.*)

Complications

Tissue hypoxia, metabolic acidosis, and respiratory and cardiac arrest are among possible complications.

Assessment findings

Because acute respiratory failure in COPD is life-threatening, you probably won't have time to conduct an in-depth patient interview. Instead, you'll rely on family members or the patient's medical records to discover the precipitating incident.

On inspection, you'll note cyanosis of the oral mucosa, lips, and nail beds; nasal flaring; and ashen skin. You may observe the patient yawning and using accessory muscles to breathe. He may appear restless, anxious, depressed, lethargic, agitated, or confused. Additionally, he usually exhibits tachypnea, which signals impending respiratory failure.

Palpation may reveal cold, clammy skin and asymmetrical chest movement, which suggests pneumothorax. If tactile fremitus is present, you'll notice that it decreases over an obstructed bronchi or pleural effusion but increases over consolidated lung tissue.

Percussion – especially in patients with COPD – reveals hyperresonance. If acute respiratory failure results from atelectasis or pneumonia, percussion usually produces a dull or flat sound.

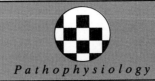

Pathophysiology

MECHANICS OF ACUTE RESPIRATORY FAILURE

Three major malfunctions account for impaired gas exchange and subsequent acute respiratory failure. They include alveolar hypoventilation, ventilation-perfusion mismatch, and intrapulmonary (right-to-left) shunting.

Alveolar hypoventilation
Decreased oxygen saturation may result when chronic airway obstruction reduces alveolar minute ventilation. In such cases, PaO_2 levels fall and $PaCO_2$ levels rise. Hypoxia results.

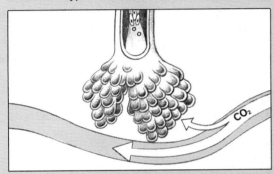

Ventilation-perfusion mismatch
The most common cause of hypoxemia, imbalances in ventilation and perfusion occur when conditions such as pulmonary embolism or adult respiratory distress syndrome interrupt normal gas exchange in a specific lung region. Either too little ventilation with normal blood flow or too little blood flow with normal ventilation may cause the imbalance. Whichever happens, the result is the same: PaO_2 levels fall.

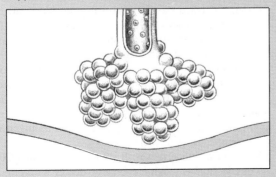

Right-to-left shunting
Untreated ventilation or perfusion imbalances can lead to right-to-left shunting in which blood passes from the heart's right side to its left without being oxygenated.

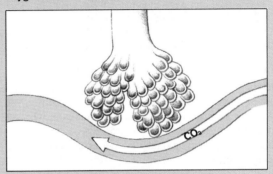

Implications
The hypoxemia and hypercapnia characteristic of respiratory failure stimulate strong compensatory responses by all body systems, including the respiratory, cardiovascular, and central nervous systems.

In response to hypoxemia, for example, the sympathetic nervous system triggers vasoconstriction, increases peripheral resistance, and boosts the heart rate.

The body responds to hypercapnia with cerebral depression, hypotension, circulatory failure, and an increased heartbeat and cardiac output. Hypoxemia or hypercapnia (or both) cause the brain's respiratory control center to first increase respiratory depth (tidal volume) and then to increase the respiratory rate. As respiratory failure worsens, intercostal, supraclavicular, and suprasternal retractions may also occur.

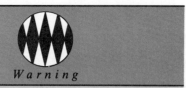

IDENTIFYING RESPIRATORY FAILURE

Use the following measurements to identify respiratory failure:
• vital capacity less than 15 cc/kg
• tidal volume less than 3 cc/kg
• negative inspiratory force under −25 cm H_2O
• respiratory rate more than twice the normal rate
• diminished PaO_2 despite increased FIO_2
• elevated $PaCO_2$ with pH lower than 7.25.

Auscultation typically discloses diminished breath sounds. In patients with pneumothorax, breath sounds may be absent. In other cases of respiratory failure, you may hear such adventitious breath sounds as wheezes (in asthma) and rhonchi (in bronchitis). If you hear crackles, suspect pulmonary edema as the cause of respiratory failure.

Diagnostic tests
• *ABG analysis* is the key to diagnosis (and subsequent treatment) of acute respiratory failure in patients with COPD. Progressively deteriorating ABG values and pH—compared with the patient's "normal" values—strongly suggest acute respiratory failure. In patients with essentially normal lung tissue, a pH below 7.35 usually indicates acute respiratory failure. In patients with COPD, the pH deviation from the normal value is even lower.
• *Chest X-rays* identify underlying pulmonary diseases or conditions, such as emphysema, atelectasis, lesions, pneumothorax, infiltrates, and effusions.
• *Electrocardiography* (ECG) can demonstrate arrhythmias. Common ECG patterns point to cor pulmonale and myocardial hypoxia.
• *Pulse oximetry* reveals a decreasing SaO_2.
• *Blood tests,* such as a white blood cell count, detect underlying causes. Abnormally low hematocrit and decreased hemoglobin levels signal blood loss, which indicates decreased oxygen-carrying capacity.
• *Serum electrolyte findings* vary. Hypokalemia may result from compensatory hyperventilation, the body's attempt to correct alkalosis; hypochloremia usually occurs in metabolic alkalosis.

• *Pulmonary artery catheterization* helps to distinguish pulmonary and cardiovascular causes of acute respiratory failure and monitors hemodynamic pressures.

Additional tests, such as a blood culture, Gram stain, and sputum culture, may identify the pathogen. (See *Identifying respiratory failure.*)

Treatment
Acute respiratory failure in patients with COPD constitutes an emergency. The patient will need cautious oxygen therapy (nasal prongs or a Venturi mask) to raise his PaO_2. If significant respiratory acidosis persists, mechanical ventilation with an endotracheal or a tracheostomy tube may be necessary. High-frequency ventilation may be initiated if the patient doesn't respond to conventional mechanical ventilation. Treatment routinely includes antibiotics (for infection), bronchodilators and, possibly, corticosteroids.

If the patient also has cor pulmonale and decreased cardiac output, fluid restrictions and administration of positive enotropic agents, vasopressors, and diuretics may be ordered. (See *Caring for the patient with acute respiratory failure in COPD.*)

Nursing diagnoses
• Altered nutrition: Less than body requirements
• Altered tissue perfusion
• Anxiety
• Fatigue
• Fear
• Impaired gas exchange
• Impaired skin integrity
• Impaired verbal communication
• Ineffective airway clearance
• Ineffective breathing pattern
• Sensory or perceptual alterations

Nursing interventions
• Orient the patient to the treatment unit. Most patients with acute respiratory failure receive intensive care. Acquainting the patient with procedures, sounds, and sights helps to minimize his anxiety.
• To reverse hypoxemia, administer oxygen at appropriate concentrations to maintain PaO_2 at a minimum pressure range of 50 to 60 mm Hg. The patient with COPD usually requires only small amounts of supplemental oxygen. Watch for a positive response—such as improved breathing, color, and ABG values.
• Maintain a patent airway. If your patient retains CO_2, encourage him to cough and breathe deeply with pursed lips. If he's alert, have him use an incentive spirometer.

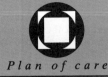

Plan of care

CARING FOR THE PATIENT WITH ACUTE RESPIRATORY FAILURE IN C.O.P.D.

After reviewing your assessment findings, you'll be ready to select nursing diagnoses and construct a plan of care. To prepare you to do this for a COPD patient in acute respiratory failure, assume that you're caring for James Smart, age 68.

Patient history
Mr. Smart is a retired clothing manufacturer whose acute respiratory failure was precipitated by bronchitis and complicated by emphysema. It was diagnosed about 5 years ago.

Thin and frail, Mr. Smart became ill soon after returning from a holiday with his son's family. His three grandsons were all sick with the flu.

Mr. Smart's history shows a pattern of bronchial infections after a cold or other respiratory disease. For his emphysema, he uses nebulizer treatments and takes bronchodilating medications daily. Occasionally, his doctor prescribes corticosteroids. He tells you that his blood pressure has been high for years, despite continuing attempts to control it with diet and medications.

Assessment findings
Mr. Smart's vital signs are ominous. His oral temperature is 100.2° F (38.9° C), and he's diaphoretic. His pulse rate is rapid (132 beats/minute), thready, and irregular. His respiratory rate is 48 breaths/minute, and his blood pressure registers 148/98 mm Hg.

On inspection, you see a thin, barrel-chested man close to exhaustion from his efforts to breathe. You note his ashen color

and circumoral and capillary bed cyanosis. You observe his obvious effort to keep his head elevated at about 90 degrees while seated in bed. He uses all accessory muscles of the chest and abdomen and purses his lips slightly with each exhalation. He has +1 pitting edema to his feet, bilaterally. You observe him picking at his sheets and pajamas. He appears extremely restless, and he changes his answers to simple questions.

Chest auscultation discloses diffuse crackles and diminished breath sounds to the lung bases, bilaterally. You can hear crowing stridor without a stethoscope.

A review of initial diagnostic test results shows the following:
• ABG values (room air)—PaO_2, 41 mm Hg; $PaCO_2$, 59 mm Hg; pH, 7.27; and SaO_2, 89%
• chest X-ray—positive for diffuse infiltrates and findings common to COPD
• red blood cell count—7.5 million/mm^3; white blood cell count—11,400/mm^3
• erythrocyte sedimentation rate—elevated; thrombocytosis evident
• theophylline level—15.2 μg/ml
• blood urea nitrogen and serum creatinine levels—elevated
• serum glucose level—141 mg/dl
• electrocardiogram—shows atrial fibrillation with occasional multifocal premature ventricular contractions.

Repeated ABG analyses were done after oxygen administration and nebulizer treatments. A specimen of purulent, blood-tinged sputum (aspirated by nasotracheal suctioning) was sent to the laboratory for culture and sensitivity testing.

Nursing diagnoses
Base your nursing diagnoses on your main assessment findings. For Mr. Smart, you choose:

• Ineffective breathing pattern, ineffective airway clearance, and impaired gas exchange related to emphysema and respiratory tract infection
• Anxiety and ineffective individual coping related to dyspnea, loss of control, and fear of dying
• Activity intolerance and self-care deficit related to hypoxia, strenuous breathing, and anxiety
• Risk for infection related to recent history, low-grade fever, and static secretions.

Expected outcomes
You'll act quickly to define immediate care goals for Mr. Smart during his acute illness. He will:
• improve his breathing pattern, airway clearance, and gas exchange to restore optimal respiratory status
• decrease his anxiety and use coping mechanisms to minimize his fear
• increase his activity tolerance and improve his ability to perform self-care
• decrease his risk of infection.

Implementation
What care measures will you take first during the acute phase of Mr. Smart's illness? You see airway patency and optimal gas exchange as your initial priority.

To improve breathing and gas exchange
• Assess Mr. Smart's respiratory status every 15 minutes until his breathing stabilizes. Check his respiratory rate and pattern. Assess his use of accessory muscles to breathe. You may want to use pulse oximetry to monitor oxygenation progress.
• Administer oxygen, bronchodilators, and nebulizer treatments, as ordered.
• Allow Mr. Smart to sit upright, or supply an overbed table and pil-

(continued)

CARING FOR THE PATIENT WITH ACUTE RESPIRATORY FAILURE IN C.O.P.D. *(continued)*

lows for support if a forward-leaning position eases his breathing.
• Monitor chest X-ray and ABG results. Report abnormal findings.
• Avoid giving central nervous system depressants, such as narcotics, to relieve discomfort; assess Mr. Smart's level of consciousness every few hours until his condition stabilizes.
• Perform chest physiotherapy as ordered to mobilize secretions and minimize airway obstruction.
• Increase Mr. Smart's fluid intake to 3,000 ml daily, if possible, to help liquefy secretions.
• Position a nasopharyngeal airway in one nostril to facilitate suctioning if Mr. Smart cannot mobilize secretions on his own.
• Keep a tracheostomy tray, a fresh tube, and sodium bicarbonate at Mr. Smart's bedside during the acute phase of illness when tracheal edema, pulmonary collapse, and spontaneous pneumothorax remain threats.

To reduce anxiety and promote coping
• Assess Mr. Smart's anxiety level. Observable indicators include irritability, restlessness, verbalization of fear and frustration, and facial expressions, such as grimacing.
• Explore the effectiveness of Mr. Smart's previous coping mechanisms (to establish baseline data).

• Keep Mr. Smart's room neat, organized, and open. Provide lightweight but warm clothing and bed linens to prevent feelings of suffocation.
• Approach Mr. Smart from the side. Speak confidently but quietly while providing a serene, reassuring environment.
• Before proceeding with medications, tests, or procedures, provide a full explanation of what will happen.
• Encourage Mr. Smart to exercise some control of his situation by helping plan some of his own care each day.

To increase activity tolerance and self-care
• Maintain activity restrictions and promote rest.
• Reinforce Mr. Smart's use of controlled breathing techniques while he receives oxygen.
• Assist Mr. Smart with self-care until his condition stabilizes. Give complete bath and mouth care; turn him every 2 hours; offer a bedpan and urinal, as needed; and screen all telephone calls that may sap his energy. Keep the call button within easy reach, and answer all calls promptly.
• Permit visitors when Mr. Smart can tolerate the activity.
• Provide small, frequent meals that are easy to chew and swallow. Keep sherbet and gelatin handy for snacking.
• Allow Mr. Smart to use the bed controls, wash his face, brush his teeth, and perform other self-care measures as his condition stabilizes.

To decrease the risk of superinfection
• Implement universal precautions and reverse isolation to avoid transmitting nosocomial infections.
• Prevent stasis of respiratory secretions. Provide chest physiotherapy, spirometry, increased fluids, and expectorants, as ordered.
• Monitor body temperature rectally; oxygen therapy and labored breathing will interfere with accurate oral assessment.
• Administer antibiotics, as ordered, and obtain sputum specimens for repeated cultures to assess treatment effectiveness.

Evaluation
By the end of Mr. Smart's first 24 hours in the hospital, you'll reassess his condition and evaluate your care plan. If his breathing is less labored, if his anxiety and fear decrease, if his color improves and his stamina increases, and if clinical findings point to a stabilizing condition, you'll know that your care plan is on track.
   You know, too, that respiratory arrest, pulmonary collapse, cor pulmonale, and congestive heart failure are all possible and probable for a man in his condition. Though you'll reduce the frequency of your assessments from every hour to once every shift, you'll watch carefully for further improvement. If Mr. Smart has relapsing illness or shows no further improvement, you'll reevaluate and adjust your care plan to accommodate new findings.

If he's intubated and lethargic, reposition him every 1 to 2 hours. Use postural drainage and chest physiotherapy to help clear secretions.
• Observe the patient closely for respiratory arrest. Auscultate chest sounds. Monitor ABG values, and report any changes immediately. Notify the doctor of any deterioration in oxygen saturation levels detected by pulse oximetry.
• Watch for treatment complications, especially oxygen toxicity and adult respiratory distress syndrome.

• Frequently monitor vital signs. Note and report an increasing pulse rate, rising or falling respiratory rate, declining blood pressure, or febrile state.
• Monitor and record serum electrolyte levels carefully. Take steps to correct imbalances. Monitor fluid balance by recording the patient's intake and output and daily weight.
• Check the cardiac monitor for arrhythmias.
• Perform oral hygiene measures frequently.
• Apply soft wrist restraints for the confused patient if needed. This will prevent him from disconnecting the

oxygen setup. However, remember that these restraints can increase anxiety, fear, and agitation.
• Position the patient for comfort and optimal gas exchange. Place the call button within the patient's reach.
• Maintain the patient in a normothermic state to reduce his body's demand for oxygen.
• Pace patient care activities to maximize the patient's energy level and provide needed rest.

If the patient requires *mechanical ventilation:*
• Check ventilator settings, cuff pressures, and ABG values often to ensure correct fraction of inspired oxygen (FIO_2) settings, which are determined by ABG levels. Draw blood samples for ABG analysis 20 to 30 minutes after every change in the FIO_2 setting or as ordered.
• Suction the trachea as needed after oxygenation. Observe for any change in sputum quality, consistency, and color. Provide humidification to liquefy secretions.
• Watch for complications of mechanical ventilation, such as reduced cardiac output, pneumothorax or other barotrauma, increased pulmonary vascular resistance, diminished urine output, increased intracranial pressure, and GI bleeding.
• Routinely assess endotracheal (ET) tube position and patency. Make sure the tube is placed properly and taped securely. Immediately after intubation, check for accidental intubation of the esophagus or the mainstem bronchus, which may have occurred during ET tube insertion. Also be alert for transtracheal or laryngeal perforation; aspiration; broken teeth; nosebleeds; vagal reflexes, such as bradycardia; arrhythmias; and hypertension.
• After tube placement, watch for complications, such as tube displacement, herniation of the tube's cuff, respiratory infection, and tracheal malacia and stenosis.
• Prevent infection by using sterile technique while suctioning and by changing ventilator tubing every 24 hours.
• Prevent tracheal erosion that can result from an overinflated artificial airway cuff compressing the tracheal wall's vasculature. Use the minimal-leak technique and a cuffed tube with high residual volume (low pressure cuff), a foam cuff, or a pressure-regulating valve on the cuff. Measure cuff pressure every 8 hours.
• Implement measures to prevent tissue necrosis. Position and maintain the nasotracheal tube midline within the nostrils and provide meticulous care. Periodically loosen the tape securing the tube to prevent skin breakdown. Reposition endotracheal tubing from side to side and retape as needed. Make sure that the ventilator tubing has adequate support.

• Monitor for signs of stress ulcers, which are common in intubated patients—especially those in the intensive care unit. Inspect gastric secretions for blood, especially if the patient has a nasogastric tube or reports epigastric tenderness, nausea, or vomiting. Also monitor hemoglobin and hematocrit levels, and check all stools for blood. Administer antacids or histamine receptor antagonists, as ordered.
• Help the patient communicate without words. Offer him a pen and tablet, a word chart, or an alphabet board.

Patient teaching
• If applicable, teach the patient about the effects of smoking. Provide resources to help him stop smoking.
• Describe all tests and procedures to the patient and his family. Discuss the reasons for suctioning, chest physiotherapy, blood tests and, if used, soft wrist restraints.
• If the patient is intubated or has a tracheostomy, explain why he can't speak. Suggest alternative means of communication.
• Identify reportable signs of respiratory infection.

ADULT RESPIRATORY DISTRESS SYNDROME

A form of pulmonary edema, adult respiratory distress syndrome (ARDS) can quickly lead to acute respiratory failure. Also known as shock, stiff, white, wet, or Da Nang lung, ARDS may follow direct or indirect lung injury.

Increased permeability of the alveolocapillary membranes allows fluid to accumulate in the lung interstitium, alveolar spaces, and small airways, causing the lung to stiffen. This impairs ventilation, reducing oxygenation of pulmonary capillary blood. Difficult to recognize, the disorder can prove fatal within 48 hours of onset if not promptly diagnosed and treated. (See *What happens in ARDS,* pages 630 and 631.)

Although this four-stage syndrome can progress to intractable and fatal hypoxemia, patients who recover may have little or no permanent lung damage.

In some patients, the syndrome may coexist with disseminated intravascular coagulation (DIC). Whether ARDS stems from DIC or develops independently remains unclear. Patients with three concurrent ARDS risk factors have an 85% probability of developing ARDS.

Causes
Trauma is the most common cause of ARDS, possibly because trauma-related factors, such as fat emboli, sep-

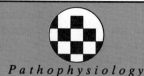

Pathophysiology

WHAT HAPPENS IN A.R.D.S.

These illustrations depict the process and progress of ARDS.

1. The body responds to insult

Injury reduces normal blood flow to the lungs, allowing platelets to aggregate. These platelets release substances, such as serotonin (S), bradykinin (B) and, especially, histamine (H), that inflame and damage the alveolar membrane and later increase capillary permeability. At this early stage, signs and symptoms of ARDS are undetectable.

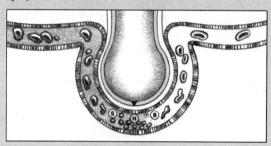

2. Fluid shift causes symptoms

Histamines and other inflammatory substances increase capillary permeability, allowing fluid to shift into the interstitial space. As a result, the patient may experience tachypnea, dyspnea, and tachycardia.

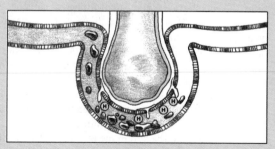

3. Pulmonary edema results

As capillary permeability increases, proteins and more fluid leak out, increasing interstitial osmotic pressure and causing pulmonary edema. At this stage, the patient may experience increased tachypnea, dyspnea, and cyanosis. Hypoxia (usually unresponsive to increased FIO_2), decreased pulmonary compliance, and crackles and rhonchi also may develop.

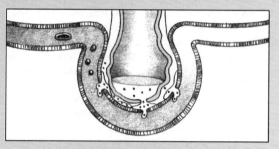

4. Alveoli collapse

Fluid in the alveoli and decreased blood flow damage surfactant in the alveoli, reducing the cells' ability to produce more. Without surfactant, alveoli collapse, impairing gas exchange. Look for thick, frothy sputum and marked hypoxemia with increased respiratory distress.

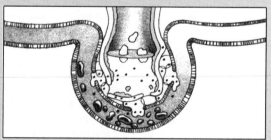

sis, shock, pulmonary contusions, and multiple transfusions, increase the likelihood that microemboli will develop.

Other common causes of ARDS include anaphylaxis, aspiration of gastric contents, diffuse pneumonia (especially viral), drug overdose (for example, heroin, aspirin, and ethchlorvynol), idiosyncratic drug reaction (to ampicillin and hydrochlorothiazide), inhalation of noxious gases (such as nitrous oxide, ammonia, and chlorine), near-drowning, and oxygen toxicity.

Less common causes of ARDS include coronary artery bypass grafting, hemodialysis, leukemia, acute miliary

WHAT HAPPENS IN A.R.D.S.   *(continued)*

5. Gas exchange slows
The patient breathes faster, but sufficient O_2 can't cross the alveolocapillary membrane. CO_2, however, crosses more easily and is lost with every exhalation. Both O_2 and CO_2 levels in the blood decrease. Look for increased tachypnea, hypoxemia, and hypocapnia.

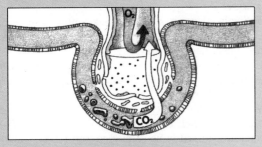

6. Metabolic acidosis occurs
Pulmonary edema worsens. Meanwhile, inflammation leads to fibrosis, which further impedes gas exchange. The resulting hypoxemia leads to metabolic acidosis. At this stage, look for increased $PaCO_2$, decreased pH and PaO_2, decreased HCO_3 levels, and mental confusion.

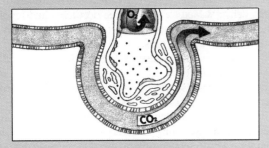

tuberculosis, pancreatitis, thrombotic thrombocytopenic purpura, uremia, and venous air embolism.

Complications
Severe ARDS can lead to metabolic and respiratory acidosis and ensuing cardiac arrest.

Assessment findings
As you conduct your assessment, be alert for the patient's particular stage of ARDS. Each has its typical signs.

In *Stage I,* the patient may complain of dyspnea, especially on exertion. Respiratory and pulse rates are normal to high. Auscultation may reveal diminished breath sounds.

In *Stage II,* respiratory distress becomes more apparent. The patient may use accessory muscles to breathe and appear pallid, anxious, and restless. He may have a dry cough with thick, frothy sputum and bloody, sticky secretions. Palpation may disclose cool, clammy skin. Tachycardia and tachypnea may accompany elevated blood pressure. Auscultation may detect basilar crackles. (Stage II signs and symptoms may be incorrectly attributed to other causes, such as multiple trauma.)

In *Stage III,* you'll observe the patient struggle to breathe. Vital signs check reveals tachypnea (more than 30 breaths/minute), tachycardia with arrhythmias (usually premature ventricular contractions), and a labile blood pressure. Inspection may reveal a productive cough and pale, cyanotic skin. Auscultation may disclose crackles and rhonchi. The patient will need intubation and ventilation.

In *Stage IV,* the patient has acute respiratory failure with severe hypoxia. His mental status is deteriorating, and he may become comatose. His skin appears pale and cyanotic. Spontaneous respirations are not evident. Bradycardia with arrhythmias accompanies hypotension. Metabolic and respiratory acidosis develop. When ARDS reaches this stage, the patient is at high risk for fibrosis. Pulmonary damage becomes life-threatening.

Diagnostic tests
• *Arterial blood gas (ABG) analysis* (with the patient breathing room air) initially shows a reduced PaO_2 (less than 60 mm Hg) and a decreased $PaCO_2$ (less than 35 mm Hg). Hypoxemia despite increased supplemental oxygen is the hallmark of ARDS. The resulting blood pH usually reflects respiratory alkalosis. As ARDS worsens, ABG values show respiratory acidosis (increasing $PaCO_2$ [more than 45 mm Hg]) and metabolic acidosis (decreasing HCO_3 levels [less than 22 mEq/liter]) and declining PaO_2 despite oxygen therapy.
• *Pulmonary artery catheterization* helps identify the cause of pulmonary edema by measuring pulmonary capillary wedge pressure (PCWP). This procedure also allows collection of samples of pulmonary artery, mixed venous blood that show decreased oxygen saturation, reflecting tissue hypoxia. Normal PCWP values in ARDS are 12 mm Hg or less.
• *Serial chest X-rays* in early stages show bilateral infiltrates. In later stages, findings demonstrate lung fields with a ground-glass appearance and, eventually (with irreversible hypoxemia), "whiteouts" of both lung fields.

Differential diagnosis must rule out cardiogenic pulmonary edema, pulmonary vasculitis, and diffuse pulmonary hemorrhage. Etiologic tests may involve sputum analyses (including Gram stain and culture and sensitivity); blood cultures (to identify infectious organisms); toxicology tests (to screen for drug ingestion); and various serum amylase tests (to rule out pancreatitis).

Treatment

Therapy focuses on correcting the cause of the syndrome, if possible, and preventing progression of life-threatening hypoxemia and respiratory acidosis. Supportive care consists of administering humidified oxygen by a tight-fitting mask, which facilitates the use of continuous positive airway pressure (CPAP). However, this therapy alone seldom fulfills the ARDS patient's ventilatory requirements. If the patient's hypoxemia doesn't subside with this treatment, he may require intubation, mechanical ventilation, and positive end-expiratory pressure (PEEP). Other supportive measures include fluid restriction, diuretic therapy, and correction of electrolyte and acid-base imbalances.

When a patient with ARDS needs mechanical ventilation, sedatives, narcotics, or neuromuscular blocking agents (such as vecuronium) may be ordered to minimize restlessness (and thereby oxygen consumption and carbon dioxide production) and to facilitate ventilation.

When ARDS results from fatty emboli or a chemical injury, a short course of high-dose corticosteroids may help if given early. Treatment with sodium bicarbonate may be necessary to reverse severe metabolic acidosis. And fluids and vasopressors may be needed to maintain blood pressure. Nonviral infections require treatment with antimicrobial drugs.

Nursing diagnoses
- Altered nutrition: Less than body requirements
- Altered tissue perfusion
- Anxiety
- Decreased cardiac output
- Fatigue
- Fear
- Impaired gas exchange
- Impaired physical mobility
- Impaired verbal communication
- Risk for impaired skin integrity
- Risk for infection

Nursing interventions
- Frequently assess the patient's respiratory status. Be alert for inspiratory retractions. Note respiratory rate, rhythm, and depth. Watch for dyspnea and accessory muscle use. Listen for adventitious or diminished breath sounds. Check for clear, frothy sputum (indicating pulmonary edema).
- Evaluate and document the patient's level of consciousness, noting confusion or mental sluggishness.
- Be alert for signs of treatment-induced complications, including arrhythmias, DIC, GI bleeding, infection, malnutrition, paralytic ileus, pneumothorax, pulmonary fibrosis, renal failure, thrombocytopenia, and tracheal stenosis.
- Maintain a patent airway by suctioning. Use sterile, nontraumatic technique. Ensure adequate humidification to help liquefy tenacious secretions.
- Closely monitor heart rate and blood pressure. Watch for arrhythmias that may result from hypoxemia, acid-base disturbances, or electrolyte imbalance.
- With pulmonary artery catheterization, know the desired PCWP level; check readings often, and watch for decreasing mixed venous oxygen saturation. Change dressings according to hospital guidelines, using strict aseptic technique.
- Monitor serum electrolyte levels, and correct imbalances. Measure intake and output. Weigh the patient daily.
- Check ventilator settings frequently, and drain condensation from the tubing promptly to ensure maximum oxygen delivery. Monitor ABG levels; document and report changes in SaO_2, as well as metabolic and respiratory acidosis and PaO_2 changes.
- Be prepared to administer CPAP to the patient with severe hypoxemia.
- Give sedatives, as ordered, to reduce restlessness. Monitor and record the patient's response to medication.
- Because PEEP may lower cardiac output, check for hypotension, tachycardia, and decreased urine output. To maintain PEEP, suction only as needed. High-frequency jet ventilation and pressure-controlled ventilation may also be required.
- Reposition the patient often.
- Record any increase in secretions, temperature, or hypotension that may indicate a deteriorating condition.
- Monitor the patient's nutritional intake and record caloric intake. Administer tube feedings and parenteral nutrition, as ordered. Plan patient care to allow periods of uninterrupted sleep. To promote health and prevent fatigue, arrange for alternate periods of rest and activity.
- Maintain joint mobility by performing passive range-of-motion (ROM) exercises. If possible, help the patient perform active ROM exercises.

• Provide meticulous skin care. To prevent skin break-down, reposition the endotracheal tube from side to side every 24 hours.
• Provide emotional support. Answer the patient's and family's questions as fully as possible, to allay their fears and concerns.
• Watch for and immediately report all respiratory changes in the patient with injuries that may adversely affect the lungs—especially in the first few days after the injury when the patient's condition may appear to be improving.
• Provide alternative communication means for the patient on mechanical ventilation.

Patient teaching
• Explain the disorder to the patient and his family. Tell them what signs and symptoms may occur, and review the treatment that may be required.
• Orient the patient and his family to the unit and hospital surroundings. Provide them with simple explanations and demonstrations of treatments.
• Tell the recuperating patient that recovery will take some time and that he'll feel weak for a while. Urge him to share his concerns with the staff.

ASTHMA
A chronic reactive airway disorder, asthma involves episodic, reversible airway obstruction resulting from bronchospasms, increased mucus secretions, and mucosal edema. Signs and symptoms range from mild wheezing and dyspnea to life-threatening respiratory failure. Signs and symptoms of bronchial airway obstruction may or may not persist between acute episodes.

Although this common respiratory condition can strike at any age, about half of all patients with asthma are under age 10. In this age-group, asthma affects twice as many boys as girls. About one-third of patients experience asthma's onset between ages 10 and 30; in this group, incidence is the same in both sexes. Hereditary factors are also important: About one-third of all patients with asthma share the disease with at least one immediate family member.

Asthma may result from sensitivity to specific external allergens (extrinsic) or from internal, nonallergenic factors (intrinsic). Allergens that cause *extrinsic asthma* (atopic asthma) include pollen, animal dander, house dust or mold, kapok or feather pillows, food additives containing sulfites, and any other sensitizing substance. Extrinsic asthma begins in children and is commonly accompanied by other manifestations of atopy (Type I,

immunoglobulin E [IgE]-mediated allergy), such as eczema and allergic rhinitis.

In *intrinsic asthma* (nonatopic asthma), no extrinsic substance can be identified. Most episodes are preceded by a severe respiratory tract infection (especially in adults). Irritants, emotional stress, fatigue, endocrine changes, temperature and humidity variations, and exposure to noxious fumes may aggravate intrinsic asthma attacks. In many asthmatics, especially children, intrinsic and extrinsic asthma coexist.

Causes and pathophysiology
In asthma, the tracheal and bronchial linings overreact to various stimuli, causing episodic smooth-muscle spasms that severely constrict the airways. Mucosal edema and thickened secretions further block the airways.

IgE antibodies, attached to histamine-containing mast cells and receptors on cell membranes, initiate intrinsic asthma attacks. When exposed to an antigen, such as pollen, the IgE antibody combines with the antigen. On subsequent exposure to the antigen, mast cells degranulate and release mediators.

These mediators cause the bronchoconstriction and edema of an asthma attack. As a result, expiratory airflow decreases, trapping gas in the airways and causing alveolar hyperinflation. Atelectasis may develop in some lung regions. The increased airway resistance initiates labored breathing. (See *What happens in asthma,* page 622.)

Several factors may contribute to bronchoconstriction. These include hereditary predisposition; sensitivity to allergens or irritants, such as pollutants; viral infections; aspirin, beta blockers, nonsteroidal anti-inflammatory drugs, and other drugs; tartrazine (a yellow food dye); psychological stress; cold air; and exercise.

Complications
Asthma can produce status asthmaticus and respiratory failure. (See *How status asthmaticus progresses,* page 623.)

Assessment findings
An asthma attack may begin dramatically, with simultaneous onset of severe, multiple symptoms, or insidiously, with gradually increasing respiratory distress. Typically, the patient reports exposure to a particular allergen followed by a sudden onset of dyspnea and wheezing, and tightness in the chest accompanied by a cough that produces thick, clear or yellow sputum.

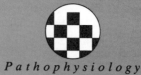

Pathophysiology

WHAT HAPPENS IN ASTHMA

These drawings show the pathophysiologic processes that occur during an asthma attack.

1. When the patient inhales a substance to which he's hypersensitive, abnormal (IgE) antibodies stimulate mast cells in the lung interstitium to release both histamine (H) and the slow-reacting substance of anaphylaxis (SRS-A). At this early stage, the patient has no detectable signs or symptoms.

2. Histamine attaches to receptor sites in the larger bronchi, where it causes swelling in smooth muscles. Mucous membranes become inflamed, irritated, and swollen. The patient may experience dyspnea, prolonged expiration, and increased respiratory rate.

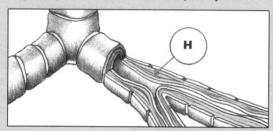

3. SRS-A attaches to receptor sites in the smaller bronchi and causes swelling of smooth muscle there. It also causes fatty acids called prostaglandins to travel by way of the bloodstream to the lungs, where they enhance histamine's effects. Listen to the patient's cough for wheezing. The higher the pitch, the narrower the bronchial lumen.

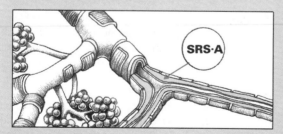

4. Histamine stimulates the mucous membranes to secrete excessive mucus, further narrowing the bronchial lumen (see top right). Goblet cells secrete

a viscous mucus that's difficult to cough up. Listen for coughing, rhonchi, high-pitched wheezing, and increased respiratory distress.

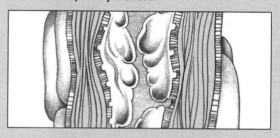

5. On inhalation, the narrowed bronchial lumen can still expand slightly, allowing air to reach the alveoli. On exhalation, increased intrathoracic pressure closes the bronchial lumen completely. Air can get in but can't get out. Check for barrel chest, hyperresonance to percussion, and wheezing cessation.

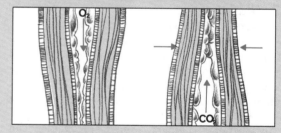

6. Mucus fills the lung bases, inhibiting alveolar ventilation. Blood, shunted to alveoli in other lung parts, still can't compensate for diminished ventilation. Respiratory acidosis results. Look for signs of hypoxemia: reduced PaO_2 (despite increased FIO_2), elevated $PaCO_2$, and decreased serum pH.

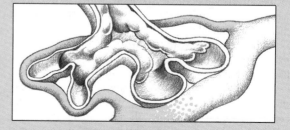

DETERMINING ASTHMA'S SEVERITY

Signs/symptoms during acute phase	Diagnostic test results	Other assessment findings
Mild asthma • Brief wheezing, coughing, dyspnea with activity • Infrequent nocturnal coughing or wheezing • Adequate air exchange • Intermittent, brief (<1 hour) wheezing, coughing, or dyspnea once or twice a week • Asymptomatic between attacks	**Mild asthma** • FEV_1 or peak flow 80% of normal values • pH normal or increased • Pao_2 normal or decreased • $Paco_2$ normal or decreased • Chest X-ray normal	**Mild asthma** • One attack per week (or none) • Positive response to bronchodilator therapy within 24 hours • No signs of asthma between episodes • No sleep interruption • No hyperventilation • Minimal evidence of airway obstruction • Minimal or no increase in lung volume
Moderate asthma • Respiratory distress at rest • Hyperpnea • Marked coughing and wheezing • Air exchange normal or below normal • Exacerbations that may last several days	**Moderate asthma** • FEV_1 or peak flow 60% to 80% of normal values; may vary 20% to 30% with symptoms • pH generally elevated • Pao_2 increased • $Paco_2$ generally decreased • Chest X-ray that shows hyperinflation	**Moderate asthma** • Symptoms occurring more than two times weekly • Coughing and wheezing between episodes • Diminished exercise tolerance • Possible sleep interruption • Increased lung volumes
Severe asthma • Marked respiratory distress • Marked wheezing or absent breath sounds • Pulsus paradoxus >10 mm Hg • Chest wall contractions • Continuous symptoms • Frequent exacerbations	**Severe asthma** • FEV_1 or peak flow less than 60% of normal values; may normally vary 20% to 30% with routine medications and up to 50% with exacerbations • pH normal or reduced • Pao_2 decreased • $Paco_2$ normal or increased • Chest X-ray that may show hyperinflation	**Severe asthma** • Frequent severe attacks • Daily wheezing • Poor exercise tolerance • Frequent sleep interruption • Bronchodilator therapy doesn't completely reverse airway obstruction • Markedly increased lung volumes

The patient may complain of feeling suffocated. He may be visibly dyspneic and able to speak only a few words before pausing for breath. You may also observe accessory respiratory muscle use. He may sweat profusely, and you may note an increased anteroposterior thoracic diameter.

Percussion may produce hyperresonance. Palpation may reveal vocal fremitus. Auscultation may disclose tachycardia, tachypnea, mild systolic hypertension, harsh respirations with both inspiratory and expiratory wheezes, prolonged expiratory phase of respiration, and diminished breath sounds.

Cyanosis, confusion, and lethargy indicate the onset of life threatening status asthmaticus and respiratory failure.

Diagnostic tests

• *Pulmonary function studies* reveal signs of airway obstructive disease (decreased flow rates and forced expiratory volume in 1 second [FEV_1]), low-normal or decreased vital capacity, and increased total lung and residual capacities. Despite abnormal findings during asthmatic episodes, pulmonary function may be normal between attacks.

Typically, the patient has decreased PaO_2 and $PaCO_2$. However, in severe asthma, $PaCO_2$ may be normal or increased, indicating severe bronchial obstruction. In fact, FEV_1 will probably be less than 25% of the predicted value. Initiating treatment tends to improve the airflow. However, even when the asthma attack appears controlled, the spirometric values (FEV_1 and forced expiratory flow between 25% and 75% of vital capacity) remain abnormal, necessitating frequent arterial blood gas (ABG) analyses or pulse oximetry measurements. Residual volume remains abnormal for up to 3 weeks after the attack.

• *Serum IgE levels* may rise from an allergic reaction.

• *Complete blood count with differential* reveals increased eosinophil count.

• *Chest X-rays* can diagnose or monitor the progress of asthma. X-rays may show hyperinflation with areas of focal atelectasis.

• *ABG analysis* detects hypoxemia and guides treatment.

• *Skin testing* may identify specific allergens. Test results are read in 1 to 2 days to detect an early reaction and then again after 4 or 5 days to reveal a late reaction.

• *Bronchial challenge testing* evaluates the clinical significance of allergens identified by skin testing.

COPING WITH ASTHMA

Use these guidelines to help your patient cope with asthma at home:
• Teach the parents and child about triggers for an attack. Evaluate their home to detect triggers and help minimize them.
• Assess the child's compliance with the medication regimen, and suggest ways to improve it.
• Teach the parents and child how to use inhalers with spacer devices. First, show them how to set up the device and stress the need for a tight seal around the mouthpiece. After demonstrating its use, watch the child use it. (He should press down to release medication into the chamber, inhale slowly, hold his breath for 5 seconds, exhale, and repeat the sequence again.) Explain the need to clean the mouthpiece with warm running water once a day and to dry it completely before replacing it in its case.
• Instruct the parents to replace the mouthpiece every 6 months and the reservoir bag every 2 to 3 weeks or as needed. If the bag develops a hole or tear, tell them to replace it immediately.
• Suggest keeping a spare device available.
• Discuss the signs of an impending attack, and identify measures to minimize it.
• If the child must take theophylline, advise the parents to call the doctor if adverse reactions occur and to return for follow-up laboratory tests.
• If the child must take a corticosteroid, monitor for cushingoid effects. If such effects occur, tell the parents not to discontinue the drug abruptly but to gradually reduce the dosage.
• Encourage the parents to let the child perform whatever activities he feels comfortable doing.
• Recommend community resources, such as the American Lung Association or the Asthma and Allergy Foundation of America.

Treatment

The best treatment for asthma is prevention by identifying and avoiding precipitating factors, such as environmental allergens or irritants. Usually, such stimuli can't be removed entirely. Desensitization to specific antigens may be more helpful in children than in adults with bronchial asthma.

Drug therapy, which usually includes bronchodilators, is most effective when begun soon after the onset of signs and symptoms. Drugs used include rapid-acting epi-nephrine, terbutaline, aminophylline, theophylline and theophylline-containing oral preparations, oral sympathomimetics, corticosteroids, and aerosolized sympathomimetics such as albuterol. ABG measurements help determine the severity of an asthma attack and the patient's response to treatment.

Low-flow oxygen may be required, as may antibiotics if infection exists. Fluid replacement may also be needed.

Status asthmaticus must be treated promptly to prevent progression to fatal respiratory failure. The patient with increasingly severe asthma that doesn't respond to drug therapy is usually admitted to the intensive care unit for treatment with corticosteroids, epinephrine, sympathomimetic aerosol sprays, and I.V. aminophylline. He'll need frequent ABG analysis and pulse oximetry to assess respiratory status, particularly after ventilator therapy or a change in oxygen concentration. The patient may require endotracheal intubation and mechanical ventilation if his $PaCO_2$ rises.

Nursing diagnoses
• Anxiety
• Fear
• Impaired gas exchange
• Ineffective airway clearance
• Ineffective breathing pattern
• Knowledge deficit

Nursing interventions
During an acute attack:
• Maintain respiratory function and relieve bronchoconstriction while allowing mucus plug expulsion.
• Control exercise-induced asthma by having the patient sit down, rest, and use diaphragmatic and pursed-lip breathing until shortness of breath subsides.
• Find out if the patient has a nebulizer and if he has used it. He should have access to an albuterol inhaler at all times. Instruct him to take no more than two or three puffs every 4 hours. If he needs the nebulizer before 4 hours pass, however, let him use it and call the doctor for further instruction. (Excessive use can weaken the patient's response and mask inflammation. Rarely, extended overuse can lead to cardiac arrest and death.)
• Reassure the patient during an asthma attack, and stay with him. Place him in semi-Fowler's position and encourage diaphragmatic breathing. Help him to relax.
• Listen to the patient's concerns, and answer his questions. Suggest relaxing care measures and activities.
• Watch for complications, such as status asthmaticus.
• As ordered, administer humidified oxygen by nasal cannula at 2 liters/minute to ease breathing and to increase SaO_2. Later, adjust oxygen according to the pa-

tient's vital functions and ABG measurements.
• As ordered, administer drugs and I.V. fluids. Continue epinephrine or a sympathomimetic. Give aminophylline I.V. as a loading dose. Follow with I.V. drip administration. Because young patients and those who smoke or take barbiturates have increased aminophylline metabolism, they require a larger dose. Monitor the drip rate. When possible, use an I.V. infusion pump. Simultaneously, give a loading dose of a corticosteroid I.V. or I.M.
• Combat dehydration with I.V. fluids until the patient can tolerate oral fluids, which help loosen secretions.

During long-term care:
• Supervise the patient's drug regimen. Make sure he knows how to use a metered-dose inhaler properly. Use of a spacer device may help optimize drug delivery.
• When the patient is using a theophylline bronchodilator, monitor plasma drug levels because oral absorption of theophylline may vary.
• Long-term corticosteroid therapy may cause cushingoid effects. Minimize them by alternate-day dosage or use of orally inhalable beclomethasone, flunisolide, or triamcinolone acetonide. Ipratropium may also be used.
• Because of their respiratory depressant effect, sedatives and narcotics are not recommended.

Patient teaching
• Teach the patient and his family about diaphragmatic and pursed-lip breathing and relaxation exercises. (For more information, see *Coping with asthma*.)
• Teach the patient how to use an oral inhaler or turbo-inhaler. Advise him about adverse reactions to his medications, and tell him to notify his doctor if they occur.
• Encourage the patient to eat a well-balanced diet to prevent respiratory infection and fatigue.

PULMONARY EDEMA
Marked by an accumulation of fluid in extravascular spaces of the lung, pulmonary edema is a common complication of cardiac disorders. The disorder may occur as a chronic condition, or it may develop quickly and rapidly become fatal.

Causes and pathophysiology
Pulmonary edema usually results from left ventricular failure caused by arteriosclerotic, cardiomyopathic, hypertensive, or valvular heart disease. The disorder stems from either of two mechanisms: increased pulmonary capillary hydrostatic pressure or decreased colloid osmotic pressure. Normally, the two pressures are in balance. When this balance changes, pulmonary edema results.

If pulmonary capillary hydrostatic pressure increases, the compromised left ventricle requires increased filling pressures to maintain adequate output; these pressures are transmitted to the left atrium, pulmonary veins, and pulmonary capillary bed. This forces fluids and solutes from the intravascular compartment into the interstitium of the lungs. As the interstitium overloads with fluid, fluid floods the peripheral alveoli and impairs gas exchange.

If colloid osmotic pressure decreases, the natural pulling force that contains intravascular fluids is lost — nothing opposes the hydrostatic force. Thus, fluid flows freely into the interstitium and alveoli, resulting in pulmonary edema.

Other factors that may predispose the patient to pulmonary edema include:
• barbiturate or opiate poisoning
• congestive heart failure
• infusion of excessive volumes of I.V. fluids or an overly rapid infusion
• impaired pulmonary lymphatic drainage (from Hodgkin's disease or obliterative lymphangitis after radiation)
• inhalation of irritating gases
• mitral stenosis and left atrial myxoma (which impair left atrial emptying)
• pneumonia
• pulmonary veno-occlusive disease.

Complications
Acute pulmonary edema may progress to respiratory and metabolic acidosis with subsequent cardiac or respiratory arrest.

Assessment findings
The history may include a predisposing factor for pulmonary edema. The patient typically complains of a persistent cough. He may report getting a cold and being dyspneic on exertion. He may experience paroxysmal nocturnal dyspnea and orthopnea.

On inspection, you may note restlessness and anxiety. With severe pulmonary edema, the patient's breathing may be visibly labored and rapid. His cough may sound intense and produce frothy, bloody sputum. In advanced stages, the patient's level of consciousness decreases.

Typical palpation findings include neck vein distention. In acute pulmonary edema, the skin feels sweaty, cold, and clammy. Auscultation may reveal crepitant crackles and a diastolic (S_3) gallop. In severe pulmonary edema, you may hear wheezing as the alveoli and bron-

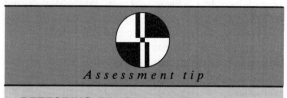

Assessment tip

DETECTING DANGER SIGNS

If you detect inspiratory crackles, dry cough, or dyspnea, notify the doctor immediately. Chest X-ray results may not be available until 24 hours after you've assessed the patient. Don't wait for X-ray findings if you suspect pulmonary edema.

chioles fill with fluid. The crackles become more diffuse. (See *Detecting danger signs.*)

Additional findings include worsening tachycardia, falling blood pressure, thready pulse, and decreased cardiac output. In advanced pulmonary edema, breath sounds diminish.

Diagnostic tests

Clinical features of pulmonary edema permit a working diagnosis. Diagnostic tests provide the following information:

• *Arterial blood gas (ABG) analysis* usually shows hypoxia with variable $PaCO_2$, depending on the patient's degree of fatigue. ABG results may also identify metabolic acidosis.

• *Chest X-rays* show diffuse haziness of the lung fields and, usually, cardiomegaly and pleural effusion.

• *Pulse oximetry* may reveal decreasing SaO_2 levels.

• *Pulmonary artery catheterization* identifies left ventricular failure (indicated by elevated pulmonary artery wedge pressures). These findings help to rule out adult respiratory distress syndrome, in which wedge pressure usually remains normal.

• *Electrocardiography* may disclose evidence of previous or current myocardial infarction.

Treatment

Treatment aims to reduce extravascular fluid, to improve gas exchange and myocardial function and, if possible, to correct underlying disease. High concentrations of oxygen can be administered by cannula or mask. (Typically, the patient with pulmonary edema doesn't tolerate a mask.) If the patient's arterial oxygen levels remain too low, assisted ventilation can improve oxygen delivery to the tissues and usually improves his acid-base balance. A bronchodilator, such as aminophylline, may de-

crease bronchospasm and enhance myocardial contractility. Diuretics, such as furosemide, ethacrynic acid, and bumetanide, increase urination, which helps to mobilize extravascular fluid.

Treatment of myocardial dysfunction includes positive inotropic agents, such as digitalis and amrinone, to enhance contractility. Pressor agents may be given to enhance contractility and to promote vasoconstriction in peripheral vessels.

Antiarrhythmics may also be given, particularly in arrhythmias related to decreased cardiac output. Occasionally, arterial vasodilators, such as nitroprusside, can decrease peripheral vascular resistance, preload, and afterload.

Morphine may reduce anxiety and dyspnea and dilate the systemic venous bed, promoting blood flow from pulmonary circulation to the periphery.

Other treatments include rotating tourniquets and phlebotomy (both reduce preload). Phlebotomy will also remove hemoglobin, which may worsen the patient's hypoxemia.

Nursing diagnoses

• Altered tissue perfusion
• Anxiety
• Fear
• Fluid volume excess
• Impaired gas exchange
• Knowledge deficit

Nursing interventions

• Help the patient relax to promote oxygenation, control bronchospasm, and enhance myocardial contractility.

• Reassure the patient, who will be frightened by his inability to breathe normally. Provide emotional support to his family as well.

• Place him in high Fowler's position to enhance lung expansion.

• Administer oxygen, as ordered.

• Assess the patient's condition frequently, and document his responses to treatment. Monitor ABG and pulse oximetry values, oral and I.V. fluid intake, urine output and, in the patient with a pulmonary artery catheter, pulmonary end-diastolic and capillary wedge pressures. Check the cardiac monitor often. Report changes immediately.

• Watch for complications of treatment, such as electrolyte depletion. Also watch for complications of oxygen therapy and mechanical ventilation.

• Monitor vital signs every 15 to 30 minutes while administering nitroprusside in dextrose 5% in water by I.V.

drip. During use, protect the solution from light by wrapping the bottle or bag with aluminum foil. Discard unused nitroprusside solution after 4 hours. Watch for arrhythmias in patients receiving digitalis and for marked respiratory depression in those receiving morphine.
• Carefully record the time morphine is given and the amount administered.

Patient teaching
• Urge the patient to comply with the prescribed medication regimen to avoid future episodes of pulmonary edema.
• Explain all procedures to the patient and his family.
• Emphasize reporting early signs of fluid overload.
• Explain the reasons for sodium restrictions. List high-sodium foods and drugs.
• Review all prescribed medications with the patient. If he takes digoxin, show him how to monitor his own pulse rate and warn him to report signs of toxicity. Encourage consumption of potassium-rich foods to lower the risk of toxicity and cardiac arrhythmias. If he takes a vasodilator, teach him the signs of hypotension and emphasize the need to avoid alcohol.
• Discuss ways to conserve physical energy.

COR PULMONALE
Also called right ventricular hypertrophy, cor pulmonale occurs at the end stage of various chronic disorders that affect lung function or structure (except those stemming from congenital heart disease or diseases that affect the left side of the heart).

Invariably, cor pulmonale follows certain disorders of the lungs, pulmonary vessels, chest wall, or respiratory control center. Because cor pulmonale usually occurs late in chronic obstructive pulmonary disease (COPD) and other irreversible diseases, the prognosis is poor.

About 85% of patients with cor pulmonale have COPD. About 25% of patients with bronchial COPD eventually develop cor pulmonale. The disorder accounts for about 25% of all types of heart failure, and it's most common in patients who smoke and who have COPD. Cor pulmonale affects middle-aged and elderly men more often than women, but the incidence in women is increasing.

In children, cor pulmonale may be a complication of cystic fibrosis, hemosiderosis, upper airway obstruction, scleroderma, extensive bronchiectasis, neurologic diseases that affect respiratory muscles, or abnormalities of the respiratory control center.

Causes and pathophysiology
In cor pulmonale, pulmonary hypertension increases the heart's work load. To compensate, the right ventricle hypertrophies to force blood through the lungs. However, the compensatory mechanism begins to fail, and larger amounts of blood remain in the right ventricle at the end of diastole. This causes ventricular dilation. In response to hypoxia, the bone marrow produces more red blood cells, resulting in polycythemia. Then, the blood's viscosity increases, further aggravating pulmonary hypertension, increasing the right ventricle's work load, and causing heart failure.

Cor pulmonale may result from:
• disorders that affect pulmonary parenchyma (such as pulmonary fibrosis, pneumoconiosis, cystic fibrosis, periarteritis nodosa, and tuberculosis)
• pulmonary diseases that affect the airways (such as COPD and bronchial asthma)
• vascular diseases (such as vasculitis, pulmonary emboli, or external vascular obstruction resulting from a tumor or an aneurysm)
• chest wall abnormalities, including thoracic deformities (such as kyphoscoliosis and pectus excavatum)
• other external factors, including obesity, living at a high altitude, and neuromuscular disorders (such as muscular dystrophy and poliomyelitis).

Complications
Cor pulmonale eventually may lead to biventricular failure. Depending on the severity of cor pulmonale, hepatomegaly, edema, ascites, and pleural effusions may develop. Because of polycythemia, the risk of thromboembolism also increases.

Assessment findings
As long as the heart can compensate for the increased pulmonary vascular resistance, your patient will report signs and symptoms associated with the underlying disorder, occurring mostly in the respiratory system. The patient is most likely to complain of a chronic productive cough, exertional dyspnea, wheezing respirations, fatigue, and weakness.

Cor pulmonale progresses with dyspnea (even at rest) that worsens on exertion, tachypnea, orthopnea, edema, weakness, and right upper quadrant discomfort. Chest examination typically discloses characteristics of the underlying lung disease.

On inspection, you may find such signs of cor pulmonale (and right ventricular failure) as dependent edema and distended neck veins. Drowsiness and alterations in consciousness may also occur.

Warning

CHECK OXYGEN CONCENTRATIONS

If your patient with cor pulmonale needs oxygen, double-check his condition. If he also has underlying COPD, don't administer high concentrations of oxygen. This could precipitate respiratory depression.

Palpation may disclose tachycardia and a weak pulse (from decreased cardiac output); an enlarged and tender liver; hepatojugular reflux; and a prominent parasternal or epigastric cardiac impulse.

Chest auscultation yields various findings, depending on the cause of cor pulmonale. If the patient also has COPD, auscultation may detect crackles, rhonchi, and diminished breath sounds. With disease secondary to upper airway obstruction or damage to the respiratory control center, auscultation findings may be normal except for a right ventricular lift, a gallop rhythm, and a loud pulmonic component of S_2.

If the patient has tricuspid insufficiency, you'll hear a pansystolic murmur at the lower left sternal border. The murmur's intensity increases when the patient inhales, distinguishing it from a murmur caused by mitral valve disease. Also, you may hear a right ventricular early murmur that increases on inspiration and can be heard at the left sternal border or over the epigastrium. You may also auscultate a systolic pulmonary ejection sound.

Diagnostic tests
• *Pulmonary artery catheterization* shows increased right ventricular and pulmonary artery pressures, resulting from increased pulmonary vascular resistance. Both right ventricular systolic and pulmonary artery systolic pressures will be over 30 mm Hg. Pulmonary artery diastolic pressure will be higher than 15 mm Hg.
• *Echocardiography* or *angiography* demonstrates right ventricular enlargement.
• *Chest X-rays* reveal large central pulmonary arteries and right ventricular enlargement.
• *Arterial blood gas (ABG) analysis* detects decreased PaO_2 — usually less than 70 mm Hg and never more than 90 mm Hg.

• *Electrocardiography (ECG)* discloses arrhythmias, such as premature atrial and ventricular contractions and atrial fibrillation during severe hypoxia. The ECG may also show right bundle-branch block, right axis deviation, prominent P waves and inverted T wave in right precordial leads, and right ventricular hypertrophy.
• *Pulmonary function tests* provide values consistent with underlying pulmonary disease.
• *Hematocrit* is typically over 50%.
• *Serum hepatic enzyme levels* show an elevated serum level of aspartate aminotransferase (formerly SGOT) with hepatic congestion and decreased liver function.
• *Serum bilirubin level* may be elevated if liver dysfunction and hepatomegaly are present.

Treatment
Therapy for the patient with cor pulmonale aims to reduce hypoxemia, increase exercise tolerance and, when possible, correct the underlying condition.

Besides bed rest, treatment may include digitalis glycosides, such as digoxin, and antibiotics for an underlying respiratory tract infection. (Usually, sputum culture and sensitivity tests determine which antibiotic the patient receives.) To treat primary pulmonary hypertension, the patient may receive a potent pulmonary artery vasodilator, such as diazoxide, nitroprusside, or hydralazine.

The patient may need oxygen administered by mask or cannula in concentrations ranging from 24% to 40%, depending on PaO_2 values. In acute disease, therapy may also include mechanical ventilation. (See *Check oxygen concentrations.*)

The patient may benefit from a low-sodium diet, restricted fluid intake and, possibly, a diuretic (furosemide, for example) to reduce edema.

Occasionally, the patient with cor pulmonale may require phlebotomy to decrease red blood cell mass. Anticoagulation with small doses of heparin can decrease the risk for thromboembolism.

Depending on the underlying cause, some treatment variations may be indicated. For example, the patient may need a tracheotomy if he has an upper airway obstruction. Or he may require corticosteroids if he has vasculitis or an autoimmune disorder.

Nursing diagnoses
• Activity intolerance
• Fluid volume excess
• Knowledge deficit
• Risk for injury

Nursing interventions

• Listen to the patient's fears and concerns about his illness. Remain with him when he feels severe stress and anxiety. Encourage him to identify actions and care measures that promote comfort and relaxation. Include him in care-related decisions whenever possible.

• Plan a nutritious diet carefully with the patient and the staff dietitian. Because the patient may tire easily, provide small, frequent feedings rather than three heavy meals. Avoid scheduling respiratory treatments immediately before meals.

• Prevent fluid retention by limiting the patient's fluid intake to 1,000 to 2,000 ml daily and by providing a low-sodium diet. Clarify the need for restricting fluids, especially if the patient has underlying COPD. (Most patients with COPD are encouraged to drink up to 10 glasses of water daily.)

• Monitor serum potassium levels closely if the patient takes a diuretic. Low serum potassium levels can potentiate the risk of arrhythmias associated with digitalis therapy.

• Be alert for complaints that signal digitalis toxicity, such as anorexia, nausea, vomiting, and seeing a yellow halo around an object. Monitor for cardiac arrhythmias.

• Reposition the bedridden patient often to prevent atelectasis.

• Provide meticulous respiratory care, including oxygen therapy and, for COPD patients, pursed-lip breathing exercises. Encourage the patient to rinse his mouth after respiratory therapies.

• Periodically, measure ABG levels and watch for signs of respiratory failure: change in pulse rate; deep, labored respirations; and increased fatigue produced by exertion.

• Pace patient care activities to avoid patient fatigue.

Patient teaching

• Before the patient's discharge, make sure he understands the importance of maintaining a low-sodium diet, weighing himself daily, and immediately reporting edema. Teach him to detect edema by pressing the skin over his shins with one finger, holding it for 1 to 2 seconds, and then checking for a finger impression. He should report a weight gain of 2 to 3 lb (0.9 to 1.4 kg) over 1 to 2 days to his doctor or nurse at once.

• Instruct the patient to schedule frequent rest periods and to perform his breathing exercises regularly.

• Because pulmonary infection usually exacerbates cor pulmonale (and COPD), advise the patient to watch for and immediately report early signs of infection, such as increased sputum production, change in sputum color, increased coughing or wheezing, chest pain, fever, and tightness in the chest. Tell the patient to avoid crowds, and people known to have infections, especially during the flu season.

• Warn the patient to avoid using nonprescription medications, such as sedatives, that may depress ventilatory drive. Teach him to check his radial pulse before taking digoxin or any digitalis glycoside. Instruct the patient to notify the doctor if he detects a pulse rate change.

• Urge the patient to discuss influenza and pneumonia immunizations with the doctor. Assist him to obtain the vaccines, if appropriate.

• Instruct the patient to add potassium-rich foods to his daily diet if he takes a potassium-wasting diuretic.

• If the patient needs suctioning or supplemental oxygen therapy at home, refer him to a social service agency that can help him obtain the equipment and care. As needed, arrange for follow-up examinations.

• If appropriate, discuss smoking cessation programs with the patient. Encourage him to quit smoking.

ATELECTASIS

Alveolar clusters (lobules) or lung segments that expand incompletely may produce a partial or complete lung collapse. Known as atelectasis, this phenomenon effectively removes certain regions of the lung from gas exchange. This allows unoxygenated blood to pass unchanged through these regions and produces hypoxia.

Atelectasis may be chronic or acute. The disorder occurs to some degree in many patients undergoing upper abdominal or thoracic surgery. The prognosis depends on prompt removal of any airway obstruction, relief of hypoxia, and reexpansion of the collapsed lung.

Causes

Atelectasis can result from bronchial occlusion by mucus plugs (a special problem in patients with chronic obstructive pulmonary disease), bronchiectasis, or cystic fibrosis. Mucus plugs may also affect lung expansion in patients who smoke heavily (smoking increases mucus production and damages cilia). The disorder may also result from occlusion caused by foreign bodies, bronchogenic carcinoma, and inflammatory lung disease.

Other causes include idiopathic respiratory distress syndrome of the newborn (hyaline membrane disease), oxygen toxicity, and pulmonary edema, in which changes in alveolar surfactant cause increased surface tension and permit complete alveolar deflation.

External compression, which inhibits full lung expansion, or any condition that makes deep breathing painful may also cause atelectasis. Such compression or pain may result from upper abdominal surgical incisions, rib fractures, pleuritic chest pain, tight chest dressings, and obesity (which elevates the diaphragm and reduces tidal volume).

What's more, lung collapse or reduced expansion may accompany prolonged immobility (which promotes ventilation of one lung area over another) or mechanical ventilation (which supplies constant small tidal volumes without intermittent deep breaths). Central nervous system depression (resulting from drug overdose, for example) eliminates periodic sighing and predisposes the patient to progressive atelectasis.

Complications
Atelectasis may cause hypoxemia and acute respiratory failure. Additionally, static secretions from atelectasis may lead to pneumonia.

Assessment findings
Clinical effects vary with the causes of lung collapse, the degree of hypoxia, and the underlying disease. If atelectasis affects a small lung area, the patient's symptoms may be minimal and transient. However, with massive collapse, the patient may report severe symptoms—for example, dyspnea and pleuritic chest pain.

Inspection may disclose decreased chest wall movement, cyanosis, diaphoresis, substernal or intercostal retractions, and anxiety.

Palpation may detect decreased fremitus and mediastinal shift to the affected side. Percussion may disclose dullness or flatness over lung fields. Auscultation findings may include crackles during the last part of inspiration and decreased (or absent) breath sounds with major lung involvement. Auscultation may also disclose tachycardia.

Diagnostic tests
• *Chest X-rays* are the primary diagnostic tool, although extensive areas of "microatelectasis" may exist without abnormalities appearing on the films. In widespread atelectasis, X-ray findings define characteristic horizontal lines in the lower lung zones. With segmental or lobar collapse, the films reveal characteristic dense shadows (commonly associated with hyperinflation of neighboring lung zones).
• *Bronchoscopy* may rule out an obstructing neoplasm or a foreign body if the cause of atelectasis can't be determined.
• *Arterial blood gas (ABG) analysis* may detect respiratory acidosis and hypoxemia resulting from atelectasis.
• *Pulse oximetry* may show deteriorating SaO_2 levels.

Treatment
Incentive spirometry, chest percussion, postural drainage, and frequent coughing and deep-breathing exercises may improve oxygenation in the patient with atelectasis. If these measures fail, bronchoscopy may help remove secretions. Humidity and bronchodilator medications can improve mucociliary clearance and dilate airways. These drugs may be administered by nebulizer or by a face mask device that establishes continuous positive airway pressure. Alternatively, intermittent positive-pressure breathing therapy may be prescribed.

If the patient has atelectasis secondary to an obstructing neoplasm, he may need surgery or radiation therapy. To minimize the risk for atelectasis after thoracic and abdominal surgery, the patient requires analgesics to facilitate deep breathing.

Nursing diagnoses
• Anxiety
• Fear
• Impaired gas exchange
• Ineffective airway clearance
• Ineffective breathing pattern
• Knowledge deficit
• Risk for infection

Nursing interventions
• Encourage the patient recovering from surgery (or other patients at high risk for atelectasis) to perform coughing and deep-breathing exercises every 1 to 2 hours. To minimize pain during these exercises, hold a pillow tightly over the patient's incisional area. Teach the patient how to do this for himself. *Gently* reposition the patient often, and help him walk as soon as possible. Administer adequate analgesics to control pain.
• Monitor mechanical ventilation. Maintain tidal volume at 10 to 15 cc/kg of the patient's body weight to ensure adequate lung expansion. Use the sigh mechanism on the ventilator, if appropriate, to intermittently increase tidal volume at the rate of 3 to 4 sighs/hour.
• Help the patient use an incentive spirometer to encourage deep breathing.
• Humidify inspired air, and encourage adequate fluid intake to mobilize secretions. Use postural drainage and chest percussion to remove secretions.
• Provide suctioning, as needed, for the intubated or uncooperative patient. Administer sedatives with care because these medications depress respirations and the cough reflex. They also suppress sighs. Keep in mind that the patient will cooperate minimally with treatment (or not at all) if he has pain.

• Assess breath sounds and respiratory status frequently. Report any changes immediately.
• Offer ample reassurance and emotional support because the patient's limited breathing capacity may frighten him.

Patient teaching
• Teach the patient how to use the spirometer. Urge him to use it every 1 to 2 hours.
• Show the patient and his family how to perform postural drainage and percussion. Instruct the patient to maintain each position for 10 minutes and then perform chest percussion. Let him know when to cough. Also, teach coughing and deep-breathing techniques to promote ventilation and mobilize secretions.
• Encourage the patient to stop smoking or to lose weight, or to do both, if needed. Refer him to appropriate support groups for help.
• Demonstrate comfort measures to promote relaxation and conserve energy. Advise the patient and his family to alternate periods of rest and activity to promote energy and prevent fatigue.

RESPIRATORY ACIDOSIS
This acid-base disturbance is characterized by reduced alveolar ventilation and manifested by hypercapnia ($PaCO_2$ greater than 45 mm Hg). (See *What happens in respiratory acidosis,* pages 644 and 645.) Respiratory acidosis can be acute (resulting from sudden failure in ventilation) or chronic (resulting from long-term pulmonary disease).

The prognosis depends on the severity of the underlying disturbance and the patient's general clinical condition.

Causes
Factors that predispose a patient to respiratory acidosis include:
• *drugs,* such as narcotics, anesthetics, hypnotics, and sedatives, which depress the respiratory control center's sensitivity
• *central nervous system (CNS) trauma,* such as medullary injury, which may impair ventilatory drive
• *chronic metabolic alkalosis,* which may occur when respiratory compensatory mechanisms attempt to normalize pH by decreasing alveolar ventilation
• *neuromuscular diseases,* such as Guillain-Barré syndrome, myasthenia gravis, and poliomyelitis, in which respiratory muscles fail to respond properly to respiratory drive, reducing alveolar ventilation.

In addition, respiratory acidosis can result from an airway obstruction or parenchymal lung disease that interferes with alveolar ventilation or from chronic obstructive pulmonary disease (COPD), asthma, severe adult respiratory distress syndrome, chronic bronchitis, large pneumothorax, extensive pneumonia, and pulmonary edema.

Complications
Acute or chronic respiratory acidosis can produce shock and cardiac arrest.

Assessment findings
The patient may initially complain of headache and dyspnea. He may also have a predisposing condition for respiratory acidosis. On inspection, you may see that he's dyspneic and diaphoretic. He may report nausea and vomiting.

Palpation may detect bounding pulses. Auscultation may reveal rapid, shallow respirations, tachycardia and, possibly, hypotension.

Ophthalmoscopic examination may uncover papilledema. And neurologic examination may disclose a level of consciousness (LOC) ranging from restlessness, confusion, and apprehension to somnolence, with a fine or flapping tremor (asterixis) and depressed reflexes.

Diagnostic tests
• *Arterial blood gas (ABG) analysis* confirms respiratory acidosis when $PaCO_2$ is above the normal 45 mm Hg; pH is typically below the normal range of 7.35 to 7.45; and HCO_3 levels are normal in acute respiratory acidosis but elevated in chronic respiratory acidosis.

Treatment
Effective treatment aims to correct the source of alveolar hypoventilation. If alveolar ventilation is significantly reduced, the patient may need mechanical ventilation until the underlying condition can be treated. This includes bronchodilators, oxygen, and antibiotics in COPD; drug therapy for conditions such as myasthenia gravis; removal of foreign bodies from the airway in cases of obstruction; antibiotics for pneumonia; dialysis to eliminate toxic drugs; and correction of metabolic alkalosis.

Dangerously low pH levels (less than 7.15) can produce profound CNS and cardiovascular deterioration and may require administration of I.V. sodium bicarbonate. In chronic lung disease, elevated CO_2 levels may persist despite treatment.

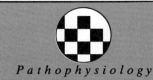

Pathophysiology

WHAT HAPPENS IN RESPIRATORY ACIDOSIS

These illustrations explain the basic pathophysiology of respiratory acidosis.

1. Pulmonary ventilation diminishes

When pulmonary ventilation decreases, retained carbon dioxide (CO_2) in the red blood cells combines with water (H_2O) to form excess carbonic acid (H_2CO_3). The H_2CO_3 dissociates to release free hydrogen (H^+) and bicarbonate ions (HCO_3^-). In this condition, ABG studies show increased $PaCO_2$ (over 45 mm Hg) and reduced blood pH (below 7.35).

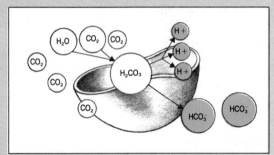

2. Oxygen saturation drops

As pH falls and 2,3-diphosphoglycerate (2,3-DPG) increases in red blood cells, 2,3-DPG alters hemoglobin (Hb) so it releases oxygen (O_2). This reduced Hb, which is strongly basic, picks up H^+ and CO_2, eliminating some free H^+ and excess CO_2. At this stage, arterial oxygen saturation (SaO_2) levels decrease, and the Hb dissociation curve shifts to the right.

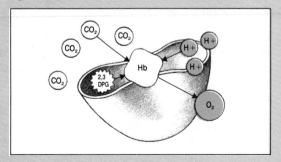

3. Respiratory rate rises

Whenever $PaCO_2$ increases, CO_2 levels increase in all tissues and fluids, including the medulla and cerebrospinal fluid. CO_2 reacts with H_2O to form H_2CO_3, which dissociates into H^+ and HCO_3^-. Elevated $PaCO_2$ and H^+ have a potent stimulatory effect on the medulla, increasing respirations to blow off CO_2. Look for rapid, shallow respirations and diminishing $PaCO_2$ levels.

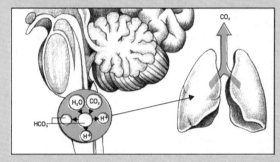

4. Blood flows to brain

The free H^+ and excess CO_2 dilate cerebral blood vessels and increase blood flow to the brain, causing cerebral edema and depressed CNS activity. At this stage, the patient experiences headache, confusion, lethargy, nausea, and vomiting.

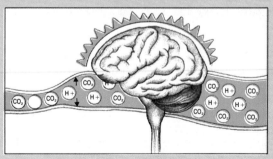

WHAT HAPPENS IN RESPIRATORY ACIDOSIS
(continued)

5. Kidneys compensate
As respiratory mechanisms fail, increasing $PaCO_2$ stimulates the kidneys to retain HCO_3^- and sodium ions (Na^+) and to excrete H^+. As a result, more sodium bicarbonate ($NaHCO_3$) is available to buffer free H^+. Ammonium ions (NH_4^+) are also excreted to remove H^+. A patient in this condition will have increased urine acidity and ammonium levels, elevated serum pH and HCO_3^- levels, and shallow, depressed respirations.

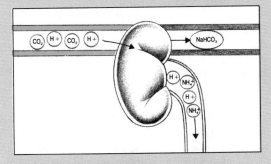

6. Acid-base balance fails
As H^+ concentration overwhelms compensatory mechanisms, H^+ ions move into the cells and potassium ions (K^+) move out. Without sufficient O_2, anaerobic metabolism produces lactic acid. Electrolyte imbalance and acidosis critically depress brain and cardiac function. ABG values in a patient in this condition show elevated $PaCO_2$ and decreased PaO_2 and pH levels. The patient will experience hyperkalemia, arrhythmias, tremors, decreased level of consciousness and, possibly, coma.

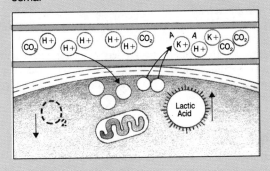

Nursing diagnoses
- Decreased cardiac output
- Fear
- Impaired gas exchange
- Ineffective airway clearance
- Risk for fluid volume deficit

Nursing interventions
- Be prepared to treat or remove the underlying cause, such as an airway obstruction.
- Be alert for critical changes in the patient's respiratory, CNS, and cardiovascular functions. Report any such changes immediately. Also report variations in ABG levels and electrolyte status.
- Maintain adequate hydration by administering I.V. fluids.
- Give oxygen (only at low concentrations in patients with COPD) if the PaO_2 level drops.
- Give aerosolized or I.V. bronchodilators. Monitor and record the patient's response to these medications.
- Start mechanical ventilation if hypoventilation cannot be corrected immediately. Continuously monitor ventilator settings.
- Maintain a patent airway and provide adequate humidification if acidosis requires mechanical ventilation.
- Perform tracheal suctioning regularly and chest physiotherapy, if ordered.
- To detect developing respiratory acidosis, closely monitor patients with COPD and chronic CO_2 retention for signs of acidosis. Also, administer oxygen at low flow rates and closely monitor all patients who receive narcotics and sedatives.
- Reassure the patient as much as possible, depending on his LOC. Allay the fears and concerns of family members by keeping them informed about the patient's status.

Patient teaching
- Instruct the patient who's recovering from a general anesthetic to turn, cough, and perform deep-breathing and coughing exercises frequently to prevent respiratory acidosis.
- If the patient receives home oxygen therapy for COPD, stress the importance of maintaining the dose at the ordered flow rate.
- Explain the reasons for ABG analysis. Discuss the blood-drawing technique and tell him that he may feel slight discomfort from the needle stick.
- Alert the patient to possible adverse reactions of prescribed medications. Tell him to call the doctor if any signs and symptoms occur.

RESPIRATORY ALKALOSIS

Marked by a decrease in $PaCO_2$ (less than 35 mm Hg) and a rise in blood pH above 7.45, respiratory alkalosis results from alveolar hyperventilation. Uncomplicated respiratory alkalosis leads to a decrease in hydrogen ion concentration, which raises the blood pH. Hypocapnia occurs when the lungs eliminate more CO_2 than the body produces at the cellular level. In the acute stage, respiratory alkalosis is also called hyperventilation syndrome.

Causes

Predisposing conditions to respiratory alkalosis include:
• congestive heart failure
• central nervous system (CNS) injury to the respiratory control center
• extreme anxiety
• fever
• overventilation during mechanical ventilation
• pulmonary embolism
• salicylate intoxication (early).

Complications

In extreme respiratory alkalosis, related cardiac arrhythmias may fail to respond to conventional treatment. Seizures may also occur.

Assessment findings

The patient history may reveal a predisposing factor associated with respiratory alkalosis. The patient may complain of light-headedness or paresthesia (numbness and tingling in his arms and legs).

On inspection, he may seem anxious with visibly rapid breathing. In severe respiratory alkalosis, tetany may be apparent with visible twitching and flexion of the wrists and ankles.

Auscultation may reveal tachycardia and deep, rapid breathing.

Diagnostic tests

• *Arterial blood gas (ABG) analysis* confirms respiratory alkalosis and rules out compensation for metabolic acidosis. $PaCO_2$ falls below 35 mm Hg; blood pH rises in proportion to a fall in $PaCO_2$ in the acute stage but drops toward normal in the chronic stage. The HCO_3 level is normal in the acute stage but below normal in the chronic stage.

• *Serum electrolyte studies* detect metabolic acid-base disorders.

Treatment

In respiratory alkalosis, treatment attempts to eradicate the underlying condition—for example, by removing ingested toxins or by treating fever, sepsis, or CNS disease. In severe respiratory alkalosis, the patient may need to breathe into a paper bag, which helps relieve acute anxiety and increase CO_2 levels. If respiratory alkalosis results from anxiety, sedatives and tranquilizers may help the patient.

Prevention of hyperventilation in patients receiving mechanical ventilation requires monitoring ABG levels and adjusting dead-space or minute ventilation volume.

Nursing diagnoses

• Anxiety
• Fatigue
• Fear
• Impaired gas exchange
• Ineffective breathing pattern

Nursing interventions

• Watch for and report changes in neurologic, neuromuscular, and cardiovascular functioning.
• Remember that twitching and cardiac arrhythmias may be associated with alkalemia and electrolyte imbalances. Monitor ABG and serum electrolyte levels closely. Report any variations immediately.
• Stay with the patient during periods of extreme stress and anxiety. Offer reassurance and maintain a calm, quiet environment.
• If the patient is coping with anxiety-induced respiratory alkalosis, help him identify factors that precipitate anxiety. Also help him find coping mechanisms and activities that promote relaxation.

Patient teaching

• Explain all care procedures to the patient. Allow ample time to answer his questions.
• Instruct the patient in anxiety-reducing techniques, such as guided imagery, meditation, or even yoga. Teach him how to counter hyperventilation with a controlled-breathing pattern.

PNEUMOTHORAX

An accumulation of air or gas between the parietal and visceral pleurae characterizes pneumothorax. The amount of air or gas trapped in the intrapleural space determines the degree of lung collapse. The most common types of pneumothorax are open, closed, and tension, and many factors contribute to pneumothorax. (See *What causes pneumothorax?*)

Causes and pathophysiology

Open pneumothorax—also called an open or sucking chest wound—results when atmospheric air (positive pressure) flows directly into the pleural cavity (negative pressure). As the air pressure in the pleural cavity becomes positive, the lung collapses on the affected side, resulting in substantially decreased total lung capacity, vital capacity, and lung compliance. The resulting ventilation-perfusion imbalances lead to hypoxia. Types of open pneumothorax include penetrating pneumothorax and traumatic pneumothorax.

Closed pneumothorax occurs when air enters the pleural space from within the lung, causing increased pleural pressure and preventing lung expansion during normal inspiration. Closed pneumothorax may be called traumatic pneumothorax when blunt chest trauma causes lung tissue to rupture, which results in air leakage.

Spontaneous pneumothorax, another type of closed pneumothorax, is more common in men than in women. It's common in older patients with chronic pulmonary disease, but it may occur in healthy, tall, young adults. Both types of closed pneumothorax can result in a collapsed lung with hypoxia and decreased total lung capacity, vital capacity, and lung compliance. The total amount of lung collapse can range from 5% to 95%.

In *tension pneumothorax*, air in the pleural space is under higher pressure than air in adjacent lung and vascular structures. The air cannot escape, and the accumulating pressure causes the lung to collapse. As air continues to accumulate and intrapleural pressures rise, the mediastinum shifts away from the affected side and decreases venous return. This forces the heart, trachea, esophagus, and great vessels to the unaffected side, compressing the heart and the contralateral lung. Without immediate treatment, this emergency can rapidly become fatal.

Complications

Extensive pneumothorax or tension pneumothorax can lead to fatal pulmonary and circulatory impairment.

Assessment findings

The patient history reveals sudden, sharp, pleuritic pain. The patient may report that chest movement, breathing, and coughing exacerbate the pain. He may also report shortness of breath.

WHAT CAUSES PNEUMOTHORAX?

The conditions and procedures listed below may trigger pressure changes that cause open, closed, or tension pneumothorax.

Open pneumothorax
• Penetrating chest injury, such as a gunshot or knife wound
• Insertion of a central venous catheter
• Chest surgery
• Transbronchial biopsy
• Thoracentesis or closed pleural biopsy

Closed pneumothorax
• Blunt chest trauma
• Air leakage from ruptured, congenital blebs adjacent to the visceral pleural space
• Rupture of emphysematous bullae
• Rupture resulting from barotrauma caused by high intrathoracic pressures during mechanical ventilation
• Tubercular or cancerous lesions that erode into the pleural space
• Interstitial lung disease, such as eosinophilic granuloma

Tension pneumothorax
• Penetrating chest wound treated with an airtight dressing
• Lung or airway puncture by a fractured rib associated with positive-pressure ventilation
• Mechanical ventilation (after chest injury) that forces air into the pleural space through damaged areas
• High-level positive end-expiratory pressure that causes alveolar blebs to rupture
• Chest tube occlusion or malfunction

Inspection typically reveals asymmetrical chest wall movement with overexpansion and rigidity on the affected side. The patient may appear cyanotic. In tension pneumothorax, he may have distended neck veins and pallor, and he may exhibit anxiety. (Test results may confirm increased central venous pressure.)

Palpation may reveal crackling beneath the skin, indicating subcutaneous emphysema (air in tissues) and decreased vocal fremitus. In tension pneumothorax, palpation may disclose tracheal deviation away from the affected side and a weak and rapid pulse. Percussion may demonstrate hyperresonance on the affected side, and auscultation may disclose decreased or absent breath sounds over the collapsed lung. The patient may be hypotensive with tension pneumothorax. Spontaneous pneumothorax that releases only a small amount of air into the pleural space may cause no signs and symptoms.

Diagnostic tests
• *Chest X-rays* reveal air in the pleural space and, possibly, a mediastinal shift, which confirms the diagnosis.
• *Arterial blood gas studies* may show hypoxemia, possibly accompanied by respiratory acidosis and hypercapnia. SaO_2 levels may fall initially but typically return to normal within 24 hours.

Treatment
Typically, treatment is conservative for spontaneous pneumothorax with no signs of increased pleural pressure (indicating tension pneumothorax), with lung collapse less than 30%, and with no dyspnea or other indications of physiologic compromise. Such treatment consists of bed rest; careful monitoring (blood pressure and pulse and respiratory rates); oxygen administration; and, possibly, aspiration of air with a large-bore needle attached to a syringe.

If more than 30% of the lung collapses, treatment to reexpand the lung includes placing a thoracostomy tube in the second or third intercostal space in the midclavicular line. The thoracostomy tube then connects to an underwater seal or to low-pressure suction.

Recurring spontaneous pneumothorax requires thoracotomy and pleurectomy. These procedures prevent recurrence by causing the lung to adhere to the parietal pleura. Traumatic and tension pneumothorax require chest tube drainage; traumatic pneumothorax may also require surgical repair. Analgesics may be prescribed.

Nursing diagnoses
• Altered tissue perfusion
• Anxiety
• Fear
• Impaired gas exchange
• Ineffective breathing pattern
• Knowledge deficit
• Pain
• Risk for infection

Nursing interventions
• Listen to the patient's fears and concerns. Offer reassurance as appropriate. Remain with the patient during periods of extreme stress and anxiety. Encourage him to identify actions and care measures that promote comfort and relaxation, and be sure to perform these measures and encourage the patient and his family to do so as well. Include the patient and his family in care-related decisions whenever possible.

• Keep the patient as comfortable as possible, and administer analgesics as necessary. The patient with pneumothorax usually feels most comfortable sitting upright.
• Watch for complications signaled by pallor, gasping respirations, and sudden chest pain. Carefully monitor vital signs at least every hour for indications of shock, increasing respiratory distress, or mediastinal shift. Listen for breath sounds over both lungs.
• Watch for signs of tension pneumothorax (especially if the patient has chest tubes inserted). These include falling blood pressure and rising pulse and respiratory rates, which could be fatal without prompt treatment.

For chest tube insertion:
• To facilitate chest tube insertion, place the patient in high Fowler's or semi-Fowler's position or supine. Or have him lie on his unaffected side with his arms overhead. During chest tube insertion, urge him to control the urge to cough and gasp. However, once the chest tube is placed, encourage him to cough and breathe deeply (at least once an hour) to facilitate lung expansion.
• Change the dressings around the chest tube insertion site at least every 24 hours. Keep the insertion site clean, and watch for signs of infection. Be careful not to reposition or dislodge the tube. If the tube dislodges, immediately place a petroleum gauze dressing over the opening to prevent rapid lung collapse; however, use extreme caution. If the lung has a hole or tear (evidenced by bubbling in the water-seal chamber), tension pneumothorax may be created by a tight dressing placement.
• Watch for continuing air leakage (bubbling). This indicates the lung defect's failure to heal, which may necessitate surgery. Also, watch for increasing subcutaneous emphysema by checking around the neck or at the tube's insertion site for crackling beneath the skin. For the patient receiving mechanical ventilation, watch for difficulty in breathing in time with the ventilator. Also watch for pressure changes on the ventilator gauges.

For thoracotomy:
• Urge the patient to control coughing and gasping during the procedure.
• Monitor vital signs frequently after thoracotomy. Also, for the first 24 hours, assess respiratory status by checking breath sounds hourly. Observe the chest tube site for leakage, and note the amount and color of drainage. Walk the patient, as ordered (usually on the first postoperative day), to promote deep inspiration and lung expansion.

Patient teaching
• Reassure the patient. Explain what pneumothorax is, what causes it, and all diagnostic tests and procedures.

If the patient is having surgery or chest tubes inserted, explain why he needs these procedures. Reassure him that the chest tubes will make him more comfortable.
• Encourage the patient to perform deep-breathing exercises every hour when awake.
• Discuss the potential for recurrent spontaneous pneumothorax and review its signs and symptoms. Emphasize the need for immediate medical intervention if these should occur.

HEMOTHORAX

This disorder occurs when blood enters the pleural cavity—from damaged intercostal, pleural, mediastinal vessels (or occasionally from the lung's parenchymal vessels). Depending on the amount of blood and the underlying cause of bleeding, hemothorax can cause varying degrees of lung collapse. About 25% of patients with chest trauma (blunt or penetrating) experience hemothorax. Pneumothorax (air in the pleural cavity) commonly accompanies hemothorax.

Causes

Hemothorax usually results from either blunt or penetrating chest trauma. Less often, it occurs as a consequence of thoracic surgery, pulmonary infarction, neoplasm, dissecting thoracic aneurysm, or anticoagulant therapy.

Complications

Hemothorax may result in mediastinal shift, ventilatory compromise, lung collapse and, without successful intervention, cardiopulmonary arrest.

Assessment findings

The patient history typically reflects recent trauma. In addition, the patient may complain of chest pain and sudden difficulty breathing, which may be mild to severe, depending on the amount of blood in the pleural cavity.

Inspection typically discloses a patient with tachypnea, dusky skin color, diaphoresis, and hemoptysis (bloody, frothy sputum). If hemothorax progresses to respiratory failure, the patient may show restlessness, anxiety, cyanosis, and stupor. As the chest rises and falls, you may notice that the affected side may expand and stiffen; the unaffected side may rise with the patient's gasping respirations.

Percussion may disclose dullness over the affected side of the chest; auscultation may detect decreased or absent breath sounds over the affected side, tachycardia, and hypotension.

Diagnostic tests

• *Thoracentesis* performed for diagnosis and therapy may yield blood or serosanguineous fluid. Fluid specimens may be sent to the laboratory for analysis.
• *Chest X-rays* display pleural fluid and detect mediastinal shift.
• *Arterial blood gas (ABG) analysis* documents respiratory failure.
• *Hemoglobin levels* may be decreased, depending on blood loss.

Treatment

In hemothorax, treatment aims to stabilize the patient's condition, stop the bleeding, evacuate blood from the pleural cavity, and reexpand the affected lung. Mild hemothorax usually clears in 10 to 14 days, requiring only observation for further bleeding. In severe hemothorax, treatment includes thoracentesis to remove blood and other fluids from the pleural cavity and then insertion of a chest tube into the sixth intercostal space in the posterior axillary line. The diameter of a typical chest tube is large to prevent clots from blocking it. Suction may also be used. If the chest tube doesn't improve the patient's condition, the surgeon may need to perform a thoracotomy to evacuate blood and clots and control bleeding.

Autotransfusion may be used if the patient's blood loss approaches or exceeds 1,000 ml. (See *Using autotransfusion for chest wounds,* page 650.)

Other treatment measures include oxygen therapy, I.V. therapy to restore fluid volume, and administration of analgesics.

Nursing diagnoses
• Altered tissue perfusion
• Anxiety
• Fluid volume deficit
• Impaired gas exchange
• Ineffective breathing pattern
• Pain
• Risk for infection

Nursing interventions
• Listen to the patient's fears and concerns. Offer reassurance as appropriate. Remain with the patient during periods of stress and anxiety. Encourage him to identify actions and care measures that promote comfort and relaxation. Be sure to perform these measures and encourage the patient and his family to do so as well. Include the patient and his family in care-related decisions whenever possible.

USING AUTOTRANSFUSION FOR CHEST WOUNDS

Used most often in patients with chest wounds—especially those that involve hemothorax—autotransfusion collects, filters, and reinfuses a patient's own blood. The procedure may also be used whenever two or three units of pooled blood can be recovered—for example, in cardiac or orthopedic surgery.

Autotransfusion eliminates the patient's risk for transfusion reaction or blood-borne disease, such as cytomegalovirus, hepatitis, and human immunodeficiency virus. It is contraindicated in patients with sepsis or cancer.

How autotransfusion works

A large-bore chest tube connected to a closed drainage system is used to collect the patient's blood from a wound or chest cavity. This blood passes through a filter, which catches most potential thrombi, including clumps of fibrin and damaged red blood cells (RBCs). The filtered blood passes into a collection bag. From the bag, the blood is reinfused immediately. Or it may be processed in a commercial cell washer that reduces anticoagulated whole blood to washed RBCs for later infusion.

Assisting with autotransfusion

• Set up the blood collection system as you would any closed chest drainage system. Attach the collection bag according to the manufacturer's instructions.
• If ordered, inject an anticoagulant, such as heparin or acid-citrate-dextrose solution, into the self-sealing port on the connector of the patient's drainage tubing.
• During reinfusion, monitor the patient for complications, such as blood clotting, hemolysis, coagulopathies, thrombocytopenia, particulate and air emboli, sepsis, and citrate toxicity (from the acid-citrate-dextrose solution).

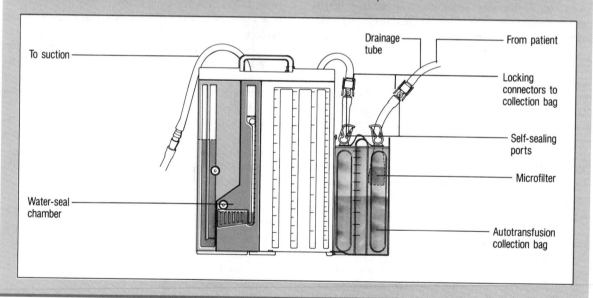

To suction

Water-seal chamber

Drainage tube

From patient

Locking connectors to collection bag

Self-sealing ports

Microfilter

Autotransfusion collection bag

• As ordered, give oxygen by face mask or nasal cannula.
• Administer blood transfusions, as ordered, using a large-bore needle.
• To treat shock, give I.V. fluids and blood transfusions, as ordered. Use a central venous pressure line to monitor treatment progress.
• Monitor ABG levels often. Also check hemoglobin levels and hematocrit, white blood cell count, and coagulation studies to determine blood replacement needs.
• Watch for complications signaled by pallor and gasping respirations.

• Monitor the patient's vital signs diligently. Watch for increasing pulse and respiratory rates and falling blood pressure, which may indicate shock or massive bleeding. Be prepared to get the patient ready for surgery.
• Give pain medication, as ordered, and record its effectiveness.
• Assist with thoracentesis.
• Observe chest tube drainage carefully. Record the volume, color, and character of drainage at least hourly. Immediately report a chest tube that's warm and full of blood and a rapidly rising bloody fluid level in the drain-

age collection chamber. The patient may need emergency surgery.
• Follow your institution's policy for milking the chest tube. If you can see bloody drainage or clots, milking may be permitted to keep the tube patent.
• Keep petroleum gauze at the bedside in case the chest tube dislodges. If it does, place the gauze over the chest tube site, taking care not to cover the wound so tightly that tension pneumothorax results.
• Don't clamp the chest tube; this may create tension pneumothorax.
• Change the chest tube dressing as necessary and according to hospital policy. Watch for signs of infection at the insertion site.
• Avoid all tubing kinks, tape all chest tube connections, and tape the tube securely to the patient's chest.

Patient teaching
• Explain all procedures to the patient and his family to allay their fears. Encourage the patient to ask questions about his care. Answer all questions as honestly as you can.
• If appropriate, provide preoperative and postoperative teaching. Explain and prepare the patient and his family for mechanical ventilation if necessary.
• Encourage the patient to perform deep-breathing exercises every hour whenever he's awake to promote gas exchange.
• Instruct the patient not to cough during thoracentesis.
• Discuss the rationale for chest tube therapy with the patient and his family.
• Instruct the patient to breathe deeply every hour when awake.

PNEUMONIA
An acute infection of the lung parenchyma that often impairs gas exchange, pneumonia can be classified in several ways. Based on microbiological etiology, it may be viral, bacterial, fungal, protozoal, mycobacterial, mycoplasmal, or rickettsial in origin.

Based on location, pneumonia may be classified as bronchopneumonia, lobular pneumonia, or lobar pneumonia. Bronchopneumonia involves distal airways and alveoli; lobular pneumonia, part of a lobe; and lobar pneumonia, an entire lobe.

Finally, the infection can be classified as one of three types—primary, secondary, or aspiration pneumonia. Primary pneumonia results directly from inhalation or aspiration of a pathogen, such as bacteria or a virus; it includes pneumococcal and viral pneumonia. Secondary

pneumonia may follow initial lung damage from a noxious chemical or other insult (superinfection) or may result from hematogenous spread of bacteria from a distant area. Aspiration pneumonia results from inhalation of foreign matter, such as vomitus or food particles, into the bronchi. (See *Understanding types of pneumonia,* pages 652 and 653.)

Pneumonia occurs in both sexes and at all ages. More than 3 million cases of pneumonia occur annually in the United States. The infection carries a good prognosis for patients with normal lungs and adequate immune systems. In debilitated patients, however, bacterial pneumonia ranks as the leading cause of death. Pneumonia is also the leading cause of death from infectious disease in the United States.

Causes and pathophysiology
In bacterial pneumonia, which can occur in any part of the lungs, an infection initially triggers alveolar inflammation and edema. Capillaries become engorged with blood, causing stasis. As the alveolocapillary membrane breaks down, alveoli fill with blood and exudate, resulting in atelectasis. In severe bacterial infections, the lungs assume a heavy, liverlike appearance, as in adult respiratory distress syndrome (ARDS).

Viral infection, which typically causes diffuse pneumonia, first attacks bronchiolar epithelial cells, causing interstitial inflammation and desquamation. It then spreads to the alveoli, which fill with blood and fluid. In advanced infection, a hyaline membrane may form. As with bacterial infection, severe viral infection may clinically resemble ARDS.

In aspiration pneumonia, aspiration of gastric juices or hydrocarbons triggers similar inflammatory changes and also inactivates surfactant over a large area. Decreased surfactant leads to alveolar collapse. Acidic gastric juices may directly damage the airways and alveoli. Particles with the aspirated gastric juices may obstruct the airways and reduce airflow, which in turn, leads to secondary bacterial pneumonia.

Certain predisposing factors increase the risk of pneumonia. For bacterial and viral pneumonia, these include chronic illness and debilitation, cancer (particularly lung cancer), abdominal and thoracic surgery, atelectasis, common colds or other viral respiratory infections, chronic respiratory disease (chronic obstructive pulmonary disease, asthma, bronchiectasis, cystic fibrosis), influenza, smoking, malnutrition, alcoholism, sickle cell disease, tracheostomy, exposure to noxious gases, aspiration, and immunosuppressive therapy.

UNDERSTANDING TYPES OF PNEUMONIA

Characteristics	Diagnostic tests	Treatment
Viral pneumonias		
Influenza • Prognosis poor even with treatment • 50% mortality from cardiopulmonary collapse • Signs and symptoms include cough (initially nonproductive; later, purulent sputum), marked cyanosis, dyspnea, high fever, chills, substernal pain and discomfort, moist crackles, frontal headache, myalgia.	• *Chest X-ray:* diffuse bilateral bronchopneumonia radiating from hilus • *White blood cell (WBC) count:* normal to slightly elevated • *Sputum smears:* no specific organisms	• Supportive treatment for respiratory failure includes endotracheal intubation and ventilator assistance; for fever, hypothermia blanket or antipyretics; for influenza A, amantadine.
Adenovirus • Insidious onset • Generally affects young adults • Good prognosis; usually clears with no residual effects • Signs and symptoms include sore throat, fever, cough, chills, malaise, small amounts of mucoid sputum, retrosternal chest pain, anorexia, rhinitis, adenopathy, scattered crackles, and rhonchi.	• *Chest X-ray:* patchy distribution of pneumonia, more severe than indicated by physical examination • *WBC count:* normal to slightly elevated	• Treatment aims to relieve symptoms.
Respiratory syncytial virus • Most prevalent in infants and children • Complete recovery in 1 to 3 weeks • Signs and symptoms include listlessness, irritability, tachypnea with retraction of intercostal muscles, slight sputum production, fine moist crackles, fever, severe malaise and, possibly, cough or croup.	• *Chest X-ray:* patchy bilateral consolidation • *WBC count:* normal to slightly elevated	• Supportive treatment includes humidified air, oxygen, and antimicrobials (often given until viral cause is confirmed).
Measles (rubeola) • Signs and symptoms include fever, dyspnea, cough, small amounts of sputum, coryza, rash, and cervical adenopathy.	• *Chest X-ray:* reticular infiltrates, sometimes with hilar lymph node enlargement • *Lung tissue specimen:* characteristic giant cells	• Supportive treatment includes bed rest, adequate hydration, antimicrobials and, if necessary, assisted ventilation.
Chicken pox (varicella) • Uncommon in children, but present in 30% of adults with varicella • Signs and symptoms include characteristic rash, cough, dyspnea, cyanosis, tachypnea, pleuritic chest pain, and hemoptysis and rhonchi 1 to 6 days after onset of rash.	• *Chest X-ray:* more extensive pneumonia than indicated by physical examination, and bilateral, patchy, diffuse, nodular infiltrates • *Sputum analysis:* predominant mononuclear cells and characteristic intranuclear inclusion bodies	• Supportive treatment includes adequate hydration and, in critically ill patients, oxygen therapy.
Cytomegalovirus • Difficult to distinguish from other nonbacterial pneumonias • In adults with healthy lung tissue, resembles mononucleosis and is generally benign; in neonates, occurs as devastating multisystemic infection; in immunocompromised hosts, varies from clinically inapparent to fatal infection • Signs and symptoms include fever, cough, shaking chills, dyspnea, cyanosis, weakness, and diffuse crackles.	• *Chest X-ray:* in early stages, variable patchy infiltrates; later, bilateral, nodular, and more predominant in lower lobes • *Percutaneous aspiration of lung tissue, transbronchial biopsy, or open lung biopsy:* typical intranuclear and cytoplasmic inclusions on microscopic examination (the virus can be cultured from lung tissue)	• Supportive treatment includes adequate hydration and nutrition, oxygen therapy, and bed rest.

UNDERSTANDING TYPES OF PNEUMONIA *(continued)*

Characteristics	Diagnostic tests	Treatment
Bacterial pneumonias		
Streptococcus • Caused by *Streptococcus pneumoniae* • Signs and symptoms include sudden onset of a single, shaking chill, and sustained temperature of 102° to 104° F (38.9° to 40° C); often preceded by upper respiratory tract infection.	• *Chest X-ray:* areas of consolidation, often lobar • *WBC count:* elevated • *Sputum culture:* possibly gram-positive *S. pneumoniae*	• Antimicrobial therapy consists of penicillin G or, if the patient is allergic to penicillin, erythromycin; therapy begun after obtaining culture specimen but without waiting for results and continues for 7 to 10 days.
Klebsiella • More likely in patients with chronic alcoholism, pulmonary disease, and diabetes • Signs and symptoms include fever and recurrent chills; cough producing rusty, bloody, viscous sputum (currant jelly); cyanosis of lips and nail beds from hypoxemia; shallow, grunting respirations.	• *Chest X-ray:* typically, but not always, consolidation in the upper lobe that causes bulging of fissures • *WBC count:* elevated • *Sputum culture and Gram stain:* possibly gram-negative cocci *Klebsiella*	• Antimicrobial therapy consists of an aminoglycoside and, in serious infections, a cephalosporin.
Staphylococcus • Commonly occurs in patients with viral illness, such as influenza or measles, and in those with cystic fibrosis • Signs and symptoms include a temperature of 102° to 104° F, recurrent shaking chills, bloody sputum, dyspnea, tachypnea, and hypoxemia.	• *Chest X-ray:* multiple abscesses and infiltrates; frequently empyema • *WBC count:* elevated • *Sputum culture and Gram stain:* possibly gram-positive staphylococci	• Antimicrobial therapy consists of nafcillin or oxacillin for 14 days if staphylococci are penicillinase-producing. • A chest tube drains empyema.
Aspiration pneumonia		
• Results from vomiting and aspiration of gastric or oropharyngeal contents into trachea and lungs • Noncardiogenic pulmonary edema possible with damage to respiratory epithelium from contact with gastric acid • Subacute pneumonia possible with cavity formation • Lung abscess possible if foreign body present • Signs and symptoms include crackles, dyspnea, cyanosis, hypotension, and tachycardia.	• *Chest X-ray:* location of areas of infiltrates (suggests diagnosis)	• Antimicrobial therapy consists of penicillin G or clindamycin. • Supportive therapy includes oxygen therapy, suctioning, coughing, deep breathing, adequate hydration, and I.V. corticosteroids.

Aspiration pneumonia is more likely to occur in elderly or debilitated patients, those receiving nasogastric tube feedings, and those with an impaired gag reflex, poor oral hygiene, or a decreased level of consciousness.

Complications

Without proper treatment, pneumonia can lead to such life-threatening complications as septic shock, hypoxemia, and respiratory failure. The infection can also spread within the patient's lungs, causing empyema or lung abscess. Or it may spread by way of the bloodstream or by cross-contamination to other parts of the body, causing bacteremia, endocarditis, pericarditis, or meningitis.

Assessment findings

In bacterial pneumonia, the patient may report pleuritic chest pain, a cough, excessive sputum production, and chills.

On assessment, you may note that the patient has a fever. During inspection, you may observe that the patient is shaking and coughs up sputum. Creamy yellow sputum suggests staphylococcal pneumonia; green sputum denotes pneumonia caused by *Pseudomonas* organisms; and sputum that looks like currant jelly indicates pneumonia caused by *Klebsiella*. (Clear sputum means that the patient doesn't have an infective process.)

In advanced cases of all types of pneumonia, you'll hear dullness when you percuss. Auscultation may disclose crackles, wheezing, or rhonchi over the affected lung area, as well as decreased breath sounds and decreased vocal fremitus.

Diagnostic tests

• *Chest X-rays* disclose infiltrates, confirming the diagnosis.
• *Sputum specimen* for Gram stain and culture and sensitivity tests shows acute inflammatory cells.
• *White blood cell count* indicates leukocytosis in bacterial pneumonia and a normal or low count in viral or mycoplasmal pneumonia.
• *Blood cultures* reflect bacteremia and help determine the causative organism.
• *Arterial blood gas (ABG) levels* vary, depending on the severity of pneumonia and the underlying lung state.
• *Bronchoscopy* or *transtracheal aspiration* allows the collection of material for culture. *Pleural fluid culture* may also be obtained.
• *Pulse oximetry* may show a reduced SaO_2 level.

Treatment

The patient needs antimicrobial therapy based on the causative agent. Therapy should be reevaluated early in the course of treatment.

Supportive measures include humidified oxygen therapy for hypoxia, bronchodilator therapy, antitussives, mechanical ventilation for respiratory failure, a high-calorie diet and adequate fluid intake, bed rest, and an analgesic to relieve pleuritic chest pain. A patient with severe pneumonia on mechanical ventilation may need positive end-expiratory pressure to maintain adequate oxygenation.

Nursing diagnoses

• Altered nutrition: Less than body requirements
• Anxiety
• Impaired gas exchange
• Ineffective airway clearance
• Pain
• Risk for fluid volume deficit
• Risk for infection

Nursing interventions

• Maintain a patent airway and adequate oxygenation. Measure the patient's ABG levels, especially if he's hypoxic. Administer supplemental oxygen if his PaO_2 falls below 55 to 60 mm Hg. If he has an underlying chronic lung disease, give oxygen cautiously. (See *Caring for a patient with pneumonia*.)
• In severe pneumonia that requires endotracheal intubation or a tracheostomy with or without mechanical ventilation, provide thorough respiratory care and suction often, using sterile technique, to remove secretions.
• Obtain sputum specimens as needed. Use suction if the patient can't produce a specimen. Collect the specimens in a sterile container and deliver them promptly to the microbiology laboratory.
• Administer antibiotics, as ordered, and pain medication, as needed. Administer I.V. fluids and electrolyte replacement, if needed, for fever and dehydration.
• Provide a high-calorie, high-protein diet of soft foods to offset the calories the patient uses to fight the infection. If necessary, supplement oral feedings with nasogastric (NG) tube feedings or parenteral nutrition.
• To prevent aspiration during NG tube feedings, elevate the patient's head, check the tube position, and administer the feeding slowly. Don't give large volumes at one time because this could cause vomiting.

If the patient has an endotracheal tube, inflate the tube cuff before feeding. Keep his head elevated for at least ½ hour after feeding.
• Monitor the patient's fluid intake and output.
• To control the spread of infection, dispose of secretions properly. Tell the patient to sneeze and cough into a disposable tissue, and tape a waxed bag to the side of the bed for used tissues.
• Provide a quiet, calm environment, with frequent rest periods. Make sure the patient has diversionary activities appropriate to his age.
• Listen to the patient's fears and concerns, and remain with him during periods of severe stress and anxiety. Encourage him to identify actions and care measures that promote comfort and relaxation.
• Whenever possible, include the patient in decisions about his care.
• Include the family in all phases of the patient's care, and encourage them to visit.

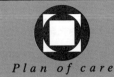

Plan of care

CARING FOR A PATIENT WITH PNEUMONIA

To give a patient with pneumonia the best chance for recovery, you need to develop a comprehensive plan of care. Here's one such plan, developed for 72-year-old Audrey Peters.

Patient history
Mrs. Peters has been receiving radiation treatment for metastatic breast cancer. She's come to the emergency department complaining of shortness of breath.

Mrs. Peters states that she feels "short of breath even when I'm watching television" and complains of a frequent cough that keeps her awake at night. She tells you she's been "feeling poorly" for the past 3 days with generalized fatigue and says she has lost about 6 lb (2.7 kg) over the past week because of a lack of appetite. She recalls an episode of shaking chills a few days before this visit, but although she's been feverish, she hasn't experienced any further chills.

Assessment findings
You begin with a respiratory assessment, noting that Mrs. Peters has a productive cough with rust-colored sputum. Her respiratory rate at rest is 26 breaths/minute. She uses accessory muscles to breathe, especially when turning in bed. When you percuss her chest, you find dullness over the left lung base. Palpation reveals increased vocal fremitus, and auscultation detects decreased breath sounds with inspiratory crackles at the left lung base.

Next, you take Mrs. Peters' temperature, which is 100.2° F (37.9° C). She has a heart rate of 110 beats/minute. You also note

that she has no tolerance for activity and becomes dyspneic with log-rolling.

Chest X-rays show left base consolidation, and Gram staining and culture and sensitivity tests are being run on sputum specimens. A white blood cell count is elevated to 18,000/mm³. Pulse oximetry reveals that Mrs. Peters has an SaO_2 level of 88% on room air.

Nursing diagnoses
Based on Mrs. Peters' low SaO_2 level, recent weight loss, and chronic disease state, you determine that promoting optimal gas exchange is a priority to avert acute respiratory failure. You also note that several other problems worsen Mrs. Peters' situation. You devise the following nursing diagnoses:
• Impaired gas exchange related to pulmonary infection and inflammation
• Ineffective airway clearance related to thick secretions and fatigue
• Altered nutrition: Less than body requirements, related to increased metabolic demands and anorexia
• Risk for fluid volume deficit related to hyperthermia, tachypnea, and decreased oral intake
• Anxiety related to breathlessness.

Expected outcomes
Based on these diagnoses, you set the following goals for Mrs. Peters. Within 3 days, she should:
• have increased aeration in the left lung base and decreased dullness on percussion and maintain adequate ventilation
• maintain a patent airway, demonstrate adequate expectoration of sputum, have a decreased quantity of produced sputum, and demonstrate controlled coughing technique; also have a decreased

respiratory rate and expend less breathing effort at rest
• show no further evidence of weight loss and tolerate oral, tube, or I.V. feedings without adverse reactions
• show no signs of dehydration, increase fluid intake to exceed output, and express an understanding of the need to maintain adequate fluid intake
• practice appropriate relaxation techniques and exhibit decreased anxiety.

Implementation
To reach these outcomes, you'll need to take the following steps.

To improve Mrs. Peters' gas exchange
• Administer oxygen, bronchodilators, and antibiotics as ordered.
• Assess her respiratory status every 2 to 4 hours, looking for signs and symptoms of respiratory distress.
• Auscultate for adventitious breath sounds every 2 to 4 hours.
• Monitor ABG and pulse oximetry results.
• Place the patient in semi-Fowler's position to promote lung expansion.

To improve airway clearance
• Provide chest physiotherapy, including vibration and postural drainage, every 4 hours as tolerated (given the primary diagnosis of metastatic breast cancer, don't perform percussion until conferring with the doctor).
• Encourage coughing and deep-breathing exercises every hour while Mrs. Peters is awake.
• Stagger care activities to provide uninterrupted rest periods.
• Advise intake of 2,000 to 3,000 ml of fluids per day to liquefy secretions.

(continued)

CARING FOR A PATIENT WITH PNEUMONIA *(continued)*

To improve nutrition
• Provide Mrs. Peters with a high-calorie, high-protein diet of soft foods.
• Supplement oral feedings with NG tube feedings or parenteral nutrition, if necessary.

To increase fluid volume
• Monitor Mrs. Peters' fluid intake and output.

• Assess her for such signs of dehydration as low urine output, dry skin, and sunken eyes.
• Administer fluids—if necessary, I.V. fluids—as prescribed.

To decrease anxiety
• Encourage Mrs. Peters to express her fears and concerns.
• Assure her that you'll be nearby.
• Include her in care decisions whenever possible.
• Teach her relaxation techniques,

and encourage her to practice them often.

Evaluation
You've met your goals if Mrs. Peters shows improved gas exchange after her pulmonary infection and inflammation have resolved; improved airway clearance, with decreased secretions and increased energy; improved nutrition, with a gradual increase in weight; improved hydration; and reduced anxiety.

Patient teaching

• Explain all procedures (especially intubation and suctioning) to the patient and his family.
• Emphasize the importance of adequate rest to promote full recovery and prevent a relapse. Explain that the doctor will advise the patient when he can resume full activity and return to work.
• Review the patient's medication. Stress the need to take the entire course of medication, even if he feels better, to prevent a relapse.
• Teach the patient procedures to clear lung secretions, such as deep-breathing and coughing exercises, as well as home oxygen therapy. Explain deep breathing and pursed-lip breathing.
• Urge the patient to drink 2 to 3 qt (2 to 3 liters) of fluid a day to maintain adequate hydration and keep mucus secretions thin for easier removal.
• Teach the patient and his family about chest physiotherapy. Explain that postural drainage, percussion, and vibration help to mobilize and remove mucus from the lungs.
• Urge all bedridden and postoperative patients to perform deep-breathing and coughing exercises frequently. Position such patients properly to promote full aeration and drainage of secretions.
• Advise patients to avoid using antibiotics indiscriminately for minor infections. Doing so could result in upper airway colonization with antibiotic-resistant bacteria. If pneumonia develops, the organisms that produce the pneumonia may require treatment with more toxic antibiotics.
• Encourage the high-risk patient to ask his doctor about an annual influenza vaccination and the pneumococcal pneumonia vaccination, which the patient would receive only once.

• Urge the patient to avoid irritants that stimulate secretions, such as cigarette smoke, dust, and significant environmental pollution. If necessary, refer him to community programs or agencies that can help him stop smoking.
• Discuss ways to avoid spreading the infection to others. Remind the patient to sneeze and cough into tissues and to dispose of the tissues in a waxed or plastic bag. Advise him to wash his hands thoroughly after handling contaminated tissues.

PULMONARY EMBOLISM

An obstruction of the pulmonary arterial bed, pulmonary embolism occurs when a mass—such as a dislodged thrombus—lodges in a pulmonary artery branch, partially or completely obstructing it. This causes a ventilation-perfusion mismatch, resulting in hypoxemia, as well as intrapulmonary shunting.

Pulmonary embolism strikes about 500,000 adults each year in the United States, causing 50,000 deaths. The prognosis varies. Although the pulmonary infarction that results from embolism may be so mild as to be asymptomatic, massive embolism (more than 50% obstruction of pulmonary arterial circulation) and infarction can cause rapid death.

Causes and pathophysiology

In most patients, pulmonary embolism results from a dislodged thrombus (blood clot) that originates in the leg veins. More than half of such thrombi arise in the deep veins of the legs; usually multiple thrombi arise. Other, less common sources of thrombi include the pelvic, renal, and hepatic veins, the right side of the heart, and the upper extremities.

Such thrombus formation results from vascular wall damage, venous stasis, or hypercoagulability of the blood. Trauma, clot dissolution, sudden muscle spasm, intravascular pressure changes, or a change in peripheral blood flow can cause the thrombus to loosen or fragmentize. Then, the thrombus—now called an embolus—floats to the heart's right side and enters the lung through the pulmonary artery. There, the embolus may dissolve, continue to fragmentize, or grow.

By occluding the pulmonary artery, the embolus prevents alveoli from producing enough surfactant to maintain alveolar integrity. As a result, alveoli collapse and atelectasis develops. If the embolus enlarges, it may clog most or all pulmonary vessels and cause death.

Rarely, pulmonary embolism results from other types of emboli, including bone, air, fat, amniotic fluid, tumor cells, or a foreign object, such as a needle, a catheter part, or talc (from drugs intended for oral administration that are injected I.V. by addicts).

The risk increases with long-term immobility, chronic pulmonary disease, congestive heart failure or atrial fibrillation, thrombophlebitis, polycythemia vera, thrombocytosis, cardiac arrest, defibrillation, cardioversion, autoimmune hemolytic anemia, sickle cell disease, varicose veins, recent surgery, age over 40, osteomyelitis, pregnancy, lower-extremity fractures or surgery, burns, obesity, vascular injury, cancer, and oral contraceptive use. (See *Who's at risk for pulmonary embolism?*)

Complications

If the embolus totally obstructs the arterial blood supply, pulmonary infarction (lung tissue death) occurs, a complication that affects about 10% of pulmonary embolism patients. It's more likely to occur if the patient has chronic cardiac or pulmonary disease.

Other complications include emboli extension, which blocks further vessels; hepatic congestion and necrosis; pulmonary abscess; shock and adult respiratory distress syndrome; massive atelectasis; venous overload; ventilation-perfusion mismatch; and death from massive embolism.

Assessment findings

The patient's history may reveal a predisposing condition. He may also complain of shortness of breath for no apparent reason, as well as pleuritic or anginal pain. The severity of these symptoms depends on the extent of damage. The signs and symptoms produced by small or fragmented emboli depend on their size, number, and location. If the embolus totally occludes the main pul-

WHO'S AT RISK FOR PULMONARY EMBOLISM?

Many disorders and treatments heighten the risk for pulmonary embolism. At particular risk are surgical patients. For example, the anesthetic used during surgery can injure lung vessels, and surgery itself or prolonged bed rest can promote venous stasis, which compounds the risk.

Predisposing disorders
• Lung disorders, especially chronic types
• Cardiac disorders
• Infection
• Diabetes mellitus
• History of thromboembolism, thrombophlebitis, or vascular insufficiency
• Sickle cell disease
• Autoimmune hemolytic anemia
• Polycythemia
• Osteomyelitis
• Long-bone fracture
• Manipulation or disconnection of central lines

Venous stasis
• Prolonged bed rest or immobilization
• Obesity
• Age over 40
• Burns
• Recent childbirth
• Orthopedic casts

Venous injury
• Surgery, particularly of the legs, pelvis, abdomen, or thorax
• Leg or pelvic fractures or injuries
• I.V. drug abuse
• I.V. therapy

Increased blood coagulability
• Cancer
• Use of high-estrogen oral contraceptives

monary artery, the patient will have severe signs and symptoms.

When you begin your assessment, you may find that the patient is tachycardic. He may also have a low-grade fever. If circulatory collapse has occurred, he'll have a weak, rapid pulse rate and hypotension.

On inspection, you may note a productive cough, possibly producing blood-tinged sputum. Less commonly, you may observe chest splinting, massive hemoptysis, leg edema and, with a large embolus, cyanosis, syncope, and distended neck veins. If you observe restlessness—

a sign of hypoxia—the patient may have circulatory collapse.

Palpation may reveal a warm, tender area in the extremities, a possible area of thrombosis. On auscultation, you may hear transient pleural friction rub and crackles at the embolus site. You may also note an S_3 and S_4 gallop, with increased intensity of the pulmonic component of S_2.

In pleural infarction, the patient's history may include heart disease and left ventricular failure. He may complain of sudden, sharp pleuritic chest pain accompanied by progressive dyspnea. On inspection, you may note that the patient has a fever and is coughing up blood-tinged sputum. Auscultation may reveal a pleural friction rub.

Diagnostic tests

• *Lung perfusion scan (lung scintiscan)* can show a pulmonary embolus.
• *Ventilation scan,* usually performed with a lung perfusion scan, confirms the diagnosis.
• *Pulmonary angiography* may show a pulmonary vessel filling defect or an abrupt vessel ending, both of which indicate pulmonary embolism. Although the most definitive test, it's only used if the diagnosis can't be confirmed any other way and anticoagulant therapy would put the patient at significant risk.
• *Electrocardiography (ECG)* helps distinguish pulmonary embolism from myocardial infarction. If the patient has an extensive embolism, the ECG shows right axis deviation, right bundle-branch block, tall peaked P waves, depressed ST segments, T-wave inversions (a sign of right ventricular heart strain), and supraventricular tachyarrhythmias.
• *Chest X-ray* helps rule out other pulmonary diseases, although it's inconclusive in the 1 to 2 hours after embolism. It may also show areas of atelectasis, an elevated diaphragm, pleural effusion, a prominent pulmonary artery and, occasionally, the characteristic wedge-shaped infiltrate that suggests pulmonary infarction.
• *Arterial blood gas (ABG) analysis* sometimes reveals decreased PaO_2 and $PaCO_2$ levels from tachypnea.
• *Thoracentesis* may rule out empyema, a sign of pneumonia, if the patient has pleural effusion.
• *Magnetic resonance imaging* can identify blood flow changes that point to an embolus or identify the embolus itself.

Treatment

The goal of treatment is to maintain adequate cardiovascular and pulmonary function until the obstruction resolves and to prevent any recurrence. (Most emboli resolve within 10 to 14 days.)

Treatment for an embolism caused by a thrombus generally consists of oxygen therapy, as needed, and anticoagulation with heparin to inhibit new thrombus formation. The patient on heparin therapy needs daily coagulation studies (partial thromboplastin time [PTT]). The patient may also receive warfarin for 3 to 6 months, depending on his risk factors. This patient's prothrombin time (PT) will be monitored daily and then biweekly.

If the patient has a massive pulmonary embolism and shock, he may need fibrinolytic therapy with urokinase, streptokinase, or alteplase. Initially, these thrombolytic agents dissolve clots within 12 to 24 hours. Seven days later, these drugs lyse clots to the same degree as heparin therapy alone.

If the embolus causes hypotension, the patient may need a vasopressor. A septic embolus requires antibiotic therapy, not anticoagulants, and evaluation for the infection's source, most likely endocarditis.

If the patient can't take anticoagulants or develops recurrent emboli during anticoagulant therapy, he'll need surgery. Surgery consists of vena caval ligation, plication, or insertion of a device (umbrella filter) to filter blood returning to the heart and lungs. Angiographic demonstration of pulmonary embolism should take place before surgery.

To prevent postoperative venous thromboembolism, the patient may require a vascular compression device applied to his legs. Or he can receive a combination of heparin and dihydroergotamine, which is more effective than heparin alone.

If the patient has a fat embolus, he'll need oxygen therapy. He may also need mechanical ventilation, corticosteroids and, if pulmonary edema arises, diuretics.

Nursing diagnoses

• Altered nutrition: Less than body requirements
• Altered tissue perfusion
• Anxiety
• Decreased cardiac output
• Diversional activity deficit
• Fear
• Impaired gas exchange
• Ineffective airway clearance
• Knowledge deficit
• Pain
• Risk for injury

Nursing interventions

• As ordered, give oxygen by nasal cannula or mask. If the patient has worsening dyspnea, check his ABG levels. If breathing is severely compromised, provide endotracheal intubation with assisted ventilation, as ordered.

• Administer heparin, as ordered, by I.V. push or by continuous drip. Monitor coagulation studies daily. Effective heparin therapy raises PTT to about 2 to 2½ times normal.

During heparin therapy, watch closely for epistaxis, petechiae, and other signs of abnormal bleeding. Also check the patient's stools for occult blood. Don't administer I.M. injections.

• After the patient stabilizes, encourage him to move about, and assist with isometric and range-of-motion exercises. Check his temperature and the color of his feet to detect venous stasis. *Never* vigorously massage his legs; that could cause thrombi to dislodge.

• If the patient needs surgery, make sure he ambulates as soon as possible afterward to prevent venous stasis.

• Provide the patient with adequate nutrition and fluids to promote healing.

• Watch for possible anticoagulant treatment complications, including gastric bleeding, cerebrovascular accident, and hemorrhage.

• If the patient has pleuritic chest pain, administer the ordered analgesic.

• If needed, provide incentive spirometry to help the patient with deep breathing. Provide tissues and a bag for easy disposal of tissues.

• Provide the patient with diversional activities to promote rest and relieve restlessness.

Patient teaching

• Explain all procedures and treatments to the patient and his family.

• Teach the patient and his family the signs and symptoms of thrombophlebitis and pulmonary embolism.

• Teach the patient on anticoagulant therapy the signs of bleeding he should watch for (bloody stools, blood in urine, large bruises).

• Tell the patient he can help prevent bleeding by shaving with an electric razor and by brushing his teeth with a soft toothbrush.

• Make sure the patient understands the importance of taking his medication exactly as ordered. Tell him not to take any other medications, especially aspirin, without asking the doctor.

• Stress the importance of follow-up laboratory tests, such as PT, to monitor anticoagulant therapy.

• Tell the patient that he must inform all his health care providers—including dentists—that he's receiving anticoagulant therapy.

• Instruct the patient taking warfarin not to significantly vary the amount of vitamin K he takes in daily. Doing so could interfere with anticoagulation stabilization.

• To prevent pulmonary emboli in a high-risk patient, encourage him to walk and exercise his legs, and to wear support or antiembolism stockings. Also, tell him not to cross or massage his legs.

SARCOIDOSIS

A multisystemic, granulomatous disorder, sarcoidosis characteristically produces lymphadenopathy, pulmonary infiltration, and skeletal, liver, eye, or skin lesions.

Sarcoidosis occurs most commonly in young adults ages 20 to 40. In the United States, sarcoidosis occurs predominantly among blacks and affects twice as many women as men. Acute sarcoidosis usually resolves within 2 years. Chronic, progressive sarcoidosis, which is uncommon, is associated with pulmonary fibrosis and progressive pulmonary disability.

Causes and pathophysiology

The cause of sarcoidosis is unknown, but several possibilities exist. The disease may result from a hypersensitivity response—possibly from T-cell imbalance—to such agents as atypical mycobacteria, fungi, and pine pollen. The incidence is slightly higher within families, suggesting a genetic predisposition. Or chemicals may trigger the disease (zirconium or beryllium lead to illnesses that resemble sarcoidosis).

Although the exact mechanism of the disease is unknown, research suggests a T-cell problem and, more specifically, a lymphokine production problem. In other granulomatous diseases, such as tuberculosis, granuloma formation occurs from inadequate pathogen clearance by macrophages. These macrophages require the help of T cells that secrete lymphokines, which, in turn, activate less effective macrophages to become aggressive phagocytes. Lack of lymphokine secretion by T cells may help explain granuloma formation in sarcoidosis.

Complications

Sarcoidosis can eventually lead to pulmonary fibrosis, with resultant pulmonary hypertension and cor pulmonale.

Assessment findings

The patient may report pain in her wrists, ankles, and elbows; general fatigue and a feeling of malaise; and unexplained weight loss. She may also complain of breathlessness and shortness of breath on exertion and have a nonproductive cough and substernal pain.

On inspection, you may observe erythema nodosum, subcutaneous skin nodules with maculopapular eruptions, and punched-out lesions on the fingers and toes. You may also note weakness and cranial or peripheral nerve palsies. When you inspect the nose, you may see extensive nasal mucosal lesions. Inspection of the eyes commonly reveals anterior uveitis. Glaucoma and blindness occasionally occur in advanced disease.

You may be able to palpate bilateral hilar and right paratracheal lymphadenopathy and splenomegaly, and you may hear such arrhythmias as premature beats on auscultation.

Diagnostic tests

A positive Kveim-Siltzbach skin test points to sarcoidosis. In this test, the patient receives an intradermal injection of an antigen prepared from human sarcoidal spleen or lymph nodes from patients with sarcoidosis. If she has active sarcoidosis, granuloma develops at the injection site in 2 to 6 weeks. When coupled with a skin biopsy at the injection site that shows discrete epithelioid cell granuloma, the test confirms the disease.

Several other tests support the diagnosis:
• *Chest X-rays* demonstrate bilateral hilar and right paratracheal adenopathy, with or without diffuse interstitial infiltrates. Occasionally, they show large nodular lesions in lung parenchyma.
• *Lymph node, skin,* or *lung biopsy* discloses noncaseating granulomas with negative cultures for mycobacteria and fungi.
• *Pulmonary function tests* indicate decreased total lung capacity and compliance, and reduced diffusing capacity.
• *Arterial blood gas (ABG) studies* show decreased PaO_2.
• *Tuberculin skin test, fungal serologies, sputum cultures* (for mycobacteria and fungi), and *biopsy cultures* are negative and help rule out infection.

Treatment

Asymptomatic sarcoidosis requires no treatment. However, sarcoidosis that causes ocular, respiratory, central nervous system, cardiac, or systemic symptoms (such as fever and weight loss) requires treatment with systemic or topical corticosteroids. So does sarcoidosis that produces hypercalcemia or destructive skin lesions. Such therapy usually continues for 1 to 2 years, but some pa-

tients may need lifelong therapy. A patient with hypercalcemia also requires a low-calcium diet and protection from direct exposure to sunlight.

If the patient has a significant response to the tubercular skin tests, showing tuberculosis reactivation, she'll need isoniazid therapy.

Nursing diagnoses
• Activity intolerance
• Altered nutrition: Less than body requirements
• Anxiety
• Dysfunctional grieving
• Fear
• Impaired gas exchange
• Knowledge deficit
• Risk for infection

Nursing interventions
• Watch for and report any complications. Also note any abnormal laboratory results (anemia, for example) that could alter patient care.
• If the patient has arthralgia, administer analgesics, as ordered. Record signs of progressive muscle weakness.
• Provide a nutritious, high-calorie diet and plenty of fluids. If the patient has hypercalcemia, speak to the dietitian about a low-calcium diet. Weigh the patient regularly to detect weight loss.
• Monitor the patient's respiratory function. Check chest X-rays for the extent of lung involvement, and note and record any increase in or bloody sputum. If the patient has pulmonary hypertension or end-stage cor pulmonale, monitor ABG levels, watch for arrhythmias, and administer oxygen, as needed.
• Because corticosteroids may induce or worsen diabetes mellitus, test the patient's urine for glucose and acetone at least every 12 hours at the beginning of corticosteroid therapy. Also, watch for other adverse effects, such as fluid retention, electrolyte imbalance (especially hypokalemia), moon face, hypertension, and personality changes.

During or after corticosteroid withdrawal (particularly if the patient has an infection or another stressor, such as emotional stress or an underlying condition), watch for and report vomiting, orthostatic hypotension, hypoglycemia, restlessness, anorexia, malaise, and fatigue. Remember that the patient on long-term or high-dose therapy is vulnerable to infection.
• Listen to the patient's fears and concerns, and remain with her during periods of extreme stress and anxiety. Encourage her to identify actions and care measures that will help make her comfortable and relaxed. Then try to

perform these measures, and encourage the patient to do so, too.
• Whenever possible, include the patient in care decisions, and include the family in all phases of the patient's care.

Patient teaching

• When preparing the patient for discharge, stress the need for compliance with the prescribed steroid therapy. Emphasize the importance of not skipping doses.
• Instruct the patient to take steroids with food.
• Make sure the patient understands the need for regular, careful follow-up examinations and treatment.
• Teach the patient to wear a medical identification bracelet or necklace indicating her corticosteroid therapy.
• Discuss the patient's increased vulnerability to infection, and review ways to minimize exposure to illness.
• Refer the patient with failing vision to community support and resource groups, including the American Foundation for the Blind, if necessary.

LUNG ABSCESS

An infection accompanied by pus accumulation and tissue destruction, a lung abscess is a localized lung infection. The abscess often has a well-defined border.

A lung abscess begins when bacteria localize in the lungs, usually from obstruction. This causes colliquative necrosis and lung destruction. Hematogenous bacterial spread may result in multiple abscesses throughout the lungs.

Effective antibiotic therapy has greatly decreased the incidence of lung abscesses.

Causes

Lung abscesses occur secondary to a localized area of pneumonia or in a necrotic area from a neoplasm that can't drain. Other causes include necrotizing infections from pyogenic bacteria, mycobacteria, fungi, and parasites; cavitary infarction from embolism, septic embolism, or vasculitis; cavitary cancer from primary bronchogenic carcinoma or metastatic cancers; infected cysts; and necrotic lesions from silicosis or coal worker's pneumoconiosis.

Complications

Chronic lung abscess may cause localized bronchiectasis, empyema and, rarely, massive hemorrhage.

Assessment findings

The patient has a history of coughing, sometimes with bloody, purulent, or foul-smelling or foul-tasting sputum; pleuritic chest pain; and dyspnea. He may also complain of a headache, a generalized feeling of malaise, and anorexia with resulting weight loss.

Inspection may show chills and fever, along with malaise and diaphoresis. You may also observe clubbing of the fingers.

On percussion, you'll note areas of dullness over affected lung tissue. When you auscultate the chest, you may hear crackles and decreased and cavernous breath sounds.

Diagnostic tests

• *Chest X-rays* show a localized infiltrate with one or more clear spaces that usually contain air and fluid. Earlier, the abscess may look like a solid mass until the liquefied material drains into a bronchus.
• *Percutaneous aspiration* of an abscess provides specimen cultures for identification of the causative organism.
• *Blood* and *sputum cultures* and *Gram stain* help determine the causative organism.
• *White blood cell count* is elevated (above 10,000/mm^3).
• *Computed tomography scan* helps differentiate the type of lesion.

If an abscess fails to close within 4 to 6 weeks after appropriate treatment and the patient's condition permits, bronchoscopy can provide a culture for identification of the causative organism and may indicate a drainage obstruction. (Bronchoscopy's use in initial evaluation is controversial.)

Treatment

Until X-rays show that the abscess has healed or stabilized, treatment consists of prolonged antibiotic therapy. Such therapy often lasts for months, even though signs and symptoms usually disappear in a few weeks. Failure of an abscess to improve with antibiotic treatment suggests a possible underlying neoplasm or another cause of obstruction.

Postural drainage may help drain necrotic material into the upper airways, where the patient can cough it up. Oxygen therapy may relieve hypoxemia.

The patient with massive hemoptysis, localized cancer, or bronchiectasis may need lesion resection or removal of the diseased lung section.

All patients also need rigorous follow-up and serial chest X-rays.

Nursing diagnoses
• Altered nutrition: Less than body requirements
• Anxiety
• Fatigue
• Fear
• Impaired gas exchange
• Ineffective airway clearance
• Knowledge deficit
• Pain
• Risk for infection

Nursing interventions
• Administer antibiotics as ordered and pain medication as needed. Record the patient's response.
• Perform chest physiotherapy, as ordered. Encourage the patient to perform deep-breathing and coughing exercises to loosen secretions.
• Keep in mind that excessive coughing and procedures to drain secretions, such as chest physiotherapy, may tire the patient. Encourage frequent rest periods and provide a calm, quiet environment. Encourage family visits, but emphasize the patient's need for rest.
• Ensure that the patient drinks enough fluids to help loosen secretions.
• To control the spread of infection, dispose of secretions properly. Make sure the patient has tissues, and tape a waxed bag to the side of the bed for used tissues.
• Provide a high-calorie diet. To conserve the patient's energy and avoid overexertion, give the patient small, frequent meals.
• To prevent lung abscess in the unconscious patient and in the patient with seizures, take steps to prevent aspiration of secretions. Suction the patient and position him to promote drainage of secretions. Give good mouth care.
• Listen to the patient's fears and concerns, and remain with him during periods of extreme stress and anxiety. Encourage him to identify care measures and actions that will make him comfortable and relaxed. Then, try to perform these measures, and encourage the patient to do so, too.
• Whenever possible, include the patient in care decisions, and include the family in all phases of the patient's care.

Patient teaching
• Explain all tests and procedures to the patient.
• Teach the patient and his family how to perform chest physiotherapy to promote removal of secretions.
• Teach the patient how to cough and deep breathe, and encourage him to do so often. Tell him to cough secretions into tissues, deposit them in the bedside receptacle,

and then wash his hands to prevent the spread of infection.
• Encourage the patient to maintain good oral hygiene.
• Advise the patient to follow a nutritious, high-calorie diet. Suggest that he eat small, frequent meals.
• Instruct the patient to drink plenty of fluids to loosen secretions.

PULMONARY HYPERTENSION
In both the rare primary form and the more common secondary form, pulmonary hypertension is indicated by a resting systolic pulmonary artery pressure (PAP) above 30 mm Hg and a mean PAP above 18 mm Hg.

Primary or idiopathic pulmonary hypertension is characterized by increased PAP and increased pulmonary vascular resistance, both without an obvious cause. This form is most common in women between ages 20 and 40 and is usually fatal within 3 to 4 years; mortality is highest in pregnant women.

Secondary pulmonary hypertension results from existing cardiac or pulmonary disease or both. The prognosis in secondary pulmonary hypertension depends on the severity of the underlying disorder.

Causes and pathophysiology
Although the cause of primary pulmonary hypertension remains unknown, the tendency for the disease to occur within families points to a hereditary defect. It also occurs more commonly in those with collagen disease and is thought to result from altered immune mechanisms. In primary pulmonary hypertension, the intimal lining of the pulmonary arteries thickens for no apparent reason. This narrows the artery and impairs distensibility, increasing vascular resistance.

Secondary pulmonary hypertension results from hypoxemia and can stem from any of the following:
• *Alveolar hypoventilation.* This can result from diseases that cause alveolar destruction, such as chronic obstructive pulmonary disease (the most common cause in the United States), sarcoidosis, diffuse interstitial pneumonia, malignant metastases, and scleroderma. Or it can stem from obesity or kyphoscoliosis, which don't damage lung tissue but prevent the chest wall from expanding sufficiently to let air into the alveoli.

Either way, the decreased ventilation that results increases pulmonary vascular resistance. Hypoxemia resulting from this ventilation-perfusion mismatch also causes vasoconstriction, further increasing vascular resistance. The result: pulmonary hypertension.

• *Vascular obstruction.* Such obstruction can arise from pulmonary embolism or vasculitis. It can also result from disorders that cause obstructions of small or large pulmonary veins, such as left atrial myxoma, idiopathic veno-occlusive disease, fibrosing mediastinitis, and mediastinal neoplasm.

• *Primary cardiac disease.* Such disease may be congenital or acquired. Congenital defects that cause left-to-right shunting include patent ductus arteriosus and an atrial or a ventricular septal defect. This shunting into the pulmonary artery reroutes blood through the lungs twice, causing pulmonary hypertension.

Acquired cardiac diseases, such as rheumatic valvular disease and mitral stenosis, result in left ventricular failure that diminishes the flow of oxygenated blood from the lungs. This increases pulmonary vascular resistance and right ventricular pressure.

Complications

Pulmonary hypertension may ultimately lead to cor pulmonale, cardiac failure, and cardiac arrest.

Assessment findings

The patient with primary pulmonary hypertension may have no signs or symptoms until lung damage becomes severe. (In fact, the disorder may not be diagnosed until an autopsy.)

Usually, a patient with pulmonary hypertension complains of increasing dyspnea on exertion, weakness, syncope, and fatigue. He may also have difficulty breathing, feel short of breath, and report that breathing causes pain. Such signs may result from left ventricular failure.

Inspection may show signs of right ventricular failure, including ascites and neck vein distention. The patient may appear restless and agitated and have a decreased level of consciousness (LOC). He may even be confused and have memory loss. You may observe decreased diaphragmatic excursion and respiration, and the point of maximal impulse may be displaced beyond the midclavicular line.

On palpation, you may also note signs of right ventricular failure, such as peripheral edema. The patient typically has an easily palpable right ventricular lift and a reduced carotid pulse. He may also have a palpable and tender liver and tachycardia.

Auscultation findings are specific to the underlying disorder but may include a systolic ejection murmur, a widely split S_2 sound, and S_3 and S_4 sounds. You may also hear decreased breath sounds and loud tubular sounds. The patient may have decreased blood pressure.

Diagnostic tests

• *Arterial blood gas (ABG) studies* reveal hypoxemia (decreased PaO_2).

• *Electrocardiography,* in right ventricular hypertrophy, shows right axis deviation and tall or peaked P waves in inferior leads.

• *Cardiac catheterization* discloses increased PAP, with a systolic pressure above 30 mm Hg. It may also show an increased pulmonary capillary wedge pressure (PCWP) if the underlying cause is left atrial myxoma, mitral stenosis, or left ventricular failure; otherwise, PCWP is normal.

• *Pulmonary angiography* detects filling defects in pulmonary vasculature, such as those that develop with pulmonary emboli.

• *Pulmonary function tests* may show decreased flow rates and increased residual volume in underlying obstructive disease; in underlying restrictive disease, they may show reduced total lung capacity.

• *Radionuclide imaging* allows assessment of right and left ventricular functioning.

• *Open lung biopsy* may determine the type of disorder.

• *Echocardiography* allows the assessment of ventricular wall motion and possible valvular dysfunction. It can also demonstrate right ventricular enlargement, abnormal septal configuration consistent with right ventricular pressure overload, and a reduction in left ventricular cavity size.

• *Perfusion lung scan* may produce normal or abnormal results, with multiple patchy and diffuse filling defects that don't suggest pulmonary thromboembolism.

Treatment

Oxygen therapy decreases hypoxemia and resulting pulmonary vascular resistance. For patients with right ventricular failure, treatment also includes fluid restriction, digitalis to increase cardiac output, and diuretics to decrease intravascular volume and extravascular fluid accumulation. Vasodilators and calcium channel blockers can reduce myocardial work load and oxygen consumption. Bronchodilators and beta-adrenergic agents may also be prescribed.

For a patient with secondary pulmonary hypertension, treatment must also aim to correct the underlying cause. If that's not possible and the disease progresses, the patient may need a heart-lung transplant.

Nursing diagnoses

• Activity intolerance
• Anxiety
• Decreased cardiac output

POTASSIUM-RICH FOODS

Teach the patient taking a potassium-wasting diuretic that the following foods can help meet his need for increased potassium:

- apricots
- bananas
- cantaloupe
- dried fruits
- grapefruit
- greens
- honeydew melon
- mushrooms

- nuts
- oranges
- peanut butter
- potato
- raw vegetables
- tomatoes
- winter squash.

- Fear
- Impaired gas exchange
- Knowledge deficit

Nursing interventions

- Administer oxygen therapy, as ordered, and observe the patient's response. Report any signs of increasing dyspnea so the doctor can adjust treatment accordingly.
- Monitor ABG levels for acidosis and hypoxemia. Report any change in the patient's LOC immediately.
- When caring for a patient with right ventricular failure, especially one receiving diuretics, record weight daily, carefully measure intake and output, and explain all medications and diet restrictions. Check for increasing neck vein distention, which may signal fluid overload.
- Monitor the patient's vital signs, especially his blood pressure and heart rate. If hypotension or tachycardia develops, notify the doctor. If the patient has a pulmonary artery catheter, monitor his PAP and PCWP, as ordered, and report any changes.
- Make sure the patient alternates periods of rest and activity to reduce his body's oxygen demand and prevent fatigue.
- Arrange for diversional activities. The type of activity—whether active or passive—depends on the patient's physical condition.
- Before discharge, help the patient adjust to the limitations imposed by this disorder.
- Listen to the patient's fears and concerns, and remain with him during periods of extreme stress and anxiety. Answer any questions he may have as best you can. Encourage him to identify care measures and activities that will make him comfortable and relaxed. Then try to perform these measures, and encourage the patient to do so, too.

- Include the patient in care decisions, and include the patient's family in all phases of his care.

Patient teaching

- Teach the patient what signs and symptoms to report to his doctor (increasing shortness of breath, swelling, increasing weight gain, increasing fatigue).
- Fully explain the medication regimen.
- If the patient smokes, encourage him to stop, and give him the names of programs to help him stop smoking.
- If necessary, go over diet restrictions the patient should follow to maintain a low-sodium diet.
- Teach the patient taking a potassium-wasting diuretic which foods are high in potassium. (See *Potassium-rich foods.*)
- Warn the patient not to overexert himself, and suggest frequent rest periods between activities.
- If the patient needs special equipment for home use, such as oxygen equipment, refer him to the social service department.

PLEURAL EFFUSION AND EMPYEMA

Normally, the pleural space contains a small amount of extracellular fluid that lubricates the pleural surfaces. But if fluid builds up from either increased production or inadequate removal, pleural effusion results. An accumulation of pus and necrotic tissue in the pleural space results in empyema, a type of pleural effusion. Blood (hemothorax) and chyle (chylothorax) may also collect in this space.

The incidence of pleural effusion increases with congestive heart failure (the most common cause) parapneumonia, cancer, and pulmonary embolism.

Causes and pathophysiology

A transudative pleural effusion—an ultrafiltrate of plasma containing a low concentration of protein—may result from congestive heart failure, hepatic disease with ascites, peritoneal dialysis, hypoalbuminemia, and disorders that increase intravascular volume.

The effusion stems from an imbalance of osmotic and hydrostatic pressures. Normally, the balance of these pressures in parietal pleural capillaries causes fluid to move into the pleural space; balanced pressure in visceral pleural capillaries promotes reabsorption of this fluid. But when excessive hydrostatic pressure or decreased osmotic pressure causes excessive fluid to pass across intact capillaries, a transudative pleural effusion results.

Exudative pleural effusions can result from tuberculosis, subphrenic abscess, pancreatitis, bacterial or fungal pneumonitis or empyema, cancer, parapneumonia, pulmonary embolism (with or without infarction), collagen disease (lupus erythematosus and rheumatoid arthritis), myxedema, intra-abdominal abscess, esophageal perforation, and chest trauma.

Such an effusion occurs when capillary permeability increases, with or without changes in hydrostatic and colloid osmotic pressures, allowing protein-rich fluid to leak into the pleural space.

Empyema usually stems from an infection in the pleural space. The infection may be idiopathic or may be related to pneumonitis, carcinoma, perforation, penetrating chest trauma, or esophageal rupture.

Complications
Large pleural effusions may result in atelectasis, infection, and hypoxemia.

Assessment findings
The patient's history characteristically shows underlying pulmonary disease. If he has a large amount of effusion, he'll typically complain of dyspnea. If he has pleurisy, he may report pleuritic chest pain. If he has empyema, he may also complain of a general feeling of malaise.

Inspection may indicate that the trachea has deviated away from the affected side. With empyema, the patient may also have a fever.

On palpation, you may note decreased tactile fremitus with a large amount of effusion. Percussion may disclose dullness over the effused area that doesn't change with respiration.

When you auscultate the chest, you may hear diminished or absent breath sounds over the effusion and a pleural friction rub during both inspiration and expiration. (This pleural friction rub is transitory, however, and disappears as fluid accumulates in the pleural space.) You'll also hear bronchial breath sounds, sometimes with the patient's pronunciation of the letter E sounding like the letter A.

Diagnostic tests
Thoracentesis allows analysis of aspirated fluid and may show the following:
• Transudative effusion usually has a specific gravity below 1.015 and contains less than 3 g/dl of protein.
• Exudative effusion has a ratio of protein in the fluid to serum of more than or equal to 0.5, pleural fluid lactate dehydrogenase (LDH) of greater than or equal to 200 IU,
and a ratio of LDH in pleural fluid to LDH in serum of more than or equal to 0.6.
• Aspirated fluid in empyema contains acute inflammatory white blood cells and microorganisms and shows leukocytosis.
• Fluid in empyema and rheumatoid arthritis—which can be the cause of an exudative pleural effusion—shows an extremely decreased pleural fluid glucose level.
• Pleural effusion that results from esophageal rupture or pancreatitis usually has fluid amylase levels higher than serum levels.

Aspirated fluid may also be tested for lupus erythematosus cells, antinuclear antibodies, and neoplastic cells. Plus, it may be analyzed for color and consistency; acid-fast bacillus, fungal, and bacterial cultures; and triglycerides (in chylothorax).

Other diagnostic tests may also be ordered. A negative tuberculin skin test helps rule out tuberculosis as a cause. If thoracentesis doesn't provide a definitive diagnosis in exudative pleural effusion, a pleural biopsy can help confirm tuberculosis or cancer.

Treatment
Depending on the amount of fluid present, symptomatic effusion may require thoracentesis to remove fluid or careful monitoring of the patient's own reabsorption of the fluid. Chemical pleurodesis—the instillation of a sclerosing agent, such as tetracycline, bleomycin, or nitrogen mustard through the chest tube to create adhesions between the two pleurae—may prevent recurrent effusions.

The patient with empyema needs one or more chest tubes inserted after thoracentesis. These tubes allow purulent material to drain. He may also need decortication (surgical removal of the thick coating over the lung) or rib resection to allow open drainage and lung expansion. He'll also require parenteral antibiotics and, if he has hypoxia, oxygen administration.

Hemothorax requires drainage to prevent fibrothorax formation.

Nursing diagnoses
• Anxiety
• Impaired gas exchange
• Ineffective breathing pattern
• Knowledge deficit
• Risk for infection

Nursing interventions
• During thoracentesis, remind the patient to breathe normally and avoid sudden movements, such as cough-

ing or sighing. Monitor his vital signs, and watch for syncope. Also be alert for bradycardia, hypotension, pain, pulmonary edema, and cardiac arrest—indications that fluid is being removed too quickly. Reassure the patient throughout the procedure.

• After thoracentesis, watch for respiratory distress and signs of pneumothorax (sudden onset of dyspnea and cyanosis).

• Allow enough time between premedications and the procedure. Postoperative sedatives and analgesics aren't nearly as effective.

• Administer oxygen and, in empyema, antibiotics, as ordered. Record the patient's response to these care measures.

• Use an incentive spirometer to promote deep breathing, and encourage the patient to perform deep-breathing exercises to promote lung expansion.

• Provide meticulous chest tube care, and use aseptic technique for changing dressings around the tube insertion site in the patient with empyema. Ensure tube patency by watching for bubbles in the underwater-seal chamber. Record the amount, color, and consistency of any tube drainage.

• Follow your hospital's policy for milking the tube. Keep petroleum gauze at the bedside in case of chest tube dislodgment.

• Don't clamp the chest tube; this may cause tension pneumothorax.

• If the patient has open drainage through a rib resection or intercostal tube, use secretion precautions. The patient will usually need weeks of such drainage to obliterate the space, so make home health nurse referrals if he'll be discharged with the tube in place.

• Throughout therapy, listen to the patient's fears and concerns and remain with him during periods of extreme stress and anxiety. Encourage him to identify care measures and actions that will make him comfortable and relaxed. Then try to perform these measures, and encourage the patient to do so, too.

Patient teaching
• Explain all tests and procedures to the patient, including thoracentesis, and answer any questions he may have.

• Before thoracentesis, tell the patient to expect a stinging sensation from the local anesthetic and a feeling of pressure when the needle is inserted. Instruct him to tell you immediately if he feels uncomfortable or has trouble breathing during the procedure.

• If the patient developed pleural effusion because of pneumonia or influenza, tell him to seek medical attention promptly whenever he gets a chest cold.

• Teach the patient the signs and symptoms of respiratory distress. If any of these develop, tell him to notify his doctor.

• Fully explain the medication regimen, including adverse effects. Emphasize the importance of completing the prescribed drug regimen.

• If the patient smokes, urge him to stop.

PLEURISY
Also called pleuritis, pleurisy is an inflammation of the visceral and parietal pleurae that line the inside of the thoracic cage and envelop the lungs. The disorder causes the pleurae to become swollen and congested, hampering pleural fluid transport and increasing friction between the pleural surfaces.

Causes
Pleurisy can result from pneumonia, tuberculosis, viruses, systemic lupus erythematosus, rheumatoid arthritis, uremia, Dressler's syndrome, cancer, pulmonary infarction, and chest trauma.

Complications
Extensively inflamed pleural membranes may result in permanent adhesions that can restrict lung expansion. The inflammation can also stimulate excessive production and hinder reabsorption of pleural fluid, leading to pleural effusion.

Assessment findings
The patient may report a sudden, sharp, stabbing pain that worsens on inspiration, the result of inflammation or irritation of sensory nerve endings in the parietal pleura that rub against one another during respiration. He may tell you that the pain is so severe it limits his movement on the affected side during breathing. He may also have dyspnea. Other symptoms vary, depending on the underlying pathologic process.

When you auscultate the chest, you may hear a characteristic pleural friction rub—a coarse, creaky sound heard during late inspiration and early expiration—directly over the area of pleural inflammation. Palpation over the affected area may reveal coarse vibration.

Diagnostic tests
Although diagnosis generally rests on the patient's history and your respiratory assessment, diagnostic tests

help rule out other causes and pinpoint the underlying disorder. Electrocardiography rules out coronary artery disease as the source of the patient's pain, and chest X-rays can identify pneumonia.

Treatment
Symptomatic treatment includes anti-inflammatory agents, analgesics, and bed rest. Severe pain may require an intercostal nerve block of two or three intercostal nerves. Pleurisy with pleural effusion calls for thoracentesis as both a diagnostic and a therapeutic measure.

Nursing diagnoses
• Activity intolerance
• Anxiety
• Impaired gas exchange
• Ineffective airway clearance
• Ineffective breathing pattern
• Pain

Nursing interventions
• Assess the patient for pain every 3 hours, and administer antitussives and pain medication. Make sure you don't overmedicate. Pain relief allows for maximum chest expansion.
• Encourage the patient to take deep breaths and to cough. To minimize pain, apply firm pressure at the site of the pain while the patient coughs.
• Position the patient in high-Fowler's position to help lung expansion. Lying him on the affected side may aid in splinting.
• Assess the patient's respiratory status at least every 4 hours to detect early signs of compromise. Also monitor for such complications as fever, increased dyspnea, and changes in breath sounds.
• Plan your care to allow the patient as much uninterrupted rest as possible.
• Pain may impair the patient's mobility, so help him perform active and passive range-of-motion exercises to prevent contractures and promote muscle strength.
• If the patient needs thoracentesis, remind him to breathe normally and avoid sudden movements, such as coughing or sighing, during the procedure. Monitor his vital signs, and watch for syncope. Also watch for bradycardia, hypotension, pain, pulmonary edema, and cardiac arrest—indications that fluid is being removed too quickly. Reassure the patient throughout the procedure.

After thoracentesis, watch for respiratory distress and signs of pneumothorax (sudden onset of dyspnea and cyanosis).

• Throughout therapy, listen to the patient's fears and concerns, and answer any questions he may have. Remain with him during periods of extreme stress and anxiety. Encourage him to identify actions and care measures that will help make him comfortable and relaxed. Then try to perform these measures, and encourage the patient to do so, too.
• Whenever possible, include the patient in care decisions, and include the family in all phases of the patient's care.

Patient teaching
• Explain all procedures to the patient and his family.
• If the patient requires thoracentesis, explain the procedure. Tell him to expect a stinging sensation from the local anesthetic and a feeling of pressure as the needle is inserted. Instruct him to tell you immediately if he feels uncomfortable or has trouble breathing during the procedure.
• If the patient about to be discharged receives a perscription for a narcotic analgesic for pain, warn him about the dangers of overuse. Explain that the drug depresses coughing and respiration and decreases alertness. Also, teach him about the drug's other possible adverse effects, and tell him to call his doctor if such effects occur.
• Teach the patient how to splint and perform deep-breathing exercises.
• Emphasize the need for regular rest periods.
• Teach the patient the signs and symptoms of possible complications, such as increased shortness of breath, fever, increasing fatigue, or any change in the quality or quantity of secretions. Tell him to call his doctor if such signs or symptoms occur.
• Reassure the patient that the pain should subside after several days.

CHRONIC DISORDERS

Several factors can lead to chronic respiratory disorders. For instance, a genetic defect leads to cystic fibrosis, whereas damage to the bronchial wall results in bronchiectasis. Environmental factors cause emphysema and chronic bronchitis, infection causes pulmonary tuberculosis, and occupational hazards lead to silicosis, asbestosis, berylliosis, and coal worker's pneumoconiosis.

CYSTIC FIBROSIS

A chronic, progressive, inherited disease, cystic fibrosis affects the exocrine (mucus-secreting) glands. The disease is transmitted as an autosomal recessive trait and is the most common fatal genetic disease of white children. When both parents are carriers of the recessive gene, they have a 25% chance of transmitting the disease with each pregnancy.

Cystic fibrosis increases the viscosity of bronchial, pancreatic, and other mucus gland secretions, obstructing glandular ducts. The accumulation of thick, tenacious secretions in the bronchioles and alveoli causes respiratory changes, eventually leading to severe atelectasis and emphysema.

The disease also causes characteristic GI effects in the intestines, pancreas, and liver. Obstruction of the pancreatic ducts results in a deficiency of trypsin, amylase, and lipase, which prevents the conversion and absorption of fat and protein in the intestinal tract. This interferes with the digestion of food and the absorption of fat-soluble vitamins (A, D, E, and K). In the pancreas, fibrotic tissue, multiple cysts, thick mucus, and fat replace the acini (small, saclike swellings normally found in this gland), producing signs of pancreatic insufficiency (insufficient insulin production, abnormal glucose tolerance, and glycosuria).

The incidence of cystic fibrosis is highest in people of northern European ancestry (about 1 in 2,000 live births). The disease is less common in African Americans (1 in 17,000 live births), Native Americans, and people of Asian ancestry. It occurs with equal frequency in both sexes.

Cystic fibrosis is incurable. But as medical research seeks to find better treatment, life expectancy has greatly increased. One-half of all patients with cystic fibrosis today are over age 28. Many survive to age 40, and a few have survived to age 50 or older.

Causes and pathophysiology

Cystic fibrosis is inherited as an autosomal recessive trait. The responsible gene is on chromosome 7. Researchers have found that most cases of cystic fibrosis arise from a mutation in this gene that causes it to encode a single amino acid, resulting in an abnormal protein that adversely affects membrane transport.

The defective protein resembles other transmembrane transport proteins. However, it lacks a phenylalanine that appears in proteins produced by normal genes. Researchers speculate that this abnormal protein may interfere with chloride transport by preventing adenosine triphosphate from binding to the protein or by interfering with activation by protein kinases. This leads to dehydration and mucosal thickening in the respiratory and intestinal tracts and may explain the characteristic elevated sweat chloride levels that occur in cystic fibrosis.

However, this abnormal protein is only the major defect in the cystic fibrosis gene. Other gene mutations remain to be found.

Complications

Cystic fibrosis can cause bronchiectasis, pneumonia, atelectasis, hemoptysis, dehydration, distal intestinal obstructive syndrome, malnutrition, gastroesophageal reflux, nasal polyps, rectal prolapse, and cor pulmonale. Other, inevitable complications that occur as the disease progresses include hepatic disease, diabetes, pneumothorax, arthritis, pancreatitis, and cholecystitis.

A deficiency of fat-soluble vitamins can lead to clotting problems, retarded bone growth, and delayed sexual development. Males may experience azoospermia; females may experience secondary amenorrhea.

Hypochloremia and hyponatremia from increased sodium and chloride concentrations in sweat can induce cardiac arrhythmias and potentially fatal shock, especially in hot weather, when sweating is profuse.

Biliary obstruction and fibrosis may prolong neonatal jaundice. In some patients, cirrhosis and portal hypertension may lead to esophageal varices, episodes of hematemesis and, occasionally, hepatomegaly.

Assessment findings

A neonate with cystic fibrosis shows meconium ileus—a failure to excrete meconium, the dark green mucilaginous material found in the intestine at birth. Your assessment of such an infant may reveal signs of intestinal obstruction, such as abdominal distention, vomiting, constipation, and dehydration.

Other signs, which may be apparent soon after birth or years later, include major aberrations in sweat gland and GI functions (sweat gland dysfunction ranks as the most consistent abnormality). The patient may also complain of frequent upper respiratory tract infections, dyspnea, paroxysmal cough, frequent bouts of pneumonia, and other types of severe respiratory dysfunction.

A young child typically has a history of poor weight gain and poor growth, despite a healthy appetite. The parents may describe the child's stools as frequent, bulky, foul-smelling, and pale.

Inspection of the child may reveal a barrel chest, cyanosis, and clubbing of the fingers and toes. He may cough up tenacious, yellow-green sputum. Palpation may show a distended abdomen. On auscultation, you may hear wheezy respirations and crackles.

Diagnostic tests

According to the Cystic Fibrosis Foundation, a definitive diagnosis requires:
• two clearly positive sweat tests, using pilocarpine solution (a sweat inducer), and the presence of an obstructive pulmonary disease, confirmed pancreatic insufficiency or failure to thrive, or a family history of cystic fibrosis
• chest X-rays that show early signs of lung obstruction
• stool specimen analysis that shows the absence of trypsin, suggesting pancreatic insufficiency.

The following test results may support the diagnosis:
• Deoxyribonucleic acid (DNA) testing can now locate the presence of the Delta F 508 deletion (found in about 70% of cystic fibrosis patients, although the disease can cause more than 100 other mutations). This test can also be used for carrier detection and prenatal diagnosis in families with a previously affected child.
• If pulmonary exacerbation exists, pulmonary function tests can reveal decreased vital capacity, elevated residual volume due to air entrapments, and decreased forced expiratory volume in 1 second.
• A liver enzyme test may reveal hepatic insufficiency.
• A sputum culture may reveal organisms that patients typically and chronically colonize, such as *Pseudomonas* and *Staphylococcus*.
• A serum albumin level helps assess nutritional status.
• Electrolyte analysis assesses for dehydration.

Treatment

Because cystic fibrosis has no cure, treatment aims to help the patient lead as normal a life as possible. Specific treatments depend on the organ systems involved.
• To combat electrolyte loss through sweat, the patient should generously salt his food and, during hot weather, take salt supplements.
• Oral pancreatic enzymes taken with meals and snacks offsets pancreatic enzyme deficiencies. Such supplements improve absorption and digestion and help satisfy hunger on a reasonable caloric intake. The patient should also follow a diet that's low in fat and high in protein and calories and includes vitamin A, D, E, and K supplements.
• To manage pulmonary dysfunction, the patient should undergo chest physiotherapy, nebulization to loosen secretions followed by postural drainage, and breathing exercises several times daily to help remove lung secretions. But he shouldn't receive antihistamines, which dry mucous membranes, making mucus expectoration difficult.

A patient with pulmonary infection needs intermittent nebulization, chest physiotherapy, and postural drainage to relieve obstruction and loosen and remove mucopurulent secretions. In acute cases, he also needs aggressive treatment with broad-spectrum antibiotics and oxygen therapy as needed.

Dornase alfa, a pulmonary enzyme given by aerosol nebulizer, helps to thin airway mucus, improving lung function and reducing the risk of pulmonary infection.
• In advanced stages of cystic fibrosis, the patient may require heart-lung transplantation.

Since the discovery of the basic genetic defect of cystic fibrosis, new treatments have been explored in some centers. Experimental treatments include drugs, such as amiloride, and gene therapy. Researchers have targeted the lungs for gene therapy because the most serious pathology occurs there. They hope to insert corrected genetic material into lung stem cells, which produce new lung cells. Lung stem cells might be reached through an aerosolized delivery system currently under study.

Nursing diagnoses

• Altered nutrition: Less than body requirements
• Altered tissue perfusion
• Anxiety
• Fear
• Impaired gas exchange
• Ineffective airway clearance
• Ineffective breathing pattern
• Ineffective family coping

Nursing interventions

• Give medications, as ordered. Administer pancreatic enzymes with meals and snacks.
• Perform chest physiotherapy, including postural drainage and chest percussion designed for all lobes, several times a day, as ordered.
• Administer oxygen therapy, as ordered. Check SaO_2 levels using pulse oximetry.
• Provide a well-balanced, high-calorie, high-protein diet. Include plenty of fats, which, though difficult for the patient to digest, are nutritionally necessary. Give him enzyme capsules to help combat most of the effects of fat malabsorption. Include vitamin A, D, E, and K supplements if laboratory analysis indicates any deficiencies.
• Make sure the patient receives plenty of liquids to prevent dehydration, especially in warm weather.
• Provide exercise and activity periods for the patient to promote health. Encourage him to perform breathing exercises to help improve his ventilation.
• Provide the young child with play periods, and enlist

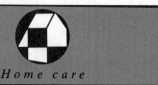

Home care

MANAGING CYSTIC FIBROSIS

To help your patient manage cystic fibrosis at home, use the following as a guide:
• Review breathing exercises and treatments with the patient and his family.
• Evaluate the patient's and family's techniques for performing chest physiotherapy (CPT); reinstruct them if needed.
• Encourage the use of CPT in the morning, before eating, after nebulization treatments, and before bedtime; recommend increasing CPT frequency whenever mucus becomes more abundant than usual.
• Advise the patient not to eat for 1 hour before CPT.
• Teach the patient to avoid tight or restrictive clothing around his chest, neck, or stomach. Suggest that he wear a light shirt or gown to prevent friction during CPT.
• Help the family find alternatives to cupped hands for CPT, such as using a small, lightweight plastic bowl or cup.
• Stress the importance of supplemental enzyme therapy; evaluate the patient's compliance and suggest ways to improve it.
• Emphasize the need for a well-balanced, high-calorie, high-protein diet; assist with meal planning and food selection as needed.
• Help the patient and family obtain necessary equipment, supplies, and medications.
• Provide referrals to local community agencies and the Cystic Fibrosis Foundation as needed.

the help of the physical therapy department. Some pediatric hospitals have play therapists, who provide essential playtime for young patients.
• Provide emotional support to the parents of children with cystic fibrosis. Because it's an inherited disease, the parents may feel enormous guilt. Encourage them to discuss their fears and concerns, and answer their questions as honestly as possible.
• Be flexible with care and visiting hours during hospitalization to allow the child to continue schoolwork and friendships.
• Include the family in all phases of the child's care. If the child is an adolescent, he may want to perform much of his own treatment protocol. Encourage him to do so. (See *Managing cystic fibrosis.*)

Patient teaching
• Inform the patient and his family about the disease, and thoroughly explain all treatment measures. Make sure they know about tests that can determine if family members carry the cystic fibrosis gene.
• Teach the patient and his family about all the medications the patient may be receiving. Explain possible adverse reactions, and urge them to notify the doctor if these reactions occur.
• Instruct the patient and his family about aerosol therapy, including intermittent nebulizer treatments before postural drainage. Tell them that these treatments help to loosen secretions and dilate the bronchi.
• If the doctor prescribes aerobic exercises, teach the patient how to do them, and review their importance in maintaining respiratory muscle and cardiopulmonary function and in improving activity tolerance.
• Teach the patient and his family signs of infection and sudden changes in the patient's condition that they should report to the doctor. These include increased coughing, decreased appetite, sputum that thickens or contains blood, shortness of breath, and chest pain.
• Advise the parents of a child with the disease not to be overly protective. Instead, help them explore ways to enhance their child's quality of life and to foster responsibility and independence in him from an early age. Stress the importance of good communication so that the child may express his fears and concerns.

EMPHYSEMA
The most common cause of death from respiratory disease in the United States, emphysema is one of several diseases usually labeled collectively as chronic obstructive pulmonary disease (COPD).

Emphysema appears to be more prevalent in men than in women; about 65% of patients with well-defined emphysema are men; about 35% are women. Postmortem findings reveal few adult lungs without some degree of emphysema.

Causes and pathophysiology
Emphysema may be caused by a deficiency of alpha$_1$-antitrypsin and by cigarette smoking. Recurrent inflammation associated with the release of proteolytic enzymes from lung cells causes abnormal, irreversible enlargement of the air spaces distal to the terminal bronchioles. This leads to the destruction of alveolar walls, which results in a breakdown of elasticity. (See *What happens in emphysema.*)

Complications

In emphysema, complications may include recurrent respiratory tract infections, cor pulmonale, and respiratory failure. Peptic ulcer disease strikes between 20% and 25% of patients with COPD. Additionally, alveolar blebs and bullae may rupture, leading to spontaneous pneumothorax or pneumomediastinum.

Assessment findings

The patient history may disclose that the patient is a long-time smoker. The patient may report shortness of breath and a chronic cough. The history may also reveal anorexia with resultant weight loss and a general feeling of malaise.

Inspection may show a barrel-chested patient who breathes through pursed lips and also uses accessory muscles. You may notice peripheral cyanosis, clubbed fingers and toes, and tachypnea.

Palpation may reveal decreased tactile fremitus and decreased chest expansion. Percussion may detect hyperresonance. On auscultation, you may hear decreased breath sounds, crackles and wheezing during inspiration, a prolonged expiratory phase with grunting respirations, and distant heart sounds.

Diagnostic tests

• *Chest X-rays* in advanced disease may show a flattened diaphragm, reduced vascular markings at the lung periphery, overaeration of the lungs, a vertical heart, enlarged anteroposterior chest diameter, and large retrosternal air space.
• *Pulmonary function tests* typically indicate increased residual volume and total lung capacity, reduced diffusing capacity, and increased inspiratory flow.
• *Arterial blood gas analysis* usually shows reduced PaO_2 and normal $PaCO_2$ until late in the disease.
• *Electrocardiography* may reveal tall, symmetrical P waves in leads II, III, and aV_F; vertical QRS axis; and signs of right ventricular hypertrophy late in the disease.
• *Red blood cell count* usually demonstrates an increased hemoglobin level late in the disease when the patient has persistent severe hypoxia.

Treatment

Emphysema management usually includes bronchodilators, such as aminophylline, to promote mucociliary clearance; antibiotics to treat respiratory tract infection; and immunizations to prevent influenza and pneumococcal pneumonia.

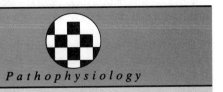

Pathophysiology

WHAT HAPPENS IN EMPHYSEMA

In normal, healthy breathing, air moves in and out of the lungs to meet metabolic needs. Any change in airway size compromises the lungs' ability to circulate sufficient air.

In a patient with emphysema, recurrent pulmonary inflammation damages and eventually destroys the alveolar walls, creating large air spaces. This breakdown leaves the alveoli unable to recoil normally after expanding and results in bronchiolar collapse on expiration. This traps air within the lungs.

Associated pulmonary capillary destruction, however, usually allows a patient with severe emphysema to match ventilation to perfusion and thus avoid cyanosis.

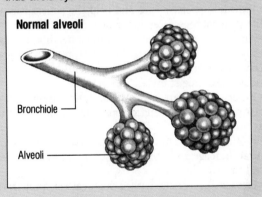

Normal alveoli

Bronchiole —

Alveoli —

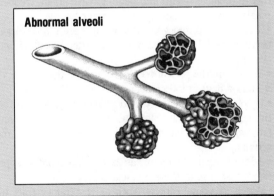

Abnormal alveoli

Other treatment measures include adequate hydration and (in selected patients) chest physiotherapy to mobilize secretions.

Some patients may require oxygen therapy (at low settings) to correct hypoxia. They may also require transtracheal catheterization to receive oxygen at home. Counseling about avoiding smoking and air pollutants is necessary.

Nursing diagnoses
• Activity intolerance
• Altered nutrition: Less than body requirements
• Anxiety
• Fatigue
• Fear
• Impaired gas exchange
• Ineffective airway clearance
• Ineffective breathing pattern
• Knowledge deficit

Nursing interventions
• Provide supportive care and help the patient adjust to life-style changes necessitated by a chronic illness.
• Answer the patient's questions about his illness as honestly as possible. Encourage him to express his fears and concerns about his illness. Remain with him during periods of extreme stress and anxiety.
• Include the patient and his family in care-related decisions. Refer the patient to appropriate support services as needed.
• If ordered, perform chest physiotherapy, including postural drainage and chest percussion and vibration, several times daily.
• Provide the patient with a high-calorie, protein-rich diet to promote health and healing. Give small, frequent meals to conserve energy and prevent fatigue.
• Schedule respiratory treatments at least 1 hour before or after meals. Provide mouth care after bronchodilator therapy.
• Make sure the patient receives adequate fluids (at least 3 liters a day) to loosen secretions.
• Encourage daily activity, and provide diversionary activities as appropriate. To conserve energy and prevent fatigue, assist the patient to alternate periods of rest and activity.
• Administer medications, as ordered. Record the patient's response to these medications.
• Watch for complications, such as respiratory tract infections, cor pulmonale, spontaneous pneumothorax, respiratory failure, and peptic ulcer disease.

Patient teaching
• Advise the patient to avoid crowds and people with known infections, and to obtain influenza and pneumococcus immunizations.
• For the patient receiving home oxygen therapy, explain the rationales for oxygen therapy and proper use of equipment. If the patient requires a transtracheal catheter, instruct him about catheter care, precautions, and follow-up.
• Teach the patient and family members how to perform postural drainage and chest percussion. Instruct them to maintain each position for about 10 minutes and then perform percussion and cough. Also, teach the patient coughing and deep-breathing techniques to promote good ventilation and mobilize secretions.
• Review the patient's medications and explain the rationale, dosage, and adverse effects related to the prescribed drug. Advise him to report adverse reactions to the doctor immediately. Show him how to use an inhaler correctly, if appropriate.
• Encourage the patient to eat high-calorie, protein-rich foods. Urge him to drink plenty of fluids to prevent dehydration and to help loosen secretions.
• If the patient smokes, encourage him to stop. Provide him with smoking cessation resources or counseling, if necessary.
• Urge the patient to avoid respiratory irritants such as automobile exhaust fumes, aerosol sprays, and industrial pollutants.
• Warn the patient that exposure to blasts of cold air may precipitate bronchospasm. Suggest that he avoid cold, windy weather or that he cover his mouth and nose with a scarf or mask if he must go outside.
• If appropriate, describe signs and symptoms of peptic ulcer disease. Instruct the patient to check his stools every day for blood and to notify the doctor if he has persistent nausea, vomiting, heartburn, indigestion, constipation, diarrhea, or bloody stools.
• Inform the patient about signs and symptoms that suggest ruptured alveolar blebs and bullae. Explain the seriousness of possible spontaneous pneumothorax. Urge him to notify the doctor if he feels sudden, sharp pleuritic pain that's exacerbated by chest movement, breathing, or coughing.

CHRONIC BRONCHITIS
A form of chronic obstructive pulmonary disease, chronic bronchitis is marked by excessive production of tracheobronchial mucus that's sufficient to cause a cough for at least 3 months each year for 2 consecutive years.

The severity of the disease is linked to the amount of cigarette smoke or other pollutants inhaled and the duration of the inhalation. A respiratory tract infection typically exacerbates the cough and related symptoms. However, few patients with chronic bronchitis develop significant airway obstruction. About 20% of men have chronic bronchitis.

Causes and pathophysiology

Cigarette smoking is the most common cause of chronic bronchitis, although some studies suggest a genetic predisposition to the disease as well.

The disease is directly correlated to heavy pollution and is more prevalent in people exposed to organic or inorganic dusts and noxious gases. Children of parents who smoke are at higher risk for respiratory tract infections that can lead to chronic bronchitis.

Chronic bronchitis results in hypertrophy and hyperplasia of the bronchial mucous glands, increased goblet cells, ciliary damage, squamous metaplasia of the columnar epithelium, and chronic leukocytic and lymphocytic infiltration of bronchial walls. Additional effects include widespread inflammation, airway narrowing, and mucus within the airways—all producing resistance in the small airways and, in turn, a severe ventilation-perfusion imbalance. (See *What happens in chronic bronchitis.*)

Complications

Chronic bronchitis can lead to cor pulmonale, pulmonary hypertension, right ventricular hypertrophy, and acute respiratory failure.

Assessment findings

The patient's history typically reflects a longtime smoker who has frequent upper respiratory tract infections. Usually, the patient seeks treatment for a productive cough and exertional dyspnea. He may describe his cough as initially prevalent in the winter months but gradually becoming a year-round problem with increasingly severe episodes. He also typically reports progressively worsening dyspnea that takes increasingly longer to subside.

Inspection usually reveals a cough, producing copious gray, white, or yellow sputum. The patient may appear cyanotic. And he may use accessory respiratory muscles for breathing (a "blue bloater"). Vital signs usually include tachypnea; other typical findings include a substantial weight gain.

Palpation may disclose pedal edema and neck vein distention. Auscultation findings include wheezing, prolonged expiratory time, and rhonchi.

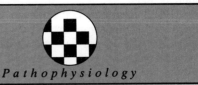

Pathophysiology

WHAT HAPPENS IN CHRONIC BRONCHITIS

In chronic bronchitis, irritants inhaled for a prolonged period inflame the tracheobronchial tree. The inflammation leads to increased mucus production and a narrowed or blocked airway.

As inflammation continues, the mucus-producing goblet cells undergo hypertrophy, as do the ciliated epithelial cells that line the respiratory tract. Hypersecretion from the goblet cells blocks the free movement of the cilia, which normally sweep dust, irritants, and mucus from the airways.

As a result, the airway stays blocked, and mucus and debris accumulate in the respiratory tract.

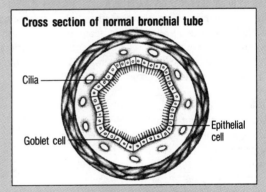

Cross section of normal bronchial tube

Cilia

Goblet cell

Epithelial cell

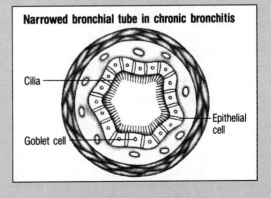

Narrowed bronchial tube in chronic bronchitis

Cilia

Goblet cell

Epithelial cell

Diagnostic tests
• *Chest X-rays* may show hyperinflation and increased bronchovascular markings.
• *Pulmonary function tests* demonstrate increased residual volume, decreased vital capacity and forced expiratory flow, and normal static compliance and diffusing capacity.
• *Arterial blood gas (ABG) analysis* displays decreased PaO_2 and normal or increased $PaCO_2$.
• *Sputum culture* may reveal many microorganisms and neutrophils.
• *Electrocardiography* may detect atrial arrhythmias; peaked P waves in leads II, III, and aV_F, and, occasionally, right ventricular hypertrophy.

Treatment
The most effective treatment is for the patient to stop smoking and to avoid air pollutants as much as possible. Antibiotics can be used to treat recurring infections. Bronchodilators may relieve bronchospasm and facilitate mucus clearance. Adequate fluid intake is essential, and chest physiotherapy may be needed to mobilize secretions. Ultrasonic or mechanical nebulizer treatments may help to loosen and mobilize secretions. Occasionally, the patient will respond to corticosteroid therapy. Diuretics may be used to treat edema, and oxygen may be necessary to treat hypoxia.

Nursing diagnoses
• Altered family processes
• Altered nutrition: Less than body requirements
• Anxiety
• Fatigue
• Fear
• Impaired gas exchange
• Ineffective breathing pattern
• Knowledge deficit

Nursing interventions
• Answer the patient's questions, and encourage him and his family to express their concerns about the illness. Include the patient and his family in care decisions. Refer them to other support services as appropriate.
• Assess for changes in baseline respiratory function. Evaluate sputum quality and quantity, restlessness, increased tachypnea, and altered breath sounds. Report changes immediately.
• As needed, perform chest physiotherapy, including postural drainage and chest percussion and vibration for involved lobes, several times daily.

• Weigh the patient three times weekly, and assess for edema.
• Provide the patient with a high-calorie, protein-rich diet. Offer small, frequent meals to conserve the patient's energy and prevent fatigue.
• Make sure the patient receives adequate fluids (at least 3 liters a day) to loosen secretions.
• Schedule respiratory therapy at least 1 hour before or after meals. Provide mouth care after bronchodilator inhalation therapy.
• Encourage daily activity, and provide diversional activities, as appropriate. To conserve the patient's energy and prevent fatigue, help him to alternate periods of rest and activity.
• Administer medications, as ordered, and note the patient's response to them.

Patient teaching
• Advise the patient to avoid crowds and people with known infections, and to obtain influenza and pneumococcus immunizations.
• If the patient is receiving home oxygen therapy, explain the treatment rationale. Show him how to operate the equipment.
• Teach the patient and family how to perform postural drainage and chest percussion. Instruct the patient to maintain each position for 10 minutes before a caregiver performs percussion and the patient coughs. Also teach the patient coughing and deep-breathing techniques to promote good ventilation and to remove secretions.
• Review all medications, including dosage, adverse effects, and purposes for the prescriptions. Teach the patient how to use an inhaler. Advise him to report any adverse reactions to the doctor immediately.
• Encourage the patient to eat high-calorie, protein-rich meals and to drink plenty of fluids to prevent dehydration and help loosen secretions.
• If the patient smokes, encourage him to stop. Provide him with smoking-cessation resources or counseling if necessary.
• Urge the patient to avoid inhaled irritants, such as automobile exhaust fumes, aerosol sprays, and industrial pollutants.
• Warn the patient that exposure to blasts of cold air may precipitate bronchospasm. Suggest that he avoid cold, windy weather or that he cover his mouth and nose with a scarf or mask if he must go outside.
• If the patient takes theophylline, warn him that cigarette or marijuana smoking significantly increases plasma clearance of theophylline. Also, patients who quit smoking should notify the doctor because they may ex-

perience the onset of adverse effects of higher blood levels of theophylline.

• If appropriate, describe the signs and symptoms of peptic ulcer disease. Instruct the patient to check his stools every day for blood and to notify the doctor if he has persistent nausea, vomiting, heartburn, indigestion, constipation, diarrhea, or bloody stools.

BRONCHIECTASIS

Marked by chronic abnormal dilation of the bronchi and destruction of the bronchial walls, bronchiectasis can occur throughout the tracheobronchial tree, or it may be confined to one segment or lobe. It's usually bilateral and involves the basilar segments of the lower lobes.

The disease has three forms: cylindrical (fusiform), varicose, and saccular (cystic). It affects people of both sexes and all ages. With antibiotics available to treat acute respiratory tract infections, the incidence of bronchiectasis has dramatically decreased over the past 20 years. Its incidence is highest among Inuit populations in the Northern Hemisphere and the Maoris of New Zealand. Bronchiectasis is irreversible.

Causes and pathophysiology

Bronchiectasis results from conditions associated with repeated damage to bronchial walls and with abnormal mucociliary clearance, which causes a breakdown of supporting tissue adjacent to the airways. Such conditions include:
• cystic fibrosis
• immune disorders (agammaglobulinemia, for example)
• recurrent, inadequately treated bacterial respiratory tract infections (such as tuberculosis)
• complications of measles, pneumonia, pertussis, or influenza
• obstruction (by a foreign body, a tumor, or stenosis) with recurrent infection
• inhalation of corrosive gas or repeated aspiration of gastric juices
• congenital anomalies (rare), such as bronchomalacia, congenital bronchiectasis, and Kartagener's syndrome (bronchiectasis, sinusitis, and dextrocardia), and various rare disorders, such as immotile cilia syndrome.

In the patient with bronchiectasis, sputum stagnates in the dilated bronchi and leads to secondary infection, characterized by inflammation and leukocytic accumulations. Additional debris collects in and occludes the bronchi. Building pressure from the retained secretions induces mucosal injury.

Complications

Advanced bronchiectasis may produce chronic malnutrition and amyloidosis, right ventricular failure, and cor pulmonale.

Assessment findings

Patient complaints commonly include frequent bouts of pneumonia or a history of coughing up blood or blood-tinged sputum. The patient typically reports a chronic cough that produces copious, foul-smelling, mucopurulent secretions (up to several cups daily). He may also report dyspnea, weight loss, and malaise.

Inspection of the patient's sputum may show a cloudy top layer, a central layer of clear saliva, and a heavy, thick, purulent bottom layer. In advanced disease, the patient may have clubbed fingers and toes and cyanotic nail beds.

If the patient also has a complicating condition, such as pneumonia or atelectasis, percussion may detect dullness over lung fields. Auscultation may reveal coarse crackles during inspiration over involved lobes or segments, and occasional wheezes. With complicating atelectasis or pneumonia, you may hear diminished breath sounds during auscultation.

Diagnostic tests

• *Bronchography* may be ordered for patients who are considering surgery or for those with recurrent or severe hemoptysis. In bronchography, a radiopaque contrast medium outlines the bronchial walls, allowing X-ray images to display the location and extent of disease.
• *Chest X-rays* show peribronchial thickening, atelectatic areas, and scattered cystic changes that suggest bronchiectasis.
• *Bronchoscopy* helps to identify the source of secretions or the bleeding site in hemoptysis.
• *Sputum culture* and a *Gram stain* identify predominant pathogens.
• *Complete blood count* can detect anemia and leukocytosis.
• *Pulmonary function studies* detect decreased vital capacity, expiratory flow, and hypoxemia; these tests also help evaluate disease severity, therapeutic effectiveness, and the patient's suitability for surgery.

Depending on the patient and his condition, additional tests may include urinalysis and electrocardiography. If the health care team suspects cystic fibrosis as the underlying cause of bronchiectasis, a sweat electrolyte test may be ordered.

Treatment

Antibiotic therapy (oral or I.V.) for 7 to 10 days—or until sputum production decreases—is the principal treatment. Bronchodilators and postural drainage and chest percussion help remove secretions if the patient has bronchospasm and thick, tenacious sputum. Occasionally, bronchoscopy may be used to remove secretions. Oxygen therapy may be used for hypoxia. Segmental resection or lobectomy may be recommended for severe hemoptysis.

The only cure for bronchiectasis is the surgical removal of the affected lung portion. However, the patient with bronchiectasis affecting both lungs probably won't benefit from surgery.

Nursing diagnoses

- Altered nutrition: Less than body requirements
- Anxiety
- Fatigue
- Impaired gas exchange
- Ineffective airway clearance
- Ineffective breathing pattern

Nursing interventions

- Provide supportive care, and help the patient adjust to the life-style changes that irreversible lung damage necessitates.
- Administer antibiotics, as ordered, and record the patient's response to this medication.
- Give oxygen as needed, and assess gas exchange by monitoring arterial blood gas values, as ordered.
- Perform chest physiotherapy, including postural drainage and chest percussion for involved lobes, several times a day, especially in the early morning and before bedtime.
- Provide a warm, quiet, comfortable environment. Also, help the patient to alternate rest and activity periods.
- Provide well-balanced, high-calorie meals for the patient. Offer small, frequent meals to prevent fatigue.
- Make sure the patient receives adequate hydration to help thin secretions and promote easier removal.
- Give frequent mouth care to remove foul-smelling sputum. Provide the patient with tissues and a waxed bag in which to dispose of the contaminated tissues.
- Watch for developing complications, such as right ventricular failure and cor pulmonale.
- After surgery, give meticulous postoperative care. Monitor vital signs, encourage deep breathing and position changes every 2 hours, and provide chest-tube care.

Patient teaching

- Show family members how to perform postural drainage and percussion. Also, teach the patient coughing and deep-breathing techniques to promote good ventilation and assist in secretion removal. Instruct him to maintain each postural drainage position for 10 minutes. Then direct the caregiver in performing percussion and instructing the patient to cough.
- If appropriate, advise the patient to stop smoking because it stimulates secretions and irritates the airways. Refer the patient to a local smoking-cessation group.
- Instruct the patient to avoid air pollutants and people with known upper respiratory tract infections.
- Direct the patient to take medications (especially antibiotics) exactly as ordered. Make sure he knows the adverse effects associated with his medications. Instruct him to notify the doctor if any of these effects occur.
- Teach the patient to dispose of all secretions properly to avoid spreading the infection to others. Advise him to wash his hands thoroughly after disposing of contaminated tissues.
- Urge the patient to keep up-to-date in his immunization schedule to prevent childhood diseases.
- Encourage the patient to rest as much as possible.
- Discuss dietary measures. Encourage the patient to follow a balanced, high-protein diet. Suggest that he eat small, frequent meals. Explain that milk products may increase the viscosity of secretions.
- Encourage the patient to drink plenty of fluids to thin secretions and to aid expectoration.
- If the patient needs surgery, offer complete preoperative and postoperative instructions. Forewarn the patient if he will have an I.V. line and chest tubes. Explain the reason for these procedures.

TUBERCULOSIS

An acute or chronic infection, tuberculosis is characterized by pulmonary infiltrates and by formation of granulomas with caseation, fibrosis, and cavitation. The American Lung Association estimates that active disease afflicts nearly 14 of every 100,000 persons.

The disease is twice as common in men as in women and four times as common in nonwhites as in whites. But incidence is highest in people who live in crowded, poorly ventilated, unsanitary conditions, such as those in some prisons, tenement houses, and homeless shelters. The typical newly diagnosed tuberculosis patient is a single, homeless, nonwhite man. With proper treatment, the prognosis is usually excellent.

Causes and pathophysiology

Tuberculosis results from exposure to *Mycobacterium tuberculosis* and, sometimes, other strains of mycobacteria. Transmission occurs when an infected person coughs or sneezes, spreading infected droplets.

When a person without immunity inhales these droplets, the bacilli lodge in the alveoli, causing irritation. The immune system responds by sending leukocytes, lymphocytes, and macrophages to surround the bacilli, and the local lymph nodes swell and become inflamed. If the encapsulated bacilli (tubercles) and the inflamed nodes rupture, the infection contaminates the surrounding tissue and may spread through the blood and lymphatic circulation to distant sites—a process called hematogenous dissemination. This same phagocytic cycle occurs whenever the bacilli spread.

After exposure to *M. tuberculosis,* roughly 5% of infected people develop active tuberculosis within 1 year; in the remainder, microorganisms cause a latent infection. The host's immunologic defense system usually destroys the bacillus or walls it up in a tubercle. But the live, encapsulated bacilli may lie dormant within the tubercle for years, reactivating later to cause active infection.

The risk for tuberculosis is higher in the following:
• Black and Hispanic men between ages 25 and 44
• those in close contact with a newly diagnosed tuberculosis patient
• those who have had tuberculosis before
• people with multiple sexual partners
• recent immigrants from Africa, Asia, Mexico, and South America
• gastrectomy patients
• people affected with silicosis, diabetes, malnutrition, cancer, Hodgkin's disease, or leukemia
• drug and alcohol abusers
• patients in mental institutions
• nursing home residents, who are ten times more likely to contract tuberculosis than anyone in the general population
• those receiving treatment with immunosuppressants or corticosteroids
• people with weak immune systems or diseases that affect the immune system, especially those with acquired immunodeficiency syndrome.

Complications

Tuberculosis can cause massive pulmonary tissue damage, with inflammation and tissue necrosis eventually leading to respiratory failure. Bronchoplural fistulas can develop from lung tissue damage, resulting in pneumothorax. The disease can also lead to hemorrhage, pleural effusion, and pneumonia. Small mycobacterial foci can infect other body organs, including the kidneys and the central nervous and skeletal systems.

Assessment findings

The patient with a primary infection may complain of weakness and fatigue, anorexia and weight loss, and night sweats. The patient with reactivated tuberculosis may report chest pain and a cough that produces blood or mucopurulent or blood-tinged sputum. He may also have a low-grade fever.

When you percuss, you may note dullness over the affected area, a sign of consolidation or the presence of pleural fluid. On auscultation, you may hear crepitant crackles, bronchial breath sounds, wheezes, and whispered pectoriloquy.

Diagnostic tests

• *Chest X-rays* show nodular lesions, patchy infiltrates (mainly in upper lobes), cavity formation, scar tissue, and calcium deposits. However, they may not help distinguish between active and inactive tuberculosis.
• A *tuberculin skin test* reveals that the patient has been infected with tuberculosis at some point, but it doesn't indicate active disease. In this test, intermediate-strength purified protein derivative or 5 tuberculin units (0.1 ml) are injected intradermally on the forearm and read in 48 to 72 hours. A positive reaction (equal to or more than a 10-mm induration) develops within 2 to 10 weeks after infection with the tubercle bacillus in both active and inactive tuberculosis.
• *Stains* and *cultures*—of sputum, cerebrospinal fluid, urine, drainage from abscess, or pleural fluid—show heat-sensitive, nonmotile, aerobic, acid-fast bacilli.
• *Computed tomography* or *magnetic resonance imaging scans* allow the evaluation of lung damage or confirm a difficult diagnosis.
• *Bronchoscopy* may be performed if the patient can't produce an adequate sputum specimen.

Several of these tests may need to be performed to distinguish tuberculosis from other diseases that may mimic it (such as lung carcinoma, lung abscess, pneumoconiosis, and bronchiectasis).

Treatment

Antitubercular therapy with daily oral doses of isoniazid or rifampin (with ethambutol added in some cases) for at least 9 months usually cures tuberculosis. After 2 to 4 weeks, the disease is no longer infectious, and the patient can resume his normal activities while continuing to take medication.

The patient with atypical mycobacterial disease or drug-resistant tuberculosis may require second-line drugs, such as capreomycin, streptomycin, para-amino-salicylic acid, pyrazinamide, and cycloserine.

Nursing diagnoses
• Altered nutrition: Less than body requirements
• Anxiety
• Fear
• Impaired gas exchange
• Ineffective airway clearance
• Knowledge deficit
• Risk for injury

Nursing interventions
• Administer ordered antibiotics and antitubercular agents.
• Isolate the infectious patient in a quiet, well-ventilated room until he's no longer contagious. Provide diversional activities and check on him frequently. Make sure the call button is nearby.
• Place a covered trash can nearby, or tape a waxed bag to the bedside for used tissues. Tell the patient to wear a mask when outside his room. Visitors and hospital personnel should also wear masks in the patient's room.
• Make sure the patient gets plenty of rest. Provide for periods of rest and activity to promote health as well as conserve energy and reduce oxygen demand.
• Provide the patient with well-balanced, high-calorie foods, preferably in small, frequent meals to conserve energy. (Small, frequent meals may also encourage the anorexic patient to eat more.) Record the patient's weight weekly. If he needs oral supplements, consult with the dietitian.
• Watch for adverse reactions to the medications.
• Administer isoniazid with food. This drug can cause hepatitis or peripheral neuritis, so monitor levels of aspartate aminotransferase (formerly SGOT) and alanine aminotransferase (formerly SGPT). To prevent or treat peripheral neuritis, give pyridoxine (vitamin B_6) as ordered.
• If the patient receives ethambutol, watch for signs of optic neuritis; report them to the doctor, who will probably discontinue the drug. Check the patient's vision monthly and give this medication with food.
• If the patient receives rifampin, watch for signs of hepatitis, purpura, and a flulike syndrome, as well as other complications, such as hemoptysis. Monitor liver and kidney function tests throughout therapy.

• Perform chest physiotherapy, including postural drainage and chest percussion, several times a day.
• Give the patient supportive care, and help him adjust to the changes he may have to make during his illness. Include the patient in care decisions, and let the family take part in the patient's care whenever possible.

Patient teaching
• Show the patient and his family how to perform postural drainage and chest percussion. Also, teach the patient coughing and deep-breathing techniques. Instruct him to maintain each position for 10 minutes and then to perform percussion and cough.
• Teach the patient the adverse effects of his medication, and tell him to report them immediately. Emphasize the importance of regular follow-up examinations, and instruct the patient and his family concerning the signs and symptoms of recurring tuberculosis. Stress the need to follow long-term treatment faithfully.
• Advise anyone exposed to an infected patient to receive tuberculin tests and, if ordered, chest X-rays and prophylactic isoniazid.
• Warn the patient taking rifampin that the drug will temporarily make his body secretions appear orange; reassure him that this effect is harmless. If the patient is a woman, warn her that oral contraceptives may be less effective while she's taking rifampin.
• Teach the patient the signs and symptoms that require medical assessment: increased cough, hemoptysis, unexplained weight loss, fever, and night sweats.
• Stress the importance of eating high-calorie, high-protein, balanced meals.
• Explain respiratory and universal precautions to the hospitalized patient. Before discharge, tell him that he must take precautions to prevent spreading the disease—such as wearing a mask around others—until his doctor tells him he's no longer contagious. He should tell all health care providers he sees, including his dentist and eye doctor, that he has tuberculosis so that they can institute infection-control precautions.
• Teach the patient other specific precautions to avoid spreading the infection. Tell him to cough and sneeze into tissues and to dispose of the tissues properly. Stress the importance of washing his hands thoroughly in hot, soapy water after handling his own secretions. Also, instruct him to wash his eating utensils separately in hot, soapy water.
• Emphasize the importance of scheduling and keeping follow-up appointments.
• Refer the patient to such support groups as the American Lung Association.

SILICOSIS

The most common form of pneumoconiosis, silicosis is a progressive disease characterized by nodular lesions, which frequently progress to fibrosis. It's classified according to the severity of the pulmonary disease and the rapidity of its onset and progression, although it usually occurs as a simple asymptomatic illness.

Those who work around silica dust, such as foundry workers, boiler scalers, and stonecutters, have the highest incidence of the disease. Silica in its pure form occurs in the manufacture of ceramics (flint) and building materials (sandstone). It occurs in mixed form in the production of construction materials (cement). It's also found in powder form (silica flour) in paints, porcelain, scouring soaps, and wood fillers, and in the mining of gold, lead, zinc, and iron.

Sand blasters, tunnel workers, and others exposed to high concentrations of respirable silica may develop acute silicosis after 1 to 3 years. Those exposed to lower concentrations of free silica can develop accelerated silicosis, usually after about 10 years of exposure.

The prognosis is good unless the disease progresses to the complicated fibrotic form.

Causes and pathophysiology

Silicosis results from the inhalation and pulmonary deposition of respirable crystalline silica dust, mostly from quartz. The risk depends on the concentration of dust in the atmosphere, the percentage of respirable free silica particles in the dust, and the duration of exposure. Although particles up to 10 microns in diameter can be inhaled, the disease-causing particles deposited in the alveolar space usually have a diameter of only 1 to 3 microns.

Nodules result when alveolar macrophages ingest silica particles, which they can't process. As a result, the macrophages die and release proteolytic enzymes into surrounding tissue. The enzymes inflame the tissue, attracting other macrophages and fibroblasts. These produce fibrous tissue to wall off the reaction, resulting in a nodule, which has an onionskin appearance.

These nodules develop adjacent to the terminal and respiratory bronchioles. Although frequently accompanied by bullous changes in both lobes, nodules concentrate in upper lung lobes. If the disease doesn't progress, the patient may experience only minimal physiologic disturbances, with no disability. Occasionally, however, the fibrotic response accelerates, engulfing and destroying a large lung area.

Complications

Silicosis may progress to massive areas of pulmonary fibrosis, which may continue to grow even though the patient is no longer exposed to dust. Pulmonary fibrosis in turn may result in cor pulmonale, ventricular or respiratory failure, and pulmonary tuberculosis.

Assessment findings

The patient has a history of long-term industrial exposure to silica dust. He may complain of dyspnea on exertion, which he's likely to attribute to "being out of shape" or "slowing down." If the disease has progressed to the chronic and complicated state, the patient may report a dry cough, especially in the morning.

When you inspect the patient, you may note decreased chest expansion and tachypnea. If he has advanced disease, he may also act lethargic and look confused. You may percuss areas of increased and decreased resonance. On auscultation, you may hear fine to medium crackles, diminished breath sounds, and an intensified ventricular gallop on inspiration—a hallmark of cor pulmonale.

Diagnostic tests

• *Chest X-rays* in simple silicosis show small, discrete, nodular lesions distributed throughout both lung fields, although they typically concentrate in the upper lung zones. The hilar lung nodes may appear enlarged and show eggshell calcification. In complicated silicosis, X-rays show one or more conglomerate masses of dense tissue.

• *Pulmonary function tests* demonstrate reduced forced vital capacity (FVC) in complicated silicosis. If the patient has obstructive disease (emphysematous silicosis areas), he'll have reduced forced expiratory volume in 1 second (FEV_1). A patient with complicated silicosis also has reduced FEV_1 but has a normal or high ratio of FEV_1 to FVC. When fibrosis destroys alveolar walls and obliterates pulmonary capillaries or when it thickens the alveolocapillary membrane, the diffusing capacity for carbon monoxide falls below normal. Both restrictive and obstructive disease reduce maximal voluntary ventilation.

• *Arterial blood gas analysis* reveals a normal PaO_2 in simple silicosis, although it may drop significantly below normal in late stages or complicated disease. The patient has normal $PaCO_2$ in the early stages of the disease, but hyperventilation may cause it to drop below normal. If restrictive lung disease develops—particularly if the patient is hypoxic and has severe alveolar ventilatory impairment—it may rise above normal.

Treatment

The goal is to relieve respiratory symptoms, manage hypoxia and cor pulmonale, and prevent respiratory tract infections and irritations. Treatment includes careful observation for the development of tuberculosis.

Daily bronchodilating aerosols and increased fluid intake (at least 3 qt [3 liters] daily) relieve respiratory signs and symptoms. Steam inhalation and chest physiotherapy (such as controlled coughing and segmental bronchial drainage) with chest percussion and vibration help clear secretions.

In severe cases, the patient may need oxygen by cannula, mask, or mechanical ventilation (if he can't maintain arterial oxygenation). Respiratory tract infection warrants prompt antibiotic administration.

Nursing diagnoses

- Altered family processes
- Altered nutrition: Less than body requirements
- Anxiety
- Fatigue
- Fear
- Impaired gas exchange
- Ineffective breathing pattern
- Knowledge deficit

Nursing interventions

- Assess for changes in baseline respiratory functioning, including changes in sputum quality and quantity, restlessness, increased tachypnea, and changes in breath sounds. Report any changes to the doctor immediately.
- Perform chest physiotherapy, including postural drainage and chest percussion and vibration designed for involved lobes, several times a day.
- Provide the patient with a high-calorie, high-protein diet, preferably in small, frequent meals.
- Schedule respiratory therapy at least 1 hour before or after meals. Provide mouth care after bronchodilator therapy.
- Make sure the patient receives enough fluids to loosen secretions.
- Encourage daily activity, and provide the patient with diversional activities, as appropriate. To conserve his energy, alternate periods of rest and activity.
- Administer medication, as ordered. Monitor the patient for desired response and for adverse reactions.
- Watch for complications, such as pulmonary fibrosis, right ventricular hypertrophy, and cor pulmonale.
- Help the patient adjust to the life-style changes associated with a chronic illness. Answer his questions, and encourage him to express his concerns about his illness.

Stay with him during periods of extreme stress and anxiety. Include the patient and his family in care decisions whenever possible.

Patient teaching

- Advise the patient to avoid crowds and people with known infections. He should also receive influenza and pneumococcus immunizations.
- Teach the patient receiving home oxygen therapy the reasons for treatment and the proper use of the equipment. If he needs a transtracheal catheter, teach him catheter care and precautions.
- Show the patient and his family how to perform postural drainage and chest percussion. Also, teach the patient coughing and deep-breathing techniques, explaining that they'll help him breathe and help remove secretions. Tell him to remain in each position for 10 minutes. Percussion and coughing should follow.
- Thoroughly explain all medications.
- Encourage the patient to follow a high-calorie, high-protein diet, and to drink plenty of fluids to prevent dehydration and help loosen secretions.
- If the patient smokes, encourage him to quit, and, if necessary, refer him to resources that can help.
- Warn the patient of the risk of tuberculosis, and advise him to be tested, as ordered.
- Refer the patient and his family to other support services as appropriate.
- If you have a patient at risk for silicosis, teach him the importance of wearing a mask and using other protective devices to reduce his risk.

ASBESTOSIS

This disorder is characterized by diffuse interstitial pulmonary fibrosis, resulting from prolonged exposure to airborne asbestos particles. Asbestosis may develop many years (about 15 to 20) after regular exposure to asbestos ceases. Asbestos exposure also causes pleural plaques and mesotheliomas of the pleura and the peritoneum. A potent co-carcinogen, asbestos heightens a cigarette smoker's risk for lung cancer. In fact, an asbestos worker who smokes is 90 times more likely to develop lung cancer than a smoker who never worked with asbestos.

Asbestos-related diseases may also develop in family members of asbestos workers from exposure to stray fibers shaken off the workers' clothing at home. Furthermore, asbestosis may develop in the general public from exposure to fibrous asbestos dust in public buildings, such as schools and factories, or waste piles from a nearby asbestos plant.

Causes and pathophysiology

A form of pneumoconiosis, asbestosis follows prolonged inhalation of respirable asbestos fibers (about 50 microns long and 0.5 micron wide). The inhaled fibers travel down the airway and penetrate respiratory bronchioles and alveolar walls. They become encased in a brown, iron-rich, proteinlike sheath (ferruginous bodies or asbestosis bodies) in sputum or lung tissue. Interstitial fibrosis may develop in lower lung zones, causing pathologic changes in lung parenchyma and pleurae. Raised hyaline plaques may form in the parietal pleura and the diaphragm and in pleura adjacent to the pericardium.

Complications

Asbestosis may progress to pulmonary fibrosis with respiratory failure and cardiovascular complications, including pulmonary hypertension and cor pulmonale.

Assessment findings

The patient typically relates a history of occupational, family, or neighborhood exposure to asbestos fibers. The average exposure time is about 10 years. He may report exertional dyspnea. With extensive fibrosis, he may report dyspnea even at rest. In advanced disease, the patient may complain of a dry cough (may be productive in smokers), chest pain (often pleuritic), and recurrent respiratory tract infections.

Inspection findings may include tachypnea and clubbing of the fingers. With auscultation, you may hear characteristic dry crackles in the lung bases.

Diagnostic tests

• *Chest X-rays* may show fine, irregular, and linear diffuse infiltrates. If the patient has extensive fibrosis, X-rays may disclose lungs with a honeycomb or ground-glass appearance. Films may also show pleural thickening and pleural calcification, bilateral obliteration of costophrenic angles and, in later disease stages, an enlarged heart with a classic "shaggy" border.
• *Pulmonary function tests* may identify decreased vital capacity, forced vital capacity (FVC), and total lung capacity; decreased or normal forced expiratory volume in 1 second (FEV_1); a normal ratio of FEV_1 to FVC; and reduced diffusing capacity for carbon monoxide when fibrosis destroys alveolar walls and thickens the alveolocapillary membrane.

• *Arterial blood gas analysis* may reveal decreased PaO_2 and $PaCO_2$ from hyperventilation.

Treatment

Chest physiotherapy techniques, such as controlled coughing and postural drainage with chest percussion and vibration, may be implemented to relieve respiratory signs and symptoms and, in advanced disease, manage hypoxia and cor pulmonale.

Aerosol therapy, inhaled mucolytics, and increased fluid intake (at least 3 liters daily) may also help relieve respiratory symptoms. Hypoxia requires oxygen administration by cannula or mask (1 to 2 liters/minute), or by mechanical ventilation if the patient's arterial oxygen level can't be maintained above 40 mm Hg.

Diuretic agents, digitalis preparations, and salt restriction may be necessary for patients with cor pulmonale. Respiratory tract infections require prompt antibiotic therapy.

Nursing diagnoses

• Altered family processes
• Altered nutrition: Less than body requirements
• Anxiety
• Fatigue
• Fear
• Impaired gas exchange
• Ineffective breathing pattern
• Knowledge deficit

Nursing interventions

• Provide supportive care, and help the patient adjust to life-style changes necessitated by chronic illness.
• Be alert for changes in baseline respiratory function. Also watch for changes in sputum quality and quantity, restlessness, increased tachypnea, and changes in breath sounds. Report these immediately.
• Perform chest physiotherapy, including postural drainage and chest percussion and vibration for involved lobes, several times daily.
• Weigh the patient three times weekly.
• Provide high-calorie, high-protein foods. Offer small, frequent meals to conserve the patient's energy and prevent fatigue.
• Make sure the patient receives adequate fluids to loosen secretions.
• Schedule respiratory therapy at least 1 hour before or after meals. Provide mouth care after inhalational bronchodilator therapy.

• Encourage daily activity, and provide diversions as appropriate. Help conserve the patient's energy and prevent fatigue by alternating rest and activity.
• Administer medication, as ordered, and note the patient's response.
• Watch for complications, such as pulmonary hypertension and cor pulmonale.

Patient teaching
• Advise the patient to avoid crowds and people with known infections, and to obtain influenza and pneumococcus immunizations.
• If the patient receives home oxygen therapy, explain why he needs it, and show him how to operate the equipment.
• If the patient has a transtracheal catheter, teach him how to care for it. Review precautions for catheter use, and urge him to schedule appointments for follow-up care.
• Teach the patient and his family how to perform chest physiotherapy.
• Review the patient's medication regimen with him.
• Encourage the patient to follow a high-calorie, high-protein diet to meet increased energy requirements. Also, tell him to drink plenty of fluids to prevent dehydration and to help loosen secretions.
• If the patient smokes, encourage him to stop. Provide him with information or counseling, as appropriate.
• Inform the public, as appropriate, about the health hazard from asbestos exposure and ways to prevent asbestosis.

BERYLLIOSIS

A type of pneumoconiosis, berylliosis is a systemic granulomatous disease that mainly affects the lungs. It occurs in two forms: acute nonspecific pneumonitis and chronic noncaseating granulomatous disease with interstitial fibrosis, which may cause death from respiratory failure and cor pulmonale. In about 10% of patients with acute berylliosis, chronic disease develops 10 to 15 years after exposure.

Most patients with chronic interstitial disease have only slight to moderate disability from impaired lung function and other symptoms. With each acute exacerbation, though, the prognosis worsens.

This occupational disease can affect workers in beryllium alloy, ceramics, foundry, grinder, cathode ray tube, gas mantle, missile, and nuclear reactor industries. It's associated with the milling and use of beryllium, but not with beryl ore mining.

Also known as beryllium poisoning or beryllium disease, berylliosis may also affect beryllium workers' families (from beryllium dust shaken off clothing) and others who live near beryllium alloy sites.

Causes
Inhaling beryllium dusts, fumes, and mists causes berylliosis; the pattern of disease depends on the amount inhaled. Beryllium may also be absorbed through the skin. How the element exerts its toxic effect isn't known.

Complications
Berylliosis may progress to pulmonary scarring with pneumothorax, blebs, and respiratory failure. Pulmonary hypertension and cor pulmonale may also occur.

Assessment findings
The history reveals occupational, family, or neighborhood exposure to beryllium dust, fumes, or mists. The history may also include an itchy rash that has disappeared.

Depending on the time between exposure and the patient's initial symptoms (usually 2 weeks from exposure), inspection may disclose a rash, caused by absorption of beryllium through broken skin, or a "beryllium ulcer," caused by beryllium accidentally implanted in the skin.

Inspection of the nasal mucosa may reveal swelling and ulceration, which can progress to septal perforation, tracheitis, and bronchitis (dry cough).

In acute disease, which develops rapidly (within 3 days) or a few weeks after exposure, the patient may report chest tightness and substernal pain. He may have a dry cough and tachycardia.

In chronic berylliosis, the history may disclose progressively worsening dyspnea. Patient complaints may include mild chest pain and a dry, unproductive cough. Tachypnea may accompany coarse crackles and decreased breath sounds.

Diagnostic tests
• *Chest X-rays* in acute berylliosis suggest pulmonary edema, demonstrating an acute miliary process or a patchy acinous filling and diffuse infiltrates with prominent peribronchial markings. Findings in chronic berylliosis include reticulonodular infiltrates, hilar adenopathy, and large coalescent infiltrates in both lungs.
• *Pulmonary function studies* demonstrate decreased vital capacity, forced vital capacity, residual volume to total lung capacity ratio, diffusing capacity for carbon mon-

oxide, and compliance. These decreased values occur as fibrosis stiffens the lungs.

• *Arterial blood gas analysis* indicates diminished PaO$_2$ and PaCO$_2$.

• *In vitro lymphocyte transformation test,* if positive, confirms the diagnosis. The test is also used to monitor workers' occupational exposure to beryllium.

• *Beryllium patch test,* if positive, establishes a patient's hypersensitivity to beryllium but doesn't confirm the disease.

• *Tissue biopsy* and *spectrographic analysis,* if positive, support but don't confirm the diagnosis.

• *Urinalysis* may identify beryllium excreted in urine, indicating exposure to the metal. Differential diagnosis must rule out sarcoidosis and granulomatous infections.

Treatment

A beryllium ulcer requires excision or curettage. Acute berylliosis requires prompt corticosteroid therapy. If the patient has hypoxia, he may need oxygen delivered by nasal cannula or mask (usually 1 to 2 liters/minute). If he has severe respiratory failure, he may need mechanical ventilation if the PaO$_2$ falls below 40 mm Hg.

The patient with chronic berylliosis usually receives corticosteroid therapy to attempt to alter the disease's progression; maintenance therapy may be lifelong.

Respiratory symptoms may respond to bronchodilators, increased fluid intake (at least 3 liters daily), and chest physiotherapy. Diuretic agents, digitalis preparations, and sodium restriction may help the patient with cor pulmonale.

Nursing diagnoses

• Altered family processes
• Altered nutrition: Less than body requirements
• Anxiety
• Fatigue
• Fear
• Impaired gas exchange
• Ineffective breathing pattern
• Knowledge deficit

Nursing interventions

• Help the patient adjust to life-style changes necessitated by chronic illness.
• Provide high-calorie, high-protein foods. Offer small, frequent meals to conserve the patient's energy and prevent fatigue.
• Make sure the patient receives adequate fluids to loosen and remove secretions.

• Schedule respiratory therapy at least 1 hour before or after meals.
• Perform chest physiotherapy several times daily.
• Encourage daily activity. Provide diversional activities as appropriate. To conserve the patient's energy and prevent fatigue, alternate periods of rest and activity.
• Administer medication, as ordered. Note the patient's response, and monitor him for adverse reactions.
• Watch for complications, such as pulmonary hypertension and cor pulmonale.

Patient teaching

• Advise the patient to avoid crowds and people with known infections, and to obtain influenza and pneumococcus immunizations.
• If the patient receives home oxygen therapy, explain its purpose, and teach him how to operate the equipment.
• Teach the patient and his family how to perform chest physiotherapy with postural drainage and chest percussion. Advise the patient to maintain each position for about 10 minutes and then to perform percussion and cough. Also teach him coughing and deep-breathing techniques to promote good ventilation and to remove secretions.
• Explain the patient's medication regimen to him and his family. Discuss the dosage, adverse effects, and purposes of the prescribed drugs.
• Encourage the patient to follow a high-calorie, protein-rich diet to promote health. Advise him to drink plenty of fluids to prevent dehydration and to help loosen secretions.
• If the patient smokes, encourage him to stop. Provide him with further information or refer him for counseling.
• Inform appropriate patient groups about the health risks posed by berylliosis. Discuss ways to prevent the disease and minimize exposure.

COAL WORKER'S PNEUMOCONIOSIS

Also known as black lung, coal miner's disease, miner's asthma, anthracosis, and anthracosilicosis, coal worker's pneumoconiosis is a progressive nodular pulmonary disease. The disease occurs in two forms: simple and complicated. With the simple form, the patient has characteristically limited lung capacity. In this patient, complicated coal worker's pneumoconiosis (also known as progressive massive fibrosis) may develop. In the complicated form, fibrous tissue masses form in the lungs.

A person's risk for coal worker's pneumoconiosis depends on various factors, including how long he has been exposed to coal dust (usually 15 or more years), the intensity of his exposure (dust count and size of inhaled particles), his proximity to the mine site, the silica content of the coal (anthracite has the highest silica content), and his susceptibility. The highest incidence of this disease is among anthracite miners in the eastern United States.

Causes and pathophysiology

Inhalation and prolonged retention of respirable coal dust particles (less than 5 microns wide) cause coal worker's pneumoconiosis. In the simple form, macules (coal dust–laden macrophages) form around terminal and respiratory bronchioles and are surrounded by a halo of dilated alveoli. At the same time, supporting tissues atrophy and harden, causing permanent small-airway dilation (focal emphysema). Simple coal worker's pneumoconiosis may progress to the complicated form — most likely if the disease begins after a relatively short exposure.

Complicated coal worker's pneumoconiosis may involve one or both lungs. Fibrous tissue masses enlarge and coalesce, grossly distorting pulmonary structures as the disease progressively destroys vessels, alveoli, and airways.

Complications

Pulmonary hypertension, cor pulmonale, and pulmonary tuberculosis can complicate coal worker's pneumoconiosis. In cigarette smokers, chronic bronchitis and emphysema can also complicate the disease.

Assessment findings

Whether the patient has simple or complicated coal worker's pneumoconiosis, the patient history will disclose exposure to coal dust. In the simple form, the patient is typically asymptomatic, especially if he's a nonsmoker.

If the patient has complicated coal worker's pneumoconiosis, the patient history may reveal exertional dyspnea and a cough. This patient may state that he occasionally coughs up inky-black sputum (from avascular necrosis and cavitation).

Additionally, the patient may report a productive cough with milky, gray, clear, or coal-flecked sputum or yellow, green, or thick sputum with recurrent bronchial and pulmonary infections.

Inspection may reveal a barrel chest. Percussion may uncover hyperresonant lungs with areas of dullness. On auscultation, you'll hear diminished breath sounds, crackles, rhonchi, and wheezes.

Diagnostic tests

• *Chest X-rays* in simple coal worker's pneumoconiosis show small opacities (less than 10 mm in diameter). These opacities may inhabit all lung zones but appear more prominent in the upper lung zones. In complicated coal worker's pneumoconiosis, X-rays may show one or more large opacities (1 to 5 cm in diameter). Some may exhibit cavitation.

• *Pulmonary function studies* indicate a vital capacity that's normal in simple coal worker's pneumoconiosis but decreased in the complicated form; decreased forced expiratory volume in 1 second (FEV_1) in the complicated form; and a normal ratio of FEV_1 to forced vital capacity.

The ratio of residual volume to total lung capacity is normal in the simple form but decreased in the complicated form. Diffusing capacity for carbon monoxide — significantly below normal in the complicated form — reflects alveolar septal destruction and pulmonary capillary obliteration.

• *Arterial blood gas analysis* typically shows normal PaO_2 in simple coal worker's pneumoconiosis but decreased PaO_2 in complicated disease. $PaCO_2$ is normal in the simple form (possibly decreasing in hyperventilation) but may increase if the patient is hypoxic and has severely impaired alveolar ventilation.

Treatment

Appropriate treatment aims to relieve respiratory symptoms, manage hypoxia and cor pulmonale, and avoid respiratory tract irritants and infections. Treatment also includes observation for developing tuberculosis.

Respiratory signs and symptoms may be relieved by bronchodilator therapy with theophylline or aminophylline (if bronchospasm is reversible), oral or inhaled sympathomimetics (such as metaproterenol), corticosteroids (such as oral prednisone or aerosolized beclomethasone), or inhalable cromolyn sodium. Chest physiotherapy may be used to mobilize and remove secretions.

Other measures include increased fluid intake (at least 3 qt [3 liters] daily) and respiratory therapy with aerosolized preparations, inhaled mucolytics, and intermittent positive-pressure breathing or incentive spirometry. Diuretic agents, digitalis preparations, and sodium restriction may be ordered to treat cor pulmonale.

In serious illness, oxygen may be administered by cannula or mask (usually 1 to 2 liters/minute) if the patient has chronic hypoxia, or by mechanical ventilation if PaO_2 falls below 40 mm Hg.

Respiratory tract infections require prompt administration of antibiotics.

Nursing diagnoses

- Altered family processes
- Altered nutrition: Less than body requirements
- Anxiety
- Fatigue
- Fear
- Impaired gas exchange
- Ineffective breathing pattern
- Knowledge deficit

Nursing interventions

- Help the patient adjust to life-style changes necessitated by chronic illness. Answer his questions, and encourage him to express his concerns. Include the patient and his family in care-related decisions.
- Assess for changes in baseline respiratory function. Be alert for changes in sputum quality and quantity. Watch for restlessness, increased tachypnea, and changes in breath sounds. Report these changes immediately.
- Provide the patient with high-calorie, high-protein foods, and offer small, frequent meals to conserve his energy and prevent fatigue.
- Make sure the patient receives adequate fluids to loosen secretions.
- Perform chest physiotherapy, including postural drainage and chest percussion and vibration, several times daily.
- Schedule respiratory therapy at least 1 hour before or after meals. Provide mouth care after inhalation therapy.
- If the patient requires incentive spirometry, assist him to a comfortable sitting or semi-Fowler's position to promote optimal lung expansion.
- Encourage daily activity. Provide diversional activities as appropriate. To conserve the patient's energy and prevent fatigue, alternate periods of rest and activity.
- Administer medications, as ordered. Record the patient's response.
- Watch for complications, such as pulmonary hypertension, cor pulmonale, and tuberculosis.

Patient teaching

- Advise the patient to avoid crowds and people with known infections, and to obtain influenza and pneumococcus immunizations.
- If the patient receives home oxygen therapy, explain its purpose. Teach him how to use the equipment.
- Teach the patient and his family how to perform chest physiotherapy with postural drainage and chest percussion. Advise the patient to maintain each position for about 10 minutes and then to perform percussion and coughing exercises. Also teach him coughing and deep-breathing techniques to promote good ventilation and to remove secretions.
- Show the patient how to use an incentive spirometer properly, and tell him why he needs it.
- Explain the patient's medication regimen to him and his family. Discuss the dosages, adverse effects, and purposes of prescribed drugs.
- Encourage the patient to follow a high-calorie, high-protein diet, and to drink plenty of fluids to prevent dehydration and help loosen secretions.
- If the patient smokes, urge him to stop. Provide him with further information, or refer him for counseling.
- As appropriate, provide information about coal worker's pneumoconiosis, including prevention. Educate workers and employers concerning the importance of wearing effective respirators in the workplace.

SELECTED REFERENCES

Avery, M.E., and First, L.R. *Pediatric Medicine*, 2nd ed. Baltimore: Williams & Wilkins Co., 1994.

Farzan, S., et al. *A Concise Handbook of Respiratory Diseases*, 3rd ed. East Norwalk, Conn.: Appleton & Lange, 1992.

Illustrated Manual of Nursing Practice, 2nd ed. Springhouse, Pa.: Springhouse Corp., 1994.

Isselbacher, K., et al. *Harrison's Principles of Internal Medicine*, 13th ed. New York: McGraw-Hill Book Co., 1995.

Kaliner, M.A., et al. "Asthma Therapy: Into the 1990s," *Patient Care* 26(1):69-100, January 15, 1992.

Kyle, J.M., et al. "Exercise-Induced Pulmonary Syndromes," *Medical Clinics of North America* 78(2):413-21, March 1994.

Madden, C.M., et al. "Thoracic Sarcoidosis: The Usual and Unusual," *Applied Radiology* 23(10):37-45, October 1994.

Rakel, R.E., ed. *Conn's Current Therapy 1996*. Philadelphia: W.B. Saunders Co., 1996.

Sahashi, K., et al. "Significance of Interleukin 6 in Patients with Sarcoidosis," *Chest: The Cardiopulmonary Journal* 106(1):158-60, July 1994.

Taylor, C.M., and Sparks, S.M. *Nursing Diagnosis Reference Manual*, 3rd ed. Springhouse, Pa.: Springhouse Corp., 1995.

Tierney, L., et al. *Current Medical Diagnosis and Treatment 1995*. East Norwalk, Conn.: Appleton & Lange, 1995.

9 NEUROLOGIC DISORDERS

INTRODUCTION

The nervous system, the body's communications network, coordinates and organizes the functions of all other body systems. This intricate network has three main divisions:
• the *central nervous system (CNS),* the control center, made up of the brain and the spinal cord
• the *peripheral nervous system,* which includes nerves that connect the CNS to remote body parts and which relays and receives messages from these parts
• the *autonomic nervous system,* which regulates the involuntary function of the internal organs.

Fundamental unit

The *neuron,* the nervous system's fundamental unit, is a highly specialized conductor cell that receives and transmits electrochemical nerve impulses. It has a special, distinguishing structure. Delicate, threadlike nerve fibers extend from the central cell body and transmit signals: *Axons* carry impulses away from the cell body; *dendrites* carry impulses to it. Most neurons have multiple dendrites but only one axon.

Sensory (afferent) neurons transmit impulses from special receptors to the spinal cord or the brain. *Motor (efferent) neurons* transmit impulses from the CNS to regulate activity of muscles or glands. And *interneurons (connecting* or *association neurons)* shuttle signals through complex pathways between sensory and motor neurons. Interneurons account for 99% of all the neurons in the nervous system and include most of the neurons in the brain itself. (See *Structure of the neuron,* page 688.)

Intricate control system

This intricate network of interlocking receptors and transmitters, with the brain and spinal cord, forms a dynamic control system—a "living computer"—that controls and regulates every mental and physical function. From birth to death, the nervous system efficiently organizes the body's affairs—controlling the smallest action, thought, or feeling; monitoring communication and the instinct for survival; and allowing introspection, wonder, and abstract thought. The brain, the center of this central system, is a large, soft mass of nervous tissue that is housed within the cranium and protected and supported by the meninges.

The fragile brain and spinal cord are protected by bone (the skull and vertebrae), which cushions cerebrospinal fluid, and three membranes:
• the *dura mater,* or outer sheath, made of tough white fibrous tissue

• the *arachnoid membrane,* the delicate and lacelike middle layer
• the *pia mater,* the inner meningeal layer, consisting of fine blood vessels held together by connective tissue. This membrane is thin and transparent and clings to the brain and spinal cord surfaces, carrying branches of the cerebral arteries deep into the brain's fissures and sulci.

Between the dura mater and the arachnoid membrane is the *subdural space;* between the pia mater and the arachnoid membrane is the *subarachnoid space.* Within the subarachnoid space and the brain's four ventricles is *cerebrospinal fluid (CSF),* a liquid comprising water and traces of organic materials (especially protein), glucose, and minerals.

CSF is formed from blood in capillary networks called *choroid plexi,* which are located primarily in the brain's lateral ventricles. CSF is eventually reabsorbed into the venous blood through the *arachnoid villi,* in dural sinuses on the brain's surface.

The *cerebrum,* the largest portion of the brain, houses the nerve center that controls sensory and motor activities and intelligence. The outer layer of the cerebrum, the *cerebral cortex,* consists of neuron cell bodies, or gray matter; the inner layers consist of axons, or white matter, plus basal ganglia, which control motor coordination and steadiness. The cerebral surface is deeply convoluted, furrowed with elevations (gyri) and depressions (sulci).

The *longitudinal fissure* divides the cerebrum into two hemispheres connected by a wide band of nerve fibers called the *corpus callosum,* which allows the hemispheres to share learning and intellect. These two hemispheres don't share equally—one always dominates, giving one side control over the other. Because motor impulses descending from the brain through the pyramidal tract cross in the medulla, the right hemisphere controls the left side of the body; the left hemisphere, the right side of the body. Several fissures divide the cerebrum into lobes, each of which is associated with specific functions. (See *A look at the lobes,* page 689.)

The *thalamus,* a relay center below the corpus callosum, further organizes cerebral function by transmitting impulses to and from appropriate areas of the cerebrum. Besides its primary relay function, the thalamus is responsible for primitive emotional response, such as fear, and for distinguishing pleasant stimuli from unpleasant ones.

The *hypothalamus,* which lies beneath the thalamus, is an autonomic center that has connections with the brain, the spinal cord, the autonomic nervous system, and the pituitary gland. It regulates temperature, appetite, blood pressure, breathing, sleep patterns, and pe-

STRUCTURE OF THE NEURON

Consisting of nerve fibers, dendrites, and axons, the neuron receives and transmits electrochemical nerve impulses.

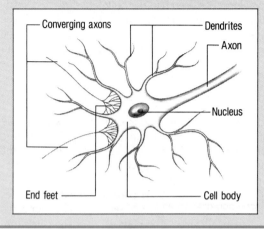

ripheral nerve discharges that occur with behavioral and emotional expression. It also partially controls pituitary gland secretion and stress reaction.

Base of the brain

Beneath the cerebrum, at the base of the brain, is the *cerebellum*. It's responsible for coordinating muscle movements with sensory impulses and maintaining muscle tone and equilibrium.

The *brain stem* houses cell bodies for most of the cranial nerves and includes the *midbrain*, the *pons*, and the *medulla oblongata*. With the thalamus and the hypothalamus, the brain stem makes up a nerve network called the *reticular formation*, which acts as an arousal mechanism. It also relays nerve impulses between the spinal cord and other parts of the brain. The midbrain is the reflex center for the third and fourth cranial nerves and mediates pupillary reflexes and eye movements. The pons helps regulate respirations. It's also the reflex center for the fifth through eighth cranial nerves and mediates chewing, taste, saliva secretion, hearing, and equilibrium. The medulla oblongata influences cardiac, respiratory, and vasomotor functions.

Blood flow to the brain

Four major arteries—two *vertebral* and two *carotid*—supply the brain with oxygenated blood. These arteries originate in or near the aortic arch. The two ver-

tebral arteries (branches of the subclavians) converge to become the basilar artery, which supplies the posterior brain. The common carotids, which supply 85% to 90% of the brain's blood supply, branch into the two internal carotids, which divide further to supply the anterior brain and the middle brain. These arteries interconnect through the *circle of Willis* at the base of the brain. This anastomosis ensures continual circulation to the brain despite interruption of any of the brain's major vessels.

Spinal cord: Conductor pathway

Extending downward from the brain, through the vertebrae, to the second lumbar vertebra is the *spinal cord*, a two-way conductor pathway between the brain stem and the peripheral nervous system. The spinal cord is also the reflex center for activities that don't require brain control, such as a knee-jerk reaction to a reflex hammer.

The spinal cord contains a mass of gray matter divided into horns that are made up mostly of neuron cell bodies, which relay sensations and are needed for voluntary or reflex motor activity. The white matter surrounding the outer part of these horns consists of myelinated nerve fibers grouped functionally in vertical columns called *tracts*. (See *Inside the spinal cord*, page 690.)

The *sensory*, or *ascending*, *tracts* carry sensory impulses up the spinal cord to the brain, while *motor*, or *descending*, *tracts* carry motor impulses down the spinal cord. The brain's motor impulses reach a descending tract and continue through the peripheral nervous system by *upper motor neurons*. These neurons originate in the brain and form two major systems:
• The *pyramidal system* (corticospinal tract) is responsible for fine, skilled movements of skeletal muscle. An impulse in this system originates in the frontal lobe's motor cortex and travels downward to the pyramids of the medulla, where it crosses to the opposite side of the spinal cord.
• The *extrapyramidal system* (extracorticospinal tract) controls gross motor movements. An impulse traveling in this system originates in the frontal lobe's motor cortex and is mediated by basal ganglia, the thalamus, cerebellum, and reticular formation before descending to the spinal cord.

Reaching outlying areas

Messages transmitted through the spinal cord reach outlying areas through the peripheral nervous system, which originates in 31 pairs of segmentally arranged spinal nerves attached to the spinal cord. Spinal nerves

are numbered according to their point of origin in the cord:
- 8 cervical — C1 to C8
- 12 thoracic — T1 to T12
- 5 lumbar — L1 to L5
- 5 sacral — S1 to S5
- 1 coccygeal.

On the cross section of the spinal cord, you'll see that these spinal nerves are attached to the spinal cord by two roots:
- the *anterior,* or *ventral, root* which consists of motor fibers that relay impulses from the cord to glands and muscles
- the *posterior,* or *dorsal, root* which consists of sensory fibers that relay sensory information from receptors to the cord. The posterior root has a swelling on it — the posterior root ganglion — which is made up of sensory neuron cell bodies.

After leaving the vertebral column, each spinal nerve separates into *rami* (branches), which distribute peripherally with extensive but organized overlapping. This overlapping reduces the chance of lost sensory or motor function from interruption of a single spinal nerve.

Two functional systems

The *somatic (voluntary) nervous system* is activated by will but can also function independently. It's responsible for all conscious and higher mental processes and for subconscious and reflex actions, such as shivering.

The *autonomic (involuntary) nervous system* regulates functions of the unconscious level to control involuntary body functions, such as digestion, respiration, and cardiovascular function. It's usually divided into two antagonistic systems. The *sympathetic nervous system* controls energy expenditure, especially in stressful situations, by releasing the adrenergic catecholamine norepinephrine. The *parasympathetic nervous system* helps conserve energy by releasing the cholinergic neurohormone acetylcholine. These antagonistic systems balance each other to support homeostasis.

Assessing neurologic function

A complete neurologic assessment helps confirm a suspected neurologic disorder. It establishes a clinical baseline and can offer lifesaving clues to rapid deterioration. Neurologic assessment includes:
- *Patient history.* In addition to the usual information, try to elicit the patient's and his family's perception of the disorder. Use the interview to make observations that help evaluate mental status and behavior.

A LOOK AT THE LOBES

Several fissures divide the cerebrum into hemispheres and lobes; each lobe has a specific function. The *fissure of Sylvius* (lateral sulcus) separates the temporal lobe from the frontal and parietal lobes. The *fissure of Rolando* (central sulcus) separates the frontal lobes from the parietal lobe. The *parieto-occipital fissure* separates the occipital lobe from the two parietal lobes.

Lobes and their functions

The *frontal lobe* controls voluntary muscle movements and contains motor areas (including the motor area for speech, or Broca's area). It's the center for personality, behavioral, and intellectual functions, such as judgment, memory, and problem solving; for autonomic functions; and for cardiac and emotional responses.

The *temporal lobe* is the center for taste, hearing, and smell, and in the brain's dominant hemisphere, interprets spoken language. The *parietal lobe* coordinates and interprets sensory information from the opposite side of the body. The *occipital lobe* interprets visual stimuli.

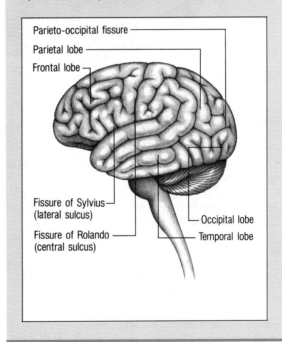

- *Physical examination.* Pay particular attention to obvious abnormalities that may signal serious neurologic problems, for example, fluid draining from the nose or ears.

INSIDE THE SPINAL CORD

A cross section of the spinal cord shows an internal H-shaped mass of gray matter divided into horns, which consist primarily of neuron cell bodies. Cell bodies in the *posterior,* or *dorsal, horn* primarily relay sensations; those in the *anterior,* or *ventral, horn* are needed for voluntary or reflex motor activity. The illustration shows the major components of the spinal cord.

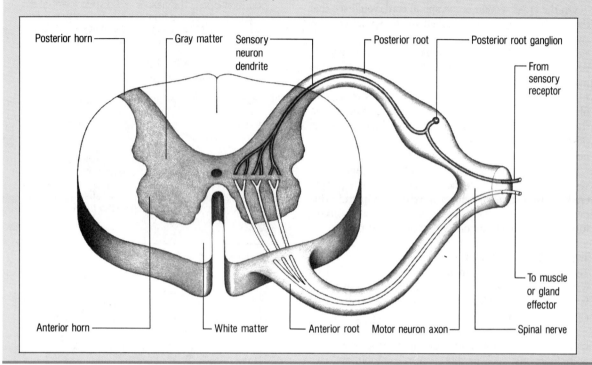

Posterior horn — Gray matter   Sensory neuron dendrite — Posterior root — Posterior root ganglion — From sensory receptor

Anterior horn — White matter — Anterior root   Motor neuron axon — To muscle or gland effector — Spinal nerve

• *Neurologic examination.* Determine cerebral, cerebellar, motor, sensory, and cranial nerve function.

Obviously, time doesn't always allow for a complete neurologic examination during bedside assessment. Therefore, you'll need to set priorities. For example, typical ongoing bedside assessment focuses on level of consciousness, pupillary response, motor function, reflexes, and vital signs. However, when time permits, a complete neurologic examination can provide valuable information regarding total neurologic function.

Mental status, intellect, and behavior

Mental status and behavior are good indicators of cerebral function. Note the patient's appearance, mannerisms, posture, facial expression, grooming, and tone of voice. Check for orientation to time, place, and person, and for memory of recent and past events. To test intellect, ask the patient to count backward from 100 by 7s,

to read aloud, or to interpret a common proverb, and see how well he understands and follows commands. But if you make such checks frequently, vary your questions to avoid a programmed response.

Level of consciousness

The single most valuable indicator of neurologic function, level of consciousness (LOC) can vary from alertness (response to verbal stimulus) to coma (failure to respond even to painful stimulus). It's best to document the patient's exact response to the stimulus: "patient pulled away in response to nail bed pressure" rather than just to write "stuporous."

The Glasgow Coma Scale (GCS), which assesses eye opening as well as verbal and motor responses, won't help you detect early changes in LOC, but it will alert you to life-threatening changes. And although the scale doesn't determine a patient's exact LOC, it does provide an easy way to describe his overall neurologic status and to detect and interpret changes from the baseline. (See *Using the Glasgow Coma Scale,* page 692.)

In this test, each response receives a numerical value. For instance, if the patient readily responds verbally and is oriented to time, place, and person, he scores a 5; if he's totally unable to respond verbally, he scores a 1. If the patient is intubated or has a tracheostomy, assess and score appropriately, such as 5T (T meaning tracheostomy). A score of 15 for all three parts is normal; 7 or less indicates a coma; 3 – the lowest score possible – usually points to brain death. Although the GCS is useful, it's not a substitute for a complete neurologic assessment.

Assessing motor function

The patient's inability to perform the following simple tests, or demonstration of tics, tremors, or other abnormalities during such testing, suggests cerebellar dysfunction.
• Ask the patient to touch his nose with each index finger, alternating hands. Repeat this test with his eyes closed.
• Instruct the patient to tap the index finger and thumb of each hand together rapidly.
• Have the patient draw a figure eight in the air with his foot.
• To test tandem walk, ask the patient to walk heel to toe in a straight line.
• To test balance, perform the Romberg test: Ask the patient to stand with his feet together, eyes closed, and arms at his sides without losing balance.

Motor function is a good indicator of LOC and can also point to central or peripheral nervous system damage. During all tests of motor function, watch for differences between right and left side functions.
• To check gait, ask the patient to walk while you observe posture, balance, and coordination of leg movement and arm swing.
• To check muscle tone, palpate muscles at rest and in response to passive flexion. Look for flaccidity, spasticity, and rigidity. Measure muscle size, and look for involuntary movements, such as rapid jerks, a tremor, or contractions.
• To evaluate muscle strength, have the patient grip your hands and squeeze. Then, ask him to push against your palm with his foot. Compare muscle strength on each side, using a 5-point scale (5 is normal strength, 0 is complete paralysis). Also, test the patient's ability to extend and flex the neck, elbows, wrists, fingers, toes, hips, and knees; to extend the spine; to contract and relax the abdominal muscles; and to rotate the shoulders.

• Rate reflexes on a 4-point scale (4 is hyperactive reflex, 0 is absent reflex). Before testing reflexes, see that the patient is comfortable and relaxed. Then, to test superficial reflexes, stroke the skin of the abdominal, gluteal, plantar, and scrotal regions with a moderately sharp object that won't puncture the skin. A normal reflex is flexion in response to this stimulus. To test deep reflexes, use a reflex hammer to briskly tap the biceps, the triceps, and the brachioradialis, patellar, and Achilles tendon regions. Normal response is rapid muscle extension and contraction.

Assessing sensory function

Impaired or absent sensation in the trunk or extremities can point to brain, spinal cord, or peripheral nerve damage. Be sure to determine the extent of sensory dysfunction because this helps locate neurologic damage. For instance, localized dysfunction indicates local peripheral nerve damage; dysfunction over a single dermatome (an area served by 1 of the 31 pairs of spinal nerves) indicates damage to the nerve's dorsal root; and dysfunction extending over more than one dermatome suggests brain or spinal cord damage.

In assessing sensory function, always test both sides of symmetrical areas; for instance, test both arms, not just one. Reassure the patient that the test won't be painful.
• *Superficial pain perception:* Lightly press the point of an open safety pin against the patient's skin. Don't press hard enough to scratch or puncture the skin.
• *Thermal sensitivity:* Ask the patient to tell you what he feels when you place a test tube filled with hot water and one filled with cold water against his skin.
• *Tactile sensitivity:* Ask the patient to close his eyes and tell you what he feels when touched lightly on hands, wrists, arms, thighs, lower legs, feet, and trunk with a wisp of cotton.
• *Sensitivity to vibration:* Place the base of a vibrating tuning fork against the patient's wrists, elbows, knees, or other bony prominences. Hold it in place, and ask the patient to tell you when it stops vibrating.
• *Position sense:* Move the patient's toes or fingers up, down, and to the side. Ask the patient to tell you the direction of movement.
• *Discriminatory sensation:* Ask the patient to close his eyes and identify familiar textures (velvet, burlap) or objects placed in his hand, or numbers and letters traced on his palm.
• *Two-point discrimination:* Using calipers or other sharp objects, touch the patient in two places simultaneously. Ask if he can feel one or two points.

USING THE GLASGOW COMA SCALE

To quickly assess a patient's level of consciousness and to uncover baseline changes, use the Glasgow Coma Scale. This assessment tool grades consciousness in relation to eye opening and motor and verbal responses. A decreased reaction score in one or more categories warns of impending neurologic crisis. A patient who scores 7 or less is comatose and probably has severe neurologic damage.

If the patient has an endotracheal tube or a tracheostomy tube and is unable to respond verbally, use the abbreviation "T" to score this patient. For example, if the patient scores a 5 for best verbal response but he has a tracheostomy tube in place, this score is noted as 5T.

Test	Patient's reaction	Score
Eye opening response	Opens spontaneously	4
	Opens to verbal command	3
	Opens to pain	2
	No response	1
Best motor response	Obeys verbal command	6
	Localizes painful stimuli	5
	Flexion-withdrawal	4
	Flexion-abnormal (decorticate rigidity)	3
	Extension (decerebrate rigidity)	2
	No response	1
Best verbal response	Oriented and converses	5
	Disoriented and converses	4
	Inappropriate words	3
	Incomprehensible sounds	2
	No response	1
Total		**3 to 15**

Localizing cranial nerve function

By using the simple tests that follow, you can reliably localize cranial nerve dysfunction:

• *Olfactory nerve (I)*. Have the patient close his eyes and, using each nostril separately, try to identify common nonirritating smells, such as cinnamon, coffee, and peppermint.

• *Optic nerve (II)*. Examine the patient's eyes with an ophthalmoscope if you've been trained to do so, and have him read a Snellen eye chart or a newspaper. To test peripheral vision, ask him to cover one eye and fix his other eye on a point directly in front of him. Then, ask if he can see you wiggle your finger to his far right or left.

• *Oculomotor nerve (III)*. Compare the size and shape of the patient's pupils and the equality of pupillary response to a small light in a darkened room.

• *Trochlear nerve (IV)* and *abducens nerve (VI)*. To assess for conjugate and lateral eye movement, ask the patient to follow your finger with his eyes as you slowly move it from his far left to his far right.

• *Trigeminal nerve (V)*. To test facial sensory response, stroke the patient's jaws, cheeks, and forehead with a cotton applicator, the point of a pin, or test tubes filled with hot or cold water. Because testing for a blink reflex is irritating to the patient, it's not commonly done. If you must test for this response (it may be decreased in patients who wear contact lenses), touch the cornea lightly with a wisp of cotton or tissue, and avoid repeating the test, if possible. To test for jaw jerk, ask the patient to hold his mouth slightly open and then tap the middle of his chin with a reflex hammer. The jaw should jerk closed.

• *Facial nerve (VII)*. To test upper and lower facial motor function, ask the patient to raise his eyebrows, wrinkle his forehead, or show his teeth. To test sense of taste, ask him to identify the taste of well-known salty, sour, sweet, and bitter substances, which you have placed on his tongue.

• *Acoustic nerve (VIII)*. Ask the patient to identify common sounds, such as a ticking clock. With a tuning fork, test for air and bone conduction, if you've been taught how to perform this procedure.

• *Glossopharyngeal nerve (IX).* To test the gag reflex, touch a tongue blade to each side of the patient's pharynx.

• *Vagus nerve (X).* Observe ability to swallow, and watch for symmetrical movements of soft palate when the patient says, "Ah."

• *Spinal accessory nerve (XI).* To test shoulder muscle strength, palpate the patient's shoulders, and ask him to shrug against a resistance.

• *Hypoglossal nerve (XII).* To test tongue movement, ask the patient to stick out his tongue. Inspect it for a tremor, atrophy, and lateral deviation. To test for strength, ask the patient to move his tongue from side to side while you hold a tongue blade against it.

Testing for a definitive diagnosis

A firm diagnosis of many neurologic disorders can require a wide range of diagnostic tests. If possible, non-invasive tests are done first and may include the following:

• *Skull X-rays.* This test identifies skull malformations, fractures, erosion, or thickening that may indicate tumors or increased intracranial pressure (ICP).

• *Computed tomography (CT) scan.* This series of X-rays of slices of the brain produces a three-dimensional effect. It's used to identify intracranial tumors, hemorrhage, arteriovenous malformation, and cerebral atrophy, calcification, edema, and infarction. If a contrast medium is used, this is an invasive procedure.

• *Magnetic resonance imaging (MRI).* Because it views the CNS in greater detail than a CT scan, MRI is far better for detecting lesions of the brain stem, posterior fossa, and spinal cord. The diagnostic test of choice for early detection of cerebral infarction and brain tumors, MRI has the ability to demonstrate demyelination disorders such as multiple sclerosis, intraluminal clots and blood flow in arteriovenous malformations, and aneurysms. It's contraindicated for patients with large metal clips because the magnet may dislodge the clip.

• *Magnetic resonance angiography (MRA).* This noninvasive test evaluates cerebral vessels. It maximizes the signals in vessels that have flow. When performed with a contrast medium (gadolinium-DPTA), this test allows better differentiation of structures than MRI and provides clearer views of areas of abnormal contrast.

• *EEG.* This test records electrical activity in the brain. Abnormalities may result from a seizure, a psychological or metabolic disorder, a tumor, mental retardation, or a drug overdose.

• *Visual evoked potentials.* This test exposes the eyes to alternating patterned and unpatterned stimuli, stimulating the visual pathways to the brain. It helps evaluate optic neuropathies and optic nerve lesions.

• *Brain stem auditory evoked potentials.* Using such auditory stimuli as clicks, this test stimulates the brain's auditory pathways, which can help diagnose posterior fossa tumors, demyelinating disease, and conductive hearing loss. It can be used on alert or comatose patients.

• *Somatosensory evoked potentials.* In this test, a peripheral nerve receives an electrical stimulus to evaluate impulse transmission from the nerve to the cerebral cortex.

Invasive tests may include:

• *Lumbar puncture.* In this test, a needle is inserted into the subarachnoid space of the spinal cord, usually between L3 and L4 (or L4 and L5), allowing measurement of CSF pressure and aspiration of CSF for analysis. This specimen is used to detect infection or hemorrhage, to determine cell count, and to determine glucose, protein, and globulin levels. Lumbar puncture is usually contraindicated in patients with hydrocephalus or known increased ICP because a rapid reduction in pressure may cause brain herniation.

• *Myelography.* After a lumbar puncture and CSF removal, a radiopaque dye is instilled. X-rays show spinal abnormalities and determine spinal cord compression related to back pain or extremity weakness.

• *Arteriography (cerebral angiography).* A catheter is inserted into the femoral or another artery and is indirectly threaded to the carotid artery. Then a radiopaque dye is injected, allowing X-ray visualization of cerebral vessels. Sometimes the catheter is threaded directly into the brachial or carotid artery. This test can reveal cerebrovascular abnormalities and spasms plus arterial changes due to tumor, arteriosclerosis, hemorrhage, aneurysm, or blockage from a cerebrovascular accident.

• *Ventriculography.* Air is introduced into the lateral ventricle through an opening in the skull. X-rays are then taken and are used to identify tumors or anomalies that affect the ventricular system.

• *Brain scan.* A scanner measures gamma rays produced by a radioisotope injected I.V. Isotope uptake and distribution in the brain can reveal masses or vascular lesions.

• *Positron emission tomography (PET) scan.* This test provides colorimetric information about the brain's metabolic activity by detecting how quickly tissues consume radioactive isotopes. It can help detect cerebral dysfunction caused by tumors, seizures, transient ischemic attacks, head trauma, some mental illnesses, Alzheimer's disease, Parkinson's disease, and multiple sclerosis.

• *ICP monitoring.* Continuous ICP monitoring is common in intensive care units with patients at risk for increased

ICP. A pressure sensor can be placed in the ventricles (intraventricular catheter), subarachnoid space (subarachnoid bolt), epidural space (epidural sensor), or brain parenchyma (intraparenchymal monitor). The sensor transmits ICP changes to a transducer, which converts the impulse to electrical or light signals. A recording device converts the signals to visible tracings that can be seen on an oscilloscope or transferred to graph paper.
• *Electromyography.* A needle inserted into selected muscles at rest and during voluntary contraction picks up nerve impulses and measures nerve conduction time. This test is used to detect lower motor neuron disorders and nerve damage.

CONGENITAL DISORDERS

Neurologic disorders present at birth may stem from a variety of maternal or fetal causes. Some, such as cerebral palsy, result from prenatal, perinatal, or postnatal central nervous system (CNS) damage. Others, such as hydrocephalus, result from cerebrospinal fluid dysfunction. A weakness in the arterial wall may cause cerebral aneurysm. Embryonic neural tube defects during the first trimester of pregnancy can lead to spinal cord malformations.

CEREBRAL PALSY

The most common crippling disease in children, cerebral palsy comprises several neuromuscular disorders resulting from prenatal, perinatal, or postnatal CNS damage. Although nonprogressive, these disorders may become more obvious as an affected infant grows older.

The three major types of cerebral palsy—spastic (affecting about 70% of children with cerebral palsy), athetoid (affecting about 20%), and ataxic (affecting about 10%)—sometimes occur in mixed forms. Motor impairment may be minimal (sometimes apparent only during physical activities such as running) or severely disabling. Associated defects, such as seizures, speech disorders, and mental retardation, are common. The prognosis varies. In mild impairment, proper treatment may make a near-normal life possible.

Cerebral palsy occurs in an estimated 7,000 live births every year. Incidence is highest in premature infants and in those who are small for gestational age. Cerebral palsy is slightly more common in boys than in girls and occurs more often in whites.

Causes
Cerebral palsy usually stems from conditions that result in cerebral anoxia, hemorrhage, or other damage. Conditions that cause these problems can occur before, during, or after birth.

Prenatal causes include Rh factor or ABO blood type incompatibility, maternal infection (especially rubella in the first trimester), maternal diabetes, irradiation, anoxia, toxemia, malnutrition, abnormal placental attachment, and isoimmunization.

During parturition, conditions that may cause cerebral palsy include trauma during delivery, depressed maternal vital signs from general or spinal anesthesia, asphyxia from cord around the neck, prematurity, prolonged or unusually rapid labor, and multiple births (infants born last in a multiple birth have an especially high rate of cerebral palsy).

Postnatal causes include infections, such as meningitis and encephalitis, head trauma, poisoning, and any condition that results in cerebral thrombus or embolus.

Complications
Cerebral palsy may produce complicating conditions, including seizure disorders (in about 25% of these patients); speech, vision, and hearing problems; language and perceptual deficits; mental retardation (in up to 40% of patients); dental problems; and respiratory difficulties, such as poor swallowing and gag reflexes.

Assessment findings
Maternal or patient history often reveals the possible cause of cerebral palsy. Patients who have mixed forms of the disorder may display a combination of clinical findings. (See *When to suspect cerebral palsy.*)

Generally, inspection reveals a child with retarded growth and development. If you observe the patient eating, you may notice that he has difficulty chewing and swallowing. Other findings vary, depending on the type of cerebral palsy.

In *spastic cerebral palsy,* inspection may reveal underdevelopment of affected limbs and the characteristic scissors gait: Typically, the child walks on his toes, crossing one foot in front of the other. Neurologic examination may reveal hyperactive deep tendon reflexes and increased stretch reflexes, rapid alternating muscle contraction and relaxation, and weakness. Muscle contraction in response to manipulation with a tendency toward contractures also occurs.

In *athetoid cerebral palsy,* inspection may disclose involuntary movements, such as grimacing, wormlike writhing, dystonia, and sharp jerks that impair voluntary movement. Usually, the arms are affected more severely than the legs; involuntary facial movements may make speech difficult. These characteristic athetoid movements may become more severe during stress, decrease with relaxation, and disappear during sleep.

The history of a patient with *ataxic cerebral palsy* chronicles a lack of leg movement during infancy and a wide gait noticed when the child began to walk. Neurologic examination may reveal disturbed balance, incoordination (especially of the arms), hypoactive reflexes, nystagmus, weakness, and tremors. Ataxia makes sudden or fine movements almost impossible.

The patient's history and physical examination findings, including results of the neurologic assessment, confirm the diagnosis of cerebral palsy.

Diagnostic tests
Appropriate tests are performed to diagnose conditions associated with cerebral palsy and to determine the degree of visual, auditory, and mental impairment. For example, an EEG may be performed to identify the source of seizure activity.

Treatment
Cerebral palsy can't be cured, but proper treatment can help affected children reach their full potential within the limits set by this disorder. Such treatment requires a comprehensive and cooperative effort, involving doctors, nurses, teachers, psychologists, the child's family, and occupational, physical, and speech therapists. Home care is often possible. Children with milder forms of cerebral palsy should attend a regular school; severely afflicted children may need special education classes.

Treatment usually includes:
• braces or splints and special appliances, such as adapted eating utensils and a low toilet seat with arms to help these children perform activities independently
• range-of-motion exercises to minimize contractures
• phenytoin, phenobarbital, or another anticonvulsant to control seizures
• sometimes muscle relaxants or neurosurgery to decrease spasticity
• orthopedic surgery to correct contractures (most often part of the treatment in spastic cerebral palsy). Children with this form are especially prone to developing equinous deformity because the heel cord shortens. Achilles tendon lengthening is commonly performed to improve foot function. Muscle transfer procedures are performed to improve function of the wrist or other joints.

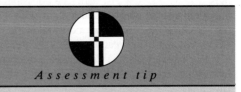

Assessment tip

WHEN TO SUSPECT CEREBRAL PALSY
Early detection—essential for effective treatment—requires careful clinical observation during infancy and precise neurologic assessment. Suspect cerebral palsy whenever an infant:
• has difficulty sucking or keeping the nipple or food in his mouth
• seldom moves voluntarily or has arm or leg tremors with voluntary movement
• crosses his legs when lifted from behind rather than pulling them up or bicycling like a normal infant
• has legs that are hard to separate, making diaper changing difficult
• persistently uses only one hand or, as he gets older, uses his hands well but not his legs.

Nursing diagnoses
• Altered nutrition: Less than body requirements
• Altered thought processes
• Body image disturbance
• Impaired physical mobility
• Knowledge deficit
• Risk for altered parenting
• Risk for impaired skin integrity
• Self-esteem disturbance
• Sensory or perceptual alterations

Nursing interventions
• Because a child with cerebral palsy may be hospitalized for orthopedic surgery and for treatment of other complications, provide emotional support to the child and his family. Answer their questions and be available to them during periods of adjustment.
• To help the child deal with activities of daily living, speak slowly and distinctly. Encourage the child to ask for things he wants. Listen patiently and don't rush him.
• Give all care in an unhurried manner to avoid increasing muscle spasticity.
• Allow the child and his family to participate in care decisions as much as possible. This will improve the child's self-esteem and body image and also help the family continue the care plan at home.
• Plan an adequate diet to meet the child's high energy needs. During meals, maintain a quiet, unhurried at-

mosphere with as few distractions as possible. The child may need special utensils and a chair with a solid footrest. Stroking the throat may aid swallowing.
• Give frequent mouth care and dental care.
• Reduce muscle spasms that increase postoperative pain by moving and turning the child carefully after surgery. Give analgesics as ordered.
• If the child wears a brace, help him apply it as needed. Every day, inspect the skin for areas of pallor or redness that indicate prolonged pressure. Also, provide meticulous skin care and daily massage for the area under the brace. Allow him to wear a T-shirt (provided it doesn't ride up under the brace) to help maintain skin integrity and promote comfort.
• Administer ordered medications as required and perform prescribed exercises to maintain muscle tone.
• Care for associated hearing and visual disturbances, as necessary.

Patient teaching
• Determine how much the child and his parents already know about the disorder and any associated conditions. Reinforce the doctor's explanation, and clear up any misconceptions they may have.
• Teach parents and, if appropriate, the child about any prescribed medications. Provide written information about potential adverse reactions and when to notify the doctor.
• Instruct parents to inspect the skin daily for pressure areas from braces. Explain the need to massage skin areas under the brace.
• Teach the child to place food far back in his mouth to facilitate swallowing. Also, explain the need to chew food thoroughly, drink through a straw, and suck on lollipops to develop muscle control needed to minimize drooling.
• Explain the importance of good nutrition for patients with this disorder. If possible, arrange for the dietitian to instruct the parents and the child.
• As appropriate, teach parents how to perform prescribed exercises to maintain muscle tone and joint function.
• Emphasize to parents the importance of giving the child opportunities for learning. If appropriate, tell parents about summer camps for handicapped children and the Special Olympics. Explain that these activities can help the child realize that he isn't the only person with this handicap. Refer the family to community support groups, such as the local chapter of the United Cerebral Palsy Association.

HYDROCEPHALUS
An excessive accumulation of cerebrospinal fluid (CSF) within the ventricular spaces of the brain, hydrocephalus is most common in neonates. It can also occur in adults as a result of injury or disease. In infants, hydrocephalus enlarges the head; in both infants and adults, resulting compression can damage brain tissue. With early detection and surgical intervention, the prognosis improves but remains guarded.

Causes
Hydrocephalus may result from an obstruction in CSF flow (noncommunicating hydrocephalus) or from faulty absorption of CSF (communicating hydrocephalus).

In noncommunicating hydrocephalus, the obstruction occurs most frequently between the third and fourth ventricles, at the aqueduct of Sylvius, but it can also occur at the outlets of the fourth ventricle (foramina of Luschka and Magendie) or, rarely, at the foramen of Monro. This obstruction may result from faulty fetal development (myelomeningocele, congenital arachnoid cysts), infection (syphilis, granulomatous diseases, meningitis), tumor, cerebral aneurysm, or a blood clot.

In communicating hydrocephalus, faulty reabsorption of CSF may result from surgery to repair a myelomeningocele, adhesions between meninges at the base of the brain, or meningeal hemorrhage.

Complications
Potential complications of hydrocephalus include mental retardation, impaired motor function, and vision loss. Death may result from increased intracranial pressure (ICP) in people of all ages; infants may also die of infection and malnutrition.

Assessment findings
The patient's history may disclose the cause of hydrocephalus. In an infant, inspection may reveal an enlarged head that is clearly disproportionate to the infant's growth, an unmistakable sign of hydrocephalus. If an assessment of the infant occurs immediately after the start of hydrocephalus, the head may appear normal in size with bulging fontanels.

Other characteristic findings noted on inspection include distended scalp veins; thin, fragile, and shiny scalp skin; and underdeveloped neck muscles. (See *The infant with hydrocephalus*.)

In severe hydrocephalus, the infant's parents may report a high-pitched, shrill cry; irritability; anorexia; and episodes of projectile vomiting. Inspection may reveal depression of the roof of the eye orbit, displacement of the eyes downward, and prominent sclera (sunset sign). Neurologic examination may demonstrate abnormal muscle tone of the legs.

In adults and older children with a fused cranium, the patient history may uncover signs of increased ICP, including frontal headaches, nausea, and vomiting that may be projectile. If the patient or parents report that these symptoms cause wakening or occur on awakening, hydrocephalus should be suspected. The patient may also report diplopia and restlessness. Neurologic examination may detect a decreased level of consciousness, ataxia, and impaired intellect. Neurologic impairment may also cause incontinence.

Diagnostic tests
• *Skull X-rays* show thinning of the skull with separation of sutures and widening of the fontanels.
• *Angiography, computed tomography scan,* and *magnetic resonance imaging* differentiate between hydrocephalus and intracranial lesions and can also demonstrate the Arnold-Chiari deformity, which occurs with hydrocephalus. (See *Arnold-Chiari syndrome,* page 698.)

Treatment
Surgical correction is the only treatment for hydrocephalus. Surgery is performed either to remove an obstruction to CSF flow or to implant a shunt to divert CSF flow. Usually, such surgery involves insertion of a ventriculoperitoneal shunt, which drains excess CSF fluid from the brain's lateral ventricle into the peritoneal cavity.

If a concurrent abdominal problem exists, the doctor may use a ventriculoatrial shunt, which drains fluid from the brain's lateral ventricle into the right atrium of the heart, where the fluid makes its way into the venous circulation.

Nursing diagnoses
• Altered cerebral tissue perfusion
• Altered family processes
• Altered growth and development
• Altered nutrition: Less than body requirements
• Anxiety
• Body image disturbance
• Impaired skin integrity
• Pain
• Risk for infection

Nursing interventions
• Provide emotional support, and encourage the patient (if appropriate) and family to express their concerns. An older child about to undergo shunt surgery may focus on

THE INFANT WITH HYDROCEPHALUS

Characteristic changes of hydrocephalus in infants include marked head enlargement; distended scalp veins; thin, shiny, and fragile-looking scalp skin; and underdeveloped neck muscles.

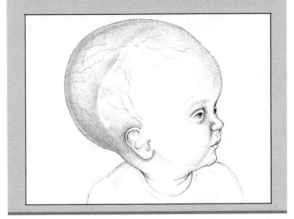

associated hair loss and the visibility of a mechanical device. To help him deal with this change in body image, introduce him to other children with similar problems.
• Encourage maternal-infant bonding when possible. When caring for the infant yourself, hold him on your lap for feeding, stroke and cuddle him, and speak soothingly.
• Check fontanels for tension or fullness, and measure and record head circumference. On the patient's chart, draw a picture showing where to measure the head so that other staff members measure it in the same place, or mark the forehead with ink.
• Elevate the head of the bed to 30 degrees to help alleviate increasing ICP.
• Administer oxygen as ordered. Have suction equipment at the bedside, and suction as necessary.
   Before surgery to insert a shunt:
• Provide small, frequent feedings, if necessary, to ensure adequate nutrition. To help lessen vomiting, decrease movement during and immediately after meals.
• Feed the infant slowly. To lessen strain from the weight of the infant's head on your arm while holding him during feeding, place his head, neck, and shoulders on a pillow.
• To prevent aspiration after feeding and hypostatic pneumonia, place the infant on his side and reposition every 2 hours, or prop him up in an infant seat.

ARNOLD-CHIARI SYNDROME

Hydrocephalus is frequently accompanied by the Arnold-Chiari syndrome, especially when a myelomeningocele is also present. In this condition, which may exist apart from hydrocephalus, an elongation or tonguelike downward projection of the cerebellum and medulla extends through the foramen magnum into the cervical portion of the spinal canal, impairing CSF drainage from the fourth ventricle.

In addition to signs and symptoms of hydrocephalus, infants with this syndrome may have nuchal rigidity, noisy respirations, irritability, vomiting, weak sucking reflex, and a preference for hyperextension of neck.

Treatment requires surgery to insert a shunt like that used in hydrocephalus. Surgical decompression of the cerebellar tonsils at the foramen magnum is sometimes indicated.

• To prevent skin breakdown, make sure the infant's earlobe is flat, and place a foam rubber pad under his head.
• When turning the infant, move his head, neck, and shoulders with his body, to reduce strain on his neck.
• Monitor the infant closely for signs of neurologic complications, such as seizure activity, irregular respirations, and bradycardia. Notify the doctor of these changes.
• Check the infant's growth and development periodically.

After shunt surgery:
• Place the infant on the side opposite the operative site, with his head level with his body unless the doctor's orders specify otherwise.
• Monitor intake and output, and administer I.V. fluids as ordered.
• Check temperature, pulse rate, blood pressure, and level of consciousness. Also check fontanels for fullness daily. Watch for vomiting, which may be an early sign of increased ICP and shunt malfunction.
• Watch for signs of infection, especially meningitis: fever, stiff neck, irritability, or tense fontanels. Also watch for redness, swelling, and other signs of local infection over the shunt tract. Check dressing often for drainage. Use strict aseptic technique when changing dressing.
• Be alert for other postoperative complications, including adhesions, paralytic ileus, migration, peritonitis, and intestinal perforation (with peritoneal shunt).
• Carefully titrate analgesics to provide pain relief but still permit adequate neurologic assessment.

Patient teaching
• Determine how much the patient (if appropriate) and his family know about the disorder, its treatment, and possible complications. Reinforce the doctor's explanation, as needed.
• Help parents set goals consistent with the patient's ability and potential. Teach them to focus on their child's strengths, not his weaknesses.
• Provide preoperative teaching, as appropriate. Be sure the patient (if appropriate) and his parents understand the surgical procedure and the desired outcome. Also teach them about postoperative care measures.
• Discuss special education programs with the parents, and emphasize the infant's needs for sensory stimulation appropriate for his age.
• Instruct them to watch for signs of shunt malfunction, infection, and paralytic ileus.
• Tell them that shunt insertion requires periodic surgery to lengthen the shunt as the child grows older and that surgery may also be required to correct malfunction or to treat infection.

CEREBRAL ANEURYSM

This localized dilation of a cerebral artery results from a weakness in the arterial wall. Its most common form is the saccular (berry) aneurysm, a saclike outpouching in a cerebral artery. (See *Comparing aneurysm types.*) Cerebral aneurysms commonly rupture, causing subarachnoid hemorrhage. Sometimes bleeding also spills into the brain tissue and subsequently forms a clot. This may result in potentially fatal increased intracranial pressure (ICP) and brain tissue damage.

Most cerebral aneurysms occur at bifurcations of major arteries in the circle of Willis and its branches. An aneurysm can produce neurologic symptoms by exerting pressure on the surrounding structures, such as the cranial nerves. (See *Common sites of cerebral aneurysm*, page 700.)

Cerebral aneurysms are much more common in adults than in children. Incidence is slightly higher in women than in men, especially women in their late 40s or early to middle 50s, but cerebral aneurysm may occur at any age. In about 20% of patients, multiple aneurysms occur.

The prognosis is usually guarded but depends on the patient's age and neurologic condition, other diseases, and the extent and location of the aneurysm. About half the patients who suffer subarachnoid hemorrhages die immediately. With new and better treatment, the prognosis is improving.

COMPARING ANEURYSM TYPES

Saccular (berry) aneurysm
- Most common type
- Secondary to congenital weakness of media
- Usually occurs at major vessel bifurcations
- Occurs at the circle of Willis
- Has a neck or stem
- Has a sac that may be partly filled with a blood clot

Fusiform (spindle-shaped) aneurysm
- Occurs with atherosclerotic disease
- Characterized by irregular vessel dilation
- Develops on internal carotid or basilar arteries
- Rarely ruptures
- Produces brain and cranial nerve compression or CSF obstruction

Mycotic aneurysm
- Rare
- Associated with septic emboli that occur secondary to bacterial endocarditis
- Develops when emboli lodge in arterial lumen, causing arteritis; the arterial wall weakens and dilates

Dissecting aneurysm
- Caused by arteriosclerosis, head injury, syphilis, or trauma during angiography
- Develops when blood is forced between layers of arterial walls, stripping intima from the underlying muscle layer

Traumatic aneurysm
- Develops in the carotid system
- Associated with fractures and intimal damage
- May thrombose spontaneously

Giant aneurysm
- Similiar to saccular, but larger — 1⅛″ (3 cm) or more in diameter
- Behaves like a space-occupying lesion, producing cerebral tissue compression and cranial nerve damage
- Associated with hypertension

Charcot-Bouchard aneurysm
- Microscopic
- Associated with hypertension
- Involves basal ganglia or brain stem

Causes

Cerebral aneurysm results from a congenital defect of the vessel wall, head trauma, hypertensive vascular disease, advancing age, infection, or atherosclerosis, which can weaken the vessel wall.

Complications

Potentially fatal complications after rupture of an aneurysm include subarachnoid hemorrhage and brain tissue infarction. Cerebral vasospasm, probably the most common cause of death after rupture, occurs in about 40% of all patients after subarachnoid hemorrhage occurs.

Other possible complications include rebleeding, which usually occurs within the first 7 days but can occur anytime within the first 6 months; meningeal irritation from blood in the subarachnoid space; and hydrocephalus, which can occur weeks or even months after rupture if blood obstructs the fourth ventricle.

Assessment findings

Most cerebral aneurysms produce no symptoms until rupture occurs. History information may have to be obtained from a family member if the patient is unconscious or severely neurologically impaired.

Usually, the patient history reveals the sudden onset of an unusually severe headache that is accompanied by nausea, vomiting and, commonly, loss of consciousness. The patient or family member may report that the rupture was preceded by a period of activity, such as exercise, labor and delivery, or sexual intercourse. The patient also may have a history of hypertension, infection, or head injury.

Other findings vary with the location of the aneurysm and the extent and severity of hemorrhage. Bleeding causes meningeal irritation, which can result in nuchal rigidity, back and leg pain, fever, restlessness, irritability, occasional seizures, and blurred vision. If the aneurysm is adjacent to the oculomotor nerve, ptosis and vision disturbances, such as diplopia and vision loss, may occur. If the bleeding extends into the brain tissue, hemiparesis, unilateral sensory deficits, dysphagia, visual defects, and altered consciousness may occur. Additional findings may result from complications. (See *What to watch for after a ruptured aneurysm*, page 701.)

To better describe the condition of patients with ruptured cerebral aneurysm, the following grading system has been developed:

• *grade I (minimal bleeding)*. Patient is alert, with no neurologic deficit; he may have a slight headache and nuchal rigidity.

COMMON SITES OF CEREBRAL ANEURYSM

Cerebral aneurysms usually arise at arterial bifurcations in the circle of Willis and its branches. The illustration below shows the most common aneurysm sites around this circle.

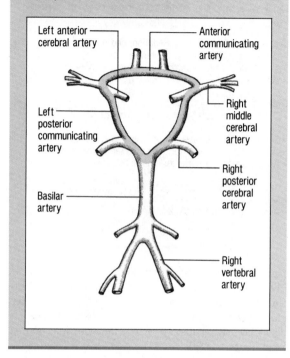

• *grade II (mild bleeding).* Patient is alert with a mild to severe headache, nuchal rigidity and, possibly, third-nerve palsy.
• *grade III (moderate bleeding).* Patient is confused or drowsy, with nuchal rigidity and, possibly, a mild focal deficit.
• *grade IV (severe bleeding).* Patient is stuporous, with nuchal rigidity and, possibly, mild to severe hemiparesis.
• *grade V (moribund [often fatal]).* If nonfatal, patient is in deep coma or decerebrate.

Diagnostic tests

The following tests help establish a diagnosis, which usually follows aneurysmal rupture:
• *Angiography* confirms the aneurysm's location and displays the vessels' condition.
• *Lumbar puncture* can detect blood in the cerebrospinal fluid (CSF), but this procedure is contraindicated if the patient shows signs of increased ICP.

• *Computed tomography scan* locates the clot and identifies hydrocephalus, areas of infarction, and the extent of blood spillage within the cisterns around the brain.
• *Magnetic resonance imaging* and *magnetic resonance angiography* show the extent of bleeding and the vessels' condition.

Treatment

If indicated, initial emergency treatment includes oxygenation and ventilation. Then, to reduce the risk of rebleeding, the doctor may attempt to repair the aneurysm. Usually, surgical repair (by clipping, ligating, or wrapping the aneurysm neck with muscle) takes place as soon as the patient's condition allows after the initial bleeding.

After surgical repair, the patient's condition depends on the extent of damage from the initial bleeding and the degree of success in treating the resulting complications. Surgery can't improve the patient's neurologic condition unless it removes a hematoma or reduces the compression effect.

When surgical correction poses too much risk (in very elderly patients and those with heart, lung, or other serious diseases), when the aneurysm is in a particularly dangerous location, or when vasospasm necessitates a delay in surgery, the patient may receive conservative treatment, including:
• bed rest in a quiet, darkened room (may last for 4 to 6 weeks) if immediate surgery isn't possible
• avoidance of coffee, other stimulants, and aspirin
• codeine or another analgesic, as needed
• hydralazine or another antihypertensive, if needed
• a vasoconstrictor to maintain blood pressure at the optimum level (20 to 40 mm Hg above normal), if needed
• corticosteroids to reduce cerebral edema
• phenobarbital or another sedative to relax the patient
• nimodipine or another calcium channel blocker to decrease vasospasm.

Nursing diagnoses

• Altered nutrition: Less than body requirements
• Altered thought processes
• Anxiety
• Impaired gas exchange
• Impaired physical mobility
• Ineffective breathing pattern
• Knowledge deficit
• Pain
• Risk for impaired skin integrity
• Risk for injury
• Sensory or perceptual alterations

WHAT TO WATCH FOR AFTER A RUPTURED ANEURYSM

If your patient survives a ruptured cerebral aneurysm, monitor him closely for rebleeding, cerebral vasospasm, and acute hydrocephalus—life-threatening complications. This chart lists the signs and symptoms of each complication, and tells when it is most likely to occur and how it should be treated.

Complication	Signs and symptoms	Onset	Treatment
Rebleeding	Deterioration of neurologic status, decrease in level of consciousness (LOC), intensifying headache	7 to 10 days after rupture	Sedation, bed rest, avoidance of Valsalva's maneuver
Cerebral vasospasm	Decrease in LOC, motor weakness or paralysis, visual deficits, changes in vital signs (particularly respiratory patterns)	Several hours to 7 days after rupture	• Intravascular volume expanders • Induced hypertensive therapy • Calcium channel blockers
Hydrocephalus	Mental changes, gait disturbances, general mental and physical deterioration	Several hours to 7 days after rupture	Cerebrospinal fluid drainage via intraventricular catheter

Nursing interventions

During initial treatment after hemorrhage:
• Maintain a patent airway because the patient may need supplementary oxygen. Position the patient to promote pulmonary drainage and prevent upper airway obstruction. Following hospital policy, suction the airway as needed to remove secretions and to prevent hypoxia and vasodilation from carbon dioxide accumulation. Suction in less than 20 seconds to avoid increased ICP.
• Provide frequent nose and mouth care.

If surgery is delayed:
• Impose aneurysm precautions to minimize the risk of rebleeding and to avoid increased ICP. Such precautions include bed rest in a quiet, darkened room (keep the head of the bed flat or elevated less than 30 degrees, as ordered); limited visitors; avoidance of coffee and other stimulants; avoidance of Valsalva's maneuver and other strenuous physical activity; and restricted fluid intake.
• Watch for these danger signs of an enlarging aneurysm, rebleeding, intracranial clot, vasospasm, or other complication: decreased level of consciousness (LOC), unilateral enlarged pupil, onset or worsening of hemiparesis or motor deficit, increased blood pressure, slowed pulse rate, worsening or sudden onset of a headache, renewed or persistent vomiting, and renewed or worsening nuchal rigidity. Intermittent signs, such as restlessness, extremity weakness, and speech alterations, can also indicate increasing ICP.
• Administer hydralazine or another antihypertensive agent, as ordered, and carefully monitor blood pressure.

Report any significant change in blood pressure, but especially note a rise in systolic pressure. If this occurs, notify the doctor immediately.

For preoperative and postoperative interventions and conservative treatment:
• Provide emotional support to the patient and his family. To minimize stress, encourage the patient to use relaxation techniques. Encourage him to express his concerns if he's able.
• Turn the patient often. Encourage deep breathing and leg movement. Assist with active range-of-motion exercises; if the patient is paralyzed, perform passive range-of-motion exercises.
• Monitor arterial blood gas levels, LOC, and vital signs often, and accurately measure intake and output. Avoid taking temperature rectally because vagus nerve stimulation may cause cardiac arrest.
• Give fluids, as ordered, and monitor I.V. infusions to avoid overhydration, which may increase ICP.
• If the patient has facial weakness, assist him during meals; assess his gag reflex, and place the food in the unaffected side of his mouth.
• If the patient can't swallow, insert a nasogastric tube, as ordered, and give all tube feedings slowly. Prevent skin breakdown by taping the tube so it doesn't press against the nostril.
• If the patient can eat, provide a high-bulk diet (including such foods as bran, salads, and fruit) to prevent straining during defecation, which can increase ICP. Obtain an order for a stool softener or a mild laxative, and administer it as ordered. Don't force fluids. Implement a

UNDERSTANDING ENCEPHALOCELE

An encephalocele is a congenital saclike protrusion of the meninges and brain through a defective opening in the skull. Usually, it's in the occipital area, but it may also occur in the parietal, nasopharyngeal, or frontal area.

Clinical effects
Varying clinical effects of encephalocele depend on the defect's location and the degree of tissue involvement. Visual defects may occur because optic tracks are stretched or absent. Often, paralysis and hydrocephalus accompany encephalocele.

Treatment
Surgery is performed during infancy to place protruding tissues back in the skull, excise the sac, and correct associated craniofacial abnormalities.
    Always handle an infant with encephalocele carefully and avoid pressure on the sac. Both before and after surgery, watch for signs of increased intracranial pressure (bulging fontanels). As the child grows older, teach his parents to watch for developmental deficiencies that may signal mental retardation.

bowel elimination program based on previous habits. If the patient is receiving steroids, check the stool for blood.
• If the patient has third or facial nerve palsy, administer artificial tears to the affected eye, and tape the eye shut at night to prevent corneal damage.
• Raise the bed's side rails to protect the patient from injury. If possible, avoid using restraints because these can cause agitation and raise ICP.
• If appropriate, perform postoperative craniotomy care: Inspect the patient's head dressing for bleeding and CSF drainage; position the patient so that the neck is in a straight line to prevent interference with cerebral drainage by neck flexion; monitor ICP as ordered; and maintain adequate respiratory function and brain oxygenation, using supplementary oxygen and mechanical ventilation, as ordered.
• Monitor the patient for postoperative complications, including sudden hemiplegia, psychological problems (disorientation, amnesia, Korsakoff's syndrome, personality impairment), fluid and electrolyte disturbances, and GI bleeding.

Patient teaching
• Teach the patient, if possible, and his family about his condition. Encourage family members to adopt a realistic

attitude, but don't discourage hope. Answer questions honestly.
• Explain all tests, neurologic examinations, treatments, and procedures to the patient even if he's unconscious.
• Warn the patient who will be treated conservatively to avoid all unnecessary physical activity.
• If surgery will be performed, provide preoperative teaching if the patient's condition permits. Be sure the patient, if possible, and the family understand the surgery and its possible complications. Reinforce the doctor's explanations as necessary.
• Before discharge, make a referral to a home health care nurse or a rehabilitation center when necessary.
• Teach family members to recognize and immediately report signs of rebleeding, such as headache, nausea, vomiting, and changes in LOC (irritability, restlessness).

SPINAL CORD DEFECTS
Defective embryonic neural tube closure during the first trimester of pregnancy results in various malformations of the spine. These defects usually occur in the lumbosacral area, but they're occasionally found in the sacral, thoracic, and cervical areas. If the skull doesn't fuse properly, the meninges and brain tissue can protrude. (See *Understanding encephalocele.*)
    The most common and least severe spinal cord defect, *spina bifida occulta* is an incomplete closure of one or more vertebrae without protrusion of the spinal cord or meninges. However, in more severe forms of spina bifida, such as spina bifida cystica, incomplete closure of one or more vertebrae causes protrusion of the spinal contents in an external sac or a cystic lesion.
    Spina bifida cystica has two classifications: myelomeningocele (meningomyelocele) and meningocele. In myelomeningocele, the external sac contains meninges, cerebrospinal fluid (CSF), and a portion of the spinal cord or nerve roots distal to the conus medullaris. When the spinal nerve roots end at the sac, motor and sensory functions below the sac are terminated. In meningocele, less severe than myelomeningocele, the sac contains only meninges and CSF. Meningocele may produce no neurologic symptoms. (See *Types of spinal cord defects.*)
    Spina bifida is relatively common: In the United States, about 12,000 infants each year are born with some form of spina bifida. Incidence is highest in people of Welsh or Irish ancestry.
    The prognosis varies with the degree of accompanying neurologic defect. It's worst in patients with large open lesions, neurogenic bladders (which predispose to infection and renal failure), or total paralysis of the legs. Be-

TYPES OF SPINAL CORD DEFECTS

There are three major types of spinal cord defects. Spina bifida occulta is characterized by a depression or raised area and a tuft of hair over the defect. In myelomeningocele, an external sac contains menin- ges, CSF, and a portion of the spinal cord or nerve roots. In meningocele, an external sac contains only meninges and CSF.

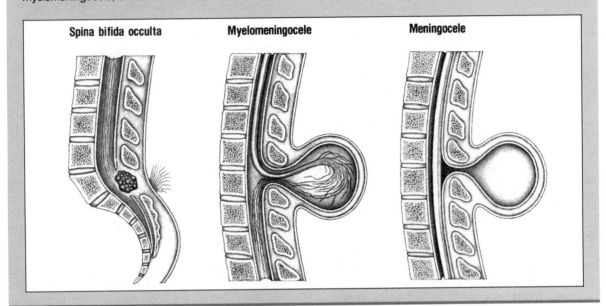

Spina bifida occulta   **Myelomeningocele**   **Meningocele**

cause such features are usually absent in spina bifida occulta and meningocele, the prognosis is much better for these patients, and many of them can lead normal lives.

Causes and pathophysiology

Normally, about 20 days after conception, the embryo develops a neural groove in the dorsal ectoderm. This groove rapidly deepens as the two edges fuse to form the neural tube. By about day 23, this tube is completely closed except for an opening at each end. Theoretically, if the posterior portion of the neural tube fails to close by the fourth week of gestation, or if it closes and then splits open from a cause such as an abnormal increase in CSF later in the first trimester, a spinal cord defect results.

The exact cause of spinal cord defects is not known. Viruses, radiation, and other environmental factors may be responsible for such defects. However, spinal cord defects occur in offspring of women who have previously had children with similiar defects, so genetic factors may also be responsible.

Complications

Spinal cord defects can lead to infection, paralysis, hydrocephalus and, if the disorder remains untreated, death.

Assessment findings

The history of the infant's mother may reveal environmental factors that could have placed the infant at risk for development of spinal cord defects.

Inspection of the neonate with spina bifida occulta often reveals a depression or dimple; a tuft of hair; soft, fatty deposits; port wine nevi; or a combination of these abnormalities over the spinal defect. Palpation may reveal a depression or raised area along the spine over the defect. In many cases, neurologic status is normal because spina bifida occulta doesn't always cause neurologic dysfunction.

In spina bifida cystica, inspection reveals a saclike protrusion over the spinal cord. Transillumination of the protruding sac can sometimes distinguish between meningocele (light typically crosses through the sac) and myelomeningocele (light doesn't cross the sac).

Depending on the defect's location, effects of myelomeningocele may include permanent neurologic dysfunction. Neurologic examination may reveal flaccid or spastic paralysis and bowel and bladder incontinence.

Other assessment findings are often related to associated disorders. These findings may include trophic skin disturbances (ulcerations, cyanosis), clubfoot, knee contractures, hydrocephalus (in about 90% of patients) and, possibly, mental retardation, Arnold-Chiari syndrome (in which part of the brain protrudes into the spinal canal), and curvature of the spine.

Diagnostic tests
• *Spinal X-rays* show the bone defect in spina bifida and can also demonstrate associated hydrocephalus in meningocele and myelomeningocele.
• *Myelography* differentiates spina bifida from other spinal abnormalities, especially spinal cord tumors.
• *Cephalic measurements* and *computed tomography scan* demonstrate associated hydrocephalus in meningocele and myelomeningocele.
• *Urinalysis* and *urine cultures* may also be done.

Treatment
Care of the patient with a severe spinal defect requires a team approach, including the neurosurgeon, orthopedist, urologist, pediatrician, nurse, social worker, occupational and physical therapists, and family members. Specific measures depend on the severity of the neurologic deficit.

Spina bifida occulta requires little or no treatment. If indicated, surgery is performed soon after birth to release the tethered spinal cord and prevent further neurologic deterioration.

Initial treatment for spina bifida cystica includes surgical closure of the defect as soon as possible after birth, if possible within 48 hours. Then the child's growth and development are continually assessed throughout life. If the protruding sac is large, plastic surgery is required for skin grafting over the lesion. Surgery doesn't reverse the neurologic deficit. Usually, a shunt is necessary to relieve associated hydrocephalus. If hydrocephalus isn't apparent at the time of the initial surgery, the child must be frequently reassessed for its occurrence because hydrocephalus occurs in about 80% of children with myelomeningocele.

After surgery, supportive measures are required to promote independence and prevent further complications. Orthopedic, rehabilitation, and urologic consultations help determine the extent of the child's disabilities. Rehabilitation measures, which may be necessary throughout the child's life, may include:
• waist supports, leg braces, walkers, crutches, and other orthopedic appliances
• diet and bowel training to manage fecal incontinence
• neurogenic bladder management to reduce urinary stasis, possibly intermittent catheterization, and antispasmodics, such as bethanechol or propantheline.

Nursing diagnoses
• Altered growth and development
• Altered parenting
• Altered tissue perfusion
• Altered urinary elimination
• Bowel incontinence
• Impaired physical mobility
• Impaired skin integrity
• Risk for infection
• Risk for injury

Nursing interventions
• Provide psychological support and encourage a positive attitude. Help parents work through their feelings of guilt, anger, and helplessness.
  Before surgery:
• Prevent infection by cleaning the defect gently with sterile 0.9% sodium chloride solution or other solutions, as ordered. Inspect the defect often for signs of infection, and keep it covered with sterile dressings moistened with sterile 0.9% sodium chloride solution. Don't use ointments on the defect, since they may cause skin maceration. Administer prophylactic antibiotic, as ordered. Prevent skin breakdown by placing sheepskin or a foam pad under the infant and positioning the child in the prone position for the first days after surgery. Keep skin clean, and apply lotion to knees, elbows, chin, and other pressure areas. Give antibiotics, as ordered.
• Position the child on his abdomen with the head of the bed slightly elevated to prevent contamination of the sac with urine or feces. If necessary, use pediatric fecal-incontinence bags to protect skin integrity.
• Observe the child for signs of meningitis, including irritability, fever, feeding intolerance, and seizures. Notify the doctor if any of these signs occurs.
• Hold and cuddle the infant, but avoid placing pressure on the sac. When holding him on your lap, position him on his abdomen.
• Provide adequate time for parent-infant bonding.
• Measure head circumference daily, and watch for signs of hydrocephalus and meningeal irritation, such as fever

and nuchal rigidity. Be sure to mark the spot for head measurement so that you get accurate readings.
• Minimize contractures with passive range-of-motion exercises and casting. To prevent hip dislocation, moderately abduct the hips with a pad between the knees or with sandbags and ankle rolls.
• Monitor intake and output. Watch for signs of decreased skin turgor, dryness, or other signs of dehydration. Provide meticulous perineal care to prevent infection.
• Ensure adequate nutrition.

After surgery:
• Monitor the patient's vital signs often. Watch for signs of shock (decreased blood pressure, tachycardia, lethargy), infection (malaise, elevated temperature, alteration in feeding pattern), and increased intracranial pressure (projectile vomiting). Frequently assess the infant's fontanels. Remember that before age 2, infants don't show typical signs of increased intracranial pressure, since suture lines aren't fully closed. In infants, the most telling sign is bulging fontanels.
• Use aseptic technique when caring for the wound. Change the dressing regularly, as ordered, or whenever it becomes soiled with urine or feces. Report any signs of drainage, wound rupture, and infection.
• If a muscle flap has been used to close the defect site, place the patient in a prone position during the first 48 hours after surgery.
• Usually, the child can't wear a diaper or a shirt until after the surgical correction because it will irritate the sac, so keep him warm in an infant Isolette.
• Watch for hydrocephalus, which often follows such surgery. Measure the child's head circumference, and monitor the infant's fontanel size and sutures.
• If a shunt is in place to decrease hydrocephalus, observe the site for redness or swelling. Stay alert for fever and neurologic changes.
• If leg casts have been applied to treat deformities, look for signs that the child is outgrowing the cast. Check distal pulses to ensure adequate circulation. Petal the cast edges with plastic to prevent softening and skin irritation. Use a cool-air blow-dryer to dry skin under the cast. Periodically check for foul odor and other indications of skin breakdown.

Patient teaching
• Teach parents how to recognize early signs of complications, such as hydrocephalus, pressure ulcers, and urinary tract infection.
• To help maintain adequate bladder function, teach parents Credé's maneuver, intermittent catheterization and, if necessary, conduit hygiene. Stress the importance of increased fluid intake to help prevent frequent urinary tract infections and, possibly, renal failure. Encourage parents to begin a bladder training routine with their child by age 3.
• To help prevent constipation and bowel obstruction, stress the need for increased fluid intake, a high-bulk diet, exercise, and use of a stool softener, as ordered. If possible, teach parents to help empty their child's bowel by telling him to bear down and giving a glycerin suppository, as needed. Explain the problems associated with incomplete bowel elimination, especially for children with myelomeningocele, and encourage parents to begin a bowel-training program when the child is a toddler.
• Teach parents to recognize developmental lags early (a possible result of hydrocephalus). If present, stress the importance of follow-up IQ assessment to help plan realistic educational goals. The child may need to attend a school with special facilities. Also, stress the need for stimulation to ensure maximum mental development. Help parents plan activities appropriate to their child's abilities.
• Refer parents for genetic counseling, and suggest that amniocentesis be performed in future pregnancies. For more information and names of support groups, refer parents to the Spina Bifida Association of America.

PAROXYSMAL DISORDERS

Characterized by a marked, usually episodic increase in symptoms, paroxysmal disorders affecting the neurologic system include headache and epilepsy.

HEADACHE
The most common patient complaint, headache usually occurs as a symptom of an underlying disorder. Unless the underlying disorder is serious, headache rarely necessitates hospitalization.

Ninety percent of all headaches are classified as vascular, muscle contraction, or a combination of the two; 10% are caused by underlying intracranial, systemic, or psychological disorders. Migraine headaches, probably the most intensively studied, are throbbing, vascular headaches that usually begin to appear in childhood or adolescence and recur throughout adulthood. Affecting up to 10% of Americans, they're more common in females than in males and have a strong familial incidence. The patient with a migraine headache usually needs to be hospitalized only if nausea and vomiting are severe enough to induce dehydration and possible shock.

Causes and pathophysiology
Most chronic headaches result from tension—muscle contraction—which may be caused by emotional stress, fatigue, menstruation, or environmental stimuli (noise, crowds, bright lights). Other possible causes include glaucoma; inflammation of the eyes or mucosa of the nasal or paranasal sinuses; diseases of the scalp, teeth, extracranial arteries, or external or middle ear; and muscle spasms of the face, neck, or shoulders.

Headaches also may be caused by vasodilators (nitrates, alcohol, histamine), systemic disease, hypoxia, hypertension, head trauma and tumors, intracranial bleeding, abscess, or aneurysm.

Although their cause is unknown, migraine headaches are believed to be associated with constriction and dilation of intracranial and extracranial arteries. Certain biochemical abnormalities are thought to occur during a migraine attack. These include local leakage of a vasodilator polypeptide through the dilated arteries and a decrease in the plasma level of serotonin.

Headache pain may emanate from the pain-sensitive structures of the skin, scalp, muscles, arteries, veins; cranial nerves V, VII, IX, and X; and cervical nerves 1, 2, and 3. Intracranial mechanisms of headache include traction or displacement of arteries, venous sinuses, or venous tributaries, and inflammation or direct pressure on the cranial nerves with afferent pain fibers.

Complications
Potential complications of headache include worsening of already existing hypertension, photophobia, emotional lability, and motor weakness.

Assessment findings
The patient's history pinpoints the headache's location, characteristics, onset, and duration. Typically, findings indicate whether the headache is bilateral or unilateral; how often it occurs; how it feels (for example, dull, aching, steady, burning, or penetrating pain); whether it's continuous or intermittent; and how long the patient has been experiencing this type of headache.

The patient's history also may reveal precipitating factors (such as tension, menstruation, loud noises, menopause, or alcohol) and aggravating factors (for example, coughing, sneezing, or sunlight). In addition, the history may indicate whether the headache interferes with daily activities; if the patient has any associated symptoms, such as nausea, vomiting, weakness, facial pain, and

scotomas; and if the patient has allergies, takes headache-inducing medications, or has a family history of headaches.

During physical examination of the head and neck, inspection may reveal signs of infection; palpation may detect defects, crepitus, or tender spots (especially after trauma); and auscultation may detect bruits. If the patient has no underlying problem, physical, neurologic, and ophthalmoscopic examination findings should be normal.

The history of a patient with a *migraine headache* usually reveals that the headache began with a unilateral, pulsating pain, which gradually became more generalized. The patient—usually female, with a compulsive or perfectionist personality—may report that the headache was preceded by a scintillating scotoma, hemianopia, unilateral paresthesias, or speech disorders. (This aura is thought to result from vasoconstriction and ischemia in the cerebral cortex and, possibly, in the retina.)

Most migraine headaches last from 2 hours to several days and are accompanied by irritability, anorexia, nausea, vomiting, and photophobia. Ninety percent of patients report a family history of migraine headaches.

During a migraine attack, the patient may appear pale. (See *Clinical features of migraine headaches.*)

The patient with *muscle-contraction* or *traction-inflammatory vascular headache* may complain of a dull, persistent ache; tender spots on the head and neck; and a feeling of tightness around the head—with a characteristic "hatband" distribution—that begins in the forehead, the temple, or the back of the neck. The patient may describe the pain as severe and unrelenting.

If the headache results from intracranial bleeding, neurologic examination may reveal neurologic deficits, such as paresthesias and muscle weakness. If the patient with intracranial bleeding has received treatment for the headache before your assessment, she may report that narcotics failed to relieve the pain. If the patient reports that the pain is most severe when she awakens and decreases somewhat when she lifts her head to an upright position, the pain may be caused by a tumor. Either of these symptoms indicates the need for further testing.

Diagnostic tests
The doctor's initial impression of the patient's condition determines which diagnostic tests will be performed. Such tests may include skull X-rays (including cervical, spine, and sinus), EEG, computed tomography scan, and lumbar puncture.

CLINICAL FEATURES OF MIGRAINE HEADACHES

Migraine headaches occur in four basic types: common, classic, hemiplegic and ophthalmoplegic, and basilar artery. The following chart compares the signs and symptoms that characterize each migraine type.

Type	Signs and symptoms
Common migraine **(most prevalent; affects 85% of patients)** Usually occurs on weekends and holidays	• Prodromal symptoms (fatigue, nausea and vomiting, and fluid imbalance) precede headache by about a day. • Most prominent feature is sensitivity to light and noise. • Headache pain (unilateral or bilateral, aching or throbbing) lasts longer than in classic migraine.
Classic migraine **(affects 10% of patients)** Usually occurs in compulsive personalities and within families	• Prodromal symptoms include visual disturbances, such as zigzag lines and bright lights (most common), sensory disturbances (tingling of face, lips, and hands), or motor disturbances (staggering gait). • Headaches are recurrent and periodic.
Hemiplegic and ophthalmoplegic migraine **(rare)** Usually occurs in young adults	• Pain is severe and unilateral. • Extraocular muscle palsies (involving third cranial nerve) and ptosis occur. • With repeated headaches, permanent third cranial nerve injury is possible. • In hemiplegic migraine, neurologic deficits (hemiparesis, hemiplegia) may persist after headache subsides.
Basilar artery migraine Occurs in young women before their menstrual periods	• Prodromal symptoms usually include partial vision loss followed by vertigo, ataxia, dysarthria, tinnitus and, sometimes, tingling of fingers and toes, lasting from several minutes to almost an hour. • Headache pain characterized by severe occipital throbbing and vomiting may occur.

Treatment

Depending on the type of headache, analgesics—ranging from aspirin to codeine or meperidine—may provide relief. A tranquilizer, such as diazepam, may help during acute attacks.

Other treatment measures include identification and elimination of causative factors and, possibly, psychotherapy for headaches caused by emotional stress. Chronic tension headaches may also require muscle relaxants.

For migraine headache, ergotamine preparations (taken alone or with caffeine) and other drugs, such as metoclopramide or naproxen, work best when taken early in the course of an attack. For acute migraine attacks or cluster headaches, sumatriptan is the drug of choice for many clinicians.

If nausea and vomiting make oral administration impossible, many of these drugs may be given as rectal suppositories. If migraine headaches occur more than two or three times a month, the doctor may order preventive drugs, such as propranolol and cyproheptadine.

Nursing diagnoses
• Anxiety
• Knowledge deficit
• Pain

Nursing interventions
• Encourage the patient to discuss her problems. Listen to her and provide emotional support, especially during periods of physical and emotional stress.
• Have the patient perform relaxation techniques to prevent or ease headache. If possible, provide her with a warm bath to promote relaxation.
• To decrease the severity of the pain, keep the patient's room dark and quiet. Place ice packs on the patient's forehead, or a cold cloth over her eyes.
• Administer ordered medications as required to relieve pain or to prevent a migraine headache. Also administer medications, such as antidepressants, barbiturates, and tranquilizers, as ordered, to help the patient cope with stress and anxiety.

Patient teaching

• Using the history as a guide, help the patient understand what precipitates her headaches so she can avoid exacerbating factors.
• Teach the patient how to perform relaxation techniques. Explain that education in relaxation techniques and biofeedback may help her to change her attitude toward stress and can help her decrease the frequency of vascular and muscle-contraction headaches.
• Encourage the patient to exercise regularly. Explain that regular exercise promotes relaxation.
• If the patient experiences migraine headaches, instruct her to take the prescribed medication at the onset of migraine symptoms. Also advise her to prevent dehydration by drinking plenty of fluids after nausea and vomiting subside; to avoid long intervals between meals; and to awaken at the same time every day (in some patients a disruption in normal sleeping patterns can precipitate a headache).
• Encourage the patient who experiences migraine headaches to keep a record of activities and events that take place just before an attack; this can help identify a pattern that precedes the onset of a migraine.
• Refer patients who experience migraine headaches to the National Headache Foundation. This organization provides a list of doctors and clinics in the United States that specialize in the care of patients with headache.

EPILEPSY

Also known as seizure disorder, epilepsy is a condition of the brain characterized by a susceptibility to recurrent seizures. Seizures are paroxysmal events associated with abnormal electrical discharges of neurons in the brain. In most patients, this condition doesn't affect intelligence. Epilepsy probably affects 0.5% to 2% of the population and usually occurs in patients under age 20. However, about 80% of patients have good seizure control with strict adherence to prescribed treatment.

Causes

About half the cases of epilepsy are idiopathic. No specific cause can be found, and the patient has no other neurologic abnormality. Nonidiopathic epilepsy may be caused by:
• genetic abnormalities, such as tuberous sclerosis and phenylketonuria
• perinatal injuries
• metabolic abnormalities, such as hypocalcemia, hypoglycemia, and pyridoxine deficiency
• brain tumors or other space-occupying lesions

• infections, such as meningitis, encephalitis, or brain abscess
• traumatic injury, especially if the dura mater was penetrated
• ingestion of toxins, such as mercury, lead, or carbon monoxide
• cerebrovascular accident.

Researchers also have detected hereditary EEG abnormalities in some families, and certain seizure disorders appear to have a familial incidence.

Complications

Associated complications may occur during a seizure. These include anoxia from airway occlusion by the tongue or vomitus and traumatic injury. Such traumatic injury could result from a fall at the onset of a generalized tonic-clonic seizure, from the rapid, jerking movements that occur during or after a generalized tonic-clonic seizure, or from a fall or sudden movement sustained while the patient is confused or has an altered level of consciousness.

Assessment findings

Depending on the type and cause of the seizure, signs and symptoms vary. (See *Differentiating among seizure types.*) Physical findings may be normal if the assessment is performed when the patient isn't having a seizure and the cause is idiopathic. If the seizure is associated with an underlying problem, the patient's history and physical examination should reveal signs and symptoms of that problem unless the seizure was caused by a brain tumor, which may produce no other symptoms.

In many cases, the patient's history reveals that seizure occurrence is unpredictable and unrelated to activities. Occasionally, a patient may report precipitating factors or events—for example, that the seizures always take place at a particular time, such as during sleep, or after a particular circumstance, such as lack of sleep or emotional stress. The patient may also report nonspecific changes, such as headache, mood changes, lethargy, and myoclonic jerking, occurring up to several hours before the onset of a seizure.

Patients who experience a generalized seizure may describe an aura, which represents the beginning of abnormal electrical discharges within a focal area of the brain. Typical auras may include a pungent smell, GI distress (nausea or indigestion), a rising or sinking feeling in the stomach, a dreamy feeling, an unusual taste, or a visual disturbance, such as a flashing light, that precedes seizure onset by a few seconds or minutes.

DIFFERENTIATING AMONG SEIZURE TYPES

The hallmark of epilepsy is recurring seizures, which can be classified as partial or generalized. Some patients may be affected by more than one type.

Partial seizures

Arising from a localized area in the brain, these seizures cause specific symptoms. In some patients, partial seizure activity may spread to the entire brain, causing a generalized seizure. Partial seizures include simple partial (jacksonian motor-type and sensory-type), complex partial (psychomotor or temporal lobe), and secondarily generalized partial seizures.

Simple partial (jacksonian motor-type) seizure

This type begins as a localized motor seizure, which is characterized by a spread of abnormal activity to adjacent areas of the brain. Typically, the patient experiences a stiffening or jerking in one extremity, accompanied by a tingling sensation in the same area. For example, the seizure may start in the thumb and spread to the entire hand and arm. The patient seldom loses consciousness, although the seizure may secondarily progress to a generalized tonic-clonic seizure.

Simple partial (sensory-type) seizure

Perception is distorted in this type of seizure. Symptoms can include hallucinations, flashing lights, tingling sensations, a foul odor, vertigo, or déjà vu (the feeling of having experienced something before).

Complex partial seizure

Symptoms of this seizure type are variable but usually include purposeless behavior. The patient may experience an aura and exhibit overt signs, including a glassy stare, picking at his clothes, aimless wandering, lip-smacking or chewing motions, and unintelligible speech. A seizure may last for a few seconds or as long as 20 minutes. Afterward, mental confusion may last for several minutes; as a result, an observer may mistakenly suspect intoxication with alcohol or drugs, or psychosis. The patient has no memory of his actions during the seizure.

Secondarily generalized partial seizure

This type of seizure can be either simple or complex and can progress to generalized seizures. An aura may precede the progression. Loss of consciousness occurs immediately or within 1 or 2 minutes of the start of the progression.

Generalized seizures

As the term suggests, these seizures cause a generalized electrical abnormality within the brain. They include several distinct types.

Absence (petit mal) seizure

This type occurs most often in children, although it may affect adults as well. It usually begins with a brief change in level of consciousness, indicated by blinking or rolling of the eyes, a blank stare, and slight mouth movements. The patient retains his posture and continues preseizure activity without difficulty. Typically, a seizure lasts from 1 to 10 seconds. The impairment is so brief that the patient is sometimes unaware of it. If not properly treated, these seizures can recur as often as 100 times a day. An absence seizure may progress to a generalized tonic-clonic seizure.

Myoclonic seizure

Also called bilateral massive epileptic myoclonus, this seizure type is marked by brief, involuntary muscular jerks of the body or extremities, which may occur in a rhythmic manner, and a brief loss of consciousness.

Generalized tonic-clonic (grand mal) seizure

Typically, this seizure begins with a loud cry, precipitated by air rushing from the lungs through the vocal cords. The patient falls to the ground, losing consciousness. The body stiffens (tonic phase) and then alternates between episodes of muscle spasm and relaxation (clonic phase). Tongue biting, incontinence, labored breathing, apnea, and subsequent cyanosis may also occur. The seizure stops in 2 to 5 minutes, when abnormal electrical conduction of the neurons is completed. The patient then regains consciousness but is somewhat confused and may have difficulty talking. If he can talk, he may complain of drowsiness, fatigue, headache, muscle soreness, and arm or leg weakness. He may fall into a deep sleep after the seizure.

Akinetic seizure

Characterized by a general loss of postural tone and a temporary loss of consciousness, this type occurs in young children. Sometimes it is called a drop attack because it causes the child to fall.

The patient may describe the effect the seizures have on his life-style, activities of daily living, and coping mechanisms. The patient may also have a history of status epilepticus. (See *Understanding status epilepticus*, page 710.)

If you observe the patient during a seizure, be sure to note the type of seizure he's experiencing. Otherwise,

UNDERSTANDING STATUS EPILEPTICUS

A continuous seizure state unless interrupted by emergency interventions, status epilepticus can occur in all seizure types. The most life-threatening example is *generalized tonic-clonic status epilepticus,* a continuous generalized tonic-clonic seizure without intervening return of consciousness.

Status epilepticus, always an emergency, is accompanied by respiratory distress. It can result from abrupt withdrawal of antiepileptic medications, hypoxic or metabolic encephalopathy, acute head trauma, or septicemia secondary to encephalitis or meningitis.

Emergency treatment for status epilepticus usually consists of diazepam, phenytoin, or phenobarbital; dextrose 50% I.V. (when seizures are secondary to hypoglycemia); and thiamine I.V. (in the presence of chronic alcoholism or withdrawal).

details of what occurs during a seizure—obtained from a family member or friend, if necessary—may help to identify the seizure type.

Diagnostic tests

• *EEG.* Paroxysmal abnormalities may confirm the diagnosis of epilepsy by providing evidence of the continuing tendency to have seizures. A negative EEG doesn't rule out epilepsy because the paroxysmal abnormalities occur intermittently. The EEG also helps guide the prognosis and can help to classify the disorder.

• *Computed tomography scan* and *magnetic resonance imaging.* These tests provide density readings of the brain and may indicate abnormalities in internal structures.

Other helpful tests include serum glucose and calcium studies, skull X-rays, lumbar puncture, brain scan, and cerebral angiography.

Treatment

Typically, treatment for epilepsy consists of drug therapy specific to the type of seizure. The most commonly pre-

scribed drugs include phenytoin, carbamazepine, phenobarbital, and primidone administered individually for generalized tonic-clonic seizures and complex partial seizures. Valproic acid, clonazepam, and ethosuximide are commonly prescribed for absence (petit mal) seizures. Lamotrigine is also prescribed as adjunct therapy for partial seizures.

If drug therapy fails, treatment may include surgical removal of a demonstrated focal lesion to attempt to bring an end to seizures. Surgery is also performed when epilepsy results from an underlying problem, such as intracranial tumors, a brain abscess or cyst, and vascular abnormalities.

Nursing diagnoses

• Anxiety
• Fear
• Ineffective individual coping
• Knowledge deficit
• Risk for injury
• Social isolation

Nursing interventions

• Provide emotional support. Encourage the patient and family to express their fears and concerns. Suggest counseling to help them cope.

• If the patient is taking anticonvulsants, constantly monitor him for signs and symptoms of toxicity, such as slurred speech, ataxia, lethargy, dizziness, drowsiness, nystagmus, irritability, nausea, and vomiting.

• When administering phenytoin I.V., use a large vein, administer at a slow rate (not to exceed 50 mg/minute), and monitor the patient frequently.

• Prepare the patient for surgery, if necessary. Provide preoperative and postoperative care appropriate for the type of surgery the patient will undergo.

Patient teaching

• Provide adequate patient support by developing an understanding of epilepsy and the myths and misconceptions that surround it. Answer any questions the patient and his family may have about the condition. Help them cope by dispelling some of the myths—for example, that epilepsy is contagious. Assure them that epilepsy is controllable for most patients who follow a prescribed regimen of medication and that most patients maintain a normal life-style.

• Explain to the patient and family the need for compliance with the prescribed drug schedule. Assure the patient that anticonvulsant drugs are safe when taken as ordered. Reinforce dosage instructions and find methods to help the patient remember to take medications. Stress the importance of taking the medication regularly at a scheduled time. Caution the patient to monitor the amount of medication left so that he doesn't run out of it.

• Teach the patient about the medication's possible adverse effects—drowsiness, lethargy, hyperactivity, confusion, visual and sleep disturbances—all of which indicate the need for dosage adjustment. Tell him that phenytoin therapy may lead to hyperplasia of the gums, which may be relieved by conscientious oral hygiene. Instruct the patient to report adverse reactions immediately.

• Explain the importance of having anticonvulsant blood levels checked at regular intervals even if the seizures are under control.

• Instruct the patient to eat regular meals and to check with his doctor before dieting. Explain that maintaining adequate glucose levels provides the necessary energy for central nervous system neurons to work normally.

• Teach the patient the following measures to help him control and decrease the occurrence of seizures:

—Take the exact dose of medication at the times prescribed. Missing doses, doubling doses, or taking extra doses can cause a seizure.

—Eat balanced, regular meals. Low blood glucose levels (hypoglycemia) and inadequate vitamin intake can lead to seizures.

—Be alert for odors that may trigger an attack. Advise the patient and his family to inform the doctor of any strong odors they notice at the time of a seizure.

—Limit alcohol intake. In fact, the patient should check with the doctor to find out whether he should drink *any* alcoholic beverages.

—Get enough sleep. Excessive fatigue can precipitate a seizure.

—Treat a fever early during an illness. If the patient can't reduce a fever, he should notify the doctor.

—Learn to control stress. If appropriate, suggest learning relaxation techniques, such as deep-breathing exercises.

—Avoid trigger factors, for example, flashing lights, hyperventilation, loud noises, heavy musical beats, video games, and television.

• If the patient is a candidate for surgery, provide appropriate preoperative teaching. Explain the care that the patient can expect postoperatively.

• Know which social agencies in your community can help epileptic patients. Refer the patient to the Epilepsy Foundation of America for general information and to the state motor vehicle department for information about a driver's license.

• Finally, teach the patient's family how to care for the patient during a seizure. This is especially important if the patient experiences generalized tonic-clonic seizures, which may necessitate first aid. Instruct the family to:

—avoid restraining the patient during a seizure

—help the patient to a lying position, loosen any tight clothing, and place something flat and soft, such as a pillow, jacket, or hand, under his head

—clear the area of hard objects

—avoid forcing anything into the patient's mouth if his teeth are clenched—a tongue blade or spoon could lacerate mouth and lips or displace teeth, precipitating respiratory distress

—protect the patient's tongue, if his mouth is open, by placing a soft object (such as folded cloth) between his teeth

—turn his head to the side to provide an open airway

—reassure the patient after the seizure subsides by telling him that he's all right, orienting him to time and place, and informing him that he's had a seizure.

BRAIN AND SPINAL CORD DISORDERS

Impaired cerebral circulation, inflammation, and infection are among the many causes of brain and spinal cord disorders that can lead to neurologic dysfunction.

CEREBROVASCULAR ACCIDENT

Also known as stroke, cerebrovascular accident (CVA) is a sudden impairment of cerebral circulation in one or more of the blood vessels supplying the brain. CVA interrupts or diminishes oxygen supply and commonly causes serious damage or necrosis in brain tissues. The sooner circulation returns to normal after CVA, the better chances are for complete recovery. However, about half of those who survive CVA remain permanently disabled and experience a recurrence within weeks, months, or years.

CVA is the third most common cause of death in the United States today and the most common cause of neurologic disability. It strikes 500,000 persons each year; half of them die as a result. Although it mostly affects older adults, it can strike people of any age and occurs most commonly in men, especially blacks.

TRANSIENT ISCHEMIC ATTACK: A WARNING SIGN OF C.V.A.

A transient ischemic attack (TIA) is a recurrent episode of neurologic deficit, lasting from seconds to hours, that clears within 12 to 24 hours. It's usually considered a warning sign of an impending thrombotic CVA. In fact, TIAs have been reported in 50% to 80% of patients who have had a cerebral infarction from such thrombosis. The age of onset varies. Incidence rises dramatically after age 50 and is highest among blacks and men.

In TIA, microemboli released from a thrombus may temporarily interrupt blood flow, especially in the small distal branches of the brain's arterial tree. Small spasms in those arterioles may impair blood flow and also precede TIA. Predisposing factors are the same as for thrombotic CVAs.

Clinical features
The most distinctive characteristics of TIAs are the transient duration of neurologic deficits and the complete return of normal function. The signs and symptoms of TIA correlate with the location of the affected artery. They include double vision, speech deficits (slurring or thickness), unilateral blindness, staggering or uncoordinated gait, unilateral weakness or numbness, falling because of weakness in the legs, and dizziness.

Treatment
During an active TIA, treatment aims to prevent a completed stroke and consists of aspirin or anticoagulants to minimize the risk of thrombosis. After or between attacks, preventive treatment includes carotid endarterectomy or cerebral microvascular bypass.

CVAs are classified according to their course of progression. The least severe is the transient ischemic attack (TIA), which results from a temporary interruption of blood flow, most often in the carotid and vertebrobasilar arteries. (See *Transient ischemic attack: A warning sign of CVA*.) A progressive stroke, or stroke-in-evolution (thrombus-in-evolution), begins with a slight neurologic deficit and worsens in a day or two. In a completed stroke, neurologic deficits are at the maximum at the onset.

Causes
Major causes of CVA include cerebral thrombosis, embolism, and hemorrhage.

Thrombosis is the most common cause of CVA in middle-aged and elderly people. CVA results from obstruction of a blood vessel. Typically, the main site of the obstruction is the extracerebral vessels, but sometimes it's intracerebral.

Embolism, the second most common cause of CVA, can occur at any age, especially among patients with a history of rheumatic heart disease, endocarditis, posttraumatic valvular disease, myocardial fibrillation and other cardiac arrhythmias, or after open-heart surgery. It usually develops rapidly—in 10 to 20 seconds—and without warning. Most often the left middle cerebral artery is the embolus site.

Hemorrhage, the third most common cause of CVA, like embolism, may occur suddenly at any age. Such hemorrhage results from chronic hypertension or aneurysms, which cause sudden rupture of a cerebral artery.

Factors that increase the risk of CVA include a history of TIAs, atherosclerosis, hypertension, arrhythmias, electrocardiogram changes, rheumatic heart disease, diabetes mellitus, gout, postural hypotension, cardiac enlargement, high serum triglyceride levels, lack of exercise, use of oral contraceptives, smoking, and a family history of cerebrovascular disease.

Complications
Among the many possible complications of CVA are unstable blood pressure from loss of vasomotor control; fluid imbalances; malnutrition; sensory impairment, including vision problems; and infections, such as pneumonia. Altered level of consciousness (LOC), aspiration, contractures, and pulmonary emboli also may occur.

Assessment findings
Clinical features of CVA vary with the artery affected (and, consequently, the portion of the brain it supplies), the severity of the damage, and the extent of collateral circulation that develops to help the brain compensate for a decreased blood supply.

When assessing a patient who may have experienced a CVA, remember this: If the CVA occurs in the left hemisphere, it produces signs and symptoms on the right side. If it occurs in the right hemisphere, signs and symptoms appear on the left side. However, a CVA that causes cranial nerve damage produces signs of cranial nerve dysfunction on the same side as the hemorrhage.

The patient's history, obtained from a family member or friend if necessary, may uncover one or more risk factors for CVA. The history may also reveal either a sudden onset of hemiparesis or hemiplegia or a gradual onset of dizziness, mental disturbances, or seizures. The patient or a family member may also report that the patient lost consciousness or suddenly developed aphasia. Speaking with the patient during the history may reveal communication problems, such as dysarthria, dysphasia or aphasia, and apraxia.

Neurologic examination identifies most of the physical findings associated with CVA. These may include unconsciousness or changes in LOC, such as a decreased attention span, difficulties with comprehension, forgetfulness, and a lack of motivation. If conscious, the patient may exhibit anxiety along with communication and mobility difficulties. Inspection may reveal related urinary incontinence.

Motor function tests and muscle strength tests often show a loss of voluntary muscle control and hemiparesis or hemiplegia on one side of the body. In the initial phase, flaccid paralysis with decreased deep tendon reflexes may occur. These reflexes return to normal after the initial phase, along with an increase in muscle tone and, in some cases, muscle spasticity on the affected side.

Vision testing often reveals hemianopia on the affected side of the body and, in patients with left-sided hemiplegia, problems with visual-spatial relations.

Sensory assessment may reveal sensory losses, ranging from slight impairment of touch to the inability to perceive the position and motion of body parts. The patient also may have difficulty interpreting visual, tactile, and auditory stimuli. (See *Understanding neurologic deficits in CVA*, page 714.)

Diagnostic tests
• *Cerebral angiography* details disruption or displacement of the cerebral circulation by occlusion or hemorrhage. It's the test of choice for examination of the entire cerebral artery.
• *Digital subtraction angiography* evaluates the patency of the cerebral vessels and identifies their position in the head and neck. It also detects and evaluates lesions and vascular abnormalities.
• *Computed tomography (CT) scan* detects structural abnormalities, edema, and lesions, such as nonhemorrhagic infarction and aneurysms. Thus, it differentiates CVA from imitative disorders, such as primary metastatic tumor and subdural, intracerebral, or epidural hematoma.

Patients with TIA commonly have a normal CT scan.
• *Positron emission tomography* provides data on cerebral metabolism and cerebral blood flow changes, especially in ischemic stroke.
• *Single-photon emission tomography* identifies cerebral blood flow and helps diagnose cerebral infarction.
• *Magnetic resonance imaging (MRI)* and *magnetic resonance angiography (MRA)* allow evaluation of the lesion's location and size without exposing the patient to radiation. MRI doesn't distinguish hemorrhage, tumor, and infarction as well as CT scanning, but it provides superior images of the cerebellum and the brain stem.
• *Transcranial Doppler studies* evaluate the velocity of blood flow through major intracranial vessels, which can indicate the vessels' diameter.
• *Cerebral blood flow studies* measure blood flow to the brain and help detect abnormalities.
• *Ophthalmoscopy* may show signs of hypertension and atherosclerotic changes in the retinal arteries.
• *EEG* may detect reduced electrical activity in an area of cortical infarction. This test proves especially useful when CT scan results are inconclusive. It can also differentiate seizure activity from CVA.
• *Oculoplethysmography* indirectly measures ophthalmic blood flow and carotid artery blood flow.

Appropriate baseline laboratory studies include urinalysis, coagulation studies, complete blood count, serum osmolality, and tests for electrolyte, glucose, triglyceride, creatinine, and blood urea nitrogen levels.

Treatment
Medical management of CVA commonly includes physical rehabilitation, dietary and drug regimens to help decrease risk factors, possibly surgery, and care measures to help the patient adapt to specific deficits, such as speech impairment and paralysis.

Depending on the CVA's cause and extent, the patient may undergo a craniotomy to remove a hematoma, endarterectomy to remove atherosclerotic plaques from the inner arterial wall, or extracranial-intracranial bypass to circumvent an artery that's blocked by occlusion or stenosis. Ventricular shunts may be necessary to drain cerebrospinal fluid.

Medications useful in CVA include:
• anticonvulsants, such as phenytoin or phenobarbital, to treat or prevent seizures
• stool softeners, such as dioctyl sodium sulfosuccinate, to avoid straining, which increases intracranial pressure (ICP)
• corticosteroids, such as dexamethasone, to minimize associated cerebral edema

UNDERSTANDING NEUROLOGIC DEFICITS IN C.V.A.

CVA can leave one patient with mild hand weakness and another with complete unilateral paralysis. In both patients, the functional loss reflects damage to the brain area normally perfused by the occluded or ruptured artery. But the damage doesn't stop there. The resulting hypoxia and ischemia produce edema that affects distal parts of the brain, causing further neurologic deficits.

Most CVAs occur in the anterior cerebral circulation and cause symptoms from damage in the middle cerebral artery, internal carotid artery, or anterior cerebral artery. CVAs can also occur in the posterior circulation. These originate in the vertebral arteries and result in signs and symptoms caused by damage to the vertebral or basilar artery and posterior cerebral artery, resulting in higher mortality. Described below are the signs and symptoms that accompany CVA at the following sites.

Middle cerebral artery
The patient may experience aphasia, dysphasia, reading difficulty (dyslexia), writing inability (dysgraphia), visual field cuts, and hemiparesis on the affected side (more severe in the face and arm than in the leg).

Internal carotid artery
The patient may complain of headaches. Expect to find weakness, paralysis, numbness, sensory changes, and visual disturbances, such as blurring on affected side. You may also detect altered level of consciousness, bruits over the carotid artery, aphasia, dysphasia, and ptosis.

Anterior cerebral artery
You may note confusion, weakness, and numbness (especially of the arm) on the affected side, paralysis of the contralateral foot and leg with accompanying footdrop, incontinence, loss of coordination, impaired motor and sensory functions, and personality changes (flat affect, distractibility).

Vertebral or basilar artery
The patient may complain of numbness around the lips and mouth and dizziness. You may note weakness on the affected side; visual deficits, such as color blindness, lack of depth perception, and diplopia; poor coordination; dysphagia; slurred speech; amnesia; and ataxia.

Posterior cerebral artery
The patient may experience visual field cuts, sensory impairment, dyslexia, coma, and cortical blindness from ischemia in the occipital area. Usually, paralysis is absent.

• anticoagulants, such as heparin, warfarin, and ticlopidine, to reduce the risk of thrombotic stroke
• analgesics, such as codeine, to relieve headache that may follow hemorrhagic CVA. Usually, aspirin is contraindicated in hemorrhagic CVA because it increases bleeding tendencies, but it may be useful in preventing TIAs.

Nursing diagnoses
• Altered cerebral tissue perfusion
• Anxiety
• Bathing or hygiene self-care deficit
• Dressing or grooming self-care deficit
• Impaired gas exchange
• Impaired physical mobility
• Impaired verbal communication
• Ineffective airway clearance
• Powerlessness
• Risk for aspiration
• Risk for impaired skin integrity
• Risk for infection
• Risk for injury
• Self-esteem disturbance
• Sensory or perceptual alterations
• Toileting self-care deficit
• Total incontinence

Nursing interventions
• During the acute phase, provide continuing neurologic assessment, respiratory support, continuous monitoring of vital signs, careful positioning to prevent aspiration and contractures, management of GI problems, and careful monitoring of fluid, electrolyte, and nutritional intake. Patient care must also prevent complications, such as infection.
• Maintain a patent airway and oxygenation. Loosen constricting clothes. Watch for ballooning of the cheek with respiration. The side that balloons is the side affected by the stroke. If the patient is unconscious, he could aspirate saliva, so keep him in a lateral position to allow secretions to drain naturally or suction secretions, as needed. Insert an artificial airway, and start

mechanical ventilation or supplemental oxygen, if necessary.

• Check vital signs and neurologic status as ordered, record observations, and report any significant changes to the doctor. Monitor blood pressure, LOC, pupillary changes, motor function (voluntary and involuntary movements), sensory function, speech, skin color, temperature, signs of increased ICP, and nuchal rigidity or flaccidity. Remember, if CVA is impending, blood pressure rises suddenly, pulse rate is rapid and bounding, and the patient may complain of headache.

• Watch for signs of pulmonary emboli, such as chest pains, shortness of breath, dusky color, tachycardia, fever, and changed sensorium. If the patient is unresponsive, monitor his arterial blood gas levels often and alert the doctor to increased partial pressure of carbon dioxide or decreased partial pressure of oxygen.

• Maintain fluid and electrolyte balance. If the patient can take liquids orally, offer them as often as fluid limitations permit. Administer I.V. fluids, as ordered; never give too much too fast because this can increase ICP.

• Offer the urinal or bedpan every 2 hours. If the patient is incontinent, he may need an indwelling urinary catheter, but this should be avoided, if possible, because of the risk of infection.

• Ensure adequate nutrition. Check for gag reflex before offering small oral feedings of semisolid foods. Place the food tray within the patient's visual field. Have the patient sit upright and tilt his head slightly forward when eating. If the patient has dysphagia or one-sided facial weakness, provide him with semisoft foods and tell him to chew on the unaffected side of his mouth. If oral feedings aren't possible, insert a nasogastric tube for tube feedings, as ordered.

• Manage GI problems. Be alert for signs that the patient is straining at stool because this increases ICP. Modify the patient's diet; administer stool softeners, as ordered; and give laxatives, if necessary. If the patient vomits (usually during the first few days), keep him positioned on his side to prevent aspiration.

• Provide careful mouth care. Clean and irrigate the patient's mouth to remove food particles. Care for his dentures, as needed.

• Provide meticulous eye care. Remove secretions with a cotton ball and 0.9% sodium chloride solution. Instill eyedrops, as ordered. Patch the patient's affected eye if he can't close his eyelid.

• Position the patient, and align his extremities correctly. Use high-topped sneakers to prevent footdrop and contracture, and a convoluted foam, flotation, or pulsating mattress to prevent pressure ulcers. To decrease the possibility of pneumonia, turn the patient at least every 2 hours. Elevate the affected hand to control dependent edema, and place it in a functional position.

• Assist the patient with exercise. Perform range-of-motion (ROM) exercises for both the affected and unaffected sides. Teach and encourage the patient to use his unaffected side to exercise his affected side.

• Give medications, as ordered, and watch for and report adverse reactions.

• Establish and maintain communication with the patient. If he's aphasic, set up a simple method of communicating basic needs. Then remember to phrase your questions so he'll be able to answer using this system. Repeat yourself quietly and calmly (remember, he isn't deaf) and use gestures if necessary to help him understand. Even the unresponsive patient can hear, so don't say anything in his presence you wouldn't want him to hear and remember.

• Provide psychological support, and establish rapport with the patient. Set realistic short-term goals. Spend time with him, involve his family in his care when possible, and explain his deficits and strengths. Remember that building rapport may be difficult because of the mood changes that may result from brain damage or as a reaction to being dependent.

• Protect the patient from injury. For example, keep the bed's side rails up at all times; pad the rails if the patient tends to bang them with his feet or arms.

• If surgery is necessary, provide preoperative and postoperative care. Monitor vital signs, fluid and electrolyte balance, and intake and output. Care for the operative area, provide pain relief, and watch for complications from the surgery.

Patient teaching

• Teach the patient and his family about the disorder. Explain the diagnostic tests, treatments, and the rehabilitation the patient will undergo.

• If surgery is scheduled, provide preoperative teaching. Be sure the patient and family understand the surgery and its possible effects.

• If necessary, teach the patient to comb his hair, dress, and wash. With the aid of a physical and an occupational therapist, obtain appliances, such as hand bars by the toilet and ramps, as needed. If speech therapy is indicated, encourage the patient to begin as soon as possible. To reinforce teaching, involve the patient's family in all aspects of rehabilitation. With their cooperation and support, devise a realistic discharge plan, and let them help decide when the patient can return home.

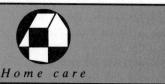

RECOVERING FROM A C.V.A.

For a patient with a cerebrovascular accident (CVA), follow these guidelines to promote his recovery at home:
• Assess the patient's self-care ability, and determine the availability of capable support people.
• Refer the patient for physical, occupational, and speech therapy, as needed. Reinforce the therapists' instructions about exercise, mobility, and activities of daily living.
• Obtain appropriate assistive devices. If the patient has difficulty speaking, suggest a talking board or a pad and pencil.
• Reinforce caregiver teaching about rehabilitation, and encourage the patient to be as independent as possible.
• Review all medication information with caregivers; instruct them to call the doctor if adverse reactions occur.
• Teach caregivers to recognize signs of an impending CVA.
• Help caregivers minimize safety hazards in the environment.
• Suggest options for caregiver support and help. Refer the patient and family to local support groups and national organizations for more information.
• Review emergency measures with the patient and caregivers.
• Emphasize the need to attend all follow-up visits.

• Prepare the patient and family for home care. (See *Recovering from a CVA.*)
• If a special diet, such as a weight loss diet for an obese patient, is prescribed, have the dietitian teach the patient about the diet. Reinforce the explanations as needed.
• Teach the patient and, if needed, a family member about the schedule, dosage, actions, and adverse effects of prescribed drugs. Make sure the patient taking aspirin realizes that he can't substitute acetaminophen for aspirin.
• To decrease the risk of another CVA, teach the patient and family about the need to correct risk factors. For example, if the patient smokes, refer him to a stop-smoking program. Teach the importance of maintaining an ideal weight and the need to control such diseases as diabetes and hypertension. Teach all patients the importance of following a low-cholesterol, low-salt diet; increasing activity; avoiding prolonged bed rest; and minimizing stress.

MENINGITIS

In this disorder, the brain and the spinal cord meninges become inflamed. Such inflammation may involve all three meningeal membranes — the dura mater, the arachnoid membrane, and the pia mater.

For most patients, meningitis follows the onset of respiratory symptoms: In about 50% of patients, it develops over 1 to 7 days; in about 20% of patients, in 1 to 3 weeks. In about 25% of patients, meningitis is unheralded by respiratory symptoms; it has a sudden onset, causing serious illness within 24 hours.

The prognosis is good and complications are rare, especially if the disease is recognized early and the infecting organism responds to antibiotics. However, mortality in untreated meningitis is 70% to 100%. The prognosis is poorer for infants and elderly people.

Causes

Meningitis can be caused by bacteria, viruses, protozoa, or fungi. It most commonly results from bacterial infection, usually due to *Neisseria meningitidis, Haemophilus influenzae, Streptococcus pneumoniae,* or *Escherichia coli.* Sometimes, no causative organism can be found.

In most patients, the infection that causes meningitis is secondary to another bacterial infection, such as bacteremia (especially from pneumonia, empyema, osteomyelitis, and endocarditis), sinusitis, otitis media, encephalitis, myelitis, or brain abscess. Meningitis may also follow a skull fracture, a penetrating head wound, lumbar puncture, or ventricular shunting procedures.

Meningitis caused by a virus is called aseptic viral meningitis. (See *Understanding aseptic viral meningitis.*)

Infants, children, and elderly people have the highest risk of developing meningitis. Other risk factors include malnourishment, immunosuppression (as from radiation therapy), and central nervous system trauma.

Complications

Potential complications of meningitis include visual impairment, optic neuritis, cranial nerve palsies, deafness, personality change, headache, paresis or paralysis, endocarditis, coma, vasculitis, and cerebral infarction. Children may develop sensory hearing loss, epilepsy, mental retardation, hydrocephalus, or subdural effusions.

Assessment findings

The cardinal signs of meningitis are those of infection and of increased intracranial pressure (ICP).

The patient history may detail headache, stiff neck and back, malaise, photophobia, chills and, sometimes, vomiting, twitching, and seizures. The patient or a family

UNDERSTANDING ASEPTIC VIRAL MENINGITIS

A benign syndrome, aseptic viral meningitis is characterized by headache, fever, vomiting, and meningeal symptoms. It results from some form of virus infection, including enteroviruses (most common), arboviruses, herpes simplex virus, mumps virus, or lymphocytic choriomeningitis virus.

Assessment findings

The history of a patient with aseptic viral meningitis usually shows that the disease began suddenly with a fever up to 104° F (40° C), alterations in consciousness (drowsiness, confusion, stupor), and neck or spine stiffness, which is slight at first. (The patient experiences such stiffness when bending forward.) The patient history may also reveal a recent illness.

Other signs and symptoms may include headaches, nausea, vomiting, abdominal pain, poorly defined chest pain, and sore throat.

The patient history and knowledge of seasonal epidemics are essential in differentiating among the many forms of aseptic viral meningitis. Negative bacteriologic cultures and CSF analysis showing pleocytosis and increased protein suggest the diagnosis. Isolation of the virus from CSF confirms it.

Supportive treatment

Management of aseptic meningitis includes bed rest, maintenance of fluid and electrolyte balance, analgesics for pain, and exercises to combat residual weakness. Isolation isn't necessary. Careful handling of excretions and good hand-washing technique prevent the spread of the disease.

---

member may also report altered level of consciousness (LOC), such as confusion and delirium. Vital signs may reveal fever. (Vomiting and fever occur more often in children than in adults.) In addition, the history for an infant may list fretfulness and refusal to eat.

In *pneumococcal meningitis,* the patient history may uncover a recent lung, ear, or sinus infection or endocarditis. It may also reveal the presence of other conditions, such as alcoholism, sickle cell disease, basal skull fracture, recent splenectomy, or organ transplant.

In *H. influenzae meningitis,* the patient history may reveal a recent respiratory tract or ear infection.

Physical findings vary, depending on the severity of the meningitis. You may note opisthotonos (a spasm in which the back and extremities arch backward so that the body rests on the head and heels), a sign of meningeal irritation. In *meningococcal meningitis,* you may also see a petechial, purpuric, or ecchymotic rash on the lower part of the body.

Neurologic examination may uncover other indications of meningeal irritation, including positive Brudzinski's and Kernig's signs (see *Two telltale signs of meningitis,* page 718) and exaggerated and symmetrical deep tendon reflexes. It may also reveal altered LOC, ranging from confusion or delirium to deep stupor or coma.

Vision testing may demonstrate diplopia and other visual problems. Ophthalmoscopic examination may show papilledema (another sign of increased ICP), although this is rare.

Diagnostic tests

• *Lumbar puncture* shows typical cerebrospinal fluid (CSF) findings associated with meningitis (elevated CSF pressure, cloudy or milky white CSF, high protein level, positive Gram stain and culture that usually identifies the infecting organism, unless it's a virus, and depressed CSF glucose concentration).
• *Chest X-rays* are especially important because they may reveal pneumonitis or lung abscess, tubercular lesions, or granulomas secondary to fungal infection. *Sinus and skull films* may help identify the presence of cranial osteomyelitis, paranasal sinusitis, or skull fracture.
• *White blood cell count* usually indicates leukocytosis and serum electrolyte levels often are abnormal.
• *Computed tomography scan* can rule out cerebral hematoma, hemorrhage, or tumor.

Treatment

Medical management of meningitis includes appropriate antibiotic therapy and vigorous supportive care.

Usually, I.V. antibiotics are given for at least 2 weeks, followed by oral antibiotics. Such antibiotics include penicillin G, ampicillin, or nafcillin. However, if the patient is allergic to penicillin, anti-infective therapy includes tetracycline, chloramphenicol, or kanamycin. Other drugs include a cardiac glycoside, such as digoxin, to control arrhythmias, mannitol to decrease cerebral edema, an anticonvulsant (usually given I.V.) or a sedative to reduce restlessness, and aspirin or acetaminophen to relieve headache and fever.

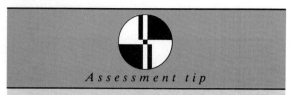

TWO TELLTALE SIGNS OF MENINGITIS

A positive response to the following tests helps establish a diagnosis of meningitis.

Brudzinski's sign

To test for this sign, place the patient in a dorsal recumbent position, then put your hands behind his neck and bend it forward. Pain and resistance may indicate meningeal inflammation, neck injury, or arthritis. But if the patient also flexes the hips and knees in response to this manipulation, chances are he has meningitis.

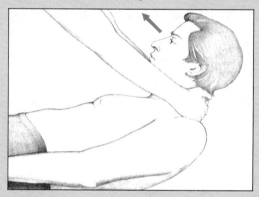

Kernig's sign

To test for this sign, place the patient in a supine position. Flex his leg at the hip and knee, then straighten the knee. Pain or resistance points to meningitis.

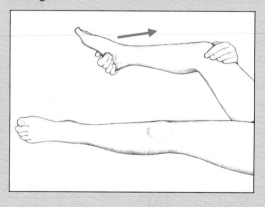

Supportive measures consist of bed rest, hypothermia, and fluid therapy to prevent dehydration. Isolation is necessary if nasal cultures are positive. Treatment includes appropriate therapy for any coexisting conditions, such as endocarditis or pneumonia.

To prevent meningitis, prophylactic antibiotics are sometimes used after ventricular shunting procedures, skull fracture, or penetrating head wounds, but this use is controversial.

Nursing diagnoses
• Anxiety
• Hyperthermia
• Impaired gas exchange
• Pain
• Risk for fluid volume deficit
• Risk for impaired skin integrity

Nursing interventions
• Maintain respiratory isolation for 24 hours after the start of antibiotic therapy. Discharges from the nose and the mouth are considered infectious. Follow strict aseptic technique when treating patients with head wounds or skull fractures.
• Continually assess the patient's clinical status, including neurologic function and vital signs. Monitor for changes in LOC and signs of increased ICP (plucking at the bedcovers, vomiting, seizures, a change in motor function and vital signs). Also watch for signs of cranial nerve involvement (ptosis, strabismus, diplopia).
• Watch for signs of deterioration. Be especially alert for a temperature increase, deteriorating LOC, onset of seizures, and altered respirations, all of which may signal an impending crisis.
• Obtain arterial blood gas measurements, as ordered, and administer oxygen, as required, to maintain partial pressure of oxygen at desired levels. If necessary, maintain the patient on mechanical ventilation and care for his endotracheal tube or tracheostomy.
• Monitor fluid balance. Maintain adequate fluid intake to avoid dehydration, but avoid fluid overload because of the danger of cerebral edema. Measure central venous pressure and intake and output accurately.
• Administer prescribed medications, and note their effects. Also watch for adverse reactions.
• Position the patient carefully to prevent joint stiffness and neck pain. Turn him often, according to a planned positioning schedule. Assist with range-of-motion exercises.

• Maintain adequate nutrition. You may need to provide small, frequent meals, or to supplement these meals with nasogastric tube or parenteral feedings.

• To prevent constipation and minimize the risk of increased ICP resulting from straining at stool, give the patient a mild laxative or stool softener, as ordered.

• Provide mouth care regularly.

• Ensure the patient's comfort, and maintain a quiet environment. Darkening the room may decrease photophobia. Relieve headache with a nonnarcotic analgesic, such as aspirin or acetaminophen, as ordered. (Narcotics interfere with accurate neurologic assessment.)

• Provide reassurance and support. The patient may be frightened by his illness and frequent lumbar punctures. If he's delirious or confused, attempt to reorient him often. Reassure the family that the delirium and behavior changes caused by meningitis usually disappear. However, if a severe neurologic deficit appears permanent, refer the patient to a rehabilitation program as soon as the acute phase of this illness has passed.

Patient teaching

• Inform the patient and his family of the contagion risks, and tell them to notify anyone who comes into close contact with the patient. Such people require antimicrobial prophylaxis and immediate medical attention if fever or other signs of meningitis develop.

• To help prevent the development of meningitis, teach patients with chronic sinusitis or other chronic infections the importance of proper medical treatment.

ENCEPHALITIS

A severe inflammation of the brain, encephalitis is characterized by intense lymphocytic infiltration of brain tissues and the leptomeninges. This causes cerebral edema, degeneration of the brain's ganglion cells, and diffuse nerve cell destruction.

Encephalitis is usually caused by a mosquito-borne or, in some areas, a tick-borne virus. However, transmission by means other than arthropod bites may occur through ingestion of infected goat's milk and accidental injection or inhalation of the virus.

Eastern (equine) encephalitis may produce permanent neurologic damage and is often fatal. It occurs in the eastern regions of North, Central, and South America. Western (equine) encephalitis occurs throughout the western hemisphere; California encephalitis, throughout the United States; St. Louis encephalitis, in Florida and in the western and southern United States; and Venezuelan encephalitis, in South America.

Between World War I and the Depression, a type of encephalitis known as lethargic encephalitis, von Economo's disease, or sleeping sickness occurred with some regularity. The causative virus was never clearly identified, and the disease is rare today. Even so, the term sleeping sickness persists and is often mistakenly used to describe other types of encephalitis as well.

Causes

Encephalitis usually results from infection with arboviruses specific to rural areas. In urban areas, encephalitis is most frequently caused by enteroviruses (coxsackievirus, poliovirus, and echovirus). Other causes include herpesvirus, mumps virus, adenoviruses, and demyelinating diseases after measles, varicella, rubella, or vaccination.

Complications

Potential complications associated with viral encephalitis include bronchial pneumonia, urine retention, urinary tract infection, pressure ulcers, and coma. Epilepsy, parkinsonism, and mental deterioration may also occur.

Assessment findings

Depending on the severity of the disease, all forms of viral encephalitis have similar clinical features. The severity of arbovirus encephalitis may range from subclinical to rapidly fatal necrotizing disease. Herpes encephalitis also produces signs and symptoms that vary from subclinical to acute and often fatal fulminating disease.

If encephalitis is the primary illness, the patient may be acutely ill when he seeks treatment because the nonspecific symptoms that occur before the onset of acute neurologic symptoms are not recognized as signs of encephalitis. Thus, patient history may include reports of systemic symptoms, such as headache, muscle stiffness, malaise, sore throat, and upper respiratory tract symptoms that existed for several days before the onset of neurologic symptoms.

After neurologic symptoms occur, patient history may reveal the sudden onset of altered levels of consciousness, from lethargy or drowsiness to stupor. The patient or a family member may also report the occurrence of seizures, which may be the only presenting sign of encephalitis.

On neurologic examination, the patient may be confused, disoriented, or hallucinating. He may also demonstrate tremors, cranial nerve palsies, exaggerated deep tendon reflexes, absent superficial reflexes, and paresis or paralysis of the extremities. The patient may also complain of a stiff neck when the head is bent forward.

Vital signs usually reveal fever. The patient may also be nauseated and vomiting.

If the cerebral hemispheres are involved, assessment findings may include aphasia; involuntary movements identified on inspection; ataxia; sensory defects, such as disturbances of taste and smell; and poor memory retention.

Diagnostic tests

During an encephalitis epidemic, diagnosis is readily made from clinical findings and patient history. However, sporadic cases are difficult to distinguish from other febrile illnesses, such as gastroenteritis or meningitis. The following tests help establish a diagnosis:
• *Blood analysis* or, rarely, *cerebrospinal fluid (CSF) analysis* identifies the virus and confirms the diagnosis. The common viruses that also cause herpes, measles, and mumps are easier to identify than arboviruses. Arboviruses and herpesviruses can be isolated by inoculating young mice with a specimen taken from the patient.
• *Serologic studies* in herpes encephalitis may show rising titers of complement-fixing antibodies. In some types of encephalitis, serologic tests of blood may be diagnostic.
• *Lumbar puncture* discloses CSF pressure elevated in all forms of encephalitis. Despite inflammation, *CSF analysis* findings often reveal clear fluid. White blood cell count and protein levels in CSF are slightly elevated, but the glucose level remains normal.
• *EEG* reveals abnormalities such as generalized slowing of waveforms.
• *Computed tomography scan* may be ordered to check for temporal lobe lesions that indicate herpesvirus and to rule out cerebral hematoma.

Treatment

The antiviral agent vidarabine is effective only against herpes encephalitis and only if it's administered before the onset of coma.

Treatment of all other forms of encephalitis is supportive. Drug therapy includes reduction of intracranial pressure (ICP) with I.V. mannitol and corticosteroids (to reduce cerebral inflammation and resulting edema); phenytoin or another anticonvulsant, usually given I.V.; sedatives for restlessness; and aspirin or acetaminophen to relieve headache and reduce fever.

Other supportive measures include adequate fluid and electrolyte intake to prevent dehydration and appropriate antibiotics for associated infections, such as pneumonia or sinusitis; maintenance of the patient's airway; admin-istration of oxygen to maintain arterial blood gas levels; and maintenance of nutrition, especially during periods of coma. Isolation is unnecessary.

Nursing diagnoses
• Altered nutrition: Less than body requirements
• Altered thought processes
• Anxiety
• Hyperthermia
• Impaired gas exchange
• Impaired physical mobility
• Knowledge deficit
• Pain
• Risk for fluid volume deficit
• Risk for impaired skin integrity

Nursing interventions
• During the acute phase of the illness, assess neurologic function often. Observe level of consciousness and signs of increased ICP (increasing restlessness, plucking at the bedcovers, vomiting, seizures, and changes in pupil size, motor function, and vital signs). Also watch for cranial nerve involvement (ptosis, strabismus, diplopia), abnormal sleep patterns, and behavior changes.
• Maintain adequate fluid intake to prevent dehydration, but avoid fluid overload, which may increase cerebral edema. Measure and record intake and output accurately.
• As ordered, give vidarabine by slow I.V. infusion only. Watch for adverse reactions, such as tremors, dizziness, hallucinations, anorexia, nausea, vomiting, diarrhea, pruritus, rash, and anemia; also watch for adverse effects of other drugs. Check the infusion sites often to prevent problems such as infiltration and phlebitis.
• Carefully position the patient to prevent joint stiffness and neck pain, and turn him often. Assist with range-of-motion exercises.
• Maintain adequate nutrition. Give the patient small, frequent meals or supplement these meals with nasogastric tube or parenteral feedings.
• To prevent constipation and minimize the risk of increased ICP resulting from straining at stool, give a mild laxative or stool softener.
• Provide good mouth care.
• Maintain a quiet environment. Darkening the room may decrease headache. If the patient naps during the day and is restless at night, plan daytime activities to minimize napping and promote sleep at night.
• If the patient has seizures, take precautions to protect the patient from injury during the seizures.

• Provide emotional support and reassure the patient and his family because the patient is apt to be frightened by the illness and frequent diagnostic tests.

• If the patient is delirious or confused, attempt to reorient him often. Providing a calendar or a clock in the patient's room may be helpful.

Patient teaching

• Teach the patient and his family about the disease and its effects. Explain the diagnostic tests and treatment measures. Be sure to explain procedures to the patient even if he's comatose.

• Explain to the patient and his family that behavior changes caused by encephalitis usually disappear, but permanent problems sometimes occur. If a neurologic deficit is severe and appears permanent, refer the patient to a rehabilitation program as soon as the acute phase has passed.

BRAIN ABSCESS

Intracranial, or brain, abscess is a free or encapsulated collection of pus typically found in the frontal, parietal, temporal, or occipital lobes. Less commonly, it occurs in the cerebellum or basal ganglia. Brain abscess can vary in size and may occur singly or in multiple areas. It has a relatively low incidence. Although it can occur at any age, it's most common in people between ages 10 and 35 and is rare in elderly people.

Untreated brain abscess is usually fatal; with treatment, the prognosis is only fair, and about 30% of patients develop focal seizures. Multiple metastatic abscesses secondary to systemic or other infections have the poorest prognosis.

Causes and pathophysiology

Brain abscess is usually secondary to some other infection, most commonly otitis media, sinusitis, dental abscess, and mastoiditis. It may result from pyogenic bacteria, such as *Staphylococcus aureus, Streptococcus viridans,* and *Streptococcus hemolyticus.* (At least 50% of brain abscesses result from mastoid or ear infections.)

It may also occur secondary to subdural empyema; bacterial endocarditis; bacteremia; pulmonary or pleural infection; pelvic, abdominal, and skin infections; and cranial trauma, such as a penetrating head wound or compound skull fracture. Penetrating head trauma or bacteremia usually leads to staphylococcal infection; pulmonary disease, to streptococcal infection.

Brain abscesses develop on the same side of the brain as the primary infection. Pus may be free at first, causing inflammatory necrosis and edema; but, over several weeks, the brain tissue surrounds the abscess with a thick capsule. The resulting mass produces clinical effects similar to those of a brain tumor.

Brain abscess occurs in about 2% of children with congenital heart disease, possibly because the hypoxic brain is a good culture medium for bacteria.

Complications

Without treatment, the encapsulated abscess breaks, spreading satellite abscesses to white brain matter and ventricles and producing empyema and meningitis. Even with treatment, hemiparesis, focal seizures, cranial nerve palsies, and visual defects may occur.

Assessment findings

Signs and symptoms depend on the location of the abscess; alterations in intracranial dynamics, such as edema and brain shift; and the presence of infection. Most patients have symptoms for 2 weeks or less before seeking treatment.

Typically, the patient reports a recent, current, or recurrent infection—especially of the middle ear, mastoid, nasal sinuses, heart, or lungs—or a history of congenital heart disease. The patient also may complain of nausea, vomiting, and a constant, intractable headache that is worse in the morning. In addition, the patient or his family may report a change in the patient's level of consciousness (LOC), such as increased irritability or decreased alertness. Some patients may be drowsy; others may be stuporous.

Neurologic examination confirms alteration in LOC. It also may reveal that the patient is confused or disoriented and has signs of a focal neurologic disorder. Focal symptoms may include:

• in temporal lobe abscess, auditory-receptive dysphasia, central facial weakness, hemiparesis

• in cerebellar abscess, dizziness, coarse nystagmus, gaze weakness on lesion side, tremor, ataxia

• in frontal lobe abscess, expressive dysphasia, hemiparesis with unilateral motor seizure, drowsiness, inattention, mental function impairment.

Besides decreased LOC and vomiting, other signs of increased intracranial pressure (ICP) may be seen, including abnormal pupillary response and depressed respirations. Additional assessment findings may include signs of an infection, such as fever, bradycardia, and pallor. (If the abscess is encapsulated, these signs may not appear.)

Diagnostic tests

EEG, computed tomography (CT) scan and, occasionally, arteriography (which highlights abscess by a halo) help locate the site. CT scan helps locate the abscess.

CSF analysis can help confirm infection, but most doctors agree that lumbar puncture is usually too risky because it can release the increased ICP and provoke cerebral herniation.

Other tests include culture and sensitivity of drainage to identify the causative organism, skull X-rays, radioisotope scan and, rarely, ventriculography to further help identify the location of the lesion and its effects on brain tissue.

Treatment

Therapy consists of antibiotics to combat the underlying infection and surgical aspiration, drainage, or removal of the abscess after craniotomy. However, surgery is delayed until the abscess becomes encapsulated (CT scan helps determine this) and is contraindicated in patients with congenital heart disease or another debilitating cardiac condition.

After surgery, serial CT scans are performed to ensure that the infection has been eradicated. Administration of a penicillinase-resistant antibiotic, such as nafcillin or methicillin, for at least 2 to 3 weeks before surgery can reduce the risk of spreading infection.

Other treatment during the acute phase is palliative and supportive and includes mechanical ventilation, administration of I.V. fluids with diuretics (urea, mannitol), and glucocorticoids (dexamethasone) to combat increased ICP and cerebral edema. Anticonvulsants, such as phenytoin and phenobarbital, help prevent seizures.

If multiple abscesses are present, treatment usually consists of antimicrobial therapy alone.

Nursing diagnoses

- Altered thought processes
- Anxiety
- Decreased adaptive capacity: Intracranial
- Impaired physical mobility
- Pain
- Risk for altered body temperature
- Risk for impaired skin integrity
- Risk for injury
- Sensory or perceptual alterations

Nursing interventions

- Frequently assess neurologic status, especially LOC, speech, and motor, sensory, and cranial nerve functions.

- Watch for signs of increased ICP (decreased LOC, vomiting, abnormal pupil response, and depressed respirations), which may lead to cerebral herniation with signs such as fixed and dilated pupils, widened pulse pressure, tachycardia, and abnormal respirations.
- Monitor vital signs continuously.
- Monitor fluid intake and output carefully because fluid overload can contribute to cerebral edema.
- Provide emotional support. Encourage the patient and family to express their concerns, and answer their questions honestly.
- If surgery is scheduled, prepare the patient as required.
  After surgery:
- Monitor the patient's neurologic status continuously as well as vital signs and intake and output.
- Monitor the patient for increasing ICP (altered LOC, abnormal respiratory and vasomotor responses) and meningitis (nuchal rigidity, headaches, chills, sweats).
- Be sure to change a dressing when it becomes damp, using aseptic technique and noting the amount of drainage. Never allow bandages to remain damp.
- To promote drainage and prevent reaccumulation of the abscess, make sure to position the patient on the operative side.
- If the patient remains stuporous or comatose for an extended period, give meticulous skin care to prevent pressure ulcers, and position him to preserve joint function and prevent contractures.
- Ambulate the patient as soon as possible to prevent complications of immobility.
- Encourage the patient to be as independent as possible. Point out actions that he can perform successfully.

Patient teaching

- Explain the disorder to the patient and his family. Be sure they understand the diagnostic tests and treatments that will be performed. Explain all procedures to the patient even if he's comatose.
- If surgery is necessary, explain the procedure to the patient and answer his questions.
- If the patient requires isolation because of postoperative drainage, make sure he and his family understand this precaution.
- Inform the family that the residual infection may occur again even after seemingly successful treatment.
- Teach the patient and his family about prescribed medications. Explain that antimicrobial therapy may be necessary for several weeks after the patient is discharged from the hospital. Anticonvulsant therapy is also usually prescribed indefinitely because epilepsy is a complication of brain abscess. Be sure the patient and his family

understand the importance of taking the medication as prescribed and not skipping doses.

• To prevent brain abscess, stress the need for treatment of otitis media, mastoiditis, dental abscess, and other infections. Administer prophylactic antibiotics, as ordered, after a compound skull fracture or penetrating head wound.

HUNTINGTON'S DISEASE

In this disease (also called Huntington's chorea, hereditary chorea, chronic progressive chorea, or adult chorea), degeneration in the cerebral cortex and basal ganglia causes chronic progressive chorea (dancelike movements) and mental deterioration, ending in dementia.

Huntington's disease usually strikes people between ages 25 and 55 (the average age is 35); however, 2% of cases occur in children, and 5%, as late as age 60. Death usually results 10 to 15 years after onset, from heart failure or pneumonia. Because the disease is hereditary, it's prevalent in areas where affected families have lived for several generations.

Recent genetic studies have identified a marker for the gene linked to Huntington's disease, opening the way for the development of a predictive test for those at risk for the disease.

Causes

The cause of Huntington's disease is unknown. Because it's transmitted as an autosomal dominant trait, either sex can transmit and inherit it. Each child of a parent with this disease has a 50% chance of inheriting it; however, the child who doesn't inherit it can't pass it on to his own children.

Complications

Potential complications include choking, aspiration, pneumonia, heart failure, and infections.

Assessment findings

Assessment findings vary, depending on disease progression. The patient history usually shows a family history of the disorder, along with emotional and mental changes.

The onset of Huntington's disease is insidious. The patient eventually becomes totally dependent through intellectual decline, emotional disturbances, and loss of musculoskeletal control.

In the early stages, the patient is described as being clumsy, irritable, or impatient and subject to fits of anger and periods of suicidal depression, apathy, or elation. As the disease progresses, family members may report that the patient's judgment and memory have became impaired. Hallucinations, delusions, and paranoid thinking may occur. (In late stages, emotional symptoms may decrease, but eventually dementia does occur.) The family describes a gradual loss of intellectual ability, although the patient seems to be aware that his symptoms are the result of the disease. (Keep in mind that the dementia doesn't always progress at the same rate as the chorea.)

The patient may be described as having a ravenous appetite, especially for sweets. In late stages, the patient history may note loss of bladder and bowel control.

Inspection usually reveals choreic movements. These movements are rapid, often violent, and purposeless. In the early stages, they're unilateral and more prominent in the face and arms than in the legs. As the disease progresses, the choreic movements progress from mild fidgeting to grimacing, tongue smacking, dysarthria (indistinct speech), athetoid movements (especially of the hands) related to emotional state, and torticollis. In later stages, the movements involve the entire body musculature. Writhing and twitching are constant, speech becomes unintelligible, chewing and swallowing are difficult, and ambulation is impossible. In these late stages, the patient may appear emaciated and exhausted.

Diagnostic tests

Positron emission tomography and deoxyribonucleic acid analysis can detect Huntington's disease, but no reliable confirming test exists.

Helpful tests include pneumoencephalography, which shows characteristic butterfly dilation of the brain's lateral ventricles, and computed tomography scan, which shows brain atrophy.

Treatment

Because there is no known cure for Huntington's disease, treatment is supportive, protective, and based on the patient's symptoms. Tranquilizers, as well as chlorpromazine, haloperidol, or imipramine, help control choreic movements, but they can't stop mental deterioration. They also alleviate discomfort and depression. However, tranquilizers increase patient rigidity. To control choreic movements without rigidity, choline may be prescribed.

Psychotherapy to decrease anxiety and stress may also be helpful. The patient may require institutionalization because of mental deterioration.

Nursing diagnoses

• Altered health maintenance
• Anxiety

- Chronic low self-esteem
- Impaired physical mobility
- Impaired verbal communication
- Risk for aspiration
- Risk for infection
- Risk for injury
- Self-care deficit
- Total incontinence

Nursing interventions

- Provide psychological support to the patient and his family, and listen to their fears and concerns. Stay with the patient during especially stressful periods. Answer questions honestly.
- Identify the patient's self-care deficits each time he's admitted to the hospital. Then provide physical support by attending to his basic needs, such as hygiene, skin care, bowel and bladder care, and nutrition. Increase this support as mental and physical deterioration make him increasingly immobile.
- Administer medications as ordered. Monitor the patient for desired effects and adverse reactions.
- Encourage the patient to remain as independent as possible. To help him do this, give short, explicit directions. Provide demonstrations, and give the patient ample time to perform the tasks that he's capable of performing.
- To help improve the patient's body image, allow him to participate in his care as much as possible. Encourage his efforts to adapt to the changes that he's experiencing.
- If the patient has difficulty speaking, provide him with communication aids, such as an alphabet board. Allow him sufficient time to communicate.
- Stay alert for possible suicide attempts. Take suicide precautions. Control the patient's environment to protect him from suicide or other self-inflicted injury. Pad the side rails of the bed, but avoid restraints, which may cause the patient to injure himself with violent, uncontrolled movements.
- If the patient has difficulty walking, provide a walker to help him maintain his balance. If his choreic movements are violent enough to cause injury, pad the bed rails and be sure the patient is secure if he's sitting in a chair or wheelchair.
- If the patient is confined to bed, turn him every 2 hours. Post a turning schedule at the bedside.
- Minimize the patient's risk of infection by washing your hands before providing care and helping the patient wash his hands before and after meals and after using the bathroom, bedpan, or urinal.

- Monitor the patient's temperature and his white blood cell count so that infection can be detected and treated early.
- Elevate the head of the bed whenever the patient eats to reduce the risk of aspiration. Stay with him while he's eating, and instruct him to eat only small amounts of food at one time.
- Provide the incontinent patient with bladder elimination devices, such as an indwelling urinary catheter and body-worn drainage devices as appropriate. If the patient has bowel incontinence, provide incontinence aids, such as pad and pants or bed protector pads.

Patient teaching

- Teach the patient and his family about the disease. Explain the diagnostic tests and any required treatments.
- Teach the family how to perform home care.
- Encourage affected families to receive genetic counseling. All affected family members should realize that each of their offspring has a 50% chance of inheriting this disease.
- Refer the patient and his family to appropriate community organizations such as home health care agencies, the social service department, psychiatric counseling, and long-term care facilities.
- For more information about this degenerative disease, refer the patient and family to the Huntington's Disease Society of America.

PARKINSON'S DISEASE

Named for the English doctor who first accurately described the disease in 1817, Parkinson's disease characteristically produces progressive muscle rigidity, akinesia, and involuntary tremors. Deterioration progresses for an average of 10 years, culminating in death, which usually results from aspiration pneumonia or some other infection.

Also called parkinsonism, paralysis agitans, or shaking palsy, Parkinson's disease is one of the most common crippling diseases in the United States. It affects men more often than women and usually occurs in middle age or later. This disease strikes 1 in every 100 persons over age 60. Because of increased patient longevity, this amounts to roughly 60,000 new cases diagnosed annually in the United States alone.

Causes

The cause of Parkinson's disease is unknown in most cases. However, studies of the extrapyramidal brain nuclei (corpus striatum, globus pallidus, substantia nigra) have established that in this disease, a dopamine deficiency prevents affected brain cells from performing their normal inhibitory function within the central nervous system.

Some cases of Parkinson's disease are caused by exposure to toxins, such as manganese dust and carbon monoxide, that destroy cells in the substantia nigra.

Complications
Common complications associated with Parkinson's disease include injury from falls, food aspiration because of impaired voluntary movements, urinary tract infections, and skin breakdown, as the patient becomes less mobile.

Assessment findings
The patient history notes the cardinal symptoms of Parkinson's disease, which include muscle rigidity and akinesia, and an insidious tremor, commonly known as unilateral pill-roll tremor, that begins in the fingers. Although the patient often can't pinpoint exactly when tremors began, he typically reports their increase during stress or anxiety and decrease with purposeful movement and sleep. He may also report dysphagia.

The patient may complain that he becomes fatigued when he tries to perform activities of daily living and that he experiences muscle cramps of the legs, neck, and trunk. He may also mention oily skin, increased perspiration, insomnia, and mood changes. You may note dysarthria and find that the patient speaks in a high-pitched monotone.

Inspection may reveal drooling, a masklike facial expression, and difficulty walking. The patient's gait often lacks normal parallel motion and may be retropulsive or propulsive. In addition, the patient may demonstrate a loss of posture control when he walks. Typically, the patient who loses posture control walks with the body bent forward. These signs result from akinesia.

You may note another result of akinesia: oculogyric crises (eyes fixed upward, with involuntary tonic movements) or blepharospasm (eyelids closed). You may also discover that the patient takes a long time to initiate movement to perform a purposeful action.

In addition to gait changes, musculoskeletal and neurologic assessment may point to muscle rigidity that results in resistance to passive muscle stretching. Such rigidity may be uniform (lead-pipe rigidity) or jerky (cogwheel rigidity). The patient may also pivot with difficulty and easily lose his balance.

As you assess this patient, keep in mind that Parkinson's disease itself doesn't impair the intellect but that a coexisting disorder, such as arteriosclerosis, may.

Diagnostic tests
Although urinalysis may reveal decreased dopamine levels, laboratory test results usually have little value in identifying Parkinson's disease.

Computed tomography scan or magnetic resonance imaging may be performed to rule out other disorders, such as intracranial tumors.

Treatment
No cure exists for Parkinson's disease, so treatment aims to relieve symptoms and keep the patient functional as long as possible. Treatment consists of drugs, physical therapy and, in severe disease unresponsive to drugs, stereotaxic neurosurgery.

Drug therapy usually includes levodopa, a dopamine replacement that is most effective for the first few years after it's initiated. The drug is given in increasing doses until signs and symptoms are relieved or adverse reactions appear. Because adverse effects can be serious, levodopa is frequently given in combination with carbidopa (a dopa-decarboxylase inhibitor) to halt peripheral dopamine synthesis. The patient may receive bromocriptine as an additive to reduce the levodopa dose. When levodopa proves ineffective or too toxic, alternative drug therapy includes anticholinergics (such as trihexyphenidyl or benztropine) and antihistamines (such as diphenhydramine).

Antihistamines may help decrease tremors because of their central anticholinergic and sedative effects. Anticholinergics may be used to control tremors and rigidity. They may also be used in combination with levodopa.

Amantadine, an antiviral agent, is used early in treatment to reduce rigidity, tremors, and akinesia.

When drug therapy fails, stereotaxic neurosurgery sometimes offers an effective alternative. In this procedure, electrical coagulation, freezing, radioactivity, or ultrasound destroys the ventrolateral nucleus of the thalamus to prevent involuntary movement. Such neurosurgery is most effective in comparatively young, otherwise healthy people with unilateral tremor or muscle rigidity. Like drug therapy, neurosurgery is a palliative measure that can only relieve symptoms.

Physical therapy complements drug treatment and neurosurgery to maintain the patient's normal muscle tone and function. Appropriate physical therapy includes both active and passive range-of-motion exercises, routine daily activities, walking, and baths and massage to help relax muscles.

Tricyclic antidepressants may be given to decrease the depression that often accompanies the disease.

Nursing diagnoses
- Altered nutrition: Less than body requirements
- Bathing or hygiene self-care deficit
- Body image disturbance
- Chronic low self-esteem
- Constipation
- Dressing or grooming self-care deficit
- Feeding self-care deficit
- Impaired physical mobility
- Impaired social interaction
- Impaired verbal communication
- Relocation stress syndrome
- Risk for injury

Nursing interventions
- Provide emotional and psychological support to the patient and his family. Listen to their concerns, and answer their questions. To promote independence, encourage the patient to participate in care decisions and to perform as much of his own care as possible. (See *Planning care for a Parkinson's patient.*)
- Monitor drug treatment so dosage can be adjusted to minimize adverse reactions. Report adverse reactions.
- If the patient has surgery, watch for signs of hemorrhage and increased intracranial pressure by frequently checking level of consciousness and vital signs.
- Encourage independence by helping the patient recognize the activities of daily living that he can perform. Provide assistive devices as appropriate. For example, to help the patient turn himself in bed, tie a rope to the foot of the bed and extend it to the patient so that he can grasp it and pull himself to a sitting position.
- To help the patient with severe tremors achieve partial control of his body, have him sit on a chair and use its arms to steady himself.
- Remember that fatigue may cause him to depend more on others, so provide rest periods between activities.
- Help the patient overcome problems related to eating and elimination. For example, if he has difficulty eating, offer supplementary feedings or small, frequent meals to increase caloric intake. Help establish a regular bowel elimination routine by encouraging him to drink at least 2,000 ml of liquids daily and eat high-bulk foods. He may need an elevated toilet seat to assist him from a standing to a sitting position.
- Work with the physical therapist to develop a program of daily exercises to increase muscle strength, decrease muscle rigidity, prevent contractures, and improve coordination. The program should include stretching exercises, swimming, use of a stationary bicycle, and postural exercises.
- Provide frequent warm baths and massage to help relax muscles and relieve muscle cramps.
- Protect the patient from injury by using the bed's side rails and assisting the patient as necessary when he walks and eats.
- To decrease the possibility of aspiration, have the patient sit in an upright position when eating. Keep in mind that these patients are often silent aspirators. Even they don't realize that they are aspirating.
- Provide the patient with a semisolid diet, which is easier to swallow than a diet consisting of solids and liquids.

Patient teaching
- Teach the patient and his family about the disease, its progressive stages, and the treatments that may help the patient. Explain the actions of prescribed medications and possible adverse effects.
- If appropriate, show the family how to prevent pressure ulcers and contractures by proper positioning.
- Explain household safety measures, such as installing or using side rails in halls and stairs and removing throw rugs from frequently traveled floors to prevent patient injury.
- Explain the importance of daily bathing to the patient with oily skin and increased perspiration.
- To make dressing easier, teach the patient to wear clothing fitted with zippers or Velcro fasteners rather than buttons.
- To improve communication, instruct the patient to make a conscious effort to speak, to speak slowly, to take a few deep breaths before he begins to speak, and to think about what he wants to say before he begins to speak.
- If appropriate, advise the patient how to eat. Tell him to place food on the tongue, close the lips, chew first on one side and then the other, then lift the tongue up and back and make a conscious effort to swallow. Because these patients eat slowly, allow them plenty of time to eat.
- Refer the patient and his family to the National Parkinson Foundation, the American Parkinson Disease Association, or the United Parkinson Foundation for more information.

MYELITIS AND ACUTE TRANSVERSE MYELITIS

Inflammation of the spinal cord (myelitis) can result from several diseases. Poliomyelitis affects the cord's gray matter and produces motor dysfunction; leukomye-

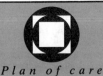

Plan of care

PLANNING CARE FOR A PARKINSON'S PATIENT

How would you go about planning effective care for a Parkinson's patient? Well, you can begin by considering that you're caring for Isadore Garber, a 73-year-old retired architect. Mr. Garber is admitted to your unit after tripping on a rug, losing his balance, and falling in his bathroom at home. He sustained a concussion and had a brief loss of consciousness.

Patient history

Mr. Garber's wife brought him to the hospital. You get most of the history from her because Mr. Garber is slow to answer your questions. You find that he has a 6-year history of Parkinson's disease after many years of good health.

The disease began with fine tremors in his right hand. These tremors seriously hampered him in his work, which involved making detailed construction drawings. Mr. Garber used to walk about seven city blocks from the train stop to his office, but the walk became difficult because of tiredness and progressive weakness of the trunk. His cognition, perception, and memory have deteriorated, and normal conversation has become difficult to maintain, especially when he has to stop to wipe his mouth or swallow excess saliva.

Mr. Garber has been taking increasing doses of carbidopa-levodopa (Sinemet) and amantadine (Symmetrel) for relief from his symptoms for nearly 6 years. Within the past 9 months, selegiline (Eldepryl) has been added to his regimen.

His only other medical condition is benign prostatic hyperplasia.

Assessment findings

You begin your assessment by checking Mr. Garber's vital signs.

He is afebrile with an oral temperature of 97.2° F (36.2° C). His pulse is bounding and regular at 82 beats/minute. His respirations are shallow and easy at 20 breaths/minute. His sitting blood pressure is 110/58 mm Hg, and it drops to 106/52 mm Hg after he stands for 1 minute. He admits to feeling lightheaded on arising from time to time.

Inspection of Mr. Garber reveals a tall, thin man with many raised, sclerotic white patches of dry skin on his flushed head and face. He has difficulty straightening his trunk and head while seated and complains that sitting up straight hurts him. Both hands and arms tremble when he extends them. His face is expressionless. When asked to walk the length of the room, he bolts to an upright position, veers to the left, and shuffles forward with his head bent down, eyes lowered to the floor.

His abdomen feels distended, and he admits to a problem with constipation. At the same time, he adds that he sometimes has to stand at the toilet for several minutes before his urine stream starts.

All laboratory reports are unremarkable. He is scheduled for a computed tomography (CT) scan of the head later this day. A follow-up study with magnetic resonance imaging may be necessary pending the results of the CT scan. A 24-hour Holter monitor will be placed on Mr. Garber tomorrow to rule out any probability of syncope secondary to cardiac arrhythmias.

Nursing diagnoses

Based on your assessment findings and Mrs. Garber's information, you formulate the following nursing diagnoses:
• Impaired physical mobility related to weakness, posture, rigidity, and gait disturbance

• Self-care deficit related to weakness and tremors
• Altered nutrition: Less than body requirements, related to difficulty in chewing and swallowing and to medications
• Constipation related to inadequate food intake and reduced physical activity
• Impaired verbal communication related to slowness of speech, memory loss, decreased volume, inability to move facial muscles, and adverse medication reactions.

Expected outcomes

You define several immediate care goals for Mr. Garber. He will:
• improve his strength and flexibility and maintain a steady gait
• participate in self-care activities of daily living with minimal weakness and tremors
• increase his intake of food, liquids, and nutrients
• gain weight
• establish a regular pattern for elimination
• improve communication.

Implementation

Keep in mind that your care for Mr. Garber will be repetitious and must be delivered with patience. You'll need to take the following steps.

To improve strength and flexibility
• Assess Mr. Garber's level of baseline strength in all major muscle groups.
• Prepare a full range of progressive exercises to do each day, such as walking, stationary bicycling, swimming, and stretching. Include isotonic exercises to tone the muscles for posture.
• Retrain Mr. Garber to walk. Instruct him to swing his arms, keep his head up, look to the horizon, and use a slow, broad-based gait. He

(continued)

PLANNING CARE FOR A PARKINSON'S PATIENT (continued)

may need a walker during the initial training period.
• Encourage Mr. Garber to take a hot bath or shower on arising to help him relax his muscles and enhance limb flexibility.

To improve self-care
• Establish a baseline of Mr. Garber's normal routine, then assist him with all fine-motor skills.
• Encourage Mr. Garber to work with the physical and occupational therapists to retrain his muscles with the use of assistive devices for self-care, such as an extended-length shoe horn; eating utensils with wide, bent handles; an extra-soft-bristled toothbrush; a palm-held hairbrush; Velcro shirt and pants closures; and well-fitting slip-on shoes and slippers.
• Praise Mr. Garber for his accomplishments with self-care, no matter how small.
• Add pull belts to each side rail of

the bed so he can pull himself from side to side during rest periods.

To promote nutritional intake, weight gain, and regular elimination
• Offer a menu based on his favorite foods; limit the daily consumption of caffeine and chocolate.
• Allow for an extended eating time with warming trays available to rewarm foods to keep them palatable.
• Provide a clear, tasteless, odorless thickening agent for all liquids, including water.
• Offer handkerchiefs or an expectorant cup so Mr. Garber can rid his mouth of excess saliva.
• Encourage Mr. Garber to take meals in an upright, seated position to discourage swallowing difficulties.
• Provide assistive devices, such as curved-handled utensils, raised plate borders, and a nonspill "sippy" cup.
• Provide a raised toilet seat to make it easier for Mr. Garber to raise or lower himself on the toilet.

• Offer frequent mouth care and treatment of any gingival or glottis infection.
• Weigh the patient weekly to track weight gain.
• Encourage intake of fluids, fruit, and fiber, as tolerated.

To improve communication
• Remind Mr. Garber to sit close to and face his listener and to speak slowly and deliberately.
• Place frequent reminders of orientation around Mr. Garber's room.
• Involve Mrs. Garber in speech therapy sessions for her husband.

Evaluation
You've met your care goals if Mr. Garber regularly practices his exercises and daily living routines with reduced difficulty, if he can communicate clearly, if his nutrition and weight gain are adequate, if he has no avoidable infections, and if his elimination is easier and more regular.

---

litis affects only the white matter and produces sensory dysfunction. These types of myelitis can attack any level of the spinal cord, causing partial destruction or scattered lesions.

Acute transverse myelitis, which affects the entire thickness of the spinal cord, produces both motor and sensory dysfunction. This form of myelitis, which has a rapid onset, is the most devastating.

The prognosis depends on the severity of cord damage and prevention of complications. If spinal cord necrosis occurs, the prognosis for complete recovery is poor. Even without necrosis, residual neurologic deficits usually persist after recovery. Patients who develop spastic reflexes early in the course of the illness are more likely to recover than those who don't.

Causes
Myelitis may result from poliovirus, herpes zoster, herpesvirus B, or rabies virus; disorders that cause meningeal inflammation, such as syphilis, abscesses and other suppurative conditions, and tuberculosis; smallpox or polio vaccination; parasitic and fungal infections; and chronic adhesive arachnoiditis.

Certain toxic agents (carbon monoxide, lead, and arsenic) can cause a type of myelitis in which acute inflammation (followed by hemorrhage and, possibly, necrosis) destroys the entire circumference (myelin, axis cylinders, and neurons) of the spinal cord.

Acute transverse myelitis has several causes. It often follows acute infectious diseases, such as measles and pneumonia (the inflammation occurs after the infection has subsided), and primary infections of the spinal cord itself, such as syphilis and acute disseminated encephalomyelitis. Acute transverse myelitis can accompany demyelinating diseases, such as acute multiple sclerosis, and inflammatory and necrotizing disorders of the spinal cord, such as hematomyelia.

Complications
Common complications include hypertension, urinary tract infection, urolithiasis, pneumonia, skeletal and smooth-muscle deformities, myocarditis, and paralytic ileus.

Assessment findings
In all types of myelitis, the extent of neurologic deficit depends on the level of the spinal cord affected.

In poliomyelitis, assessment findings vary with the type. In *abortive poliomyelitis,* the patient may report headache, vomiting, diarrhea, constipation, and sore throat. Vital signs may reveal fever. Neurologic assessment is normal. Signs of central nervous system involvement are absent.

In *nonparalytic poliomyelitis,* the patient history notes complaints of headache, neck, back, and extremity pain as well as vomiting, abdominal pain, lethargy, and irritability. Palpation may disclose continuous muscle spasms in the extensor muscles of the neck and back and often in the hamstring and other muscles. The muscles may also be tender on palpation. A vital signs check detects fever.

In *paralytic poliomyelitis,* patient history may reveal that the patient had a fever and a minor respiratory illness several days before development of poliomyelitis. The patient usually explains that the fever returned accompanied by cramping muscle pain and spasm and twitching in the affected parts.

These patients may develop spinal poliomyelitis, bulbar poliomyelitis, or both. In *spinal poliomyelitis,* neurologic assessment finds weakness or paralysis of the muscles supplied by the spinal nerves affected. Paralysis of one leg commonly occurs in children under age 5. In patients ages 5 to 15, weakness of one arm and paraplegia are common. In adults, quadriplegia is more likely. You'll also find deep tendon reflexes diminished or lost, often asymmetrically, in areas of involvement.

In *bulbar poliomyelitis,* the patient may report difficulty chewing, inability to swallow or expel saliva, and regurgitation of fluids through the nose. As the patient speaks, you may notice a nasal voice and dysphonia. Neurologic assessment may reveal weakness of the facial, sternocleidomastoid, and trapezius muscles.

In *myelitis caused by herpesvirus type 2 infection in the genital and perineal region,* neurologic examination usually finds a paralyzed sphincter (bladder or anal).

In *acute transverse myelitis,* patient history reveals a rapid onset with motor and sensory dysfunction below the level of spinal cord damage appearing in 1 to 2 days. The patient may report that he had a respiratory tract infection just before the onset of the disorder.

Neurologic examination may reveal flaccid paralysis of the legs, which the patient occasionally reports as beginning in just one leg. This paralysis is often accompanied by loss of sensory and sphincter function. The patient may explain that sensory loss followed pain in the legs or trunk.

Reflexes may be absent in the early stages but may reappear later. Neurologic examination almost always reveals normal arm function. Transverse myelitis rarely involves the arms. If spinal cord damage is severe, the patient may experience shock (hypotension and hypothermia).

Diagnostic tests
Diagnostic evaluation must rule out spinal cord tumor and identify any underlying infection.
• *White blood cell count* may be normal or slightly elevated.
• *Cerebrospinal fluid analysis* may show normal or increased lymphocyte and protein levels without isolating the causative agent.
• *Throat washings* may reveal the causative virus in patients suspected of having poliomyelitis.
• *Computed tomography scan* or *magnetic resonance imaging* is useful to rule out spinal cord tumor.

Treatment
In myelitis, treatment is supportive and focused on relieving the patient's symptoms. An underlying bacterial infection requires appropriate treatment.

Nursing diagnoses
• Anxiety
• Body image disturbance
• Impaired physical mobility
• Knowledge deficit
• Pain
• Risk for infection

Nursing interventions
• Provide psychological support to the patient and his family. Encourage them to express their concerns, and answer their questions honestly. Allow the patient to participate in care planning as appropriate.
• Maintain the patient in a comfortable position as much as possible.
• Prevent contracture development in a patient with paralysis by using footboards and light splints. Perform passive range-of-motion exercises.
• Frequently assess vital signs. Watch carefully for signs of shock (hypotension and diaphoresis).
• Perform comfort measures, such as massage for the patient with muscle spasms. Administer analgesics, as ordered.
• Watch for signs of urinary tract infection if the patient has an indwelling urinary catheter.
• Prevent skin infections and pressure ulcers with meticulous skin care. Check pressure points often and keep the patient's skin clean and dry; use a low-air-loss bed,

foam pad, or other pressure-relieving device. Turn the patient every 2 hours.
• Initiate rehabilitation as soon as the patient passes the acute stage of the disorder. For example, as soon as the fever subsides, begin early mobilization and active exercises as directed by the physical therapist.
• If the patient has trouble dealing with body image changes, point out to him the actions that he performs well, providing encouragement and support whenever possible.
• Watch for problems that can develop, such as respiratory muscle paralysis in the patient with bulbar poliomyelitis. Provide oxygen and mechanical ventilation as necessary.

Patient teaching
• Explain the disorder to the patient and his family. Tell them about diagnostic tests. Be sure that the patient and his family understand the possible problems that may follow the acute phase of the disorder.
• Explain the treatments, such as physical therapy and bowel and bladder training, to help the patient recover as much independence as possible.
• As appropriate, refer the patient and his family to the social service department and to home health care agencies for assistance with care after discharge.

ALZHEIMER'S DISEASE

This progressive degenerative disorder of the cerebral cortex (especially the frontal lobe) accounts for more than half of all cases of dementia. An estimated 5% of people over age 65 have a severe form of this disease, and 12% suffer from mild to moderate dementia. Because this is a primary progressive dementia, the prognosis for a patient with this disease is poor.

Typically, patients die of debilitating brain disease 2 to 15 years after the onset of symptoms. The average duration of the illness before death is 8 years.

Causes and pathophysiology
The cause of Alzheimer's disease is unknown. However, several factors are thought to be closely connected to this disease. These include neurochemical factors, such as deficiencies of the neurotransmitters acetylcholine, somatostatin, substance P, and norepinephrine; viral factors, such as slow-growing central nervous system viruses; trauma; and genetic factors.

Researchers believe that up to 70% of Alzheimer's cases stem from a genetic abnormality. Recently, they located the abnormality on chromosome 21. They've also isolated a genetic substance (amyloid) that causes brain damage typical of Alzheimer's disease. The brain tissue of patients with this dementia has three distinguishing features: neurofibrillary tangles, neuritic plaques, and granulovascular degeneration.

Complications
In this disorder, complications include injury from the patient's own violent behavior or from wandering or unsupervised activity; pneumonia and other infections, especially if the patient doesn't receive enough exercise; malnutrition and dehydration, especially if the patient refuses or forgets to eat; and aspiration.

Assessment findings
As you assess this patient, keep in mind that the onset of this disorder is insidious and that initial changes are almost imperceptible but gradually progress to serious problems. The patient history is almost always obtained from a family member or caregiver.

Typically, the patient history shows initial onset of very small changes, such as forgetfulness and subtle memory loss without loss of social skills and behavior patterns. It also reveals that over time the patient began experiencing recent memory loss and had difficulty learning and remembering new information. The history also may reveal a general deterioration in personal hygiene and appearance and an inability to concentrate.

Depending on the severity of the disease, the patient history may reveal that the patient experiences several of the following problems: difficulty with abstract thinking and activities that require judgment; progressive difficulty in communicating; and a severe deterioration of memory, language, and motor function that in the more severe cases finally results in coordination loss and an inability to speak or write. He may also perform repetitive actions and experience restlessness; negative personality changes, such as irritability, depression, paranoia, hostility, and combativeness; nocturnal awakenings; and disorientation.

The person giving the history may explain that the patient is suspicious and fearful of imaginary people and situations, misperceives his environment, misidentifies objects and people, and complains of stolen or misplaced objects.

He also may report that the patient seems overdependent on caregivers and has difficulty using correct words and may often substitute meaningless words. He may report that conversations with the patient drift off into nonsensical phrases. The patient's emotions may be described as labile. Also, the patient may laugh or cry inappropriately, and have mood swings, sudden angry outbursts, and sleep disturbances.

Neurologic examination confirms many of the problems revealed during the history. In addition, it often reveals an impaired sense of smell (usually an early symptom), impaired stereognosis (inability to recognize and understand the form and nature of objects by touching them), gait disorders, tremors, and loss of recent memory. The patient with Alzheimer's also has a positive snout reflex. (See *Snout reflex.*)

If the patient is in the final stages, he typically has urinary or fecal incontinence and may twitch and have seizures.

Diagnostic tests

Alzheimer's disease is diagnosed by exclusion. Various tests, such as those described below, are performed to rule out other disorders. However, the diagnosis cannot be confirmed until death, when pathologic findings come to light at autopsy.
• *Positron emission tomography* measures the metabolic activity of the cerebral cortex and may help confirm early diagnosis.
• *Computed tomography scan* in some patients shows progressive brain atrophy in excess of that which occurs in normal aging.
• *Magnetic resonance imaging* may permit evaluation of the condition of the brain and rule out intracranial lesions as the source of dementia.
• *EEG* allows evaluation of the brain's electrical activity and may show slowing of the brain waves in the late stages of the disease. This diagnostic test also helps identify tumors, abscesses, and other intracranial lesions that might cause the patient's symptoms.
• *Cerebrospinal fluid analysis* may help determine if the patient's signs and symptoms stem from a chronic neurologic infection.
• *Cerebral blood flow studies* may detect abnormalities in blood flow to the brain.

Treatment

No cure or definitive treatment exists for Alzheimer's disease. Therapy consists of cerebral vasodilators, such as ergoloid mesylates, isoxsuprine, and cyclandelate to enhance the brain's circulation; hyperbaric oxygen to increase oxygenation to the brain; psychostimulators, such as methylphenidate, to enhance the patient's mood; and antidepressants if depression seems to exacerbate the patient's dementia.

Most other drug therapies being tried are experimental. These include choline salts, lecithin, physostigmine,

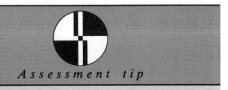

Assessment tip

SNOUT REFLEX

When results are positive in an adult, the snout reflex test suggests organic brain disease.

The test involves tapping or stroking the patient's lips or the area just under the nose. Grimacing or puckering the lips is a positive sign for Alzheimer's disease in an adult. A positive result in early infancy is normal.

tacrine, enkephalins, and naloxone, which may slow the disease process.

Nursing diagnoses
• Altered nutrition: Less than body requirements
• Altered thought processes
• Bathing or hygiene self-care deficit
• Constipation
• Dressing or grooming self-care deficit
• Feeding self-care deficit
• Impaired verbal communication
• Ineffective family coping
• Knowledge deficit
• Risk for trauma
• Toileting self-care deficit

Nursing interventions
• Establish an effective communication system with the patient and his family to help them adjust to the patient's altered cognitive abilities.
• Provide emotional support to the patient and his family. Encourage them to talk about their concerns. Listen carefully to them, and answer their questions honestly and completely.
• Because the patient may misperceive his environment, use a soft tone and a slow, calm manner when speaking to him.
• Allow the patient sufficient time to answer your questions because his thought processes are slow, impairing his ability to communicate verbally.
• Administer ordered medications to the patient and note their effects.
• If the patient has trouble swallowing, crush tablets and open capsules and mix them with a semisoft food. Al-

TEACHING PATIENTS ABOUT ALZHEIMER'S DISEASE

Counsel family members to expect progressive deterioration in the patient with Alzheimer's disease. To help them plan future patient care, discuss the stages of this relentless and inevitably progressive disease.

Bear in mind that family members may refuse to believe that the disease is advancing. So be sensitive to their concerns and, if necessary, review the information again when they're more receptive.

Forgetfulness
The patient becomes forgetful, especially of recent events. He frequently loses everyday objects, such as keys. Aware of his loss of function, he may compensate by relinquishing tasks that might reveal his forgetfulness. Because his behavior isn't disruptive and may be attributed to stress, fatigue, or normal aging, he usually doesn't consult a doctor at this stage.

Confusion
The patient has increasing difficulty at activities that require planning, decision making, and judgment, such as managing personal finances, driving a car, and performing his job. However, he does retain everyday skills, such as personal grooming. Social withdrawal occurs when the patient feels overwhelmed by a changing environment and his inability to cope with multiple stimuli. Travel is difficult and tiring. As he becomes aware of his progressive loss of function, he may become severely depressed.

Safety becomes a concern when the patient forgets to turn off appliances or to recognize unsafe situations, such as boiling water. At this point, the family may need to consider day care or a supervised residential facility.

Decline in activities of daily living
The patient at this stage loses his ability to perform daily activities, such as eating or washing, without direct supervision. Weight loss may occur. He withdraws from the family and increasingly depends on the primary caregiver. Communication becomes difficult as his understanding of written and spoken language declines. Agitation, wandering, pacing, and nighttime awakening are linked to his inability to cope with a multisensory environment. He may mistake his mirror image for a real person (pseudohallucination). Caregivers must be constantly vigilant, which may lead to physical and emotional exhaustion. They may also be angry and feel a sense of loss.

Total deterioration
In the final stage of Alzheimer's disease, the patient no longer recognizes himself, his body parts, or other family members. He becomes bedridden, and his activity consists of small, purposeless movements. Verbal communication stops, although he may scream spontaneously. Complications of immobility may include pressure ulcers, urinary tract infections, pneumonia, and contractures.

---

ways check with the pharmacist before crushing tablets or opening capsules because some drugs should not be altered.

• Protect the patient from injury by providing a safe, structured environment. Provide rest periods between activities because these patients tire easily.

• Encourage the patient to exercise, as ordered, to help maintain mobility.

• Encourage patient independence and allow ample time for the patient to perform tasks.

• Encourage sufficient fluid intake and adequate nutrition. Provide assistance with menu selection, and allow the patient to feed himself as much as he can. Provide a well-balanced diet with adequate fiber. Avoid stimulants, such as coffee, tea, cola, and chocolate. Give the patient semisolid foods if he has dysphagia. Insert and care for a nasogastric tube or a gastrostomy tube for feeding, as ordered.

• Because the patient may be disoriented or neuromuscular functioning may be impaired, take the patient to the bathroom at least every 2 hours, and make sure he knows the location of the bathroom.

• Assist the patient with hygiene and dressing as necessary. Many patients with Alzheimer's disease are incapable of performing these tasks.

Patient teaching
• Teach the patient's family about the disease. Explain that the cause of the disease is unknown. Review the signs and symptoms of the disease with them. Be sure to explain that the disease progresses but at an unpredictable rate and that the patient will eventually suffer complete memory loss and total physical deterioration. (See *Teaching patients about Alzheimer's disease.*)

• Review the diagnostic tests that will be performed and the treatment the patient will require.

• Advise the family to provide the patient with exercise. Suggest physical activities, such as walking or light housework, that occupy and satisfy the patient.

• Stress the importance of diet. Instruct the family to limit the number of foods on the patient's plate so he won't have to make decisions. If the patient has coordination problems, tell the family to cut his food and to provide finger foods, such as fruit and sandwiches. Suggest using plates with rim guards, built-up utensils, and cups with lids and spouts.

• Encourage the family to allow the patient as much independence as possible while ensuring his and others' safety. Tell them to create a routine for all the patient's activities, which will avoid confusion. If the patient becomes belligerent, advise the family to remain calm and to try distracting him.

• Refer the family to support groups, such as the Alzheimer's Association. Set up an appointment with the social service department, which will help the family assess its needs.

REYE'S SYNDROME

An acute childhood illness, Reye's syndrome causes fatty infiltration of the liver with concurrent hyperammonemia, encephalopathy, and increased intracranial pressure (ICP). In addition, fatty infiltration of the kidneys, brain, and myocardium may occur. Reye's syndrome affects children from infancy to adolescence and occurs equally in boys and girls. It affects whites over age 1 more often than blacks.

Reye's syndrome almost always follows within 1 to 3 days of an acute viral infection, such as an upper respiratory tract infection, type B influenza, or varicella (chicken pox).

The prognosis depends on the severity of central nervous system depression. Previously, mortality was as high as 90%. Today, though, increased awareness of Reye's syndrome, early detection, and prompt, aggressive treatment have reduced mortality to about 5%. Death is usually a result of cerebral edema or respiratory arrest. Most comatose patients who survive have some residual brain damage, such as developmental and neuropsychological difficulties.

Causes and pathophysiology

The cause is unknown, but viral and toxic agents, especially salicylates, have been implicated. Studies performed between 1980 and 1985 proved a relation between aspirin administration during a viral infection and onset of Reye's syndrome. Since this finding was published, pediatric use of aspirin has declined, and Reye's syndrome has become less common.

In this disease, damaged hepatic mitochondria disrupt the urea cycle, which normally changes ammonia to urea for its excretion from the body. This results in hyperammonemia, hypoglycemia, and an increase in serum short-chain fatty acids, leading to encephalopathy. As the ammonia level increases, the brain, a secondary site of urea metabolism, swells markedly. At the same time, fatty infiltration occurs in renal tubular cells, neuronal tissue, and muscle tissue, including the heart.

Complications

Increased ICP is the worst complication of Reye's syndrome. The child's ICP is commonly so fragile that even standard nursing care, such as turning and bathing the child, may precipitate a large increase in ICP.

Other possible complications include respiratory alkalosis and subsequent impaired gas exchange, respiratory arrest, and decreased cardiac output.

Assessment findings

The severity of the child's signs and symptoms varies with the degree of encephalopathy and cerebral edema.

Most commonly, the patient history reveals a viral infection followed by a brief period of several days during which the child seems to recover. Later, he develops intractable vomiting and progressive changes in level of consciousness, from drowsiness and lethargy to stupor and coma.

Vital signs may include a low-grade fever or normal temperature, slight tachycardia, rapid respirations, and a normal blood pressure. Inspection may reveal diaphoresis and a child who appears healthy but may be agitated, confused, or combative. Jaundice is usually absent. The liver is not usually palpable.

Neurologic examination usually is normal except for hyperreflexia. Signs of increased ICP are rare. Pupils are usually reactive, and ophthalmoscopic examination reveals no evidence of papilledema.

If the child is assessed late in the disease, respiratory distress (progressing from hyperventilation to Cheyne-Stokes and apneic respirations) is usually evident. Then as the child passes into coma, he may develop unilateral or bilateral fixed and dilated pupils (with severe encephalopathy), seizures, and decorticate or decerebrate posturing.

Diagnostic tests

• *Laboratory tests* disclose elevated serum ammonia levels; normal or (in 15% of cases) low serum glucose levels; and increased serum fatty acid and lactate levels. Liver function studies indicate aspartate aminotransfer-

ase (formerly SGOT) and alanine aminotransferase (formerly SGPT) at twice the normal levels. Bilirubin levels are normal. Coagulation studies demonstrate increased prothrombin time and partial thromboplastin time.
• *Liver biopsy* reveals fatty droplets uniformly distributed throughout liver cells.
• *Cerebrospinal fluid (CSF) analysis* shows a white blood cell count of less than 10/mm³; coma causes increased CSF pressure.

Treatment
In Reye's syndrome, treatment depends on the disease's stage and must be started as soon as Reye's syndrome is diagnosed because the disease progresses rapidly. Initially, therapy consists of I.V. administration of glucose to prevent onset of coma. Other treatments include airway maintenance, adequate oxygenation, and control of cerebral edema. (See *Reye's syndrome: Stages and treatment.*)

Nursing diagnoses
• Altered cerebral tissue perfusion
• Anxiety
• Fear
• Impaired gas exchange
• Impaired physical mobility
• Ineffective breathing pattern
• Risk for impaired skin integrity

Nursing interventions
• Provide emotional and psychological support to the child, as appropriate, and his family. Listen to their concerns, and stay with them during periods of acute stress.
• Continuously monitor vital signs, and assess the child's level of consciousness. Watch for increasing lethargy. Immediately report any signs of coma. Also continuously assess the child for loss of reflexes and signs of flaccidity.
• Anticipate the possible need for intubation and mechanical ventilation to help control increasing ICP and to maintain adequate oxygenation. Keep the necessary supplies available. If mechanical ventilation is begun, be prepared to administer a paralyzing agent, such as pancuronium I.V., and an analgesic, as ordered.
• Keep the head of the bed elevated at a 30-degree angle to increase venous outflow and decrease ICP.
• Monitor ICP and report changes.
• Monitor cardiovascular status with a pulmonary artery catheter or central venous line.
• Administer ordered I.V. fluids and medications as directed. Monitor the child for the desired effect. As or-

dered, give mannitol I.V., thiopental I.V., or glycerol by nasogastric tube to control ICP.
• Maintain seizure precautions during the acute stage; seizures may occur at any time.
• Hyperventilate the child with 100% oxygen before suctioning to forestall precipitous falls in partial pressure of oxygen in arterial blood (PaO_2) and increases in partial pressure of carbon dioxide in arterial blood ($PaCO_2$), either of which may lead to sudden changes in ICP.
• Provide good skin care, and perform range-of-motion exercises.
• If the child begins to recover from the illness, reorient him as often as necessary because he usually can't remember anything that occurred during the acute stage of the illness. Be sure to explain all procedures to the child to decrease his anxiety. Encourage the parents to bring familiar things from home and to spend as much time as possible with their child.

Patient teaching
• Teach the family and, as appropriate, the child, about the disorder, its signs and symptoms, the diagnostic tests, and the treatments that are necessary. Discuss the prognosis with the parents. Reinforce teaching as necessary.
• Advise the parents to give nonsalicylate analgesics and antipyretics, such as acetaminophen.
• Refer the parents to the National Reye's Syndrome Foundation.

GUILLAIN-BARRÉ SYNDROME
This disorder is an acute, rapidly progressive, and potentially fatal form of polyneuritis that causes segmented demyelination of peripheral nerves. Guillain-Barré syndrome occurs equally in both sexes, usually between the ages of 30 and 50. It affects about 2 of every 100,000 people.

The clinical course of Guillain-Barré syndrome has three phases. The *acute phase* begins when the first definitive symptom develops; it ends 1 to 3 weeks later, when no further deterioration is noted. The *plateau phase* lasts for several days to 2 weeks and is followed by the *recovery phase,* which is believed to coincide with remyelination and axonal process regrowth. The recovery phase extends over 4 to 6 months; however, patients with severe disease may take up to 2 to 3 years to recover, and recovery may not be complete. The disorder is also known as infectious polyneuritis, Landry-Guillain-Barré syndrome, or acute idiopathic polyneuritis.

REYE'S SYNDROME: STAGES AND TREATMENT

Each stage of Reye's syndrome presents its own set of signs and symptoms, which require appropriate medical treatments and nursing interventions, as outlined below.

Signs and symptoms	Treatment	Nursing interventions
Stage I Vomiting, lethargy, hepatic dysfunction	• Give glucose I.V. to help decrease the possibility of coma. • Give I.V. fluids at two-thirds of maintenance dose and an osmotic diuretic or furosemide administered to decrease ICP and cerebral edema. • Give vitamin K to decrease hypoprothrombinemia; if unsuccessful, give fresh-frozen plasma.	• Obtain serum ammonia, blood glucose, and plasma osmolality values every 4 to 8 hours to monitor patient progress. • Monitor fluid intake and output to prevent fluid overload. Maintain urine output at 1 ml/kg/hour, plasma osmolality at 290 mOsm/kg, and blood glucose levels at 150 mg/dl. (Goal: Keep glucose levels high, osmolality normal to high, and ammonia levels low.) Also, restrict protein intake.
Stage II Hyperventilation, delirium, hepatic dysfunction, hyperactive reflexes	• Continue baseline treatment.	• Institute seizure precautions. • Be prepared for invasive supportive therapy, such as intubation.
Stage III Coma, hyperventilation, decorticate rigidity, hepatic dysfunction	• Continue baseline treatment and supportive care.	• Continue seizure precautions. • Monitor ICP. • Perform endotracheal intubation and institute mechanical ventilation to control $PaCO_2$ levels. Administering a paralyzing agent, such as pancuronium I.V., may help maintain ventilation. • Administer mannitol I.V., thiopental I.V. or glycerol by nasogastric tube to help control ICP. • When ventilating the patient, maintain $PaCO_2$ between 20 and 30 mm Hg and PaO_2 between 80 and 100 mm Hg. • Insert a pulmonary artery catheter or central venous pressure catheter to monitor cardiovascular status.
Stage IV Deepening coma; decerebrate rigidity; large, fixed pupils; minimal hepatic dysfunction	• Continue baseline and supportive care. • If all previous measures fail, some pediatric centers use barbiturate coma, decompressive craniotomy, hypothermia, or exchange transfusion.	• Check the patient for loss of reflexes and signs of flaccidity. • Give the family the extra support they need, considering their child's poor prognosis.
Stage V Seizures, loss of deep tendon reflexes, flaccidity, respiratory arrest, ammonia level above 300 mg/dl	• Continue baseline and supportive care. The prognosis is very poor at this stage; usually the child does not recover.	• Help the family to face the patient's impending death.

Causes and pathophysiology

The precise cause of Guillain-Barré syndrome is unknown, but it's thought to be a cell-mediated immunologic attack on peripheral nerves in response to a virus. Risk factors include surgery, rabies or swine influenza vaccination, viral illness, Hodgkin's or some other malignant disease, and lupus erythematosus.

The major pathologic effect is segmental demyelination of the peripheral nerves, which prevents normal transmission of electrical impulses along the sensorimotor nerve roots. (See *Understanding sensorimotor nerve degeneration*, page 736.)

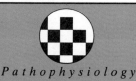

Pathophysiology

UNDERSTANDING SENSORIMOTOR NERVE DEGENERATION

Guillain-Barré syndrome attacks the peripheral nerves so that they can't transmit messages to the brain correctly. Here's what goes wrong.

The myelin sheath degenerates for unknown reasons. This sheath covers the nerve axons and conducts electrical impulses along the nerve pathways. With degeneration comes inflammation, swelling, and patchy demyelination. As this disorder destroys myelin, the nodes of Ranvier (at the junctures of the myelin sheaths) widen. This delays and impairs impulse transmission along both the dorsal and the ventral nerve roots.

Because the dorsal nerve roots handle sensory function, the patient may experience sensations such as tingling and numbness when the nerve root is impaired. Similarly, because the ventral roots are responsible for motor function, impairment causes varying weakness, immobility, and paralysis.

Complications

Because of the patient's inability to use his muscles, complications can occur. These include thrombophlebitis, pressure ulcers, contractures, muscle wasting, aspiration, respiratory tract infections, and life-threatening respiratory and cardiac compromise.

Assessment findings

Most patients seek treatment when the disease is in the acute stage. Typically, the history reveals that the patient experienced a minor febrile illness (usually an upper respiratory tract infection or, less often, GI infection) 1 to 4 weeks before his current symptoms.

The patient may report feelings of tingling and numbness (paresthesia) in the legs. If the disease has progressed further, he may report that the tingling and numbness began in the legs and progressed to the arms, the trunk and, finally, the face. The paresthesia usually precedes muscle weakness but tends to vanish quickly; in some patients, it may never occur. Some patients may also report stiffness and pain in the calves, such as a severe charley horse, and in the back.

Neurologic examination uncovers muscle weakness (the major neurologic sign) and sensory loss, usually in the legs. If the disease has progressed, the weakness and sensory loss may also be present in the arms. Keep in mind that the disease progresses rapidly and that symptoms may progress beyond the legs within 24 to 72 hours. (See *Testing for thoracic sensation.*)

If the cranial nerves are affected—as they often are—the patient may have difficulty talking, chewing, and swallowing. Subsequent cranial nerve testing may reveal paralysis of the ocular, facial, and oropharyngeal muscles.

Remember that muscle weakness sometimes develops in the arms first (descending type), rather than in the legs (ascending type) or in the arms and legs simultaneously. Remember, too, that in milder forms of this disease, muscle weakness may affect only the cranial nerves or may not occur at all. Neurologic examination may reveal a loss of position sense and diminished or absent deep tendon reflexes.

Diagnostic tests

• *Cerebrospinal fluid (CSF) analysis* may show a normal white blood cell count, an elevated protein count, and, in severe disease, increased CSF pressure. The CSF protein level begins to rise several days after the onset of signs and symptoms, peaking in 4 to 6 weeks, probably resulting from widespread inflammatory disease of the nerve roots.
• *Electromyography* may demonstrate repeated firing of the same motor unit instead of widespread sectional stimulation.
• *Electrophysiologic testing* may reveal marked slowing of nerve conduction velocities.

Treatment

In Guillain-Barré syndrome, treatment is primarily supportive and may require endotracheal intubation or tracheotomy if the patient has difficulty clearing secretions. Mechanical ventilation is necessary if the patient has respiratory difficulties.

Continuous electrocardiogram monitoring is necessary to identify cardiac arrhythmias. Propranolol may be administered to treat tachycardia and hypotension. Atropine may be administered to treat bradycardia. Marked hypotension may require volume replacement.

Plasmapheresis produces a temporary reduction in circulating antibodies. Now an accepted form of therapy, it is most effective when performed during the first few weeks of the disease. The patient may receive three to five plasma exchanges.

Nursing diagnoses

- Altered nutrition: Less than body requirements
- Altered urinary elimination
- Anxiety
- Fear
- Impaired gas exchange
- Impaired physical mobility
- Impaired verbal communication
- Ineffective breathing pattern

Nursing interventions

- Monitor the patient's vital signs and level of consciousness.
- Continually assess the patient's respiratory function. If respiratory muscles are weak, take serial vital capacity recordings. Use a spirometer with a mouthpiece or a face mask for bedside testing.
- Auscultate breath sounds, turn and position the patient, and encourage coughing and deep breathing. Begin respiratory support at the first sign of dyspnea (in adults, vital capacity less than 800 ml; in children, less than 12 ml/kg of body weight) or decreasing partial pressure of oxygen in arterial blood (PaO_2).
- Monitor pulse oximetry to keep oxygen saturation above 93%.
- Obtain arterial blood gas measurements as ordered. Because neuromuscular disease results in primary hypoventilation with hypoxemia and hypercapnia, watch for PaO_2 below 70 mm Hg, which signals respiratory failure. Be alert for confusion and tachypnea—signs of rising partial pressure of carbon dioxide in arterial blood.
- If respiratory failure becomes imminent, establish an emergency airway with an endotracheal tube. Be prepared to begin and maintain mechanical ventilation.
- Provide meticulous skin care to prevent skin breakdown and contractures. Establish a strict turning schedule, inspect the skin (especially sacrum, heels, and ankles) for breakdown, and reposition the patient every 2 hours. Use alternating pressure pads at points of contact.
- Perform passive range-of-motion exercises within the patient's pain limits, possibly using a Hubbard tank. Remember that the proximal muscle group of the thighs, shoulders, and trunk will be the most tender and will cause the most pain on passive movement and turning. When the patient's condition stabilizes, change to gentle stretching and active assistance exercises.
- To prevent aspiration, test the gag reflex, and elevate the head of the bed before giving the patient anything to eat. If the gag reflex is absent, give nasogastric feedings until the reflex returns.

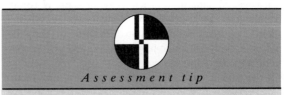

Assessment tip

TESTING FOR THORACIC SENSATION

When Guillain-Barré syndrome progresses rapidly, test for ascending sensory loss by touching the patient or pressing his skin lightly with a pin every hour. Move systematically from the iliac crest (T12) to the scapula, occasionally substituting the blunt end of the pin to test the patient's ability to discriminate between sharp and dull.

Using an indelible pen, mark on the patient the level of diminished sensation to measure any change. If diminished sensation ascends to T8 or higher, the patient's intercostal muscle function (and consequently respiratory function) will probably be impaired.

As Guillain-Barré syndrome subsides, sensory and motor weakness descend to the lower thoracic segments, heralding a return of intercostal and extremity muscle function.

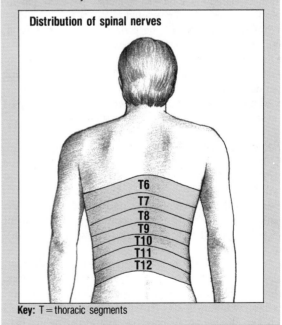

Distribution of spinal nerves

T6
T7
T8
T9
T10
T11
T12

Key: T = thoracic segments

- As the patient regains strength and can tolerate a vertical position, be alert for postural hypotension. Monitor blood pressure and pulse rate during tilting periods and, if necessary, apply toe-to-groin elastic bandages or an abdominal binder to prevent postural hypotension.

• Inspect the patient's legs regularly for signs of thrombophlebitis (localized pain, tenderness, erythema, edema, positive Homans' sign). To prevent thrombophlebitis, apply antiembolism stockings and give prophylactic anticoagulants, as ordered.

• If the patient has facial paralysis, give eye and mouth care every 4 hours. Protect the corneas with isotonic eyedrops and conical eye shields.

• Watch for urine retention. Measure and record intake and output every 8 hours, and offer the bedpan every 3 to 4 hours. Encourage adequate fluid intake (2,000 ml/day) unless contraindicated. If urine retention develops, begin intermittent catheterization, as ordered. Because the abdominal muscles are weak, the patient may need manual pressure on the bladder (Credé's method) before he can urinate.

• To prevent and relieve constipation, offer prune juice and a high-bulk diet. If necessary, give daily or alternate-day suppositories (glycerin or bisacodyl) or enemas, as ordered.

• If the patient is unable to communicate because of paralysis, tracheostomy, or intubation, try to establish some form of communication—for example, have the patient blink his eyes, once for yes and twice for no.

• Provide diversions for the patient, such as television, family visits, or listening to tapes.

• Provide emotional support to the patient and his family. Listen to their concerns. Stay with the patient during periods of severe stress.

• Administer medications as ordered. Analgesics may be prescribed to relieve muscle stiffness and spasm.

Patient teaching

• Explain the disease and its signs and symptoms to the patient and his family. Explain the diagnostic tests that will be performed.

• Explain the treatments that are ordered, and tell the patient why they're necessary. For example, if the patient loses his gag reflex, tell him tube feedings are necessary to maintain nutritional status.

• Advise the family to help the patient maintain mental alertness, fight boredom, and avoid depression. Suggest that they plan frequent visits, read books to the patient, or borrow library books on tape for him.

• Before discharge, prepare an appropriate home care plan. Teach the patient how to transfer from bed to wheelchair, from wheelchair to toilet or to tub, and how to walk short distances with a walker or a cane.

• Instruct the family how to help the patient eat, compensating for facial weakness, and how to help him avoid skin breakdown.

• Emphasize the importance of establishing a regular bowel and bladder elimination routine.

• Tell the patient to schedule physical therapy sessions.

NEUROMUSCULAR DISORDERS

In these disorders—myasthenia gravis, amyotrophic lateral sclerosis, and multiple sclerosis—a neurologic problem causes muscle degeneration.

MYASTHENIA GRAVIS

This disorder produces sporadic, but progressive weakness and abnormal fatigability of striated (skeletal) muscles. Muscle weakness is exacerbated by exercise and repeated movement but improved by anticholinesterase drugs. Usually, myasthenia gravis affects muscles innervated by the cranial nerves (face, lips, tongue, neck, and throat), but it can affect any muscle group. It commonly accompanies immune and thyroid disorders. In fact, 15% of myasthenic patients have thymomas. When the disease involves the respiratory system, it may be life-threatening.

Myasthenia gravis follows an unpredictable course of recurring exacerbations and periodic remissions. No cure is known. However, drug treatment has improved the prognosis and allows patients to lead relatively normal lives except during exacerbations.

Myasthenia gravis affects 2 to 20 persons per 100,000. It occurs at any age, but incidence is highest in women ages 18 to 25 and in men ages 50 to 60. About three times as many women as men develop this disease.

About 20% of infants born to myasthenic mothers have transient (or occasionally persistent) myasthenia. Spontaneous remissions occur in about 25% of patients.

Causes

Myasthenia gravis is thought to be an autoimmune disorder. For an unknown reason, the patient's blood cells and thymus gland produce antibodies that block, destroy, or weaken the neuroreceptors that transmit nerve impulses, causing a failure in transmission of nerve impulses at the neuromuscular junction. (See *Impaired transmission in myasthenia gravis.*)

Complications

In myasthenia gravis, complications include respiratory distress, pneumonia, and chewing and swallowing dif-

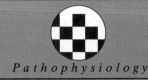

Pathophysiology

IMPAIRED TRANSMISSION IN MYASTHENIA GRAVIS

During normal neuromuscular transmission, a motor nerve impulse travels to a motor nerve terminal, stimulating the release of a chemical neurotransmitter called acetylcholine (ACh).

When ACh diffuses across the synapse, ACh receptor sites in the motor end plate react and depolarize the muscle fiber. The depolarization spreads through the muscle fiber, causing muscle contraction.

In myasthenia gravis, however, antibodies attach to the ACh receptor sites. The antibodies block, destroy, and weaken these sites, leaving them insensitive to ACh, thereby blocking neuromuscular transmission.

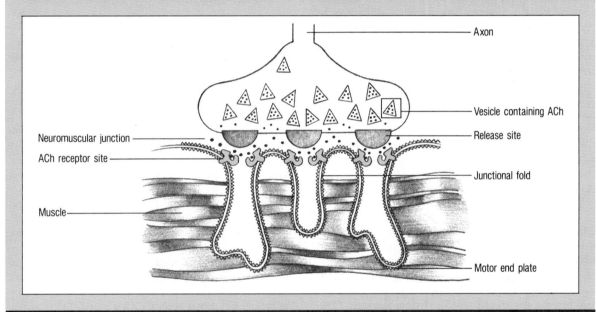

ficulties, possibly leading to choking and food aspiration.

Assessment findings

Depending on the muscles involved and the severity of the disease, assessment findings may vary. Muscle weakness is progressive, and eventually some muscles may lose function entirely.

Expect the patient to complain of extreme muscle weakness and fatigue. The muscles most often initially involved are those innervated by the cranial nerves; thus, the patient often mentions ptosis and diplopia (the most common sign and symptom). She may also report that chewing and swallowing are difficult, that her jaw hangs open (especially when she's tired), and that her head bobs. She may also say that she must tilt her head back to see properly. Some patients (about 15%) report weakness of arm or hand muscles and, rarely, a patient may report leg weakness.

The patient usually notes that symptoms are milder on awakening and worsen as the day progresses and that short rest periods temporarily restore muscle function. On questioning, she may report that symptoms become more intense during menses and after emotional stress, prolonged exposure to sunlight or cold, or infections.

On inspection, the patient may have a sleepy, mask-like expression (caused by involvement of the facial muscles) and a drooping jaw if she's tired. Inspection may also confirm ptosis. Auscultation may reveal hypoventilation if the respiratory muscles are involved.

Respiratory muscle involvement may lead to decreased tidal volume, making breathing difficult; this may predispose the patient to pneumonia and other respiratory tract infections. Progressive weakness of the diaphragm and the intercostal muscles may eventually lead to severe respiratory distress and myasthenic crisis.

Diagnostic tests

• A positive *Tensilon test* confirms a diagnosis of myasthenia gravis. This test shows temporarily improved muscle function after an I.V. injection of edrophonium (or, occasionally, neostigmine). In myasthenic patients, muscle function improves within 30 to 60 seconds and lasts up to 30 minutes. However, long-standing ocular muscle dysfunction often fails to respond to such testing. The Tensilon test can also differentiate a myasthenic crisis from a cholinergic crisis, which is caused by acetylcholine overactivity at the neuromuscular junction, possibly caused by anticholinesterase overdose.

• *Electromyography* measures the electrical potential of muscle cells and helps differentiate nerve disorders from muscle disorders.

• *Nerve conduction studies* measure the speed at which electrical impulses travel along a nerve and also help distinguish nerve disorders from muscle disorders.

• *Chest X-rays* or *computed tomography scan* may identify a thymoma.

Treatment

Measures to relieve symptoms may include anticholinesterase drugs, such as neostigmine and pyridostigmine. These drugs counteract fatigue and muscle weakness and allow about 80% of normal muscle function. However, they become less effective as the disease worsens. Corticosteroids may also help to relieve symptoms.

Some patients may undergo plasmapheresis if medications prove ineffective. This procedure will remove acetylcholine-receptor antibodies and temporarily lessen the severity of symptoms.

Patients with thymomas require thymectomy, which leads to remission in adult-onset myasthenia in about 40% of patients if done in the first 2 years after diagnosis.

Acute exacerbations that cause severe respiratory distress (myasthenic crisis) necessitate emergency treatment. Tracheotomy, ventilation with a positive-pressure ventilator, and vigorous suctioning to remove secretions usually bring improvement in a few days. Because anticholinesterase drugs aren't effective in myasthenic crisis,

they're discontinued until respiratory function begins to improve. Such a crisis requires immediate hospitalization and vigorous respiratory support.

Nursing diagnoses

• Anxiety
• Bathing or hygiene self-care deficit
• Chronic low self-esteem
• Dressing or grooming self-care deficit
• Fatigue
• Feeding self-care deficit
• Impaired gas exchange
• Impaired physical mobility
• Ineffective airway clearance
• Toileting self-care deficit

Nursing interventions

• Provide psychological support. Listen to the patient's concerns, and answer questions honestly. Encourage the patient to participate in her own care.

• Establish an accurate neurologic and respiratory baseline. Thereafter, regularly monitor tidal volume, vital capacity, and inspiratory force.

• Be alert for signs of impending myasthenic crisis (increased muscle weakness, respiratory distress, difficulty in talking or chewing). The patient may need a ventilator and frequent suctioning to remove accumulating secretions.

• Administer medications at evenly spaced intervals, and give them on time, as ordered, to prevent relapses. Be prepared to give atropine for anticholinesterase overdose or toxicity.

• Plan exercise, meals, patient care, and activities to make the most of energy peaks. For example, administer the patient's medication 20 to 30 minutes before meals to facilitate chewing or swallowing.

• When swallowing is difficult, give soft, semisolid foods (applesauce, mashed potatoes) instead of liquids to lessen the risk of choking.

• After a severe exacerbation, try to increase social activity as soon as possible.

• If surgery is scheduled, prepare the patient according to hospital policy.

Patient teaching

• Help the patient plan daily activities to coincide with energy peaks.

• Stress the need for frequent rest periods throughout the day. Emphasize that periodic remissions, exacerbations, and day-to-day fluctuations are common.

• Teach the patient how to recognize adverse effects and signs and symptoms of toxicity of anticholinesterase drugs (headaches, weakness, sweating, abdominal cramps, nausea, vomiting, diarrhea, excessive salivation, and bronchospasm) and corticosteroids (decreased or blurred vision; increased thirst; frequent urination; rectal bleeding, burning, or itching; restlessness; depression).

• Warn the patient to avoid strenuous exercise, stress, infection, and needless exposure to the sun or cold weather. All of these things may worsen signs and symptoms. Wearing an eye patch or glasses with one frosted lens may help the patient with diplopia.

• Teach the patient with swallowing difficulties to eat semisolid foods and to avoid alcohol because it increases weakness. Tell her that eating warm (not hot) foods can help ease swallowing.

• If surgery is scheduled, provide preoperative teaching. Explain to the patient that before surgery, her chest will be cleaned and shaved and she'll receive a general anesthetic. Tell her that depending on where the surgeon makes the incision, she may awaken from surgery with a chest tube or a drain in place. Also tell her that she may require intubation and mechanical ventilation after surgery and that she'll have antimyasthenic drugs administered I.V. or I.M. until she's well enough to take them orally. Explain that these medications will be progressively withdrawn so that the doctor can assess her muscle strength after surgery.

• For information and an opportunity to meet patients with myasthenia gravis who lead productive lives, refer the patient to the Myasthenia Gravis Foundation.

AMYOTROPHIC LATERAL SCLEROSIS

Also known as Lou Gehrig's disease (after a well-known baseball player who died of it in 1941), this disease is the most common motor neuron disease of muscular atrophy. Amyotrophic lateral sclerosis (ALS) is a chronic, progressive, and debilitating disease that is invariably fatal. It's characterized by progressive degeneration of the anterior horn cells of the spinal cord and cranial nerves and of the motor nuclei in the cerebral cortex and corticospinal tracts.

Generally, ALS affects people ages 40 to 70. Most patients with ALS succumb after about 3 years, but some may live as long as 10 to 15 years. Death usually results from a complication, such as aspiration pneumonia or respiratory failure.

Reportedly, more than 30,000 Americans have ALS; about 5,000 more are newly diagnosed each year. ALS is about three times more common in men than in women.

Causes

The exact cause of ALS is unknown, but about 10% of ALS patients inherit the disease as an autosomal dominant trait. ALS may also be caused by a virus that creates metabolic disturbances in motor neurons or by immune complexes, such as those formed in autoimmune disorders.

Precipitating factors that can cause acute deterioration include severe stress, such as myocardial infarction, traumatic injury, viral infections, and physical exhaustion.

Complications

Common complications of ALS include respiratory tract infections, such as pneumonia, respiratory failure, and aspiration, and complications of physical immobility, such as pressure ulcers and contractures.

Assessment findings

Signs and symptoms of ALS depend on the location of the affected motor neurons and the severity of the disease. Keep in mind that muscle weakness, atrophy, and fasciculations are the principal symptoms of the disorder, the disease may begin in any muscle group, and eventually, all muscle groups become involved. Unlike other degenerative disorders, such as Alzheimer's disease, ALS doesn't affect mental function.

The patient history may reveal other family members with ALS if the problem was inherited. In the early disease stages, the patient may report asymmetrical weakness first noticed in one limb. He also usually reports fatigue and easy cramping in the affected muscles. Inspection may reveal fasciculations in the affected muscles if these muscles are not concealed by adipose tissue and muscle atrophy. Fasciculations and atrophy are most obvious in the feet and hands.

As the disease progresses, the patient may report progressive weakness in muscles of the arms, legs, and trunk. Inspection reveals atrophy and fasciculations. Neurologic examination often reveals brisk and overactive stretch reflexes. Muscle strength tests confirm the reported muscle weakness.

When the disease progresses to involve the brain stem and the cranial nerves, the patient has difficulty talking, chewing, swallowing and, ultimately, breathing. In these patients, auscultation may reveal decreased breath sounds.

In some patients (about 25%), muscle weakness begins in the musculature supplied by the cranial nerves. When this occurs, initial patient history reveals difficulty talking, swallowing, and breathing. Occasionally, the patient may report choking. Inspection may reveal some shortness of breath and, occasionally, drooling.

Diagnostic tests

Although no diagnostic tests are specific to this disease, the following tests may aid in its diagnosis:
• *Electromyography* may show abnormalities of electrical activity of involved muscles.
• *Muscle biopsy* may disclose atrophic fibers interspersed among normal fibers.
• *Nerve conduction studies* are usually normal.
• *Cerebrospinal fluid analysis* reveals increased protein content in one-third of patients.
• Other studies, such as *computed tomography scan* and *EEG*, may help rule out other disorders, including multiple sclerosis, spinal cord neoplasms, syringomyelitis, myasthenia gravis, and progressive muscular dystrophy.

Treatment

ALS has no cure. Treatment, which is supportive and based on the patient's symptoms, may include diazepam, dantrolene, or baclofen for spasticity, and quinidine for relief of painful muscle cramps that occur in some patients. I.V. or intrathecal administration of thyrotropin-releasing hormone temporarily improves motor function in some patients but has no long-term benefits. Rehabilitative measures can help patients function effectively for a longer period, and mechanical ventilation can help them survive longer.

Nursing diagnoses

• Altered nutrition: Less than body requirements
• Anticipatory grieving
• Anxiety
• Bathing or hygiene self-care deficit
• Dressing or grooming self-care deficit
• Feeding self-care deficit
• Hopelessness
• Impaired physical mobility
• Impaired verbal communication
• Ineffective airway clearance
• Ineffective breathing pattern
• Ineffective family coping
• Knowledge deficit
• Risk for impaired skin integrity
• Risk for infection
• Toileting self-care deficit

Nursing interventions

• Provide emotional and psychological support to the patient and his family. Stay with the patient during periods of severe stress and anxiety. Keep in mind that because mental status remains intact while progressive physical degeneration takes place, the patient acutely perceives every change in his condition.
• Implement a rehabilitation program designed to help the patient maintain his independence as long as possible.
• Have the patient perform active exercises and range-of-motion exercises on unaffected muscles to help strengthen these muscles. Stretching exercises are also helpful.
• Depending on the patient's muscular capacity, assist with bathing, personal hygiene, and transfers from wheelchair to bed. Help establish a regular bowel and bladder elimination routine.
• To prevent skin breakdown, provide good skin care when the patient's mobility decreases. Turn him often, keep his skin clean and dry, and use pressure-reducing devices such as an alternating air mattress.
• Help the patient obtain equipment, such as a walker or a wheelchair, when this becomes necessary.
• If the patient can't talk, provide an alternate means of communication, such as message boards, eye blinks for yes and no, or a computer.
• Administer ordered medications, as necessary, to relieve the patient's symptoms. Crush tablets and mix them with semisolid food for the patient who has dysphagia.
• Have the patient with breathing difficulty perform deep-breathing and coughing exercises. Suctioning, chest physiotherapy, and incentive spirometry can also prove helpful.
• If the patient chooses to use mechanical ventilation to assist his breathing, provide necessary care. Carefully assess the patient with respiratory involvement for infection because respiratory complications may be fatal.
• If the patient has trouble swallowing, give him soft, semisolid foods and position him upright during meals. Have suctioning equipment available to prevent aspiration. Use a soft cervical collar to help the patient hold his head upright if he has difficulty doing so. Gastrostomy and nasogastric tube feedings may be necessary if he can no longer swallow.

Patient teaching

• Teach the patient and his family about ALS and its signs and symptoms. Explain that this is a progressive, incurable disease, but reassure the patient that treatments exist to make him more comfortable and to help him stay independent and live at home as long as possible. (See *Modifying the home for a patient with ALS.*)

• Teach the patient who has trouble chewing to cut up his food or mince food in a blender or food processor. Suggest adding baby cereal to minced foods to help thicken them.

• Urge the caregiver to take breaks from patient care; recommend agencies or support personnel for respite care.

• Refer the patient and family to a local ALS support group. Prepare them for his eventual death and help them grieve.

MULTIPLE SCLEROSIS

This chronic disease is caused by progressive demyelination of the white matter of the brain and spinal cord. These sporadic patches of demyelination in the central nervous system cause widespread and varied neurologic dysfunction. (See *When myelin breaks down,* page 744.)

Characterized by exacerbations and remissions, multiple sclerosis (MS) is a major cause of chronic disability in young adults ages 20 to 40. The prognosis varies. MS may progress rapidly, causing death within months or disability by early adulthood. However, about 70% of patients lead active, productive lives with prolonged remissions.

The incidence of MS is highest in women and among people in northern urban areas and higher socioeconomic groups. A family history of MS increases the risk.

Causes

The exact cause of MS is unknown but may be a slow-acting viral infection, an autoimmune response of the nervous system, or an allergic response. Other possible factors include trauma, anoxia, toxins, nutritional deficiencies, vascular lesions, and anorexia nervosa, all of which may help destroy axons and the myelin sheath.

Emotional stress, overwork, fatigue, pregnancy, or acute respiratory tract infections may precede the onset of this illness. Genetic factors may also be involved.

Complications

In MS, complications include injuries from falls, urinary tract infections, constipation, joint contractures, pressure ulcers, rectal distention, and pneumonia.

Assessment findings

Clinical findings in MS correspond to the extent and site of myelin destruction, the extent of remyelination, and the adequacy of subsequent restored synaptic transmission. Symptoms may be transient or may last for hours or weeks. They may vary from day to day, be unpredictable, and be difficult for the patient to describe.

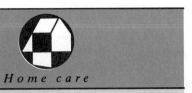

Home care

MODIFYING THE HOME FOR A PATIENT WITH A.L.S.

To help your patient with ALS live safely at home, follow these guidelines:

• Explain basic safety precautions, such as keeping stairs and pathways free of clutter; using nonskid mats in the bathroom and in place of loose throw rugs; keeping stairs well lighted; installing handrails in stairwells and shower, tub, and toilet areas; and removing electrical and telephone cords from traffic areas.

• Discuss the need for rearranging the furniture, moving items in or out of the patient's care area, and obtaining such equipment as a hospital bed, a commode, or oxygen equipment.

• Recommend devices to ease the patient's and caregiver's work, such as extra pillows or a wedge pillow to help the patient sit up, a draw sheet to help him move up in bed, a lap tray for eating, or a bell for calling the caregiver.

• Help the patient adjust to changes in his environment. Encourage independence.

• Advise the patient to keep a suction machine handy to reduce the fear of choking due to secretion accumulation and dysphagia. Teach him to suction himself.

The patient history commonly reveals initial visual problems and sensory impairment, such as paresthesia. After the initial episode, findings may vary widely and include blurred vision or diplopia, urinary problems, emotional lability and, possibly, dysphagia.

As the patient speaks, you may notice poorly articulated speech. Neurologic examination and muscle function tests may reveal muscle weakness of the involved area and spasticity, hyperreflexia, intention tremor, gait ataxia, and paralysis, ranging from monoplegia to quadriplegia. Visual examination may reveal nystagmus, scotoma, optic neuritis, or ophthalmoplegia.

Diagnostic tests

This difficult diagnosis may require years of testing and observation. The following tests help diagnose MS:

• *EEG* shows abnormalities in one-third of patients.

• *Cerebrospinal fluid analysis* reveals elevated immunoglobulin G (IgG) levels but normal total protein levels.

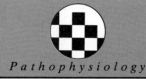

Pathophysiology

WHEN MYELIN BREAKS DOWN

Myelin plays a key role in speeding electrical impulses to the brain for interpretation. A lipoprotein complex formed of glial cells or oligodendrocytes, the myelin sheath protects the neuron's long nerve fiber (the axon), much like the insulation on an electrical wire. Its high electrical resistance and low capacitance allow the myelin sheath to permit sufficient conduction of nerve impulses from one node of Ranvier to the next.

However, myelin is susceptible to injury, for example, by hypoxemia, toxic chemicals, vascular insufficiency, and autoimmune responses. As a result, the myelin sheath becomes inflamed and the membrane layers break down into smaller components that become well-circumscribed plaques (filled with microglial elements, macroglia, and lymphocytes). This process is called demyelination.

The damaged myelin sheath impairs normal conduction, causing partial loss or dispersion of the action potential and consequent neurologic dysfunction.

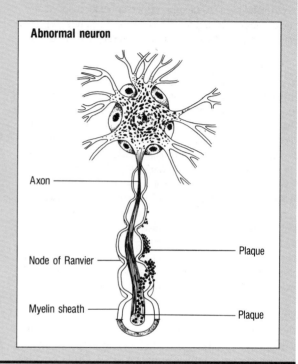

Abnormal neuron

Axon

Node of Ranvier

Myelin sheath

Plaque

Plaque

Such elevated IgG levels are significant only when serum gamma globulin levels are normal, and they reflect hyperactivity of the immune system due to chronic demyelination. The white blood cell count may be slightly increased.

• *Evoked potential studies* demonstrate slowed conduction of nerve impulses in 80% of MS patients.

• *Computed tomography scan* may disclose lesions within the brain's white matter.

• *Magnetic resonance imaging* is the most sensitive method of detecting MS lesions. More than 90% of patients with MS show multifocal white matter lesions when this test is performed. It is also used to evaluate disease progression.

Other tests, such as neuropsychological tests, may help rule out other disorders.

Treatment

The aim of treatment is to shorten exacerbations and, if possible, relieve neurologic deficits, so the patient can resume a normal life-style.

Because MS is thought to have allergic and inflammatory causes, corticotropin, prednisone, or dexamethasone is used to reduce the associated edema of the myelin sheath during exacerbations. Corticotropin and corticosteroids seem to relieve symptoms and hasten remission but don't prevent future exacerbations.

Other useful drugs include chlordiazepoxide to mitigate mood swings, baclofen or dantrolene to relieve spasticity, and bethanechol or oxybutynin to relieve urine retention and minimize urinary frequency and urgency.

During acute exacerbations, supportive measures include bed rest, comfort measures such as massages, prevention of fatigue and pressure ulcers, bowel and bladder training (if necessary), treatment of bladder infections with antibiotics, physical therapy, and counseling.

Nursing diagnoses

- Activity intolerance
- Altered nutrition: Less than body requirements
- Altered thought processes
- Altered urinary elimination
- Chronic low self-esteem
- Constipation
- Fatigue
- Impaired physical mobility
- Knowledge deficit
- Risk for infection
- Risk for injury

Nursing interventions

- Provide emotional and psychological support for the patient and the family, and answer their questions honestly. Stay with them during crisis periods. Encourage the patient by suggesting ways to help him cope with his disease.
- Assist with physical therapy. Increase patient comfort with massages and relaxing baths. Make sure the water isn't too hot because it may temporarily intensify otherwise subtle symptoms. Assist with active, resistive, and stretching exercises to maintain muscle tone and joint mobility, decrease spasticity, improve coordination, and boost morale. Provide rest periods between exercises because fatigue may contribute to exacerbations.
- Administer medications, as ordered, and watch for adverse reactions. For instance, dantrolene may cause muscle weakness and decreased muscle tone.
- Promote emotional stability. Help the patient establish a daily routine to maintain optimal functioning. Her activity level is regulated by her tolerance level. Encourage regular rest periods to prevent fatigue and daily physical exercise.
- Keep the bedpan or urinal readily accessible because the need to void is immediate.
- Evaluate the need for bowel and bladder training during hospitalization. Encourage adequate fluid intake and regular urination. Eventually, the patient may require urinary drainage by self-catheterization or, in men, condom catheter.

Patient teaching

- Educate the patient and her family about this chronic disease. Emphasize the need to avoid stress, infections, and fatigue, and to maintain independence by developing new ways of performing daily activities. Be sure to tell the patient to avoid exposure to infections.
- Emphasize the importance of exercise. Tell the patient that walking exercise may improve her gait. If her motor dysfunction causes coordination or balance problems, teach her to walk with a wide base of support. If she has trouble with position sense, tell her to watch her feet while walking. If she's still in danger of falling, a walker or a wheelchair may be required.
- Stress the importance of taking rest periods, preferably lying down.
- Teach the importance of eating a nutritious, well-balanced diet that contains sufficient roughage to prevent constipation.
- Provide bowel and bladder training, if necessary. Also, teach the patient how to use suppositories to establish a regular bowel elimination schedule.
- Inform the patient that exacerbations are unpredictable, necessitating physical and emotional adjustments in lifestyle.
- Refer the patient to the social service department, when appropriate, and to a local chapter of the National Multiple Sclerosis Society.

PERIPHERAL NERVE DISORDERS

This group of disorders includes trigeminal neuralgia and Bell's palsy.

TRIGEMINAL NEURALGIA

Also known as tic douloureux, trigeminal neuralgia is a painful disorder of one or more branches of the fifth cranial (trigeminal) nerve. This nerve affects chewing movements and sensations of the face, scalp, and teeth. On stimulation of a trigger zone, the patient experiences paroxysmal attacks of excruciating facial pain, probably produced by an interaction or short-circuiting of touch and pain fibers.

The disease occurs mostly in people over age 40 (about 25% more women than men) and on the right side of the face more often than the left. Trigeminal neuralgia can subside spontaneously, with remissions lasting from several months to years.

Causes

Although the cause remains unknown, trigeminal neuralgia may reflect an afferent reflex phenomenon located centrally in the brain stem or more peripherally in the sensory root of the trigeminal nerve. Such neuralgia may also be related to compression of the nerve root by posterior fossa tumors, middle fossa tumors, or vascular lesions, although such lesions usually will produce simultaneous loss of sensation. Occasionally, trigeminal neuralgia results from multiple sclerosis or herpes zoster.

Complications

In this disorder, pain may be so severe and incapacitating that the patient fails to care for herself properly. This leads to complications, such as excessive weight loss, depression, and social isolation.

Assessment findings

Typically, the patient reports a searing or burning pain that occurs in lightninglike jabs and lasts from 1 to 15 minutes (usually 1 to 2 minutes). The pain is localized in an area innervated by a division of the trigeminal nerve and initiated by a light touch to a hypersensitive area, such as the tip of the nose, the cheeks, or the gums. The patient may also report that although attacks can occur at any time, they may follow a draft of air, exposure to heat or cold, eating, smiling, talking, or drinking hot or cold beverages.

Between attacks, most patients report that they are free of pain, although some may complain of a constant, dull ache. Keep in mind that all patients fear the next attack and that the frequency of attacks varies greatly, from many times a day to several times a month or year.

On inspection, you may observe the patient favoring (splinting) the affected area. If she has a painful attack during the assessment, you may notice that to ward off the attack, she may hold her face immobile when talking. She may also leave the affected side of her face unwashed (if male, also unshaven), or protect it with a coat or shawl. When asked where the pain occurs, she points to — but never touches — the affected area. Witnessing a typical attack helps to confirm the diagnosis.

Neurologic assessment shows no impairment of sensory or motor function. If sensory impairment is found, a space-occupying lesion may be the cause.

Diagnostic tests

Skull X-rays, computed tomography scan, and magnetic resonance imaging are performed to rule out sinus or tooth infections, and tumors. If the patient has trigeminal neuralgia, these test results are normal.

Treatment

Oral administration of carbamazepine or phenytoin may temporarily relieve or prevent pain because they reduce the transmission of nerve impulses at affected nerve terminals. Narcotics may be helpful during the acute pain episode.

Before surgery is performed, nonsurgical treatment — injecting small amounts of glycerol into the subarachnoid space — may be tried. If this treatment fails, the procedure of choice is percutaneous electrocoagulation of nerve rootlets under local anesthesia. An alternative is a percutaneous radio frequency procedure, which causes partial root destruction and relieves pain. One to three treatments are usually necessary. The procedure causes partial numbness of the face.

Microsurgery for vascular decompression of the trigeminal nerve involves an intracranial approach. This major procedure requires postoperative management similar to that for craniotomy. Its advantage is that it preserves normal sensation in the face.

Nursing diagnoses

• Altered nutrition: Less than body requirements
• Anxiety
• Knowledge deficit
• Pain

Nursing interventions

• Provide emotional support, and encourage the patient to express her concerns. Promote independence through self-care and maximum physical activity. Encourage the patient to stay as active as possible, and explain that this will improve her sense of well-being and help her cope with the pain.
• Observe and record the characteristics of each attack, including the patient's protective mechanisms.
• Provide small, frequent meals at room temperature to maintain adequate nutrition.
• Recognize which factors may precipitate an attack, and urge the patient to avoid stimulation (air, heat, cold) of trigger zones (lips, cheeks, gums).
• If the patient is receiving carbamazepine, watch for cutaneous and hematologic reactions (such as erythematous and pruritic rashes, urticaria, photosensitivity, exfoliative dermatitis, leukopenia, agranulocytosis, eosinophilia, aplastic anemia, thrombocytopenia) and, possibly, urine retention and transient drowsiness. Complete blood count and liver function tests should be monitored weekly for the first 3 months of carbamazepine therapy, then monthly.

• If the patient is receiving phenytoin, watch for adverse reactions, including ataxia, skin eruptions, gingival hyperplasia, and nystagmus.
• After any neurosurgical procedure, check neurologic and vital signs frequently.
• After trigeminal microsurgery, if the patient elects to have this procedure, provide all care required for the patient who has had a craniotomy. This includes fluid, respiratory, pain, and neurologic management.

Patient teaching
• Teach the patient about trigeminal neuralgia, the procedures ordered, and the treatments she's chosen. Be sure the patient knows the complications that may occur. Reinforce the doctor's explanations, as necessary.
• Warn the patient to immediately report fever, sore throat, mouth ulcers, easy bruising, or petechial or purpuric hemorrhage because these may signal thrombocytopenia or aplastic anemia and may require discontinuation of drug therapy.
• If the patient is losing weight because of poor appetite due to the pain, help her select foods that are high in calories and nutrients, so that she can get more nourishment with less chewing. Suggest that she eat many frequent, small meals instead of three large ones. To minimize jaw movements when eating, suggest that she puree foods and eat soft or liquid foods, such as soups, custards, and stews.
• Teach the patient about prescribed medications. Be sure that she understands the desired and adverse effects to watch for and that she knows when to notify the doctor if adverse reactions occur.
• Teach the patient how to ward off neuralgia attacks. For example, tell the patient to protect her trigger zones from such stimuli as wind and temperature changes by wearing a scarf or turning up her coat collar. If brushing the teeth is painful, suggest trying a water-powered dental device because this will reduce jaw movement.
• If the patient will undergo craniotomy, provide extensive preoperative teaching so that she fully understands the procedure and the postoperative treatment. Counsel the patient to review her options with the doctor carefully and to ask about potential complications, such as facial numbness and paralysis.

BELL'S PALSY
In this disorder, impulses from the seventh cranial nerve — the nerve responsible for motor innervation of the facial muscles — are blocked. The conduction block results from an inflammatory reaction around the nerve (usually at the internal auditory meatus) and produces unilateral facial weakness or paralysis.

Although Bell's palsy affects all age-groups, it occurs most often in people ages 20 to 60 years. Onset is rapid. In 80% to 90% of patients, the disorder subsides spontaneously, with complete recovery in 1 to 8 weeks; however, recovery may be delayed in elderly people. If recovery is partial, contractures may develop on the paralyzed side of the face. The disorder may recur on the same or the opposite side of the face.

Causes
Bell's palsy results from an unknown cause, possibly ischemia, viral disease such as herpes simplex or herpes zoster, local traumatic injury, or autoimmune disease.

Complications
Potential complications of Bell's palsy include corneal ulceration and blindness because the eye will not close; impaired nutrition secondary to paralysis of the lower face; and long-term psychosocial problems because of the patient's altered body image.

Assessment findings
The patient history may reveal that pain occurred on the affected side around the angle of the jaw or behind the ear for a few hours or days before the onset of weakness. The patient may also report difficulty eating on the affected side because of relaxation of the facial muscle. When you speak with the patient, you may notice that he has difficulty speaking clearly, which also may result from facial muscle relaxation.

On inspection, you may find that the mouth droops (causing the patient to drool saliva from the corner of his mouth) on the affected side and the forehead appears smooth.

Neurologic assessment may reveal that taste perception is distorted over the affected anterior portion of the tongue and that the patient is unable to raise his eyebrow, smile, show his teeth, or puff out his cheek. In addition, the patient's ability to close his eye on the weak side is markedly impaired. With any attempt to close the eye, the eye rolls upward (Bell's phenomenon) and shows excessive tearing. Although Bell's phenomenon occurs in normal people, in Bell's palsy, incomplete eye closure makes this upward motion obvious. (See *Facial paralysis in Bell's palsy*, page 748.)

Diagnostic tests
Diagnosis is based on clinical presentation. After 10 days, electromyography helps predict the level of ex-

FACIAL PARALYSIS IN BELL'S PALSY

Unilateral facial paralysis typifies Bell's palsy. The paralysis produces a distorted appearance and an inability to wrinkle the forehead, close the eyelid, smile, show the teeth, or puff out the cheek.

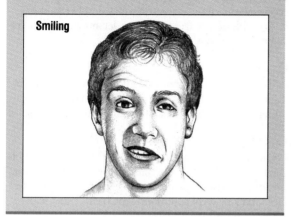

Smiling

pected recovery by distinguishing temporary conduction defects from a pathologic interruption of nerve fibers.

Treatment

Appropriate treatment consists of prednisone, an oral corticosteroid that reduces facial nerve edema and improves nerve conduction and blood flow. Prednisone treatment is especially helpful when begun in the first week after the disorder's onset. After the 14th day of prednisone therapy, electrotherapy may help prevent facial muscle atrophy.

Analgesics are used to control facial pain and discomfort. Heat may also be applied to the affected side to provide comfort.

If the patient fails to recover from facial paralysis, surgery that involves exploration of the facial nerve may be necessary.

Nursing diagnoses

- Altered nutrition: Less than body requirements
- Anxiety
- Body image disturbance
- Knowledge deficit
- Pain

Nursing interventions

- Provide psychological support to the patient. Reassure him that he has not had a stroke. Tell him that spon-

taneous recovery usually occurs within 8 weeks. This should help decrease his anxiety and help him adjust to the temporary change in his body image.

- During treatment with prednisone, watch for steroid adverse reactions, especially GI distress and fluid retention. If GI distress is troublesome, an antacid given concomitantly usually provides relief. If the patient has diabetes, prednisone must be used with caution and necessitates frequent monitoring of serum glucose levels.
- To reduce pain, apply moist heat to the affected side of the face, as ordered. Be careful to avoid burning the patient's skin.
- To help maintain muscle tone, massage the patient's face with a gentle upward motion two to three times daily for 5 to 10 minutes, or have him massage his face himself.
- Apply a facial sling, if necessary, to improve lip alignment. Also, give the patient frequent and complete mouth care, taking special care to remove residual food that collects between the cheeks and gums.
- Provide a soft, nutritionally balanced diet, eliminating hot foods and fluids. Arrange for privacy at mealtimes to reduce embarrassment.
- If surgery is necessary, provide the patient with complete preoperative and postoperative care.

Patient teaching

- Teach the patient about Bell's palsy, its signs and symptoms, and its treatments.
- Advise the patient to protect his affected eye by covering it with an eyepatch, especially when outdoors. Tell him to keep warm and avoid exposure to dust and wind. When exposure is unavoidable, instruct him to cover his face.
- When the patient is ready for active exercises, teach him to exercise the facial muscles by grimacing in front of a mirror.
- To prevent excessive weight loss, help the patient cope with difficulty in eating and drinking. Instruct him to chew on the unaffected side of his mouth and to eat semisolid foods.

SELECTED REFERENCES

Betz, C., et al. *Family-Centered Nursing Care of Children,* 2nd ed. Philadelphia: W.B. Saunders Co., 1994.

Clinical Laboratory Tests: Values and Implications, 2nd ed. Springhouse, Pa.: Springhouse Corp., 1995.

Cunningham, F.G., et al. *Williams Obstetrics,* 19th ed. East Norwalk, Conn.: Appleton & Lange, 1993.

Fischbach, F. *A Manual of Laboratory and Diagnostic Tests,* 4th ed. Philadelphia: J.B. Lippincott Co., 1992.

Illustrated Manual of Nursing Practice, 2nd ed. Springhouse, Pa.: Springhouse Corp., 1994.

Isselbacher, K., et al., eds. *Harrison's Principles of Internal Medicine,* 13th ed. New York: McGraw-Hill Book Co., 1995.

Meissner, J.E. "Caring for Patients with Meningitis," *Nursing95* 25(7):50-51, July 1995.

Neils, J., et al. "Decline in Homophone Spelling Associated with Loss of Semantic Influence on Spelling in Alzheimer's Disease," *Brain and Language* 49(1):27-49, April 1995.

Oleske, D.M., et al. "Epidemiology of Injury in People with Alzheimer's Disease," *Journal of the American Geriatrics Society* 43(7):741-46, July 1995.

Rakel, R.E., ed. *Conn's Current Therapy 1996.* Philadelphia: W.B. Saunders Co., 1996.

Smeltzer, S., and Bare, B. *Brunner and Suddarth's Textbook of Medical-Surgical Nursing,* 8th ed. Philadelphia: J.B. Lippincott Co., 1996.

Taylor, C.M., and Sparks, S.M. *Nursing Diagnosis Reference Manual,* 3rd ed. Springhouse, Pa.: Springhouse Corp., 1995.

Tierney, L., et al. *Current Medical Diagnosis and Treatment 1995.* East Norwalk, Conn.: Appleton & Lange, 1995.

10   MUSCULOSKELETAL DISORDERS

INTRODUCTION

A complex of muscles, tendons, ligaments, bones, and other connective tissue, the musculoskeletal system gives the body form and shape. It also protects vital organs, allows movement, stores calcium and other minerals, and provides the site for hematopoiesis.

Muscles

The body contains three major muscle types: skeletal (voluntary, striated), visceral (involuntary, smooth), and cardiac. This chapter focuses on skeletal muscle, which is attached to bone.

Viewed through a microscope, skeletal muscle appears as long bands or striations. (See *Looking inside a muscle*, page 752.) Skeletal muscle functions voluntarily; its contraction can be controlled at will. Muscle develops when existing musculoskeletal fibers hypertrophy. Exercise, nutrition, sex, and genetics account for muscle strength and size in individuals.

Tendons

These bands of fibrous connective tissue attach muscle to the periosteum, which is the fibrous membrane covering the bone. Tendons enable bones to move when skeletal muscles contract.

Ligaments

Dense, strong, flexible bands of fibrous connective tissue, ligaments attach one bone to another. Ligaments of concern in a musculoskeletal assessment are those that connect the joint ends (articular ends) of the bones. These ligaments either limit or facilitate movement and provide structural stability.

Bones

The human skeleton contains 206 bones consisting of inorganic minerals and salts, such as calcium and phosphate, embedded in a framework of collagen fibers. Classified by shape and location, bones may be long (such as the humerus, radius, femur, and tibia), short (such as the carpals and tarsals), flat (such as the scapula, ribs, and skull), irregular (such as the vertebrae and mandible), or sesamoid (such as the patella).

Bones of the *axial skeleton* (the head and the trunk) include the facial and cranial bones, hyoid bone, vertebrae, ribs, and sternum. Bones of the *appendicular skeleton* (the extremities) include the clavicle, scapula, humerus, radius, ulna, metacarpals, pelvic bone, femur, patella, fibula, tibia, and metatarsals. (See *Looking inside a bone*, page 753.)

Bone function

Bones perform an anatomic (or mechanical) and a physiologic function. They protect internal tissues and organs (for example, 33 vertebrae surround and protect the spinal cord); they stabilize and support the body; and they provide a surface for muscle, ligament, and tendon attachments (which facilitates "levered action" when the muscles contract). They also produce red blood cells in the marrow (hematopoiesis), and they store minerals (about 99% of the body's calcium).

Bone formation

A 3-month-old fetus has a beginning skeletal structure composed entirely of cartilage. By fetal age 6 months, much of this cartilage has become bony skeleton, although some bones harden (ossify) only after birth—most notably the carpals and tarsals. The changes result from endochondral ossification, a process by which bone-forming cells (osteoblasts) produce a collagenous material (osteoid) that hardens (ossifies).

Two types of bone cells (or osteocytes)—osteoblasts and osteoclasts—participate in a continuous process known as remodeling, whereby bone is created and destroyed. *Osteoblasts* deposit new bone, and *osteoclasts* increase long-bone diameter by resorbing previously deposited bone. These activities promote longitudinal bone growth, which continues until the epiphyseal growth plates, located at the bone ends, close during adolescence.

Researchers are currently studying the endocrine system's role in bone formation. The hormone estrogen plays a significant role not only in regulating calcium uptake and release but also in regulating osteoblastic activity. Researchers think that decreased estrogen levels may lead to diminished osteoblastic activity.

A patient's age, race, and sex affect bone mass, structural integrity (ability to withstand stress), and bone loss. For example, blacks commonly have denser bones than whites, and men typically have denser bones than women. Bone density and structural integrity decrease after age 30 in women and after age 45 in men. Thereafter, the bone matrix undergoes a relatively steady quantitative loss.

Cartilage

A dense connective tissue, cartilage consists of fibers embedded in a strong, gel-like substance. Cartilage is avascular and lacks innervation.

Cartilage may be fibrous, hyaline, or elastic. *Fibrous cartilage* forms the symphysis pubis and the intervertebral disks. *Hyaline cartilage* covers the articular bone

LOOKING INSIDE A MUSCLE

The human body has about 600 skeletal muscles, each classified by the kind of movement for which it's responsible. For example, flexors facilitate flexion; adductors, adduction; circumductors, circumduction; and external rotators, rotation.

Each muscle contains cell groups called muscle fibers that extend the length of the muscle. The perimysium—a sheath of connective tissue—binds the fibers into a bundle, or fasciculus. A stronger sheath, the epimysium, binds fasciculi together to form the fleshy part of the muscle. Extending beyond the muscle, the epimysium becomes a tendon.

A plasma membrane—the sarcolemma—surrounds each muscle fiber. Within the sarcoplasm (cytoplasm) of the muscle fiber lie tiny myofibrils. Arranged lengthwise, myofibrils contain still finer filament-like fibers—about 1,500 myosin (thick) and about 3,000 actin (thin) fibers.

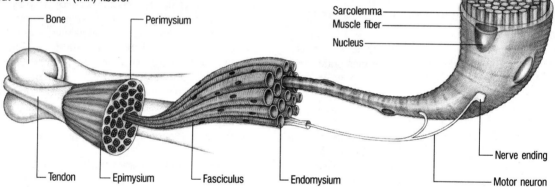

surfaces (where one or more bones meet at a joint); connects the ribs to the sternum; and appears in the trachea, bronchi, and nasal septum. *Elastic cartilage* is located in the auditory canal, the external ear, and the epiglottis.

Cartilage supports and shapes various structures, such as the auditory canal and the intervertebral disks. It also cushions and absorbs shock, preventing direct transmission to the bone.

Joints

The junction of two or more bones is a joint. Major kinds of human joints are classified by the extent of their movement. *Synarthrodial joints,* such as cranial sutures, permit no movement. In this joint type, a thin layer of fibrous connective tissue separates the bones. *Amphiarthrodial joints,* such as the symphysis pubis, allow slight movement. A hyaline cartilage separates the bones in

this kind of joint. *Diarthrodial joints,* such as the ankle, wrist, knee, hip, and shoulder, permit free movement.

Separating the bones that form a diarthrodial joint is a cavity lined by a synovial membrane that secretes a viscous lubricating substance called synovial fluid. The membrane is encased in a fibrous joint capsule. This capsule—along with ligaments, tendons, and muscles—helps to stabilize the joint.

Shape and motion are other criteria used to further classify joints: for example, ball-and-socket joints, hinge joints, and pivot joints.

Bursae

Located at friction points and around joints between tendons, ligaments, and bones, these small synovial fluid sacs act as cushions, decreasing stress on adjacent struc-

LOOKING INSIDE A BONE

The human skeleton contains 206 bones: 80 from the axial skeleton and 126 from the appendicular skeleton.

Bone consists of layers of calcified matrix containing spaces occupied by osteocytes (bone cells). Bone layers (lamellae) are arranged concentrically around central canals (haversian canals). Small cavities (lacunae) lying between the lamellae contain osteocytes. Tiny canals (canaliculi) connect the lacunae. They form the structural units of bone and provide nutrients to bone tissue.

A typical long bone has a diaphysis (main shaft) and an epiphysis (end). The epiphyses are separated from the diaphysis by cartilage at the epiphyseal line. Beneath the epiphyseal articular surface lies the articular cartilage, which cushions the joint.

Internal characteristics

Each bone consists of an outer layer of dense, compact bone containing haversian systems (osteons) and an inner layer of spongy (cancellous) bone consisting of thin plates, called trabeculae, that interlace to form a latticework. Red marrow fills the spaces between the trabeculae of some bones. Cancellous bone doesn't contain haversian systems.

Compact bone is located in the diaphyses of long bones and the outer layers of short, flat, and irregular bones. Cancellous bone fills central regions of the epiphyses and the inner portions of short, flat, and irregular bones. Periosteum—specialized fibrous connective tissue—consists of an outer fibrous layer and an inner, bone-forming layer. Endosteum (tissue) lines the medullary cavity (inner surface of bone, which contains the marrow).

Blood reaches bone by way of arterioles in haversian canals; vessels in Volkmann's canals, which enter bone matrix from the periosteum; and vessels within the bone ends and within the marrow. In children, the periosteum is thicker than in adults and has an increased blood supply to assist new bone formation around the shaft (diaphysis).

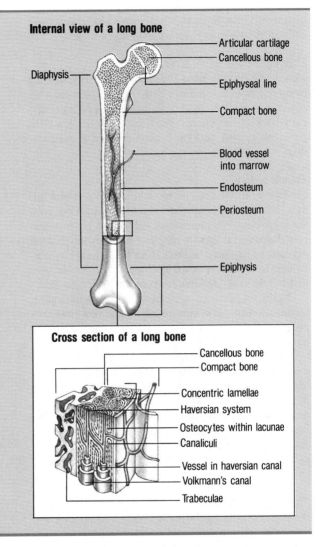

Internal view of a long bone

- Articular cartilage
- Cancellous bone
- Diaphysis
- Epiphyseal line
- Compact bone
- Blood vessel into marrow
- Endosteum
- Periosteum
- Epiphysis

Cross section of a long bone

- Cancellous bone
- Compact bone
- Concentric lamellae
- Haversian system
- Osteocytes within lacunae
- Canaliculi
- Vessel in haversian canal
- Volkmann's canal
- Trabeculae

tures. Examples of bursae include the shoulder's subacromial bursa and the knee's prepatellar bursa.

Skeletal movement

Although skeletal movement results primarily from muscle contractions, other musculoskeletal structures play a role. To contract, a skeletal muscle (richly supplied with blood vessels and nerves) needs an impulse from the nervous system and oxygen and nutrients from the circulatory system.

A skeletal muscle contraction applies force to the tendon. The force pulls the bone toward, away from, or around a second bone, depending on the type of muscle contracted. Usually, one bone moves less than the other. The muscle-tendon attachment to the more stationary bone is called the origin. The muscle-tendon attachment to the more movable bone is called the insertion site. The origin usually lies on the proximal end of the bone; the insertion site, on the distal end.

In skeletal movement, the bones act as levers, and the joints act as fulcrums, or fixed points. Each bone's function is partially determined by the location of the fulcrum, which establishes the relationship between resistance (a force to be overcome) and effort (a force to be resisted). (See *Basic joint movements.*) Most movement calls for muscle groups rather than one muscle.

Musculoskeletal assessment

Musculoskeletal disorders typically affect patients facing prolonged immobilization, elderly people, patients with concurrent medical conditions, or victims of traumatic injury. For these patients, you'll need to obtain a complete history and perform a careful physical examination.

Patient history

Compile a full medical, social, family, and personal history. Ask about general daily activity, occupation, diet, sexual activity, and elimination habits, and try to assess how the patient's disorder may alter his body image. Find out how he functions at home. Can he perform daily activities? Does he have trouble getting around? Does he need assistive devices? Can family members help with his care?

Obtain an accurate account of the musculoskeletal problem. When did symptoms begin, and how have they progressed? Was the patient or a family member previously treated for the same problem?

Assess the location, duration, and intensity of pain. Evaluate past and current responses to treatment. For instance, if the patient takes anti-inflammatory agents or other medications for arthritis, ask about their effectiveness. Does he require more or less medication than before? Has he tried other forms of treatment? In addition, ask the patient if muscle weakness, fatigue, or tissue or joint swelling accompanies the current musculoskeletal problem.

Physical examination

Data collected during the physical examination will help determine the diagnosis and establish a basis for planning and evaluating treatment. Perform a head-to-toe assessment, simultaneously evaluating muscle and joint function of each body area. Observe the patient's gait and coordination. Inspect and palpate his muscles, joints, and bones.

Evaluate the patient's posture — the attitude or position that his body parts assume in relation to one another and to the external environment. Inspect spinal curvature and knee positioning. Inspect the patient's overall body symmetry as he assumes different positions and makes various movements. Note marked discrepancies in side-to-side size, shape, and motion.

Expect to perform inspection and palpation simultaneously during the musculoskeletal assessment. Evaluate the patient's muscle tone, mass, and strength. Take care to palpate his muscles gently. Never force movement when the patient reports pain or appears injured. Look carefully for localized edema, a change in pigmentation, reddening of pressure points, point tenderness, and deformities.

Check mobility and gait. To evaluate range of motion, ask the patient to abduct, adduct, and flex affected muscles. Palpate arterial pulses for symmetry and for arterial blood return to fingertips and toes. Press momentarily on the toenails of both feet, and compare the time needed for normal color to return. Palpate for fine crepitus over joints.

Check neurovascular status, including motion sensation and circulation. Measure and record discrepancies in muscle circumference or length.

Diagnostic tests

• *X-rays* are probably the most useful diagnostic tool for evaluating structural or functional changes in musculoskeletal diseases.

• *Myelography,* an invasive procedure, may be used to evaluate abnormalities of the spinal canal and cord. The study entails injecting a radiopaque contrast medium into the subarachnoid space of the spine. Then, serial X-rays show how the contrast medium moves through the subarachnoid space. Displacement of the contrast medium indicates a space-occupying lesion.

• *Arthrography* also involves injecting contrast medium to show the shape and integrity of a joint capsule.

• *Arthroscopy* is the visual examination of the interior of a joint with a fiber-optic endoscope.

• *Bone scan* — accomplished with injected radioisotopes — identifies areas of increased bone activity or active bone formation.

• *Magnetic resonance imaging* (MRI) produces images of soft tissues. An MRI scan can detect lesions of the spinal cord and white matter.

• *Computed tomography scan* can detect herniated disks, spinal stenosis, and tumors by identifying variations in tissue density.

Other useful tests include bone and muscle biopsies, electromyography, microscopic examination of synovial fluid, and laboratory analyses of urine and blood to identify systemic abnormalities.

Treatment and nursing care

Depending on the patient's disorder, therapy and care measures usually involve relieving pain and managing

BASIC JOINT MOVEMENTS

Diarthrodial joints permit 13 angular and circular motions. (You'll evaluate all of them in a musculoskeletal assessment.) The shoulder demonstrates circumduction; the elbow, flexion and extension; the arm, abduction and adduction; the jaw, retraction and protraction; the hand, pronation and supination; the hip, internal and external rotation; and the foot, eversion and inversion.

Circumduction
Moving in a circular manner

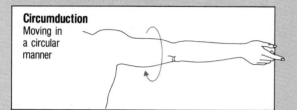

Flexion
Bending, decreasing the joint angle

Extension
Straightening, increasing the joint angle

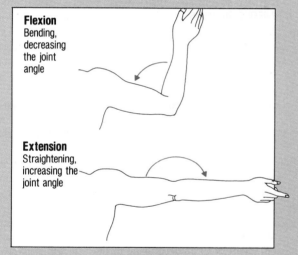

Abduction
Moving away from midline

Adduction
Moving toward midline

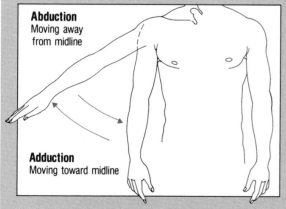

Retraction and protraction
Moving backward and forward

Pronation
Turning downward

Supination
Turning upward

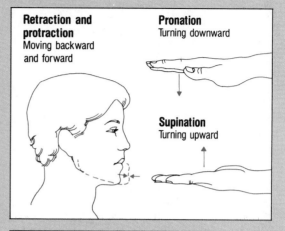

Internal rotation
Turning toward midline

External rotation
Turning away from midline

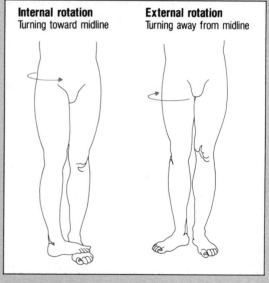

Eversion
Turning outward

Inversion
Turning inward

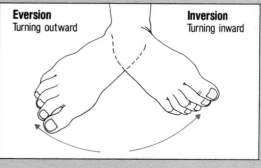

KINDS OF TRACTION

Your patient may need traction—the manual or mechanical application of a steady pulling force—to reduce a fracture, minimize muscle spasms, immobilize a bone, or align a joint. The kind of traction he has—skin, skeletal, or manual—depends on his musculoskeletal disorder.

Skin traction
This involves indirect application of a pulling force to the skeletal system through skin and soft tissues. A common example is Buck's traction, which uses pulleys and weights to improve body alignment.

Skeletal traction
The direct application of traction to bones is known as skeletal traction. It may be accomplished by traversing the affected bone with a pin (Steinmann's pin) or wire (Kirschner wire) or by gripping the bone with calipers or a tonglike device (Gardner-Wells tongs or halo vest). This kind of traction can immobilize healing bones, such as the vertebrae.

Manual traction
Used in an emergency, manual traction is the direct application of pulling force to a body part by hand. It may be used, for instance, to realign a broken bone after an accident.

at least one of the following: traction, casts, braces, splints, crutches, or intermittent range-of-motion (ROM) devices. Of equal importance is the nursing care provided to prevent complications of immobility.

Controlling pain

Analgesics, including patient-controlled analgesia delivery devices, can relieve pain and promote mobility. Analgesics delivered by an epidural catheter are gaining popularity for postoperative pain management. And preservative-free morphine administered epidurally can relieve pain for up to 12 hours.

Other measures include transcutaneous electrical nerve stimulation (TENS) units. These external devices provide dermal stimulation of nerve pathways to manage acute or chronic pain. Relaxation achieved by progressive muscle relaxation, deep breathing, biofeedback, and dissociative visualization techniques may also be helpful.

Coping with traction, casts, and other devices

• If the patient must use *traction devices,* explain how traction works. (See *Kinds of traction.*) Define his activity limits, and estimate how long he will be in traction. Also discuss whether he can remove the traction devices and when, and teach active ROM exercises.

• Check neurovascular status to prevent nerve damage. Also, make sure that the patient has a firm mattress, that his traction ropes remain whole and unfrayed, that they stay on the pulley's center track, and that traction weights hang freely. Thoroughly investigate any patient complaints.

• Check for signs of infection (odor, local inflammation and drainage, fever) at pin sites if the patient is in skeletal traction. Also check hospital policy regarding pin site care measures, such as cleaning and protection.

• If the patient must have a cast, remember that it provides immobility without adding too much weight. A good cast fits snugly, not constrictively. It has a smooth inner surface and smooth edges to prevent pressure or skin irritation. However, check skin integrity frequently.

• Forewarn the patient that a wet cast takes between 24 and 48 hours to dry. To prevent indentations, caution him not to squeeze the cast with his fingers, not to cover or walk on the cast until it dries, and not to bump a damp cast on a hard surface because dents in the cast can exert pressure on underlying areas. Warn the patient that he may feel a transient sensation of heat under the cast as it's applied and, possibly, as it dries.

• If the patient needs a cast on any part of the arm or leg, emphasize that he must keep that body part above heart level for 24 hours after cast application. This helps to minimize swelling in the extremity.

• Until the cast dries completely, have the patient watch for and immediately report persistent pain in the casted body part or in an area distal to the cast. Other danger signs and symptoms include edema, changes in skin color, coldness, and tingling or numbness in this area. If any of these complications occurs, tell the patient to position the casted body part above heart level and notify the doctor.

• If the patient doesn't stay in the hospital after the cast is applied, instruct him to report any drainage through the cast or any odor that may indicate infection. Warn against inserting foreign objects under the cast, getting it wet, pulling out its padding, or scratching inside it. Suggest that he blow air from a hair dryer (cool setting) into the cast to relieve itching. Tell him to seek immediate attention for a broken cast.

• Instruct the patient to exercise the joints above and below the cast to prevent stiffness and contractures.

• If the patient needs *a brace, a splint,* or *a sling,* explain that these devices provide alignment, immobilization, and pain relief for musculoskeletal disorders. Splints and slings are typically used for short-term immobilization.

• As needed, show the patient and family members how to apply a brace, splint, or sling for optimal benefit. Also teach proper crutch-walking, if needed.

• Inform the patient how long he will need to use the device, and list activity limitations. If the patient has a brace, check with his orthotist about proper care.

Coping with immobility

An immobilized patient requires meticulous care to prevent complications. Without constant care, a bedridden patient is more susceptible to skin breakdown caused by increased pressure on tissues over bony prominences. He's especially vulnerable to cardiopulmonary complications.

• To prevent pressure ulcers, turn the patient regularly, and massage areas over bony prominences. Place a flotation pad, a sheepskin pad, an alternating-air-current mattress, or a convoluted foam mattress under bony prominences. Be sure to show the patient how to use a Balkan frame with a trapeze to move about in bed.

• Increase fluid intake to minimize the risk of renal calculi.

• Perform passive ROM exercises on the patient's affected side, as ordered, to prevent contractures. And instruct the patient in active ROM exercises on the unaffected side. Apply footboards or high-topped sneakers to prevent footdrop.

• Because most bedridden patients involuntarily perform Valsalva's maneuver when using the upper arms and trunk to move, instruct the patient to exhale instead of holding his breath as he turns. This will prevent possible cardiac complications from increased intrathoracic pressure.

• Emphasize the importance of coughing and deep breathing. And teach the patient to use an incentive spirometer, if ordered.

• Because constipation commonly occurs in bedridden patients, establish a bowel elimination program (fluids, fiber, laxatives, stool softeners), as needed. Monitor the effectiveness of the bowel regimen, and document bowel movements.

• Provide a diet high in proteins, carbohydrates, and vitamins to enhance healing.

Rehabilitation

Restoring the patient's former good health isn't always possible. If this is the case with your patient, help him adjust to a modified life-style. During hospitalization, promote independence by letting him perform as many tasks as he can by himself. If necessary, refer him to a community facility for continued rehabilitation.

CONGENITAL DISORDERS

Arising before or at birth, congenital disorders of the musculoskeletal system include clubfoot, congenital hip dysplasia, muscular dystrophy, and osteogenesis imperfecta.

CLUBFOOT

Also known as talipes, clubfoot is the most common congenital disorder of the lower extremities. The affected patient has a deformed talus and shortened Achilles tendon, which combine to give the foot a characteristic clublike appearance.

Clubfoot is classified according to the orientation of the deformed foot. In talipes equinovarus, the foot points downward (equinus) and inward (varus), and the front of the foot curls toward the heel (forefoot adduction). See *Recognizing clubfoot*, page 758, for descriptions of other variations.

The deformity usually is obvious at birth, allowing an early diagnosis. But clubfoot that causes only subtle deformity must be distinguished from apparent clubfoot, such as metatarsus varus (pigeon toe). Such apparent clubfoot results when a fetus maintains a position in utero that gives his feet the appearance of clubfoot; unlike true clubfoot, it can usually be corrected without surgery. Inversion of the feet, another type of apparent clubfoot, may result from the peroneal type of progressive muscular atrophy or dystrophy.

Clubfoot typically affects both feet. It may be associated with other birth defects, such as myelomeningocele, spina bifida, or arthrogryposis. The deformity occurs about once in every 1,000 live births and is twice as common in boys as in girls. Treated promptly, it can be corrected.

Causes

Clubfoot appears to result from a combination of genetic factors and environmental conditions that arise in utero. The mechanism of genetic transmission remains unknown, but researchers are convinced that such a mechanism exists. The sibling of a child born with clubfoot has a 1 in 35 chance of being affected. The child of a

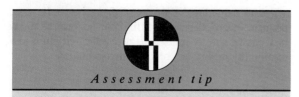

Assessment tip

RECOGNIZING CLUBFOOT

Clubfoot may have various specific names, depending on the orientation of the deformity, as shown in the illustrations below.

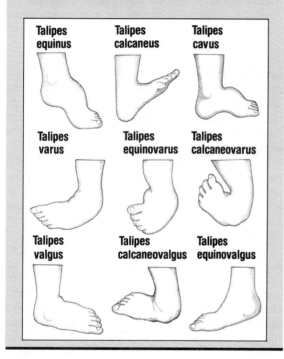

Talipes equinus

Talipes calcaneus

Talipes cavus

Talipes varus

Talipes equinovarus

Talipes calcaneovarus

Talipes valgus

Talipes calcaneovalgus

Talipes equinovalgus

parent with clubfoot has a 1 in 10 chance of inheriting the disorder.

Among children who have no family history of clubfoot, the anomaly may be linked to arrested development during the 10th to 12th week of gestation, when the feet form. Researchers also suspect muscle abnormalities, which lead to variations in tendon length and insertion points, as possible causes.

Clubfoot may arise in older children secondary to paralysis, poliomyelitis, or cerebral palsy. In these instances, treatment for clubfoot must be accompanied by treatment of the underlying disorder.

Complications

The feet may retain some deformity despite treatment.

Assessment findings

The patient may have a family history of clubfoot. Older patients may have a history of a related primary disorder, such as poliomyelitis or cerebral palsy.

Inspection usually reveals the deformity, which may vary greatly in severity. It may be only mildly apparent, or it may be so severe that the neonate's toes touch the inside of the ankle. In all patients, the talus is deformed, the Achilles tendon shortened, and the calcaneus somewhat shortened and flattened. Depending on the degree of varus deformity, the calf muscles are shortened and underdeveloped, with soft-tissue contractures at the site of the deformity.

In the patient with true clubfoot, the foot is tight in its deformed position and resists efforts to push it back into position. In a normal neonate, the dorsum of the foot can be made to touch the outer side of the shin.

Diagnostic tests

X-rays show the talus superimposed on the calcaneus. The metatarsals have a ladderlike appearance.

Treatment

Correction of clubfoot requires three stages: correcting the deformity, maintaining the correction until the foot regains normal muscle balance, and observing the foot closely for several years to prevent the deformity from recurring.

In neonates, corrective treatment begins at once. An infant's foot contains large amounts of cartilage, and the muscles, ligaments, and tendons are supple. The ideal time to begin treatment is in the first few weeks after birth when the foot is most malleable. Deformities are usually corrected sequentially: first forefoot adduction, then varus (or inversion), then equinus (or plantar flexion). Trying to correct all three deformities at once creates a misshapen, rocker-bottomed foot.

Correction begins by manipulating the foot appropriately and casting the foot in that position. The procedure is repeated several times until the foot assumes a normal or nearly normal shape (usually in about 3 months).

The Denis Browne splint, a device that consists of two padded, metal footplates connected by a flat, horizontal bar, is sometimes used as a follow-up measure (when the foot is large enough) to help promote bilateral correction and strengthen the foot muscles.

More than half of all patients who have clubfoot—even those who receive conservative treatment—also need surgical correction. Typically, the doctor orders surgery if 3 months of casting hasn't corrected the condition or if the forefoot dorsiflexes and the hindfoot remains in equinus. Surgical correction may involve tenotomy, tendon transfer, stripping of the plantar fascia, and capsulotomy. If the patient has a severe deformity that persists into later life, surgery may involve wedge resection, osteotomy, or talectomy. The patient must wear a cast to preserve the correction. Clubfoot severe enough to require surgical correction usually can't be corrected completely.

After corrective treatment, proper alignment must be maintained actively, through exercise, splints, and orthopedic shoes. The patient may need to wear a device, such as a polypropylene above-the-knee splint, at night and during naps and a prewalker clubfoot shoe during the day.

Nursing diagnoses
• Body image disturbance
• Fear
• Impaired physical mobility
• Knowledge deficit
• Risk for impaired skin integrity
• Risk for injury

Nursing interventions
• Look for exaggerated positions in a neonate's feet and, if he seems to have a deformity, gently try to manipulate his foot. In apparent clubfoot, the foot will move easily. Avoid excessive force when manipulating a clubfoot.
• After application of a cast, elevate the child's feet with pillows. Check the toes every 1 to 2 hours for temperature, color, sensation, motion, and capillary refill time; watch for edema.
• Insert plastic petals over the top edges of a new cast while it's still wet to keep urine from soaking and softening the cast. After the cast dries, petal the edges with adhesive tape to keep out plaster crumbs and prevent skin irritation. (See *How to petal a cast.*) Care for the skin under the cast edges every 4 hours. After washing and drying the skin, rub it with alcohol. Don't use oils or powders because they tend to macerate the skin.
• If the doctor uses wedging maneuvers to reshape the existing cast (rather than recasting), check circulatory status frequently; it may be compromised by increased pressure on tissues and blood vessels. The equinus correction places considerable strain on ligaments, blood vessels, and tendons.
• After surgery, elevate the child's feet with pillows to decrease swelling and pain. Report signs of discomfort or pain immediately. Try to locate the source of pain—it may result from cast pressure rather than the incision. If bleeding develops under the cast, circle the location,

HOW TO PETAL A CAST

Rough cast edges can be cushioned by petaling them with adhesive tape or moleskin. To do this, first cut several 4″ × 2″ (10.2 × 5 cm) strips. Round off one end of each strip to keep it from curling. Then, making sure the rounded end of the strip is on the outside of the cast, tuck the straight end just inside the cast edge.

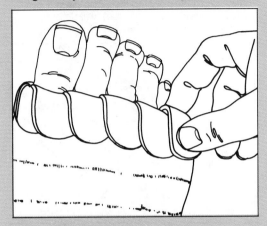

Smooth the moleskin with your finger until you're sure it's secured inside and out. Repeat the procedure, overlapping the moleskin pieces until you've gone all the way around the cast edge.

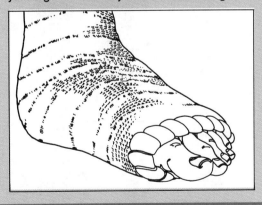

and mark the time on the cast. If bleeding spreads, report it to the doctor.
• Perform range-of-motion exercises at least once every shift, unless contraindicated, to prevent contractures and muscle atrophy.
• Encourage the patient (if he's old enough) and his family to express their concerns about his disorder and his

DEGREES OF HIP DYSPLASIA

Normally, the head of the femur fits snugly into the acetabulum, allowing the hip to move properly. In congenital hip dysplasia, flattening of the acetabulum prevents the head of the femur from rotating adequately. The child's hip may be unstable, subluxated (partially dislocated), or completely dislocated, with the femoral head lying totally outside the acetabulum. The degree of dysplasia—and the child's age—will determine the treatment choice.

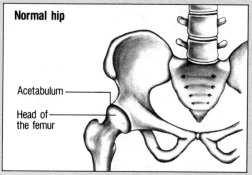

Normal hip

Acetabulum

Head of the femur

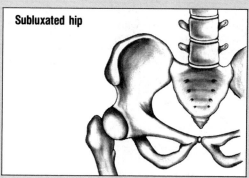

Subluxated hip

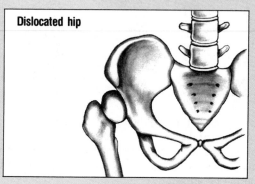

Dislocated hip

appearance. Answer their questions, and offer reassurance and support when necessary.

Patient teaching

• Explain the disorder to the patient (if he's old enough) and to his family. Make sure they understand that clubfoot demands immediate therapy and orthopedic supervision throughout the growth process.

• Before a child in a clubfoot cast goes home, teach the family cast care and the signs of circulatory impairment.

• Stress to parents that correcting this defect takes time and patience. Teach them exercises that they and the child can do at home to help maintain the correction. Urge parents to apply corrective shoes and splints when the child takes naps and goes to sleep at night.

• After an older child has had his foot placed in a cast, warn him and his parents to avoid letting the cast wear thin and get soft around the foot area. If it does, much of the correction may be lost.

• If appropriate, explain to an older child and his parents that surgery may improve the clubfoot enough to ensure adequate function. However, the affected calf muscle will remain slightly underdeveloped.

DEVELOPMENTAL DYSPLASIA OF THE HIP

The most common disorder affecting the hip joints of children under age 3, developmental dysplasia of the hip (DDH) occurs when structures in the hip joint articulate abnormally. The condition may be unilateral or bilateral. It occurs in three forms of varying severity:

• unstable hip dysplasia, in which the hip is positioned normally but the ligaments around the hip are loose, predisposing it to dislocation, especially by manipulation

• subluxation or incomplete dislocation, in which the head of the femur is partially displaced and rides on the edge of the acetabulum

• complete dislocation, in which the head of the femur lies completely outside the acetabulum. (See *Degrees of hip dysplasia*.)

About 60% to 70% of affected infants are female. Dislocation is ten times more common after breech delivery than after normal cephalic delivery. It also may be more common among large neonates and twins. With prompt treatment, the prognosis is good.

Causes

Experts are uncertain about the cause of DDH. Some theorize that the hormones that relax maternal ligaments in preparation for labor may also relax the ligaments around the infant's hip joint.

Complications

If treatment doesn't begin until after the child reaches age 2, DDH may cause degenerative hip changes, lordosis, joint malformation, and soft-tissue damage. A unilateral dislocation, which shortens one of the child's legs, can result in functional scoliosis.

Untreated DDH can lead to crippling osteoarthritis and a progressive limp by the time the patient reaches early adulthood.

Assessment findings

The patient may have a history of a breech delivery, or she may have been a large neonate or one of twins. An older child may have a history of delayed walking or, as the child begins to walk, limited abduction on the dislocated side.

When you inspect an affected infant in the supine position, you may observe extra thigh folds on the side of subluxation or dislocation. Extra folds may also appear when the child lies prone. The buttock fold on the affected side appears higher. You may also discover dysplasia by palpation.

In complete dysplasia, the hip rides above the acetabulum, making the child's knees uneven. An older child will have one leg shorter than the other.

A child with bilateral dysplasia may sway from side to side when walking, a sign called "duck waddle." Unilateral dysplasia may cause a limp. (See *Ortolani's and Trendelenburg's signs,* page 762.)

Diagnostic tests

• *X-rays* reveal the location of the femur head and a shallow acetabulum and allow monitoring of the progress of the disorder or treatment. However, X-rays are difficult to interpret because the femoral head is not evident until ossification begins at age 3 to 4 months.
• *Ultrasonography* can define the relationship between the head of the femur and the acetabulum without the use of ionizing radiation.

Treatment

The earlier an infant receives treatment, the better her chances of normal development. Treatment for older children depends on their age.

Infants younger than age 3 months receive gentle manipulation to reduce the dislocation, followed by placement of a splintlike brace or harness (such as the Frejka pillow or the Pavlik harness) to maintain the hips in a flexed and abducted position. The infant must wear the appliance continuously for 2 to 3 months and then wear a night splint for another month so the joint capsule can tighten and stabilize in correct alignment.

If treatment doesn't begin until after age 3 months, it may include bilateral skin traction (Bryant's traction). Skeletal traction may be necessary if the child has started walking. Both treatments aim to reduce the dislocation by gradually abducting the hips.

If traction fails, gentle closed reduction under general anesthesia can further abduct the hips; the infant then wears a spica cast for 4 to 6 months. If closed reduction fails, the doctor may perform open reduction and apply a spica cast for about 6 months, or he may perform an osteotomy.

Treatment for children ages 2 to 5 is difficult; it includes skeletal traction and subcutaneous adductor tenotomy. Treatment begun after age 5 usually fails to restore satisfactory hip function.

Nursing diagnoses

• Altered nutrition: Less than body requirements
• Constipation
• Fear
• Fluid volume deficit
• Impaired physical mobility
• Knowledge deficit
• Risk for impaired skin integrity
• Risk for injury

Nursing interventions

• When transferring the child immediately after application of a spica cast, use your palms to avoid making dents in the cast. Such dents can cause pressure ulcers. Remember that the cast needs 24 to 48 hours to dry naturally. Don't use heat to make it dry faster; that will also make it more fragile.
• Use strips of plastic sheet to protect the edges of the cast from moisture around the perineum and buttocks. Cut the strips long enough to cover the outside of the cast, then overlap them around the edge and tuck each one about a finger length beneath the edge. Using overlapping strips of tape, tack the corner of each strip to the outside of the cast. Remove the plastic under the cast every 4 hours; then wash, dry, and retuck it. Disposable diapers folded lengthwise over the perineum may also be used.
• Position the child either on a Bradford frame elevated on blocks, with a bedpan under the frame, or on pillows to support the child's legs. Keep the cast dry, and change the child's diapers often.

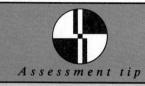

Assessment tip

ORTOLANI'S AND TRENDELENBURG'S SIGNS

Two signs can help you assess for developmental dysplasia of the hip.

Ortolani's sign
Place the infant on his back, with his hips flexed in a neutral position. Grasp his legs just below the knees with the long fingers of each hand extending down the lateral side of the thigh to the greater trochanter.

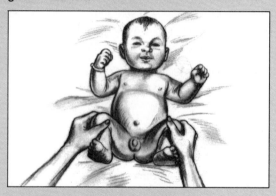

Then, gently abduct the hips from a neutral position. If you exert slight pressure upward and inward beneath the greater trochanter with your long finger, the dislocated head of the femur may slip *into* the acetabulum with a palpable click.

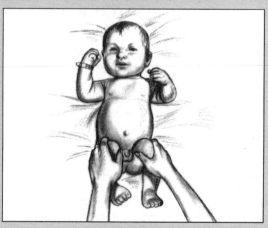

Trendelenburg's sign
Have the child rest her weight on the side of the dislocation and lift her other knee (as shown). Her pelvis drops on the normal side because of the weak abductor muscles in the affected hip. (Also note how the spine curves in this position.) However, when the child stands with her weight on the normal side and lifts the other knee, the pelvis remains horizontal or is elevated.

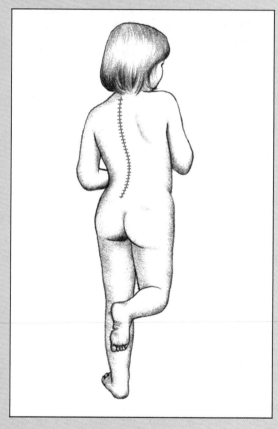

• Wash and dry the skin under the cast edges every 2 to 4 hours, and rub it with alcohol. Don't use oils or powders; they can macerate the skin.
• Turn the child every 2 hours during the day and every 4 hours at night. Check color, sensation, and motion in her legs and feet, and examine all her toes. Notify the doctor if they're dusky or cool or if you suspect they are numb.
• Shine a flashlight under the cast every 4 hours to check for foreign objects and crumbs of food. Check the cast daily for odors, which may indicate infection. Record temperature daily.
• If a child complains of itching, she may benefit from diphenhydramine. Or you may use a hair dryer to blow cool air at the cast edges.
• Provide adequate nutrition and fluid intake to avoid renal calculi and constipation.
• Provide adequate stimuli to promote growth and development.
• Encourage the parents to stay with their child as much as possible for the first few days after a cast or splintlike brace is applied. Their presence will calm and reassure her while she adapts to newly restricted movement.
• Assure the parents that the child will adjust to this restriction and return to normal sleeping, eating, and playing behavior in a few days.
• If the patient is in Bryant's traction, make sure that the amount of weight is sufficient to lift her buttocks slightly off the bed.
• Maintain the patient's skin integrity.
• Monitor respiratory status and watch for aspiration.

Patient teaching
• Explain possible causes of DDH, and reassure the parents that early, prompt treatment usually results in complete correction.
• Teach the parents how to splint or brace the hips correctly. Stress the need for frequent checkups.
• If the patient is using a Bradford frame, teach the parents how to apply the traction and how to care for the child while she's in traction. Remind them to keep her from bearing weight on her legs while she rests between periods of traction.
• If the child's hips are abducted in a froglike position (which prevents sitting in a high chair), encourage the parents to let her sit at a table (by seating her on pillows on a chair), to put her on the floor for short periods of play, and to let her play with other children her age.
• If the doctor orders it, instruct the parents to remove braces and splints while bathing the infant. Tell them

they need to replace them immediately afterward.
• Stress the importance of cleanliness; the parents should bathe and change the child frequently and wash her perineum with warm water and soap at each diaper change.
• Tell the parents to watch for signs that the child is outgrowing the cast, such as cyanosis, cool extremities, and pain.
• If the child wears a Pavlik harness or spica cast, urge the parents to modify a commercially manufactured car seat to ensure the child's safety when riding in a car.
• Tell the parents that treatment for DDH may be prolonged and will require patience.
• Teach the parents to recognize signs of respiratory distress.

MUSCULAR DYSTROPHY
A group of hereditary disorders, muscular dystrophy is characterized by progressive symmetrical wasting of skeletal muscles but no neural or sensory defects. Four main types of muscular dystrophy occur: Duchenne's (pseudohypertrophic) muscular dystrophy, which accounts for 50% of all cases; Becker's (benign pseudohypertrophic) muscular dystrophy; facioscapulohumeral (Landouzy-Dejerine) dystrophy; and limb-girdle (Erb's) dystrophy.

Depending on the type, the disorder may affect vital organs and lead to severe disability, even death. Early in the disease, muscle fibers necrotize and regenerate in various states. Over time, regeneration slows and degeneration dominates. Fat and connective tissue replace muscle fibers, causing weakness.

Duchenne's and Becker's muscular dystrophies affect males almost exclusively; the incidence of Duchenne's in males is 13 to 33 per 100,000, and of Becker's, about 1 to 3 per 100,000. The remaining two types affect both sexes about equally.

The prognosis varies. Duchenne's muscular dystrophy typically begins during early childhood and causes death within 10 to 15 years. Patients with Becker's muscular dystrophy usually live into their 40s. Facioscapulohumeral and limb-girdle dystrophies usually don't shorten life expectancy.

Causes
Muscular dystrophy is caused by various genetic mechanisms. The basic defect can be mapped genetically to band Xp 21. Duchenne's and Becker's muscular dystrophies are X-linked recessive, and facioscapulohumeral dystrophy is autosomal dominant. Limb-girdle dystrophy

may be inherited in several ways but usually is autosomal recessive.

Exactly how these inherited defects cause progressive muscle weakness isn't known. They may create an abnormality in the intracellular metabolism of muscle cells. The abnormality may be related to an enzyme deficiency or dysfunction or to an inability to synthesize, absorb, or metabolize an unknown substance vital to muscle function.

Complications

Duchenne's and Becker's muscular dystrophies lead to crippling disability and contractures. Progressive skeletal deformity and thoracic muscle weakness inhibit pulmonary function, increasing the risk of pneumonia and other respiratory infections. These diseases can also lead to such cardiac problems as arrhythmias and hypertrophy; sudden heart failure may cause death. Most patients with Duchenne's or Becker's muscular dystrophy die from respiratory complications.

Complications from other types of dystrophy vary with the site and severity of muscle involvement.

Assessment findings

The patient's family history may point to evidence of genetic transmission. If another family member has muscular dystrophy, its clinical characteristics can indicate the type of dystrophy the patient has and how he may be affected.

The patient may complain of progressive muscle weakness. The onset and characteristics of the increasing weakness vary with the type of dystrophy involved.

Duchenne's muscular dystrophy begins insidiously. Onset typically occurs when the child is between ages 3 and 5. Weakness begins in the pelvic muscles and interferes with the child's ability to run, climb, and walk. The disease progresses rapidly; by age 12, the child usually can't walk.

Signs and symptoms of Becker's muscular dystrophy resemble those of Duchenne's, but they progress more slowly. They start after age 5, but the patient can still walk well beyond age 15 — sometimes into his 40s.

Facioscapulohumeral dystrophy — a slowly progressive and relatively benign form of muscular dystrophy — typically begins before the child reaches age 10. However, symptoms may develop during adolescence. Early symptoms include weakness of eye, face, and shoulder muscles. The patient may complain that he's unable to raise his arms over his head or close his eyes completely. The patient or the patient's parents may notice other early signs, including an inability to pucker the lips or whistle, abnormal facial movements, and the absence of facial movements when laughing or crying. Pelvic muscles weaken as the disease progresses.

Limb-girdle dystrophy follows a similarly slow course and commonly causes only slight disability. Onset usually occurs when the child is between ages 6 and 10 but may occur in early adulthood. Muscle weakness first appears in the upper arm and pelvic muscles.

Inspection reveals the effects of muscle weakness and eventually muscle wasting. Findings vary according to the type of dystrophy. Early in Duchenne's and Becker's muscular dystrophies, you may notice that the patient has a wide stance and a waddling gait. He may also display Gowers' sign when rising from a sitting or supine position (see *Observing Gowers' sign*).

During the initial stage, you may notice muscle hypertrophy. As the disease progresses, however, most muscles atrophy. The calves remain enlarged because of fat infiltration into the muscle. As abdominal and paravertebral muscles weaken, you may observe posture changes. The patient develops lordosis and a protuberant abdomen. Weakened thoracic muscles may cause scapular "winging" or flaring when the patient raises his arms. Bone outlines become prominent as surrounding muscles atrophy. In later stages, you may note contractures and pulmonary signs, such as tachypnea and shortness of breath.

A patient with facioscapulohumeral dystrophy may develop a pendulous lower lip, and the nasolabial fold may disappear. Diffuse facial flattening leads to a masklike expression. Infants can't suckle. The scapulae develop a winglike appearance, and the patient can't raise his arms above his head.

With limb-girdle dystrophy, you may note winging of the scapulae, lordosis with abdominal protrusion, a waddling gait, poor balance, and an inability to raise the arms. (See *Detecting muscular dystrophy*, page 766.)

Diagnostic tests

Several tests help confirm the diagnosis:
• *Muscle biopsy* shows fat and connective tissue deposits and confirms the diagnosis. It also shows degeneration and necrosis of muscle fibers and, in Duchenne's and Becker's dystrophies, a deficiency of the muscle protein dystrophin.
• *Electromyography* typically demonstrates short, weak bursts of electrical activity in affected muscles.
• *Urine creatinine, serum creatine phosphokinase (CPK), lactate dehydrogenase, alanine aminotransferase (formerly SGPT) and aspartate aminotransferase (formerly SGOT) levels* are elevated. CPK levels rise before muscle weak-

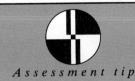

Assessment tip

OBSERVING GOWERS' SIGN

Because Duchenne's and Becker's muscular dystrophies weaken pelvic and lower extremity muscles, the patient must use his upper body to maneuver from a prone to an upright position.

Lying on his stomach with his arms stretched in front of him, the patient raises his head, backs into a crawling position and on into a half-kneel.

Then stooping, he braces his legs with his hands at the ankles and walks his hands (one after the other) up his legs until he pushes himself upright.

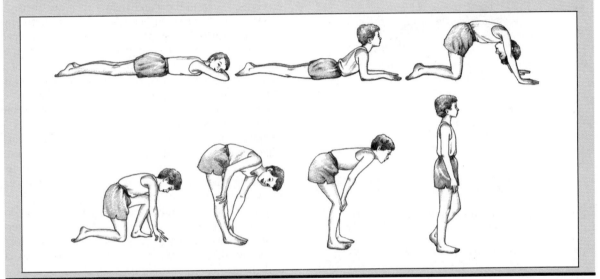

ness becomes severe, providing an early indicator of Duchenne's and Becker's muscular dystrophies. These diagnostic tests are also useful for genetic screening because unaffected carriers also show elevated enzyme levels.

• *Amniocentesis* can't detect muscular dystrophy definitively, but because it reveals the sex of the fetus, it may be recommended for pregnant patients known to carry the gene for Duchenne's or Becker's muscular dystrophy.

• *Genetic testing* can detect the gene defect that leads to muscular dystrophy in some families.

Treatment

Currently, no treatment can stop the progressive muscle impairment. However, orthopedic appliances, exercise, physical therapy, and surgery to correct contractures can help preserve the patient's mobility and independence.

Nursing diagnoses

• Activity intolerance
• Altered nutrition: More than body requirements
• Body image disturbance
• Constipation
• Impaired physical mobility
• Ineffective breathing pattern
• Ineffective family coping
• Ineffective individual coping
• Self-care deficit

Nursing interventions

• If a patient with Duchenne's or Becker's muscular dystrophy develops respiratory involvement, encourage coughing and deep-breathing exercises.
• Help the patient to preserve joint mobility and prevent muscle atrophy by encouraging and assisting with active and passive range-of-motion exercises.

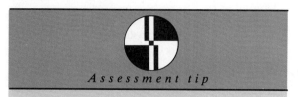

DETECTING MUSCULAR DYSTROPHY

In muscular dystrophy, the trapezius muscle typically rises, creating a stepped appearance at the shoulder's point.

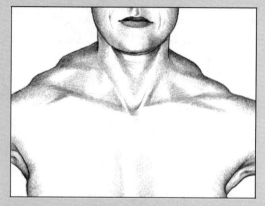

From the posterior view, the scapulae ride over the lateral thoracic region, giving them a winged appearance. In Duchenne's and Becker's dystrophies, this winglike sign appears when the patient raises his arms, whereas in other dystrophies, the sign is obvious without arm raising. (In fact, the patient can't raise his arms.)

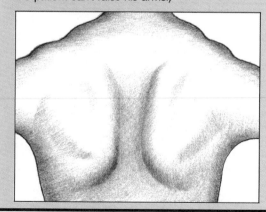

• The patient may need splints, braces, grab bars, and overhead slings. For comfort and to prevent footdrop, use a footboard or high-topped shoes and a foot cradle.

• Because inactivity may cause constipation, encourage adequate fluid intake, increase dietary bulk, and obtain an order for a stool softener. Because the patient is prone to obesity from reduced physical activity, provide him with a low-calorie, high-protein, high-fiber diet.
• Allow the patient plenty of time to perform even simple physical tasks.

Patient teaching
• Encourage communication between the family members and the patient to help them handle emotional strain and cope with changes in body image.
• Encourage the patient and his family to express their concerns. Listen to them and answer their questions.
• Help a child with Duchenne's muscular dystrophy maintain peer relationships and realize his intellectual potential by encouraging his parents to keep him in a regular school as long as possible.
• Teach the patient and his parents ways to maintain his mobility and independence for as long as possible.
• Inform the patient and his parents about possible complications and steps they can take to prevent them.
• Explain the possibility of respiratory tract infections, what signs to watch for, and what to do if the patient develops a respiratory infection. Urge the patient and his parents to report signs of infection to the doctor at once.
• When the patient becomes confined to a wheelchair, help him and his family to see the chair as a way to preserve his independence. Have an occupational therapist teach the patient about his wheelchair and other supportive devices that can help him with activities of daily living.
• Help the patient and his family plan a low-calorie, high-protein, high-fiber diet to prevent obesity caused by reduced physical activity.
• Advise the patient to avoid long periods of bed rest and inactivity; if necessary, he should limit television viewing and other sedentary activities.
• If desired, refer adult patients for sexual counseling.
• Refer the patient for appropriate physical therapy, vocational rehabilitation, social services, and financial assistance. Suggest the Muscular Dystrophy Association as a source of information and support.
• Refer family members who carry the muscular dystrophy trait to genetic counseling so they understand the risk of transmitting this disorder.

OSTEOGENESIS IMPERFECTA
Also called brittle bones, osteogenesis imperfecta is a hereditary disease of bones and connective tissue. It causes

fragile bones, thin skin, blue sclera, poor teeth, hypermobility of the joints, and progressive deafness.

The disease occurs in many forms. In the rare congenital form, in which fractures are present at birth, the patient usually dies during the first few days or weeks after birth. In the late-appearing form (osteogenesis imperfecta tarda), the child appears normal at birth but develops recurring fractures—mostly of the extremities—after age 1.

Some children with osteogenesis imperfecta tarda have gross multiple fractures and deformities; others have an increased tendency to fracture but no significant deformities. Some have multiple fractures during childhood, improve after puberty, and then begin to fracture more frequently later in life, particularly during pregnancy and then again after menopause.

Causes and pathophysiology
Osteogenesis imperfecta may result from autosomal dominant or recessive inheritance. Clinical signs may result from defective osteoblastic activity and defective mesenchymal collagen (embryonic connective tissue) and its derivatives (sclera, bones, and ligaments). The reticulum fails to differentiate into mature collagen or may cause collagen to develop abnormally, leading to immature and coarse bone formation. Cortical bone thinning also occurs.

Complications
A third of patients become deaf by ages 30 to 40 because of osteosclerosis, pressure on the auditory nerve, and neurogenic deafness. Other complications include scoliosis, multiple deformities, and dwarfism.

Assessment findings
The patient has a history of repeated fractures that result from even slight trauma. He may complain of a progressive hearing loss.

In congenital and delayed osteogenesis imperfecta, inspection may show a bilaterally bulging skull, triangle-shaped head and face, prominent eyes, and blue sclera. You may also observe thin, translucent skin; signs of possible subcutaneous hemorrhages; and discolored (blue-gray or yellow-brown) teeth, which break easily and are prone to cavities. Other findings include poorly developed (atrophied) skeletal muscles and hypermobility of the joints.

You may notice that the patient is short. In congenital osteogenesis, epiphyseal fractures result in deformities and stunted growth.

Diagnostic tests
• *X-rays* show evidence of multiple old fractures and skeletal deformities. A skull X-ray shows wide sutures with small, irregularly shaped islands of bone (wormian bones) between them. These findings can help differentiate osteogenesis imperfecta from child abuse.
• *Serum calcium* and *serum phosphorus levels* are normal.
• *DNA analysis* may reveal the diagnosis in some families.

Treatment
Because no cure currently exists, treatment aims to prevent deformities through the use of traction, immobilization, or both, and to aid normal development and rehabilitation. Limb deformities may be corrected by multiple osteotomies and rod placement.

Other measures include assessing for and treating scoliosis, a common complication, and promoting preventive dental care and repair of dental caries.

Patients with mild osteogenesis imperfecta may need little treatment after age 15, when the fracture rate begins to decrease. Women, however, will need special attention during pregnancy and after menopause, when their tendency to fracture may return.

Nursing diagnoses
• Altered growth and development
• Impaired physical mobility
• Knowledge deficit
• Pain
• Risk for infection
• Risk for injury
• Sensory or perceptual alterations

Nursing interventions
• Emphasize the importance of coughing and deep breathing, and teach the patient how to use an incentive spirometer, if ordered.
• If the patient has a cast, monitor his circulatory, motor, and sensory abilities.
• Monitor skin condition, especially over bony prominences and areas under pressure from a cast or brace.
• If the patient is in skeletal traction, check for signs of infection (odor, fever, local inflammation, and drainage) at pin sites. Care for the pin sites with peroxide or povidone-iodine, or as the doctor orders.
• Provide a high-protein, high-carbohydrate, high-vitamin diet to enhance healing.
• Administer analgesics, as ordered, and monitor the patient's response.

• Monitor dental and hearing needs.
• Encourage the patient and his parents to express their concerns about the disorder, and answer any questions they may have. Involve them in all phases of care.

Patient teaching

• Teach the patient and his parents how to recognize a fracture and how to splint it correctly.
• If the patient needs a cast, explain that it may dry in 24 to 48 hours. To avoid making indentations in it while it's still wet, tell the patient to avoid squeezing it with his fingers, covering it, walking on it, and bumping it on hard surfaces. Doing so could cause dents that can press against the underlying skin. Tell the patient that he'll feel a transient sensation of heat under the cast while it's drying.
• Teach the patient and his parents how to care for the cast. Instruct them to report any odors or drainage through the cast; these signs may indicate infection. Warn them against inserting foreign objects under the cast, getting it wet, pulling out its padding, or scratching inside it. Tell the patient to seek immediate treatment for a broken cast.
• Instruct the patient to exercise the joints above and below the cast to prevent stiffness and contractures.
• If the patient needs a brace, splint, sling, or traction for alignment or immobilization, explain why he needs the appliance, and show him and his family how to apply it properly. Tell them how long the appliance should be worn, and advise them of any activity restrictions. If the patient has a brace, check with his orthotist about proper care. Encourage the patient to refer further questions to his doctor.
• If the patient needs a cast or brace, teach him and his family how to assess for skin breakdown.
• Teach proper crutch-walking, as necessary.
• Stress the importance of meticulous dental hygiene and routine dental checkups. Also stress the importance of routine hearing tests to detect hearing loss.
• Emphasize the importance of sound nutrition (which helps to heal bones) and immunizations.
• Advise parents to encourage their child to develop interests that don't require strenuous physical activity and to develop his fine-motor skills. Success at these activities will promote the child's self-esteem.
• Teach the child to assume some responsibility for precautions during physical activity to help foster his independence.
• Refer the family for genetic counseling.

JOINT DISORDERS

Painful and disabling, joint disorders attack the body's centers of mobility. Causes of joint disorders may range from chronic conditions to acute infections. No matter what the cause, however, they all need a team treatment approach that emphasizes patient participation.

This section covers septic arthritis, gout, neuropathic arthropathy, and osteoarthritis.

SEPTIC ARTHRITIS

Also known as infectious arthritis, pyogenic septic arthritis is a medical emergency. It arises when bacteria invade a joint and cause the synovial lining to become inflamed. If the organisms enter the joint cavity, effusion and pyogenesis follow, with eventual destruction of bone and cartilage.

The disorder usually affects a single joint. It most often develops in a large joint but can strike any joint, including the spine and small peripheral joints. Migratory polyarthritis sometimes precedes localization of joint inflammation.

Septic arthritis can lead to ankylosis and even fatal septicemia. However, prompt antibiotic therapy and aspiration or drainage of the joint cure most patients.

Causes

In most cases of septic arthritis, bacteria spread from a primary site of infection, usually in adjacent bone or soft tissue, through the bloodstream to the joint. Common infecting organisms include:
• four strains of gram-positive cocci — *Staphylococcus aureus, Streptococcus pyogenes, Streptococcus pneumoniae,* and *Streptococcus viridans*
• two strains of gram-negative cocci — *Neisseria gonorrhoeae* and *Haemophilus influenzae*
• various gram-negative bacilli, including *Escherichia coli, Salmonella,* and *Pseudomonas.*

Rarely, fungi or mycobacteria cause the infection. Anaerobic organisms, such as gram-positive cocci, may infect adults and children over age 2. *H. influenzae* most often infects children under age 2.

Various factors can predispose a person to septic arthritis. Any concurrent bacterial infection (of the genitourinary or upper respiratory tract, for example) or serious chronic illness (such as cancer, renal failure, rheumatoid arthritis, septic lupus erythematosus, diabetes, or cirrhosis) heightens susceptibility. Conse-

OTHER TYPES OF ARTHRITIS: CHARACTERISTICS AND TREATMENT

You may care for patients with several other types of arthritis besides septic arthritis. The information below will help you differentiate among those types.

Traumatic arthritis
This disorder results from blunt, penetrating, or repeated trauma or from forced inappropriate motion of a joint or ligament. Clinical effects may include swelling, pain, tenderness, joint instability, and internal bleeding.

Treatment includes analgesics, anti-inflammatory drugs, application of cold followed by heat and, if needed, compression dressings, splints, joint aspiration, casting or, possibly, surgery.

Schönlein-Henoch purpura
A vasculitic syndrome, this condition is marked by palpable purpura, abdominal pain, renal disease, and arthralgia that most commonly affects the knees and ankles. It produces swollen, warm, tender joints without joint erosion or deformity.

Most patients have microscopic hematuria and proteinuria 4 to 8 weeks after onset. Incidence is highest in children and young adults, occurring most often in the spring after a respiratory tract infection. Treatment may include corticosteroids.

Hemophilic arthritis
This disorder may arise when the patient is between ages 1 and 5 and tends to recur until about age 10. It produces transient or permanent joint changes. Attacks typically are precipitated by trauma, but they may be spontaneous.

Hemophilic arthritis usually affects only one joint at a time—most commonly the knee, elbow, or ankle—and tends to recur in the same joint. Initially, the patient may feel only mild discomfort; later, he may experience warmth, swelling, tenderness, and severe pain with adjacent muscle spasms that prompt him to hold the extremity in a flexed position. Mild hemophilic arthritis may cause limited stiffness that subsides within a few days.

Severe hemophilic arthritis may be accompanied by fever and leukocytosis; severe, prolonged, or repeated bleeding may lead to chronic hemophilic joint disease.

Treatment includes I.V. infusion of the deficient clotting factor, bed rest with the affected extremity elevated, application of ice packs, analgesics, and possibly joint aspiration. Physical therapy includes progressive range-of-motion and muscle-strengthening exercises to restore motion and to prevent contractures and muscle atrophy.

Intermittent hydrarthrosis
Benign and very rare, this condition is characterized by regular, recurrent joint effusions. It most commonly affects the knee. The patient may have difficulty moving the affected joint but have no other arthritic symptoms.

The cause of intermittent hydrarthrosis is unknown; it may be linked to familial tendencies, allergies, or menstruation. Onset is usually at or soon after puberty. No effective treatment exists.

---

quently, alcoholics and elderly persons run an increased risk of developing septic arthritis.

Susceptibility also increases among patients with immune system depression or a history of immunosuppressive therapy. I.V. drug abuse can also lead to septic arthritis. Other predisposing factors include recent articular trauma, joint surgery, intra-articular injections, and local joint abnormalities.

Complications
Septic arthritis may cause infection of the bone (osteomyelitis) or other adjacent structures and a loss of joint cartilage that leads to joint destruction.

Assessment findings
The patient may have a history of a known infection outside the involved joint, an immunosuppressive condition, or I.V. drug abuse. He may complain of an abrupt onset of intense pain in the affected joint. He may also have fever and chills if he has a systemic infection. These findings can help differentiate septic arthritis from other types. (See *Other types of arthritis: Characteristics and treatment.*)

Inspection may show that the patient prefers to keep the affected joint flexed. This position eases pain by minimizing intra-articular pressure. You may observe redness and edema over the affected joint and severely reduced range of motion (ROM), both active and passive.

On palpation, you'll usually note warmth and extreme tenderness over the involved joint.

Diagnostic tests
• *Arthrocentesis* allows the collection of a synovial fluid specimen.
• *Synovial fluid analysis* shows gross pus or watery, cloudy fluid of decreased viscosity, typically with 50,000/mm³ or more white blood cells (WBCs) containing primarily neutrophils. It may also show a lower glu-

cose level than a simultaneous 6-hour postprandial blood glucose level.

• *Gram stain* or *culture of the fluid* — or a *biopsy of the synovial membrane* — confirms the diagnosis and identifies the causative organism.

• *Blood cultures* may be positive and confirm the diagnosis even when the synovial culture is negative.

• *X-rays* may be normal for several weeks and usually don't aid the diagnosis; however, radiographic changes may appear as early as a week after infection. These can include distention of the joint capsule, narrowing of the joint space (indicating cartilage damage), and erosion of bone (joint destruction).

• *Radioisotope joint scan* may be used for less accessible joints, such as spinal articulations, and may help detect infection or inflammation. However, the test by itself isn't diagnostic. Joint bone scans are invariably positive but are useful only in occult sepsis (as in vertebral osteomyelitis).

• *Countercurrent immunoelectrophoresis* measures bacterial antigens in body fluids and helps to guide treatment.

• *Gas chromatography,* which defines microorganisms, helps to identify the causative agent.

• *WBC count* may be elevated, with many polymorphonuclear cells.

• *Erythrocyte sedimentation rate* is increased.

Treatment

Parenteral antibiotic therapy should begin right away. Empiric coverage may include a penicillinase-resistant penicillin (such as ticarcillin with clavulanic acid) or a second-generation cephalosporin (such as cefazolin), typically with gentamicin added for gram-negative coverage. Treatment may be modified as needed when sensitivity studies of the infecting organism become available.

I.V. antibiotic therapy continues for 4 to 6 weeks, possibly longer. The patient may need an implantable I.V. device, such as a Hickman catheter or an implanted infusion port, for home use.

Treatment of septic arthritis requires monitoring of progress through frequent analysis of joint fluid cultures, synovial fluid leukocyte counts, and glucose determinations. Bioassays or bactericidal assays of synovial fluid and bioassays of blood may confirm clearing of the infection.

Codeine or propoxyphene can be given for pain, if needed. (Aspirin misleadingly reduces swelling and may mask fever, hindering accurate monitoring of progress.)

The affected joint may be immobilized with a splint or put into traction until the patient can tolerate move-

ment. As the infection resolves, the doctor will add exercise to the treatment regimen to restore strength and mobility.

Needle aspiration (arthrocentesis) to remove grossly purulent joint fluid may be repeated daily until the fluid appears normal. If cultures remain positive or the WBC count remains elevated, the patient may need arthroscopic surgical drainage to remove resistant infection. (Septic arthritis of the hip requires open surgical drainage.)

Reconstructive surgery is warranted only for severe joint damage and only after all signs of active infection have disappeared. This usually takes several months. The patient will most likely undergo arthroplasty or joint fusion. Prosthetic replacement remains controversial because it may exacerbate the infection; however, it has been used successfully when the femoral head or acetabulum has sustained damage.

Nursing diagnoses

• Anxiety
• Fear
• Impaired physical mobility
• Knowledge deficit
• Pain
• Risk for infection
• Self-care deficit

Nursing interventions

• Practice strict aseptic technique with all procedures. Dispose of soiled linens and dressings properly. Prevent contact between immunosuppressed patients and infected patients.

• Watch for such signs of joint inflammation as heat, redness, swelling, pain, and drainage. Monitor vital signs and fever pattern.

• Check splints or traction regularly. Keep the joint in proper alignment, but prevent prolonged immobilization. Start ROM exercises as soon as ordered. Begin with passive ROM and isometric exercises, then add active ROM exercises. Once acute inflammation resolves, the patient may resume weight bearing on the affected joint.

• Monitor pain levels, and provide medication accordingly, especially before exercise. (The pain of septic arthritis tends to be underestimated.) Administer narcotics and analgesics for acute pain and heat or ice packs for moderate pain. Monitor the patient's response.

• Carefully evaluate the patient's condition after joint aspiration.

• Encourage the patient to perform as much self-care as his immobility and pain allow. Give him time to perform these activities at his own pace.

• Throughout therapy, encourage the patient to express his concerns, and answer any questions he may have. Offer support and encouragement when appropriate. Whenever possible, include the patient and his family in care decisions.

Patient teaching

• Explain all treatments, tests, and procedures to the patient. Warn him that needle aspiration will be extremely painful.

• Discuss all prescribed medications and any adverse reactions they may cause. Tell the patient to call his doctor if these symptoms occur. Explain why therapy must be closely monitored.

• Instruct the patient and his family about the prescribed exercise regimen. Make sure they understand how to perform each exercise and the importance of rest periods to avoid tiring the patient.

• If the patient needs surgery, explain preoperative and postoperative procedures to him and his family.

• If the patient needs home I.V. therapy, explain the procedure to him and his family.

GOUT

Also known as gouty arthritis, this metabolic disease is marked by monosodium urate deposits that cause red, swollen, and acutely painful joints. Gout may affect any joint but mostly affects those in the feet, especially the great toe, ankle, and midfoot.

Primary gout typically occurs in men over age 30 and in postmenopausal women who take diuretics. It follows an intermittent course that may leave patients symptom-free for years between attacks.

In asymptomatic patients, serum urate levels rise but produce no symptoms. In symptom-producing gout, the first acute attack strikes suddenly and peaks quickly. Although it may involve only one or a few joints, this attack causes extreme pain. Mild, acute attacks usually subside quickly yet tend to recur at irregular intervals. Severe attacks may persist for days or weeks.

Intercritical periods are the symptom-free intervals between attacks. Most patients have a second attack between 6 months and 2 years after the first; in some patients, however, the second attack is delayed for 5 to 10 years. Delayed attacks, which may be polyarticular, are more common in untreated patients. These attacks tend to last longer and produce more symptoms than initial

episodes. A migratory attack strikes various joints and the Achilles tendon sequentially and may be associated with olecranon bursitis.

Eventually, *chronic polyarticular gout* sets in. This final, unremitting stage of the disease (also known as tophaceous gout) is marked by persistent painful polyarthritis. An increased concentration of uric acid leads to urate deposits — called tophi — in cartilage, synovial membranes, tendons, and soft tissue.

Tophi form in the fingers, hands, knees, feet, ulnar sides of the forearms, pinna of the ear, Achilles tendon and, rarely, in such internal organs as the kidneys and myocardium. Renal involvement may adversely affect renal function.

Patients who receive treatment for gout have a good prognosis.

Causes

Although the underlying cause of primary gout remains unknown, in many patients the disease results from decreased renal excretion of uric acid. In a few patients, gout is linked to a genetic defect in purine metabolism that causes overproduction of uric acid (hyperuricemia).

Secondary gout develops during the course of another disease, such as obesity, diabetes mellitus, hypertension, polycythemia, leukemia, myeloma, sickle cell anemia, and renal disease. Secondary gout can also follow treatment with such drugs as hydrochlorothiazide or pyrazinamide.

Complications

Potential complications include renal disorders, such as renal calculi; circulatory problems, such as atherosclerotic disease, cardiovascular lesions, cerebrovascular accident, coronary thrombosis, and hypertension; and infection that develops with tophi rupture and nerve entrapment.

Assessment findings

Patient history may reveal that the patient has a sedentary life-style and a history of hypertension and renal calculi. He may report waking during the night with pain in his great toe or another location in the foot. He may complain that initially moderate pain has grown intense so that eventually he can't bear the weight of bedsheets or the vibrations of a person walking across the room. He may report accompanying chills and a mild fever.

Inspection typically reveals a swollen, dusky red or purple joint with limited movement. You may also notice tophi, especially in the outer ears, hands, and feet. (See

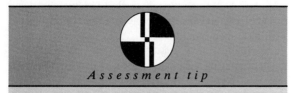

Assessment tip

RECOGNIZING GOUTY TOPHI

In advanced gout, urate crystal deposits develop into hard, irregular, yellow-white nodules called tophi. These bumps commonly protrude from the great toe and the pinna.

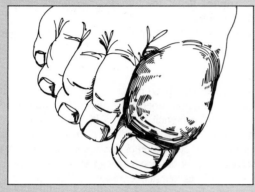

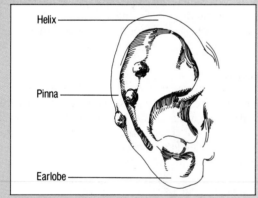

Helix

Pinna

Earlobe

Recognizing gouty tophi.) Late in the chronic stage of gout, the skin over the tophi may ulcerate and release a chalky white exudate or pus. Chronic inflammation and tophaceous deposits prompt secondary joint degeneration. Then erosions, deformity, and disability may develop.

Palpation may reveal warmth over the joint and extreme tenderness. The vital signs assessment may disclose fever and hypertension. If the patient has a fever, possible occult infection must be investigated.

Diagnostic tests

• *Needle aspiration* of synovial fluid (arthrocentesis) or of tophaceous material for examination under polarized light microscopy reveals needlelike intracellular crystals of sodium urate. Monosodium urate monohydrate crystals in synovial fluid that's been taken from an inflamed joint or tophus establishes the diagnosis. If test results identify calcium pyrophosphate crystals, the patient probably has pseudogout, a disease similar to gout. (See *Understanding pseudogout.*)
• *Serum uric acid levels* may be normal. However, the higher the level (especially when it's above 10 mg/dl) the more likely a gout attack.
• *Urine uric acid levels* are high in about 20% of gout patients.
• *X-ray studies* initially produce normal results. However, in chronic gout, X-ray findings show damage to the articular cartilage and subchondral bone. Outward displacement of the overhanging margin from the bone contour characterizes gout.

Treatment

Correct management has three goals:
• First, terminate the acute attack.
• Next, treat hyperuricemia to reduce urine uric acid levels.
• Finally, prevent recurrent gout and renal calculi.

Treatment of an acute attack consists of bed rest; immobilization and protection of the inflamed, painful joints; and local application of cold. Analgesics, such as acetaminophen, relieve the pain associated with mild attacks. Acute inflammation, however, requires nonsteroidal anti-inflammatory drugs or intramuscular corticotropin. Colchicine, oral or parenteral, or intra-articular corticosteroids are occasionally necessary to treat acute attacks.

Treatment of chronic gout involves decreasing the serum uric acid level to less than 6.5 mg/dl. This may be accomplished with various medications after a 24-hour urinalysis determines whether the patient overexcretes or underexcretes uric acid. If he overexcretes uric acid, he may be given allopurinol (in reduced doses if he has decreased renal function). If he underexcretes uric acid, he may be treated with probenecid or sulfinpyrazone (if he has no history of renal calculi). Taken once or twice daily, colchicine effectively prevents acute gout attacks, although it doesn't affect uric acid levels.

Adjunctive therapy emphasizes avoiding alcohol (especially beer and wine) and sparing use of purine-rich foods, such as anchovies, liver, sardines, kidneys, sweetbreads, and lentils. Obese patients should begin a weight-loss program because weight reduction will decrease uric acid levels and stress on painful joints as well.

Nursing diagnoses
- Anxiety
- Impaired physical mobility
- Ineffective individual coping
- Knowledge deficit
- Pain
- Risk for injury
- Sleep pattern disturbance

Nursing interventions
- To diffuse anxiety and promote coping mechanisms, encourage the patient to express his concerns about his condition. Listen supportively. Include him and his family in care-related decisions and all phases of care. Answer the patient's questions about his disorder as honestly as possible.
- Urge the patient to perform as much self-care as his immobility and pain allow. Provide him with adequate time to perform these activities at his own pace.
- Encourage bed rest, but use a bed cradle to keep bed linens off of sensitive, inflamed joints.
- Carefully evaluate the patient's condition after joint aspiration. Provide emotional support during diagnostic tests and procedures.
- Give pain medication, as needed, especially during acute attacks. Monitor the patient's response to this medication. Apply cold packs to inflamed joints to ease discomfort and reduce swelling.
- To promote sleep, administer pain medication at times that allow for maximum rest. Provide the patient with sleep aids, such as an extra pillow, a bath, or a back rub.
- Help the patient identify techniques and activities that promote rest and relaxation. Encourage him to perform them.
- Administer anti-inflammatory medication and other drugs, as ordered. Watch for adverse reactions. Be alert for GI disturbances if he takes colchicine.
- When forcing fluids, record intake and output accurately. Be sure to monitor serum uric acid levels regularly. As ordered, administer sodium bicarbonate or other agents to alkalinize the patient's urine.
- Provide a nutritious, but purine-poor diet.
- Watch for acute gout attacks 24 to 96 hours after surgery. Even minor surgery can trigger an attack. Before and after surgery, administer colchinine to help prevent gout attacks, as ordered.

UNDERSTANDING PSEUDOGOUT

Also known as calcium pyrophosphate disease, pseudogout results when calcium pyrophosphate crystals collect in periarticular joint structures.

Signs and symptoms
Like true gout, pseudogout causes sudden joint pain and swelling—most commonly of the knee, wrist, ankle, or other peripheral joints.

Pseudogout attacks are self-limiting and triggered by stress, trauma, surgery, severe dieting, thiazide therapy, or alcohol abuse. Associated symptoms resemble those of rheumatoid arthritis.

Establishing a diagnosis
Diagnosis of pseudogout hinges on joint aspiration and synovial biopsy to detect calcium pyrophosphate crystals. X-rays show calcium deposits in the fibrocartilage and linear markings along the bone ends. Blood tests may detect an underlying endocrine or metabolic disorder.

Relief for pressure and inflammation
Management of pseudogout may include aspirating the joint to relieve pressure; instilling corticosteroids and administering analgesics, salicylates, phenylbutazone, or other nonsteroidal anti-inflammatory drugs to treat inflammation; and, if appropriate, treating the underlying disorder.

Without treatment, pseudogout leads to permanent joint damage in about half of those it affects—most of whom are elderly people.

Patient teaching
- Urge the patient to drink plenty of fluids (up to 2 liters a day) to prevent renal calculi.
- Explain all treatments, tests, and procedures. Warn the patient before his first needle aspiration that it will be painful.
- Make sure the patient understands the rationale for evaluating serum uric acid levels periodically.
- Teach the patient relaxation techniques to use. Encourage him to perform them regularly.
- Instruct the patient to avoid purine-rich foods because these substances raise the urate level.
- Discuss the principles of gradual weight reduction with an obese patient. Explain the advantages of a diet containing moderate amounts of protein and little fat.
- If the patient receives allopurinol, probenecid, or other drugs, instruct him to report any adverse reactions immediately. (Reactions may include nausea, vomiting, drowsiness, dizziness, urinary frequency, and dermatitis.) Warn the patient taking probenecid or sulfinpyra-

zone to avoid aspirin or any other salicylate. Their combined effect causes urate retention.
• Inform the patient that long-term colchicine therapy is essential during the first 3 to 6 months of treatment with uricosuric drugs or allopurinol. Stress the importance of compliance.
• Urge the patient to control hypertension, especially if he has tophaceous renal deposits. Keep in mind that diuretics are not advised for the gout patient; alternative antihypertensives are preferred.

NEUROPATHIC ARTHROPATHY

Most common in men over age 40, neuropathic arthropathy (also called Charcot's arthropathy) is a progressively degenerative disease of peripheral and axial joints that results from impaired sensory innervation. Trauma or disease results in loss of sensation in the joint, which damages the supporting ligaments. Eventually, the affected joint disintegrates.

The specific joints affected vary. Diabetes mellitus usually attacks joints and bones of the feet. Tabes dorsalis affects large, weight-bearing joints, such as the knee, hip, ankle, or lumbar and dorsal vertebrae. Syringomyelia involves the shoulder, elbow, or cervical intervertebral joint. Neuropathic arthropathy caused by intra-articular corticosteroid injections may develop in the hip or knee joint.

Causes

In adults, the most common cause of neuropathic arthropathy is diabetes mellitus. Other causes include syringomyelia (which progresses to neuropathic arthropathy in about one of four patients), myelopathy of pernicious anemia, spinal cord trauma, paraplegia, hereditary sensory radicular neuropathy, and Charcot-Marie-Tooth disease. Rarely, tabes dorsalis, amyloidosis, peripheral nerve injury, myelomeningocele (in children), leprosy, or alcoholism cause neuropathic arthropathy.

Frequent intra-articular injection of corticosteroids has also been linked to neuropathic arthropathy. The analgesic effect of the corticosteroids may mask symptoms and allow continuous damaging stress to accelerate joint destruction.

Complications

Neuropathic arthropathy can lead to joint subluxation or dislocation, pathologic fractures, infection, pseudogout, or neurovascular compression.

Assessment findings

The patient's history may reveal an insidious onset, underlying neurologic disease, previous pathologic fractures, trauma and swelling in the affected area, and progressively worsening symptoms. Even with marked swelling over the joints, the patient may report no pain.

Inspection and other physical assessment techniques disclose extreme joint swelling, increased joint range of motion, joint deformity and instability, dislocation or subluxation, and loss of muscle tone around the joint.

Palpation may detect warmth or tenderness over the involved joints and loose objects and abnormal calcification in the joint. (The joint may feel like a "bag of bones.")

Diagnostic tests

• *X-rays* confirm the diagnosis and allow evaluation of damage. Early in the disease, soft-tissue swelling or effusion may be the only overt effect. Late in the disease, X-rays may display articular fracture, subluxation, and cartilaginous erosion; periosteal new bone formation; and excessive growth of marginal loose bodies (osteophytosis). Bone resorption also may be evident.
• *Vertebral examination* shows narrowed disk spaces, vertebral deterioration, and osteophyte formation, leading to ankylosis and deforming kyphoscoliosis.
• *Synovial biopsy* detects bony fragments and bits of calcified cartilage.
• *Neuromuscular tests* may reveal motor and sensory deficits and diminished deep tendon reflexes.

Treatment

Pain relief—the immediate treatment goal—may be achieved with analgesics, nonsteroidal anti-inflammatory drugs (NSAIDs), and joint immobilization (crutches, splints, braces, and weight-bearing restrictions). Surgical correction, such as joint fusion or amputation, may be necessary in severe disease although surgical treatment has a high failure rate because of nonunion, infection, or dislocation.

Nursing diagnoses

• Anxiety
• Fear
• Impaired physical mobility
• Risk for impaired skin integrity
• Risk for injury
• Self-care deficit

Nursing interventions

• Assist the patient to overcome anxiety and fear by expressing his feelings and concerns about his disorder. Listen, offering support and encouragement when appropriate. Include the patient and his family in all phases of his care. Answer questions as honestly as you can.

• Encourage the patient to perform as much self-care as his immobility and pain allow. Recognize that he may need extra time to perform activities at his own pace.

• Maintain neutral joint alignment. Apply splints and restrict weight bearing, as ordered.

• Assess the patient's pain pattern, and give analgesics, as needed. Monitor his response.

• Check sensory perception, range of motion, alignment, joint swelling, and the status of underlying disease.

• Assess the patient's skin regularly for breakdown.

Patient teaching

• Teach the patient joint protection techniques. Advise him to avoid physical stress that could cause pathologic fractures and to take safety precautions to avoid falls. Tell him to remove throw rugs and clutter from passageways.

• Instruct the patient to report severe joint pain, swelling, or instability. Suggest applying warm compresses to relieve local pain and tenderness.

• Teach the patient how to use crutches or other orthopedic devices. Stress the importance of proper fitting and regular professional readjustment of such devices. Forewarn him that impaired sensation might allow these aids to cause tissue damage without causing discomfort.

• Explain all treatments, tests, and procedures.

• Review prescribed medications and possible adverse reactions. Tell the patient to notify his doctor if adverse reactions persist.

• Urge the patient to continue with regular treatment of the underlying disease.

• As necessary, refer the patient to an occupational therapist or a home health nurse to help him cope with activities of daily living.

OSTEOARTHRITIS

The most common form of arthritis, osteoarthritis causes deterioration of the joint cartilage and formation of reactive new bone at the margins and subchondral areas of the joints. This chronic degeneration results from a breakdown of chondrocytes, most often in the hips and knees.

Osteoarthritis occurs equally in both sexes. More than half of people over age 30 have some features of primary osteoarthritis. And nearly all people over age 60 have radiographic evidence of the disorder, although fewer than half experience symptoms.

Depending on the site and severity of joint involvement, disability can range from minor limitation of the fingers to near immobility in persons with hip or knee disease. Progression rates vary; joints may remain stable for years in the early stage of deterioration.

Causes and pathophysiology

Primary osteoarthritis may be related to aging, although researchers don't understand why. This form of the disease seems to lack any predisposing factors. In some patients, however, it may be hereditary.

Secondary osteoarthritis usually follows an identifiable event—most commonly a traumatic injury or a congenital abnormality such as hip dysplasia. Endocrine disorders (such as diabetes mellitus), metabolic disorders (such as chondrocalcinosis), and other types of arthritis also can lead to secondary osteoarthritis. (See What happens in osteoarthritis, page 776.)

Complications

Osteoarthritis may cause flexion contractures, subluxation and deformity, ankylosis, bony cysts, gross bony overgrowth, central cord syndrome (with cervical spine osteoarthritis), nerve root compression, and cauda equina syndrome.

Assessment findings

The patient usually complains of gradually increasing signs and symptoms. He may report a predisposing event, such as a traumatic injury. Most commonly, the patient has a deep, aching joint pain, particularly after he exercises or bears weight on the affected joint. Rest may relieve the pain.

Additional complaints include stiffness in the morning and after exercise, aching during changes in weather, a "grating" feeling when the joint moves, contractures, and limited movement. These symptoms tend to be worse in patients with poor posture, obesity, or occupational stress.

Inspection may reveal joint swelling, muscle atrophy, deformity of the involved areas, and gait abnormalities (when arthritis affects the hips or knees). Osteoarthritis of the interphalangeal joints produces hard nodes on the distal and proximal joints. Painless at first, these nodes eventually become red, swollen, and tender. The fingers may become numb and lose their dexterity. (See Signs of osteoarthritis, page 777.)

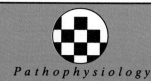

Pathophysiology

WHAT HAPPENS IN OSTEOARTHRITIS

The characteristic breakdown of articular cartilage is a gradual response to aging or predisposing factors, such as joint abnormalities or traumatic injury. The illustrations below will help you understand how osteoarthritis progresses.

Normal anatomy

Normally, bones fit together. Cartilage—a smooth, fibrous tissue—cushions the end of each bone, and synovial fluid fills the joint space. This fluid lubricates the joint and eases movement, much like brake fluid functions in a car.

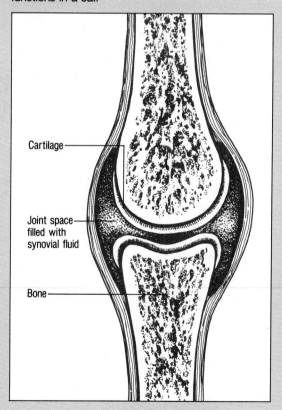

Cartilage

Joint space filled with synovial fluid

Bone

Early stage

Cartilage may begin to break down long before symptoms surface. In early osteoarthritis, the patient typically has no symptoms or has a mild, dull ache when he uses the joint. Rest relieves the discomfort. Or he may feel stiffness in the affected joint, especially in the morning. The stiffness usually lasts 15 minutes or less.

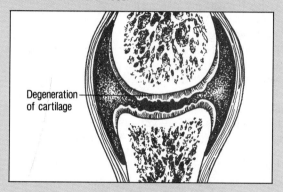

Degeneration of cartilage

Later stage

As the disease progresses, whole sections of cartilage may disintegrate, osteophytes (bony spurs) form, and fragments of cartilage and bone float freely in the joint. More common now, pain may be present even during rest. It typically worsens throughout the day. Movement becomes increasingly limited, and stiffness may persist even after limbering exercises.

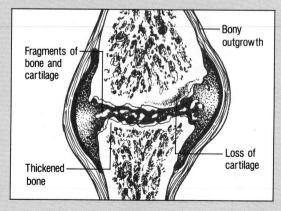

Fragments of bone and cartilage

Thickened bone

Bony outgrowth

Loss of cartilage

Palpation may reveal joint tenderness and warmth without redness, grating with movement, joint instability, muscle spasms, and limited movement.

Diagnostic tests

• *X-rays* of the affected joint may help confirm the diagnosis; however, findings may be normal in the early stages. X-ray studies may require many views and typically show a narrowing of the joint space or margin, cyst-like bony deposits in the joint space and margins, sclerosis of the subchondral space, joint deformity caused by degeneration or articular damage, bony growths at weight-bearing areas, and joint fusion in patients with erosive, inflammatory osteoarthritis.
• *Synovial fluid analysis* can rule out inflammatory arthritis.
• *Radionuclide bone scan* can also rule out inflammatory arthritis by showing normal uptake of the radionuclide.
• *Arthroscopy* identifies soft-tissue swelling by showing internal joint structures.
• *Magnetic resonance imaging* produces clear cross-sectional images of the affected joint and adjacent bones. Scan results also show disease progression.
• *Neuromuscular tests* may disclose reduced muscle strength (reduced grip strength, for example).

Treatment

To relieve pain, improve mobility, and minimize disability, treatment includes medications, rest, physical therapy, assistive mobility devices and, possibly, surgery.

Medications include aspirin and other salicylates and such nonsteroidal anti-inflammatory drugs as piroxicam, tolmetin, naproxen, indomethacin, fenoprofen, ibuprofen, and diclofenac. In some patients, intra-articular injections of corticosteroids may be necessary. Such injections, given every 4 to 6 months, may delay nodal development in the hands.

Adequate rest is essential and should be balanced with activity. Physical therapy includes massage, moist heat, paraffin dips for the hands, supervised exercise to decrease muscle spasms and atrophy, and protective techniques for preventing undue joint stress. Some patients may reduce stress and increase stability by using crutches, braces, a cane, a walker, a cervical collar, or traction. Weight reduction may help an obese patient.

In some instances, a patient with severe disability or uncontrollable pain may undergo surgery, including:
• *arthroplasty (partial or total)* — replacement of deteriorated part of joint with prosthetic appliance
• *arthrodesis* — surgical fusion of bones, used primarily in the spine (laminectomy)

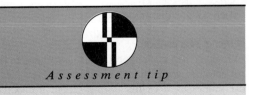

Assessment tip

SIGNS OF OSTEOARTHRITIS

Heberden's nodes appear on the dorsolateral aspect of the distal interphalangeal joints. Usually hard and painless, these bony and cartilaginous enlargements typically occur in middle-aged and elderly osteoarthritis patients. Bouchard's nodes, similar to Heberden's nodes but less common, appear on the proximal interphalangeal joints.

Heberden's nodes

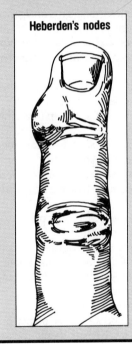

Bouchard's nodes

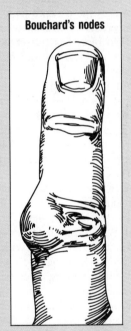

• *osteoplasty* — scraping and lavage of deteriorated bone from the joint
• *osteotomy* — excision or cutting of a wedge of bone (usually in the lower leg) to change alignment and relieve stress.

Nursing diagnoses

• Anxiety
• Body image disturbance
• Impaired physical mobility
• Ineffective individual coping
• Pain

• Self-care deficit
• Sleep pattern disturbance

Nursing interventions

• Provide emotional support and reassurance to help the patient cope with limited mobility. Give the patient opportunities to voice his feelings about immobility and nodular joints. Include him and his family in all phases of his care. Answer questions as honestly as you can.
• Encourage the patient to perform as much self-care as his immobility and pain allow. Provide him with adequate time to perform activities at his own pace.
• To help promote sleep, adjust pain medications to allow for maximum rest. Provide the patient with normal sleep aids, such as a pillow, bath, or back rub.
• Assess the patient's pain pattern, and give analgesics as needed. Monitor his response.
• Help him identify techniques and activities that promote rest and relaxation. Encourage him to perform them.
• Administer anti-inflammatory medication and other drugs, as ordered. Watch for adverse reactions.
• For joints in the hand, provide hot soaks and paraffin dips to relieve pain, as ordered.
• For lumbosacral spinal joints, provide a firm mattress (or bed board) to decrease morning pain.
• For cervical spinal joints, adjust the patient's cervical collar to avoid constriction; watch for irritated skin with prolonged use.
• For the hip, use moist heat pads to relieve pain. Administer antispasmodic drugs, as ordered.
• For the knee, assist with prescribed range-of-motion (ROM) exercises twice daily to maintain muscle tone. Also help perform progressive resistance exercises to increase the patient's muscle strength.
• Provide elastic supports or braces if needed.
• Check crutches, cane, braces, or walker for proper fit. A patient with unilateral joint involvement should use an orthopedic appliance (such as a cane or walker) on the normal side.

Patient teaching

• Instruct the patient to plan for adequate rest during the day, after exertion, and at night. Encourage him to learn and use energy conservation methods, such as pacing, simplifying work procedures, and protecting joints.
• Instruct him to take medications exactly as prescribed. Tell him which adverse reactions to report immediately.
• Advise against overexertion. Tell him that he should take care to stand and walk correctly, to minimize weight-bearing activities, and to be especially careful when stooping or picking up objects.
• Tell the patient to wear well-fitting support shoes and to repair worn heels.
• Tell him to have safety devices installed at home, such as grab bars in the bathroom.
• Teach him to do ROM exercises, performing them as gently as possible.
• Advise maintaining proper body weight to minimize strain on joints.
• Teach the patient how to use crutches or other orthopedic devices properly. Stress the importance of proper fitting and regular professional readjustment of such devices. Warn that impaired sensation might allow tissue damage from these aids without discomfort.
• Recommend using cushions when sitting. Also suggest using an elevated toilet seat. Both reduce stress when rising from a seated position.
• Positively reinforce the patient's efforts to adapt. Point out improving or stabilizing physical functioning.
• As necessary, refer the patient to an occupational therapist or a home health nurse to help him cope with activities of daily living.

BONE DISORDERS

Disorders affecting bone structure and function include osteomyelitis, osteoporosis, Legg-Calvé-Perthes disease, Osgood-Schlatter disease, Paget's disease, hallux valgus, kyphosis, herniated disk, and scoliosis.

OSTEOMYELITIS

A pyogenic bone infection, osteomyelitis may be chronic or acute. The disease commonly results from combined traumatic injury — usually minor but severe enough to cause a hematoma — and acute infection originating elsewhere in the body. Although osteomyelitis usually remains a local infection, it can spread through the bone to the marrow, cortex, and periosteum.

Typically a blood-borne disease, *acute osteomyelitis* most often affects rapidly growing children, particularly boys. The rarer *chronic osteomyelitis* is characterized by multiple draining sinus tracts and metastatic lesions. The incidence of both types of osteomyelitis is declining, except in drug abusers.

In children, the most common disease sites include the lower end of the femur and the upper end of the tibia, humerus, and radius. In adults, the disease commonly localizes in the pelvis and vertebrae and usually results from contamination related to surgery or trauma.

The prognosis for a patient with acute osteomyelitis is good if he receives prompt treatment. The prognosis for a patient with chronic osteomyelitis (more prevalent in adults) is poor.

Causes and pathophysiology

Infection causes osteomyelitis. Bacterial pyogens are the most common agents, but the disease also may result from fungi or viruses. The most common pyogenic organism in osteomyelitis is *Staphylococcus aureus*; others include *Streptococcus pyogenes, Pseudomonas aeruginosa, Escherichia coli,* and *Proteus vulgaris.*

Typically, these organisms find a culture site in a recent hematoma or a weakened area, such as a site of local infection (as in furunculosis). From there, they spread directly to bone. As the organisms grow and produce pus within the bone, pressure builds within the rigid medullary cavity and forces the pus through the haversian canals. A subperiosteal abscess forms, depriving the bone of its blood supply and eventually causing necrosis.

In turn, necrosis stimulates the periosteum to create new bone (involucrum). The old, dead bone (sequestrum) detaches and works its way out through an abscess or the sinuses. By the time the body processes sequestrum, osteomyelitis is chronic.

Complications

Osteomyelitis may lead to chronic infection, skeletal deformities, joint deformities, disturbed bone growth (in children), differing leg lengths, and impaired mobility.

Assessment findings

The patient's history may reveal a previous injury, surgery, or primary infection. The patient may complain of a sudden, severe pain in the affected bone and related chills, nausea, and malaise. He may describe the pain as unrelieved by rest and worse with motion.

The patient's vital signs may show tachycardia and a fever. Inspection may reveal swelling and restricted movement over the infection site. The patient may refuse to use the affected area. Palpation may detect tenderness and warmth over the infection site.

Usually, chronic and acute osteomyelitis have similar clinical features. However, chronic infection can persist intermittently for years, flaring up spontaneously after minor trauma. Sometimes the only sign of chronic infection is persistent pus drainage from an old pocket in a sinus tract.

Diagnostic tests

• *White blood cell (WBC) count* shows leukocytosis if the patient has osteomyelitis.
• *Erythrocyte sedimentation rate* rises in osteomyelitis.
• *Blood culture* can identify the pathogen.
• *X-rays* may show bone involvement only after the disease has been active for some time, usually 2 to 3 weeks.
• *Bone scans* can detect early infection.

Diagnosis must rule out poliomyelitis, rheumatic fever, myositis, and bone fractures.

Treatment

To decrease internal bone pressure and prevent infarction, treatment for acute osteomyelitis begins even before confirming the diagnosis. After drawing samples for blood culture, you'll typically administer high doses of I.V. antibiotics (usually a penicillinase-resistant agent, such as nafcillin or oxacillin). The infected site may be drained surgically to relieve pressure and remove sequestrum. Usually, the infected bone is immobilized with a cast or traction or by complete bed rest. The patient receives analgesics and I.V. fluids as needed. (See *Planning care for the patient with osteomyelitis,* pages 780 and 781.)

If an abscess forms, treatment includes incision and drainage, followed by a culture of the drainage. Anti-infective therapy may include systemic antibiotics; intracavitary instillation of antibiotics through closed-system continuous irrigation with low intermittent suction; limited irrigation with a blood drainage system equipped with suction (such as a Hemovac); or local application of packed, wet, antibiotic-soaked dressings.

Some patients may receive hyperbaric oxygen therapy to increase the activity of naturally occurring WBCs. Additional measures include using free tissue transfers and local muscle flaps to fill in dead space and increase blood supply.

Chronic osteomyelitis also may require surgery: sequestrectomy to remove dead bone and saucerization to promote drainage and decrease pressure. The typical patient reports great pain and requires prolonged hospitalization. Unrelieved chronic osteomyelitis in an arm or a leg may require amputation.

Nursing diagnoses

• Activity intolerance
• Anxiety
• Fear
• Fluid volume excess
• Impaired physical mobility

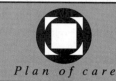

Plan of care

PLANNING CARE FOR THE PATIENT WITH OSTEOMYELITIS

When planning care, keep in mind that osteomyelitis commonly affects patients who've had an earlier traumatic injury. Consider, for instance, that you're caring for John Haas, a 28-year-old construction worker.

Patient history

When you meet Mr. Haas, he's angry. Last year a construction accident injured his left leg. He followed his doctor's instructions and seemed to recover well. But a few months ago, he bumped his leg. An ulcer developed, and it didn't go away—not even with repeated antibiotics and topical soaks. He tells you his leg is so swollen and painful that he can't work or even walk without a cane.

Mr. Haas tells you he played football in school and in a neighborhood league for about 10 years. He's had knee injuries, shin splints, sprained ankles, and bruised bones. But they all got better. This leg ulcer persists.

Assessment findings

Mr. Haas's oral temperature is 99.8° F (37.7° C). His blood pressure is 162/96 mm Hg. His pulse rate is irregular and rapid at 95 beats/minute. He breathes deeply and his respiratory rate is 24 breaths/minute.

Inspection reveals a stocky man, who weighs 240 lb (109 kg) and is 5'10" (178 cm) tall. His left lower leg appears red and slightly blue over the mid-tibia. Here the skin is taut and shiny. He can't bear any weight on the leg. You defer palpation of the leg when Mr. Haas asks you not to touch it.

Early test findings indicate a white blood cell count of 13,300/mm³. (Blood samples for culture are expected to confirm *Staphylococcus aureus* infection.) And X-rays of the left tibia show a large, irregular cavity filled with necrotic material.

The tentative diagnosis is osteomyelitis with sequestered, purulent osseous tissue in the cavity. Mr. Haas's doctor intends to remove the diseased tissue surgically, so Mr. Haas will need I.V. antibiotics now and heparin, analgesics, and stool softeners after surgery. He'll also need immobilization.

Nursing diagnoses

Using your assessment findings, you select these nursing diagnoses:
• Pain related to inflammation and swelling over the left tibia
• Impaired physical mobility related to non-weight-bearing on the left leg and postoperative bed rest
• Risk for injury related to possible deep vein thrombosis (DVT) developing during bed rest
• Ineffective individual coping with osteomyelitis.

Expected outcomes

You next devise care goals for Mr. Haas. He will:
• experience relief of left leg pain
• adapt to impaired mobility and participate in rehabilitation
• learn how to prevent DVT
• develop coping skills and comply with therapy.

Implementation

To ensure the best outcome for Mr. Haas, take these steps:

To relieve leg pain

• Handle the affected leg with extreme care when moving Mr. Haas

in bed, changing dressings, or applying the immobilizer.
• Place bed linens over a cradle to keep weight off the legs.
• Support the left knee and foot during elevation of the left leg.
• Provide warm soaks and wound treatment, as ordered; keep dressings as nonrestrictive as possible.
• Provide analgesics before Mr. Haas has severe pain or before each treatment or dressing change.
• Teach him to perform relaxation techniques, such as guided imagery and distraction. Help him practice these techniques.

To promote mobility and participation in rehabilitation

• Allow full upper-body assistance with activities of daily living.
• Encourage Mr. Haas to use an overbed trapeze while on bed rest.
• Provide a diet high in protein and vitamins C and D to promote healing and muscle strength.
• Explain the rationale for every treatment. Encourage his questions.
• Use pillows or towel rolls to maintain proper positioning and body alignment during strict bed rest.
• Encourage participation in physical therapy as soon as possible.

To reduce the risk of DVT

• During bed rest, assess circulation in both legs (from thigh to toe) every 4 hours. Record the findings.
• Administer heparin. Monitor partial thromboplastin time daily.
• Encourage Mr. Haas to change position at least every 2 hours.
• Place him on an air or a foam mattress to decrease pressure on skin.
• Supply at least 2,500 ml of fluids daily to decrease blood viscosity.
• Assist Mr. Haas with passive and active range-of-motion exercises for the legs as soon as possible.
• Discourage any positioning that would impede blood flow.

PLANNING CARE FOR THE PATIENT WITH OSTEOMYELITIS
(continued)

To improve coping and compliance
• Explain all treatments and procedures. Encourage questions. Let Mr. Haas help plan therapy schedules.
• Inform Mr. Haas that he may need to take medication after discharge. Point out that compliance can speed recovery and a return to work and normal activities.
• Involve Mr. Haas's family in all teaching related to treatment after discharge. Urge them to create a positive home environment.
• Assist Mr. Haas to plan and follow a weight-reduction diet and an exercise program when possible. These activities help strengthen damaged bone.
• Teach him to recognize signs of a recurrent infection. Instruct him to report any warmth, redness, or swelling of the left leg to his doctor as soon as possible.

• Encourage Mr. Haas to schedule and keep regular, follow-up appointments with his doctor.

Evaluation
To evaluate your care, consider if the infection is subsiding. Is Mr. Haas's wound draining sufficiently to heal properly? Does he have signs of DVT? Does he say that his pain is relieved? Is he able and willing to participate in self-care? Is he complying with therapy while in the hospital?

• Impaired tissue integrity
• Knowledge deficit
• Pain

Nursing interventions
• Focus care on controlling infection, protecting the bone from injury, and providing support.
• Encourage the patient to verbalize his concerns about his disorder. Offer support and encouragement. Include the patient and his family in all phases of his care. Answer questions as honestly as you can.
• Encourage the patient to perform as much self-care as his condition allows. Allow him adequate time to perform these activities at his own pace.
• Help the patient identify care techniques and activities that promote rest and relaxation. Encourage him to perform them.
• Use strict aseptic technique when changing dressings and irrigating wounds.
• If the patient is in skeletal traction for compound fractures, cover the pin insertion points with small, dry dressings. Tell the patient not to touch the skin around the pins and wires.
• Provide a diet high in protein and vitamin C to promote healing.
• Assess vital signs, wound appearance, and new pain (which may indicate secondary infection) daily.
• Carefully monitor drainage and suctioning equipment. Keep containers nearby that are filled with the irrigant being instilled. Monitor the amount of solution instilled and drained.
• Support the affected limb with firm pillows. Keep it level with the body; don't let it sag.

• Provide thorough skin care. Turn the patient gently every 2 hours, and watch for signs of developing pressure ulcers.
• Provide complete cast care. Support the cast with firm pillows, and petal the edges with pieces of adhesive tape or moleskin to smooth rough edges. Check circulation and drainage: If a wet spot appears on the cast, circle it with a marking pen, and note the time of appearance (on the cast). Be aware of how much drainage to expect. Keep in mind that one drop of blood can cause a 3″ (7.6 cm) stain on the cast. Check the circled spot at least every 4 hours. Assess increasing drainage and report as appropriate. Monitor vital signs for excessive blood loss.
• Protect the patient from mishaps, such as jerky movements and falls, which may threaten bone integrity. Tell him to report sudden pain, unusual bone sensations and noises (crepitus), or deformity immediately. Watch for any sudden malpositioning of the limb, which may indicate fracture.
• Assess the patient's pain pattern. Give analgesics, as needed. Monitor his response.

Patient teaching
• Explain all test and treatment procedures.
• Review prescribed medications. Discuss possible adverse reactions to drug administration, and instruct the patient to report them to the doctor.
• Before surgery, explain all preoperative and postoperative procedures to the patient and his family.
• Teach the patient techniques for promoting rest and relaxation. Encourage him to perform them.
• Before discharge, teach the patient how to protect and clean the wound site and, most importantly, how to recognize signs of recurring infection (elevated temperature, redness, localized heat, and swelling).

• Urge the patient to schedule follow-up examinations and to seek treatment for possible sources of recurrent infection—blisters, boils, sties, and impetigo.
• As necessary, refer the patient to an occupational therapist or a home health nurse to help him manage the activities of daily living.

OSTEOPOROSIS

In this metabolic bone disorder, the rate of bone resorption accelerates, and the rate of bone formation decelerates. The result: decreased bone mass. Bones affected by this disease lose calcium and phosphate and become porous, brittle, and abnormally vulnerable to fracture. Osteoporosis may be primary or secondary to an underlying disease.

Primary osteoporosis can be classified as idiopathic, type I, or type II. Idiopathic osteoporosis affects children and adults. Type I (or postmenopausal) osteoporosis usually affects women ages 51 to 75. Related to the loss of estrogen's protective effect on bone, type I osteoporosis results in trabecular bone loss and some cortical bone loss. Vertebral and wrist fractures are common. Type II (or senile) osteoporosis occurs most commonly between ages 70 and 85. Trabecular and cortical bone loss and consequent fractures of the proximal humerus, proximal tibia, femoral neck, and pelvis characterize type II osteoporosis.

Causes

The cause of primary osteoporosis is unknown. However, clinicians suspect these contributing factors:
• mild but prolonged negative calcium balance resulting from inadequate dietary intake
• declining gonadal adrenal function
• faulty protein metabolism caused by estrogen deficiency
• a sedentary life-style.

Secondary osteoporosis may result from prolonged therapy with steroids or heparin, bone immobilization or disuse (as occurs with hemiplegia), alcoholism, malnutrition, rheumatoid arthritis, liver disease, malabsorption, scurvy, lactose intolerance, hyperthyroidism, osteogenesis imperfecta, and Sudeck's atrophy (localized in hands and feet, with recurring attacks).

Complications

Bone fractures are the major complication of osteoporosis. They occur most commonly in the vertebrae, the femoral neck, and the distal radius.

Assessment findings

The history may typically disclose a postmenopausal patient or one with a condition known to cause secondary osteoporosis. The patient (usually an elderly woman) may report that she bent down to lift something, heard a snapping sound, and felt a sudden pain in her lower back. Or she may say that the pain developed slowly over several years. If the patient has vertebral collapse, she may describe a backache and pain radiating around the trunk. Any movement or jarring aggravates the pain.

Inspection may reveal that the patient has a humped back and a markedly aged appearance. She may report a loss of height. (See *Detecting height loss*.)

Palpation may reveal muscle spasm. The patient may also have decreased spinal movement with flexion more limited than extension.

Diagnostic tests

Differential diagnosis must exclude other causes of rarefying bone disease, especially those that affect the spine, such as metastatic carcinoma and advanced multiple myeloma.
• *X-ray studies* show characteristic degeneration in the lower thoracolumbar vertebrae. The vertebral bodies may appear flatter and denser than usual. Loss of bone mineral appears in later disease.
• *Serum calcium, phosphorus,* and *alkaline phosphatase levels* remain within normal limits.
• *Parathyroid hormone levels* may be elevated.
• *Transiliac bone biopsy* allows direct examination of osteoporotic changes in bone cells.
• *Computed tomography scan* allows accurate assessment of spinal bone loss.
• *Bone scans* that use a radionuclide agent display injured or diseased areas as darker portions.

Treatment

To control bone loss, prevent additional fractures, and control pain, treatment focuses on a physical therapy program of gentle exercise and activity and drug therapy to slow disease progress. Other treatment measures include supportive devices and, possibly, surgery.

Estrogen may be prescribed within 3 years after menopause to decrease the rate of bone resorption. Sodium fluoride may be given to stimulate bone formation. Calcium and vitamin D supplements may help to support normal bone metabolism. Calcitonin may be used to reduce bone resorption and slow the decline in bone mass.

Etidronate is the first agent proved to restore lost bone. Studies show that etidronate used for 2 weeks every 4 months increases bone mass.

Weakened vertebrae should be supported, usually with a back brace. Surgery (open reduction and internal fixation) can correct pathologic fractures of the femur. Colles' fracture requires reduction and immobilization (with a cast) for 4 to 10 weeks.

Nursing diagnoses

- Altered nutrition: Less than body requirements
- Body image disturbance
- Impaired physical mobility
- Knowledge deficit
- Pain
- Risk for impaired skin integrity
- Risk for injury
- Self-care deficit

Nursing interventions

- Design your care plan to consider the patient's fragility. Focus on careful positioning, ambulation, and prescribed exercises.
- Provide emotional support and reassurance to help the patient cope with limited mobility. Give her opportunities to voice her feelings. If possible, arrange for her to interact with others who have similar problems.
- Include the patient and her family in all phases of care. Answer questions as honestly as you can.
- Encourage the patient to perform as much self-care as her immobility and pain allow. Allow her adequate time to perform these activities at her own pace.
- Check the patient's skin daily for redness, warmth, and new sites of pain, which may indicate new fractures.
- Provide the patient with activities that involve mild exercise; help her to walk several times daily. As appropriate, perform passive range-of-motion exercises, or encourage her to perform active exercises. Make sure she attends scheduled physical therapy sessions.
- Impose safety precautions. Keep side rails up on the patient's bed. Move the patient gently and carefully at all times. Discuss with ancillary hospital personnel how easily an osteoporotic patient's bones can fracture.
- Provide a balanced diet rich in nutrients that support skeletal metabolism: vitamin D, calcium, and protein.
- Administer analgesics and heat to relieve pain, as ordered. Assess the patient's response.

Patient teaching

- Explain all treatments, tests, and procedures. For example, if the patient is undergoing surgery, explain all

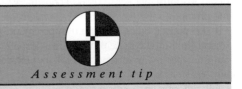

Assessment tip

DETECTING HEIGHT LOSS

Typically, a patient with osteoporosis loses height gradually. A condition known as dowager's hump (shown below) develops when repeated vertebral fractures increase the spinal curvature. (Although a hallmark of osteoporosis, this malformation may occur apart from the disease.)

Reduced thoracic and abdominal volumes, decreased exercise tolerance, pulmonary insufficiency, and abdominal protrusion may accompany height loss.

To assess height loss, have the patient stand with arms raised laterally and parallel to the floor. A measured difference exceeding 1½" (3.8 cm) between the patient's height and the distance across the outstretched arms (from longest fingertip to longest fingertip) suggests height loss.

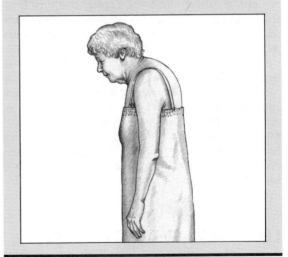

preoperative and postoperative procedures and treatments to the patient and her family.

- Make sure the patient and her family clearly understand the prescribed drug regimen. Tell them how to recognize significant adverse reactions. Instruct them to report them immediately.
- Teach the patient taking estrogen to perform breast self-examination. Tell her to perform this examination at least once a month and to report any lumps right away. Emphasize the need for regular gynecologic examina-

tions. Also instruct her to report abnormal vaginal bleeding promptly.

• If the patient takes a calcium supplement, encourage liberal fluid intake to help maintain adequate urine output and thereby avoid renal calculi, hypercalcemia, and hypercalciuria.

• Tell the patient to report any new pain sites immediately, especially after trauma.

• Advise the patient to sleep on a firm mattress and· to avoid excessive bed rest.

• Teach the patient how to use a back brace properly, if appropriate.

• Thoroughly explain osteoporosis to the patient and her family. If they don't understand the disease process, they may feel needless guilt, thinking that they could have acted to prevent bone fractures.

• Demonstrate proper body mechanics. Show the patient how to stoop before lifting anything and how to avoid twisting movements and prolonged bending.

• Encourage the patient to install safety devices, such as grab bars and railings, at home.

• Advise the patient to eat a diet rich in calcium. Give her a list of calcium-rich foods. Explain that type II osteoporosis may be prevented by adequate dietary calcium intake and regular exercise. Hormonal and fluoride treatments also may help prevent osteoporosis.

• Explain that secondary osteoporosis may be prevented by effectively treating underlying disease, early mobilization after surgery or trauma, decreased alcohol consumption, careful observation for signs of malabsorption, and prompt treatment of hyperthyroidism.

• Reinforce the patient's efforts to adapt, and show her how her condition is improving or stabilizing. As necessary, refer her to an occupational therapist or a home health nurse to help her cope with activities of daily living.

LEGG-CALVÉ-PERTHES DISEASE

Also called coxa plana, Legg-Calvé-Perthes disease is an avascular necrosis of the femoral head. Vascular interruption leads eventually to a flattened femoral head. Typically a unilateral condition, this disease occurs bilaterally in 15% of patients. It occurs most commonly in boys ages 4 to 10 and tends to recur in families.

The disease usually runs its four-stage course in 3 to 4 years. In the first stage, vascular interruption causes necrosis of the femoral head (usually in several months to a year). In the second stage, which may take 1 to 3 years, a new blood supply causes bone resorption and deposition of new bone cells. Deformity may result from pressure on the weakened area. In the third stage, new bone replaces necrotic bone and the femoral head gradually reforms. This process takes 1 to 3 years. The final, or residual, stage involves healing and regeneration, which fixes the joint's shape.

Causes
What causes this disease isn't known, but metabolic, infectious, or traumatic factors may be involved.

Complications
Legg-Calvé-Perthes disease may lead to permanent disability. It also may lead to premature osteoarthritis later in life from misalignment of the acetabulum and the flattened femoral head.

Assessment findings
The patient may have a family history of the disease. Typically, he has a limp that becomes progressively worse. He may complain of persistent pain in the groin, anterior thigh, or knee that's aggravated by activity and relieved by rest. These symptoms appear during the second stage, when bone resorption and deformity begin.

Inspection may disclose muscle atrophy in the upper thigh and slight shortening of the affected leg. Palpation may reveal restricted hip abduction and internal rotation and adductor muscle spasm in the affected hip.

Diagnostic tests
• *Range-of-motion tests* help to differentiate between Legg-Calvé-Perthes disease (restriction of only the abduction and rotation of the hip) and infection or arthritis (restriction of all motion).

• *X-rays* of the hip confirm the diagnosis. Findings vary with the disease's stage.

• *Magnetic resonance imaging* and *bone scan* reveal classic involvement of the anterolateral portion of the femoral head and can aid early diagnosis.

• *Aspiration and culture of synovial fluid* rule out joint sepsis.

Treatment
The aim of treatment is to retain the femoral head's normal shape. Typically, this is accomplished by containing the femoral head within the acetabulum to protect it from further stress and damage.

Methods of containing the femoral head include prolonged use of braces and casts and surgical correction. The use of braces and casts allows weight bearing while maintaining the femur in an abducted position to keep the head contained by the acetabulum. Conservative therapy lasts 2 to 4 years. Analgesics help relieve pain.

Surgical containment involves osteotomy and subtrochanteric derotation, which returns the femoral head to its normal shape and full range of motion. Proper placement of the epiphysis thus allows remolding with ambulation. Postoperatively, the patient requires a spica cast for about 2 months.

Surgical containment requires shorter treatment periods and less emphasis on compliance when compared with prolonged bracing or casting. However, controversy exists as to which containment method works best.

Nursing diagnoses
• Altered nutrition: Risk for more than body requirements
• Anxiety
• Diversional activity deficit
• Knowledge deficit
• Pain
• Risk for impaired skin integrity
• Self-care deficit

Nursing interventions
• Maintain adequate fluid balance, and provide a diet sufficient for growth. But make sure the diet doesn't cause excessive weight gain, which could make cast replacement necessary, interfering with corrective positioning.
• Provide diversional activity for the child, alternating periods of rest and play. Arrange for tutoring for a school-age child, if possible.
• Allow the patient to perform as much self-care as his immobility and pain allow. Give him time to perform these activities at his own pace.
• Provide thorough cast care. While the cast is still wet, turn the child every 2 to 3 hours to expose the cast to air. Use the palms of your hands rather than your fingers against the wet cast to avoid making depressions in it that could lead to pressure ulcers.
• After the cast dries, petal it with tape or moleskin. Change the petals as they become soiled. Protect the cast with a plastic cover during each bowel movement.
• Watch for complications. Check the child's toes for color, temperature, swelling, sensation, and motion; report dusky, cool, numb toes immediately. Check the skin under the cast with a flashlight every 4 hours while the patient is awake.
• Follow a consistent plan of washing, drying (use alcohol), and rubbing the skin under cast or brace edges to improve circulation and prevent skin breakdown. Never use oils or powders under the cast because they encourage skin breakdown and soften the cast. Check under

the cast daily for odors to detect skin breakdown or wound problems. Report persistent soreness.
• Administer analgesics, as ordered, and assess the patient's response.
• Relieve itching by using a hair dryer (set on cool) at the cast edges. This technique also decreases dampness from perspiration. If itching becomes excessive, obtain an order for an antipruritic.
• Provide emotional support to the child and his parents, and encourage them to express their concerns. Include them in all phases of care.

Patient teaching
• Explain all treatments, tests, and procedures to the patient and his family.
• Make sure that the patient and his family understand the rationale for braces and know how to apply and remove them properly.
• Teach the patient and his parents proper cast care. Tell them never to insert an object under the cast to scratch an itchy area. Discuss how to recognize signs of skin breakdown. Offer tips on ways to ease home management of the bedridden child. Tell parents which special supplies they'll need: pajamas and trousers a size larger than usual (opened at the side seam, with Velcro fasteners), a bedpan, adhesive tape, a moleskin and, possibly, a hospital bed.
• After the cast is removed, show the patient and his family how to gradually debride dry, scaly skin by applying lotion after bathing.
• Stress the need for follow-up care to monitor rehabilitation and for home tutoring and socialization to promote normal growth and development.
• As necessary, refer the patient to an occupational therapist or a home health nurse to help him cope with activities of daily living.

OSGOOD-SCHLATTER DISEASE
In the past, experts defined Osgood-Schlatter disease as osteochondritis caused by incomplete separation of the epiphysis of the tibial tubercle from the tibial shaft. Recently, however, researchers have concluded that it's a mechanical inefficiency of the extensor mechanism that causes tendinitis of the knee. It can affect one or both knees and is most common in active adolescent boys.

Causes
Osgood-Schlatter disease may result from traumatic avulsion of the proximal tibial tuberosity at the patellar tendon insertion.

Complications

This disease can cause irregular growth and partial avascular necrosis of the proximal tibial epiphysis. Without treatment, symptoms persist until the epiphyseal line of the upper end of the tibia closes.

Assessment findings

The patient may complain of constant aching, pain, swelling, and tenderness below the kneecap that worsens during activity. On inspection, you may see obvious soft-tissue swelling, and you may palpate localized heat and tenderness. Palpation may also reveal decreased flexibility and restriction in the hamstrings, triceps surae, and quadriceps muscle.

Another assessment technique involves forcing the tibia into internal rotation while slowly extending the patient's knee from 90 degrees of flexion. At about 30 degrees, such flexion produces pain that subsides immediately after externally rotating the tibia.

Diagnostic tests

X-ray findings may be normal or may show epiphyseal separation and soft-tissue swelling for up to 6 months after onset; eventually, they may show bone fragmentation.

Treatment

Essentially, treatment initially involves ice, nonsteroidal anti-inflammatory drugs, and avoidance of exercises that demand quadriceps contraction. In mild cases, simple restriction of predisposing activities (bicycling, running) may relieve symptoms. Rehabilitation exercises aim to treat inflexibility and to strengthen weak ankle dorsiflexion.

If the patient doesn't respond to this treatment, he may have his affected leg immobilized for 6 to 8 weeks with a reinforced elastic knee support, plaster cast, or splint. He won't have his leg fully immobilized unless his pain doesn't respond to more conservative treatment or he doesn't comply with treatment. Rarely, conservative measures fail and the patient needs surgery.

Nursing diagnoses

- Fear
- Impaired physical mobility
- Noncompliance
- Pain
- Self-care deficit

Nursing interventions

- Assess daily for limitation of movement.
- Administer analgesics, as needed, and assess the patient's response to them.
- Make sure the knee support or splint isn't too tight. If the patient has a cast, keep it dry and clean. Petal it to avoid skin irritation.
- Provide the patient with crutches, if needed.
- Monitor for muscle atrophy.
- If the patient needs surgery, monitor his circulation, sensation, and pain afterward, and watch for excessive bleeding.
- Encourage the patient to perform as much self-care as his immobility and pain allow. Give him time to perform these activities at his own pace. Whenever possible, include the family in the patient's care.
- Encourage the patient to express his concerns, and answer any questions. Remember that limiting normal activities is hard for an active teenager. Reassure him that restrictions are temporary.

Patient teaching

- Teach the patient about the prescribed exercise program, and stress the importance of following it. Make sure he understands his exercises and knows when and how often to do them.
- Teach the patient to use crutches, if needed.
- Stress the importance of protecting the injured knee by avoiding trauma and repeated flexion (from running, contact sports, and bicycling, for example).
- If the patient needs surgery, explain all preoperative and postoperative procedures and treatments to the patient and his family.

PAGET'S DISEASE

Also known as osteitis deformans, this slowly progressive metabolic bone disease is characterized by an initial phase of excessive bone resorption (osteoclastic phase), followed by a reactive phase of excessive abnormal bone formation (osteoblastic phase). The new bone structure, which is chaotic, fragile, and weak, causes painful deformities of the external contour and the internal structures.

Paget's disease usually affects one or several skeletal areas (most commonly the spine, pelvis, femur, and skull). Occasionally, the patient will have widely distributed skeletal deformity. In about 5% of patients, the involved bone will undergo malignant changes.

The disease can be fatal, particularly when associated with congestive heart failure (widespread disease creates a continuous need for high cardiac output), bone sarcoma, or giant cell tumors.

Paget's disease occurs worldwide but only rarely in Asia, the Middle East, Africa, and Scandinavia. In the United States, it affects about 2.5 million people over age 40, primarily men.

Causes

Although the disease's exact cause isn't known, one theory suggests that a slow or dormant viral infection (possibly mumps) causes a dormant skeletal infection, which surfaces many years later as Paget's disease.

Complications

Involved sites may fracture easily after only minor trauma. These fractures heal slowly and usually incompletely. Vertebral collapse or vascular changes that affect the spinal cord could lead to paraplegia. Bony impingement on the cranial nerves may cause blindness and hearing loss with tinnitus and vertigo.

Other complications include osteoarthritis, sarcoma, hypertension, renal calculi, hypercalcemia, gout, congestive heart failure, and a waddling gait (from softened pelvic bones).

Assessment findings

Clinical effects vary. The patient with early disease may be asymptomatic. As the disease progresses, he may report severe, persistent pain. If abnormal bone impinges on the spinal cord or sensory nerve root, he may complain of impaired mobility and pain increasing with weight bearing.

If the patient's head is involved, inspection may reveal characteristic cranial enlargement over the frontal and occipital areas. The patient may comment that his hat size has increased, and he may have headaches. Other deformities include kyphosis (spinal curvature caused by compression fractures of affected vertebrae) accompanied by a barrel-shaped chest and asymmetrical bowing of the tibia and femur, which typically reduces height. Palpation may detect warmth and tenderness over affected sites.

Diagnostic tests

• *X-ray studies* performed before overt symptoms develop show bone expansion and increased bone density.
• *Bone scans* (more sensitive than X-rays) clearly show early pagetic lesions (the radioisotope concentrates in areas of active disease).
• *Bone biopsy* may show bone tissue that has a characteristic mosaic pattern.

• *Red blood cell count* indicates anemia.
• *Serum alkaline phosphatase level* – an index of osteoblastic activity and bone formation – is elevated.
• *A 24-hour urinalysis* demonstrates elevated hydroxyproline levels. Hydroxyproline, an amino acid excreted by the kidneys, provides an index of osteoblastic hyperactivity.

Treatment

If the patient is asymptomatic, treatment isn't needed. The patient with symptoms requires drug therapy.

The hormone calcitonin may be given subcutaneously or intramuscularly. Although the patient will require long-term maintenance therapy with calcitonin, noticeable improvement occurs after the first few weeks of treatment. The patient also may receive oral etidronate to retard bone resorption (and relieve bone lesions) and to reduce serum alkaline phosphatase and urinary hydroxyproline excretion. Etidronate produces improvement after 1 to 3 months.

Plicamycin (a cytotoxic antibiotic used to decrease serum calcium, urinary hydroxyproline, and serum alkaline phosphatase levels) produces remission of symptoms within 2 weeks and biochemically detectable improvement in 1 to 2 months. However, plicamycin may destroy platelets or compromise renal function. So it's usually given only to patients who have severe disease, who require rapid relief, or who don't respond to other treatment.

Self-administration of calcitonin and etidronate helps patients with Paget's disease lead nearly normal lives. Even so, these patients may need surgery to reduce or prevent pathologic fractures, correct secondary deformities, and relieve neurologic impairment. To decrease the risk of excessive bleeding caused by hypervascular bone, drug therapy with calcitonin and etidronate or plicamycin must precede surgery. Joint replacement is difficult because methyl methacrylate (a glulike bonding material) doesn't set properly on bone affected by Paget's disease. Other treatments vary according to symptoms. Aspirin, indomethacin, or ibuprofen typically controls pain.

Nursing diagnoses

• Impaired home maintenance management
• Impaired physical mobility
• Knowledge deficit
• Pain
• Risk for impaired skin integrity
• Risk for injury

Nursing interventions

• Assess the patient's pain level daily to evaluate the effectiveness of analgesic therapy. Watch for new areas of pain or newly restricted movements—which may indicate new fracture sites—and sensory or motor disturbances, such as difficulty in hearing, seeing, or walking.

• Monitor serum calcium and alkaline phosphatase levels.

• If bed rest confines the patient for prolonged periods, prevent pressure ulcers with meticulous skin care. Reposition the patient frequently, and use a flotation mattress. Provide high-topped sneakers or a footboard to manage footdrop.

• Monitor intake and output. Encourage adequate fluid intake to minimize renal calculi formation.

Patient teaching

• Help the patient adjust to the life-style changes imposed by Paget's disease. Teach him to pace activities and, if necessary, to use assistive devices.

• Encourage the patient to follow a recommended exercise program. Urge him to avoid both immobilization and excessive activity.

• Suggest a firm mattress or a bed board to minimize spinal deformities.

• Explain all medications to the patient. Instruct him to use analgesic medications cautiously.

• To prevent falls at home, urge the patient to remove throw rugs and other small obstacles from the floor.

• Emphasize the importance of regular checkups, including the eyes and ears, to assess for complications.

• Demonstrate how to inject calcitonin properly and how to rotate injection sites. Caution the patient that adverse reactions may occur (including nausea, vomiting, local inflammatory reaction at the injection site, facial flushing, itchy hands, and fever). Reassure him that these reactions are usually mild and occur infrequently.

• Tell the patient receiving etidronate to take this medication with fruit juice 2 hours before or after meals (milk or other calcium-rich fluids impair absorption), to divide the daily dosage to minimize adverse reactions, and to watch for and report stomach cramps, diarrhea, fractures, and new or increasing bone pain.

• Instruct the patient receiving plicamycin to watch for signs of infection, easy bruising, bleeding, and temperature elevation. Urge him to schedule and report for regular follow-up laboratory tests.

• Refer the patient and his family to community support resources, such as a home health care agency and the Paget's Disease Foundation.

HALLUX VALGUS

A common, painful foot condition, hallux valgus involves lateral deviation of the great toe at the metatarsophalangeal joint. It occurs with medial enlargement of the first metatarsal head and bunion formation (bursa and callus formation at the bony prominence).

In congenital hallux valgus, abnormal bony alignment (an increased space between the first and second metatarsal known as metatarsus primus varus) causes bunion formation. In acquired hallux valgus, bony alignment is normal at the outset of the disorder.

Hallux valgus is more common in women.

Causes

Hallux valgus may be congenital or familial but is more often acquired from degenerative arthritis or prolonged pressure on the foot, especially from narrow-toed, high-heeled shoes, which compress the forefoot.

Complications

Deformity and pain may impair mobility.

Assessment findings

The patient may have a family history of hallux valgus, degenerative arthritis, or both. She may report prolonged pressure on the foot and chronic pain over a bunion. If she has marked hallux valgus, she may complain of pain over the second or third metatarsal heads because they're bearing more weight than they should.

Inspection shows a laterally deviated great toe, frequently associated with bunion formation. In an advanced stage, a flat, splayed forefoot may develop, with severely curled toes (hammertoes) and formation of a small bunion on the fifth metatarsal (see *Hammertoe*). On palpation, you'll note the characteristic tender bunion covered by deformed, hard, erythematous skin and palpable bursa, often distended with fluid.

Diagnostic tests

X-rays confirm the diagnosis by showing medial deviation of the first metatarsal and lateral deviation of the great toe.

Treatment

In the very early stages of acquired hallux valgus, proper shoes and foot care may eliminate the need for further treatment. Other useful measures for early management include felt pads to protect the bunion, foam pads or other devices to separate the first and second toes at night, and a supportive pad and exercises to strengthen the metatarsal arch. Early treatment is vital in patients predisposed to foot problems, such as those with rheumatoid arthritis.

If the disease progresses to severe deformity with disabling pain, the patient will need a bunionectomy. After surgery, the toe is immobilized in its corrected position one of two ways: with a soft compression dressing (which may cover the entire foot or just the great toe and the second toe and serves as a splint) or with a short cast (such as a light slipper spica cast).

The patient may need crutches or controlled weight bearing. Depending on the extent of the surgery, some patients walk on their heels a few days afterward; others must wait 4 to 6 weeks to bear weight on the affected foot. Supportive treatment may include physical therapy, such as warm compresses, soaks, and exercises, and analgesics to relieve pain and stiffness.

Nursing diagnoses
- Anxiety
- Fear
- Knowledge deficit
- Pain
- Risk for impaired mobility
- Risk for impaired skin integrity
- Self-care deficit

Nursing interventions
- Encourage the patient to perform as much self-care as her immobility and pain allow. Give her time to perform these activities at her own pace.
- Administer analgesics to relieve pain, as ordered.
- Before surgery, assess the foot's neurovascular status (temperature, color, sensation, blanching sign).
- After bunionectomy, apply ice to reduce swelling. Increase negative venous pressure and reduce edema by elevating the foot or supporting it with pillows.
- Record the neurovascular status of the patient's toes, including her ability to move them (taking into account the inhibiting effect of the dressing). Perform this check every hour for the first 24 hours, then every 4 hours. Report any change in neurovascular status to the doctor immediately.
- Prepare the patient for walking by having her dangle her foot over the bedside briefly before she gets up. This increases venous pressure gradually.
- Encourage the patient to express her concerns about her limited mobility, and offer support when appropriate. Answer any questions she may have. Give her positive reinforcement for her attempts to adapt to her condition, and point out how her condition is improving. Whenever possible, include the patient in care decisions.

HAMMERTOE

In this disorder, the toe assumes a clawlike position caused by hyperextension of the metatarsophalangeal joint, flexion of the proximal interphalangeal joint, and hyperextension of the distal interphalangeal joint, usually under pressure from hallux valgus displacement. This causes a painful corn on the back of the interphalangeal joint and on the bone end, and a callus on the sole of the foot, both of which make walking painful. Hammertoe may be mild or severe and can affect one toe or all five.

Hammertoe can be congenital and familial, or acquired from repeatedly wearing short, narrow shoes, which puts pressure on the end of the long toe. Acquired hammertoe is usually bilateral and commonly develops in children who rapidly outgrow their shoes and socks.

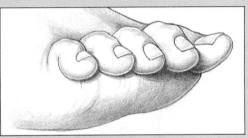

Treatment
In young children or adults with early deformity, repeated foot manipulation and splinting of the affected toe relieve discomfort and may correct the deformity. Other treatment includes protection of protruding joints with felt pads, corrective footwear (open-toed shoes and sandals, or special shoes that conform to the shape of the foot), a metatarsal arch support, and exercises, such as passive manual stretching of the proximal interphalangeal joint. Severe deformity requires surgical fusion of the proximal interphalangeal joint in a straight position.

Patient teaching
- If the patient needs crutches after surgery, teach her how to use them. Make sure she has a proper cast shoe or boot to protect the cast or dressing.
- Before discharge, instruct the patient to limit activities, to rest frequently with her feet elevated — especially when she feels pain or has edema — and to wear wide-toed shoes and sandals after the dressings are removed.

DEPICTING KYPHOSIS

The patient with kyphosis exhibits excessive vertebral curvature in the thoracic spine.

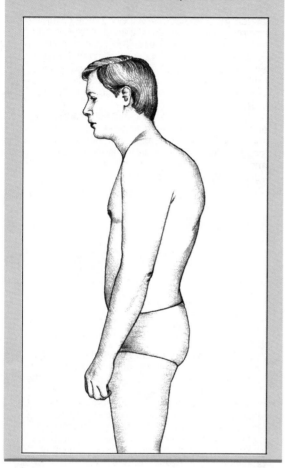

• Teach the patient proper foot care, including cleanliness and massages. Show her how to cut her toenails straight across to prevent ingrown nails and infection.
• Demonstrate exercises the patient can do at home to strengthen her foot muscles, such as standing at the edge of a step on her heel, then raising and inverting the top of her foot.
• Stress the importance of follow-up care and prompt medical attention for painful bunions or corns.
• If the patient needs surgery, explain all preoperative and postoperative procedures and treatments.

KYPHOSIS

Once known as roundback, kyphosis is an anteroposterior spinal curve that causes the back to bow, commonly at the thoracic level but sometimes at the thoracolumbar or sacral level. (See *Depicting kyphosis*.) The normal spine has a slightly convex shape, but excessive thoracic kyphosis is abnormal.

Kyphosis may occur in children and adults. Symptomatic adolescent kyphosis affects more girls than boys and is most common between ages 12 and 16.

Disk lesions (Schmorl's nodes) may develop in this disorder. These small fingers of nuclear material (from the nucleus pulposus) protrude through the cartilage plates and into the spongy bone of the vertebral bodies. If the protrusion destroys the anterior portions of cartilage, bridges of new bone may form at the intervertebral space and cause ankylosis.

Causes

Adolescent kyphosis (Scheuermann's disease, juvenile kyphosis, vertebral epiphysitis) is the most common form. No one knows what causes this disease, although some think it results from growth retardation or a vascular disturbance in the vertebral epiphysis (usually at the thoracic level) during rapid growth periods. Other suspected causes include infection, inflammation, aseptic necrosis, and disk degeneration, with the subsequent stress of weight bearing on compromised vertebrae, resulting in the thoracic hump seen in adolescents with kyphosis.

Adult kyphosis (adult roundback) may result from aging and associated intervertebral disk degeneration, atrophy, and vertebral collapse from osteoporosis. The condition also may result from such endocrine disorders as hyperparathyroidism and Cushing's disease or from prolonged steroidal therapy. Additional possible causes include arthritis, Paget's disease, poliomyelitis, compression fractures of the thoracic vertebrae, metastatic tumor, plasma cell myeloma, or tuberculosis.

In both children and adults, kyphosis may result from poor posture. Rarely, congenital kyphosis occurs. This usually severe condition produces cosmetic deformity and reduces pulmonary function.

Complications

Kyphosis may result in pulmonary complications or neurologic damage, such as spastic paraparesis secondary to spinal cord compression or herniated nucleus pulposus.

Assessment findings

Adolescents with kyphosis may report a history of excessive athletic activity. Adults with kyphosis may have an associated primary condition. Patients in either group may have poor posture.

In about half of affected adolescents, kyphosis may produce mild pain at the apex of the spinal curve. Some patients complain of fatigue, tenderness, or stiffness in the involved area or along the entire spine. Adult patients may also report pain, a weak back, and fatigue.

Inspection may reveal poor posture and increased thoracic curvature when the patient stands or bends forward. You may notice varying degrees of curvature and in some patients, compensatory lordosis (increased lumbar curvature). In adolescent and adult forms of kyphosis that are not due to poor posture alone, the spinal curve will not straighten when the patient lies down.

During palpation, you'll rarely discover local tenderness in adult patients (unless the patient also has senile osteoporosis with recent compression fracture). However, local tenderness is common in adolescent patients.

Diagnostic tests

Adolescent kyphosis must be distinguished from tuberculosis and other inflammatory or neoplastic diseases that cause vertebral collapse. The severe pain, bone destruction, and systemic symptoms common with these diseases help to rule out a diagnosis of kyphosis.

X-ray studies may show vertebral wedging, Schmorl's nodes, irregular end plates and, possibly, a 10- to 20-degree scoliotic curve.

Treatment

For kyphosis caused by poor posture alone, treatment may consist of therapeutic exercises, bed rest on a firm mattress (with or without traction), and a brace to correct the spinal curve until the patient stops growing.

Corrective exercises include pelvic tilt to decrease lumbar lordosis, hamstring stretch to overcome muscle contractures, and thoracic hyperextension to flatten the kyphotic curve. Exercises may be performed with or without the brace. Lateral X-rays (every 4 months) can evaluate the success of correction. Gradual weaning from the brace can begin after the spine reaches full skeletal maturity and after X-rays demonstrate maximum curve correction and decreased vertebral wedging.

Other treatment for adolescent and adult kyphosis includes management of the underlying disease and spinal arthrodesis to relieve symptoms. Surgery is rarely necessary unless kyphosis causes neurologic damage, a spinal curve over 60 degrees, or intractable and disabling back pain in a skeletally mature patient.

Preoperative measures may include traction. Corrective surgery may involve a posterior spinal fusion (with spinal instrumentation, iliac bone grafting, and plaster casting for immobilization) or an anterior spinal fusion (followed by casting) if kyphosis produces a spinal curve over 70 degrees.

Nursing diagnoses
- Anxiety
- Body image disturbance
- Diversional activity deficit
- Pain
- Risk for impaired skin integrity
- Risk for injury

Nursing interventions
- After surgery, check the patient's neurovascular status every 2 to 4 hours for the first 48 hours, and report any changes immediately. Turn the patient often, using the logroll method.
- If patient-controlled analgesia is not used, offer an analgesic every 3 to 4 hours.
- Maintain fluid balance and monitor for ileus.
- Check the patient's neurologic status every 2 hours.
- Maintain adequate ventilation and oxygenation.
- Encourage family support. For an adolescent patient, suggest that family members supply diversional activities. For an adult patient, arrange for alternating periods of rest and activity.
- If the patient requires a brace, check its condition daily. Look for worn or malfunctioning parts. Carefully assess how the brace fits the patient. Keep in mind that weight changes may alter proper fit.
- Give meticulous skin care. Check the skin at the cast edges several times daily; use heel and elbow protectors to prevent skin breakdown. Remove antiembolism stockings, if ordered, at least three times a day for at least 30 minutes. Change dressings as ordered.
- Provide emotional support. Urge the patient and family members to voice their concerns, and answer their questions honestly. Expect more mood changes and depression in the adolescent patient than in the adult patient. Keep communication lines open. Offer frequent encouragement and reassurance.
- Assess the patient's readiness to make decisions, and include him in care-related decisions. As possible, include the family in all phases of patient care.
- Assist during suture removal and new cast application (usually about 10 days after surgery). Encourage gradual

ambulation (usually beginning with a tilt table in the physical therapy department). As needed, arrange for follow-up care with a social worker and a home health nurse.

Patient teaching
• For the adolescent patient with kyphosis caused by poor posture, outline the fundamentals of good posture, and demonstrate prescribed exercises. Have the patient perform a return demonstration if appropriate. Suggest bed rest to relieve severe pain. Encourage him to use a firm mattress, preferably with a bed board.
• If the patient has a cast, provide detailed, written cast care instructions at discharge. Tell him to immediately report pain, burning, skin breakdown, loss of feeling, tingling, numbness, or cast odor. Urge him to drink plenty of liquids to avoid constipation and to report any illness (especially abdominal pain or vomiting) immediately. Show him how to use proper body mechanics to minimize strain on the spine. Warn him not to lie on his stomach or on his back with his legs flat.
• If the patient is discharged with a brace, explain its purpose and tell him how and when to wear it. Make sure he understands how to check it daily for proper fit and function. Teach him to perform proper skin care. Advise against using lotions, ointments, or powders that can irritate the skin where it comes in contact with the brace. Warn that only the doctor or orthotist should adjust the brace.

HERNIATED DISK
Also known as a herniated nucleus pulposus or a slipped disk, a herniated disk occurs when all or part of the nucleus pulposus—an intervertebral disk's gelatinous center—extrudes through the disk's weakened or torn outer ring (anulus fibrosus). The resultant pressure on spinal nerve roots or on the spinal cord itself causes back pain and other symptoms of nerve root irritation.

About 90% of herniations affect the lumbar (L) and lumbosacral spine; 8% occur in the cervical (C) spine and 1% to 2% in the thoracic spine. The most common site for herniation is the L4-L5 disk space. Other sites include L5-S1, L2-L3, L3-L4, C6-C7, and C5-C6.

Lumbar herniation usually develops in people ages 20 to 45 and cervical herniation in those age 45 or older. Herniated disks affect more men than women.

Causes and pathophysiology
Herniated disks may result from severe trauma or strain, or they may be related to intervertebral joint degenera-

tion. In an elderly person with degenerative disk changes, minor trauma may cause herniation. A person with a congenitally small lumbar spinal canal or with osteophytes along the vertebrae may be more susceptible to nerve root compression with a herniated disk. This person is also more likely to exhibit neurologic symptoms. (See *How a herniated disk develops.*)

Complications
Neurologic deficits (most common) and bowel and bladder problems (with lumbar herniations) are complications of herniated disk.

Assessment findings
Initially, the patient may seek relief for usually unilateral, low back pain radiating to the buttocks, legs, and feet. Typically, he may report a previous traumatic injury or back strain.

When herniation follows trauma, the patient may tell you that the pain began suddenly, subsided in a few days, and then recurred at shorter intervals and progressive intensity. He may then describe sciatic pain that began as a dull ache in the buttocks and that grows with Valsalva's maneuver, coughing, sneezing, or bending. He may also complain of accompanying muscle spasms and may add that the pain subsides with rest.

Inspection may reveal a patient with limited ability to bend forward and a posture favoring the affected side. In later stages, you may observe muscle atrophy. Palpation may disclose tenderness over the affected region.

Tissue tension assessment may reveal radicular pain from straight leg raising (with lumbar herniation) and increased pain from neck movement (with cervical herniation).

Thorough assessment of the patient's peripheral vascular status—including posterior tibial and dorsalis pedis pulses and skin temperature of the arms and legs—may help to rule out ischemic disease as the cause of leg pain or numbness. (See *Two tests for a herniated disk*, page 794.)

Diagnostic tests
• *X-ray studies* of the spine are essential to show degenerative changes and to rule out other abnormalities. Films may not show a herniated disk because even marked disk prolapse may show up as normal on an X-ray.
• *Myelography* pinpoints the level of the herniation.
• *Computed tomography scan* detects bone and soft-tissue abnormalities. It can also show spinal canal compression that results from herniation.

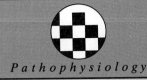

Pathophysiology

HOW A HERNIATED DISK DEVELOPS

A spinal disk has two parts: the soft center called the nucleus pulposus and the tough, fibrous, surrounding ring called the anulus fibrosus. The nucleus pulposus acts as a shock absorber, distributing the mechanical stress applied to the spine when the body moves.

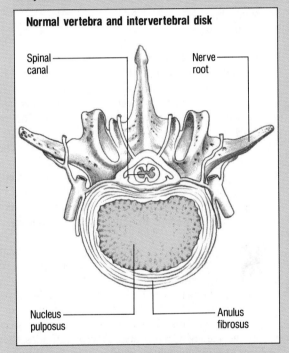

Normal vertebra and intervertebral disk

Spinal canal

Nerve root

Nucleus pulposus

Anulus fibrosus

Physical stress—usually a twisting motion—can cause the anulus fibrosus to tear or rupture, allowing the nucleus pulposus to push through (herniate) into the spinal canal. This process allows the vertebrae to move closer together as the disk compresses. This, in turn, causes pressure on the nerve roots as they exit between the vertebrae. Pain and, possibly, sensory and motor loss follow.

A herniated disk can also occur with intervertebral joint degeneration. If the disk has begun to degenerate, minor trauma may cause herniation.

Herniation occurs in three stages: protrusion, extrusion, and sequestration.

Protrusion
The nucleus pulposus presses against the anulus fibrosus.

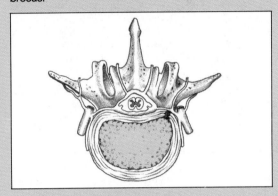

Extrusion and sequestration
The nucleus pulposus bulges forcefully through the anulus fibrosus, pushing against the nerve root. Then, the anulus fibrosus gives way as the disk's core bursts through to press against the nerve root.

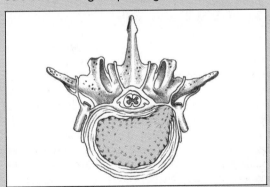

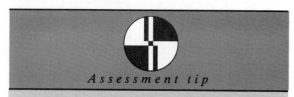

Assessment tip

TWO TESTS FOR A HERNIATED DISK

The straight-leg-raising test and its variant, La-sègue's test, are perhaps the best tests for a herniated disk.

Straight-leg-raising test
Have the patient lie in the supine position. Place one hand on the patient's ilium to stabilize the pelvis and the other hand under the patient's ankle. Slowly raise the patient's leg. If the patient complains of posterior leg (sciatic) pain—*not back pain*—suspect a herniated disk.

Lasègue's test
To do this test, have the patient lie supine with his thigh and knee flexed (to a 90-degree angle). Resistance and pain as well as loss of ankle or knee-jerk reflex indicate spinal root compression.

• *Magnetic resonance imaging* defines tissues in areas usually obscured by bone on other imaging tests, such as those done with X-rays.
• *Electromyography* confirms nerve involvement by measuring the electrical activity of muscles innervated by the herniated disk.
• *Neuromuscular tests* can detect sensory and motor loss and leg muscle weakness as well.

Treatment
Unless neurologic impairment progresses rapidly, initial treatment is conservative, consisting of bed rest (possibly with pelvic traction) for several weeks; supportive devices (such as a brace); heat or ice applications; and exercise. Nonsteroidal anti-inflammatory drugs reduce inflammation and edema at the injury site. Steroidal drugs, such as dexamethasone, may be prescribed for the same purpose. Muscle relaxants (diazepam or methocarbamol) may help also.

A herniated disk that fails to respond to conservative treatment may require surgery. The most common procedure, laminectomy, involves removing a portion of the lamina and the protruding nucleus pulposus. If laminectomy doesn't alleviate pain and disability, the patient may undergo spinal fusion to stabilize the spine. Lam-

inectomy and spinal fusion may be performed concurrently.

Percutaneous automated diskectomy is another alternative. Guided by X-ray visualization, the doctor suctions out the disk portion that causes pain. Typically used for smaller, less severe disk abnormalities, this procedure succeeds about 50% of the time.

Nursing diagnoses
• Activity intolerance
• Anxiety
• Fear
• Impaired physical mobility
• Pain
• Risk for injury
• Self-care deficit

Nursing interventions
• Assess the patient's pain. With the patient and the doctor, plan a pain-control regimen, using such methods as relaxation, transcutaneous electrical nerve stimulation, distraction, heat or ice application, traction, bracing, or positioning in addition to analgesics and muscle relaxants. Give pain medications, as ordered, and assess the patient's response.
• Offer supportive care, careful patient teaching, and encouragement to help the patient cope with the discomfort and frustration of chronic back pain and impaired mobility. Include the patient and his family in all phases of his care.
• Encourage the patient to verbalize his concerns about his disorder. Answer any questions the patient may have as honestly as you can.
• Encourage the patient to perform as much self-care as his immobility and pain allow. Provide him with adequate time to perform these activities at his own pace.
• Help the patient identify and perform activities that promote rest and relaxation.
• If the patient will undergo myelography, question him carefully about allergies to iodides, iodine-containing substances, or seafood because such allergies may indicate sensitivity to a radiopaque contrast agent used in the test. Monitor intake and output. Watch for seizures and an allergic reaction.
• If the patient is in traction, ensure that the pelvic straps are properly positioned and that the weights are suspended. Periodically remove the traction to inspect skin. Also, remember to monitor for deep vein thrombosis.
• During conservative treatment, watch for any deterioration in neurologic status (especially during the first 24

hours after admission), which may indicate an urgent need for surgery. Use antiembolism stockings, as prescribed, and encourage the patient to move his legs, as allowed. Provide high-topped sneakers or a footboard to prevent footdrop. Work closely with the physical therapy department to ensure a consistent regimen of leg- and back-strengthening exercises. Give plenty of fluids to prevent urinary stasis. Remind the patient to cough, breathe deeply, or blow into bottles or an incentive spirometer to avoid pulmonary complications. Provide thorough skin care. Assess bowel function, and provide a fracture bedpan for the patient on complete bed rest.

• After laminectomy, microdiskectomy, or spinal fusion, enforce bed rest, as ordered. If the patient has a blood drainage system (Hemovac) in use, check the tubing frequently for patency and a secure vacuum seal. Empty the system at the end of each shift, as ordered, and record the amount and color of drainage. Report colorless moisture on dressings (possible cerebrospinal fluid leakage) or excessive drainage immediately. Check the neurovascular status of the patient's legs (color, motion, temperature, sensation).

• Monitor vital signs, and check for bowel sounds and abdominal distention. Use the logrolling technique to turn the patient. Administer analgesics, as ordered, especially about 30 minutes before initial attempts to sit or walk. Assist the patient during his first attempt to walk. Provide a straight-backed chair, and allow him to sit in it briefly.

Patient teaching

• Teach the patient about treatments, which may include bed rest and pelvic traction; heat application to the area to decrease pain; an exercise program; medications to decrease pain, inflammation, and muscle spasms; and surgery.

• Before myelography, reinforce previous explanations of the need for this test, and tell the patient to expect some pain. Assure him that he'll receive a sedative before the test, if needed, to keep him as calm and comfortable as possible. After the test, urge the patient to remain in bed with his head elevated (especially if metrizamide was used) and to drink plenty of fluids.

• If surgery is required, explain all preoperative and postoperative procedures and treatments to the patient and his family.

• Prepare the patient for discharge. (See *Coping with a herniated disk.*)

Home care

COPING WITH A HERNIATED DISK

Follow these guidelines for a home care patient with a herniated disk.

• Discuss all medications with the patient and his caregiver. Describe adverse reactions, especially those that require immediate attention. If the patient must take a muscle relaxant, tell him to avoid activities that require alertness until he develops a tolerance to the drug's sedative effects.

• Refer the patient to an occupational therapist.

• Teach him relaxation techniques.

• Encourage the patient to maintain an appropriate body weight, and discuss proper nutrition.

• Reinforce proper body mechanics; instruct the patient to lie on his side, not his abdomen. Recommend an extra firm mattress or a bed board.

• If the patient must wear a brace, advise him to prevent skin breakdown by not using lotions, ointments, or powders on areas where the brace touches the skin. Suggest rubbing alcohol or tincture of benzoin on these areas to toughen the skin. Tell him to keep the skin dry and clean and to wear a snug-fitting T-shirt under the brace.

SCOLIOSIS

In this lateral curvature of the spine, the vertebrae rotate into the convex part of the curve. This rotation causes rib prominence along the thoracic spine and waistline asymmetry in the lumbar spine. Although scoliosis can affect the spine at any level, right thoracic curves are most common.

Idiopathic scoliosis affects fewer than 1% of school-age children and arises most commonly during the growth spurt between ages 10 and 13. It affects boys and girls equally; however, spinal curve progression is more common in girls.

The disorder can be classified as nonstructural or structural. In *nonstructural scoliosis,* the spinal curve appears flexible, straightening temporarily when the patient leans sideways. In contrast, *structural scoliosis* is a fixed deformity that doesn't correct itself when the patient leans sideways.

Scoliosis is also classified by age of onset as infantile, juvenile, or adolescent. *Infantile scoliosis* is most common in boys ages 1 to 3. It may resolve spontaneously or it may progress and require treatment. *Juvenile scoliosis* affects boys and girls ages 3 to 10 about equally. This disorder usually requires long-term follow-up and treatment during the peak growing years. *Adolescent scoliosis* occurs after age 10 and during adolescence.

Causes

Nonstructural scoliosis is commonly related to leg-length discrepancies, poor posture, paraspinal inflammation, or acute disk disease.

Structural scoliosis has no known cause, but it may stem from a congenital or a neuromuscular problem. The disorder affects otherwise healthy children for no known reason.

In congenital structural scoliosis, the vertebrae or the rib cage develops abnormally before birth, making the spine more likely to curve. Common abnormalities include wedge-shaped and block (unseparated) vertebrae. Spinal abnormalities can occur separately or together to cause abnormal curvature. Sometimes multiple spinal abnormalities balance each other, making treatment unnecessary.

Neuromuscular scoliosis may be caused by spinal muscles weakened by Duchenne's muscular dystrophy (marked by a long C-shaped spinal curve), polio, cerebral palsy, or spinal muscular atrophy.

Some types of scoliosis fit no specific category, such as that resulting from neurofibromatosis (Recklinghausen's disease). Traumatic scoliosis may derive from vertebral fractures or disk disease. Degenerative scoliosis may develop in older patients with osteoporosis and degenerative joint disease of the spine.

Complications

Untreated or inadequately treated extreme spinal curvature can eventually result in debilitating back pain and severe deformity. Thoracic curves exceeding 60 degrees may decrease pulmonary function; those exceeding 80 degrees heighten the patient's risk for cor pulmonale in middle age.

Assessment findings

The patient history may reveal a family history of scoliosis. Typically, the disorder is detected during a community or school scoliosis screening program or as part of a routine checkup. A parent may notice that the child's hemlines look uneven, pant legs appear unequal in length, or one hip rises higher than the other. Scoliosis rarely produces symptoms until it's well established; then symptoms include backache, fatigue, and dyspnea.

Inspection may reveal signs of scoliosis. (See *Testing for scoliosis.*) For example, to assess thoracic (or trunk) alignment, hold a plumb line (a string with an attached weight) while the patient stands with her back toward you. The plumb line should fall perpendicularly from the center of her head to the cervical spine at C7, through the coccyx (between the gluteal folds), to an area between the feet. Any other angle suggests scoliosis.

Diagnostic tests

• *Spinal X-ray studies,* including anterior, posterior, and lateral views taken with the patient standing upright and bending, confirm scoliosis and help determine the degree of curvature and flexibility of the spine. X-rays also help determine skeletal maturity, predict remaining bone growth, and show whether the patient has nonstructural or structural scoliosis.
• *Bone growth studies,* though not diagnostic, may help to determine skeletal maturity.

Treatment

The severity of the deformity and potential spine growth determine appropriate treatment, which may include close observation, exercise, a brace, surgery, or a combination of these. Therapy aims to begin early, while spinal deformity remains subtle. A mild curve of less than 20 degrees should be monitored by X-ray studies and an examination every 3 months. If the curve progresses between 5 degrees and 10 degrees and if the patient is still growing, the doctor may recommend a brace. An exercise program that includes sit-up pelvic tilts, spine hyperextension, push-ups, and breathing exercises may strengthen torso muscles.

A 20- to 40-degree curve requires management with spinal exercises and a brace to prevent the curve from progressing. Lateral electrical surface stimulation (LESS) to stimulate the spinal muscles may be helpful and can be used while the patient sleeps. Electrodes lead to a battery pack, and the device stimulates the paraspinal muscles with a mild electrical charge. This current "pulls" muscles away from the curve, theoretically preventing the curve progression.

Usually, a brace halts progression in most patients but doesn't reverse the established curvature. Such devices passively strengthen the patient's spine by applying asymmetrical pressure to skin, muscles, and ribs. Braces can be adjusted as the patient grows and can be worn until bone growth is complete.

A curve of 40 degrees or more requires surgery (spinal fusion with instrumentation) because such a lateral curve continues to progress at the rate of 1 degree a year even after the patient reaches skeletal maturity.

Surgery corrects lateral curvature by posterior spinal fusion and internal stabilization with various rods and

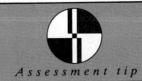

Assessment tip

TESTING FOR SCOLIOSIS

If you're assessing your patient for an abnormal spinal curve, use this screening test for scoliosis. Have the patient remove her shirt and stand as straight as she can with her back to you. Instruct her to distribute her weight evenly on each foot. While the patient does this, observe both sides of her back from neck to buttocks. Look for these signs:
• uneven shoulder height and shoulder blade prominence
• unequal distance between the arms and the body
• asymmetrical waistline
• uneven hip height
• a sideways lean.

   With the patient's back still facing you, ask the patient to do the "forward-bend" test. In this test the patient places her palms together and slowly bends forward, remembering to keep her head down. As she complies, check for these signs:
• asymmetrical thoracic spine or prominent rib cage (rib hump) on either side
• asymmetrical waistline.

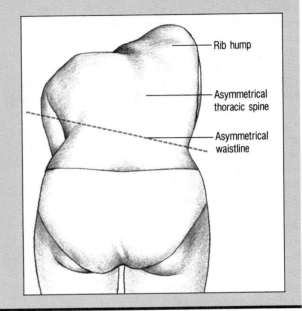

Rib hump

Asymmetrical thoracic spine

Asymmetrical waistline

spinal hardware, depending on the patient's condition and the surgeon's preference.

After spinal fusion, the patient may need to wear a brace until the spine heals and stabilizes. Periodic follow-up examinations are needed for several months.

Nursing diagnoses
• Anxiety
• Body image disturbance
• Fear
• Impaired physical mobility
• Knowledge deficit
• Pain
• Risk for injury

Nursing interventions
• Provide emotional support, along with meticulous skin and cast care and patient teaching.
• Encourage the patient to verbalize her concerns about the disorder, and answer her questions honestly. Include the patient and her family in all phases of her care.

• Encourage the patient to perform as much self-care as her immobility and pain allow. Provide her with adequate time to perform these activities at her own pace.
• If the patient needs a brace, enlist the help of a physical therapist, a social worker, and an orthotist.
• If the patient needs a body cast, remember that its application can be traumatic because it's done on a special frame with the patient's head and face covered throughout the procedure.
• Check the skin around the cast edge daily. Keep the cast clean and dry. Petal the edges of the cast.
• After corrective surgery, provide the patient with pain medications, as ordered, and assess the patient's response to them.
• Check sensation, movement, color, and blood supply in all extremities every 2 to 4 hours for the first 48 hours; then several times a day to detect neurovascular deficit (a serious complication following spinal surgery). Logroll the patient often.
• Measure intake, output, and urine specific gravity to monitor effects of blood loss, which may be substantial.

• Monitor abdominal distention and bowel sounds.

• Encourage deep-breathing exercises to avoid pulmonary complications.

• Promote active range-of-motion (ROM) arm exercises to help maintain muscle strength. Remember that any exercise, even brushing the hair or teeth, is helpful. Encourage the patient to perform quadriceps-setting, calf-pumping, and active ROM exercises with the feet.

• Watch for skin breakdown and signs and symptoms of cast syndrome (nausea, abdominal pressure, and vague abdominal pain), which may result from hyperextension of the spine.

• Remove antiembolism stockings for 30 minutes daily.

• To help prevent depression that may result from altered body image and immobility, encourage the patient to wear her own clothes, wash her hair, and use makeup.

• If the patient underwent surgery with spinal instrumentation (such as a Harrington rod), if she's discharged in a cast, or if she must have bed rest, arrange for a social worker and a home health nurse to provide home care.

• If you work in a school, screen children routinely for scoliosis during physical examinations.

Patient teaching

• If the patient needs a brace, explain what it does and how to care for it (for example, how to check the screws for tightness and pad the uprights to prevent excessive wear on clothing). Suggest loose-fitting, oversized clothes for greater comfort.

• Instruct the patient to wear the brace 23 hours a day and to remove it only for bathing and exercise.

• To prevent skin breakdown, advise the patient not to use lotions, ointments, or powders on areas where the brace contacts the skin. Instead, suggest rubbing alcohol or tincture of benzoin to toughen the skin. Tell her to keep the skin dry and clean and to wear a snug T-shirt under the brace.

• Advise the patient to increase activities gradually and to avoid vigorous sports. Emphasize the importance of conscientiously performing prescribed exercises. Recommend swimming during the 1 hour out of the brace but strongly warn against diving.

• Instruct the patient to turn her whole body instead of just her head when looking to the side. To make reading easier, suggest holding a book so she can look straight ahead at it instead of down. If she finds this difficult, help her to obtain prism glasses.

• If the patient has a cast, make sure she and her family understand proper cast care. Explain cast syndrome. Also warn the patient not to insert or let anything get under the cast and to immediately report cracks in the cast, pain, burning, skin breakdown, numbness, or odor.

• If the patient is having surgery, explain preoperative and postoperative procedures. After surgery, make sure she knows how to recognize complications and measures to take to prevent them. Before discharge, check with the surgeon about activity limitations and make sure the patient understands them.

• Discuss all prescribed medications with the patient and any adverse reactions. Advise the patient to notify the doctor if these reactions persist.

• Teach the patient relaxation techniques to promote rest and relaxation, and encourage her to perform them.

MUSCLE AND CONNECTIVE TISSUE DISORDERS

Diseases that affect the skeletal muscles and connective tissues invariably cause discomfort and restrict movement. Common among these disorders are tendinitis and bursitis, Achilles tendon contracture, carpal tunnel syndrome, and torticollis.

TENDINITIS AND BURSITIS

In tendinitis, inflammation affects the tendons and tendon-muscle attachments to bone, usually in the shoulder rotator cuff, hip, Achilles tendon, hamstring, or elbow. (See *Understanding epicondylitis.*) Although this disorder is more common in older people, tendinitis can afflict anyone who performs an activity that overstresses a tendon or repeatedly stresses a joint. (See *Anatomy of a joint: A look at tendons and bursae,* page 800.) The disorder causes localized pain around the affected area and restricts joint movement. Initially, swelling results from fluid accumulation. Then, as the disorder progresses, calcium deposits form in and around the tendon, causing further swelling and immobility.

Bursitis is a painful inflammation of one or more bursae. These closed sacs hold lubricating synovial fluid and facilitate the movement of muscles and tendons over bony prominences. Bursitis causes sudden or gradual pain and limits joint motion. Usually, the disorder occurs in the subdeltoid, subacromial, olecranon, trochanteric, calcaneal, or prepatellar bursae. It may be septic, calcific, acute, or chronic.

Causes

Tendinitis commonly results from trauma (such as strain during a sports activity), another musculoskeletal disorder (rheumatic diseases, congenital defects), postural malalignment, abnormal body development, or hypermobility. In calcific tendinitis, calcium deposits in the tendon cause proximal weakness and, if calcium erodes into adjacent bursae, acute calcific bursitis.

Bursitis usually results from recurring trauma that stresses or pressures a joint or from an inflammatory joint disease, such as rheumatoid arthritis or gout. Chronic bursitis follows attacks of acute bursitis or repeated trauma and infection. Common stressors include repetitive kneeling, such as that done by carpet layers (knee), jogging in worn-out shoes on hard asphalt surfaces (ankle or foot), and prolonged sitting with crossed legs on hard surfaces (hip). Septic bursitis may result from wound infection or from bacterial invasion of the skin over the bursa.

Complications

Untreated tendinitis can produce scar tissue and subsequent disability. As calcium erodes into adjacent tissue, acute calcific bursitis may flare up. Untreated bursitis can cause extreme pain and restricted joint movement.

Assessment findings

In *tendinitis,* the patient history may reveal traumatic injury or strain associated with athletic activity. Or the patient may report a concurrent musculoskeletal disorder. The patient with tendinitis may report palpable tenderness over the affected site, referred tenderness in the related segment, or both.

In tendinitis of the *shoulder,* the patient history may disclose restricted shoulder movement (especially abduction) and localized pain that's most severe at night and often interferes with sleep. Significantly, the patient with this disorder may say that heat aggravates shoulder pain rather than provides relief. In tendinitis of the *elbow* (epicondylitis), the patient usually complains of tenderness over the lateral epicondyle and pain when grasping objects or twisting the elbow. In tendinitis of the *hamstring,* the patient may have pain in the posterolateral aspect of the knee and palpable tenderness when he flexes his knee at a 90-degree angle. In tendinitis of the *foot,* the patient may complain of pain over the Achilles tendon and on dorsiflexion. Palpation may reveal crepitus when the patient moves his foot.

In *bursitis,* the patient typically recalls an unusual strain or injury 2 to 3 days before his pain began. The pain, which can develop suddenly or gradually, may limit

UNDERSTANDING EPICONDYLITIS

Also known as tennis elbow, epicondylitis is one of several activity-related joint disorders. It occurs when the forearm extensor supinator tendon fibers become inflamed at their common attachment to the lateral humeral epicondyle.

Epicondylitis may produce acute or subacute pain. It probably begins as a partial tear and is common among tennis players or persons whose activities require a forceful grasp, wrist extension against resistance, or frequent forearm rotation.

Signs and symptoms

The patient may initially have elbow pain that gradually increases, radiating to the forearm and back of the hand whenever he grasps an object or twists his elbow. Rarely, the elbow may be red, swollen, warm, or restricted in range of motion. The patient may have tenderness over the involved lateral or medial epicondyle or over the head of the radius.

Selective tissue tension assessment may reproduce the pain by wrist extension and supination with lateral involvement or by flexion and pronation with medial epicondyle involvement. Neuromuscular test results may reveal a weak grasp.

Treatment

The patient may receive a local injection of a corticosteroid and anesthetic and systemic nonsteroidal anti-inflammatory drugs, such as aspirin or ibuprofen, to relieve pain. Supportive treatment includes:
• immobilization with a splint from the distal forearm to the elbow, which may relieve pain in 2 to 3 weeks
• heat therapy with warm compresses, short wave diathermy, or ultrasound (alone or with diathermy)
• physical therapy to detach the tendon from the chronically inflamed periosteum
• possibly, a "tennis elbow strap" wrapped snugly around the forearm about 1" (2.5 cm) below the epicondyle to relieve the strain on affected forearm muscles and tendons.

Should medical and supportive measures fail, surgical release of the tendon at the epicondyle may be necessary.

movement. The patient's work or leisure activity may involve a repetitive action. Usually you can palpate tenderness over the site and, in severe bursitis, swelling.

Other symptoms vary according to the affected site and may include impaired arm abduction (subdeltoid bursitis) or pain when attempting to climb stairs (prepatellar bursitis).

ANATOMY OF A JOINT: A LOOK AT TENDONS AND BURSAE

Tendons, like stiff rubber bands, hold the muscles in place and allow them to move the bones. Bursae are located at friction points around joints and between tendons, cartilage, or bone. Bursae keep these body parts lubricated so they move freely.

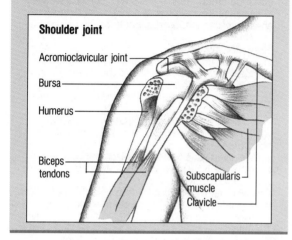

Shoulder joint

Acromioclavicular joint

Bursa

Humerus

Biceps tendons

Subscapularis muscle

Clavicle

Diagnostic tests

• *X-rays* may appear normal at first in tendinitis, but later, bony fragments, osteophyte sclerosis, or calcium deposits may appear. In early bursitis, X-rays also usually appear normal, except in calcific bursitis, where films show calcium deposits in the joint.
• *Arthrography* results are usually normal in tendinitis with minor irregularities on the tendon undersurface.
• *Ultrasonography* can help diagnose bursitis by identifying inflamed tissue.
• *Arthrocentesis* detects microorganisms and other causes of inflammation if joint infection is suspected.

Additionally, the patient may have various blood tests and urinalyses to rule out other disorders.

Treatment

To relieve pain, treatment involves resting the joint (by immobilization); nonsteroidal anti-inflammatory drugs; cold, heat, or ultrasound applications; possible injection of a local anesthetic (such as lidocaine) and corticosteroids for immediate relief; and extended-release corticosteroids, such as triamcinolone or prednisolone, for longer relief.

Until the patient can perform range-of-motion exercises easily, treatment also includes oral anti-inflammatory agents and short-term analgesics. Supplementary measures involve fluid removal by aspiration, physical therapy to preserve motion and prevent frozen joints, and heat and cold therapies. Rarely, calcific tendinitis requires surgical removal of calcium deposits. Long-term control of chronic bursitis and tendinitis may require life-style changes.

Nursing diagnoses
• Anxiety
• Impaired physical mobility
• Knowledge deficit
• Pain
• Self-care deficit

Nursing interventions
• Assess the severity of the patient's pain. Also assess the range of motion in the affected joint to determine the effectiveness of the treatment.
• Encourage the patient to verbalize his concerns about his disorder. Listen, answer his questions, and offer support and encouragement. Include the patient and his family in all phases of his care.
• Encourage the patient to perform as much self-care as his immobility and pain allow. Provide him with adequate time to perform these activities at his own pace.
• Give medications, as ordered, and assess the patient's response to them.
• Before injecting corticosteroids or local anesthetics, ask the patient if he has any drug allergies.
• Assist with intra-articular injection. Scrub the patient's skin thoroughly with povidone-iodine (or a comparable solution), and shave the injection site, if necessary. After the injection, massage the area to ensure penetration through the tissue and joint space. Apply ice intermittently for about 4 hours to minimize pain. Avoid applying heat to the area for 2 days.

Patient teaching
• Instruct the patient to take anti-inflammatory agents with milk to minimize GI distress. Direct him to report any signs or symptoms of GI distress immediately.
• Help the patient identify and perform activities that promote rest and relaxation.
• Teach the patient how to perform strengthening exercises, and encourage him to follow the prescribed exercise regimen. To maintain joint mobility and prevent muscle atrophy, urge him to perform exercises or physical therapy regularly when he is free of pain.

• Advise the patient to wear a sling during the first few days of an attack of subdeltoid bursitis or tendinitis to support the arm and protect the shoulder, particularly at night. Demonstrate how to apply and wear the sling to relieve weight on the shoulder. To protect the shoulder during sleep, a splint may be worn instead of a sling. Instruct the patient to remove the splint during the day.
• Tell a patient with sports-related bursitis or tendinitis to evaluate his sports equipment, shoes, and playing surfaces.
• If the patient has Achilles tendinitis, recommend that he wear cushioned shoes, lose excess weight, and choose non-weight-bearing activities, such as swimming.
• If the patient needs cold treatments to relieve swelling and pain, show him how to use a commercial cold pack or how to make an ice pack. If he needs heat applications, show him how to apply dry and moist heat. With either therapy, caution him to limit treatments to 20 minutes to prevent skin damage.
• To prevent recurrence, teach the patient to use proper body mechanics to minimize joint stress.

ACHILLES TENDON CONTRACTURE

This shortening of the Achilles tendon (also known as the tendo calcaneus or heel cord) causes foot pain and strain, with limited ankle dorsiflexion.

Causes

Achilles tendon contracture may reflect a congenital structural anomaly or a muscular reaction to chronic poor posture, especially in women who wear high-heeled shoes or joggers who land on the balls of their feet instead of their heels. Other causes include paralytic conditions, such as poliomyelitis or cerebral palsy.

Complications

Untreated Achilles tendon contracture can produce increasing pain and immobility.

Assessment findings

The history may reveal that the patient has a paralytic condition affecting the legs or that he's a runner. He may complain of foot pain, which he describes as spasmodic and most pronounced during dorsiflexion of the foot. If the patient has footdrop (fixed equinus), he may be unable to place his heel on the ground. (This condition is caused by contracture of the flexor foot muscle.)

A simple test confirms Achilles tendon contracture: Have the patient keep his knee flexed as you position his foot in dorsiflexion. With Achilles tendon contracture, gradual knee extension will force the foot into plantar flexion.

Diagnostic tests

A physical examination and patient history suggest Achilles tendon contracture.

Treatment

Conservative measures may help correct Achilles tendon contracture. Among them are raising the inside heel of the shoe in the reflex type of contracture; gradually lowering the heels of shoes (sudden lowering can aggravate the problem) and stretching exercises if the cause is high-heeled shoes; or using support braces or casting to prevent footdrop in a paralyzed patient. Alternatives include using wedged plaster casts or stretching the tendon by manipulation. Analgesics may relieve pain.

With fixed footdrop, treatment may include surgery (Z-tenotomy) to cut the tendon and allow further stretching. After surgery, a short leg cast maintains the foot in 90-degree dorsiflexion for 6 weeks. Some patients begin partial weight bearing after 2 weeks.

Nursing diagnoses

• Altered tissue perfusion
• Impaired physical mobility
• Pain
• Risk for impaired skin integrity
• Risk for injury

Nursing interventions

• After surgery to lengthen the Achilles tendon, elevate the casted foot to decrease venous pressure and edema. Raise the foot of the bed or support the foot with pillows.
• Check and document the neurovascular status of the toes (temperature, color, sensation, capillary refill time, toe mobility) every hour for the first 24 hours, then every 4 hours. If you detect any changes, increase the elevation of the patient's legs and notify the surgeon immediately.
• Prepare the patient for ambulation by having him dangle his foot over the side of the bed briefly (5 to 15 minutes) before he gets out of bed. This lets venous pressure increase gradually. Assist the patient in walking, as ordered (usually within 24 hours of surgery), using crutches and a non-weight-bearing or touch-down gait.
• Protect the patient's skin with moleskin or by petaling the edges of the cast.
• To prevent Achilles tendon contracture in paralyzed patients, apply support braces, universal splints, casts, or high-topped sneakers. Make sure the weight of the sheets doesn't keep paralyzed feet in plantar flexion.

LOCATING THE CARPAL TUNNEL

The carpal tunnel lies between the longitudinal tendons of the hand-flexing forearm muscles (not shown) and the transverse carpal ligament. Note the median nerve and flexor tendons passing through the tunnel on their way from the forearm to the hand.

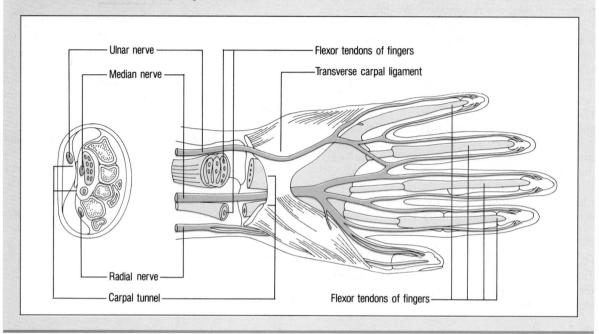

- Ulnar nerve
- Median nerve
- Flexor tendons of fingers
- Transverse carpal ligament
- Radial nerve
- Carpal tunnel
- Flexor tendons of fingers

• Administer analgesics, as ordered, for pain.

Patient teaching
• Before discharge, teach the patient how to care for the cast. Advise him to elevate his foot regularly when sitting or whenever the foot throbs or swells.
• Make sure he understands exercise and walking recommendations.
• Teach meticulous foot care, and urge the patient to seek immediate medical care for foot problems. Warn women against wearing high-heeled shoes constantly, and suggest regular foot (dorsiflexion) exercises.
• Teach the patient about prescribed analgesics and reportable adverse effects.

CARPAL TUNNEL SYNDROME

The most common nerve entrapment syndrome, carpal tunnel syndrome results from compression of the median nerve in the wrist, where it passes through the carpal tunnel. (See *Locating the carpal tunnel.*)

The median nerve controls motions in the forearm, wrist, and hand, such as turning the wrist toward the body, flexing the index and middle fingers, and many thumb movements. It also supplies sensation to the index, middle, and ring fingers. Compression of this nerve causes loss of movement and sensation in the wrist, hand, and fingers. Carpal tunnel syndrome usually occurs in women between ages 30 and 60 and may pose a serious occupational health problem. It may also occur in people who move their wrists continuously—for example, butchers, computer operators, and concert pianists. Any strenuous use of the hands—sustained grasping, twisting, or flexing—aggravates the condition.

Causes
The exact cause of carpal tunnel syndrome is unknown. However, the syndrome may result from amyloidosis or from an edema-producing condition, such as diabetes, rheumatoid arthritis, pregnancy, premenstrual fluid retention, renal failure, and heart failure.

Repetitive wrist motions involving excessive flexion or extension also cause the carpal tunnel structures (tendons, for example) to swell and press the median nerve against the transverse carpal ligament. Dislocation or an acute sprain may damage the median nerve. Some experts think that a vitamin B_6 deficiency contributes to carpal tunnel syndrome.

Complications

Continued use of the affected wrist may increase tendon inflammation, compression, and neural ischemia. Wrist function will decrease. Untreated carpal tunnel syndrome can produce permanent nerve damage with loss of movement and sensation.

Assessment findings

The history may disclose that the patient's occupation or hobby requires strenuous or repetitive use of the hands. It may reveal a hormonal condition, wrist injury, rheumatoid arthritis, or another condition that causes swelling in carpal tunnel structures.

The patient may complain of weakness, pain, burning, numbness, or tingling in one or both hands. Paresthesia may affect the thumb, forefinger, middle finger, and half of the ring finger. She may report that the paresthesia worsens at night and in the morning (because of vasodilation and venous stasis). She may also report that the pain spreads to the forearm and, in severe cases, as far as the shoulder. She can usually relieve the pain by shaking her hands vigorously or dangling her arms at her sides. Inspection and palpation may show that the patient can't make a fist; her fingernails may be atrophied, with surrounding dry, shiny skin. (See *Eliciting signs of carpal tunnel syndrome.*)

Diagnostic tests

• *Electromyography* detects a median nerve motor conduction delay of more than 5 milliseconds.
• *Digital electrical stimulation* discloses median nerve compression by measuring the length and intensity of stimulation from the fingers to the median nerve in the wrist.
• *Motor function tests* of the median nerve indicate nerve compression and carpal tunnel syndrome because movement is delayed after electrical stimulation.
• *Neuromuscular testing* reveals decreased sensation to light touch or pinpricks in the affected fingers.

Treatment

Initially conservative, treatment includes splinting the wrist for 1 to 2 weeks, possible occupational changes,

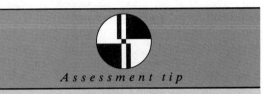

Assessment tip

ELICITING SIGNS OF CARPAL TUNNEL SYNDROME

Two simple tests—for Tinel's sign and Phalen's sign—may confirm carpal tunnel syndrome. The tests prove that certain wrist movements compress the median nerve, causing pain, burning, numbness, or tingling in the hand and fingers.

Tinel's sign
Lightly percuss the transverse carpal ligament over the median nerve where the patient's palm and wrist meet. If this action produces discomfort, such as numbness or tingling, shooting into the palm and fingers, the patient has Tinel's sign.

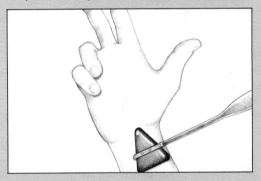

Phalen's sign
If flexing the patient's wrist for about 30 seconds causes the patient to feel subsequent pain or numbness in her hand or fingers, she has Phalen's sign. The more severe the carpal tunnel syndrome, the more rapidly the symptoms develop.

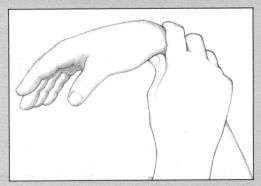

and correction of any underlying disorder. Medications such as nonsteroidal anti-inflammatory drugs (NSAIDS) taken orally and corticosteroids given by injection are the most commonly prescribed agents. NSAIDs, such as indomethacin, mefenamic acid, phenylbutazone, or piroxicam, typically accompany corticosteroid and splinting therapy. They help control pain and reduce inflammation. Corticosteroid injections will reduce inflammation almost immediately, but only temporarily. If the doctor suspects a vitamin B_6 deficiency, he may prescribe pyridoxine.

When conservative treatment fails, the only alternative is surgical decompression of the nerve by sectioning the entire transverse carpal tunnel ligament. Neurolysis (freeing the nerve fibers) may also be necessary.

Nursing diagnoses
• Altered role performance
• Anxiety
• Impaired physical mobility
• Pain
• Self-care deficit

Nursing interventions
• Encourage the patient to express her concerns. Listen and offer your support and encouragement.
• Have her perform as much self-care as her immobility and pain allow. Provide her with adequate time to perform these activities at her own pace.
• Administer mild analgesics, as needed. Encourage the patient to use her hands as much as possible; however, if the condition has impaired her dominant hand, you may have to help her eat and bathe.
• After surgery, monitor vital signs, and regularly check the color, sensation, and motion of the affected hand.

Patient teaching
• Teach the patient how to apply a splint. Advise her not to make it too tight. Show her how to remove the splint to perform gentle range-of-motion exercises (which should be done daily).
• Advise the patient who is about to be discharged to occasionally exercise her hands in warm water. If she's using a sling, tell her to remove it several times a day to exercise her elbow and shoulder.
• If the patient requires surgery, explain preoperative and postoperative care procedures fully.
• Suggest occupational counseling for the patient who has to change jobs because of carpal tunnel syndrome.
• Review the prescribed medication regimen. Emphasize that drug therapy may require 2 to 4 weeks before max-

imum effectiveness is achieved. If the regimen includes indomethacin, mefenamic acid, phenylbutazone, or piroxicam, advise taking the drug with foods or antacids to avoid stomach upset. List possible adverse reactions. Instruct the patient which adverse reactions require immediate medical attention.
• If the patient is pregnant, advise her to avoid NSAIDs because their effects on the fetus aren't known.

TORTICOLLIS
In this neck deformity, also known as wryneck, spastic or shortened sternocleidomastoid neck muscles cause the head to tilt to the affected side and the chin to rotate to the opposite side. The disorder may be congenital or acquired. Congenital (muscular) torticollis mostly affects infants after difficult delivery (breech presentation), firstborn infants, and girls. Acquired torticollis usually develops either before age 10 or after age 40. It may be acute, spasmodic, or hysterical.

Causes
Possible causes of *congenital torticollis* include malposition of the head in utero, prenatal injury, fibroma, interrupted blood supply, or fibrotic rupture of the sternocleidomastoid muscle with hematoma and scar formation. *Acute torticollis* results from muscular damage caused by inflammatory diseases, such as myositis, lymphadenitis, and tuberculosis, and from cervical spinal injuries that produce scar tissue contractures. *Spasmodic torticollis* results from rhythmic muscle spasms caused by an organic central nervous system (CNS) disorder (probably irritation of the nerve root by arthritis or osteomyelitis). *Hysterical torticollis* results from a psychogenic inability to control the neck muscles.

Complications
Permanent contracture may complicate torticollis.

Assessment findings
In acquired torticollis, the history usually reveals gradual onset of painful neck deformity. It may disclose an organic CNS disorder or an inflammatory disorder that causes muscle damage. The patient may complain of recurring and unilateral neck muscle stiffness and pain followed by a drawing sensation and a momentary twitching or contraction that pulls the head to the side.

If the patient is an infant with suspected congenital torticollis, inspection may reveal an enlarged sternocleidomastoid muscle visible at birth and for several weeks afterward. The muscle slowly shrinks (or regresses) over

6 months, although incomplete regression can cause permanent contracture. In severe deformity, the infant's face and head flatten from sleeping on the affected side; this asymmetry gradually worsens.

Palpation detects an enlarged, firm, and tender sternocleidomastoid muscle in both congenital and acquired torticollis.

Diagnostic tests
X-rays of the cervical spine do not reveal bone or joint disease but may detect an associated disorder.

Treatment
In congenital torticollis, treatment aims to stretch the shortened neck muscle. Nonsurgical treatment for an infant includes passive neck stretching and proper positioning during sleep. For an older child, treatment involves active stretching exercises. Surgical correction should be done during preschool years and only if other therapies fail.

Treatment of acquired torticollis aims to correct the underlying condition. In the acute form, application of heat, cervical traction, and gentle massage may help relieve pain. Stretching exercises and a neck brace may relieve symptoms of the spasmodic and hysterical forms.

In elderly patients with acquired torticollis, treatment may include carbidopa-levodopa, carbamazepine, and haloperidol.

Nursing diagnoses
- Anxiety
- Body image disturbance
- Fear
- Impaired tissue integrity
- Pain

Nursing interventions
- To aid early diagnosis of congenital torticollis, observe the infant for limited neck movement. Thoroughly assess her degree of discomfort.
- Prepare the patient for surgery, if necessary, by shaving her neck to the hairline on the affected side. Also prepare her for possible immobilization with a brace.
- After corrective surgery, monitor the patient closely for nausea or signs of respiratory complications, especially if she's in cervical traction. Keep suction equipment available to manage possible aspiration.
- If the patient has an immobilization device, such as a brace, monitor circulation, sensation, and color around the device. Inspect the skin around the device for signs of breakdown.

- Provide emotional support for the patient and family to relieve their anxiety caused by fear, pain, an altered body image, and limitations imposed by treatments.
- Assist the patient to begin stretching exercises, as ordered, as soon as she can tolerate them.

Patient teaching
- Teach parents how to perform stretching exercises with the child. Suggest placing toys or hanging mobiles on the side of the crib opposite the affected side of the child's neck. This will encourage the child to move her head and stretch her neck in that direction.
- Before discharge, emphasize to the patient or her parents the importance of continuing daily heat applications, massages, and stretching exercises, as prescribed. Explain that physical therapy is essential to recovery.

SELECTED REFERENCES
Avery, M.E., and First, L. *Pediatric Medicine*, 2nd ed. Baltimore: Williams & Wilkins Co., 1994.

Folcik, M.A., et al. *Traction Assessment and Management*. St. Louis: Mosby–Year Book, Inc., 1994.

Illustrated Manual of Nursing Practice, 2nd ed. Springhouse, Pa.: Springhouse Corp., 1994.

Isselbacher, K., et al., eds. *Harrison's Principles of Internal Medicine*, 13th ed. New York: McGraw-Hill Book Co., 1995.

Long, B.C., et al. *Medical-Surgical Nursing: A Nursing Process Approach,* 3rd ed. St. Louis: Mosby–Year Book, Inc., 1993.

Mader, J.T., et al. "Long-Bone Osteomyelitis: Diagnosis and Management," *Hospital Practice* 29(10):71-79, October 15, 1994.

Maher, A.B., et al., eds. *Orthopedic Nursing*. Philadelphia: W.B. Saunders Co., 1994.

Rakel, R.E., ed. *Conn's Current Therapy 1996.* Philadelphia: W.B. Saunders Co., 1996.

Taylor, C.M., and Sparks, S.M. *Nursing Diagnosis Reference Manual,* 3rd ed. Springhouse, Pa.: Springhouse Corp., 1995.

Tierney, L., et al. *Current Medical Diagnosis and Treatment 1995.* East Norwalk, Conn.: Appleton & Lange, 1995.

Zupan, A., et al. "Long-lasting Effects of Electrical Stimulation upon Muscles of Patients Suffering from Progressive Muscular Dystrophy," *Clinical Rehabilitation* 9(2):102-09, May 1995.

11   RENAL AND UROLOGIC DISORDERS

INTRODUCTION

Because renal and urologic disorders affect more than 8 million Americans, you'll undoubtedly encounter such patients often. To give them the best possible care, you need to know about normal anatomy and physiology. (See *Reviewing renal and urologic anatomy*, pages 808 and 809.) You'll also need to know the causes, complications, and typical assessment findings for specific renal and urologic disorders. Furthermore, your familiarity with diagnostic tests and treatments will enable you to explain them to the patient and answer his questions.

Kidneys and homeostasis

By producing and eliminating urine, the kidneys maintain homeostasis. These vital organs regulate the volume, electrolyte concentration, and acid-base balance of body fluids; detoxify the blood and eliminate wastes; regulate blood pressure; and aid in erythropoiesis.

The kidneys eliminate wastes from the body through urine formation (by glomerular filtration, tubular reabsorption, and tubular secretion) and excretion. Glomerular filtration, the process of filtering the blood flowing through the kidneys, depends on the permeability of the capillary walls, vascular pressure, and filtration pressure. The normal glomerular filtration rate (GFR) is about 120 ml/minute.

Clearance measures function

Clearance, the volume of plasma that can be cleared of a substance per unit of time, depends on how renal tubular cells handle a substance that has been filtered by the glomerulus.
• If the tubules don't reabsorb or secrete the substance, clearance equals the GFR.
• If the tubules reabsorb it, clearance is less than the GFR.
• If the tubules secrete it, clearance exceeds the GFR.
• If the tubules reabsorb and secrete it, clearance is less than, equal to, or greater than the GFR.

The most accurate measure of glomerular function is creatinine clearance. That's because creatinine is only filtered by the glomerulus and not reabsorbed by the tubules.

The transport of filtered substances in tubular reabsorption or secretion may be active (requiring energy expenditure) or passive (requiring no expenditure). For example, energy is required to move sodium across tubular cells (active transport), but none is required to move urea (passive transport). The amount of reabsorption or secretion of a substance depends on the maximum tubular transport capacity for that substance — that is, the most of a substance that can be reabsorbed or secreted in a minute without saturating the system.

Fluid and acid-base balance

Hormones partially control water regulation by the kidneys. Hormonal control depends on the response of osmoreceptors to changes in osmolality. The two hormones involved are antidiuretic hormone (ADH), produced by the pituitary gland, and aldosterone, produced by the adrenal cortex. ADH alters the collecting tubules' permeability to water. When plasma concentration of ADH is high, the tubules are most permeable to water, so a greater amount of water is reabsorbed, creating a high concentration but small volume of urine. The reverse holds true if ADH concentration is low.

Aldosterone, however, regulates sodium and water reabsorption from the distal tubules. A high plasma aldosterone concentration promotes sodium and water reabsorption from the tubules and decreases sodium and water excretion in the urine; a low plasma aldosterone concentration promotes sodium and water excretion.

Aldosterone also helps control the distal tubular secretion of potassium. Other factors that determine potassium secretion include the amount of potassium ingested, the number of hydrogen ions secreted, the level of intracellular potassium, the amount of sodium in the distal tubule, and the GFR.

The countercurrent mechanism is the method by which the kidneys concentrate urine. This mechanism is composed of a multiplication system and an exchange system, which occur in the renal medulla by way of the limbs of the loop of Henle and the vasa recta. It achieves active transport of sodium and chloride between the loop of Henle and the medullary interstitial fluid. Failure of this mechanism produces polyuria and nocturia.

To regulate acid-base balance, the kidneys secrete hydrogen ions, reabsorb sodium and bicarbonate ions, acidify phosphate salts, and synthesize ammonia — all of which keep the blood at its normal pH of 7.37 to 7.43.

Blood pressure regulation

The kidneys help regulate blood pressure by synthesizing and secreting renin in response to an actual or perceived decline in the volume of extracellular fluid. Renin, in turn, acts on a substrate to form angiotensin I, which is converted to the more potent angiotensin II. Angiotensin II raises arterial blood pressure by peripheral vasoconstriction and stimulation of aldosterone secretion. The resulting increase in the aldosterone level promotes the reabsorption of sodium and water to correct the fluid deficit and renal ischemia.

(Text continues on page 810.)

REVIEWING RENAL AND UROLOGIC ANATOMY

The kidneys are located retroperitoneally in the lumbar area, with the right kidney a little lower than the left because of the liver mass above it. The left kidney is slightly longer than the right and closer to the midline. The kidneys assume different locations with changes in body position. The coverings of the kidneys consist of the fibrous (or true) capsule, perirenal fat, renal fascia, and pararenal fat.

Structure of the kidney
The gross structure of each kidney includes the lateral and medial margins, the hilus, the renal sinus, and renal parenchyma. The hilus, located at the medial margin, is the indentation where the blood and lymph vessels enter the kidney and the ureter emerges. The hilus leads to the renal sinus, a spacious cavity filled with adipose tissue, branches of the renal vessels, calyces, the renal pelvis, and the ureter. The renal sinus is surrounded by parenchyma, which consists of a cortex and a medulla.

The cortex, or outermost layer of the kidney, contains the glomeruli (parts of the nephron), cortical arches (areas that separate the medullary pyramids from the renal surface), columns of Bertin (areas that separate the pyramids from one another), and medullary rays of Ferrein (long, delicate processes from the bases of the pyramids that mix with the cortex).

The medulla contains the pyramids (cone-shaped structures of parenchymal tissue), papillae (apical ends of the pyramids through which urine oozes into the minor calyces), and Bellini's ducts (collecting ducts in the pyramids that empty into the papillae).

The ureters are a pair of retroperitoneally located, mucosa-lined, fibromuscular tubes that transport urine from the renal pelvis to the urinary bladder. Although the ureters have no sphincters, their oblique entrance into the bladder creates a mucosal fold that produces a sphincterlike action during bladder contraction.

Structure of the bladder
The gross structure of the bladder includes the fundus (large, central, posterosuperior portion of the bladder), the apex (anterosuperior region), the body (posteroinferior region containing the ureteral orifices), and the urethral orifice, or neck (most inferior portion of the bladder). The three orifices compose a triangular area called the trigone.

The adult urinary bladder is a spherical, muscular sac, with a normal capacity of 300 to 500 ml. It's located anterior and inferior to the peritoneal cavity and posterior to the pubic bones.

Functional units
The functional units of each kidney are its 1 to 3 million nephrons. Each nephron consists of the renal corpuscle and the tubular system.

The renal corpuscle includes the glomerulus (a network of minute blood vessels) and Bowman's capsule (an epithelial sac surrounding the glomerulus that is part of the tubular system). The renal corpuscle has a vascular pole, where the afferent arteriole enters and the efferent arteriole emerges, and a urinary pole that narrows to form the beginning of the tubular system.

The tubular system includes the proximal convoluted tubule, the loop of Henle, and the distal convoluted tubule. The last portion of the nephron consists of the collecting duct.

Vasculature
Renal arteries branch into five segmental arteries that supply different areas of the kidneys. The segmental arteries then branch into several divisions from which the afferent arterioles and vasa recta arise. Renal veins follow a similar branching pattern, characterized by stellate vessels and segmental branches, and empty into the inferior vena cava. The tubular system receives its blood supply from a peritubular capillary network of vessels.

The ureters receive their blood supply from the renal, vesical, gonadal, and iliac arteries and the abdominal aorta. The ureteral veins follow the arteries and drain into the renal vein. The bladder receives blood through vesical arteries. Vesical veins unite to form the pudendal plexus, which empties into the iliac veins. A rich lymphatic system drains the renal cortex, the kidneys, the ureters, and the bladder.

Innervation
The kidneys are innervated by sympathetic branches from the celiac plexus, upper lumbar splanchnic and thoracic nerves, and intermesenteric and superior hypogastric plexuses, which form a plexus around the kidneys. Similar numbers of sympathetic and parasympathetic nerves from the renal plexus, superior hypogastric plexus, and intermesenteric plexus innervate the ureters. Nerves that arise from the inferior hypogastric plexus innervate the bladder. The parasympathetic nerve supply to the bladder controls urination.

REVIEWING RENAL AND UROLOGIC ANATOMY *(continued)*

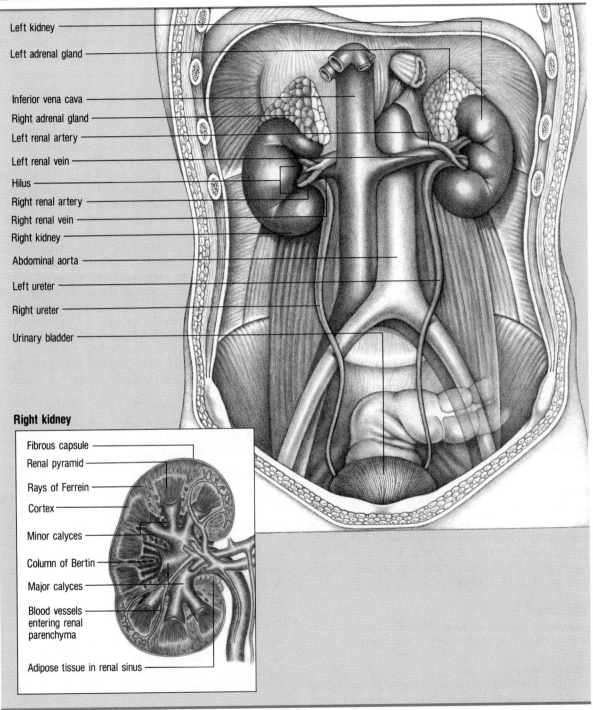

Left kidney

Left adrenal gland

Inferior vena cava

Right adrenal gland

Left renal artery

Left renal vein

Hilus

Right renal artery

Right renal vein

Right kidney

Abdominal aorta

Left ureter

Right ureter

Urinary bladder

Right kidney

Fibrous capsule

Renal pyramid

Rays of Ferrein

Cortex

Minor calyces

Column of Bertin

Major calyces

Blood vessels entering renal parenchyma

Adipose tissue in renal sinus

CAUSES OF COMMON RENAL AND UROLOGIC SYMPTOMS

Symptom	Possible cause
Dribbling	Prostatic enlargement, urethral strictures, ectopic ureter
Dysuria	Infection
Edema	Nephrotic syndrome, renal failure
Frequency	Infection, diabetes mellitus, excess fluid intake
Hematuria	Glomerular diseases, renal or urologic trauma, neoplasms, renal calculi
Hesitancy	Prostatic enlargement, sphincter dyssynergia
Incontinence	Infection, renal or urologic neoplasms, prolapsed uterus, neurogenic bladder, excess fluid intake
Nocturia	Infection, cardiovascular fluid shift when prone
Oliguria	Renal failure, renal or urologic neoplasms, vascular insufficiency
Proteinuria	Glomerular diseases, infection
Pyuria	Infection
Renal colic	Thrombi, emboli, renal calculi
Urgency	Infection, prostatic disease

Other renal functions

The kidneys secrete erythropoietin in response to decreased oxygen tension in the renal blood supply. Erythropoietin then acts on the bone marrow to increase the production of red blood cells (RBCs). Renal tubular cells synthesize active vitamin D and help regulate calcium balance and bone metabolism.

Assessment

Assessment requires an accurate patient history, a thorough physical examination, and certain laboratory data.

Patient history

Ask the patient about symptoms that pertain specifically to a renal or urologic problem, such as urinary frequency or urgency. (See *Causes of common renal and urologic symptoms.*) Also ask about any systemic diseases that can produce renal or urologic dysfunction, such as hypertension, diabetes mellitus, or bladder infections. Family history may suggest a genetic predisposition to certain renal diseases, such as polycystic kidney disease. Finally, ask which medications the patient has been taking; abuse of analgesics or antibiotics may cause nephrotoxicity.

Physical examination

Carefully observe the patient's overall appearance. Examine his skin for color, turgor, intactness, and texture; his mucous membranes for color, secretions, odor, and intactness; his eyes for periorbital edema and vision; his general activity for motion, gait, and posture; his muscle movement for motor function and general strength; and his mental status for level of consciousness, orientation, and response to stimuli.

Next, assess the patient for distinctive changes in vital signs that renal disease can cause: hypertension from fluid and electrolyte imbalances and renin-angiotensin system hyperactivity; a strong, fast, irregular pulse due to fluid and electrolyte imbalances; hyperventilation to compensate for metabolic acidosis; and increased susceptibility to infection from decreased resistance. Palpation and percussion may reveal little because, unless the kidneys and bladder are enlarged, they may be hard to palpate, especially if the patient is obese or in pain.

Relevant diagnostic tests

If the patient needs invasive tests, such as cystoscopy, excretory urography, and renal angiography, explain each procedure to allay his anxiety and encourage cooperation. (See *Invasive diagnostic tests in renal and urologic disorders.*) Afterward, observe the patient closely for complications, such as hypersensitivity to the contrast medium and hemorrhage, and document your findings. Monitor vital signs, intake and output, and general status.

Various laboratory tests analyze serum levels of chemical substances, such as uric acid, creatinine, and blood urea nitrogen. Tests also determine urine characteristics, including the presence of RBCs, white blood cells, casts, and bacteria; specific gravity and pH; and physical properties, such as clarity, color, and odor.

Noninvasive renal and urologic monitoring includes:
• *Intake and output assessment.* Measuring intake and output helps assess the patient's hydration status but isn't a valid evaluation of renal function because urine output varies with different types of renal disorders. To provide

INVASIVE DIAGNOSTIC TESTS IN RENAL AND UROLOGIC DISORDERS

Invasive diagnostic tests allow the assessment of renal and urologic disorders. Below you'll find the purpose for invasive tests your patient may undergo, along with nursing considerations for each test.

Cystoscopy

In this test, the doctor visualizes the inside of the bladder with a fiber-optic scope.

Before the procedure, give a sedative or apply a local anesthetic (such as lidocaine gel), as ordered. Afterward, offer increased fluids and administer analgesics. Watch for hematuria and signs of perforation, hemorrhage, and infection.

Cystometry

In this test, sterile water or carbon dioxide is used to evaluate intravesical pressure, sensation, and capacity in response to filling.

Before the procedure, observe the patient's voiding and catheterize him for residual urine. During the procedure, document the patient's verbalized sensations and signs of media leakage. Ask him to cough during the test to increase abdominal pressure and determine the effect on intravesical pressure. Afterward, remove the catheter. Again observe the patient's voiding and catheterize him for residual urine.

Excretory urography

In this test, X-rays and a contrast medium are used to allow visualization of the renal parenchyma, renal pelves, ureters, and bladder.

Before the procedure, ask the patient about previous reactions to contrast media and allergies to shellfish or iodine. Adequately hydrate him. Afterward, watch for signs of a hypersensitivity reaction (chills, dyspnea, fever, increased pulse rate, pruritus, and urticaria). Also watch for hematomas at the injection site.

Nephrotomography

After I.V. injection of a contrast medium, tomography is used to visualize the parenchyma, calyces, and pelves in layers.

Before the test, ask the patient about previous reactions to contrast media and allergies to shellfish or iodine. Adequately hydrate him. After the test, watch for signs of a hypersensitivity reaction.

Renal angiography

This test calls for the injection of a contrast medium into a catheter in the femoral artery or vein, allowing the visualization of the arterial tree, capillaries, and venous drainage of the kidneys.

Before the procedure, ask the patient about previous reactions to contrast media and allergies to shellfish or iodine. Adequately hydrate him. Afterward, offer increased fluids, and watch for signs of a hypersensitivity reaction. Watch for hematomas and hemorrhage at the injection site as well as for nephrotoxicity.

Renal scan

This procedure determines renal function by showing the appearance and disappearance of radioisotopes within the kidneys.

Before the procedure, ask the patient about previous reactions to contrast media and allergies to shellfish or iodine. Adequately hydrate him. After the procedure, offer increased fluids and watch for signs of a hypersensitivity reaction. Dispose of urine, following hospital guidelines.

Renal biopsy

During this procedure, a specimen is obtained to develop a histologic diagnosis and determine therapy and the prognosis.

Before the procedure, make sure the patient's clotting times, prothrombin times, and platelet count are recorded on his chart and that he has undergone excretory urography. Place him in the prone position with his side slightly elevated on a towel or pillow, and clean the skin over the biopsy site.

During the procedure, help the patient maintain the correct position. Tell him to lie still and hold his breath if the biopsy is done at the bedside. In many cases, it's done in the operating room.

Afterward, instruct the patient to breathe normally. Apply gentle pressure to the bandage site. Watch for hemorrhage and hematoma at the biopsy site; also watch for hematuria. Enforce bed rest for 24 hours after the procedure, and offer increased fluids.

Voiding cystourethrography

In this test, X-rays and a contrast medium are used to determine the size and shape of the bladder and urethra.

Before the procedure, ask the patient about previous reactions to contrast media and allergies to shellfish or iodine. Adequately hydrate him. Catheterize him during the procedure. Afterward, offer him increased fluids and watch for signs of a hypersensitivity reaction.

Videourodynamic studies

A combination of fluoroscopy and complex cystometry, this procedure documents voiding dysfunction.

Follow the nursing procedures described above for cystometry and voiding cystourethrography.

the most useful and accurate information, use calibrated containers, establish baseline values for the patient, compare measurement patterns, and validate intake and output measurements by weighing the patient daily. Also, monitor all fluid losses, including blood, emesis, diarrhea, and wound and stoma drainage.

• *Specimen collection.* Meticulous collection is vital for valid laboratory data. If the patient collects the specimen, explain how to clean the meatal orifice properly.

The culture specimen should be caught midstream in a sterile container; a urinalysis specimen should be collected in a clean container, preferably at the first voiding of the day. Begin a 24-hour specimen collection after discarding the first voiding; such specimens commonly require special handling or preservatives. When obtaining a urine specimen from a catheterized patient, don't take the specimen from the collection bag; instead, aspirate a sample through the collection port in the catheter, using a sterile needle and a syringe.

Send all urine specimens to the laboratory as soon as possible to avoid degradation and altered values. Unless contraindicated and whenever possible, refrigerate urine until testing can be done.

• *X-rays.* A plain film of the abdomen assesses the size, shape, and position of the kidneys, ureters, and bladder and the possible areas of calcification.

Treatment
Intractable renal or urologic dysfunction may require urinary diversion, dialysis, or kidney transplantation.

Urinary diversion is the creation of an abnormal outlet for excreting urine. Several methods of urinary diversion may be performed: ileal conduit, cutaneous ureterostomy, ureterosigmoidostomy, continent diversions, and bladder augmentation or substitution procedures.

In dialysis, a semipermeable membrane, osmosis, and diffusion imitate normal kidney function by eliminating excess body fluids, maintaining or restoring plasma electrolyte and acid-base balances, and removing waste products and dialyzable toxins from the blood. Dialysis most often is used for patients with acute or chronic renal failure. The most common types are peritoneal dialysis and hemodialysis.

In peritoneal dialysis, a dialysis solution (dialysate) is infused into the peritoneal cavity. Substances then diffuse through the peritoneal membrane. Waste products remain in the solution and are removed.

Hemodialysis separates solutes in an external receptacle by differential diffusion through a cellophane membrane placed between the blood and the dialysate. Because the blood must actually pass out of the body into a dialysis machine, hemodialysis requires an access route to the blood supply by an arteriovenous fistula or cannula or by a bovine or synthetic graft. When caring for a patient with such vascular access routes, monitor the patency of the access route, prevent infection, and promote safety and adequate function. After dialysis, watch for complications, which may include headache, vomiting, agitation, and twitching.

Patients with end-stage renal disease may benefit from kidney transplantation, despite its limitations: a shortage of donor kidneys, the chance of transplant rejection, and the lifelong need for medications and follow-up care. After transplantation, maintain fluid and electrolyte balance, prevent infection, monitor for rejection, and promote psychological well-being.

CONGENITAL RENAL DISORDERS

Although present at birth, congenital disorders may not cause signs and symptoms until much later in life. These disorders include medullary sponge kidney and polycystic kidney disease.

MEDULLARY SPONGE KIDNEY
In this disorder, the collecting ducts in the renal pyramids dilate, and cavities, clefts, and cysts form in the medulla. Medullary sponge kidney may affect only a single pyramid in one kidney or all pyramids in both kidneys. Although an affected kidney may be of normal size, it's usually somewhat enlarged and spongy.

Because this disorder normally is asymptomatic and benign, it's commonly overlooked until the patient reaches adulthood. Although found in both sexes and in all age-groups, it's usually diagnosed in adolescents and adults ages 30 to 50. It occurs in about 1 in every 5,000 persons. The prognosis usually is good.

This disorder is unrelated to medullary polycystic disease, a hereditary disorder. These conditions are similar only in the presence and location of the cysts.

Causes
Medullary sponge kidney may be transmitted as an autosomal dominant trait (but sometimes as a recessive trait). It's generally considered a congenital abnormality.

Complications

In 50% to 60% of patients, complications include formation of calcium oxalate calculi, which lodge in the dilated cystic collecting ducts or pass through a ureter, and infection from duct dilation (in 20% to 30% of patients). Hypertension and renal failure seldom occur, except in patients with severe infection or nephrolithiasis. Secondary impairment of renal function from obstruction and infection occurs in about 10% of patients.

Assessment findings

Clinical features usually appear only as a result of complications and seldom occur before young adulthood. The patient may complain of severe colic, hematuria, burning on urination, urgency, and frequency—all signs and symptoms of a lower urinary tract infection (UTI). He also may report signs and symptoms of pyelonephritis—sudden onset of chills, fever, dull flank pain, and costovertebral angle tenderness.

Diagnostic tests

Excretory urography, usually the key to diagnosis, typically reveals a characteristic flowerlike appearance of the pyramidal cavities when they fill with contrast material. It also may show renal calculi.

Urinalysis is normal unless complications develop, such as an increased white blood cell count and casts with infection, and an increased red blood cell count with hematuria. It may show hypercalciuria or a slight reduction in concentrating ability.

Diagnosis must distinguish medullary sponge kidney from renal tuberculosis, renal tubular acidosis, and healed papillary necrosis. If infection is suspected, calculi should be evaluated.

Treatment

Treatment focuses on preventing or treating complications caused by calculi and infection. Specific measures include increasing fluid intake and monitoring renal function and urine output. If new symptoms develop, the patient needs immediate evaluation.

Because medullary sponge kidney is benign, surgery seldom is necessary, except to remove calculi during acute obstruction. Only serious, uncontrollable infection or hemorrhage necessitates nephrectomy.

Nursing diagnoses

• Altered urinary elimination
• Pain
• Risk for infection
• Risk for injury

Nursing interventions

• Limit the patient's dietary calcium intake to prevent calculus formation.
• When the patient is hospitalized for calculi, strain all urine, and give analgesics to relieve pain.
• Before diagnostic tests that use a contrast medium, ask about previous allergic reaction to shellfish, iodine, or contrast media. If the patient has had such a reaction, the doctor may cancel the test, do a limited study without a contrast medium, or pretreat the patient with antihistamines or steroids.
• If infection occurs, administer the prescribed antibiotic either I.V. or by mouth.
• Provide at least 2,000 ml of fluids daily by mouth (or parenterally if the patient has difficulty swallowing).

Patient teaching

• Explain the disorder to the patient and his family. Stress that the condition is benign and the prognosis is good, but warn them to watch for and report any signs of calculus passage or UTI.
• Explain all tests and demonstrate how to collect a clean-catch urine specimen for culture and sensitivity tests.
• To prevent UTI, instruct the patient to bathe often and use proper toilet hygiene.

POLYCYSTIC KIDNEY DISEASE

This inherited disorder is characterized by multiple, bilateral, grapelike clusters of fluid-filled cysts that enlarge the kidneys, compressing and eventually replacing functioning renal tissue. (See *Polycystic kidney*, page 814.) The disease affects males and females equally and appears in two distinct forms. The rare infantile form causes stillbirth or early neonatal death. The adult form has an insidious onset but usually becomes obvious between ages 30 and 50; rarely, it may not cause symptoms until the patient is in his 70s. Renal deterioration is more gradual in adults than in infants, but in both age-groups, the disease progresses relentlessly to fatal uremia.

The prognosis in adults is extremely variable. Progression may be slow, even after symptoms of renal insufficiency appear. Once uremic symptoms develop, polycystic disease usually is fatal within 4 years unless the patient receives dialysis.

Causes

Although both types of polycystic kidney disease are genetically transmitted, the incidence in two distinct age-groups and the different inheritance patterns suggest

POLYCYSTIC KIDNEY

The kidney in the cross-section below has multiple areas of cystic damage. Each indentation represents a cyst.

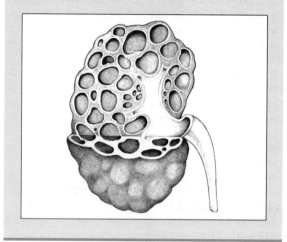

two unrelated disorders. The infantile type appears to be inherited as an autosomal recessive trait; the adult type, as an autosomal dominant trait.

Complications
A few infants with this disease survive for 2 years and then die of hepatic complications or renal, congestive heart, or respiratory failure. In adults, this disease may cause recurrent hematuria, life-threatening retroperitoneal bleeding from cyst rupture, proteinuria, and colicky abdominal pain from the ureteral passage of clots or calculi. In most cases, about 10 years after symptoms appear, progressive compression of kidney structures by the enlarging mass produces renal failure.

Assessment findings
Inspection of the neonate with infantile polycystic disease reveals pronounced epicanthal folds, a pointed nose, a small chin, and floppy, low-set ears (Potter facies). The infant also exhibits huge, bilateral, symmetrical masses on his flanks that are tense and can't be transilluminated.

Characteristically, the infant also shows signs of respiratory distress, congestive heart failure and, eventually, uremia and renal failure. Accompanying hepatic fibrosis and intrahepatic bile duct abnormalities may cause portal hypertension and bleeding varices as well.

The patient with adult polycystic kidney disease commonly is asymptomatic while in his 30s and 40s, but he may report polyuria, urinary tract infections (UTIs), and other nonspecific symptoms. Your assessment may show hypertension.

Later assessment reveals overt symptoms caused by the enlarging kidney mass, such as lumbar pain, widening girth, and a swollen or tender abdomen. The patient states that abdominal pain usually is worsened by exertion and relieved by lying down. In advanced stages, palpation easily reveals grossly enlarged kidneys.

Diagnostic tests
In a patient with polycystic disease, the following laboratory test results are typical:
• *Excretory* or *retrograde urography* reveals enlarged kidneys, with elongation of the pelvis, flattening of the calyces, and indentations caused by cysts. Excretory urography of the neonate shows poor excretion of contrast medium.
• *Ultrasonography, tomography,* and *radioisotopic scans* show kidney enlargement and cysts; tomography, computed tomography, and magnetic resonance imaging show multiple areas of cystic damage.
• *Urinalysis* and *creatinine clearance tests* — nonspecific tests that evaluate renal function — indicate abnormalities.

Diagnosis must rule out renal tumors.

Treatment
Polycystic kidney disease can't be cured. The primary goal of treatment is to preserve renal parenchyma and prevent pyelonephritis. Progressive renal failure requires treatment similar to that for other types of renal disease, including dialysis or, rarely, kidney transplantation.

When adult polycystic kidney disease is discovered in the asymptomatic stage, careful monitoring is required, including urine cultures and creatinine clearance tests every 6 months. When urine culture detects infection, the patient needs prompt and vigorous antibiotic treatment, even if he has no symptoms.

As renal impairment progresses, selected patients may undergo dialysis, transplantation, or both. Cystic abscess or retroperitoneal bleeding may necessitate surgical drainage; intractable pain (an uncommon symptom) also may require surgery. Nephrectomy usually isn't recommended because this disease occurs bilaterally and the infection could recur in the remaining kidney.

Nursing diagnoses

• Altered family processes
• Altered tissue perfusion
• Fatigue
• Fluid volume deficit
• Ineffective individual coping
• Pain
• Risk for infection
• Risk for injury
• Self-care deficit

Nursing interventions

• Provide supportive care to minimize any associated symptoms.
• Carefully assess the patient's life-style and physical and mental state. Determine how rapidly the disease is progressing. Use this information to plan individualized patient care.
• Encourage the patient to rest, and help with activities of daily living when the patient has abdominal pain. Offer analgesics as needed.
• Acquaint yourself with all aspects of end-stage renal disease, including dialysis and transplantation, so that you can provide appropriate care and patient teaching as the disease progresses.
• Administer antibiotics, as ordered, for UTI. Provide adequate hydration during antibiotic therapy.
• Screen urine for blood, cloudiness, and calculi or granules. Report any of these findings immediately.
• Use universal precautions when handling all blood and body fluids.
• Before beginning excretory urography and other procedures that use an iodine-based contrast medium, ask the patient if he's ever had an allergic reaction to iodine or shellfish. Even if he says no, watch for a possible allergic reaction after the procedures.
• If the patient requires peritoneal dialysis, position him carefully, elevating the head of the bed to reduce pressure on the diaphragm and aid respiration. Be alert for signs of infection, such as cloudy drainage, elevated temperature and, rarely, bleeding. If pain occurs, reduce the amount of dialysate. Periodically monitor the diabetic patient's blood glucose levels, and administer insulin, as ordered. Watch for complications, such as peritonitis, atelectasis, hypokalemia, pneumonia, and shock.
• If the patient requires hemodialysis, check the blood access site (arteriovenous fistula or subclavian or femoral catheter) every 2 hours for patency and signs of clotting. Don't use the arm with the shunt or fistula for measuring blood pressure or drawing blood. Weigh the patient before beginning dialysis.

• During hemodialysis, monitor vital signs, clotting times, blood flow, vascular access site function, and arterial and venous pressures. Watch for complications, such as septicemia, embolism, hepatitis, and rapid fluid and electrolyte losses.
• After hemodialysis, monitor vital signs and check the vascular access site. Also, weigh the patient and watch for signs of fluid and electrolyte imbalances.
• Allow the patient to verbalize his fears and concerns about the progressive disorder.

Patient teaching

• Discuss the patient's prognosis, including possible treatments, such as dialysis or transplantation; also answer any questions.
• Explain all diagnostic procedures to the patient or to his family if he's an infant. Also review any treatments, such as dialysis.
• Discuss prescribed medications and their possible adverse effects. Stress the need to take medications exactly as prescribed, even if symptoms are minimal or absent.
• Refer the young adult patient or the parents of an infant with polycystic kidney disease for genetic counseling. Parents will probably have many questions about the risk to other offspring.

ACUTE RENAL DISORDERS

These disorders have a sudden onset. They range from acute renal failure and acute pyelonephritis to renal calculi and renal vein thrombosis.

ACUTE RENAL FAILURE

About 5% of all hospitalized patients develop acute renal failure—the sudden interruption of renal function resulting from obstruction, reduced circulation, or renal parenchymal disease. This condition is classified as prerenal, intrarenal, or postrenal, and normally passes through three distinct phases—oliguric, diuretic, and recovery. It's usually reversible with medical treatment. If not treated, it may progress to end-stage renal disease, uremia, and death.

Causes

The three types of acute renal failure each have separate causes. Prerenal failure results from conditions that diminish blood flow to the kidneys. Between 40% and 80% of all cases of acute renal failure are caused by prerenal

CAUSES OF ACUTE RENAL FAILURE

Acute renal failure can be classified as prerenal, intrarenal, or postrenal. All conditions that lead to prerenal failure impair renal perfusion, resulting in decreased glomerular filtration rate and increased proximal tubular reabsorption of sodium and water. Intrarenal failure results from damage to the kidneys themselves; postrenal failure, from obstruction of urine flow.

Prerenal failure	Intrarenal failure	Postrenal failure
Cardiovascular disorders • Arrhythmias • Cardiac tamponade • Cardiogenic shock • Congestive heart failure • Myocardial infarction **Hypovolemia** • Burns • Dehydration • Diuretic abuse • Hemorrhage • Hypovolemic shock • Trauma **Peripheral vasodilation** • Antihypertensive drugs • Sepsis **Renovascular obstruction** • Arterial embolism • Arterial or venous thrombosis • Tumor **Severe vasoconstriction** • Disseminated intravascular coagulation • Eclampsia • Malignant hypertension • Vasculitis	**Acute tubular necrosis** • Ischemic damage to renal parenchyma from unrecognized or poorly treated prerenal failure • Nephrotoxins—analgesics (such as phenacetin), anesthetics (such as methoxyflurane), antibiotics (such as gentamicin), heavy metals (such as lead), radiographic contrast media, organic solvents • Obstetric complications—eclampsia, postpartum renal failure, septic abortion, uterine hemorrhage • Pigment release—crush injury, myopathy, sepsis, transfusion reaction **Other parenchymal disorders** • Acute glomerulonephritis • Acute interstitial nephritis • Acute pyelonephritis • Bilateral renal vein thrombosis • Malignant nephrosclerosis • Papillary necrosis • Periarteritis nodosa • Renal myeloma • Sickle cell disease • Systemic lupus erythematosus • Vasculitis	**Bladder obstruction** • Anticholinergic drugs • Autonomic nerve dysfunction • Infection • Tumor **Ureteral obstruction** • Blood clots • Calculi • Edema or inflammation • Necrotic renal papillae • Retroperitoneal fibrosis or hemorrhage • Surgery (accidental ligation) • Tumor • Uric acid crystals **Urethral obstruction** • Prostatic hyperplasia or tumor • Strictures

azotemia. Intrarenal failure (also called intrinsic or parenchymal renal failure) results from damage to the kidneys themselves, usually from acute tubular necrosis. Postrenal failure results from bilateral obstruction of urine outflow. (See *Causes of acute renal failure.*)

Complications

Ischemic acute tubular necrosis can lead to renal shutdown. Electrolyte imbalance, metabolic acidosis, and other severe effects follow as the patient becomes increasingly uremic and renal dysfunction disrupts other body systems. If left untreated, the patient will die. Even with treatment, the elderly patient is particularly susceptible to volume overload, precipitating acute pulmonary edema, hypertensive crisis, hyperkalemia, and infection.

Assessment findings

The patient's history may include a disorder that can cause renal failure, and he may have a recent history of fever; chills; GI problems, such as anorexia, nausea, vomiting, diarrhea, and constipation; and central nervous system problems, such as headache.

The patient may appear irritable, drowsy, and confused or demonstrate other alterations in his level of consciousness. In advanced stages, seizures and coma may occur. Depending on the stage of renal failure, his urine output may be oliguric (less than 400 ml/24 hours) or anuric (less than 100 ml/24 hours).

Inspection may uncover evidence of bleeding abnormalities, such as petechiae and ecchymoses. Hematemesis may occur. The skin may be dry and pruritic and, rarely, you may note uremic frost. Mucous membranes may be dry, and the patient's breath may have a uremic odor. If the patient has hyperkalemia, muscle weakness may occur.

Auscultation may detect tachycardia and, possibly, an irregular rhythm. Bibasilar crackles may be heard if the patient has congestive heart failure (CHF).

Palpation and percussion may reveal abdominal pain, if pancreatitis or peritonitis occurs, and peripheral edema, if the patient has CHF.

Diagnostic tests

Blood test results indicating acute intrarenal failure include elevated blood urea nitrogen, serum creatinine, and potassium levels, and low blood pH, bicarbonate, hematocrit, and hemoglobin levels.

Urine specimens show casts, cellular debris, decreased specific gravity and, in glomerular diseases, proteinuria and urine osmolality close to serum osmolality. The urine sodium level is less than 20 mEq/liter if oliguria results from decreased perfusion and more than 40 mEq/liter if it results from an intrarenal problem. A creatinine clearance test measures the glomerular filtration rate and allows for an estimate of the number of remaining functioning nephrons.

Other studies that help determine the cause of renal failure include kidney ultrasonography, plain films of the abdomen, kidney-ureter-bladder radiography, excretory urography, renal scan, retrograde pyelography, computed tomography scans, and nephrotomography.

An electrocardiogram (ECG) shows tall, peaked T waves; a widening QRS complex; and disappearing P waves if hyperkalemia is present.

Treatment

Supportive measures include a diet high in calories and low in protein, sodium, and potassium, with supplemental vitamins and restricted fluids. Meticulous electrolyte monitoring is essential to detect hyperkalemia. If hyperkalemia occurs, acute therapy may include hypertonic glucose-and-insulin infusions and sodium bicarbonate—all administered I.V.—and sodium polystyrene sulfonate (Kayexalate) by mouth or enema to remove potassium from the body.

If measures fail to control uremic symptoms, the patient may require hemodialysis or peritoneal dialysis. Early initiation of diuretic therapy during the oliguric phase may benefit the patient.

Nursing diagnoses

- Altered family processes
- Altered nutrition: Less than body requirements
- Altered oral mucous membrane
- Decreased cardiac output
- Fear
- Fluid volume deficit
- Fluid volume excess
- Impaired skin integrity
- Risk for infection
- Risk for injury

Nursing interventions

- Measure and record intake and output of all fluids, including wound drainage, nasogastric tube output, and diarrhea.
- Follow universal precautions during care because the patient with acute renal failure is highly susceptible to infection. Don't allow staff members or visitors with upper respiratory tract infections to come into contact with the patient. Also use universal precautions when handling all blood and body fluids.
- Be sure to weigh the patient daily. You also may need to measure abdominal girth every day. Mark the skin with indelible ink so that measurements can be taken in the same place.
- Evaluate all drugs the patient may be taking to identify those that may affect or be affected by renal function.
- Assess hematocrit and hemoglobin levels and replace blood components, as ordered. *Don't use whole blood if the patient is prone to CHF and can't tolerate extra fluid volume.* Packed red blood cells deliver the necessary blood components without added volume.
- Monitor vital signs. Watch for and report signs of pericarditis (pleuritic chest pain, tachycardia, and pericardial friction rub), inadequate renal perfusion (hypotension), and acidosis.
- Maintain proper electrolyte balance. Strictly monitor potassium levels. Watch for symptoms of hyperkalemia (malaise, anorexia, paresthesia, muscle weakness, and ECG changes), and report them immediately. Avoid administering medications that contain potassium.
- Assess the patient frequently, especially during emergency treatment to lower potassium levels. If he receives hypertonic glucose-and-insulin infusions, monitor potassium and glucose levels. If you give sodium polystyrene sulfonate rectally, make sure the patient doesn't retain it and become constipated. This can lead to bowel perforation.
- Maintain nutritional status. Provide a diet high in calories and low in protein, sodium, and potassium, with

vitamin supplements. Give the anorexic patient small, frequent meals.

• Prevent complications of immobility by encouraging frequent coughing and deep breathing and by performing passive range-of-motion exercises. Help the patient walk as soon as possible. Add lubricating lotion to his bath water to combat skin dryness.

• Provide mouth care frequently to lubricate dry mucous membranes. If stomatitis occurs, use an antibiotic solution, if ordered, and have the patient swish it around in his mouth before swallowing.

• Monitor for GI bleeding by testing all stools for occult blood, using the guaiac test. Administer medications carefully, especially antacids and stool softeners.

• Provide meticulous perineal care to reduce the risk of ascending urinary tract infection in women and to protect skin integrity caused by frequent loose, irritating stools, particularly when sodium polystyrene sulfonate is used.

• Use appropriate safety measures, such as side rails and restraints, because the patient with central nervous system involvement may become dizzy or confused.

• If the patient requires hemodialysis, check the blood access site (arteriovenous fistula or subclavian or femoral catheter) every 2 hours for patency and signs of clotting. Don't use the arm with the shunt or fistula for measuring blood pressure or drawing blood. Weigh the patient before beginning dialysis.

During dialysis, monitor vital signs, clotting times, blood flow, vascular access site function, and arterial and venous pressures. Watch for complications, such as septicemia, embolism, hepatitis, and rapid fluid and electrolyte losses.

After dialysis, monitor vital signs, check the vascular access site, weigh the patient, and watch for signs of fluid and electrolyte imbalances.

• If the patient requires peritoneal dialysis, position him carefully, elevating the head of the bed to reduce pressure on the diaphragm and aid respiration. Be alert for signs of infection, such as cloudy drainage, elevated temperature and, rarely, bleeding. If pain occurs, reduce the amount of dialysate. Periodically monitor the diabetic patient's blood glucose levels, and administer insulin, as ordered. Watch for complications, such as peritonitis, atelectasis, hypokalemia, pneumonia, and shock.

• Provide emotional support to the patient and his family.

• Administer any prescribed medications after hemodialysis is completed. Many medications are removed from the blood during treatment.

• Assess the patient's ability to resume normal activities of daily living, and plan for the gradual resumption of activity.

Patient teaching

• Reassure the patient and his family by clearly explaining all diagnostic tests, treatments, and procedures.

• Tell the patient about his prescribed medications, and stress the importance of complying with the regimen.

• Stress the importance of following the prescribed diet and fluid allowance.

• Instruct the patient to weigh himself daily and report changes of 3 lb or more immediately.

• Advise the patient against overexertion. If he becomes dyspneic or short of breath during normal activity, tell him to report it to his doctor.

• Teach the patient how to recognize edema, and tell him to report this finding to the doctor.

ACUTE PYELONEPHRITIS

Also called acute infective tubulointerstitial nephritis, acute pyelonephritis is one of the most common renal diseases. In this disorder, sudden inflammation is caused by bacterial invasion. It occurs mainly in the interstitial tissue and the renal pelvis and occasionally in the renal tubules. It may affect one or both kidneys. With treatment and continued follow-up care, the prognosis is good and extensive permanent damage is rare.

Pyelonephritis occurs more often in women than in men, probably because the shorter urethra and the proximity of the urinary meatus to the vagina and rectum allow bacteria to reach the bladder more easily. Women also lack the antibacterial prostatic secretions that men produce.

Typically, the infection spreads from the bladder to the ureters and then to the kidneys, commonly through vesicoureteral reflux. Vesicoureteral reflux may result from congenital weakness at the junction of the ureter and the bladder. Bacteria refluxed to intrarenal tissues may create colonies of infection within 24 to 48 hours.

Causes

Acute pyelonephritis results from bacterial infection of the kidneys. Infecting bacteria usually are normal intestinal and fecal flora that grow readily in urine. The most common causative organism is *Escherichia coli,* but *Proteus, Pseudomonas, Staphylococcus aureus,* and *Streptococcus faecalis* (enterococcus) also may cause such infections.

Infection also may result from procedures that involve the use of instruments (such as catheterization, cystoscopy, and urologic surgery) or from a hematogenic infection (such as septicemia and endocarditis).

Pyelonephritis may result from an inability to empty the bladder (for example, in patients with neurogenic bladder), from urinary stasis, or from urinary obstruction caused by tumors, strictures, or benign prostatic hyperplasia. Incidence increases with age and is higher in the following groups:
• *Sexually active women.* Intercourse increases the risk of bacterial contamination.
• *Pregnant women.* About 5% of pregnant women develop asymptomatic bacteriuria; if untreated, about 40% of these women develop pyelonephritis.
• *People with obstructive diseases.* Resulting hydronephrosis increases the risk of urinary tract infection (UTI), which can lead to pyelonephritis.
• *People with neurogenic bladder.* Seen in diabetes, spinal cord injury, multiple sclerosis, and tabes dorsalis, neurogenic bladder causes incomplete emptying and urinary stasis. Frequent catheterization increases the risk of introducing bacteria. Glycosuria may support bacterial growth in urine.
• *People with other renal diseases.* Compromised renal function increases susceptibility to acute pyelonephritis.

Complications
Associated complications include secondary arteriosclerosis, calculus formation, further renal damage, renal abscesses with possible metastasis to other organs, septic shock, and chronic pyelonephritis. (See *Chronic pyelonephritis.*)

Assessment findings
A patient with acute pyelonephritis commonly looks quite ill. She usually complains of pain over one or both kidneys, urinary urgency and frequency, burning during urination, dysuria, nocturia, and hematuria (usually microscopic but possibly gross). Palpating the flank area may increase pain. Urine may appear cloudy and have an ammonia-like or fishy odor. Other common symptoms include a temperature of 102° F (38.9° C) or higher, shaking chills, anorexia, and general fatigue.

The patient usually reports that symptoms developed rapidly over a few hours or a few days. Although these symptoms may disappear within days, even without treatment, residual bacterial infection is likely and may cause recurrence of symptoms.

CHRONIC PYELONEPHRITIS

A persistent kidney inflammation, chronic pyelonephritis can scar the kidneys and lead to chronic renal failure. Its etiology may be bacterial, metastatic, or urogenous. This disease most frequently occurs in patients who are predisposed to recurrent acute pyelonephritis—for instance, those with urinary obstructions or vesicoureteral reflux.

Assessment and diagnosis
Patients with chronic pyelonephritis may have a childhood history of unexplained fevers or bedwetting. Clinical signs and symptoms include flank pain, anemia, low urine specific gravity, proteinuria, leukocytes in urine, and hypertension. Uremia seldom develops unless structural abnormalities exist in the excretory system. Intermittent bacteriuria may occur.

When no bacteria are found in the urine, diagnosis depends on excretory urography (the patient's renal pelvis may appear small and flattened) and renal biopsy.

Treatment
Effective treatment of chronic pyelonephritis requires control of hypertension, elimination of the obstruction (when possible), and long-term antimicrobial therapy.

Diagnostic tests
Diagnosis requires a urinalysis and culture and sensitivity testing. Typical findings include:
• *Pyuria.* Urine sediment reveals leukocytes singly, in clumps, and in casts and, possibly, a few red blood cells.
• *Significant bacteriuria.* Urine culture reveals more than 100,000 organisms/mm³ of urine.
• *Low specific gravity and osmolality.* These findings result from a temporarily decreased ability to concentrate urine.
• *Slightly alkaline urine pH.*
• *Proteinuria, glycosuria, and ketonuria.* These conditions occur less frequently.

Blood tests and X-rays also help in the evaluation of acute pyelonephritis. A complete blood count shows an elevated white blood cell count (up to 40,000/mm³) and an elevated neutrophil count. The erythrocyte sedimentation rate also is elevated.

Kidney-ureter-bladder radiography may reveal calculi, tumors, or cysts in the kidneys and the urinary tract. Excretory urography may show asymmetrical kidneys, possibly indicating a high frequency of infection.

Treatment

Appropriate treatment centers on antibiotic therapy appropriate to the specific infecting organism after identification by urine culture and sensitivity studies. For example, enterococcus requires treatment with ampicillin, penicillin G, or vancomycin. *Staphylococcus* requires penicillin G or, if the bacterium is resistant, a semisynthetic penicillin, such as nafcillin, or a cephalosporin. *Escherichia coli* may be treated with sulfisoxazole, nalidixic acid, or nitrofurantoin; *Proteus,* with ampicillin, sulfisoxazole, nalidixic acid, or a cephalosporin; and *Pseudomonas,* with gentamicin, tobramycin, or carbenicillin.

When the infecting organism can't be identified, therapy usually consists of a broad-spectrum antibiotic, such as ampicillin or cephalexin. Antibiotics must be prescribed cautiously for elderly patients because of the combined effects of aging and pyelonephritis on renal function. Antibiotics also are used with caution in pregnant patients. In these patients, urinary analgesics, such as phenazopyridine, can help relieve pain.

Symptoms may disappear after several days of antibiotic therapy. Although urine usually becomes sterile within 48 to 72 hours, the course of such therapy ranges from 10 to 14 days. Follow-up treatment includes reculturing urine 1 week after drug therapy stops and then periodically for the next year to detect residual or recurring infection. A patient with an uncomplicated infection usually responds well to therapy and doesn't suffer reinfection.

If infection results from obstruction or vesicoureteral reflux, antibiotics may be less effective and surgery may be necessary to relieve the obstruction or correct the anomaly. A patient at high risk for recurring urinary tract and kidney infections—for example, a patient with a long-term indwelling catheter or on maintenance antibiotic therapy—requires lengthy follow-up care.

Nursing diagnoses

• Altered tissue perfusion
• Fluid volume excess
• Impaired physical mobility
• Pain
• Risk for infection
• Self-care deficit

Nursing interventions

• Administer antipyretics for fever.
• Force fluids to achieve a urine output of more than 2,000 ml/day. This helps empty the bladder of contaminated urine and is the best way to prevent calculus formation. Don't encourage intake of more than 2 to 3 liters because this may decrease the effectiveness of the antibiotics.
• Provide an acid-ash diet to prevent calculus formation.
• Observe strict sterile technique during catheter insertion and care.
• Be sure to refrigerate or culture a urine specimen within 30 minutes of collection to prevent overgrowth of bacteria.

Patient teaching

• Instruct a female patient to avoid bacterial contamination by wiping the perineum from front to back after bowel movements.
• Teach proper technique for collecting a clean-catch urine specimen.
• Stress the need to complete the prescribed antibiotic regimen, even after symptoms subside. Encourage long-term follow-up care for a high-risk patient.
• Advise routine checkups for a patient with a history of UTIs. Teach her to recognize signs and symptoms of infection, such as cloudy urine, burning on urination, and urinary urgency and frequency, especially when accompanied by a low-grade fever and back pain.

ACUTE POSTSTREPTOCOCCAL GLOMERULONEPHRITIS

Also called acute glomerulonephritis, acute poststreptococcal glomerulonephritis is relatively common. This disorder, a bilateral inflammation of the glomeruli, follows a streptococcal infection of the respiratory tract or, less often, a skin infection such as impetigo. Most common in boys ages 3 to 7, it can occur at any age. Up to 95% of children and 70% of adults recover fully; the rest, especially elderly patients, may progress to chronic renal failure within months.

Causes

Acute poststreptococcal glomerulonephritis results from the entrapment and collection of antigen-antibody complexes (produced as an immunologic mechanism in response to a group A beta-hemolytic streptococcus) in the glomerular capillary membranes, inducing inflammatory damage and impeding glomerular function. Sometimes the immune complement further damages the glomerular membrane. The damaged and inflamed glomeruli lose the ability to be selectively permeable, allowing red blood cells and proteins to filter through as the glomerular filtration rate (GFR) falls. Uremic poisoning may result.

Complications

Children usually have few complications. However, renal function progressively deteriorates in 33% to 50% of adults who contract sporadic acute poststreptococcal glomerulonephritis, often in the form of glomerulosclerosis accompanied by hypertension. The more severe the disorder, the more likely that complications will follow.

Assessment findings

In most cases, acute poststreptococcal glomerulonephritis begins within 1 to 3 weeks after an untreated streptococcal infection in the respiratory tract. The patient—or the patient's parents—may report decreased urination, smoky or coffee-colored urine, and fatigue. The patient also may experience shortness of breath, dyspnea, and orthopnea. These symptoms of pulmonary edema point to congestive heart failure (CHF) resulting from hypervolemia.

Assessment findings may show oliguria (with output less than 400 ml/24 hours) and mild to moderate periorbital edema. Findings also may reveal mild to severe hypertension resulting from either sodium or water retention (caused by decreased GFR) or inappropriate renin release.

An elderly patient may complain of vague, nonspecific symptoms, such as nausea, malaise, and arthralgia. Auscultation reveals bibasilar crackles if CHF is present.

Diagnostic tests

Abnormal blood values (elevated electrolyte, blood urea nitrogen [BUN], and creatinine levels and decreased serum protein levels) and the presence of red blood cells, white blood cells, mixed cell casts, and protein in the urine indicate renal failure. (The proteinuria in an elderly patient usually is not as pronounced.) Urine frequently contains high levels of fibrin-degradation products and C3 protein.

Elevated antistreptolysin-O titers (in 80% of patients), elevated streptozyme and anti-DNase B titers, and low serum complement levels verify recent streptococcal infection. A throat culture may show group A beta-hemolytic streptococci.

Kidney-ureter-bladder X-rays show bilateral kidney enlargement. A renal biopsy may be necessary to confirm the diagnosis or assess renal tissue status.

Treatment

Therapy aims to relieve symptoms and prevent complications. Vigorous supportive care includes bed rest, fluid and dietary sodium restrictions, and correction of electrolyte imbalances (possibly with dialysis, although this seldom is necessary).

Treatment may include loop diuretics, such as metolazone or furosemide, to reduce extracellular fluid overload, and vasodilators, such as hydralazine or nifedipine. If the patient has a documented staphylococcal infection, antibiotics are recommended for 7 to 10 days; otherwise, their use is controversial.

Nursing diagnoses

- Altered nutrition: Less than body requirements
- Altered role performance
- Decreased cardiac output
- Fatigue
- Fluid volume excess
- Impaired gas exchange
- Impaired physical mobility
- Pain
- Risk for infection
- Risk for injury
- Self-care deficit

Nursing interventions

- Acute poststreptococcal glomerulonephritis usually resolves within 2 weeks, so nursing care primarily is supportive.
- Provide bed rest during the acute phase. Perform passive range-of-motion exercises for the patient on bed rest. Allow the patient to resume normal activities *gradually* as symptoms subside.
- Check the patient's vital signs and electrolyte values. Assess renal function daily through serum creatinine and BUN levels and urine creatinine clearance tests. Immediately report signs of acute renal failure (oliguria, azotemia, and acidosis).
- Monitor intake and output and daily weight. Report peripheral edema or the formation of ascites.
- Consult the dietitian about a diet high in calories and low in protein, sodium, potassium, and fluids.
- Protect the debilitated patient against secondary infection by providing good nutrition and good hygienic technique, and preventing contact with infected people.
- Provide emotional support for the patient and his family. Encourage the patient to verbalize his concerns about his inability to perform in his expected role. Assure him that the activity restrictions are temporary.

Patient teaching
• Stress to the patient, or his parents if the patient is a child, that follow-up examinations are necessary to detect chronic renal failure. Emphasize the need for regular blood pressure, urine protein, and renal function assessments during the convalescent months to detect recurrence. Explain that after acute poststreptococcal glomerulonephritis, gross hematuria may recur during nonspecific viral infections and abnormal urinary findings may persist for years.
• If the patient is scheduled for dialysis, explain the procedure fully.
• Advise a patient with a history of chronic upper respiratory tract infections to report signs and symptoms of infection, such as fever and sore throat, immediately.
• Encourage a pregnant patient with a history of acute poststreptococcal glomerulonephritis to have frequent medical evaluations because pregnancy further stresses the kidneys and increases the risk of chronic renal failure.
• Explain to the patient taking diuretics that he may experience orthostatic hypotension and dizziness when he changes positions quickly.

ACUTE TUBULAR NECROSIS

The most common cause of acute renal failure in critically ill patients, acute tubular necrosis (also called acute tubulointerstitial nephritis) accounts for about 75% of all cases of acute renal failure. This disorder injures the tubular segment of the nephron, causing renal failure and uremic syndrome. Mortality can be as high as 70%, depending on complications from underlying diseases. Nonoliguric forms of acute tubular necrosis have a better prognosis.

Causes

Acute tubular necrosis results from ischemic or nephrotoxic injury, most commonly in debilitated patients, such as the critically ill or those who've undergone extensive surgery. In ischemic injury, disruption of blood flow to the kidneys may result from circulatory collapse, severe hypotension, trauma, hemorrhage, dehydration, cardiogenic or septic shock, surgery, anesthetics, or transfusion reactions. Nephrotoxic injury may follow ingestion or inhalation of certain chemicals, such as aminoglycoside antibiotics and radiographic contrast agents, or it may result from a hypersensitivity reaction of the kidneys.

Specifically, acute tubular necrosis can result from any of the following:

• diseased tubular epithelium that allows leakage of glomerular filtrate across the membranes and reabsorption of filtrate into the blood
• obstructed urine flow from the collection of damaged cells, casts, red blood cells (RBCs), and other cellular debris within the tubular walls
• ischemic injury to glomerular epithelial cells, resulting in cellular collapse and decreased glomerular capillary permeability
• ischemic injury to vascular endothelium, eventually resulting in cellular swelling, sludging, and tubular obstruction.

Complications

Nephrotoxic acute tubular necrosis doesn't damage the basement membrane of the nephron, so it's potentially reversible. However, ischemic acute tubular necrosis can damage the epithelial and basement membranes and can cause lesions in the renal interstitium. Infections (frequently septicemia) can complicate up to 70% of all cases and are the leading cause of death. GI hemorrhage, fluid and electrolyte imbalance, and cardiovascular dysfunction may occur during the acute phase or not until the recovery phase. Neurologic complications occur commonly in elderly patients and occasionally in younger patients. Hypercalcemia may occur during the recovery phase.

Assessment findings

The patient's history may include an ischemic or a nephrotoxic injury that can cause acute tubular necrosis. The signs of acute tubular necrosis may be obscured by the patient's primary disease.

You may first note that the patient's urine output may be oliguric (less than 400 ml/24 hours); occasionally, in severe cases, urine output may be less than 100 ml/24 hours for several days.

Inspection may reveal evidence of bleeding abnormalities such as petechiae and ecchymoses. Hematemesis may occur. The skin may be dry and pruritic and, rarely, a uremic frost may be present. Mucous membranes also may be dry, and the breath may have a uremic odor. If hyperkalemia is present, muscle weakness may occur.

The patient may exhibit evidence of central nervous system involvement, such as lethargy, somnolence, confusion, disorientation, asterixis, agitation, myoclonic muscle twitching and, possibly, seizures.

Auscultation may reveal tachycardia and, possibly, an irregular rhythm. Rarely, a pericardial friction rub can be heard, indicating pericarditis. Bibasilar crackles may occur if congestive heart failure (CHF) is present.

Palpation and percussion may reveal abdominal pain, if pancreatitis or peritonitis occurs, and peripheral edema, if CHF is present.

Fever and chills can signal the onset of infection.

Diagnostic tests

Diagnosis usually doesn't occur until the condition reaches an advanced stage. The most significant laboratory test findings are urine sediment, containing RBCs and casts, and dilute urine with a low specific gravity (1.010), low osmolality (less than 400 mOsm/kg), and high sodium level (40 to 60 mEq/liter).

Blood studies reveal elevated blood urea nitrogen and serum creatinine levels, decreased serum protein levels, anemia, defects in platelet adherence, metabolic acidosis, and hyperkalemia.

An electrocardiogram may show arrhythmias (from electrolyte imbalances). With hyperkalemia, it also may show a widening QRS complex, disappearing P waves, and tall, peaked T waves.

Treatment

Acute tubular necrosis requires vigorous supportive measures during the acute phase until normal renal function resumes. Initial treatment may include administration of diuretics and infusion of a large volume of fluids to flush tubules of cellular casts and debris and to replace fluid loss. This treatment carries a risk of fluid overload. Long-term fluid management requires daily replacement of projected and calculated losses (including insensible loss).

Other appropriate measures to control complications include transfusion of packed RBCs for anemia and administration of antibiotics for infection. A patient with hyperkalemia may require emergency I.V. administration of 50% glucose, regular insulin, and sodium bicarbonate. Sodium polystyrene sulfonate may be given by mouth or by enema to reduce extracellular potassium levels. Peritoneal dialysis or hemodialysis may be needed for a catabolic patient.

Nursing diagnoses

- Altered nutrition: Less than body requirements
- Altered role performance
- Altered tissue perfusion
- Decreased cardiac output
- Fatigue
- Fluid volume excess
- Impaired gas exchange
- Pain
- Risk for infection
- Risk for injury
- Self-care deficit

Nursing interventions

- Maintain fluid balance, and watch for fluid overload, a common complication of therapy. Accurately record intake and output, including wound drainage, nasogastric tube output, and peritoneal dialysis and hemodialysis balances. Weigh the patient at the same time every day.
- Monitor hemoglobin and hematocrit levels, and administer blood products as needed. Use fresh packed cells instead of whole blood, especially in an elderly patient, to prevent fluid overload and CHF.
- Maintain electrolyte balance. Monitor laboratory test results and report imbalances. Restrict foods that contain sodium and potassium, such as bananas, prunes, orange juice, and baked potatoes. Check for potassium content in prescribed medications (for example, potassium penicillin).
- Provide adequate calories and essential amino acids while restricting protein intake to maintain an anabolic state. Total parenteral nutrition (TPN) may be indicated for a severely debilitated or catabolic patient. If the patient is receiving TPN, keep his skin meticulously clean.
- Use aseptic technique, particularly when handling catheters, because the debilitated patient is vulnerable to infection. Immediately report fever, chills, delayed wound healing, or flank pain if the patient has an indwelling catheter.
- Watch for complications. If anemia worsens, causing pallor, weakness, or lethargy with decreased hemoglobin, administer RBCs, as ordered. For acidosis, give sodium bicarbonate or assist with dialysis in severe cases, as ordered. Watch for hypotension, which diminishes renal perfusion and decreases urine output.
- Perform passive range-of-motion exercises. Provide good skin care, and apply lotion or bath oil to prevent dry skin. Help the patient walk as soon as possible, but make sure he doesn't become exhausted.
- To prevent acute tubular necrosis, make sure every patient is well hydrated before surgery or after X-rays that use a contrast medium. Administer mannitol, as ordered, to a high-risk patient before and during these procedures. Carefully monitor a patient receiving a blood transfusion, and discontinue the transfusion immediately if early signs of transfusion reaction (fever, rash, and chills) occur.
- Provide emotional support to the patient and his family. Encourage the patient to verbalize his concerns about his inability to perform his expected role. Assure him that activity restrictions are temporary.

SITES OF RENAL INFARCTION

Infarction, most often resulting from renal blood vessel occlusion, affects the renal cortex, but it can extend into the medulla.

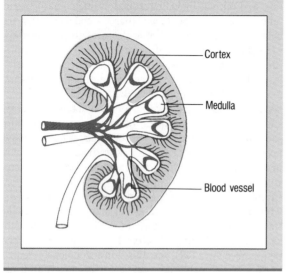

Cortex

Medulla

Blood vessel

Patient teaching
• Teach the patient the signs of infection, and tell him to report them to the doctor immediately. Remind him to stay away from crowds and any infected person.
• Review the prescribed diet, including dietary restrictions, and stress the importance of adhering to it.
• Teach the patient how to cough and perform deep breathing to prevent pulmonary complications.
• Fully explain each procedure to the patient and his family as often as necessary, and help them set goals that are realistic for the patient's prognosis.

RENAL INFARCTION

Caused by renal blood vessel occlusion, renal infarction is the formation of a coagulated, necrotic area in one or both kidneys. The location and size of the infarction depend on the site of occlusion. The embolism reduces the blood flow rate to renal tissue and leads to ischemia. The degree of blood flow reduction determines whether the insult is acute or chronic as arterial narrowing progresses. (See *Sites of renal infarction.*) Residual renal function depends on the extent of the damage from the infarction.

Causes
In 75% of patients, renal infarction results from renal artery embolism secondary to mitral stenosis, infective endocarditis, atrial fibrillation, microthrombi in the left ventricle, rheumatic valvular disease, or recent myocardial infarction.

Less common causes of renal infarction include atherosclerosis (with or without thrombus formation), thrombus from flank trauma, sickle cell anemia, scleroderma, polyarteritis nodosa, and arterionephrosclerosis.

Complications
Renovascular hypertension commonly occurs several days after infarction. It results from reduced blood flow, which stimulates the renin-angiotensin mechanism.

Assessment findings
The patient's recent history usually includes onset of hypertension in a previously normotensive person. The patient commonly complains of severe, sharp, unrelenting upper abdominal pain or of gnawing flank pain; flank or costovertebral tenderness; fever; anorexia; nausea; and vomiting. A bruit may be auscultated in the epigastrium. The affected kidney is small and not palpable. The contralateral kidney may feel enlarged when palpated. Muscle weakness or tetany also may be present. Urine output may be increased.

Diagnostic tests
A firm diagnosis requires appropriate diagnostic tests, including the following:
• *Urinalysis* reveals proteinuria and gross microscopic hematuria.
• *Urine enzyme levels,* especially lactate dehydrogenase (LDH) and alkaline phosphatase, often are elevated for about 48 hours after infarction because of tissue destruction.
• *Serum enzyme levels,* especially aspartate aminotransferase (formerly SGOT), alkaline phosphatase, and LDH, are elevated. Blood studies also may reveal leukocytosis and an increased erythrocyte sedimentation rate.
• *Captopril test* result is positive in renovascular hypertension, and is useful in differentiating this form of hypertension from essential hypertension before more invasive tests are done.
• *Excretory urography* shows diminished or absent excretion of contrast medium, indicating vascular occlusion.
• *Isotopic renal scan,* a benign, noninvasive technique, demonstrates absent or reduced blood flow to the kidneys.

• *Renal arteriography* gives proof of an existing infarction. This high-risk test is used only as a last resort.
• *Computed tomography* locates the exact areas of occlusion and the extent of the infarction.

Treatment

Infection in the infarcted area or significant hypertension may require surgical removal of the occlusion or nephrectomy. Surgery to establish collateral circulation to the area can relieve renovascular hypertension. Persistent hypertension may respond to antihypertensives and a low-sodium diet. Other treatments may include the early administration of intra-arterial streptokinase to lyse blood clots, catheter embolectomy, and heparin therapy.

Nursing diagnoses

• Altered nutrition: Less than body requirements
• Fluid volume excess
• Pain
• Risk for infection

Nursing interventions

• Give ordered pain medication to provide comfort.
• Monitor intake and output, vital signs (particularly blood pressure), electrolyte levels, and daily weight. Watch for signs of fluid overload, such as dyspnea and tachycardia.
• Provide the prescribed low-sodium diet. Consult the dietitian to provide well-balanced meals.
• Monitor for further bleeding from thrombolytic drugs, if used, and further infarction caused by clot breakdown.
• Give emotional support to the patient and his family.

Patient teaching

• Explain diagnostic tests and treatments, and discuss self-care measures. (See *Living with renal infarction*.)
• Encourage a follow-up visit, which usually includes excretory urography or a renal scan to assess regained renal function and possibly a cardiovascular workup.

RENAL CALCULI

Although they may form anywhere in the urinary tract, renal calculi most commonly develop in the renal pelvis or calyces. Calculi formation occurs when substances that normally are dissolved in the urine (such as calcium oxalate and calcium phosphate) precipitate. Renal calculi vary in size and may be solitary or multiple. (See *Variations in renal calculi*, page 826.)

About 1 in 1,000 Americans require hospitalization for renal calculi. They're more common in men than in women and rare in blacks and children.

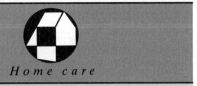

Home care

LIVING WITH RENAL INFARCTION

Follow these guidelines to help your patient learn to live with renal infarction:
• Explain a low-sodium diet, and encourage the patient to follow it.
• Instruct the patient to eat natural foods and to avoid frozen or prepared meals, spicy or salty snacks, carbonated beverages, luncheon meats, and cheese. Explain that many regional and ethnic foods are high in sodium and monosodium glutamate. Show him how to read food labels.
• Teach the patient how to buy and use a home blood pressure monitor. Tell him how often to take his blood pressure (daily or biweekly) and when to report it to the doctor.
• Teach the patient about his medications, including which adverse effects require calling his doctor. Caution him not to mix antihypertensives, diuretics, and over-the-counter drugs.

Causes

Renal calculi are particularly prevalent in certain geographic areas, such as the southeastern United States (called the "stone belt"), possibly because a hot climate promotes dehydration and concentrates calculus-forming substances or because of regional dietary habits. Although the exact cause of renal calculi is unknown, predisposing factors include:
• *Dehydration.* Decreased water excretion concentrates calculus-forming substances.
• *Infection.* Infected, scarred tissue may be a site for calculus development. In addition, infected calculi (usually magnesium ammonium phosphate or staghorn calculi) may develop if bacteria serve as the nucleus in calculus formation. Struvite calculus formation commonly results from *Proteus* infections, which may lead to destruction of renal parenchyma.
• *Changes in urine pH.* Consistently acidic or alkaline urine may provide a favorable medium for calculus formation, especially for magnesium ammonium phosphate or calcium phosphate calculi.
• *Obstruction.* Urinary stasis allows calculus constituents to collect and adhere, forming calculi. Obstruction

VARIATIONS IN RENAL CALCULI

Renal calculi vary in size and type. Small calculi may remain in the renal pelvis or pass down the ureter. A staghorn calculus (a cast of the calyceal and pelvic collecting system) may develop from a stone that stays in the kidney.

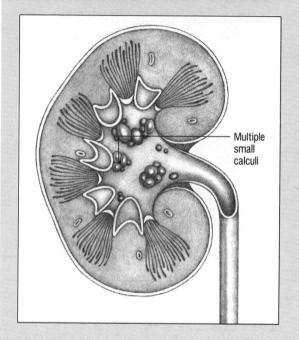

Multiple small calculi

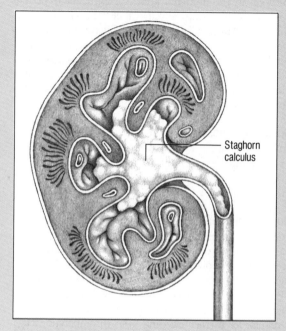

Staghorn calculus

also encourages infection, which compounds the obstruction.

• *Immobilization.* Immobility from spinal cord injury or other disorders allows calcium to be released into the circulation and, eventually, to be filtered by the kidneys.

• *Metabolic factors.* Hyperparathyroidism, renal tubular acidosis, elevated uric acid (usually with gout), defective metabolism of oxalate, a genetically caused defect in metabolism of cystine, and excessive intake of vitamin D or dietary calcium may predispose a person to renal calculi.

Complications

Calculi may either remain in the renal pelvis and damage or destroy renal parenchyma, or enter the ureter; large calculi in the kidneys cause pressure necrosis. In certain locations, calculi cause obstruction, with resultant hydronephrosis, and tend to recur. Intractable pain and serious bleeding also can result from calculi and the damage they cause.

Assessment findings

Typically, assessment findings vary with the size, location, and cause of the calculi. The key symptom of renal calculi is severe pain, which usually results from obstruction—large, rough calculi occlude the opening to the ureteropelvic junction and increase the frequency and force of peristaltic contractions. The patient usually reports that the pain travels from the costovertebral angle to the flank and then to the suprapubic region and external genitalia (classic renal colic pain). Pain intensity fluctuates and may be excruciating at its peak.

The patient with calculi in the renal pelvis and calyces may complain of more constant, dull pain. He also may report back pain (from calculi causing obstruction within a kidney) and severe abdominal pain (from calculi traveling down a ureter). The patient with severe pain also typically complains of nausea, vomiting and, possibly, fever and chills.

You may note hematuria (when calculi abrade a ureter), abdominal distention and, rarely, anuria (from bilateral obstruction or, in the patient with one kidney, unilateral obstruction).

Diagnostic tests
Diagnosis is based on clinical features and the following tests:
• *Kidney-ureter-bladder (KUB) radiography* reveals most renal calculi.
• *Excretory urography* helps confirm the diagnosis and determine the size and location of calculi.
• *Kidney ultrasonography* — easily performed, noninvasive, and nontoxic — detects obstructive changes, such as unilateral or bilateral hydronephrosis and radiolucent calculi not seen on the KUB radiography.
• *Urine culture* of a midstream specimen may indicate pyuria, a sign of urinary tract infection.
• A *24-hour urine collection* is evaluated for calcium oxalate, phosphorus, and uric acid excretion levels. Three separate collections, along with blood samples, are needed for accurate testing.
• *Calculus analysis* shows mineral content.
  Other diagnostic test results may suggest the cause of calculus formation.
• *Serial blood calcium and phosphorus levels* detect hyperparathyroidism and show an increased calcium level in proportion to normal serum protein levels.
• *Blood protein levels* determine the level of free calcium unbound to protein.
• If increased, *blood uric acid levels* may indicate gout.
  Appendicitis, cholecystitis, peptic ulcer, and pancreatitis must be ruled out as potential sources of pain before the diagnosis can be confirmed.

Treatment
Because 90% of renal calculi are smaller than 5 mm in diameter, treatment usually involves encouraging their natural passage through vigorous hydration (more than 3 liters/day). Other treatment measures include administration of antimicrobial agents for infection (varying with the cultured organism); analgesics, such as meperidine or morphine, for pain; and diuretics to prevent urinary stasis and further calculus formation (thiazides decrease calcium excretion into the urine). Methenamine mandelate is given to suppress calculus formation when infection is present.
  Measures to prevent recurrence include a low-calcium diet, often combined with oxalate-binding cholestyramine, for absorptive hypercalciuria; parathyroidectomy for hyperparathyroidism; administration of allopurinol for uric acid calculi; and daily oral doses of ascorbic acid to acidify the urine.

Calculi too large for natural passage may require removal. A calculus lodged in the ureter may be removed by inserting a cystoscope through the urethra and then manipulating the calculus with catheters or retrieval instruments. Extraction of calculi from other areas, such as the kidney calyx or renal pelvis, may necessitate a flank or lower abdominal approach. Two other methods, percutaneous ultrasonic lithotripsy and extracorporeal shock wave lithotripsy, shatter the calculus into fragments for removal by suction or natural passage.
  Cystine calculi are difficult to treat without surgical intervention or invasive procedure. If electrohydraulic ultrasound isn't effective, the calculi are surgically removed.

Nursing diagnoses
• Altered urinary elimination
• Pain
• Risk for infection

Nursing interventions
• To aid diagnosis, maintain a 24- to 48-hour record of urine pH, using nitrazine pH paper. Strain all urine through gauze or a tea strainer, and save all solid material recovered for analysis.
• To facilitate spontaneous passage of calculi, encourage the patient to walk, if possible. Also force fluids to maintain a urine output of 3 to 4 liters/day (urine should be very dilute and colorless).
• If the patient can't drink the required amount of fluid, give supplemental I.V. fluids. Record intake and output and daily weight to assess fluid status and renal function.
• Medicate the patient generously for pain when he's passing a calculus.
• To help acidify urine, offer fruit juices, especially cranberry juice.
• If the patient had calculi surgically removed, he'll probably have an indwelling catheter or a nephrostomy tube. Unless one of his kidneys was removed, expect bloody drainage from the catheter. Never irrigate the catheter without a doctor's order. Check dressings regularly for bloody drainage, and know how much drainage to expect. Immediately report excessive drainage or a rising pulse rate, symptoms of hemorrhage. Use sterile technique when changing dressings or providing catheter care.
• Watch for signs of infection, such as a rising fever or chills, and give antibiotics, as ordered.

Patient teaching
• Encourage increased fluid intake. If appropriate, show the patient how to check his urine pH, and instruct him to keep a daily record. Tell him to immediately report symptoms of acute obstruction, such as pain or an inability to void.
• Urge the patient to follow a prescribed diet and comply with drug therapy to prevent recurrence of calculi. For example, if a hyperuricemic condition caused the patient's calculi, teach him which foods are high in purine.
• If surgery is necessary, supplement and reinforce the doctor's teaching. The patient is apt to be fearful, especially if he needs a kidney removed, so emphasize that the body can adapt well to one kidney. If he's having an abdominal or flank incision, teach deep-breathing and coughing exercises.

RENAL VEIN THROMBOSIS

Clotting in the renal vein, or renal vein thrombosis, produces renal congestion, engorgement, and, sometimes, infarction. Thrombosis may affect both kidneys and occurs in an acute or a chronic form.

Chronic thrombosis usually impairs renal function, causing nephrotic syndrome. If thrombosis affects both kidneys, the prognosis is poor. Thrombosis that affects only one kidney, or gradual progression that allows development of collateral circulation, may preserve partial renal function. The disorder occurs in people of all ages, including infants.

The acute form usually can be recognized and treated before nephrotic syndrome occurs.

Causes

Renal vein thrombosis often results from a tumor that obstructs the renal vein (usually hypernephroma). Other causes include thrombophlebitis of the inferior vena cava (which may result from abdominal trauma) or blood vessels of the legs, congestive heart failure, periarteritis, and pregnancy or retroperitoneal fibrosis that causes increased venous compression.

Oral contraceptives and cancers that cause hypercoagulability heighten the risk of renal vein thrombosis. In infants, thrombosis usually follows diarrhea that causes severe dehydration.

Chronic renal vein thrombosis often is a complication of other glomerulopathic diseases, such as amyloidosis, diabetic nephropathy, and membranoproliferative glomerulonephritis.

Complications

Thrombosis that occurs abruptly and causes extensive damage may precipitate rapidly fatal renal infarction. Disseminated intravascular coagulation also may occur.

Assessment findings

Symptoms vary, depending on the severity and abruptness of occlusion. A patient with a rapid onset of venous obstruction may report severe lumbar pain and tenderness in the epigastric region and the costovertebral angle. You may note fever, chills, nausea, vomiting, hematuria, ipsilateral lower leg edema, and oliguria when the obstruction is bilateral. The kidneys enlarge and become easily palpable. Hypertension occasionally develops.

When onset is gradual, as often occurs in elderly patients, the patient may have a history of recurrent pulmonary emboli. He may also have newly developed or worsening hypertension. He usually complains of nausea and vomiting. Peripheral edema, usually without pain— a sign of venous congestion— may be palpable.

Diagnostic tests

• *Excretory urography* provides reliable diagnostic evidence. In acute renal vein thrombosis, the kidneys appear enlarged and excretory function diminishes or is absent in the affected kidney. Contrast medium seems to "smudge" necrotic renal tissue. In chronic renal thrombosis, the test may show ureteral indentations that result from collateral venous channels.
• *Renal arteriography* and *biopsy* may confirm the diagnosis.
• *Venography* confirms the presence of the occluding thrombosis.
• *Urinalysis* reveals hematuria, oliguria, proteinuria (more than 2 g/day in chronic disease), and casts.
• *Blood studies* show leukocytosis, hypoalbuminemia, hyperlipidemia, and thrombocytopenia.

Treatment

Gradual thrombosis that affects only one kidney may be treated effectively with anticoagulant therapy (heparin or warfarin), particularly if it's long term and if the thrombus extends into the vena cava. Thrombolytic therapy, using streptokinase or alteplase, also has proved effective.

Surgery must be performed within 24 hours of thrombosis, but even then it has limited success because thrombi may extend into the small veins. Extensive intrarenal bleeding and severe hypertension in an atrophic kidney may necessitate nephrectomy.

A patient who survives abrupt thrombosis with extensive renal damage will develop nephrotic syndrome and require treatment for renal failure, such as dialysis and, possibly, transplantation. An infant with renal vein thrombosis may either recover completely after rehydration and heparin therapy or surgery, or suffer irreversible kidney damage. Bilateral damage can be fatal.

Nursing diagnoses
- Altered nutrition: Less than body requirements
- Altered tissue perfusion
- Decreased cardiac output
- Fluid volume deficit
- Pain
- Risk for injury

Nursing interventions
- Give analgesics to relieve pain and promote comfort.
- Assess renal function regularly. Monitor vital signs, intake and output, daily weight, and electrolyte levels.
- Administer diuretics for edema, as ordered, and enforce dietary restrictions on sodium and potassium intake.
- Monitor closely for signs of pulmonary emboli, such as bibasilar crackles and dyspnea.
- If you give heparin by continuous I.V. infusion, frequently monitor partial thromboplastin time to determine the patient's response to the drug. Follow protocols for heparin infusion, and watch for infiltration to avoid tissue damage and a drop in heparin's therapeutic blood levels.
- During anticoagulant or thrombolytic therapy, watch for and report signs of internal bleeding, such as tachycardia, hypotension, hematuria, bleeding from the nose or gums, ecchymoses, petechiae, and tarry stools.

Patient teaching
- Teach the patient about any medications he's taking. If he's on maintenance warfarin therapy, caution him to avoid trauma and to use an electric razor and a soft toothbrush.
- Warn him to avoid aspirin and aspirin-containing products because they aggravate bleeding tendencies.
- Instruct him to plan his diet to maintain a consistent amount of vitamin K because varying levels can interfere with effective anticoagulation. Also teach him how to reduce sodium and potassium in his diet.
- Teach him the signs of bleeding, and tell him to immediately report any findings to the doctor.

CHRONIC RENAL DISORDERS

Ranging from nephrotic syndrome and chronic glomerulonephritis to chronic renal failure, chronic renal disorders develop slowly and persist for a long time.

NEPHROTIC SYNDROME
Although not a disease in itself, nephrotic syndrome is characterized by marked proteinuria, hypoalbuminemia, hyperlipidemia, and edema. It results from a glomerular defect that affects the vessels' permeability and indicates renal damage. The prognosis is highly variable, depending on the underlying cause, but age plays no part in progression or prognosis. Some forms of nephrotic syndrome may eventually progress to end-stage renal failure.

Causes
About 75% of nephrotic syndrome cases result from primary (idiopathic) glomerulonephritis. Causes include the following:
- *Lipid nephrosis (nil lesions)* is the main cause of nephrotic syndrome in children under age 8. The glomeruli appear normal by light microscopy. Some tubules may contain increased lipid deposits.
- *Membranous glomerulonephritis* is the most common lesion in adult idiopathic nephrotic syndrome. It's characterized by the appearance of immune complexes, seen as dense deposits, within the glomerular basement membrane and by the uniform thickening of the basement membrane. It eventually progresses to renal failure.
- *Focal glomerulosclerosis* can develop spontaneously at any age, can occur after kidney transplantation, or can result from heroin injection. Ten percent of children and up to 20% of adults with nephrotic syndrome develop this condition. Lesions initially affect some of the deeper glomeruli, causing hyaline sclerosis. Involvement of the superficial glomeruli occurs later. These lesions usually cause slowly progressive deterioration in renal function, although remissions may occur in children.
- *Membranoproliferative glomerulonephritis* causes slowly progressive lesions to develop in the subendothelial region of the basement membrane. This disorder may follow infection, particularly streptococcal infection, and occurs primarily in children and young adults.

Other causes of nephrotic syndrome include metabolic diseases, such as diabetes mellitus; collagen-vascular disorders, such as systemic lupus erythematosus and

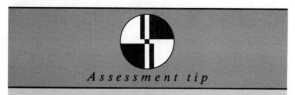

Assessment tip

EVALUATING EDEMA

To assess pitting edema, press firmly for 5 to 10 seconds over a bony surface, such as the subcutaneous part of the tibia, fibula, sacrum, or sternum. Then remove your finger and note how long the depression remains. Document your observation on a scale from +1 (barely detectable depression) to +4 (persistent pit as deep as 1" [2.5 cm]).

In severe edema, tissue swells so much that fluid can't be displaced, making pitting impossible. The surface feels rock-hard, and subcutaneous tissue becomes fibrotic. Brawny edema eventually may develop.

+1 pitting edema

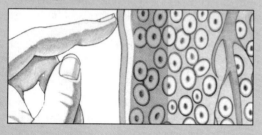

+4 pitting edema

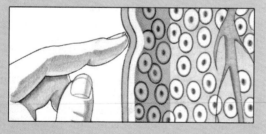

Brawny edema

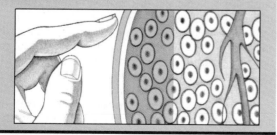

periarteritis nodosa; circulatory diseases, such as congestive heart failure, sickle cell anemia, and renal vein thrombosis; nephrotoxins, such as mercury, gold, and bismuth; infections, such as tuberculosis and enteritis; allergic reactions; pregnancy; hereditary nephritis; and certain neoplastic diseases, such as multiple myeloma.

All of these diseases increase glomerular protein permeability, which leads to increased urinary excretion of protein, especially albumin, and subsequent hypoalbuminemia.

Complications
Major complications include malnutrition, infection, coagulation disorders, thromboembolic vascular occlusion (especially in the lungs and legs), and accelerated atherosclerosis. Hypochromic anemia can develop from excessive urinary excretion of transferrin. Acute renal failure may occur.

Assessment findings
The patient may complain of lethargy and depression. Your assessment may reveal two common problems: periorbital edema, which occurs primarily in the morning and is more common in children, and mild to severe dependent edema of the ankles or sacrum. (See *Evaluating edema.*) You may note orthostatic hypotension, ascites, swollen external genitalia, signs of pleural effusion, anorexia, and pallor.

Diagnostic tests
Consistent, heavy proteinuria (levels over 3.5 mg/dl for 24 hours) strongly suggests nephrotic syndrome. Examination of urine also reveals an increased number of hyaline, granular, and waxy, fatty casts as well as oval fat bodies.

Serum values that support the diagnosis include increased levels of cholesterol, phospholipids (especially low-density and very-low-density lipoproteins), and triglycerides, and decreased albumin levels.

Histologic identification of the lesion necessitates a renal biopsy.

Treatment
Effective treatment of nephrotic syndrome requires correction of the underlying cause, if possible. Supportive treatment consists of a nutritious diet of 0.6 g of protein/kg of body weight, with restricted sodium intake, diuretics for edema, and antibiotics for infection.

Some patients respond to an 8-week course of a corticosteroid, such as prednisone, followed by maintenance therapy. Others respond better to a combination of prednisone and azathioprine or cyclophosphamide. Treatment for hyperlipidemia frequently is unsuccessful.

Nursing diagnoses
- Altered nutrition: Less than body requirements
- Altered tissue perfusion
- Body image disturbance
- Fluid volume excess
- Risk for infection
- Risk for injury

Nursing interventions
- Frequently check urine for protein. Urine that contains protein appears frothy.
- Document the location and character of the patient's edema.
- Measure blood pressure while the patient is supine and also while he's standing. Immediately report a drop in systolic or diastolic pressure exceeding 20 mm Hg.
- After a renal biopsy, watch for bleeding and signs of shock.
- Monitor intake and output and weigh the patient each morning after he voids and before he eats. Make sure he's wearing the same kind of clothing each time you weigh him.
- Ask the dietitian to plan a low-sodium diet with moderate amounts of protein.
- Monitor plasma albumin and transferrin concentrations to evaluate overall nutritional status.
- Provide meticulous skin care to combat the edema that usually occurs with nephrotic syndrome. Use a reduced-pressure mattress or padding to help prevent pressure ulcers.
- To avoid thrombophlebitis, encourage activity and exercise and provide antiembolism stockings, as ordered.
- Offer the patient and his family reassurance and support, especially during the acute phase, when edema is severe and the patient's body image changes.

Patient teaching
- If the patient is taking immunosuppressants, teach him and his family to report even mild signs of infection. If he's undergoing long-term corticosteroid therapy, teach him and his family to report muscle weakness and mental changes.

   To prevent GI complications, suggest to the patient that he take steroids with an antacid or with cimetidine or ranitidine. Explain that adverse effects of steroids will subside when therapy stops, but warn the patient not to discontinue the drug abruptly or without a doctor's consent.

- Stress the importance of adhering to the special diet.
- If the doctor prescribes antiembolism stockings for home use, show the patient how to safely apply and remove them.

CHRONIC GLOMERULONEPHRITIS
A slowly progressive disease, chronic glomerulonephritis is characterized by inflammation of the glomeruli, which results in sclerosis, scarring and, eventually, renal failure. This condition normally remains subclinical until the progressive phase begins. By the time it produces symptoms, chronic glomerulonephritis usually is irreversible.

Causes
Common causes of chronic glomerulonephritis include primary renal disorders, such as membranoproliferative glomerulonephritis, membranous glomerulopathy, focal glomerulosclerosis, rapidly progressive glomerulonephritis, and, less often, poststreptococcal glomerulonephritis. Systemic disorders that may cause chronic glomerulonephritis include systemic lupus erythematosus, Goodpasture's syndrome, and hemolytic-uremic syndrome.

Complications
Chronic glomerulonephritis can cause contracted, granular kidneys and lead to end-stage renal failure. It also can produce severe hypertension, leading to cardiovascular complications, including cardiac hypertrophy and congestive heart failure (CHF), which may speed the development of advanced renal failure, eventually necessitating dialysis or kidney transplantation.

Assessment findings
This disorder usually develops insidiously and without symptoms, often over many years. But when it becomes suddenly progressive, your assessment may reveal edema and hypertension.

   In late stages, the patient may complain of nausea, vomiting, pruritus, dyspnea, malaise, fatigue, and mild to severe edema. Your assessment may show severe hypertension and associated cardiac complications.

Diagnostic tests
The following findings support a diagnosis of chronic glomerulonephritis:
- *Urinalysis* shows proteinuria, hematuria, cylindruria, and red blood cell casts.

• *Blood studies* reveal rising blood urea nitrogen and serum creatinine levels in advanced renal insufficiency as well as a decrease in hemoglobin.

• *X-rays* exhibit symmetrically contracted kidneys with normal pelves and calyces.

• *Renal biopsy* establishes the underlying disease and provides data to plan therapy.

Treatment

Appropiate treatment is essentially nonspecific and symptomatic. Goals include controlling hypertension with antihypertensives and a sodium-restricted diet, correcting fluid and electrolyte imbalances through restrictions and replacement, reducing edema with loop diuretics such as furosemide, and preventing CHF. Treatment also may include antibiotics for symptomatic urinary tract infections (UTIs), dialysis, or kidney transplantation.

Nursing diagnoses

• Altered nutrition: Less than body requirements
• Fatigue
• Fluid volume excess
• Impaired skin integrity
• Risk for infection

Nursing interventions

• Monitor vital signs, intake and output, and daily weight to evaluate fluid retention. Observe for signs of fluid, electrolyte, and acid-base imbalances.

• Ask the dietitian to help the patient plan low-sodium, high-calorie meals with adequate protein.

• Provide good skin care to help prevent complications of pruritus, edema, and friability.

• Help the patient adjust to his illness by encouraging him to express his feelings and ask questions.

Patient teaching

• Instruct the patient to take prescribed antihypertensives and diuretics as scheduled, even if he feels better. Advise him to take diuretics in the morning so that his nightly sleep won't be disturbed.

• Teach him the signs of infection, particularly those of UTI, and warn him to report them immediately. Tell him to avoid contact with people who have communicable illnesses.

• Urge compliance with the prescribed diet.

• Stress the importance of keeping all follow-up examinations to assess renal function.

CYSTINURIA

An inborn error of amino acid transport in the kidneys and intestine, cystinuria allows excessive urinary excretion of cystine and other dibasic amino acids. This results in recurrent cystine renal calculus formation.

The most common defect of amino acid transport, cystinuria occurs in about 1 in 15,000 live births. Onset of symptoms commonly occurs between ages 10 and 30 (although it can occur in infants as young as age 1 or in adults well into their 30s). With proper treatment, the prognosis is good.

Causes and pathophysiology

Cystinuria is inherited as an autosomal recessive trait. It affects both sexes but is more severe in males. For some unknown reason, it's more common in people of short stature.

The condition arises when impaired renal tubular reabsorption of dibasic amino acids (cystine, lysine, arginine, and ornithine) causes excessive amino acid concentration and excretion in the urine. When cystine concentration exceeds its solubility, cystine precipitates and forms crystals, precursors of cystine calculi. Excessive excretion of the other three amino acids produces no ill effects.

Complications

Cystine calculi can obstruct and destroy the tissue in the kidneys and ureters. Although infections occur frequently, treatment almost always prevents long-lasting effects.

Assessment findings

A patient with cystine calculi will typically complain of dull flank pain from renal parenchymal and capsular distention; of nausea, vomiting, and abdominal distention from acute renal colic (caused by smooth-muscle spasm and hyperperistalsis or paralytic ileus); of hematuria; and of tenderness at the costovertebral angle.

Renal calculi also may cause urinary tract obstruction, with resultant secondary infection. A patient will report chills, fever, burning, itching, dysuria, urinary frequency, and foul-smelling urine. In prolonged ureteral obstruction, assessment shows a visible or palpable flank mass.

Diagnostic tests

The following diagnostic tests confirm cystinuria:

• *Chemical analysis of calculi* shows cystine crystals with a variable amount of calcium. Pure cystine calculi are radiolucent on X-ray, but most contain some calcium.

These calculi are light yellow or brownish yellow and granular, and may be large.

• *Blood studies* may show an elevated white blood cell count, especially if the patient has a urinary tract infection (UTI), and elevated clearance of cystine, lysine, arginine, and ornithine.

• *Urinalysis* with amino acid chromatography indicates aminoaciduria, consisting of cystine, lysine, arginine, and ornithine. Urine pH normally is less than 5.0.

• *Microscopic examination of urine* shows hexagonal, flat cystine crystals. When glacial acetic acid is added to chilled urine, cystine crystals resemble benzene rings.

• *Cyanide-nitroprusside test* result is positive. In cystinuria, a urine specimen made alkaline by adding ammonia turns magenta when nitroprusside is added.

Confirming tests also include *excretory urography* to determine renal function and *kidney-ureter-bladder radiography* to detect the size and location of calculi. But because cystine calculi are translucent, these tests can only confirm a diagnosis if other minerals are deposited on the calculus or if an obstruction is present.

Treatment

No effective treatment exists to decrease cystine excretion. Increasing fluid intake to maintain a minimum 24-hour urine volume of 3,000 ml and reduce urine cystine concentration is the primary means of diluting excess cystine and preventing cystine calculus formation.

Sodium bicarbonate and an alkaline-ash diet (high in vegetables and fruit and low in protein) alkalinize urine, thereby increasing cystine solubility. However, this therapy may provide a favorable environment for formation of calcium phosphate calculi.

Penicillamine also can increase cystine solubility, but it should be used with caution because of its toxicity and the high incidence of allergic reactions.

Dissolving cystine calculi may take up to 12 months (in 40% of patients). Irrigating agents, such as tromethamine or acetylcysteine, have been effective. Or electrohydraulic ultrasonography may be used to break the calculi into fragments that can be passed.

Treatment also may include surgical removal of calculi, when necessary, and appropriate measures to prevent and treat UTI.

Nursing diagnoses

• Altered urinary elimination
• Knowledge deficit
• Pain
• Risk for infection

Nursing interventions

• Carefully monitor sodium bicarbonate administration because metabolic alkalosis may develop. Estimate the arterial bicarbonate level by subtracting 2 from the serum carbon dioxide level.

• Watch for cardiac and neuromuscular problems associated with low potassium levels.

• If irrigating agents are used, the patient will need a percutaneous nephrostomy tube and access for drainage. Stop the irrigation if intrarenal pressures increase or if fever and extreme pain occur.

• To prevent high intrarenal pressures, check and regulate the solution flow whenever the patient changes position.

• Keep the patient on bed rest and apply antiembolism stockings during irrigations to reduce the risk of emboli.

Patient teaching

• Emphasize the need for an increased, evenly spaced fluid intake, even through the night.

• Teach the patient the signs and symptoms of renal calculi and UTI, and tell him to report them immediately.

• Teach the patient how to check and record urine pH and when to report the results.

• Encourage the patient to adhere to the recommended diet.

• Explain to the patient receiving penicillamine that it may cause an allergic or serum sickness–type reaction. Describe this and other possible adverse effects, including severe proteinuria, neutropenia, tinnitus, and taste impairment.

• Explain that periodic serum and urine evaluations will be necessary to monitor for drug effectiveness.

RENOVASCULAR HYPERTENSION

When systemic blood pressure rises because of stenosis of the major renal arteries or their branches or because of intrarenal atherosclerosis, renovascular hypertension occurs. This narrowing (sclerosis) may be partial or complete, and the resulting blood pressure elevation may be benign or malignant. About 5% to 15% of patients with high blood pressure display renovascular hypertension.

Causes and pathophysiology

In about 95% of patients, renovascular hypertension results from either atherosclerosis (especially in older men) or fibromuscular diseases of the renal artery wall layers (for example, medial fibroplasia and, less commonly, intimal and subadventitial fibroplasia). Other causes include arteritis, anomalies of the renal arteries, embolism, trauma, tumor, and dissecting aneurysm.

Stenosis or a renal artery occlusion stimulates the affected kidney to release renin, an enzyme that converts angiotensinogen (a plasma protein) to angiotensin I. As angiotensin I circulates through the lungs and liver, it converts to angiotensin II, which causes peripheral vasoconstriction, increased arterial pressure and aldosterone secretion and, eventually, hypertension. (See *What happens in renovascular hypertension.*)

Complications
Renovascular hypertension can lead to such significant complications as congestive heart failure, myocardial infarction, cerebrovascular accident and, occasionally, renal failure.

Assessment findings
In the early stages, the patient may complain of flank pain. During your assessment, you may note reduced urine output, elevated blood pressure, and a systolic bruit over the epigastric vein in the upper abdomen on auscultation.

As the disorder progresses, the patient may report headache, nausea, anorexia, fatigue, palpitations, tachycardia, and anxiety. If renal failure occurs, you may notice alterations in the patient's level of consciousness and pitting edema. Auscultation may reveal bibasilar crackles.

Diagnostic tests
An isotopic renal blood flow scan and rapid-sequence excretory urography are needed to identify renal blood flow abnormalities and discrepancies of kidney size and shape. Renal arteriography reveals the actual arterial stenosis or obstruction.

In addition, samples from the right and left renal veins are obtained for comparison of plasma renin levels with those in the inferior vena cava (split renal vein renins). Increased renin levels from the involved kidney that exceed levels from the uninvolved kidney by a ratio of 1.5:1.0 or greater implicate the affected kidney and determine whether surgery can reverse hypertension.

Laboratory evaluation of serum samples shows hypokalemia, hyponatremia or hypernatremia, and elevated blood volume. Elevated blood urea nitrogen (BUN) and serum creatinine levels signal the onset of renal failure. Urine studies may reveal albuminuria and high specific gravity.

A positive captopril test can differentiate renovascular hypertension from essential hypertension before more invasive tests are done.

Treatment
Angioplasty is the treatment of choice for all patients except those with osteal lesions or complete occlusion. Other surgical techniques include renal artery bypass, endarterectomy, arterioplasty and, as a last resort, nephrectomy. Surgery is effective in up to 95% of cases in restoring adequate circulation and controlling severe hypertension. It also can improve severely impaired renal function.

Symptomatic measures include antihypertensives, diuretics, and a sodium-restricted diet.

Nursing diagnoses
- Altered nutrition: Less than body requirements
- Altered thought processes
- Altered urinary elimination
- Anxiety
- Decreased cardiac output
- Fluid volume excess
- Pain
- Risk for injury

Nursing interventions
- Prepare the patient for diagnostic tests. For example, adequately hydrate him before tests that use a contrast medium, and make sure he's not allergic to the medium used. Watch for complications after excretory urography or arteriography.
- Accurately monitor and record intake and output and daily weight. Weigh the patient at the same time each day (before a meal) and when he's wearing the same clothing.
- Frequently assess urine specific gravity, BUN, serum creatinine, and protein levels.
- Check blood pressure in both arms regularly, with the patient lying down and standing. A drop of 20 mm Hg or more in either systolic or diastolic pressure on arising may necessitate a dosage adjustment in antihypertensive medications.
- Administer drugs as ordered. Adequately medicate the patient for pain to decrease anxiety and increase comfort.
- Maintain fluid and sodium restrictions.
- If the patient is anorexic, offer appetizing, high-calorie meals to ensure adequate nutrition.
- If a nephrectomy is necessary, reassure the patient that his remaining kidney will be adequate for renal function.

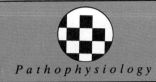

Pathophysiology

WHAT HAPPENS IN RENOVASCULAR HYPERTENSION

The kidneys normally play a key role in maintaining blood pressure and volume by vasoconstriction and regulation of sodium and fluid levels. In renovascular hypertension, these regulatory mechanisms fail.

Certain conditions, such as renal artery stenosis and tumors, reduce blood flow to the kidneys. This causes juxtaglomerular cells to continuously secrete renin.
  In this stage, be alert for flank pain, systolic bruit in the epigastric vein or upper abdomen, reduced urine output, and elevated renin levels.

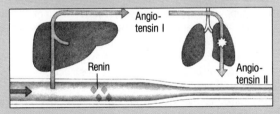

In the liver, renin and angiotensinogen combine to form angiotensin I, which converts to angiotensin II in the lungs. This potent vasoconstrictor heightens peripheral resistance and blood pressure.
  Check for headache, nausea, anorexia, elevated renin levels, and hypertension.

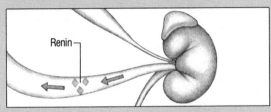

Angiotensin II acts directly on the kidneys, causing them to reabsorb sodium and water.
  Assess for hypertension, diminished urine output, albuminuria, hypokalemia, and hypernatremia.

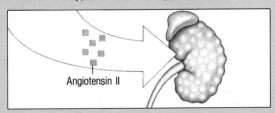

Angiotensin II stimulates the adrenal cortex to secrete aldosterone. This also causes the kidneys to retain sodium and water, elevating blood volume and pressure.
  Expect worsening symptoms.

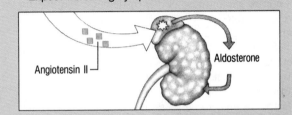

Intermittent pressure diuresis causes excretion of sodium and water, reduced blood volume, and decreasing cardiac output.
  Check for blood pressure that rises slowly, drops (but not as low as before), and then rises again. Headache, high urine specific gravity, hyponatremia, fatigue, and heart failure also occur.

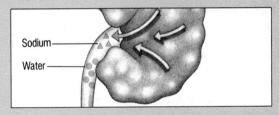

High aldosterone levels cause further sodium retention. But they can't curtail renin secretion. Excessive aldosterone and angiotensin II can damage renal tissue, leading to renal failure. Expect to find hypertension, pitting edema, anemia, decreased level of consciousness, and elevated blood urea nitrogen and serum creatinine levels.

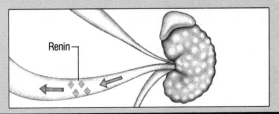

• Provide good postoperative care: Watch for bleeding and hypotension. If the sutures around the renal vessels slip, the patient can quickly go into shock because kidneys receive 25% of cardiac output. Report and record the number and amount of dressing reinforcements. Monitor vital signs and report hypotension, which can precipitate acute renal failure.
• Provide a quiet, stress-free environment, if possible.
• Encourage cardiovascular fitness, and work with the doctor and patient to develop a beneficial program.

Patient teaching
• Help the patient and his family understand renovascular hypertension, and emphasize the importance of following the prescribed treatment regimen.
• Describe the purpose of diagnostic tests, and explain each procedure. If the patient is scheduled for surgery, explain the procedure and postoperative care.
• Familiarize the patient with his medications, and encourage him to take them as ordered. Suggest taking diuretics in the morning so that sleep patterns won't be disturbed.
• Suggest regular blood pressure screenings.
• Explain the purpose of a low-sodium diet, and stress the importance of following it. Also stress the need to restrict fluids, if appropriate.
• Encourage the patient to perform stress-relieving exercises.

HYDRONEPHROSIS
An abnormal dilation of the renal pelvis and the calyces of one or both kidneys, hydronephrosis is caused by an obstruction of urine flow in the genitourinary tract. Although a partial obstruction and hydronephrosis may not produce symptoms initially, the pressure built up behind the area of obstruction eventually results in symptoms of renal dysfunction.

Causes and pathophysiology
Almost any type of obstructive uropathy can lead to hydronephrosis. The most common causes are benign prostatic hyperplasia, urethral strictures, and calculi. Less common causes include strictures or stenosis of the ureter or bladder outlet; congenital abnormalities; bladder, ureteral, or pelvic tumors; blood clots; and neurogenic bladder.

If the obstruction is in the urethra or bladder, hydronephrosis usually is bilateral; if the obstruction is in a ureter, hydronephrosis usually is unilateral. Obstructions distal to the bladder cause the bladder to dilate and

act as a buffer zone, delaying hydronephrosis. Total obstruction of urine flow with dilation of the collecting system ultimately causes complete cortical atrophy and cessation of glomerular filtration.

Complications
The most common complication of an obstructed kidney is life-threatening infection (pyelonephritis) caused by urinary stasis that exacerbates renal damage. If hydronephrosis results from acute obstructive uropathy, the patient may develop paralytic ileus. Untreated bilateral hydronephrosis can lead to renal failure, a life-threatening condition.

Assessment findings
The patient's history and chief complaint will vary, depending on the cause of the obstruction. For example, a patient may have no symptoms or complain of only mild pain and slightly decreased urine flow. Or he may report severe, colicky renal pain or dull flank pain that radiates to the groin and gross urinary abnormalities, such as hematuria, pyuria, dysuria, alternating oliguria and polyuria, and anuria.

A patient with hydronephrosis also may report nausea, vomiting, abdominal fullness, pain on urination, dribbling, and urinary hesitancy. Pain on only one side, usually in the flank area, may signal a unilateral obstruction.

Diagnostic tests
Excretory urography, retrograde pyelography, renal ultrasonography, and renal function studies confirm the diagnosis. Visualization tests show concave (early stage) or convex (later stage) calyces as dilation progresses.

If the disease is extensive, tests will show atrophied distal and proximal tubules and obstructions. Urine studies will confirm the inability to concentrate urine, a decreased glomerular filtration rate and, possibly, pyuria if infection is present.

Treatment
The goals of treatment are to preserve renal function and prevent infection through surgical removal of the obstruction. Surgery includes dilatation for a urethral stricture or prostatectomy for benign prostatic hyperplasia.

If renal function has already been affected, therapy may include a diet low in protein, sodium, and potassium. This diet is designed to stop the progression of renal failure before surgery.

Inoperable obstructions may necessitate decompression and drainage of the kidney, using a nephrostomy tube placed temporarily or permanently in the renal pelvis. Concurrent infection requires appropriate antibiotic therapy.

Nursing diagnoses
- Altered nutrition: Less than body requirements
- Altered urinary elimination
- Anxiety
- Fluid volume deficit
- Pain
- Risk for infection

Nursing interventions
- Administer prescribed pain medication as needed.
- Monitor renal function studies daily, including blood urea nitrogen, serum creatinine, and serum potassium levels. Specific gravity tests can be done at the bedside.
- Postoperatively, closely monitor intake and output, vital signs, and fluid and electrolyte status. Watch for a rising pulse rate and cold, clammy skin, which can indicate impending hemorrhage and shock.

 Keep in mind that postobstructive diuresis may cause the patient to lose great volumes of dilute urine over hours or days. If this occurs, administer I.V. fluids at a constant rate, as ordered, plus an amount of I.V. fluid equal to a percentage of hourly urine, to safely replace intravascular volume. (See *Understanding postobstructive diuresis.*)
- Consult with a dietitian to provide a diet consistent with the treatment plan that contains foods the patient will eat.
- If a nephrostomy tube has been inserted, frequently check it for bleeding and patency. Irrigate the tube only as ordered, and don't clamp it. Provide meticulous skin care to the area surrounding the tube; if urine leaks, provide a protective skin barrier to decrease excoriation. Observe for signs of infection.
- Allow the patient to express his fears and anxieties, and help him find effective coping strategies.

Patient teaching
- Explain hydronephrosis to the patient and his family. Also explain the purpose of diagnostic tests and how they're performed.
- If the patient is scheduled for surgery, explain the procedure and postoperative care.
- If the patient will be discharged with a nephrostomy tube in place, teach him how to care for it, including how to thoroughly clean the skin around the insertion site.

UNDERSTANDING POSTOBSTRUCTIVE DIURESIS

Polyuria—urine output that exceeds 2,000 ml in an 8-hour period—and excessive electrolyte losses characterize postobstructive diuresis. Although usually self-limiting, this condition can cause vascular collapse, shock, and death if not treated with fluid and electrolyte replacement.

 Prolonged pressure of retained urine damages renal tubules, limiting their ability to concentrate urine. Removing the obstruction relieves the pressure, but tubular function may not significantly improve for days or weeks, depending on the patient's condition.

 Although diuresis typically abates in a few days, it persists if serum creatinine levels remain high. When these levels approach the normal range (0.7 to 1.4 mg/dl), diuresis usually subsides.

- If the patient must take antibiotics after discharge, tell him to take all of the prescribed medication, even if he feels better.
- To prevent the progression of hydronephrosis to irreversible renal disease, urge an older male patient (especially a patient with a family history of benign prostatic hyperplasia or prostatitis) to have routine medical checkups. Teach him to recognize and report symptoms of hydronephrosis, such as colicky pain or hematuria, or urinary tract infection.

RENAL TUBULAR ACIDOSIS
A syndrome that causes persistent dehydration, hyperchloremia, hypokalemia, metabolic acidosis, and nephrocalcinosis, renal tubular acidosis results from the kidneys' inability to conserve bicarbonate. This disorder is classified as distal (Type I, or classic renal tubular acidosis) or proximal (Type II).

 Distal renal tubular acidosis occurs in two forms:
- *Primary distal renal tubular acidosis* is most prevalent in women, older children, adolescents, and young adults. The disease may result from a hereditary defect. Occasionally, it may occur for unknown reasons.
- *Secondary distal renal tubular acidosis* has been linked to many renal or systemic conditions, such as starvation, malnutrition, and hepatic cirrhosis, and to several genetically transmitted disorders.

 Proximal renal tubular acidosis results from defective reabsorption of bicarbonate in the proximal tubule. This causes bicarbonate to flood the distal tubule, which normally secretes hydrogen ions, and leads to impaired formation of titratable acids and ammonium for excretion. Metabolic acidosis ultimately results.

Proximal renal tubular acidosis also occurs in two forms:
• In *primary proximal renal tubular acidosis,* the reabsorptive defect is idiopathic and is the only disorder present.
• In *secondary proximal renal tubular acidosis,* the reabsorptive defect may be one of several and is due to proximal tubular cell damage from a disease, such as Fanconi's syndrome.

Renal tubular acidosis affects people of all ages, including infants. The prognosis usually is good but depends on the severity of renal damage that precedes treatment.

Causes
Distal renal tubular acidosis is caused by the distal tubule's inability to secrete hydrogen ions against established gradients across the tubular membrane. This results in decreased excretion of titratable acids and ammonium, increased loss of potassium and bicarbonate in the urine, and systemic acidosis.

Type I is transmitted as an autosomal dominant trait, and Type II probably is transmitted as an autosomal recessive trait but also may be autosomal dominant or X-linked.

Complications
This syndrome can result in pyelonephritis. Prolonged acidosis causes mobilization of calcium from bone and, eventually, hypercalciuria, predisposing the patient to the formation of renal calculi. Lack of calcium stunts growth in children and causes osteomalacia in adults.

Assessment findings
Parents of infants with renal tubular acidosis will report that the infant is vomiting and has anorexia, constipation, occasional fever, and polyuria. Inspection reveals lethargy, weakness, tissue wasting, and growth retardation, as well as signs of dehydration (poor skin turgor and dry, cracked lips), rickets (irritability, delayed closure of fontanels, and bowed legs), and nephrocalcinosis (hematuria and low abdominal or flank pain).

Older children may have urinary tract infections (UTIs), rickets, and growth problems. Adults may complain of frequent UTIs and also may show signs of osteomalacia.

Diagnostic tests
Demonstration of impaired urine acidification with systemic metabolic acidosis confirms distal renal tubular acidosis. Demonstration of bicarbonate wasting due to impaired reabsorption confirms proximal renal tubular acidosis.

An ammonium chloride loading test helps determine the type of renal tubular acidosis. If the urine pH stays above 5.5 after oral administration of ammonium chloride, despite systemic acidosis, distal renal tubular acidosis is present; if the urine pH falls below 5.5, proximal renal tubular acidosis is present.

Other relevant laboratory results show:
• decreased serum bicarbonate, potassium, and phosphorus levels
• increased serum chloride and alkaline phosphatase levels
• alkaline pH, with low titratable acid and ammonium content in urine, increased urine bicarbonate and potassium levels, and low specific gravity.

In later stages, X-rays may show nephrocalcinosis.

Treatment
Supportive treatment requires replacement of substances being excreted abnormally, especially bicarbonate. Treatment may include sodium bicarbonate tablets or Shohl's solution to control acidosis, oral potassium for dangerously low potassium levels, and vitamin D for bone disease. If pyelonephritis occurs, antibiotics may be prescribed as well.

Treatment for renal calculi secondary to nephrocalcinosis varies and may include supportive therapy until the calculi pass or until surgery for severe obstruction is performed.

Nursing diagnoses
• Altered growth and development
• Altered nutrition: Less than body requirements
• Altered parenting
• Altered urinary elimination
• Fluid volume deficit
• Ineffective family coping
• Pain
• Risk for infection

Nursing interventions
• Monitor laboratory test values, especially potassium levels to detect hypokalemia.
• Administer potassium, sodium bicarbonate or Shohl's solution, vitamin D preparations, or antibiotics, as ordered.

• Consult with the dietitian to ensure an appetizing diet that is nutritionally adequate.
• Test urine for pH and strain it for calculi.
• If surgery is performed to eliminate an obstruction, watch for signs of postoperative hemorrhage and shock secondary to hypovolemia.
• If the patient is an infant or a child, encourage the parents to express their concerns and fears. Offer support as needed.

Patient teaching
• Explain all diagnostic tests. If the patient is scheduled for surgery, explain the procedure and postoperative care.
• If rickets develops, explain the condition and its treatment to the patient and his family.
• Urge compliance with all medication instructions. Emphasize that the prognosis for the disorder and bone lesion healing is directly related to the adequacy of treatment.
• Review the signs and symptoms of calculi (hematuria and low abdominal or flank pain). Tell the patient or parents to report any suspicious findings immediately.
• Instruct the patient with low potassium levels to eat foods with a high potassium content, such as bananas, baked potatoes, orange juice, and prune juice.
• Because renal tubular acidosis may be caused by a genetic defect, encourage family members to seek genetic counseling or screening for this disorder.

CHRONIC RENAL FAILURE
Usually the end result of a gradually progressive loss of renal function, chronic renal failure also occasionally results from a rapidly progressive disease of sudden onset that gradually destroys the nephrons and eventually causes irreversible renal damage. Few symptoms develop until after more than 75% of glomerular filtration is lost. Then the remaining normal parenchyma deteriorates progressively, and symptoms worsen as renal function decreases.

Chronic renal failure may progress through the following stages:
• reduced renal reserve (glomerular filtration rate [GFR] 35% to 50% of normal)
• renal insufficiency (GFR 20% to 35% of normal)
• renal failure (GFR 20% to 25% of normal)
• end-stage renal disease (GFR less than 20% of normal).

This syndrome is fatal without treatment, but maintenance dialysis or a kidney transplant can sustain life.

Causes
Chronic renal failure may result from:
• *chronic glomerular disease,* such as glomerulonephritis
• *chronic infections,* such as chronic pyelonephritis or tuberculosis
• *congenital anomalies,* such as polycystic kidney disease
• *vascular diseases,* such as renal nephrosclerosis or hypertension
• *obstructive processes,* such as calculi
• *collagen diseases,* such as systemic lupus erythematosus
• *nephrotoxic agents,* such as long-term aminoglycoside therapy
• *endocrine diseases,* such as diabetic neuropathy.

Complications
If this condition continues unchecked, uremic toxins accumulate and produce potentially fatal physiologic changes in all major organ systems.

Even if the patient can tolerate life-sustaining maintenance dialysis or a kidney transplant, he may still have anemia, peripheral neuropathy, cardiopulmonary and GI complications, sexual dysfunction, and skeletal defects.

Assessment findings
The patient's history may include a disease or condition that can cause renal failure; however, he may not have any symptoms for a long time. Symptoms usually occur by the time the GFR is 20% to 35% of normal, and almost all body systems are affected. Assessment findings will reflect involvement of each system, although many findings reflect involvement of more than one system.
• *Renal.* In certain fluid and electrolyte imbalances, the kidneys cannot retain salt, and hyponatremias occur. The patient may complain of dry mouth, fatigue, and nausea. You may note hypotension, loss of skin turgor, and listlessness that may progress to somnolence and confusion. Later, as the number of functioning nephrons decreases, so does the kidneys' capacity to excrete sodium and potassium. Urine output decreases, and the urine is very dilute, with casts and crystals present. Accumulation of potassium causes muscle irritability and then muscle weakness, irregular pulses, and life-threatening cardiac arrhythmias as serum potassium levels increase. Sodium retention causes fluid overload, and edema is palpable. Metabolic acidosis also occurs.
• *Cardiovascular.* When the cardiovascular system is involved, you'll note hypertension and an irregular pulse. Life-threatening cardiac arrhythmias can occur. With pericardial involvement, you may auscultate a pericardial friction rub. Heart sounds may be distant if pericardial effusion is present. Bibasilar crackles may be

auscultated, and peripheral edema may be palpated if congestive heart failure occurs.

• *Respiratory*. Pulmonary changes include reduced pulmonary macrophage activity with increased susceptibility to infection. If pneumonia is present, lung sounds may be decreased over areas of consolidation. Bibasilar crackles indicate pulmonary edema. With pleural involvement, the patient may complain of pleuritic pain, and you may auscultate a pleural friction rub. Kussmaul's respirations occur with metabolic acidosis.

• *GI*. With inflammation and ulceration of GI mucosa, inspection of the mouth may reveal gum ulceration and bleeding and, possibly, parotitis. The patient may complain of hiccups, a metallic taste in the mouth, anorexia, nausea, and vomiting caused by esophageal, stomach, or bowel involvement. You may note a uremic fetor (ammonia smell) to the breath. Abdominal palpation and percussion may elicit pain.

• *Skin*. Inspection of the skin typically reveals a pallid, yellowish bronze color. The skin is dry and scaly with purpura, ecchymoses, petechiae, uremic frost (most often in critically ill or terminal patients), and thin, brittle fingernails with characteristic lines. The hair is dry and brittle and may change color and fall out easily. The patient usually complains of severe itching.

• *Neurologic*. You may note that the patient has alterations in the level of consciousness that may progress from mild behavior changes, shortened memory and attention span, apathy, drowsiness, and irritability to confusion, coma, and seizures. The patient may complain of hiccups, muscle cramps, fasciculations, and twitching, which are caused by muscle irritability. He also may complain of restless leg syndrome. One of the first signs of peripheral neuropathy, this syndrome causes pain, burning, and itching in the legs and feet that may be relieved by voluntarily shaking, moving, or rocking them. This condition eventually progresses to paresthesia, motor nerve dysfunction (usually bilateral footdrop), and, unless dialysis is initiated, flaccid paralysis.

• *Endocrine*. Children with chronic renal failure exhibit growth retardation, even with elevated growth hormone levels. Adults may have a history of infertility, decreased libido, and, in women, amenorrhea, and, in men, impotence.

• *Hematologic*. Inspection may reveal purpura, GI bleeding and hemorrhage from body orifices, easy bruising, ecchymoses, and petechiae caused by thrombocytopenia and platelet defects.

• *Musculoskeletal*. The patient may have a history of pathologic fractures and complain of bone and muscle pain caused by calcium-phosphorus imbalance and con-

sequent parathyroid hormone imbalances. You may note gait abnormalities or, possibly, that the patient is no longer able to ambulate. Children may have impaired bone growth and bowed legs from rickets.

Diagnostic tests

The following laboratory findings aid in the diagnosis and monitoring of chronic renal failure:

• *Blood studies* show elevated blood urea nitrogen, serum creatinine, sodium, and potassium levels; decreased arterial pH and bicarbonate levels; low hemoglobin and hematocrit; decreased red blood cell (RBC) survival time; mild thrombocytopenia; platelet defects; and metabolic acidosis. They also show increased aldosterone secretion (related to increased renin production) and increased blood glucose levels similar to those that occur in diabetes mellitus (a sign of impaired carbohydrate metabolism). Hypertriglyceridemia and decreased high-density lipoprotein levels are common.

• *Arterial blood gas analysis* reveals metabolic acidosis.

• *Urine specific gravity* becomes fixed at 1.010; urinalysis may show proteinuria, glycosuria, RBCs, leukocytes, and casts and crystals, depending on the cause.

• *X-ray studies*, including kidney-ureter-bladder radiography, excretory urography, nephrotomography, renal scan, and renal arteriography, show reduced kidney size.

• *Renal biopsy* allows histologic identification of underlying pathology.

• *Electroencephalography* shows changes that indicate metabolic encephalopathy.

Treatment

Conservative treatment aims to correct specific symptoms. A low-protein diet reduces the production of end-products of protein metabolism that the kidneys can't excrete. (However, a patient receiving continuous peritoneal dialysis should have a high-protein diet.) A high-calorie diet prevents ketoacidosis and the negative nitrogen balance that results in catabolism and tissue atrophy. The diet also should restrict sodium and potassium.

Maintaining fluid balance requires careful monitoring of vital signs, weight changes, and urine volume (if not anuric). Fluid retention can be reduced with loop diuretics such as furosemide (if some renal function remains) and with fluid restriction. Digitalis in small doses may be used to mobilize the fluids causing the edema; antihypertensives may be used to control blood pressure and associated edema.

Antiemetics taken before meals may relieve nausea and vomiting, and cimetidine or ranitidine may decrease gastric irritation. Methylcellulose or docusate can help prevent constipation.

Anemia necessitates iron and folate supplements; severe anemia requires infusion of fresh frozen packed cells or washed packed cells. Transfusions relieve anemia only temporarily. Synthetic erythropoietin (epoetin alfa) stimulates the division and differentiation of cells within the bone marrow to produce RBCs.

Drug therapy commonly relieves associated symptoms. An antipruritic, such as trimeprazine or diphenhydramine, can relieve itching, and aluminum hydroxide gel can lower serum phosphate levels. The patient also may benefit from supplementary vitamins (particularly B vitamins and vitamin D) and essential amino acids.

Careful monitoring of serum potassium levels is necessary to detect hyperkalemia. Emergency treatment for severe hyperkalemia includes dialysis therapy and administration of 50% hypertonic glucose I.V., regular insulin, calcium gluconate I.V., sodium bicarbonate I.V., and cation exchange resins, such as sodium polystyrene sulfonate. Cardiac tamponade resulting from pericardial effusion may require emergency pericardial tap or surgery.

Intensive dialysis and thoracentesis can relieve pulmonary edema and pleural effusion.

Hemodialysis or peritoneal dialysis (particularly the newer techniques — continuous ambulatory peritoneal dialysis and continuous cyclic peritoneal dialysis) can help control most manifestations of end-stage renal disease. Altering the dialysate can correct fluid and electrolyte disturbances. However, maintenance dialysis itself may produce complications, including serum hepatitis (hepatitis B) from numerous blood transfusions, protein wasting, refractory ascites, and dialysis dementia.

Nursing diagnoses
- Altered family processes
- Altered nutrition: Less than body requirements
- Altered oral mucous membrane
- Altered sexuality patterns
- Altered thought processes
- Altered tissue perfusion
- Decreased cardiac output
- Fluid volume excess
- Impaired gas exchange
- Impaired tissue integrity
- Ineffective family coping
- Pain
- Powerlessness
- Risk for infection
- Risk for injury

Nursing interventions
The widespread clinical effects of chronic renal failure require meticulous and carefully coordinated supportive care.
- Provide good skin care. Bathe the patient daily, using superfatted soaps, oatmeal baths, and skin lotion to ease pruritus. Give good perineal care, using mild soap and water. Pad the bed side rails to guard against ecchymoses. Turn the patient often, and use a convoluted foam or low-pressure mattress to prevent skin breakdown.
- Provide good oral hygiene. Brush the patient's teeth often with a soft brush or sponge tip to reduce breath odor. Hard candy and mouthwash minimize metallic taste in the mouth and alleviate thirst.
- Offer small, palatable, nutritious meals. Try to provide favorite foods within dietary restrictions, and encourage intake of high-calorie foods.
- Monitor the patient for hyperkalemia. Observe for cramping of the legs and abdomen and for diarrhea. As potassium levels rise, watch for muscle irritability and a weak pulse rate. Monitor the electrocardiogram for tall, peaked T waves; widening QRS complex; prolonged PR interval; and disappearance of P waves, indicating hyperkalemia.
- Carefully assess the patient's hydration status. Check for jugular vein distention, and auscultate the lungs for crackles. Carefully measure daily intake and output, including all drainage, emesis, diarrhea, and blood loss. Record daily weight, presence or absence of thirst, axillary sweat, tongue dryness, hypertension, and peripheral edema.
- Monitor for bone or joint complications. Prevent pathologic fractures by turning the patient carefully and ensuring his safety. Perform passive range-of-motion exercises for the bedridden patient.
- Encourage the patient to perform deep-breathing and coughing exercises to prevent pulmonary congestion. Auscultate for crackles, rhonchi, and decreased breath sounds. Be alert for clinical signs of pulmonary edema (such as dyspnea and restlessness). Administer diuretics and other medications, as ordered.
- Maintain strict aseptic technique. Use a micropore filter during I.V. therapy, watch for signs of infection (listlessness, high fever, and leukocytosis), and warn the outpatient to avoid contact with infected people during the cold and flu season.
- Carefully observe and document seizure activity. Infuse sodium bicarbonate for acidosis and sedatives or anticonvulsants for seizures, as ordered. Pad the bed side rails and keep an oral airway and suction setup at the bedside. Periodically assess neurologic status, and check

for Chvostek's and Trousseau's signs, indicators of low serum calcium levels.

• Observe for signs of bleeding. Watch for prolonged bleeding at puncture sites and at the vascular access site used for hemodialysis. Monitor hemoglobin and hematocrit, and check stool, urine, and vomitus for blood.

• Report signs of pericarditis, such as a pericardial friction rub and chest pain. Also watch for the disappearance of friction rub, with a drop of 15 to 20 mm Hg in blood pressure during inspiration (paradoxical pulse)—an early sign of pericardial tamponade.

• Schedule medication administration carefully. Give iron before meals, aluminum hydroxide gels after meals, and antiemetics (as necessary) a half hour before meals. Administer antihypertensives at appropriate intervals. If the patient requires a rectal infusion of sodium polystyrene sulfonate for dangerously high potassium levels, apply an emollient to soothe the perianal area. Be sure the sodium polystyrene sulfonate enema is expelled; otherwise, it will cause constipation and won't lower potassium levels. Recommend antacid cookies as an alternative to aluminum hydroxide gels needed to bind GI phosphate. Don't give magnesium products because poor renal excretion can lead to toxic levels.

• If the patient requires dialysis, check the vascular access site every 2 hours for patency and the arm used for adequate blood supply and intact nerve function (check temperature, pulse rate, capillary refill, and sensation). If a fistula is present, feel for a thrill and listen for a bruit. Use a gentle touch to avoid occluding the fistula. Report signs of possible clotting. Don't use the arm with the vascular access site to take blood pressure readings, draw blood, or give injections because these procedures may rupture the fistula or occlude blood flow.

• Withhold the 6 a.m. (or morning) dose of antihypertensive on the morning of dialysis, and instruct the outpatient to do the same.

• Check the patient's hepatitis antigen status. If he's a carrier of hepatitis B, use universal precautions.

• After dialysis, check for disequilibrium syndrome, a result of sudden correction of blood chemistry abnormalities. Symptoms range from a headache to seizures. Also check for excessive bleeding from the dialysis site, and apply a pressure dressing or an absorbable gelatin sponge, as indicated. Monitor blood pressure carefully after dialysis.

Patient teaching

• Teach the patient how to take his medications and what adverse effects to watch for. Suggest that he take diuretics in the morning so that his sleep won't be disturbed.

• Instruct the anemic patient to conserve energy by resting frequently.

• Tell the patient to report leg cramps or excessive muscle twitching. Stress the importance of keeping follow-up appointments to have his electrolyte levels monitored.

• Tell the patient to avoid high-sodium and high-potassium foods. Encourage adherence to fluid and protein restrictions. To prevent constipation, stress the need for exercise and sufficient dietary fiber.

• If the patient is having dialysis, remember that he and his family are under extreme stress. The hospital will probably offer a course on dialysis; if not, you'll need to teach the patient and his family. Topics to cover include reason for the procedure; complications; signs and symptoms of the related disease; how to check for bleeding, electrolyte imbalance, and changes in blood pressure; diet; exercise; and use of equipment.

• Refer the patient and his family for counseling if they need help coping with chronic renal failure.

• Demonstrate how to care for the shunt, fistula, or other vascular access device and how to perform meticulous skin care. Discourage activity that might cause the patient to bump or irritate the access site.

• Suggest that the patient wear a medical identification bracelet or carry pertinent information with him.

LOWER URINARY TRACT DISORDERS

These disorders, which affect the bladder, the ureters, and the urethra, include lower urinary tract infection (UTI), vesicoureteral reflux, neurogenic bladder, and congenital anomalies of the ureter, bladder, and urethra.

LOWER URINARY TRACT INFECTION

The two forms of lower UTI are cystitis (infection of the bladder) and urethritis (infection of the urethra). They're nearly 10 times more common in females than in males (except in elderly males) and affect 10% to 20% of all females at least once. UTI is prevalent in girls.

In adult males and in children, lower UTIs typically are associated with anatomic or physiologic abnormalities and therefore need close evaluation. Most UTIs respond readily to treatment, but recurrence and resistant bacterial flare-up during therapy are possible.

REVIEWING U.T.I. RISK FACTORS

Certain factors increase the risk of UTI. They include natural anatomic variations, trauma or invasive procedures, urinary tract obstructions, and urine reflux.

Natural anatomic variations
Females are more prone to UTI than males because the female urethra is shorter than the male urethra (about 1" to 2" [2.5 to 5 cm] compared with 7" to 8" [18 to 20 cm]). It's also closer to the anus, allowing bacterial entry into the urethra from the vagina, perineum, or rectum or from a sexual partner.

Pregnant women are especially prone to UTIs because of hormonal changes. Also, the enlarged uterus displaces the bladder and exerts greater pressure on the ureters, increasing their length. This restricts urine flow, allowing bacteria to linger longer in the urinary tract.

In men, release of prostatic fluid serves as an antibacterial shield. Men lose this protection around age 50 when the prostate gland begins to enlarge. This enlargement, in turn, may promote urine retention.

Trauma or invasive procedures
Fecal matter, sexual intercourse, and instruments, such as catheters and cystoscopes, can introduce bacteria into the urinary tract to trigger infection.

Obstructions
A narrowed ureter or calculi lodged in the ureters or the bladder can obstruct urine flow. Slowed urine flow allows bacteria to remain and multiply, risking damage to the kidneys.

Reflux
Vesicourethral reflux results when pressure inside the bladder (caused by coughing or sneezing) pushes a small amount of urine from the bladder into the urethra. When the pressure returns to normal, the urine flows back into the bladder, bringing bacteria from the urethra with it.

In vesicoureteral reflux, urine flows from the bladder back into one or both ureters. The vesicoureteral valve normally shuts off reflux. However, damage can prevent the valve from doing its job.

Other risk factors
Urinary stasis can promote infection, which, if undetected, can spread to the entire urinary system. And because urinary tract bacteria thrive on sugars, diabetes also is a risk factor.

Causes
Most lower UTIs result from ascending infection by a single gram-negative, enteric bacterium, such as *Escherichia coli, Klebsiella, Proteus, Enterobacter, Pseudomonas,* and *Serratia.* In a patient with neurogenic bladder, an indwelling urinary catheter, or a fistula between the intestine and bladder, a lower UTI may result from simultaneous infection with multiple pathogens.

Studies suggest that infection results from a breakdown in local defense mechanisms in the bladder that allows bacteria to invade the bladder mucosa and multiply. These bacteria can't be readily eliminated by normal urination.

Bacterial flare-up during treatment usually is caused by the pathogen's resistance to the prescribed antimicrobial therapy. Even a small number of bacteria (fewer than 10,000/ml) in a midstream urine specimen obtained during treatment casts doubt on the effectiveness of treatment.

In almost all patients, recurrent lower UTIs result from reinfection by the same organism or by some new pathogen. In the remaining patients, recurrence reflects persistent infection, usually from renal calculi, chronic bacterial prostatitis, or a structural anomaly that's a source of infection. The high incidence of lower UTI among females probably occurs because natural anatomic features facilitate infection. (See *Reviewing UTI risk factors.*)

Complications
If untreated, chronic UTI can seriously damage the urinary tract lining. Infection of adjacent organs and structures (for example, pyelonephritis) also may occur. When this happens, the prognosis is poor.

Assessment findings
The patient may complain of urinary urgency and frequency, dysuria, bladder cramps or spasms, itching, a feeling of warmth during urination, nocturia, and urethral discharge (in men). Other complaints include low back pain, malaise, nausea, vomiting, pain or tenderness over the bladder, chills, and flank pain. Inflammation of the bladder wall also causes hematuria and fever.

Diagnostic tests

The following tests are used to diagnose lower UTI:

• *Microscopic urinalysis* showing red blood cell and white blood cell counts greater than 10 per high-power field suggests lower UTI.

• *Clean-catch urinalysis* revealing a bacterial count of more than 100,000/ml confirms UTI. Lower counts don't necessarily rule out infection, especially if the patient is urinating frequently, because bacteria require 30 to 45 minutes to reproduce in urine. Clean-catch collection is preferred to catheterization, which can reinfect the bladder with urethral bacteria.

• *Sensitivity testing* determines the appropriate antimicrobial drug. If the patient history and physical examination warrant, a blood test or a stained smear of uretheral discharge can rule out venereal disease.

• *Voiding cystourethrography* or *excretory urography* may detect congenital anomalies that predispose the patient to recurrent UTI.

Treatment

Appropriate antimicrobials are the treatment of choice for most initial lower UTIs. A 7- to 10-day course of antibiotics is standard, but studies suggest that a single dose or a 3- to 5-day regimen may be sufficient to render the urine sterile. (Elderly patients may still need 7 to 10 days of antibiotics to fully benefit from treatment.) If a culture shows that urine still isn't sterile after 3 days of antibiotic therapy, bacterial resistance probably has occurred, and a different antimicrobial will be prescribed.

A single dose of amoxicillin or co-trimoxazole may be effective for females with acute, uncomplicated UTI. A urine culture taken 1 to 2 weeks later will indicate whether the infection has been eradicated. Recurrent infections from infected renal calculi, chronic prostatitis, or structural abnormalities may necessitate surgery. Prostatitis also requires long-term antibiotic therapy. In patients without these predisposing conditions, long-term, low-dose antibiotic therapy is the treatment of choice.

Nursing diagnoses

• Altered urinary elimination
• Pain
• Risk for infection
• Sexual dysfunction
• Sleep pattern disturbance

Nursing interventions

• Watch for GI disturbances from antimicrobial therapy. If ordered, administer nitrofurantoin macrocrystals with milk or meals, to prevent such distress.

• If sitz baths don't relieve perineal discomfort, apply warm compresses sparingly to the perineum, but be careful not to burn the patient. Apply topical antiseptics on the urethral meatus, as necessary.

• Collect all urine specimens for culture and sensitivity testing carefully and promptly.

Patient teaching

• Explain the nature and purpose of antimicrobial therapy. Emphasize the importance of completing the prescribed course of therapy or, with long-term prophylaxis, of strictly adhering to the ordered dosage.

• Familiarize the patient with prescribed medications and their possible adverse effects. If antibiotics cause GI distress, explain that taking nitrofurantoin macrocrystals with milk or a meal can help prevent such problems. If therapy includes phenazopyridine, warn the patient that this drug turns urine red-orange and stains clothing.

• Explain that an uncontaminated midstream urine specimen is essential for accurate diagnosis. Before collection, teach the female patient to clean the perineum properly and to keep the labia separated during urination.

• Suggest warm sitz baths for relief of perineal discomfort.

• To prevent recurrent lower UTIs, teach a female patient to carefully wipe the perineum from front to back and to thoroughly clean it with soap and water after bowel movements. If she's infection-prone, she should urinate immediately after sexual intercourse. Tell her never to postpone urination and to empty her bladder completely.

• Tell the male patient that prompt treatment of predisposing conditions, such as chronic prostatitis, will help prevent recurrent UTIs.

• Urge the patient to drink about 2,000 ml (at least eight glasses) of fluids a day during treatment. More or less than this amount may alter the antimicrobial's effect. Be aware that the elderly patient may resist this suggestion because it causes him to make frequent trips, possibly up and down the stairs, to urinate.

• Explain that fruit juices, especially cranberry juice, and oral doses of vitamin C may help acidify urine and enhance certain medications' action.

VESICOURETERAL REFLUX

In vesicoureteral reflux, urine flows from the bladder back into the ureters and eventually into the renal pelvis or the parenchyma. When the bladder empties only part of what has been stored, urinary tract infection (UTI) may result. This disorder is most common during infancy in boys and during early childhood (ages 3 to 7) in girls. Primary vesicoureteral reflux that results from congenital anomalies is most common in females and rare in blacks. Up to 25% of asymptomatic siblings of children with diagnosed primary vesicoureteral reflux also show reflux. Secondary vesicoureteral reflux occurs in adults.

Causes

In patients with vesicoureteral reflux, incompetence of the ureterovesical junction and shortening of intravesical ureteral musculature allow backflow of urine into the ureters when the bladder contracts during voiding.

Primary vesicoureteral reflux may result from congenital anomalies of the ureters or bladder, including short or absent intravesical ureters, ureteral ectopia lateralis (greater-than-normal lateral placement of ureters), ureteral duplication, ureterocele, and a gaping or golf-hole ureteral orifice.

Secondary vesicoureteral reflux starts with a competent ureterovesical junction that has been damaged by bladder outlet obstruction, iatrogenic injury, trauma, or inadequate detrusor muscle buttress in the bladder. The last problem has several causes: congenital paraureteral bladder diverticulum, acquired diverticulum (from outlet obstruction), flaccid neurogenic bladder, and high intravesical pressure from outlet obstruction or an unknown cause.

Vesicoureteral reflux also may result from cystitis, with inflammation of the intravesical ureter, which causes edema and intramural ureter fixation. This usually leads to reflux in people with congenital ureteral or bladder anomalies or other predisposing conditions.

Complications

Recurrent UTIs can lead to acute or chronic pyelonephritis and renal damage due to renal scarring, hypertension, or calculi.

Assessment findings

The patient with vesicoureteral reflux typically reports symptoms and shows signs of UTI: urinary frequency and urgency, burning on urination, hematuria, foul-smelling urine and, in infants, dark, concentrated urine. With upper urinary tract involvement, the patient usually complains of high fever, chills, flank pain, painful urination, vomiting, and malaise. In children, fever, non-specific abdominal pain, and diarrhea may be the only clinical effects.

In male infants, palpation may reveal a hard, thickened bladder (felt as a hard mass deep in the pelvis) if posterior urethral valves are causing an obstruction. Rarely, children with minimal symptoms remain undiagnosed until puberty or adulthood, when they begin to show clear signs of renal impairment, such as anemia, hypertension, and lethargy.

Diagnostic tests

The following studies are pertinent to the diagnosis of vesicoureteral reflux:

• *Clean-catch urinalysis* shows a bacterial count over 100,000/ml, sometimes without pyuria. Microscopic examination may reveal red blood cells and white blood cells and an increased urine pH when infection is active. Specific gravity less than 1.010 demonstrates inability to concentrate urine.
• *Elevated levels of serum creatinine* (more than 1.2 mg/dl) and *blood urea nitrogen* (more than 18 mg/dl) demonstrate advanced renal dysfunction.
• *Voiding cystourethrography* identifies and determines the degree of reflux and shows when reflux occurs. It also may pinpoint the causative anomaly. In this procedure, contrast material is instilled into the bladder, and X-rays are taken before, during, and after voiding.
• *Catheterization of the bladder* after the patient voids determines the amount of residual urine.
• *Excretory urography* may show a dilated lower ureter, a ureter visible for its entire length, hydronephrosis, calyceal distortion, and renal scarring.
• *Cystoscopy,* with instillation of a solution containing methylene blue or indigo carmine dye, may confirm the diagnosis. After the bladder is emptied and refilled with clear sterile water, color-tinged fluid from either ureter positively confirms reflux.
• *Radioisotope scanning* and *renal ultrasonography* also may be used to detect reflux and screen the upper urinary tract for damage secondary to infection and other renal abnormalities.

Treatment

The goal of treatment in a patient with vesicoureteral reflux is to prevent pyelonephritis and renal dysfunction through antibiotic therapy and, when necessary, vesicoureteral reimplantation. Appropriate surgery creates a normal valve effect at the junction by reimplanting the ureter into the bladder wall at a more oblique angle.

Antibiotics usually are effective for reflux that is secondary to infection, reflux related to neurogenic bladder, and, in children, reflux related to a short intravesical ureter (which disappears spontaneously with growth). Reflux related to infection usually subsides after the infection is cured; however, 80% of females with vesicoureteral reflux will have recurrent UTIs within a year. Recurrent infection requires long-term prophylactic antibiotic therapy and careful patient follow-up (voiding cystourethrography and excretory urography every 4 to 6 months) to track the degree of reflux.

UTI that recurs despite prophylactic antibiotic therapy necessitates vesicoureteral reimplantation. In the patient with neurogenic bladder, other treatments may be more effective in preventing reflux. These patients may benefit from transurethral sphincterotomy (to relieve the obstructed outlet) or from bladder capacity augmentation (to decrease intravesical pressure).

After surgery (as after antibiotic therapy), close medical follow-up is necessary (excretory urography every 2 to 3 years and urinalysis once a month for a year), even if symptoms haven't recurred.

Nursing diagnoses
• Altered urinary elimination
• Fluid volume excess
• Impaired tissue integrity
• Pain
• Risk for infection

Nursing interventions
• If the patient is a child, encourage a parent to be present during diagnostic tests and procedures so that the child won't be frightened.
• Explain postoperative care to surgical patients and their parents, as appropriate: Males will have a suprapubic catheter; females, an indwelling catheter; and both sexes, one or two ureteral catheters or splints brought out of the bladder through a small abdominal incision. Both types of catheters keep the bladder empty and prevent pressure from stressing the surgical wound. Ureteral catheters drain urine directly from the renal pelvis and stent the anastomosis site. After complicated reimplantations, all catheters remain in place for 7 to 10 days.
• Postoperatively, closely monitor fluid intake and output. Give analgesics and antibiotics, as ordered. Make sure the catheters are patent and draining well. Maintain sterile technique during catheter care, and watch for fever, chills, and flank pain, which suggest a blocked catheter.
• After bladder augmentation, catheterize the patient every 2 to 3 hours at first. Gradually increase the time between catheterizations to allow the augmented bladder to expand. Irrigate for mucous sediment as needed.

Patient teaching
• Explain all diagnostic tests and procedures to the patient and his parents, if the patient is a child.
• Tell the surgical patient that he'll be able to move and walk with the catheters, but that he must be careful not to dislodge them.
• To ensure complete bladder emptying, teach the patient with vesicoureteral reflux to double-void (void once and then try to void again in a few minutes). Also, because his natural urge to void may be impaired, advise him to try to void every 2 to 3 hours, even if he doesn't feel the urge.
• Instruct the patient or his parents to watch for and report recurring signs of UTI: painful, frequent, burning urination and foul-smelling urine.
• If the patient is taking antimicrobial drugs, make sure he understands the importance of completing the prescribed therapy or maintaining low-dose prophylaxis.
• Before discharging the patient, stress the importance of close follow-up care and adequate daily fluid intake.

NEUROGENIC BLADDER
All types of bladder dysfunction caused by an interruption of normal bladder innervation by the nervous system are referred to as neurogenic bladder. (Other names for this disorder include neuromuscular dysfunction of the lower urinary tract, neurologic bladder dysfunction, and neuropathic bladder.) Neurogenic bladder can be hyperreflexic (hypertonic, spastic, or automatic) or flaccid (hypotonic, atonic, or autonomous).

An upper motor neuron lesion (at or above T12) causes spastic neurogenic bladder, with spontaneous contractions of detrusor muscles, increased intravesical voiding pressure, bladder wall hypertrophy with trabeculation, and urinary sphincter spasms. A lower motor neuron lesion (at or below S2 to S4) causes flaccid neurogenic bladder with decreased intravesical pressure, increased bladder capacity and residual urine retention, and poor detrusor contraction.

Causes
At one time, neurogenic bladder was thought to result primarily from spinal cord injury; now it appears to stem from a host of underlying conditions, including:
• *cerebral disorders,* such as cerebrovascular accident, brain tumor (meningioma and glioma), Parkinson's dis-

ease, multiple sclerosis, dementia, and incontinence associated with aging
- *spinal cord disease or trauma,* such as spinal stenosis (causing cord compression) or arachnoiditis (causing adhesions between the membranes covering the cord), cervical spondylosis, spina bifida, myelopathies from hereditary or nutritional deficiencies and, rarely, tabes dorsalis
- *disorders of peripheral innervation,* including autonomic neuropathies resulting from endocrine disturbances, such as diabetes mellitus (most common)
- *metabolic disturbances,* such as hypothyroidism, porphyria, or uremia (infrequent)
- *acute infectious diseases,* such as Guillain-Barré syndrome and transverse myelitis
- *heavy metal toxicity*
- *chronic alcoholism*
- *collagen diseases,* such as systemic lupus erythematosus
- *vascular diseases,* such as atherosclerosis
- *distant effects of certain cancers,* such as primary oat cell carcinoma of the lung
- *herpes zoster*
- *sacral agenesis.*

Complications
Incontinence, residual urine retention, urinary tract infection (UTI), calculus formation, and renal failure can complicate neurogenic bladder.

Assessment findings
The patient's history includes a condition or disorder that can cause neurogenic bladder. The patient will have some degree of incontinence and will experience changes in initiation or interruption of micturition or an inability to completely empty the bladder. He also may have a history of frequent UTIs. Other assessment findings may be present, depending on the site and extent of the spinal cord lesion. For example, with spinal cord lesions at the upper thoracic (cervical) level, hyperactive autonomic reflexes (autonomic dysreflexia) result when the bladder is distended. You may note severe hypertension, bradycardia, vasodilation (blotchy skin) above the level of the lesion, piloerection, and profuse sweating, and the patient may complain of a headache.

With *hyperreflexic neurogenic bladder,* the patient may have involuntary or frequent scanty urination, without a feeling of bladder fullness and, possibly, spontaneous spasms of the arms and legs. Anal sphincter tone may be increased. Tactile stimulation of the abdomen, thighs, or genitalia may precipitate voiding and spontaneous contractions of the arms and legs.

With *flaccid neurogenic bladder,* the patient may have overflow incontinence and diminished anal sphincter tone. Palpation and percussion reveal a greatly distended bladder. However, the patient may not experience the accompanying feeling of bladder fullness because of sensory impairment.

Diagnostic tests
The following diagnostic tests will help assess bladder function:
- *Voiding cystourethrography* evaluates bladder neck function, vesicoureteral reflux, and continence.
- *Urodynamic studies* allow the evaluation of how urine is stored in the bladder, how well the bladder empties urine, and the rate of movement of urine out of the bladder during voiding. These studies consist of four components:
  —*Urine flow study (uroflow)* shows diminished or impaired urine flow.
  —*Cystometry* evaluates bladder nerve supply, detrusor muscle tone, and intravesical pressures during bladder filling and contraction.
  —*Urethral pressure profile* determines urethral function with respect to length of the urethra and outlet pressure resistance.
  —*Sphincter electromyelography* correlates the neuromuscular function of the external sphincter with bladder muscle function during bladder filling and contraction. This evaluates how well the bladder and urinary sphincter muscles work together.
- *Videourodynamic studies* correlate visual documentation of bladder function with pressure studies.
- *Retrograde urethrography* reveals strictures and diverticula. This test may not be done routinely.

Treatment
The goals of treatment are to maintain the integrity of the upper urinary tract, control infection, and prevent urinary incontinence through evacuation of the bladder, drug therapy, surgery or, less often, nerve blocks and electrical stimulation.

Techniques for bladder evacuation include Valsalva's maneuver and intermittent self-catheterization. Tapping over the bladder can also initiate voiding but, even when performed properly, this practice isn't always successful and doesn't always eliminate the need for catheterization.

The patient can perform Valsalva's maneuver himself by sitting on the toilet and forcefully exhaling (while keeping his mouth closed). This helps the bladder release urine and promotes complete emptying.

Intermittent self-catheterization — more effective than either tapping or Valsalva's maneuver — is a major advance in treatment because it completely empties the bladder without the risks of an indwelling catheter. A male can perform this procedure more easily, but a female can learn self-catheterization with the help of a mirror. Intermittent self-catheterization, along with a bladder retraining program, is especially useful in patients with flaccid neurogenic bladder. Anticholinergics and alpha-adrenergic stimulators can help the patient with hyperreflexic neurogenic bladder until intermittent self-catheterization is performed.

Drug therapy for neurogenic bladder may include terazosin and phenoxybenzamine to facilitate bladder emptying and propantheline, methantheline, flavoxate, dicyclomine, imipramine, and pseudoephedrine to facilitate urine storage.

When conservative treatment fails, surgery may correct the structural impairment through transurethral resection of the bladder neck, urethral dilation, external sphincterotomy, or urinary diversion procedures. Implantation of an artificial urinary sphincter may be necessary if permanent incontinence follows surgery.

Nursing diagnoses
• Altered urinary elimination
• Body image disturbance
• Fluid volume deficit
• Impaired skin integrity
• Knowledge deficit
• Risk for infection
• Sensory alteration
• Sexual dysfunction

Nursing interventions
• Nursing care for patients with neurogenic bladder varies with the underlying cause and the method of treatment. (See *Planning care for the patient with neurogenic bladder.*)
• Use strict aseptic technique during insertion of an indwelling urinary catheter (a temporary measure to drain the incontinent patient's bladder). Don't interrupt the closed drainage system for any reason. Obtain urine specimens with a syringe and small-bore needle inserted through the aspirating port of the catheter itself (below the junction of the balloon instillation site). Irrigate in the same manner, if ordered.
• Clean the catheter insertion site with soap and water at least twice a day. Don't allow the catheter to become encrusted. Keep the drainage bag below the tubing and below the level of the bladder. Clamp the tubing or empty the bag before transferring the patient to a wheelchair or stretcher, to prevent accidental urine reflux if the drainage container doesn't have an antireflux valve. If urine output is considerable, empty the bag more often than once every 8 hours because bacteria can multiply in standing urine and migrate up the catheter and into the bladder.
• When the patient is on an intermittent self-catheterization and bladder retraining program, regulate fluid intake at 1,500 ml/day to maintain sufficient amounts of urine. Adjust this amount for the pediatric patient, based on urodynamic study findings. For females, the goal is urine retention because no acceptable urinary incontinence devices are on the market. Males can use an external device when bladder function returns. Reevaluate the patient when urine volume returned with catheterization is 300 ml every 6 hours between independent voidings; at that point, you may need to reduce the frequency of the catheterizations. In a patient with neurogenic bladder, catheterization can be stopped when the amount of postvoiding residual urine is consistently less than 100 ml.
• Watch for signs of infection (fever or cloudy or foul-smelling urine). Try to keep the patient as mobile as possible, or perform passive range-of-motion exercises, if necessary.
• If a urinary diversion procedure, such as catheter drainage or insertion of a suprapubic catheter, is to be performed, consult with an enterostomal therapist and coordinate the care plans.
• Neurogenic bladder can produce emotional turmoil. Suggest a support group at a local rehabilitation center or hospital.

Patient teaching
• Explain all diagnostic tests clearly so that the patient understands the procedure, the time involved, and the possible results. Assure him that the lengthy diagnostic process is necessary to identify the most effective treatment plan. After the treatment plan is chosen, explain it to him in detail.
• Encourage the patient to drink plenty of fluids every day to prevent calculus formation and infection from urinary stasis.
• Before discharge, teach the patient and his family evacuation techniques, as necessary (for example, tapping or intermittent self-catheterization). Also teach him how to care for the catheter, if appropriate.
• Discuss sexual activities. The incontinent patient will feel embarrassed and worried about sexual function, so provide emotional support.

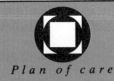

Plan of care

PLANNING CARE FOR THE PATIENT WITH NEUROGENIC BLADDER

How can you best care for a patient with neurogenic bladder? Your assessment findings can help you identify nursing diagnoses and plan, implement, and evaluate your care. The following case illustrates how the nursing process can work.

Patient history
Tom Murray, a married, 40-year-old construction worker, fell off a two-story scaffold and sustained a spinal cord lesion at S1. That injury resulted in Mr. Murray's becoming a paraplegic. His rehabilitation is progressing well, and he seems to be accepting his disability. But he has hyperreflexic neurogenic bladder. He initially had an indwelling urinary catheter, but it was removed because it resulted in several urinary tract infections (UTIs). Mr. Murray's problems have increased since the catheter was removed. When he tries to void, he produces only a small amount of urine; then he becomes incontinent, producing a larger volume. He says, "I feel terrible. Can't you do something?" But he also tells you, "I don't want to be stuck with a catheter for the rest of my life."

Assessment findings
When you palpate Mr. Murray's bladder, it feels distended, even though he says he has no feeling of fullness. This stimulation triggers the micturition reflex and causes him to void. Even though he voids a large amount, a postvoiding catheterization shows residual urine in his bladder.

Every time this happens, Mr. Murray becomes frustrated. "I can't go home like this," he says.

"I'll never be able to leave the house."

He's adamant about not having an indwelling catheter because it will interfere with his sex life.

Nursing diagnoses
Before formulating nursing diagnoses, you think carefully about Mr. Murray's case. You know that he's highly motivated to return home and resume as normal a life as possible, including his sex life. All that stands in his way is the incontinence problem, and he says that he's willing to learn intermittent self-catheterization. So, based on your assessment, you decide that Mr. Murray has the following problems:
• Altered urinary elimination related to spinal cord injury
• Body image disturbance related to loss of urinary continence
• Knowledge deficit related to managing urinary continence
• Risk for infection related to intermittent self-catheterization
• Sexual dysfunction related to continuous indwelling urinary catheterization.

Expected outcomes
To regulate Mr. Murray's altered urinary elimination patterns, you set the following expected outcomes. Mr. Murray will:
• achieve urinary continence
• maintain sufficient fluid intake.
To improve Mr. Murray's knowledge deficit, he will:
• demonstrate skill in performing intermittent self-catheterization
• identify the signs of UTI.

Implementation
To implement the care plan, you'll take the following steps:
• Provide at least 1,500 ml of fluid each day to ensure sufficient urine output.

• Start the following bladder evacuation procedure. At regular intervals (usually every 2 hours initially), stimulate the skin of the abdomen, thighs, or genitalia to initiate bladder contractions and trigger voiding. Or use tapping to empty the bladder. Teach the patient how to perform these techniques.

Next, teach Mr. Murray to perform intermittent self-catheterization to drain residual urine. Have him wash his hands and then sit on the toilet or the edge of the bed. Show him how to insert a clean catheter into the urethra and advance it into the bladder until urine returns. After draining the urine into the toilet or a container, he should remove the catheter and wash, rinse, and dry it. Show him how to measure the drainage, and teach him which unusual characteristics may indicate infection.

If the amount of urine returned is consistently under 100 ml, increase the interval between catheterizations; if it's more than 300 ml, decrease the interval. Explain to the patient that he should follow these guidelines at home.
• Provide the patient with a list of local stores that carry the supplies he'll need.

Evaluation
Your teaching has been successful if Mr. Murray can correctly demonstrate tactile stimulation and tapping, and if he's proficient in performing self-catheterization and caring for the equipment. He also should be drinking adequate amounts of fluids and know the signs of infection he needs to report to the doctor.

Once he can regulate his urinary elimination pattern, Mr. Murray's outlook on living with his symptoms and on his sexuality should improve.

• Demonstrate good hand-washing technique, and encourage meticulous cleaning of the drainage site.
• Teach the patient the signs of UTI, and warn him to report them immediately.

CONGENITAL ANOMALIES OF THE URETER, BLADDER, AND URETHRA

Among the most common birth defects, congenital anomalies of the ureter, bladder, and urethra occur in about 5% of all births. Some of these abnormalities are obvious at birth; others aren't recognized until they produce symptoms. Obstructions and malformations that necessitate surgery have a good prognosis.

Causes
The cause of these anomalies is unknown. For information about their pathophysiology, see *Reviewing congenital urologic anomalies.*

Complications
Mild to severe infections, hematuria, and calculi can complicate any anomaly that prevents urine from flowing freely from the body.

Assessment findings
In *duplicated ureter,* the patient may report persistent or recurrent urinary tract infection (UTI); urinary frequency and urgency; burning on urination; diminished urine output; and flank pain, fever, and chills. These signs and symptoms are associated with vesicoureteral reflux, ectopic ureters, and ureterocele.

In *retrocaval ureter (preureteral vena cava),* the patient may complain of right flank pain, recurrent UTI, and hematuria. If renal calculi occur, the patient may complain of severe pain that travels from the costovertebral angle to the flank and then to the suprapubic area and the external genitalia. Infants may cry uncontrollably.

In *ectopic orifice of the ureter,* symptoms are rare when the ureteral orifice opens between the trigone and bladder neck. Incontinence (dribbling) occurs in about 50% of female patients; they may complain of back pain or severe abdominal pain accompanied by anuria, nausea, and vomiting if obstruction occurs. Male patients may complain of flank pain and urinary frequency and urgency.

In *stricture or stenosis of the ureter,* the patient may have back pain accompanied by anuria, nausea, and vomiting if obstruction occurs.

In *ureterocele,* the patient may report signs of obstruction and persistent or recurrent UTI.

In *exstrophy of the bladder,* which is obvious at birth, urine seeps onto the abdominal wall from abnormal ureteral orifices. You'll also observe excoriation of the surrounding skin and ulceration of the exposed bladder mucosa. Infection and associated abnormalities also are characteristic.

In *congenital bladder diverticulum,* the patient may report fever, urinary frequency, and painful urination. UTI may occur, particularly cystitis in males.

Hypospadias usually is associated with chordee, making normal urination with the penis elevated impossible. The patient may exhibit an absence or deficit of the ventral prepuce and ambiguous genitalia. Vaginal discharge may occur in females.

In mild cases of *epispadias,* the orifice appears along the dorsum of the glans; in severe cases, it appears along the dorsum of the penis. In females, you'll see a bifid clitoris and a short, wide urethra. Total urinary incontinence occurs when the urethral opening is proximal to the sphincter.

Diagnostic tests and treatments
In *duplicated ureter,* diagnostic tests may include excretory urography, cystoscopy, voiding cystourethrography, and retrograde pyelography. Surgery may be necessary for obstruction, reflux, or severe renal damage.

In *retrocaval ureter,* excretory or retrograde urography demonstrates superior ureteral enlargement with spiral appearance. Treatment involves surgical resection and anastomosis of the ureter with the renal pelvis or reimplantation into the bladder.

In *ectopic orifice of the ureter,* diagnostic tests include excretory urography, urethroscopy, vaginoscopy, voiding cystourethrography, and retrograde urethrography. Treatment consists of resection and ureteral reimplantation into the bladder for incontinence.

In *stricture or stenosis of the ureter,* diagnostic tests include ultrasonography, excretory and retrograde urography, renography, and voiding cystourethrography. Treatment consists of surgical repair of the stricture. Nephrectomy may be necessary for severe renal damage, based on radionuclide studies.

In *ureterocele,* voiding cystourethrography, excretory urography, cystography, and cystoscopy may help diagnose the disorder. Excretory urography and cystography may show a thin, translucent mass. Cystoscopy helps assess the location of ureteral orifices and the changes on the submucosal tunnel. Treatment involves surgical ex-

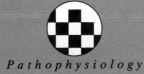

Pathophysiology

REVIEWING CONGENITAL UROLOGIC ANOMALIES

The most common malformations are duplicated ureter, retrocaval ureter, ectopic orifice of the ureter, stricture or stenosis of the ureter, ureterocele, exstrophy of the bladder, congenital bladder diverticulum, hypospadias, and epispadias.

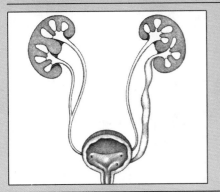

Duplicated ureter
Referred to as either complete or incomplete, duplicated ureter is the most common ureteral anomaly. A *complete* duplicated ureter consists of a double collecting system with two separate pelves, each with its own ureter and orifice. An *incomplete* duplicated ureter (Y type) has two separate ureters that join before entering the bladder.

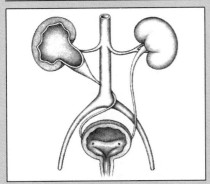

Retrocaval ureter (preureteral vena cava)
In this anomaly, the right ureter passes behind the inferior vena cava before entering the bladder. Compression of the ureter between the vena cava and the spine causes dilation and elongation of the pelvis, hydroureter, hydronephrosis, and fibrosis and stenosis of the ureter in the compressed area. Although rare in either sex, retrocaval ureter has a higher incidence in males.

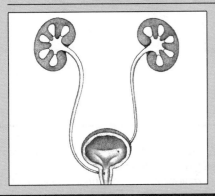

Ectopic orifice of ureter
In this anomaly, the openings of single or duplicated ureters are displaced. In females, ectopic ureters usually are part of a duplicated anomaly, and the ureters open into the urethra, vestibule, or vagina beyond the external urethral sphincter. In males, ectopic ureters occur more often with a single system and commonly open into the prostatic urethra, seminal vesicles, vas deferens, or epididymis.

(continued)

REVIEWING CONGENITAL UROLOGIC ANOMALIES *(continued)*

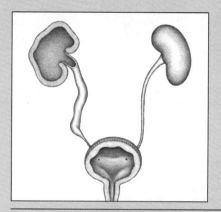

Stricture or stenosis of ureter
The most common site for stricture or stenosis is the distal ureter above the ureterovesical junction; less common, the ureteropelvic junction; rare, the midureter. This anomaly is discovered during infancy in 25% of patients and before puberty in most. It's more common in males than in females by a 5:2 ratio.

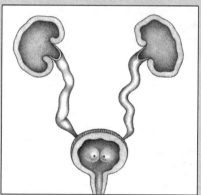

Ureterocele
In this anomaly, the submucosal ureter bulges into the bladder. It can be unilateral, bilateral, or ectopic with resulting hydroureter and hydronephrosis.

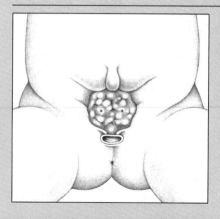

Exstrophy of bladder
In exstrophy of the bladder, the absence of the lower anterior abdominal wall and anterior bladder wall allows the posterior bladder wall to protrude onto the abdomen. In males, associated disorders include epispadias and undescended testes; in females, cleft clitoris, separated labia, and stenotic vagina. Skeletal and intestinal anomalies also are possible.

cision or resection of the ureterocele and reimplantation of the ureter.

In *exstrophy of the bladder,* diagnosis requires a radio-nuclide scan and renal ultrasonography. Buccal smears and karotyping may be necessary.

In infants, treatment includes surgical closure of the

REVIEWING CONGENITAL UROLOGIC ANOMALIES *(continued)*

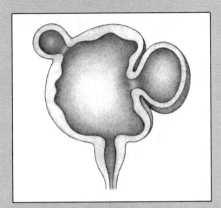

Congenital bladder diverticulum
A circumscribed pouch or sac (diverticulum) of the bladder wall can occur anywhere in the bladder but usually arises lateral to the ureteral orifice. A large diverticulum at the orifice can cause reflux.

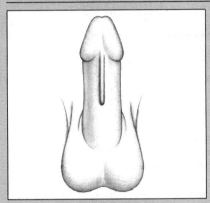

Hypospadias
In this anomaly, the urethral opening is on the ventral surface of the penis or, in females (rare), within the vagina. Hypospadias occurs in 1 of 300 live male births. A genetic factor is suspected in less severe cases.

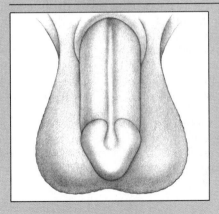

Epispadias
This rare disorder involves a urethral opening on the dorsal surface of the penis; in females, a fissure of the upper wall of the urethra. Epispadias occurs more commonly in males than in females and often accompanies bladder exstrophy.

defect and bladder and urethral reconstruction to allow pubic bone fusion and normal continence and renal function. Additional measures may include bladder recon-

struction with the use of an artificial urinary sphincter and reconstruction of a functional penis in males. Alternative treatment includes protective dressing and diapering. Urinary diversion eventually is necessary for most patients:

In *congenital bladder diverticulum,* excretory urography shows a diverticulum obstructing the ureteral entry to the bladder. Voiding cystourethrography shows vesicoureteral reflux in the ureter, and cystoscopy confirms the diverticulum. Surgery may be necessary to correct the reflux.

If *hypospadias* is mild, it requires no treatment. Buccal smears and karotyping may be necessary when sexual identification is questionable. If the anomaly is severe, surgical repair usually is necessary before the child reaches school age.

In *epispadias,* surgical repair in several stages is almost always necessary.

Nursing diagnoses
• Altered family processes
• Altered parenting
• Altered urinary elimination
• Fluid volume deficit
• Impaired skin integrity
• Knowledge deficit
• Pain
• Risk for infection

Nursing interventions
• Because these anomalies aren't always obvious at birth, carefully evaluate the neonate's urogenital function. Document the amount and color of urine, voiding pattern, strength of stream, and any indications of infection, such as fever and urine odor.
• In all children, watch for signs of obstruction, such as dribbling, oliguria or anuria, an abdominal mass, hypertension, fever, bacteriuria, and pyuria.
• Monitor renal function daily; record intake and output.
• Follow strict aseptic technique in handling cystostomy tubes or indwelling urinary catheters.
• Make sure that ureteral, suprapubic, or urethral catheters remain in place and don't become contaminated. Document the type, color, and amount of drainage.
• Apply a nonadherent film of plastic wrap over the exposed mucosa of the neonate with bladder exstrophy. Don't use heavy clamps on the umbilical cord—this only causes more trauma and excoriation of the bladder surface. Don't diaper the infant. Instead, place him in an incubator, and direct a stream of saline mist onto the bladder to keep it moist. Use warm water and mild soap to keep the surrounding skin clean; rinse well. Keep the area as dry as possible to prevent excoriation.

• Provide reassurance and emotional support to the parents. Allow them to express their concerns and fears. When possible, allow them to participate in their child's care to promote normal bonding.
• As appropriate, suggest or arrange for genetic counseling.

Patient teaching
• Before discharge, teach the parents about the particular anomaly and its treatment. Also teach them how to care for their child at home.
• Teach the parents how to clean around drainage tubes and how to apply sterile dressings if necessary.
• Discuss signs of infection to watch for and report to the doctor.

GENITAL DISORDERS

These disorders affect the testes, the prostate, and the epididymis. Nonspecific genitourinary infections also affect other areas, such as the urethra, vagina, and cervix.

UNDESCENDED TESTES
In this congenital disorder also known as cryptorchidism, one or both testes remain in the abdomen, in the inguinal canal, or at the external ring instead of descending into the scrotum. The disorder may occur bilaterally but usually affects only the right testis; it may be categorized as true or ectopic. True undescended testes remain along the path of normal descent, whereas ectopic testes deviate from that path.

Because the testes normally descend into the scrotum in the seventh gestational month, cryptorchidism affects more premature neonates (about 30%) than full-term neonates (about 3%). In about 80% of affected neonates, the testes descend spontaneously during the first year; in the rest, they may or may not descend later.

The prognosis for recovery is excellent because one or both testes usually descend spontaneously. If this doesn't occur, orchiopexy (fixation of a viable testis to the scrotum) can readily correct the disorder.

Causes
No one knows exactly how the testes descend into the scrotum. Some experts think that hormones play a role. Likely suspects include androgenic hormones from the placenta, the maternal or fetal adrenal glands, or the immature fetal testis. Other possible causes include mater-

nal progesterone or gonadotropic hormones from the maternal pituitary gland.

A popular but unsubstantiated theory links undescended testes to a defective gubernaculum, the fibromuscular band that connects the testes to the scrotal floor. In the normal male fetus, testosterone stimulates the gubernaculum's formation. This band probably helps pull the testes into the scrotum by shortening as the fetus grows. Thus, cryptorchidism may result from inadequate testosterone levels or from a defect in the testes or the gubernaculum.

Complications

Bilateral cryptorchidism that persists into adolescence prevents spermatogenesis and results in sterility, even though testosterone levels remain normal. Other complications of untreated cryptorchidism include increased testicular vulnerability to trauma and an increased risk for testicular cancer.

Assessment findings

In a patient with unilateral cryptorchidism, the scrotum on the affected side may appear underdeveloped. Occasionally, the scrotum on the unaffected side will be enlarged, whereas the testis in the scrotum on the affected side will be unpalpable.

Diagnostic tests

The following laboratory tests determine sex in questionable situations:
• *Buccal smear* identifies gender (by showing a male sex chromatin pattern).
• *Serum gonadotropin analysis* confirms existing testes by evaluating hormone levels in circulation.

Treatment

If the testes don't descend spontaneously by age 1, surgical correction (orchiopexy) may be needed to secure the testes to the scrotum. Commonly performed before the patient reaches age 4, orchiopexy prevents sterility, injury related to abnormal testicular positioning, and harmful psychological effects.

In some patients, human chorionic gonadotropin given intramuscularly may stimulate descent. This therapy is ineffective if the testes lie in the abdomen or if the patient also has an inguinal hernia.

Nursing diagnoses
• Knowledge deficit
• Pain
• Risk for injury

Nursing interventions
• Offer emotional support and reassurance. Encourage the parents to express their concerns about their child's condition.
• After orchiopexy, monitor the patient's vital signs and his intake and output. Watch for urine retention. Also check his dressings. If he's old enough to understand and cooperate, encourage him to do coughing and deep-breathing exercises.
• Keep the operative site clean. If the surgeon applied a rubber band to keep the testis in place, maintain the rubber band's tension while ensuring that the band isn't too tight.
• If the patient is an infant or a child, encourage his parents to participate in such postoperative care as bathing and feeding.
• If the patient is an older child or an adult, urge him to care for himself as much as possible.

Patient teaching
• If the patient is a neonate, review the causes of cryptorchidism and available treatments with his parents. Discuss the disorder's effect on reproduction if left untreated. Emphasize that testicular descent may occur spontaneously, especially in premature infants.
• If the patient is undergoing orchiopexy, explain the surgery to the parents. Also explain it to the patient in terms he can understand. Tell him that a rubber band may be taped to his thigh for about 1 week after surgery, to keep the testis in place. Inform him that his scrotum may swell but should not be painful.
• Tell the patient to wipe from front to back after a bowel movement. Explain that this helps to keep the operative site clean.
• Caution the patient to avoid rough play that can cause groin injury until the doctor approves strenuous activities.
• Suggest wearing comfortable, soft, loose-fitting clothes to prevent friction and swelling.
• Instruct the parents to notify the doctor if the child reports or appears to have severe pain.
• If the patient is an adult undergoing orchiopexy, explain that the procedure won't improve fertility or diminish his risk of developing testicular cancer. Teach him how to perform a self-examination when testicular palpation is possible.

TESTICULAR TORSION

In this condition, the spermatic cord twists with the rotation of a testis or the mesorchium (the mesentery be-

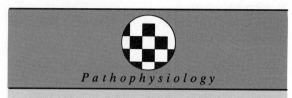

P a t h o p h y s i o l o g y

WHAT HAPPENS IN TESTICULAR TORSION

In extravaginal torsion, rotation of the spermatic cord above the testis causes strangulation and, eventually, infarction of the testis.

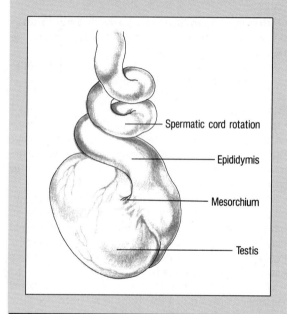

- Spermatic cord rotation
- Epididymis
- Mesorchium
- Testis

tween the testis and epididymis), strangulating the testis.

Occurring unilaterally about 90% of the time, testicular torsion is most common in males ages 12 to 18 (although it may occur at any age). With early detection and prompt treatment, the prognosis is good.

Causes

The tunica vaginalis normally envelops the testis and attaches to the epididymis and spermatic cord. In *intravaginal torsion* (the most common type of testicular torsion in adolescents), testicular twisting may result from abnormal positioning of the testis in the tunica or from a narrowing of the mesentery support. In *extravaginal torsion* (most common in neonates), loose attachment of the tunica vaginalis to the scrotal lining causes spermatic cord rotation above the testis. (See *What hap-*

pens in testicular torsion.) A sudden, forceful contraction of the cremaster muscle may precipitate this condition.

Complications

Without prompt treatment, complete testicular infarction followed by testicular atrophy may occur.

Assessment findings

The patient may report excruciating pain in the affected testis or iliac fossa. Pain increases when the scrotum is elevated. Inspection reveals tense, tender swelling in the scrotum or inguinal canal and hyperemia of the overlying skin.

Diagnostic tests

- *Doppler ultrasonography* helps distinguish testicular torsion from strangulated hernia, undescended testes, and epididymitis.
- *Testicular scan*, using technetium 99m pertechnetate, allows a definitive diagnosis.

Treatment

A vascular emergency, testicular torsion must be treated within 4 hours of initial pain. Treatment consists of immediate surgical repair by orchiopexy (fixation of a viable testis to the scrotum) or orchiectomy (excision of a nonviable testis). Analgesics relieve pain postoperatively.

Nursing diagnoses

- Pain
- Risk for infection
- Risk for injury
- Self-esteem disturbance

Nursing interventions

- Offer reassurance, and keep the patient comfortable before and after surgery. Administer pain medication, as ordered.
- Monitor voiding, and apply a covered ice bag to the surgical site to reduce edema.
- Protect the wound from contamination. Otherwise, allow as many normal daily activities as possible.

Patient teaching

- Explain the surgical procedure and postoperative care. Even if the testis must be removed, reassure the patient that sexual function and fertility should be unaffected.
- Recommend that the patient routinely wear a scrotal support when exercising.

PROSTATITIS

An inflammation of the prostate gland, prostatitis occurs in several forms. *Acute prostatitis* most often results from gram-negative bacteria and is easily recognized and treated. *Chronic prostatitis*, which affects up to 35% of men over age 50 and is the most common cause of recurrent urinary tract infection (UTI) in men, is harder to recognize. Other classifications include *granulomatous prostatitis* (also called tuberculous prostatitis), *nonbacterial prostatitis*, and *prostatodynia* (painful prostate).

Causes

About 80% of bacterial prostatitis cases result from infection by *Escherichia coli*. The rest result from infection by *Klebsiella, Enterobacter, Proteus, Pseudomonas, Serratia, Streptococcus, Staphylococcus*, and diphtheroids, which are contaminants from the anterior urethra's normal flora.

Infection probably spreads to the prostate gland by the hematogenous route or from ascending urethral infection, invasion of rectal bacteria by way of the lymphatic vessels, or reflux of infected bladder urine into prostate ducts. Less commonly, infection may result from urethral procedures performed with instruments, such as cystoscopy and catheterization, or from infrequent or excessive sexual intercourse.

Chronic prostatitis usually results from bacterial invasion from the urethra. Granulomatous prostatitis occurs secondary to a miliary spread of *Mycobacterium tuberculosis*. Nonbacterial prostatitis is probably caused by the protozoa *Mycoplasma, Ureaplasma, Chlamydia*, or *Trichomonas vaginalis*, or some viruses. The cause of prostatodynia is unknown.

Complications

UTI is the most common complication of prostatitis. An untreated infection can progress to prostatic abscess, acute urine retention from prostatic edema, pyelonephritis, and epididymitis.

Assessment findings

The patient with acute prostatitis may report sudden fever, chills, low back pain, myalgia, perineal fullness, arthralgia, frequent urination, urinary urgency, dysuria, nocturia, and transient erectile dysfunction. Some degree of urinary obstruction also may occur, and the urine may appear cloudy. The bladder may feel distended when palpated. When palpated rectally, the prostate is markedly tender, indurated, swollen, firm, and warm.

Clinical features of chronic bacterial prostatitis vary. Although some patients are asymptomatic, this condition usually elicits the same urinary symptoms as the acute form but to a lesser degree. Other possible signs and symptoms include hemospermia, persistent urethral discharge, and painful ejaculation that's responsible for some sexual dysfunction. The prostate may feel soft, and crepitation may be evident if prostatic calculi are present.

Digital examination in granulomatous prostatitis may reveal a stony, hard induration of the prostate (mimicking carcinoma or a calculus). This finding may suggest prostatitis if the patient has a history of pulmonary or GI tuberculosis or has been receiving intravesical therapy for superficial bladder cancer.

With nonbacterial prostatitis, the patient usually complains of dysuria, mild perineal or low back pain, and frequent nocturia. With prostatodynia, he may complain of perineal, low back, or pelvic pain.

Diagnostic tests

Although a urine culture often can identify the causative infectious organism, and characteristic rectal examination findings suggest prostatitis (especially in the acute phase), firm diagnosis depends on comparison of bacterial growth in specimens obtained by the Meares and Stamey technique.

This test requires four specimens: one collected when the patient starts voiding (voided bladder one [VB1]); another midstream (VB2); another after the patient stops voiding and the doctor massages the prostate to produce secretions (expressed prostate secretions [EPS]); and a final voided specimen (VB3). A significant increase in colony count of the prostatic specimens (EPS and VB3) confirms prostatitis.

In granulomatous prostatitis, demonstration of *M. tuberculosis* in the urine or a tissue biopsy from the prostate confirms the diagnosis.

In nonbacterial prostatitis, smears of prostatic secretions reveal inflammatory cells, but often no causative organism. In prostatodynia, urine cultures are negative and no inflammatory cells are present in smears of prostatic secretions. Urodynamic evaluation may reveal detrusor hyperreflexia and pelvic floor myalgia from chronic spasms.

Treatment

Systemic antibiotic therapy, guided by sensitivity studies, is the treatment of choice for acute prostatitis. Aminoglycosides, in combination with penicillins or cephalosporins, may be most effective for severe cases. Cotrimoxazole is given to prevent chronic prostatitis; it's also used to combat infections with *E. coli*. Other drugs used for *E. coli* infections include carbenicillin, nitrofurantoin, erythromycin, and tetracycline.

If drug therapy is unsuccessful, treatment may include transurethral resection of the prostate. Successful resection must remove all infected tissue. Usually not performed on young adults, this procedure may lead to retrograde ejaculation and sterility. Total prostatectomy is curative but may cause impotence and incontinence.

Treatment for granulomatous prostatitis consists of antitubercular drug combinations. Minocycline, doxycycline, or erythromycin is used for nonbacterial prostatitis for 4 weeks, but antibiotic therapy isn't repeated if symptoms don't subside.

Supportive therapy includes bed rest, adequate hydration, and administration of analgesics, antipyretics, and stool softeners, as necessary. If symptoms are present in chronic prostatitis, treatment may consist of sitz baths and regular sexual intercourse (the patient should use condoms during the treatment phase) or ejaculation to promote drainage of prostatic secretions. Regular prostatic massage for several weeks or months is effective in some patients. Anticholinergics and analgesics may help relieve the symptoms of nonbacterial prostatitis. Alpha-adrenergic blocking agents and muscle relaxants may be used for prostatodynia.

Nursing diagnoses
• Altered sexuality patterns
• Altered urinary elimination
• Ineffective individual coping
• Pain
• Risk for infection
• Self-esteem disturbance
• Sexual dysfunction

Nursing interventions
• Administer analgesics for pain, as ordered.
• Ensure bed rest and adequate hydration.
• Provide stool softeners and administer sitz baths, as ordered. Avoid rectal examination because it may precipitate bleeding.
• As necessary, prepare to assist with suprapubic needle aspiration of the bladder or a suprapubic cystostomy.
• If transurethral resection of the prostate is performed, monitor the patient postoperatively for signs of hypovolemia (decreased blood pressure, increased pulse rate, and pale, clammy skin).
• Check the catheter every 15 minutes for the first 2 to 3 hours after surgery for patency, urine color and consistency, and excessive urethral meatus bleeding.

• If a three-way continuous bladder irrigation is being performed, keep the solution flow rate sufficient to maintain patency and keep the return light pink. Watch for fluid overload from absorption of the irrigating fluid into the systemic circulation. Palpate for bladder distention. If the solution stops or the patient complains of pain, irrigate the catheter with 0.9% sodium chloride, using a 50-ml syringe.
• Watch for septic shock, the most serious complication of prostatic surgery. Immediately report severe chills, sudden fever, tachycardia, hypotension, or other signs of shock. Start rapid infusion of I.V. antibiotics, as ordered. Watch for pulmonary embolism, congestive heart failure, and acute renal failure. Continuously monitor vital signs and central venous pressure.
• Administer belladonna and opium suppositories or other anticholinergics, as ordered, to relieve painful bladder spasms that commonly occur after transurethral resection.

Patient teaching
• Familiarize the patient with any prescribed drugs and their possible adverse effects. Tell him to take the drugs exactly as ordered and to complete the prescribed drug regimens.
• Tell the patient to immediately report adverse drug reactions, such as rash, nausea, vomiting, fever, chills, and GI irritation.
• Instruct him to drink at least eight glasses of water a day (about 2 liters).
• If the patient has chronic prostatitis, recommend that he stay sexually active and ejaculate regularly to promote drainage of prostatic secretions. Tell him to use a condom during sexual intercourse when he's having a bout of prostatitis.

If the patient is scheduled for transurethral resection of the prostate:
• Tell him that after catheter removal, he may have urinary frequency, dribbling, and occasional hematuria. Reassure him that he'll gradually regain urinary control. Explain this to the family so that they can offer reassurance as well.
• Reinforce prescribed limits on activity. Warn the patient not to lift, exercise strenuously, or take long automobile rides because these increase bleeding tendency. Also caution him to abstain from sexual activity for several weeks after discharge.
• Instruct the patient to take oral antibiotics exactly as prescribed and for as long as prescribed. Also review the indications for using gentle laxatives.

• Urge the patient to seek medical care immediately if he can't void, if he passes bloody urine, or if he develops a fever.

EPIDIDYMITIS

Infection of the epididymis, the testis' cordlike excretory duct, is one of the most common infections of the male reproductive tract. It usually affects adults and is rare before puberty.

Causes

Epididymitis usually results from pyogenic organisms, such as staphylococci, *Escherichia coli*, streptococci, chlamydia, *Neisseria gonorrhoeae*, and *Treponema pallidum*. Infection usually results from established urinary tract infection (UTI) or prostatitis extending to the epididymis through the lumen of the vas deferens. Rarely, epididymitis is secondary to a distant infection, such as pharyngitis or tuberculosis, that spreads through the lymphatic system or, less commonly, the bloodstream.

Trauma may reactivate a dormant infection or initiate a new one. In addition, epididymitis is a complication of prostatectomy and may also result from chemical irritation by extravasation of urine through the vas deferens.

Complications

Epididymitis may spread to the testis itself, causing orchitis (see *Orchitis*). Bilateral epididymitis may cause sterility (see *How epididymitis can decrease fertility*, page 860).

Assessment findings

The patient may complain of unilateral, dull, aching pain radiating to the spermatic cord, lower abdomen, and flank, and of an extremely heavy feeling in the scrotum. He also may have erythema, a high fever, and malaise and may exhibit a characteristic waddle—an attempt to protect the groin and scrotum during walking. An acute hydrocele may occur as a reaction to the inflammatory process.

Diagnostic tests

Diagnosis requires the following laboratory tests:
• *Urinalysis.* Increased white blood cell (WBC) count indicates infection.
• *Urine culture and sensitivity tests.* Findings may identify the causative organism.
• *Serum WBC count.* A count of more than 10,000/mm³ indicates infection. If orchitis also is present, the diagnosis must be made cautiously because symptoms mimic

ORCHITIS

An infection of the testes, orchitis is a serious complication of epididymitis. It also may result from mumps, which may lead to sterility, or, less often, another systemic infection.

Signs and symptoms
Its typical effects include unilateral or bilateral tenderness and redness, sudden onset of pain, and swelling of the scrotum and testes. Nausea and vomiting also occur. Sudden cessation of pain indicates testicular ischemia, which may cause permanent damage to one or both testes. Hydrocele also may be present.

Treatment
Appropriate treatment consists of immediate antibiotic therapy or, in mumps orchitis, injection of 20 ml of lidocaine near the spermatic cord of the affected testis, which may relieve swelling and pain. Although corticosteroid use is experimental, such drugs may be used to treat nonspecific granulomatous orchitis. Severe orchitis may require surgery to incise and drain the hydrocele and to improve testicular circulation. Other treatments are similar to those for epididymitis.

To prevent mumps orchitis, suggest prepubertal males receive the mumps vaccine (or gamma globulin injection after contracting mumps).

those of testicular torsion, a condition that requires urgent surgical intervention.

Treatment

Therapy aims to reduce pain and swelling and combat infection. It must begin immediately, particularly in bilateral epididymitis, because sterility is always a threat.

During the acute phase, treatment consists of bed rest, scrotal elevation with towel rolls or adhesive strapping, broad-spectrum antibiotics, and analgesics. An ice bag applied to the area may reduce swelling and relieve pain (heat is contraindicated because it may damage germinal cells, which are viable only at or below normal body temperature). When pain and swelling subside and permit walking, an athletic supporter may prevent pain. Corticosteroids may be prescribed to help counteract inflammation, but their use is controversial.

When epididymitis is refractory to antibiotic therapy, epididymectomy under local anesthesia is necessary.

In an older patient undergoing prostatectomy, bilateral vasectomy may be necessary to prevent epididymitis as

HOW EPIDIDYMITIS CAN DECREASE FERTILITY

To understand how infection occurs, review normal anatomy shown in the diagram below. Male reproductive cells, called spermatozoa (sperm), are produced in the testes—a complex system of coiled tubules. The immature sperm swim out of the testes into a long, coiled duct, called the epididymis, where the maturing process continues. From here, they pass into the vas deferens, where they become fully mature. The vas deferens terminates in the prostatic urethra.

Epididymitis can inhibit the normal development of sperm, decreasing fertility. Here's how. The sperm leave the body through the urethra when ejaculation occurs. In epididymitis, bacteria from other parts of the urogenital system, such as the urethra, travel backward through the reproductive tract to invade the epididymis. Here, these infecting organisms can interfere with sperm development, decreasing the patient's fertility.

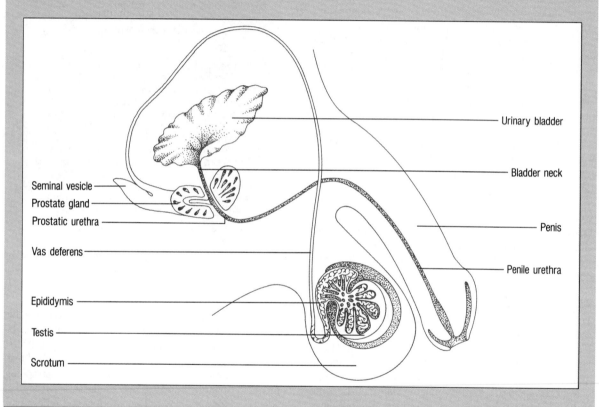

a postoperative complication. However, antibiotics alone may prevent it.

Nursing diagnoses
• Altered sexuality patterns
• Altered urinary elimination
• Knowledge deficit
• Pain
• Risk for infection
• Sexual dysfunction

Nursing interventions
• Watch closely for signs of abscess formation (a localized, hot, red, tender area) or extension of the infection into the testes. Closely monitor temperature, and ensure adequate fluid intake.
• Because the patient usually is very uncomfortable, administer analgesics as necessary. Allow him to rest in bed, legs slightly apart, with testes elevated on a towel roll. Suggest that he wear nonconstrictive, lightweight

clothing until the swelling subsides. Apply ice packs as needed for comfort.

• Administer antibiotics and antipyretics, as ordered. If epididymitis is secondary to a sexually transmitted disease (STD), treat the patient and his sexual partner with appropriate antibiotics.

• If the patient faces the possibility of sterility, suggest supportive counseling as necessary.

Patient teaching

• If the patient will be taking antibiotics after discharge, emphasize the importance of completing the prescribed regimen, even after symptoms subside.

• Suggest that the patient wear a scrotal support while sitting, standing, or walking.

• If epididymitis is secondary to an STD, encourage the patient to use a condom during sexual intercourse and to notify sexual partners so that they can be adequately treated for infection.

BENIGN PROSTATIC HYPERPLASIA

Although most men over age 50 have some prostatic enlargement, in benign prostatic hyperplasia (BPH), the prostate gland enlarges sufficiently to compress the urethra and cause some overt urinary obstruction. BPH begins with changes in periurethral glandular tissue. As the prostate enlarges, it may extend into the bladder and obstruct urine outflow by compressing or distorting the prostatic urethra. BPH also may cause a diverticulum musculature that retains urine when the rest of the bladder empties. Depending on the size of the enlarged prostate, the age and health of the patient, and the extent of the obstruction, BPH may be treated surgically or symptomatically.

Causes

Recent evidence suggests a link between BPH and hormonal activity. As men age, production of androgenic hormones decreases, causing an imbalance in androgen and estrogen levels and high levels of dihydrotestosterone, the main prostatic intracellular androgen. Other theoretical causes include neoplasm, arteriosclerosis, inflammation, and metabolic or nutritional disturbances.

Complications

Because BPH causes urinary obstruction, a patient may have one or more of the following complications:

• urinary stasis, urinary tract infection (UTI), or calculi
• bladder wall trabeculation
• detrusor muscle hypertrophy

• bladder diverticuli and saccules
• urethral stenosis
• hydronephrosis
• paradoxical (overflow) incontinence
• acute or chronic renal failure
• acute postobstructive diuresis.

Assessment findings

Clinical features of BPH depend on the extent of prostatic enlargement and on the lobes affected. Characteristically, the patient complains of a group of symptoms known as "prostatism": decreased urine stream caliber and force, an interrupted stream, urinary hesitancy, and difficulty starting urination, which results in straining and a feeling of incomplete voiding.

As the obstruction increases, the patient may report frequent urination with nocturia, dribbling, urine retention, incontinence and, possibly, hematuria.

Physical examination reveals a visible midline mass above the symphysis pubis, which represents an incompletely emptied bladder. Palpation discloses a distended bladder; rectal palpation, an enlarged prostate.

Diagnostic tests

The following tests help to confirm this diagnosis:

• *Excretory urography* may indicate urinary tract obstruction, hydronephrosis, calculi or tumors, and filling and emptying defects in the bladder.

• *Elevated blood urea nitrogen* and *serum creatinine levels* suggest impaired renal function.

• *Urinalysis* and *urine culture* show hematuria, pyuria, and, when the bacterial count exceeds 100,000/mm^3, UTI.

When symptoms are severe, cystourethroscopy is the definitive diagnostic measure and helps to determine the best surgical procedure. It can show prostate enlargement, bladder wall changes, calculi, and a raised bladder.

A prostate-specific antigen test may be performed to rule out prostatic cancer.

Treatment

Conservative therapy includes prostatic massages, sitz baths, short-term fluid restriction (to prevent bladder distention) and, if infection develops, antimicrobials. Regular sexual intercourse may help relieve prostatic congestion. Treatment with terazosin and finasteride has also proven effective.

Surgery is the only effective therapy for relief of acute urine retention, hydronephrosis, severe hematuria, and recurrent UTI, or for palliative relief of intolerable symptoms. A transurethral resection may be performed if the prostate weighs less than 2 oz (57 g).

In this procedure, a resectoscope removes tissue with a wire loop and an electric current. For high-risk patients, continuous drainage with an indwelling urinary catheter alleviates urine retention. Other transurethral procedures include vaporization of the prostate or a prostate incision with a scalpel or laser.

Other procedures involve open surgical removal of the prostate. One of the following operations may be appropriate:
• *Suprapubic (transvesical) prostatectomy* is the most common and is especially useful when prostatic enlargement remains within the bladder area.
• *Perineal prostatectomy* usually is performed for a large gland in an older patient. The operation commonly results in impotence and incontinence.
• *Retropubic (extravesical) prostatectomy* allows direct visualization; potency and continence usually are maintained.

Less frequently performed procedures include balloon dilatation, ultrasound needle ablation, and use of stents.

Nursing diagnoses
• Altered urinary elimination
• Pain
• Risk for infection
• Sexual dysfunction

Nursing interventions
• Prepare the patient for diagnostic tests and surgery, as appropriate.
• Monitor and record the patient's vital signs, intake and output, and daily weight. Watch closely for signs of postobstructive diuresis (such as increased urine output and hypotension), which may lead to serious dehydration, lowered blood volume, shock, electrolyte losses, and anuria.
• Administer antibiotics, as ordered, for UTI, urethral procedures that involve instruments, and cystoscopy.
• If urine retention occurs, try to insert an indwelling urinary catheter. If the catheter can't be passed transurethrally, assist with suprapubic cystostomy. Watch for rapid bladder decompression.
• Avoid giving a patient with BPH decongestants, tranquilizers, alcohol, antidepressants, or anticholinergics because these drugs can worsen the obstruction.

After *prostatic surgery:*
• Maintain patient comfort, and watch for and prevent postoperative complications. Observe for signs of shock and hemorrhage. Check the catheter frequently (every 15 minutes for the first 2 to 3 hours) for patency and urine color; check the dressings for bleeding.
• Postoperatively, many urologists insert a three-way catheter and establish continuous bladder irrigation. Keep the solution flowing at a rate sufficient to maintain patency and ensure that returns are clear and light pink. Watch for fluid overload from absorption of the irrigating fluid into the systemic circulation. If a regular catheter is used, observe it closely. If drainage stops because of clots, irrigate the catheter, as ordered, usually with 80 to 100 ml of 0.9% sodium chloride solution, while maintaining strict aseptic technique.
• Watch for septic shock, the most serious complication of prostatic surgery. Immediately report severe chills, sudden fever, tachycardia, hypotension, or other signs of shock. Start rapid infusion of I.V. antibiotics, as ordered. Watch for pulmonary embolism, congestive heart failure, and acute renal failure. Monitor vital signs, central venous pressure, and arterial pressure.
• Administer belladonna and opium suppositories or other anticholinergics, as ordered, to relieve bladder spasms that may occur after transurethral resection.
• Make the patient comfortable after an open procedure: Administer suppositories (except after perineal prostatectomy), and give analgesics to control incisional pain. Change dressings frequently.
• Continue infusing I.V. fluids until the patient can drink enough on his own (2,000 to 3,000 ml/day) to maintain adequate hydration.
• Administer stool softeners and laxatives, as ordered, to prevent straining. *Don't* check for fecal impaction because a rectal examination may cause bleeding.

Patient teaching
• After the catheter is removed, the patient may experience urinary frequency, dribbling and, occasionally, hematuria. Reassure him and his family that he'll gradually regain urinary control.
• Reinforce prescribed limits on activity. Warn the patient against lifting, performing strenuous exercises, and taking long automobile rides for at least 1 month after surgery because these activities increase bleeding tendency. Also caution him not to have sexual intercourse for at least several weeks after discharge.
• Teach the patient to recognize the signs of UTI. Urge him to immediately report these signs to the doctor because infection can worsen the obstruction.
• Instruct the patient to follow the prescribed oral antibiotic regimen, and tell him the indications for using gentle laxatives.

• Urge the patient to seek medical care immediately if he can't void at all, if he passes bloody urine, or if he develops a fever.

NONSPECIFIC GENITOURINARY INFECTIONS

These infections, which include nongonococcal urethritis in males and mild vaginitis or cervicitis in females, have similar manifestations. Nonspecific genitourinary infections have become more prevalent since the mid-1960s and are more widespread than gonorrhea. The prognosis is good if sexual partners are treated simultaneously.

Causes

Nonspecific genitourinary infections are spread primarily through sexual intercourse. In males, nongonococcal urethritis commonly results from *Chlamydia trachomatis* or *Ureaplasma urealyticum*. It also may result from bacteria, such as staphylococci, diphtheroids, coliform organisms, and *Gardnerella vaginalis*. Less frequently, infection may be related to preexisting strictures, neoplasms, and chemical or traumatic inflammation.

Although less is known about nonspecific genitourinary infections in females, chlamydial or corynebacterial organisms and *G. vaginalis* (which causes bacterial vaginosis) also may cause these infections.

Complications

Untreated nonspecific genitourinary infections may cause infertility. In males, nongonococcal urethritis can lead to acute epididymitis.

Assessment findings

One week to 1 month after intercourse with an infected partner, a male with nongonococcal urethritis may report a mucopurulent urethral discharge and variable dysuria. Hematuria occasionally occurs. Subclinical urethritis may be found on physical examination, especially if the patient's sex partner has been diagnosed with a nonspecific genitourinary infection.

A female with a nonspecific genitourinary infection may report a persistent vaginal discharge or acute or recurrent cystitis for which no underlying cause can be found. She also may have cervicitis with inflammatory erosion. Both males and females with nonspecific genitourinary infections may be asymptomatic but show signs of urethral, vaginal, or cervical infection on physical examination.

Diagnostic tests

In males, examination of smears of prostatic or urethral secretions shows excessive polymorphonuclear leukocytes but few, if any, specific organisms. In females, cervical or urethral smears show similar results. Epithelial cells covered with bacteria confirm infection.

Treatment

Therapy for both sexes consists of 500 mg of oral metronidazole twice a day for 7 days or a single 2-g dose. For females, treatments also may include application of a vaginal cream and, occasionally, cryosurgery.

Nursing diagnoses
• Altered sexuality patterns
• Risk for infection
• Sexual dysfunction

Nursing interventions

No interventions other than patient teaching are needed.

Patient teaching
• Tell the female patient to clean the pubic area before applying vaginal medication and to avoid using tampons during treatment.
• Be sure the patient follows the dosage schedule.
• To prevent nonspecific genitourinary infections, advise the patient to abstain from sexual intercourse with infected partners, to use condoms during sexual activity, to follow appropriate hygienic measures afterward, and to void before and after intercourse.
• Advise the patient to inform all prior sexual partners so that they can be treated.
• Encourage adequate fluid intake.
• Advise the female patient not to insert foreign objects in the vagina, not to use douches and hygiene sprays routinely, and not to wear tight-fitting pants, panty hose, nylon panties, or panty liners.

SELECTED REFERENCES

Davis, V.M. "Electric Stimulation: Does Nursing Have a Role in the Treatment of Adult Urinary Incontinence," *Urologic Nursing* 15(2):69-70, June, 1995.

Karlowicz, K.A., ed. *Urologic Nursing: Principles and Practices.* Philadelphia: W.B. Saunders Co., 1995.

Tanagho, E.A., and McAninch, J.W., eds. *Smith's General Urology,* 14th ed. East Norwalk, Conn.: Appleton & Lange, 1995.

Taylor, C.M., and Sparks, S.M. *Nursing Diagnosis Reference Manual,* 3rd ed. Springhouse, Pa.: Springhouse Corp., ·1995.

12 GASTROINTESTINAL DISORDERS

INTRODUCTION

As the site of digestion, the GI system has the critical task of supplying essential nutrients to fuel the brain, heart, lungs, and other tissues. GI function also profoundly affects the quality of life by its impact on overall health. A malfunction along the GI tract or in one of the accessory GI organs can produce far-reaching metabolic effects, eventually threatening life itself.

Anatomy and physiology

The GI system has two major components: the alimentary canal and the accessory organs. The *alimentary canal*, or GI tract, consists essentially of a hollow muscular tube that begins in the mouth and ends at the anus. It includes the oral cavity, pharynx, esophagus, stomach, small intestine, and large intestine. *Accessory glands and organs* aiding GI function include the salivary glands, liver, biliary duct system (gallbladder and bile ducts), and pancreas.

Together, the GI tract and accessory organs serve two major functions: digestion, the breaking down of food and fluids into simple chemicals that can be absorbed into the bloodstream and transported throughout the body, and the elimination of waste products from the body through defecation.

Cellular anatomy

The GI tract wall consists of several layers. The *innermost layer (tunica mucosa, or mucosa)* contains epithelial and surface cells and loose connective tissue. In the small intestine, epithelial cells elaborate into millions of fingerlike projections (villi) that vastly increase their absorptive surface area. These cells also secrete gastric and protective juices and absorb nutrients. Surface cells overlie connective tissue (lamina propria), supported by a thin layer of smooth muscle (muscularis mucosa).

The *submucosa (tunica submucosa)* encircles the mucosa. It's composed of loose connective tissue, blood and lymphatic vessels, and a nerve network (the submucosal, or Meissner's, plexus). Around this layer lies the *tunica muscularis,* composed of skeletal muscle in the mouth, pharynx, and upper esophagus, and of longitudinal and circular smooth-muscle fibers elsewhere in the GI tract. During peristalsis, longitudinal fibers shorten the lumen's length and circular fibers reduce the lumen's diameter. At points along the tract, circular fibers thicken to form sphincters. Between the two muscle layers of the tunica muscularis lies another nerve network, the myenteric, or Auerbach's, plexus. The stomach wall contains a third muscle layer.

The GI tract's outer covering—known as the *tunica adventitia* in the esophagus and rectum, the *tunica serosa* elsewhere—consists of connective tissue protected by epithelium. Also called the visceral peritoneum, this layer covers most of the abdominal organs and is contiguous with an identical layer (parietal peritoneum) lining the abdominal cavity. The visceral peritoneum becomes a double-layered fold around the blood vessels, nerves, and lymphatics supplying the small intestine and attaches the jejunum and ileum to the posterior abdominal wall to prevent twisting. A similar mesenteric fold attaches the transverse colon to the posterior abdominal wall.

Digestion and elimination

Digestion starts in the oral cavity, where chewing (mastication), salivation (the beginning of starch digestion), and swallowing (deglutition) all take place.

When a person swallows a food bolus, the upper esophageal (hypopharyngeal) sphincter relaxes, allowing food to enter the esophagus. In the esophagus, peristaltic waves activated reflexively by the glossopharyngeal nerve propel food down toward the stomach. As food moves through the esophagus, glands in the esophageal mucosal layer secrete mucus, which lubricates the bolus and protects the esophageal mucosal layer from being damaged by poorly chewed foods.

In the stomach

By the time the food bolus is on its way to the stomach, the cephalic phase of digestion has already begun. In this phase, the stomach secretes digestive juices (hydrochloric acid and pepsin) in response to stimuli from the person's smelling, tasting, chewing, or thinking of food. When food enters the stomach through the cardiac sphincter, the stomach wall distends, initiating the gastric phase of digestion. In this phase, stomach wall distention stimulates the antral mucosa of the stomach to release gastrin. Gastrin, in turn, stimulates the stomach's motor functions and gastric juice secretion. These highly acidic digestive secretions (pH of 0.9 to 1.5) consist mainly of pepsin, hydrochloric acid, intrinsic factor, and proteolytic enzymes.

The stomach has three major motor functions: storing food, mixing food by peristaltic contractions with gastric juices, and slowly parceling this food (now called chyme) into the small intestine for further digestion and absorption. Except for alcohol, little food absorption normally occurs in the stomach.

In the small intestine

Nearly all digestion and absorption takes place in the 20' (6 m) of the small intestine coiled in the abdomen in three major sections: the duodenum, jejunum, and ileum. The *duodenum* extends from the stomach and contains the ampulla of Vater (hepatopancreatic ampulla or Oddi's sphincter), an opening that drains bile from the common duct and pancreatic enzymes from the main pancreatic duct.

The *jejunum* follows the duodenum and leads to the *ileum*. The small intestine ends in the right lower abdominal quadrant at the ileocecal valve, a sphincter that empties nearly nutrient-free chyme into the large intestine. Peristaltic contractions and various digestive secretions break down carbohydrates, proteins, and fats and enable the intestinal mucosa to absorb these nutrients, along with water and electrolytes, into the bloodstream for use by the body.

In the large intestine

By the time chyme passes through the small intestine and enters the *ascending colon* of the large intestine, it has been reduced to mostly indigestible substances. From the ascending colon, chyme passes through the *transverse colon* and *descending colon* to the rectum, and finally into the *anal canal,* where it's expelled.

Although the large intestine produces no hormones or digestive enzymes, it is the site of the absorptive process. Through blood and lymph vessels in the submucosa, the proximal half of the large intestine absorbs all but about 100 ml of the remaining water in the colon plus large amounts of sodium and chloride. The large intestine also harbors the bacteria *Escherichia coli, Enterobacter aerogenes, Clostridium welchii,* and *Lactobacillus bifidus,* which help synthesize vitamin K and break down cellulose into usable carbohydrates. Bacterial action also produces flatus, which helps propel feces toward the rectum. In addition, the mucosa produces alkaline secretions from tubular glands composed of goblet cells. This alkaline mucus lubricates the intestinal walls as food pushes through and protects the mucosa from acidic bacterial action.

In the lower part of the descending colon, long and relatively sluggish contractions cause propulsive waves known as mass movements. These movements, which normally occur several times a day, propel intestinal contents into the rectum and produce the urge to defecate.

Accessory organs of digestion

Allied to the GI tract are the liver, biliary duct system, and pancreas, which contribute hormones, enzymes, and bile vital to digestion. These organs deliver their secretions to the duodenum through the ampulla of Vater.

Liver

Performing complex and important functions related to digestion and nutrition, the liver is the body's largest gland. Weighing 3 lb (1.4 kg), the liver is highly vascular and enclosed in a fibrous capsule in the right upper abdominal quadrant. It plays an important role in carbohydrate metabolism, detoxifies various endogenous and exogenous toxins in plasma, and synthesizes plasma proteins, nonessential amino acids, and vitamin A. The liver also stores essential nutrients, such as iron and vitamins K, D, and B_{12}. What's more, it secretes bile and removes ammonia from body fluids, converting it to urea for excretion in urine.

Bile, a greenish liquid composed of water, cholesterol, bile salts, electrolytes, and phospholipids, is important in fat breakdown and intestinal absorption of fatty acids, cholesterol, and other lipids. When bile salts are absent from the intestinal tract, lipids are excreted and fat-soluble vitamins are absorbed poorly. Bile also aids in excretion of conjugated bilirubin (an end product of hemoglobin degradation) from the liver and thereby prevents jaundice.

The liver recycles about 80% of bile salts into bile, combining them with bile pigments (biliverdin and bilirubin—the breakdown products of red blood cells) and cholesterol. The liver metabolizes digestive end products by regulating blood glucose levels. When glucose is being absorbed through the intestine (anabolic state), the liver stores glucose as glycogen. When glucose isn't being absorbed or when blood glucose levels fall (catabolic state), the liver mobilizes glucose to restore blood levels necessary for brain function.

The liver's functional unit, the *lobule,* consists of a plate of hepatic cells (hepatocytes) that encircle a central vein and radiate outward. The plates of hepatocytes are separated from each other by *sinusoids,* which constitute the liver's capillary system. Lining the sinusoids are reticuloendothelial macrophages (Kupffer's cells), which remove bacteria and toxins that have entered the blood through the intestinal capillaries.

The sinusoids carry oxygenated blood from the hepatic artery and nutrient-rich blood from the portal vein. Unoxygenated blood leaves through the central vein and flows through hepatic veins to the inferior vena cava. Bile, recycled from bile salts in the blood, leaves through bile ducts (canaliculi) that merge into right and left hepatic ducts to form the common hepatic duct. This common duct joins the cystic duct from the gallbladder to form the common bile duct to the duodenum.

Gallbladder
This pear-shaped organ, 3" to 4" (8 to 10 cm) long, is joined to the liver's ventral surface by the cystic duct. It stores and concentrates bile produced by the liver. Its customary 30- to 50-ml storage capacity can increase up to tenfold. Secretion of the hormone cholecystokinin causes gallbladder contraction and relaxation of the ampulla of Vater, releasing bile into the common bile duct for delivery to the duodenum. When the ampulla of Vater closes, bile shunts to the gallbladder for storage.

Pancreas
Somewhat flat and 6" to 9" (15 to 23 cm) long, the pancreas lies behind the stomach. Its head and neck extend into the curve of the duodenum, and its tail lies against the spleen.

The pancreas performs both exocrine and endocrine functions. Its exocrine function involves scattered cells that secrete more than 1,000 ml of digestive enzymes daily. Lobules and lobes (acini) of enzyme-producing cells release their secretions into ducts that merge into the pancreatic duct. This duct runs the length of the pancreas and joins the bile duct from the gallbladder before entering the duodenum. Vagal stimulation and release of the hormones secretin and cholecystokinin control the rate and amount of pancreatic secretion.

The endocrine function of the pancreas involves the islets of Langerhans, which are located between the acinar cells. Over 1 million of the islets house two cell types: beta and alpha. Beta cells secrete insulin to promote carbohydrate metabolism; alpha cells secrete glucagon, which stimulates glycogenolysis in the liver. Both hormones flow directly into the blood, their release stimulated by blood glucose levels.

GI assessment
Your assessment of the patient with suspected GI disease must include a thorough history and physical examination.

History
Begin with a careful history that includes occupation, family history, alcohol consumption, recent exposure to infections, recent abdominal injury, and recent travel. The medical history should include previous hospital admissions; any surgery (including recent tooth extraction); any recent blood or plasma transfusions; a family history of ulcers, colitis, or cancer; and any current medications, such as aspirin, steroids, or anticoagulants.

Next, have the patient describe his chief complaint in his own words. Was the onset of symptoms abrupt or insidious? Did they follow a recent abdominal injury? Does he have abdominal pain, indigestion, heartburn, or rectal bleeding? How long has he had his symptoms? What relieves them or makes them worse?

Has the patient recently experienced nosebleeds or difficulty in swallowing? Does he bruise or bleed easily? Has he had any recent weight loss or gain? Has he noticed any loss of appetite? Can he tolerate fatty foods? Is he on a special diet? Does he drink alcoholic beverages or smoke? How much and how often? Ask about bowel habits. Does he regularly use laxatives or enemas? If he experiences nausea and vomiting, what does the vomitus look like? Does changing his position relieve nausea?

Next, try to define and locate any pain. Ask the patient to describe the pain. Is it dull, sharp, burning, aching, spasmodic, intermittent? Where is it located? How long does it last? When does it occur? Does it radiate? What relieves it? (Also see *Emergency signals,* page 868.)

Inspection
Observe the patient's appearance and note the appropriateness of his behavior. Severe infection, drug toxicity, hepatic disease, and changes in fluid and electrolyte balance may cause abnormal behavior. Begin your visual inspection by observing the following:
• *Skin.* Look for loss of turgor, jaundice, cyanosis, pallor, diaphoresis, petechiae, spider angiomas, bruises, edema, oily or dry texture, and decreased axillary or pubic hair (may indicate hepatic disease).
• *Head.* Note the color of sclerae, sunken eyes, dentures, caries, lesions, breath odor, and tongue color, swelling, or dryness.
• *Chest.* Inspect the shape of the chest, and assess the rate, rhythm, and quality of respirations.
• *Abdomen.* Check the size and shape, noting distention, contour, visible masses, and protrusions. Note abdominal scars or fistulae, excessive skin folds (may indicate wasting), and abnormal respiratory movements (may indicate inflammation of the diaphragm).

Auscultation, palpation, and percussion
Auscultation provides helpful clues to GI abnormalities. For example, absent bowel sounds over the area to the lower right of the umbilicus may indicate peritonitis. High-pitched sounds that coincide with colicky pain may indicate small-bowel obstruction. Less intense, low-pitched rumbling noises may accompany minor irrita-

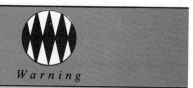

Warning

EMERGENCY SIGNALS

When assessing any patient with a GI problem, stay alert for the signs and symptoms described below, which may signal an emergency.

Abdominal pain
• Progressive, severe, or colicky pain that persists without improvement for more than 6 hours
• Acute pain associated with hypertension
• Acute pain in an elderly patient (such a patient may have minimal tenderness, even with a ruptured abdominal organ or appendicitis)
• Severe pain with guarding and a history of recent abdominal surgery
• Pain accompanied by evidence of free intraperitoneal air (gas) or mediastinal gas on X-ray
• Disproportionately severe pain under benign conditions (soft abdomen with normal physical findings)

Vomitus and stools
• Vomitus containing fresh blood
• Vomiting or heaving that's prolonged, with or without obstipation (intractable constipation)
• Bloody or black, tarry stools

Abdominal tenderness
• Abdominal tenderness and rigidity, even when the patient is distracted
• Rebound tenderness

Other signs
• Fever
• Tachycardia
• Hypotension
• Dehydration

If you note any of these signs or symptoms, notify the doctor and assess the patient for deterioration, such as signs of shock. Intervene, as necessary, by providing oxygen therapy and I.V. fluids, as ordered. Place the patient on a cardiac monitor if appropriate. Provide emotional support.

tion. A venous hum over the patient's abdomen suggests portal hypertension. A pleural friction rub may indicate a liver abscess or neoplastic disease.

Palpate the parotid glands. Enlargement may occur in alcohol-induced liver damage. Palpate the abdomen after auscultation to help detect tenderness, muscle guarding, organ enlargement, and abdominal masses. Note muscle tone (boardlike rigidity points to peritonitis; transient rigidity suggests severe pain) and tenderness (rebound tenderness may indicate peritoneal inflammation; tenderness at the liver's edge may indicate hepatic disease).

Percussion helps detect air, fluid, and solid matter in the abdomen.

Diagnostic tests
After physical assessment, a range of tests can identify GI, liver, or gallbladder malfunction.
• *Barium swallow* allows examination of the pharynx and esophagus to detect strictures, ulcers, tumors, polyps, diverticula, hiatal hernia, esophageal webs, motility disorders, and (sometimes) achalasia.
• In an *upper GI series*, swallowed barium sulfate proceeds into the esophagus, stomach, and small intestine to reveal abnormalities. The barium outlines stomach walls and delineates ulcer craters and filling defects. It can help diagnose gastritis, cancer, hiatal hernia, diverticula, strictures, and (most commonly) gastric and duodenal ulcers.
• *Small-bowel series*, an extension of the upper GI series, visualizes barium flowing through the small intestine to the ileocecal valve. It helps to diagnose sprue, obstruction, motility disorders, malabsorption syndrome, Hodgkin's disease, lymphosarcoma, ischemia, bleeding, and inflammation.
• *Barium enema (lower GI X-ray)* allows visualization of the colon, permitting easier identification of lesions in this area than is possible in a small-bowel series.
• *Stool specimen* is useful in suspected GI bleeding, infection, or malabsorption. Guaiac test for occult blood, microscopic stool examination for ova and parasites, and fat analysis require several specimens.
• In *upper GI endoscopy*, insertion of a fiber-optic scope allows direct visual inspection of the esophagus, stomach and, sometimes, duodenum; proctosigmoidoscopy permits inspection of the rectum and distal sigmoid colon; colonoscopy, inspection of the descending, transverse, and ascending colon.
• *Peritoneoscopy* visualizes the serosal lining, liver, gallbladder, spleen, and other organs; it's useful in determining the cause of unexplained hepatomegaly and in detecting ascites or an abdominal mass.
• *Gastric analysis* examines gastric secretions and analyzes acid content.
• *Esophageal acidity test* assesses lower sphincter competence by measuring intraesophageal pH with an electrode attached to a manometric catheter. This sensitive test is used for patients who complain of persistent heart-

burn and helps to discriminate GI problems from those in other systems.

• In an *acid perfusion test*, 0.9% sodium chloride and acidic solutions are perfused separately into the esophagus through a nasogastric tube to distinguish pain caused by the backflow of acidic juices into the esophagus from pain caused by angina pectoris or other disorders.

• *Duodenal drainage* diagnoses cholelithiasis, choledocholithiasis, biliary obstruction, hepatic cirrhosis, and pancreatic disease and differentiates types of jaundice. It permits measurement of bile flow and the collection of specimens, which are examined for mucus, blood, cholesterol crystals, pancreatic enzymes, cancer cells, bacteria, and calcium bilirubinate.

• *Peritoneal fluid analysis* includes examination of peritoneal fluid for gross appearance; erythrocyte and leukocyte counts; cytologic studies; microbiological studies for bacteria and fungi; and determinations of protein, glucose, amylase, ammonia, and alkaline phosphatase levels.

• *Portal and hepatic vein manometry* can locate obstructions in the extrahepatic portion of the portal vein and in the portal inflow system and can detect pressure in the presinusoidal vessels.

• *Percutaneous or transvenous liver biopsy* can determine the cause of unexplained hepatomegaly, hepatosplenomegaly, cholestasis, or persistently abnormal liver function tests. This test is also useful in suspected systemic infiltrative disease (sarcoidosis, for example) and suspected primary or metastatic hepatic tumors.

• In *gallbladder ultrasonography*, sound waves are used to visualize the gallbladder and locate obstructions, calculi, and tumors.

• *Abdominal X-ray,* also called flatplate of the abdomen or kidney-ureter-bladder radiography, helps detect and evaluate tumors, renal calculi, abnormal gas collection, and other abdominal disorders.

• *Liver function studies* measure serum enzyme levels and other substances.

• *Oral cholecystography* confirms gallbladder disease through radiographic examination of the gallbladder after administration of a contrast medium.

• *Endoscopic retrograde cholangiopancreatography* directly visualizes the proximal duodenum. This test helps determine the cause of jaundice; evaluate tumors and inflammation of the pancreas, gallbladder, and liver; and locate obstructions in the pancreatic duct and hepatobiliary tree.

• *I.V. cholangiography,* also called T-tube cholangiography or postoperative cholangiography, visualizes the intra-

hepatic and extrahepatic bile ducts and locates obstructing lesions in the major ducts.

• *Percutaneous transhepatic cholangiography* differentiates obstructive from intrahepatic types of jaundice and detects hepatic dysfunction and calculi.

• *Angiography* demonstrates hepatic arterial circulation (deranged in cirrhosis) and helps diagnose primary or secondary hepatic tumors.

• *Radioisotope liver scan* can detect such abnormalities as tumors, cysts, and abscesses.

• *Computed tomography scan* produces in-depth images (three-dimensional) of the biliary tract, the liver, and the pancreas to help distinguish between obstructive and nonobstructive jaundice; to identify abscesses, cysts, pseudocysts, hematomas, and tumors; and to diagnose and evaluate pancreatitis.

MOUTH AND ESOPHAGEAL DISORDERS

Although any GI disorder can cause serious signs and symptoms, disorders of the mouth and esophagus often lead to dysphagia, predisposing the patient to nutritional deficiencies and to respiratory and cardiovascular complications.

STOMATITIS AND OTHER ORAL INFECTIONS

A common infection, stomatitis may occur in children or adults, alone or as part of a systemic disease. This inflammation of the oral mucosa may also extend to the buccal mucosa, lips, and palate. The two main types are acute herpetic stomatitis and aphthous stomatitis.

Acute herpetic stomatitis is usually self-limiting; however, it may be severe and, in neonates, generalized and potentially fatal. This type of stomatitis is common in children between ages 1 and 3.

Aphthous stomatitis is common in girls and female adolescents and usually heals spontaneously, without a scar, in 10 to 14 days. Other oral infections include gingivitis, periodontitis, and Vincent's angina. (See *Understanding oral infections*, page 870.)

Causes

Acute herpetic stomatitis is caused by the herpes simplex virus. The cause of aphthous stomatitis is unknown, but

UNDERSTANDING ORAL INFECTIONS

Diseases and causes	Assessment findings	Treatment
Gingivitis • Early sign of hypovitaminosis, diabetes, blood dyscrasias • Occasionally related to the use of oral contraceptives	• Inflammation with painless swelling, redness, change of normal contours, bleeding, and peritoneal pocket (gum detachment from the teeth)	• Removal of irritating factors (calculus, faulty dentures) • Good oral hygiene, regular dental checkups, vigorous chewing • Oral or topical corticosteroids
Periodontitis • Progression of gingivitis • Early sign of hypovitaminosis, diabetes, blood dyscrasias • Occasionally related to use of oral contraceptives • Dental factors: calculus, poor oral hygiene, malocclusion; major cause of tooth loss after middle age	• Acute onset of bright red gum inflammation, painless swelling of interdental papillae, easy bleeding • Loosening of teeth, typically without inflammatory symptoms, progressing to loss of teeth and alveolar bone • Acute systemic infection (fever, chills)	• Scaling, root planing, and curettage for infection control • Periodontal surgery to prevent recurrence • Good oral hygiene, regular dental checkups, vigorous chewing
Vincent's angina • Also called trench mouth and necrotizing ulcerative gingivitis • Fusiform bacillus or spirochete infection • Predisposing factors: stress, poor oral hygiene, insufficient rest, nutritional deficiencies, smoking, immunosuppressant therapy	• Sudden onset of painful, superficial, bleeding gingival ulcers (rarely, on buccal mucosa) covered with a gray-white membrane • Ulcers become punched-out lesions after slight pressure or irritation • Malaise, fever, excessive salivation, bad breath, pain on swallowing or talking, enlarged submaxillary lymph nodes	• Removal of devitalized tissue with ultrasonic scaler • Antibiotics (oral penicillin or erythromycin) for infection • Analgesics, as needed • Hourly mouth rinses (with equal amounts of hydrogen peroxide and water) • Soft, nonirritating diet; rest; no smoking • With treatment, improvement common within 24 hours
Glossitis • Streptococcal infection • Irritation or injury, jagged teeth, ill-fitting dentures, biting during seizures, alcohol, spicy foods, smoking, sensitivity to toothpaste or mouthwash • Vitamin B deficiency, anemia • Skin conditions: lichen planus, erythema multiforme, pemphigus vulgaris	• Reddened, ulcerated, or swollen tongue (may obstruct airway) • Painful chewing and swallowing • Speech difficulty • Painful tongue without inflammation	• Treatment of underlying cause • Topical anesthetic mouthwash or systemic analgesics (aspirin or acetaminophen) for painful lesions • Good oral hygiene, regular dental checkups, vigorous chewing • Avoidance of hot, cold, or spicy foods and alcohol
Candidiasis • Also called thrush • *Candida albicans* • Predisposing factors: denture use, diabetes mellitus, immunosuppressant therapy	• Cream-colored or bluish white pseudomembranous patches on the tongue, mouth, or pharynx • Pain, fever, lymphadenopathy	• Hydrogen peroxide and normal saline mouthwashes • Clotrimazole tablets dissolved in the mouth five times/day • Nystatin troches (100,000 units) dissolved in the mouth four times/day • Varied local or systemic antifungal therapies

autoimmune and psychosomatic causes are under investigation. Predisposing factors associated with aphthous stomatitis include stress, fatigue, anxiety, febrile states, trauma, and overexposure to the sun.

Complications
Stomatitis may be complicated by nutritional deficiencies if painful oral lesions cause dysphagia or make chewing difficult.

Assessment findings

The patient with acute herpetic stomatitis usually reports symptoms of sudden onset, including mouth pain, malaise, lethargy, anorexia, irritability, and a fever that may last 1 to 2 weeks. He may also complain of bleeding gums and extreme tenderness of the oral mucosa.

On inspection, the gums typically appear swollen with papulovesicular ulcers evident in the mouth and throat. Eventually these ulcers become punched-out lesions with reddened areolae. The pain usually disappears 2 to 4 days before healing of ulcers is complete. Palpation commonly reveals submaxillary lymphadenitis. If the patient is a child, be sure to inspect his hands; thumb sucking can spread the viral infection to the hands.

In aphthous stomatitis, typical complaints are burning and tingling of the oral mucosa and painful ulcers. Mouth inspection reveals a slight swelling of the mucous membrane and single or multiple shallow ulcers with whitish centers and red borders, measuring about 2 to 5 mm in diameter. These ulcers appear and heal at one site but then reappear at another.

Diagnostic tests

Although diagnosis depends on physical examination, the following tests may help to identify the type of infection:

• *Smear of ulcer exudate* allows identification of the causative organism in Vincent's angina.
• *Viral cultures* may be performed on fluid and herpetic vesicles in acute herpetic stomatitis.

Treatment

For both acute herpetic and aphthous stomatitis, treatment is conservative, focusing on symptom relief until the infection resolves.

For acute herpetic stomatitis, symptom management includes nonantiseptic warm-water mouth rinses and topical medications to relieve pain and reduce inflammation.

Topical anesthetic solutions that may be used include lidocaine viscous or dyclonine. Topical corticosteroids may also be prescribed. Acyclovir may be ordered to manage herpetic stomatitis. Supplementary treatments to ease symptoms until the infection subsides include a soft, pureed, or liquid diet and, in severe cases of stomatitis, I.V. fluids and bed rest.

For aphthous stomatitis, a topical anesthetic coating agent, such as kaolin and milk of magnesia, is the primary treatment. The coating helps to relieve severe oral pain while preventing further irritation.

Nursing diagnoses

• Altered nutrition: Less than body requirements
• Altered oral mucous membrane
• Knowledge deficit
• Pain
• Risk for infection

Nursing interventions

• If the patient's mouth hurts, show him how to clean his teeth with sponges instead of a toothbrush. Suggest that he rinse with hydrogen peroxide or normal saline mouthwash to soothe irritated mucosa, debride oral structures, and prevent superinfection.
• Administer prescribed analgesics to relieve painful stomatitis. If ordered, apply a topical coating or swishing agent to relieve pain.
• If the patient has difficulty chewing or swallowing, contact the dietitian and develop a meal plan based on soft, liquid, or pureed foods. A change in food consistency often eases discomfort while maintaining adequate nutrition. Icy cold drinks also may be well tolerated. In severe cases, supplement oral foods with I.V. fluid or nasogastric feedings.

Patient teaching

• Teach the patient about the infection and its expected course. For the patient with herpetic stomatitis, emphasize the importance of good oral hygiene to prevent the spread of infection.
• Show the patient, or his parents, how to apply ordered topical medications. Discuss recommended dietary changes and adverse effects of prescribed medications.
• Caution the patient to avoid antiseptic and glycerine-containing mouthwashes while he has stomatitis because these irritate mouth ulcers.
• Advise the patient with aphthous stomatitis to avoid precipitating factors, such as stress and fatigue.

GASTROESOPHAGEAL REFLUX

Popularly known as heartburn, gastroesophageal reflux is the backflow of gastric or duodenal contents, or both, into the esophagus and past the lower esophageal sphincter (LES), without associated belching or vomiting. Reflux may or may not cause symptoms or pathologic changes. Persistent reflux may cause reflux esophagitis, an inflammation of the esophageal mucosa. The prognosis varies with the underlying cause.

Causes

Normally, gastric contents don't back up into the esophagus because the LES creates enough pressure around the lower end of the esophagus to close it. Reflux occurs when LES pressure is deficient or pressure within the stomach exceeds LES pressure. When this happens, the LES relaxes, allowing gastric contents to regurgitate into the esophagus. Any of the following predisposing factors may lead to reflux:

• pyloric surgery (alteration or removal of the pylorus), which allows reflux of bile or pancreatic juice
• nasogastric intubation for more than 4 days
• any agent that lowers LES pressure: food, alcohol, cigarettes, anticholinergics (atropine, belladonna, propantheline), other drugs (morphine, diazepam, calcium channel blockers, and meperidine)
• hiatal hernia with incompetent sphincter
• any condition or position that increases intra-abdominal pressure.

Complications

Reflux esophagitis, the primary complication of gastric reflux, can lead to other sequelae, including esophageal stricture, esophageal ulcer, and replacement of the normal squamous epithelium with columnar epithelium (Barrett's epithelium). A patient with severe reflux esophagitis may also develop anemia from chronic low-grade bleeding of inflamed mucosa.

Pulmonary complications may develop if the patient experiences reflux of gastric contents into his throat and subsequent aspiration. Reflux aspiration may lead to chronic pulmonary disease.

Assessment findings

The patient complains of heartburn that typically occurs 1 to 2 hours after eating. It often worsens with vigorous exercise, bending, or lying down. He may report relief from antacids or sitting upright. If asked, he may recall regurgitating without associated nausea or belching. This symptom is often described as a feeling of warm fluid traveling up the throat, followed by a sour or bitter taste in the mouth if the fluid reaches the pharynx.

Although heartburn is the most common feature of reflux, the patient may report any of the following signs and symptoms:

• a feeling of fluid accumulation in the throat without a sour or bitter taste. This is caused by hypersecretion of saliva.
• odynophagia, possibly followed by a dull substernal ache. This symptom may indicate severe, long-term reflux dysphagia from esophageal spasm, stricture, or esophagitis.
• bright red or dark brown blood in vomitus
• chronic pain that may mimic angina pectoris, radiating to the neck, jaw, and arm. This pain may be associated with esophageal spasm and result from reflux esophagitis.
• nocturnal hypersalivation, a rare symptom that the patient says awakens him with coughing, choking, and a mouthful of saliva.

In children, assessment findings may identify failure to thrive and forceful vomiting caused by esophageal irritation. Keep in mind that vomiting may cause aspiration pneumonia.

Diagnostic tests

Although a careful history and physical examination are essential to the diagnosis, the following tests help to confirm it:

• *Esophageal acidity test,* a standard test for acid reflux, is the most sensitive and accurate measure of gastroesophageal reflux.
• *Gastroesophageal scintillation testing* may also detect reflux.
• *Esophageal manometry* evaluates the resting pressure of the LES and determines sphincter competence.
• *Acid perfusion test* confirms esophagitis.
• *Esophagoscopy* and *biopsy* allow visualization and tissue sampling of the esophagus. These tests help to evaluate the extent of the disease and confirm pathologic changes in the mucosa.
• *Barium swallow with fluoroscopy* reveals normal findings except in patients with advanced disease. In children, *barium esophagography* under fluoroscopic control may show reflux.

Treatment

Effective management relieves symptoms by reducing reflux through gravity, strengthening the LES with drug therapy, neutralizing gastric contents, and reducing intra-abdominal pressure. Treatment should also include reviewing how the patient's life-style or dietary habits may affect his LES pressure and reflux symptoms. (See *Factors affecting LES pressure.*) In mild cases, diet therapy may reduce symptoms sufficiently so that no other treatment is required. Positional therapy, which relieves symptoms by reducing intra-abdominal pressure, is especially useful in infants and children with uncomplicated cases.

For intermittent reflux, antacids given 1 hour before and 3 hours after meals and at bedtime may be effective.

Drug therapy may also include cholinergic drugs, such as bethanechol, to increase LES pressure, and histamine-receptor antagonists, such as cimetidine or ranitidine, to reduce gastric acidity. Metoclopramide and sucralfate have also been used with beneficial results.

Surgery is usually reserved for patients with refractory symptoms or serious complications. Indications for surgery include pulmonary aspiration, hemorrhage, esophageal obstruction or perforation, intractable pain, incompetent LES, or associated hiatal hernia. Surgical procedures reduce reflux by creating an artificial closure at the gastroesophageal junction. Several surgical approaches are currently available, including Belsey's repair, Hill's repair, and the Nissen procedure; all of these procedures involve wrapping the gastric fundus around the esophagus. Other surgical procedures include a vagotomy or pyloroplasty (which may be combined with an antireflux regimen) to modify gastric contents.

Nursing diagnoses
• Altered nutrition: Less than body requirements
• Anxiety
• Knowledge deficit
• Pain
• Risk for aspiration

Nursing interventions
• Offer the patient emotional and psychological support to help him cope with pain and discomfort.
• In consultation with a dietitian, develop a diet for the patient that takes his food preferences into account but, at the same time, helps to minimize his reflux symptoms. If the patient is obese, place him on a weight reduction diet, as ordered.
• To reduce intra-abdominal pressure, have the patient sleep in a reverse Trendelenburg position (with the head of the bed elevated 6″ to 12″ [15 to 31 cm]). He should also avoid lying down immediately after meals and late-night snacks.
• After surgery, provide care as you would for any patient who has undergone a laparotomy. Pay particular attention to the patient's respiratory status because the surgical procedure is performed close to the diaphragm. Administer prescribed analgesics, oxygen, and I.V. fluids. Monitor his intake and output and check his vital signs. If surgery was performed using a thoracic approach, watch and record chest tube drainage. If needed, provide chest physiotherapy.

FACTORS AFFECTING L.E.S. PRESSURE

Various dietary and life-style elements can increase or decrease lower esophageal sphincter (LES) pressure. Take these into account as you plan the patient's treatment program.

What increases LES pressure
• Protein
• Carbohydrate
• Nonfat milk
• Low-dose ethanol

What decreases LES pressure
• Fat
• Whole milk
• Orange juice
• Tomatoes
• Antiflatulent (simethicone)
• Chocolate
• High-dose ethanol
• Cigarette smoking
• Lying on right or left side
• Sitting

Patient teaching
• Teach the patient about the causes of gastroesophageal reflux, and review his antireflux regimen of medication, diet, and positional therapy.
• Discuss recommended dietary changes. Advise him to sit upright after meals and snacks, and to eat small, frequent meals. Explain that he should eat meals at least 2 to 3 hours before lying down. Tell him to avoid highly seasoned food, acidic juices, alcoholic drinks, bedtime snacks, and foods high in fat or carbohydrates because these reduce LES pressure.
• Instruct him to avoid situations or activities that increase intra-abdominal pressure, such as bending, coughing, vigorous exercise, obesity, constipation, and wearing tight clothing. Caution him to refrain from using any substance that reduces sphincter control, including cigarettes, alcohol, fatty foods, and certain drugs.
• Encourage compliance with his drug regimen. Review the desired drug actions and potential adverse effects.

TRACHEOESOPHAGEAL FISTULA AND ESOPHAGEAL ATRESIA

Among the most serious congenital anomalies in neonates, tracheoesophageal fistula and esophageal atresia may develop separately but usually occur together. In tra-

TYPES OF TRACHEOESOPHAGEAL ANOMALIES

The American Academy of Pediatrics classifies tracheoesophageal anomalies as follows:

Type A (7.7%)
Esophageal atresia without fistula

Type B (0.8%)
Esophageal atresia with tracheoesophageal fistula to the proximal segment

Type C (86.5%)
Esophageal atresia with fistula to the distal segment only

Type D (0.7%)
Esophageal atresia with fistula to both segments

Type E or H (4.2%)
Tracheoesophageal fistula without atresia

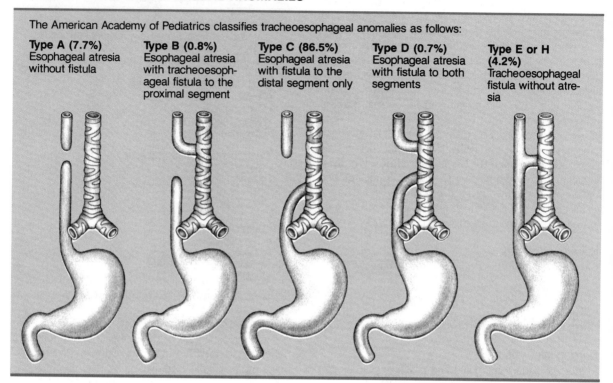

cheoesophageal fistula, an abnormal connection develops between the trachea and the esophagus. In esophageal atresia, the esophagus is closed off at some point.

Both disorders are surgical emergencies, requiring immediate diagnosis and correction. Sometimes, they coexist with other serious anomalies, such as congenital heart disease, imperforate anus, genitourinary abnormalities, and intestinal atresia.

Congenital malformations of the esophagus occur in about 1 in 4,000 live births. These malformations have numerous anatomic variations. (See *Types of tracheoesophageal anomalies.*) They are classified in the following ways:

• In Type C tracheoesophageal fistula with esophageal atresia—by far the most common esophageal malformation—the upper section of the esophagus terminates in a blind pouch (which has no fistula). The lower section ascends from the stomach and connects with the trachea by a short fistulous tract.

• In Type A atresia, both esophageal segments are blind pouches, and neither has a fistulous connection to the airway.

• In Type E (also known as Type H or tracheoesophageal fistula without atresia), the fistula may occur anywhere between the level of the cricoid cartilage and the midesophagus. The fistula, which may be as small as a pinpoint, is usually higher in the trachea than in the esophagus.

• In Types B and D, the upper portion of the esophagus opens into the trachea. (In Type D an additional fistula connects the trachea and the esophagus at a lower level.) Infants with either anomaly may experience life-threatening aspiration of saliva or food.

Causes

Tracheoesophageal fistula and esophageal atresia result from failure of the embryonic esophagus and trachea to develop and separate correctly.

Complications

These anomalies must be treated or the infant will die. Immediate complications include aspiration of secretions into the lungs, leading to respiratory distress, cessation of breathing, or pneumonia.

Assessment findings

Both the maternal history and the patient history should be included in the assessment. In most patients, the maternal history reveals hydramnios. About one-third of these infants are born prematurely.

On inspection, the neonate with Type C tracheoesophageal fistula with esophageal atresia usually appears to swallow normally. Soon after swallowing, however, he begins to cough, struggle, and become cyanotic. Unless suctioned, he will aspirate fluids returning from the blind pouch of the esophagus and stop breathing. Inspection may disclose drooling from the mouth with possible bubbling through the nostrils. Stomach distention may be apparent upon inspection and palpation.

An infant with Type A esophageal atresia appears normal at birth. However, inspection reveals excessive drooling, even though he appears to swallow normally. As secretions fill the esophageal sac and overflow into the oropharynx, the infant develops mucus in the oropharynx, causing increased drooling. If the infant is inspected during feeding, he typically regurgitates and aspirates, causing respiratory distress and cessation of breathing unless he is suctioned.

With Type E tracheoesophageal fistula, the patient history may reveal frequent episodes of pneumonitis, pulmonary infection, and abdominal distention. Upon inspection, the child may look normal and not drool excessively because the esophagus doesn't end in a blind pouch. However, if he's inspected while drinking, he's likely to cough, choke, and become cyanotic as excessive mucus builds up in his oropharynx. Inspection and palpation may also disclose abdominal distention, particularly when the infant cries. Crying may force air from the trachea through the fistula into the esophagus, causing some air to settle in the stomach. If the fistula is small, the presence of a congenital malformation may not be suspected initially, delaying diagnosis for as long as a year.

In both Type B (proximal fistula) and Type D (fistula to both segments), inspection initially reveals a normal-appearing neonate who begins to aspirate saliva into the airway. Aspiration may lead to bacterial pneumonitis.

Diagnostic tests

The following tests help to confirm and classify tracheoesophageal fistula and esophageal atresia:

• *A radiopaque #8 or #10 French catheter passed through the nose* confirms the presence of a blind pouch in the proximal esophagus if it meets an obstruction between 4″ and 5″ (10 and 13 cm) distal to the nostrils.

• *Chest X-ray* demonstrates the catheter position in the esophagus and can also show a dilated, air-filled upper esophageal pouch; pneumonia in the right upper lobe of the lung; or bilateral pneumonitis. Both pneumonia and pneumonitis suggest aspiration.

• *Abdominal X-ray* shows gas in the bowel in a distal fistula (Type C) but none in a proximal fistula (Type B) or in atresia without fistula (Type A).

• *Cinefluorography* allows visualization on a fluoroscopic screen. After a #10 or #12 French catheter is passed through the patient's nostril into the esophagus, a small amount of contrast medium is instilled to define the tip of the upper pouch. Findings help differentiate between overflow aspiration from a blind end (atresia) and aspiration due to passage of liquids through a tracheoesophageal fistula.

• *Bronchoscopy* with telescopic endoscopy also can confirm the diagnosis in most patients.

Treatment

Tracheoesophageal fistula and esophageal atresia require surgical correction and are usually emergencies. The type of surgery and when it's performed depend on several factors: the nature of the anomaly, the patient's general condition, and the presence of coexisting congenital defects.

Depending on what type of anomaly the child has, a sump tube may be placed in the esophageal pouch until surgery is performed. This procedure removes accumulated secretions, decreasing the possibility of aspiration. A gastrostomy tube may be placed to decompress the stomach. The child's respiratory status must be closely monitored.

Both before and after surgery, positioning varies according to the doctor's preferences and the child's anatomy: The child may be placed supine, with his head low to facilitate drainage or with his head elevated to prevent aspiration.

To correct gastroesophageal reflux and esophageal atresia, a thoracotomy is performed and the fistula is ligated, after which the upper and the lower segments of the esophagus are anastomosed. In patients who are poor surgical risks, such as those born prematurely or those with other congenital defects, correction of combined tracheoesophageal fistula and esophageal atresia is done in two stages. The first stage consists of gastrostomy (for gastric decompression, prevention of reflux, and feeding) and closure of the fistula. One to two months later, the esophagus is anastomosed.

Correction of esophageal atresia alone requires anastomosis of the proximal and distal esophageal segments in one or two stages. End-to-end anastomosis often produces postoperative stricture; end-to-side anastomosis is less likely to do so. If the esophageal ends are widely separated, treatment may include a colonic interposition (grafting a piece of the colon) or elongation of the proximal segment of the esophagus by bougienage. About 10 days after surgery, and again 1 month and 3 months later, X-rays are required to evaluate the effectiveness of surgical repair.

Nursing diagnoses
• Altered nutrition: Less than body requirements
• Anxiety (parental)
• Ineffective airway clearance
• Pain
• Risk for aspiration
• Risk for infection

Nursing interventions
• Provide emotional and psychological support to the parents. Stay with them during periods of extreme stress. Encourage them to participate in the infant's care and to hold and touch him as much as possible to facilitate bonding.
• Monitor the infant's respiratory status continuously. Administer oxygen and perform chest physiotherapy and suctioning, as needed. Provide a humid environment. Observe the infant closely for signs of airway obstruction, such as an anxious facial expression and an increased respiratory rate.
• To prevent aspiration, be sure the infant is given nothing by mouth. Perform suction of the nasopharynx until a sump tube can be placed in the esophageal pouch. Irrigate the sump tube as necessary to ensure patency.
• Position the infant as ordered to prevent aspiration.
• Comfort the infant by stroking his back gently and by careful handling. Administer pain medications as ordered. Once the sump tube is in place a pacifier can be given to help satisfy the infant's sucking needs.
• Administer antibiotics and parenteral fluids, as ordered. Keep accurate intake and output records.
• Maintain gastrostomy tube feedings, as ordered. Such feedings initially consist of dextrose and water (not more than a 5% solution); later, add a proprietary formula

(first diluted and then full strength). If the infant develops gastric atony, use an iso-osmolar formula.

After corrective surgery:
• Monitor the patient's respiratory status. He may be on mechanical ventilation for the first few days after surgery. If so, maintain the setting as ordered.
• Keep the infant in the position ordered, and carefully administer I.V. fluids to maintain electrolyte and fluid balance.
• Administer prescribed medications, such as analgesics for pain and antibiotics for pneumonia.
• Provide care for the gastrostomy to prevent reflux and provide feedings. Maintain adequate nutrition through gastrostomy feedings or if the infant's condition allows, oral feedings. Oral feedings can usually resume 8 to 10 days postoperatively. If gastrostomy or oral feedings are impossible because of intolerance or decreased intestinal motility, provide total parenteral nutrition, as ordered.
• When the sump pump is removed after surgery, suction the infant as necessary. Be very gentle, and perform the procedure quickly to prevent removal of oxygen from the area and to prevent trauma.
• If the patient has chest tubes postoperatively, check them frequently for patency. Maintain proper suction, measure and mark drainage periodically, and milk the tubing, as necessary.
• Observe the patient carefully for signs of postoperative complications, such as abnormal esophageal motility, recurrent fistulas, pneumothorax, esophageal stricture, reflux esophagitis, recurrent bronchitis, hiatal hernia, and failure to thrive. Esophageal motility dysfunction or hiatal hernia may develop after surgical correction of esophageal atresia.

Patient teaching
• Teach the parents about the disorder. Reinforce the doctor's explanation as necessary. Explain the diagnostic tests and the type of corrective surgery required.
• Teach the parents how to care for their infant at home. Be sure they understand how to position, hold, and feed the child. Refer them to the social service department and local home health care agencies, as necessary.

CORROSIVE ESOPHAGITIS AND STRICTURE

Accidental or intentional ingestion of a caustic chemical produces corrosive esophagitis. Similar to a burn, this injury is characterized by esophageal inflammation and damage. It may be temporary or lead to permanent stricture (narrowing or stenosis) of the esophagus, which is correctable only through surgery. In children, household chemical ingestion is accidental; in adults, it's usually a suicide attempt or gesture.

The type and amount of chemical ingested determine the severity and location of the damage. The corrosive agent may damage only the mucosa or submucosa or injure all esophageal layers. Tissue damage occurs in three phases: an acute phase, marked by edema and inflammation; a latent phase, characterized by ulceration, exudation, and tissue sloughing; and a chronic phase of diffuse scarring.

Causes
Ingestion of lye or other strong alkalies is the most common cause of corrosive esophagitis. Less often, strong acids, such as toilet bowl cleaners or hydrochloric acid, are ingested.

Complications
Severe injury can quickly lead to esophageal perforation, mediastinitis, and death from infection, shock, or massive hemorrhage (if the aorta is perforated). In less severe cases, secondary infection can occur 3 to 4 days after ingestion. Stricture of the esophagus may occur within weeks of the ingestion or, less commonly, several years later.

Assessment findings
In corrosive esophagitis and stricture, assessment findings depend on the cause and severity of the injury. Usually, the patient's history reveals a recent chemical ingestion. He may report gagging at the time of ingestion and intense pain in his mouth and anterior chest. Other common complaints include a marked increase in salivation and an inability to swallow. If he's unable to speak, suspect laryngeal damage.

On inspection, you may notice tachypnea and drooling. The patient's mouth may show obvious mucosal burns of the lips and oropharynx, with whitened membranes and edema of the soft palate and uvula. If the patient vomits, inspect the vomitus for blood and pieces of esophageal tissue. These findings signal severe damage. As part of the inspection, smell the patient; an identifiable odor will be apparent if ammonia or formaldehyde was ingested.

Palpation may reveal crepitation, an indication of esophageal perforation and mediastinitis and, possibly, destruction of the entire esophagus.

In severe cases, auscultation may disclose marked hypotension.

Diagnostic tests
The following two tests may be ordered to assess the severity of esophageal damage:
• *Endoscopy* may be used to determine the extent of the injury in patients with a history of chemical ingestion and an oropharynx that appears abnormal. However, endoscopy use is controversial because of the risk of perforating the damaged esophagus.
• *Barium swallow* is usually performed 1 week after chemical ingestion and every 3 weeks thereafter, as ordered. Although this test is useful for identifying segmental spasm or fistula, it may not reveal mucosal injury. The test is contraindicated if esophageal perforation is suspected.

Treatment
An immediate priority is to identify the type and amount of chemical ingested. Sometimes, this can be done by examining the empty containers of the ingested material or by calling the local poison control center.

Conservative treatment includes monitoring the patient's condition and administering medications as ordered. Drug therapy may include narcotics for pain relief; corticosteroids, such as prednisone or hydrocortisone, to reduce inflammation and inhibit fibrosis; and a broad-spectrum antibiotic, such as ampicillin, to protect the patient taking a corticosteroid against infection by his own mouth flora. If the patient has burns of the oral mucosa, topically applied agents, such as lidocaine viscous or dyclonine, can provide temporary pain relief and coat the burned area. This protects the area from further injury.

If an esophageal stricture develops, bougienage is performed. In this procedure, a slender, flexible, cylindrical instrument called a bougie is passed into the esophagus to dilate it. If stricture is untreatable with bougienage, surgery is required. Immediate surgery is necessary if the patient develops esophageal perforation. Some patients require corrective surgery, which may involve transplanting a piece of the colon to repair the damaged esophagus. Even after surgery, stricture may recur at the site of the anastomosis.

Supportive treatment includes I.V. therapy (to replace fluids) or total parenteral nutrition if the patient can't swallow. As the patient's condition improves, nutrition can gradually progress to clear liquids, then to a soft diet.

Nursing diagnoses
• Altered nutrition: Less than body requirements
• Altered oral mucous membrane

- Anxiety
- Pain
- Risk for infection

Nursing interventions

- Support the patient and the family emotionally. Stay with them during periods of severe crisis.
- Don't induce vomiting or lavage because this will expose the esophagus and oropharynx to injury a second time. Avoid performing gastric lavage because the caustic chemical may cause further damage to the mucous membrane of the GI lining.
- Depending on the severity of the injury, provide vigorous support of vital functions, such as oxygen, mechanical ventilation, I.V. fluid administration, and treatment for shock as needed.
- Carefully observe and record intake and output.
- Administer analgesics, corticosteroids, and antibiotics, as ordered.
- Monitor the patient for complications. Watch for the development of fever, which may signal a secondary infection. Observe him for a return of dysphagia, which may indicate esophageal stricture and can occur within weeks of chemical ingestion.
- Provide parenteral nutrition as ordered until the patient can tolerate oral foods.
- Stay with the patient when he first tries eating. If his esophagus was not destroyed, he can usually attempt eating in 3 to 4 days after the acute phase subsides.
- If surgery is scheduled, provide appropriate preoperative and postoperative care.
- Because the adult who has ingested a corrosive agent has usually done so with suicidal intent, encourage and assist him and his family to seek psychological counseling. Make appropriate referrals.
- When the patient is a child, look for signs of abuse or neglect. Notify the authorities if you see such signs.

Patient teaching

- Teach the patient and his family about the damage to the esophagus and necessary treatments to relieve symptoms and repair the injury. Make sure they understand potential complications, such as esophageal perforation and infection.
- Warn the patient not to swallow topical medications, especially if he's allowed nothing by mouth.
- Teach parents whose child ingested a chemical to take safety precautions, such as locking accessible cabinets and keeping all corrosive agents out of a child's reach.

- Discuss and encourage long-term follow-up because these patients have an increased risk of squamous cell carcinoma of the esophagus.

MALLORY-WEISS SYNDROME

Characterized by mild to massive and usually painless bleeding, Mallory-Weiss syndrome results from a tear in the mucosa or submucosa of the cardia or lower esophagus. Such a tear, usually singular and longitudinal, results from prolonged or forceful vomiting.

Sixty percent of these tears involve the cardia; 15%, the terminal esophagus; and 25%, the region across the esophagogastric junction. Mallory-Weiss syndrome is most common in men over age 40, especially alcoholics.

Causes

Forceful or prolonged vomiting is the direct cause of Mallory-Weiss syndrome. The tear in the gastric mucosa probably occurs when the upper esophageal sphincter fails to relax during vomiting. This lack of sphincter coordination seems more common after excessive intake of alcohol. Other factors or conditions that may increase intra-abdominal pressure and predispose a person to esophageal tearing include coughing, straining during bowel movements, trauma, seizures, childbirth, hiatal hernia, esophagitis, gastritis, and atrophic gastric mucosa.

Complications

Hypovolemia may develop if bleeding is excessive. Rarely, massive bleeding, usually from a tear on the gastric side near the cardia, quickly leads to fatal shock.

Assessment findings

Typically, the history will reveal a recent bout of forceful vomiting, followed by vomiting of bright red blood. The patient may describe this bleeding as mild to massive and may complain of accompanying epigastric or back pain. He also may report passing large amounts of blood rectally a few hours to several days after normal vomiting. Be alert for a history of hiatal hernia or alcoholism.

Diagnostic tests

- *Fiber-optic endoscopy* of esophageal tears confirms Mallory-Weiss syndrome. In most patients, lesions appear as recently produced, erythematous, longitudinal cracks in the mucosa. In older tears, lesions appear as raised, white streaks surrounded by erythema.

• *Angiography* (selective celiac arteriography) can determine the bleeding site but not the cause. This procedure may be used when endoscopy isn't available.
• *Serum hematocrit* helps quantify blood loss.

Treatment

Because GI bleeding usually stops spontaneously, treatment often consists of supportive measures and careful observation. However, treatment must be geared to the severity of bleeding. In some patients, blood transfusion is necessary. If severe bleeding continues, other treatments may include:
• angiography, with infusion of a vasoconstrictor (vasopressin) into the superior mesenteric artery or direct infusion into a vessel that leads to the bleeding artery.
• endoscopy with electrocoagulation or heater probe for hemostasis.
• transcatheter embolization or thrombus formation with an autologous blood clot or other hemostatic material (insertion of artificial material, such as shredded absorbable gelatin sponge, or, less often, the patient's own clotted blood through a catheter into the bleeding vessel to aid thrombus formation).
• surgery to suture each laceration (rare).

Nursing diagnoses

• Altered nutrition: Less than body requirements
• Anxiety
• Risk for fluid volume deficit

Nursing interventions

• Provide support for the patient, particularly if bleeding has frightened him.
• Keep the patient warm and monitor vital signs, urine output, and overall clinical status.
• Monitor the patient's hemoglobin and hematocrit levels and his red blood cell count.
• Insert a large-bore (14G to 18G) I.V. line, and start a temporary infusion of 0.9% sodium chloride solution, as ordered, in case transfusion is necessary.
• Draw blood for coagulation studies (prothrombin time, partial thromboplastin time, and platelet count), and typing and cross matching. As ordered, keep units of matched blood on hand. Transfuse blood if ordered.
• Avoid giving the patient medications that may cause nausea or vomiting.
• If surgery is necessary, prepare the patient for the scheduled surgery.

Patient teaching

• Explain the disorder and its treatment.
• Advise the patient to avoid alcohol, aspirin, and other substances irritating to the GI tract.
• Encourage an alcoholic patient to join a support group, such as Alcoholics Anonymous, or refer him for counseling.

ESOPHAGEAL DIVERTICULA

Occurring as hollow outpouchings of the esophageal wall, esophageal diverticula develop in three main areas: just above the upper esophageal sphincter (Zenker's diverticulum, the most common type), near the midpoint of the esophagus (a midesophageal diverticulum), and just above the lower esophageal sphincter (an epiphrenic diverticulum, the rarest type). Diverticula may involve one or more layers of the mucosa.

Generally, esophageal diverticula occur later in life, but they can also affect infants and children. The disorder is three times more common in men than in women. Epiphrenic diverticula usually occur in middle-aged men. Zenker's diverticulum usually occurs in men over age 60.

Causes

Esophageal diverticula are due to either primary muscular abnormalities that may be congenital or to inflammatory processes adjacent to the esophagus. Zenker's diverticulum results from developmental muscle weakness of the posterior pharynx above the border of the cricopharyngeal muscle. The pressure of swallowing aggravates this weakness, as does contraction of the pharynx before relaxation of the sphincter, resulting in development of diverticula.

A midesophageal diverticulum may be a response to scarring and pulling on esophageal walls by an external inflammatory process, such as tuberculosis, or by traction from old adhesions. Another cause may be propulsion associated with esophageal motor abnormalities, such as diffuse esophageal spasm. An epiphrenic diverticulum probably results from traction and pulsation or from esophageal motor disturbances, such as diffuse esophageal spasm and achalasia.

Complications

Regurgitation of saliva or food particles may lead to aspiration, causing pulmonary complications, such as bronchitis, bronchiectasis, and lung abscess. The disorder may also lead to esophageal perforation.

Assessment findings

In the early stage of Zenker's diverticulum, the patient may report recent weight loss, which he may attribute to difficulty eating. The patient history may reveal dysphagia and regurgitation of saliva and food particles soon after eating. In the later stage, the esophageal opening may be almost completely blocked. The patient may describe regurgitation of food particles he consumed several days earlier. He may also hear gurgling sounds in his neck when he's swallowing liquids.

Other signs and symptoms of a Zenker's diverticulum include nocturnal coughing, a bad taste in the mouth and, rarely, bleeding. Halitosis may be obvious. Inspection may reveal a swelling at the side of the neck caused by food trapped in the diverticulum.

Midesophageal and epiphrenic diverticula usually produce no symptoms in early stages. In later stages, the patient may complain of dysphagia and heartburn.

Diagnostic tests

- *Barium swallow* usually confirms the diagnosis by showing a characteristic outpouching.
- *Esophagoscopy* may rule out another lesion as the cause of the problem. However, the procedure must be performed with extreme care because it risks rupturing the diverticulum by passing the scope into it rather than into the lumen of the esophagus, a special danger with Zenker's diverticulum.

Treatment

For Zenker's diverticulum, treatment is usually palliative, including a bland diet, thorough chewing, and drinking water after eating to flush out the sac. However, severe symptoms or a large diverticulum require surgery to remove the sac or facilitate drainage. An esophagomyotomy may be necessary to prevent recurrence.

A midesophageal or an epiphrenic diverticulum typically requires no therapy because it usually produces no symptoms or complications. If symptoms occur, treatment includes antacids and an antireflux regimen. If the diverticulum becomes very large and causes symptoms, surgical removal may be indicated. Distal myotomy is usually performed if the diverticulum is associated with esophageal motor abnormalities.

If surgery is necessary, then, depending on the patient's nutritional status, treatment may also include insertion of a nasogastric tube (passed carefully to prevent perforation) and tube feedings to prepare for the stress of surgery.

Nursing diagnoses

- Altered nutrition: Less than body requirements
- Anxiety
- Impaired swallowing
- Knowledge deficit
- Pain
- Risk for aspiration

Nursing interventions

- Support the patient emotionally, especially if he's upset and concerned about his symptoms.
- Regularly assess the patient's nutritional status (weight, caloric intake, physical appearance).
- If the patient regurgitates food and mucus, protect him from aspiration by positioning him carefully (head elevated or turned to one side). To prevent aspiration, tell him to empty any visible outpouching in the neck by massage or postural drainage before retiring.
- If the patient has dysphagia, record well-tolerated foods and note circumstances that ease swallowing. If necessary, provide a "blenderized" diet, with vitamin or protein supplements.
- If the patient with a midesophageal or an epiphrenic diverticulum has discomfort, administer ordered antacids and provide antireflux care: Keep his head elevated; maintain him in an upright position for 2 hours after eating; provide small, frequent meals; control chronic coughing; and advise him to avoid constrictive clothing.
- If surgery is scheduled, perform required preoperative and postoperative care.

Patient teaching

- Teach the patient about his disorder. Explain necessary diagnostic tests and treatments.
- Emphasize the need to chew food thoroughly to prevent food particles from becoming trapped in the diverticulum.
- If surgery is necessary, provide complete preoperative teaching. Make sure the patient understands the surgical approach, its desired effects, and possible complications.

HIATAL HERNIA

Commonly producing no symptoms, hiatal hernia (hiatus hernia) is a defect in the diaphragm that permits a portion of the stomach to pass through the diaphragmatic opening into the chest. Three types of hiatal hernia can occur. They include a sliding hernia, a paraesophageal (rolling) hernia, or a mixed hernia. (A mixed hernia includes features of the sliding and the rolling hernias.) See *Types of hiatal hernia*.

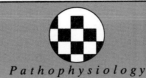

Pathophysiology

TYPES OF HIATAL HERNIA

To provide the most effective nursing care, you'll need to be able to distinguish between the types of hiatal hernia.

In a sliding hernia, both the stomach and the gastroesophageal junction slip up into the chest, so the gastroesophageal junction is above the diaphragmatic hiatus. This type of hernia causes symptoms if the lower esophageal sphincter (LES) is incompetent, which permits gastric reflux and heartburn.

In a paraesophageal or rolling hernia, a part of the greater curvature of the stomach rolls through the diaphragmatic defect. This type of hernia usually doesn't cause gastric reflux and heartburn because the closing mechanism of the LES is unaffected. However, it may cause displacement or stretching of the stomach or lead to strangulation of the herniated portion.

Sliding hiatal hernia

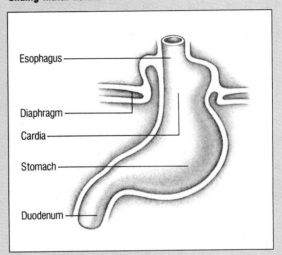

Esophagus
Diaphragm
Cardia
Stomach
Duodenum

Normal stomach

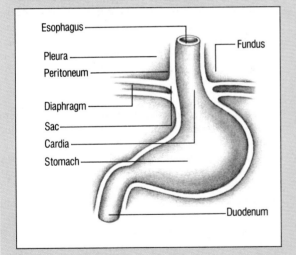

Esophagus
Pleura
Peritoneum
Diaphragm
Sac
Cardia
Stomach
Fundus
Duodenum

Paraesophageal or rolling hernia

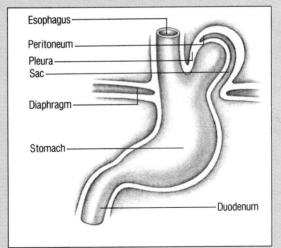

Esophagus
Peritoneum
Pleura
Sac
Diaphragm
Stomach
Duodenum

The incidence of this disorder increases with age. By the sixth decade of life, about 60% of people have hiatal hernias. However, most have no symptoms; the hernia is an incidental finding during a barium swallow. Or it may be detected by tests that follow the discovery of occult blood. The prevalence is higher in women than in men (especially the paraesophageal type).

Causes

In a sliding hernia, the muscular collar around the esophageal and diaphragmatic junction loosens, permitting the lower portion of the esophagus and the upper portion of the stomach to rise into the chest when intra-abdominal pressure increases. This muscle weakening may be associated with normal aging, or it may be secondary to esophageal carcinoma, kyphoscoliosis, trauma, or surgery. A sliding hernia may also result from certain diaphragmatic malformations that may cause congenital weakness.

The exact cause of a paraesophageal hiatal hernia is not fully understood. One assumption holds that the stomach is not properly anchored below the diaphragm, permitting the upper portion of the stomach to slide through the esophageal hiatus when intra-abdominal pressure increases.

Increased intra-abdominal pressure can be caused by conditions such as ascites, pregnancy, obesity, constrictive clothing, bending, straining, coughing, Valsalva's maneuver, and extreme physical exertion.

Complications

If the hiatal hernia is associated with gastroesophageal reflux, the esophageal mucosa may become irritated, leading to esophagitis, esophageal ulceration, hemorrhage, peritonitis, and mediastinitis. Aspiration of refluxed fluids may lead to respiratory distress, aspiration pneumonia, or cardiac dysfunction from pressure on the heart and lungs.

Other complications include esophageal stricture and incarceration, in which a large portion of the stomach is caught above the diaphragm. Incarceration may lead to perforation, gastric ulcer, and strangulation and gangrene of the herniated stomach portion.

Assessment findings

When a sliding hernia causes symptoms, the patient typically complains of heartburn, indicating an incompetent lower esophageal sphincter (LES) and gastroesophageal reflux. The patient history usually reveals that heartburn occurs from 1 to 4 hours after eating and is aggravated by reclining, belching, or conditions that increase intra-abdominal pressure. Heartburn may be accompanied by regurgitation or vomiting. The patient may complain of retrosternal or substernal chest pain (typically after meals or at bedtime), reflecting reflux of gastric contents, distention of the stomach, and spasm.

Keep in mind that the patient with a paraesophageal hernia is usually asymptomatic. Because this type of hernia doesn't disturb the closing mechanism of the LES, it doesn't usually cause gastric reflux and reflux esophagitis. Symptoms, when present, usually stem from incarceration of a stomach portion above the diaphragmatic opening. The symptomatic patient may report a feeling of fullness after eating or, if the hernia interferes with breathing, a feeling of breathlessness or suffocation. She may also complain of chest pain resembling angina pectoris.

During the history, be attentive for the following signs and symptoms of possible complications:
• dysphagia, especially after ingestion of very hot or cold foods, alcoholic beverages, or a large amount of food (may indicate esophagitis, esophageal ulceration, or stricture)
• bleeding, which may be mild or massive, frank or occult (may indicate esophagitis or erosion of the gastric pouch).

Severe pain and shock are signs of incarceration, in which a large portion of the stomach is caught above the diaphragm (usually occurs in paraesophageal hernia). Incarceration requires immediate surgery because it can lead to perforation or strangulation and gangrene of the herniated stomach portion.

Diagnostic tests

• *Chest X-ray* occasionally shows an air shadow behind the heart in a large hernia; infiltrates in the lower lung lobes if the patient has aspirated the refluxed fluids.
• *Barium swallow with fluoroscopy* is the most specific test for detecting a hiatal hernia. The hernia may appear as an outpouching containing barium at the lower end of the esophagus. (Small hernias are difficult to recognize.) This study also shows diaphragmatic abnormalities.
• *Serum hemoglobin* and *hematocrit levels* may be decreased in patients with paraesophageal hernia.
• *Endoscopy* and *biopsy* differentiate between hiatal hernia, varices, and other small gastroesophageal lesions. These tests also identify the mucosal junction and the edge of the diaphragm indenting the esophagus and can rule out cancer that otherwise may remain undetected.
• *Esophageal motility studies* reveal esophageal motor or lower esophageal pressure abnormalities before surgical repair of the hernia.
• *pH studies* assess for reflux of gastric contents.

• *Acid perfusion test* indicates that heartburn results from esophageal reflux when hydrochloric acid perfusion through a nasogastric (NG) tube provokes this symptom.

Treatment

Therapy aims to relieve symptoms by minimizing or correcting the incompetent LES (if present) and to manage and prevent complications. Drugs, activity modifications, and diet changes reduce gastroesophageal reflux.

Probably the best treatment for intermittent reflux, antacids neutralize refluxed fluids. Intensive antacid therapy may call for hourly dosing; however, the choice of antacids should take into account the patient's bowel function. Histamine-receptor antagonists also modify the acidity of the fluid refluxed into the esophagus.

Drug therapy to strengthen LES tone may consist of a cholinergic agent, such as bethanechol. Metoclopramide has also been used to stimulate smooth-muscle contraction, increase LES tone, and decrease reflux after eating.

Other measures to reduce intermittent reflux include restricting any activity that increases intra-abdominal pressure and discouraging smoking because it stimulates gastric acid production. Modifying the diet to include smaller, more frequent meals and to eliminate spicy or irritating foods also may help to reduce reflux.

Rarely, surgery is required when symptoms persist despite medical treatment or if complications develop. Indications for surgery include esophageal stricture, significant bleeding, pulmonary aspiration, or incarceration or strangulation of the herniated stomach portion. Techniques vary, but most forms of surgery create an artificial closing mechanism at the gastroesophageal junction to strengthen the barrier function of the LES. The surgeon may use an abdominal or a thoracic approach.

Rare postsurgical complications may include mucosal erosion, ulcers, and bleeding of the gastric pouch; pressure on the left lung due to the size and placement of the pouch; and formation of a volvulus.

A sliding hernia without an incompetent sphincter rarely produces reflux or symptoms and thus requires no treatment. But a large rolling hernia should be surgically repaired (even if it produces no symptoms) because of the high risk of complications, especially strangulation.

Nursing diagnoses

• Altered nutrition: Less than body requirements
• Impaired swallowing
• Pain
• Risk for aspiration

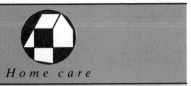

Home care

LIVING WITH HIATAL HERNIA

Follow these guidelines to help your patient live with hiatial hernia:
• Explain that the patient will need medications for hiatal hernia indefinitely, even after surgery.
• Teach her about dietary changes to reduce reflux. For example, instruct her to eat small, frequent, bland meals.
• Tell her to avoid alcohol, hot spices, and other beverages and foods that worsen her symptoms.
• Suggest that she lie down for 2 hours after eating, and elevate the head of the bed on 6″ (15-cm) blocks.
• Instruct her to avoid activities that increase intra-abdominal pressure, such as coughing, wearing restrictive clothing, and straining.

Nursing interventions

• Prepare the patient for diagnostic tests. After endoscopy, watch for signs of perforation (falling blood pressure, rapid pulse, shock, sudden pain) caused by the endoscope.
• Administer prescribed antacids and other medications, and monitor patient response.
• To reduce intra-abdominal pressure and prevent aspiration, have the patient sleep in a reverse Trendelenburg position (with the head of the bed elevated 6″ to 12″ [15 to 31 cm]). Tell her not to lie down right after eating.
• If surgery is necessary, prepare the patient, and provide appropriate preoperative and postoperative care.

Patient teaching

• Teach the patient about her disorder. (See *Living with hiatal hernia*.) Explain significant symptoms, diagnostic tests, and prescribed treatments.
• Teach the patient about her prescribed medications.

STOMACH, INTESTINAL, AND PANCREATIC DISORDERS

Acute or chronic inflammation is commonly associated with disorders of the stomach, intestines, and pancreas. In addition, the GI mucosa lining the stomach and intestines may be damaged by ulceration, herniation, or the development of diverticula.

GASTRITIS

An inflammation of the gastric mucosa, gastritis may be acute or chronic. Acute gastritis, the most common stomach disorder, produces mucosal reddening, edema, and superficial surface erosion. Chronic gastritis is common among elderly people and people with pernicious anemia. It's often present as chronic atrophic gastritis, in which all stomach mucosal layers are inflamed, with a reduced number of chief and parietal cells. However, acute or chronic gastritis can occur at any age.

Causes

Acute gastritis has numerous causes, including:
• chronic ingestion of irritating foods, such as hot peppers (or an allergic reaction to them), or alcohol
• drugs, such as aspirin and other nonsteroidal anti-inflammatory agents (in large doses), cytotoxic agents, caffeine, corticosteroids, antimetabolites, phenylbutazone, and indomethacin
• ingested poisons, especially DDT, ammonia, mercury, carbon tetrachloride, or corrosive substances
• endotoxins released from infecting bacteria, such as staphylococci, *Escherichia coli,* or salmonella.

Acute gastritis also may develop in acute illnesses, especially when the patient has major trauma; burns; severe infection; hepatic, renal, or respiratory failure; or major surgery.

Chronic gastritis may be associated with peptic ulcer disease or gastrostomy because these conditions cause chronic reflux of pancreatic secretions, bile, and bile acids from the duodenum into the stomach. Recurring exposure to irritating substances, such as drugs, alcohol, smoking, or environmental agents, also may lead to chronic gastritis. Chronic gastritis may occur with pernicious anemia, renal disease, or diabetes mellitus.

Bacterial infection with *Helicobacter pylori* can cause acute or chronic gastritis.

Complications

Although gastritis usually resolves when the causative agent is removed, persistent or untreated disease can lead to hemorrhage, shock, obstruction, perforation, peritonitis, and gastric cancer.

Assessment findings

The patient history may reveal one or more causative agents. After exposure to the offending substance, the patient with acute gastritis typically reports rapid onset of symptoms, such as epigastric discomfort, indigestion, cramping, anorexia, nausea, hematemesis, and vomiting. The patient's symptoms may last from a few hours to a few days.

The patient with chronic gastritis may describe similar symptoms or he may only experience mild epigastric discomfort. Or his complaints may be vague. For example, he may report an intolerance for spicy or fatty foods or have mild epigastric pain that's relieved by eating. Patients with chronic atrophic gastritis are often asymptomatic.

On inspection, the patient may appear normal or show signs of distress, such as fatigue, grimacing, or restlessness, depending on symptom severity. If gastric bleeding has occurred, he may appear pale, and his vital signs may reveal tachycardia and hypotension. Inspection and palpation may disclose abdominal distention, tenderness, and guarding. Auscultation may reveal increased bowel sounds.

Diagnostic tests

• *Gastroscopy* (commonly with biopsy) confirms gastritis when it is performed before lesions heal (usually within 24 hours). Biopsy reveals the inflammatory process. If the procedure fails to stimulate acid production, it also confirms achlorhydria. In patients with pernicious anemia, gastroscopy also fails to detect the intrinsic factor. This procedure is contraindicated after ingestion of a corrosive agent.
• *Laboratory analyses* can detect occult blood in vomitus or stools (or both) if the patient has gastric bleeding.
• *Hemoglobin and hematocrit levels* are decreased if the patient has developed anemia from bleeding.

Treatment

An immediate therapeutic priority is to eliminate the cause of gastritis. For example, bacterial gastritis is treated with antibiotics; ingested poisons are neutralized with the appropriate antidote. Once the associated disease is treated or the offending agent is eradicated or neutralized, the gastric mucosa usually will begin to heal.

Treatment for acute gastritis is symptomatic and supportive. Healing usually occurs within a few hours to a few days after the cause has been eliminated. Histamine antagonists, such as cimetidine, ranitidine, or famotidine, may be ordered to block gastric secretion. Antacids, such as aluminum hydroxide and magnesium hydroxide, may be used as buffering agents. Some patients also require analgesics.

When gastritis causes massive bleeding, treatment includes blood replacement; iced saline lavage, possibly with norepinephrine; angiography with vasopressin infused in 0.9% sodium chloride solution; and, sometimes, surgery.

A last resort, surgery is performed only if more conservative treatments fail. Vagotomy and pyloroplasty have been used with limited success. Rarely, partial or total gastrectomy may be required.

Because patients with chronic gastritis may be asymptomatic or have only vague complaints, no specific treatment may be necessary, except for avoiding aspirin and spicy foods. If symptoms develop or persist, antacids may be taken. If pernicious anemia is the underlying cause, vitamin B_{12} is administered parenterally.

Nursing diagnoses
• Altered nutrition: Less than body requirements
• Ineffective individual coping
• Knowledge deficit
• Pain
• Risk for fluid volume deficit

Nursing interventions
• Provide physical and emotional support to the patient to help him manage his symptoms.
• If the patient is vomiting, give antiemetics and, as ordered, replace I.V. fluids. Monitor fluid intake and output and electolyte levels.
• Monitor the patient for returning symptoms as food is reintroduced after he has received nothing by mouth. At this time, provide a bland diet that takes into account his food preferences.
• Offer smaller, more frequent servings to reduce the amount of irritating gastric secretions. Help the patient identify specific foods that cause gastric upset. Then, eliminate them from his diet.
• Administer prescribed medications, as ordered, and monitor the patient's response.
• If pain or nausea interferes with the patient's appetite, administer pain medications or antiemetics about 1 hour before meals.
• If surgery is necessary, prepare the patient preoperatively and provide appropriate postoperative care.

Patient teaching
• Teach the patient about the disorder. Explain the relationship between his symptoms and the causative agents so that he'll understand the need to modify his diet or life-style. Be attentive to his questions, and inform him about diagnostic tests and treatments.

• If the patient is scheduled for surgery, reinforce the doctor's explanation of the procedure and provide preoperative teaching.
• Give the patient a list of irritating foods to avoid, such as spicy or highly seasoned foods, alcohol, and caffeine. Be sure he understands that these changes are lifelong measures to prevent recurrence of gastritis. If necessary, refer him to the dietitian for further instruction.
• If the patient smokes, encourage him to quit by pointing out that this habit can cause or aggravate symptoms by irritating the gastric mucosa. Refer him to a smoking-cessation program.
• If appropriate, help the patient identify the need for stress reduction. Teach him stress-reduction techniques, such as meditation, deep breathing, progressive relaxation, and guided imagery.
• Urge the patient to seek immediate attention for recurring symptoms, such as hematemesis, nausea, or vomiting.
• To prevent recurrence, stress the importance of taking prophylactic medications as ordered. To reduce gastric irritation, advise the patient to take steroids with milk, food, or antacids. Instruct him to take antacids between meals and at bedtime and to avoid aspirin-containing compounds.
• Teach family members the importance of supporting the patient as he makes the necessary dietary and life-style changes.

GASTROENTERITIS
A self-limiting disorder, gastroenteritis (intestinal flu, traveler's diarrhea, viral enteritis, food poisoning) is an inflammation of the stomach and small intestine. The bowel reacts to any of the varied causes of gastroenteritis with hypermotility, producing severe diarrhea and secondary depletion of intracellular fluid.

A major cause of morbidity and mortality in underdeveloped nations, gastroenteritis occurs in persons of all ages. In the United States, this disorder ranks second to the common cold as a cause of lost work time and fifth as the cause of death among young children. It also can be life-threatening in elderly and debilitated persons.

Causes
Gastroenteritis has many possible causes, including:
• bacteria, such as *Staphylococcus aureus*, *Salmonella*, *Shigella*, *Clostridium botulinum*, *C. perfringens*, and *Escherichia coli*
• amoebae, especially *Entamoeba histolytica*

PREVENTING TRAVELER'S DIARRHEA

If the patient travels, especially to developing nations, discuss precautions that he can take to reduce his chances of getting traveler's diarrhea. Inform him that traveler's diarrhea is caused by inadequate sanitation and occurs after ingestion of bacteria-contaminated food or water. These organisms attach to the lining of the small intestine, where they release a toxin that causes diarrhea and cramps.

To minimize this risk, advise him to:
• drink water (or brush his teeth with water) only if it's chlorinated. Chlorination protects the water supply from bacterial contaminants, such as *Escherichia coli.*
• avoid beverages in glasses that may have been washed in contaminated water.
• refuse ice cubes if they may have been made from contaminated water.
• drink only beverages made with boiled water, such as coffee or tea, or those contained in bottles or cans.
• sanitize impure water by adding 2% tincture of iodine (5 drops/liter of clear water; 10 drops/liter of cloudy water) or by adding liquid laundry bleach (about 2 drops/liter of clear water; 4 drops/liter of cloudy water).
• avoid uncooked vegetables, fresh fruits with no peel, salads, unpasteurized milk, and other dairy products.
• beware of foods offered by street vendors.

If traveler's diarrhea occurs despite precautions, bismuth subsalicylate, diphenoxylate with atropine, or loperamide can be used to relieve the symptoms.

• parasites, such as *Ascaris, Enterobius,* and *Trichinella spiralis*
• viruses, such as adenoviruses, echoviruses, and coxsackieviruses
• ingestion of toxins, such as poisonous plants or toadstools
• drug reactions from antibiotics
• food allergens.

Complications

In most patients, the disorder resolves with no sequelae. However, persistent or untreated gastroenteritis can cause severe dehydration and loss of crucial electrolytes, which can lead to shock, vascular collapse, renal failure and, rarely, death. Typically, infants, elderly persons, and debilitated patients are at greatest risk because of their immature or impaired immune systems.

Assessment findings

Patient history commonly reveals the acute onset of diarrhea accompanied by abdominal pain and discomfort. The patient may complain of cramping, nausea, and vomiting. He may also report malaise, fatigue, anorexia, fever, abdominal distention, and rumbling in his lower abdomen. If diarrhea is severe, he may experience rectal burning, tenesmus, and bloody mucoid stools.

Investigate the patient's history to try to determine the cause of his signs and symptoms. Ask about ingestion of contaminated food or water. The cause may be apparent if the patient reports that others who ingested the same food or water have similar signs and symptoms. Also ask about the health of other family members and about his recent travels. (For more information, see *Preventing traveler's diarrhea.*)

Inspection may reveal slight abdominal distention. On palpation, the patient's skin turgor may be poor, a sign of dehydration. Auscultation may disclose hyperactive bowel sounds and, if the patient is dehydrated, orthostatic hypotension or generalized hypotension. Temperature may be normal or elevated.

Diagnostic tests

Laboratory studies identify the causative bacteria, parasites, or amoebae. These studies include Gram's stain, stool culture (by direct rectal swab), or blood culture.

Treatment

Medical management is usually supportive, consisting of bed rest, nutritional support, increased fluid intake and, occasionally, antidiarrheal therapy. If gastroenteritis is severe or affects a young child or an elderly or debilitated person, hospitalization may be required. Treatment may include I.V. fluid and electrolyte replacement and administration of antidiarrheals, antiemetics, and antimicrobials.

Antidiarrheals, such as bismuth subsalicylate, are typically used as the first line of defense against diarrhea. If necessary, other antidiarrheals, such as camphorated opium tincture (paregoric), diphenoxylate with atropine, and loperamide may be ordered.

Antiemetics (oral, I.M., or rectal suppository), such as prochlorperazine or trimethobenzamide, may be prescribed for severe vomiting. However, these medications should be avoided in patients with viral or bacterial gastroenteritis.

Specific antibiotic administration is restricted to patients who have bacterial gastroenteritis, as identified by diagnostic testing.

Nursing diagnoses
• Altered nutrition: Less than body requirements
• Diarrhea
• Pain
• Risk for fluid volume deficit

Nursing interventions
• Plan your care to allow uninterrupted rest periods for the patient. Rest usually helps to relieve the patient's symptoms, increase his resistance, and conserve his strength.
• If the patient is nauseated, advise him to avoid quick movements, which can increase the severity of nausea.
• If the patient can tolerate oral fluid intake, replace lost fluids and electrolytes with broth, ginger ale, and lemonade, as tolerated. Vary his diet to make eating more enjoyable, and allow some choice of foods. Warn him to avoid milk and milk products, which may provoke recurrence.
• Monitor fluid status carefully. Take vital signs at least every 4 hours, weigh the patient daily, monitor for fluid and electrolyte balance, and record intake and output.
• Watch for signs of dehydration, such as dry skin and mucous membranes, fever, and sunken eyes.
• If dehydration occurs, administer oral and I.V. fluids, as ordered. If necessary, a potassium supplement may be added to the I.V. solution. If the patient is receiving a potassium supplement, be especially alert for the development of hyperkalemia.
• Administer medications, as ordered. Correlate dosages and routes with the patient's meals and activities (for example, give antiemetics 30 to 60 minutes before meals).
• Wash your hands thoroughly after giving care to avoid spreading infection, and use blood and body fluid precautions whenever handling vomitus or stools.
• To ease anal irritation caused by diarrhea, clean the area carefully and apply a repellent cream, such as petroleum jelly. Warm sitz baths and application of witch hazel compresses can also soothe irritation.
• If food poisoning is probable, contact public health authorities so they can interview patients and food handlers and take samples of the suspected contaminated food.

Patient teaching
• Teach the patient about gastroenteritis, describing its symptoms and varied causes. Explain why a stool specimen may be necessary for diagnosis. Discuss the purpose of prescribed treatments.

• Instruct the patient to wait until his diarrhea subsides and then to start drinking unsweetened fruit juice, tea, bouillon, or other clear broths, and eating bland soft foods, such as cooked cereal, rice, or applesauce. Tell him to avoid foods that are spicy, greasy, or high in roughage, such as whole-grain products or raw fruits or vegetables. Explain that these foods can precipitate recurrent diar-

• Carefully review the proper use of all prescribed medications with the patient, making sure that he fully understands the desired effects of the drugs and their possible adverse effects.
• Teach preventive measures. If the patient expects to travel, advise him to pay close attention to what he eats and drinks, especially in developing nations. Review proper hygiene measures to prevent recurrence. Instruct the patient to thoroughly cook foods, especially pork; to refrigerate perishable foods, such as milk, mayonnaise, potato salad, and cream-filled pastry; to always wash his hands with warm water and soap before handling food, especially after using the bathroom; to clean utensils thoroughly; and to eliminate flies and roaches in the home.

PEPTIC ULCERS
Occurring as circumscribed lesions in the mucosal membrane, peptic ulcers can develop in the lower esophagus, stomach, duodenum, or jejunum. The major forms are duodenal ulcer and gastric ulcer; both are chronic conditions.

Duodenal ulcers, which account for about 80% of peptic ulcers, affect the proximal part of the small intestine. These ulcers, which occur most commonly in men between ages 20 and 50, follow a chronic course characterized by remissions and exacerbations. About 5% to 10% of patients with duodenal ulcers develop complications that necessitate surgery.

Gastric ulcers, which affect the stomach mucosa, are most common in middle-aged and elderly men, especially among those who are poor and undernourished. This kind of ulcer also tends to occur in chronic users of aspirin or alcohol.

Causes
Recently, researchers identified a bacterial infection with *Helicobacter pylori* (formerly known as *Campylobacter pylori*) as a leading cause of peptic ulcer disease. They also found that *H. pylori* releases a toxin that promotes mucosal inflammation and ulceration.

In a peptic ulcer resulting from *H. pylori,* acid seems to be mainly a contributor to the consequences of the bacterial infection rather than the dominant cause. Other risk factors include the use of certain medications—nonsteroidal anti-inflammatory drugs (NSAIDs), for example—and pathologic hypersecretory states—Zollinger-Ellison syndrome, for example.

Investigators think drug therapy, in particular with salicylates and other NSAIDs, reserpine, or caffeine, may erode the mucosal lining. They believe that NSAIDs can cause a gastric ulcer by inhibiting prostaglandins (the fatty acids that mediate and suppress ulceration).

These substances are present in large quantities in the gastric mucosa, where they inhibit injury by stimulating secretion of gastric mucus and gastric and duodenal mucosal bicarbonate.

Prostaglandins also promote gastric mucosal blood flow, maintain the integrity of the gastric mucosal barrier, and help renew the epithelium after a mucosal injury. When an agent, such as an NSAID, inhibits prostaglandin production, an ulceration can occur.

Glucocorticoids also predispose the patient to ulcer formation. These drugs inhibit prostaglandin synthesis, increase gastric acid and pepsin secretion, reduce gastric mucosal blood flow, and decrease cytoprotective mucus production. Because these drugs also decrease gastric pain, they may mask signs of ulcer development until hemorrhage or perforation actually occurs.

Certain illnesses – in particular, pancreatitis, hepatic disease, Crohn's disease, preexisting gastritis, and Zollinger-Ellison syndrome – are believed to have a strong association with ulcer development.

Although research continues to unveil the exact mechanisms of ulcer formation, several predisposing factors are acknowledged. They include:

• *Blood type.* For unknown reasons, gastric ulcers commonly strike people who have type A blood. Duodenal ulcers tend to afflict people who have type O blood, perhaps because these people don't secrete blood group antigens in their saliva and other body fluids. These special blood group antigens are mucopolysaccharides, which scientists think may serve to protect the mucosa.

• *Genetic factors.* Duodenal ulcers are about three times more common in first-degree relatives of duodenal ulcer patients than in the general population.

• *Exposure to irritants.* Like certain other drugs, alcohol inhibits prostaglandin secretion, triggering a mechanism much like the one caused by NSAIDs.

Cigarette smoking also appears to encourage ulcer formation. Smoking evidently inhibits pancreatic secretion of bicarbonate by a mechanism involving nicotine. It also may accelerate the emptying of gastric acid into the duodenum and promote mucosal breakdown.

• *Trauma.* Critical illness, shock, or severe tissue injury from extensive burns or from intracranial surgery may lead to a stress ulcer.

• *Psychogenic factors.* Emotional stress may stimulate long-term overproduction of gastric secretions that aid in ulcer production by eroding stomach, duodenal, and esophageal tissue.

• *Normal aging.* The pyloric sphincter may wear down in the course of normal aging, which, in turn, permits the reflux of bile into the stomach. This appears to be a common contributor to the development of gastric ulcers in elderly persons.

Complications

Erosion of the mucosa can cause GI hemorrhage, which can progress to hypovolemic shock, perforation, and obstruction. Obstruction of the pylorus may cause the stomach to distend with food and fluid and result in abdominal or intestinal infarction.

Penetration, in which the ulcer crater extends beyond the duodenal walls into attached structures, such as the pancreas, biliary tract, liver, or gastrohepatic omentum, occurs fairly frequently in duodenal ulcer.

Assessment findings

Typically, the patient describes periods of exacerbation and remission of his symptoms, with remissions lasting longer than exacerbations. Investigation of the patient's history may reveal possible causes or predisposing factors, such as smoking, use of aspirin or other medications, or associated disorders. (See *Planning care for the peptic ulcer patient.*)

The patient with a gastric ulcer may report a recent loss of weight or appetite. He may explain that he doesn't feel like eating or that he has developed an aversion to food because eating causes discomfort. He may have pain in the left epigastrium, which he describes as heartburn or indigestion. His discomfort may be accompanied by a feeling of fullness or distention. Commonly, the onset of pain signals the start of an attack.

The patient's history will help distinguish between a gastric or a duodenal ulcer. Ask the patient whether his pain worsens after eating or is relieved by it. In the patient with a gastric ulcer, eating often triggers or aggravates pain. Conversely, food often relieves the pain of a duodenal ulcer. Also inquire whether the patient has experienced nocturnal pain that disrupts his sleep. The patient with duodenal ulcer reports waking up because of pain; the patient with gastric ulcer does not.

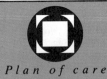

Plan of care

PLANNING CARE FOR THE PEPTIC ULCER PATIENT

When your patient has a peptic ulcer, devising an effective plan of care can be a challenge. However, the challenge can grow if your patient happens to be a health care professional. Consider, for instance, the challenge of caring for Beverly Baxter, RN, a hard-working 36-year-old who has recently suffered a relapse of peptic ulcer symptoms. Despite her education, she faces the same difficulty as any other patient in modifying her diet and life-style. To relieve her present exacerbation and prevent recurrence, Ms. Baxter needs a carefully constructed care plan, such as this one.

Patient history

Ms. Baxter tells you that recurrent, gnawing gastric pain started many years ago when she was finishing nursing school exams and going through a divorce. Often, she would awaken during the night with severe stomach pain and take several doses of antacids before her symptoms would subside several hours later.

Ms. Baxter explains that she placed herself on a bland diet. She started taking over-the-counter cimetidine at that point. Although it made her slightly drowsy, she continued to take it with excellent results. She vowed then to stop smoking and has never restarted.

Recently, Ms. Baxter completed her BSN and transferred to her hospital's emergency department. For the last year, she has been working overtime and weekends. She describes her diet as "mostly eat-and-run—whatever I can grab out of the vending machines at work." She also drinks six to eight cups of black coffee every day. Occasionally, she would vomit "coffee-ground" material—a warning sign that first prompted her to seek care.

Assessment findings

Your assessment begins with Ms. Baxter's vital signs. She is afebrile at 97.4° F (36.3° C). Her pulse rate is 72 beats/minute and slightly irregular. Her respirations are 19 breaths/minute and shallow. She insists that her blood pressure of 98/52 mm Hg is normal for her.

On inspection, you note that Ms. Baxter looks pale and thin. She sits in a knee-chest position to ease her epigastric pain. Her nasogastric (NG) tube, connected to suction, drains blood and mucus. You observe that her lips are dry and cracked.

Upon auscultation of the lungs, you note clear fields bilaterally. Palpation of the epigastric region reveals acute tenderness and rigidity.

Initial laboratory findings show a loss of sodium and potassium from her prolonged vomiting. Hematocrit and hemoglobin levels are reduced from blood loss, though not dangerously so. As soon as her condition is stable, Ms. Baxter will undergo gastroscopy to pinpoint the bleeding site.

Nursing diagnoses

As you review your assessment findings, you begin to develop your plan of care, taking into account how Ms. Baxter's stressful life-style and poor eating habits may be exacerbating her symptoms. You arrive at the following nursing diagnoses:
• Pain related to irritation of the mucosa of the stomach
• Anxiety related to working conditions and emotional stress
• Altered nutrition: Less than body requirements, related to vomiting, inadequate diet, and antacid use
• Risk for injury related to complications from blood loss, dehydration, or obstruction
• Noncompliance related to nonacceptance of personal and physical limitations.

Expected outcomes

You set immediate and long-term goals with Ms. Baxter. You must work together to:
• reduce pain
• relieve stress and anxiety
• achieve rehydration, food tolerance, increased physical strength, and return to adequate nutritional status
• avoid injury from complications
• demonstrate future compliance with diet, stress reduction, and medications.

Implementation

As you review your initial goals, you define the steps needed to implement your anticipated outcomes.

To reduce pain
• Determine how Ms. Baxter responds to pain; have her rate her pain on a scale of 1 to 10 both before and after analgesics.
• Assess for nonverbal signs of pain; document type and time of pain.
• After NG tube removal, instruct Ms. Baxter to drink about 3 qt (3 liters) of water daily to dilute the contents of her stomach.
• Administer and document the effectiveness of all medications, including antibiotics prescribed after confirmation of *Helicobacter pylori;* histamine-receptor antagonists to decrease hydrochloric acid formation; analgesics (not aspirin-based) to relieve pain; mucosal barriers to protect the excoriated stomach lining; and anticholinergics to inhibit gastric acid release.

(continued)

PLANNING CARE FOR THE PEPTIC ULCER PATIENT
(continued)

• Provide small, nonirritating meals that are not highly spiced or too hot in temperature; encourage slow eating and careful chewing before swallowing.
• Teach Ms. Baxter relaxation techniques to divert her attention from discomfort and to reduce anxiety associated with pain.

To reduce stress and anxiety
• Encourage Ms. Baxter to ask questions about her hospitalization and treatment regimen.
• Instruct her to list factors that will aggravate her condition. Then elicit methods she has used in the past to successfully cope with them.
• Suggest that she consult a psychologist to begin stress-reduction therapy. Encourage her to continue to practice stress-reduction measures at work and at home.
• Maintain a calm, confident manner when speaking with her.
• Provide for rest and comfort; keep the environment free of excessive stimulation.
• Encourage visits from family and friends who have a nurturing relationship with Ms. Baxter.

To restore adequate nutritional status and increase strength
• Assess Ms. Baxter's skin and mucosa for signs of dehydration; administer parenteral nutrition to improve fluid balance until the NG tube is removed.
• Administer antiemetics if she remains nauseated after the NG tube is removed.
• Provide frequent oral care and keep ice chips near her bedside.
• Monitor her weight daily until stabilized, then twice weekly; measure her height accurately.

• Correct nutritional deficiencies, including vitamins, minerals, proteins, and carbohydrates.
• Offer small, frequent meals that are not highly spiced or too hot in temperature. Encourage Ms. Baxter to drink fluids with meals.
• Encourage Ms. Baxter to select foods she likes, but discourage her dependence on caffeine.
• Provide a quiet, relaxed atmosphere during meals.
• Assist Ms. Baxter with activities of daily living, as needed, and encourage early ambulation. Schedule rest periods throughout the day.
• Monitor intake and output; complete a calorie count if Ms. Baxter doesn't finish her meals.

To avoid injury
• Encourage compliance with planned treatments.
• Observe for, and review with Ms. Baxter, signs of hemorrhage: hematemesis, melena, dyspnea, tachycardia, light-headedness, and mental confusion.
• Watch for and discuss with Ms. Baxter the signs of stomach wall perforation: excruciating abdominal pain, tender rigid abdomen with rebound tenderness, tachycardia, and dyspnea.
• Be alert for signs of obstruction, and review these with Ms. Baxter: new onset of nausea and vomiting, abdominal distention, and fetid breath.
• Monitor and record vital signs every 4 hours.
• Record the following laboratory values daily: complete blood count, electrolyte levels, and occult blood in stools.

To promote compliance
• Assess Ms. Baxter's willingness to comply. Anticipate whether all treatments will be acceptable to her.

• Introduce Ms. Baxter to other health care workers who have successfully managed peptic ulcers and reduced occupational stress.
• Encourage one-on-one meetings between Ms. Baxter and key personnel in the dietary, psychology, social services, and medical departments. Promote an atmosphere of trust.
• Suggest that Ms. Baxter meet with her department head and human resources personnel to devise less stressful approaches to her job.
• Emphasize the importance of keeping scheduled follow-up visits and seeking prompt medical attention if symptoms recur.

Evaluation
Because Ms. Baxter is a nurse, you may assume that she'll automatically recognize signs of her disease in the future and comply with self-care measures, such as stress reduction and diet therapy. However, to ensure a successful outcome, you'll need to provide Ms. Baxter with the same teaching and encouragement as any patient with peptic ulcer disease.

You may wish to reevaluate Ms. Baxter at 3, 6, and 12 months, when you can reassess her work-related behavior. Encourage her to continue to use relaxation techniques at home or on breaks at work. You'll also need to evaluate the effectiveness of her medical regimen and the success of dietary modifications.

Your goals will be met if you've reduced Ms. Baxter's pain, instructed her in stress management, and corrected her fluid and nutritional status. Ms. Baxter also should be able to recognize and avoid potential complications and comply with dietary measures, relaxation methods, and medications.

The patient with a duodenal ulcer may have epigastric pain that he describes as sharp, gnawing, or burning. Alternatively, he may describe the pain as boring or aching and poorly defined. Or he may liken it to a sensation of hunger, abdominal pressure, or fullness. Typically, pain occurs 90 minutes to 3 hours after eating. Because eating often reduces the pain of a duodenal ulcer, the patient may report a recent weight gain. Vomiting and other digestive disturbances are rare in these patients.

If the patient is anemic from blood loss, you may notice pallor on inspection. Palpation in the midline and midway between the umbilicus and the xiphoid process may disclose epigastric tenderness. Auscultation may reveal hyperactive bowel sounds.

Diagnostic tests

• *Barium swallow* or *upper GI and small-bowel series* may reveal the presence of the ulcer. This is the initial test performed on a patient whose symptoms are not severe.
• *Upper GI endoscopy* or *esophagogastroduodenoscopy* confirms the presence of an ulcer and permits cytologic studies and biopsy to rule out *H. pylori* or cancer. Endoscopy is the major diagnostic test for peptic ulcers.
• *Upper GI tract X-rays* reveal mucosal abnormalities.
• *Laboratory analysis* may detect occult blood in stools.
• *Serologic testing* may disclose clinical signs of infection, such as an elevated white blood cell count.
• *Gastric secretory studies* show hyperchlorhydria.
• *Carbon 13 (^{13}C) urea breath test* results reflect activity of *H. pylori*. (*H. pylori* contains the enzyme urease, which breaks down orally administered urea containing the radioisotope ^{13}C before it's absorbed systemically. Low levels of ^{13}C in exhaled breath point to *H. pylori* infection.)

Treatment

Medical management is essentially symptomatic, emphasizing drug therapy, physical rest, dietary changes, and stress reduction. For patients with severe symptoms or complications, surgery may be required.

Drug therapy aims to eradicate *H. pylori*, reduce gastric secretions, protect the mucosa from further damage, and relieve pain. Medications may include:
• bismuth and two other antimicrobial agents, usually tetracycline or amoxicillin and metronidazole
• antacids to reduce gastric acidity
• histamine-receptor antagonists, such as cimetidine or ranitidine, to reduce gastric secretion for short-term therapy (up to 8 weeks)
• coating agents, such as sucralfate, for duodenal ulcers. Sucralfate forms complexes with proteins at the base of an ulcer, making a protective coat that prevents further digestive action of acid and pepsin.
• sedatives and tranquilizers, such as chlordiazepoxide and phenobarbital, for patients with gastric ulcers
• anticholinergics, such as propantheline, to inhibit the vagus nerve effect on the parietal cells and to reduce gastrin production and excessive gastric activity in duodenal ulcers. (These drugs are usually contraindicated in gastric ulcers.)

Standard therapy also includes physical rest and decreased activity, which help decrease the amount of gas-tric secretion. Diet therapy may consist of eating six small meals daily (or even small hourly meals) rather than three regular meals. Although some doctors prescribe a milk and cream or bland diet, the value of these measures is controversial.

If GI bleeding occurs, emergency treatment begins with passage of a nasogastric (NG) tube to allow for iced saline lavage, possibly containing norepinephrine. Gastroscopy allows visualization of the bleeding site and coagulation by laser or cautery to control bleeding. This therapy allows surgery to be postponed until the patient's condition stabilizes.

Surgery is indicated for perforation, unresponsiveness to conservative treatment, suspected cancer, and other complications. The type of surgery chosen for peptic ulcers depends on the location and extent of the disorder. Major operations include bilateral vagotomy, pyloroplasty, and gastrectomy. (For more information, see *Types of peptic ulcer surgery*, page 892.)

Nursing diagnoses

• Activity intolerance
• Altered nutrition: Less than body requirements
• Anxiety
• Fluid volume deficit
• Pain
• Risk for injury
• Sleep pattern disturbance

Nursing interventions

• Support the patient emotionally and offer reassurance.
• Administer prescribed medications, and monitor the patient for the desired effects. Also watch for adverse reactions. Most medications should alleviate the patient's discomfort, so ask if his pain is relieved.
• Provide six small meals or small hourly meals as ordered. Advise the patient to eat slowly, chew thoroughly, and have small snacks between meals.
• Schedule the patient's care so that he can get plenty of rest.
• Continuously monitor the patient for complications: hemorrhage (sudden onset of weakness, fainting, chills, dizziness, thirst, the desire to defecate, and passage of loose, tarry, or even red stools); perforation (acute onset of epigastric pain followed by lessening of the pain and the onset of a rigid abdomen, tachycardia, fever, or rebound tenderness); obstruction (feeling of fullness or heaviness, copious vomiting containing undigested food after meals); and penetration (pain radiating to the back, night distress). If any of the above occurs, notify the doctor immediately.

TYPES OF PEPTIC ULCER SURGERY

Surgery		Indications	Effects
Vagotomy Truncal (total abdominal vagotomy)		• Recurrent ulcer disease • Acid reduction	• Completely severs both vagus nerves at the esophageal base • Destroys gastric, intestinal, and gallbladder motility • Stops acid production • Causes impaired emptying and diarrhea
Selective vagotomy		• Recurrent ulcer disease • Acid reduction	• Severs vagus nerve • Destroys vagal innervation of stomach (but retains abdominal innervation) • Reduces acid production • Impairs gastric motility
Highly selective (parietal cell vagotomy)		• Recurrent ulcer disease • Acid reduction	• Severs only the parietal cell branches of vagus nerve • Denervates acid-producing cells but doesn't affect motility
Pyloroplasty		• Pyloric stricture or obstruction (may be combined with vagotomy to reduce gastric secretion and motility)	• Enlarges pylorus by removing sphincter • Improves drainage; eliminates obstruction • Facilitates neutralization without inhibiting gastric secretion • Increases gastric emptying
Gastrectomy Billroth I (gastroduodenostomy, hemigastrectomy)		• Gastric ulcer • Pyloric obstruction • Hemorrhage	• Resects antrum and connects gastric remnant to proximal duodenum • Destroys antral function and pyloric sphincter • Reduces gastric secretion; increases emptying • May cause bile reflux, steatorrhea, dumping syndrome, weight loss, vomiting, and anemia
Billroth II (gastrojejunostomy)		• Duodenal ulcer • Pyloric obstruction	• Resects antrum • Attaches gastric remnant to proximal jejunum (retains duodenum) • Destroys antral function • Allows digestive secretions of liver and pancreas to mix in duodenum • Duodenum serves as afferent loop; proximal jejunum as efferent loop • Reduces gastric secretion; increases emptying • Commonly causes steatorrhea, dumping syndrome, weight loss, vomiting, and anemia
Total gastrectomy (esophagojejunostomy)		• Ulcer disease • Perforation • Gastric cancer	• Resects stomach from lower esophageal sphincter to duodenal bulb; anastomoses duodenum and esophagus • Destroys gastric function; ingested materials pass from esophagus to duodenum
Gastric resection (antrectomy)		• Recurrent ulcers • Perforation	• Removes stomach portion • Varies, depending on stomach portion removed (for example, antrectomy alters digestive function)

After surgery:

• Keep the NG tube (inserted in the operating room) patent. If the tube isn't functioning, don't reposition it; you may damage the suture line or anastomosis. Notify the surgeon promptly.

• Monitor intake and output, including NG tube drainage. Also, check bowel sounds. Allow the patient nothing by mouth until peristalsis resumes and the NG tube is removed or clamped.

• Replace fluids and electrolytes. Assess for signs of dehydration, sodium deficiency, and metabolic alkalosis, which may occur secondary to gastric suction. Provide parenteral nutrition, if ordered. This is usually given if the patient isn't allowed to eat for a week or more.

• Control postoperative pain with narcotics and analgesics, as ordered.

• Watch for complications—hemorrhage; shock; iron, folate, or vitamin B_{12} deficiency anemia; and dumping syndrome.

Patient teaching

• Teach the patient about peptic ulcer disease, and help him to recognize its signs and symptoms. Explain scheduled diagnostic tests and prescribed therapies. Review symptoms associated with complications, and urge him to notify the doctor if any of these occur. Emphasize the importance of complying with treatment, even after his symptoms are relieved.

• Review the proper use of prescribed medications, discussing the desired actions and possible adverse reactions of each drug.

• Instruct the patient to take antacids 1 hour after meals. If he follows a sodium-restricted diet, advise him to take only low-sodium antacids. Caution him that antacids may cause changes in bowel habits (diarrhea with magnesium-containing antacids, constipation with aluminum-containing antacids).

• Check all medications the patient is using. Antacids inhibit the absorption of many other drugs, including digoxin. Work out a schedule for taking medications.

• Warn against excessive intake of coffee and alcoholic beverages during exacerbations.

• Encourage the patient to make appropriate life-style changes. Explain that emotional tension can precipitate an ulcer attack and prolong healing. Help the patient identify anxiety-producing situations, and teach him to perform relaxation techniques, such as distraction and meditation.

• If the patient smokes, urge him to stop because smoking stimulates gastric acid secretion. Refer him to a smoking-cessation program.

• Tell the patient to read labels of nonprescription medications and to avoid preparations that contain corticosteroids, aspirin, or other nonsteroidal anti-inflammatory drugs, such as ibuprofen. Explain that these drugs inhibit mucus secretion and therefore leave the GI tract vulnerable to injury from gastric acid. Advise him to use alternative analgesics, such as acetaminophen. Caution him to avoid systemic antacids, such as sodium bicarbonate, because they're absorbed into the circulation and can cause an acid-base imbalance.

• Tell the patient that, although cimetidine, famotidine, and other histamine-receptor antagonists are available over-the-counter, he should not take them without consulting his doctor. These drugs may duplicate prescribed medications or suppress important symptoms.

• To avoid dumping syndrome after gastric surgery, advise the patient to lie down after meals; to drink fluids between meals rather than with meals; to avoid eating large amounts of carbohydrates; and to eat four to six small, high-protein, low-carbohydrate meals daily.

ULCERATIVE COLITIS

An inflammatory, commonly chronic disease, ulcerative colitis causes ulcerations of the mucosa in the colon. It usually begins in the rectum and sigmoid colon and may extend upward into the entire colon; it rarely affects the small intestine, except for the terminal ileum. Ulcerative colitis produces congestion, edema (leading to mucosal friability), and ulcerations. Severity ranges from a mild, localized disorder to a fulminant disease that can cause many complications.

Ulcerative colitis occurs primarily in young adults, especially women; it is also more prevalent among Jews and higher socioeconomic groups. The incidence of the disease is unknown; however, some studies indicate that as many as 1 out of 1,000 persons are affected. Onset of symptoms seems to peak between ages 15 and 20 and again between ages 55 and 60.

Causes

Although the etiology of ulcerative colitis is unknown, it may be related to an abnormal immune response in the GI tract, possibly associated with genetic factors. Stress was once thought to be a cause of ulcerative colitis. Studies show that, although it's not a cause, stress can increase the severity of an attack. Although no specific organism has been linked to the disease, infection hasn't been ruled out as a cause.

Complications

Ulcerative colitis may lead to a variety of complications, depending on the severity and site of inflammation. Nutritional deficiencies are the most common complication, but the disease can also lead to perineal sepsis with anal fissure, anal fistula, perirectal abscess, hemorrhage, and toxic megacolon. A patient with ulcerative colitis has an increased risk of various arthritis types (forty times more prevalent in this group than in the general population) and cancer (if the disease has persisted more than 10 years since childhood).

Other complications include coagulation defects resulting from vitamin K deficiency, erythema nodosum on the face and arms, pyoderma gangrenosum on the legs and ankles, uveitis, pericholangitis, sclerosing cholangitis, cirrhosis, possible cholangiocarcinoma, ankylosing spondylitis, loss of muscle mass, strictures, pseudopolyps, stenosis, and perforated colon, leading to peritonitis and toxemia.

Assessment findings

Usually, the patient's history will reveal periods of remission and exacerbation of symptoms. During an exacerbation, the patient generally reports mild cramping, lower abdominal pain, and recurrent bloody diarrhea—as often as 10 to 25 times daily. She may also experience nocturnal diarrhea. During these periods, she may complain of fatigue, weakness, anorexia, weight loss, nausea, and vomiting.

On inspection, the patient's stools may appear liquid, with visible pus and mucus. Check for blood in the stools—a cardinal sign of ulcerative colitis. Abdominal distention may be present in fulminant disease. Palpation may disclose abdominal tenderness. A rectal examination may reveal perianal irritation, hemorrhoids, and fissures. Rarely, rectal fistulas and abscesses may be evident.

Diagnostic tests

• *Sigmoidoscopy* confirms rectal involvement in most cases by showing increased mucosal friability, decreased mucosal detail, and thick inflammatory exudate.
• *Colonoscopy* may determine the extent of the disease and also evaluate the strictured areas and pseudopolyps. This test is not performed when the patient has active signs and symptoms.
• *Biopsy,* performed during colonoscopy, can help confirm the diagnosis.
• *Barium enema* evaluates the extent of the disease and detects complications, such as strictures and carcinoma.

This study is not performed in a patient with active signs and symptoms.
• *Stool specimen analysis* reveals blood, pus, and mucus, but no pathogenic organisms.
• *Other supportive laboratory tests* show decreased serum levels of potassium, magnesium, hemoglobin, and albumin, as well as leukocytosis and increased prothrombin time. Erythrocyte sedimentation rate elevation correlates with the severity of the attack.

Treatment

The goals of treatment are to control inflammation, replace nutritional losses and blood volume, and prevent complications. Supportive treatment includes dietary therapy, bed rest, I.V. fluid replacement, and medications. Blood transfusions or iron supplements may be needed to correct anemia.

Dietary measures depend on disease severity. Patients with severe disease usually receive total parenteral nutrition and are allowed nothing by mouth. Parenteral nutrition also is used for patients awaiting surgery or showing signs of dehydration and debilitation from excessive diarrhea. The goals of parenteral nutrition are to rest the intestinal tract, decrease stool volume, and restore positive nitrogen balance.

The patient with moderate signs and symptoms may receive Ensure or another brand of elemental feeding to provide adequate nutrition with minimal bowel stimulation. A low-residue diet may be ordered for the patient with mild signs and symptoms. As signs and symptoms subside, the diet may gradually advance to include a greater variety of foods.

Drug therapy to control inflammation includes corticotropin and adrenal corticosteroids, such as prednisone, prednisolone, and hydrocortisone; sulfasalazine, which has anti-inflammatory and antimicrobial properties, may also be used. Antispasmodics, such as tincture of belladonna, and antidiarrheals, such as diphenoxylate and atropine, are used only for the patient with frequent, troublesome diarrhea whose ulcerative colitis is otherwise under control. These drugs may precipitate massive dilation of the colon (toxic megacolon) and are generally contraindicated.

Surgery, the treatment of last resort, is performed if the patient has toxic megacolon, if she fails to respond to drugs and supportive measures, or if she finds signs and symptoms unbearable.

The most common surgical technique is proctocolectomy with ileostomy. Total colectomy and ileorectal anastomosis is done less often because of its mortality rate (2% to 5%). This procedure removes the entire colon and anastomoses the rectum and the terminal ileum. It requires observation of the remaining rectal stump for any signs of cancer or colitis.

Pouch ileostomy, in which a pouch is created from a small loop of the terminal ileum and a nipple valve is formed from the distal ileum, is gaining popularity. The resulting stoma opens just above the pubic hairline; the pouch empties through a catheter inserted in the stoma several times a day. In ulcerative colitis, colectomy to prevent colon cancer is controversial.

Ileoanal reservoir is a newer surgery that preserves the anal sphincter and provides the patient with a reservoir made from the ileum and attached to the anal opening. The procedure is performed in two steps. First, the rectal mucosa is excised. An abdominal colectomy is performed; then a reservoir is constructed and attached. After that, a temporary loop ileostomy is created to allow the new rectal reservoir to heal. Finally, the loop ileostomy is closed after a 3- or 4-month waiting period. Stools from the reservoir are similar to the stools from an ileostomy.

Nursing diagnoses
• Activity intolerance
• Altered nutrition: Less than body requirements
• Body image disturbance
• Diarrhea
• Pain
• Risk for fluid volume deficit
• Risk for impaired skin integrity

Nursing interventions
• Support the patient emotionally. Stay with her when she's acutely distressed. Spend a few minutes with her several times a day, and listen to her concerns. Offer reassurance when appropriate.
• Provide diet therapy as ordered. Monitor the fluid and electrolyte status of the patient on total parenteral nutrition. Change dressings, and assess for inflammation at the insertion site. Check urine every 6 hours for glucose and acetone.
• Provide frequent mouth care for the patient who is allowed nothing by mouth. Regardless of the prescribed diet, monitor intake and calorie count. Record intake and output, noting the frequency and volume of stools.
• Monitor hemoglobin and hematocrit levels and give blood transfusions, as ordered.
• Administer medications, as ordered, and monitor the patient for desired effects. Note any adverse reactions, such as those from prolonged corticosteroid therapy. Be aware that such therapy may mask infection.

• Watch for signs of dehydration (poor skin turgor, furrowed tongue) and electrolyte imbalances, especially signs of hypokalemia (muscle weakness, paresthesia) and hypernatremia (tachycardia, fever, dry tongue).
• Schedule care to allow for frequent rest periods. These patients are often very tired and weak.
• After each bowel movement, thoroughly clean the skin around the rectum and apply a soothing and protective agent, such as petroleum jelly, to the irritated area. Provide an air mattress to help prevent skin breakdown.
• Watch closely for signs of complications, such as a perforated colon and peritonitis (fever, severe abdominal pain, abdominal rigidity and tenderness, cool clammy skin), and toxic megacolon (abdominal distention, decreased bowel sounds).
• If surgery will be performed, provide preoperative care as required. Do a bowel preparation, if ordered. This usually involves keeping the patient on a clear-liquid diet, using cleansing enemas, and administering an antimicrobial agent, such as neomycin.
• After surgery, provide all necessary postoperative care. Monitor vital signs, intake and output, fluid and electrolyte levels, and respiratory status. Change dressings and maintain skin integrity. Provide comfort measures.
• If the postoperative patient has a nasogastric tube, keep the tube patent. After removal of the tube, provide a clear-liquid diet as ordered, and gradually advance to a low-residue diet, as tolerated.

Patient teaching
• Teach the patient about the disorder and review its signs and symptoms. Explain diagnostic tests and ordered treatments.
• Discuss all prescribed dietary changes, and help the patient understand how these measures will decrease her symptoms. If she's placed on parenteral nutrition or a very restricted diet, reassure her that she will be able to progress to a more advanced diet as her symptoms resolve. In general, caution the patient to avoid GI stimulants, such as caffeine, alcohol, and smoking.
• Review the patient's medications with her. Explain the desired actions, dosage, and adverse reactions.
• If the patient is scheduled for surgery, reinforce the doctor's explanation of the procedure and its possible complications. As part of preoperative teaching, describe the stoma and explain how it differs from normal anatomy. Provide additional patient information as needed (available from the United Ostomy Association). Arrange for a visit by an enterostomal therapist and, ideally, a recovered ileostomate.

• After a proctocolectomy and ileostomy, teach stoma care. After a pouch ileostomy, demonstrate procedures to insert the catheter and care for the stoma.
• Emphasize the need for regular physical examinations because of the increased risk of colorectal cancer.

NECROTIZING ENTEROCOLITIS

Characterized by diffuse or patchy intestinal necrosis, necrotizing enterocolitis is accompanied by sepsis in about one-third of cases. Sepsis usually involves *Escherichia coli, Clostridium, Salmonella, Pseudomonas,* or *Klebsiella.* Initially, necrosis is localized, occurring anywhere along the intestine, but most often it is right-sided (in the ileum, ascending colon, or rectosigmoid). With early detection, the survival rate is 60% to 80%. If diffuse bleeding occurs, the disorder usually results in disseminated intravascular coagulation.

Necrotizing enterocolitis is most common in premature infants (less than 34 weeks' gestation) and those of low birth weight (less than 5 lb [2.3 kg]). It is related to 2% of all infant deaths, with onset usually occurring from 1 to 14 days after birth.

Necrotizing enterocolitis has become more prevalent in some areas, possibly because of the higher incidence and survival of premature infants and of neonates who have low birth weights. One in ten infants who develops this disorder is full-term. Among premature and low-birth-weight infants in intensive care nurseries, the incidence varies from about 1% to 12%.

Causes

The exact cause of necrotizing enterocolitis is unknown. Possible predisposing factors include birth asphyxia, postnatal hypotension, respiratory distress, hypothermia, umbilical vessel catheterization, or patent ductus arteriosus. The disorder may also be a response to significant prenatal stress, such as premature rupture of membranes, placenta previa, maternal sepsis, toxemia of pregnancy, or breech or cesarean birth.

According to a current theory, necrotizing enterocolitis develops when the infant suffers perinatal hypoxemia that results when blood from the gut is shunted to more vital organs. Subsequent mucosal ischemia provides an ideal medium for bacterial growth. Hypertonic formula may increase bacterial activity because—unlike breast milk—it lacks protective immune activity and contributes to the production of hydrogen gas. As the bowel swells and breaks down, gas-forming bacteria invade damaged areas, producing free air in the intestinal wall and resulting in perforation and peritonitis.

Complications

Perforation, the major complication of necrotizing enterocolitis, requires surgery. Infants who survive acute necrotizing enterocolitis may develop recurrent disease or mechanical and functional abnormalities of the intestine. In surgical patients, these complications may develop as late as 3 months postoperatively.

Assessment findings

The maternal and patient histories may reveal one or more predisposing factors. Just before the onset of necrotizing enterocolitis, the infant may experience temperature instability, bradycardia, apnea, and lethargy or irritability. You may notice an increase in gastric aspirates, bile-stained vomitus, or bloody diarrhea. On inspection, the abdomen may appear distended. Suspect gastric retention if the abdomen feels tense or rigid on palpation. A taut abdomen, with red or shiny skin, may indicate peritonitis.

Diagnostic tests

• *Stool cultures* may identify the infecting organism, and *stool analysis* may identify occult blood.
• *Anteroposterior and lateral abdominal X-rays* confirm the diagnosis. These X-rays show nonspecific intestinal dilation and, in later stages of necrotizing enterocolitis, pneumatosis cystoides intestinalis (gas or air in the intestinal wall).
• *Blood studies* show several abnormalities. Platelet count may fall below 50,000/mm³, and serum sodium levels are decreased. Arterial blood gas levels show metabolic acidosis, indicating sepsis. Bilirubin levels are elevated because of infection-induced breakdown of erythrocytes. Blood cultures identify the infecting organism. Clotting studies and hemoglobin levels identify disseminated intravascular coagulation.
• *Abdominal X-rays* monitor the disorder's progress.

Treatment

Medical management is supportive, with successful treatment dependent on early detection. At the first signs of necrotizing enterocolitis, oral feedings are discontinued for about 7 to 10 days to rest the injured bowel. I.V. fluids, including total parenteral nutrition, maintain fluid and electrolyte balance and nutrition during this time. To aid bowel decompression, a nasogastric (NG) tube is placed and connected to suction. If coagulation studies indicate a need for transfusion, the infant usually receives dextran to promote hemodilution, increase mesenteric blood flow, and reduce platelet aggregation.

Antibiotic therapy consists of parenteral administration of an aminoglycoside or ampicillin to suppress bacterial flora and prevent bowel perforation. (These drugs can also be administered through an NG tube, if necessary.)

Surgery is indicated if the patient develops any of the following: signs of perforation (free intraperitoneal air on X-ray or symptoms of peritonitis); respiratory insufficiency (caused by severe abdominal distention); progressive and intractable acidosis; or disseminated intravascular coagulation.

Surgery removes all necrotic and acutely inflamed bowel, then creates a temporary colostomy or ileostomy. The procedure must leave at least 12″ (30.5 cm) of bowel, or the infant may suffer from malabsorption or chronic vitamin B_{12} deficiency.

Nursing diagnoses
• Altered nutrition: Less than body requirements
• Fluid volume deficit
• Risk for infection

Nursing interventions
• Provide psychological support for the parents, and remain with them during stressful periods. Answer their questions about their child's condition.
• Monitor the patient continuously. Administer I.V. fluids and, if necessary, total parenteral nutrition, as ordered. Monitor fluid and electrolyte levels, acid-base balance, and intake and output.
• Administer prescribed antibiotics; observe the infant for adverse reactions.
• Take axillary temperatures to avoid perforating the bowel.
• Promptly dispose of soiled diapers to prevent cross-contamination. Wash your hands wih soap and water after diaper changes.
• Be alert for signs and symptoms of gastric distention and perforation including apnea, bradycardia, cardiovascular shock, edema, erythema, increasing abdominal tenderness, involuntary abdominal rigidity, rag-doll limpness, a sudden drop in body temperature, or sudden listlessness. If any of these signs or symptoms occur, notify the doctor immediately.
• If surgery is necessary, provide appropriate preoperative care.

After surgery:
• Gently suction secretions and frequently assess respirations.
• Replace fluids lost through drainage from the NG tube and stoma. Include drainage losses in output records.

• Weigh the infant daily. A daily weight gain of 0.35 to 0.7 oz (9.9 to 19.9 g) indicates a good response to therapy.
• Because of the infant's small abdomen, the suture line is near the stoma; therefore, keeping the suture line clean can be a problem. Good skin care is essential because the immature infant's skin is fragile and vulnerable to excoriation, and the active enzymes in bowel secretions are corrosive.
• Improvise tiny colostomy bags from urine collection bags, medicine cups, or condoms. Karaya gum may be used to make a seal.
• Watch for wound disruption, infection, and excoriation. Also monitor for signs and symptoms of intestinal malfunction from stricture or short-gut syndrome. Such complications usually develop 1 month after the infant resumes normal feedings.

Patient teaching
• Explain the disorder to the parents, helping them to understand necessary tests and treatments. Try to prepare them for potential deterioration in their infant's condition. Be honest and explain all treatments, such as why feedings are withheld.
• If the infant is scheduled for a temporary colostomy or ileostomy, reinforce the doctor's explanation of the surgery and explain why it's necessary. Reassure the parents that they will be able to participate in their infant's physical care once his condition is no longer critical, and encourage them to do so.
• Before discharge, refer the parents to community resources and home health care agencies, as needed.
• Encourage mothers whose infants are at risk for development of necrotizing enterocolitis to breast-feed. Point out that breast milk contains live macrophages that fight infection, and its low pH inhibits the growth of many organisms. Ideally, breast-feeding should begin immediately postpartum because colostrum (fluid secreted before the milk) contains high concentrations of maternal immunoglobulin A, which directly protects the infant gut from infection and which the infant lacks for several days postpartum.
• If the mother plans to express breast milk for later use, instruct her to store it in plastic—not glass—containers because leukocytes adhere to glass. Tell mothers they may refrigerate their milk for 48 hours but shouldn't freeze or heat it because doing so destroys antibodies.

CROHN'S DISEASE

A type of inflammatory bowel disease, Crohn's disease may affect any part of the GI tract but usually involves the terminal ileum. The disease extends through all layers of the intestinal wall and may involve regional lymph nodes and the mesentery.

Crohn's disease is most prevalent in adults ages 20 to 40. It is two to three times more common in Jews and least common in blacks. The disease is not considered a predisposing factor for colon or rectal cancer.

Crohn's disease has a varied nomenclature. When it affects only the small bowel, it is also known as regional enteritis. If the disorder also involves the colon or only affects the colon, it is known as Crohn's disease of the colon. (Crohn's disease of the colon also has been termed granulomatous colitis—an inaccurate term because not all patients develop granulomas.)

Causes and pathophysiology

Although researchers are still probing the etiology of Crohn's disease, possible causes include lymphatic obstruction, infection, allergies, and other immune disorders, such as altered immunoglobulin A production and increased suppressor T-cell activity. Genetic factors may also play a role: Crohn's disease sometimes occurs in monozygotic twins, and 10% to 20% of patients with the disease have one or more affected relatives. However, no simple pattern of inheritance has been identified.

Inflammation spreads slowly and progressively, beginning with lymphadenia and obstructive lymphedema in the submucosa, where Peyer's patches develop in the intestinal mucosa. Lymphatic obstruction causes edema, with mucosal ulceration and development of fissures, abscesses and, sometimes, granulomas. The mucosa may acquire a characteristic "cobblestone" look.

As the disease progresses, fibrosis occurs, thickening the bowel wall and narrowing the lumen. Serositis (serosal inflammation) also develops, causing inflamed bowel loops to adhere to other diseased or normal loops. This may result in bowel shortening. Because inflammation usually occurs segmentally, the bowel may become a patchwork of healthy and diseased segments. Eventually, the diseased parts of the bowel become thicker, more narrow, and shorter.

Complications

Anal fistula, resulting from severe diarrhea and enzymatic corrosion of the perineal area, is the most common complication. A perineal abscess may also develop during the active inflammatory state. Fistulas may develop to the bladder or vagina or even to the skin in an old scar area. Other complications include intestinal obstruction, nutritional deficiencies (caused by malabsorption and maldigestion) and, rarely, peritonitis.

Assessment findings

Generally, the patient reports signs and symptoms of gradual onset, marked by periods of remission and exacerbation. Because signs and symptoms may be intermittent, he may have postponed seeking medical attention for some time.

The patient typically complains of fatigue, fever, abdominal pain, diarrhea (usually without obvious bleeding) and, occasionally, weight loss. Questioning may reveal that his diarrhea worsens after emotional upset or after ingestion of poorly tolerated foods, such as milk, fatty foods, and spices.

The patient with regional enteritis, often a young adult, may report similar signs and symptoms as well as anorexia, nausea, and vomiting. Typically, this patient describes his abdominal pain as steady, colicky, or cramping. It usually occurs in the right lower abdominal quadrant.

On inspection, the patient's stool may appear soft or semiliquid, without gross blood (a distinguishing clinical feature from the bloody diarrhea seen in ulcerative colitis). Palpation may reveal tenderness in the right lower abdominal quadrant; it may also disclose an abdominal mass, indicating adherent loops of bowel.

Diagnostic tests

• *Laboratory analysis* to detect occult blood in stools is usually positive.

• *Small-bowel X-rays* may show irregular mucosa, ulceration, and stiffening.

• *Barium enema* that reveals the string sign (segments of stricture separated by normal bowel) supports the diagnosis. This test may also show fissures and narrowing of the lumen.

• *Sigmoidoscopy* and *colonoscopy* may show patchy areas of inflammation, thus helping to rule out ulcerative colitis. These studies may also reveal the characteristic coarse irregularity (cobblestone appearance) of the mucosal surface. When the colon is involved, discrete ulcerations may be evident.

• *Biopsy,* performed during sigmoidoscopy or colonoscopy, reveals granulomas in up to half of all specimens.

• *Laboratory test findings* indicate increased white blood cell count and erythrocyte sedimentation rate. Other findings include hypokalemia, hypocalcemia, hypomagnesemia, and decreased hemoglobin levels.

Treatment

Effective management of Crohn's disease requires drug therapy and significant life-style changes, including physical rest and dietary restrictions. In debilitated patients, treatment includes total parenteral nutrition to maintain nutrition while resting the bowel.

Drug therapy, designed to combat inflammation and relieve symptoms, may include:
• corticosteroids, such as prednisone, to reduce signs and symptoms of diarrhea, pain, and bleeding by decreasing inflammation
• immunosuppressant agents, such as azathioprine, to suppress the body's response to antigens
• sulfasalazine to reduce inflammation
• metronidazole to treat perianal complications
• antidiarrheals, such as diphenoxylate and atropine, to combat diarrhea (contraindicated in patients with significant bowel obstruction)
• narcotics to control pain and diarrhea.

Life-style changes, such as stress reduction and reduced physical activity, help to rest the bowel, giving it time to heal. Also essential are dietary changes that decrease bowel activity while still providing adequate calories and nutrition. Dietary modifications include elimination of high-fiber foods (no fruits or vegetables) and foods that irritate the mucosa (such as dairy products, and spicy and fatty foods). Foods that stimulate excessive intestinal activity (such as carbonated or caffeinated beverages) also should be avoided. Vitamins may be prescribed to compensate for the bowel's inability to absorb them.

If complications develop, surgery may be required. Indications for surgery include bowel perforation, massive hemorrhage, fistulas, or acute intestinal obstruction. Colectomy with ileostomy is often necessary in patients with extensive disease of the large intestine and rectum.

Nursing diagnoses
• Altered gastrointestinal tissue perfusion
• Altered nutrition: Less than body requirements
• Body image disturbance
• Chronic low self-esteem
• Diarrhea
• Hopelessness
• Ineffective individual coping
• Pain
• Risk for fluid volume deficit
• Risk for impaired skin integrity

Nursing interventions
• Provide emotional support to the patient and his family. Listen to the patient's concerns, and help him cope with body image disturbance.
• Record fluid intake and output (including the amount of stools), and weigh the patient daily. Watch for dehydration, and maintain fluid and electrolyte balance. Be alert for signs of intestinal bleeding (bloody stools); check stools for occult blood.
• Schedule patient care to include rest periods throughout the day.
• Provide the patient with a diet that is high in protein, calories, and vitamins. Also try providing frequent small meals throughout the day rather than three large meals.
• Carefully monitor the patient on total parenteral nutrition, and provide meticulous site care.
• If the patient is receiving steroids, watch for adverse reactions, such as GI bleeding. Remember that steroids can mask signs of infection.
• Monitor hemoglobin and hematocrit levels. Give iron supplements and blood transfusions, as ordered.
• Administer medications as ordered. Monitor the patient to ensure that medications are producing desired effects without adverse reactions.
• Provide good patient hygiene and meticulous oral care if the patient is restricted to nothing by mouth. After each bowel movement, provide careful skin care. Always keep a clean, covered bedpan within the patient's reach. Ventilate the room to eliminate odors.
• Monitor the patient for complications. Watch for fever and pain on urination, which may signal bladder fistula. Abdominal pain, fever, and a hard, distended abdomen may indicate intestinal obstruction.
• If the patient is scheduled for surgery, provide appropriate preoperative care. Before ileostomy, arrange for a visit by an enterostomal therapist.
• After surgery, frequently check the patient's I.V. line and nasogastric tube for proper functoning. Monitor vital signs and fluid intake and output. Maintain acid-base balance. Watch for wound infection and provide meticulous stoma care.

Patient teaching
• Teach the patient about the disease, its symptoms, and its complications. Explain ordered diagnostic tests; make sure he's aware of all pretest dietary restrictions or other pretest guidelines. Answer his questions.
• Emphasize the importance of adequate rest. Explain that limiting physical activity helps to reduce intestinal motility and promote healing.

• Encourage the patient to identify and reduce sources of stress in his life. If stress clearly aggravates his disease, teach him stress-management techniques or refer him for counseling.

• Be sure the patient understands prescribed dietary changes. Emphasize the need for a restricted diet, which may be trying, especially for a young patient. Refer him to a dietitian for further instruction, if necessary.

• Give the patient a list of foods to avoid, including milk products, spicy or fried high-residue foods, raw vegetables and fruits, and whole-grain cereals. Advise him to avoid carbonated, caffeinated, or alcoholic beverages (because they increase intestinal activity) and extremely hot or cold foods or fluids (because they increase flatus). Remind him to take supplemental vitamins, if prescribed.

• Teach the patient about prescribed medications, their desired effects, and possible adverse reactions. Urge him to call his doctor if adverse reactions occur.

• If the patient smokes, encourage him to quit, and assist him in joining a smoking-cessation program. Point out that smoking can aggravate his disease by altering bowel motility.

• Instruct the patient to notify his doctor if he experiences signs and symptoms of complications, such as fever, fatigue, weakness, a rapid heart rate, abdominal cramping or pain, vomiting, or acute diarrhea.

• If the patient is scheduled for surgery, provide preoperative teaching. Reinforce the doctor's explanation of the surgery, and mention possible complications.

• Postoperatively, teach stomal care to the patient and his family. Realize that ileostomy changes the patient's body image, so provide reassurance and emotional support. Refer him and his family to the local chapter of the National Foundation for Ileitis and Colitis for further support. If the patient has an ostomy, put him in touch with the United Ostomy Association.

PSEUDOMEMBRANOUS ENTEROCOLITIS

An acute inflammation and necrosis of the small and large intestines, pseudomembranous enterocolitis usually affects the mucosa but may extend into the submucosa and, rarely, other layers. This rare condition, marked by severe diarrhea, can be fatal in 1 to 7 days from severe dehydration and from toxicity, peritonitis, or perforation.

Causes

What triggers the acute inflammation and necrosis characteristic of this disorder is unknown; however, *Clostridium difficile* may produce a toxin that plays a role in its development. The disease typically occurs in patients who are undergoing treatment with broad-spectrum antibiotics or who have received such therapy in the past 4 weeks. Nearly all broad-spectrum antibiotics, especially clindamycin, ampicillin, and the cephalosporins, have been linked with its onset. Possible exceptions are vancomycin and aminoglycosides.

Pseudomembranous enterocolitis may also occur postoperatively in debilitated patients undergoing abdominal surgery. Whatever the cause, the necrosed mucosa is replaced by a pseudomembrane filled with staphylococci, leukocytes, mucus, fibrin, and inflammatory cells.

Complications

Severe dehydration, electrolyte imbalance, hypotension, shock, colonic perforation, and peritonitis are among the potentially fatal complications associated with this disorder.

Assessment findings

The patient's history usually reveals current or recent antibiotic treatment. Typically, the patient reports the sudden onset of copious, watery or, rarely, bloody diarrhea; abdominal pain; and fever. Palpation may reveal abdominal tenderness.

Careful consideration of the patient history is essential because the abrupt onset of enterocolitis and the emergency situation it creates may make diagnosis difficult.

Diagnostic tests

A rectal biopsy through sigmoidoscopy confirms pseudomembranous enterocolitis. Stool cultures can identify *C. difficile*.

Treatment

If the patient is receiving broad-spectrum antibiotic treatment, the first priority is immediate discontinuation of the offending drug. Usually, the patient is then treated with oral metronidazole or oral vancomycin. Metronidazole generally is used first; if it's ineffective, vancomycin is given. Anion exchange resins, such as cholestyramine, which bind the toxin produced by *C. difficile,* may be ordered for patients with mild pseudomembranous enterocolitis. However, patient response to this treatment has proven inferior to that with oral vancomycin or metronidazole.

Supportive treatments maintain fluid and electrolyte balance and combat hypotension and shock with vasopressors, such as dopamine and norepinephrine.

Nursing diagnoses
• Diarrhea
• Fluid volume deficit
• Pain

Nursing interventions
• Monitor vital signs, skin color, and level of consciousness. Immediately report signs of shock.
• Record fluid intake and output, including fluid lost in stools. Watch for dehydration (poor skin turgor, sunken eyes, and decreased urine output). If ordered, administer I.V. therapy to maintain fluid and electrolyte balance.
• Check serum electrolyte levels daily, and watch for clinical signs of hypokalemia (especially malaise) and a weak, rapid, irregular pulse.
• Administer medications as ordered. Monitor the patient for the desired effects and for adverse reactions.
• Keep the patient as comfortable as possible. Administer analgesics, if necessary, to decrease abdominal pain and antipyretics to control high fever. Teach the patient how to perform relaxation techniques, such as distraction or guided imagery, to help him cope with abdominal pain.
• Keep a bedpan within the patient's reach to help prevent embarrassing accidents.

Patient teaching
• Teach the patient about the disorder and its possible causes; discuss signs and symptoms, ordered diagnostic tests, and treatments.
• Review prescribed medications, explaining their desired effects, potential adverse reactions, and proper administration.
• Point out that because pseudomembranous enterocolitis recurs in about 20% of cases, the patient must immediately report symptoms of recurrence. Reassure him that a second course of therapy resolves the disorder.
• If the disorder was antibiotic-related, instruct the patient to caution doctors who might prescribe similar medications in the future.

IRRITABLE BOWEL SYNDROME

A common condition, irritable bowel syndrome (spastic colon, spastic colitis, mucous colitis) is marked by chronic or periodic diarrhea alternating with constipation. It is accompanied by straining and abdominal cramps.

Irritable bowel syndrome occurs mostly in women, with symptoms first emerging before age 40. The prognosis is good.

Causes
Although the precise etiology is unclear, irritable bowel syndrome involves a change in bowel motility, reflecting an abnormality in the neuromuscular control of intestinal smooth muscle. (See *What happens in irritable bowel syndrome*, page 902.)

Contributing or aggravating factors include anxiety and stress. Initial episodes occur early in life; psychological stress probably causes most exacerbations. Irritable bowel syndrome may also result from dietary factors, such as fiber, fruits, coffee, alcohol, or foods that are cold, highly seasoned, or laxative in nature. Other possible triggers include hormones, laxative abuse, and allergy to certain foods or drugs.

Complications
Irritable bowel syndrome is associated with a higher-than-normal incidence of diverticulitis and colon cancer. Although complications are usually few, the disorder may lead (rarely) to chronic inflammatory bowel disease.

Because symptoms mimic those of acute abdomen, misdiagnosis occasionally results in the performance of unnecessary surgery.

Assessment findings
Typically, the patient reports a history of chronic constipation, diarrhea, or both. She may complain of lower abdominal pain (usually in the left lower quadrant) that is often relieved by defecation or passage of gas. She may report bouts of diarrhea, which typically occur during the day. This symptom alternates with constipation or normal bowel function.

The patient may describe her stools as small with visible mucus. Or she may have small, pasty, and pencil-like stools instead of diarrhea. Other common complaints include dyspepsia, abdominal bloating, heartburn, faintness, and weakness.

During the patient history, investigate possible contributing psychological factors, such as a recent stressful life change, that may have triggered or aggravated symptoms.

On inspection, the patient may seem anxious and fatigued, but otherwise normal. Auscultation may reveal normal bowel sounds. Palpation typically discloses a relaxed abdomen. Occasionally, percussion reveals tympany over a gas-filled bowel.

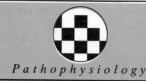

Pathophysiology

WHAT HAPPENS IN IRRITABLE BOWEL SYNDROME

Typically, the patient with irritable bowel syndrome has a normal-appearing GI tract. However, careful examination of the colon may reveal functional irritability—an abnormality in colonic smooth-muscle function marked by excessive peristalsis and spasms, even during remission.

Intestinal function

To understand what happens in irritable bowel syndrome, consider how smooth muscle controls bowel function. Normally, segmental muscle contractions mix intestinal contents while peristalsis propels the contents through the GI tract. Motor activity is most propulsive in the proximal (stomach) and the distal (sigmoid) portions of the intestine. Activity in the rest of the intestines is slower, permitting nutrient and water absorption.

In irritable bowel syndrome, the autonomic nervous system, which innervates the large intestine, fails to produce the alternating contractions and relaxations that propel stools smoothly toward the rectum.

The result is constipation or diarrhea or both.

Constipation

Some patients have spasmodic intestinal contractions, which set up a partial obstruction by trapping gas and stools. This causes distention, bloating, gas pain, and constipation.

Diarrhea

Other patients have dramatically increased intestinal motility. Usually triggered by eating or by cholinergic stimulation, the small intestine's contents speed into the large intestine, dumping watery stools and causing mucosal irritation, which results in diarrhea.

Mixed symptoms

If further spasms trap liquid stools, the intestinal mucosa absorbs water from the stools, leaving them dry, hard, and difficult to pass. The result: a pattern of alternating diarrhea and constipation.

Diagnostic tests

Because no definitive test exists to confirm irritable bowel syndrome, the diagnosis typically involves studies to rule out other, more serious, disorders, such as diverticulitis or colon cancer. The most frequently performed tests include the following:

• *Barium enema* may reveal colonic spasm and a tubular appearance of the descending colon. It also rules out certain other disorders, such as diverticula, tumors, and polyps.

• *Sigmoidoscopy* may disclose spastic contractions.

• *Stool examination* for occult blood, parasites, and pathogenic bacteria is negative.

Treatment

The aim of therapy is to control symptoms through dietary changes, stress management, and life-style modifications. Medications are reserved for severe symptoms and, if used, are discontinued as the patient learns to control her symptoms through diet and stress reduction.

The type of dietary therapy depends on the patient's symptoms. If she has diarrhea, an elimination diet may help determine whether her symptoms result from food intolerance. In this type of diet, certain foods, such as citrus fruits, coffee, corn, dairy products, tea, and wheat, are sequentially eliminated. Then, each food is gradually reintroduced to identify which foods, if any, trigger the patient's symptoms.

Other dietary changes include elimination of sorbitol, an artificial sweetener that may cause diarrhea, abdominal distention, and bloating. Also helpful is dietary elimination of nonabsorbable carbohydrates, such as beans and cabbage, and lactose-containing foods, all of which can cause flatulence.

To control diarrhea, bran may be added to increase dietary bulk. By increasing the time the stool remains in the bowel, bran helps to promote stool formation.

If the patient has constipation and abdominal pain, her diet should contain at least 15 to 20 grams daily of bulky foods, such as wheat bran, oatmeal, oat bran, rye cereals, prunes, dried apricots, and figs. These foods help to minimize the effect of nonpropulsive colonic contractions that may trap stool or retard its passage, causing abdominal pain. The patient should also increase her water intake to at least eight glasses a day.

Counseling to help the patient understand the relationship between stress and her illness is essential, as is instruction in stress-management techniques.

Drug therapy, if required, may include:

• anticholinergic, antispasmodic drugs, such as propantheline bromide, to reduce intestinal hypermotility

• antidiarrheals, such as diphenoxylate and atropine, to control diarrhea

• laxatives for constipation

• antiemetics, such as metoclopramide, to relieve heartburn, epigastric discomfort, and after-meal fullness
• simethicone to relieve belching and bloating from gas in the stomach and intestines
• mild tranquilizers, such as diazepam, prescribed for a short time to help reduce psychological stress associated with irritable bowel syndrome
• tricyclic antidepressants, if depression accompanies the disorder.

Nursing diagnoses
• Body image disturbance
• Constipation
• Diarrhea
• Ineffective individual coping

Nursing interventions
Because the patient with irritable bowel syndrome isn't hospitalized, nursing interventions almost always focus on patient teaching.

Patient teaching
• Explain the disorder to the patient, and reassure her that irritable bowel syndrome can be relieved. Point out, however, that the condition is chronic with no known cure.
• Help the patient understand ordered diagnostic tests. Review all pretest guidelines. Explain that diagnostic tests cannot specifically diagnose irritable bowel syndrome but do rule out other disorders.
• Review the patient's dietary plan, then suggest ways to implement it. Help her schedule meals; the GI tract works best if meals are eaten at regular intervals. Show her how to keep a daily record of her symptoms and food intake, carefully noting which foods trigger symptoms. Advise her to eat slowly and carefully to prevent swallowing air, which causes bloating, and to increase her intake of dietary fiber.
• Encourage the patient to drink 8 to 10 glasses of water or other compatible fluids daily. Point out that this will help regulate the consistency of her stools and promote balanced hydration. Caution her to avoid beverages associated with GI discomfort, such as carbonated or caffeinated drinks, fruit juices, and alcohol.
• Discuss the proper use of prescribed drugs, reviewing their desired effects and possible adverse reactions.
• Help the patient to implement life-style changes that will reduce stress. Teach her to set priorities in her daily activities, and, if possible, to delegate some responsibilities to other family members. Encourage her to schedule more time for rest and relaxation. Provide instruction in

relaxation techniques, such as guided imagery or deep-breathing exercises, and advise her to perform them regularly. If appropriate, instruct her to seek professional counseling for stress management.
• Remind the patient that regular exercise is important to relieve stress and promote regular bowel function; even a 20- or 30-minute walk each day is helpful.
• Discourage smoking. If the patient smokes, warn her that this habit can aggravate her symptoms by altering bowel motility.
• Explain the need for regular physical examinations. For patients over age 40, emphasize the need for colorectal cancer screening, including annual proctosigmoidoscopy and rectal examinations.

CELIAC DISEASE
Relatively uncommon, celiac disease (idiopathic steatorrhea, nontropical sprue, gluten enteropathy, celiac sprue) is characterized by poor food absorption and intolerance of gluten, a protein in wheat and wheat products. With treatment (eliminating gluten from the patient's diet), the prognosis is good, but residual bowel changes may persist in adults.

Celiac disease affects twice as many females as males and is more common among relatives, especially siblings. The incidence in the general population is about 1 in 3,000. This disease primarily affects whites of northwestern European ancestry; it's rare among Blacks, Jews, Asians, and people of Mediterranean ancestry. Although it may occur in adults, it usually affects children, most commonly between 9 and 18 months old.

Causes
Several theories attempt to explain the causes of celiac disease, but a genetic predisposition is undoubtedly important. Celiac disease may also result from an intramucosal enzyme defect that produces an inability to digest gluten. Resulting tissue toxicity produces rapid cell turnover, increases epithelial lymphocytes, and damages surface epithelium of the small bowel. Another theory holds that the disease involves an abnormal immune response. According to research findings, the presence of human leukocyte antigen (HLA)-B8 may be the primary determinant of celiac disease.

The primary dysfunction, malabsorption of gluten, results from atrophy of the villi in the small bowel and a decrease in the activity and amount of enzymes in the surface epithelium. Atrophy of intestinal villi leads to malabsorption of fat, carbohydrates, and protein. It also causes loss of calories, fat-soluble vitamins, and essential minerals and electrolytes.

Complications
Celiac disease can be fatal if not detected and properly treated because patients become malnourished and debilitated, making them vulnerable to infection and secondary adrenal insufficiency.

In severe cases, complications include anemia from malabsorption of iron, vitamin B_6, or vitamin B_{12}, which, if untreated, can lead to syncope, congestive heart failure, and angina.

Bleeding disorders can result from vitamin K deficiency. Rarely, ulceration of the jejunum or ileum occurs. Patients also have a higher-than-usual incidence of intestinal lymphoma.

Assessment findings
Both the patient history and the family history should be investigated. If the patient is a child, the history may reveal that symptoms emerged during the first year of life, shortly after gluten-containing cereal was introduced into the diet. The family history may disclose that siblings, parents, or other relatives have had obscure digestive complaints, such as intermittent diarrhea or, in children, failure to thrive and gain weight.

Symptoms are varied but typically include recurrent attacks of diarrhea, steatorrhea, abdominal distention from flatulence, stomach cramps, weakness, anorexia and, occasionally, increased appetite without weight gain. The patient or her parents may report bulky, foul-smelling stools. The patient may experience mood changes and irritability. Women may report amenorrhea.

On inspection, the patient may have a distended abdomen or appear malnourished. In children, you may notice a potbelly and obvious muscle wasting. Skin inspection may show dryness or rashes, such as eczema, psoriasis, dermatitis herpetiformis, or acne rosacea. Other findings on inspection include generalized fine, sparse, prematurely gray hair; brittle nails; and localized hyperpigmentation on the face, lips, or mucosa.

Sometimes, the patient denies diarrhea or steatorrhea but complains of bone pain, especially in the lower back, rib cage, and pelvis. This symptom may indicate compression fractures in adults or rickets in children caused by calcium loss and vitamin D deficiency. The patient may also have a history of seizures or paresthesia.

Diagnostic tests
Because celiac disease produces clinical effects in many body systems, a variety of tests may be ordered.

• *Small-bowel biopsy* showing histologic changes confirms the diagnosis. Histologic changes reveal a mosaic pattern of alternating flat and bumpy areas on the bowel surface (reflecting an almost total absence of villi) and an irregular, blunt, and disorganized network of blood vessels. These changes appear most prominently in the jejunum.
• *Upper GI series,* followed by a *small-bowel series,* demonstrates protracted barium passage. The barium shows up in a segmented, coarse, scattered, and clumped pattern; the jejunum shows generalized dilation.
• *Glucose tolerance test* shows poor glucose absorption.
• *D-xylose tolerance test* discloses low urine and blood levels of xylose (less than 3 g over 5 hours); however, renal disease may cause a false-positive result.
• *Serum carotene levels* are low, indicating malabsorption. (Because the body neither stores nor manufactures carotene, the patient must ingest carotene for several days before the test.)
• *Stool specimen analysis,* after a 72-hour stool collection, shows excess fat.
• *Hemoglobin and hematocrit levels,* as well as *white blood cell and platelet counts,* may be decreased.
• *Albumin, sodium, potassium, cholesterol,* and *phospholipid levels* are reduced; *prothrombin time* is commonly decreased.

Treatment
Elimination of gluten from the patient's diet is the required — and lifelong — treatment. About 80% of patients improve after this exclusion, but full return to normal absorption and bowel histology may not occur for months or may never occur. The gluten-free diet is high in protein but low in carbohydrates and fat. Depending on individual tolerance, the diet initially consists of proteins and gradually expands to include other foods.

Supportive treatment may include supplemental iron, vitamin B_{12}, and folic acid; reversal of electrolyte imbalance (by I.V. infusion, if necessary); I.V. fluid replacement for dehydration; corticosteroids (prednisone, hydrocortisone) to treat accompanying adrenal insufficiency; vitamin K for hypoprothrombinemia; and, when necessary, parenteral nutrition.

Nursing diagnoses
• Altered nutrition: Less than body requirements
• Diarrhea
• Fluid volume deficit

Nursing interventions

• Observe the patient's nutritional status and progress by daily calorie counts and weight checks. Also, evaluate tolerance to new foods. In the early stages, offer small, frequent meals to counteract anorexia.

• Assess the patient's fluid status: Record intake, urine output, and number of stools (may exceed 10 per day). Watch for signs of dehydration, such as dry skin and mucous membranes and poor skin turgor.

• Check serum electrolyte levels. Watch for signs of hypokalemia (weakness, lethargy, rapid pulse, nausea, and diarrhea) and of low calcium levels (impaired blood clotting, muscle twitching, and tetany).

• Monitor prothrombin time and hemoglobin and hematocrit levels. Protect the patient from bleeding and bruising. Administer vitamin K, iron, folic acid, and vitamin B_{12}, as ordered. Early in the treatments, give hematinic supplements as ordered. Use the Z-track method to give iron I.M. If the patient can tolerate oral iron, give it between meals, when absorption is best. Dilute oral iron preparations, and give them through a straw to prevent staining the teeth.

• Insert a nasogastric tube to relieve abdominal distention, if ordered, and attach the tube to intermittent suction. Monitor drainage, noting color, consistency, and amount.

• Protect the patient with osteomalacia from injury by keeping the side rails up and assisting with ambulation, as necessary.

• Give steroids, as ordered. Monitor the patient for desired effects and assess regularly for cushingoid adverse reactions, such as hirsutism and muscle weakness.

• Provide a gluten-free diet for the patient.

• Assess the patient's acceptance and understanding of the disease, and encourage regular reevaluation.

Patient teaching

• Explain the disorder to the patient or, if the patient is a young child, to the parents. Review the signs and symptoms as well as required diagnostic tests and treatments.

• Emphasize the importance of a gluten-free diet. Reassure the family that the patient usually begins to improve dramatically within a few days of beginning the diet. If the patient is a child, tell the parents that her weight should return to within the normal range for her age within 6 months to 1 year after starting the diet.

• Reinforce specific dietary guidelines. Advise elimination of gluten-containing foods, such as wheat, barley, rye, and oats, as well as foods made from these grains, such as breads and baked goods. Suggest substitution of corn, rice, or soybean flour. Refer the patient to a dietitian, who can develop a meal plan and suggest ways to obtain gluten-free food. Point out that health food stores are usually a good source for these foods.

• Urge the patient or her parents to carefully read food labels to avoid products with hidden gluten content. For example, grains are typically used as fillers. In particular, caution them to avoid foods containing "vegetable protein."

DIVERTICULAR DISEASE

In this disorder, bulging pouches (diverticula) in the GI wall push the mucosal lining through the surrounding muscle. The most common site for diverticula is in the sigmoid colon, but they may develop anywhere, from the proximal end of the pharynx to the anus. Other typical sites are the duodenum, near the pancreatic border or the ampulla of Vater, and the jejunum. Diverticular disease of the stomach is rare and may be a precursor of peptic or neoplastic disease. Diverticular disease of the ileum (Meckel's diverticulum) is the most common congenital anomaly of the GI tract. (See *Meckel's diverticulum*, page 906.)

Diverticular disease has two clinical forms. In *diverticulosis*, diverticula are present but don't cause symptoms. In *diverticulitis*, a far more serious disorder, diverticula become inflamed and may cause complications, such as obstruction, infection, and hemorrhage.

Most common in adults age 45 and older, diverticular disease affects 30% of adults over age 60. Diverticulosis is less common in nations where the diet contains abundant natural bulk and fiber.

Causes and pathophysiology

A diverticulum develops when high intraluminal pressure is exerted on areas of weakness, such as points where blood vessels enter the intestine, causing a break in the muscular continuity of the GI wall. The pressure in the intestinal lumen forces the intestine out, creating a pouch (diverticulum).

Diet, especially highly refined foods, may be a contributing factor. Lack of fiber reduces fecal residue, narrows the bowel lumen, and leads to higher intra-abdominal pressure during defecation.

Diverticulitis occurs when retained undigested food mixed with bacteria accumulates in the diverticulum, forming a hard mass (fecalith). This substance cuts off the blood supply to the diverticulum's thin walls, increasing its susceptibility to attack by colonic bacteria. Inflammation follows bacterial infection.

MECKEL'S DIVERTICULUM

A congenital abnormality, Meckel's diverticulum occurs when a blind tube, like the appendix, opens into the distal ileum near the ileocecal valve. This disorder results when the intra-abdominal portion of the yolk sac fails to close completely during fetal development. It occurs in about 2% of the population, mostly in males.

Complications

Uncomplicated Meckel's diverticulum produces no symptoms, but complications cause melena and abdominal pain, especially around the umbilicus. The lining of the diverticulum may be either gastric mucosa or pancreatic tissue. This disorder may lead to peptic ulceration, perforation, and peritonitis and may resemble acute appendicitis.

Meckel's diverticulum may also cause bowel obstruction when a fibrous band that connects the diverticulum to the abdominal wall, the mesentery, or other structures snares a loop of the intestine. This may cause intussusception into the diverticulum, or volvulus near the diverticular attachment to the back of the umbilicus or another intra-abdominal structure.

Meckel's diverticulum should be considered in patients with GI obstruction or hemorrhage, especially when routine GI X-rays are negative.

Treatment

Treatment is surgical resection of the inflamed bowel and antibiotic therapy if infection occurs.

Complications

Diverticulitis causes most complications. In severe diverticulitis, the diverticula can rupture, producing abscesses or peritonitis. Diverticular rupture occurs in up to 20% of such patients.

Diverticulitis also may lead to intestinal obstruction, resulting from edema or spasm related to inflammation, or, in chronic diverticulitis, from fibrosis and adhesions that narrow and seal the bowel's lumen.

Other complications include rectal hemorrhage or portal pyemia (generalized septicemia with abscess formation) from artery or vein erosion. Occasionally, the inflamed colon segment may produce a fistula by adhering to the bladder or other organs.

In elderly patients, a rare complication of diverticulosis (without diverticulitis) is hemorrhage from colonic diverticula, usually in the right colon. Such hemorrhage is usually mild to moderate and easily controlled. Occasionally, bleeding may be life-threatening.

Assessment findings

Usually, the patient with diverticulosis is symptom-free. Occasionally, the history may reveal intermittent pain in the left lower abdominal quadrant, which may be relieved by defecation or the passage of flatus. The patient may report alternating bouts of constipation and diarrhea. The assessment usually reveals no clinical findings. Rarely, palpation may disclose abdominal tenderness in the left lower quadrant.

The patient with diverticulitis may have a history of diverticulosis, diagnosed incidentally on radiography of the GI tract. Investigation of his dietary history commonly reveals low fiber consumption. He may report recent consumption of foods containing seeds or kernels, such as tomatoes, nuts, popcorn, or strawberries, or indigestible roughage, such as celery or corn. Seeds and undigested roughage can block the neck of a diverticulum, causing diverticulitis.

The patient with diverticulitis typically complains of moderate pain in the left lower abdominal quadrant, which he may describe as dull or steady. Straining, lifting, or coughing may aggravate his pain. Other signs and symptoms include mild nausea, gas, and intermittent bouts of constipation, sometimes accompanied by rectal bleeding. Some patients report diarrhea.

On inspection, the patient with diverticulitis may appear distressed. Palpation may confirm his reports of left lower quadrant abdominal pain. He may have a low-grade fever.

In acute diverticulitis, the patient may report muscle spasms and show signs of peritoneal irritation. Palpation may reveal guarding and rebound tenderness. Rectal examination may disclose a tender mass if the inflamed area is close to the rectum.

Diagnostic tests

Various tests may establish the diagnosis, determine complications, and rule out other disorders, such as cancer.
• *Barium studies* confirm the diagnosis. An upper GI series confirms or rules out diverticulosis of the esophagus and upper bowel; a barium enema confirms or rules out diverticulosis of the lower bowel. Barium-filled diverticula can be single, multiple, or clustered like grapes and may have a wide or narrow mouth. Barium outlines, but doesn't fill, diverticula blocked by impacted feces. In patients with acute diverticulitis, a barium enema may rupture the bowel, so this procedure isn't done before the acute phase resolves.
• *Radiography* may reveal colonic spasm if irritable bowel syndrome accompanies diverticular disease.

• *Biopsy* rules out cancer; however, a colonoscopic biopsy isn't recommended during acute diverticular disease because of the strenuous bowel preparation it requires.

• *Blood studies* may show leukocytosis and an elevated erythrocyte sedimentation rate in diverticulitis, especially if the diverticula are infected.

• *Stool tests* detect occult blood in 20% of patients with diverticulitis.

Treatment

Patient management depends on the type of diverticular disease and the severity of symptoms. Asymptomatic diverticulosis generally requires no treatment. Intestinal diverticulosis that causes pain, mild GI distress, constipation, or difficult defecation may respond to a liquid or bland diet, stool softeners, and occasional doses of mineral oil. These measures relieve symptoms, minimize irritation, and lessen the risk of progression to diverticulitis. After pain subsides, patients also benefit from a high-residue diet and bulk medication, such as psyllium.

Treatment of mild diverticulitis without signs of perforation must prevent constipation and combat infection. Therapy may include bed rest, a liquid diet, stool softeners, a broad-spectrum antibiotic, meperidine to control pain and relax smooth muscle, and an antispasmodic, such as propantheline, to control muscle spasms.

For more severe diverticulitis, treatment consists of the above measures and I.V. therapy. A nasogastric (NG) tube to relieve intra-abdominal pressure is usually required, and the patient is allowed nothing by mouth.

Patients who hemorrhage need blood replacement and careful monitoring of fluid and electrolyte balance. Such bleeding usually stops spontaneously. If it continues, angiography for catheter placement and infusion of vasopressin into the bleeding vessel is effective. Rarely, surgery may be required.

A colon resection to remove a diseased segment of intestine may be required to treat diverticulitis that is unresponsive to medical treatment or that causes severe recurrent attacks in the same area.

Nursing diagnoses

• Altered gastrointestinal tissue perfusion
• Anxiety
• Constipation
• Diarrhea
• Fluid volume deficit
• Pain

Nursing interventions

• Keep in mind that diverticulitis, which produces more serious symptoms and complications, usually requires more interventions than diverticulosis.

• If the patient is anxious, provide psychological support. Listen to his concerns and offer reassurance, when appropriate.

• Administer medications (antibiotics, stool softeners, antispasmodics), as ordered. Monitor the patient for the desired effects, and observe for possible adverse reactions. If pain is severe, also administer analgesics, such as meperidine, as ordered.

• Inspect all stools carefully for color and consistency. Note the frequency of bowel movements.

• Maintain bed rest for the patient with acute diverticulitis. Don't permit him to perform any actions that increase intra-abdominal pressure, such as lifting, straining, bending, or coughing.

• Maintain the diet as ordered. The patient experiencing an acute attack is usually maintained on a liquid diet. If the patient's symptoms are severe, or if he experiences nausea and vomiting or abdominal distention, insert an NG tube and attach it to intermittent suction, as ordered. Make sure this patient receives nothing by mouth, and administer ordered I.V. fluids. As symptoms subside, gradually advance the diet.

• Monitor the patient for signs and symptoms of complications. Watch for temperature elevation, increasing abdominal pain, blood in stools, and leukocytosis.

• If diverticular bleeding occurs, the patient may require angiography and catheter placement for vasopressin infusion. If so, inspect the insertion site frequently for bleeding, check pedal pulses often, and keep the patient from flexing his legs at the groin. Also watch for vasopressin-induced fluid retention (apprehension, abdominal cramps, seizures, oliguria, or anuria) and severe hyponatremia (hypotension; rapid, thready pulse; cold, clammy skin; and cyanosis).

• If surgery is scheduled, provide routine preoperative care. Also perform any special required procedures, such as administering antibiotics or providing a specific diet for several days preoperatively.

After colon resection:
• Watch for signs of infection. Provide meticulous wound care because perforation may have already infected the area. Check drainage sites frequently for signs of infection (pus on dressing, foul odor) or fecal drainage. Change dressings as necessary.

• Encourage coughing and deep breathing to prevent atelectasis.

• Watch for such signs of postoperative bleeding as hypotension or decreased hemoglobin and hematocrit levels.
• Record intake and output accurately. Administer I.V. fluids and medications, as ordered.
• Keep the NG tube patent. If it dislodges, notify the surgeon at once; don't attempt to reposition it yourself. After the NG tube is removed, advance the patient's diet as ordered, and note how he tolerates diet changes.
• If the patient has a colostomy, care for it and give him an opportunity to express his feelings.

Patient teaching
• In uncomplicated diverticulosis, patient teaching focuses on bowel and dietary habits.
• Explain what diverticula are and how they form. Teach the patient about necessary diagnostic tests and prescribed treatments.
• Be sure the patient understands the desired actions and possible adverse effects of his prescribed medications.
• Review recommended dietary changes. Encourage the patient to drink 2 to 3 liters of fluid daily. Emphasize the importance of dietary roughage and the harmful effects of constipation and straining during a bowel movement. Advise him to increase his intake of foods high in undigestible fiber, such as fresh fruits and vegetables, whole grain breads, and wheat or bran cereals. Warn that a high-fiber diet may temporarily cause flatulence.
• Advise the patient to relieve constipation with stool softeners or bulk-forming cathartics. Instruct him to take bulk-forming cathartics with plenty of water; if swallowed dry, they may absorb enough moisture in the mouth and throat to swell and obstruct the esophagus or trachea.
• Teach the patient to notify the doctor if he experiences a temperature above 101° F (38.3° C); abdominal pain that is severe or that lasts for more than 3 days; or blood in his stools. Emphasize that these symptoms indicate complications.
• Provide preoperative teaching to the patient needing surgery. Reinforce the doctor's explanation of the surgery, and discuss possible complications.
• Postoperatively, teach the patient to care for his colostomy, as needed. Arrange for a visit by an enterostomal therapist.

APPENDICITIS

The most common major surgical disease, appendicitis is an inflammation of the vermiform appendix, a small, fingerlike projection attached to the cecum just below the ileocecal valve. Although the appendix has no known function, it does regularly fill and empty itself of food. Appendicitis occurs when the appendix becomes inflamed from ulceration of the mucosa or obstruction of the lumen.

Appendicitis may occur at any age and affects both sexes equally; however, between puberty and age 25, it's more prevalent in men. Since the advent of antibiotics, the incidence and death rate of appendicitis have declined. If untreated, this disease is invariably fatal.

Causes
Appendicitis probably results from an obstruction of the appendiceal lumen, caused by a fecal mass, stricture, barium ingestion, or viral infection. This obstruction sets off an inflammatory process that can lead to infection, thrombosis, necrosis, and perforation.

Complications
The most common and perilous complication of appendicitis occurs when the appendix ruptures or perforates. When this happens, the infected contents spill into the abdominal cavity, causing peritonitis. Other complications include appendiceal abscess and pyelophlebitis.

Assessment findings
During the initial phase of appendicitis, the patient typically complains of abdominal pain. Pain may be generalized, but within a few hours, becomes localized in the right lower abdomen (McBurney's point). He may also report anorexia, nausea, and one or two episodes of vomiting. Later signs and symptoms include malaise, constipation, or diarrhea (rare). He may have a low-grade fever.

Inspection typically shows a patient who walks bent over to reduce right lower quadrant pain. When sleeping or lying supine, he may keep his right knee bent up to decrease pain.

Auscultation usually reveals normal bowel sounds. Initially, palpation and percussion disclose no localized abdominal findings except for diffuse tenderness in the midepigastrium and around the umbilicus. Later, palpation may disclose tenderness in the right lower abdominal quadrant that worsens when the patient is asked to cough or upon gentle percussion. Rebound tenderness and spasm of the abdominal muscles are also usually present.

If the appendix is positioned retrocecally or in the pelvis, abdominal tenderness may be completely absent; instead, rectal or pelvic examination reveals tenderness in the flank.

Keep in mind that abdominal rigidity and tenderness worsen as the condition progresses. Sudden cessation of abdominal pain signals perforation or infarction.

Diagnostic tests
A finding of a moderately elevated white blood cell count, with increased numbers of immature cells, supports the diagnosis. The use of an enema containing a radiographic contrast agent (a diatrizoate meglumine and diatrizoate sodium solution) may aid the diagnosis. The radiologist attempts to fill the appendix with the contrast agent; failure of the organ to fill indicates appendicitis.

Diagnosis must rule out illnesses with similar symptoms: bladder infection, diverticulitis, gastritis, ovarian cyst, pancreatitis, renal colic, and uterine disease.

Treatment
Appendectomy is the only effective treatment. If peritonitis develops, treatment involves GI intubation, parenteral replacement of fluids and electrolytes, and administration of antibiotics.

Nursing diagnoses
• Altered gastrointestinal tissue perfusion
• Altered nutrition: Less than body requirements
• Impaired skin integrity
• Pain
• Risk for fluid volume deficit

Nursing interventions
• Make sure the patient with suspected or known appendicitis receives nothing by mouth until surgery is performed. Administer I.V. fluids to prevent dehydration. Never administer cathartics or enemas because they may rupture the appendix.
• Don't administer analgesics until the diagnosis is confirmed because they mask symptoms. Once the diagnosis is confirmed, analgesics may be given.
• Place the patient in Fowler's position to reduce pain. (This is also helpful postoperatively.) Never apply heat to the right lower abdomen; this may cause the appendix to rupture.
• Once the diagnosis is confirmed, provide preoperative care, such as administering prescribed preoperative medications.

After appendectomy:
• Monitor vital signs and intake and output.
• Give analgesics, as ordered.
• Administer I.V. fluids, as necessary, to maintain fluid and electrolyte balance.

• Document bowel sounds, passing of flatus, or bowel movements — signs of peristalsis. These signs in a patient whose nausea and boardlike abdominal rigidity have subsided indicate readiness to resume oral fluids.
• Watch closely for possible surgical complications, such as an abscess or wound dehiscence.
• If peritonitis occurs, nasogastric drainage may be necessary to decompress the stomach and reduce nausea and vomiting. If so, record drainage, and provide good mouth and nose care.

Patient teaching
• Explain what happens in appendicitis.
• Help the patient understand the required surgery and its possible complications. If time allows, provide preoperative teaching.
• Teach the patient how to care for the incision. If he has a surgical dressing, demonstrate how to change it properly. Instruct him to observe the incision daily and to report any swelling, redness, bleeding, drainage, and warmth at the site.
• Review the proper use of all prescribed medications. Be sure the patient knows how to administer each drug and understands the desired effects and possible adverse reactions.
• Discuss postoperative activity limitations with the patient. Caution him to avoid lifting heavy objects for 6 weeks after surgery. Explain that this precaution prevents strain on abdominal muscles until healing is complete. Tell him to follow the doctor's orders for driving and returning to work.

PERITONITIS
An acute or chronic disorder, peritonitis is an inflammation of the peritoneum, the membrane that lines the abdominal cavity and covers the visceral organs. Such inflammation may extend throughout the peritoneum or be localized as an abscess. Peritonitis commonly decreases intestinal motility and causes intestinal distention with gas. Mortality is about 10%, with bowel obstruction the usual cause of death.

Causes
Although the GI tract normally contains bacteria, the peritoneum is sterile. In peritonitis, however, bacteria invade the peritoneum. Generally, such infection results from inflammation and perforation of the GI tract, allowing bacterial invasion. Usually, this is a result of appendicitis, diverticulitis, peptic ulcer, ulcerative colitis, volvulus, strangulated obstruction, abdominal neoplasm,

or a stab wound. Peritonitis can also result from chemical inflammation after rupture of a fallopian tube, ovarian cyst, or the bladder; perforation of a gastric ulcer; or released pancreatic enzymes.

In both bacterial and chemical inflammation, fluid containing protein and electrolytes accumulates in the peritoneal cavity and makes the transparent peritoneum opaque, red, inflamed, and edematous. Because the peritoneal cavity is so resistant to contamination, such infection is often localized as an abscess instead of disseminated as a generalized infection.

Complications
Peritonitis can lead to abscess formation, septicemia, respiratory compromise, bowel obstruction, and shock.

Assessment findings
The patient's symptoms depend on when the disorder is assessed—early or late in its course. In the early phase, he may report vague, generalized abdominal pain. If peritonitis is localized, he may describe pain over a specific area (usually over the site of inflammation); if the peritonitis is generalized, he may complain of diffuse pain over the abdomen.

As the disorder progresses, the patient typically reports increasingly severe and constant abdominal pain. Pain often increases with movement and respirations. Occasionally, pain may be referred to the shoulder or the thoracic area. Other signs and symptoms include abdominal distention, anorexia, nausea, vomiting, and an inability to pass feces and flatus.

Assessment of vital signs may reveal fever, tachycardia (a response to the fever), and hypotension. On inspection, the patient usually appears acutely distressed. He may lie very still in bed, often with his knees flexed to try to alleviate abdominal pain. He tends to breathe shallowly and move as little as possible to minimize pain. If he loses excessive fluid, electrolytes, and proteins into the abdominal cavity, you may observe excessive sweating, cold skin, pallor, abdominal distention, and signs of dehydration, such as dry mucous membranes.

Early in peritonitis, auscultation usually discloses bowel sounds; as the inflammation progresses, these sounds tend to disappear. Abdominal rigidity is usually felt on palpation. If peritonitis spreads throughout the abdomen, palpation may disclose general tenderness; if peritonitis stays in a specific area, you may detect local tenderness. Rebound tenderness may also be present.

Diagnostic tests
The following tests support the diagnosis:
• *White blood cell count* shows leukocytosis (commonly more than 20,000/mm^3).
• *Abdominal X-rays* demonstrate edematous and gaseous distention of the small and large bowel. With perforation of a visceral organ, the X-ray shows air in the abdominal cavity.
• *Chest X-ray* may reveal elevation of the diaphragm.
• *Paracentesis* discloses the nature of the exudate and permits bacterial culture so appropriate antibiotic therapy can be instituted.

Treatment
To prevent peritonitis, early treatment of GI inflammatory conditions and preoperative and postoperative antibiotic therapy are important. After peritonitis develops, emergency treatment must combat infection, restore intestinal motility, and replace fluids and electrolytes.

Antibiotic therapy depends on the infecting organism but usually includes administration of cefoxitin with an aminoglycoside or penicillin G and clindamycin with an aminoglycoside. To decrease peristalsis and prevent perforation, the patient should receive nothing by mouth; instead, he requires supportive fluids and electrolytes parenterally.

Supplementary treatment includes administration of an analgesic, such as meperidine; nasogastric (NG) intubation to decompress the bowel; and possible use of a rectal tube to facilitate the passage of flatus.

The treatment of choice, surgery eliminates the cause of peritonitis. Surgery, which is necessary as soon as the patient's condition is stable enough to tolerate it, aims to eliminate the source of infection by evacuating the spilled contents and inserting drains.

The surgical procedure varies with the cause of peritonitis. For example, if appendicitis is the cause, an appendectomy is performed; if the colon is perforated, a colon resection may be performed. Occasionally, abdominocentesis may be necessary to remove accumulated fluid. Irrigation of the abdominal cavity with antibiotic solutions during surgery may be appropriate.

Nursing diagnoses
• Altered gastrointestinal tissue perfusion
• Altered nutrition: Less than body requirements
• Fear
• Fluid volume deficit
• Pain

Nursing interventions

• Provide psychological support, and offer encouragement when appropriate.
• Administer prescribed medications, such as analgesics and antibiotics, as ordered; monitor the patient for desired effects and possible adverse reactions.
• Maintain parenteral fluid and electrolyte administration, as ordered. Monitor fluid volume by checking skin turgor, mucous membranes, urine output, weight, vital signs, amount of NG tube drainage, and amount of I.V. infusion. Accurately record intake and output, including NG tube drainage.
• Maintain bed rest, and place the patient in semi-Fowler's position to help him breathe deeply with less pain and thus prevent pulmonary complications.
• Counteract mouth and nose dryness due to fever, dehydration, and NG intubation with regular hygiene and lubrication.

After surgery:
• Place the patient in Fowler's position to promote drainage (through drainage tube) by gravity. Move him carefully because the slightest movement will intensify the pain. Keep the bed's side rails up and implement other safety measures if fever and pain disorient the patient.
• Immediately after surgery, monitor the patient's pain, vital signs, level of consciousness, respiratory status, bowel signs and abdominal distention, incisional drainage, urine output, NG tube drainage, and I.V. fluid intake at least once every hour, or as ordered.
• Allow the patient nothing by mouth, as ordered, until NG tube suction is discontinued. Administer parenteral feedings as ordered.
• If necessary, administer ordered blood transfusions.
• Encourage and assist ambulation, as ordered, usually on the first postoperative day.
• Frequently assess for peristaltic activity by listening for bowel sounds and checking for flatus, bowel movements, and a soft abdomen. When peristalsis resumes, and temperature and pulse rate become normal, gradually decrease parenteral fluids and increase oral fluids. If the patient has an NG tube in place, clamp it for short intervals. If nausea or vomiting doesn't result, begin oral fluids, as ordered and tolerated.
• Watch for signs of dehiscence (the patient may complain that "something gave way") and abscess formation (continued abdominal tenderness and fever).
• If necessary, refer the patient to the hospital's social service department or a home health care agency that can help him obtain needed services during convalescence.

Patient teaching

• Teach the patient about peritonitis, its cause (in his case), and necessary treatments. If time allows, before surgery, reinforce the doctor's explanation of the procedure and its possible complications. Tell him how long he can expect to be hospitalized; many patients remain hospitalized for 2 weeks or more after surgery.
• Provide teaching before surgery. Include coughing and deep-breathing instructions. Review postoperative care procedures.
• Instruct the patient to report any swelling, drainage, bleeding, redness, warmth, or odor from the incision. Teach him how to care for the incision, including how to change the dressing and how to irrigate the wound, if necessary.
• Discuss the proper use of prescribed medications, reviewing their correct administration, desired effects, and possible adverse reactions.
• Review diet and activity limitations with the patient (depending on his type of surgery). Typically, he must avoid lifting for at least 6 weeks postoperatively.

INTESTINAL OBSTRUCTION

Commonly a medical emergency, intestinal obstruction is the partial or complete blockage of the small- or large-bowel lumen. Complete obstruction in any part of the bowel, if untreated, can cause death within hours from shock and vascular collapse. Intestinal obstruction is most likely after abdominal surgery or in persons with congenital bowel deformities.

Causes and pathophysiology

Intestinal obstruction results from mechanical or nonmechanical (neurogenic) blockage of the lumen. Causes of mechanical obstruction include adhesions and strangulated hernias (usually associated with small-bowel obstruction); carcinomas (usually associated with large-bowel obstruction); foreign bodies, such as fruit pits, gallstones, or worms; compression of the bowel wall from stenosis; intussusception; volvulus of the sigmoid or cecum; tumors; or atresia.

Nonmechanical obstruction usually results from paralytic ileus, the most common of all intestinal obstructions. Paralytic ileus is a physiologic form of intestinal obstruction that usually develops in the small bowel after abdominal surgery. Other nonmechanical causes of obstruction include electrolyte imbalances; toxicity, such as that associated with uremia or generalized infection; neurogenic abnormalities, such as spinal cord lesions; and thrombosis or embolism of mesenteric vessels.

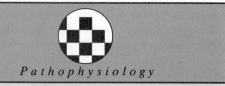

Pathophysiology

EFFECTS OF INTESTINAL OBSTRUCTION

Intestinal obstruction develops in three forms:
• *Simple.* Blockage prevents intestinal contents from passing, with no other complications.
• *Strangulated.* Blood supply to part or all of the obstructed section is cut off, in addition to blockage of the lumen.
• *Close-looped.* Both ends of a bowel section are occluded, isolating it from the rest of the intestine.

In all three forms, the physiologic effects are similar: When intestinal obstruction occurs, fluid, air, and gas collect near the site. Peristalsis increases temporarily as the bowel tries to force its contents through the obstruction, injuring intestinal mucosa and causing distention at and above the site of the obstruction.

Because distention blocks venous blood flow, normal absorptive processes cease. As a result, the bowel begins to secrete water, sodium, and potassium into the fluid pooled in the lumen. Obstruction in the upper intestine results in metabolic alkalosis from dehydration and loss of gastric hydrochloric acid. Obstruction in the lower intestine causes slower dehydration and loss of intestinal alkaline fluids, resulting in metabolic acidosis.

Ultimately, intestinal obstruction may lead to ischemia, necrosis, and death.

Although intestinal obstruction may occur in several forms, the underlying pathophysiology is similar. (See *Effects of intestinal obstruction.*)

Complications

Intestinal obstruction can lead to perforation, peritonitis, septicemia, secondary infection, metabolic alkalosis or acidosis, hypovolemic or septic shock and, if untreated, death.

Assessment findings

Investigation of the patient's history often reveals predisposing factors, such as surgery (especially abdominal surgery), radiation therapy, or gallstones. The history may also disclose certain illnesses, such as Crohn's disease, diverticular disease, or ulcerative colitis, that can lead to obstruction. Family history may reveal colorectal cancer among one or more relatives. *Caution:* If the patient reports a recent change in bowel habits or blood in his stools, colon cancer may be the cause of obstruction.

Hiccups are a common complaint in all types of bowel obstruction. Other specific assessment findings depend on the cause of obstruction—mechanical or nonmechanical—and its location in the bowel.

Mechanical obstruction of the small bowel

The patient may complain of colicky pain, nausea, vomiting, and constipation. If obstruction is complete, he may report vomiting of fecal contents. This results from vigorous peristaltic waves that propel bowel contents toward the mouth instead of the rectum.

Inspection may reveal a distended abdomen, the hallmark of all types of mechanical obstruction. Auscultation may detect bowel sounds, borborygmi, and rushes (occasionally loud enough to be heard without a stethoscope). Palpation may disclose abdominal tenderness. Rebound tenderness may be noted in patients with obstruction that results from strangulation with ischemia.

Mechanical obstruction of the large bowel

In this patient, a history of constipation is common, with a more gradual onset of signs and symptoms than in small-bowel obstruction. Several days after constipation begins, the patient may report the sudden onset of colicky abdominal pain, producing spasms that last less than 1 minute and recur every few minutes.

The patient history may reveal constant hypogastric pain, nausea, and, in the later stages, vomiting. He may describe his vomitus as orange-brown and foul-smelling, which is characteristic of large-bowel obstruction. On inspection, the abdomen may appear dramatically distended, with visible loops of large bowel. Auscultation may reveal loud, high-pitched borborygmi.

Partial obstruction usually causes similar signs and symptoms, in a milder form. Leakage of liquid stools around the partial obstruction is common.

Nonmechanical obstruction

The patient with a nonmechanical form of obstruction, such as paralytic ileus, usually describes diffuse abdominal discomfort instead of colicky pain. Typically, he also reports frequent vomiting, which may consist of gastric and bile contents but, rarely, fecal contents. He may also complain of constipation and hiccups.

If obstruction results from vascular insufficiency or infarction, the patient may complain of severe abdominal pain. On inspection, the abdomen is distended. Early in the disease, auscultation discloses decreased bowel sounds; this sign disappears as the disorder progresses.

Diagnostic tests

Various tests help to establish the diagnosis and pinpoint complications.

• *Abdominal X-rays* confirm intestinal obstruction and reveal the presence and location of intestinal gas or fluid. In small-bowel obstruction, a typical "stepladder" pattern emerges, with alternating fluid and gas levels apparent in 3 to 4 hours. In large-bowel obstruction, barium enema reveals a distended, air-filled colon or a closed loop of sigmoid with extreme distention (in sigmoid volvulus).

• *Serum sodium, chloride,* and *potassium levels* may fall because of vomiting.

• *White blood cell counts* may be normal or slightly elevated if necrosis, peritonitis, or strangulation occurs.

• *Serum amylase level* may increase, possibly from irritation of the pancreas by a bowel loop.

• *Hemoglobin concentration* and *hematocrit* may increase, indicating dehydration.

• *Sigmoidoscopy, colonoscopy,* or a *barium enema* may help determine the cause of obstruction; however, these tests are contraindicated if perforation is suspected.

Treatment

Surgery is usually the treatment of choice. One important exception is paralytic ileus in which nonoperative therapy is usually attempted first. The type of surgery depends on the cause of blockage. For example, if a tumor is obstructing the intestine, a colon resection with anastomosis is performed; if adhesions are obstructing the lumen, these are lysed.

Surgical preparation is often lengthy, taking as long as 6 to 8 hours. It includes correction of fluid and electrolyte imbalances; decompression of the bowel to relieve vomiting and distention; treatment of shock and peritonitis; and administration of broad-spectrum antibiotics. Often, decompression is begun preoperatively with passage of a nasogastric (NG) tube attached to continuous suction. This tube relieves vomiting, reduces abdominal distention, and prevents aspiration. In strangulating obstruction, preoperative therapy also usually requires blood replacement and I.V. fluids.

Postoperative care involves careful patient monitoring and interventions geared to the type of surgery. Total parenteral nutrition may be ordered if the patient has a protein deficit from chronic obstruction, postoperative or paralytic ileus, or infection.

Nonsurgical treatment may be attempted in some patients with partial obstruction, particularly those who suffer recurrent partial obstruction or who developed it after surgery or a recent episode of diffuse peritonitis.

Nonsurgical treatment usually includes decompression with an NG tube attached to low-pressure continuous suction; correction of fluid and electrolyte deficits; administration of broad-spectrum antibiotics; and, occasionally, total parenteral nutrition. Rarely, a long nasointestinal tube is used for decompression.

Throughout nonsurgical treatment, the patient's condition must be closely monitored. If he fails to improve or his condition deteriorates, surgery is required.

Another indication for nonsurgical treatment is nonmechanical obstruction from adynamic ileus (paralytic ileus). Most of these cases occur postoperatively and disappear spontaneously in 2 or 3 days. However, if the disorder doesn't resolve in 48 hours, treatment consists of decompression with an NG tube attached to low-pressure continuous suction. Oral intake is restricted until bowel function resumes; then, the diet is gradually advanced.

In the patient with paralytic ileus, decompression occasionally responds to colonoscopy or rectal tube insertion. When paralytic ileus develops secondary to another illness, such as severe infection or electrolyte imbalance, the primary problem must also be treated. Again, if conservative treatment fails, surgery is required.

In both surgical and nonsurgical treatment, drug therapy includes antibiotics and analgesics or sedatives, such as meperidine or phenobarbital (but not opiates because they inhibit GI motility).

Nursing diagnoses

• Altered gastrointestinal tissue perfusion
• Altered nutrition: Less than body requirements
• Constipation
• Fluid volume deficit
• Pain

Nursing interventions

• Because intestinal obstruction may be fatal and often causes overwhelming pain and distress, patients require skillful supportive care and keen observation.

• Allow the patient nothing by mouth, as ordered, but be sure to provide frequent mouth care to help keep mucous membranes moist. Look for signs of dehydration (thick, swollen tongue; dry, cracked lips; dry oral mucous membranes). If surgery won't be performed, he may be allowed a small amount of ice chips. Avoid using lemon-glycerin swabs, which can increase mouth dryness.

• Insert an NG tube to decompress the bowel, as ordered. Attach to low-pressure, intermittent suction. Monitor drainage for color, consistency, and amount. Irrigate the tube, if necessary, with 0.9% sodium chloride solution to maintain patency.

• If ordered, assist with insertion of a weighted nasointestinal tube, such as a Miller-Abbott, Cantor, or Harris tube. If a weighted tube has been inserted, check periodically to make sure it's advancing. Help the patient turn from side to side (or walk around, if he can) to facilitate passage of the tube.

• Begin and maintain I.V. therapy, as ordered. Monitor intake and output. Maintain fluid and electrolyte balance by monitoring electrolyte, blood urea nitrogen, and creatinine levels. Provide I.V. fluids to keep levels within normal ranges.

• Monitor vital signs frequently. A drop in blood pressure may indicate reduced circulating blood volume due to blood loss from a strangulated hernia. Remember, as much as 10 liters of fluid can collect in the small bowel, drastically reducing plasma volume. Observe closely for signs of shock (pallor, rapid pulse, and hypotension). Provide blood replacement therapy, as necessary.

• Administer analgesics, broad-spectrum antibiotics, and other medications as ordered. Monitor the patient for the desired effects and for adverse reactions.

• Keep in mind that analgesics may be withheld until a diagnosis is confirmed. To ease discomfort, help the patient to change positions frequently. Continually assess his pain. Remember, colicky pain that suddenly becomes constant could signal perforation.

• Watch for signs of metabolic alkalosis (changes in sensorium; slow, shallow respirations; hypertonic muscles; tetany) or acidosis (shortness of breath on exertion; disorientation; and, later, deep, rapid breathing, weakness, and malaise). Watch for signs and symptoms of secondary infection, such as fever and chills.

• Monitor urine output carefully to assess renal function, circulating blood volume, and possible urine retention due to bladder compression by the distended intestine. If you suspect bladder compression, catheterize the patient for residual urine immediately after he has voided. Also measure abdominal girth frequently to detect progressive distention.

• Keep the patient in semi-Fowler's or Fowler's position as much as possible. These positions help to promote pulmonary ventilation and ease respiratory distress from abdominal distention. Listen for bowel sounds, and watch for other signs of resuming peristalsis (passage of flatus and mucus through the rectum).

• If surgery is scheduled, prepare the patient as required.

• After surgery, provide all necessary postoperative care. Care for the surgical site, maintain fluid and electrolyte balance, relieve pain and discomfort, maintain respiratory status, and monitor intake and output.

Patient teaching

• Teach the patient about his disorder, focusing on his type of intestinal obstruction, its cause, and signs and symptoms. Listen to his questions and take time to answer them.

• Explain necessary diagnostic tests and treatments. Make sure the patient understands that these procedures are necessary to relieve the obstruction and reduce pain. Instruct him in pretest guidelines; for example, advise him to lie on his left side for about a half hour before X-rays are taken.

• Prepare the patient and his family for the possibility of surgery. Provide preoperative teaching and reinforce the doctor's explanation of the surgery. Demonstrate techniques for coughing and deep breathing, and teach the patient how to use incentive spirometry.

• Tell the patient what to expect postoperatively. After surgery, if he has a colostomy or ileostomy, teach him how to care for it, and arrange for an enterostomal therapist to visit him. Also review incisional care. Provide emotional support and positive reinforcement before and after the surgery.

• Discuss postoperative activity limitations and point out why these restrictions are necessary.

• Review the proper use of prescribed medications, focusing on their correct administration, desired effects, and possible adverse reactions.

• Emphasize the importance of following a structured bowel regimen, particularly if the patient had a mechanical obstruction from fecal impaction. Encourage him to eat a high-fiber diet and to exercise daily.

• Reassure the patient who had an obstruction from paralytic ileus that recurrence is unlikely. However, remind him to report any recurrence of abdominal pain, abdominal distention, nausea, or vomiting.

INGUINAL HERNIA

When part of an internal organ protrudes through an abnormal opening in the containing wall of its cavity, a hernia results. In an inguinal hernia—the most common type—the large or small intestine, omentum, or bladder protrudes into the inguinal canal.

Hernias can be reducible (if the hernia can be manipulated back into place with relative ease); incarcerated (if the hernia can't be reduced because adhesions have formed in the hernial sac); or strangulated (if part of the herniated intestine becomes twisted or edematous, causing serious complications).

Inguinal hernias can be direct (herniation through an area of muscle weakness in the inguinal canal) or indirect (herniation through the inguinal ring). Indirect hernias, the more common form, can develop at any age but are especially prevalent in infants under age 1. This form is three times more common in males.

Causes

Inguinal hernias result from abdominal muscles weakened by congenital malformation, traumatic injury, or aging; or from increased intra-abdominal pressure (due to heavy lifting, exertion, pregnancy, obesity, excessive coughing, or straining with defecation).

Inguinal hernia is a common congenital malformation that may occur in males during the seventh month of gestation. Normally, at this time, the testicle descends into the scrotum, preceded by the peritoneal sac. If the sac closes improperly, it leaves an opening through which the intestine can slip, causing a hernia.

Complications

Inguinal hernia may lead to incarceration or strangulation. Strangulation may seriously interfere with normal blood flow and peristalsis, possibly leading to intestinal obstruction and necrosis.

Assessment findings

The patient history may reveal precipitating factors, such as weight lifting, recent pregnancy, or excessive coughing. Usually, the patient reports the appearance of a lump in the inguinal area when he stands or strains. He may also complain of sharp, steady groin pain, which tends to worsen when tension is placed on the hernia and improve when the hernia is reduced.

If the patient has a large hernia, inspection may reveal an obvious swelling in the inguinal area. If he has a small hernia, the affected area may simply appear full. As part of your inspection, have the patient lie down. If the hernia disappears, it is reducible. Also ask him to perform Valsalva's maneuver; while he does so, inspect the inguinal area for characteristic bulging.

Auscultation should reveal bowel sounds. The absence of bowel sounds may indicate incarceration or strangulation. Palpation helps to determine the size of an obvious hernia. It also can disclose the presence of a hernia in a male patient. (See *Detecting inguinal hernia*.)

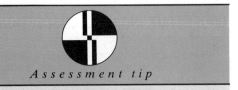

Assessment tip

DETECTING INGUINAL HERNIA

To detect a hernia in a male patient, ask him to stand, keeping the leg on the side to be examined slightly flexed and resting his weight on the other leg.

Insert an index finger into the lower part of the scrotum and invaginate the scrotal skin so that the finger advances through the external inguinal ring (about 1½″ to 2″ [about 4 to 5 cm]). Tell the patient to cough.

If you feel pressure against your fingertip, an indirect hernia exists; if you feel pressure against the side of your finger, a direct hernia exists.

Diagnostic tests

Although assessment findings are the cornerstone of diagnosis, suspected bowel obstruction requires X-rays and a white blood cell count (may be elevated).

Treatment

The choice of therapy depends on the type of hernia. For a reducible hernia, temporary relief may result from moving the protruding organ back into place. Afterward, a truss may be applied to keep the abdominal contents from protruding through the hernial sac. (A truss is a firm pad, with a belt attached, that is placed over the hernia to keep it reduced.) Although a truss can't cure a hernia, the device is especially helpful for an elderly or a debilitated patient, for whom any surgery is potentially hazardous.

Herniorrhaphy is the preferred surgical treatment for infants, adults, and otherwise healthy elderly patients. This procedure replaces hernial sac contents into the abdominal cavity and seals the opening. Another effective procedure is hernioplasty, which reinforces the weakened area with steel mesh, fascia, or wire.

A strangulated or necrotic hernia requires bowel resection. Rarely, an extensive resection may require a temporary colostomy.

Nursing diagnoses
• Activity intolerance
• Altered gastrointestinal tissue perfusion
• Pain
• Risk for injury

UNDERSTANDING INTUSSUSCEPTION

In intussusception, a bowel segment invaginates and is propelled along by peristalsis, pulling in more bowel. In this illustration, a portion of the cecum invaginates and is propelled into the large intestine. Intussusception typically produces edema, hemorrhage from venous engorgement, incarceration, and obstruction.

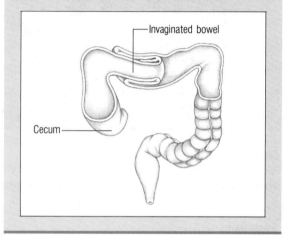

Invaginated bowel

Cecum

Nursing interventions

• Apply a truss only after a hernia has been reduced. For best results, apply it in the morning before the patient gets out of bed. Assess the skin daily and apply powder for protection because the truss may be irritating.
• Watch for and immediately report signs of incarceration and strangulation. Don't try to reduce an incarcerated hernia; doing so may perforate the bowel. If severe intestinal obstruction arises because of hernial strangulation, tell the doctor immediately. A nasogastric (NG) tube may be inserted promptly to empty the stomach and relieve pressure on the hernial sac.
• When surgery is scheduled, closely monitor vital signs and provide routine preoperative preparation. If necessary, administer I.V. fluids and analgesics for pain, as ordered. Control fever with acetaminophen or tepid sponge baths, as ordered. Place the patient in Trendelenburg's position to reduce pressure on the hernia site.
• After surgery, provide routine postoperative care. Don't allow the patient to cough, but do encourage deep breathing and frequent turning. Apply ice bags to the scrotum to reduce swelling and relieve pain; elevating the scrotum on rolled towels also reduces swelling. Administer

analgesics as necessary. In males, a jock strap or suspensory bandage may be used to provide support.

Patient teaching

• Explain what an inguinal hernia is and how it is usually treated. Point out that elective surgery is the treatment of choice and far safer than waiting until hernial complications develop, necessitating emergency surgery. Warn the patient that a strangulated hernia can require extensive bowel resection, involving a protracted hospital stay and, possibly, a colostomy.
• Teach the patient who will not undergo surgery to watch for signs of incarceration or strangulation. Tell him that severe pain, nausea, vomiting, and diarrhea may indicate complications. Warn him and his family that shock, high fever, and bloody stools are signs of complete obstruction and must be reported at once. Tell them that immediate surgery is needed if complications occur.
• If the patient uses a truss, instruct him to bathe daily and apply liberal amounts of cornstarch or baby powder to prevent skin irritation. Warn against applying the truss over clothing, which reduces its effectiveness and may cause slippage. Point out that wearing a truss doesn't cure a hernia and may be uncomfortable.
• If surgery is scheduled, provide preoperative teaching. Reinforce the doctor's explanation of the surgery and its possible complications. Reassure the patient that he'll have no tubes or drains after surgery unless his hernia was complicated by strangulation or incarceration.
• Tell the postoperative patient that he'll probably be able to return to work or school and resume all normal activities within 2 to 4 weeks. Remind him to obtain his doctor's permission before returning to work or completely resuming his normal activities.
• Before discharge, warn the patient against lifting or straining. Instruct him to watch for signs of infection (oozing, tenderness, warmth, or redness) at the incision site. Tell him to keep the incision clean and covered until the sutures are removed.
• Inform the postoperative patient that the risk of recurrence depends on the success of the surgery, his general health, and his life-style.

INTUSSUSCEPTION

Considered a pediatric emergency, intussusception occurs when a portion of the bowel telescopes or invaginates into an adjacent bowel portion. (See *Understanding intussusception.*) Because this disorder leads to bowel obstruction and other serious complications, it can be fatal, especially if treatment is delayed for more than 24 hours.

Intussusception is most common in infants and occurs three times more often in males than in females; about 87% of children with intussusception are under age 2; about 70% of these children are between 4 and 11 months old.

Causes
In infants, intussusception usually arises from unknown causes. In older children, polyps, hemangioma, lymphosarcoma, lymphoid hyperplasia, Meckel's diverticulum, or alterations in intestinal motility may trigger the process. In adults, intussusception most commonly results from benign or malignant tumors (65% of patients); other possible causes include polyps, Meckel's diverticulum, gastroenterostomy with herniation, or an appendiceal stump.

In addition, studies suggest that intussusception may be linked to viral infections because seasonal peaks are noted—in the spring and summer, coinciding with peak incidence of enteritis, and in the midwinter, coinciding with peak incidence of respiratory tract infections.

Complications
Without prompt treatment, strangulation of the intestine may occur, with gangrene, shock, perforation, and peritonitis. These complications can be fatal.

Assessment findings
If the patient is an infant or a child, the history may reveal intermittent attacks of colicky pain. Typically, this pain causes the child to scream, draw his legs up to his abdomen, turn pale and diaphoretic and, possibly, grunt. Parents may report that the child vomits, initially, stomach contents, and later, bile-stained or fecal material. Parents may describe the child's "currant jelly" stools, which contain a mixture of blood and mucus.

Inspection and palpation may reveal a distended, tender abdomen, with some guarding over the intussusception site. A sausage-shaped abdominal mass may be palpable in the right upper quadrant or in the midepigastrium if the transverse colon is involved. Rectal examination may show bloody mucus.

In the adult patient, the history may reveal nonspecific, chronic, and intermittent symptoms, such as colicky abdominal pain and tenderness, vomiting, diarrhea (occasionally constipation), bloody stools, and weight loss. He may describe abdominal pain that's localized in the right lower quadrant, radiates to the back, and increases with eating. The abdomen may be distended. Palpation may help pinpoint the tender area in the right lower quadrant.

In the adult patient, excruciating pain, abdominal distention, and tachycardia are signs that severe intussusception has led to strangulation.

Diagnostic tests
The following tests help to confirm the diagnosis:
• *Barium enema* confirms colonic intussusception when it shows the characteristic coiled-spring sign; it also delineates the extent of intussusception.
• *Upright abdominal X-rays* may show a soft-tissue mass and signs of complete or partial obstruction, with dilated loops of bowel.
• *White blood cell count* up to 15,000/mm³ indicates obstruction; more than 15,000/mm³, strangulation; more than 20,000/mm³, bowel infarction.

Treatment
In children, therapy may include hydrostatic reduction or surgery. Surgery is indicated for children with recurrent intussusception, for those who show signs of shock or peritonitis, and for those in whom symptoms have been present longer than 24 hours. In adults, surgery is always the treatment of choice.

During hydrostatic reduction, the radiologist drips a barium solution into the rectum through a catheter from a height of not more than 3' (0.9 m); fluoroscopy traces the progress of the barium. If the procedure is successful, the barium backwashes into the ileum, and the mass disappears. If not, the procedure is stopped, and the patient is prepared for surgery.

During surgery, manual reduction is attempted first. After compressing the bowel above the intussusception, the doctor attempts to milk the intussusception back through the bowel. However, if manual reduction fails, or if the bowel is gangrenous or strangulated, the doctor will perform a resection of the affected bowel segment.

Nursing diagnoses
• Altered gastrointestinal tissue perfusion
• Anxiety
• Fear
• Knowledge deficit
• Pain
• Risk for fluid volume deficit
• Risk for infection

Nursing interventions
• Offer reassurance and emotional support to the patient and, if the patient is a child, to his parents. Because this condition is considered a pediatric emergency, parents are often unprepared for their child's hospitalization and

WHAT HAPPENS IN VOLVULUS

Although volvulus may occur anywhere in a bowel segment long enough to twist, the most common site, as this illustration depicts, is the sigmoid colon. Here, a counterclockwise twist has occluded the colon, causing edema within the closed loop and obstruction at both its proximal and distal ends.

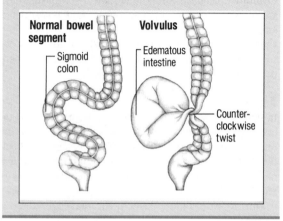

Normal bowel segment
— Sigmoid colon

Volvulus
— Edematous intestine
— Counterclockwise twist

possible surgery. Similarly, the child is unprepared for an abrupt separation from his parents and familiar environment.

• Monitor vital signs before and after surgery. A change in temperature may indicate sepsis; infants may become hypothermic at the onset of infection. Rising pulse rate and falling blood pressure may signal peritonitis.

• Check intake and output. Administer I.V. fluids, as ordered. Watch for signs of dehydration and bleeding. If the patient is in shock, give blood or plasma, as ordered.

• A nasogastric (NG) tube is inserted to decompress the intestine and minimize vomiting. Monitor tube drainage, and replace volume lost, as ordered.

• Monitor the patient who has undergone hydrostatic reduction for passage of stools and barium, a sign that the reduction has been successful. Keep in mind that a few patients have a recurrence of intussusception; this usually occurs within the first 36 to 48 hours after the hydrostatic reduction.

After surgery:

• Monitor NG tube drainage for color, consistency, and amount; check fluid and electrolyte balance. Frequently assess the patient for return of bowel sounds. Administer analgesics, broad-spectrum antibiotics, and I.V. fluids, as ordered.

• Provide meticulous wound care. Most incisions heal without complications. However, closely check the incision for inflammation, drainage, or suture separation. Encourage the patient to cough productively by turning him from side to side. Take care to splint the incision when he coughs and, if appropriate, teach him to do so himself. Make sure he takes 10 deep breaths an hour.

• Oral fluids may be reintroduced postoperatively when bowel sounds and peristalsis resume, NG tube drainage is minimal, the abdomen remains soft, and vomiting doesn't occur when the NG tube is clamped briefly for a trial period. When the patient tolerates oral fluids well, the tube can be removed and the patient's diet gradually returned to normal, as tolerated.

• Check for abdominal distention after the patient resumes a normal diet.

Patient teaching

• Depending on the patient's age, explain what happens in intussusception to him or his parents. Review required diagnostic tests and treatments. If hydrostatic reduction by barium enema will be attempted, be sure the patient or his parents understand the procedure. Let them know that surgery will be necessary if the procedure isn't successful.

• If surgery is required, provide preoperative teaching. Reinforce the doctor's explanation of the surgery and its possible complications.

• To minimize the stress of hospitalization, encourage parents to participate in their child's care as much as possible. Be flexible about visiting hours.

VOLVULUS

Marked by sudden onset of severe abdominal pain, volvulus is a twisting of the intestine at least 180 degrees on itself. Volvulus results in blood vessel compression and causes obstruction both proximal and distal to the twisted loop. (For more information, see *What happens in volvulus.*)

Volvulus occurs in a bowel segment long enough to twist. The most common area, particularly in adults, is the sigmoid colon; the small bowel is a common site in children. Other common sites include the stomach and cecum.

Causes

In volvulus, twisting may result from an anomaly of bowel rotation in utero, an ingested foreign body, or an adhesion. Volvulus secondary to meconium ileus may occur in patients with cystic fibrosis. In some patients, however, the cause is unknown.

Complications
Without immediate treatment, volvulus can lead to strangulation of the twisted bowel loop, ischemia, infarction, perforation, and fatal peritonitis.

Assessment findings
The patient with volvulus complains of severe abdominal pain and may report bilious vomiting. If the patient is an infant, the parents may report increased vomiting of feedings. The history may also reveal the passage of bloody stools.

On inspection, the patient appears to be in pain. Abdominal inspection and palpation may reveal distention and a palpable mass.

Diagnostic tests
• *X-rays.* Abdominal X-rays may show multiple distended bowel loops and a large bowel without gas; in midgut volvulus, abdominal X-rays may be normal.
• *Barium enema.* In cecal volvulus, barium fills the colon distal to the section of cecum; in sigmoid volvulus, barium may twist to a point; and, in adults, take on an "ace of spades" configuration.
• *White blood cell count.* In strangulation, the count is greater than 15,000/mm³; in bowel infarction, greater than 20,000 mm³.

Treatment
The severity and location of the volvulus determine therapy. For children with midgut volvulus, surgery is required. For adults with sigmoid volvulus, nonsurgical treatment includes proctoscopy to check for infarction and reduction by careful insertion of a flexible sigmoidoscope to deflate the bowel. Success of nonsurgical reduction is indicated by expulsion of gas and immediate relief of abdominal pain.

If the bowel is distended but viable, surgery consists of detorsion (untwisting); if the bowel is necrotic, surgery includes resection and anastomosis. Prolonged total parenteral nutrition and I.V. administration of antibiotics are usually necessary. Sedatives may be needed.

Nursing diagnoses
• Altered gastrointestinal tissue perfusion
• Altered nutrition: Less than body requirements
• Pain
• Risk for fluid volume deficit
• Risk for infection

Nursing interventions
• Provide psychological support. Listen to the patient's concerns, and offer reassurance; take time to answer his questions.
• Administer analgesics and broad-spectrum antibiotics, as ordered. Monitor the patient for desired effects and potential adverse reactions before and after surgery.
• Monitor vital signs, intake and output, and fluid and electrolyte balance.
• Administer I.V. fluids, as ordered.
• Insert a nasogastric (NG) tube and connect to low-pressure intermittent suction, if ordered, to relieve abdominal distention.
• Provide appropriate preoperative care, if surgery will be performed.
   After surgical correction of volvulus:
• Monitor vital signs, watching for temperature changes (a sign of sepsis), and a rapid pulse rate and falling blood pressure (signs of shock and peritonitis). If ordered, administer total parenteral nutrition. Carefully monitor fluid intake and output (including stools), electrolyte levels, and complete blood count. Be sure to measure and record drainage from the NG tube and any surgical drains.
• When bowel sounds and peristalsis resume, begin oral feedings with clear liquids, as ordered. Before removing the NG tube, clamp it for a trial period, and watch for abdominal distention. When solid food can be tolerated, gradually expand the diet.
• Encourage frequent coughing and deep breathing. Reposition the patient often, and suction him, as needed.
• Keep the dressings clean and dry. Record any excessive or unusual drainage. Later, check for incisional inflammation and suture separation.

Patient teaching
• Explain what happens in volvulus, using teaching aids, if available. Review its signs and symptoms, and possible complications. Discuss necessary diagnostic procedures and treatments.
• Reinforce the doctor's explanation of scheduled surgery and its possible complications. Provide preoperative teaching.
• If the patient is a child, encourage the parents to participate in his care to minimize the stress of hospitalization.
• If surgery was extensive, or if the patient's condition requires it, refer him and his family to the social service department and a local home health care agency.

HIRSCHSPRUNG'S DISEASE

A congenital disorder of the large intestine, Hirschsprung's disease (congenital megacolon, aganglionic megacolon) is characterized by the absence or marked reduction of parasympathetic ganglion cells in the colorectal wall. This disorder impairs intestinal motility and causes severe, intractable constipation.

Without prompt treatment, an infant with colonic obstruction may die within 24 hours from enterocolitis that leads to severe diarrhea and hypovolemic shock. With prompt treatment, the prognosis is good.

Hirschsprung's disease occurs in 1 in 2,000 to 1 in 5,000 live births. It's up to seven times more common in males than in females (although the aganglion intestinal segment is usually shorter in males than in females) and is more prevalent in whites. Total aganglionosis of the large intestine affects both sexes equally. Although clinical effects usually appear shortly after birth, mild symptoms may not be recognized until adolescence or early adulthood.

Causes

Hirschsprung's disease is believed to be caused by a congenital, usually familial, defect. The disease may coexist with other congenital anomalies, particularly trisomy 21 and anomalies of the urinary tract, such as megaloureter. Women with Hirschsprung's disease are at higher risk for having affected children.

Symptoms result when the aganglionic bowel segment contracts without the reciprocal relaxation needed to propel the feces forward. In 90% of patients, this aganglionic segment is in the rectosigmoid area, but it occasionally extends to the entire colon and parts of the small intestine.

Complications

Disease progression causes most complications, such as nutritional deficiencies, severe diarrhea, enterocolitis, and hypovolemic shock. In infants, the main cause of death is enterocolitis, caused by fecal stagnation that leads to bacterial overgrowth, production of bacterial toxins, intestinal irritation, profuse diarrhea, hypovolemic shock, and perforation.

Assessment findings

In a neonate with Hirschsprung's disease, the history commonly reveals failure to pass meconium within the first 24 to 48 hours after birth and vomiting of bile-stained or fecal contents. The family history may disclose that siblings, parents, or other relatives have had difficulty passing stools.

On inspection, the infant may have abdominal distention, causing him to breathe rapidly and, possibly, grunt. A fecal mass may be felt on palpation. Rectal examination reveals a rectum without stools; then, when the examining finger is withdrawn, an explosive gush of malodorous gas and liquid stools occurs.

In more advanced disease, the patient may have a history of anorexia, nausea, and lethargy. Inspection may show evidence of dehydration, such as pallor, loss of skin turgor, dry mucous membranes, and sunken eyes. In patients with severe disease, failure to grow is characterized by wasted extremities and loss of subcutaneous tissue, with a large protuberant abdomen.

The older infant, child, or adult usually complains of intractable constipation (usually requiring laxatives and enemas). In adolescents and adults, the examination also reveals poor physical condition as well as the symptoms described above.

Adult megacolon, though rare, usually affects men. The patient with this disorder may report a history of chronic, intermittent constipation, with possible rectal bleeding. On inspection, this patient appears in poor physical condition and has a distended abdomen.

Diagnostic tests

• *Rectal biopsy* showing absence of ganglion cells provides definitive diagnosis. Suction aspiration, using a small tube inserted into the rectum, may be performed initially.
• *Full-thickness surgical biopsy* (under general anesthesia) may be performed if findings from suction aspiration are inconclusive.
• *Barium enema* in older infants, children, and adults shows a narrow segment of distal colon with a sawtooth appearance and a funnel-shaped segment above it to help confirm the diagnosis and identify the extent of intestinal involvement. Significantly, infants with Hirschsprung's disease retain barium longer than the usual 12 to 24 hours, so delayed films are often helpful when other characteristic signs are absent.
• *Rectal manometry* detects failure of the internal anal sphincter to relax and contract.
• *Upright plain films of the abdomen* show marked colonic distention.

Treatment

Surgery to restore normal defecation is the treatment of choice. The most effective surgical procedure involves pulling the normal ganglionic segment through to the anus. Before surgery, a preliminary bowel prep with an antibiotic, such as neomycin or nystatin, is necessary.

Corrective surgery in an infant is usually delayed until the child is at least 10 months old and better able to withstand it. Management of an infant until the time of surgery consists of daily colonic lavage to empty the bowel. If total obstruction is present in the neonate, a temporary colostomy or ileostomy is necessary to decompress the colon.

Nursing diagnoses
• Altered nutrition: Less than body requirements
• Constipation
• Fluid volume deficit
• Knowledge deficit
• Risk for altered parenting
• Risk for impaired skin integrity
• Risk for infection

Nursing interventions
• Provide psychological support to the patient and his family. Because an infant with Hirschsprung's disease needs surgery and hospitalization so early in life, parents may have difficulty establishing an emotional bond with their child. To promote bonding, encourage them to participate in their child's care as much as possible.
• Monitor vital signs and intake and output, and maintain fluid and electrolyte balance.
• Keep the patient in an upright position. The infant can be placed in an infant seat.
• Observe the patient for signs of complications, such as fever, bloody diarrhea, and vomiting; notify the doctor immediately if any of these occur.
• Initiate and maintain I.V. therapy, as ordered. Administer antibiotics and monitor the patient for desired effects and possible adverse reactions.
• If ordered, insert a nasogastric (NG) tube connected to low-pressure, intermittent suction. Note the color, consistency, and amount of drainage.
• Provide adequate nutrition.
• If shock occurs, provide transfusions as ordered.

After colostomy or ileostomy:
• Place the infant in a heated incubator, with the temperature set at 98° to 99° F (36.6° to 37.2° C), or in a radiant warmer. Monitor vital signs, watching for sepsis and enterocolitis (increased respiratory rate with abdominal distention).
• Carefully monitor and record fluid intake and output (including drainage from an ileostomy or a colostomy) as well as electrolyte levels. An ileostomy is especially likely to cause excessive electrolyte losses. Also measure and record NG tube drainage, and replace fluids and electro-

lytes, as ordered. Check the stools carefully for excess water—a sign of fluid loss.
• Provide total parenteral nutrition, if ordered.
• Check the urine for specific gravity, glucose (total parenteral nutrition may lead to osmotic diuresis), and blood.
• To prevent aspiration pneumonia and skin breakdown, turn and reposition the patient often. Also, suction the nasopharynx frequently.
• Keep the area around the stoma clean and dry, and cover it with dressings or a colostomy or ileostomy appliance to absorb drainage. To prevent infection, use aseptic technique until the wound heals. Watch for prolapse, discoloration, or excessive bleeding (slight bleeding is common). To prevent excoriation, use a powder, such as karaya gum, or a protective stoma disk.
• Begin oral feedings, as ordered, when bowel sounds resume. An infant may best tolerate predigested formulas.

Before final corrective surgery:
• If a colostomy or an ileostomy isn't performed, perform colonic lavage at least once a day with 0.9% sodium chloride solution to evacuate the colon. Keep in mind that ordinary enemas and laxatives won't clean it adequately. Keep accurate records of how much lavage solution is instilled. Repeat lavage until the return solution is completely free of fecal particles.
• Administer antibiotics for bowel preparation, as ordered.

After final corrective surgery:
• Keep the wound clean and dry, and check for significant inflammation (some inflammation is normal). Don't use a rectal thermometer or suppository until the wound has healed. After 3 to 4 days, the infant will have a first bowel movement—a liquid stool—that will probably create discomfort. Record the number of stools.
• Check the urine for blood, especially in a boy; extensive surgical manipulation may cause bladder trauma.
• Watch for signs of possible anastomotic leaks (sudden development of abdominal distention unrelieved by gastric aspiration, temperature spike, extreme irritability), which may lead to pelvic abscess.
• Begin oral feedings when active bowel sounds resume and NG tube drainage decreases. As an additional check, clamp the NG tube for brief, intermittent periods, as ordered. If abdominal distention develops, the patient isn't ready to begin oral feedings. Begin oral feedings with clear fluids, increasing bulk as tolerated.

Patient teaching

• Explain the disorder to the patient and the parents. Be sure they understand necessary diagnostic tests and treatments.
• Before surgery, provide appropriate preoperative teaching to the patient or the parents. Reinforce the doctor's explanation of the procedure and its possible complications, as necessary.
• Instruct the patient or the parents, as appropriate, to recognize signs of fluid loss and dehydration (decreased urine output, sunken eyes, poor skin turgor) and of enterocolitis (sudden, marked abdominal distention, vomiting, diarrhea, fever, lethargy).
• Before discharge, if possible, make sure the parents or the adult patient consults an enterostomal therapist for valuable tips on colostomy or ileostomy care.
• If the patient is a child, instruct the parents to watch for foods that increase the number of stools and to avoid offering these foods. Reassure them that their child will, in time, probably gain sphincter control and eat a normal diet. But warn them that complete continence may take years to develop, and constipation may recur.

PANCREATITIS

Inflammation of the pancreas, or pancreatitis, occurs in acute and chronic forms and may stem from edema, necrosis, or hemorrhage. In men, the disorder is commonly associated with alcoholism, trauma, or peptic ulcer; in women, with biliary tract disease. The prognosis is good when pancreatitis follows biliary tract disease but poor when it follows alcoholism. Mortality reaches 60% when pancreatitis is associated with necrosis or hemorrhage.

Causes and pathophysiology

The most common causes of pancreatitis are biliary tract disease and alcoholism, but the disorder can also result from abnormal organ structure, metabolic or endocrine disorders (such as hyperlipidemia or hyperparathyroidism), pancreatic cysts or tumors, penetrating peptic ulcers, or trauma (blunt or iatrogenic, resulting from surgical manipulation). This disorder also can develop after the use of certain drugs, such as glucocorticoids, sulfonamides, thiazides, and oral contraceptives.

Pancreatitis may result as a complication of renal failure and kidney transplantation or endoscopic retrograde cholangiopancreatography (ERCP). Heredity may be a predisposing factor and, in some patients, emotional or neurogenic factors are involved.

Regardless of the cause, pancreatitis involves autodigestion: The enzymes normally excreted by the pancreas digest pancreatic tissue.

Complications

If pancreatitis damages the islets of Langerhans, diabetes mellitus may occur. Fulminant pancreatitis causes massive hemorrhage and total destruction of the pancreas, resulting in diabetic acidosis, shock, or coma. Respiratory complications include adult respiratory distress syndrome, atelectasis, pleural effusion, and pneumonia. Proximity of the inflamed pancreas to the bowel may cause paralytic ileus. Other complications include GI bleeding, pancreatic abscess, pseudocysts and, rarely, cancer.

Assessment findings

Commonly, the patient describes intense epigastric pain centered close to the umbilicus and radiating to the back, between the tenth thoracic and sixth lumbar vertebrae. He typically reports that this pain is aggravated by eating fatty foods, consuming alcohol, or lying in a recumbent position. He may also complain of weight loss, with nausea and vomiting.

Investigation may uncover predisposing factors, such as alcoholism, biliary tract disease, or pancreatic disease. Other medical problems, such as peptic ulcer disease or hyperlipidemia, may be discovered.

Assessment of vital signs may reveal decreased blood pressure, tachycardia, and fever. These signs, if present, indicate respiratory complications. Other signs of respiratory complications are dyspnea or orthopnea. Observe the patient for changes in behavior and sensorium; these signs may be related to alcohol withdrawal or indicate hypoxia or impending shock.

Abdominal inspection may disclose generalized jaundice, Cullen's sign (bluish periumbilical discoloration), and Turner's sign (bluish flank discoloration). Inspection of stools may reveal steatorrhea, a sign of chronic pancreatitis.

During abdominal palpation, you may note tenderness, rigidity, and guarding. If you hear a dull sound while percussing, suspect pancreatic ascites. If bowel sounds are absent or decreased on abdominal auscultation, suspect paralytic ileus.

Diagnostic tests

• *Serum amylase and lipase levels* are elevated — the diagnostic hallmarks that confirm acute pancreatitis. Characteristically, serum amylase reaches peak levels in 24 hours after onset of pancreatitis, then returns to normal within 48 to 72 hours, despite continued symptoms. Amylase levels are also dramatically elevated in urine, ascites, and pleural fluid. Urine amylase levels and serum lipase levels remain elevated longer than serum amylase levels.

• *Supportive laboratory studies* include elevated white blood cell count and serum bilirubin level. In many patients, hypocalcemia occurs and appears to be associated with the severity of the disease. Blood and urine glucose tests may reveal transient glucosuria and hyperglycemia. In chronic pancreatitis, significant laboratory findings include elevations in serum alkaline phosphatase, amylase, and bilirubin levels. Serum glucose levels may be transiently elevated. Stools contain elevated lipid and trypsin levels.

• *Abdominal and chest X-rays* differentiate pancreatitis from other diseases that cause similar symptoms and detect pleural effusions.

• *Computed tomography scan* and *ultrasonography* reveal an increased pancreatic diameter; these tests also identify pancreatic cysts and pseudocysts.

• *ERCP* shows the anatomy of the pancreas; identifies ductal system abnormalities, such as calcification or strictures; and differentiates pancreatitis from other disorders, such as pancreatic cancer.

Treatment

The goals are to maintain circulation and fluid volume, relieve pain, and decrease pancreatic secretions. Emergency treatment for shock (the most common cause of death in early stage pancreatitis) consists of vigorous I.V. replacement of electrolytes and proteins. Metabolic acidosis secondary to hypovolemia and impaired cellular perfusion requires vigorous fluid volume replacement. Blood transfusions may be needed if shock occurs. Food and fluids are withheld to allow the pancreas to rest and to reduce pancreatic enzyme secretion.

In acute pancreatitis, nasogastric (NG) tube suctioning is usually required to decrease gastric distention and suppress pancreatic secretions. Prescribed medications may include:

• meperidine to relieve abdominal pain (this drug causes less spasm at the ampulla of Vater than opiates, such as morphine)

• antacids to neutralize gastric secretions

• histamine antagonists, such as cimetidine or ranitidine, to decrease hydrochloric acid production

• antibiotics, such as clindamycin or gentamicin, to treat bacterial infections

• anticholinergics to reduce vagal stimulation, decrease GI motility, and inhibit pancreatic enzyme secretion

• insulin to correct hyperglycemia, if present.

Once the crisis begins to resolve, oral low-fat, low-protein feedings are gradually implemented. Alcohol and caffeine are eliminated from the diet. If the crisis occurred during treatment with glucocorticoids, oral contraceptives, or thiazide diuretics, these drugs are discontinued.

Surgery usually isn't indicated in acute pancreatitis. However, if complications occur, such as pancreatic abscess or pseudocyst, surgical drainage may be necessary. If biliary tract obstruction causes acute pancreatitis, a laparotomy may be required.

For chronic pancreatitis, treatment depends on the cause. Nonsurgical measures are appropriate if the patient isn't a suitable candidate for surgery or if he refuses this treatment. Measures to prevent and relieve abdominal pain are similar to those used in acute pancreatitis. Meperidine usually is the drug of choice; however, pentazocine also effectively relieves pain. Treatments for diabetes mellitus may include dietary modification, insulin replacement, or antidiabetic agents. Malabsorption and steatorrhea are treated with pancreatic enzyme replacement.

Surgical intervention relieves abdominal pain, restores pancreatic drainage, and reduces the frequency of acute pancreatic attacks. Surgical drainage is required for an abscess or pseudocyst. If biliary tract disease is the underlying cause, cholecystectomy or choledochotomy is performed. A sphincterotomy is indicated to enlarge a pancreatic sphincter that has become fibrotic. To relieve obstruction and allow drainage of pancreatic secretions, pancreaticojejunostomy (anastomosis of the jejunum with the opened pancreatic duct) may be required.

Nursing diagnoses

• Altered nutrition: Less than body requirements
• Fluid volume deficit
• Hopelessness
• Ineffective breathing pattern
• Pain

Nursing interventions

• Assess the patient's level of pain. As ordered, administer meperidine or other analgesics. Evaluate and document effectiveness of pain medications; watch for adverse reactions.
• Maintain the NG tube for drainage or suctioning.
• Restrict the patient to bed rest, and provide a quiet and restful environment.

• Place the patient in a comfortable position that also allows maximal chest expansion, such as Fowler's position.
• Assess pulmonary status at least every 4 hours to detect early signs of respiratory complications.
• Monitor fluid and electrolyte balance and report any abnormalities. Maintain an accurate record of intake and output. Weigh the patient daily and record his weight.
• Keep water and other beverages at the bedside, and encourage the patient to drink plenty of fluids.
• Evaluate the patient's present nutritional status and metabolic requirements.
• Provide I.V. fluids and parenteral nutrition, as ordered. As soon as the patient can tolerate it, provide a diet high in carbohydrates, low in proteins, and low in fat.
• Monitor serum glucose levels and administer insulin, as ordered.
• Watch for signs of calcium deficiency: tetany, cramps, carpopedal spasm, and seizures. If you suspect hypocalcemia, keep airway and suction apparatus handy and pad the bed's side rails.
• Don't confuse thirst due to hyperglycemia (indicated by serum glucose levels up to 350 mg/dl and glucose and acetone in the urine) with dry mouth due to NG intubation and anticholinergics.
• If the patient has chronic pancreatitis, allow him to express feelings of anger, depression, and sadness related to his condition, and help him to cope with these feelings. Encourage him to use appropriate physical outlets to express his emotions, such as pounding a punching bag or throwing pillows.
• Counsel the patient to contact a self-help group, such as Alcoholics Anonymous, if needed.

Patient teaching
• Emphasize the importance of avoiding factors that precipitate acute pancreatitis, especially alcohol.
• Refer the patient and his family to the dietitian. Stress the need for a diet high in carbohydrates and low in protein and fats. Caution the patient to avoid caffeinated beverages and irritating foods.
• Point out the need to comply with pancreatic enzyme replacement therapy. Instruct the patient to take the enzymes with meals or snacks to help digest food and to promote fat and protein absorption. Advise him to watch for and report any of the following signs and symptoms: fatty, frothy, foul-smelling stools; abdominal distention; cramping; and skin excoriation.
• If the patient has chronic pain, teach a family member how to give I.M. injections, as ordered.

LIVER DISORDERS

Because the liver performs well over 100 functions, many of them essential for life, hepatic diseases and their complications tend to be life-threatening, especially in advanced cases of cirrhosis, liver abscess, and hepatic encephalopathy.

VIRAL HEPATITIS

A fairly common systemic disease, viral hepatitis is marked by hepatic cell destruction, necrosis, and autolysis, leading to anorexia, jaundice, and hepatomegaly. In most patients, hepatic cells eventually regenerate with little or no residual damage, allowing ready recovery. However, old age and serious underlying disorders make complications more likely. The prognosis is poor if edema and hepatic encephalopathy develop.

More than 70,000 cases are reported annually in the United States. Today, five types of viral hepatitis are recognized:
• *Type A* (infectious or short-incubation hepatitis). The incidence of this type is rising among homosexuals and in persons with immunosuppression related to human immunodeficiency virus (HIV) infection.
• *Type B* (serum or long-incubation hepatitis). Also increasing among HIV-positive individuals, this type accounts for 5% to 10% of posttransfusion hepatitis cases in the United States.
• *Type C*. This type accounts for about 20% of all viral hepatitis and for most posttransfusion hepatitis cases.
• *Type D* (also called delta hepatitis). This type is responsible for about 50% of fulminant hepatitis, which has an extremely high mortality rate. In the United States, type D is confined to persons frequently exposed to blood and blood products, such as I.V. drug users and hemophiliacs.
• *Type E* (formerly grouped with Type C under the name type non-A, non-B hepatitis). Type E primarily occurs among patients who have recently returned from an endemic area (India, Africa, Asia, or Central America); it's more common in young adults and more severe in pregnant women.

Causes
The five major forms of viral hepatitis result from infection with the causative viruses: A, B, C, D, or E.

Type A hepatitis is highly contagious and is usually transmitted by the fecal-oral route, commonly within institutions or families. However, it may also be transmitted parenterally. Hepatitis A usually results from ingestion of contaminated food, milk, or water. Outbreaks of this type are often traced to ingestion of seafood from polluted water.

Type B hepatitis, once thought to be transmitted only by the direct exchange of contaminated blood, is now known to be transmitted also by contact with contaminated human secretions and feces. As a result, nurses, doctors, laboratory technicians, and dentists are frequently exposed to type B hepatitis, often as a result of wearing defective gloves. Transmission of this type also occurs during intimate sexual contact and through perinatal transmission.

Although specific viruses defined as type C hepatitis have been isolated, only a small percentage of patients have tested positive for them — reflecting, perhaps, poor specificity of the test. Usually, this type is transmitted through transfused blood from asymptomatic donors.

Type D hepatitis is found only in patients with an acute or a chronic episode of hepatitis B. Type D infection requires the presence of the hepatitis B surface antigen; the type D virus depends on the double-shelled type B virus to replicate. For this reason, type D infection cannot outlast a type B infection.

Type E hepatitis is a new form of hepatitis that is transmitted enterically, much like type A. Because this virus is inconsistently shed in feces, detection is difficult.

Complications

The most feared complication, life-threatening fulminant hepatitis develops in about 1% of patients, causing unremitting liver failure with encephalopathy. It progresses to coma and commonly leads to death within 2 weeks.

Complications may be specific to the type of hepatitis:
• Chronic active hepatitis may occur as a late complication of hepatitis B.
• During the prodromal stage of acute hepatitis B, a syndrome resembling serum sickness, characterized by arthralgia or arthritis, rash, and angioedema, may occur. This syndrome may cause misdiagnosis of hepatitis B as rheumatoid arthritis or lupus erythematosus.
• Primary liver cancer may develop after infection with hepatitis B or C.
• Type D hepatitis can cause a mild or asymptomatic form of type B hepatitis to flare into severe, progressive chronic active hepatitis and cirrhosis.
• Weeks to months after apparent recovery from acute hepatitis A, relapsing hepatitis may develop.

Rarely, hepatitis may lead to pancreatitis, myocarditis, atypical pneumonia, aplastic anemia, transverse myelitis, or peripheral neuropathy.

Assessment findings

Investigate the patient's history for the source of transmission. For example, you may learn that he was recently exposed to individuals with hepatitis A or B; underwent recent blood transfusions or used I.V. drugs; or had hemodialysis for renal failure. Look for evidence of recent ear piercing or tattooing (significant because contaminated instruments can transmit hepatitis); travel to a foreign country where hepatitis is endemic; or living conditions that are, or were, overcrowded.

Be sure to ask about alcohol consumption, which holds paramount significance in suspected cirrhosis. Remember, the alcoholic often deliberately underestimates how much he drinks, so you may need to interview family members as well.

Also check the patient's employment history; you may turn up occupational exposure. For instance, he may work in a hospital or laboratory, where the risk of viral exposure from contaminated instruments or waste could be high. Also probe the patient's background for possible exposure to toxic chemicals, such as carbon tetrachloride, which can cause nonviral hepatitis.

Assessment findings are similar for the different types of hepatitis. Typically, signs and symptoms progress in several stages. In the prodromal (preicteric) stage, the patient generally complains of easy fatigue and anorexia, possibly with mild weight loss. He may also report generalized malaise, depression, headache, weakness, arthralgia, myalgia, photophobia, and nausea with vomiting. He may describe changes in his senses of taste and smell.

Vital signs assessment may reveal fever, with a temperature of 100° to 102° F (37.8° to 38.9° C). As the prodromal stage draws to a close, usually within 1 to 5 days before the onset of the clinical jaundice stage, inspection of urine and stool specimens may reveal dark-colored urine and clay-colored stools.

If the patient has progressed to the clinical jaundice stage, he may report pruritus, abdominal pain or tenderness, and indigestion. Early in this stage, he may complain of anorexia; later, his appetite may return. Inspection of the sclerae, mucous membranes, and skin may show jaundice, which can last for 1 to 2 weeks. Jaundice indicates that the damaged liver is unable to remove bilirubin from the blood; however, its presence doesn't indicate disease severity. Occasionally, hepatitis occurs without jaundice.

During the clinical jaundice stage, skin inspection may detect rashes, erythematous patches, or hives, especially if the patient has hepatitis B or C. Palpation may disclose abdominal tenderness in the right upper quadrant, an enlarged and tender liver and, in some cases, splenomegaly and cervical adenopathy.

If you assess the patient during the recovery or posticteric stage, you'll find most symptoms are decreasing or have subsided. On palpation, you may notice a decrease in liver enlargement. The recovery phase generally lasts from 2 to 12 weeks — sometimes longer in patients with hepatitis B, C, or E.

Diagnostic tests

In suspected viral hepatitis, a hepatitis profile is routinely performed. This study identifies antibodies specific to the causative virus, establishing the type of hepatitis:

• *Type A.* Detection of an antibody to hepatitis A (anti-HAV) confirms the diagnosis.
• *Type B.* The presence of hepatitis B surface antigens (HBsAg) and hepatitis B antibodies (anti-HBs) confirms the diagnosis.
• *Type C.* Diagnosis depends on serologic testing for the specific antibody 1 or more months after the onset of acute illness. Until then, the diagnosis is principally established by obtaining negative test results for hepatitis A, B, and D.
• *Type D.* Detection of intrahepatic delta antigens or immunoglobulin (Ig) M antidelta antigens in acute disease (or IgM and IgG in chronic disease) establishes the diagnosis.
• *Type E.* Detection of hepatitis E antigens supports the diagnosis; however, the diagnosis may also consist of ruling out hepatitis C.

Additional findings from liver function studies support the diagnosis:

• *Serum aspartate aminotransferase (formerly SGOT) and serum alanine aminotransferase (formerly SGPT) levels* are increased in the prodromal stage of acute viral hepatitis.
• *Serum alkaline phosphatase levels* are slightly increased.
• *Serum bilirubin levels* are elevated. Levels may continue to be high late in the disease, especially if the patient has severe disease.
• *Prothrombin time* is prolonged (more than 3 seconds longer than normal indicates severe liver damage).
• *White blood cell counts* commonly reveal transient neutropenia and lymphopenia followed by lymphocytosis.
• *Liver biopsy* is performed if chronic hepatitis is suspected. (This study is performed for acute hepatitis only if the diagnosis is questionable.)

Treatment

No specific drug therapy has been developed for hepatitis, with the exception of hepatitis C, which has been treated with interferon alfa with some success. Instead, the patient is advised to rest in the early stages of the illness and combat anorexia by eating small, high-calorie, high-protein meals. (Protein intake should be reduced if signs of precoma — lethargy, confusion, mental changes — develop.) Large meals are usually better tolerated in the morning because many patients experience nausea late in the day.

In acute viral hepatitis, hospitalization usually is required only for those patients with severe symptoms or complications. Parenteral nutrition may be required if the patient has persistent vomiting and is unable to maintain oral intake.

Antiemetics (trimethobenzamide or benzquinamide) may be given a half hour before meals to relieve nausea and prevent vomiting; phenothiazines have a cholestatic effect and should be avoided. For severe pruritus, the resin cholestyramine, which sequesters bile salts, may be given.

Nursing diagnoses

• Activity intolerance
• Altered nutrition: Less than body requirements
• Risk for infection

Nursing interventions

• Observe appropriate isolation precautions to prevent transmission of the disease. (See *Isolation precautions for viral hepatitis.*) Make sure that visitors also observe these precautions.
• Provide rest periods throughout the day. Schedule treatments and tests so that the patient can rest between activities.
• Because inactivity may make the patient anxious, include diversional activities as part of his care. Suggest television programs of interest to him. Gradually add activities to his schedule as he begins to recover.
• To help the patient maintain an adequate diet, don't overload his meal tray. Too much food may only diminish his appetite. Also take care not to overmedicate him, which may cause loss of appetite. Determine his food preferences and try to include favorite foods in his meal plan.
• Administer supplemental vitamins and commercial feedings, as ordered. If symptoms are severe and the patient can't tolerate oral intake, provide I.V. therapy and parenteral nutrition, as ordered.

ISOLATION PRECAUTIONS FOR VIRAL HEPATITIS

To prevent transmission of infectious hepatitis, you'll need to observe isolation precautions—and discuss them with your patient to promote his cooperation. Depending on the type of hepatitis, enteric or universal precautions are observed.

Enteric precautions

If the patient has hepatitis A or E, the hospital staff will exercise *enteric precautions:*
• The patient may have a private room (necessary only for a patient with fecal incontinence or poor hygiene). Staff members will wear gowns (when fecal soiling is likely) and gloves (for contact with feces or feces-soiled items).
• Hospital staff members will double-bag fecally contaminated bed linens in isolation bags and label any fecal specimens "Enteric precautions."
• Whenever hospital staff members transport the patient, they'll use added protection (moisture-resistant pads for a fecally incontinent patient, for example).
• At home, the patient should use meticulous hygiene after a bowel movement—starting with thorough hand washing, for example. Furthermore, he shouldn't handle food or share food or hand towels.

Universal precautions

If the patient has hepatitis B, C, or D, the hospital staff will observe *universal (blood and body fluid) precautions:*
• The patient may have a private room (necessary only for a patient with poor hygiene), and staff members will wear gowns and gloves (for direct contact with blood or body fluids).
• Staff members will dispose of needles and syringes in prominently labeled, puncture-resistant containers and won't recap needles and syringes. They'll double-bag dressings and tissues and dispose of them in the hospital's designated area for contaminated refuse.
• If bed linens are contaminated with blood or body fluids, the staff will double-bag them in isolation bags. And they'll label specimens "Blood and body fluid precautions."
• The patient must avoid sexual relations until the doctor confirms the danger of contagion is past.

Teaching the patient

After discussing isolation measures, educate the patient about the mode of transmission, incubation period, diagnostic tests, prophylaxis, and those at high risk for his type of hepatitis.

• Provide adequate fluid intake. The patient should consume at least 4 liters of liquid daily to maintain adequate hydration. To help him meet or exceed this goal, provide him with fruit juices, soft drinks, ice chips, and water.
• Administer antiemetics, as ordered. Observe the patient for the desired effects and note any adverse reactions.
• Record weight daily, and keep accurate intake and output records. Observe the feces for color, consistency, and amount. Also note the frequency of defecation.
• Watch for signs of complications, such as changes in level of consciousness, ascites, edema, dehydration, respiratory problems, myalgia, and arthralgia.
• Report all cases of hepatitis to health officials. Ask the patient to name anyone he came in contact with recently.

Patient teaching

• Teach the patient about the disease, its signs and symptoms, and recommended treatments.
• Explain all necessary diagnostic tests. Review any special preparation that may be required. Point out that the findings from these tests, together with his symptoms, help to establish his diagnosis.

• Educate the patient about the importance of rest and a proper diet to help the liver heal and minimize complications.
• Stress that complete recovery takes time. Point out that the liver takes 3 weeks to regenerate and up to 4 months to return to normal functioning. Advise the patient to avoid contact sports until his liver returns to its normal size. Instruct him to check with his doctor before performing any strenuous activity.
• Review measures to prevent spread of the disease. Stress the importance of thorough and frequent hand washing. Tell the patient not to share food, eating utensils, or toothbrushes. If he has hepatitis A or E, warn him not to contaminate food or water with fecal matter, because the disease is transmitted via the fecal-oral route. If he has hepatitis B, C, or D, explain that transmission occurs through exchange of blood or body fluids that contain blood. Therefore, while he is infected, he shouldn't donate blood or have sexual relations. Also advise him to take extra care to avoid cutting himself.
• Emphasize the importance of good nutrition in promoting liver regeneration. Instruct the patient to eat a high-calorie, high-protein diet. Advise him to eat several small meals rather than three large meals. Also stress the importance of drinking adequate fluids every day.

• Tell the patient who is recuperating at home to weigh himself every day and to report any weight loss greater than 5 lb (2.3 kg) to his doctor.

• Warn the patient to abstain from alcohol while he has this disease. If necessary, explain that, because alcohol is detoxified in the liver, its consumption could put undue stress on the liver during the illness.

• Explain to the patient and his family that anyone exposed to the disease through contact with him should receive prophylaxis as soon as possible after exposure. Immune globulin is given for hepatitis A. It may also be given for hepatitis C and E, but its effectiveness for these types of hepatitis has not been proven. Hepatitis B vaccine is given for hepatitis B or D.

• Tell the patient to check with the doctor before taking any medication—even nonprescription drugs—because some medications can precipitate a relapse.

• Stress the need for continued medical care. Advise the patient to see the doctor again about 2 weeks after the diagnosis is made. Mention that he'll probably have follow-up visits every month for up to 6 months after diagnosis. Also explain that if chronic hepatitis develops, he'll always have to visit the doctor regularly so that the disease can be monitored.

CIRRHOSIS

A chronic hepatic disease, cirrhosis is characterized by diffuse destruction and fibrotic regeneration of hepatic cells. As necrotic tissue yields to fibrosis, this disease alters liver structure and normal vasculature, impairs blood and lymph flow, and ultimately causes hepatic insufficiency.

Cirrhosis is the ninth most common cause of death in the United States and, among patients ages 35 to 55, the fourth leading cause of death. The disease, which can occur at any age, occurs in four main types: Laënnec's, postnecrotic, biliary, and cardiac. Laënnec's cirrhosis, the most common type, is most prevalent among malnourished alcoholic men; it accounts for more than half of all cirrhosis cases in the United States. Postnecrotic cirrhosis is more common in women than in men and is the most common type worldwide.

Causes

The factors that lead to the development of cirrhosis are not clearly defined. A genetic factor appears to be important, with familial tendencies to develop cirrhosis or possess a sensitivity to alcohol in some individuals. However, many alcoholics don't develop cirrhosis, whereas others develop the disease even though their nutritional status is adequate.

Cirrhosis has a diverse etiology, reflecting the varied clinical types:

• Laënnec's cirrhosis (alcoholic, nutritional, or portal cirrhosis) stems from chronic alcoholism and malnutrition.

• Postnecrotic cirrhosis usually results as a complication of viral hepatitis. This type also may occur after exposure to liver toxins, such as arsenic, carbon tetrachloride, or phosphorus.

• Biliary cirrhosis results from prolonged biliary tract obstruction or inflammation.

• Cardiac cirrhosis is associated with protracted venous congestion in the liver caused by right ventricular failure.

• In addition, some patients develop idiopathic cirrhosis, with no known cause.

Complications

Depending on the amount of liver damage, cirrhosis can lead to such complications as portal hypertension, bleeding esophageal varices, hepatic encephalopathy, hepatorenal syndrome, and death. (See *What happens in portal hypertension.*)

Assessment findings

Signs and symptoms are similar for all types, regardless of the cause. However, clinical manifestations vary depending on when in the course of the disease the patient seeks treatment.

In the early stage, the patient may experience only vague signs and symptoms, but typically he complains of abdominal pain, diarrhea, fatigue, nausea, and vomiting. Later, as the disease progresses, he may complain of chronic dyspepsia, constipation, pruritus, and weight loss. He may report a tendency for easy bleeding, such as frequent nosebleeds, easy bruising, or bleeding gums.

During the history, you may uncover alcoholism or other diseases or conditions, such as acute viral hepatitis, biliary tract disorders, congestive heart failure, recent blood transfusions, or viral infections.

In a head-to-toe approach, inspection reveals these common signs: telangiectasis on the cheeks; spider angiomas on the face, neck, arms, and trunk; gynecomastia; umbilical hernia; distended, abdominal blood vessels; ascites; testicular atrophy; palmar erythema; clubbed fingers; thigh and leg edema; ecchymosis; and jaundice.

In the early phase of the disease, palpation finds the liver to be large and firm with a sharp edge. Later, scar tissue causes the liver to decrease in size; at this point,

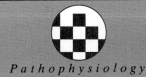

Pathophysiology

WHAT HAPPENS IN PORTAL HYPERTENSION

Portal hypertension—elevated pressure in the portal vein—occurs when blood flow meets increased resistance. The disorder, a common result of cirrhosis, may also stem from mechanical obstruction and occlusion of the hepatic veins (Budd-Chiari syndrome).

As pressure in the portal vein rises, blood backs up into the spleen and flows through collateral channels to the venous system, bypassing the liver. Consequently, portal hypertension produces splenomegaly with thrombocytopenia, dilated collateral veins (esophageal varices, hemorrhoids, or prominent abdominal veins), and ascites.

Bleeding esophageal varices: The first sign
In many patients, the first sign of portal hypertension is bleeding from esophageal varices—dilated tortuous veins in the submucosa of the lower esophagus. Esophageal varices commonly cause massive hematemesis, requiring emergency care to control hemorrhage and prevent hypovolemic shock.

Care for the patient who has portal hypertension with esophageal varices focuses on careful monitoring for signs and symptoms of hemorrhage and subsequent hypotension, compromised oxygen supply, and altered level of consciousness.

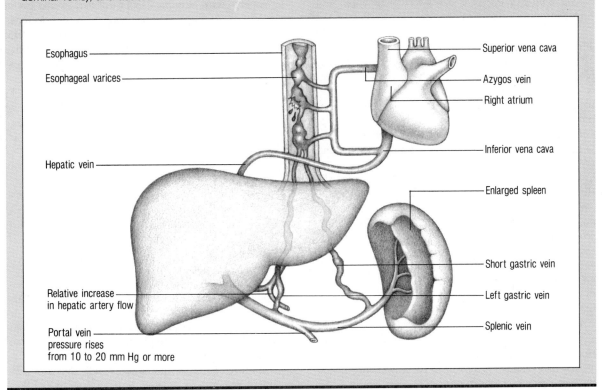

Esophagus
Esophageal varices
Hepatic vein
Relative increase in hepatic artery flow
Portal vein pressure rises from 10 to 20 mm Hg or more

Superior vena cava
Azygos vein
Right atrium
Inferior vena cava
Enlarged spleen
Short gastric vein
Left gastric vein
Splenic vein

if the liver is palpable, its edge is nodular. Palpation also reveals an enlarged spleen.

Diagnostic tests
A thorough workup consisting of diagnostic and laboratory tests is required to confirm the diagnosis, establish the type of cirrhosis, and pinpoint complications.

• *Liver biopsy.* The definitive test for cirrhosis, biopsy detects hepatic tissue destruction and fibrosis.

• *Abdominal X-rays.* Films show liver size and cysts or gas within the biliary tract or liver; liver calcification; and massive ascites.

• *Computed tomography and liver scans.* These studies determine liver size, identify liver masses, and visualize hepatic blood flow and obstruction.

• *Esophagogastroduodenoscopy.* This study reveals bleeding esophageal varices, stomach irritation or ulceration, or duodenal bleeding and irritation.

• *Blood studies.* Liver enzymes (alanine aminotransferase [formerly SGPT], aspartate aminotransferase [formerly SGOT]), total serum bilirubin, and indirect bilirubin levels are elevated. Total serum albumin and protein levels decrease; prothrombin time is prolonged. Hemoglobin, hematocrit, and serum electrolyte levels decrease. Vitamins A, C, and K are deficient.

• *Urine and stool studies.* Urine levels of bilirubin and urobilinogen increase; fecal urobilinogen levels fall.

Treatment

Therapy aims to remove or alleviate the underlying cause of cirrhosis, prevent further liver damage, and prevent or treat complications. Vitamins and nutritional supplements promote healing of damaged hepatic cells and improve the patient's nutritional status. Sodium consumption is usually restricted to 500 mg/day and liquid intake is limited to 1,500 ml/day to help manage ascites and edema.

Drug therapy requires special caution because the cirrhotic liver can't detoxify harmful substances efficiently. Antacids may be prescribed to reduce gastric distress and decrease the potential for GI bleeding. Potassium-sparing diuretics, such as furosemide, may be used to reduce ascites and edema. However, diuretics require careful monitoring because fluid and electrolyte imbalance may precipitate hepatic encephalopathy. Vasopressin may be indicated for esophageal varices. Alcohol is prohibited and sedatives should be avoided.

In patients with ascites, paracentesis may be used as a palliative treatment to relieve abdominal pressure. However, surgical intervention may be required to divert ascites into venous circulation; if so, a peritoneovenous shunt is used. Shunt insertion results in weight loss, decreased abdominal girth, increased sodium excretion from the kidneys, and improved urine output.

To control bleeding from esophageal varices or other GI hemorrhage, nonsurgical measures are attempted first. These include gastric intubation and esophageal balloon tamponade. In gastric intubation, a tube is inserted and the stomach is lavaged until the contents are clear. If the bleeding is assessed as a gastric ulcer, antacids and histamine antagonists are administered.

In esophageal balloon tamponade, bleeding vessels are compressed to stanch blood loss from esophageal varices. Several forms of balloon tamponade are available, including the Sengstaken-Blakemore method, the esophagogastric tube method, and the Minnesota tube method.

Sclerotherapy is performed if the patient continues to experience repeated hemorrhagic episodes despite conservative treatment. A sclerosing agent is injected into the oozing vessels. This agent traumatizes epithelial tissue, which causes thrombosis and leads to sclerosis. If bleeding from the varices doesn't stop within 2 to 5 minutes, a second injection is given below the bleeding site. Sclerotherapy also may be performed prophylactically on nonbleeding varices.

As a last resort, portal-systemic shunts may be used for patients with bleeding esophageal varices and portal hypertension. Surgical shunting procedures decrease portal hypertension by diverting a portion of the portal vein blood flow away from the liver. These procedures are seldom performed because they can result in bleeding, infection, and shunt thrombosis.

Massive hemorrhage requires blood transfusions. To maintain blood pressure, crystalloid or colloid volume expanders are administered until the blood is available.

Nursing diagnoses

• Activity intolerance
• Altered nutrition: Less than body requirements
• Altered thought processes
• Fluid volume excess
• Hopelessness
• Risk for impaired skin integrity
• Risk for injury

Nursing interventions

• Monitor vital signs, intake and output, and electrolyte levels to determine fluid volume status.
• To assess fluid retention, measure and record abdominal girth every shift. Weigh the patient daily and document his weight.
• Administer diuretics, potassium, and protein or vitamin supplements, as ordered. Restrict sodium and fluid intake, as ordered.
• Provide or assist with oral hygiene before and after meals.
• Determine food preferences and provide them within the patient's prescribed diet limitations. Offer frequent, small meals.

• Observe and document the degree of sclerae and skin jaundice.

• Give the patient frequent skin care, bathe him without soap, and massage him with emollient lotions. Keep his fingernails short. Handle him gently; turn and reposition him often to keep the skin intact.

• Observe for bleeding gums, ecchymoses, epistaxis, and petechiae. Constantly remain with the patient during hemorrhagic episodes.

• Inspect stools for amount, color, and consistency. Test stools and vomitus for occult blood.

• Increase the patient's exercise tolerance by decreasing fluid volumes and providing rest periods before exercise.

• Address the patient by name and tell him your name. Mention time, place, and date frequently throughout the day. Place a clock and a calendar where he can easily see them.

• Use appropriate safety measures to protect the patient from injury. Avoid physical restraints if possible.

• Watch for signs of anxiety, epigastric fullness, restlessness, and weakness.

• Observe closely for signs of behavioral or personality changes. Report increasing stupor, lethargy, hallucinations, or neuromuscular dysfunction. Arouse the patient periodically to determine level of consciousness. Watch for asterixis, a sign of developing encephalopathy.

• Allow the patient to express his feelings about having cirrhosis. Offer psychological support and encouragement, when appropriate. Offer him and his family a realistic evaluation of his present health status and communicate hope for the immediate future.

Patient teaching

• To minimize the risk of bleeding, warn the patient against taking nonsteroidal anti-inflammatory drugs, straining to defecate, and blowing his nose or sneezing too vigorously. Suggest using an electric razor and a soft toothbrush.

• Advise the patient that rest and good nutrition conserve energy and decrease metabolic demands on the liver. Urge him to eat frequent, small meals. Teach him to alternate periods of rest and activity to reduce oxygen demand and prevent fatigue.

• Tell the patient how he can conserve energy while performing activities of daily living. For example, suggest that he sit on a bench while bathing or dressing.

• Stress the need to avoid infections and abstain from alcohol. Refer the patient to Alcoholics Anonymous, if appropriate.

LIVER ABSCESS

A relatively uncommon but life-threatening disorder, liver abscess occurs when bacteria or protozoa destroy hepatic tissue. The damage produces a cavity, which fills with infectious organisms, liquefied hepatic cells, and leukocytes. Necrotic tissue then walls off the cavity from the rest of the liver.

Liver abscess carries a mortality rate of 30% to 50%. This rate soars to more than 80% with multiple abscesses and to more than 90% with complications. Liver abscess affects both sexes and all age-groups, although it's slightly more prevalent in hospitalized children (because of a high rate of immunosuppression) and in women (most commonly those between ages 40 and 60).

Causes

An amoebic abscess (the most common cause) results from infection with the protozoa *Entamoeba histolytica,* the organism that causes amebic dysentery. Amoebic liver abscesses usually occur singly, in the right lobe.

In pyogenic liver abscesses, the common infecting organisms are *Escherichia coli, Klebsiella, Salmonella, Staphylococcus,* and enterococcus. Such organisms may invade the liver directly after a liver wound, or they may spread from the lungs, skin, or other organs by the hepatic artery, portal vein, or biliary tract. (See *How liver abscess develops,* page 932.) Though multiple pyogenic abscesses are usual, a singular abscess may occur.

Certain illnesses or conditions also may lead to abscess development; these include cholecystitis, colon cancer, diverticulitis, peritonitis, regional enteritis, infective endocarditis, pelvic inflammatory disease, pneumonia, trauma, and septicemia.

Complications

Without treatment, liver abscess usually leads to death. Complications include abscess rupture into the peritoneum, pleura, or pericardium.

Assessment findings

The clinical manifestations of a liver abscess depend on the degree of involvement. Some patients are acutely ill; in others, the abscess is recognized only at autopsy, after death from another illness. Onset of symptoms of a pyogenic abscess is usually sudden; in an amoebic abscess, onset is more insidious.

The patient may report right abdominal and shoulder pain, chills, fever, diaphoresis, nausea, vomiting, and weight loss. If the abscess extends through the diaphragm, she may complain of dyspnea and chest pain

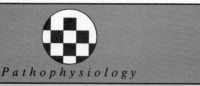

Pathophysiology

HOW LIVER ABSCESS DEVELOPS

With its rich vasculature and lymphatic supply, the liver offers several routes of entry for infectious bacteria. Pathogenic invaders, which may arise from distant infections in the GI tract or elsewhere, can spread to the liver via the biliary tract, the portal venous system, or the hepatic arterial or lymphatic systems.

Abscess formation
Usually, the liver destroys these bacteria but, occasionally, some infiltrate hepatic defenses. As these bacteria multiply and release toxins, they destroy adjacent hepatocytes. A necrotic wall forms, enclosing and protecting the bacteria.

At the same time, leukocytes swarm into the infected area, creating an abscess. The abscessed cavity fills with fluid containing living and dead leukocytes, liquefied hepatic cells, and bacteria, causing a life-threatening disease.

Lower mortality
In the past, liver abscess was virtually always fatal. It was hard to diagnose because of its vague clinical features and ineffective diagnostic tools. It was also difficult to treat because surgical techniques to drain the abscess were inadequate.

With the recent advent of sophisticated liver-scanning techniques, including computed tomography, and more effective surgical drainage procedures, survival has greatly improved.

(symptoms of pleural effusion); if she has developed anemia, she may report fatigue.

Inspection may detect jaundice, a sign of liver damage. On palpation, the liver may feel enlarged, indicating hepatic disease.

Diagnostic tests
• *Liver scan* showing filling defects at the abscess area more than ¾" (2 cm), together with characteristic clinical features, confirms the diagnosis.
• *Hepatic ultrasonography* may indicate defects caused by the abscess but is less definitive than a liver scan.
• *Computed tomography (CT) scan* verifies the diagnosis after a liver scan or hepatic ultrasonography.
• *Chest X-ray* shows the diaphragm on the right side as raised and fixed.

• *Blood tests* demonstrate elevated levels of serum aspartate aminotransferase (formerly SGOT), serum alanine aminotransferase (formerly SGPT), alkaline phosphatase, and bilirubin. Serum albumin level is decreased. White blood cell count is elevated (usually more so in pyogenic than in amoebic abscess).
• *Blood cultures* and *percutaneous liver aspiration* may help identify the causative organism in pyogenic abscess.
• *Stool cultures* and *serologic* and *hemagglutination tests* can isolate *Entamoeba histolytica* in amoebic abscess.

Treatment
If the organism causing the liver abscess is unknown, long-term antibiotic therapy begins immediately with aminoglycosides, cephalosporins, clindamycin, or chloramphenicol. If cultures demonstrate that the infectious organism is *Escherichia coli*, treatment includes ampicillin; if *Entamoeba histolytica,* it includes emetine, chloroquine hydrochloride, chloroquine phosphate, or metronidazole. The therapy continues for 2 to 4 months. Surgery is usually avoided, but it may be required for a single pyogenic abscess or for an amoebic abscess that fails to respond to antibiotics. Placement of drains (using CT or ultrasonography), particularly in large abscesses, reduces the need for abdominal surgery.

Nursing diagnoses
• Altered nutrition: Less than body requirements
• Knowledge deficit
• Pain
• Risk for impaired skin integrity
• Risk for infection

Nursing interventions
• Provide supportive care, monitor vital signs (especially respirations), and maintain fluid and nutritional intake.
• Assess the patient's pain level and administer analgesics, as ordered. Monitor and document the drug's effectiveness and adverse reactions (if any occur). Apply heat or cold, as ordered, to minimize or relieve pain. Help the patient into a comfortable position, using pillows to splint or support painful areas.
• Administer anti-infectives and antibiotics, as ordered, and watch for possible adverse effects.
• Wash your hands before and after providing patient care. Wear gloves to maintain asepsis when providing direct care, such as dressing changes.
• Obtain and record the patient's weight at the same time every day to ensure the most accurate readings.
• Inspect the patient's skin every shift; document skin condition and report any changes.

• Watch carefully for complications of abdominal surgery, such as hemorrhage and infection.

Patient teaching
• Explain all diagnostic and surgical procedures to the patient.
• Stress the importance of compliance with antibiotic drug therapy. Review the medication's purpose, correct use, potential adverse effects, and any special considerations.
• Teach the patient how to perform skin care. Advise her to use nonirritating soap; pat rather than rub her skin dry; inspect skin on a regular basis; and avoid prolonged exposure to environmental elements, such as the sun and wind.

FATTY LIVER

A common clinical finding, fatty liver (steatosis) is the accumulation of triglycerides and other fats in hepatic cells. In severe fatty liver, fat constitutes as much as 40% of the liver's weight (as opposed to 5% in a normal liver), and the weight of the liver may increase from 3⅓ lb (1.5 kg) to as much as 11 lb (5 kg).

Minimal fatty changes are temporary and asymptomatic; severe or persistent changes may cause liver dysfunction. Fatty liver is usually reversible by simply eliminating the cause; however, this disorder can result in recurrent infection or sudden death from fat emboli in the lungs.

Causes and pathophysiology
Chronic alcoholism is the most common cause of fatty liver in the United States and Europe, with the severity of hepatic disease directly related to the amount of alcohol consumed. Other causes include malnutrition (especially protein deficiency), obesity, diabetes mellitus, jejunoileal bypass surgery, Cushing's syndrome, Reye's syndrome, pregnancy, large doses of hepatotoxins (such as I.V. tetracycline), carbon tetrachloride intoxication, prolonged I.V. total parenteral nutrition, and DDT poisoning.

Whatever the cause, fatty infiltration of the liver probably results from mobilization of fatty acids from adipose tissues or altered fat metabolism.

Complications
Without treatment, this disease can lead to permanent liver damage, portal hypertension, metabolic disturbances, disseminated intravascular coagulation, renal failure, coma, and death.

Assessment findings
Clinical features of fatty liver vary with the degree of lipid infiltration; many patients are asymptomatic.

The patient history may uncover predisposing factors, such as alcoholism, malnutrition, biliary stasis, hepatic necrosis, diabetes mellitus, or obesity.

The patient may complain of right upper quadrant pain (with massive or rapid infiltration). Less common symptoms are nausea or vomiting and, rarely, menstrual disorders.

On inspection, you may note jaundice, edema, and ascites. With ascites, the patient may also have an emaciated chest and thin extremities. Rarely, inspection may detect transient gynecomastia or spider angiomas. Abdominal palpation may reveal a large, tender liver (hepatomegaly) and splenomegaly, indicating cirrhosis.

Diagnostic tests
A liver biopsy confirms excessive fat in the liver.

The following results in liver function studies support the diagnosis:
• albumin – low
• globulin – usually elevated
• cholesterol – usually elevated
• total bilirubin – elevated
• alkaline phosphatase – elevated
• aminotransferase – usually low
• prothrombin time – may be prolonged.

Other diagnostic findings may include anemia, leukocytosis, elevated white blood cell count, albuminuria, hyperglycemia or hypoglycemia, and deficiencies of iron, folic acid, and vitamin B_{12}.

Treatment
Management is essentially supportive and consists of correcting the underlying condition or eliminating its cause. For instance, when fatty liver results from I.V. total parenteral nutrition, decreasing the rate of carbohydrate infusion may correct the disease. In alcoholic fatty liver, abstinence from alcohol and a proper diet can begin to correct liver changes within 4 to 8 weeks. Such correction requires comprehensive patient teaching.

Nursing diagnoses
• Altered nutrition: Less than body requirements
• Fluid volume excess
• Knowledge deficit
• Pain

Nursing interventions

• Assess the patient's pain and administer analgesics, as ordered. Monitor and record the drug's effectiveness and watch for adverse effects.

• Apply heat or cold, as ordered, to minimize or relieve pain.

• Help the patient into a comfortable position, and use pillows to splint or support the painful areas.

• Assess for malnutrition, especially protein deficiency, in the patient with chronic illness. Encourage the patient to eat a nutritious diet.

• Weigh the patient at the same each day to determine weight loss. Restrict oral liquid intake to 2 qt (2 liters) daily. Provide sugarless hard candies to decrease thirst and improve taste.

Patient teaching

• Suggest counseling for alcoholics. Provide emotional support for their families as well. If necessary, refer them to support groups, such as Alcoholics Anonymous and Al-Anon.

• Teach the diabetic patient and his family about proper care, such as the purpose of insulin injections, diet, and exercise. Refer him to a public health nurse or to group classes, as necessary, to promote compliance with treatment. Emphasize the need for long-term medical supervision, and urge immediate reporting of any changes in the patient's health.

• Instruct the obese patient and his family about proper diet. Warn against fad diets, which often are nutritionally unsound. Recommend medical supervision for those more than 20% overweight. Encourage attendance at group diet and exercise programs and, if necessary, suggest behavior modification programs to correct eating habits. Be sure to follow up on your patient's progress, and provide positive reinforcement for any weight loss.

• Explain the reasons for liquid and dietary restrictions to help the patient comply.

• Advise the patient receiving hepatotoxins and those who risk occupational exposure to DDT to watch for and immediately report signs of toxicity.

• Emphasize that fatty liver is reversible only if the patient strictly follows the therapeutic program; otherwise, he risks permanent liver damage.

HEPATIC ENCEPHALOPATHY

A neurologic syndrome, hepatic encephalopathy (hepatic coma, portal-systemic encephalopathy) develops as a complication of aggressive fulminant hepatitis or chronic hepatic disease. Most common in patients with cirrhosis, this syndrome may be acute and self-limiting or chronic and progressive. In advanced stages, the prognosis is extremely poor despite vigorous treatment.

Causes and pathophysiology

Most experts attribute this syndrome to ammonia intoxication of the brain, but the precise etiology is unknown. Normally, the ammonia produced by protein breakdown in the bowel is metabolized to urea in the liver. When portal blood shunts past the liver, ammonia directly enters the systemic circulation and is carried to the brain. Such shunting may result from the collateral venous circulation that develops in portal hypertension or from surgically created portal-systemic shunts. Cirrhosis further compounds this problem because impaired hepatocellular function prevents conversion of ammonia that reaches the liver.

Other factors that may lead to rising ammonia levels include excessive protein intake, sepsis, excessive accumulation of nitrogenous body wastes (from constipation or GI hemorrhage), and bacterial action on protein and urea to form ammonia.

Certain other factors heighten the brain's sensitivity to ammonia intoxication: fluid and electrolyte imbalance (especially metabolic alkalosis), hypoxia, azotemia, impaired glucose metabolism, infection, and administration of sedatives, narcotics, and general anesthetics.

Complications

Hepatic encephalopathy can lead to irreversible coma and death.

Assessment findings

Clinical features vary, depending on the severity of neurologic involvement. The disorder usually progresses through four stages, but the patient's symptoms can fluctuate from one stage to another.

In the *prodromal stage,* early symptoms are typically overlooked because they're so subtle. The patient's history, obtained from the patient or from a family member or caregiver, may reveal slight personality changes, such as agitation, belligerence, disorientation, or forgetfulness. The patient may also have trouble concentrating or thinking clearly. He may report feeling fatigued or drowsy. He may have slurred or slowed speech. On inspection, you may observe a slight tremor.

In the *impending stage,* the patient undergoes continuing mental changes. He may be confused and disoriented as to time, place, and person. Inspection continues to reveal tremors that have progressed to asterixis (liver flap, flapping tremor). The hallmark of hepatic encephalopathy, asterixis refers to quick, irregular extensions and flexions of the wrists and fingers, when the wrists are held out straight and the hands flexed upward. On inspection, you may observe lethargy and aberrant behavior. Some patients demonstrate apraxia. When asked, the patient is unable to reproduce a simple design, such as a star.

In the *stuporous stage,* the patient shows marked mental confusion. On inspection, he appears drowsy and stuporous. Yet he can still be aroused and is often noisy and abusive when aroused. Hyperventilation, muscle twitching, and asterixis are also evident.

In the *comatose stage,* the patient cannot be aroused and is obtunded with no asterixis. Seizures, though uncommon, may occur. Palpation may reveal hyperactive reflexes and demonstrate a positive Babinski's sign. The patient often has fetor hepaticus (musty odor of the breath and urine). Fetor hepaticus may occur in other stages also. Eventually this stage progresses to coma; it's usually fatal.

Diagnostic tests
• *Serum ammonia levels in venous and arterial samples* are elevated and, together with characteristic clinical features, highly suggest hepatic encephalopathy.
• *Electroencephalography* shows slowing waves as the disease progresses.

Treatment
Therapy aims to eliminate the underlying cause of the disorder and lower serum ammonia levels to stop progression of encephalopathy. In mild cases, treating the underlying cause of the encephalopathy may reverse the symptoms. In most patients, though, the toxic products, often ammonia, must also be eliminated from the body.

Treatments to eliminate ammonia from the GI tract include sorbitol-induced catharsis to produce osmotic diarrhea, continuous aspiration of blood from the stomach, reduction of dietary protein intake, and administration of lactulose to reduce serum ammonia levels.

Lactulose traps ammonia in the bowel and promotes its excretion. It's effective because bacterial enzymes change lactulose to lactic acid, thereby rendering the colon too acidic for bacterial growth. At the same time, the resulting increase in free hydrogen ions prevents diffusion of ammonia through the mucosa; lactulose promotes conversion of systemically absorbable ammonia to ammonium, which is poorly absorbed and can be excreted. Lactulose syrup may be given orally. In acute hepatic coma, lactulose may be administered by retention enema.

Lactulose therapy requires careful monitoring of fluid and electrolyte balance.

Although it's now considered a second-line treatment because of potential toxicity, neomycin may be given to suppress bacterial flora (preventing them from converting amino acids into ammonia). Neomycin is administered orally or by retention enema. Although neomycin is nonabsorbable at recommended dosages of 3 to 4 g/day, an amount that exceeds 4 g/day may produce irreversible hearing loss and nephrotoxicity.

Treatment may also include potassium supplements (80 to 120 mEq/day, given by mouth or I.V.) to correct alkalosis (from increased ammonia levels), especially if the patient is taking diuretics. Salt-poor albumin may be used to maintain fluid and electrolyte balance, replace depleted albumin levels, and restore plasma.

Other treatments that have been tried, usually with little success, are hemodialysis and exchange transfusions.

Nursing diagnoses
• Altered nutrition: Less than body requirements
• Altered thought processes
• Fluid volume deficit

Nursing interventions
• Frequently assess and record the patient's level of consciousness. Continually orient him to place and time. Remember to keep a daily record of the patient's handwriting to monitor the progression of neurologic involvement.
• Promote rest, comfort, and a quiet atmosphere. Discourage stressful exercise.
• Monitor intake, output, and fluid and electrolyte balance. Check the patient's weight, and measure abdominal girth daily. Watch for, and immediately report, signs of anemia (decreased hemoglobin), alkalosis (increased serum bicarbonate), GI bleeding (melena, hematemesis), and infection. Monitor the patient's serum ammonia level for signs of improvement.
• Administer medications, as ordered. Monitor the patient for the desired effects, and watch for adverse reactions.
• Ask the dietary department to provide the specified low-protein diet, with carbohydrates supplying most of the calories. Provide good mouth care. As ordered, provide parenteral nutrition to the semicomatose or comatose patient.
• Use appropriate safety measures to protect the patient from injury. Avoid physical restraints, if possible.
• Don't give the semicomatose or comatose patient sedatives because they deepen the coma. Protect the co-

matose patient's eyes from corneal injury by using artificial tears or eye patches.

• Provide emotional support for the patient's family in the terminal stage of encephalopathy.

Patient teaching

• Teach the patient, if he's still able to understand, and his family about the disease and its treatment. Repeat explanations of each treatment before you perform it. Be sure to explain all procedures even if the patient is comatose.

• If the patient has chronic encephalopathy, be sure that he and his family understand the mental and physical effects that the illness will eventually have on the patient. Alert them to signs of complications or worsening symptoms. Advise them when to notify the doctor.

• As the patient begins to recover, inform him about the low-protein diet. Emphasize that recovery from so severe an illness takes time. Review how to use medications.

GALLBLADDER AND DUCT DISORDERS

Diseases of the gallbladder and biliary tract are common and often painful conditions that usually require surgery and may be life-threatening. They are often associated with inflammation and deposition of calculi.

CHOLELITHIASIS, CHOLECYSTITIS, AND RELATED DISORDERS

The leading biliary tract disease, cholelithiasis is the formation of stones or calculi (gallstones) in the gallbladder. The prognosis is usually good with treatment unless infection occurs. Then the prognosis depends on the infection's severity and its response to antibiotics.

The formation of gallstones can give rise to a number of related disorders:

• In *cholecystitis,* the gallbladder becomes acutely or chronically inflamed, usually because a gallstone becomes lodged in the cystic duct, causing painful gallbladder distention. The acute form is most common during middle age; the chronic form, among elderly persons. The prognosis is good with treatment.

• In *choledocholithiasis,* gallstones pass out of the gallbladder and lodge in the common bile duct, causing par-

tial or complete biliary obstruction. The prognosis is good unless infection occurs.

• In *cholangitis,* the bile duct becomes infected; this disorder is commonly associated with choledocholithiasis and may follow percutaneous transhepatic cholangiography. Nonsuppurative cholangitis usually responds rapidly to antibiotic treatment. Suppurative cholangitis has a poor prognosis unless surgery to correct the obstruction and drain the infected bile is performed promptly.

• In *gallstone ileus,* a gallstone obstructs the small bowel. Typically, the gallstone travels through a fistula between the gallbladder and small bowel and lodges at the ileocecal valve. This condition is most common in elderly persons. The prognosis is good with surgery.

Generally, gallbladder and duct diseases occur during middle age. Between ages 20 and 50, they're six times more common in women, but the incidence in men and women equalizes after age 50. The incidence rises with each succeeding decade.

Causes

These related disorders all stem from a common cause: formation of calculi. Although the exact cause of gallstone formation is unknown, abnormal metabolism of cholesterol and bile salts clearly plays an important role. (See *How gallstones form.*)

A number of risk factors have been identified that predispose a person to calculi formation. These include:

• a high-calorie, high-cholesterol diet, associated with obesity

• elevated estrogen levels from oral contraceptive use, postmenopausal hormone-replacement therapy, or pregnancy

• the use of clofibrate

• diabetes mellitus, ileal disease, hemolytic disorders, hepatic disease, or pancreatitis.

The type of disorder that develops depends on where in the gallbladder or biliary tract the calculi collect. For example, cholelithiasis results when gallstones form and remain in the gallbladder. Cholecystitis, choledocholithiasis, cholangitis, and gallstone ileus usually develop after a gallstone lodges in a duct or in the small bowel, causing an obstruction. (See *Where calculi collect,* page 938.)

Acute cholecystitis also may result from conditions that alter the gallbladder's ability to fill or empty. These conditions include trauma, reduced blood supply to the gallbladder, prolonged immobility, chronic dieting, adhesions, prolonged anesthesia, and narcotic abuse.

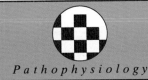
Pathophysiology

HOW GALLSTONES FORM

Bile is made continuously by the liver and is concentrated and stored in the gallbladder until needed by the duodenum to help digest fat. Changes in the composition of bile or in the absorptive ability of the gallbladder epithelium allow gallstones to form. The following explains the physiology of gallstone formation and tells you what to look for.

1. Certain conditions (such as age, obesity, and estrogen imbalance) cause the liver to secrete bile that is abnormally high in cholesterol or lacking the proper concentration of bile salts.
  Signs and symptoms are undetectable at this phase.

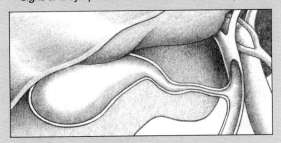

2. When the gallbladder concentrates this bile, inflammation may or may not occur. Excessive water and bile salts are reabsorbed, making the bile less soluble. Cholesterol, calcium, and bilirubin precipitate into gallstones.
  Look for nausea, belching, and pain in the right upper quadrant, especially after a fatty meal.

3. Fat entering the duodenum causes the intestinal mucosa to secrete the hormone cholecystokinin, which stimulates the gallbladder to contract and empty. If a calculus lodges in the cystic duct, the gallbladder contracts but can't empty.
  Look for severe pain, nausea, and vomiting.

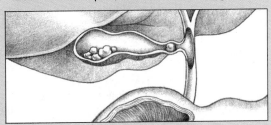

4. If a calculus lodges in the common bile duct, the flow of bile into the duodenum becomes obstructed. Bilirubin is absorbed into the blood, causing jaundice.
  Look for jaundice, biliary colic, clay-colored stools, and fat intolerance.

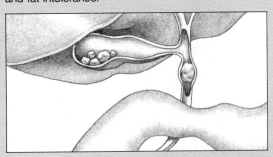

5. Biliary stasis and ischemia of the tissue surrounding the calculus can also cause irritation and inflammation of the common bile duct.
  Look for jaundice, high fever, chills, and an increased eosinophil count.

6. Inflammation can progress up the biliary tree and lead to infection of any of the bile ducts. This causes scar tissue, edema, cirrhosis, portal hypertension, and variceal hemorrhage.
  Look for fever, an increased white blood cell count, ascites, increased prothrombin time, bleeding tendencies, confusion, and coma.

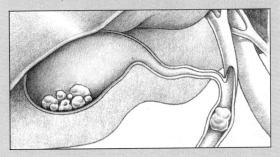

WHERE CALCULI COLLECT

Possible locations for calculi include these sites.

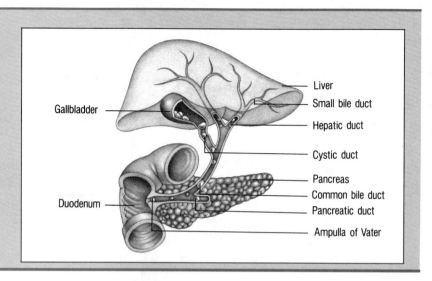

Liver
Small bile duct
Hepatic duct
Cystic duct
Pancreas
Common bile duct
Pancreatic duct
Ampulla of Vater
Gallbladder
Duodenum

Complications

Each of these disorders produces its own set of complications:

• *Cholelithiasis* may lead to any of the disorders associated with gallstone formation: cholangitis, cholecystitis, choledocholithiasis, and gallstone ileus.

• *Cholecystitis* can progress to gallbladder complications, such as empyema, hydrops or mucocele, or gangrene. Gangrene may lead to perforation, resulting in peritonitis, fistula formation, pancreatitis, limy bile, and porcelain gallbladder. Other complications include chronic cholecystitis and cholangitis.

• *Choledocholithiasis* may lead to cholangitis, obstructive jaundice, pancreatitis, and secondary biliary cirrhosis.

• *Cholangitis* may progress to septic shock and death, especially in the suppurative form.

• *Gallstone ileus* may cause bowel obstruction, which can lead to intestinal perforation, peritonitis, septicemia, secondary infection, and septic shock.

Assessment findings

Although gallbladder disease may produce no symptoms (even when X-rays reveal gallstones), acute cholelithiasis, acute cholecystitis, and choledocholithiasis produce symptoms of a classic gallbladder attack.

In a gallbladder attack, the patient typically complains of sudden onset of severe steady or aching pain in the midepigastric region or the right upper abdominal quadrant. He may describe this pain as radiating to his back, between the shoulder blades, or over the right shoulder blade, or just to the shoulder area. This type of pain is known as biliary colic and is the most characteristic symptom of gallbladder disease. It's often severe enough to send him to the emergency department.

Often, the patient reports that the attack followed eating a fatty meal or a large meal after fasting for an extended time. The attack may have occurred in the middle of the night, suddenly awakening him. He may also report nausea, vomiting, and chills; a low-grade fever may be assessed.

The patient may report a history of milder GI symptoms that preceded the acute attack. He may have experienced these symptoms for some time before seeking treatment. Such symptoms may include indigestion, vague abdominal discomfort, belching, and flatulence after eating meals or snacks rich in fats.

During an acute attack, inspection confirms that the patient is in severe pain and reveals pallor, diaphoresis, and exhaustion. If he has chronic cholecystitis, inspection of the skin, sclerae, and oral mucous membranes may confirm jaundice; inspection of urine and stool specimens may reveal dark-colored urine and clay-colored stools.

Tachycardia may be noted on palpation. Light palpation of the abdomen may disclose tenderness over the gallbladder, which increases on inspiration. If a calculus-filled gallbladder without ductal obstruction is palpated, a painless, sausagelike mass can be felt. Auscultation may reveal hypoactive bowel sounds if the patient has acute cholecystitis.

If the patient has cholangitis, he may report a history of choledocholithiasis and classic symptoms of biliary colic. On inspection, jaundice and pain may be evident. He may also have a spiking fever with chills.

In gallstone ileus, the patient may complain of colicky pain, which may persist for several days, sometimes with nausea and vomiting. You may note abdominal distention on inspection. Auscultation may reveal absent bowel sounds if the patient has a complete bowel obstruction.

Diagnostic tests

Ultrasonography and X-rays detect gallstones. Specific procedures include the following:
• *Plain abdominal X-rays* identify gallstones if they contain enough calcium to be radiopaque. X-rays are also helpful in identifying porcelain gallbladder, limy bile, and gallstone ileus.
• *Ultrasonography of the gallbladder* confirms cholelithiasis in most patients and distinguishes between obstructive and nonobstructive jaundice; calculi as small as 2 mm can be detected.
• *Oral cholecystography* confirms the presence of gallstones, although this test is gradually being replaced by ultrasonography.
• *Technetium-labeled iminodiacetic acid scan of the gallbladder* indicates cystic duct obstruction and acute or chronic cholecystitis if the gallbladder can't be seen.
• *Percutaneous transhepatic cholangiography,* imaging performed under fluoroscopic control, supports the diagnosis of obstructive jaundice and visualizes calculi in the ducts.
• *Blood studies* may reveal elevated levels of serum alkaline phosphatase, lactate dehydrogenase, aspartate aminotransferase (formerly SGOT), icteric index, and total bilirubin. The white blood cell count is slightly elevated during a cholecystitis attack.

Treatment

Surgery, usually elective, remains the most common treatment for gallbladder and duct disease. Surgery is usually recommended if the patient has symptoms frequent enough to interfere with his regular routine, if he has any complications of gallstones, or if he has had a previous attack of cholecystitis.

Procedures may include cholecystectomy (laparoscopic or abdominal), cholecystectomy with operative cholangiography, choledochostomy, or exploration of the common bile duct.

If the patient's gallstones are radiolucent and consist all or in part of cholesterol, he may undergo gallstone dissolution therapy. In this procedure, the doctor uses oral chenodeoxycholic acid or ursodeoxycholic acid to partially or completely dissolve gallstones. But this treatment has several limitations, including the need for prolonged treatment, its dissolution of only small calculi, the high incidence of adverse reactions, and the frequency of calculus re-formation after treatment ends.

Other, more direct methods may be used to remove the gallstones. One of these is insertion of a percutaneous transhepatic biliary catheter under fluoroscopic guidance, which permits visualization of the calculi and their removal using a basket-shaped tool, called a Dormia basket. Another calculus-removal technique is endoscopic retrograde cholangiopancreatography (ERCP). In this procedure, the calculi are removed with a balloon or basketlike tool passed through an endoscope. Both of these techniques permit decompression of the biliary tree, allowing bile to flow.

Another technique, lithotripsy, breaks up gallstones using ultrasonic waves. It's been used successfully in some patients with radiolucent calculi. This outpatient procedure is contraindicated in patients with a pacemaker or an automatic implantable defibrillator.

If the patient is asymptomatic or has recovered from a first attack of biliary colic, noninvasive treatment may be attempted. This treatment includes a low-fat diet with replacement of the fat-soluble vitamins A, D, E, and K and administration of bile salts to facilitate digestion and vitamin absorption.

During an acute attack, narcotics relieve pain. (Meperidine is preferred over morphine, which may constrict the sphincter and cause biliary spasm.) Antispasmodics and anticholinergics relax smooth muscles and decrease ductal tone and spasm, and antiemetics reduce nausea and vomiting. A nasogastric (NG) tube may also be inserted and connected to intermittent low-pressure suction to relieve vomiting.

In patients with severe acute cholecystitis, I.V. fluids and I.V. antibiotic therapy are often given before surgery. Cholestyramine may be given if the patient has obstructive jaundice with severe itching from accumulation of bile salts in the skin.

Nonsuppurative cholangitis usually responds quickly to antibiotic therapy. Suppurative cholangitis requires antibiotic therapy, prompt surgical correction of the obstruction, and drainage of the infected bile.

Nursing diagnoses
• Altered gastrointestinal tissue perfusion
• Altered nutrition: Less than body requirements
• Pain
• Risk for fluid volume deficit
• Risk for infection

Nursing interventions
• If the patient will be managed without invasive procedures, provide a low-fat diet and smaller, more frequent meals to help prevent attacks of biliary colic. Also replace vitamins A, D, E, and K, and administer bile salts, as ordered.
• As ordered, administer narcotics and anticholinergics if the patient has pain, and antiemetics if he has nausea and vomiting. Monitor him for the desired effects, and watch for possible adverse reactions.
• If the patient vomits or has nausea, stay with him, assess his vital signs, monitor intake and output, and withhold food and fluids.
• If the patient has cholangitis, give antibiotics as ordered and watch for desired effects and adverse reactions. Also monitor vital signs, and watch for signs of severe toxicity, including confusion, septicemia, and septic shock.
• After percutaneous transhepatic biliary catheterization or ERCP to remove gallstones, assess vital signs. Allow the patient nothing by mouth until the gag reflex returns. Monitor intake and output, keeping in mind that urine retention can be a problem. Observe the patient for complications, including cholangitis and pancreatitis.
• If surgery is scheduled, provide appropriate preoperative care. Usually, this includes insertion of an NG tube.
   After surgery:
• Be alert for signs of bleeding, infection, or atelectasis. Evaluate the incision site for bleeding. Serosanguineous and bile drainage is common during the first 24 to 48 hours if the patient has a wound drain, such as a Jackson-Pratt or Penrose drain. If, after a choledochostomy, a T-tube drain is placed in the duct and attached to a drainage bag, make sure the drainage tube has no kinks. Also make sure the connecting tubing from the T tube is well secured to the patient to prevent dislodgment. Measure and record drainage daily (200 to 300 ml is normal).
• If the patient underwent laparoscopic cholecystectomy, assess for "free-air" pain caused by carbon dioxide insufflation. Encourage ambulation soon after the procedure to promote gas absorption.
• Monitor intake and output. Provide appropriate I.V. fluid intake. Allow the patient nothing by mouth for 24 to 48 hours or until bowel sounds resume and nausea and vomiting cease (postoperative nausea may indicate a full urinary bladder). Administer antiemetics, as ordered, for postoperative nausea and vomiting. Monitor NG tube drainage for color, amount, and consistency.
• When peristalsis resumes, remove the NG tube and begin a clear liquid diet. Advance the diet as tolerated by the patient. If he doesn't void within 8 hours (or if he voids an inadequate amount—based on I.V. fluid intake), percuss over the symphysis pubis for bladder distention (especially in patients receiving anticholinergics). Avoid catheterization, if possible.
• Encourage leg exercises every hour. The patient should ambulate in the evening or morning after surgery. Encourage hourly coughing and deep breathing. Discourage sitting in a chair. Provide elastic stockings to support leg muscles and promote venous blood flow, thus preventing stasis and possible clot formation. Have the patient rest in slight Fowler's position as much as possible to direct any abdominal drainage into the pelvic cavity rather than allowing it to accumulate under the diaphragm.
• Evaluate the location, duration, and character of any pain. Report sudden pain that the patient describes as a tearing of the incision (possible wound dehiscence) as well as chest or back pain. Administer adequate medication to relieve pain, especially before such activities as deep breathing and ambulation, which increase pain. Abdominal distention is common sometime during the second and third postoperative days and may aggravate pain. Abdominal distention resolves spontaneously as bowel function resumes.

Patient teaching
• Teach the patient about the disease and the reasons for his symptoms.
• Explain scheduled diagnostic tests, reviewing pretest instructions and necessary aftercare.
• If a low-fat diet is prescribed, suggest ways to implement it. If necessary, ask the dietitian to reinforce your instructions. Be sure the patient understands how dietary changes help to prevent biliary colic.
• Review the proper use of prescribed medications, explaining their desired effects. Point out possible adverse effects, especially those that warrant a call to the doctor.
• Reinforce the doctor's explanation of the ordered treatment, such as surgery, ERCP, or lithotripsy. Be sure the patient fully understands the possible complications, if any, associated with his treatments.
   Before and after surgery:
• Teach the patient to breathe deeply, cough, expectorate, and perform leg exercises that are necessary after sur-

gery. Also teach splinting, repositioning, and ambulation techniques.

• Explain the procedures that will be performed before, during, and after surgery to help ease the patient's anxiety and ensure his cooperation. Teach the patient who will be discharged with a T tube how to empty it, change the dressing, and provide skin care.

• Upon discharge (usually 4 to 7 days after traditional surgery), advise the patient against heavy lifting or straining for 6 weeks. Urge him to walk daily. Tell him that food restrictions are unnecessary unless he has an intolerance to a specific food or some underlying condition (diabetes, atherosclerosis, obesity) that requires such restriction.

• After laparoscopic surgery, tell the patient he may return to work within 3 to 7 days if no complications develop.

ANORECTAL DISORDERS

These disorders, which commonly cause pain and bleeding, include hemorrhoids, anorectal abscess, anorectal stricture, pilonidal disease, anal fissure, and proctitis, among others.

HEMORRHOIDS

Often painful, hemorrhoids are varicosities in the superior or inferior hemorrhoidal venous plexus. Dilation and enlargement of the superior plexus produce mucosa-covered, internal hemorrhoids that bulge into the rectal lumen and may prolapse during defecation. Dilation and enlargement of the inferior plexus produce skin-covered, external hemorrhoids that may protrude from the rectum. External hemorrhoids are more likely to be thrombotic than internal hemorrhoids. Generally, the incidence of hemorrhoids peaks between ages 20 and 50 and affects both sexes.

Causes

Hemorrhoids probably result from increased intravenous pressure in the hemorrhoidal plexus. Predisposing factors include occupations that require prolonged standing or sitting; straining due to constipation, diarrhea, coughing, sneezing, or vomiting; heart failure; hepatic disease, such as cirrhosis, amoebic abscesses, or hepatitis; alcoholism; anorectal infections; loss of muscle tone due to old age, rectal surgery, or episiotomy; anal intercourse; and pregnancy.

Complications

Local infection or thrombosis of hemorrhoids may occur. Rarely, hemorrhoids cause severe or recurrent bleeding, leading to secondary anemia with significant pallor, fatigue, and weakness.

Assessment findings

Typically, the patient notices and reports intermittent rectal bleeding after defecation. He may report bright red blood on his stools or toilet paper—a sign that the fragile mucosa covering the hemorrhoid was injured during defecation. He also may complain of anal itching (the result of poor anal hygiene) or describe a vague feeling of anal discomfort when bleeding occurs.

If the hemorrhoids are thrombosed, the patient usually complains of rectal pain, which may be accompanied by anal pruritus and mucus discharge. If external hemorrhoids are thrombosed, he may be aware of a large subcutaneous lump in the anal area.

Inspection of the anal area confirms the presence of external hemorrhoids. If the external hemorrhoids are thrombosed, they appear on inspection as blue swellings at the anus. Although internal hemorrhoids usually aren't seen on inspection, they will be obvious if they have prolapsed.

Palpation reveals anal tenderness. Digital rectal examination may detect internal hemorrhoids.

Diagnostic tests

Anoscopy and flexible sigmoidoscopy confirm internal hemorrhoids and rule out other possible causes of symptoms, such as rectal polyps or anal fistulas.

Treatment

Hemorrhoids generally require only conservative treatment designed to ease pain, combat swelling and congestion, and regulate bowel habits. To reduce local pain and swelling, local anesthetic agents (lotions, creams, or suppositories), astringents, or cold compresses may be applied, followed by warm sitz baths or thermal packs. A steroid preparation, such as hydrocortisone, can relieve itching or inflammation.

Stool softeners help prevent straining during defecation. If the patient has a mildly prolapsed internal hemorrhoid, manual reduction may be attempted. Rarely, the patient with chronic, profuse bleeding may require a blood transfusion.

Several outpatient procedures may be used to treat hemorrhoids. A sclerosing solution may be injected to induce scar formation and decrease prolapse. Elastic band ligation is even more effective than sclerotherapy.

Hemorrhoidectomy, still the most effective method with less need for further therapy, is indicated for patients with severe bleeding, intolerable pain, pruritus, and large prolapse. This surgery, which removes the hemorrhoid through cauterization or excision, can now also be performed on an outpatient basis.

Nursing diagnoses
• Constipation
• Knowledge deficit
• Pain
• Risk for infection

Nursing interventions
• If hemorrhoidectomy is scheduled, prepare the patient for surgery. Administer an enema, as ordered (usually 2 to 4 hours before surgery), and record the results. Shave and clean the perianal area.

Postoperative care:
• Watch the patient closely for signs of prolonged rectal bleeding, acute hemorrhage, and hypovolemic shock. Monitor the patient's vital signs every 2 to 4 hours while he is in the hospital. Also monitor and record intake and output. Assess for signs of fluid volume deficit, such as dry mucous membranes and feelings of faintness or weakness.
• Check the dressing regularly, and immediately report any excessive bleeding or drainage. If bleeding is excessive, you may be asked to insert a balloon-tipped catheter into the patient's rectum and inflate the balloon. This will exert pressure on the hemorrhagic area and reduce blood loss.
• Make sure the patient voids within 24 hours after surgery. If necessary, help stimulate voiding with massage and warm sitz baths; catheterize him only if other measures fail to induce urination.
• Clean the perianal area with warm water and a mild soap to prevent infection and irritation, then gently pat the area dry. After spreading petroleum jelly on the wound site to prevent skin irritation, apply a wet dressing (a 1:1 solution of cold water and witch hazel) to the perianal area.
• As necessary, provide the patient with analgesics and sitz baths or hot compresses, which can help prevent rectoanal spasms and reduce local pain, swelling, and inflammation.
• As soon as the patient can resume oral feeding, administer a bulk-forming or stool-softening laxative, as ordered, to ease defecation and ensure the passage of stools shortly after surgery.

Patient teaching
• Teach the patient about hemorrhoidal development, predisposing factors, and tests.
• If conservative treatment is ordered, teach the patient measures to relieve hemorrhoidal discomfort. Suggest that he apply cold packs to the anorectal region for 3 to 4 hours at the onset of pain, followed by warm sitz baths. Recommend nonprescription remedies, such as witch hazel soaks or dibucaine ointment. Advise him to use dibucaine ointment only temporarily; if his pain continues for more than 5 days, he must notify the doctor. Point out that this ointment may mask worsening symptoms and cause him to delay seeking attention for a more serious disorder.
• Encourage the patient to eat a high-fiber diet to promote regular bowel movements. To avoid venous congestion, remind him not to sit on the toilet longer than necessary.
• If the patient has had surgery, provide tips on avoiding constipation. Encourage adequate intake of dietary fiber and fluids. Advise the patient to increase the amount of raw vegetables, fruits, and whole grain cereals in his diet.
• Instruct the patient to check with his doctor about when he can begin using stool softeners to prevent constipation. Warn against using a stool softener too soon after hemorrhoidectomy because a firm stool acts as a natural anal dilator to prevent anal stricture from the scar tissue.
• Emphasize the need for good anal hygiene. Caution against vigorous wiping with washcloths and using harsh soaps. Encourage the use of medicated astringent pads and toilet paper made without dyes or perfumes.
• To reduce postoperative pain and swelling, encourage sitz baths. Instruct the patient to watch for and report increased rectal bleeding, purulent drainage, fever, constipation, or rectal spasm.

ANORECTAL ABSCESS AND FISTULA
A localized infection, anorectal abscess appears as a collection of pus due to inflammation of the soft tissue. As the abscess produces more pus, a fistula may form, creating an abnormal opening in the anal skin.

A fistula usually forms in the soft tissue beneath the muscle fibers of the sphincters (especially the external sphincter), extending into the perianal skin. The internal (primary) opening of the abscess or fistula is usually near the anal glands and crypts; the external (secondary) opening, in the perianal skin. In severe cases, this opening may communicate with the rectum.

Causes

The inflammatory process that leads to abscess may begin with an abrasion or tear in the lining of the anal canal, rectum, or perianal skin and subsequent infection with *Escherichia coli*, staphylococci, or streptococci. Such trauma may result from abrasive contact with certain objects, such as enema tips, ingested eggshells, fishbones, or very hard stools. An abscess may also develop after infection of submucosal hematomas, sclerosed hemorrhoids, or anal fissures.

Other causes include obstruction of glands in the anal area, extension of cryptitis, infection in the apocrine glands, or folliculitis in the perianal region. Certain systemic illnesses also may lead to abscess formation, including ulcerative colitis and Crohn's disease.

Complications

Anorectal abscess may lead to anorectal fistula. Either disorder can cause perineal cellulitis, scar tissue formation, and anal stricture. Rarely, peritonitis develops from internal abscess rupture.

Assessment findings

Signs and symptoms depend on the severity of the infection and whether or not the abscess is a chronic condition. Assessment findings also vary according to the type of abscess. (See *Types of anorectal abscess.*)

Usually, the first symptom the patient reports is rectal pain, which he usually describes as throbbing. Occasionally, diarrhea precedes the onset of rectal pain. The patient may also state that he can't sit comfortably because of the development of a hard, painful lump on one side.

If the anorectal abscess is a chronic condition, the patient may report discharge or bleeding and anal pruritus. If he also has an anal fistula, anal pruritus and purulent discharge are commonly reported.

Depending on the infection's severity, the patient may also complain of fever, chills, nausea, vomiting, and malaise.

Inspection may reveal an erythematous lump or swelling in the anal area. If the patient has a fistula, its external opening may be visible as a pink or red, elevated, discharging sinus or ulcer on the skin near the anus. Palpation usually reveals tenderness over the reddened or swollen area.

Digital examination of the patient with a fistula may detect a palpable, indurated tract and a depression or ulcer in the midline anteriorly or at the dentate line posteriorly.

TYPES OF ANORECTAL ABSCESS

Although perianal abscess is the most common form of anorectal abscess, don't overlook the possibility of other types. Assessment findings usually help to distinguish among the four types of anorectal abscesses.

Perianal abscess
This abscess, which occurs in 80% of patients, appears on inspection as a red, tender, localized oval swelling close to the anus. Pus may drain from the abscess. The patient may report that sitting or coughing increases his pain. Digital examination reveals no abnormalities.

Ischiorectal abscess
This abscess, which affects 15% of patients, involves the entire perianal region on the affected side of the anus. Palpation reveals tenderness. The abscess may not produce drainage. Digital examination detects a tender induration bulging into the anal canal.

Submucosal or high intermuscular abscess
About 5% of patients have this form of abscess, which may cause a dull, aching pain in the rectum. The abscess may produce tenderness and, occasionally, induration. Digital examination reveals a smooth swelling of the upper part of the anal canal or lower rectum.

Pelvirectal abscess
The patient with this rare abscess typically reports malaise and myalgia. He also has a fever, but no local anal or external rectal signs or pain. Digital examination detects a tender mass high in the pelvis, perhaps extending into one of the ischiorectal fossae.

Diagnostic tests

Sigmoidoscopy, barium enema, and colonoscopy may be performed to rule out other conditions.

Treatment

Anorectal abscesses require surgical incision and drainage, usually under caudal anesthesia. Fistulas require fistulotomy—removal of the fistula and associated granulation tissue—under caudal anesthesia. If the fistula tract is epithelialized, treatment requires fistulectomy—removal of the fistulous tract—followed by insertion of drains, which remain in place for 48 hours. Fistulas that result from an intestinal disorder, such as Crohn's disease, are usually treated conservatively because surgery is often not successful.

Nursing diagnoses
• Pain
• Risk for infection

Nursing interventions
• Before surgery, apply ice and witch hazel soaks, and provide sitz baths to help ease the patient's discomfort.
• After the incision to drain the anorectal abscess, provide adequate medication for pain relief, as ordered. Examine the wound frequently to assess proper healing. Healing should be complete in 4 to 5 weeks for perianal fistulas and 12 to 16 weeks for deeper wounds.
• Dispose of soiled dressings properly.
• Note the time of the first postoperative bowel movement. Anticipating pain, the patient may suppress the urge to defecate; the resulting constipation would increase pressure at the wound site. Such a patient benefits from a stool-softening laxative, such as psyllium.

Patient teaching
• Explain the disorder to the patient. If diagnostic tests are scheduled, review their purpose and required preparation and aftercare.
• Emphasize that complete recovery takes time. Offer encouragement.
• Teach the patient that a diet high in fiber and fluids promotes regular bowel movements, which helps to prevent irritation of an existing abscess. Explain that straining during a bowel movement can increase abscess discomfort.
• Stress the importance of perianal cleanliness at all times, especially after bowel movements or any contact with a foreign body. Tell the patient that good hygiene helps prevent infection.
• Provide appropriate preoperative teaching if surgery will be performed. Be sure the patient understands the procedure and its possible complications.
• After surgery, reinforce the importance of diet and perianal cleanliness. Teach the patient about prescribed medications, such as analgesics or stool softeners. Also show him how to perform sitz baths, if these are ordered to promote comfort.

POLYPS
Arising as masses of tissue above the mucosal membrane, polyps may develop in the rectum or colon, where they protrude into the GI tract. Polyps are classified according to tissue type: They include common polypoid adenomas, villous adenomas, familial polyposis, focal polypoid hyperplasia, and juvenile polyps (hamarto-

mas). Polyps also may be described by their appearance: They may be pedunculated (attached by a stalk to the intestinal wall) or sessile (attached to the intestinal wall with a broad base and no stalk).

Most polyps are benign. However, villous and familial polyps show a marked inclination to become malignant. Indeed, a striking feature of familial polyposis is its frequent association with rectosigmoid adenocarcinoma.

Villous adenomas are most prevalent in men over age 55; common polypoid adenomas, in white women between ages 45 and 60. The incidence in both sexes rises after age 70. Juvenile polyps occur most commonly in children under age 10 and are characterized by rectal bleeding.

Causes
Polyps are caused by unrestrained cell growth in the upper epithelium. Risk factors include heredity, age, infection, and diet.

Complications
Slow bleeding from polyps can result in anemia. Occasionally, a polyp may grow large enough to cause bowel obstruction. Polyps can also be complicated by gross rectal bleeding or intussusception. Polypoid adenomas are believed to give rise to most colorectal cancers.

Assessment findings
In many patients, assessment findings are minimal because these patients have no obvious symptoms. Usually, polyps are discovered incidentally during a digital examination or rectosigmoidoscopy. Rarely, the patient history reveals obvious rectal bleeding and diarrhea.

Diagnostic tests
• *Proctosigmoidoscopy* or *colonoscopy with biopsy* confirms the diagnosis.
• *Stool analyses* detect occult blood in the stools of about 5% of patients with polyps.
• *Hemoglobin and hematocrit levels* may decrease in rectal bleeding.

Treatment
The therapeutic regimen depends on the type and size of the polyps and their location within the rectum or colon. Polypectomy may be performed if the polyp is pedunculated. This procedure uses an electrocautery snare inserted through a sigmoidoscope or a colonoscope. Even large, pedunculated polyps can be removed by this method. Sessile polyps usually require abdominal surgery for removal. Some benign polyps are not removed

but are monitored periodically for changes by routine sigmoidoscopy or colonoscopy.

Depending on the extent of GI involvement, familial polyposis requires total abdominoperineal resection with a permanent ileostomy or subtotal colectomy with an ileoproctostomy. Juvenile polyps are prone to autoamputation; if this doesn't occur, snare removal during colonoscopy is the treatment of choice.

Nursing diagnoses
• Anxiety
• Pain
• Risk for infection

Nursing interventions
• Offer psychological support to the patient, as necessary, because he probably fears a diagnosis of cancer. Listen to his concerns and offer reassurance.
• After polypectomy, monitor the patient for signs of complications, such as bleeding, infection, and perforation. Watch for decreased hemoglobin and hematocrit levels, rectal bleeding, mucopurulent rectal drainage, and abdominal pain and discharge. If the patient is hospitalized, watch for and record the first bowel movement, which may not occur for 2 to 3 days. Provide sitz baths for 3 days.
• If abdominal surgery is necessary, prepare the patient for the type of scheduled surgery.
• After abdominal surgery, provide appropriate postoperative care. Monitor vital signs, intake and output, and fluid and electrolyte balance. Provide I.V. therapy, and administer pain medications, as needed. Monitor the surgical site for healing, and change the dressing, as ordered.
• If the patient has an ileostomy or another type of stoma, provide stoma care, and arrange for an enterostomal therapist to visit the patient.

Patient teaching
• Teach the patient about polyps. Explain monitoring procedures, such as sigmoidoscopy and colonoscopy, that will be performed periodically. Stress the need for periodic monitoring of benign polyps. Instruct him to report any rectal bleeding.
• If polypectomy is scheduled, explain the procedure and its possible complications. Emphasize the need for follow-up care to monitor for any new growth.
• If abdominal surgery is scheduled, provide appropriate preoperative teaching. Show the patient how to cough and deep-breathe. Teach him how to splint his incision. Review his postoperative care plan, including the use of

analgesics to relieve pain. Discuss the proper use of other medications, including their desired effects and possible adverse reactions. If necessary, teach him how to perform stoma care.

ANORECTAL STRICTURE, STENOSIS, OR CONTRACTURE

A narrowing of the anal canal, anorectal stricture results from intraluminal inflammation or scarring. Stenosis or contracture prevents sphincter dilation.

Causes
Anorectal stricture results from scarring after anorectal surgery or inflammation, radiation to the pelvic area, inadequate postoperative care, or laxative abuse.

Complications
Severe bleeding and infection are the most common complications.

Assessment findings
The patient typically reports a history of anorectal surgery, radiation to the pelvic area, or laxative abuse. He may describe excessive straining to have a bowel movement and a feeling of incomplete bowel evacuation. Other clinical features are pain, bleeding, and pruritus.

Inspection reveals narrowing of the anal canal; digital examination discloses anal tenderness and tightness.

Diagnostic tests
Visual inspection and digital examination confirm the diagnosis. No diagnostic tests are performed for this disorder.

Treatment
The aim of therapy is to alleviate the underlying cause. For example, if inflammation is the cause of stricture, correction of the underlying inflammatory process is necessary. If laxative abuse is the cause, this habit must be corrected to prevent recurrence.

Surgical removal of scar tissue is usually the most effective treatment. Digital or instrumental dilatation may be beneficial; however, it may cause additional tears and splits of the anal mucosa. Balloon dilatation also may be successful.

Nursing diagnoses
• Anxiety
• High risk for infection

- Pain
- Risk for infection

Nursing interventions
- Provide psychological support. Patients with elimination problems often are very anxious. Listen to the patient's fears and concerns.
- After dilatation, provide the patient with a high-fiber diet to help keep the sphincter dilated.
- If surgery is scheduled, provide appropriate preoperative care.

  After surgery:
- Check vital signs often until the patient is stable. Watch for signs of hemorrhage (excessive bleeding on the perianal dressing). If surgery was performed under spinal anesthesia, record the first leg movement, and keep the patient lying flat for 6 to 8 hours after surgery.
- When the patient's condition is stable, resume a normal diet, and record the time of the first bowel movement. Administer stool softeners, as ordered. Give analgesics, provide sitz baths, and change the perianal dressing, as ordered.

Patient teaching
- Teach the patient about the disorder, explaining its probable cause and the treatment plan. If he will undergo dilatation, point out that this procedure may need to be repeated. If he's scheduled for surgery to remove adhesions, provide appropriate preoperative teaching.
- Review the proper use of prescribed medications, focusing on their desired effects and possible adverse reactions.
- Stress the benefits of a high-fiber diet to the patient. Have the dietitian review the dietary plan with him.
- Discuss proper perineal care with the patient, stressing the importance of good hygiene.

PILONIDAL DISEASE
In this disorder, a lesion called a coccygeal or pilonidal cyst develops in the sacral area. The cyst—which usually contains hair—becomes infected and commonly produces an abscess, a draining sinus, or a fistula. Generally, a pilonidal cyst produces no symptoms until it becomes infected. The incidence is highest among hirsute, white men ages 18 to 30.

Causes
Pilonidal disease may develop congenitally from a tendency to hirsutism, or it may be acquired from stretching or irritation of the sacrococcygeal area (intergluteal fold)

from prolonged rough exercise (such as horseback riding), heat, excessive perspiration, or constricting clothing.

Complications
Pain and discomfort associated with pilonidal disease can cause psychosocial complications for the patient, such as impaired social interaction and difficulty performing work-related activities. This is most likely if his life-style or occupation requires vigorous activity that irritates the cyst, causing increased pain.

Assessment findings
Investigation of the patient history may turn up one or more predisposing factors for pilonidal disease. Typically, the patient complains of localized pain, tenderness, swelling, and heat over the affected area. He may also describe continuous or intermittent purulent drainage. If the infection is severe enough, signs and symptoms include chills, fever, headache, and malaise.

On inspection, you may detect a series of openings along the midline, with thin, brown, foul-smelling drainage or a protruding tuft of hair. Palpation of the area may produce purulent drainage, if the drainage is not already continuous.

Diagnostic tests
Cultures of discharge from the infected cyst may show staphylococci or skin bacteria; the discharge doesn't usually contain bowel bacteria.

Treatment
Conservative measures consist of incision and drainage of abscesses, regular extraction of protruding hairs, and sitz baths (four to six times daily). However, persistent infections may result in abscess formation and require surgical excision of the infected area.

After excision of a pilonidal abscess, the patient requires regular follow-up care to monitor wound healing. The surgeon may periodically palpate the wound during healing with a cotton-tipped applicator, curette excess granulation tissue, and extract loose hairs to promote wound healing from the inside out and to prevent dead cells from collecting in the wound. Complete healing may take several months.

Nursing diagnoses
- Impaired social interaction
- Pain
- Risk for infection

Nursing interventions

• Before incision and drainage of a pilonidal abscess, reassure the patient that he'll receive analgesics to ease discomfort. If surgery will be performed, provide appropriate preoperative care.

After surgery:

• Monitor vital signs often until the patient is stable; check compression dressings for signs of excessive bleeding, such as large amounts of blood on the perianal dressing. Change the dressing as directed, using sterile technique to avoid infection.

• Administer analgesics and provide sitz baths, as needed, to relieve discomfort and maintain hygiene.

• Provide stool softeners, as ordered, and record the time of the first bowel movement. When the patient's condition is stable, resume a normal diet.

• Encourage the patient to walk within 24 hours.

Patient teaching

• Teach the patient about pilonidal disease, and explain his treatment plan. Reassure him that the disorder usually resolves completely with proper treatment.

• Before surgery, reinforce the doctor's explanation of the procedure, and answer the patient's questions.

• After surgery or incision and drainage, instruct the patient to wear a gauze sponge over the site once the dressing has been removed. Explain that the protective covering will provide ventilation and prevent friction from clothing from irritating the wound. Recommend the continued use of sitz baths, followed by air-drying instead of towel drying.

• Review the proper use of prescribed medications, usually analgesics and antibiotics. Teach the patient about the desired action of each drug and any adverse reactions that he should report to his doctor.

RECTAL PROLAPSE

The circumferential protrusion of one or more layers of the mucous membrane through the anus, rectal prolapse occurs in two forms. Partial (mucosal) prolapse involves rectal mucosa up to the internal sphincter; complete prolapse involves both the rectal mucosa and the rectal wall.

More common in women than in men, rectal prolapse is most common after age 40. It also occurs in children — typically between ages 1 and 3 — especially those with cystic fibrosis.

Causes

Increased intra-abdominal pressure — for example, from straining during defecation — usually triggers rectal prolapse. Other causes include relaxed anal sphincters and weak pelvic muscles that can result from neurologic disorders, injury, tumors, aging, and chronic wasting diseases, such as tuberculosis or cystic fibrosis.

Complications

Rectal prolapse may lead to rectal ulceration, bleeding, and incontinence.

Assessment findings

The patient may report tissue protrusion from the rectum, which occurs during defecation or some type of exertion, such as walking. She may also report one or more of the following problems: a persistent sensation of rectal fullness, mucus discharge, bloody diarrhea, fecal incontinence and, occasionally, lower abdominal pain.

Inspection distinguishes between complete and partial prolapse. Complete prolapse involves a protruding rectal mass that exposes the full thickness of the bowel wall and, possibly, a protruding sphincter muscle with mucosa falling into bulky, concentric folds. Partial prolapse involves a partly protruding mucosa and a smaller mass of radial mucosal folds. If necessary, ask the patient to squat before you inspect the prolapse. Sometimes, the prolapse is obvious only when the patient squats.

Diagnostic tests

Physical examination confirms the diagnosis.

Treatment

The type of therapy depends on the symptoms and the underlying cause. Eliminating the cause (straining or coughing) may be the only treatment needed. In a child, prolapsed tissue usually diminishes as the child grows. In an older patient, a sclerosing agent may be injected to cause a fibrotic reaction that fixes the rectum in place. Severe or chronic prolapse requires surgical repair by strengthening or tightening the sphincters with wire or by resecting prolapsed tissue anteriorly or rectally.

Nursing diagnoses

• Anxiety
• Constipation
• Knowledge deficit
• Pain
• Risk for infection

Nursing interventions

• Provide psychological support to the patient. She's likely to be upset and anxious about her condition.

• Before surgery, give appropriate care. After surgery, monitor the patient's vital signs and intake and output. Administer pain medications, as needed, and watch for desired effects and possible adverse reactions. Also watch for immediate complications (hemorrhage) and later ones (pelvic abscess, fever, pus drainage, pain, rectal stenosis, constipation, or pain on defecation).

Patient teaching
• Explain what causes rectal prolapse. Review treatment options and answer questions the patient may have.
• Help the patient prevent constipation. Explain the role of diet and stool softeners. If she has severe prolapse and incontinence, advise her to wear a perianal pad.
• Teach perineum strengthening exercises: Have the patient lie down, with her back flat on the mattress; then ask her to pull in her abdomen and squeeze while taking a deep breath. Or have her repeatedly squeeze and relax her buttocks while sitting on a chair.
• If the patient will be treated with a sclerosing agent, explain that the injected medication will cause fibrosis, which will fix the rectum in place.
• If surgery will be performed, review the operation and possible complications, as needed. Be sure that the patient understands that surgery may not correct the prolapse and that it may cause fecal incontinence.
• Teach the patient about prescribed medications, reviewing their desired and possibly adverse effects.

ANAL FISSURE

An anal fissure is a laceration or crack in the lining of the anus that extends to the circular muscle. Acute fissures usually heal spontaneously or with minimal treatment. Chronic fissures recur and may require surgery. The prognosis is good, especially with fissurectomy and good anal hygiene.

Posterior fissure, the most common form, is equally prevalent in males and females. Anterior fissure, the rarer type, is 10 times more common in females.

Causes
Posterior fissure results from the passage of large, hard stools that stretch the anal lining beyond its limits. Anterior fissure usually results from strain on the perineum during childbirth or, rarely, from stricture caused by scar tissue. Diarrhea and spasm may cause anal fissures. Some anal fissures develop secondary to proctitis, Crohn's disease, trauma, anal tuberculosis, or cancer.

Complications
Rare complications include abscess, fistula, septicemia, and hemorrhage. Chronic fissure may produce scar tissue that hampers normal bowel evacuation.

Assessment findings
Typically, the patient complains of pain, which he describes as tearing, cutting, or burning, during or immediately after a bowel movement. He may also report blood on his underclothes or toilet paper.

In the patient with chronic fissure, additional signs and symptoms may include dysuria, pruritus, and urinary frequency or urine retention. This patient may also complain of painful anal sphincter spasms that result from ulceration of "sentinel pile" (swelling at the lower end of the fissure).

Gentle traction on the perianal skin can create sufficient eversion to visualize the fissure directly. Digital rectal examination permits palpation of the fissure. Keep in mind that a digital examination can elicit pain and bleeding.

Diagnostic tests
Anoscopy showing longitudinal tears helps to confirm the diagnosis. If the patient has painless or multiple fissures, barium enema and sigmoidoscopy are performed to rule out inflammatory bowel disease.

Treatment
Management of an acute fissure aims to provide local pain relief with analgesics, sitz baths, and bulk-producing agents, such as psyllium. Soft stools prevent further tearing and decrease pain associated with defecation. Intra-anal application of isosorbide dinitrate ointment over 6 to 12 weeks is successful in most patients. If further treatment is required, the fissure may be removed by surgical excision (fissurectomy).

Nursing diagnoses
• Constipation
• Diarrhea
• Pain

Nursing interventions
• Provide hot sitz baths, warm soaks, and local anesthetic ointment to relieve pain.
• Administer pain medications, stool softeners, and bulk-forming laxatives, as ordered. Monitor the patient for the desired effects and potential adverse reactions.
• In addition to stool softeners and laxatives, provide the patient with a low-residue diet and adequate fluids to

soften stools and prevent straining during defecation.
• If diarrhea occurs, control it with diphenoxylate or other antidiarrheals.
• If surgery is necessary, provide preoperative care, as appropriate. Postoperatively, monitor the patient's vital signs and continue with the regimen (including sitz baths) established before surgery.

Patient teaching
• Teach about the disorder, explaining how a fissure develops and what can be done to prevent recurrence.
• If rectal examination will be performed, discuss the procedure with the patient. Help him to understand that, although the examination may be painful, it will help the doctor confirm the presence of a fissure.
• Stress the need to drink fluids to prevent hard stools.
• If surgery is necessary, reinforce the doctor's explanation of the procedure and review any possible complications. Provide appropriate preoperative teaching.

PROCTITIS

An inflammation of the rectal mucosa, proctitis has a good prognosis unless massive bleeding occurs.

Causes
Proctitis may develop secondary to rectal gonorrhea, candidiasis, or syphilis, or nonspecific sexually transmitted infections. The most common causative pathogens are *Neisseria gonorrhoeae*, chlamydiae, and herpesvirus.

Other causes include chronic constipation, habitual laxative use, emotional upset, radiation therapy, endocrine dysfunction, rectal surgery, rectal medications, allergies, vasomotor disturbance that interferes with normal muscle control, and food poisoning.

Complications
Proctitis can lead to ulcerations, crypt abscesses, bleeding, fissures, and fistulas. Submucosal inflammation with fibrosis may occur, leading to stricture.

Assessment findings
The patient typically complains of these key symptoms: constipation, a feeling of rectal fullness, and cramps in the left abdomen. The history may also reveal tenesmus producing a few bloody or mucoid stools.

Diagnostic tests
• *Sigmoidoscopy* in acute proctitis shows edematous, bright red or pink rectal mucosa that is shiny, thick, friable, and possibly ulcerated. In chronic proctitis, sigmoidoscopy shows thickened mucosa, loss of vascular pattern, and stricture of the rectal lumen.
• *Biopsy* is performed to rule out cancer.
• *Bacteriologic and viral analyses* detect the cause.

Treatment
Therapy aims to remove the underlying cause of proctitis, such as fecal impaction or laxative abuse. Anti-infective medications are given for infection. Corticosteroids (in enema or suppository form) may reduce inflammation as may sulfasalazine, mesalamine, or similar agents. Tranquilizers may relieve emotional stress.

Nursing diagnoses
• Anxiety
• Knowledge deficit
• Pain

Nursing interventions
• Offer emotional support and reassurance during rectal examinations and treatment, as appropriate.
• Administer anti-infective medications, sulfasalazine, and tranquilizers, as ordered. Provide soothing enemas, steroid foam, or steroid suppositories, as ordered, to relieve pain. Monitor the patient's response.

Patient teaching
• Explain proctitis and its treatment to help the patient understand the disorder and prevent its recurrence.
• Instruct the patient to watch for and report anal bleeding and other persistent signs and symptoms.
• Review prescribed medications.
• Teach the patient how to administer steroid enemas, foam, or suppositories, as needed.
• If constipation adds to symptoms, teach about fluid intake, a high-fiber diet, and stool softeners.

SELECTED REFERENCES

Betz, C., et al., eds. *Family-Centered Nursing Care of Children*, 2nd ed. Philadelphia: W.B. Saunders Co., 1994.

Fischbach, F.A. *A Manual of Laboratory and Diagnostic Tests*, 4th ed. Philadelphia: J.B. Lippincott Co., 1992.

Illustrated Manual of Nursing Practice, 2nd ed. Springhouse, Pa.: Springhouse Corp., 1994.

Isselbacher, K., et al., eds. *Harrison's Principles of Internal Medicine*, 13th ed. New York: McGraw-Hill Book Co., 1995.

Rakel, R.E., ed. *Conn's Current Therapy 1996*. Philadelphia: W.B. Saunders Co., 1996.

Tierney, L., et al. *Current Medical Diagnosis and Treatment 1995*. East Norwalk, Conn.: Appleton & Lange, 1995.

13   METABOLIC DISORDERS

INTRODUCTION

A complex progression of chemical changes, cell metabolism determines the final use of nutrients by the body. Cell metabolism has two main phases: catabolism and anabolism. In *catabolism,* the body breaks down complex substances into simple constituents for energy production or excretion. In *anabolism,* the tissue-building phase, simple substances combine to form more complex substances; this process produces new cellular material and stores energy. Both phases are accomplished by a chemical process that uses energy.

At the cellular level, metabolism provides energy in the form of adenosine triphosphate (ATP), a compound that's essential for cells to function. Three basic nutrients — carbohydrates, proteins, and fats — supply the energy needed for metabolism; vitamins and minerals must also contribute to the process.

Basal metabolism refers to the energy that the resting body needs to maintain life. To maintain an activity level, a person needs energy above and beyond the basal metabolic rate. Activity levels are expressed as kilocalories used per minute. One kilocalorie (kcal) equals the amount of heat required to raise 1 kg of water 1° C at atmospheric pressure. This unit is used in the study of metabolism and to express the energy value of foods.

Activity levels are also expressed as metabolic equivalents of a task (METs). METs refer to the amount of oxygen used per kilogram of body weight per minute. One MET equals 3.5 cc oxygen/kg/minute. A person at rest expends approximately 1 MET.

Carbohydrate metabolism

Composed of carbon, hydrogen, and oxygen, carbohydrates provide the primary source of energy, yielding 4 kcal/g. Experts recommend that carbohydrates make up about 55% of a person's daily dietary intake.

Ingested as starches (complex carbohydrates) and sugars (simple carbohydrates), carbohydrates are the chief protein-sparing ingredients in a nutritionally sound diet. Carbohydrates are absorbed primarily as glucose; some are absorbed as fructose and galactose and converted to glucose by the liver. A body cell may metabolize glucose to produce the energy needed to maintain cell life or may store it as glycogen.

Most of the energy produced by glucose metabolism goes toward forming the ATP found in the cytoplasm and nucleoplasm of all body cells. ATP is the principal storage form of immediately available energy for cell reactions. Complex carbohydrates, such as rice, pasta, and legumes, provide more energy than simple carbohydrates, such as sugar, ice cream, and candy.

The liver synthesizes glycogen (glycogenesis) from glucose, then reconverts glycogen to glucose (glycogenolysis) as needed. The liver can also transform excess glucose into fatty acids (lipogenesis) that may be stored as adipose tissue (fat).

Excessive carbohydrate intake — especially of simple carbohydrates — can cause obesity, predisposing the patient to many disorders, including hypertension.

Protein metabolism

Proteins are complex organic compounds containing carbon, hydrogen, oxygen, and nitrogen atoms. They consist of amino acids joined by peptide bonds. One gram of protein yields 4 kcal. Proteins should make up about 15% of the daily caloric intake. The body needs protein for growth, maintenance, and repair of all tissue as well as for efficient performance of regulatory mechanisms.

Different proteins consist of different numbers and kinds of amino acids (organic compounds necessary for nitrogen balance but not synthesized in the body). Some amino acids are supplied by food (called essential amino acids), and the others can be produced by the body (called nonessential amino acids). Not all protein food sources are identical in quality. Complete proteins, such as those found in poultry, fish, meat, eggs, milk, and cheese, can maintain body tissue and promote a normal growth rate. Incomplete proteins, such as vegetables and grains, lack essential amino acids.

The body must break down dietary protein into amino acids and peptides for absorption. Amino acids pass unchanged through the intestinal wall and travel by the portal vein through the liver and into the general circulation; from there, each tissue type absorbs the specific amino acid it needs to make its protein.

The collected amino acids derived from protein digestion, absorption, and endogenous tissue breakdown form a reserve metabolic pool, which ensures the availability of a balanced mixture of amino acids to meet the energy needs of various organs and tissues.

The body doesn't store protein. This nutrient has a limited life span and constantly undergoes change (synthesis, degradation to amino acids, and resynthesis into new tissue proteins). The rate of protein turnover varies in different tissues. When the usual sources (available carbohydrate or fat) cannot meet the energy demands of the body, the body uses protein precursors to generate energy.

In a healthy person, if caloric intake is adequate and protein intake exceeds the minimum requirement, nitrogen intake should equal nitrogen excretion, producing nitrogen balance. Positive nitrogen balance occurs when nitrogen intake exceeds its output—for example, during pregnancy or growth periods. Negative nitrogen balance occurs when nitrogen output exceeds intake. Negative balance may result from inadequate dietary protein intake, which causes tissue to break down to supply energy; inadequate quality of ingested dietary protein; or excessive tissue breakdown after stress, injury, immobilization, or disease.

Fat metabolism

Like carbohydrates, fats consist of carbon, hydrogen, and oxygen. However, fats have a smaller proportion of oxygen than carbohydrates and also differ in their structure and properties. The major fats are the glycerides (primarily triglycerides), phospholipids, and cholesterol. Glycerides, the end product of fat digestion, are used by body cells for energy. Phospholipids, formed by the liver, make up 95% of all blood lipids and serve several functions:

• assisting in the transport of fatty acids through the intestinal mucosa into the lymph
• providing protective insulation of nerve fibers as the myelin sheath
• participating in phosphate tissue reactions
• forming thromboplastin and some structural body elements.

Also formed by the liver, cholesterol contributes to the formation of cholic acid, which produces the bile salts necessary for fat digestion. It also contributes to the synthesis of provitamin D, helps form hormones (especially the adrenocortical steroids and the steroid sex hormones), and helps produce the water-resistant quality of the skin. Together with phospholipids in the body cells, cholesterol helps form the insoluble cell membrane needed to maintain physical cellular integrity.

Fats are insoluble in water. However, when proteins combine with fats and phospholipids, the resulting lipoproteins can move through the aqueous medium of the blood. Lipoproteins contain proteins, triglycerides, cholesterol, phospholipids, and traces of related materials, including fat-soluble vitamins and steroid sex hormones. The percentage of protein determines the density of a lipoprotein. For example, a high-density lipoprotein contains a higher percentage of protein than a low-density lipoprotein.

One gram of fat yields 9 kcal. Fats should make up about 30% of the daily caloric intake—5% to 10% less than the amount ingested by the average American. Saturated fats should account for only about one-third of total fat consumption, and a person should consume no more than 300 mg of cholesterol per day. A major source

of energy, fats give taste and flavor to food. They have a high satiety value, reduce gastric motility, and remain in the stomach longer than other foods, thereby delaying the onset of hunger sensations.

Dietary fat carries fat-soluble vitamins. The absorption of vitamin A and its precursor carotene requires fat.

Fats not used for energy are synthesized into other lipids in the liver or stored as adipose tissue in subcutaneous tissue and in the abdominal cavity, where they insulate the body (reducing body heat loss in cold weather) and provide padding and protection for vital organs. When the body needs energy, adipose tissue releases fatty acids and glycerol into the circulation.

Role of vitamins and minerals

Essential for normal metabolism, growth, and development, these biologically active organic compounds contribute to enzyme reactions that facilitate the metabolism of amino acids, fats, and carbohydrates. Although each person requires relatively small amounts of vitamins, inadequate vitamin intake leads to deficiency states or disorders. (For more information on vitamins, see the appendix "Nutritional disorders.")

Equally essential to good nutrition, minerals participate in various physiologic activities, including:
• metabolism of many enzymes
• membrane transfer of essential compounds
• maintenance of acid-base balance (stable concentration of hydrogen ions in the body) and osmotic pressure (pressure on a semipermeable membrane separating a solution from a solvent)
• nerve impulse transmission
• muscle contractility.

Minerals also contribute indirectly to the growth process; although requirements for individual minerals vary, the greatest overall need occurs from birth to puberty.

Maintaining homeostasis

A critical component of metabolism is fluid and electrolyte balance. Water—body fluid's essential component—and electrolytes serve many functions within the body. For instance, water helps regulate body temperature, transports nutrients and gases, conveys wastes to excretion sites, and helps maintain cell shape (through its high surface tension). Electrolytes—chemical compounds that dissociate in solution into charged particles (ions)—carry an electric charge that conducts the electric current necessary for normal cell function.

Body fluids account for about 57% of total body weight in an average (154-lb [70-kg]) adult and about 75% in an average infant. Adipose tissue contains less water than any other tissue in the body, so obese persons and women, who usually have a greater proportion of adipose tissue than men, have a lower percentage of body fluids.

Fluid balance

The term *fluid balance* describes fluid homeostasis: a total body water content that remains relatively constant. But fluid balance also means a relatively constant fluid distribution between the body's main fluid compartments: intracellular fluid (ICF) and extracellular fluid (ECF).

Two-thirds of body fluid is ICF (contained within the cells); the other third is ECF (found outside the cells). The ECF is mainly found in two compartments: the vascular compartment (fluid in the blood vessels) and the interstitial compartment (fluid surrounding the cells). Small amounts of ECF are also found in dense connective tissue, bone, and transcellular spaces, such as gut lumen; cerebrospinal fluid; and intraocular fluid. However, these are not usually clinically significant.

For health and optimal growth and development, the patient must maintain both *external fluid balance* (steady-state fluid and electrolyte exchange between his body and the environment) and *internal fluid balance* (steady-state fluid and electrolyte exchange between fluid compartments). The body gains and loses water each day, with infants exchanging a greater amount than adults. To maintain body fluid volume, gains and losses must balance each other.

Regulation of fluids and electrolytes

Physical processes, such as diffusion, active transport, and osmotic pressure, affect the movement of solutes and water through both the ICF and ECF compartments. Both compartments normally have equal concentrations of solutes (particles), so no *net* water movement occurs from one compartment to the other. Although water does move back and forth, each compartment's volume remains the same.

However, if one compartment's fluid concentration (osmolality) exceeds the other's, water moves between compartments by osmosis, creating a fluid imbalance. For example, if extracellular water loss exceeds electrolyte loss (or if electrolyte gain exceeds water gain), ECF osmolality rises. This fluid would contain more solutes per liter than normal and would thus have a higher osmolality than the ICF. Because cell membranes don't allow free solute passage, water would leave cells and pass, by osmosis, into the ECF. Cell shrinkage and disrupted function would result.

Conversely, if ECF gains more water than it gains solutes (or loses more electrolytes than water), its osmolality declines and water moves from the ECF into the more concentrated ICF. (See *Comparing fluid tonicity,* page 954.)

Internal regulation

Internal factors also alter fluid and electrolyte status. These factors and the regulating organs and hormones that maintain fluid and electrolyte balance are discussed below:

• *Stretch receptors in atrial walls.* These respond to increased fluid volume. The increased volume heightens sodium ion excretion, thereby increasing water excretion. It stimulates receptors that signal the brain to diminish sympathetic nervous system signals to the kidneys, thereby raising urine output. It also stimulates receptors that signal the posterior pituitary gland to inhibit secretion of antidiuretic hormone (ADH), causing the kidneys to increase urine output. And it raises arterial pressure and stimulates baroreceptors that increase the glomerular filtration rate, also causing greater urine output.

• *Osmoreceptors in the hypothalamus.* Hypothalamic osmoreceptors are stimulated by increased ECF osmolarity, causing the posterior pituitary gland to secrete ADH.

• *Pituitary gland.* The pituitary gland stores and releases ADH and corticotropin. ADH increases water reabsorption in the distal tubules and collecting ducts of the kidneys. Corticotropin influences production and release of adrenocortical hormones, such as aldosterone.

• *Kidneys.* The kidneys regulate fluid and electrolyte excretion and secretion. They also control ECF by regulating concentration of specific electrolytes, osmolarity of body fluids, ECF volume, blood volume, and pH.

• *Parathyroid glands.* These glands release parathyroid hormone, which regulates calcium. Diminished serum calcium levels spur parathyroid hormone secretion, causing increased calcium reabsorption in the kidneys.

• *Lungs.* The lungs remove about 400 ml of water daily through exhalation. Lung abnormalities, such as hyperpnea, increase water loss. The lungs also play an important role in maintaining acid-base balance.

• *Heart and blood vessels.* The heart pumps blood through the kidneys, creating enough pressure for urine to form. If this pumping action fails, renal perfusion and, consequently, fluid and electrolyte balance are affected.

• *Adrenal glands.* By secreting aldosterone, the adrenal glands have an important effect on fluid and electrolyte balance. Increased aldosterone secretion enhances renal reabsorption of sodium and water and loss of potassium. Decreased aldosterone secretion reduces renal reabsorp-

COMPARING FLUID TONICITY

Isotonic fluid
An isotonic fluid has a concentration of dissolved particles, or tonicity, equal to that of intracellular fluid (ICF). When isotonic fluids, such as dextrose 5% in water or 0.9% sodium chloride solution, enter the circulation, they cause no net water movement across the semipermeable cell membrane. And because osmotic pressure is the same inside and outside the cells, the cells don't swell or shrink.

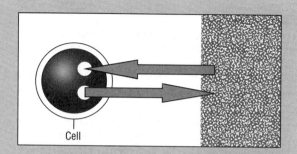

Hypertonic fluid
This type of fluid has a concentration greater than that of ICF. When you rapidly infuse a hypertonic solution, such as 3% sodium chloride or dextrose 50% in water, into a patient's body, water rushes out of the cells to the area of greater concentration and the cells shrivel. Dehydration can also make extracellular fluid (ECF) hypertonic, which also leads to cell shrinkage.

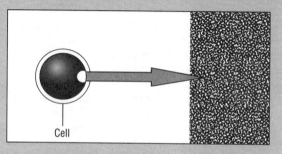

Hypotonic fluid
A hypotonic fluid has a concentration less than that of ICF. When you infuse a hypotonic solution, such as 0.45% sodium chloride, into the body, water diffuses into the ICF, causing the cell to swell. Inappropriate use of I.V. fluids or severe electrolyte losses make body fluids hypotonic. For example, a patient with a sodium deficit after gastric suction may have hypotonic ECF.

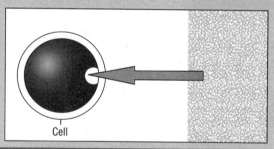

tion of sodium and water and enhances potassium retention. Another adrenocortical hormone, cortisol, if secreted in large amounts, results in retention of sodium and water and loss of potassium.

Role of electrolytes
Electrolytes dissociate in solution into electrically charged particles called ions. Because they conduct electric current, they permit cellular excitability. Ions can have a negative charge (anions) or a positive charge (cations). The composition of electrolytes in body fluids is electrically balanced so that the cations (sodium, potassium, calcium, and magnesium) equal the anions (chloride, bicarbonate, sulfate, phosphate, proteinate, and carbonic acid and other organic acids). Although these particles are present in relatively low concentrations, any deviation from their normal levels can have profound physiologic effects.

Because cell membranes separate the ICF and ECF, the two compartments maintain very different ion concentrations. ICF contains large quantities of potassium and phosphates but very little sodium and chloride. ECF contains mostly sodium and chloride but very little potassium and phosphates.

Elevated electrolyte levels can result from either an electrolyte gain (from increased intake or decreased output) without a corresponding water gain, or from reduced body water (from excessive loss or diminished intake) without a corresponding electrolyte loss. Reduced electrolyte levels can occur from an electrolyte loss (from reduced intake or increased loss) without a corresponding water loss, or from increased body water without a corresponding electrolyte gain.

Six electrolytes play important roles in maintaining metabolic balance: sodium, chloride, potassium, phosphate, calcium, and magnesium.

Acid-base balance

Primarily through the complex chemical regulation of carbonic acid by the lungs and of base bicarbonate by the kidneys, the body maintains the hydrogen ion concentration (pH) to keep the ECF pH between 7.35 and 7.45. Maintaining the pH within this normal narrow range is critical for the functioning of important physiologic processes.

Disturbances in acid-base balance can cause a lowered pH (acidosis) or an increased pH (alkalosis) and can produce serious and even lethal consequences. Such disturbances generally stem from:
• conditions that change the concentration of acids or bases at a rate that exceeds the body's normal homeostatic mechanisms
• abnormal conditions that impair the functioning of the body's homeostatic mechanisms
• nutritional deficiency or excess, disease, injury, or metabolic disturbance.

Assessing homeostasis

Evaluation consists of a patient history, a physical examination, and various diagnostic tests.

History and physical examination

In assessing fluid, electrolyte, and acid-base balance, focus on key signs and symptoms. Consider the patient's age, medication history, intake and output, and any predisposing illnesses, such as diabetes mellitus. Address questions about changes in mental status to the patient's partner or family.

For patients with fluid and electrolyte disorders, signs and symptoms frequently include changes in fluid intake and output, weight, skin and mucous membranes, vital signs, and level of consciousness (LOC), plus neuromuscular and GI changes, thirst, and jugular vein distention.

For patients with acid-base disorders, signs and symptoms typically include changes in LOC; muscle tone or strength; respiratory depth, rate, and rhythm; pulse rate and rhythm; skin; and urine output.

Diagnostic tests

In fluid and electrolyte and acid-base disorders, diagnostic tests can provide valuable information. Tests may include measurement of serum electrolytes, serum glucose, carbon dioxide content, serum osmolality, serum proteins, blood urea nitrogen (BUN), serum creatinine, BUN-creatinine ratio, hematocrit, urine sodium, urine chloride, urine potassium, urine calcium, urine phosphate (phosphorus), and urine magnesium.

Arterial blood gas measurements are the major diagnostic tool for identifying an acid-base imbalance. Other tests include mixed venous blood gas measurement, transcutaneous blood gas measurement, pulse oximetry, anion gap, and serum potassium, chloride, and total carbon dioxide measurements.

METABOLIC ANOMALIES

Some metabolic anomalies, such as phenylketonuria, are inherited; others, such as hypoglycemia, are acquired. Many can be treated with dietary changes.

GLYCOGEN STORAGE DISEASES

Consisting of at least eight, and possibly twelve, distinct errors of metabolism, glycogen storage diseases alter the synthesis or degradation of glycogen, the form in which glucose is stored in the body. All such metabolic errors are inherited.

Normally, muscle and hepatic cells store glycogen. Muscle glycogen is used in muscle contraction; liver glycogen can be converted into free glucose, which can then diffuse out of the hepatic cells to increase blood glucose levels.

Glycogen storage diseases manifest primarily as dysfunctions of the liver, the heart, or the musculoskeletal system. Signs and symptoms vary from mild and easily controlled hypoglycemia to severe organ involvement.

Causes

Almost all glycogen storage diseases (Types Ia and Ib through Types V and VII) are transmitted as autosomal recessive traits. Precise transmission of Type VI is unknown. However, phosphorylase *b* kinase deficiency (Type VIII) is an X-linked recessive trait.

Each glycogen storage disease reflects deficient activity of specific enzymes involved in the synthesis and storage of glycogen. This can cause glycogen to accumulate abnormally in the liver, heart, skeletal muscle, brain, and kidneys.

Complications
Severe involvement of the liver, heart, skeletal muscle, brain, and kidneys can lead to organ failure and death.

Assessment findings
Typically, the history of a patient with liver glycogen storage disease (Types Ia, Ib, III, and VI, and phosphorylase *b* kinase deficiency) reveals rapid onset of hypoglycemia when food is withheld. Palpation reveals hepatomegaly, a cardinal sign.

In a patient with Type Ia disease, the history may also disclose symptomatic hypoglycemia and lactic acidosis, usually occurring during the first 12 months of life; growth retardation (after normal growth for the first few months of life); delayed adolescence; and bleeding (especially epistaxis).

Inspection of a patient with Type Ia disease may reveal a protuberant abdomen due to an enlarged liver; thin extremities; small superficial vessels visible in the skin due to impaired platelet function; full cheeks, round face; short stature; and xanthomas over extensor surfaces of the arms and legs due to hyperlipidemia. Ophthalmoscopic examination may demonstrate bilateral, yellow lesions in the fundi. Palpation may detect hepatomegaly and, possibly, kidney enlargement. Motor system assessment may indicate poor muscle tone.

A patient with muscle glycogen storage disease (Types V and VII) may report the onset of pain and muscle cramps during and after strenuous exercise. Physical assessment often detects marked hypotonia.

Patients with glycogen storage disease with individualized pathophysiology (Types II and IV) may have a history of failure to thrive and motor weakness. Physical assessment findings vary according to the disease type and the patient's age. For example, in patients with Type II disease, auscultation may detect signs of heart failure in infancy. In patients with Type IV disease, palpation may detect hepatomegaly. (See *Classifying glycogen storage diseases.*)

Diagnostic tests
• *Liver biopsy* confirms diagnosis of Type Ia disease by showing normal glycogen synthetase and phosphorylase enzyme activities but reduced or absent glucose-6-phosphatase activity. Glycogen structure is normal, but amounts are elevated.
• *Laboratory studies* of plasma demonstrate low glucose levels but high levels of free fatty acids, triglycerides, cho-

lesterol, and uric acid in Type Ia disease. Serum analysis reveals elevated pyruvic acid levels and elevated lactic acid levels. Prenatal diagnoses are available for Types II, III, and IV.
• *Injection of glucagon or epinephrine* increases pyruvic and lactic acid levels but doesn't increase blood glucose levels in patients with Type Ia disease. Glucose tolerance test curve typically shows depletional hypoglycemia and reduced insulin output.

Treatment
For both Type Ia and Ib, the goals of treatment include maintaining glucose homeostasis and preventing secondary consequences of hypoglycemia through frequent feedings and constant nocturnal nasogastric (NG) tube feedings. Dietary treatment calls for a regimen of about 60% carbohydrate intake, with low fat and normal amounts of protein and calories; carbohydrates should contain glucose or glucose polymers only, such as raw cornstarch.

Therapy for Types III and VI includes frequent feedings. Carbohydrates should make up about 50% of the total daily dietary intake. A larger percentage of protein (than in Type Ia) can be ingested to increase calorie consumption.

Types V and VII require no treatment except avoidance of strenuous exercise. No treatment — or, possibly, dietary management (as in Type III) — may be necessary for phosphorylase *b* kinase deficiency. No effective treatment exists for Types II and IV.

Nursing diagnoses
• Activity intolerance
• Body image disturbance
• Decreased cardiac output
• Knowledge deficit
• Risk for infection

Nursing interventions
In Type I disease:
• Watch for and report signs of infection (fever, chills, myalgia, purulent drainage) and of hepatic encephalopathy (mental confusion, stupor, asterixis, coma) due to increased blood ammonia levels. Also monitor for hypoglycemia and lactic acidosis.
• As warranted, plan care to provide sufficient rest periods balanced with tolerated activity. Provide safety measures for the patient with muscle weakness.
• Help the patient and family obtain psychosocial support, as needed, to deal with the poor prognosis, body image disturbances, and life-style adaptations.

CLASSIFYING GLYCOGEN STORAGE DISEASES

Most glycogen storage diseases fall into two broad categories: liver and muscle. Disease Types Ib, III, VI, and VIII are characterized by abnormal amounts of glycogen in liver tissue; Types V and VII, by abnormal amounts of glycogen in muscle tissue. Some diseases, such as Types II and IV, have individualized pathophysiologies. This chart compares the various types.

Type	Clinical features	Diagnostic test results
Liver glycogen storage disease		
Ib *(pseudo Type I)* Deficiency of glucose-6-phosphatase (G6P) microsomal translocase	• Similar to, but more severe than Type Ia; neutropenia; recurrent pyogenic infections	• *Liver biopsy:* G6P activity low in presence of detergent
III *(Cori)* Absence of debranching enzyme (amylo-1,6-glucosidase) (*Note:* predominant cause of glycogen storage disease in Israel)	• *Young children:* massive hepatomegaly, which may disappear by puberty; growth retardation; moderate splenomegaly; hypoglycemia • *Adults:* progressive myopathy; occasionally, moderate cardiomegaly, cirrhosis, muscle wasting, hypoglycemia	• *Liver biopsy:* deficient debranching activity; increased glycogen concentration, with abnormal glycogen structure • *Laboratory tests* (in children only): elevated serum transaminase; increased erythrocyte glycogen
VI *(Hers)* Deficiency of hepatic phosphorylase	• Mild symptoms, such as hepatomegaly or hypoglycemia (similar to those of Type III)	• *Liver biopsy:* absent phosphorylase; increased glycogen concentration with normal structure
VIII Phosphorylase *b* kinase deficiency (*Note:* formerly Type VI; sometimes designated as Type VIa or Type IX)	• Mild hepatomegaly • Mild hypoglycemia • Possible growth retardation	• *Liver biopsy:* deficient phosphorylase *b* kinase activity; increased liver glycogen • *Blood study:* deficient phosphorylase *b* kinase in leukocytes
Muscle glycogen storage disease		
V *(McArdle)* Deficiency of muscle phosphorylase	• *Children:* mild or no symptoms • *Adults:* muscle cramps and pain during strenuous exercise, possibly resulting in myoglobinuria and renal failure • *Older patients:* significant muscle weakness and wasting	• *Serum lactate:* no increase in venous levels in sample drawn from extremity after ischemic exercise; increased creatinine phosphokinase with exercise • *Muscle biopsy:* lack of phosphorylase activity; increased glycogen content with normal structure
VII Deficiency of muscle phosphofructokinase	• Muscle cramps during strenuous exercise, resulting in myoglobinuria and possible renal failure • Reticulocytosis; mild hemolytic anemia, sometimes without muscle involvement	• *Serum lactate:* no increase in venous levels in sample drawn from extremity after ischemic exercise • *Muscle biopsy:* deficient phosphofructokinase; marked rise in glycogen concentration with normal structure • *Blood studies:* low erythrocyte phosphofructokinase activity; reduced erythrocyte half-life

(continued)

CLASSIFYING GLYCOGEN STORAGE DISEASES *(continued)*

Type	Clinical features	Diagnostic test results
Disease with individualized pathophysiology		
II *(Pompe)* Absence of alpha-1,4-glucosidase (acid maltase); lysosomal storage disease	• *Infants:* massive cardiomegaly, profound hypotonia and, occasionally, endocardial fibroelastosis (usually fatal in first 2 to 3 years) • *Some infants and young children:* muscle weakness and wasting, variable organ involvement; no cardiac symptoms (slower progression, variable length of survival) • *Adults:* muscle weakness without organomegaly (slowly progressive, may develop pulmonary insufficiency)	• *Muscle biopsy:* increased concentration of glycogen with normal structure; alpha-1,4-glucosidase deficiency • *Electrocardiogram (in infants):* large QRS complexes in all leads; inverted T waves; shortened PR interval • *Electromyography (in adults):* muscle fiber irritability; myotonic discharges • *Amniocentesis:* alpha-1,4-glucosidase deficiency • *Placenta or umbilical cord examination:* alpha-1,4-glucosidase deficiency
IV *(Andersen)* Deficiency of branching enzyme (amylo-1,4-1,6-transglucosidase)	• *Infants:* hepatosplenomegaly, ascites, extreme muscle hypotonia; failure to thrive; usually fatal before age 2 from cirrhosis	• *Liver biopsy:* deficient branching enzyme activity; glycogen molecule has longer outer branches

In Type IV disease:

• Monitor for signs of hepatic failure (nausea, vomiting, irregular bowel function, clay-colored stools, right upper quadrant pain, jaundice, dehydration, electrolyte imbalance, edema, and changes in mental status, progressing to coma).

In Types II, III, and IV disease:

• Offer parents reassurance and emotional support. Recommend and arrange for genetic counseling, if appropriate.

• Monitor patients for signs of heart failure.

Patient teaching

• Before discharge, teach the patient with Type I disease and his family about dietary treatment, especially the need for carbohydrate foods containing mainly starch. Teach them to sweeten foods with glucose only.

• Also instruct the patient and the family how to insert an NG tube, use a pump with alarm capacity, monitor blood glucose, and recognize and report symptoms of hypoglycemia, including fatigue, headache, hunger, malaise, and a rapid heart rate.

• Also teach the patient and family to recognize and report signs of infection, including fever and chills, malaise, myalgia, and purulent drainage.

• Explain test procedures, which may include liver or muscle biopsy, electromyography, and electroencephalography.

• Inform the patient with Type III disease, Type VI disease (if warranted), or phosphorylase *b* kinase deficiency about the need for frequent feedings. Tell him to ingest adequate calories (mainly from carbohydrates) and protein (eggs, nuts, fish, meat, poultry, and cheese).

• Advise the patient with Type V or Type VII disease to avoid strenuous exercise. Help him to accept the physical limitations imposed by his disease.

HYPOGLYCEMIA

Potentially dangerous, hypoglycemia is an abnormally low blood glucose level. It occurs when glucose burns up too rapidly, when the glucose release rate falls behind tissue demands, or when excessive insulin enters the bloodstream. When the brain is deprived of glucose, as with oxygen deprivation, its functioning becomes deranged. With prolonged glucose deprivation, tissue damage — or even death — may occur.

Hypoglycemia may be classified as reactive, pharmacologic, or fasting. *Reactive hypoglycemia* results from the reaction to the disposition of meals. Blood glucose levels typically fall 2 to 4 hours after a meal.

Pharmacologic hypoglycemia results in response to a drug that does one of the following: increases the amount of insulin circulating in the blood, enhances insulin action, or impairs the liver's glucose-producing capacity. Blood glucose levels may fall slowly or rapidly.

Fasting hypoglycemia causes discomfort during periods of abstinence from food. Blood glucose levels fall gradually. Signs and symptoms do not occur until 5 hours or more after a meal. This rare type of hypoglycemia occurs most often during the night.

Manifestations of hypoglycemia tend to be vague and depend on how quickly the patient's glucose levels drop. Gradual onset of hypoglycemia produces predominantly central nervous system (CNS) signs and symptoms; a more rapid decline in plasma glucose levels results predominantly in adrenergic signs and symptoms. (See *What happens in acute hypoglycemia,* page 960.)

Causes and pathophysiology
Reactive hypoglycemia may take several forms. Most commonly, it results from alimentary hyperinsulinism caused by dumping syndrome. Fructose or galactose ingestion may cause hypoglycemia in patients with fructose intolerance or galactosemia. Reactive hypoglycemia may also occur secondary to imminent onset of Type II diabetes mellitus or impaired glucose tolerance. In some patients, reactive hypoglycemia may have no known cause (idiopathic reactive).

Pharmacologic hypoglycemia most commonly results from the use of insulin or oral sulfonylureas. Other causes include the use of beta blockers and excessive alcohol ingestion.

Fasting hypoglycemia most commonly results from hepatic disease or a tumor. Insulinomas, small islet cell tumors in the pancreas, secrete excessive amounts of insulin, which inhibits hepatic glucose production. These tumors are usually benign (in 90% of patients). Extrapancreatic tumors, though uncommon, can also cause hypoglycemia by increasing glucose utilization and inhibiting glucose output. Such tumors occur primarily in the mesenchyma, liver, adrenal cortex, GI system, and lymphatic system. They may be benign or malignant.

Among nonendocrine causes of fasting hypoglycemia are severe hepatic diseases, including hepatitis, cancer, cirrhosis, and liver congestion associated with heart failure. All of these conditions reduce the uptake and release of glycogen from the liver.

Some endocrine causes include destruction of pancreatic islet cells; adrenocortical insufficiency, which contributes to hypoglycemia by reducing the production of cortisol and cortisone needed for gluconeogenesis; and pituitary insufficiency, which reduces corticotropin and growth hormone levels.

Hypoglycemia is at least as common in infants and children as it is in adults. Usually, infants develop hypoglycemia because of an increased number of cells per unit of body weight and because of increased demands on stored liver glycogen to support respirations, thermoregulation, and muscular activity. In full-term neonates, hypoglycemia may occur 24 to 72 hours after birth and is usually transient. In neonates who are premature or small for gestational age, onset of hypoglycemia is much more rapid—it can occur as soon as 6 hours after birth—because of their small, immature livers, which produce much less glycogen. Maternal disorders that can produce hypoglycemia in neonates within 24 hours after birth include diabetes mellitus, toxemia, erythroblastosis, and glycogen storage diseases.

Complications
Prolonged or severe hypoglycemia (blood glucose levels of 20 mg/dl or less) can cause permanent brain damage and may be fatal.

Assessment findings
The history of a patient with suspected hypoglycemia should note the pattern of food intake for the preceding 24 hours, as well as drug and alcohol use. The medical or surgical history may note the existence of causative factors, such as gastrectomy or hepatic disease.

A patient with reactive hypoglycemia may report adrenergic symptoms, such as diaphoresis, anxiety, hunger, nervousness, and weakness, indicating a rapid decline in his blood glucose levels. A patient with fasting hypoglycemia may report signs and symptoms of CNS disturbance, such as dizziness, headache, clouding of vision, restlessness, and mental status changes, indicating a slow decline in blood glucose levels. With prolonged glucose deprivation, the patient's history (obtained from family or friends, if necessary) may reveal seizures, decreasing level of consciousness (LOC), and coma. A patient with pharmacologic hypoglycemia may experience a rapid or slow decline in blood glucose levels.

Inspection may reveal adrenergic signs, such as diaphoresis, pallor, and tremor; or CNS signs, such as restlessness, loss of fine-motor skills, and altered LOC. Palpation may detect tachycardia.

Infants and children with hypoglycemia generally exhibit vague symptoms, such as refusal to feed or a weak or high-pitched cry. Inspection may reveal tremor, twitching, sweating, limpness, seizures, and coma.

Diagnostic tests
Glucometer readings provide quick screening methods for determining blood glucose levels. Laboratory testing confirms the diagnosis by showing decreased blood glucose values.

Pathophysiology

WHAT HAPPENS IN ACUTE HYPOGLYCEMIA

Normally, homeostatic mechanisms maintain blood glucose levels within narrow limits (60 to 120 mg/dl). The body burns available glucose and stores the rest as glycogen in the liver and muscles. When the glucose level drops, the liver converts glycogen back to glucose (glycogenolysis) or makes new glucose from noncarbohydrate sources, such as amino acids or fatty acids (gluconeogenesis).

Hormones maintain the delicate balance between glucose production and use. But this balance is upset when a patient has hypoglycemia. The flowchart below shows the events that lead to central and autonomic nervous system reactions associated with hypoglycemia.

Acute hypoglycemia
Blood glucose drops rapidly.

Cells break down fatty and amino acids into adenosine triphosphate (ATP) for energy.

Brain cells can't use ATP for energy.

Neuroglycopenia
Early glucose deprivation in brain tissue causes mild cerebral dysfunction.

Headache, dizziness, restlessness, decreased mental capacity

Autonomic nervous system stimulation

Pancreas
Sympathetic nerves and epinephrine rapidly stimulate glucagon secretion; epinephrine inhibits insulin secretion.

Adrenal glands
Sympathetic nerves stimulate epinephrine secretion (rapid response). Hypothalamus stimulates pituitary gland to secrete corticotropin, which acts on the adrenal cortex to cause cortisol secretion (delayed response).

Stomach
Hypothalamus stimulates hunger; parasympathetic nerves increase gastric juices and stomach contractions.

Liver
Sympathetic nerves directly stimulate glycogenolysis; epinephrine, glucagon, cortisol, and growth hormone increase gluconeogenesis; glucagon also stimulates glycogenolysis.

Muscle
Hypothalamus stimulates pituitary to secrete growth hormone (delayed response), which— along with epinephrine and cortisol— inhibits glucagon use.

Adrenergic changes
Hunger, weakness, diaphoresis, tachycardia, pallor, anxiety, tremor, rebound hyperglycemia

The following values indicate hypoglycemia:
• full-term neonates—less than 30 mg/dl before feeding, less than 40 mg/dl after feeding
• preterm neonates—less than 20 mg/dl before feeding, less than 30 mg/dl after feeding
• children and adults—less than 40 mg/dl before meal, less than 50 mg/dl after meal.

In addition, a 5-hour glucose tolerance test may be administered to provoke reactive hypoglycemia. Following a 12-hour fast, laboratory testing to detect plasma insulin and plasma glucose levels may identify fasting hypoglycemia.

A C-peptide assay helps diagnose fasting hypoglycemia. It also differentiates fasting hypoglycemia caused by an insulinoma from fasting hypoglycemia caused by insulin injections.

Treatment

For *severe hypoglycemia* (producing confusion or coma), initial treatment is usually I.V. administration of a bolus of 25 or 50 g of glucose as a 50% solution. This is followed by a constant infusion of glucose until the patient can eat a meal. A patient who experiences adrenergic reactions without CNS symptoms may receive oral carbohydrate (parenteral therapy isn't required).

Reactive hypoglycemia requires dietary modification to help delay glucose absorption and gastric emptying. Usually, this includes small, frequent meals; avoidance of simple carbohydrates; and ingestion of high-protein meals with added fiber. The patient may also receive anticholinergic drugs to slow gastric emptying and intestinal motility and to inhibit vagal stimulation of insulin release.

For *fasting hypoglycemia*, surgery and drug therapy may be required. In patients with insulinoma, removal of the tumor is the treatment of choice. Drug therapy may include diazoxide or octreotide for inoperable insulinomas. Hormone replacement therapy may be needed for pituitary or adrenal gland insufficiency. In many cases of recurrent hypoglycemia, the only treatment needed is avoidance of fasting.

For *infants* who have hypoglycemia or who are at risk of developing it, therapy includes preventive measures. A hypertonic solution of dextrose 10% in water, calculated at 5 to 10 ml/kg of body weight, administered I.V. over 10 minutes and followed by 4 to 8 mg/kg/minute for maintenance should correct a severe hypoglycemic state in neonates. To reduce the chance of hypoglycemia in high-risk infants, feedings—of either breast milk or a solution of dextrose 5% to 10% in water—should begin as soon after birth as possible.

Nursing diagnoses
• Anxiety
• Knowledge deficit
• Noncompliance
• Risk for injury

Nursing interventions
• Watch for and report signs of hypoglycemia in high-risk patients.
• Implement measures to protect the unconscious patient, such as maintenance of a patent airway.
• Monitor infusion of hypertonic glucose (especially in the neonate) to avoid hyperglycemia, circulatory overload, and cellular dehydration.
• Measure blood glucose levels, as ordered.
• Monitor the effects of drug therapy, and watch for the development of any adverse reactions.

Patient teaching
• Explain the purpose, preparation, and procedure for any diagnostic tests.
• Emphasize the importance of preventing or promptly treating hypoglycemic episodes to avoid severe complications. Be sure the patient understands the key danger with hypoglycemia: Once it occurs, he may quickly lose his ability to think clearly. If this should happen while he's driving a car or operating machinery, a serious accident could result.
• Inform the patient that he should note what early symptoms he typically experiences with hypoglycemia. Family, friends, and co-workers should also be able to recognize the warning signs so that immediate treatment can be initiated.
• Review with the patient and family the treatment measures they should follow if the patient has a hypoglycemic episode. If the patient is conscious, he should consume a readily available source of glucose, such as five to six pieces of hard candy; 4 to 6 oz of apple juice, orange juice, cola, or other soft drink; or 1 tbs of honey or grape jelly. If the patient is unconscious, he should be given a subcutaneous injection of glucagon. Teach the patient's family how to administer glucagon. Advise the patient and family to notify the doctor if hypoglycemic episodes don't respond to treatment, or if they occur frequently.
• Emphasize to the patient the importance of carefully following the prescribed diet to prevent a rapid drop in blood glucose levels. Advise him to eat small meals throughout the day, and mention that bedtime snacks also may be necessary to keep blood glucose at an even level. Instruct the patient to avoid alcohol and caffeine

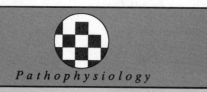

Pathophysiology

UNDERSTANDING LACTASE INSUFFICIENCY

Normally, the enzyme lactase hydrolyzes dietary lactose in the jejunum and proximal ileus. This hydrolysis splits lactose into glucose and galactose, which bind to glucose carriers and eventually pass into the portal vein. But if lactase levels are insufficient to split the lactose, a chain of effects is triggered as follows in this flowchart.

> Available lactase is insufficient to hydrolyze dietary lactose.

> Unsplit lactose remains as unabsorbed glucose in the small intestine.

> Unabsorbed glucose acts osmotically to draw in and retain intraluminal fluid, leading to diarrhea.

> Intestinal bacteria ferment the lactose, breaking it down into hydrogen, carbon dioxide, water, and organic acids.

> Accumulation of gases causes discomfort, flatulence, and distention.

because they may trigger severe hypoglycemic episodes.
• If the patient is obese and has impaired glucose tolerance, suggest ways he can restrict his caloric intake and lose weight. If necessary, help him find a weight-loss support group.
• Warn the patient with fasting hypoglycemia not to postpone or skip meals and snacks. Instruct the patient to call his doctor for instructions if he doesn't feel well enough to eat.
• Discuss life-style and personal habits to help the patient identify precipitating factors, such as poor diet,

stress, or noncompliance with diabetes mellitus treatment. Explain ways that he can change or avoid each precipitating factor identified. If necessary, teach him stress-reduction techniques, and encourage him to join a support group.
• Teach the patient about precautions to take when exercising; for example, tell him to consume extra calories and not to exercise alone or when his blood glucose level is likely to drop.
• Inform the patient that he should carry a source of fast-acting carbohydrate, such as hard candy, with him at all times. Advise him to wear a medical identification bracelet or to carry a medical identification card that describes his condition and its emergency treatment measures.
• For the patient with pharmacologic hypoglycemia from insulin or oral antidiabetic agents, review the essentials of managing diabetes mellitus, if indicated.
• If warranted, teach the patient about prescribed drug therapy or surgery.
• Because hypoglycemia is a chronic disorder, encourage the patient to see his doctor regularly.
• Encourage the patient and family to discuss their concerns about the patient's condition and treatment.

LACTOSE INTOLERANCE

Stemming from an insufficiency of the enzyme lactase, lactose intolerance is the inability to digest and absorb lactose, the main carbohydrate in milk. (See *Understanding lactase insufficiency*.)

Lactose intolerance may be congenital (rare) or acquired. In primary acquired lactose intolerance, the most common form, lactase levels start to decline between ages 2 and 3. By the time the patient reaches adolescence or early adulthood, lactase levels are decreased by about 90% of neonatal levels. This deficiency continues for life.

The incidence of lactose intolerance is high among certain ethnic groups, including Blacks, Orientals, Native Americans, Greek Cypriots, and some Ashkenazic Jews.

Causes

Both congenital and primary acquired lactose intolerance are thought to have a genetic basis.

Secondary acquired lactose intolerance may result from medical conditions, such as viral gastroenteritis, inflammatory bowel disease, celiac and sprue syndromes, and intestinal parasites, which disrupt the intestinal mucosa.

Or lactose intolerance can stem from medications that cause GI disturbances (broad-spectrum antibiotics, colchicine, and certain chemotherapeutic drugs, such as antimetabolites). Ionizing radiation to the abdomen and surgery, such as small-bowel resection (with removal of some lactase-producing mucosa) or gastrectomy (with dumping syndrome), can also cause lactose intolerance. The effects may be temporary or permanent.

Complications
Lactose intolerance with resulting diarrhea can lead to dehydration, especially in infants and young children.

Assessment findings
The patient's history may reveal a pattern of GI signs and symptoms following ingestion of milk products. This may be associated with a recent dietary change, such as a pregnant woman's increase in milk intake. Or the patient may have a history of a medical disorder or treatment that disrupts the GI mucosa.

Typically, the patient complains of diarrhea, abdominal cramping, discomfort, distention, flatulence, and borborygmus (intestinal rumbling).

Inspection may reveal abdominal distention and nonverbal signs of patient distress, such as doubling over or holding the abdomen. Rectal tissue irritation and excoriation related to diarrhea may be noted. Auscultation may detect hyperactive bowel sounds.

Diagnostic tests
• *Lactose challenge testing* is performed when lactose intolerance is suspected. In this test, the patient drinks a quart of skim milk on an empty stomach and notes any symptoms that develop within 4 hours. If the patient is lactase deficient, such symptoms as diarrhea and bloating occur within minutes to hours.
• *Lactose-free diet testing* involves eliminating lactose from the patient's diet for a period of time, such as 5 days. If he becomes asymptomatic, the diagnosis is upheld.
• *Lactose tolerance testing* is performed if the patient has a complicating disorder, such as celiac disease or gastroenteritis. In this test, a blood sample is taken after the patient has fasted overnight. Then the patient ingests a specified oral lactose load. Serum glucose levels are taken on blood samples drawn at specified intervals following lactose ingestion and on the fasting blood sample. A minimal rise (less than 20 mg/dl) in the serum glucose level and GI symptoms (cramping, flatulence, and perhaps diarrhea) confirm lactase deficiency.
• *Breath hydrogen analysis*, a more sensitive and specific noninvasive test, measures excess hydrogen exhalation, resulting from bacterial fermentation of lactose within the colon. (Hydrogen from the colon passes to the blood and then to the lungs.) Increased hydrogen content of expired air confirms lactose intolerance.
• *Small-bowel biopsy*, rarely used, determines whether lactose intolerance is primary or secondary. Only the secondary form shows abnormal epithelium.

Treatment
For an infant with temporary lactose intolerance, a lactose-free formula may be substituted for breast milk or milk-based formula. Older children and adults with temporary lactose intolerance must eliminate all milk products from the diet until the causative disorder improves.

Patients with genetic lactase deficiency must limit dietary lactose to the level they can comfortably tolerate. Some patients benefit from commercially available lactase enzyme products (LactAid, Lactrase), which may be added to milk or purchased ready to use. The commercial lactase reduces the lactose to glucose and galactose. Lactase enzyme capsules are also available.

Lactose-intolerant patients receiving tube feedings require a lactose-free formula (Resource or Ensure).

Nursing diagnoses
• Altered nutrition: Less than body requirements
• Diarrhea
• Impaired skin integrity
• Knowledge deficit
• Pain
• Risk for fluid volume deficit

Nursing interventions
• Monitor the patient's elimination patterns. Administer antidiarrheal agents, as prescribed.
• Give lactase enzyme products, as prescribed.
• Assess the patient for abdominal discomfort. Administer prescribed medication, such as anticholinergics 30 minutes to 1 hour before meals. Encourage relaxation and diversion techniques to relieve discomfort.
• Initiate patient care measures to protect the rectal skin and mucous membranes. For example, keep the area clean and dry, and apply protective cream, as needed. Apply a local anesthetic, if necessary.
• Assess the patient for signs of dehydration, such as poor skin turgor, tachycardia, decreased urine output, and hypotension. Monitor intake and output and obtain daily weight. Encourage the patient to drink about 3,000 ml of fluid daily, unless contraindicated.
• Offer emotional support and provide patient privacy.
• Refer the patient to the dietitian, as needed.

Patient teaching

• Inform the patient or family about lactose intolerance and its associated signs and symptoms, risks, and treatment, especially dietary management.

• Teach the patient and anyone who cooks or shops for him the foods that contain lactose, such as milk (whole, low-fat, skim, evaporated, condensed, buttermilk, cream), ice cream, cheese, sour cream, custards, milk-based puddings, butter, drinks prepared with chocolate or malted milk powder, cream sauces and gravies, cream-based soups, chocolate candy, instant potatoes, baked products made with milk, and frozen or canned fruits and vegetables containing lactose. Caution him to check product labels carefully for lactose content and to avoid products that list milk solids, milk sugars, whey, and casein.

• Instruct the patient with primary acquired lactose intolerance to eliminate all sources of lactose from his diet until he is free of symptoms. (This usually takes about 3 weeks.) Then describe how to increase lactose ingestion gradually until he reaches his tolerance threshold. Explain that he needs to remain on a low-lactose diet for the rest of his life, but encourage him to gradually experiment with different lactose products over the years, noting tolerance levels.

• Inform the patient that he may be better able to tolerate milk products in which a portion of the lactose has been fermented—hard cheeses and yogurt, for example. If he makes his own yogurt, suggest that he allow fermentation to continue beyond the usual time to lower lactose content. Live-culture yogurt contains its own lactase, which is activated in the duodenum and continues the lactose ingestion.

• Explain to the patient or family how to use lactase enzyme products.

• Teach the patient how to avoid vitamin D and calcium deficiencies. Lactose-free sources of vitamin D include enzyme-treated milk, saltwater fish and their oils, lactose-free margarine, eggs, and exposure to sunlight. Sources of calcium for lactose-intolerant patients include enzyme-treated milk; dark green, leafy vegetables; dried beans; canned sardines and salmon (with small edible bones); almonds; and tofu. Some patients can tolerate cheeses, such as aged natural cheddar, Gouda, and Edam, which are lower in lactose but high in calcium.

HYPERLIPOPROTEINEMIA

Marked by increased plasma concentrations of one or more lipoproteins, hyperlipoproteinemia affects lipid transport in serum. Primary hyperlipoproteinemia oc-

curs as at least five distinct metabolic disorders, all of which may be inherited. Hyperlipoproteinemia may also occur secondary to other conditions, such as diabetes mellitus.

The disorder produces varied clinical changes, from relatively mild symptoms that can be corrected by dietary management to potentially fatal pancreatitis. (See *Types of hyperlipoproteinemia.*)

Causes

The primary hyperlipoproteinemias result from genetic disorders. Types I and III are transmitted as autosomal recessive traits; Types II, IV, and V are transmitted as autosomal dominant traits. Secondary hyperlipoproteinemia results from another metabolic disorder, such as diabetes mellitus, consumption of alcohol, or ingestion of oral contraceptives.

Complications

Sequelae of hyperlipoproteinemia include coronary artery disease and pancreatitis.

Assessment findings

The history of a patient with Type I disease typically reveals recurrent attacks of severe abdominal pain similar to pancreatitis, usually preceded by fat intake. The patient may also report malaise and anorexia.

Inspection may reveal papular or eruptive xanthomas (pinkish yellow cutaneous deposits of fat) over pressure points and extensor surfaces. Ophthalmoscopic examination typically reveals lipemia retinalis (reddish white retinal vessels). Palpation may detect abdominal spasm, rigidity, or rebound tenderness, and hepatosplenomegaly, with liver or spleen tenderness. Fever may be present.

A patient with Type II disease may have a history of premature and accelerated coronary atherosclerosis, with symptoms typically developing when the patient is in his 20s or 30s. Inspection commonly reveals tendinous xanthomas (firm masses) on the Achilles tendons and tendons of the hands and feet, tuberous xanthomas, xanthelasma, and juvenile corneal arcus (opaque ring surrounding the corneal periphery).

Typically, a patient with Type III disease doesn't complain of clinical symptoms until after age 20 when severe atherosclerosis may develop. The patient's history may include such aggravating factors as obesity, hypothyroidism, and diabetes mellitus.

Inspection may reveal tuberoeruptive xanthomas (soft, inflamed, pedunculated lesions) over the elbows and knees and palmar xanthomas on the hands, partic-

TYPES OF HYPERLIPOPROTEINEMIA

The following chart compares the five forms of hyperlipoproteinemia, their causes and incidence, and diagnostic findings.

Type	Causes and incidence	Diagnostic findings
Type I (Frederickson's hyperlipoproteinemia, fat-induced hyperlipemia, idiopathic familial)	• Deficient or abnormal lipoprotein lipase, resulting in decreased or absent lipolytic activity after heparin administration • Relatively rare • Present at birth	• Chylomicrons (very-low-density lipoprotein [VLDL], low-density lipoprotein [LDL], high-density lipoprotein [HDL]) in plasma 14 hours or more after last meal • High elevated serum chylomicron and triglyceride levels; slightly elevated serum cholesterol levels • Decreased serum lipoprotein lipase levels • Leukocytosis
Type II (familial hyperbetalipoproteinemia, essential familial hypercholesterolemia)	• Deficient cell surface receptor that regulates LDL degradation and cholesterol synthesis, resulting in increased levels of plasma LDL over joints and pressure points • Onset between ages 10 and 30	• Increased plasma concentrations of LDL • Elevated serum LDL and cholesterol levels • Increased LDL levels detected by amniocentesis
Type III (familial broad-beta disease, xanthoma tuberosum)	• Primary defect involving deficient LDL receptor • Uncommon: usually occurring after age 20, possibly earlier in men	• Abnormal serum beta-lipoprotein levels • Elevated cholesterol and triglyceride levels • Slightly elevated glucose tolerance
Type IV (endogenous hypertriglyceridemia, hyperbetalipoproteinemia)	• Primary defect unknown; usually occurs with increased prevalence of obesity, diabetes, hypertension • Relatively common, especially in middle-aged men	• Elevated VLDL levels • Moderately increased plasma triglyceride levels • Normal or slightly elevated serum cholesterol levels • Mildly abnormal glucose tolerance • Family history • Early coronary artery disease
Type V (mixed hypertriglyceridemia, mixed hyperlipidemia)	• Defective triglyceride clearance causes pancreatitis; usually secondary to another disorder, such as obesity or nephrosis • Uncommon: usually occurring in late adolescence or early adulthood	• Chylomicrons in plasma • Elevated plasma VLDL levels • Elevated serum cholesterol and triglyceride levels

ularly the fingertips (orange or yellow discolorations of the palmar and digital creases).

A patient with Type IV disease may have a history of atherosclerosis and early coronary artery disease. Patient history also may include factors, such as excessive alcohol consumption, poorly controlled diabetes mellitus, and ingestion of birth control pills containing estrogen, which can precipitate severe hypertriglyceridemia. Hypertension and hyperuricemia may also be present. Inspection commonly reveals the presence of obesity.

Although not characteristic, xanthomas may be noted during exacerbations.

The history of a patient with Type V disease may reveal abdominal pain associated with pancreatitis and complaints related to peripheral neuropathy. Inspection may note eruptive xanthomas on extensor surface of the arms and legs. Ophthalmoscopic examination may reveal lipemia retinalis. Palpation may detect hepatosplenomegaly.

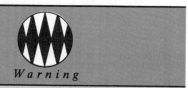

Warning

USING BILE ACID SEQUESTRANTS

Before giving the patient a bile acid sequestrant, such as cholestyramine, to lower cholesterol levels, make certain he isn't taking one of the following drugs whose absorptions are affected by bile acid sequestrants:
- beta-adrenergic blockers
- digitoxin
- diuretics
- fat-soluble vitamins
- folic acid
- thiazides
- thyroxine
- warfarin.

Diagnostic tests

Serum lipid profiles—elevated levels of total cholesterol, triglycerides, very-low-density lipoproteins (VLDL), low-density lipoproteins (LDL), or high-density lipoproteins (HDL)—indicate hyperlipoproteinemia.

Treatment

Primary treatment focuses on dietary management, including weight reduction, restriction of cholesterol and saturated animal fat intake, and inclusion of polyunsaturated vegetable oils, which reduce concentration of plasma LDL. Dietary fat should account for no more than 30% of the total caloric intake.

The second therapeutic aim is to eliminate aggravating factors, such as diabetes mellitus, alcoholism, or hypothyroidism. The patient should also reduce other risk factors that may predispose him to atherosclerosis. Self-care measures may include cessation of smoking, treatment of hypertension, maintenance of a good exercise and physical fitness program and, if the patient has diabetes mellitus, control of blood glucose levels.

Treatment may be supplemented by drug therapy (cholestyramine, clofibrate, colestipol hydrochloride, gemfibrozil, lovastatin, nicotinic acid, pravastatin sodium, probucol, or simvastatin) to lower plasma concentrations of lipoproteins, either by decreasing their production or by increasing their removal from plasma.

Type I hyperlipoproteinemia requires long-term weight reduction, with fat intake restricted to less than 20 g/

day. A 20- to 40-g/day, medium-chain triglyceride diet may be ordered to supplement caloric intake. The patient should also avoid alcoholic beverages to decrease plasma triglyceride levels. The prognosis is good with treatment; without treatment, death can result from pancreatitis.

For Type II hyperlipoproteinemia, dietary management to restore normal lipid levels and decrease the risk of atherosclerosis includes restriction of cholesterol intake to under 300 mg/day for adults and under 150 mg/day for children. Additional measures include restricting triglyceride intake to less than 100 mg/day for both children and adults. The diet should also be high in polyunsaturated fats.

If these measures don't bring cholesterol levels to within normal range, bile acid-binding resins, such as cholestyramine, are added to the regimen. (See *Using bile acid sequestrants*.) The regimen also may be supplemented with nicotinic acid or lovastatin.

If the patient can't tolerate drug therapy, surgical creation of an ileal bypass may be necessary. This surgery accelerates the loss of bile acids in the stool and often causes heterozygotes to show a moderate to marked lowering of plasma cholesterol levels.

For severely affected homozygote children, portacaval shunt may be used as a last resort to reduce plasma cholesterol levels. A continuous-flow blood cell centrifuge to perform plasma exchanges at monthly intervals may be used to lower cholesterol levels.

For Type III hyperlipoproteinemia, dietary management includes restriction of cholesterol intake to less than 300 mg/day; carbohydrates must also be restricted, and polyunsaturated fats are increased. Clofibrate and gemfibrozil help lower blood lipid levels. Weight reduction is helpful. With strict adherence to the prescribed diet, the prognosis is good.

For Type IV, weight reduction may normalize blood lipid levels without additional treatment. Long-term dietary management includes restricted cholesterol intake, increased polyunsaturated fats, and avoidance of alcoholic beverages. Some patients respond to drug therapy; for example, gemfibrozil or nicotinic acid. Clofibrate may also be helpful in treating certain patients. The prognosis remains uncertain, however, because of predisposition to premature coronary artery disease (CAD).

The most effective treatment for Type V hyperlipoproteinemia is weight reduction and long-term maintenance of a low-fat diet. Alcoholic beverages and oral contraceptives must be avoided. Nicotinic acid, clofibrate, gemfibrozil, and a 20- to 40-g/day medium-chain triglyceride diet may prove helpful. The prognosis is uncertain because of the risk of pancreatitis. Increased fat intake may cause recurrent bouts of illness, possibly leading to pseudocyst formation, hemorrhage, and death.

Nursing diagnoses
• Altered cardiopulmonary tissue perfusion
• Fear
• Health-seeking behaviors
• Knowledge deficit
• Risk for injury

Nursing interventions
• Administer antilipemics as ordered, taking measures to prevent or minimize adverse reactions. Monitor the patient for reactions, and document and report any that occur.
• Urge the patient to adhere to his diet (usually 1,000 to 1,500 calories/day) and to avoid excess sugar and alcoholic beverages, to minimize the intake of saturated fats (higher in meats, coconut oil), and to increase the intake of polyunsaturated fats (vegetable oils).
• Assist the patient with additional life-style changes. Stress the need for medically supervised exercise and cessation of smoking. Refer him to safe, effective programs and support groups, as needed.
• Assess the patient for signs and symptoms related to CAD or its sequelae.
• Encourage the patient to verbalize fears related to premature CAD. Offer support and provide a clear explanation of the treatment regimen. Refer the patient for additional counseling, if needed.

Patient teaching
• For the 2 weeks preceding serum cholesterol and serum triglyceride tests, instruct the patient to maintain a steady weight and to adhere strictly to the prescribed diet. He should also fast for 12 hours before the test.
• Caution women with elevated serum lipids to avoid oral contraceptives or drugs that contain estrogen.
• Provide the patient with written information about foods high in cholesterol and saturated fats. Refer him to a dietitian, if necessary.
• Teach the patient about the varying components of the lipid profile and the ramifications of each. Discuss various means of lowering VLDL and LDL levels while increasing HDL levels.
• Make sure the patient understands his prescribed medication regimen. Provide verbal and written information on drug name, action, dosage, adverse reactions, monitoring requirements, and signs and symptoms requiring medical evaluation.

GAUCHER'S DISEASE
The most common lipidosis, Gaucher's disease causes an abnormal accumulation of glucocerebrosides in reticuloendothelial cells. It occurs in three forms: Type I (adult), Type II (infantile), and Type III (juvenile). Type I may be diagnosed at any time between age 1 month and 80 years and is 30 times more prevalent in people of Ashkenazic Jewish ancestry. Types II and III are less common and occur mainly in non-Jewish populations. Type II can prove fatal within 9 months of onset, usually from pulmonary involvement.

Causes
Gaucher's disease results from an autosomal recessive inheritance, which causes decreased activity of the enzyme glucosylceramide β-glucosidase.

Complications
Possible complications of Gaucher's disease include neurologic impairment, portal hypertension, pathologic fractures, anemia and, in Type II, respiratory failure.

Assessment findings
A patient with Type I Gaucher's disease usually conveys visceral complaints; neurologic complaints are rare. Typically, the patient first notes an increasing left upper quadrant mass, followed by dull, aching joint pain and fever. He may report severe leg, arm, and back pain, occurring at adolescence. The patient may have a history of respiratory problems (pneumonia or cor pulmonale), pathologic fractures (particularly of the femoral head and neck), and easy bruising and bleeding.

Inspection of an older patient may reveal a yellow pallor and brown-yellow pigmentation on the face and legs. On palpation, you'll note splenomegaly, hepatomegaly and, possibly, abdominal distention from large-bowel hypotonicity. Neurologic findings are normal. Fever may be present.

The history of a patient with Type II disease emphasizes neurologic complaints with few visceral complaints. Problems usually become evident by age 3 months. Usually, the parent describes a weak cry, failure to thrive, and psychomotor retardation. Seizures and easy bruising and bleeding may also occur.

Inspection findings may include dysphagia and respiratory distress. On palpation, you may note abdominal distention. Neurologic assessment may detect motor dysfunction and spasticity, occurring at age 6 to 7 months; strabismus; muscular hypertonicity; retroflexion of the head; neck rigidity, and hyperreflexia.

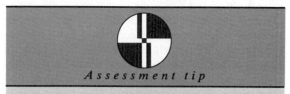

Assessment tip

UNEXPLAINED SPLENOMEGALY

Consider the possibility of Gaucher's disease in any patient with unexplained splenomegaly, especially if combined with increased serum acid phosphatase activity.

The history of a patient with Type III disease reveals both neurologic and visceral complaints, including any of the problems mentioned above. For example, the patient may report bone pain and easy bruising and bleeding. Palpation may detect hepatosplenomegaly. Neurologic assessment may reveal poor coordination and mental ability, hypertonicity, strabismus, seizures, and myoclonus. (See *Unexplained splenomegaly.*)

Diagnostic tests
• *Bone marrow aspiration* shows typical Gaucher's cells.
• *Direct assay of glucosylceramide β-glucosidase activity* in blood, bone marrow, skin, or amniotic fluid samples shows absent or deficient activity, confirming the diagnosis.
• *Liver biopsy* reveals increased glucosylceramide accumulation.

Supportive laboratory results include increased serum acid phosphatase level and decreased platelet count and serum iron level. Magnetic resonance imaging evaluates bone, liver, and spleen involvement.

Treatment
Therapy involves treating the underlying enzyme defect with alglucerase. This drug acts by replacing the missing enzyme in Type I Gaucher's disease. Imiglucerase, a new drug produced by recombinant DNA technology, acts in much the same way. Supportive treatment consists of vitamins; supplemental iron or liver extract, to prevent anemia caused by iron deficiency and to alleviate other hematologic problems; blood transfusions for anemia; splenectomy for hypersplenism; and analgesics for bone pain. Bone marrow transplantation may be performed in Gaucher's disease, but various studies of this treatment report a mortality rate ranging from 20% to 50%.

Nursing diagnoses
• Altered parenting
• Chronic pain
• Impaired gas exchange
• Knowledge deficit
• Risk for infection
• Risk for injury

Nursing interventions
• For the patient confined to bed, prevent pathologic fractures by turning him carefully. If he's ambulatory, help him when he's getting out of bed or walking.
• Observe closely for changes in pulmonary status. Plan the patient's activities within his level of tolerance. If he's on bed rest, have him turn, cough, and breathe deeply every 4 hours.
• Maintain safety precautions (including the use of padded side rails if seizure activity is a possibility). Keep the patient's call button within easy reach and the bed lowered.
• Observe for signs and symptoms of bleeding. Administer blood and blood products, as ordered, and monitor for adverse reactions.
• Maintain good hand washing, and implement measures to protect the patient from infection.
• Administer prescribed analgesics for pain. As indicated, use other pain-control techniques, including distraction, guided imagery, and meditation.
• Help the patient and family develop effective coping mechanisms. Refer them to appropriate support services.
• Recommend genetic counseling for parents who want to have another child.

Patient teaching
• Explain all diagnostic tests and procedures to the patient or family.
• Teach the patient and family supportive home care measures, including proper positioning, medication regimen, safety precautions, and nutrition guidelines. Also teach them to recognize and report status changes that require medical intervention.

AMYLOIDOSIS
A rare, chronic disease, amyloidosis results in the accumulation of an abnormal fibrillar scleroprotein (amyloid), which infiltrates body organs and soft tissues. The forms of amyloidosis may differ clinically and biochemically.

A primary disease (not associated with other disease), amyloidosis may also be familial, especially in persons of Portuguese ancestry. Amyloidosis is frequently associated with carpal tunnel syndrome. It may occur in conjunction with multiple myeloma, or it may be associated with chronic infections, tuberculosis, osteomyelitis, long-term hemodialysis, or chronic inflammatory conditions, such as rheumatoid arthritis. It may also accompany aging or Alzheimer's disease. Localized amyloidosis affects isolated organs with no evidence of systemic involvement.

Although the prognosis varies with the disease type, site, and extent of involvement, amyloidosis sometimes results in permanent—even life-threatening—organ damage. The average survival rate for a patient with generalized amyloidosis is about 1 to 4 years, although some patients live as long as 10 years or more.

Causes

The precise etiology of amyloidosis is unknown. Multiple immunobiological factors are thought to contribute to this disorder.

Complications

Renal failure is the most common cause of death associated with amyloidosis; arrhythmias resulting in sudden death also are common. Other life-threatening complications of amyloidosis include GI hemorrhage, respiratory failure, intractable heart failure, and superimposed infections.

Assessment findings

Depending on which body site is involved, amyloidosis may cause dysfunction of the heart, respiratory tract, kidneys, GI tract, skin, peripheral nerves, joints, and liver.

The patient may have a history of an associated disease or condition. He may list decreased sensations of pain and temperature; difficulty talking, swallowing, and eating due to macroglossia; and an inability to sweat. He may also have dyspnea, a cough, light-headedness with position changes, palpitations, and increased clotting time. With GI involvement, he may report abdominal pain, constipation, diarrhea, or GI bleeding. With joint involvement, he may complain of morning stiffness and fatigue.

Inspection may reveal dyspnea with respiratory involvement, and enlargement of the tongue with hindered enunciation. The patient may appear malnourished due to chronic malabsorption. With skin involvement, characteristic lesions appear as slightly raised papules or plaques found mainly in the axillary, inguinal, or anal regions; or on the face, neck, ear, or tongue. With proteinuria, edema may be evident.

Palpation may reveal abdominal tenderness and an enlarged liver. The tongue may feel stiff and firm. And you may be able to palpate small joint nodules.

On auscultation, you may discover distant heart sounds, crackles, or murmurs due to amyloid deposits in the subendocardium, endocardium, and myocardium, resulting in congestive heart failure (CHF) and valvular abnormalities. With GI involvement, bowel sounds may be decreased.

Neurologic testing may detect decreased muscle strength and, with peripheral nervous system involvement, decreased temperature and pain sensation.

Diagnostic tests

Definitive diagnosis requires histologic examination of a tissue biopsy specimen, using a polarizing or electron microscope. After appropriate tissue staining, this technique identifies amyloid deposits. Rectal mucosa biopsy and abdominal fat pad aspiration are the best screening tests because they're less hazardous than kidney or liver biopsy. Other biopsy sites include the gingiva and skin.

Other tests depend on the site of involvement; for example, electrocardiography may show low voltage and conduction or rhythm abnormalities resembling those of myocardial infarction. Echocardiography (M-mode and two-dimensional) may detect myocardial infiltration; however, only biopsy is definitive for cardiac amyloidosis. Liver function studies are usually normal except for slightly elevated serum alkaline phosphatase levels.

Treatment

No specific treatment currently exists for amyloidosis. Management is mainly supportive and conservative. It may include drugs, such as colchicine, melphalan, and prednisone, which may decrease amyloid deposits. However, the use of melphalan and prednisone is controversial: One view holds that immunosuppressants may increase amyloid deposits. Also, melphalan therapy produces bone marrow depression.

Transplantation may be useful for amyloidosis-induced renal failure. Patients with cardiac amyloidosis require conservative treatment to prevent dangerous arrhythmias. Malnutrition caused by malabsorption in end-stage GI involvement may require total parenteral nutrition. Vitamin K for coagulopathy, analgesics for musculoskeletal pain, and tracheostomy for macroglossia may also be required.

Nursing diagnoses

- Altered nutrition: Less than body requirements
- Decreased cardiac output
- Impaired skin integrity
- Impaired verbal communication
- Ineffective airway clearance
- Ineffective individual coping
- Pain
- Risk for injury

Nursing interventions

- Maintain the patient's nutrition and fluid balance; give analgesics to relieve pain; control constipation or diarrhea.
- Provide good mouth care for the patient with tongue involvement. If needed, refer him for speech therapy, provide an alternate method of communication, and alert the staff to his communication problem.
- Assess the patient's airway patency when the tongue is involved, and prevent respiratory tract compromise by gentle and adequate suctioning, when indicated. Keep a tracheostomy tray at the patient's bedside.
- When long-term bed rest is necessary, properly position the patient, and turn him often to prevent pressure ulcers. Perform range-of-motion exercises to prevent contractures.
- Provide supportive measures, such as assistance with general hygiene and comfort, when skin lesions are present.
- Monitor the patient for signs and symptoms of CHF (jugular vein distention, peripheral edema, crackles, dyspnea, and oliguria).
- Monitor electrolyte levels and coagulation studies.
- Provide a safe environment to prevent injury. Be sure to test heating pads and bath water for the patient with sensory impairment.
- Provide psychological support. Exercise patience and understanding to help the patient cope with this chronic illness. Encourage the patient to use available support systems.

Patient teaching

- Instruct the patient to move slowly when changing positions from lying or sitting to standing.
- Make sure the patient understands his medication regimen, including the names of prescribed drugs, their actions, dosages, and adverse effects.
- Teach the patient to recognize the signs and symptoms of CHF and renal failure. Tell him when to notify the doctor.

PORPHYRIAS

An umbrella term, porphyrias are metabolic disorders that affect the biosynthesis of heme (a component of hemoglobin) and cause excessive production and excretion of porphyrins or their precursors. Porphyrins, which are present in all protoplasm, play a role in energy storage and use. The classification of porphyrias depends on the site of excessive porphyrin production: They may be erythropoietic (erythroid cells in bone marrow), hepatic (in the liver), or erythrohepatic (in bone marrow and in the liver).

Causes

Porphyrias are inherited as autosomal dominant traits, except for Günther's disease, which is an autosomal recessive trait, and toxic-acquired porphyria, which usually results from lead ingestion or lead exposure. Enzymatic defects occurring in the heme synthetic pathway cause porphyrias.

Complications

Hepatic porphyrias may result in neurologic and hepatic dysfunction. Acute intermittent porphyria may result in flaccid paralysis, respiratory paralysis, and death. Erythropoietic porphyrias may cause hemolytic anemia.

Assessment findings

Clinical findings vary widely, depending on the type of porphyria. (See *Clinical variants of porphyria.*)

A patient with hepatic porphyria may complain of mild or severe abdominal pain and, possibly, nausea, vomiting, and constipation. Many patients with porphyrias also report photosensitivity. The patient history may help pinpoint precipitating factors, such as the use of certain medications, hormonal changes that occur during the menstrual and premenstrual cycles, infection, and malnutrition.

Neurologic examination may reveal paresthesia, hypoesthesia, neuritic pain, psychosis, and seizures.

Depending on the type of porphyria, inspection findings may include skin lesions (possibly associated with erythema, altered pigmentation, and edema in areas exposed to light); urine that becomes darker when left standing in light and air; and neurologic signs, such as wristdrop and footdrop. If hemolytic anemia occurs, expect to find splenomegaly on palpation.

In a patient with acute intermittent porphyria, auscultation may reveal wheezing and dyspnea, compounded by the patient's anxiety. During an acute attack, fever may occur.

CLINICAL VARIANTS OF PORPHYRIA

Porphyria	Clinical findings	Treatment
Erythropoietic porphyria		
Günther's disease • Usual onset before age 5 • Extremely rare	• Red urine (earliest, most characteristic sign); severe cutaneous photosensitivity, leading to vesicular or bullous eruptions on exposed areas and eventual scarring and ulceration • Hypertrichosis • Brown or red-stained teeth • Splenomegaly, hemolytic anemia	• Beta carotene to reduce photosensitivity • Anti-inflammatory ointments • Prednisone to reverse anemia • Packed red blood cells to inhibit erythropoiesis and excreted porphyrins • Hemin for recurrent attacks • Splenectomy for hemolytic anemia • Topical dihydroxyacetone and lawson sunscreen filter • Oral cholestyramine and charcoal to reduce intestinal reabsorption of porphyrins
Erythrohepatic porphyria		
Protoporphyria • Usually affects children • More common in males	• Photosensitive dermatitis • Hemolytic anemia • Chronic hepatic disease	• Avoidance of causative factors • Beta carotene to reduce photosensitivity
Toxic-acquired porphyria • Usually affects children • Significant mortality	• Acute, colicky pain • Anorexia, nausea, vomiting • Neuromuscular weakness • Behavioral changes • Seizures, coma	• Chlorpromazine I.V. (25 mg every 4 to 6 hours during an acute attack) to relieve pain and GI symptoms • Avoidance of lead exposure
Hepatic porphyria		
Acute intermittent porphyria • Most common form • More prevalent in females, usually between ages 15 and 40	• Colicky abdominal pain with fever, general malaise, and hypertension • Peripheral neuritis, behavior changes, possibly leading to frank psychosis • Respiratory paralysis possible	• Chlorpromazine I.V. to relieve abdominal pain and control psychic abnormalities; meperidine for severe pain • Avoidance of precipitating medications, infections, alcohol, and fasting • Hemin for recurrent attacks • High carbohydrate diet • I.V. glucose
Variegate porphyria • Onset between ages 30 and 50 • Occurs almost exclusively among South African whites • Affects males and females equally	• Skin lesions, fragile skin in exposed areas • Hypertrichosis of face and temples • Hyperpigmentation • Abdominal pain during acute attack • Neuropsychiatric manifestations	• High-carbohydrate diet • Avoidance of sunlight, or wearing of protective clothing and use of sunscreen when avoidance isn't possible • Hemin for recurrent attacks
Porphyria cutanea tarda • Most common in men ages 40 to 60 • Highest incidence in South Africans	• Facial pigmentation • Red-brown urine • Photosensitivity dermatitis • Hypertrichosis	• Avoidance of precipitating factors (alcohol, estrogen, sunlight exposure, and iron) • Phlebotomy at 2-week intervals to lower serum iron level
Hereditary coproporphyria • Rare • Affects males and females equally	• Asymptomatic or mild neurologic, abdominal, or psychiatric symptoms	• High-carbohydrate diet • Avoidance of barbiturates • Hemin for recurrent attacks

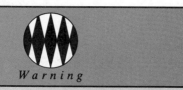

DRUGS THAT AGGRAVATE PORPHYRIA

Make sure the patient with porphyria doesn't receive any of the following drugs, which are known to precipitate signs and symptoms of porphyria:

- alcohol
- aminopyrine
- barbiturates
- carbamazepine
- carisoprodol
- chloramphenicol
- chlordiazepoxide
- danazol
- diazepam
- ergot alkaloids
- estrogens
- glutethimide
- griseofulvin
- imipramine
- meprobamate
- methsuximide
- methyldopa
- methylprylon
- pentazocine
- phenytoin
- progesterones
- sulfonamides
- tolbutamide.

Diagnostic tests

- In acute intermittent porphyria, the Watson-Schwartz test may be positive for porphobilinogen in the urine; the ion exchange chromatography test may identify aminolevulinic acid in the urine.
- In variegate porphyria, protoporphyrin and coproporphyrin may be positive in the stools. With hereditary coproporphyria, large amounts of coproporphyrin appear in the stools and, to a lesser extent, in the urine.
- Porphyria cutanea tarda results in increased excretion of uroporphyrins; the amount of fecal porphyrins varies.
- With Günther's disease, porphyrins are found in the urine, especially uroporphyrin I.
- With erythropoietic protoporphyria, fluorescent microscopy is used to confirm the diagnosis by detecting excess protoporphyrin in the red blood cells.
- A urine lead level of 0.2 mg/liter helps confirm toxic-acquired porphyria.

Other laboratory values may include increased serum iron levels in porphyria cutanea tarda. Leukocytosis, elevated bilirubin and alkaline phosphatase levels, and hyponatremia occur in acute intermittent porphyria.

Treatment

Depending on the type of porphyria, treatment may include the administration of beta carotene to reduce photosensitivity, chlorpromazine I.V. to treat mild abdominal discomfort, meperidine to treat severe pain, levulose I.V. to increase carbohydrate intake, and hemin to suppress hepatic aminolevulinic acid and porphobilinogen. Splenectomy may be performed to treat hemolytic anemia. Patients with photosensitivity are advised to avoid direct sunlight or, possibly, to use sunscreen preparations.

Nursing diagnoses

- Constipation
- Impaired gas exchange
- Impaired skin integrity
- Knowledge deficit
- Pain
- Risk for injury

Nursing interventions

- Before administering medications to the patient, make certain the drugs don't precipitate an acute attack. (See *Drugs that aggravate porphyria.*)
- Administer hemin by a large arm vein or central venous catheter, as ordered. Overdosage may result in renal shutdown.
- Provide emotional support, and encourage the patient to verbalize his concerns about his condition.

In acute intermittent porphyria:

- Provide active and passive range-of-motion exercises every 8 hours. Position the patient's body in proper alignment, using splinting as necessary. Assess respiratory status every 2 hours; respiratory depression or paralysis requires mechanical ventilation.
- Observe for signs and symptoms of decreased GI motility, resulting in distention, ileus, vomiting, and constipation.
- Take safety precautions, as indicated. For example, use padded side rails, and keep an oral airway at the bedside if seizure activity is possible.
- If the patient is experiencing an acute attack, administer comfort measures, including mouth care, skin care, and massage every 2 hours, with positioning and pulmonary hygiene. Administer analgesics, as ordered.

Patient teaching

- Warn the patient against excessive sun exposure.
- Stress the importance of wearing a medical identification bracelet or necklace.
- If the patient has toxic-acquired porphyria, discuss sources of lead, and refer him to resources that can identify such sources in the home.
- Warn the patient to avoid precipitating factors, including crash dieting; fasting; and the use of specific drugs, such as alcohol, estrogens, and barbiturates. Teach

stress-management techniques because emotional stress may also precipitate an acute attack. Discuss measures to help prevent infection, another precipitating factor.

• Encourage a high-carbohydrate diet to provide sufficient calories without taxing the liver to break down proteins.

TAY-SACHS DISEASE

The most common of the lipid storage diseases, Tay-Sachs disease results from a congenital enzyme deficiency. Tay-Sachs disease occurs in fewer than 100 infants born each year in the United States. However, it strikes persons of Ashkenazic Jewish ancestry about 100 times more often than the general population, occurring in about 1 in 3,600 live births in this ethnic group. About 1 in 30 of this group are heterozygous carriers of this defective gene. If two such carriers have children, each of their offspring has a 25% chance of having Tay-Sachs disease.

The disease is characterized by progressive mental and motor deterioration and is always fatal, usually before age 5.

Causes

Tay-Sachs disease is an autosomal recessive disorder in which the enzyme hexosaminidase A is deficient. This enzyme is necessary for metabolism of gangliosides, water-soluble glycolipids found primarily in central nervous system (CNS) tissues. Without hexosaminidase A, accumulating lipid pigments distend and progressively destroy and demyelinate CNS cells.

Complications

Starting at about age 2, the patient with Tay-Sachs disease contracts recurrent bronchopneumonia, which is usually fatal before age 5.

Assessment findings

Usually, the patient has a familial history of Tay-Sachs disease. The patient history typically reveals a normal appearance at birth (with the possible exception of an exaggerated Moro's reflex) and onset of clinical signs and symptoms between ages 5 and 6 months, followed by progressive deterioration, with psychomotor retardation, blindness, and dementia.

On inspection, the 3- to 6-month-old infant appears apathetic and displays an augmented response to loud sounds. Progressive weakness of the neck, trunk, arm, and leg muscles prevents the child from sitting up or lifting his head. He has difficulty turning over, can't grasp objects, and has progressive vision loss.

By 18 months, the infant may have a history of seizures, generalized paralysis, and spasticity. Although blind, the infant may hold his eyes wide open and roll his eyeballs. His pupils are always dilated. Decerebrate rigidity and a complete vegetative state follow.

Measurement of the head circumference may detect enlargement. Pupillary testing finds no reaction to light. Ophthalmoscopic examination may show optic nerve atrophy and a distinctive cherry-red spot on the retina.

Diagnostic tests

Serum analysis showing deficient hexosaminidase A is typically the key to diagnosis. Diagnostic screening is essential for all couples of Ashkenazic Jewish ancestry and for others with a family history of the disease. A simple blood test evaluating hexosaminidase A levels can identify carriers. If carriers wish prenatal diagnosis, amniocentesis or chorionic villus biopsy can detect hexosaminidase A deficiency and, consequently, Tay-Sachs disease in the fetus.

Treatment

Tay-Sachs disease has no known cure. Supportive treatment includes tube feedings using nutritional supplements, suctioning and postural drainage to remove secretions, skin care to prevent pressure ulcers once the child becomes bedridden, and mild laxatives to relieve neurogenic constipation. Unfortunately, anticonvulsants usually fail to prevent seizures. Because these children need round-the-clock physical care, they commonly require long-term care in special facilities.

Nursing diagnoses

• Anticipatory grieving
• Impaired physical mobility
• Ineffective airway clearance
• Ineffective family coping
• Knowledge deficit
• Risk for impaired skin integrity
• Risk for injury

Nursing interventions

• Help the family deal with their infant's inevitably progressive illness and death.
• Refer parents for genetic counseling, and stress the importance of amniocentesis in future pregnancies. Refer siblings for screening to determine if they're carriers. If they are carriers and are adults, refer them for genetic

counseling, but stress that the disease is not transmitted to offspring if they don't marry another carrier.
• Because parents may feel excessive stress or guilt about their child's illness, impending death, and the emotional and financial burden it places on them, refer them for psychological counseling, if indicated.
• Implement measures to prevent skin breakdown in the child, provide for adequate nutrition, and maintain a patent airway. Implement seizure precautions to prevent injury.

Patient teaching
• If parents plan to care for their child at home, teach them how to do suctioning, postural drainage, and tube feeding. Also teach them how to give good skin care to prevent pressure ulcers.
• Refer parents to the National Tay-Sachs and Allied Diseases Association for more information on this disease.

PHENYLKETONURIA

An inborn error in amino acid (specifically phenylalanine) metabolism, phenylketonuria (PKU) results in high serum levels of phenylalanine, increased urine concentrations of phenylalanine and its by-products, cerebral damage, and mental retardation. Also called phenylalaninemia and phenylpyruvica oligophrenia, the disorder occurs once in about 14,000 births in the United States. (About one person in 60 is an asymptomatic carrier.) It has a low incidence in Finland and among Ashkenazic Jews and American Blacks. The incidence is high among the Irish and Scottish.

Although blood phenylalanine levels approach normal at birth, they begin to rise within a few days. By the time they reach significant levels (about 30 mg/dl), cerebral damage has begun. Such irreversible damage probably is complete by age 2 or 3. However, early detection and treatment can minimize cerebral damage.

Causes and pathophysiology
PKU transmits through an autosomal recessive gene. Patients with classic PKU, the most common and clinically important of the hyperphenylalaninemias, have almost totally deficient activity of phenylalanine hydroxylase, an enzyme that acts as a catalyst in the conversion of phenylalanine to tyrosine. As a result, phenylalanine accumulates in the blood and urine, and reduced tyrosine formation results.

Complications
Phenylalanine accumulation causes mental retardation.

Assessment findings
The patient may have a family history of PKU. Typically, the history reveals no abnormalities apparent at birth, but by age 4 months, the untreated child begins to show signs of arrested brain development, including mental retardation and, later, personality disturbances (schizoid and antisocial personality patterns and uncontrollable temper). About one-third of patients have a history of seizures, which usually begin between ages 6 and 12 months. Many patients also show a precipitous decrease in IQ in their first year.

On inspection, the patient typically has a lighter complexion than unaffected siblings and may have blue eyes. He may also exhibit macrocephaly, eczematous skin lesions, or dry, rough skin. He's usually hyperactive and irritable; shows purposeless, repetitive motions; and has an awkward gait. You may also note a musty odor from the skin and urinary excretion of phenylacetic acid.

Diagnostic tests
Most states require screening for PKU at birth; the Guthrie screening test on a capillary blood sample (bacterial inhibition assay) reliably detects the disorder. However, because phenylalanine levels may be normal at birth, the infant should be evaluated after he has begun protein feedings. With PKU, levels are usually abnormally high by day 4. More quantitative fluorometric or chromatographic assays provide additional diagnostic information.

About 80% of affected children have abnormal electroencephalography patterns.

Deoxyribonucleic acid–based tests now make prenatal diagnosis of classic PKU possible.

Treatment
To prevent or minimize brain damage, phenylalanine blood levels are kept between 3 and 15 mg/dl by restricting dietary intake of the amino acid phenylalanine. During the first month of life, a special, low-phenylalanine, amino acid mixture is substituted for most of the protein in the diet, supplemented with a small amount of natural foods. Even with this special diet, slight central nervous system (CNS) dysfunction may occur. Although dietary restrictions can be relaxed after age 6 in children with classic PKU, some restriction should probably continue throughout life.

Such a diet calls for close monitoring. The body doesn't make phenylalanine, so overzealous dietary restriction can induce phenylalanine deficiency, causing lethargy, anorexia, anemia, skin rashes, diarrhea, and even death.

Nursing diagnoses

- Altered growth and development
- Family coping: Potential for growth
- Knowledge deficit
- Risk for altered parent/infant/child attachment
- Risk for disorganized infant behavior
- Risk for injury

Nursing interventions

- If the child is experiencing seizures or has some mental dysfunction, implement safety measures to prevent injury. Refer the parents and child to appropriate community resources.

  To prevent this disorder:
- Routinely screen infants for PKU because detection and control of phenylalanine intake soon after birth can prevent severe mental retardation.
- Refer classic phenylketonuric females who reach reproductive age for genetic counseling because recent research indicates that their offspring may have a higher than normal incidence of brain damage, microcephaly, and major congenital malformations (especially of the heart and CNS). Such damage may be prevented with a low-phenylalanine diet begun before conception and continued throughout pregnancy.

Patient teaching

- Teach the parents and child about PKU, and provide emotional support and counseling. (Psychological and emotional problems may result from the difficult dietary restrictions.)
- Teach the child and his parents about the critical importance of adhering to his diet. The child must avoid breads, cheese, eggs, flour, meat, poultry, fish, nuts, milk, legumes, and aspartame (Nutrasweet). He'll need frequent tests for urine phenylpyruvic acid and blood phenylalanine levels to evaluate the diet's effectiveness.
- As the child grows older and is supervised less closely, his parents have less control over what he eats. As a result, deviation from the restricted diet becomes more likely and so does the risk of further brain damage. Encourage parents to allow the child some choices in the kinds of low-protein foods he eats; this will help make him feel trusted and more responsible.
- Teach parents about normal physical and mental growth and development to help them recognize any developmental delay from excessive phenylalanine intake.

FLUID, ELECTROLYTE, AND ACID-BASE DISORDERS

The mechanisms of fluid, electrolyte, and acid-base balance maintain homeostasis by controlling body functions, such as the heart rate, hematopoiesis, blood pressure, body temperature, respiration, and glandular secretion. With prompt treatment, the prognosis for most types of homeostatic imbalance is good.

POTASSIUM IMBALANCE

A cation that's the dominant cellular electrolyte, potassium facilitates contraction of both skeletal and smooth muscles, including myocardial contraction. It figures prominently in nerve impulse conduction, acid-base balance, enzyme action, and cell membrane function. Because serum potassium level has such a narrow range (3.5 to 5 mEq/liter), a slight deviation in either direction can produce profound consequences.

Causes

Hypokalemia rarely results from a dietary deficiency because many foods contain potassium. Instead, potassium loss results from:
- excessive GI losses, such as vomiting, gastric suction, diarrhea, villous adenoma, or laxative abuse
- chronic renal disease, with tubular potassium wasting
- certain drugs, especially potassium-wasting diuretics, steroids, and certain sodium-containing antibiotics (carbenicillin)
- alkalosis or insulin effect, which causes potassium shifting into cells without true depletion of total body potassium
- prolonged potassium-free I.V. therapy
- hyperglycemia, causing osmotic diuresis and glycosuria
- Cushing's syndrome, primary hyperaldosteronism, excessive ingestion of licorice, and severe serum magnesium deficiency.

Hyperkalemia usually results from reduced excretion by the kidneys. This may be due to acute or severe chronic renal failure, oliguria due to shock or severe dehydration, or the use of potassium-sparing diuretics, such as triamterene, by patients with renal disease. Inadequate potassium excretion may also be due to hypoaldosteronism or Addison's disease.

Hyperkalemia may also result from failure to excrete excessive amounts of potassium infused I.V. or admin-

E.C.G. CHANGES IN POTASSIUM IMBALANCE

Hypokalemia and hyperkalemia can induce cardiac arrhythmias, as shown on the following electrocardiogram (ECG) strips.

HYPOKALEMIA

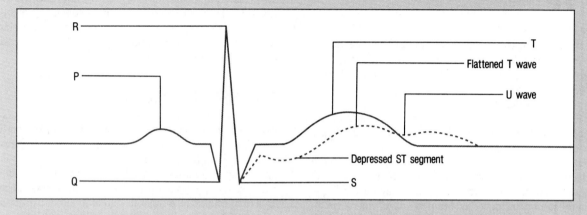

HYPERKALEMIA

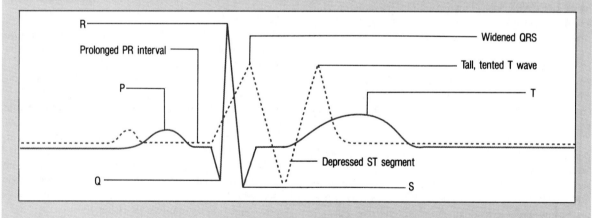

istered orally. Another cause is massive release of intracellular potassium, such as can occur with burns, crushing injuries, severe infection, or acidosis.

Complications

Potassium imbalances may result in muscle weakness and flaccid paralysis and may also lead to cardiac arrest. (For more information on cardiac effects, see *ECG changes in potassium imbalance*.)

Assessment findings

The patient's history and physical examination may reveal cardiovascular irregularities manifested by dizziness, postural hypotension, and arrhythmias.

GI complaints may include nausea and vomiting, anorexia, abdominal distention, constipation, paralytic ileus, and decreased peristalsis (with hypokalemia) or nausea, diarrhea, and abdominal cramps (with hyperkalemia).

The patient may also experience neuromuscular symptoms, such as weakness and hyporeflexia (with hypokalemia); skeletal muscle weakness, numbness, and tingling (with hyperkalemia); and flaccid paralysis or respiratory paralysis (with both imbalances).

Diagnostic tests
Serum potassium levels definitively diagnose a potassium abnormality. In hypokalemia, potassium levels are less than 3.5 mEq/liter. In hyperkalemia, levels are more than 5 mEq/liter.

Additional tests may be necessary to determine the underlying cause of the imbalance.

Treatment
Hypokalemia treatment should involve increased dietary intake of potassium or oral supplements with potassium salts. Potassium chloride is the preferred choice. Edematous patients with diuretic-induced hypokalemia should receive a potassium-sparing diuretic, such as spironolactone.

Patients with GI potassium loss or severe potassium depletion require I.V. potassium replacement therapy. If hypocalcemia is also present, treatment should include calcium replacement. (See *Administering I.V. potassium safely.*)

For *hyperkalemia*, treatment consists of withholding potassium and administering a cation exchange resin orally or by enema. Sodium polystyrene sulfonate (Kayexalate) with 70% sorbitol produces exchange of sodium ions for potassium ions in the intestine.

In an emergency, rapid infusion of 10% calcium gluconate decreases myocardial irritability and temporarily prevents cardiac arrest but doesn't correct serum potassium excess; it's also contraindicated in patients receiving digitalis.

Also as an emergency measure, sodium bicarbonate I.V. increases pH and causes potassium to shift back into the cells. Insulin and 10% to 50% glucose I.V. also move potassium back into cells. Infusions should be followed by dextrose 5% in water because infusion of 10% to 15% glucose will stimulate secretion of endogenous insulin. Hemodialysis or peritoneal dialysis also aids in removal of excess potassium; however, these are slow techniques.

Nursing diagnoses
• Constipation
• Decreased cardiac output
• Diarrhea
• Knowledge deficit
• Risk for injury

Warning

ADMINISTERING I.V. POTASSIUM SAFELY

I.V. replacement of potassium is necessary only if hypokalemia is severe or if the patient can't take supplements by mouth. Carefully monitor I.V. potassium replacement to prevent or lessen toxic effects. Follow these guidelines:
• I.V. infusion concentrations generally shouldn't exceed 40 to 60 mEq/liter. The infusion rate shouldn't exceed 40 mEq/hour (200 mEq/day), unless indicated. More concentrated potassium solutions may be used in severely fluid-restricted patients.
• Use volumetric devices whenever concentrations of more than 40 mEq/liter are infused.
• *Never* administer potassium by I.V. push or bolus; it may cause cardiac arrest.
• Monitor cardiac rhythm during rapid I.V. administration of potassium to avoid cardiac toxicity from inadvertent hyperkalemia. Report any irregularities immediately.
• Monitor serum potassium levels and evaluate signs and symptoms, such as muscle weakness.
• Monitor the I.V. site for signs and symptoms of infiltration, phlebitis, or tissue necrosis.

Nursing interventions
In hypokalemia:
• Frequently monitor serum potassium and other electrolyte levels during potassium replacement therapy to avoid overcorrection to hyperkalemia. (For more information, see *Planning care for the hypokalemic patient,* pages 978 and 979.)
• Assess intake and output carefully. Remember, the kidneys excrete 80% to 90% of ingested potassium. Never give supplementary potassium to a patient whose urine output is below 600 ml/day. Also, measure GI loss from suctioning or vomiting.
• Because of the risk of potassium toxicity, administer I.V. potassium slowly and cautiously to prevent cardiac arrhythmias and vein irritation.
• If the patient is taking a liquid oral potassium supplement, have him sip it slowly to prevent GI irritation. Give the supplement with or after meals with a full glass of water or fruit juice.
• Carefully monitor patients receiving digitalis because hypokalemia enhances the action of digitalis. Assess for

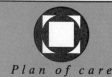

Plan of care

PLANNING CARE FOR THE HYPOKALEMIC PATIENT

How do you develop an effective plan of care for the hypokalemic patient? To prepare yourself, consider that you're caring for Amanda Long, a 62-year-old homemaker with hypertension. Her condition had been well controlled by digoxin 25 mg every day, furosemide 40 mg twice a day, and captopril 25 mg twice a day. However, with a recent bout of gastroenteritis, she has lost her appetite and has become severely dehydrated. Today, she was admitted to your unit for an evaluation of her condition and an explanation of troubling symptoms.

Patient history
Mrs. Long tells you, "I've been feeling 'under the weather' for 3 days." She confesses to taking her husband's penicillin and now reports diarrhea. Constant nausea has killed her appetite, and she's drinking only tea. Her complaints include lack of energy, along with numbness and tingling in her hands, feet, and face. She's concerned that her blood pressure is too high, and she fears she's about to have a stroke.

As her history continues, you learn that Mrs. Long has continued to take her antihypertensive medication, as prescribed, even though she hasn't eaten anything over the past 72 hours.

Assessment findings
Your assessment starts with Mrs. Long's vital signs. Her oral temperature is slightly elevated at 99.8° F (37.7° C). Her thready pulse is 54 beats/minute and very irregular; her respirations are shallow at 14 breaths/minute. Her blood pressure is 122/60 mm Hg.

You examine Mrs. Long and find that her skin is pale, dry, and leathery, and her lips and oral mucous

membranes are dry and cracked. Her skin turgor is poor. Auscultation discloses mild, diffuse crackles throughout both lung fields.

Diagnostic tests suggest that severe dehydration and ingestion of regularly scheduled medications have complicated Mrs. Long's condition. Her readings are as follows:
• serum potassium, 2.9 mEq/liter
• serum chloride, 94 mEq/liter
• total CO_2, 25 mEq/liter
• BUN, 22 mg/dl
• serum creatinine, 1.7 mg/dl
• serum digoxin, 2.8 ng/ml.

An electrocardiogram reveals atrial fibrillation with a slow ventricular response of 52 to 58 beats/minute. U waves, flattened T waves, and depressed ST segments appear throughout the tracing. Arterial blood gas analysis shows that Mrs. Long has adequate oxygenation but that she's experiencing metabolic alkalosis.

The suspected medical diagnosis is dehydration with hypokalemia complicated by digoxin toxicity.

Nursing diagnoses
Based on your assessment findings and impressions of Mrs. Long, you arrive at these nursing diagnoses:
• Fluid volume deficit and altered oral mucous membranes related to prolonged diarrhea and poor oral fluid intake
• Activity intolerance related to fatigue and weakness from dehydration, potassium loss, and arrhythmias
• Altered nutrition: Less than body requirements of potassium-rich foods and fluids, related to reduced absorption of nutrients and drug-induced potassium loss
• Knowledge deficit related to medication use during secondary illness.

Expected outcomes
You define the following immediate and long-term goals for Mrs. Long.

She will:
• have hydration restored
• increase and modify her activity levels to facilitate comfort
• improve her nutritional intake and stabilize deficits
• demonstrate understanding of diet, medications and their adverse effects, and prevention of hypokalemia and digoxin toxicity.

Implementation
To help Mrs. Long achieve her expected outcomes, you take the following steps.

To restore hydration
• Provide Mrs. Long with 2,500 to 3,000 ml of fluid daily; fluid intake may be oral or parenteral or both.
• Auscultate lung fields every 4 hours during rehydration (fluid collection in the lungs is a potential hazard).
• Record intake and output. Include all fluids, diarrhea, vomitus, and insensible losses.
• Check Mrs. Long's skin turgor and mucous membranes each shift for signs of rehydration.
• Weigh Mrs. Long daily at the same time, in the same weight clothes, and on the same scale. Record and track her weight changes during rehydration.
• Monitor urine specific gravity and serum osmolality as well as hematocrit, BUN, creatinine, and electrolyte levels daily during rehydration.
• Monitor for orthostatic hypotension.
• Provide frequent mouth care, especially before meals; offer ice chips, lubricants, and emollients for the mouth and lips.

To increase and modify activity levels
• Assess Mrs. Long's baseline activity levels at the beginning of each shift to determine her activity limits.
• Assess for signs of activity intolerance, such as increased fatigue and weakness, dyspnea on exertion,

PLANNING CARE FOR THE HYPOKALEMIC PATIENT
(continued)

dizziness, chest pain, or significant pulse rate or blood pressure changes.
• Provide frequent rest periods during the full 24-hour cycle. Limit the length of time for procedures, activities, and visitors. Assist Mrs. Long with activities of daily living, and gradually allow her to perform more physical activity each day.
• Reduce the amount of noxious stimuli to the environment; provide soft lighting, low-level music or conversation, and a comfortable and supportive bed.
• Provide warmth and measures to increase circulation when paresthesia affects Mrs. Long's extremities.
• In cooperation with physical and occupational therapy, move from providing passive to active range-of-motion exercises.
• Involve Mrs. Long in the planning and implementation of all her activities while in the hospital.

To improve nutritional intake and stabilize deficits
• Consult the dietitian, and help Mrs. Long select potassium-rich foods.
• Monitor electrolyte levels.
• Monitor Mrs. Long's dietary intake. Place her on a calorie count if her in-

take doesn't improve within 48 hours.
• Supplement her diet with oral or parenteral potassium or both. Monitor for increased nausea or gastric burning.
• Provide pleasant, balanced meals after rest periods; allow adequate time for meal completion; and ensure that Mrs. Long can tolerate the temperature, texture, and consistency of each food or liquid.

To prevent electrolyte imbalance and drug toxicity
• Assess Mrs. Long's baseline knowledge of all prescribed medications and possible associated adverse reactions; correct misconceptions and provide assurance that she can continue to self-medicate and monitor her symptoms of impending problems after discharge.
• Teach or reinforce the need for Mrs. Long to take her pulse for 1 full minute before taking her daily dose of digoxin. If her heart rate is less than 60 beats/minute, advise her to rest and retake her pulse in 30 minutes. Instruct her to report a continued low pulse rate to her doctor as soon as possible.
• Teach or reinforce the signs and symptoms associated with hypokalemia (fatigue, nausea, vomiting, anorexia, weakness, paresthesia) and digoxin toxicity (changes in heart rate, anorexia, nausea, vomiting,

headache, irritability, confusion, visual disturbances).
• Provide full dietary assistance. Use the social services and occupational therapy departments to help Mrs. Long learn how to plan and prepare a well-balanced, potassium-rich diet in the home.
• Discuss the use of potassium-sparing diuretics should diuretic therapy need to continue.
• Encourage Mrs. Long to make and keep regular outpatient appointments and to notify her doctor's office if symptoms of hypokalemia or digoxin toxicity recur.

Evaluation
You've met your goals when Mrs. Long has balanced intake and output, shows no signs of dehydration, participates in normal activities without tiring, understands her prescribed diet and medications, and complies with treatment.

Mrs. Long will need constant reassessment during her hospitalization and after discharge. Many of her symptoms will change rapidly, so you'll need to devise ongoing evaluation and innovative strategies to help her meet her goals. After she's stabilized, she'll need family or friends to support her efforts to maintain homeostasis at home.

---

signs of digitalis toxicity (anorexia, nausea, vomiting, blurred vision, and arrhythmias).
• Monitor cardiac rhythm, and report any irregularities immediately.
• Implement safety measures for the patient with muscle weakness or postural hypotension.
• Assess for abdominal distention, decreased bowel sounds, and constipation.
   In hyperkalemia:
• As in hypokalemia, frequently monitor serum potassium and other electrolyte levels, and carefully record intake and output.
• Administer sodium polystyrene sulfonate orally, or rectally by retention enema. (Encourage the patient to retain the enema for at least 30 to 60 minutes.) Watch for signs of hypokalemia with prolonged use.

• Assess for clinical effects of hypoglycemia (muscle weakness, syncope, hunger, diaphoresis) with repeated insulin and glucose treatment.
• Monitor for and report cardiac arrhythmias.
• Provide sufficient calories to prevent tissue breakdown and release of potassium into extracellular fluid.
• Assess GI functioning for abdominal distention, intestinal cramping, and diarrhea.
• Implement safety measures for the patient with muscle weakness.
• Watch for signs of hyperkalemia in predisposed patients, especially those with poor urine output or those receiving potassium supplements by mouth or I.V. Also, before giving a blood transfusion, check to see when the blood was donated; older blood cell hemolysis releases potassium. Infuse only *fresh* blood for patients with average to high serum potassium levels.

Patient teaching

• To prevent hypokalemia, instruct patients (especially those taking diuretics) to include potassium-rich foods in their diets. Such foods include oranges, bananas, tomatoes, milk, dried fruits, apricots, peanuts, and dark green, leafy vegetables.

• Emphasize the importance of taking potassium supplements as prescribed, particularly if the patient is also taking digitalis or diuretics. If appropriate, teach the patient to recognize and report signs of digitalis toxicity, such as pulse irregularities. Demonstrate the proper technique for assessing the patient's pulse.

• Make sure the patient can recognize signs of hypokalemia and hyperkalemia, including weakness and pulse irregularities. Tell him to report them to the doctor.

• To prevent hyperkalemia, teach patients who use salt substitutes containing potassium to discontinue them if urine output decreases.

SODIUM IMBALANCE

The major cation (90%) in extracellular fluid (ECF), sodium is the main factor responsible for ECF concentration. Increases or decreases in ECF sodium concentrations greatly affect ECF volume and distribution. Sodium controls the distribution of water throughout the body and regulates ECF volume. It also plays an important role in the transmission of nerve impulses and muscle contraction.

Hyponatremia refers to an excess of body water relative to sodium; it is not synonymous with sodium depletion. Sodium loss is just one state in which hyponatremia may occur. *Hypernatremia* refers to a deficit of body water relative to sodium. Thirst seems to be the major defense mechanism against hypernatremia.

Although the body requires only 2 to 4 g of sodium daily, most Americans consume 6 to 10 g daily (mostly sodium chloride, as table salt), excreting excess sodium through the kidneys and skin. Under the influence of antidiuretic hormone (ADH) and aldosterone, the kidneys primarily regulate ECF sodium balance.

Causes

Hyponatremia usually results from defective urine dilution, caused by either an excessive loss of sodium or an excessive gain of water. Specific causes of hyponatremia include:

• excessive GI loss of water and electrolytes due to vomiting, suctioning, fistulas, or diarrhea; excessive perspiration; or fever. When such losses decrease circulating fluid volume, increased secretion of ADH promotes maximum water reabsorption, which further dilutes serum sodium. Combined with too much free water intake, these factors are especially likely to cause hyponatremia.

• diuretic therapy, most commonly thiazides

• excessive drinking of water (psychogenic polydipsia); infusion of I.V. dextrose in water without other solutes, particularly during stress

• endocrine disorders, such as adrenal gland insufficiency and moderate to severe hypothyroidism

• chronic illnesses, such as cirrhosis of the liver and congestive heart failure

• syndrome of inappropriate antidiuretic hormone (SIADH) secretion, resulting from central nervous system disorders, such as head injury, cerebrovascular accident; nonmalignant pulmonary diseases, such as tuberculosis; neoplasms with ectopic ADH production, such as oat cell lung tumors; or certain drugs, such as chlorpropamide and clofibrate.

Hypernatremia results from a sodium gain in excess of water or, most commonly, by a water loss in excess of sodium. It may also result from water loss alone. Specific causes of hypernatremia include:

• severe insensible water losses that aren't replaced, such as in patients with fever, hyperventilation, or extensive burns

• severe renal water losses, as in acute diabetes insipidus

• severe vomiting and diarrhea, causing water loss that exceeds sodium loss; serum sodium levels rise, but overall ECF volume decreases

• excess adrenocortical hormones, as in Cushing's syndrome

• water loss in excess of sodium due to diaphoresis, if the patient can't drink

• administration of high-protein feedings without adequate water supplement (due to urea diuresis)

• sodium excess, such as administration of excessive amounts of hypertonic sodium chloride infusions to obtunded patients who can't drink or inadvertent introduction of hypertonic sodium chloride solution into maternal circulation during therapeutic abortion.

Thirst is such a strong drive that severe, persistent hypernatremia only occurs in persons who can't respond to thirst voluntarily, such as infants or unconscious patients. A disturbance of the thirst mechanism is rare.

Complications

States of severe hyponatremia or hypernatremia may result in seizures, coma, and permanent neurologic damage.

Hyponatremia may lead to cerebral edema, as decreased plasma osmolality causes water movement into cells. Increased brain cell volume, in turn, leads to neurologic symptoms.

Increased plasma osmolality associated with hypernatremia causes a water shift out of cells, possibly resulting in cerebral cell dehydration and neurologic symptoms.

Assessment findings

A patient with *hyponatremia* may complain initially of anorexia, nausea, abdominal cramping, headache, and exhaustion. When the serum sodium level drops further (between 120 and 125 mEq/liter), neurologic assessment may reveal lethargy, confusion, twitching, and focal weakness, which, if untreated, may progress to seizures and coma.

If hyponatremia is secondary to ECF loss, the patient may complain of dizziness. Palpation may detect dry mucous membranes, and vital signs assessment reflects orthostatic hypotension and tachycardia.

If hyponatremia is secondary to fluid gain, inspection may note edema; palpation may disclose fingerprint edema (with SIADH); further assessment may reveal hypertension and weight gain.

A patient with *hypernatremia* may complain of fatigue, restlessness, and weakness. When hypernatremia is severe, assessment of level of consciousness may reveal disorientation, which may progress to seizures and coma.

On inspection, the hypernatremic patient may have flushed skin. Palpation may reveal a dry, swollen tongue and sticky mucous membranes. The patient may have a low-grade fever.

Diagnostic tests

Serum sodium levels will be less than 135 mEq/liter with hyponatremia and more than 145 mEq/liter with hypernatremia.

Additional laboratory studies determine the etiology of the imbalance and differentiate between a true deficit and an apparent deficit due to sodium shift or to hypervolemia or hypovolemia.

Treatment

When possible, patients with sodium deficits receive oral sodium supplementation. Therapy for mild hyponatremia associated with hypervolemia usually consists of restricted water intake. If fluid restriction alone fails to normalize serum sodium levels, demeclocycline or lith-

ium, which blocks ADH action in the renal tubules, can be used to promote water excretion.

In extremely rare instances of severe symptomatic hyponatremia, when serum sodium levels fall below 110 mEq/liter, treatment may include infusion of 3% or 5% sodium chloride solution.

Treatment with an infusion of hypertonic saline solution requires careful patient monitoring in an intensive care setting for signs of circulatory overload, which is potentially fatal. (Administration of hypertonic saline solution causes water to shift out of cells, risking intravascular volume overload.) For this reason, furosemide is usually administered concurrently. The hypertonic saline solution is infused slowly, in small volumes.

If indicated, treatment must include correction of the underlying disorder; for example, hormonal therapy may be needed to treat endocrine disorders.

Primary treatment of hypernatremia associated with water deficit aims to stop the water loss with slow, oral replacement of the water deficit. If the patient can't tolerate oral replacement, treatment requires I.V. administration of salt-free solutions (such as dextrose in water) to return serum sodium levels to normal, followed by infusion of 0.45% sodium chloride solution to prevent hyponatremia.

Hypernatremia must be corrected slowly, over about 2 days, to avoid shifting water into brain cells, resulting in cerebral edema. Some clinicians recommend infusion of a hypotonic solution, such as 0.3% sodium chloride, to permit a more gradual lowering of serum sodium levels, reducing the risk of cerebral edema.

Other treatment measures may include restricted sodium intake for patients with sodium gain. Diuretics may be given to increase sodium loss in combination with oral or I.V. water replacement.

Nursing diagnoses

For hyponatremia:
• Altered thought processes
• Fatigue
• Knowledge deficit
• Risk for injury
  For hypernatremia:
• Altered oral mucous membrane
• Altered thought processes
• Knowledge deficit
• Risk for injury

Nursing interventions

For hyponatremia:

• Watch for and report extremely low serum sodium and accompanying serum chloride levels. Monitor urine specific gravity and other laboratory results. Record fluid intake and output accurately, and weigh the patient daily.

• During administration of isosmolar or hyperosmolar sodium chloride solution, watch closely for signs of hypervolemia (dyspnea, crackles, engorged neck or hand veins), and report them immediately.

• Conserve the patient's energy through rest, planning, and setting priorities; avoid unnecessary fatigue.

For hypernatremia:

• Monitor serum sodium levels. Notify the doctor of rapid decreases in levels because rapid correction of hypernatremia may lead to cerebral edema. Increases in serum sodium levels should also be reported because they may signal the need for additional treatment.

• During fluid replacement therapy, observe for signs and symptoms of cerebral edema, particularly headache, lethargy, nausea, vomiting, widening pulse pressure, decreased pulse rate, and seizures.

• Record fluid intake and output accurately, checking for body fluid loss. Weigh the patient daily.

• Assist with oral hygiene. Lubricate the patient's lips frequently with a water-based lubricant. Provide mouthwash or gargle if the patient is alert.

• Obtain a drug history to check for drugs that promote sodium retention.

For hyponatremia or hypernatremia:

• Perform frequent neurologic checks. Report deteriorating level of consciousness. Provide a safe environment for the patient with altered thought processes. If seizures are likely, pad the patient's side rails, and keep an airway at the bedside. Reorient the patient, as needed.

Patient teaching

For patients with hyponatremia:

• Refer the patient on maintenance dosage of diuretics to a dietitian for instruction about dietary sodium intake.

• Teach the patient and family the rationale for fluid restriction, if prescribed. Inform the patient of ways to minimize thirst, including the use of ice chips, ice pops, or lemon drops.

• Make sure the patient understands his medication regimen, including the drug name, action, dosage, precautions, and potential adverse effects.

For patients with hypernatremia:

• If warranted, explain the importance of sodium restriction, and teach the patient how to plan a low-sodium diet. Refer the patient to a dietitian for additional teaching.

CALCIUM IMBALANCE

Calcium plays an indispensable role in cell permeability, the formation of bones and teeth, blood coagulation, transmission of nerve impulses, and normal muscle contraction. Nearly all of the body's calcium is found in the bones. The remaining exists in serum in three forms: ionized or free calcium (the only active, or available, calcium), calcium bound to protein, and calcium complexed with citrate or other organic ions.

The maintenance of ionized calcium in the serum is critical to healthy neurologic function. The parathyroid glands regulate ionized calcium and determine its resorption into bone, absorption from the GI mucosa, and excretion in urine and feces.

Causes

Hypocalcemia may result from:

• inadequate intake of calcium and vitamin D, in which inadequate levels of vitamin D inhibit intestinal absorption of calcium

• hypoparathyroidism as a result of injury, disease, or surgery that decreases or eliminates secretion of parathyroid hormone (PTH), which is necessary for calcium absorption and normal serum calcium levels

• malabsorption or loss of calcium from the GI tract, caused by increased intestinal motility from severe diarrhea or laxative abuse. Malabsorption of calcium from the GI tract can also result from inadequate levels of vitamin D or PTH, or a reduction in gastric acidity, decreasing the solubility of calcium salts.

• severe infections or burns, in which diseased and burned tissue traps calcium from the extracellular fluid

• alkalosis, in which calcium forms a complex with bicarbonate, causing decreased ionized calcium and inducing symptoms of hypocalcemia

• pancreatic insufficiency, which may cause malabsorption of calcium and subsequent calcium loss in feces. In acute pancreatitis, hypocalcemia varies in degree with the disorder's severity. The exact cause of hypocalcemia in this instance is unknown.

• renal failure, resulting in excessive excretion of calcium (can also occur with the use of loop diuretics)

• hypomagnesemia, which causes decreased PTH secretion and blocks the peripheral action of that hormone

• hyperphosphatemia, which causes calcium levels to decrease as phosphorus levels rise

• extensive administration of citrated blood, which may result in citrate binding with calcium.

   Hypercalcemia may result from:

• hyperparathyroidism, a primary cause, which increases serum calcium levels by promoting calcium absorption from the intestine, resorption from bone, and reabsorption from the kidneys

• hypervitaminosis D, which can promote increased absorption of calcium from the intestine

• certain cancers, such as multiple myeloma, lymphoma, squamous cell carcinoma of the lung, and breast cancer, which raise serum calcium levels by destroying bone or by releasing PTH or a PTH-like substance, osteoclast-activating factor, prostaglandins and, perhaps, a vitamin D–like sterol

• multiple fractures and prolonged immobilization, which release bone calcium and raise the serum calcium level.

   Other causes of hypercalcemia include milk-alkali syndrome, renal failure, sarcoidosis, hyperthyroidism, adrenal insufficiency, thiazide diuretics, and excessive administration of calcium during cardiopulmonary arrest.

Complications

Severe hypocalcemia can lead to laryngeal spasm, seizures and, possibly, respiratory arrest. Cardiac arrhythmias may also occur.

   In hypercalcemia, serum calcium levels greater than 13.5 mg/dl may cause coma and cardiac arrest. Hypercalcemia may also lead to renal calculi.

Assessment findings

The history of a patient with *hypocalcemia* may disclose risk factors, such as hypothyroidism or renal failure. The patient may report digital and perioral paresthesia and muscle cramps. Inspection may find twitching, carpopedal spasm, tetany, and seizures. Auscultation sometimes detects cardiac arrhythmias. Also, a physical examination may uncover reliable indicators of hypocalcemia, including hyperactive reflexes, a positive Trousseau's sign, and a positive Chvostek's sign.

   A patient with *hypercalcemia* may have a history of risk factors, such as excessive ingestion of vitamin D or prolonged immobilization. He may complain of lethargy, weakness, anorexia, constipation, nausea, vomiting, and polyuria. Family members may report personality changes.

   During assessment, the patient may appear confused or, in severe cases, comatose. Neuromuscular assessment may reveal muscle weakness, with hyporeflexia and decreased muscle tone.

Diagnostic tests

• *Total serum calcium levels* will be less than 8.5 mg/dl in hypocalcemia; greater than 10.5 mg/dl in hypercalcemia.

• *Ionized serum calcium levels* less than 4.5 mg/dl confirm hypocalcemia; levels greater than 5.3 mg/dl confirm hypercalcemia. (However, because about one-half of serum calcium is bound to albumin, changes in serum protein levels must be considered when interpreting serum calcium levels.)

• *Sulkowitch's urine test* shows increased calcium precipitation in hypercalcemia.

• *Electrocardiogram (ECG)* results are significant for lengthened QT interval, prolonged ST segment, and arrhythmias in hypocalcemia. In hypercalcemia, a shortened QT interval is seen. Ventricular arrhythmias may occur with severe hypercalcemia.

Treatment

The aim of treatment is to correct acute imbalance, followed by maintenance therapy and correction of the underlying cause.

   Mild hypocalcemia may require only a diet adjustment to allow adequate intake of calcium, vitamin D, and protein, possibly with oral calcium supplements.

   Acute hypocalcemia is an emergency that needs immediate correction by I.V. administration of calcium gluconate, which is usually preferable to calcium chloride. If the hypocalcemia is related to hypomagnesemia, magnesium replacement is necessary because the hypocalcemia often doesn't respond to calcium therapy alone.

   Chronic hypocalcemia also requires vitamin D supplements to facilitate GI calcium absorption. To correct mild deficiency, the amount of vitamin D found in most multivitamin preparations is adequate. For severe deficiency, vitamin D is used in four forms: ergocalciferol (vitamin D_2), cholecalciferol (vitamin D_3), calcitriol, and dihydrotachysterol, a synthetic form of vitamin D_2.

   Treatment of hypercalcemia that produces no symptoms may consist only of managing the underlying cause. Treatment of hypercalcemia that produces symptoms primarily eliminates excess serum calcium through hydration with 0.9% sodium chloride solution, which promotes calcium excretion in urine. Loop diuretics, such as ethacrynic acid and furosemide, also promote calcium excretion. (Thiazide diuretics are contraindicated in hypercalcemia because they inhibit calcium excretion.)

Corticosteroids, such as prednisone and hydrocortisone, are helpful in treating sarcoidosis, hypervitaminosis D, and certain tumors. Mithramycin can also lower serum calcium levels and is especially effective against hypercalcemia secondary to certain tumors. Calcitonin may also be helpful in certain instances. The administration of I.V. phosphates is potentially dangerous and is used only when other treatments prove ineffective.

Nursing diagnoses

For hypocalcemia:
• Decreased cardiac output
• Impaired gas exchange
• Knowledge deficit
• Risk for injury
  For hypercalcemia:
• Altered urinary elimination
• Decreased cardiac output
• Knowledge deficit
• Risk for injury

Nursing interventions

For hypocalcemia:
• Watch for the disorder in patients at risk, such as those receiving massive transfusions of citrated blood and in those with chronic diarrhea, severe infections, and insufficient dietary intake of calcium and protein (especially elderly patients).
• Monitor serum calcium levels every 12 to 24 hours and report any decrease.
• When giving calcium supplements, frequently check pH level because an alkalotic state that exceeds 7.45 pH inhibits calcium ionization.
• Check for Trousseau's and Chvostek's signs, and report positive signs to the doctor.
• Monitor ECG results for signs of worsening hypocalcemia.
• Using a volumetric infusion pump, administer calcium gluconate I.V. slowly, in dextrose 5% in water (*never* in 0.9% sodium chloride solution, which encourages renal calcium loss). Don't infuse more than 1 g/hour except in emergencies.
• Don't add calcium gluconate I.V. to solutions containing bicarbonate; it will precipitate. When administering calcium solutions, watch for anorexia, nausea, and vomiting — possible signs of overcorrection to hypercalcemia.
• If possible, monitor the patient for ECG changes. Notify the doctor if ventricular arrhythmias or heart block develops.
• Observe the I.V. site for signs of infiltration because calcium can cause tissue sloughing.

• If the patient is receiving calcium chloride, watch for abdominal discomfort.
• Monitor the patient closely for a possible drug interaction if he's receiving digitalis with large doses of oral calcium supplements; watch for signs and symptoms of digitalis toxicity (anorexia, nausea, vomiting, yellow vision, and cardiac arrhythmias). Administer oral calcium supplements 1 to 1½ hours after meals or with milk, if GI upset occurs.
• Provide a quiet, safe, stress-free environment for the patient. Observe seizure precautions for patients with severe hypocalcemia that may lead to seizures.
• Assess the patient's respiratory rate, depth, pattern, and rhythm. Be alert for stridor, dyspnea, or crowing. For the symptomatic patient, keep a tracheostomy tray and manual resuscitation bag at the bedside in case of laryngeal spasm.
  For hypercalcemia:
• Monitor serum calcium levels frequently. Report increasing levels.
• Increase fluid intake to dilute calcium in serum and urine and to prevent renal damage and dehydration.
• Watch for signs of congestive heart failure in patients receiving 0.9% sodium chloride solution diuresis therapy.
• Administer loop diuretics (not thiazide diuretics), as ordered. Monitor intake and output, and strain urine for renal calculi. Provide acid-ash drinks, such as cranberry juice, because calcium salts are more soluble in acid than in alkali.
• Check ECG results and vital signs frequently. Observe for arrhythmias if hypercalcemia is severe.
• If the patient is receiving digitalis, watch for signs of toxicity, such as anorexia, nausea, vomiting, and an irregular pulse.
• Ambulate the patient as soon as possible. Handle the patient with chronic hypercalcemia *gently* to prevent pathologic fractures. If the patient is bedridden, reposition him frequently, and encourage range-of-motion exercises to promote circulation and prevent urinary stasis and calcium loss from bone.
• Provide a safe environment. Keep the bed's side rails raised and the bed in the lowest position with the wheels locked.
• Frequently assess the patient's level of consciousness. Orient him, as needed.

Patient teaching

For patients with hypocalcemia:
• To prevent hypocalcemia, be sure to advise all patients — especially elderly patients — to eat foods rich in

calcium, vitamin D, and protein, such as fortified milk and cheese. Explain how important calcium is for normal bone formation and blood coagulation. Discourage chronic use of laxatives.
• If the patient requires oral calcium preparations or vitamin D supplements, make sure he understands his medication regimen.

For patients with hypercalcemia:
• To prevent recurrence of hypercalcemia, suggest a low-calcium diet with increased fluid intake.
• Review nonprescription medications that are high in calcium, and advise the patient to avoid these. Also caution him not to take megadoses of vitamin D.
• Stress the importance of increased fluid intake (up to 3 liters in nonrestricted patients) to minimize the possibility of renal calculi formation.

CHLORIDE IMBALANCE

Hypochloremia and hyperchloremia are chloride imbalances. A deficient serum level of the anion chloride results in hypochloremia; an excessive serum chloride level causes hyperchloremia. A predominantly extracellular anion, chloride accounts for two-thirds of all serum anions.

Secreted by the stomach mucosa as hydrochloric acid, chloride provides an acid medium conducive to digestion and activation of enzymes. It also participates in maintaining acid-base and body water balances, influences the osmolality or tonicity of extracellular fluid (ECF), plays a role in oxygen and carbon dioxide exchange in red blood cells, and helps activate salivary amylase (which, in turn, activates the digestive process).

Causes

Hypochloremia may result from:
• decreased chloride intake or absorption, as in low dietary sodium intake, sodium deficiency, potassium deficiency, metabolic alkalosis; prolonged use of mercurial diuretics; or administration of I.V. dextrose without electrolytes
• excessive chloride loss, resulting from prolonged diarrhea or diaphoresis; or loss of hydrochloric acid in gastric secretions due to vomiting, gastric suctioning, or gastric surgery.

Hyperchloremia may result from:
• excessive chloride intake or absorption—as in hyperingestion of ammonium chloride or ureterointestinal anastomosis—allowing reabsorption of chloride by the bowel
• hemoconcentration, caused by dehydration

• compensatory mechanisms for other metabolic abnormalities, as in metabolic acidosis, brain stem injury causing neurogenic hyperventilation, and hyperparathyroidism.

Complications

Hypochloremia may result in depressed respirations, leading to respiratory arrest. Hyperchloremia may cause coma.

Assessment findings

The patient's history may reveal risk factors for hypochloremia or hyperchloremia.

When hypochloremia is associated with hyponatremia, physical assessment may detect characteristic muscle weakness and twitching because renal chloride loss always accompanies sodium loss, and sodium reabsorption is not possible without chloride.

However, if chloride depletion results from metabolic alkalosis secondary to loss of gastric secretions, chloride is lost independently of sodium. Inspection may note tetany and shallow, depressed breathing. Neuromuscular assessment may find muscle hypertonicity.

Because of the natural affinity of sodium and chloride ions, hyperchloremia usually produces clinical effects associated with hypernatremia and resulting ECF volume excess. On inspection, you may note agitation, pitting edema, and dyspnea. Vital signs may reflect tachycardia and hypertension.

When hyperchloremia is associated with metabolic acidosis (due to base bicarbonate excretion by the kidneys), inspection may reveal deep, rapid breathing. Neurologic assessment may reveal weakness, diminished cognitive ability and, ultimately, coma.

Diagnostic tests

Serum chloride levels less than 95 mEq/liter confirm hypochloremia; supportive values with metabolic alkalosis include a serum pH over 7.45 and serum carbon dioxide levels greater than 32 mEq/liter.

Serum chloride levels over 106 mEq/liter confirm hyperchloremia; with metabolic acidosis, serum pH is under 7.35 and serum carbon dioxide levels are less than 22 mEq/liter.

Treatment

For *hypochloremia,* treatment aims to correct the condition that causes excessive chloride loss and to give an oral replacement, such as salty broth.

When oral therapy isn't possible or when emergency measures are necessary, treatment may include I.V. administration of 0.9% sodium chloride solution (if hypovolemia is present) or chloride-containing drugs, such as ammonium chloride, to increase serum chloride levels, and potassium chloride for metabolic alkalosis.

For *severe hyperchloremic acidosis,* treatment consists of sodium bicarbonate I.V. to raise serum bicarbonate levels and permit renal excretion of the chloride anion because bicarbonate and chloride compete for combination with sodium. For *mild hyperchloremia,* lactated Ringer's solution is administered; it converts to bicarbonate in the liver, thus increasing base bicarbonate to correct acidosis.

In either kind of chloride imbalance, treatment must correct the underlying disorder.

Nursing diagnoses

For hypochloremia:
• Ineffective breathing pattern
• Knowledge deficit
• Risk for injury
  For hyperchloremia:
• Altered thought processes
• Fluid volume excess
• Ineffective breathing pattern
• Risk for injury

Nursing interventions

For hypochloremia:
• Monitor serum chloride levels frequently, particularly during I.V. therapy.
• Watch for signs of hyperchloremia or hypochloremia. Be alert for respiratory difficulty.
• To prevent hypochloremia, monitor laboratory results (serum electrolyte levels and arterial blood gas values) and fluid intake and output of patients who are vulnerable to chloride imbalance, particularly those recovering from gastric surgery. Record and report excessive or continuous loss of gastric secretions. Also report prolonged infusion of dextrose in water without 0.9% sodium chloride solution.
• If the patient has muscle weakness, initiate measures to prevent injury. Assist the patient with ambulation. Keep personal articles within easy reach.
  For hyperchloremia:
• Check serum electrolyte levels every 3 to 6 hours. If the patient is receiving high doses of sodium bicarbonate, watch for signs of overcorrection (metabolic alkalosis, respiratory depression) or lingering signs of hyperchloremia, which indicate inadequate treatment.
• If the patient shows altered thought processes due to hyperchloremic acidosis, provide a safe environment,

and assess neurologic status frequently for signs of deterioration.
• If sodium excess is also present, assess for signs of fluid overload.
• Assess respiratory functioning. Rapid, deep respirations, a compensatory mechanism, may accompany hyperchloremic acidosis.
• To prevent hyperchloremia, check laboratory results for elevated serum chloride or potassium imbalance if the patient is receiving I.V. solutions containing sodium chloride, and monitor fluid intake and output. Also, watch for signs of metabolic acidosis. When administering I.V. fluids containing lactated Ringer's solution, monitor flow rate according to the patient's age, physical condition, and bicarbonate level. Report any irregularities promptly.

Patient teaching

• Explain all tests and procedures to the patient and his family.
• Discuss food sources of sodium, potassium, and chloride with the patient experiencing hypochloremia.

MAGNESIUM IMBALANCE

The second most abundant intracellular cation, magnesium functions chiefly to enhance neuromuscular integration. Changes in magnesium level affect neuromuscular irritability and contractility. Magnesium also stimulates parathyroid hormone (PTH) secretion, thus regulating intracellular fluid calcium levels.

Magnesium may also regulate skeletal muscle contraction through its influence on calcium utilization by depressing acetylcholine release at synaptic junctions. In addition, it activates many enzymes for proper carbohydrate and protein metabolism, aids in cell metabolism and the transport of sodium and potassium across cell membranes, and influences sodium, potassium, calcium, and protein levels.

Causes

Hypomagnesemia most commonly results from chronic alcoholism. The deficiency may also result from malabsorption syndromes, chronic diarrhea, prolonged nasogastric suction, or postoperative complications after bowel resection. It may follow decreased intake or administration of parenteral fluids without magnesium salts, enteral or total parenteral nutrition without adequate magnesium content, increased renal excretion associated with prolonged diuretic therapy, and cisplatin, amphotericin, tobramycin, or gentamicin therapy. It may also follow excessive loss of magnesium, as in severe dehydration and diabetic acidosis; hyperaldosteronism and hypoparathyroidism; hyperparathyroidism and hypercalcemia; and excessive release of adrenocortical hormones.

Hypermagnesemia usually results from the kidneys' inability to excrete magnesium that was either absorbed from the intestines or infused. Common causes of hypermagnesemia include chronic renal insufficiency; overuse of magnesium-containing antacids, especially with renal insufficiency (see *Drugs that contain magnesium*); severe dehydration; overdose with magnesium salts; and adrenal insufficiency.

Complications
Hypomagnesemia may result in transient hypoparathyroidism, interference with the peripheral action of PTH, seizures, and confusion deteriorating to coma. Serious cardiac arrhythmias may also occur. Hypermagnesemia may cause complete heart block and respiratory paralysis.

Assessment findings
Generally, a patient with hypomagnesemia exhibits neuromuscular irritability and cardiac arrhythmias. A patient with hypermagnesemia may exhibit central nervous system and respiratory depression in addition to neuromuscular and cardiac effects. (See *Recognizing magnesium imbalance,* page 988.)

Diagnostic tests
Serum magnesium levels determine imbalance. Values less than 1.5 mEq/liter or 1.8 mg/dl confirm hypomagnesemia; values more than 2.5 mEq/liter or 3.0 mg/dl indicate hypermagnesemia.

Low levels of other serum electrolytes (especially potassium and calcium) typically coexist with hypomagnesemia. In fact, unresponsiveness to correct treatment for hypokalemia strongly suggests hypomagnesemia. Similarly, elevated levels of other serum electrolytes are associated with hypermagnesemia.

Serum magnesium levels should be evaluated in combination with serum albumin levels because low albumin levels will decrease the total magnesium while leaving the amount of free ionized magnesium unchanged.

Treatment
Therapy aims to identify and correct the underlying cause. Therapy for mild hypomagnesemia consists of dietary replacement and possibly daily oral magnesium supplements. For severe hypomagnesemia, it includes I.V.

Warning

DRUGS THAT CONTAIN MAGNESIUM
To avoid hypermagnesemia, don't give magnesium-containing drugs to a patient with renal failure or poor renal functioning. Also, instruct the patient to avoid these nonprescription medications that contain magnesium.

Antacids
• Aludrox
• Camalox
• Di-Gel
• Gaviscon
• Gelusil and Gelusil-II
• Maalox and Maalox Plus
• Mylanta and Mylanta-II
• Riopan
• Simeco
• Tempo

Laxatives
• Magnesium citrate
• Magnesium hydroxide (Phillips' Milk of Magnesia, Haley's M-O)
• Magnesium sulfate (Epsom salts)

administration of magnesium sulfate (10 to 40 mEq/liter diluted in I.V. fluid). Magnesium intoxication is a possible adverse effect. Treatment requires calcium gluconate I.V.

Therapy for hypermagnesemia includes increased fluid intake and loop diuretics, such as furosemide, with impaired renal function; calcium gluconate (10%) I.V., a magnesium antagonist, for temporary relief of serious symptoms in an emergency, along with ventilatory support; and peritoneal dialysis or hemodialysis if renal function fails or if excess magnesium can't be eliminated.

Nursing diagnoses
For hypomagnesemia:
• Altered nutrition: Less than body requirements
• Impaired swallowing
• Knowledge deficit
• Risk for injury
  For hypermagnesemia:
• Altered nutrition: More than body requirements
• Altered renal tissue perfusion

RECOGNIZING MAGNESIUM IMBALANCE

Hypomagnesemia and hypermagnesemia may produce the following neuromuscular, central nervous system, cardiovascular, and GI effects.

Dysfunction	Hypomagnesemia	Hypermagnesemia
Neuromuscular	Hyperirritability, athetoid tetany, leg and foot cramps, Chvostek's sign (facial muscle spasms induced by tapping the branches of the facial nerve)	Diminished deep tendon reflexes, muscle weakness, flaccid paralysis, respiratory muscle paralysis with high magnesium levels
Central nervous system	Mood changes, confusion, delusions, hallucinations, seizures	Drowsiness, confusion, diminished sensorium; may progress to coma
Cardiovascular	Arrhythmias	Bradycardia, weak pulse, hypotension, diffuse vasodilation, heart block, cardiac arrest with high magnesium levels
Gastrointestinal	Anorexia, nausea, vomiting	Nausea, vomiting

- Impaired gas exchange
- Knowledge deficit

Nursing interventions

For hypomagnesemia:
- Watch for and report signs of hypomagnesemia in patients at risk.
- Monitor serum electrolyte levels (including magnesium, calcium, and potassium) daily for mild deficits and every 6 to 12 hours during replacement therapy. Assess for signs associated with low serum electrolyte levels.
- Assess for dysphagia by testing the patient's ability to swallow water before giving food or medications.
- With severe hypomagnesemia, initiate seizure precautions, and take other measures to ensure patient safety if confusion is present.
- Closely monitor patients receiving digitalis because hypomagnesemia predisposes to digitalis toxicity.
- Monitor for cardiac arrhythmias.
- Monitor vital signs during I.V. replacement therapy. Infuse magnesium replacement slowly, using an I.V. controller. Watch for bradycardia, heart block, and decreased respirations. Have calcium gluconate I.V. available to reverse hypermagnesemia from overcorrection.
- Refer the alcoholic patient to a support group.

For hypermagnesemia:
- Watch for signs of the disorder in predisposed patients.
- Frequently assess level of consciousness, muscle activity, and vital signs, noting hypotension and shallow respirations.
- Monitor serum magnesium levels. Respiratory paralysis may occur when serum magnesium levels are between 10 and 15 mEq/liter.
- Keep accurate intake and output records. Provide sufficient fluids for adequate hydration and maintenance of renal function.
- Report abnormal serum electrolyte levels immediately.
- Carefully monitor a patient who receives digitalis and calcium gluconate simultaneously; calcium excess enhances digitalis action, predisposing the patient to digitalis intoxication.

Patient teaching

For patients with hypomagnesemia:
- Advise the patient to eat foods high in magnesium, such as seed grains, nuts, and legumes. Inform him that fresh meat, fish, and fresh fruits usually contain small amounts of magnesium.
- Warn a patient receiving parenteral magnesium that he may experience flushing and warmth secondary to peripheral vasodilation.
- Advise the patient to avoid laxative or diuretic abuse; this practice may result in loss of magnesium.

For patients with hypermagnesemia:
- Advise a patient with renal failure to check with his doctor before taking any nonprescription medication.
- Caution the patient not to abuse laxatives and antacids containing magnesium, particularly if he's elderly or has compromised renal function.

PHOSPHORUS IMBALANCE

The primary intracellular anion, phosphorus is critical for normal cellular functioning. It's mainly found in inorganic combination with calcium in teeth and bones.

Phosphorus has a variety of important functions, such as formation of energy-storing substances (adenosine triphosphate [ATP]) and support to bones and teeth. It also plays a role in utilization of B vitamins, acid-base homeostasis, nerve and muscle activity, cell division, and metabolism of carbohydrates, proteins, and fats.

Renal tubular reabsorption of phosphate is inversely regulated by calcium levels — an increase in phosphorus causes a decrease in calcium. An imbalance causes hypophosphatemia or hyperphosphatemia.

The incidence of hypophosphatemia varies with the underlying cause. Hyperphosphatemia is most common in children, who tend to consume more phosphorus-rich foods and beverages than adults, and in children and adults with renal insufficiency.

Causes

Rarely, mild *hypophosphatemia* results from decreased dietary intake. When combined with overuse of phosphate-binding antacids, hypophosphatemia may become severe. Decreased absorption due to such conditions as vitamin D deficiency, malabsorption syndromes, or diarrhea may also cause this condition.

More commonly, hypophosphatemia stems from respiratory alkalosis. (Prolonged, intense hyperventilation can cause severe hypophosphatemia.) Also, increased urinary excretion associated with such conditions as hyperparathyroidism, aldosteronism, renal tubular defects, and administration of mineralocorticoids, glucocorticoids, or diuretics, may lead to hypophosphatemia.

Other important causes include the use of total parenteral nutrition with inadequate phosphate content, diabetic ketoacidosis, chronic alcoholism, and alcohol withdrawal, which may lead to severe hypophosphatemia.

Hyperphosphatemia most commonly results from renal failure with decreased renal phosphorus excretion. It also may stem from overuse of laxatives with phosphates or phosphate enemas, excessive administration of phosphate supplements, and vitamin D excess with increased GI absorption.

Hyperthyroidism may be associated with hyperphosphatemia. Conditions that result in cellular destruction, such as malignant tumors (especially when treated with chemotherapy), cause phosphorus to shift out of the cell and accumulate in extracellular fluid. Respiratory acidosis may also cause such a shift.

Complications

Possible complications of hypophosphatemia include heart failure, shock, and arrhythmias. Also, rhabdomyolysis (destruction of striated muscle), seizures, and coma may occur. Hypophosphatemia also may increase susceptibility to infection.

Hyperphosphatemia may result in soft-tissue calcifications and complications resulting from hypocalcemia.

Assessment findings

A patient with chronic hypophosphatemia may have a history of anorexia, memory loss, muscle and bone pain, and fractures. With acute hypophosphatemia, the patient may complain of chest pain, muscle pain, apprehension, and paresthesia.

On inspection, you may detect a tremor and weakness in the patient's speaking voice and hand grasp. Depending on the severity of hypophosphatemia, you may note confusion, seizures, and coma. You also may detect bruises and bleeding due to platelet dysfunction.

A patient with hyperphosphatemia usually remains asymptomatic unless his condition results in hypocalcemia; then his chief complaint may be tetany. The patient may describe tingling sensations in the fingertips and around the mouth. He also may complain of muscle cramps.

If the patient has soft-tissue calcifications, inspection may reveal oliguria, conjunctivitis, and papular eruptions. Auscultation may reveal an irregular heart rate.

Diagnostic tests

• *Serum phosphorus values* less than 1.7 mEq/liter or 2.5 mg/dl confirm hypophosphatemia; results that are more than 2.6 mEq/liter or 4.5 mg/dl confirm hyperphosphatemia.
• *Urine phosphorus values* above 1.3 g/24 hours support hypophosphatemia; values under 0.9 g/24 hours support hyperphosphatemia.
• *Serum calcium values* less than 9 mg/dl support the diagnosis of hyperphosphatemia.

Treatment

The goal of treatment is to correct the underlying cause of phosphorus imbalance. In the meantime, management of hypophosphatemia consists of phosphorus replacement, with a high phosphorus diet and oral administration of phosphate salt tablets or capsules. Severe hypophosphatemia requires I.V. infusion of potassium phosphate. I.V. supplements are also required when the GI tract can't be used to administer supplements.

Hyperphosphatemia is commonly treated with aluminum, magnesium, or calcium gels or antacids, which bind with phosphorus in the intestine and increase its elimination. Reduced phosphorus intake may be used in conjunction with these phosphorus-binding antacids. Severe hyperphosphatemia may require peritoneal dialysis or hemodialysis to lower the serum phosphorus level.

Nursing diagnoses

For hypophosphatemia:
• Impaired gas exchange
• Knowledge deficit
• Pain
• Risk for injury
    For hyperphosphatemia:
• Knowledge deficit
• Risk for injury

Nursing interventions

• Carefully monitor serum electrolyte, calcium, magnesium, and phosphorus levels. Report any changes immediately. Monitor patients at risk for phosphorus imbalance.
    For hypophosphatemia:
• Record the patient's fluid intake and output accurately.
• Administer I.V. potassium phosphate slowly to prevent overcorrection to hyperphosphatemia. Administer the infusion at a rate no greater than 10 mEq/hour. Observe for signs of infiltration; potassium phosphate can cause tissue sloughing and necrosis.
• Assess the patient's renal function, and be alert for signs of hypocalcemia, such as tetany, when giving phosphate supplements. If phosphate salt tablets cause nausea, use capsules instead.
• Observe safety precautions: Keep the patient's bed in its lowest position, with the wheels locked and all four side rails raised. If seizures are possible, pad the side rails and keep an artificial airway at the patient's bedside.
• Monitor the rate and depth of respirations. Report signs of hypoxia, such as confusion and cyanosis.
• Frequently assess the patient's level of consciousness and neurologic status. Orient the patient as needed.
• Administer medication for bone pain, as ordered. Assist the patient with ambulation and activities of daily living.
    For hyperphosphatemia:
• Monitor the patient's intake and output. If urine output falls below 25 ml/hour or 600 ml/day, notify the doctor immediately; decreased output can seriously affect renal clearance of excess serum phosphorus.

• Watch for signs of hypocalcemia, such as muscle twitching and tetany, which often accompany hyperphosphatemia.
• Obtain a dietary consultation if the condition results from chronic renal insufficiency.

Patient teaching
For patients with hypophosphatemia:
• To prevent recurrence, advise the patient to follow a high-phosphorus diet containing milk and milk products, kidney, liver, turkey, dried fruits, seeds, eggs, nuts, and whole grains.
• Provide verbal and written instructions for the patient taking prescribed oral phosphate supplements.
    For patients with hyperphosphatemia:
• Make sure the patient and family understand the medication regimen, including possible adverse effects and dosage of prescribed phosphate binders.
• Encourage the patient to avoid foods with high phosphorus content. Review foods with low phosphorus content, such as vegetables.
• Stress the importance of avoiding nonprescription preparations containing phosphorus or phosphate, such as laxatives and enemas.

SYNDROME OF INAPPROPRIATE ANTIDIURETIC HORMONE SECRETION

A potentially life-threatening condition, syndrome of inappropriate antidiuretic hormone (SIADH) secretion is marked by excessive release of antidiuretic hormone (ADH), which disturbs fluid and electrolyte balance. SIADH occurs secondary to diseases that affect the osmoreceptors (supraoptic nucleus) of the hypothalamus. The prognosis depends on the underlying disorder and the patient's response to treatment. (See *What happens in SIADH.*)

Causes
Usually, SIADH results from oat cell carcinoma of the lung, which secretes excessive ADH or vasopressor-like substances. Other neoplastic diseases (such as pancreatic and prostatic cancers, Hodgkin's disease, and thymoma) may also trigger SIADH. Additional causes include:
• central nervous system (CNS) disorders, including brain tumor or abscess, cerebrovascular accident, head injury, and Guillain-Barré syndrome
• pulmonary disorders (such as pneumonia, tuberculosis, lung abscess) and positive-pressure ventilation

• drugs (for example, chlorpropamide, tolbutamide, vincristine, cyclophosphamide, haloperidol, carbamazepine, clofibrate, morphine, and thiazides)
• miscellaneous conditions (such as myxedema or psychosis).

Complications
Without prompt treatment, SIADH may lead to water intoxication, cerebral edema, and severe hyponatremia, with resultant coma and death.

Assessment findings
The patient's medical and medication histories may provide a clue to the cause of SIADH. A history of cerebrovascular disease, cancer, pulmonary disease, or recent head injury is especially significant.

Most commonly, a patient with SIADH complains of anorexia, nausea, and vomiting. Despite these symptoms, the patient may report weight gain. The patient or family also may report CNS symptoms, such as lethargy, headaches, and emotional and behavioral changes.

Inspection usually fails to reveal edema because much of the free water excess is within cellular boundaries. Palpation may detect tachycardia associated with increased fluid volume. Neurologic assessment may detect disorientation, which may progress to seizures and coma. Examination findings may also include sluggish deep tendon reflexes and muscle weakness.

Diagnostic tests
• *Serum osmolality levels* less than 280 mOsm/kg of water and *serum sodium levels* less than 123 mEq/liter confirm SIADH.
• *Urine sodium levels* more than 20 mEq/liter without diuretics support the SIADH diagnosis.
• *Renal function tests* are normal with no evidence of dehydration in SIADH.

Treatment
Based primarily on the patient's symptoms, treatment for SIADH begins with restricted water intake (500 to 1,000 ml/day). Some patients who continue to have symptoms are given a high-salt, high-protein diet or urea supplements to enhance water excretion. Or they may receive demeclocycline or lithium to help block the renal response to ADH.

Rarely, with severe water intoxication, administration of 200 to 300 ml of 3% to 5% sodium chloride solution may be needed to raise the serum sodium level. A loop diuretic may also be prescribed to reduce the risk of heart failure after the excess fluid load and the admin-

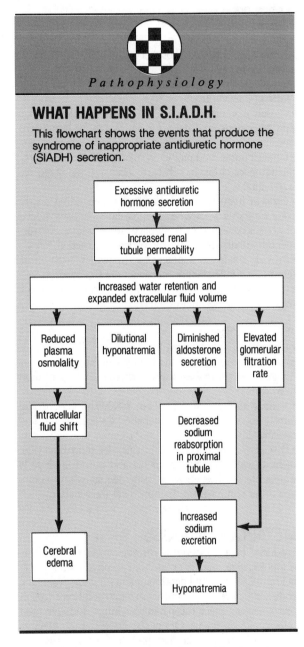

WHAT HAPPENS IN S.I.A.D.H.
This flowchart shows the events that produce the syndrome of inappropriate antidiuretic hormone (SIADH) secretion.

istration of the hypertonic sodium chloride solution. When possible, treatment should include correction of the underlying cause of SIADH. If SIADH is due to cancer, success in alleviating water retention may be obtained by surgery, irradiation, or chemotherapy.

Nursing diagnoses
• Altered thought processes
• Fluid volume excess
• Knowledge deficit
• Risk for injury

Nursing interventions
• Closely monitor and record the patient's intake and output, vital signs, and daily weight. Watch for hyponatremia.
• Restrict fluids, and provide comfort measures for thirst, including ice chips, mouth care, lozenges, and staggered water intake.
• Perform frequent neurologic checks, depending on the patient's status. Look for and report early changes in level of consciousness (LOC). Reduce unnecessary environmental stimuli and orient the patient, as needed.
• Provide a safe environment for the patient with an altered LOC. Take seizure precautions, as needed.
• Observe for signs and symptoms of heart failure, which may occur due to fluid overload.

Patient teaching
• If SIADH hasn't resolved by the time of discharge, explain to the patient and his family why he *must* restrict his fluid intake. Review ways to decrease his discomfort from thirst.
• If drug therapy is prescribed, teach the patient and family about the regimen, including dosage, action, and possible adverse effects.
• Discuss self-monitoring techniques for fluid retention, including measurement of intake and output and daily weight. Teach the patient to recognize signs and symptoms that require immediate medical intervention.

METABOLIC ACIDOSIS
Produced by an underlying disorder, metabolic acidosis is a physiologic state of excess acid accumulation and deficient base bicarbonate. Symptoms result from the body's attempts to correct the acidotic condition through compensatory mechanisms in the lungs, kidneys, and cells.

Metabolic acidosis is more prevalent among children, who are vulnerable to acid-base imbalance because their metabolic rates are faster and their ratios of water to total body weight are lower. Severe or untreated metabolic acidosis can be fatal.

Causes
Metabolic acidosis usually results from excessive burning of fats in the absence of usable carbohydrates. This can be caused by diabetic ketoacidosis, chronic alcoholism, malnutrition, or a low-carbohydrate, high-fat diet — all of which produce more keto acids than the metabolic process can handle. Other causes include:
• *anaerobic carbohydrate metabolism (lactic acidosis).* A decrease in tissue oxygenation or perfusion (as occurs with pump failure after myocardial infarction, or with pulmonary or hepatic disease, shock, or anemia) forces a shift from aerobic to anaerobic metabolism, causing a corresponding rise in lactic acid level.
• *renal insufficiency and failure (renal acidosis).* Underexcretion of metabolized acids or inability to conserve base bicarbonate results in excess acid accumulation or deficient base bicarbonate.
• *diarrhea and intestinal malabsorption.* Loss of sodium bicarbonate from the intestines causes the bicarbonate buffer system to shift to the acidic side.
• *massive rhabdomyolysis.* High quantities of organic acids added to the body with the breakdown of cells causes high anion gap acidosis.
• *poisoning and drug toxicity.* Common causative agents include salicylates, ethylene glycol, and methyl alcohol, which may produce acid-base imbalance.
• *hypoaldosteronism or use of potassium-sparing diuretics.* These conditions inhibit distal tubular secretion of acid and potassium.

Complications
If untreated, metabolic acidosis may lead to coma, arrhythmias, and cardiac arrest.

Assessment findings
The history of a patient with metabolic acidosis may point to the presence of risk factors, including associated disorders or the use of medications that contain alcohol or aspirin. Information about the patient's urine output, fluid intake, and dietary habits (including any recent fasting) may help to establish the underlying cause and severity of metabolic acidosis.

The patient's history (obtained from a family member, if necessary) also may reveal central nervous system (CNS) symptoms, such as changes in level of consciousness (LOC), ranging from lethargy, drowsiness, and confusion, to stupor and coma.

Inspection findings may include Kussmaul's respirations (as the lungs attempt to compensate by "blowing off" carbon dioxide). Underlying diabetes mellitus may cause a fruity breath odor from catabolism of fats and excretion of accumulated acetone through the lungs.

Palpation may reveal cold and clammy skin. As acidosis grows more severe, the skin feels warm and dry, indicating ensuing shock. Auscultation may detect hypotension and arrhythmias. Neuromuscular assessment may reveal diminished muscle tone and deep tendon reflexes.

Diagnostic tests

• *Arterial blood gas analysis* reveals a pH less than 7.35 to confirm metabolic acidosis, decreased partial pressure of carbon dioxide as part of the compensatory mechanism, and bicarbonate levels less than 24 mEq/liter in acute metabolic acidosis.
• *Urine pH* is 4.5 in the absence of renal disease.
• *Serum potassium levels* are usually elevated, as hydrogen ions move into the cells and potassium moves out of the cells to maintain electroneutrality.
• *Blood glucose levels* rise in diabetes.
• *Serum ketone body levels* increase in diabetes mellitus.
• *Plasma lactic acid levels* are elevated in lactic acidosis.
• *Anion gap values* more than 14 mEq/liter indicate metabolic acidosis. These values result from increased acid production or renal insufficiency. (See *Measuring the anion gap*.)

Treatment

For acute metabolic acidosis, treatment may include I.V. administration of sodium bicarbonate (when arterial pH is less than 7.2) to neutralize blood acidity. For chronic metabolic acidosis, oral bicarbonate may be given. Other treatment measures include careful evaluation and correction of electrolyte imbalances and, ultimately, correction of the underlying cause. For example, diabetic ketoacidosis requires insulin administration and fluid replacement.

Mechanical ventilation may be required to ensure adequate respiratory compensation.

Nursing diagnoses

• Altered oral mucous membrane
• Altered thought processes
• Ineffective breathing pattern
• Knowledge deficit
• Risk for injury

Nursing interventions

• Keep sodium bicarbonate ampules handy for emergency administration. Frequently monitor the patient's vital

MEASURING THE ANION GAP

The anion gap is the difference between serum cation (sodium) and serum anion (chloride and bicarbonate) concentrations. The gap is measured by determining the cation and the anion levels and then by subtracting the anion from the cation level. The process begins with normal concentration values: sodium, 140 mEq/liter; chloride, 104 mEq/liter; bicarbonate, 24 mEq/liter.

Thus, the anion gap between *measured* cations (actually sodium alone) and *measured* anions is about 12 mEq/liter (or 140 minus 128).

Concentrations of potassium, calcium, and magnesium (*unmeasured* cations), or proteins, phosphate, sulfate, and organic acids (*unmeasured* anions) are not needed to measure the anion gap. When added together, the concentration of unmeasured cations would be approximately 11 mEq/liter; of unmeasured anions, about 23 mEq/liter. Thus, the normal anion gap between unmeasured cations and anions is about 12 mEq/liter (23 minus 11) — plus or minus 2 mEq/liter for normal variation.

An anion gap over 14 mEq/liter indicates *metabolic acidosis*. It may result from the accumulation of excess organic acids (which are produced faster than they can be metabolized, as in ketoacidosis or lactic acidosis) or from renal insufficiency (because acids are not excreted sufficiently). In other types of metabolic acidosis (for example, GI or renal loss of bicarbonate), the anion gap may be normal.

signs, laboratory results, and LOC because changes can occur rapidly.
• Assess respiratory functioning. Position the patient to facilitate chest expansion; turn the stuporous patient frequently.
• In diabetic acidosis, watch for secondary changes due to hypovolemia, such as decreasing blood pressure.
• Record the patient's intake and output accurately to monitor renal function. Watch for signs of excessive serum potassium, including weakness, flaccid paralysis, and arrhythmias, possibly leading to cardiac arrest. After treatment, check for overcorrection to hypokalemia.
• Orient the patient frequently, as needed. Reduce unnecessary environmental stimuli. Ensure a safe environment for the patient who is confused. Keep the patient's bed in the lowest position with the side rails raised.
• Provide good oral hygiene. Use sodium bicarbonate washes to neutralize mouth acids, and lubricate the patient's lips with lemon and glycerin swabs.

Patient teaching

• To prevent diabetic ketoacidosis, teach the patient with diabetes how to routinely test blood glucose levels or, if otherwise prescribed, how to test urine for glucose and acetone. Encourage strict adherence to insulin or oral hypoglycemic therapy, and reinforce the need to follow the prescribed dietary therapy.

• As needed, teach the patient and family about prescribed medications, including their mechanism of action, dosage, and possible adverse effects. Provide verbal and written instructions.

METABOLIC ALKALOSIS

Always secondary to an underlying cause, metabolic alkalosis is a clinical state marked by decreased amounts of acid or increased amounts of base bicarbonate. It's usually associated with hypocalcemia and hypokalemia, which may account for signs and symptoms. With early diagnosis and prompt treatment, the prognosis is good. However, untreated metabolic alkalosis may be fatal.

Causes

Metabolic alkalosis results from the loss of acid or the increase of base.

Causes of acid loss include vomiting, nasogastric (NG) tube drainage or lavage without adequate electrolyte replacement, fistulas, and the use of steroids and certain diuretics (furosemide, thiazides, and ethacrynic acid). Hyperadrenocorticism is another cause of severe acid loss. Cushing's disease, primary hyperaldosteronism, and Bartter's syndrome, for example, all lead to the retention of sodium and chloride and urinary loss of potassium and hydrogen.

Excessive retention of base can result from excessive intake of bicarbonate of soda or other antacids (usually for treatment of gastritis or peptic ulcer), excessive intake of absorbable alkali (as in milk-alkali syndrome, often seen in patients with peptic ulcers), administration of excessive amounts of I.V. fluids with high concentrations of bicarbonate or lactate, massive blood transfusions, or respiratory insufficiency.

Complications

Untreated metabolic alkalosis may result in coma, atrioventricular arrhythmias, and death.

Assessment findings

The patient's history (obtained from a family member, if necessary) may disclose risk factors, such as excessive ingestion of alkali antacids. The history may include extracellular fluid (ECF) volume depletion, which is frequently associated with conditions leading to metabolic alkalosis (for example, vomiting or NG tube suctioning). The patient or a family member may report irritability, belligerence, and paresthesia.

Inspection may reveal the presence of tetany if serum calcium levels are borderline or low. The rate and depth of the patient's respirations may be decreased as a compensatory mechanism; however, this mechanism is limited because of the development of hypoxemia, which stimulates ventilation.

Assessment of the patient's level of consciousness may find apathy, confusion, seizures, stupor, or coma if alkalosis is severe. Neuromuscular assessment may discover hyperactive reflexes and muscle weakness if serum potassium is markedly low. Auscultation may detect cardiac arrhythmias occurring with hypokalemia.

Diagnostic tests

• *Arterial blood gas analysis* may reveal a blood pH over 7.45 and a bicarbonate level over 29 mEq/liter in metabolic alkalosis. A partial pressure of carbon dioxide over 45 mm Hg indicates attempts at respiratory compensation.

• *Serum electrolyte studies* usually show low potassium, calcium, and chloride levels in metabolic alkalosis.

• *Electrocardiogram (ECG)* findings disclose a low T wave merging with a P wave and atrial or sinus tachycardia.

Treatment

Correcting the underlying cause of metabolic alkalosis is the goal of treatment. Mild metabolic alkalosis generally requires no treatment. Rarely, therapy for severe alkalosis includes cautious I.V. administration of ammonium chloride to release hydrogen chloride and restore concentration of ECF and chloride levels. Potassium chloride and 0.9% sodium chloride solution (except with heart failure) are usually sufficient to replace losses from gastric drainage.

Electrolyte replacement with potassium chloride and discontinuing diuretics correct metabolic alkalosis resulting from potent diuretic therapy.

Oral or I.V. acetazolamide, which enhances renal bicarbonate excretion, may be prescribed to correct metabolic alkalosis without rapid volume expansion. Because acetazolamide also enhances potassium excretion, potassium administration before giving this drug may be necessary.

Nursing diagnoses
- Altered thought processes
- Decreased cardiac output
- Ineffective breathing pattern
- Knowledge deficit
- Risk for injury

Nursing interventions
- Structure the plan of care around cautious I.V. therapy, keen observation, and strict monitoring of the patient's status.
- Dilute potassium when giving the patient I.V. solutions containing potassium salts. Monitor the infusion rate to prevent damage to blood vessels; use an I.V. infusion pump. Watch for signs of phlebitis.

  When administering ammonium chloride 0.9% I.V., limit the infusion rate to 1 liter/4 hours; faster administration may cause hemolysis of red blood cells. Avoid overdosage, which may cause overcorrection to metabolic acidosis. Don't give ammonium chloride to a patient with signs of hepatic or renal disease.
- Monitor the patient's laboratory values, including pH, serum bicarbonate, serum potassium, and serum calcium. Notify the doctor if you detect significant changes or poor response to treatment.
- Monitor the ECG for arrhythmias.
- Watch closely for signs of muscle weakness, tetany, or decreased activity. Monitor the patient's vital signs frequently, and record intake and output to evaluate respiratory, fluid, and electrolyte status. Remember, respiratory rate usually decreases in an effort to compensate for alkalosis. Tachycardia may indicate electrolyte imbalance, especially hypokalemia.
- Observe seizure precautions, and provide a safe environment for the patient with altered thought processes. Assess level of consciousness frequently, and orient the patient, as needed.
- Irrigate the patient's NG tube with 0.9% sodium chloride solution instead of plain water to prevent loss of gastric electrolytes. Monitor I.V. fluid concentrations of bicarbonate or lactate.

Patient teaching
- To prevent metabolic alkalosis, warn patients against overusing alkaline agents.
- Teach patients with ulcers to recognize signs of milk-alkali syndrome, including a distaste for milk, anorexia, weakness, and lethargy.
- If potassium-wasting diuretics or potassium chloride supplements are prescribed, make sure the patient understands the medication regimen, including the purpose, dosage, and possible adverse effects.

SELECTED REFERENCES
"Gaucher's Disease Treatment Now Includes a Genetically Made Drug," *RN* 57(10):94, October 1994.

Ignatavicius, D.D., et al., eds. *Medical-Surgical Nursing: A Nursing Process Approach,* 2nd ed. Philadelphia: W.B. Saunders Co., 1995.

Illustrated Manual of Nursing Practice, 2nd ed. Springhouse, Pa.: Springhouse Corp., 1994.

Isselbacher, K., et al., eds. *Harrison's Principles of Internal Medicine,* 13th ed. New York: McGraw-Hill Book Co., 1995.

Lavery, G., et al. "Tonometry in Critical Illness," *Care of the Critically Ill* 11(1):23-27, January-February 1995.

Parker, C. "Responding Quickly to Hypoglycemia," *AJN* 94(6):46, June 1994.

Taylor, C.M., and Sparks, S.M. *Nursing Diagnosis Reference Manual,* 3rd ed. Springhouse, Pa.: Springhouse Corp., 1995.

Tierney, L., et al. *Current Medical Diagnosis and Treatment 1995.* East Norwalk, Conn.: Appleton & Lange, 1995.

Weissman, C., et al. "Metabolic Measurements in the Critically Ill," *Critical Care Clinics* 11(1):169-97, January 1995.

White, E. "Managing Hyperlipidemia," *Nursing94* 24(6):66-69, 1994.

14 ENDOCRINE DISORDERS

INTRODUCTION

The endocrine system consists of *glands,* specialized cell clusters, and *hormones,* chemical transmitters secreted by the glands in response to central nervous system (CNS) stimulation. Together with the CNS, the endocrine system regulates and integrates the body's metabolic activities and maintains internal homeostasis.

Hormonal regulation

The hypothalamus, the main integrative center for the endocrine and autonomic nervous systems, helps control some endocrine glands by neural and hormonal pathways. Neural pathways connect the hypothalamus to the posterior pituitary gland, or neurohypophysis. Neural stimulation of the posterior pituitary causes the secretion of two effector hormones: antidiuretic hormone (ADH [vasopressin]) and oxytocin.

The hypothalamus also exerts hormonal control at the anterior pituitary gland, or adenohypophysis, through releasing and inhibiting hormones and factors, which arrive by a portal system. Hypothalamic hormones stimulate the pituitary gland to release trophic hormones, such as corticotropin; thyroid-stimulating hormone (TSH); and gonadotropins, such as luteinizing hormone (LH) and follicle-stimulating hormone (FSH). Hypothalamic hormones also stimulate the pituitary gland to release or inhibit effector hormones, such as growth hormone (GH) and prolactin. Secretion of trophic hormones stimulates the adrenal cortex, thyroid gland, and gonads.

In a patient with a possible endocrine disorder, this complex hormonal sequence requires careful assessment to identify the dysfunction, which may result from defects in the gland; defects of releasing, trophic, or effector hormones; or defects of the target tissue. Hyperthyroidism, for example, may result from excessive thyrotropin-releasing hormone, TSH, or thyroid hormones.

Besides hormonal and neural controls, a negative feedback system regulates the endocrine system. (See *Feedback mechanism of the endocrine system,* page 998.) The feedback mechanism may be simple or complex. Simple feedback occurs when the level of one substance regulates secretion of a hormone. For example, a low serum calcium level stimulates parathyroid hormone (PTH) secretion from the parathyroid glands; a high serum calcium level inhibits PTH.

Complex feedback occurs through the hypothalamic-pituitary-target organ axis. For example, secretion of the hypothalamic corticotropin-releasing hormone (CRH) releases pituitary corticotropin, which, in turn, stimulates adrenal cortisol secretion. Subsequently, a rise in serum cortisol levels inhibits corticotropin by decreasing CRH secretion. Corticosteroid therapy disrupts the hypothalamic-pituitary-adrenal (HPA) axis by suppressing the hypothalamic-pituitary secretion mechanism. Because abrupt withdrawal of steroids doesn't allow time for recovery of the HPA axis to stimulate cortisol secretion, it can induce life-threatening adrenal crisis.

Hormonal effects

The *posterior pituitary* secretes oxytocin and ADH. Oxytocin stimulates contraction of the uterus and is responsible for the milk let-down reflex in lactating women. ADH controls the concentration of body fluids by altering the permeability of the distal convoluted tubules and collecting ducts of the kidneys to conserve water. ADH secretion depends on plasma osmolality as monitored by hypothalamic neurons. Hypovolemia and hypotension are the most powerful stimulators of ADH release. Other stimulators include pain, stress, trauma, nausea, morphine, tranquilizers, certain anesthetics, and positive-pressure breathing.

The *anterior pituitary* secretes prolactin, which stimulates milk secretion, and GH. GH affects most body tissues, triggering growth by increasing protein synthesis and fat mobilization and decreasing carbohydrate use.

The *thyroid gland* secretes the iodinated hormones thyroxine (T_4) and triiodothyronine (T_3). Thyroid hormones are necessary for normal growth and development and act on many tissues to increase metabolic activity and protein synthesis.

The *parathyroid glands* secrete PTH, which regulates calcium and phosphate metabolism. PTH elevates serum calcium levels by stimulating resorption of calcium and phosphate from bone, reabsorption of calcium and excretion of phosphate by the kidneys, and—by combined action with vitamin D—absorption of calcium and phosphate from the GI tract. Calcitonin, another hormone secreted by the thyroid gland, affects calcium metabolism, although its precise role in humans is unknown.

The *pancreas* produces glucagon from the alpha cells and insulin from the beta cells. Glucagon, the hormone of the fasting state, releases stored glucose from the liver to raise blood glucose levels. Insulin, the hormone of the postprandial state, facilitates glucose transport into the cells, promotes glucose storage, stimulates protein synthesis, and enhances free fatty acid uptake and storage.

The *adrenal cortex* secretes mineralocorticoids, glucocorticoids, and sex steroid hormones (androgens). Aldosterone, a mineralocorticoid, regulates the reabsorption of sodium and the excretion of potassium by the kidneys. Although affected by corticotropin, aldosterone

FEEDBACK MECHANISM OF THE ENDOCRINE SYSTEM

The hypothalamus receives regulatory information (feedback) from its own circulating hormones (simple loop) and also from target glands (complex loop).

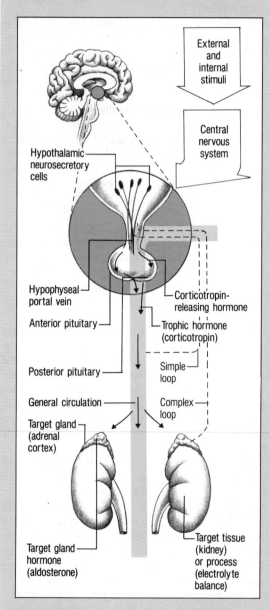

External and internal stimuli

Central nervous system

Hypothalamic neurosecretory cells

Hypophyseal portal vein

Anterior pituitary

Posterior pituitary

General circulation

Target gland (adrenal cortex)

Target gland hormone (aldosterone)

Corticotropin-releasing hormone

Trophic hormone (corticotropin)

Simple loop

Complex loop

Target tissue (kidney) or process (electrolyte balance)

is also regulated by angiotensin II, which is regulated by renin. Together, aldosterone, angiotensin II, and renin may be implicated in the pathogenesis of hypertension.

Cortisol, a glucocorticoid, stimulates gluconeogenesis, increases protein breakdown and free fatty acid mobilization, suppresses the immune response, and provides for an appropriate response to stress.

The *adrenal medulla* is an aggregate of nervous tissue that produces the catecholamines epinephrine and norepinephrine, both of which cause vasoconstriction. In addition, epinephrine causes the fight-or-flight response—dilation of bronchioles and increased blood pressure, blood glucose level, and heart rate.

The *testes* synthesize and secrete testosterone in response to gonadotropic hormones, especially LH, from the anterior pituitary gland; spermatogenesis occurs in response to FSH. The *ovaries* produce sex steroid hormones (primarily estrogen and progesterone) in response to anterior pituitary trophic hormones.

Endocrine disorders

The most common endocrine disorders include hypofunction (hormone deficiency), hyperfunction (hormone overproduction), inflammation, and tumor. The source of hypofunction and hyperfunction may be the hypothalamus, the pituitary effector glands, or the target gland. Inflammation may be acute or subacute, as in thyroiditis, but is usually chronic, often resulting in glandular hypofunction. Tumors can occur within the gland—as in thyroid carcinoma or pheochromocytoma (excessive catecholamines)—or in other areas, resulting in ectopic hormone production. Certain lung tumors, for example, secrete ADH or PTH.

Assessment

A thorough assessment can help to identify an endocrine disorder. The patient with such a disorder commonly reports fatigue, weakness, weight changes, mental status changes, polyuria, polydipsia, and abnormalities of sexual maturity and function. Careful questioning may identify insidious, vague symptoms that might otherwise go unreported. A thorough family history can uncover a familial tendency toward endocrine disorders.

Your physical examination should include a total body evaluation and complete neurologic assessment. Begin with the patient's vital signs, height, and weight. Compare these measurements with normal expected ones and the patient's baseline measurements, if available. Then, to obtain the most objective findings, inspect, palpate, and auscultate the patient.

Inspection

Systematically note the patient's overall appearance and mental and emotional status. Consider such factors as overall affect, speech, level of consciousness, orientation, appropriateness of behavior, grooming and dress, and activity level. Observe general body development, posture, body build, proportionality of body parts, and distribution of body fat and hair.

Assess overall skin color. Inspect the skin and mucous membranes for any lesions or areas of increased, decreased, or absent pigmentation. Assess the face for erythematous areas. Note facial expression, shape and symmetry of the eyes, and the presence of eyeball protrusion, incomplete lid closure, or periorbital edema. Inspect the tongue for color, size, lesions, tremor, and positioning. Stand in front of the patient and inspect the neck area for symmetry. Then check the neck while the patient holds it straight, slightly extends it, and then swallows water. Also remember to check for tracheal symmetry.

Evaluate the overall size, shape, and symmetry of the chest, noting any deformities, especially around the nipples. Inspect the external genitalia for normal development. Inspect the arms and legs for tremors, muscle development, symmetry, color, and hair distribution. Assess muscle strength. Examine the feet, noting size, deformities, lesions, marks from shoes and socks, maceration, dryness, or fissures.

Palpation

The thyroid gland and the testes are the only endocrine glands accessible to palpation. In many patients, the thyroid gland isn't palpable, but if it is, it should be smooth, finely lobulated, nontender, and either soft or firm. The gland's sections also should be palpable. The testes are palpable within the scrotal sac and are usually small, round, and firm.

Auscultation

Auscultate the thyroid gland to identify systolic bruits. These are caused by vibrations produced by accelerated blood flow through the thyroid arteries.

Diagnostic tests

Various diagnostic tests can suggest, confirm, or rule out an endocrine disorder. Endocrine function can be tested by direct, indirect, provocative, and radiographic studies.

Direct testing, the most common method of measuring endocrine function, involves measuring the hormone levels present in the blood or urine. Because the body contains only minute quantities of hormones, special techniques may be needed to obtain accurate measurements.

Common endocrine blood tests include:
• cortisol measurement to evaluate adrenocortical function
• catecholamine measurement to assess adrenal medulla function
• PTH measurement to evaluate parathyroid function
• GH radioimmunoassay to evaluate GH oversecretion
• T_4 radioimmunoassay to evaluate thyroid function and monitor iodine or antithyroid therapy
• T_3 radioimmunoassay to detect hyperthyroidism if T_4 levels are normal
• FSH and LH measurements to distinguish a primary gonadal problem from pituitary insufficiency.

Common endocrine urine studies include:
• 17-ketosteroids test to evaluate adrenocortical and gonadal function
• 17-hydroxycorticosteroids test to evaluate adrenal function
• free cortisol test
• 24-hour urine test.

Indirect testing measures the substance a particular hormone controls, not the hormone itself. Examples include these blood tests:
• oral glucose tolerance test to detect impaired glucose tolerance and hypoglycemia
• calcium measurement to detect bone and parathyroid disorders
• phosphorus test to detect parathyroid disorders and renal failure
• glycosylated hemoglobin test to monitor the degree of glucose control in diabetes mellitus over 3 months.

Provocative testing helps determine an endocrine gland's reserve function when other tests show borderline hormone levels. However, it can't pinpoint the site of the abnormality. These tests work on the principle that an underactive gland will be stimulated and an overactive gland will be suppressed, depending on the patient's suspected disorder. Examples include:
• insulin-induced hypoglycemia test to detect hypopituitarism
• TSH test to detect primary hypothyroidism.

Radiographic studies used to evaluate the endocrine system include X-rays, computed tomography scans, magnetic resonance imaging, and nuclear imaging.

PITUITARY DISORDERS

Two disorders of the pituitary gland—hypopituitarism and hyperpituitarism—cause abnormal growth. A third pituitary disorder—diabetes insipidus—causes excessive urine output. They're discussed in the following section.

HYPOPITUITARISM

A complex syndrome marked by metabolic dysfunction, sexual immaturity, and growth retardation (when it occurs in childhood), hypopituitarism results from a deficiency of the hormones secreted by the anterior pituitary gland. The disorder is also known as panhypopituitarism.

Panhypopituitarism refers to a generalized condition caused by partial or complete failure of the gland to produce all six of the vital hormones: corticotropin, thyroid-stimulating hormone (TSH), luteinizing hormone (LH), follicle-stimulating hormone (FSH), growth hormone (GH), and prolactin. Partial hypopituitarism and complete hypopituitarism occur in adults and children; in children, these diseases may cause dwarfism and pubertal delay.

Total loss of all hormones is fatal unless treated, but the prognosis is good with adequate replacement therapy and correction of the underlying causes.

Causes

The most common cause of primary hypopituitarism is a tumor. Other causes include congenital defects (hypoplasia or aplasia of the pituitary gland); pituitary infarction (most often from postpartum hemorrhage); partial or total hypophysectomy by surgery, irradiation, or chemical agents; and, rarely, granulomatous disease, such as tuberculosis. Occasionally, primary hypopituitarism has no identifiable cause.

Secondary hypopituitarism stems from a deficiency of releasing hormones produced by the hypothalamus. The process may be idiopathic or may result from infection, trauma, or tumor.

Complications

Any combination of deficits in the production of the six major hormones may occur. If the process is an evolving one (due to a hypothalamic destructive lesion), additional hormonal deficiencies may occur over time. Hypopituitarism can result in GH deficiency, TSH or corticotropin deficiency, and gonadotropin and prolactin

deficiency. Pituitary apoplexy is a medical emergency. (See *What happens in pituitary apoplexy.*) The patient's inability to cope with minor stressors can lead to a high fever, shock, coma, and death. In secondary hypopituitarism, damage to the posterior pituitary from infection, trauma, or tumor is occasionally extensive enough to cause diabetes insipidus.

Assessment findings

Physical findings depend on the specific pituitary hormones that are deficient, the patient's age, and the disorder's severity. Typically, clinical features develop slowly and don't become apparent until 75% of the pituitary gland is destroyed. Assessment findings related to specific hormonal deficiencies include the following:

• *GH deficiency.* Physical signs of GH deficiency may not be apparent in neonates. Growth retardation is usually apparent at age 6 months, although sometimes it may not be obvious until late childhood. In children, inspection reveals chubbiness from fat deposits in the lower trunk, short stature, delayed secondary tooth eruption, and delayed puberty. Growth continues at as little as half the normal rate—sometimes extending into the patient's twenties or thirties—to an average height of 4' (122 cm), with normal proportions.

Inspection of adults with GH deficiency finds more subtle signs, such as fine wrinkles near the mouth and eyes.

• *Gonadotropin (FSH and LH) deficiency.* In women, history discloses amenorrhea; dyspareunia, related to reduced vaginal secretions; infertility; and reduced libido. Inspection may discover breast atrophy, sparse or absent axillary and pubic hair, and dry skin. Men report weakness, impotence, and reduced libido. Inspection may show decreased muscle strength, testicular softening and shrinkage, and retarded secondary sexual hair growth.

• *TSH deficiency.* Patients may report cold intolerance, constipation, increased or decreased menstrual flow, and lethargy. Children will have severe growth retardation despite treatment. Inspection may find dry, pale, puffy skin and slow thought processes. Palpation may detect bradycardia.

• *Corticotropin deficiency.* Patient history discloses fatigue, nausea, vomiting, anorexia, and weight loss. During inspection you may note depigmentation of the skin and nipples. Vital signs during periods of stress may reflect hypothermia and hypotension.

• *Prolactin deficiency.* Patients commonly report absent postpartum lactation, amenorrhea, sparse or absent growth of pubic and axillary hair, and symptoms of thyroid and adrenocortical failure.

• *Panhypopituitarism.* All six pituitary hormones are at least partially deficient. This may result in a host of mental and physical abnormalities, including lethargy, psychosis, orthostatic hypotension, bradycardia, and anemia.

Diagnostic tests

In suspected hypopituitarism, evaluation must confirm hormonal deficiency caused by impairment or destruction of the anterior pituitary gland. It must also rule out disease of the target organs (adrenals, gonads, and thyroid gland) or the hypothalamus. Low serum levels of thyroxin, for example, indicate diminished thyroid gland function, but further tests are necessary to identify the source of this dysfunction as the thyroid, pituitary, or hypothalamus.

• Radioimmunoassay showing decreased plasma levels of some or all pituitary hormones (except corticotropin, which may require more sophisticated testing), accompanied by target-organ hypofunction, suggests pituitary failure and eliminates target gland disease. Failure of thyrotropin-releasing hormone administration to increase TSH or prolactin concentrations rules out hypothalamic dysfunction as the cause of hormonal deficiency.

• Gonadotropin-releasing hormone administered intravenously can distinguish between pituitary and hypothalamic causes of gonadotropin deficiency.

• Administering a dopamine antagonist, such as metoclopramide, evaluates prolactin secretory reserve. In patients with hypopituitarism, increased levels of prolactin indicate a lesion in the hypothalamus or pituitary stalk.

• Clomiphene, an estrogen antagonist, can also be used as a diagnostic agent.

• Diagnosis of dwarfism requires measurement of GH levels in the blood after administration of regular insulin to induce hypoglycemia, or of levodopa, which causes hypotension. These drugs should provoke increased GH secretion. Persistently low GH levels, despite provocative testing, confirm GH deficiency.

• Computed tomography scans, magnetic resonance imaging, or cerebral angiography confirms the presence of intrasellar or extrasellar tumors.

The following provocative tests are also used, but both require careful medical supervision because they may precipitate an adrenal crisis:

• Oral administration of metyrapone pinpoints the source of low hydroxycorticosteroid levels. The drug blocks cortisol synthesis, which should stimulate pituitary secretion of corticotropin.

• Insulin administration induces hypoglycemia and stimulates corticotropin secretion. Persistently low levels

WHAT HAPPENS IN PITUITARY APOPLEXY

Five to ten percent of patients with pituitary tumors develop pituitary apoplexy, a potentially life-threatening condition caused by hemorrhage into the tumor. Pituitary apoplexy usually occurs suddenly when rapid adenoma growth causes infarction or rupture of the tumor's thin-walled vessels. Patients with acromegaly, Cushing's disease, or large nonfunctioning tumors have a higher-than-average incidence of pituitary apoplexy.

Signs and symptoms
Assessment findings for pituitary apoplexy include:
• sudden, severe headache
• blurred vision
• diplopia
• blindness (from optic chiasma compression)
• eye deviation and pupil dilation (from oculomotor nerve paralysis)
• altered level of consciousness (possibly progressing to unconsciousness)
• nausea and vomiting
• hyperpyrexia
• nuchal rigidity.

Diagnosis and treatment
Diagnosis is based on the patient's history and test results, which may include leukocytosis, xanthochromic or frankly bloody cerebrospinal fluid (CSF), elevated CSF pressure and protein concentration, or suprasellar extension (as shown by a computed tomography scan).

Treatment is controversial, but it may involve corticosteroid administration. If visual deterioration continues, surgical evacuation of the hematoma may be performed to preserve vision.

of corticotropin indicate pituitary or hypothalamic failure.

Treatment

Replacement of hormones normally secreted by the target glands is the most effective treatment for hypopituitarism and panhypopituitarism. Hormonal replacement includes cortisol, the most important drug; thyroxine; and androgens or cyclic estrogen. Prolactin doesn't need replacement. The patient of reproductive age may benefit from FSH and human chorionic gonadotropin to boost fertility.

Somatrem, identical to GH but the product of recombinant DNA technology, has replaced growth hormones derived from human sources. It's effective for treating dwarfism, stimulating growth increases of 4″ to 6″ (10.2

to 15.2 cm) in the first year of treatment. The growth rate tapers off in subsequent years. However, after pubertal changes occur, the effects of GH therapy are limited.

Occasionally, a child becomes unresponsive to GH therapy, even with larger doses, perhaps because of antibody formation against the hormone. In such patients, small doses of androgen may again stimulate growth, but extreme caution is necessary to prevent premature closure of the epiphyses. Children with hypopituitarism may also need adrenal and thyroid hormone replacement and, as they approach puberty, sex hormones.

Nursing diagnoses
- Altered growth and development
- Altered nutrition: Less than body requirements
- Body image disturbance
- Hypothermia
- Ineffective individual coping
- Knowledge deficit
- Risk for infection
- Self-esteem disturbance
- Sensory or perceptual alterations (visual)
- Sexual dysfunction

Nursing interventions
- Until hormone replacement therapy is completed, monitor the results of all laboratory tests for hormonal deficiencies.
- Monitor patients with panhypopituitarism for anorexia. Determine food preferences and encourage the patient to maintain an adequate caloric intake. Offer frequent small meals and keep accurate records of weight loss or gain.
- Record vital signs every 4 to 8 hours, and monitor intake and output. Check eyelids, nail beds, and skin for pallor, which indicates anemia. Check neurologic status. Observe for signs of pituitary apoplexy, a medical emergency.
- Provide meticulous skin care, and use good handwashing technique to prevent infection. Combat skin dryness with alcohol-free skin care products and an emollient lotion after bathing.
- Keep the patient warm if his body temperature is low. Provide extra clothing and blankets, and adjust room temperature, if possible.
- During insulin testing, monitor closely for signs of hypoglycemia (initially, slow cerebration, tachycardia, and nervousness; later, seizures). Keep dextrose 50% in water available for I.V. administration to correct hypoglycemia rapidly.
- To prevent postural hypotension, keep the patient supine during levodopa testing.

- Institute safety precautions for patients with impaired visual acuity to decrease the risk of injury.
- Support the family in setting realistic goals for the child, based on his age and abilities.
- Provide strong emotional support for the patient who's coping with changes in body appearance and sexual functioning. Encourage verbalization of feelings, and discuss fear of rejection by others. Provide a positive, realistic assessment of the patient's situation. Encourage him to develop interests that support a positive self-image and de-emphasize appearance.
- Refer the family for psychological counseling or to appropriate community resources. Emotional stress increases as the child becomes older and more aware of his condition.

Patient teaching
- Teach the patient and his family about the limitations imposed by the disease. If the patient has dwarfism, explain that these children often look younger than their chronologic age and that they may grow in height more slowly than their peers.
- Review the treatment regimen with the patient and his family, especially long-term hormonal replacement therapy. Discuss the importance of taking the medication as ordered and of keeping regular follow-up appointments for blood studies.
- If the patient needs GH replacement, teach him and his family how to perform subcutaneous injections.
- Teach the patient and his family measures to conserve the patient's energy, manage stressful situations, and prevent infections. Stress the importance of adequate rest to avoid fatigue, a balanced diet with adequate calories and fluids, good personal hygiene and hand-washing technique, and avoidance of people with colds or other infections.
- Emphasize the importance of identifying and reporting emergency situations. If necessary, teach the family to administer steroids parenterally.

HYPERPITUITARISM
Also called acromegaly and gigantism, hyperpituitarism is a chronic, progressive disease marked by hormonal dysfunction and startling skeletal overgrowth. Although the prognosis depends on the causative factor, this disease usually reduces life expectancy.

Hyperpituitarism appears in two forms: acromegaly (rare) and gigantism. Acromegaly occurs after epiphyseal closure, causing bone thickening and transverse growth and visceromegaly. This form of hyperpituitarism occurs equally among men and women, usually between the ages of 30 and 50.

Gigantism begins before epiphyseal closure and causes proportional overgrowth of all body tissues. As the disease progresses, loss of other trophic hormones, such as thyroid-stimulating hormone, luteinizing hormone, follicle-stimulating hormone, and corticotropin, may cause dysfunction of the target organs.

Gigantism affects infants and children, causing them to grow to as much as three times the normal height for their age. As adults, they may eventually reach a height of more than 8' (243.8 cm).

Causes
In most patients, the source of excessive growth hormone (GH) secretion is a GH-producing adenoma of the anterior pituitary gland, usually macroadenoma (eosinophilic or mixed-cell). However, the etiology of the tumor itself is unclear. Occasionally, hyperpituitarism occurs in more than one family member, suggesting a genetic cause.

Complications
Prolonged effects of excessive GH secretion include arthritis, carpal tunnel syndrome, osteoporosis, kyphosis, hypertension, arteriosclerosis, heart enlargement, and congestive heart failure. Acromegaly may result in blindness and severe neurologic disturbances due to tumor compression of surrounding tissues. Both gigantism and acromegaly may also cause signs of glucose intolerance and clinically apparent diabetes mellitus, because of the insulin-antagonistic character of GH.

Assessment findings
The onset of acromegaly is gradual. The patient may report soft-tissue swelling and hypertrophy of the face and extremities at first. Then as the disease progresses, he may complain of diaphoresis, oily skin, fatigue, heat intolerance, weight gain, headaches, decreased vision, decreased libido, impotence, oligomenorrhea, infertility, joint pain (possibly from osteoarthritis), hypertrichosis, and sleep disturbances (related to obstructive sleep apnea).

Observation reveals an enlarged jaw, thickened tongue, enlarged and weakened hands, coarsened facial features, oily or leathery skin, and a prominent supraorbital ridge. You may also notice a deep, hollow-sounding voice, caused by laryngeal hypertrophy, and enlarged paranasal sinuses and tongue. Additional observations include irritability, hostility, and other psychological disturbances.

Inspection may reveal cartilaginous and connective tissue overgrowth, causing a characteristic hulking appearance and thickened ears and nose. Prognathism (projection of the jaw) becomes marked and may interfere with chewing. The fingers are thick, and the tips appear "tufted" or shaped like arrowheads on X-ray.

Gigantism develops abruptly, producing some of the same skeletal abnormalities seen in acromegaly. In infants, inspection reveals a highly arched palate, muscular hypotonia, slanting eyes, and exophthalmos. On palpation, patients commonly exhibit a characteristic moist, doughy, weak handshake.

Diagnostic tests
The following tests support a diagnosis of hyperpituitarism:
• *GH radioimmunoassay* shows increased plasma GH levels. However, because GH isn't secreted at a steady rate, a random sampling may be misleading. This test also shows increased levels of insulin-like growth factor I.
• *Glucose suppression test* offers more reliable information. Glucose normally suppresses GH secretion; therefore, a glucose infusion that fails to suppress the hormone level to below the accepted norm of 5 mg strongly suggests hyperpituitarism when combined with characteristic clinical features.
• *Skull X-ray, computed tomography scan,* or *magnetic resonance imaging* may help locate the pituitary tumor.
• *Bone X-rays* show a thickening of the cranium (especially of frontal, occipital, and parietal bones) and of the long bones as well as osteoarthritis in the spine.

Treatment
The aim of treatment is to curb overproduction of GH by removing the underlying tumor. Removal occurs by cranial or transsphenoidal hypophysectomy or pituitary radiation therapy. In acromegaly, surgery is mandatory when a tumor is compressing surrounding healthy tissue. Postoperative therapy commonly requires replacement of thyroid, cortisone, and gonadal hormones. Adjunctive treatment may include bromocriptine, which inhibits GH synthesis, and octreotide acetate, a long-acting analogue of somatostatin that suppresses GH secretion in at least two-thirds of patients with acromegaly.

Nursing diagnoses
• Activity intolerance
• Altered growth and development
• Altered oral mucous membrane
• Body image disturbance
• Impaired physical mobility

- Ineffective individual coping
- Knowledge deficit
- Pain
- Self-esteem disturbance
- Sensory or perceptual alterations (visual)
- Sexual dysfunction

Nursing interventions

- The grotesque body changes and sexual dysfunction that occur in this disorder can cause severe psychological stress. Provide emotional support to help the patient cope with an altered body image. Encourage him to verbalize his feelings, and discuss fear of rejection by others. Provide a positive, but realistic, assessment of his situation. Encourage him to develop other interests that support a positive self-image and de-emphasize appearance. Refer him and his family for counseling to help them deal with body image changes and sexual dysfunction.
- Be sensitive to any mood changes the patient may experience. Reassure him and his family that these changes result from hormonal imbalances caused by the disease and can be lessened with treatment.
- If the patient has skeletal manifestations, such as arthritis of the hands or osteoarthritis of the spine, administer analgesics and provide comfort measures. To preserve joint function, perform or assist with range-of-motion exercises. Apply heat or cold as ordered. Use pillows and splints to support painful extremities.
- Evaluate muscle weakness, especially in the patient with late-stage acromegaly, by checking the strength of his handclasp. If it's very weak, help with tasks such as cutting food. Also help him to walk, and take other safety precautions.
- Provide meticulous skin care. Keep the skin dry, and use oil-free skin cleansers and lotions.
- Monitor serum glucose levels. Observe for signs of hyperglycemia, such as sweating, fatigue, polyuria, and polydipsia.
- Remember that the tumor may cause visual problems. If the patient has hemianopia, stand where he can see you.

   After hypophysectomy:
- Monitor for signs of increased intracranial pressure (ICP) and intracranial bleeding (decreased level of consciousness, unequal pupils, decreased visual acuity, bradycardia, hypertension, and vomiting).
- Check blood glucose often. Remember, GH levels usually fall rapidly after surgery, removing an insulin-antagonist effect in many patients and possibly precipitating hypoglycemia.

- Measure intake and output hourly, and report large increases in urine output. Transient diabetes insipidus, which sometimes occurs after surgery for hyperpituitarism, can cause such increases.
- If the transsphenoidal approach is used, the patient will have nasal packing in place for several days. Keep an airway at the bedside. The patient must breathe through his mouth, so give good mouth care. Pay special attention to the mucous membranes—which usually become very dry—and the incision site under the upper lip, at the top of the gum line.
- In the transsphenoidal approach, the surgical site is packed with a piece of tissue generally taken from a mid-thigh donor site. Watch for cerebrospinal fluid leaks from the packed site and increased external nasal drainage or drainage into the nasopharynx. Additional surgery may be needed to repair the leak.
- Help the patient walk on the first or second day after surgery.

Patient teaching

- In your preoperative teaching, include an honest explanation of the procedure and its outcome, including what to expect during the recovery period. Stress the positive effects, which include limited postoperative problems and minimal pain.
- Instruct the patient to avoid vigorous coughing or sneezing in the immediate postoperative period—it can cause increased ICP.
- Teach the surgery patient to do deep breathing through his mouth because he'll have nasal packing in place.
- Before discharge, emphasize the importance of continuing hormone replacement therapy, if ordered. Make sure the patient and his family understand how and when to take the hormones, and warn against stopping them suddenly.
- If the patient is taking bromocriptine, explain that nausea, light-headedness, and postural hypotension are common at the beginning of therapy but will usually subside. Other adverse effects include constipation and nasal congestion.
- Advise the patient to wear a medical identification bracelet at all times and to bring his hormone replacement schedule with him whenever he returns to the hospital.
- Instruct the patient to have follow-up examinations at least once a year for the rest of his life because a slight chance exists that the tumor may recur.

DIABETES INSIPIDUS

A deficiency of vasopressin (also called antidiuretic hormone) causes this disorder of water metabolism characterized by excessive fluid intake and hypotonic polyuria. The disorder may start in childhood or early adulthood (median age of onset is 21) and is more common in men than in women. Incidence is slightly higher today than in the past.

In uncomplicated diabetes insipidus, with adequate water replacement, the prognosis is good, and patients usually lead normal lives. However, in cases complicated by an underlying disorder, such as cancer, the prognosis varies.

Causes and pathophysiology

The most common cause of diabetes insipidus is failure of vasopressin secretion in response to normal physiologic stimuli (pituitary or neurogenic diabetes insipidus). A less common cause is failure of the kidneys to respond to vasopressin (congenital nephrogenic diabetes insipidus).

Normally, vasopressin is synthesized in the hypothalamus and then stored by the posterior pituitary gland (neurohypophysis). Once released into the general circulation, vasopressin acts on the distal and collecting tubules of the kidneys, increasing their water permeability and causing water reabsorption. The absence of vasopressin in diabetes insipidus allows the filtered water to be excreted in the urine instead of being reabsorbed and results in the passage of large quantities of dilute fluid throughout the body.

Two types of pituitary diabetes insipidus exist: Primary pituitary diabetes insipidus (50% of patients) is familial or idiopathic in origin. The primary form may occur in neonates as a result of congenital malformation of the central nervous system (CNS), infection, trauma, or tumor.

Secondary pituitary diabetes insipidus results from intracranial neoplastic or metastatic lesions, hypophysectomy or other types of neurosurgery, a skull fracture, or head trauma—which damages the neurohypophyseal structures. The secondary form of this disease can also result from infection, granulomatous disease, and vascular lesions.

A transient form of diabetes insipidus also occurs during pregnancy, usually after the fifth or sixth month of gestation. The condition usually spontaneously reverses after delivery.

Complications

Untreated diabetes insipidus can produce hypovolemia, hyperosmolality, circulatory collapse, loss of consciousness, and CNS damage. These complications are most likely to occur if the patient has an impaired or absent thirst mechanism.

A prolonged urinary flow increase may produce chronic complications, such as bladder distention, enlarged calyceal, hydroureter, and hydronephrosis. Complications may result from underlying conditions, such as metastatic brain lesions, head trauma, and infections.

Assessment findings

The patient's history shows an abrupt onset of extreme polyuria (usually 4 to 16 liters/day of dilute urine, but sometimes as much as 30 liters/day), extreme thirst, and consumption of extraordinarily large volumes of fluid. The patient may report weight loss, dizziness, weakness, constipation, slight to moderate nocturia and, in severe cases, fatigue from inadequate rest caused by frequent voiding and excessive thirst. In children, reports of enuresis, sleep disturbances, irritability, anorexia, and decreased weight gain and linear growth are common.

On inspection, you may notice signs of dehydration, such as dry skin and mucous membranes, fever, and dyspnea. Urine is pale and voluminous. Palpation may reveal poor skin turgor, tachycardia, and decreased muscle strength. Hypotension may be present on blood pressure auscultation.

Diagnostic tests

To distinguish diabetes insipidus from other types of polyuria, the following tests may be ordered:
• *Urinalysis* reveals almost colorless urine of low osmolality (50 to 200 mOsm/kg of water, less than that of plasma) and of low specific gravity (less than 1.005).
• *Dehydration test* is a simple, reliable way to diagnose diabetes insipidus and differentiate vasopressin deficiency from other forms of polyuria. It compares urine osmolality after dehydration with urine osmolality after vasopressin administration. Fluids are withheld long enough to result in stable hourly urine osmolality values (an hourly increase of 30 mOsm/kg of water for at least 3 successive hours). After the third hour, the patient is given 5 units of aqueous vasopressin. Plasma osmolality is determined immediately before vasopressin administration, and urine osmolality is measured 30 and 60 minutes later. In diabetes insipidus, the rise in urine osmolality after vasopressin administration exceeds 9%. Patients with pituitary diabetes insipidus respond to exogenous vasopressin with decreased urine output and

increased urine specific gravity. Those patients who have nephrogenic diabetes insipidus show no response to vasopressin.

• *Plasma or urinary vasopressin evaluation* may be performed after fluid restriction or a hypertonic saline infusion.

If a patient is critically ill, diagnosis shouldn't wait for more time-consuming tests. A diagnosis may be based on the following laboratory values only:
• urine osmolality—200 mOsm/kg
• urine specific gravity—1.005
• serum osmolality—300 mOsm/kg
• serum sodium—147 mEq/liter.

Treatment
Until the cause of the patient's diabetes insipidus is identified and eliminated, administration of various forms of vasopressin or a vasopressin stimulant can control fluid balance and prevent dehydration:

• Aqueous vasopressin is a replacement agent administered by subcutaneous injection in doses of 5 to 10 units. It has a duration of action that ranges from 3 to 6 hours. This drug is used in the initial management of diabetes insipidus after head trauma or a neurosurgical procedure.

• Desmopressin acetate, a synthetic vasopressin analogue, affects prolonged antidiuretic activity and has no pressor effects. It's given intranasally in doses of 10 to 25 mcg or subcutaneously in doses of 1 to 2 mcg. (The dosage is halved for children.) The duration of action of desmopressin acetate is 12 to 24 hours, making it the drug of choice.

• Lypressin is a synthetic vasopressin replacement that's given as a short-acting nasal spray. This medication has significant disadvantages, including a variable absorption rate, nasal congestion and irritation, ulcerated nasal passages (with repeated use), substernal chest tightness, coughing, and dyspnea (after accidental inhalation of large doses).

Nursing diagnoses
• Altered growth and development
• Altered oral mucous membrane
• Altered urinary elimination
• Anxiety
• Energy field disturbance
• Fear
• Fluid volume deficit
• Hopelessness
• Ineffective family coping
• Ineffective individual coping
• Knowledge deficit
• Risk for altered parent-child attachment
• Sleep pattern disturbance

Nursing interventions
• Make sure that you keep accurate records of the patient's hourly fluid intake and urine output, vital signs, and daily weight.

• Closely monitor the patient's urine specific gravity. Also monitor his serum electrolyte and blood urea nitrogen levels.

• During dehydration testing, watch the patient for signs of hypovolemic shock. Monitor his blood pressure, pulse rate, and body weight. Also watch for changes in mental or neurologic status.

• If the patient has any complaints of dizziness or muscle weakness, institute safety precautions to help prevent injury.

• Make sure that the patient has easy access to the bathroom or bedpan.

• Provide meticulous skin and mouth care. Use a soft toothbrush and mild mouthwash to avoid trauma to the oral mucosa. If the patient has cracked or sore lips, apply petroleum jelly, as needed. Use alcohol-free skin care products, and apply emollient lotion to the patient's skin after baths.

• Use caution when administering vasopressin to a patient with coronary artery disease because the drug may cause coronary artery constriction. Closely monitor the patient's electrocardiogram, looking for changes and exacerbation of angina.

• Urge the patient to verbalize his feelings. Offer encouragement, and provide a realistic assessment of his situation.

• Help the the patient identify his strengths, and help him see how he can use these strengths to develop effective coping strategies.

• As necessary, refer the patient to a mental health professional for additional counseling.

• Advise the patient to wear a medical identification bracelet at all times. Tell him he should also always keep his medication with him.

Patient teaching
• Before the dehydration test: Tell the patient to take nothing by mouth until the test is over, and explain the need for hourly urine tests, vital sign and weight checks and, if necessary, blood tests. Explain the risks involved in the test, but reassure the patient that he'll be closely monitored.

• Instruct the patient and his family to identify and report signs of severe dehydration and impending hypovolemia.
• Tell the patient to record his weight daily, and teach him and his family how to monitor intake and output and how to use a hydrometer to measure urine specific gravity.
• Encourage the patient to maintain fluid intake during the day to prevent severe dehydration but to limit fluids in the evening to prevent nocturia.
• Inform the patient and his family about long-term hormone replacement therapy. Instruct them to take the medication as prescribed and to avoid abrupt discontinuation of the drug without the doctor's order. Teach them how to give subcutaneous or intramuscular injections and how to use nasal applicators. Discuss the drug's adverse effects and when to report them.
• Teach the parents of a child with diabetes insipidus about normal growth and development. Discuss how their child may differ. Encourage the parents to identify the child's strengths and use them to develop coping strategies. Refer the family for counseling, if necessary.

THYROID DISORDERS

Diseases of the thyroid include thyroid hormone deficiency and overproduction and gland inflammation and enlargement. With treatment, most of these disorders have a good prognosis; untreated, they progress to medical emergencies or irreversible disabilities.

HYPOTHYROIDISM IN ADULTS
In this disorder, metabolic processes slow down because of a deficiency of the thyroid hormones triiodothyronine (T_3) or thyroxine (T_4).

Hypothyroidism is classified as primary or secondary. Primary hypothyroidism stems from a disorder of the thyroid gland itself. Secondary hypothyroidism is caused by a failure to stimulate normal thyroid function or by a failure of target tissues to respond to normal blood levels of thyroid hormones. Either type may progress to myxedema, which is clinically much more severe and considered a medical emergency. (See *Managing myxedema coma,* page 1008.)

The disorder is most prevalent in women; in the United States, incidence is rising significantly in people ages 40 to 50.

Causes
Hypothyroidism results from a variety of abnormalities that lead to insufficient synthesis of thyroid hormones. Common causes of hypothyroidism include thyroid gland surgery (thyroidectomy), irradiation therapy inflammation, chronic autoimmune thyroiditis (Hashimoto's disease), or inflammatory conditions, such as amyloidosis and sarcoidosis.

The disorder may also result from pituitary failure to produce thyroid-stimulating hormone (TSH), hypothalamic failure to produce thyrotropin-releasing hormone, inborn errors of thyroid hormone synthesis, inability to synthesize thyroid hormones because of iodine deficiency (usually dietary), or the use of antithyroid medications, such as propylthiouracil.

Complications
Thyroid hormones affect almost every organ system in the body, so complications of hypothyroidism vary according to organs involved, as well as to the duration and severity of the condition.

Cardiovascular complications may include hypercholesterolemia with associated arteriosclerosis and ischemic heart disease. Poor peripheral circulation, heart enlargement, congestive heart failure, and pleural and pericardial effusions may also occur.

GI complications include achlorhydria, pernicious anemia, and adynamic colon, resulting in megacolon and intestinal obstruction.

Anemia due to the generalized suppression of erythropoietin may result in bleeding tendencies and iron deficiency anemia. Other complications include conductive or sensorineural deafness, psychiatric disturbances, carpal tunnel syndrome, benign intracranial hypertension, and impaired fertility.

Assessment findings
The patient history may reveal vague and varied symptoms that developed slowly over time. The patient may report energy loss, fatigue, forgetfulness, sensitivity to cold, unexplained weight gain, and constipation. As the disorder progresses, signs and symptoms may include anorexia, decreased libido, menorrhagia, paresthesia, joint stiffness, and muscle cramping.

Inspection reveals characteristic alterations in the patient's overall appearance and behavior. These changes include decreased mental stability (slight mental slowing to severe obtundation); and a thick, dry tongue, causing hoarseness and slow, slurred speech.

You'll probably note dry, flaky, inelastic skin; puffy face, hands, and feet; periorbital edema; and drooping

MANAGING MYXEDEMA COMA

A medical emergency, myxedema coma often has a fatal outcome. Progression is usually gradual, but when stress aggravates severe or prolonged hypothyroidism, coma may develop abruptly. Examples of severe stress are infection, exposure to cold, and trauma. Other precipitating factors include thyroid medication withdrawal and the use of sedatives, narcotics, or anesthetics.

Patients in myxedema coma have significantly depressed respirations, so their partial pressure of carbon dioxide in arterial blood may rise. Decreased cardiac output and worsening cerebral hypoxia may also occur. The patient is stuporous and hypothermic, and her vital signs reflect bradycardia and hypotension.

Lifesaving interventions

If your patient becomes comatose, begin these interventions as soon as possible:
• Maintain airway patency with ventilatory support if necessary.
• Maintain circulation through I.V. fluid replacement.

• Provide continuous electrocardiogram monitoring.
• Monitor arterial blood gas measurements to detect hypoxia and metabolic acidosis.
• Warm the patient by wrapping her in blankets. Don't use a warming blanket because it might increase peripheral vasodilation, causing shock.
• Monitor body temperature until stable with a low-reading thermometer.
• Replace thyroid hormone by administering large I.V. levothyroxine doses, as ordered. Monitor vital signs because rapid correction of hypothyroidism can cause adverse cardiac effects.
• Monitor intake and output and daily weight. With treatment, urine output should increase and body weight decrease; if not, report this to the doctor.
• Replace fluids and other substances, such as glucose. Monitor serum electrolyte levels.
• Administer corticosteroids, as ordered.
• Check for possible sources of infection, such as blood, sputum, or urine, which may have precipitated coma. Treat infections or any other underlying illness.

---

upper eyelids. Hair may be dry and sparse with patchy hair loss and loss of the outer third of the eyebrow. Nails may be thick and brittle with visible transverse and longitudinal grooves. You may also find ataxia, intention tremor, and nystagmus.

Palpation may detect rough, doughy skin that feels cool; a weak pulse and bradycardia; muscle weakness; sacral or peripheral edema; and delayed reflex relaxation time (especially in the Achilles tendon). The thyroid tissue itself may not be easily palpable unless a goiter is present.

Auscultation may show absent or decreased bowel sounds, hypotension, a gallop or distant heart sounds, and adventitious breath sounds. Percussion and palpation may detect abdominal distention or ascites.

Diagnostic tests

Hypothyroidism is confirmed when radioimmunoassay with radioactive iodine (^{131}I) shows low serum levels of thyroid hormones and when a thorough history and physical examination show characteristic signs and symptoms. A differential diagnosis requires additional tests and may reveal the following results:
• *Serum TSH levels* determine the primary or secondary nature of the disorder. An increased serum TSH level with hypothyroidism is due to thyroid insufficiency; a decreased TSH level is due to hypothalamic or pituitary insufficiency.
• *Serum antithyroid antibodies* are elevated in autoimmune thyroiditis.
• *Perchlorate discharge test* identifies disorders of iodine organification. It may provide insight into the operative mechanism of the particular thyroid disorder but is useful only when combined with other diagnostic tests.
• *Radioisotope scanning* of the thyroid tissue identifies ectopic thyroid tissue.
• *Skull X-ray, computed tomography scan,* and *magnetic resonance imaging* help locate pituitary or hypothalamic lesions that may be the underlying cause of hypothyroidism.

Treatment

In hypothyroidism, recommended treatment consists of gradual thyroid hormone replacement with synthetic hormone. Synthetic hormones include levothyroxine (T_4), liothyronine (T_3), dessicated thyroid USP, liotrix (T_3 and T_4), and thyroglobulin (T_3 and T_4). Treatment begins slowly, particularly in elderly patients, to avoid adverse cardiovascular effects; the dosage increases every 2 to 3 weeks until the desired response is obtained.

Rapid treatment may be necessary for patients with myxedema coma and those about to undergo emergency surgery (because of sensitivity to central nervous system depression). In these patients, both I.V. administration of levothyroxine and hydrocortisone therapy are warranted.

In underdeveloped areas, prophylactic iodine supplements have successfully decreased the incidence of iodine-deficient goiter.

Nursing diagnoses

- Altered cardiopulmonary tissue perfusion
- Altered nutrition: Potential for more than body requirements
- Altered thought processes
- Body image disturbance
- Chronic low self-esteem
- Colonic constipation
- Decreased cardiac output
- Fluid volume excess
- Ineffective individual coping
- Knowledge deficit
- Risk for altered body temperature
- Risk for impaired skin integrity
- Sensory or perceptual alterations (auditory)

Nursing interventions

- Routinely monitor and keep accurate records of the patient's vital signs, fluid intake, urine output, and daily weight.
- Monitor the patient's cardiovascular status. Auscultate heart and breath sounds, and watch closely for chest pain or dyspnea. Provide rest periods, and gradually increase activity to avoid fatigue and to decrease myocardial oxygen demand. Observe for dependent and sacral edema, apply antiembolism stockings, and elevate extremities to assist venous return.
- Encourage the patient to cough and breathe deeply to prevent pulmonary complications. Maintain fluid restrictions and a low-salt diet.
- Auscultate bowel sounds, check for abdominal distention, and monitor the frequency of bowel movements. Provide the patient with a high-bulk, low-calorie diet, and encourage activity to combat constipation and promote weight loss. Administer cathartics and stool softeners, as needed.
- Monitor mental and neurologic status. Observe the patient for disorientation, decreased level of consciousness, and hearing loss. If needed, reorient her to person, place, and time, and use alternative communication techniques if she has impaired hearing. Explain all procedures slowly and carefully, and avoid sedation, if possible. Provide a consistent environment to decrease confusion and frustration. Offer support and encouragement to the patient and her family.
- Provide meticulous skin care. Turn and reposition the patient every 2 hours if she's on extended bed rest. Use alcohol-free skin care products and an emollient lotion after bathing.
- Provide extra clothing and blankets for a patient with decreased cold tolerance. Dress the patient in layers, and adjust room temperature, if possible.
- During thyroid replacement therapy, watch for symptoms of hyperthyroidism, such as restlessness, sweating, and excessive weight loss.
- Encourage the patient to verbalize her feelings and fears about changes in body image and possible rejection by others. Help her identify her strengths and use them to develop coping strategies, and encourage her to develop interests that foster a positive self-image and de-emphasize appearance. Reassure the patient that her appearance will improve with thyroid replacement.

Patient teaching

- Help the patient and her family understand the patient's physical and mental changes. Teach them that hypothyroidism commonly causes mood changes and altered thought processes. Stress that these problems will probably subside with proper treatment. Urge the family to encourage and accept the patient and to help her adhere to her treatment regimen. If necessary, refer the patient and her family to a mental health professional for additional counseling.
- Instruct the patient and her family to identify and report the signs and symptoms of life-threatening myxedema. Stress the importance of obtaining prompt medical care for respiratory problems and chest pain.
- Teach the patient and family about long-term hormone replacement therapy. Emphasize that the patient needs lifelong administration if this medication is necessary, that she should take it exactly as prescribed, and that she should never abruptly discontinue it. Advise the patient always to wear a medical identification bracelet and to

carry her medication with her.

• Advise the patient and her family to keep accurate records of daily weight.

• Instruct the patient to eat a well-balanced diet that's high in fiber and fluids to prevent constipation, to restrict sodium to prevent fluid retention, and to limit calories to minimize weight gain.

• Tell the patient to schedule activities to avoid fatigue and to get adequate rest.

HYPOTHYROIDISM IN CHILDREN

A deficiency of thyroid hormone secretion during fetal development or early infancy results in congenital hypothyroidism, formerly called cretinism. Hypothyroidism occurs in about 1 in 5,000 neonates and is three times more common in girls than in boys.

Early diagnosis and treatment allow the best prognosis, and infants treated before age 3 months usually grow and develop normally. However, children with deficient thyroid activity who remain untreated beyond age 3 months and children with acquired hypothyroidism who remain untreated beyond age 2 suffer irreversible mental retardation.

Causes

In infants, hypothyroidism usually results from defective embryonic development that causes congenital absence or underdevelopment of the thyroid gland. The next most common cause is an inherited enzymatic defect in the synthesis of thyroxine (T_4), caused by an autosomal recessive gene. Less frequently, antithyroid drugs or a profound iodine deficiency during pregnancy may produce hypothroidism in infants. In children older than age 2, hypothyroidism usually results from chronic autoimmune thyroiditis.

Complications

Hypothyroidism that results from intrauterine iodine deficiency is associated with irreversible neurologic and intellectual deficiencies. If it isn't identified and treated in the first few months of life, it can cause severe mental retardation and skeletal malformations, such as dwarfism, epiphyseal degeneration, and bone and muscle dystrophy.

Children with untreated hypothyroidism may also suffer the same complications as in adult-onset hypothyroidism: life-threatening myxedema, respiratory compromise, cardiovascular dysfunction, anemias, megacolon, and intestinal obstruction.

Assessment findings

Clinical manifestations of hypothyroidism may not be visible at birth but are usually evident within the first 6 months. The parent may report feeding difficulties, constipation, somnolence, inactivity, respiratory problems, and an infrequent, hoarse cry.

Inspection of the infant with hypothyroidism may show a protruding abdomen; umbilical hernia; and slow, awkward movements. The skin is usually pale, mottled, dry, and flaky. The hair is coarse, dull, and brittle. Prolonged physiologic jaundice may also be visible. The tongue is large and protruding and may obstruct respiration, resulting in dyspnea and mouth breathing. Characteristic abnormal facial features may include a short forehead; puffy, wide-set eyes (periorbital edema); wrinkled eyelids; a broad, short, upturned nose; and a dull expression.

In the child over age 2, inspection may reveal delayed tooth eruption and early decay. Growth retardation is obvious, evidenced by short stature (due to delayed epiphyseal maturation, particularly in the legs), obesity, and a head that appears abnormally large because the arms and legs are stunted. An older child may show delayed or accelerated sexual development.

In both infants and children, palpation may detect hypotonic abdominal muscles, cold skin, a weak pulse, bradycardia, and diminished deep tendon reflexes. The thyroid tissue itself may not be palpable unless a goiter is present. Auscultation may reveal hypotension, absent or diminished bowel sounds, abnormal heart sounds, and adventitious breath sounds.

Diagnostic tests

• *Serum thyroid-stimulating hormone (TSH) level* is high and associated with low T_4 and triiodothyronine (T_3) levels in hypothyroidism. Because early detection and treatment can minimize the effects of hypothyroidism, many states require measurement of infant thyroid hormone levels at birth.

• *Thyroid scan (^{131}I uptake test)* shows decreased uptake levels and confirms the absence of thyroid tissue in children.

• *Gonadotropin levels* are increased and compatible with sexual precocity in older children. These findings may coexist with hypothyroidism.

• *X-rays* of the hip, knee, and thigh reveal the absence of the femoral or tibial epiphyseal line and delayed skeletal development that is markedly inappropriate for the child's chronologic age.

• *Skull X-ray, computed tomography scan,* and *magnetic resonance imaging* may identify a pituitary or hypothalamic lesion.
• *T₄ level,* if low and associated with a low TSH level, suggests hypothyroidism secondary to hypothalamic or pituitary disease, a rare condition.

Treatment
In infants under age 1, treatment consists of replacement therapy with oral levothyroxine, beginning with moderate doses. Dosage gradually increases to levels sufficient for lifelong maintenance. (Rapid increase may precipitate thyrotoxicity.) Doses are proportionately higher in children than in adults because children metabolize thyroid hormone more quickly.

Levothyroxine is also used to treat older children.

Nursing diagnoses
• Altered growth and development
• Altered nutrition: Less than body requirements
• Body image disturbance
• Colonic constipation
• Hypothermia
• Ineffective airway clearance
• Ineffective family coping: Compromised
• Knowledge deficit
• Self-esteem disturbance

Nursing interventions
• Keep accurate records of the infant's vital signs, weight, fluid intake, urine output, and respiratory and neurologic status.
• Monitor body temperature every 3 hours by the axillary or inguinal route. If indicated, place the infant in a warming unit. If she's in an open crib, avoid heat loss by keeping her warm with pajamas, blankets, and a stocking cap.
• Observe the infant's sucking, swallowing, gag, and cough reflexes. Have suction equipment nearby. Try different nipple types, such as a "preemie" nipple, or use a nipple shield to help prevent feeding difficulties. Place the infant in a lateral or prone position to prevent airway obstruction.
• Monitor the infant's bowel sounds and frequency of bowel movements.
• Provide meticulous skin care, using alcohol-free skin care products and emollient lotion after bathing. Turn and reposition the infant every 2 hours.
• Encourage parents to verbalize their feelings about the patient's condition. Encourage the older child to verbalize her feelings about altered body image and to discuss fear of rejection by others. Provide emotional support and a realistic assessment of the child's condition. Refer the family to community support groups and, if necessary, to a mental health professional for additional counseling.
• Encourage the child and her family to identify their strengths and use them to develop coping strategies. Assist the child to develop interests that foster a positive self-image and de-emphasize appearance. Involve the parents and child in decision making.

Patient teaching
• Inform parents that the child requires lifelong treatment with thyroid supplements. Teach them to identify and report signs of overdose: rapid pulse rate, irritability, insomnia, fever, sweating, and weight loss. Stress the need to comply with treatment to prevent further mental impairment. Reassure them that thyroid replacement, when started early, will reverse many of the effects of hypothyroidism.
• Advise the parents to have the child wear a medical identification bracelet.
• Tell parents to feed the child a high-fiber, low-calorie diet and to encourage physical activity to avoid excess weight gain and constipation.
• Teach parents about normal growth and development and their child's limitations. Advise them that she may be slower at achieving developmental milestones.
• To prevent infantile hypothyroidism, emphasize the importance of adequate nutrition during any future pregnancy, including iodine-rich foods and iodized salt. If the patient must restrict sodium, she should take an iodine supplement.

THYROIDITIS
Several disorders that involve inflammation of the thyroid gland are categorized as thyroiditis.

Hashimoto's thyroiditis (lymphadenoid goiter) is a common chronic inflammatory disease of the thyroid gland in which autoimmune factors play a prominent role. It occurs most often in middle-aged women and is the most common cause of sporadic goiter in children.

Subacute thyroiditis (granulomatous, giant cell, silent, or de Quervain's thyroiditis) is a transient inflammation of the thyroid gland.

Chronic thyroiditis with transient thyrotoxicosis (CTTT), also called silent or painless thyroiditis, is a self-limiting episode of thyrotoxicosis associated with chronic lymphocytic thyroiditis.

Pyogenic thyroiditis usually follows a pyogenic infection elsewhere in the body and is relatively uncommon.

Riedel's thyroiditis causes intense fibrosis of the thyroid and surrounding structures, leading to an induration of the tissues in the neck, and may be associated with mediastinal and retroperitoneal fibrosis. This rare disorder needs to be differentiated from thyroid neoplasm.

Causes

Each type of thyroiditis has a different etiology. Hashimoto's thyroiditis is thought to result from lymphocytic infiltration of the thyroid gland and formation of antibodies to thyroid antigens in the blood. Glandular atrophy and Graves' disease are linked to this type of thyroiditis.

Subacute thyroiditis is viral and may follow mumps, influenza, coxsackie virus, or adenovirus infections. CTTT's origin remains unclear, but current theories suggest that this variation may be caused by leakage of thyroid hormone from the gland.

Pyogenic thyroiditis stems from bacterial invasion of the thyroid gland. The most common causative microorganisms are *Staphylococcus aureus, Streptococcus hemolyticus,* and pneumococcus.

Riedel's thyroiditis is caused by fibrotic changes from an autoimmune or a subacute process.

Complications

Thyroiditis complications depend on the type of inflammation. In Hashimoto's thyroiditis, they include compression of the surrounding tissues by the goiter and malignant lymphomas of the thyroid gland (rare). Subacute thyroiditis may lead to a permanent hypothyroid or hyperthyroid condition. CTTT may cause recurrent episodes of thyrotoxicosis or several months of self-limiting hypothyroidism. In pyogenic thyroiditis, rupture of an abscess into the mediastinum, trachea, or esophagus may occur. Riedel's thyroiditis may cause hypothyroidism, tracheal or esophageal compression, necrosis of the compressed tissues, and hemorrhage.

Assessment findings

The patient's history may reveal a recent viral or bacterial infection, or a disorder such as systemic lupus erythematosus, rheumatoid arthritis, pernicious anemia, or Graves' disease. The patient may report the gradual onset of hypothyroid-like symptoms, such as sensitivity to cold, fatigue, and weight gain. Occasionally, symptoms of hyperthyroidism occur, such as heat intolerance, nervousness, and weight loss despite increased appetite. The patient may also complain of local pain or pain referred to the lower jaw, ear, or occiput; dysphagia; dyspnea; asthenia; and malaise.

On inspection, you may notice enlargement of the thyroid gland. In Hashimoto's thyroiditis, goiter is the outstanding clinical feature. The skin over the thyroid gland may be reddened, and in Riedel's thyroiditis, the neck tissues may be indurated.

Findings on palpation vary, depending on the type of thyroiditis. In Hashimoto's disease, the thyroid gland feels small, firm, and finely nodular, with a characteristic bandlike depression circling the gland and creating a butterfly shape. A small lymph node (Delphian node) found in the midline above the isthmus is palpable only in Hashimoto's thyroiditis or thyroid cancer. In the subacute form, palpation reveals pain over the thyroid and nodularity that may be unilateral but usually involves other areas of the gland. In CTTT, the thyroid is usually painless, nontender, symmetrical, and firm. You may palpate a slight to moderate enlargement. In the pyogenic form, swelling and warmth of the overlying skin suggest an infectious process. And in Riedel's thyroiditis, you'll palpate a woody, hard enlargement that feels "anchored" to surrounding structures.

Auscultation may reveal stridor due to compression of the thyroid gland on the trachea.

Diagnostic tests

Precise diagnosis depends on the type of thyroiditis:
• In Hashimoto's thyroiditis, thyroid failure is evidenced by a rise in thyroid-stimulating hormone (TSH), decreasing titers of triiodothyronine (T_3) and thyroxine (T_4), and high titers of antimicrosomal and antithyroglobulin antibodies. Histologic confirmation by fine-needle biopsy is usually performed.
• In subacute thyroiditis, thyroid hormone levels may be elevated, suppressed, or normal, depending on the phase of the disorder. Protein-bound iodine levels are elevated. During the thyrotoxic phase, TSH levels are low and fail to respond to thyrotropin-releasing hormone. TSH levels then rise in the hypothyroid phase, ^{131}I uptake is suppressed, and erythrocyte sedimentation rate (ESR), white blood cell (WBC) count, and hepatic enzyme levels also rise. Thyroid antibodies may appear transiently low in the serum. A thyroid scan may show isolated areas of function or total failure to visualize the gland.
• In CTTT, elevated T_3 and T_4, decreased ^{131}I uptake, low serum thyroid antibodies, and slightly elevated ESR are present.
• An elevated WBC count accompanying physical symptoms suggests pyogenic thyroiditis. A biopsy of the thyroid tissue for Gram stain, culture, microscopy, and

histologic examination may be performed. Radioisotope scanning and ultrasonography may be used to isolate the infected area. ^{131}I uptake and serum hormone levels are usually within normal limits.

• In Riedel's thyroiditis, ^{131}I uptake is normal or decreased. Some patients may have elevated titers of antimicrosomal antibodies, but not as high as in Hashimoto's thyroiditis.

Treatment

Appropriate treatment varies with the type of thyroiditis. Drug therapy includes levothyroxine for accompanying hypothyroidism, analgesics and anti-inflammatory drugs for mild subacute granulomatous thyroiditis, propranolol for transient hyperthyroidism, and steroids for severe episodes of acute illness. Suppurative thyroiditis requires antibiotic therapy. A partial thyroidectomy may be necessary to relieve tracheal or esophageal compression in Riedel's thyroiditis.

Nursing diagnoses

• Altered nutrition: Less than body requirements
• Body image disturbance
• Impaired swallowing
• Ineffective airway clearance
• Ineffective individual coping
• Knowledge deficit
• Pain

Nursing interventions

• Monitor the patient's respiratory status. Help him find a position that facilitates breathing, and tell him to avoid lying supine. Elevate the head of the bed 90 degrees during mealtimes and for 30 minutes afterward to decrease the risk of aspiration. Keep suction equipment available.
• Consult the dietitian to find nutritious foods that the patient can swallow easily. Be sure the patient consumes adequate calories.
• Provide frequent mouth care, and lubricate the patient's lips to prevent cracks and blisters. Provide meticulous skin care.
• Keep accurate records of vital signs, weight, fluid intake, and urine output. Measure the patient's neck circumference daily and record progressive enlargement.
• If the patient has a fever, provide comfort measures. Administer analgesics and antipyretics as ordered. Encourage the patient to drink plenty of fluids.
• Encourage the patient to verbalize his feelings and fears about body image changes and being rejected by others. Offer emotional support, and help him identify his

strengths for use in coping. Refer him to a mental health professional for additional counseling, if necessary.

After thyroidectomy:
• Monitor vital signs every 15 to 30 minutes until stable. Watch for signs of tetany secondary to accidental parathyroid injury during surgery. Keep 10% calcium gluconate available for I.V. use, if needed. Check dressings frequently for excessive bleeding. Watch for signs of airway obstruction, such as difficulty talking or increased swallowing, and keep tracheotomy equipment handy.

Patient teaching

• Teach the patient and his family to identify and report signs of respiratory distress, thyrotoxicity, hyperthyroidism, and hypothyroidism.
• Advise the patient that lifelong hormone replacement therapy is necessary after a thyroidectomy. Encourage him to wear a medical identification bracelet and to carry his medication with him at all times.

SIMPLE GOITER

Any enlargement of the thyroid gland not caused by inflammation or neoplasm is called a simple (or nontoxic) goiter. Simple goiter is classified as endemic or sporadic. Endemic goiter usually results from geographically related nutritional factors, such as iodine-depleted soil or iodine deficiency that accompanies malnutrition. Areas in the United States where this deficiency is most common are called "goiter belts" and include the Midwest, Northwest, and Great Lakes region. Sporadic goiter follows ingestion of certain drugs or foods.

Simple goiter is most common in females, especially during adolescence, pregnancy, and menopause, when the demand on the body for thyroid hormone increases. Sporadic goiter affects no particular population segment. With treatment, the patient can expect a good prognosis for either type of goiter.

Causes

Simple goiter occurs when the thyroid gland can't secrete enough thyroid hormone to meet metabolic requirements. As a result, the thyroid mass increases to compensate for inadequate hormone synthesis. Such compensation usually overcomes mild to moderate hormonal impairment. Because thyroid-stimulating hormone (TSH) levels are generally within normal limits in patients with simple goiter, goitrogenicity probably results from impaired intrathyroidal hormone synthesis and depletion of glandular iodine that increases the thyroid gland's sensitivity to TSH. However, increased levels of TSH may be transient and therefore missed.

Endemic goiter usually results from inadequate dietary intake of iodine, which leads to inadequate secretion of thyroid hormone. However, in Japan, goiter resulting from iodine excess has been found, stemming from chronic ingestion of seaweed.

Sporadic goiter commonly results from ingestion of large amounts of goitrogenic foods or use of goitrogenic drugs. Goitrogenic foods contain agents that decrease thyroxine (T_4) production. Such foods include rutabagas, cabbage, soybeans, peanuts, peaches, peas, strawberries, spinach, and radishes. Goitrogenic drugs include propylthiouracil, iodides, phenylbutazone, aminosalicylic acid, cobalt, and lithium.

Inherited defects may cause insufficient thyroxine synthesis or impaired iodine metabolism. Because families tend to congregate in one geographic area, this familial factor may contribute to endemic and sporadic goiters.

Complications

Production of excessive amounts of thyroid hormone in the goitrous state may lead to thyrotoxicosis. Complications from simple goiter are mainly mechanical, resulting from the compression and displacement of the trachea or esophagus. Superior mediastinal obstruction may occur with large retrosternal goiters. The development of thyroid cysts and hemorrhage into the cysts may add to the increasing pressure and compression of the surrounding tissues and structures. Large goiters may obstruct venous return, produce venous engorgement, and induce development of collateral circulation of the chest (rare).

Assessment findings

Diagnosis of simple goiter requires a thorough patient history and physical examination to rule out disorders with similar clinical effects, such as Graves' disease, Hashimoto's thyroiditis, and thyroid carcinomas.

The patient history may reveal ingestion of goitrogenic medications or foods, or endemic influence. The patient may complain of respiratory distress and dysphagia from compression of the trachea and esophagus, and dizziness or syncope (Pemberton's sign) when she raises her arms above her head.

Inspection shows enlargement of the thyroid gland in the anterior neck. Palpation reveals a single or multinodular, firm, irregular enlargement. Auscultation may reveal stridor caused by tracheal compression.

Diagnostic tests

• *Serum thyroid hormone levels* are usually normal. Abnormalities in triiodothyronine (T_3), T_4, and TSH levels rule out this diagnosis.
• *Thyroid antibody titers* are usually normal. Increases indicate chronic thyroiditis.
• *^{131}I uptake* is usually normal but may increase in the presence of iodine deficiency or a biosynthetic defect.
• *Urinalysis* may show low urinary excretion of iodine.
• *Radioisotope scanning* identifies thyroid neoplasms.

Treatment

The goal of treatment is to reduce thyroid hyperplasia. Exogenous thyroid hormone replacement with levothyroxine, dessicated thyroid, or liothyronine is the treatment of choice because it inhibits TSH secretion and allows the gland to rest. Small doses of iodide (Lugol's or potassium iodide solution) often relieve goiters that result from iodine deficiency. Sporadic goiter requires avoidance of known goitrogenic drugs or food. Radioiodine ablation therapy to the thyroid gland is used to destroy the autonomous foci. In rare cases of a large goiter unresponsive to treatment, a subtotal thyroidectomy may be performed to relieve pressure on surrounding structures.

Nursing diagnoses

• Altered nutrition: Less than body requirements
• Body image disturbance
• Impaired swallowing
• Ineffective airway clearance
• Ineffective individual coping
• Knowledge deficit

Nursing interventions

• Measure the patient's neck circumference daily to check for progressive thyroid gland enlargement. Check for the development of hard nodules in the gland, which may indicate cancer.
• Monitor respiratory status. Help the patient find a position that facilitates breathing, and tell her not to lie supine. Elevate the head of the bed 90 degrees during mealtimes and for 30 minutes afterward to decrease the risk of aspiration. Keep suction equipment available.
• Consult the dietitian for nutritious foods that are easy for the patient to swallow. Be sure the patient takes in adequate calories.
• Provide frequent mouth care, and lubricate the patient's lips to prevent cracks and blisters.
• Encourage the patient to verbalize feelings and fears about changes in body image and rejection by others.

OTHER FORMS OF HYPERTHYROIDISM

Besides Graves' disease, other forms of hyperthyroidism include toxic adenoma, thyrotoxicosis factitia, functioning metastatic thyroid carcinoma, TSH-secreting pituitary tumor, and subacute thyroiditis.

Toxic adenoma
A small, benign nodule in the thyroid gland, toxic adenoma secretes thyroid hormone and is the second most common cause of hyperthyroidism. The cause of toxic adenoma is unknown; its incidence is highest in elderly people.

Clinical effects are similar to those of Graves' disease except that toxic adenoma doesn't induce ophthalmopathy, pretibial myxedema, or acropachy. The presence of adenoma is confirmed by radioactive iodine (^{131}I) uptake and thyroid scan, which show a single hyperfunctioning nodule suppressing the rest of the gland.

Treatment includes ^{131}I therapy or surgery to remove the adenoma after antithyroid drugs achieve a euthyroid state.

Thyrotoxicosis factitia
This form of hyperthyroidism results from chronic ingestion of thyroid hormone for thyrotropin suppression in patients with thyroid carcinoma. It may also result from thyroid hormone abuse by persons trying to lose weight.

Functioning metastatic thyroid carcinoma
A rare disease, this carcinoma causes excess production of thyroid hormone.

TSH-secreting pituitary tumor
In this disorder, a TSH-secreting pituitary tumor causes overproduction of thyroid hormone.

Subacute thyroiditis
A virus-induced granulomatous inflammation of the thyroid, subacute thyroiditis produces transient hyperthyroidism associated with fever, pain, pharyngitis, and tenderness of the thyroid gland.

Offer emotional support. Help her identify her strengths and use them to develop coping strategies. Refer her to a mental health professional for counseling, as needed.
• If the patient takes goitrogenic drugs, monitor her for signs of sporadic goiter.

Patient teaching
• To maintain constant hormone levels, instruct the patient to take her prescribed thyroid hormone preparation at the same time each day. Teach her and her family to identify and report signs of thyrotoxicosis: increased pulse rate, palpitations, nausea, vomiting, diarrhea, sweating, tremor, agitation, and shortness of breath.
• Instruct the patient with endemic goiter to use iodized salt to supply the daily 150 to 300 mcg of iodine necessary to prevent goiter.
• Advise the patient who's at risk for simple goiter to avoid goitrogenic foods.
• Tell the patient to wear a medical identification bracelet and to carry her medication with her at all times.

HYPERTHYROIDISM
Thyroid hormone overproduction results in a metabolic imbalance in this disorder, which is also called thyrotoxicosis. Several types of hyperthyroidism exist. (See *Other forms of hyperthyroidism.*)

The most common form of hyperthyroidism is Graves' disease, which increases thyroxine (T_4) production, enlarges the thyroid gland (goiter), and causes multiple systemic changes. The incidence of Graves' disease is highest between ages 30 and 60, especially in people with family histories of thyroid abnormalities; only 5% of hyperthyroid patients are younger than age 15. With treatment, most patients can lead normal lives. However, thyrotoxic crisis or thyroid storm — an acute exacerbation of hyperthyroidism — is a medical emergency that may lead to life-threatening cardiac, hepatic, or renal failure. (See *What happens in thyrotoxic crisis,* page 1016.)

Causes
In Graves' disease, thyroid-stimulating antibodies bind to and then stimulate the thyroid-stimulating hormone (TSH) receptors of the thyroid gland. The trigger for this autoimmune disease is unclear, but in light of its various manifestations, it may not have one single cause. For example, many experts believe that Graves' disease is the result of genetic and immunologic factors. The disease's increased incidence among monozygotic twins points to an inherited factor, probably with a polygenic inheritance pattern. Graves' disease occasionally coexists with other autoimmune endocrine abnormalities, such as diabetes mellitus, thyroiditis, and hyperparathyroidism. It's also associated with the production of autoantibodies (long-acting thyroid stimulator [LATS], LATS-protector, and human thyroid adenyl cyclase stimulator), possibly caused

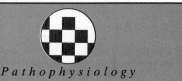

Pathophysiology

WHAT HAPPENS IN THYROTOXIC CRISIS

Also known as thyroid storm, thyrotoxic crisis is an acute manifestation of hyperthyroidism, usually occurring in patients with preexisting (though often unrecognized) thyrotoxicosis. Left untreated, it's invariably fatal.

Pathophysiology
The thyroid gland secretes the thyroid hormones triiodothyronine (T_3) and thyroxine (T_4). When it overproduces them in response to any of the precipitating factors listed below, systemic adrenergic activity increases. This results in epinephrine overproduction and severe hypermetabolism, leading rapidly to cardiac, GI, and sympathetic nervous system decompensation.

Assessment findings
Initially, the patient may have marked tachycardia, vomiting, and stupor. If left untreated, he may experience vascular collapse, hypotension, coma, and death. Other findings may include a combination of irritability and restlessness; visual disturbance, such as diplopia; tremor and weakness; angina; or shortness of breath, a cough, and swollen extremities. Palpation may disclose warm, moist flushed skin and a high fever (beginning insidiously and rising rapidly to a lethal level).

Precipitating factors
Onset is almost always abrupt, evoked by a stressful event, such as trauma, surgery, or infection. Other, less common, precipitators include:
• insulin-induced hypoglycemia or diabetic ketoacidosis
• cardiovascular accident
• myocardial infarction
• pulmonary embolism
• sudden discontinuation of antithyroid drug therapy
• initiation of radioiodine therapy
• preeclampsia
• subtotal thyroidectomy with accompanying excess intake of synthetic thyroid hormone.

by a defect in suppressor-T-lymphocyte function that allows the formation of these autoantibodies.

In a person with latent hyperthyroidism, excessive intake of iodine and, possibly, stress can precipitate clinical hyperthyroidism. Similarly, in a person with inadequately treated hyperthyroidism, stressful conditions, such as surgery, infection, toxemia of pregnancy, and diabetic ketoacidosis, can precipitate thyrotoxic crisis.

Complications
Thyroid hormones have widespread effects on almost all body tissues, so the complications of hypersecretion may be far-reaching and varied. Cardiovascular complications are most common in elderly people and include arrhythmias, especially atrial fibrillation; cardiac insufficiency; cardiac decompensation; and resistance to the usual therapeutic dose of digitalis. Additional complications include muscle weakness and atrophy; paralysis; osteoporosis; vitiligo and skin hyperpigmentation; corneal ulcers; myasthenia gravis; impaired fertility; decreased libido; and gynecomastia.

Assessment findings
The patient's history may disclose that the onset of symptoms followed a period of acute physical or emotional stress. A family history of Graves' disease is also common. The patient may report classic symptoms of nervousness, heat intolerance, weight loss despite increased appetite, excessive sweating, diarrhea, tremor, and palpitations. Symptoms suggesting nervous system involvement generally dominate in younger patients, whereas cardiovascular and myopathic symptoms are more common in older patients. The patient may also complain of difficulty concentrating; trouble climbing stairs; dyspnea on exertion and possibly at rest; anorexia; nausea and vomiting; and menstrual abnormalities.

On inspection, the patient typically appears anxious and restless. You may note fine tremors of the fingers and tongue, shaky handwriting, clumsiness, emotional instability, and mood swings (occasional outbursts to overt psychosis). The skin is flushed, and the hair is fine and soft. Premature graying and increased hair loss are common in both sexes. The nails appear fragile, and the distal nail may be separated from the nail bed (onycholysis).

Inspection also reveals pretibial myxedema over the dorsum of the legs or feet, which produces raised, thickened skin that may be itchy, hyperpigmented, and usually well demarcated from normal skin. Lesions typically look plaquelike or nodular. Generalized or localized muscle atrophy and acropachy (soft-tissue swelling with underlying bone changes where new bone formation occurs) are also visible.

Inspection of the eyes detects infrequent blinking, a characteristic stare, and lid lag, resulting from sympathetic overstimulation. Another characteristic finding is exophthalmos, which results from accumulated mucopolysaccharides and fluids in the retro-orbital tissues that force the eyeball outward. The conjunctiva and cornea may appear reddened. The patient may have an impaired upward gaze, convergence, and strabismus due to ocular muscle weakness (exophthalmic ophthalmoplegia).

On palpation, the thyroid gland may feel asymmetrical, lobular, and enlarged to three or four times its normal size. The liver may also feel enlarged. The skin is warm and moist with a velvety texture, and tachycardia with a full bounding pulse is palpable. Hyperreflexia is also present.

Auscultation of the heart may detect paroxysmal supraventricular tachycardia and atrial fibrillation (especially in elderly patients) and, occasionally, a systolic murmur at the left sternal border. Wide pulse pressures may be audible when taking blood pressure readings. Auscultation of the abdomen may detect increased bowel sounds. In Graves' disease, an audible bruit over the thyroid gland indicates thyrotoxicity, but occasionally, it may also be present in other disorders associated with a hyperplastic thyroid.

Diagnostic tests

The following laboratory test results confirm the diagnosis of hyperthyroidism:
• *Radioimmunoassay* shows increased serum triiodothyronine (T_3) and T_4 concentrations.
• *Thyroid scan* reveals increased uptake of radioactive iodine (^{131}I). (This test is contraindicated in pregnant patients.)
• *Thyrotropin-releasing hormone (TRH) stimulation test* helps confirm a diagnosis of hyperthyroidism if the TSH level fails to rise within 30 minutes after administration of TRH.

Other supportive test results show increased serum protein-bound iodine and decreased serum cholesterol and total lipid levels. Ultrasonography confirms subclinical ophthalmopathy.

Treatment

In hyperthyroidism, treatment consists of drugs, radioiodine, and surgery. Antithyroid drug therapy is used for children, young adults, pregnant women, and patients who refuse surgery or radioiodine treatment. Thyroid hormone antagonists include propylthiouracil (PTU) and methimazole, which block thyroid hormone synthesis.

Although hypermetabolic symptoms subside within 4 to 8 weeks after therapy begins, the patient must continue taking the medication for 6 months to 2 years. In many patients, concomitant propranolol is used to manage tachycardia and other peripheral effects of excessive sympathetic activity.

During pregnancy, antithyroid medication should be kept at the minimum dosage required to maintain normal maternal thyroid function and to minimize the risk of fetal hypothyroidism—even though most infants of hyperthyroid mothers are born with mild and transient hyperthyroidism. (Neonatal hyperthyroidism may even require treatment with antithyroid drugs and propranolol for 2 to 3 months.) Because exacerbation of hyperthyroidism sometimes occurs in the puerperium, continuous control of maternal thyroid function is essential. About 3 to 6 months postpartum, antithyroid drugs can be gradually decreased and thyroid function reassessed (drugs may be discontinued at that time). Mothers shouldn't breast-feed during treatment with antithyroid drugs because this may cause neonatal hypothyroidism.

Treatment with ^{131}I consists of a single oral dose and is the treatment of choice for women past reproductive age or men and women not planning to have children. (Patients of reproductive age must give informed consent for this treatment because small amounts of ^{131}I concentrate in the gonads.) During treatment, the thyroid gland picks up the radioactive element as it would regular iodine. Subsequently, the radioactivity destroys some of the cells that normally concentrate iodine and produce thyroxine, thus decreasing thyroid hormone production and normalizing thyroid size and function. In most patients, hypermetabolic symptoms diminish within 6 to 8 weeks after such treatment. However, some patients may require a second dose.

Subtotal (partial) thyroidectomy is indicated for the patient under age 40 who has a very large goiter and whose hyperthyroidism has repeatedly relapsed after drug therapy. This surgery removes part of the thyroid gland, decreasing its size and capacity for hormone production. Preoperatively, the patient may receive iodides (Lugol's or potassium iodide solution), antithyroid drugs, or high doses of propranolol to help prevent thyroid storm. If euthyroidism isn't achieved, surgery should be delayed and propranolol should be administered to decrease the risk of cardiac arrhythmias that are caused by hyperthyroidism.

Therapy for hyperthyroid ophthalmopathy includes local applications of topical medications but may require high doses of corticosteroids. A patient with severe exophthalmos that causes pressure on the optic nerve may require surgical decompression to lessen pressure on the orbital contents.

Treatment of thyrotoxic crisis includes administration of an antithyroid drug such as PTU, I.V. propranolol to block sympathetic effects, a corticosteroid to inhibit the conversion of triiodothyronine to thyroxine and to replace depleted cortisol, and an iodide to block release of the thyroid hormones. Supportive measures include nutrients, vitamins, fluid administration, and sedatives, as necessary.

Nursing diagnoses
• Altered nutrition: Less than body requirements
• Altered thought processes
• Body image disturbance
• Decreased cardiac output
• Diarrhea
• Ineffective individual coping
• Knowledge deficit
• Risk for altered body temperature
• Risk for fluid volume deficit

Nursing interventions
• Keep accurate records of vital signs, weight, fluid intake, and urine output. Measure neck circumference daily to check for progression of thyroid enlargement.
• Monitor serum electrolyte levels, and check for hyperglycemia and glycosuria. Monitor the patient's electrocardiogram for arrhythmias and ST-segment changes.
• Monitor for signs of heart failure, such as dyspnea, jugular vein distention, pulmonary crackles, and peripheral or sacral edema.
• Minimize physical and emotional stress. Try to balance rest and activity periods. Keep the patient's room cool and quiet and the lights dim. Encourage the patient to dress in loose-fitting, cotton clothing.
• Consult a dietitian to ensure a nutritious diet with adequate calories and fluids. Offer frequent, small meals.
• Monitor the frequency and characteristics of stools, and give antidiarrheal preparations, as ordered. Provide meticulous skin care to minimize skin breakdown.
• Reassure the patient and his family that mood swings and nervousness will probably subside with treatment. Encourage the patient to verbalize feelings about changes in body image. Help him identify and develop coping strategies. Offer emotional support. Refer him and his family to a mental health counselor, if necessary.
• If iodide is part of the treatment, mix it with milk, juice, or water to prevent GI distress, and give it through a straw to prevent tooth discoloration.

• Monitor the patient taking propranolol for signs of hypotension (dizziness and decreased urine output).
• If the patient is taking PTU or methimazole, monitor complete blood count results periodically to detect leukopenia, thrombocytopenia, and agranulocytosis.
• If the patient has exophthalmos or other ophthalmopathy, moisten the conjunctivae often with isotonic eyedrops.
• Avoid excessive palpation of the thyroid—this can precipitate thyroid storm.
  After thyroidectomy:
• Check often for respiratory distress, and keep a tracheotomy tray at the bedside.
• Check the dressings for spots of blood, which may indicate hemorrhage into the neck. Change dressings and perform wound care, as ordered. Also check the *back* of the dressing for drainage. Keep the patient in semi-Fowler's position, and support his head and neck with sandbags to ease tension on the incision.
• Check for dysphagia or hoarseness from possible laryngeal nerve injury.
• Watch for signs of hypocalcemia (tetany and numbness), a complication that results from accidental removal of the parathyroid glands during surgery.

Patient teaching
• Stress the importance of regular medical follow-up visits after discharge because hypothyroidism may develop 2 to 4 weeks postoperatively and after ^{131}I therapy. Advise the patient that he'll need lifelong thyroid hormone replacement. Encourage him to wear a medical identification bracelet and to carry his medication with him at all times.
• Tell the patient who's had ^{131}I therapy not to expectorate or cough freely because his saliva is radioactive for 24 hours. Stress the need for repeated measurement of serum thyroxine levels. Be sure he understands that he must not resume antithyroid drug therapy.
• Instruct the patient taking PTU or methimazole to take these drugs with meals to minimize GI distress and to avoid over-the-counter cough preparations because many contain iodine.
• Tell the patient taking propranolol to rise slowly after sitting or lying down to prevent a feeling of faintness.
• Instruct the patient taking antithyroid drugs or radioisotope therapy to identify and report symptoms of hypothyroidism.
• Advise the patient with exophthalmos or other ophthalmopathy to wear sunglasses or eyepatches to protect his eyes from light. If he has severe lid retraction, warn him to avoid sudden physical movements that might cause the

lid to slip behind the eyeball. Instruct him to report signs of decreased visual acuity.

PARATHYROID DISORDERS

The parathyroid glands regulate calcium balance, so undersecretion (hypoparathyroidism) or oversecretion (hyperparathyroidism) of parathyroid hormone can cause serious complications.

HYPOPARATHYROIDISM

A deficiency in parathyroid hormone (PTH) secretion by the parathyroid glands or the decreased action of PTH in the periphery causes hypoparathyroidism. Because the parathyroid glands primarily regulate calcium balance, hypoparathyroidism causes hypocalcemia, which produces neuromuscular symptoms ranging from paresthesia to tetany.

PTH normally maintains serum calcium levels by increasing bone resorption and by stimulating renal conversion of vitamin D to its active form, which enhances GI absorption of calcium. PTH also maintains the inverse relationship between serum calcium and phosphate levels by inhibiting phosphate reabsorption in the renal tubules. Abnormal PTH production in hypoparathyroidism disrupts this delicate balance.

Hypoparathyroidism may be acute or chronic and is classified as idiopathic, acquired, or reversible. The idiopathic and reversible forms are most common in children, and the clinical effects are usually correctable with replacement therapy. The acquired form, which is irreversible, is most common in older patients who've undergone thyroid gland surgery.

Causes

Idiopathic hypoparathyroidism may result from an autoimmune genetic disorder or the congenital absence of the parathyroid glands.

Acquired hypoparathyroidism typically results from accidental removal of or injury to one or more parathyroid glands during thyroidectomy or other neck surgery. It may also result from ischemic infarction of the parathyroids during surgery, hemochromatosis, sarcoidosis, amyloidosis, tuberculosis, neoplasms, trauma, or massive thyroid irradiation (rare).

Reversible hypoparathyroidism may result from hypomagnesemia-induced impairment of hormone secretion, from suppression of normal gland function due to hypercalcemia, or from delayed maturation of parathyroid function.

Complications

In hypoparathyroidism, complications are related to hypocalcemia. Decreased calcium levels can cause neuromuscular excitability and delayed cardiac repolarization, which may lead to heart failure. Lens calcification leads to cataract formation that may persist despite calcium replacement therapy. Papillary edema and increased intracranial pressure, irreversible calcification of basal ganglia, and bone deformities also occur. Laryngospasm, respiratory stridor, anoxia, paralysis of the vocal cords, seizures, and death may occur in severe cases of tetany. Hypoparathyroidism that develops during childhood results in malformed teeth.

Assessment findings

The patient's history may reveal neck surgery or irradiation or long-term hypomagnesemia from GI malabsorption or alcoholism.

The patient may report symptoms that reflect altered neuromuscular irritability. Acute (overt) tetany begins with a tingling in the fingertips, around the mouth and, occasionally, in the feet. The tingling spreads and becomes more severe, producing muscle tension and spasms. Pain varies with the degree of muscle tension but rarely affects the face, legs, and feet. The patient may also complain of his throat feeling constricted and of dysphagia. In chronic tetany, the patient may report difficulty in walking and a tendency to fall.

The patient may also complain of nausea, vomiting, abdominal pain, constipation or diarrhea, and personality changes, ranging from irritability and anxiety to depression, delirium, and frank psychosis.

On inspection, you may find dry skin, brittle hair, alopecia, transverse and longitudinal ridges in the fingernails, loss of eyelashes and fingernails, and stained, cracked, and decayed teeth from weakened enamel. During a tetany episode, you may observe that the hands, forearms and, less commonly, the feet may contort in a specific pattern, with thumb adduction followed by metacarpophalangeal joint flexion, interphalangeal joint extension, and wrist and elbow joint flexion.

Palpation may elicit Chvostek's and Trousseau's signs, which indicate latent tetany. (See *Eliciting signs of hypocalcemia,* page 1020.) Chvostek's sign may appear in other disorders, but only a hypocalcemic patient exhibits Trousseau's sign. You may also palpate increased deep tendon reflexes resulting from neuromuscular irritability.

ELICITING SIGNS OF HYPOCALCEMIA

When your patient complains of muscle spasms and paresthesia in his limbs, try eliciting Chvostek's and Trousseau's signs—indications of tetany associated with calcium deficiency.

Follow the procedures described below, keeping in mind the discomfort they typically cause. If you detect these signs, notify the doctor immediately. During these tests, watch the patient for laryngospasm, monitor his cardiac status, and have resuscitation equipment nearby.

Chvostek's sign

To elicit this sign, tap the patient's facial nerve just in front of the earlobe and below the zygomatic arch or between the zygomatic arch and the corner of the mouth, as shown below.

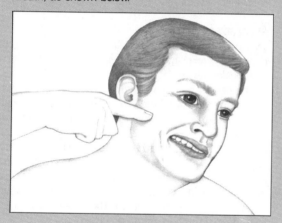

A positive response (indicating latent tetany) ranges from simple mouth-corner twitching to twitching of all facial muscles on the side tested. Simple twitching may be normal in some patients. However, a more pronounced response usually confirms Chvostek's sign.

Trousseau's sign

In this test, you occlude the brachial artery by inflating a blood pressure cuff on the patient's upper arm to a level between diastolic and systolic blood pressure. Maintain this inflation for 3 minutes while observing the patient for *carpal spasm* (shown below), which is Trousseau's sign.

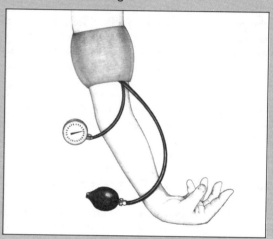

Auscultation of the apical pulse may detect cardiac arrhythmias.

Diagnostic tests

• *Radioimmunoassay* for parathyroid hormone shows diminished serum PTH concentration.
• *Blood and urine tests* reveal decreased serum and urine calcium levels, increased serum phosphate levels (more than 5.4 mg/dl), and reduced urine creatinine levels.
• *X-rays* indicate greater bone density and malformation.
• *Electrocardiogram (ECG) changes* disclose increased QT and ST intervals due to hypocalcemia.

Treatment

Because calcium absorption from the small intestine depends on the presence of activated vitamin D, treatment initially includes vitamin D, with or without supplemental calcium. Such therapy is usually lifelong, except in patients with reversible hypoparathyroidism. If the patient can't tolerate the pure form of vitamin D, alternatives include dihydrotachysterol if renal function is adequate, and calcitriol if renal function is severely compromised. However, these alternatives will only be effective if the patient has adequate PTH.

Acute, life-threatening tetany calls for immediate I.V. administration of 10% calcium gluconate, 10% calcium gluceptate, or 10% calcium chloride to raise ionized serum calcium levels. Sedatives and anticonvulsants may control muscle spasms until calcium levels rise. Chronic tetany calls for maintenance of serum calcium levels with oral calcium supplements.

Nursing diagnoses

• Altered thought processes
• Anxiety
• Body image disturbance

- Decreased cardiac output
- Impaired skin integrity
- Ineffective breathing pattern
- Ineffective individual coping
- Knowledge deficit

Nursing interventions
- Maintain a patent I.V. line. Keep emergency equipment available, including I.V. calcium gluconate and calcium chloride, an airway, a tracheotomy tray, and an endotracheal tube. If the patient receives I.V. calcium, assess the I.V. site for irritation. Maintain seizure precautions.
- Monitor serum calcium and phosphorus levels.
- Monitor the patient's ECG for increasing changes in QT intervals, heart block, and signs of decreasing cardiac output. Closely monitor the patient receiving both digitalis and calcium because calcium potentiates the effect of digitalis. Stay alert for signs of digitalis toxicity (arrhythmias, nausea, fatigue, and visual changes).
- Hyperventilation, which may stem from anxiety during a tetany episode, can worsen tetany. So can recent blood transfusions because anticoagulant in stored blood binds calcium. Keep the patient calm, and give a sedative, if prescribed. Help the patient with mild tetany rebreathe his own exhaled air by breathing into a paper bag.
- Provide meticulous skin care. Use alcohol-free skin care products and an emollient lotion after bathing.
- Institute safety precautions to minimize the risk of injury from falls. Provide support for walking.
- Encourage the patient to verbalize his feelings about body image changes and rejection by others. Offer emotional support, and help him identify his strengths and use them to develop coping strategies. Refer him to a mental health professional for additional counseling, if necessary.

Patient teaching
- Stress the importance of long-term management and follow-up care, especially periodic checks of serum calcium levels. (See *Living with hypoparathyroidism.*)
- Advise the patient that long-term replacement therapy will be necessary. Instruct him to take the medication as ordered and not to discontinue it abruptly.

HYPERPARATHYROIDISM
Characterized by overactivity of one or more of the four parathyroid glands, hyperparathyroidism results in excessive secretion of parathyroid hormone (PTH). Increased PTH levels act directly on the bone and kidney tubules, causing an increase of calcium in the extracel-

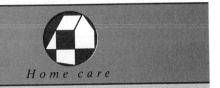

Home care

LIVING WITH HYPOPARATHYROIDISM
To help your patient learn to live with hypoparathyroidism, follow these guidelines:
- Tell the patient to take calcium supplements with or after meals and to chew the tablets well.
- Suggest that he wear a medical identification bracelet and carry his medication with him at all times.
- Teach the patient and his family to identify and report signs and symptoms of hypercalcemia, tetany, and respiratory distress.
- Teach the patient techniques for decreasing stress and avoiding fatigue.
- Advise the patient to follow a high-calcium, low-phosphorus diet. Discuss high-calcium foods, including dairy products, salmon, egg yolks, shrimp, and green, leafy vegetables. Caution him to avoid high-phosphate foods, such as spinach, rhubarb, and asparagus.

lular fluid that can't be compensated for by renal excretion or uptake into the soft tissues or skeleton.

Hyperparathyroidism is most common in women (especially those past menopause), with onset usually occurring between ages 35 and 65. The disorder is classified as primary or secondary, based on its etiology.

Causes
In primary hyperparathyroidism, one or more of the parathyroid glands enlarges, increasing PTH secretion and elevating serum calcium levels. The most common cause is a single adenoma. Other causes include a genetic disorder or multiple endocrine neoplasia.

In secondary hyperparathyroidism, excessive compensatory production of PTH stems from a hypocalcemia-producing abnormality outside the parathyroid gland, which causes a resistance to the metabolic action of PTH. Some hypocalcemia-producing abnormalities are vitamin D deficiency, chronic renal failure, or osteomalacia due to laxative abuse or phenytoin.

Complications
Untreated hyperparathyroidism damages the skeleton and kidneys from hypercalcemia. Bone and articular problems, such as chondrocalcinosis, osteoporosis, subper-

iosteal resorption, occasional severe osteopenia, erosions of the juxta-articular surface, subchondrial fractures, traumatic synovitis, and pseudogout, may occur. Renal complications include nephrolithiasis; hypercalciuria; renal calculi, colic, and insufficiency; and renal failure.

Other possible complications include peptic ulcers, cholelithiasis, cardiac arrhythmias, vascular damage, and heart failure. Severe hypercalcemia may cause parathyroid poisoning, which includes central nervous system (CNS) changes, renal failure, rapid precipitation of calcium throughout the soft tissues and, possibly, coma.

Assessment findings
The patient may report polyuria, chronic low back pain, bone tenderness, vague arm or leg pain, nausea, vomiting, anorexia, constipation, weight loss, lethargy, drowsiness, and personality changes, such as loss of initiative and memory. However, many patients are asymptomatic.

On inspection, you may note marked muscle weakness and atrophy, particularly in the legs, and joint hyperextensibility. With CNS involvement, alterations in level of consciousness, such as disorientation, stupor, and coma, may appear. Skeletal deformities of the long bones are visible. Palpation may detect hyporeflexia, and auscultation of blood pressure may reveal hypertension.

Diagnostic tests
• *Serum PTH, ionized calcium, and calcium phosphorus determinations* are the tests used most often to detect hyperparathyroidism.
• *Radioimmunoassay* confirms diagnosis by showing increased concentration of PTH, with accompanying hypercalcemia.
• *X-rays* reveal diffuse bone demineralization, bone cysts, subperiosteal resorption in long bones, and a "salt and pepper" appearance of the skull.
• *X-ray spectrophotometry* or other microscopic examinations of the bone demonstrate increased bone turnover.
• *Esophagography, thyroid scan, parathyroid thermography, ultrasonography, thyroid angiography, computed tomography scan,* and *magnetic resonance imaging* can help locate parathyroid lesions.
• *Supportive laboratory tests* reveal decreased serum phosphorus levels and elevated urine calcium and serum chloride, uric acid, creatinine, alkaline phosphatase, basal acid secretion, and serum immunoreactive gastrin levels.

In diagnosing secondary hyperparathyroidism, laboratory test findings show normal or slightly decreased serum calcium levels and variable serum phosphorus levels, especially when hyperparathyroidism is due to rickets, osteomalacia, or renal disease. Other laboratory values

and physical examination findings identify the cause of secondary hyperparathyroidism.

Treatment
Primary hyperparathyroidism may be treated by surgical removal of the adenoma or, depending on the extent of hyperplasia, removal of all but half of one gland (the remaining part is necessary to maintain normal PTH levels). Although surgery may relieve bone pain within 3 days, renal damage may be irreversible.

Preoperatively—or if surgery isn't feasible or necessary—other treatments can decrease calcium levels. Such treatments include forcing fluids; limiting dietary intake of calcium; promoting sodium and calcium excretion through forced diuresis using 0.9% sodium chloride solution (up to 6 liters in life-threatening circumstances), furosemide, or ethacrynic acid; and administering oral sodium or potassium phosphate, calcitonin, or plicamycin.

To prevent postoperative magnesium and phosphate deficiencies, the patient receives I.V. magnesium and phosphate or sodium phosphate solution given orally or by retention enema. In addition, during the first 4 or 5 days after surgery, when serum calcium falls to low-normal levels, supplemental calcium may be necessary; vitamin D or calcitriol may also be used to raise serum calcium levels.

Treatment of secondary hyperparathyroidism aims to correct the underlying cause of parathyroid hypertrophy and includes vitamin D therapy or, in the patient with renal disease, aluminum hydroxide for hyperphosphatemia. The patient with renal failure requires dialysis—possibly for the rest of her life—to lower calcium levels. In the patient with chronic secondary hyperparathyroidism, the enlarged glands may not revert to normal size and function even after calcium levels have been controlled.

Glucocorticoids are effective inhibitors of bone resorption and may be particularly useful in treating hypercalcemia associated with certain cancers.

Nursing diagnoses
• Activity intolerance
• Altered nutrition: Less than body requirements
• Altered thought processes
• Anxiety
• Body image disturbance
• Decreased cardiac output
• Fear
• Fluid volume excess
• Ineffective individual coping

- Knowledge deficit
- Pain

Nursing interventions

- Before treatment, obtain baseline serum potassium, calcium, phosphate, and magnesium levels because these values may change abruptly during treatment.
- Record intake and output during hydration to reduce serum calcium levels. Strain urine to check for renal calculi. Provide at least 3 liters of fluid a day, including cranberry or prune juice to increase urine acidity and help prevent calculus formation.
- Auscultate the lungs regularly, listening for signs of pulmonary edema in the patient receiving large amounts of 0.9% sodium chloride solution, especially if she has pulmonary or cardiac disease. Monitor the patient on digitalis for elevated serum calcium levels.
- Take safety precautions to minimize the risk of injury from a fall. Help the patient walk, keep the bed in the lowest position, and raise the side rails. Lift the immobilized patient carefully to minimize bone stress.
- Schedule care to allow the patient with muscle weakness as much rest as possible. Gradually increase activity according to her tolerance. Moderate weight-bearing activities are more beneficial than exercising in a bed or chair.
- Provide comfort measures to alleviate bone pain. Help the patient to turn, and reposition her every 2 hours. Support the affected extremities with pillows. Use extreme care when lifting the patient. Provide analgesics as ordered.
- Monitor for signs of peptic ulcer and administer antacids, as appropriate. Consult a dietitian to plan a diet with adequate calories.
- Encourage the patient to verbalize her feelings about body image changes and rejection by others. Offer emotional support, and help her to develop coping strategies. Refer her to a mental health professional for additional counseling, if necessary.

After parathyroidectomy:

- Monitor vital signs, respiratory status, and hourly urine output. Check for signs of increased neuromuscular irritability.
- Keep a tracheotomy tray and an endotracheal tube at the bedside. Maintain seizure precautions. Observe for postoperative complications, such as laryngeal nerve damage or hemorrhage.
- Check for swelling at the operative site. Place the patient in semi-Fowler's position, and support her head and neck with sandbags to decrease edema that may cause pressure on the trachea.
- Be alert for complaints of tingling in the hands and around the mouth. If these symptoms don't subside quickly, they may be prodromal signs of tetany, so keep I.V. calcium gluconate or calcium chloride available for emergency administration.
- Help the patient walk as soon as possible after surgery, even though she may find this uncomfortable. Pressure on bones speeds up bone recalcification.
- Check laboratory results for low serum calcium and magnesium levels.
- Monitor the patient's mental status and watch for listlessness. Check for muscle weakness and psychiatric symptoms in the patient with persistent hypercalcemia.

Patient teaching

- Before discharge, advise the patient of possible adverse reactions to drug therapy.
- Teach her and her family to identify and report signs of tetany, respiratory distress, and renal dysfunction.
- Emphasize the need for periodic blood tests.
- If the patient didn't have surgery to correct her hyperparathyroidism, warn her to avoid calcium-containing antacids and thiazide diuretics.
- Encourage the patient to wear a medical identification bracelet.

ADRENAL DISORDERS

The adrenal glands produce steroid hormones, epinephrine, and norepinephrine. Hyposecretion or hypersecretion of these substances results in a variety of serious disorders with complications ranging from psychiatric and sexual problems to coma and death.

ADRENAL HYPOFUNCTION

Also called adrenal insufficiency, this disorder has primary and secondary forms. Primary adrenal hypofunction (Addison's disease) originates within the adrenal gland itself and is characterized by decreased mineralocorticoid, glucocorticoid, and androgen secretion. A relatively uncommon disorder, Addison's disease occurs in people of all ages and both sexes.

Adrenal hypofunction can also occur secondary to a disorder outside the gland (such as pituitary tumor with corticotropin deficiency), but aldosterone secretion may continue intact. With early diagnosis and adequate replacement therapy, the prognosis for both primary and secondary adrenal hypofunction is good.

Adrenal crisis—also called addisonian crisis—is a critical deficiency of mineralocorticoids and glucocorticoids. A medical emergency, adrenal crisis requires immediate, vigorous treatment. (See *How adrenal crisis develops.*)

Causes

Addison's disease occurs when more than 90% of the adrenal gland is destroyed. Such massive destruction usually results from an autoimmune process in which circulating antibodies react specifically against the adrenal tissue.

Other causes of Addison's disease include tuberculosis, bilateral adrenalectomy, hemorrhage into the adrenal gland, neoplasms, and infections, such as human immunodeficiency virus, histoplasmosis, meningococcal pneumonia, and cytomegalovirus. Rarely, a familial tendency toward autoimmune disease can predispose a patient to Addison's disease, as well as to other endocrinopathies.

Secondary adrenal hypofunction that results in glucocorticoid deficiency can stem from hypopituitarism, which can cause decreased corticotropin secretion. It also can stem from abrupt withdrawal of long-term corticosteroid therapy, as when long-term exogenous corticosteroid stimulation suppresses pituitary corticotropin secretion and causes adrenal gland atrophy. In addition, it can result from removal of a nonendocrine, corticotropin-secreting tumor.

Adrenal crisis occurs in a patient with adrenal hypofunction when trauma, surgery, or other severe physiologic stress completely exhausts his body's stores of glucocorticoids.

Complications

Adrenal crisis is the most serious complication of adrenal hypofunction.

Assessment findings

The history of a patient with adrenal hypofunction may reveal synthetic steroid use, adrenal surgery, or recent infection. The patient may complain of muscle weakness, fatigue, light-headedness when rising from a chair or bed, weight loss, cravings for salty food, decreased tolerance for even minor stress, and various GI disturbances, such as nausea, vomiting, anorexia, and chronic diarrhea. He may also complain of anxiety, irritability, and confusion. He may experience reduced urine output and other symptoms of dehydration. Women may have decreased libido resulting from reduced androgen production, and amenorrhea.

On inspection, you may detect poor coordination, dry skin and mucous membranes related to dehydration, and decreased axillary and pubic hair in women. The patient with Addison's disease typically has a conspicuous bronze coloration of the skin that resembles a deep suntan, especially in the creases of the hands and over the metacarpophalangeal joints, elbows, and knees. The patient may also exhibit a darkening of scars, areas of vitiligo (an absence of pigmentation), and increased pigmentation of the mucous membranes, especially the buccal mucosa.

This abnormal coloration results from decreased secretion of cortisol (one of the glucocorticoids), which causes the pituitary gland to simultaneously secrete excessive amounts of melanocyte-stimulating hormone (MSH) and corticotropin. Secondary adrenal hypofunction doesn't cause hyperpigmentation because corticotropin and MSH levels are low.

On palpation, you may note a weak, irregular pulse. Auscultation of the patient's blood pressure demonstrates hypotension.

Diagnostic tests

The diagnosis of this disorder requires demonstration of decreased corticosteroid concentrations in plasma and an accurate classification of adrenal hypofunction as primary or secondary.

The following laboratory tests are used in diagnosing adrenal hypofunction:
• *Plasma and urine steroid testing* determine baseline levels.
• *Measurement of corticotropin levels* allows classification of the disease as primary or secondary. A high level indicates a primary adrenocortical disorder; a low level points to a secondary disorder.
• *Rapid corticotropin test* demonstrates plasma cortisol response to corticotropin. After obtaining plasma cortisol samples, an I.V. infusion of cosyntropin is administered. Plasma samples are taken 30 minutes after administration. If the plasma cortisol level doesn't rise, adrenal insufficiency is suspected. An elevated corticotropin level indicates a primary adrenocortical disorder, whereas a low corticotropin level indicates a pituitary (secondary) disorder.

In a patient with typical symptoms of Addison's disease, the following laboratory findings strongly suggest acute adrenal insufficiency:
• decreased cortisol levels in plasma (under 10 mcg/dl in the morning, with lower levels in the evening); however, this test is time-consuming, so crisis therapy shouldn't be delayed for results

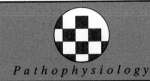

Pathophysiology

HOW ADRENAL CRISIS DEVELOPS

The most serious complication of adrenal hypofunction, adrenal crisis can occur gradually or with catastrophic suddenness, making prompt emergency treatment essential.

Also known as acute adrenal insufficiency, this potentially lethal condition usually develops in a patient who doesn't respond to hormone replacement therapy, who undergoes marked stress without adequate glucocorticoid replacement, or who abruptly stops hormonal therapy.

It can also result from trauma, bilateral adrenalectomy, or adrenal gland thrombosis after a severe infection (Waterhouse-Friderichsen syndrome).

Signs and symptoms

In adrenal crisis, signs and symptoms include profound weakness, fatigue, nausea, vomiting, hypotension, dehydration, and occasionally, high fever followed by hypothermia. If untreated, this condition can ultimately cause vascular collapse, renal shutdown, coma, and death.

The flowchart below summarizes what happens in adrenal crisis and pinpoints its warning signs and symptoms.

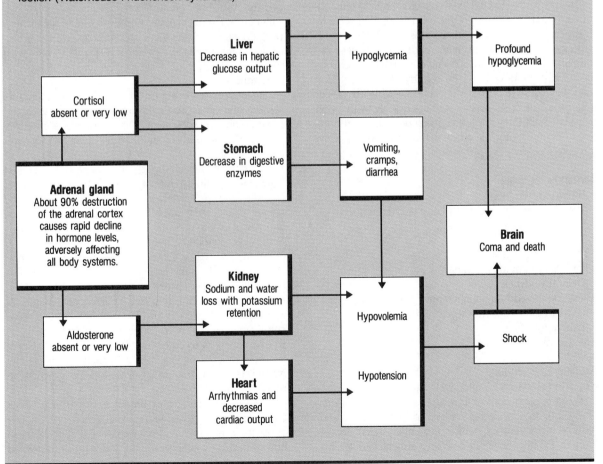

• reduced serum sodium levels
• increased serum potassium, serum calcium, and blood urea nitrogen levels
• elevated hematocrit and elevated lymphocyte and eosinophil counts.

In addition, X-rays may show a small heart and adrenal calcification.

Treatment

Lifelong corticosteroid replacement is the main treatment for all patients with primary or secondary adrenal hypofunction. In general, cortisone or hydrocortisone (which have a mineralocorticoid effect) are given. Patients with Addison's disease may also need fludrocortisone, a synthetic drug that acts as a mineralocorticoid, to prevent dangerous dehydration and hypotension. Women with Addison's disease who have muscle weakness and decreased libido may benefit from testosterone injections but risk unfortunate masculinizing effects.

Treatment for adrenal crisis is prompt I.V. bolus administration of 100 mg of hydrocortisone, followed by hydrocortisone diluted with dextrose in 0.9% sodium chloride solution and given I.V. until the patient's condition stabilizes. Up to 300 mg/day of hydrocortisone and 3 to 5 liters of I.V. 0.9% sodium chloride solution may be required during the acute stage. With proper treatment, the crisis usually subsides quickly, with blood pressure stabilizing and water and sodium levels returning to normal. After the crisis, maintenance doses of hydrocortisone preserve physiologic stability.

Nursing diagnoses

• Activity intolerance
• Altered nutrition: Less than body requirements
• Altered thought processes
• Body image disturbance
• Fluid volume deficit
• Ineffective individual coping
• Knowledge deficit
• Risk for altered body temperature
• Risk for impaired skin integrity
• Risk for infection
• Sexual dysfunction

Nursing interventions

• In adrenal crisis, monitor vital signs carefully, especially for hypotension, volume depletion, and other signs of shock. Check for decreased level of consciousness and reduced urine output, which may also signal shock. Monitor for hyperkalemia before treatment and for hy-pokalemia afterward (from excessive mineralocorticoid effect). Check for cardiac arrhythmias.
• If the patient also has diabetes mellitus, check blood glucose levels periodically because steroid replacement may necessitate adjustment of the insulin dosage.
• Record weight and intake and output carefully because the patient may have volume depletion. Until onset of mineralocorticoid effect, force fluids to replace excessive fluid loss.

For patients on maintenance steroid therapy:
• Control the environment to prevent stress. Encourage the patient to use relaxation techniques. Plan rest periods during the day, gradually increasing activities according to the patient's tolerance.
• Encourage the patient to dress in layers to retain body heat, and adjust room temperature, if possible.
• Provide good skin care. Use alcohol-free skin care products and an emollient lotion after bathing. Turn and reposition the bedridden patient every 2 hours. Avoid pressure over bony prominences.
• Use protective measures to minimize the risk of infection. Provide a private room and reverse isolation if necessary. Limit the patient's visitors, especially those with infectious conditions. Use meticulous hand-washing technique.
• Consult with a dietitian to plan a diet that maintains sodium and potassium balances and provides adequate proteins and carbohydrates. If the patient is anorexic, suggest that he eat six small meals a day to increase calorie intake.
• If the patient is receiving steroids, watch for cushingoid signs, such as fluid retention around the eyes and face. Monitor fluid and electrolyte balance, especially if the patient is receiving mineralocorticoids. Monitor weight and check blood pressure to assess body fluid status. Remember, steroids administered in the late afternoon or evening may cause central nervous system stimulation and insomnia in some patients. Check for petechiae because these patients bruise easily.
• In women receiving testosterone injections, watch for and report facial hair growth and other signs of masculinization. A dosage adjustment may be necessary.
• If the patient is receiving only glucocorticoids, observe for orthostatic hypotension or abnormal serum electrolyte levels, which may indicate a need for mineralocorticoid therapy.
• Encourage the patient to verbalize his feelings about body image changes and sexual dysfunction. Discuss fear of rejection by others and offer emotional support. Help him to develop coping strategies. Refer him to a mental

health professional for additional counseling, if necessary.

Patient teaching

• Explain that lifelong steroid therapy is necessary. Teach the patient and his family to identify and report signs and symptoms of drug overdose (weight gain and edema) or underdose (fatigue, weakness, and dizziness).
• Advise the patient that he will need to increase the dosage during times of stress (when he has a cold, for example). Warn that infection, injury, or profuse sweating in hot weather may precipitate adrenal crisis. Caution him not to withdraw the medication suddenly because this may also cause adrenal crisis.
• Instruct the patient always to carry a medical identification card stating that he takes a steroid and giving the name and dosage of the drug. Teach him and his family how to give an injection of hydrocortisone, and advise them to keep an emergency kit available containing a prepared syringe of hydrocortisone to use in times of stress.
• Instruct the patient to take steroids with antacids or meals to minimize gastric irritation. Suggest taking two-thirds of the dosage in the morning and the remaining one-third in the early afternoon to mimic diurnal adrenal secretion.
• Inform the patient and his family that the disease causes mood swings and changes in mental status, which steroid replacement therapy can correct.
• Review protective measures to decrease stress and help prevent infections. For example, the patient should get adequate rest, avoid fatigue, eat a balanced diet, and avoid people with infectious conditions. Also be sure to provide instructions for stress management and relaxation techniques.

CUSHING'S SYNDROME

The clinical manifestation of glucocorticoid (particularly cortisol) excess, Cushing's syndrome may also be caused by excess secretions of mineralocorticoids and androgens. The disorder is classified as primary, secondary, or iatrogenic, depending on its etiology, and is most common in females.

Its unmistakable signs include adiposity of the face, neck, and trunk, and purple striae on the skin. The prognosis depends on early diagnosis, identification of the underlying cause, and effective treatment.

Causes

In about 70% of patients, Cushing's syndrome results from excess production of corticotropin and consequent hyperplasia of the adrenal cortex. Corticotropin overproduction may stem from pituitary hypersecretion (Cushing's disease), a corticotropin-producing tumor in another organ (particularly bronchogenic or pancreatic carcinoma), or administration of synthetic glucocorticoids or corticotropin. In the remaining 30% of patients, Cushing's syndrome results from a cortisol-secreting adrenal tumor, which is usually benign. In infants, the usual cause of Cushing's syndrome is adrenal carcinoma.

Complications

The stimulating and catabolic effects of cortisol produce the complications of Cushing's syndrome. Increased calcium resorption from bone may lead to osteoporosis and pathologic fractures. Peptic ulcer may result from increased gastric secretions, pepsin production, and decreased gastric mucus. Dyslipidosis usually occurs. Increased hepatic gluconeogenesis and insulin resistance can cause impaired glucose tolerance. Overt diabetes mellitus occurs in fewer than 10% of patients.

Frequent infections or slow wound healing due to decreased lymphocyte production and suppressed antibody formation may occur. Suppressed inflammatory response may mask even a severe infection.

Hypertension due to sodium and water retention is common and may lead to ischemic heart disease and congestive heart failure. Menstrual disturbances and sexual dysfunction also occur. Decreased ability to handle stress may result in psychiatric problems, ranging from mood swings to frank psychosis.

Assessment findings

The patient may report using synthetic steroids. She may complain of fatigue, muscle weakness, sleep disturbances, water retention, amenorrhea, decreased libido, irritability, and emotional lability. Additionally, the patient may list various signs and symptoms that resemble those of hyperglycemia. Inspection may reveal a spectrum of characteristic signs and symptoms including thin hair, a moon-shaped face, hirsutism, acne, a buffalo humplike back, and thin extremities from muscle wasting. Other observable features may include petechiae, ecchymoses, and purplish striae; delayed wound healing; and swollen ankles. Auscultation typically reveals hypertension.

Diagnostic tests

Diagnosis of Cushing's syndrome depends on a demonstrated increase in cortisol production and the failure to suppress endogenous cortisol secretion after administration of dexamethasone. Initial screening may consist of a 24-hour urine test to determine free cortisol excretion rate and a low-dose dexamethasone test. Failure to suppress plasma and urine cortisol levels confirms the diagnosis of Cushing's syndrome.

A low-dose dexamethasone suppression test can determine if Cushing's syndrome results from pituitary dysfunction (Cushing's disease). In this diagnostic test, dexamethasone suppresses plasma cortisol levels. Failure to suppress these levels indicates that the syndrome results from an adrenal tumor or a nonendocrine, corticotropin-secreting tumor. This test can produce false-positive results.

In a stimulation test, administration of metyrapone, which blocks cortisol production by the adrenal glands, tests the ability of the pituitary gland and the hypothalamus to detect and correct low levels of plasma cortisol by increasing corticotropin production. The patient with Cushing's disease reacts to this stimulus by secreting an excess of plasma corticotropin. If the patient has an adrenal or a nonendocrine corticotropin-secreting tumor, the pituitary gland – which is suppressed by the high cortisol levels – cannot respond normally, so steroid levels remain stable or fall.

Radiologic evaluation for Cushing's syndrome seeks to locate the causative tumor in the pituitary gland or the adrenals. Tests include ultrasonography, a computed tomography scan, and magnetic resonance imaging enhanced with gadolinium.

Treatment

Management to restore hormone balance and reverse Cushing's syndrome may necessitate radiation, drug therapy, or surgery.

A patient with pituitary-dependent Cushing's syndrome with adrenal hyperplasia may require hypophysectomy or pituitary irradiation. If hypophysectomy and irradiation are unsuccessful or infeasible, bilateral adrenalectomy may be performed. A patient with a nonendocrine corticotropin-producing tumor requires excision of the tumor, followed by drug therapy with mitotane, metyrapone, or aminoglutethimide. Aminoglutethimide, cyproheptadine, and ketoconazole decrease cortisol levels and have been beneficial for many cushingoid patients. Aminoglutethimide alone, or in combination with metyrapone, may also be useful in metastatic adrenal carcinoma.

Before surgery, the patient with cushingoid symptoms requires management to control hypertension, edema, diabetes, and cardiovascular manifestations and to prevent infection. Glucocorticoid administration on the morning of surgery can help prevent acute adrenal insufficiency during surgery. Cortisol therapy is essential during and after surgery to help the patient tolerate the physiologic stress imposed by removal of the pituitary or adrenal glands. If normal cortisol production resumes, steroid therapy may gradually be tapered and eventually discontinued. However, bilateral adrenalectomy or total hypophysectomy mandates lifelong steroid replacement therapy to correct hormonal deficiencies.

Nursing diagnoses

- Activity intolerance
- Altered thought processes
- Body image disturbance
- Fluid volume excess
- Impaired skin integrity
- Ineffective individual coping
- Knowledge deficit
- Risk for infection
- Risk for injury
- Sexual dysfunction

Nursing interventions

- Keep accurate records of vital signs, fluid intake, urine output, and weight. Monitor serum electrolyte levels daily.
- Consult a dietitian to plan a diet high in protein and potassium but low in calories, carbohydrates, and sodium.
- Use protective measures to reduce the risk of infection. If necessary, provide a private room and institute reverse isolation precautions. Use meticulous hand-washing technique.
- Schedule activities around the patient's rest periods to avoid fatigue. Gradually increase activity as tolerated.
- Institute safety precautions to minimize the risk of injury from falls. Help the patient walk to avoid bumps and bruises.
- Help the bedridden patient turn and reposition herself every 2 hours. Use extreme caution while moving the patient to minimize skin trauma and bone stress. Provide frequent skin care, especially over bony prominences. Provide support with pillows and a convoluted foam mattress.
- Encourage the patient to verbalize her feelings about body image changes and sexual dysfunction. Offer emotional support and a positive, realistic assessment of her

condition. Help her to develop coping strategies. Refer her to a mental health professional for additional counseling, if necessary.

After bilateral adrenalectomy and hypophysectomy:
• Monitor urine output, and check vital signs carefully, watching for signs of hemorrhage and shock (decreased blood pressure; increased pulse rate; pallor; and cold, clammy skin). To counteract shock, give vasopressors, and increase the rate of I.V. fluids, as ordered. Because mitotane, aminoglutethimide, and metyrapone decrease mental alertness and produce physical weakness, assess neurologic and behavioral status, and warn the patient of adverse central nervous system effects. Also watch for severe nausea, vomiting, and diarrhea.
• Check laboratory reports for hypoglycemia due to removal of the source of cortisol, a hormone that maintains blood glucose levels.
• Check for abdominal distention and return of bowel sounds following adrenalectomy.
• Check regularly for signs of adrenal hypofunction—orthostatic hypotension, apathy, weakness, and fatigue—indicators that steroid replacement is inadequate.
• In the patient undergoing pituitary surgery, check for and immediately report signs of increased intracranial pressure (confusion, agitation, changes in level of consciousness, nausea, and vomiting). Monitor for signs of hypopituitarism and transient diabetes insipidus.

Patient teaching
• Advise the patient that lifelong steroid replacement will be necessary. Teach her and her family to identify and report signs of drug overdose (edema and weight gain) or underdose (fatigue, weakness, and dizziness). Warn her not to abruptly discontinue the drug because this may precipitate adrenal crisis.
• Instruct the patient to take steroids with antacids or meals to minimize gastric irritation. Advise her to take two-thirds of a dose in the morning and the remaining third in the early afternoon to mimic diurnal adrenal secretion.
• Encourage the patient to wear a medical identification bracelet and carry her medication with her at all times.
• Teach the patient protective measures to decrease stress and infections. For example, she should get adequate rest and avoid fatigue, eat a balanced diet, and avoid people with infections. Also teach her relaxation and stress-reduction techniques.

HYPERALDOSTERONISM

In this disorder, hypersecretion of the mineralocorticoid aldosterone by the adrenal cortex causes excessive reabsorption of sodium and water and excessive renal excretion of potassium. (See *Effects of excessive aldosterone,* page 1030.)

The disorder may be classified as primary, resulting from a stimulus inside the adrenal gland, or secondary, resulting from an extra-adrenal stimulus. Incidence of hyperaldosteronism is two times greater in women than in men and highest between ages 30 and 50.

Causes
Primary hyperaldosteronism (Conn's syndrome) is uncommon. In 70% of patients, it results from a small, unilateral aldosterone-producing adrenal adenoma. In the remaining 30%, the cause is either unclear, adrenocortical hyperplasia (in children), or carcinoma. Excessive ingestion of English black licorice or a similar substance can produce a syndrome similar to primary hyperaldosteronism due to the mineralocorticoid action of glycyrrhizic acid, which is present in licorice.

Secondary hyperaldosteronism results from extra-adrenal pathology, which stimulates the adrenal gland to increase production of aldosterone. For example, conditions that reduce renal blood flow (renal artery stenosis) and extracellular fluid volume or that produce a sodium deficit activate the renin-angiotensin system and, subsequently, increase aldosterone secretion. Thus, secondary hyperaldosteronism may result from conditions that induce hypertension through increased renin production (such as Wilms' tumor), from ingestion of oral contraceptives, and from pregnancy. However, this type may also result from disorders unrelated to hypertension that may or may not cause edema. For example, nephrotic syndrome, hepatic cirrhosis with ascites, and congestive heart failure (CHF) commonly induce edema; Bartter's syndrome and salt-losing nephritis don't.

Complications
Hyperaldosteronism can produce neuromuscular irritability, tetany, paresthesia, and seizures. Cardiac complications include arrhythmias, ischemic heart disease, left ventricular hypertrophy, CHF, and death. Metabolic alkalosis, nephropathy, and azotemia may also occur.

Assessment findings
The patient may complain of headache, visual disturbances, muscle weakness, fatigue, polyuria, and polydipsia. Inspection may detect intermittent flaccid paralysis, resulting from hypokalemia and, possibly, tet-

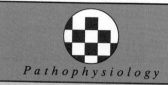

Pathophysiology

EFFECTS OF EXCESSIVE ALDOSTERONE

Excessive aldosterone secretion fosters serious electrolyte imbalances. The chart below shows what happens.

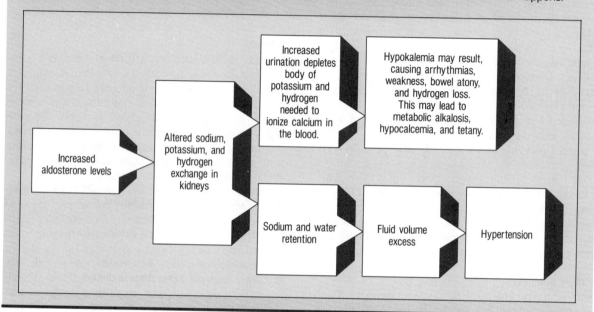

any, which may be caused by metabolic alkalosis and lead to hypocalcemia. Secondary hyperaldosteronism rarely occurs without edema.

Palpation may reveal a weak pulse, signs of muscle tonicity, and positive Chvostek's and Trousseau's signs. Auscultation of the apical pulse may detect cardiac arrhythmias. Auscultation of blood pressure reveals hypertension.

Diagnostic tests

Persistently low serum potassium levels in a nonedematous patient who isn't taking diuretics, who doesn't have obvious GI losses (from diarrhea), and who has a normal sodium intake suggest hyperaldosteronism. If hypokalemia develops in a hypertensive patient shortly after starting treatment with potassium-wasting diuretics (such as thiazides), and it persists after the diuretic has been discontinued and potassium replacement therapy has been instituted, evaluation for hyperaldosteronism is

necessary. The test results below confirm hyperaldosteronism:

• A low plasma renin level after volume depletion by diuretic administration when the patient is sitting or standing and a high plasma aldosterone level after volume expansion by salt loading confirm primary hyperaldosteronism in a hypertensive patient without edema.

• An elevated serum bicarbonate level with ensuing alkalosis commonly results from hydrogen and potassium ion loss in the distal renal tubules.

Other test findings show markedly increased urine aldosterone levels, increased plasma aldosterone levels, and increased plasma renin levels (in secondary hyperaldosteronism).

• A suppression test differentiates between primary and secondary hyperaldosteronism. The patient receives oral desoxycorticosterone acetate for 3 days while plasma aldosterone levels and urine metabolites are continuously measured. These levels decrease in secondary hyperaldosteronism but remain the same in primary. Simultaneously, renin levels are low in primary hyperaldosteronism and high in the secondary form.

Other helpful diagnostic evidence includes increased plasma volume of 30% to 50% above normal; electrocardiogram signs of hypokalemia (ST-segment depression and U waves); chest X-ray showing left ventricular hypertrophy from chronic hypertension; and localization of tumor shown on computed tomography scan, ultrasonography, or magnetic resonance imaging.

Treatment

Although treatment for primary hyperaldosteronism may include unilateral adrenalectomy, hyperaldosteronism may be controlled without surgery through administration of the potassium-sparing diuretic spironolactone and sodium restriction. Bilateral adrenalectomy reduces blood pressure for most patients with idiopathic primary hyperaldosteronism. However, some degree of hypertension usually persists, requiring treatment with spironolactone or other antihypertensive drug. Such patients also require lifelong adrenal hormone replacement.

Treatment of secondary hyperaldosteronism must include correction of the underlying cause.

Nursing diagnoses
• Altered tissue perfusion
• Altered urinary elimination
• Decreased cardiac output
• Ineffective individual coping
• Knowledge deficit
• Pain

Nursing interventions
• Keep accurate records of the patient's vital signs, fluid intake, urine output, and weight.
• Monitor serum electrolyte levels.
• Watch for signs of tetany (muscle twitching and Chvostek's sign) and for hypokalemia-induced cardiac arrhythmias, paresthesia, or weakness. Give potassium replacement, as ordered, and keep I.V. calcium gluconate available.
• Provide comfort measures to relieve headache: Administer analgesics, apply ice packs, and decrease environmental stimuli.
• Consult a dietitian to plan a low-sodium, high-potassium diet.
• Schedule activities to encourage rest, prevent fatigue, and decrease myocardial oxygen demand. Gradually increase activity as tolerated.

• After adrenalectomy, monitor for weakness, hyponatremia, rising serum potassium levels, and signs of adrenal insufficiency, especially hypotension.
• Encourage the patient to verbalize her feelings about her illness. Offer emotional support, and help her identify her strengths and use them to develop coping strategies. Refer her to a mental health professional, if necessary.

Patient teaching
• Advise the patient that she'll need long-term adrenal hormone replacement. Tell her and her family to identify and report signs of drug overdose or underdose.
• Encourage the patient to wear a medical identification bracelet and to carry her medications with her at all times.
• Instruct the patient to follow a low-sodium, high-potassium diet.
• If the patient is taking spironolactone, tell her to watch for and report signs of hyperkalemia. If the patient is a man, warn him that impotence and gynecomastia may follow long-term use.

ADRENOGENITAL SYNDROME

Excessive production of adrenal androgens causes adrenogenital syndrome, resulting in masculinization, virilization, and hermaphrodism. In rare, true hermaphrodism the person has both ovarian and testicular tissues, a uterus, and ambiguous gonads distributed in various patterns. Adrenogenital syndrome may be inherited (congenital adrenal hyperplasia [CAH]) or acquired (adrenal virilism), usually as a result of an adrenal tumor. (See *Acquired adrenal virilism,* page 1032.)

CAH is the most common adrenal disorder in infants and children; simple virilizing CAH and salt-losing CAH are the most common forms. Adrenal virilism is rare and affects females twice as often as males.

Causes and pathophysiology

CAH is transmitted as an autosomal recessive trait that causes deficiencies in the enzymes needed for adrenocortical secretion of cortisol and, possibly, aldosterone. Compensatory secretion of corticotropin produces varying degrees of adrenal hyperplasia.

In simple virilizing CAH, deficiency of the enzyme 21-hydroxylase results in underproduction of cortisol. In turn, this cortisol deficiency stimulates increased secretion of corticotropin, producing large amounts of cortisol precursors and androgens that don't require 21-hydroxylase for synthesis.

ACQUIRED ADRENAL VIRILISM

Acquired adrenal virilism results from virilizing adrenal tumors, carcinomas, or adenomas.

Clinical effects
Although acquired adrenal virilism can develop at any age, its clinical effects vary with the patient's age at onset.
• Prepubescent girls: pubic hair, clitoral enlargement; at puberty, no breast development, menses delayed or absent
• Prepubescent boys: hirsutism, macrogenitosomia precox (excessive body development with marked enlargement of genitalia). Occasionally, the penis and prostate equal those of an adult male in size; however, testicular maturation fails to occur.
• Women (especially middle-aged): dark hair on legs, arms, chest, back, and face; pubic hair extending toward navel; oily skin, sometimes with acne; menstrual irregularities; muscular hypertrophy (masculine resemblance); male pattern baldness; and atrophy of breasts and uterus
• Men: no overt signs; discovery of tumor is usually accidental

• All patients: good muscular development, taller than average during childhood and adolescence, short stature as adults due to early closure of epiphyses.

Diagnostic tests
• *Urine total 17-ketosteroids (17-KS):* greatly elevated levels, which vary daily; oral dexamethasone doesn't suppress 17-KS.
• *Dehydroepiandrosterone:* plasma levels greatly elevated
• *Serum electrolyte levels:* normal
• *X-ray of kidneys:* may show downward displacement of kidneys by tumor.

Treatment
The patient undergoes surgical excision of the tumor and metastases (if present), when possible, or radiation therapy and chemotherapy. Preoperative treatment may include glucocorticoids. With treatment, the prognosis is very good in patients with slow-growing, nonrecurring tumors. Levels of 17-hydroxyprogesterone, androstenedione, testosterone, and renin are measured to monitor therapy.

In salt-losing CAH, 21-hydroxylase is almost completely absent. Corticotropin secretion increases, causing excessive production of cortisol precursors, including salt-wasting compounds. However, plasma cortisol levels and aldosterone—both dependent on 21-hydroxylase—fall precipitously and, in combination with the excessive production of salt-wasting compounds, expedite acute adrenal crisis. Corticotropin hypersecretion stimulates adrenal androgens, possibly even more than in simple virilizing CAH, and produces masculinization.

Other rare CAH enzyme deficiencies exist and lead to increased or decreased production of affected hormones.

Complications
Unless salt-losing CAH is treated promptly, dehydration and hyperkalemia may lead to cardiovascular collapse and cardiac arrest in neonates. Other complications of adrenogenital syndrome include hypertension, hyperkalemia, infertility, adrenal tumor, tendency to develop adrenal crisis (from stress), and altered growth, external genitalia, and sexual maturity.

Assessment findings
Varying assessment findings depend on the disorder's cause and the patient's age and sex. Suspect CAH in infants hospitalized for failure to thrive, dehydration, or diarrhea, as well as in tall, sturdy-looking children with a history of episodic illnesses.

Inspection of the female neonate with simple virilizing CAH finds ambiguous genitalia (enlarged clitoris with urethral opening at the base and some labioscrotal fusion) but a normal genital tract and gonads. Inspection of an older female child with simple virilizing CAH reveals signs of progressive virilization: early appearance of pubic and axillary hair, deep voice, acne, and facial hair. Patient history notes failure to begin menstruation.

On inspection, the male neonate with simple virilizing CAH has no obvious abnormalities. However, at prepuberty, the child shows accentuated masculine characteristics, such as a deepened voice, an enlarged phallus, and frequent erections.

At puberty, the males have small testes. Both males and females with this condition may be taller than other children their age due to rapid bone and muscle growth. But because excessive androgen levels hasten epiphyseal closure, they may exhibit abnormally short adult stature.

Parents of an infant with salt-losing CAH may disclose that the child is apathetic, fails to eat, and has diarrhea. Without prompt treatment, the infant may develop fatal adrenal crisis in the first week of life (vomiting, dehydration from hyponatremia, and hyperkalemia).

Inspection of the older female with salt-losing CAH finds more complete virilization than in the simple form, even the development of male external genitalia without testes. The male child with this condition has no external genital abnormalities.

Diagnostic tests

Although ambiguous external genitalia suggest hermaphrodism, a gonadal biopsy and chromosomal studies are needed to confirm it just as the following test findings are needed to confirm adrenogenital syndrome:
• elevated levels of urine 17-ketosteroids (17-KS), which can be suppressed by administering oral dexamethasone
• increased urine metabolites of hormones, particularly pregnanetriol
• elevated levels of plasma 17-hydroxyprogesterone and dehydroepiandrosterone sulfate (DHEAS)
• hyperkalemia, hyponatremia, and hypochloremia in the presence of elevated levels of urine 17-KS and pregnanetriol, and decreased aldosterone levels, which confirm salt-losing CAH in any infant with signs and symptoms of adrenal hypofunction or adrenal crisis in the first week after birth.

Treatment

Simple virilizing CAH necessitates correction of the cortisol deficiency and inhibition of excessive pituitary corticotropin production. This is accomplished through daily administration of cortisone or hydrocortisone. Such treatment returns androgen production to normal levels. Initially, the oral hydrocortisone dosage starts at 25 to 30 mg/m²/day. Then, the dosage is reduced to 10 to 20 mg/m²/day. Infants must receive I.M. cortisone or hydrocortisone until age 18 months; after that, they may take the drug orally.

The infant with salt-losing CAH in adrenal crisis requires immediate I.V. sodium chloride and glucose infusion to maintain fluid and electrolyte balance and to stabilize vital signs. If this treatment doesn't control symptoms while diagnosis is being established, I.M. desoxycorticosterone and, occasionally, I.V. hydrocortisone are necessary. Later, maintenance therapy includes mineralocorticoid (desoxycorticosterone) and glucocorticoid (cortisone or hydrocortisone) replacement.

Based on the anatomy of the external genitalia and chromosomal evaluation, sexual assignment and reconstructive surgery may be recommended. For example, the female with masculine external genitalia requires reconstructive surgery, such as correction of the labial fusion and of the urogenital sinus. Such surgery is usually scheduled between ages 1 and 3 after the effect of cortisone therapy has been assessed.

Nursing diagnoses
• Altered growth and development
• Body image disturbance
• Ineffective family coping
• Ineffective individual coping
• Knowledge deficit
• Risk for fluid volume deficit

Nursing interventions
• When caring for an infant with adrenal crisis, keep the I.V. line patent, infuse fluids, and give steroids, as ordered. Monitor body weight, vital signs, respiratory status, urine output, and serum electrolyte levels.
• Provide protective measures to minimize external stress. Limit visitors, provide a private room, and decrease environmental stimuli.
• Monitor the patient receiving desoxycorticosterone for edema, weakness, and hypertension. Be alert for significant weight gain and rapid changes in height because normal growth is an important indicator of adequate therapy.
• Encourage the parents and the older child to verbalize their feelings about altered body image and fear of rejection by others. Offer a positive, but realistic, assessment of the patient's condition. Assist the parents and child to identify strengths and use them to develop coping strategies. Refer the family to a mental health counselor, if necessary.

Patient teaching
• Teach the parents of an infant with adrenogenital syndrome about normal growth and development and how their child may differ. Correct misconceptions about the disorder and explain treatment options. Explain how the choice of sexual assignment is made and how abnormalities are surgically corrected. Refer the family to a genetic specialist for counseling.
• Advise the parents and the child that long-term steroid therapy is necessary. Warn them not to discontinue steroids abruptly to prevent potentially fatal adrenal insufficiency.
• Teach the patient and the family to identify and report signs of drug overdose and underdose, stress, and infection, which may require altered steroid dosages.
• Instruct the patient to wear a medical identification bracelet, indicating that she's receiving prolonged steroid therapy and providing information about dosage.

• Stress the importance of continued medical follow-up throughout the child's life.

PHEOCHROMOCYTOMA

A rare disease, pheochromocytoma (also known as chromaffin tumor) is characterized by paroxysmal or sustained hypertension due to oversecretion of the catecholamines epinephrine and norepinephrine. By some estimates, about 0.5% of newly diagnosed patients with hypertension have pheochromocytoma; although this tumor is usually benign, it may be malignant in a few patients.

Pheochromocytoma affects all races and both sexes and is typically familial. Although this disorder is potentially fatal, the prognosis is generally good with treatment.

Causes

Pheochromocytoma stems from a chromaffin cell tumor of the adrenal medulla or sympathetic ganglia, more commonly in the right adrenal gland than in the left. Extra-adrenal pheochromocytomas may be located in the abdomen, thorax, urinary bladder, and neck and in association with the 9th and 10th cranial nerves.

In about 5% of patients, pheochromocytoma is inherited as an autosomal dominant trait.

Complications

Pheochromocytoma produces the same complications as those of severe, persistent hypertension: cerebrovascular accident (CVA), retinopathy, heart disease, and irreversible kidney damage. Often, the disorder is diagnosed during pregnancy when uterine pressure on the tumor induces more frequent attacks of hypertensive crisis. Such attacks can prove fatal for both mother and fetus as a result of CVA, acute pulmonary edema, cardiac arrhythmias, or hypoxia. In such patients, the risk of spontaneous abortion is high, but most fetal deaths occur during labor or immediately after birth. Cholelithiasis is often associated with this disorder.

Patients with pheochromocytoma have an increased risk of serious complications and death during invasive diagnostic testing and surgery. After adrenalectomy, severe hypotension resulting in circulatory collapse and shock may occur.

Assessment findings

The cardinal sign of pheochromocytoma is persistent or paroxysmal hypertension. The patient's history may reveal unpredictable episodes of hypertensive crisis, paroxysmal symptoms suggestive of a seizure disorder or anxiety attacks, hypertension that responds poorly to conventional treatment and, in some cases, hypotension or shock, resulting from surgery or diagnostic procedures.

The patient may describe attacks of such signs and symptoms as headache, palpitations, visual blurring, nausea, vomiting, severe diaphoresis, feelings of impending doom, and precordial or abdominal pain. The attacks may be precipitated by any activity or condition that displaces the abdominal contents, such as heavy lifting, exercise, bladder distention, or pregnancy. Severe attacks may be precipitated by the administration of opiates, histamine, glucagon, and corticotropin. Sometimes, no precipitating event is found.

The patient may also report mild to moderate weight loss caused by increased metabolism. In addition, he may have symptoms related to orthostatic hypotension: dizziness, light-headedness, or faintness when rising to an upright position.

Inspection may find tachypnea, pallor, or flushing accompanied by profuse sweating during an attack. Tremor and seizures may also occur.

During an attack, palpation may reveal moist, cool hands and feet or generalized warmth and flushing. Tachycardia is usually present. The tumor itself is rarely palpable, but when it is, palpation of the surrounding area may induce a typical acute attack and help confirm the diagnosis.

Auscultation of blood pressure reveals hypertension, the most common manifestation. Although hypertension is sustained in most patients, some lability is usually noted. During an attack, blood pressure may rise to dangerously high levels.

Diagnostic tests

Diagnosis of pheochromocytoma is usually based on the following test findings:
• Increased urinary excretion of total free catecholamine and its metabolites, vanillylmandelic acid (VMA) and metanephrine, as measured by analysis of a 24-hour urine specimen, confirms pheochromocytoma.
• Labile blood pressure necessitates urine collection during a hypertensive episode and comparison of this specimen to a baseline specimen. Direct assay of total plasma catecholamines may show levels 10 to 50 times higher than normal.
• Computed tomography (CT) scan or magnetic resonance imaging of the adrenal glands is usually successful in identifying the intra-adrenal lesions. CT scanning,

chest X-rays, or abdominal aortography may identify extra-adrenal pheochromocytomas.

Treatment

Surgical removal of the tumor is the treatment of choice. To decrease the patient's blood pressure, the alpha-adrenergic blocking agents phentolamine or phenoxybenzamine, or metyrosine (which blocks catecholamine synthesis), are administered from 1 day to 2 weeks before surgery or invasive diagnostic procedures. A beta-adrenergic blocking agent (propranolol or atenolol) may also be used after achieving alpha blockade. Prazosin, labetalol, and nifedipine may also be used.

Postoperatively, the patient may require I.V. fluids, plasma volume expanders and, possibly, transfusions if marked hypotension occurs. However, persistent hypertension in the immediate postoperative period is more common.

If surgery isn't feasible, alpha- and beta-adrenergic blocking agents—such as phenoxybenzamine and propranolol, respectively—are beneficial in controlling catecholamine effects and preventing attacks. Research is currently being done to investigate the use of a combination of chemotherapeutic agents in treating inoperable malignant adrenal tumors.

Management of acute attacks or hypertensive crisis requires administration of phentolamine by I.V. push or drip, or nitroprusside to normalize blood pressure.

Nursing diagnoses

• Altered nutrition: Less than body requirements
• Altered tissue perfusion
• Anxiety
• Fear
• Ineffective individual coping
• Knowledge deficit
• Pain
• Risk for infection
• Sensory or perceptual alterations (visual)

Nursing interventions

• To ensure the reliability of urine catecholamine measurements, keep the patient at rest, and make sure he avoids foods high in vanillin (such as coffee, nuts, chocolate, and bananas) for 2 days before urine collection of VMA. Also, be aware that some drugs—such as guaifenesin and salicylates—may interfere with the accurate determination of VMA. When possible, avoid administering these medications before the test. Collect the urine in a special receptacle, containing hydrochloric acid, that's been prepared by the laboratory. Don't schedule the test if the patient has recently been exposed to iodine-containing radiographic contrast media because they can suppress the levels of urine catecholamine.

• Monitor the patient's blood pressure—transient hypertensive attacks are possible. Tell him to report headaches, palpitations, nervousness, or other symptoms of an acute attack.

• If hypertensive crisis develops, monitor blood pressure and heart rate every 2 to 5 minutes until blood pressure stabilizes at an acceptable level.

• Administer analgesics for headache. Provide comfort measures: Decrease environmental stimuli, apply ice packs, and avoid abrupt jarring motions.

• Monitor serum glucose levels, and observe for weight loss from hypermetabolism.

• Monitor peripheral circulation, neurologic status, and renal and cardiac function for signs of adequate perfusion.

• Help the patient decrease his anxiety by encouraging him to verbalize his feelings and fears, by listening actively, and by answering his questions. Help him identify and use his strengths to develop coping strategies.

• Consult a dietitian to plan a high-protein diet that has adequate calories.

After adrenalectomy:

• The first 24 to 48 hours after surgery are the most critical. Monitor vital signs—blood pressure may rise or fall sharply. Keep the patient quiet because excitement may trigger a hypertensive episode. Postoperative hypertension is common because the stress of surgery and manipulation of the adrenal gland stimulate secretion of catecholamines. This excess secretion causes profuse sweating, so keep the room cool, and change the patient's clothing and bedding often.

• If the patient receives phentolamine, monitor his blood pressure closely. Observe and record adverse drug reactions, such as dizziness, weakness, hypotension, tachycardia, and diarrhea.

• Watch for abdominal distention and return of bowel sounds.

• Check dressings and vital signs for indications of hemorrhage (increased pulse rate, decreased blood pressure, cold and clammy skin, pallor, and unresponsiveness).

• Give analgesics for pain, as ordered, but monitor blood pressure carefully. Many analgesics, especially meperidine, can cause hypotension.

• If autosomal dominant transmission of pheochromocytoma is suspected, suggest that the family be genetically evaluated for this condition.

Patient teaching

• Provide honest and clear explanations of all procedures to allay the patient's fears.
• Teach the patient methods that help prevent paroxysmal attacks—for example, relaxation techniques to reduce anxiety, adequate fluids and fiber to avoid constipation, and adequate rest to avoid fatigue.
• Teach the patient and her family to report signs of adrenal insufficiency and adverse effects of replacement therapy. Warn against abrupt discontinuation of medication. Advise the patient that lifelong treatment is necessary.
• Encourage the patient to wear medical identification and to carry her medication with her at all times.

PANCREATIC AND OTHER DISORDERS

Endocrine imbalances can also cause insulin deficiency, gonadal abnormalities, precocious puberty, and male infertility. They are discussed in the following section.

DIABETES MELLITUS

A chronic disease of absolute or relative insulin deficiency or resistance, diabetes mellitus is characterized by disturbances in carbohydrate, protein, and fat metabolism. Insulin transports glucose into the cells for use as energy and storage as glycogen. It also stimulates protein synthesis and free fatty acid storage in the adipose tissues. Insulin deficiency compromises the body tissues' access to essential nutrients for fuel and storage.

The disorder occurs in two primary forms: Type I, insulin-dependent diabetes mellitus, and the more prevalent Type II, non-insulin-dependent diabetes mellitus. A number of secondary forms also exist, resulting from conditions such as pancreatic disease, pregnancy, hormonal or genetic syndromes, or ingestion of certain drugs or chemicals.

Diabetes mellitus is thought to affect about 5% of the population of the United States (14 million people), about half of whom are undiagnosed. Incidence is higher in males than in females and rises with age.

Causes and pathophysiology

Type I diabetes is caused by destruction of the beta cells in the pancreas. By the time the disease becomes apparent, 80% of the beta cells have been destroyed. The destructive process is autoimmune in nature. The current theory is that genetic susceptibility follows an environmental stimulus—for example, a foreign antigen such as a virus or another microorganism. This antigen provokes a normal immune response somewhere in the body, but if it's similar in chemistry and configuration to the beta cell, it also stimulates an immune attack against these cells. This attack causes an inflammatory response in the pancreas called *insulitis*.

In insulitis, the islets are infiltrated with activated T lymphocytes, and the beta cells similar to the antigen are mistaken as foreign by the immune system. Cytotoxic antibodies develop and act in concert with cell-mediated immune mechanisms to destroy the beta cells.

Type II diabetes may arise from abnormal insulin secretion, resistance to insulin action in target tissues, and inappropriate hepatic gluconeogenesis. These may be caused by primary islet cell abnormality. Acquired insulin resistance, usually obesity-related, may be required for hyperglycemia to develop.

The causes of secondary diabetes vary greatly. Physiologic or emotional stress may induce prolonged elevation of levels of stress hormones, such as cortisol, epinephrine, glucagon, and growth hormone. This, in turn, raises blood glucose and places increased demands on the pancreas. Pregnancy causes weight gain and heightened levels of estrogen and placental hormones. Certain medications have been shown to antagonize the effects of insulin, including thiazide diuretics, adrenal corticosteroids, and oral contraceptives.

Complications

Two acute metabolic complications of diabetes are diabetic ketoacidosis (DKA) and hyperosmolar nonketotic syndrome (HNKS). These life-threatening conditions require immediate medical intervention. (See *What happens in DKA and HNKS*, pages 1038 and 1039.)

Patients with diabetes mellitus also have a higher risk for various chronic illnesses affecting virtually all body systems. The most common chronic complications include cardiovascular disease, peripheral vascular disease, retinopathy, nephropathy, diabetic dermopathy, and peripheral and autonomic neuropathy.

Peripheral neuropathy usually affects the hands and feet and may cause numbness or pain. Autonomic neuropathy manifests itself in several ways, including gastroparesis (leading to delayed gastric emptying and a feeling of nausea and fullness after meals), nocturnal diarrhea, impotence, and postural hypotension.

Hyperglycemia impairs the patient's resistance to infection because the glucose content of the epidermis and urine encourages bacterial growth. The patient is susceptible to skin and urinary tract infections and vaginitis.

Infants of diabetic mothers have a two- to three-times-greater incidence of congenital malformations and fetal distress. And patients with diabetes mellitus have an increased incidence of cognitive depression.

Assessment findings
The patient with Type I diabetes usually reports rapidly developing symptoms. With Type II diabetes, the patient's symptoms are usually vague, long-standing, and develop gradually (see *Devising an effective plan for diabetic care,* pages 1040 and 1041). Patients with Type II diabetes generally report a family history of diabetes mellitus, gestational diabetes or the delivery of a baby weighing more than 9 lb (4 kg), severe viral infection, other endocrine disease, recent stress or trauma, or use of drugs that increase blood glucose levels.

Patients with both types of diabetes may report symptoms related to hyperglycemia, such as polyuria, polydipsia, polyphagia, weight loss, and fatigue. Or they may complain of weakness; vision changes; frequent skin infections; dry, itchy skin; sexual problems; and vaginal discomfort—all symptoms of hyperglycemia.

Inspection may show retinopathy or cataract formation. Skin changes, especially on the legs and feet, may represent impaired peripheral circulation. Muscle wasting and loss of subcutaneous fat may be evident in Type I diabetes; Type II is characterized by obesity, particularly in the abdominal area.

Palpation may detect poor skin turgor and dry mucous membranes related to dehydration. Decreased peripheral pulses, cool skin temperature, and decreased reflexes may also be palpable. Auscultation may reveal orthostatic hypotension. Patients with diabetic ketoacidosis may have a characteristic "fruity" breath odor because of increased acetone production.

Diagnostic tests
In nonpregnant adults, one of the following findings confirms a diagnosis of diabetes mellitus:
• symptoms of uncontrolled diabetes and a random blood glucose level equal to or above 200 mg/dl
• a fasting plasma glucose level equal to or greater than 140 mg/dl on at least two occasions
• with normal fasting glucose, a blood glucose level above 200 mg/dl at 2 hours and on at least one other occasion during the glucose tolerance test.

An ophthalmologic examination may show diabetic retinopathy. Other diagnostic and monitoring tests include urinalysis for acetone and blood testing for glyco-sylated hemoglobin (hemoglobin A), which reflects recent glucose control.

Treatment
Effective treatment of diabetes optimizes blood glucose levels and decreases complications. In Type I diabetes, goals are achieved with insulin replacement, diet, and exercise. Current forms of insulin replacement include single-dose, mixed-dose, split-mixed-dose, and multiple-dose regimens. The multiple-dose regimens may use an insulin pump. Insulin may be rapid-acting (Regular), intermediate-acting (NPH and Lente), long-acting (Ultralente), or a premixed combination of rapid-acting and intermediate-acting. Insulin may also be standard or purified, and it may be derived from beef, pork, or human sources. Purified human insulin is used commonly today. Pancreas transplantation is also an option.

Treatment for both types also requires strict adherence to a diet carefully planned to meet nutritional needs, control blood glucose levels, and reach and maintain appropriate body weight. An estimate is made of the total energy intake needed per day based on the patient's ideal body weight. Then a decision is made regarding carbohydrate, fat, and protein content, and an appropriate diet is constructed.

For the obese patient with Type II diabetes, weight reduction is a dietary goal. In Type I, the calorie allotment may be high, depending on the patient's growth stage and activity level. To be successful, the patient must follow the diet consistently and eat at regular times.

Exercise along with weight reduction and proper diet has proven useful in managing Type II diabetes. Physical activity increases insulin sensitivity, improves glucose tolerance, and promotes weight loss. Patients with Type II diabetes may also need oral antidiabetic drugs to stimulate endogenous insulin production and, possibly, increase insulin sensitivity at the cellular level.

Treatment for long-term complications may include dialysis or kidney transplantation for renal failure, photocoagulation for retinopathy, and vascular surgery for large vessel disease. Optimal blood glucose control is essential to help prevent the acute and chronic complications of diabetes.

Nursing diagnoses
• Altered nutrition: Less than body requirements
• Altered nutrition: More than body requirements
• Altered peripheral tissue perfusion
• Altered urinary elimination
• Anticipatory grieving
• Fluid volume deficit

(Text continues on page 1041.)

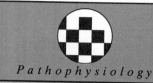

Pathophysiology

WHAT HAPPENS IN D.K.A. AND H.H.N.S.

Diabetic ketoacidosis (DKA) and hyperosmolar hyperglycemic nonketotic syndrome (HHNS) are acute complications of hyperglycemic crisis that may occur in the diabetic patient. If not treated properly, either may result in coma or death.

DKA occurs most often in patients with Type I diabetes; in fact, it may be the first evidence of previously unrecognized Type I diabetes. HHNS occurs most often in patients with Type II diabetes. But HHNS may also occur in anyone whose insulin tolerance is stressed and in patients who've undergone certain therapeutic procedures – such as peritoneal dialysis, hemodialysis, tube feedings, or total parenteral nutrition.

Acute insulin deficiency (absolute in DKA; relative in HHNS) precipitates both conditions. Causes include illness, stress, infection, and failure to take insulin (only in a patient with DKA).

Buildup of glucose

Inadequate insulin hinders glucose uptake by fat and muscle cells. Because the cells can't take in glucose to convert to energy, glucose accumulates in the blood. At the same time, the liver responds to the demands of the energy-starved cells by converting glycogen to glucose and releasing glucose into the blood, *further* increasing the blood glucose level. When this level exceeds the renal threshold, excess glucose is excreted in the urine.

Still, the insulin-deprived cells can't utilize glucose. Their response is rapid metabolism of protein, which results in loss of intracellular potassium and phosphorus and in excessive liberation of amino acids. The liver converts these amino acids into urea and glucose.

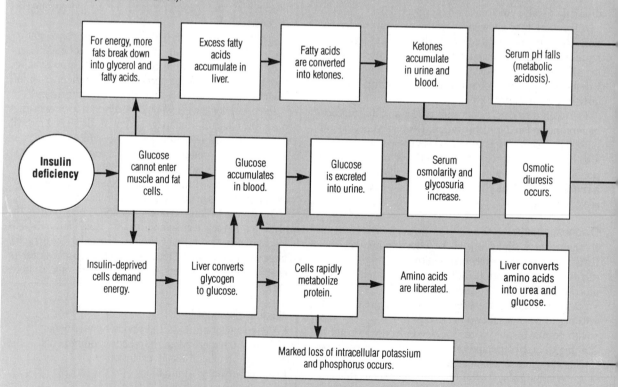

As a result of these processes, blood glucose levels are grossly elevated. The aftermath is increased serum osmolarity and glucosuria (higher in HHNS than in DKA because blood glucose levels are higher in HHNS), leading to osmotic diuresis.

A deadly cycle

The massive fluid loss from osmotic diuresis causes fluid and electrolyte imbalances and dehydration. Water loss exceeds electrolyte loss, contributing to hyperosmolarity. This, in turn, perpetuates dehydration, decreasing the glomerular filtration rate and reducing the amount of glucose excreted in the urine. This leads to a deadly cycle: Diminished glucose excretion *further* raises blood glucose levels, producing severe hyperosmolarity and dehydration and finally causing shock, coma, and death.

Further DKA complication

All these steps hold true for both DKA and HHNS. But DKA has an additional simultaneous process that leads to metabolic acidosis. The *absolute* insulin deficiency causes cells to convert fats into glycerol and fatty acids for energy. The fatty acids can't be metabolized as quickly as they're released, so they accumulate in the liver, where they're converted into ketones (ketoacids). These ketones accumulate in the blood and urine and cause *acidosis*. Acidosis leads to more tissue breakdown, more ketosis, more acidosis, and eventually shock, coma, and death.

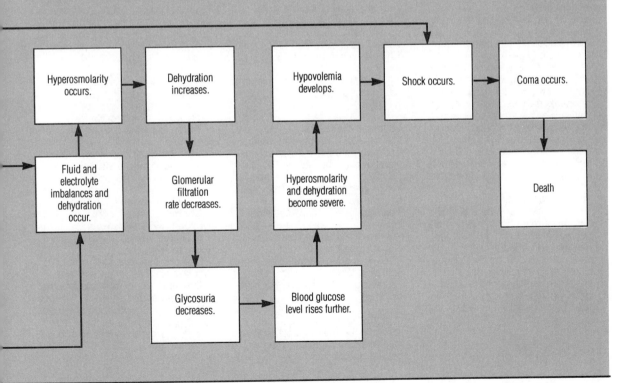

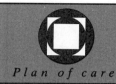

Plan of care

DEVISING AN EFFECTIVE PLAN FOR DIABETIC CARE

To help you identify nursing diagnoses using your assessment findings and to help you plan, implement, and evaluate care, consider the case of Helen Strong, a 54-year-old administrative assistant with Type II diabetes mellitus. Her diabetes had been well controlled by diet and by glyburide (10 mg) before breakfast and dinner. However, with the recent death of her mother, she has experienced stress and has gained 20 lb (9 kg). Today, she has come to the clinic for a reevaluation of her blood glucose level (it was 265 mg/dl at her last visit).

Patient history

Mrs. Strong tells you, "I feel sleepy all of the time. Does this have anything to do with my blood sugar, or am I just depressed by my mother's death?" She also reports that she urinates frequently and drinks a lot of fluid. Her doctor has recommended that she begin taking insulin. She says that she's afraid of giving herself injections, especially because her eyesight has been getting worse lately. She's concerned that she won't see well enough to perform the procedure.

Assessment findings

You examine Mrs. Strong and find her height to be 5'5" (165 cm) and her weight to be 175 lb (79.5 kg). Her skin is flushed and dry. Turgor is poor, as evidenced by tenting.

You ask Mrs. Strong for a urine specimen, which appears dilute. Urine glucose and ketone test results prove negative. However, the blood glucose level is 320 mg/dl.

Nursing diagnoses

Before identifying nursing diagnoses, consider what you've gleaned from your assessment. Mrs. Strong seems quite anxious about giving herself insulin injections. Considered with assessment and laboratory findings, her complaints point to ineffective dietary and drug control of blood glucose levels. Oral antidiabetic agents may control blood glucose for only a period and then become ineffective, causing secondary failure. In addition, obesity and stress raise insulin requirements.

Based on your assessment findings and impressions, you arrive at these nursing diagnoses:
• Knowledge deficit related to the disorder, insulin injection, and meal plan and activity requirements
• Altered nutrition: More than body requirements, related to decreased exercise and increased food intake
• Anxiety related to self-injection of insulin
• Altered family processes related to the recent death of Mrs. Strong's mother.

Expected outcomes

Because Mrs. Strong has several self-care areas to master, you devise several goals jointly. She will:
• show proficiency in giving herself insulin injections without feeling excessive anxiety
• demonstrate an understanding of insulin
• demonstrate an understanding of diabetes mellitus
• follow an adequate nutrition and activity regimen
• show signs of accepting her mother's death.

Implementation

You take the following steps to help Mrs. Strong achieve the expected outcomes.

To increase skill and decrease anxiety about insulin injection

• Provide an insulin syringe and needle, and assist Mrs. Strong to fill the syringe with the exact amount of the right medication.
• Furnish a syringe magnifier or magnifying glass to compensate for decreased visual acuity.
• Guide Mrs. Strong as she learns proper injection technique using 0.9% sodium chloride solution initially.
• Have Mrs. Strong compile a list of the insulin types and amounts she will use. Then show her how to mix the insulin and how to draw it into the syringe. Describe how to store the medication properly.
• Encourage Mrs. Strong to use sites on her abdomen (the preferred area) for insulin injections. Then, assist her until she becomes comfortable and skillful with the procedure.
• Explain the importance of rotating insulin injection sites.

To improve knowledge of insulin

• First, review why Mrs. Strong needs insulin; then explain how insulin works to control diabetes.
• Teach about the different types of insulin as they relate to Mrs. Strong.
• Describe insulin reactions. Discuss how to recognize a reaction and when to notify the doctor.

To gain an understanding of diabetes

• Explain what diabetes is and how the disease relates to dietary and exercise regimens.
• Describe the signs and symptoms of insulin deficit and excess, and state measures to take should either condition occur.
• Teach Mrs. Strong how to measure blood glucose levels at home. Have her state what she'll do if they're sig-

DEVISING AN EFFECTIVE PLAN FOR DIABETIC CARE *(continued)*

nificantly elevated or decreased. Help her to set up a daily log book to record blood glucose levels.
• Point out the danger of blood glucose levels that are too low (as well as too high). Explain that lowering her blood glucose level safely with insulin will relieve such symptoms as nocturia and fatigue.
• Explain how diabetes increases the risk for infection. Review the signs of infection and steps to take should signs occur. Be sure Mrs. Strong understands the need to report minor infections so that they don't become major ones.
• Teach proper foot care to prevent serious infections.
• Instruct Mrs. Strong to report worsening vision immediately.

To promote adequate nutrition and activity
• Give Mrs. Strong a printed copy of the diet that the doctor prescribed.

Explain how to select and vary foods to maintain consistent caloric intake.
• Help Mrs. Strong write out daily menus.
• If needed, arrange a meeting with the dietitian, who can explain important features of the diet and answer questions.
• Emphasize the importance of modifying body weight to reduce insulin resistance and, possibly, to reduce the amount of insulin required.
• Assist Mrs. Strong to plan and perform a regular exercise program.
• Stress the value of exercise to stimulate carbohydrate metabolism, aid weight control and, possibly, minimize complications. Urge Mrs. Strong to exercise the same amount each day.

To help Mrs. Strong cope with death and loss
• Encourage Mrs. Strong to express her feelings about her mother's death.

• Acknowledge her fears and concerns.
• Help her to identify and use effective coping strategies.
• If needed, refer her to a counselor who can help her work through her grief.

Evaluation
You can judge the success of your care plan by several signposts. By watching Mrs. Strong, you'll know whether she can give herself insulin properly and without anxiety. By talking with her, you'll learn how well she understands insulin and diabetes and their effects on her health. You'll also look for other indications that your plan was adequate. Ask, for example, whether Mrs. Strong's weight has stabilized at a healthful level. What exercise does she perform regularly? Chances are, if she's caring for herself effectively, she's probably dealing with her mother's death effectively as well.

• Hopelessness
• Impaired adjustment
• Impaired skin integrity
• Ineffective family coping
• Ineffective individual coping
• Knowledge deficit
• Noncompliance
• Powerlessness
• Risk for infection
• Risk for injury
• Sensory or perceptual alterations (visual)
• Sexual dysfunction

Nursing interventions
• Keep accurate records of vital signs, weight, fluid intake, urine output, and caloric intake. Monitor serum glucose and urine acetone levels.
• Monitor for acute complications of diabetic therapy, especially hypoglycemia (vagueness, slow cerebration, dizziness, weakness, pallor, tachycardia, diaphoresis, seizures, and coma); immediately give carbohydrates in the form of fruit juice, hard candy, honey, or, if the patient is unconscious, glucagon or I.V. dextrose. Also be alert for signs of HNKS (polyuria, thirst, neurologic abnor-

malities, and stupor). This hyperglycemic crisis requires I.V. fluids and insulin replacement.
• Monitor diabetic effects on the cardiovascular system, such as cerebral vascular, coronary artery, and peripheral vascular impairment, and on the peripheral and autonomic nervous systems.
• Provide meticulous skin care, especially to the feet and legs. Treat all injuries, cuts, and blisters. Avoid constricting hose, slippers, or bed linens. Refer the patient to a podiatrist.
• Observe for signs of urinary tract and vaginal infections. Encourage adequate fluid intake.
• Monitor the patient for signs of diabetic neuropathy (numbness or pain in the hands and feet, footdrop, and neurogenic bladder).
• Consult a dietitian to plan a diet with the recommended allowances of calories, protein, carbohydrates, and fats, based on the patient's particular requirements.
• Encourage the patient to verbalize his feelings about diabetes and its effects on life-style and life expectancy. Offer emotional support and a realistic assessment of his condition. Stress that with proper treatment, he can have a near-normal life-style and life expectancy. Assist the patient to develop coping strategies. Refer him and his

family to a counselor, if necessary. Encourage them to join a support group.

Patient teaching
• Stress the importance of carefully adhering to the prescribed program. Tailor your teaching to the patient's needs, abilities, and developmental stage. Discuss diet, medications, exercise, monitoring techniques, hygiene, and how to prevent and recognize hypoglycemia and hyperglycemia.
• To encourage compliance to life-style changes, emphasize how blood glucose control affects long-term health.
• Teach the patient how to care for his feet: He should wash them daily, carefully dry between his toes, and inspect for corns, calluses, redness, swelling, bruises, and breaks in the skin. Urge him to report any skin changes to the doctor. Advise him to wear comfortable, nonconstricting shoes and never to walk barefoot.
• Urge annual regular ophthalmologic examinations for early detection of diabetic retinopathy.
• Describe the signs and symptoms of diabetic neuropathy, and emphasize the need for safety precautions because decreased sensation can mask injuries.
• Teach the patient how to manage his diabetes when he has a minor illness, such as a cold, flu, or upset stomach.
• To prevent diabetes, teach people at high risk to avoid risk factors; for example, women with family histories of diabetes require counseling about contraceptive use and the risks of pregnancy. Advise genetic counseling for adult diabetic patients who are planning families.
• Teach the patient and family how to monitor the patient's diet and use food exchange lists. Show them how to read labels in the supermarket to identify fat, carbohydrate, protein, and sugar content.
• Encourage the patient and family to contact the Juvenile Diabetes Foundation, the American Association of Diabetes Educators, and the American Diabetes Association for additional information.

TURNER'S SYNDROME
Caused by a chromosomal abnormality, Turner's syndrome is the most common disorder of gonadal dysgenesis in females. It occurs in about 1 per 3,000 births; 95% of fetuses with this syndrome are spontaneously aborted. The syndrome produces characteristic signs, which are irreversible.

Causes
Turner's syndrome occurs when an X chromosome (or part of the second X chromosome) is missing from either the ovum or sperm through nondisjunction or chromosome lag. Mixed aneuploidy may result from mitotic nondisjunction.

Complications
In Turner's syndrome, complications include diabetes mellitus, thyroid disease, osteoarthritis, osteoporosis, cardiomyopathy, renal dysfunction, precocious aging, and sterility.

Assessment findings
Turner's syndrome produces characteristic signs that are obvious on inspection. At birth, 50% of infants with this syndrome measure below the third percentile in length. Commonly, they have swollen hands and feet, a wide chest, and a low hairline that becomes more obvious as they grow. They may have severe webbing of the neck, and some have coarse, enlarged, prominent ears. Gonadal dysgenesis is seen at birth. Inspection may also reveal pigmented nevi, lymphedema, hypoplasia, or malformed nails.

As the child grows, short stature is the most common physical manifestation. The patient may exhibit average to slightly below-average intelligence. Developmental problems include right-left disorientation for extrapersonal space and defective figure drawing. The patient is typically immature, socially naive, and conforming.

Auscultation of the infant's chest indicates cardiovascular malformations, such as coarctation of the aorta and ventricular septal defects.

Diagnostic tests
Turner's syndrome can be diagnosed by chromosome analysis. Differential diagnosis should rule out mixed gonadal dysgenesis, Noonan-Ehmke's syndrome, and other similar disorders.

Treatment
Cardiovascular malformations must be corrected surgically. Hormonal replacement should begin in childhood and include androgen, human growth hormone and, possibly, small doses of estrogen. Later, progesterone and estrogen can induce sexual maturation.

Nursing diagnoses
• Altered growth and development
• Body image disturbance
• Chronic low self-esteem

- Ineffective family coping
- Ineffective individual coping
- Knowledge deficit
- Sexual dysfunction

Nursing interventions

- Encourage the patient and her family to verbalize their feelings about the patient's condition and to discuss fear of rejection by others. Offer emotional support and a realistic assessment of the patient's condition.
- Assist the patient and her family to develop coping strategies. Refer them for sexual or genetic counseling (as necessary).
- Provide appropriate preoperative and postoperative care for the infant with cardiovascular malformations.

Patient teaching

- Explain the surgical procedure and its expected outcomes to the parents of the infant with cardiovascular malformations. Help them participate in the child's care and make informed decisions about treatment options. Explain all procedures, and provide ongoing information about the infant's condition.
- Teach the parents about normal growth and development and how their child may differ. Clarify any misconceptions, and explain the treatment. Suggest strategies to help the child achieve age-related skills.
- Teach the family and, if appropriate, the patient about long-term hormone replacement therapy. Stress the importance of strictly complying with therapy.

HYPOGONADISM

Resulting from decreased androgen production in males, hypogonadism usually causes infertility and inhibits the development of normal secondary sex characteristics. Primary and secondary forms exist, and the disorder is classified by the age of onset (prepuberty or postpuberty) or the location of the causative lesion. In primary (hypergonadotropic) hypogonadism, the lesion is in the testes; in secondary (hypogonadotropic) hypogonadism, the lesion is in the hypothalamic-pituitary area.

Causes and pathophysiology

Primary hypogonadism results directly from interstitial (Leydig's cell) cellular or seminiferous tubular damage due to faulty development or mechanical damage. This causes increased secretion of gonadotropins (follicle-stimulating hormone [FSH] and luteinizing hormone [LH]) by the pituitary gland in an attempt to increase the testicular functional state. It encompasses the following disorders: Klinefelter's syndrome, Reifenstein's syndrome, male Turner's syndrome, Sertoli-cell-only syndrome, anorchism, orchitis, and sequelae of irradiation.

Secondary hypogonadism results from faulty interaction within the hypothalamic-pituitary axis, resulting in failure to secrete normal levels of gonadotropins. It includes the following disorders: hypopituitarism, isolated FSH deficiency, isolated LH deficiency, prolactinomas, Kallmann's syndrome, and Prader-Willi syndrome.

Complications

Hypogonadism may lead to complications such as infertility, eunuchism (total gonadal failure), eunuchoidism (partial gonadal failure), low-grade chronic anemia, diabetes mellitus, vasomotor instability, osteoporosis, skeletal malformations due to incomplete epiphyseal closure, malignancies, and autoimmune disorders.

Assessment findings

Clinical effects of hypogonadism vary with the specific cause and the age of onset. Adults may report diminished sex drive and potency and regression of secondary sex characteristics. Young patients may have a history of delayed puberty.

Patients may have an infantile penis and small, soft, or absent testes; gynecomastia; below-average muscle development and strength; increased length of the long bones; fine, sparse facial hair; scant or absent axillary, pubic, and body hair; girdle obesity; small Adam's apple; lack of temporal recession of the hairline; kyphosis; and a high-pitched voice.

Diagnostic tests

- *Serum gonadotropin levels* increase in primary hypogonadism but decrease in secondary hypogonadism.
- *Serum testosterone levels* are low.
- *Other hormonal studies* are used to assess neuroendocrine functions, such as thyrotropin, adrenocorticotropin, growth hormone, prolactin, and vasopressin levels.
- *Chromosomal analysis* may detect the specific cause.
- *Testicular biopsy* and *semen analysis* determine sperm production, and identify impaired spermatogenesis.
- *X-rays* and *bone scans* may show delayed closure of the epiphyses and immature bone age.

Treatment

In primary hypogonadism, treatment may consist of hormone replacement, especially with testosterone, FSH, methyltestosterone, or human chorionic gonadotropin (HCG). Treatment for secondary hypogonadism is HCG

1054 ENDOCRINE DISORDERS

alone. Although fertility can't be restored after permanent testicular damage, eunuchism resulting from hypothalamic-pituitary lesions can be corrected with
gonadotropins to stimulate testicular function.

Nursing diagnoses
• Altered growth and development
• Body image disturbance
• Chronic low self-esteem
• Ineffective individual coping
• Knowledge deficit
• Sexual dysfunction

Nursing interventions
• Encourage the patient to verbalize his feelings about his
condition. Help him to develop coping strategies.
• Refer the patient to a mental health professional or for
sexual counseling, if appropriate.

Patient teaching
• Teach the patient and his family about normal growth
and development and how the patient may differ.
• Review long-term hormone therapy. Explain how to
identify and report adverse effects, such as acne and
water retention. Urge the patient to take the drugs exactly as directed and not to stop the drugs abruptly.
• Encourage the family to obtain genetic counseling.

PRECOCIOUS PUBERTY IN MALES
Boys who begin to mature sexually before age 10 exhibit
one of two forms of precocious puberty, also called iso-
sexual precocity. The most common form is true precocious puberty, characterized by early maturation of the
hypothalamic-pituitary-gonadal axis, development of
secondary sex characteristics, gonadal development, and
spermatogenesis. Pseudoprecocious puberty induces development of secondary sex characteristics without gonadal development. Boys with true precocious puberty
reportedly have fathered children as early as age 7.

In most boys with precocious puberty, sexual characteristics develop in essentially normal sequence. These
children function normally when they reach adulthood.

Causes
True precocious puberty may be idiopathic (constitutional) or cerebral (neurogenic). In some patients, idiopathic precocity may be genetically transmitted as a
dominant trait. Cerebral precocity results from pituitary
or hypothalamic intracranial lesions that cause excessive
secretion of gonadotropin.

Pseudoprecocious puberty may result from testicular
tumors (hyperplasia, adenoma, or carcinoma) or from
congenital adrenogenital syndrome. Testicular tumors
create excessive testosterone levels; adrenogenital syndrome creates high levels of adrenocortical steroids. Deficiencies of 11β-hydroxylase or 21-hydroxylase may also
cause precocious puberty in males.

Complications
Emotional disturbances may result from premature sexual development. Premature closure of the epiphyses results in stunted adult stature. Tumors of the pituitary
gland may cause compression and necrosis of surrounding tissue. Increased intracranial pressure, visual disturbances, and seizure disorders may also occur.
Malignant tumors are usually fatal.

Assessment findings
The patient's history may disclose altered growth patterns, behavior changes, family history of precocious puberty, or ingestion of hormones. Parents may note that
the child had an initial growth spurt and early muscle
development. The patient with precocity due to cerebral
lesions may report nausea, vomiting, headache, and visual disturbances.

In all patients, inspection may reveal an adult hair
pattern, penile growth, and bilateral enlarged testes. In
pseudoprecocity caused by a testicular tumor, you may
also observe acne and a discrepancy in testis size. Adrenogenital syndrome produces adult skin tone, excessive
hair (including beard), and a deepened voice. A boy with
this syndrome appears stocky and muscular; his penis
and scrotal sac appear enlarged.

In true precocious puberty, palpation may reveal bilaterally enlarged testes at an early age. The patient with
pseudoprecocity due to testicular tumors has an enlarged
testis that may be hard or may contain a palpable, isolated nodule. If adrenogenital syndrome is the cause, the
scrotal sac and prostate are enlarged, but not the testes.

Diagnostic tests
In true precocious puberty:
• *Serum luteinizing hormone, follicle-stimulating hormone,*
and *corticotropin levels* are elevated.
• *Plasma testosterone levels* increase to adult levels.
• *Ejaculate evaluation* may reveal live spermatozoa.
• *Brain scan, magnetic resonance imaging, skull X-rays,*
and *EEG* may detect central nervous system tumors.
• *Skull* and *hand X-rays* show advanced bone age.
  In pseudoprecocious puberty:
• *Chromosomal karyotype analysis* may demonstrate an

abnormal pattern of autosomes and sex chromosomes.
• *Adrenal androgen levels* are elevated.

Treatment

Boys with idiopathic precocious puberty generally require no medical treatment and, except for stunted growth, experience no physical complications in adulthood. Psychological counseling is important. Medroxyprogesterone may be used to inhibit gonadotropin secretion.

When precocious puberty is caused by tumors, the prognosis is discouraging. Brain tumors require neurosurgery but commonly resist treatment and may be fatal. Radiation therapy is used when indicated. A hypothalamic hamartoma requires a gonadotropin-releasing hormone (Gn-RH) analogue; idiopathic neurogenic precocious puberty demands a long-acting Gn-RH analogue. Testicular tumors may be treated by removing the affected testis (orchiectomy). Malignant tumors also require chemotherapy and lymphatic radiation therapy.

When precocious puberty results from an autosomal dominant disorder, treatment aims to block androgen and estrogen stimulation. Spironolactone and testolactone are sometimes used. The antifungal agent ketoconazole is currently being tested for its inhibitory effect on the biosynthesis of adrenal and gonadal steroids.

Adrenogenital syndrome that causes precocious puberty may respond to lifelong therapy with glucocorticoids (cortisol) to inhibit corticotropin production.

Nursing diagnoses

• Altered growth and development
• Body image disturbance
• Impaired adjustment
• Ineffective individual coping
• Knowledge deficit

Nursing interventions

• Encourage the child to verbalize his feelings about changes in his body. Offer emotional support, and help the child develop coping strategies. Refer him and his family to a counselor, if necessary.
• If the patient has a tumor, provide appropriate preoperative and postoperative care and emotional support.

Patient teaching

• Teach the child and his family about normal growth and development and how the patient may differ. Emphasize that the child's social and emotional development should remain consistent with his chronologic age, not with his physical development.
• Stress the importance of continuing medical follow-up care and testing.
• Teach the patient and his family to identify and report adverse effects (cushingoid symptoms) of androgen antagonistic medication.
• If the child is being treated with the luteinizing hormone-releasing hormone (LH-RH) analogues histrelin or deslorelin, instruct the parents to administer the drug in the evening to counteract the nocturnal surge of endogenous LH-RH. Teach the parents and child how to administer the drug by subcutaneous injection and to identify and report skin reactions at the injection site.
• Advise the child to wear medical identification.

PRECOCIOUS PUBERTY IN FEMALES

In girls, precocious puberty involves early pubertal changes: breast development, pubic and axillary hair growth, and menarche before age 8. In true precocious puberty, the ovaries mature, and pubertal changes progress in an orderly manner. In pseudoprecocious puberty, pubertal changes occur without ovarian maturation.

Causes

About 85% of all cases of true precocious puberty in females are constitutional, resulting from early development and activation of the endocrine glands without corresponding abnormalities. Other causes of true precocious puberty include such central nervous system (CNS) disorders as hypothalamic tumors, intracranial tumors (pinealoma, granuloma, and hamartoma), hydrocephaly, degenerative encephalopathy, tuberous sclerosis, neurofibromatosis, encephalitis, skull injuries, and meningitis.

Pseudoprecocious puberty may result from increased levels of sex hormones due to ovarian and adrenocortical tumors, adrenocortical virilizing hyperplasia, ingestion of estrogens or androgens, and increased end-organ sensitivity to low levels of circulating sex hormones.

Complications

Early signs of sexual development can cause emotional problems. If ovulation is occurring, pregnancy is possible. Short stature may result from premature epiphyseal closure. As an adult, the patient may experience excessive menstrual bleeding, causing anemia. Cystic mastitis and an increased incidence of uterine adenofibromas are also linked with this disorder. Compression of surrounding tissues by intracranial tumors may result in hemorrhage, necrosis, and increased intracranial pressure. Malignant estrogen-secreting tumors may be fatal.

Assessment findings

The patient's history shows a rapid growth spurt before age 9. Inspection may find thelarche (breast development), pubarche (pubic hair development), and menarche—all before age 8. These changes may occur independently or simultaneously.

Diagnostic tests

• *X-ray studies* of hands, wrists, knees, and hips show bone age and premature epiphyseal closure.
• *Blood analyses* of serum gonadotropin (follicle-stimulating hormone [FSH] and luteinizing hormone [LH]) and sex steroid (estradiol and progesterone) levels are in the normal adult range. Low levels of gonadotropins indicate an ovarian or adrenal tumor; high levels suggest an intracranial lesion or a human chorionic gonadotropin–secreting tumor.
• *Laboratory tests,* including vaginal smear for estrogen secretion, urinalysis for gonadotropic activity and excretion of 17-ketosteroids, and radioimmunoassay for both FSH and LH, define elevated values.
• *Ultrasonography, computed tomography (CT) scans, magnetic resonance imaging (MRI), laparoscopy,* or *exploratory laparotomy* may verify an abdominal lesion.
• *EEG, ventriculography, pneumoencephalography, CT scans, MRI,* or *angiography* can detect CNS disorders.

Treatment

Though still controversial, treatment of constitutional true precocious puberty may include medroxyprogesterone to reduce secretion of gonadotropins and prevent menstruation. Adrenogenital syndrome requires cortical or adrenocortical steroid replacement. Surgery may be needed to remove ovarian and adrenal tumors; regression of secondary sex characteristics may follow such surgery, especially in young children. Choriocarcinomas may require surgery, irradiation, or chemotherapy. Hypothyroidism requires thyroid extract or levothyroxine to decrease gonadotropic secretions.

Nursing diagnoses

• Altered growth and development
• Body image disturbance
• Impaired adjustment
• Ineffective individual coping
• Knowledge deficit

Nursing interventions

• Encourage the child and parents to verbalize their feelings about changes in the child's body image.
• Explain all diagnostic procedures, and offer honest and realistic information on the child's condition.
• Help the child to develop coping strategies.
• Refer the family to a mental health professional for additional counseling, if necessary.
• Advise parents to dress the child in age-appropriate clothing that de-emphasizes her physical development.
• Reassure the parents that precocious puberty usually doesn't precipitate precocious sexual behavior.
• If the patient requires surgery to remove a tumor, take appropriate preoperative and postoperative measures.

Patient teaching

• Teach the parents and child about normal development and how the child may differ. Explain that although the patient appears physically mature, she's not psychologically mature. Warn them that the discrepancy between physical and psychological maturity may create problems. Caution them against expecting more of her than of other children her age.
• Provide appropriate sex education. Include information on menstruation and related hygiene.
• Teach the parents and child to identify and report adverse effects of medications. Stress the importance of complying with long-term treatment.

MALE INFERTILITY

When a couple fails to achieve pregnancy after about 1 year of regular, unprotected intercourse, male infertility may be the reason. About half of the infertility problems in the United States are attributed to the male.

Causes

Some of the factors that cause male infertility include:
• varicocele—a mass of dilated and tortuous varicose veins in the spermatic cord
• semen disorders, such as volume or motility disturbances or inadequate sperm density
• proliferation of abnormal or immature sperm with variations in the size and shape of the head
• systemic disease, such as diabetes mellitus, neoplasms, hepatic and renal diseases, and viral disturbances, especially mumps orchitis
• genital infections, such as gonorrhea and herpes
• disorders of the testes, such as cryptorchidism, Sertoli-cell-only syndrome, and ductal obstruction (caused by absence or ligation of vas deferens or infection)

• genetic defects, such as Klinefelter's syndrome (chromosomal pattern XXY, eunuchoidal habitus, gynecomastia, and small testes) or Reifenstein's syndrome (chromosomal pattern 46,XY, reduced testosterone, azoospermia, eunuchoidism, and hypospadias)
• immune disorders, such as autoimmune infertility
• endocrine imbalance that disrupts pituitary gonadotropins, inhibiting spermatogenesis, testosterone production, or both (occurring in Kallmann's syndrome, panhypopituitarism, hypothyroidism, and congenital adrenal hyperplasia)
• chemicals and drugs that can inhibit gonadotropins or interfere with spermatogenesis, such as arsenic, methotrexate, medroxyprogesterone, nitrofurantoin, monoamine oxidase inhibitors, and some antihypertensives
• sexual problems, such as erectile dysfunction, ejaculatory incompetence, or low libido
• other factors, such as age, trauma to the testes, and alcohol or marijuana use.

Complications
Male infertility often causes anger, hurt, disgust, guilt, and loss of self-esteem—in both partners. Psychological distress may also be linked with male infertility.

Assessment findings
Patient history may reveal abnormal sexual development, delayed puberty, previous infertility, and a history of prolonged fever, mumps, impaired nutritional status, genital surgery or trauma, or alcohol or marijuana use. Inspection may reveal atrophied testes; empty scrotum; scrotal edema; varicocele; and penile nodes, warts, plaques, or hypospadias. The seminal vesicles may feel warm. You may feel beading or abnormal nodes on the spermatic cord and vas deferens; anteversion of the epididymis; and prostatic enlargement, nodules, swelling, or tenderness.

Diagnostic tests
The most conclusive test for male infertility is semen analysis, performed three to six times over 2 to 4 months. Other tests include gonadotropin assay to determine the integrity of the pituitary gonadal axis; serum testosterone evaluation to determine end-organ response to luteinizing hormone (LH); and testicular biopsy to clarify unexplained oligospermia and azoospermia. Vasography and seminal vesiculography may also help.

Treatment
Infertility resulting from anatomic dysfunction or infection requires correction of the underlying problem. A varicocele requires surgical repair or removal. Patients with sexual dysfunction need education, counseling, or special therapy. Decreased follicle-stimulating hormone and LH levels may respond to chorionic gonadotropin or human menopausal gonadotropin. Normal or elevated LH requires low dosages of testosterone. Low testosterone levels, decreased semen motility, and volume disturbances may respond to chorionic gonadotropin. Assisted reproduction, such as artificial insemination, may help.

Patients with oligospermia who have a normal history and physical examination, normal hormonal assays, and no signs of systemic disease require emotional support and counseling, adequate nutrition, multivitamins, and selective therapeutic agents.

Nursing diagnoses
• Body image disturbance
• Ineffective family coping
• Ineffective individual coping
• Knowledge deficit
• Self-esteem disturbance

Nursing interventions
• Encourage the couple to express their feelings, and help them develop coping strategies.
• Refer them to a mental health professional and a fertility specialist for additional counseling, if necessary.

Patient teaching
• Educate the couple about reproductive and sexual functions and about factors that may interfere with fertility.
• Urge men with oligospermia to avoid habits that may interfere with normal spermatogenesis by elevating scrotal temperature, such as wearing tight underwear, taking hot tub baths, or habitually riding a bicycle. Cool scrotal temperatures are essential for adequate spermatogenesis.

SELECTED REFERENCES
Avery, M.E., and First, L.R. *Pediatric Medicine,* 2nd ed. Baltimore: Williams & Wilkins Co., 1994.

Becker, K.L., et al., eds. *Principles and Practice of Endocrinology & Metabolism,* 2nd ed. Philadelphia: J.B. Lippincott Co., 1995.

Felig, P., et al., eds. *Endocrinology and Metabolism,* 3rd ed. New York: McGraw-Hill Book Co., 1995.

Rakel, R.E., ed. *Conn's Current Therapy 1996.* Philadelphia: W.B. Saunders Co., 1996.

Santiago, J., ed. *Therapy for Diabetes Mellitus and Related Disorders,* 2nd ed. Alexandria, Va.: American Diabetes Association, 1994.

Tierney, L., et al. *Current Medical Diagnosis and Treatment 1995.* East Norwalk, Conn.: Appleton & Lange, 1995.

15   OBSTETRIC AND GYNECOLOGIC DISORDERS

INTRODUCTION

Today, nursing care of the obstetric or gynecologic patient reflects a growing interest in improving the quality of women's health. Besides assessing, counseling, and referring these patients, you need to consider such relevant factors as the desire to have children, problems of sexual adjustment, and self-image.

Frequently, nursing care is further complicated by multiple and concurrent problems. For example, a patient with endometriosis may also have trichomonal vaginitis, dysuria, and unsuspected infertility. You can readily understand why multiple problems like these occur if you're familiar with the anatomy of the female genitalia.

External structures

Female genitalia include the following external structures, collectively known as the *vulva:* mons pubis (or mons veneris), labia majora, labia minora, clitoris, and the vestibule. The size, shape, and color of these structures — as well as pubic hair distribution, and skin texture and pigmentation — vary greatly among individuals. Furthermore, these external structures undergo distinct changes during the life cycle.

The *mons pubis* is the pad of fat over the symphysis pubis (pubic bone). It's usually covered by the base of the inverted triangular patch of pubic hair that grows over the vulva after puberty.

The *labia majora* are the two thick, longitudinal folds of fatty tissue that extend from the mons pubis to the posterior aspect of the perineum. The labia majora protect the perineum and contain large sebaceous glands that help maintain lubrication. Virtually absent in the young child, their development characteristically signals the onset of puberty. The skin of the more prominent parts of the labia majora is pigmented and darkens after puberty.

The *labia minora* are the two thin, longitudinal folds of skin that border the vestibule. Firmer than the labia majora, they extend from the clitoris to the fourchette.

The *clitoris* is the small, protuberant organ located just beneath the arch of the mons pubis. The clitoris contains erectile tissue, venous cavernous spaces, and specialized sensory corpuscles that are stimulated during coitus.

The *vestibule* is the oval space bordered by the clitoris, labia minora, and fourchette. The *urethral meatus* is located in the vestibule's anterior portion; the *vaginal meatus,* in its posterior portion. The *hymen* is the elastic membrane that partially obstructs the vaginal meatus in virgins.

Several glands lubricate the vestibule. *Skene's glands* open on both sides of the urethral meatus; *Bartholin's glands* open on both sides of the vaginal meatus.

Other anatomic structures include the *fourchette* (the posterior junction of the labia majora and labia minora) and the *perineum* (which includes the underlying muscles and fascia of the external surface of the pelvic floor that extends from the fourchette to the anus).

Internal structures

The internal female genitalia includes the vagina, cervix, uterus, fallopian tubes (or oviducts), and ovaries.

The *vagina* occupies the space between the bladder and the rectum. A muscular, membranous tube measuring about 3″ (7.6 cm), the vagina connects the uterus and the vestibule of the external genitalia. It serves as a passageway for sperm to the fallopian tubes, for the discharge of menstrual fluid, and for childbirth.

The *cervix,* or uterine neck, protrudes at least ¾″ (2 cm) into the proximal end of the vagina. A rounded, conical structure, the cervix joins the uterus and the vagina at a 45- to 90-degree angle.

The *uterus* is the hollow, pear-shaped organ in which the conceptus grows during pregnancy. The part of the uterus above the junction of the fallopian tubes is called the *fundus;* the part below this junction is called the *corpus.* The junction of the corpus and cervix forms the *lower uterine segment.*

The thick uterine wall consists of mucosal, muscular, and serous layers. The inner mucosal lining — the *endometrium* — undergoes cyclic changes to facilitate and maintain pregnancy.

The smooth muscular middle layer — the *myometrium* — interlaces the uterine and ovarian arteries and veins that circulate blood through the uterus. During pregnancy, this vascular system expands dramatically. Afterward, the myometrium contracts to constrict the vasculature and control the loss of blood.

The outer serous layer, the *parietal peritoneum,* covers all the fundus, part of the corpus, but none of the cervix. This incompleteness allows surgical entry into the uterus without incision of the peritoneum, thereby reducing the risk of peritonitis.

The *fallopian tubes,* which extend from the sides of the fundus and terminate near the ovaries, are about 3¼″ to 5½″ (8 to 14 cm) long. Through ciliary and muscular action, they carry ova from the ovaries to the uterus and facilitate the movement of sperm from the uterus toward the ovaries. Fertilization of the ovum normally occurs in a fallopian tube. The same ciliary and muscular action helps move a *zygote* (fertilized ovum) down to the uterus, where it implants in the blood-rich inner uterine lining, the endometrium.

The *ovaries* are two almond-shaped organs, one on either side of the fundus, situated behind and below the fallopian tubes. The ovaries produce ova and two primary hormones—estrogen and progesterone—in addition to small amounts of androgen. These hormones, in turn, produce and maintain secondary sex characteristics, prepare the uterus for pregnancy, and stimulate mammary gland development.

The ovaries are connected to the uterus by the utero-ovarian ligament and are divided into two parts: the *cortex,* which contains primordial and graafian follicles in various stages of development, and the *medulla,* which consists primarily of vasculature and loose connective tissue.

A normal female is born with at least 400,000 primordial follicles in her ovaries. At puberty, these ova precursors become graafian follicles, in response to the effects of pituitary gonadotropic hormones—follicle-stimulating hormone (FSH) and luteinizing hormone (LH). In the life cycle of a female, however, fewer than 500 ova eventually mature and develop the potential for fertilization.

Menstrual cycle

Maturation of the hypothalamus and the resultant increase in hormone levels initiate puberty. In the young girl, breast development—the first sign of puberty—is followed by the appearance of pubic and axillary hair and the characteristic adolescent growth spurt. The reproductive system begins to undergo a series of hormone-induced changes that result in *menarche,* onset of menstruation (or menses). Menarche usually occurs at about age 13 but may occur anytime between ages 9 and 18. Usually, initial menstrual periods are irregular and anovulatory, but after a year or so, periods generally are more regular.

Three phases

The menstrual cycle consists of three phases: menstrual, proliferative (estrogen-dominated), and secretory (progesterone-dominated). These phases correspond to the phases of ovarian function. The menstrual and proliferative phases correspond to the follicular ovarian phase; the secretory phase, to the luteal ovarian phase. (See *How the menstrual cycle reflects ovarian function.*)

The *menstrual phase* begins with day 1 of menstruation. During this phase, decreased estrogen and progesterone levels provoke shedding of most of the endometrium. When these hormone levels are low, pos-

itive feedback causes the hypothalamus to produce FSH-releasing factor and LH-releasing factor. These two factors, in turn, stimulate pituitary secretion of FSH and LH. FSH stimulates the growth of ovarian follicles; LH stimulates these follicles to secrete estrogen.

The *proliferative phase* begins with the cessation of the menstrual period and ends with ovulation. During this phase, the increased amount of estrogen secreted by the developing ovarian follicles causes the endometrium to proliferate in preparation for possible pregnancy. At about day 14 of a 28-day menstrual cycle (the average length), these high estrogen levels trigger ovulation—the rupture of one of the developing follicles and subsequent release of an ovum.

The *secretory phase* extends from the day of ovulation to about 3 days before the next menstrual period (premenstrual phase). In most women, this final phase of the menstrual cycle lasts 13 to 15 days (its length varies less than those of the menstrual and proliferative phases). After ovulation, the ruptured follicle that released the ovum remains under the influence of LH. It then becomes the *corpus luteum* and starts secreting progesterone, in addition to estrogen.

Fertilization

In the nonpregnant female, LH controls the secretions of the corpus luteum; in the pregnant female, human chorionic gonadotropin (HCG) controls them. At the end of the secretory phase, the uterine lining is ready to receive and nourish a zygote.

If fertilization doesn't occur, increasing estrogen and progesterone levels decrease FSH and LH production. Because LH is necessary to maintain the corpus luteum, a decrease in LH production causes the corpus luteum to atrophy and stop secreting estrogen and progesterone. The thickened uterine lining then begins to slough off, and menstruation begins again.

However, if fertilization and pregnancy do occur, the endometrium grows even thicker. After implantation of the zygote (about 5 or 6 days after fertilization), the endometrium becomes the *decidua.* Chorionic villi produce HCG soon after implantation, stimulating the corpus luteum to continue secreting estrogen and progesterone, a process that prevents further ovulation and menstruation.

HCG continues to stimulate the corpus luteum until the placenta—the vascular organ that develops to transport materials to and from the fetus—forms and starts producing its own estrogen and progesterone. After the placenta takes over hormonal production, secretions of the corpus luteum are no longer needed to maintain the

HOW THE MENSTRUAL CYCLE REFLECTS OVARIAN FUNCTION

Endometrial changes experienced during the menstrual cycle reflect the phases of ovarian function, as illustrated below.

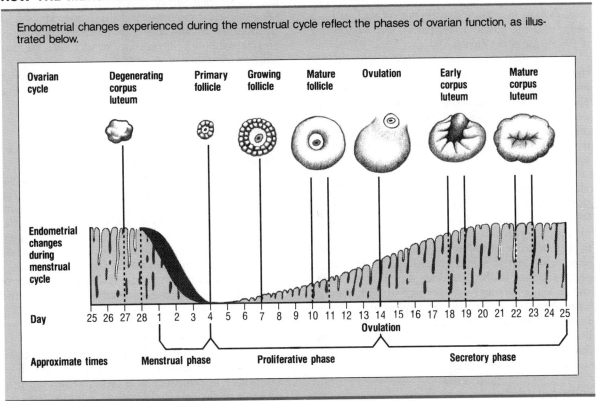

pregnancy, and the corpus luteum gradually decreases its function and begins to degenerate.

Pregnancy

Cell multiplication and differentiation begin in the zygote at the moment of conception. By about 17 days after conception, the placenta has established circulation to what is now an *embryo* (the term used for the conceptus between the 2nd and 7th weeks of pregnancy). By the end of the embryonic stage, fetal structures are formed. Further development now consists primarily of growth and maturation of already formed structures. From this point until birth, the conceptus is called a *fetus*.

The length of a normal pregnancy ranges from 240 to 300 days. Although pregnancies vary in duration, they're conveniently divided into three trimesters.

First trimester

During the first trimester, a female usually experiences physical changes, such as amenorrhea, urinary frequency, nausea and vomiting (more severe in the morning or when the stomach is empty), breast swelling and tenderness, fatigue, increased vaginal secretions, and constipation.

Within 10 days of conception, pregnancy tests, which detect HCG in the urine and serum, are usually positive. Although such positive tests strongly suggest pregnancy, a pelvic examination helps confirm it by showing Hegar's sign (cervical and uterine softening), Chadwick's sign (a bluish coloration of the vagina and cervix resulting from increased venous circulation), and an enlarged uterus.

The first trimester is a critical time during pregnancy. Rapid cell differentiation makes the developing embryo or fetus highly susceptible to the teratogenetic effects of viruses, alcohol, cigarettes, caffeine, and other drugs.

Second trimester

During the second trimester (from the 13th to the 26th week of pregnancy), uterine and fetal size increase substantially, causing weight gain, a thickening waistline, abdominal enlargement and, possibly, reddish streaks as abdominal skin stretches (striation). In addition, pigment changes may cause skin alterations, such as linea nigra, melasma (mask of pregnancy), and a darkening of the areolae of the nipples.

Other physical changes may include diaphoresis, increased salivation, indigestion, continuing constipation, hemorrhoids, nosebleeds, and some dependent edema. The breasts become larger and heavier, and about 19 weeks after the last menstrual period, they may secrete colostrum. By about the 16th to 18th week of pregnancy, the fetus is large enough for the mother to feel it move (quickening).

Third trimester

During the third trimester, the mother feels Braxton Hicks contractions—sporadic episodes of painless uterine tightening—which help strengthen uterine muscles in preparation for labor. Increasing uterine size may displace pelvic and intestinal structures, causing indigestion, protrusion of the umbilicus, shortness of breath, and insomnia. The mother may experience backaches because she walks with a swaybacked posture to counteract her frontal weight. By lying on her left side, she may help minimize the development of varicose veins, hemorrhoids, and ankle edema. This position relieves pressure on the lower vasculature.

Labor and delivery

About 2 to 4 weeks before birth, lightening—the descent of the fetal head into the pelvis—shifts the uterine position. This relieves pressure on the diaphragm and enables the mother to breathe more easily.

Onset of labor characteristically produces low back pain and passage of a small amount of bloody show (although this brownish or blood-tinged plug of cervical mucus may be passed up to 2 weeks before active labor). As labor progresses, the cervix becomes soft, then effaces and dilates; the amniotic membranes may rupture spontaneously, causing a gush or leakage of amniotic fluid. Uterine contractions become increasingly regular, frequent, intense, and longer.

Four stages

Labor is usually divided into four stages (see *Stages of labor*).

• *Stage I*, the longest stage, lasts from onset of regular contractions until full cervical dilation (4″ [10 cm]). The average duration of this stage is about 12 hours for a primigravida and 6 hours for a multigravida.

• *Stage II* lasts from full cervical dilation until delivery of the infant—about 1 to 2 hours for a primigravida, 30 minutes for a multigravida.

• *Stage III*, the time between delivery and expulsion of the placenta, usually lasts 3 to 4 minutes for a primigravida and 4 to 5 minutes for a multigravida, but may last up to 30 minutes.

• *Stage IV* constitutes a period of recovery during which homeostasis is reestablished. This final stage lasts 1 to 4 hours after expulsion of the placenta.

Assessment

In no other part of the body do so many interrelated physiologic functions occur in such proximity as in the area of the female reproductive tract. Besides the internal genitalia, the female pelvis contains the organs of the urinary and the GI systems. The reproductive tract and its surrounding area are thus the site of urination, defecation, menstruation, ovulation, copulation, impregnation, and parturition. An abnormality in one pelvic organ can readily induce an abnormality in another.

As with other body systems, thorough assessment of the reproductive system relies on an accurate history and physical examination.

History

A complete history includes information about the patient's overall patterns of health and illness, as well as any history of pregnancy or abortion. Other pertinent data include the date of the patient's last menstrual period, whether her periods are regular or irregular, and the patient's sexual history, including number of partners, frequency, satisfaction, and current method of birth control. The patient's family history, personal medical and surgical history, allergies, and habits, such as smoking or alcohol use, should also be documented.

Common chief complaints associated with gynecologic or obstetric disorders include pain, especially associated with the menstrual cycle or intercourse; abnormal vaginal discharge accompanied by burning or itching; disturbances of the menstrual cycle; infertility; and changes in patterns of urinary elimination. Many disorders produce no symptoms and may be detected only during routine physical examinations.

Physical examination

This careful examination should include the patient's thyroid gland, heart, lungs, breasts, abdomen, extremities, and pelvis. Measuring vital signs, height, and weight allows comparison with expected values to es-

STAGES OF LABOR

Labor begins with the onset of regular uterine contractions, when the head of the fetus is engaged in the mother's pelvis. It ends when the placenta is delivered.

Lightening
About 2 to 4 weeks before birth and before the onset of regular contractions, the fetal head descends into the pelvis.

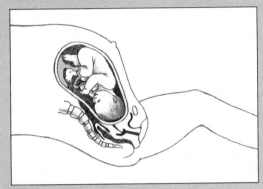

Stage I
In this stage, the onset of regular contractions and rupture of the amniotic sac proceed to full cervical dilation.

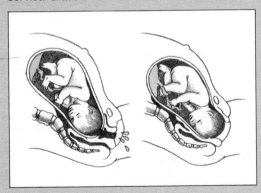

Stage II
This stage lasts from full cervical dilation until delivery of the neonate. Delivering the head and rotating the head are shown here.

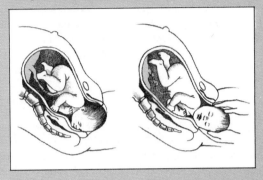

Stage III
The time between delivery and expulsion of the placenta makes up stage III.

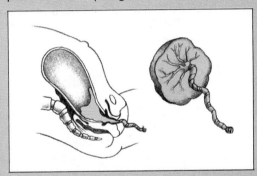

Stage IV
Reestablishment of homeostasis during this stage includes recuperation from the anesthetic (if used), normalization of vital signs, cessation of bleeding, and return of muscle tone.

tablish a baseline for the patient. Assessing nutritional status completes the examination.

Diagnostic tests
For gynecologic disorders, diagnostic tests include the following studies, which can be performed in an outpatient setting:

• *wet smear,* to examine vaginal secretions for specific organisms, such as *Trichomonas vaginalis, Candida albicans,* or *Haemophilus vaginalis,* or to evaluate semen specimens in rape or infertility cases
• *endometrial biopsy,* to assess hormonal secretions of the corpus luteum, to determine whether normal ovulation is occurring, and to check for neoplasia

• *hysteroscopy,* as an adjunct to endometrial biopsy, used with laparoscopy to directly view the uterus and to confirm uterine fibroid tumors and adhesions
• *dilatation and curettage,* to evaluate atypical bleeding and to detect carcinoma
• *echosteroscopy,* a relatively new diagnostic tool that combines ultrasonography with hysteroscopy, to visualize internal structures and detect abnormalities
• *laparoscopy,* to evaluate infertility, dysmenorrhea, and pelvic pain, and as a means of sterilization. Laparoscopy can be performed only in a hospital while the patient is under anesthesia.

GYNECOLOGIC DISORDERS

Common gynecologic complaints may arise from menstrual problems, such as premenstrual syndrome, and infections, such as vulvovaginitis and pelvic inflammatory disease. Hormonal dysfunction can lead to other gynecologic disorders, such as endometriosis and infertility. Also, the development of benign tumors can account for such disorders as ovarian cysts and uterine leiomyomas.

PREMENSTRUAL SYNDROME

Common among menstruating women, premenstrual syndrome (PMS) is characterized by a group of somatic, behavioral, cognitive, and mood symptoms that appear 1 to 10 days before menses and usually subside with its onset. Its effects range from minimal discomfort to severe, disruptive symptoms and can include anxiety, irritability, depression, and multiple somatic complaints.

Reportedly, 70% to 90% of women experience PMS sometime during their childbearing years, usually between ages 25 and 45.

Causes
Although the cause of PMS is unknown, the syndrome is generally thought to result from many causes. PMS has been linked to physiologic, psychological, and sociocultural factors. It was previously believed to result from a progesterone deficiency in the luteal phase of the ovarian cycle or from an increased estrogen-progesterone ratio. About 10% of patients with PMS have elevated prolactin levels.

Other conditions thought to contribute to PMS include abnormal carbohydrate metabolism, salt and water imbalance, nutritional and vitamin deficiencies, mental and emotional disorders, and tubal ligation. A relationship also seems to exist between PMS and changes in endorphin levels. Recent research has focused on diminished serotonin levels in the brain.

Complications
Women affected by PMS may experience psychosocial complications, such as lowered self-esteem, depression, and the inability to function in home, work, or school settings.

Assessment findings
The history may list behavioral changes, ranging from mild to severe personality changes, nervousness, hostility, irritability, agitation, sleep disturbances, fatigue, lethargy, and depression. The patient may also report breast tenderness or swelling, abdominal tenderness or bloating, joint pain, headache, edema, diarrhea or constipation, and exacerbations of skin, respiratory, or neurologic problems.

Diagnostic tests
A daily symptom calendar (in which the patient records menstrual symptoms for two to three menstrual cycles) is the single most useful tool in diagnosing PMS.

Blood studies may rule out anemia, thyroid disease, or other hormonal imbalances.

A psychological evaluation may rule out or detect an underlying psychiatric disorder.

Treatment
Education and reassurance that PMS is a real, physiologic syndrome are vital parts of treatment. Essentially, treatment aims to relieve the patient's symptoms. Initial interventions may focus on life-style changes, such as decreasing caffeine consumption; eating a low-fat, high-complex carbohydrate diet; increasing calcium intake; increasing aerobic exercise; reducing stress; and practicing relaxation techniques.

Treatment may include tranquilizers, sedatives, antidepressants, vitamins, progestins, prostaglandin inhibitors, and nonsteroidal anti-inflammatory drugs.

Nursing diagnoses
• Altered family processes
• Altered role performance
• Altered sexuality patterns
• Anxiety
• Body image disturbance
• Fluid volume excess
• Impaired social interaction

- Ineffective individual coping
- Knowledge deficit
- Pain
- Situational low self-esteem

Nursing interventions
- Encourage the patient and family to express their feelings. Offer emotional support and reassurance that the patient's mood changes are related to the disorder and can be controlled with treatment.
- Help the patient develop coping strategies. If necessary, refer her for psychological counseling, and refer her and her partner for sexual counseling.
- Consult a dietitian to provide a diet low in salt, caffeine, and fat, and high in complex carbohydrates.
- Encourage the patient to drink adequate fluids to promote diuresis and decrease bloating and edema.
- Provide comfort measures to relieve pain.

Patient teaching
- Discuss life-style changes that might help alleviate symptoms. Advise further medical consultation if severe symptoms disrupt the patient's life-style.
- Point out that self-help groups exist for women with PMS. If appropriate, help her contact such a group.

VULVOVAGINITIS
An inflammation of the vulva (vulvitis) and vagina (vaginitis), vulvovaginitis may occur at any age and affects most females at some time. Because of the proximity of these two structures, inflammation of one usually precipitates inflammation of the other. The prognosis is good with treatment.

Causes
Common causes of vaginitis (with or without consequent vulvitis) include:
- infection with *Trichomonas vaginalis,* a protozoan flagellate, usually transmitted through intercourse
- infection with *Candida albicans,* a fungus that requires glucose for growth. Incidence rises during the secretory phase of the menstrual cycle. Such infection occurs twice as often in pregnant females as in nonpregnant females. It also commonly affects users of oral contraceptives, diabetic patients, and patients receiving systemic therapy with broad-spectrum antibiotics.
- infection with *Gardnerella vaginalis,* a gram-negative bacillus
- venereal infection with *Neisseria gonorrhoeae* (gonorrhea), a gram-negative diplococcus

- viral infection with venereal warts (condylomata acuminata) or herpes simplex virus II, usually transmitted by intercourse
- vaginal mucosa atrophy in menopausal women due to decreasing estrogen levels, which predisposes these women to bacterial invasion.

Common causes of vulvitis include:
- parasitic infection (*Phthirus pubis,* crab louse)
- traumatic injury or poor personal hygiene
- chemical irritations or allergic reactions to hygiene sprays, douches, detergents, clothing, or toilet paper
- vulval atrophy in menopausal women due to decreasing estrogen levels
- retention of a foreign body, such as a tampon.

Complications
Inflammation and edema may affect the perineum. Skin breakdown may lead to secondary infection.

Assessment findings
Signs and symptoms may vary according to the infecting organism.

In *trichomonal vaginitis,* the patient may have vaginal irritation and itching along with urinary symptoms, such as burning and frequency. Inspection may reveal a vaginal discharge that is thin, bubbly, green-tinged, and malodorous.

A patient with *candidal vaginitis* may report intense vaginal itching and a thick, white, cottage-cheese-like discharge. Red, edematous mucous membranes with white flecks may be seen on the vaginal wall.

In *Gardnerella vaginitis,* inspection may disclose a gray, foul, fishy-smelling discharge.

Gonorrhea may produce no symptoms, or inspection may reveal a profuse, purulent discharge; the patient may complain of dysuria.

In *acute vulvitis,* the patient may complain of vulvar burning, pruritus, severe dysuria, and dyspareunia. Inspection may find vulvar edema and erythema.

In *herpesvirus infection,* you may note ulceration or vesicle formation on the perineum during the active phase; in chronic infection, severe edema that may involve the entire perineum.

Diagnostic tests
Diagnosis of vaginitis requires identification of the infectious organism during microscopic examination of vaginal exudate on a wet slide preparation (vaginal exudate applied to the slide is moistened by a drop of 0.9% sodium chloride solution and then a drop of potassium solution).

• In trichomonal infections, the presence of motile, flagellated trichomonads confirms the diagnosis.
• In candidal vaginitis, 10% potassium hydroxide is added to the slide; diagnosis requires identification of *C. albicans* fungi.
• In *Gardnerella* vaginitis, wet smear shows a striking absence of lactobacilli and few other bacteria.
• Gonorrhea requires a culture of vaginal exudate on Thayer-Martin or Transgrow medium to confirm the diagnosis.

Diagnosis of vulvitis or a suspected sexually transmitted disease may require a complete blood count, urinalysis, cytology screening, biopsy of chronic lesions to rule out cancer, and culture of exudate from acute lesions.

Treatment
Common therapeutic measures in vulvovaginitis include the following:
• metronidazole given orally for the patient with trichomonal vaginitis and all sexual partners (if possible) because recurrence often results from reinfection by an infected, asymptomatic male
• vaginal ointments and suppositories, such as nystatin, miconazole, or butoconazole; or oral fluconazole in a single dose for candidal vaginitis
• metronidazole for *Gardnerella* vaginitis
• systemic antibiotics (for the patient and the sexual partner), such as penicillin and probenecid (for gonorrhea) or tetracycline (for other infections).

Cold compresses or cool sitz baths may relieve pruritus in acute vulvitis; severe inflammation may require warm compresses. Other therapy includes avoiding drying soaps, wearing loose clothing to promote air circulation, and applying topical corticosteroids to reduce inflammation.

Chronic vulvitis may respond to topical hydrocortisone or antipruritics and good hygiene (especially in elderly or incontinent patients). Topical estrogen ointments may be used to treat atrophic vulvovaginitis. No cure currently exists for herpesvirus infections; however, oral and topical acyclovir decreases the duration and symptoms of active lesions.

Local treatment of genital warts usually consists of application of trichloroacetic acid.

Nursing diagnoses
• Altered sexuality patterns
• Body image disturbance
• Ineffective individual coping
• Knowledge deficit

• Pain
• Risk for impaired skin integrity
• Risk for infection

Nursing interventions
• Encourage the patient to express her feelings and help her develop effective coping strategies.
• Provide comfort measures, such as cool or warm compresses, to alleviate pain, burning, and pruritus.
• Use meticulous hand-washing technique. If necessary, use wound and skin precautions.
• Report cases of sexually transmitted diseases to the public health authorities.

Patient teaching
• Teach the patient about the correlation between sexual contact and the spread of vaginal infections. Provide information about the use of condoms to prevent or decrease the spread of sexually transmitted infections. Advise her to notify sexual partners of the need for treatment.
• Advise the patient to abstain from sexual intercourse until the infection resolves.
• Instruct her to use the entire medication prescription as ordered, even if symptoms subside.
• Teach her how to insert vaginal ointments and suppositories. Tell her to remain prone for at least 30 minutes after insertion to promote absorption. Suggest that she wear a pad to prevent staining her underclothing.
• Emphasize the need for meticulous hand washing before and after drug administration. Advise her that scratching may cause skin breakdown and secondary infections.
• Encourage good hygiene. Advise the patient with a history of recurrent vulvovaginitis to wear all-cotton underpants. Tell her to avoid wearing tight-fitting pants and panty hose.
• Warn the patient on metronidazole therapy to abstain from alcoholic beverages because the alcohol may provoke a disulfiram-type reaction. Also tell the patient that this drug may turn the urine dark brown.

OVARIAN CYSTS
Usually nonneoplastic, ovarian cysts are sacs on an ovary. These cysts contain fluid or semisolid material. Though they are usually small and produce no symptoms, they require thorough investigation as possible sites of malignant change. Common ovarian cysts include follicular cysts, lutein cysts (granulosa-lutein, corpus luteum, and theca-lutein cysts), and polycystic (or

sclerocystic) ovarian disease. Ovarian cysts can develop anytime between puberty and menopause, including during pregnancy. Granulosa-lutein cysts occur infrequently, usually during early pregnancy. The prognosis for nonneoplastic cysts is excellent.

Causes and pathophysiology

Follicular cysts are usually small and arise from follicles that overdistend instead of going through the atretic stage of the menstrual cycle. They appear semitransparent and are filled with a watery fluid visible through their thin walls. When such cysts persist into menopause, they secrete excessive amounts of estrogen in response to the hypersecretion of follicle-stimulating hormone and luteinizing hormone that normally occurs during menopause.

Granulosa-lutein cysts, which occur within the corpus luteum, are functional, nonneoplastic enlargements of the ovaries, caused by excessive accumulation of blood during menstruation.

Theca-lutein cysts are commonly bilateral and filled with clear, straw-colored fluid; they're often associated with hydatidiform mole, choriocarcinoma, or hormone therapy (with human chorionic gonadotropin [HCG] or clomiphene citrate).

Polycystic ovarian disease is part of the Stein-Leventhal syndrome and stems from endocrine abnormalities.

Complications

Possible complications include amenorrhea, oligomenorrhea, secondary dysmenorrhea, and infertility. Torsion of the ovary and fallopian tube may result in rupture of the cyst with resulting peritonitis or intraperitoneal hemorrhage, shock, and death.

Assessment findings

Small ovarian cysts (such as follicular cysts) usually don't produce symptoms unless torsion or rupture occurs. The patient may report mild pelvic discomfort, low back pain, dyspareunia, or abnormal uterine bleeding secondary to a disturbed ovulatory pattern. Inspection may reveal signs of an acute abdomen similar to signs of appendicitis (abdominal tenderness, distention, and rigidity).

Granulosa-lutein cysts that appear early in pregnancy may grow as large as 2″ to 2½″ (5.1 to 6.4 cm) in diameter and produce unilateral pelvic discomfort. If rupture occurs, massive intraperitoneal hemorrhage may result. A nonpregnant patient may report delayed menses, followed by prolonged or irregular bleeding.

Palpation may detect enlarged ovaries caused by lack of ovulation. It may also reveal large follicular cysts. Theca-lutein cysts, however, usually aren't palpable.

Diagnostic tests

Visualization of the ovary through ultrasonography, laparoscopy, or surgery (often for another condition) confirms ovarian cysts. The following tests provide additional diagnostic information:
• *HCG titers* that are extremely elevated strongly suggest theca-lutein cysts.
• *Urine 17-ketosteroid concentrations* that are slightly elevated accompany polycystic ovarian disease.
• *Basal body temperature graphs* and *endometrial biopsy* results indicate anovulation.

Direct visualization must rule out paraovarian cysts of the broad ligament, salpingitis, endometriosis, and neoplastic cysts.

Treatment

Follicular cysts generally don't require treatment because they tend to disappear spontaneously by reabsorption or silent rupture within 60 days. Follicular cysts are usually observed for one menstrual cycle; if they persist, oral contraceptives are used to accelerate involution.

Treatment for granulosa-lutein cysts that occur during pregnancy is based on the patient's symptoms because these cysts diminish during the third trimester and rarely require surgery. Theca-lutein cysts disappear spontaneously after elimination of the hydatidiform mole, destruction of choriocarcinoma, or discontinuation of HCG or clomiphene citrate therapy.

Treatment for polycystic ovarian disease may include drugs, such as hydrocortisone or clomiphene citrate, to induce ovulation or, if drug therapy fails to induce ovulation, surgical wedge resection of one-third to one-half of the ovary.

Indications for surgical intervention (cystectomy) for both diagnosis and treatment include the following: a cyst that remains after one menstrual period, a cystic mass that is larger than 3″ (or over 8 cm) or that persists longer than 8 weeks, a solid mass, or an adnexal mass after menopause.

Nursing diagnoses
• Altered sexuality patterns
• Anxiety
• Ineffective individual coping
• Knowledge deficit
• Pain

Nursing interventions

• Before surgery, watch for signs of cyst rupture, such as increasing abdominal pain, distention, and rigidity. Monitor vital signs for fever, tachypnea, or hypotension, a sign of possible peritonitis or intraperitoneal hemorrhage. Administer sedatives, as ordered, to ensure adequate preoperative rest.

• After surgery, encourage frequent movement in bed and early ambulation.

• Encourage the patient to discuss her feelings, provide emotional support, and help her develop effective coping strategies.

Patient teaching

• Carefully explain the nature of the particular cyst, the type of discomfort — if any — the patient may experience, and how long the condition may last.

• Before discharge, advise the patient to increase her at-home activity gradually — preferably over 4 to 6 weeks. Tell her to abstain from intercourse, using tampons, and douching during this time.

ENDOMETRIOSIS

When endometrial tissue appears outside the lining of the uterine cavity, endometriosis results. Such ectopic tissue is generally confined to the pelvic area, most commonly around the ovaries, uterovesical peritoneum, uterosacral ligaments, and the cul-de-sac, but it can appear anywhere in the body.

This ectopic endometrial tissue responds to normal stimulation in the same way that the endometrium does. During menstruation, the ectopic tissue bleeds, which causes inflammation of the surrounding tissues. This inflammation causes fibrosis, leading to adhesions, which produce pain and infertility.

Active endometriosis usually occurs between ages 30 and 40, especially in women who postpone childbearing; it's uncommon before age 20. Severe symptoms of endometriosis may have an abrupt onset or may develop over many years. This disorder usually becomes progressively severe during the menstrual years but tends to subside after menopause.

Causes and pathophysiology

The direct cause is unknown, but familial susceptibility or recent hysterotomy may predispose a woman to endometriosis. Although neither of these possible predisposing factors explains all the lesions in endometriosis or their location, research focuses on the following possible causes:

• *Transportation* (retrograde menstruation). During menstruation, the fallopian tubes expel endometrial fragments that implant outside the uterus.

• *Formation in situ.* Inflammation or a hormonal change triggers metaplasia.

• *Induction* (a combination of transportation and formation in situ). The endometrium chemically induces undifferentiated mesenchyma to form endometrial epithelium. (This is the most likely cause.)

• *Immune system defects.* Endometriosis may result from a specific defect in cell-mediated immunity. Researchers have documented higher titers of antibodies to endometrial antigens in patients with this disorder.

Complications

The primary complication of endometriosis is infertility. Other complications include spontaneous abortion, anemia due to excessive bleeding, and emotional problems due to infertility.

Assessment findings

The patient may complain of cyclic pelvic pain, infertility, and acquired dysmenorrhea. The patient typically reports pain in the lower abdomen, vagina, posterior pelvis, and back. This pain usually begins from 5 to 7 days before menses, reaches a peak, and lasts for 2 to 3 days. It differs from primary dysmenorrheal pain, which is more cramplike and concentrated in the abdominal midline. However, the severity of pain doesn't necessarily indicate the extent of the disease.

Other clinical features depend on the ectopic tissue site. The patient may report a history of infertility and profuse menses (oviducts and ovaries). She may complain of deep-thrust dyspareunia (ovaries and cul-de-sac); suprapubic pain, dysuria, and hematuria (bladder); painful defecation, rectal bleeding with menses, and pain in the coccyx or sacrum (rectovaginal septum and colon); nausea and vomiting that worsen before menses, and abdominal cramps (small bowel and appendix).

Palpation may detect multiple tender nodules on uterosacral ligaments or in the rectovaginal septum. These nodules enlarge and become more tender during menses. Palpation may also uncover ovarian enlargement in the presence of endometrial cysts on the ovaries or thickened, nodular adnexa (as in pelvic inflammatory disease).

Diagnostic tests

• *Laparoscopy* confirms the diagnosis and identifies the stage of the disease. A scoring and staging system created by the American Fertility Society quantifies endo-

metrial implants according to size, character and location. Stage I is minimal disease (1 to 5 points); Stage II signifies mild disease (6 to 15 points); Stage III, moderate disease (16 to 40 points); and Stage IV, severe disease (more than 40 points).
• *Barium enema* rules out malignant or inflammatory bowel disease.

Treatment

The stage of the disease and the patient's age and desire to have children determine the course of treatment.

Conservative therapy for young women who want to have children includes androgens, such as danazol, which produce a temporary remission in Stages I and II. Progestins and oral contraceptives also relieve symptoms. Newer treatment involves gonadotropin-releasing analogues, which suppress estrogen production. This causes atrophic changes in the ectopic endometrial tissue, which allows healing.

Laparoscopy, used for diagnostic purposes, can also be used therapeutically to lyse adhesions, remove small implants, and cauterize implants. Laparoscopy also permits laser vaporization of implants. This surgery is usually followed with hormonal therapy to suppress the return of endometrial implants.

When the patient has ovarian masses, surgery may be needed to rule out cancer. Conservative surgery is possible, but the treatment of choice for women who don't want to bear children or for extensive disease (Stages III and IV) is a total abdominal hysterectomy with bilateral salpingo-oophorectomy.

Minor gynecologic procedures are contraindicated immediately before and during menstruation.

Nursing diagnoses

• Anxiety
• Body image disturbance
• Chronic pain
• Ineffective individual coping
• Knowledge deficit
• Sexual dysfunction

Nursing interventions

• Encourage the patient and her partner to verbalize their feelings about the disorder and its effect on their relationship. Offer emotional support. Stress the need for open communication before and during intercourse to minimize discomfort and frustration.
• Help the patient to develop effective coping strategies. Refer her and her partner to a mental health professional for additional counseling, if necessary. Encourage her to

contact a support group, such as the Endometriosis Association.

Patient teaching

• Explain all procedures and treatment options. Clarify any misconceptions about the disorder, associated complications, and fertility.
• Advise adolescents to use sanitary napkins instead of tampons. This can help prevent retrograde flow in girls with a narrow vagina or small vaginal meatus.
• Because infertility is a possible complication, counsel the patient who wants children not to postpone childbearing.
• Advise the patient to have an annual pelvic examination and a Papanicolaou test.

UTERINE LEIOMYOMAS

The most common benign tumors in women, uterine leiomyomas are smooth-muscle tumors. Usually multiple, they generally occur in the uterine corpus, although they may appear on the cervix or on the round or broad ligament. Also known as myomas or fibromyomas, uterine leiomyomas are often called *fibroids,* but this term is misleading because leiomyomas consist of muscle cells and not fibrous tissue.

Uterine leiomyomas occur in about 20% of all women over age 35 and affect blacks three times more often than whites. Malignant tumors (leiomyosarcomas) develop from benign tumors in only about 0.1% of patients.

Causes and pathophysiology

The cause of uterine leiomyomas is unknown, but excessive levels of estrogen and growth hormone (GH) may influence tumor formation by stimulating susceptible fibromuscular elements. Large doses of estrogen and the later stages of pregnancy increase both tumor size and GH levels. Conversely, uterine leiomyomas usually shrink or disappear after menopause, when estrogen production decreases.

Complications

Possible complications include infertility, anemia from excessive bleeding, and possible intestinal obstruction if the tumors are large or twist around nearby organs. If the patient is pregnant, a leiomyoma may cause spontaneous abortion, premature labor, and dystocia.

Assessment findings

Usually, the patient's history reveals submucosal hypermenorrhea (the cardinal sign of uterine leiomyomas), although other forms of abnormal endometrial bleeding, as well as dysmenorrhea, are possible.

The patient may complain of pain if the tumors twist or degenerate after circulatory occlusion or infection or if the uterus contracts in an attempt to expel a pedunculated submucous leiomyoma. She may also report increasing abdominal girth without weight gain, a feeling of heaviness in the abdomen, constipation, and urinary frequency or urgency if the tumors press on surrounding organs. However, most women with leiomyomas are asymptomatic.

Palpation of the uterus may reveal irregular uterine enlargement, often asymptomatically. Palpation of the tumor may find a round or irregular mass.

Diagnostic tests
• *Blood studies* show anemia from abnormal bleeding.
• *Ultrasonography, dilatation and curettage,* and *submucosal hysterosalpingography* may detect submucosal leiomyomas.
• *Laparoscopy* visualizes subserous leiomyomas on the uterine surface.

Treatment
Medical management of uterine leiomyomas depends on the severity of symptoms; the size and location of the tumors; and the patient's age, parity, pregnancy status, desire to have children, and general health. Treatment options include the following:
• pelvic examination every 4 to 6 months, to monitor the growth of small leiomyomas that produce no symptoms
• surgical removal (myomectomy) of small leiomyomas that caused previous problems, threaten a future pregnancy, expand rapidly in the pelvis, bleed abnormally and persistently, produce pain or pressure, cause infertility, or enlarge beyond 3″ (8 cm). (*Note:* Myomectomy is the treatment of choice for a young woman who wants to have children.)
• hysterectomy (with preservation of the ovaries, if possible) for tumors that twist or grow large enough to cause intestinal obstruction.

If the patient is pregnant, but her uterus is no larger than a 6-month normal uterus by the 16th week of pregnancy, the outcome for the pregnancy is favorable, and surgery is usually unnecessary. However, if a pregnant woman has a leiomyomatous uterus the size of a 5- to 6-month normal uterus by the 9th week of pregnancy, spontaneous abortion will probably occur, especially with a cervical leiomyoma. If surgery is necessary, a hysterectomy is usually performed 5 to 6 months after de-

livery (when involution is complete), with preservation of the ovaries, if possible.

Nursing diagnoses
• Altered sexuality patterns
• Anxiety
• Ineffective individual coping
• Knowledge deficit
• Pain

Nursing interventions
• In a patient with severe anemia due to excessive bleeding, administer iron and blood transfusions, as ordered.
• Encourage the patient and her partner to verbalize their feelings about the disorder and its effect on their relationship. Offer emotional support.
• Help the patient develop effective coping strategies. Refer her and her partner to a mental health professional for additional counseling, if necessary.

Patient teaching
• Tell the patient to report any abnormal bleeding or pelvic pain immediately.
• If a hysterectomy or oophorectomy is indicated, explain the effects of the operation on menstruation, menopause, and sexual activity to the patient.
• Reassure the patient that she won't experience premature menopause if her ovaries are left intact.
• If the patient must have a multiple myomectomy, make sure she understands that pregnancy is still possible. However, if a hysterotomy is performed, explain that a cesarean delivery may be necessary.

FEMALE INFERTILITY
The inability to conceive after regular intercourse for at least 1 year without contraception, infertility affects 10% to 15% of all couples in the United States. Following extensive investigation and treatment, about half of infertile couples achieve pregnancy. Of the half who do not, roughly 10% have no pathologic basis for infertility; the prognosis in this group becomes extremely poor if pregnancy isn't achieved after 3 years.

Causes and pathophysiology
Female infertility may stem from functional, anatomic, or psychological causes.

Functional causes
Complex hormonal interactions determine the normal function of the female reproductive tract and require an

intact hypothalamic-pituitary-ovarian mechanism, a system that stimulates and regulates the hormones necessary for normal sexual development and function. Malfunction of this mechanism can cause infertility.

The ovary controls, and is controlled by, the hypothalamus through a system of negative and positive feedback mediated by estrogen production. Insufficient gonadotropin levels (both luteinizing and follicle-stimulating hormones) may result from infections, tumors, or neurologic disease of the hypothalamus or pituitary gland. Hypothyroidism also impairs fertility.

Anatomic causes
Possible anatomic causes of infertility include:
• *Ovarian factors* are related to anovulation and oligo-ovulation (infrequent ovulation) and are a major cause of infertility. Pregnancy or direct visualization provides irrefutable evidence of ovulation. Presumptive signs of ovulation include regular menses, cyclic changes reflected in basal body temperature readings, postovulatory progesterone levels, and endometrial changes due to the presence of progesterone. Absence of presumptive signs suggests anovulation.

Ovarian failure, in which no ova are produced by the ovaries, may result from ovarian dysgenesis or premature menopause. Amenorrhea is often associated with ovarian failure. Oligo-ovulation may result from a mild hormonal imbalance in gonadotropin production and regulation, which may be caused by polycystic ovary disease or abnormalities in the adrenal or thyroid gland that adversely affect hypothalamic-pituitary functioning.
• *Uterine abnormalities* may include congenitally absent uterus, bicornuate or double uterus, leiomyomas, or Asherman's syndrome, in which the anterior and posterior uterine walls adhere because of scar tissue formation.
• *Tubal and peritoneal factors* are due to faulty tubal transport mechanisms and unfavorable environmental influences affecting the sperm, ova, or recently fertilized ovum. Tubal loss or impairment may occur secondary to ectopic pregnancy.

In many cases, tubal and peritoneal factors result from anatomic abnormalities: bilateral occlusion of the tubes due to salpingitis (resulting from gonorrhea, tuberculosis, or puerperal sepsis); peritubal adhesions (resulting from endometriosis, pelvic inflammatory disease, use of an intrauterine device for contraception, diverticulosis, or childhood rupture of the appendix); and uterotubal obstruction due to tubal spasm.
• *Cervical factors* may include a malfunctioning cervix that produces deficient or excessively viscous mucus and is impervious to sperm, preventing entry into the uterus.

In cervical infection, viscous mucus may contain spermicidal macrophages. The possible existence of cervical antibodies that immobilize sperm is also under investigation.

Psychological causes
Relatively few cases of infertility stem from psychological problems. Occasionally, ovulation may stop under stress due to failure of luteinizing hormone release. More often, however, psychological problems result from, rather than cause, infertility.

Complications
Associated complications center on psychosocial problems.

Assessment findings
The patient's history indicates the inability to conceive after at least 1 year of regular intercourse without contraception. The patient may also report irregular, painless menses, which may indicate anovulation, or a history of pelvic inflammatory disease, which may suggest fallopian tube blockage.

Diagnostic tests
• *Basal body temperature graph* shows a sustained elevation in body temperature postovulation until just before onset of menses, indicating the approximate time of ovulation.
• *Endometrial biopsy,* done on or about day 5 after the basal body temperature elevates, provides histologic evidence that ovulation has occurred.
• *Cervical mucus evaluation* determines anovulatory or luteal phase deficiency.
• *Hysterosalpingography* provides radiologic evidence of tubal obstruction and uterine cavity abnormalities.
• *Endoscopy* confirms the results of hysterosalpingography and visualizes the endometrial cavity by hysteroscopy or explores the posterior surface of the uterus, fallopian tubes, and ovaries by culdoscopy.
• *Laparoscopy* allows visualization of the abdominal and pelvic areas.
• *Postcoital examination* examines the cervical mucus for motile sperm cells following intercourse that takes place at midcycle (as close to ovulation as possible).
• *Immunologic or antibody testing* detects spermicidal antibodies in the sera of the female.

Treatment
Identification of the underlying abnormality or dysfunction determines the appropriate treatment:

• In hyperactivity or hypoactivity of the adrenal or thyroid gland, hormonal therapy is necessary; progesterone deficiency requires progesterone replacement. Anovulation necessitates treatment with clomiphene citrate, human menopausal gonadotropins, or human chorionic gonadotropin; ovulation usually occurs several days after such administration. If mucus production decreases (an adverse effect of clomiphene citrate), small doses of estrogen to improve the quality of cervical mucus may be given concomitantly.
• Surgical restoration may correct certain anatomic causes of infertility, such as fallopian tube obstruction. Surgery may also be necessary to remove tumors located within or near the hypothalamus or pituitary gland.
• Endometriosis requires drug therapy (danazol, medroxyprogesterone, GnRh agonists, or noncyclic administration of oral contraceptives); surgical removal of areas of endometriosis; or a combination of both.
• Other options, often controversial and involving emotional and financial cost, include surrogate mothering, frozen embryos, in vitro fertilization, and gamete intrafallopian transfer.

Nursing diagnoses
• Altered sexuality patterns
• Anxiety
• Body image disturbance
• Dysfunctional grieving
• Hopelessness
• Ineffective family coping
• Ineffective individual coping
• Knowledge deficit
• Powerlessness
• Self-esteem disturbance

Nursing interventions
• Help the couple cope effectively with feelings of anxiety, hopelessness, and powerlessness by explaining all procedures thoroughly. Help boost the patients' self-esteem by encouraging them to talk about their feelings. Listen nonjudgmentally and with empathy.
• Help the couple to develop effective coping strategies. Refer them to a mental health counselor, if needed.
• Encourage the couple to join community support groups for infertile couples, if appropriate.

Patient teaching
• Teach the couple about normal reproductive anatomy and physiology and how theirs may differ.

• Explain all procedures and treatment options to help the couple make informed decisions. If surgery is required, explain what to expect after surgery.

PELVIC INFLAMMATORY DISEASE
An umbrella term, pelvic inflammatory disease (PID) refers to any acute, subacute, recurrent, or chronic infection of the oviducts and ovaries, with adjacent tissue involvement. It includes inflammation of the cervix (cervicitis), uterus (endometritis), fallopian tubes (salpingitis), and ovaries (oophoritis), which can extend to the connective tissue lying between the broad ligaments (parametritis). (See *Forms of PID: Features and test findings.*)

About 60% of cases result from overgrowth of one or more of the common bacterial species found in the cervical mucus. Early diagnosis and treatment help prevent damage to the reproductive system, as does well-planned nursing care. (See *Planning care for the patient with PID,* pages 1064 and 1065.) Untreated PID may be fatal.

Causes
PID can result from infection with aerobic or anaerobic organisms. The organisms *Neisseria gonorrhoeae* and *Chlamydia trachomatis* are the most common causes because they most readily penetrate the bacteriostatic barrier of cervical mucus.

Common bacteria found in cervical mucus include staphylococci, streptococci, diphtheroids, chlamydiae, and coliforms, including *Pseudomonas* and *Escherichia coli.* Uterine infection can result from any one or several of these organisms or may follow the multiplication of normally nonpathogenic bacteria in an altered endometrial environment. Bacterial multiplication is most common during parturition because the endometrium is atrophic, quiescent, and not stimulated by estrogen.

Risk factors include:
• any sexually transmitted infection
• multiple sex partners
• conditions or procedures, such as conization or cauterization of the cervix, that alter or destroy cervical mucus, allowing bacteria to ascend into the uterine cavity
• any procedure that risks transfer of contaminated cervical mucus into the endometrial cavity by an instrument, such as a biopsy curet or an irrigation catheter, or by tubal insufflation or abortion
• infection during or after pregnancy
• infectious foci within the body, such as drainage from a chronically infected fallopian tube, a pelvic abscess, a ruptured appendix, or diverticulitis of the sigmoid colon.

FORMS OF P.I.D.: FEATURES AND TEST FINDINGS

Clinical features	Diagnostic findings
Salpingo-oophoritis • *Acute:* sudden onset of lower abdominal and pelvic pain, usually following menses; increased vaginal discharge; fever; malaise; lower abdominal pressure and tenderness; tachycardia; pelvic peritonitis • *Chronic:* recurring acute episodes	• Blood studies show leukocytosis or a normal white blood cell (WBC) count. • X-rays may show ileus. • Pelvic examination reveals extreme tenderness. • Smear of cervical or periurethral gland exudate shows gram-negative intracellular diplococci.
Cervicitis • *Acute:* purulent, foul-smelling vaginal discharge; vulvovaginitis, with itching or burning; red, edematous cervix; pelvic discomfort; sexual dysfunction; metrorrhagia; infertility; spontaneous abortion • *Chronic:* cervical dystocia, laceration or eversion of the cervix, ulcerative vesicular lesion (when cervicitis results from herpes simplex virus 2)	• Cultures for *N. gonorrhoeae* are positive in more than 90% of patients. • Cytologic smears may reveal severe inflammation. • If cervicitis isn't complicated by salpingitis, WBC count is normal or slightly elevated; erythrocyte sedimentation rate (ESR) is elevated. • In *acute cervicitis*, cervical palpation reveals tenderness. • In *chronic cervicitis*, causative organisms are usually staphylococcus or streptococcus.
Endometritis (generally postpartum or postabortion) • *Acute:* mucopurulent or purulent vaginal discharge oozing from the cervix; edematous, hyperemic endometrium, possibly leading to ulceration and necrosis (with virulent organisms); lower abdominal pain and tenderness; fever; rebound pain; abdominal muscle spasm; thrombophlebitis of uterine and pelvic vessels (in severe forms) • *Chronic:* recurring acute episodes (increasingly common because of widespread use of intrauterine devices)	• In severe infection, palpation may reveal a boggy uterus. • Uterine and blood samples are positive for a causative organism, usually staphylococcus. • WBC count and ESR are elevated.

Complications

Possible complications of PID may include potentially fatal septicemia from a ruptured pelvic abscess, pulmonary emboli, infertility, and shock.

Assessment findings

The patient with PID may complain of profuse, purulent vaginal discharge, sometimes accompanied by low-grade fever and malaise (particularly if gonorrhea is the cause). She may also describe lower abdominal pain and vaginal bleeding. Vaginal examination may reveal pain during movement of the cervix or palpation of the adnexa.

Diagnostic tests

• *Gram stain* of secretions from the endocervix or cul-de-sac determines the causative agent.
• *Culture and sensitivity testing* aids selection of the appropriate antibiotic. Urethral and rectal secretions may also be cultured.

• *Ultrasonography, computed tomography scan,* and *magnetic resonance imaging* may help to identify and locate an adnexal or uterine mass.
• *Culdocentesis* obtains peritoneal fluid or pus for culture and sensitivity testing.

Treatment

To prevent progression of PID, antibiotic therapy begins immediately after culture specimens are obtained. Such therapy can be reevaluated as soon as laboratory results are available (usually after 24 to 48 hours). Infection may become chronic if treated inadequately.
• The preferred antibiotic therapy for PID includes I.V. doxycycline and cefoxitin for 4 to 6 days (alternative therapy includes clindamycin and gentamicin), followed by oral doxycycline for another 10 to 14 days. Outpatient therapy may consist of cefoxitin I.M. with probenecid and oral doxycycline for 14 days *or* oral ofloxacin with metronidazole or clindamycin for 14 days. The patient may also require therapy for syphilis.

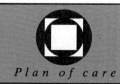

Plan of care

PLANNING CARE FOR THE PATIENT WITH P.I.D.

How can you best care for a patient with PID? To begin, use your assessment findings to help you develop nursing diagnoses and a plan of care. For instance, suppose you're caring for Vicki Hibbert, age 27, who just had a spontaneous abortion after becoming pregnant with an intrauterine device (IUD) in place.

Patient history

About 2 months ago, Ms. Hibbert discovered that she was pregnant, even though she had had an IUD contraceptive for more than 1 year. Infrequently during the year she noticed heavier than normal menstrual flow and twice experienced an annoying, milky, foul-smelling vaginal discharge that seemed to clear after several days' use of nonprescription douches and vaginal creams.

Four days before admission, she began to experience lower abdominal pain, with cramping and spotting of blood. This condition progressed over 48 hours to full menstruation-like bleeding with clot formation. She had a fever of 101° F (38.3° C). A purulent discharge and increased pain over the right ovary and fallopian tube quickly followed, associated with nausea and vomiting.

Assessment findings

Your assessment begins with Ms. Hibbert's vital signs. Her oral temperature is 103.2° F (39.4° C), and she's diaphoretic. Her pulse rate is 96 beats/minute and her respiratory rate is 28 breaths/minute. Her blood pressure is 110/66 mm Hg.

Inspection reveals a young, thin woman, grimacing with pain and splinting her lower abdomen with her hands. She states that sitting in the knee-chest position gives her the best pain relief. Her abdomen is distended and rigid and positive for rebound tenderness. She has diminished bowel sounds in all quadrants and tells you that she hasn't had a bowel movement for 4 or 5 days.

You assist with her pelvic examination and note severe tenderness when the doctor examines the right pelvis bimanually. The vaginal discharge is sent for a Papanicolaou smear and culture and sensitivity testing.

Preliminary laboratory test results disclose a white blood cell count of 16,250/ mm³. Ultrasonography reveals the displaced IUD along with endometrial congestion and early peritonitis. As a result, Ms. Hibbert is scheduled for dilatation and evacuation of the uterus, and she is immediately given I.V. penicillin G.

Nursing diagnoses

Based on your assessment findings and those of the gynecologist, you select the following nursing diagnoses:
• Pain related to swelling and suppuration in the peritoneal cavity
• Anxiety related to loss of the fetus and severe pelvic infection
• Self-esteem disturbance related to the stigma attached to reproductive system infections.

Expected outcomes

Carefully, you define immediate and long-term goals for Ms. Hibbert. She will:
• experience decreased pain and swelling in the pelvic region
• be less fearful and anxious about her immediate condition
• demonstrate increased self-esteem and understanding of contraceptive techniques.

Implementation

You plan the following interventions to help Ms. Hibbert achieve the expected goals.

To decrease pain and swelling

• Assess Ms. Hibbert's level of pain on a scale of 1 to 10, with 10 being the most severe pain. Reassess her pain level every few hours.
• Administer prescribed analgesics effective enough to override Ms. Hibbert's pain threshold. Encourage her to communicate any breakthrough pain immediately.
• Adjust Ms. Hibbert's analgesic dosage, as ordered.
• Assess her previous ways of coping with pain and stress. Suggest and help her develop alternative methods for dealing with pain: Use imagery, soft music, positioning, or other measures for comfort.
• Administer antibiotics, as ordered, to fight the infection and thereby diminish swelling.

To decrease fear and anxiety

• Explain all tests, procedures, and treatments beforehand. Answer the patient's questions and dispel any misconceptions.
• Fully explain, in layman's terms, the surgical procedure and possible complications if the procedure isn't done.
• Discuss the need for an I.V. line and administration of antibiotics and fluids.
• Allow Ms. Hibbert to perform or participate in as many activities of daily living as possible.
• Decrease her physical and emotional pain whenever possible; offer conversation, back rubs, and analgesics, and encourage loved ones and friends to visit; suggest professional counseling to help her accept the loss of the fetus.

PLANNING CARE FOR THE PATIENT WITH P.I.D. *(continued)*

To increase self-esteem
• Emphasize that the infection was not brought about through any fault of hers.
• Inform Ms. Hibbert that antibiotic treatment and surgery will restore her health.
• Encourage safe gynecologic care at home. Teach Ms. Hibbert to use mild soaps, take showers, avoid bubble baths, douche infrequently, use sanitary pads instead of tampons, and clean the perineum from front to back.
• Stress follow-up gynecologic and psychological care.
• Instruct her to report any unusual or malodorous discharge to her gynecologist.
• Advise Ms. Hibbert to encourage her sexual partner to use a condom if infection is suspected.

Evaluation
Your care will be successful if Ms. Hibbert shows a better understanding of her condition and exhibits less anxiety. You'll also know you've accomplished your goals if her self-esteem improves once she learns that she didn't cause the infection and can prevent its recurrence.

• Supplemental treatment of PID may include bed rest, analgesics, and I.V. fluids as needed.
• Development of a pelvic abscess necessitates adequate drainage. A ruptured pelvic abscess is a life-threatening condition. If this complication develops, the patient may need a total abdominal hysterectomy, with bilateral salpingo-oophorectomy.

Nursing diagnoses
• Altered sexuality patterns
• Anxiety
• Fluid volume deficit
• Ineffective individual coping
• Knowledge deficit
• Pain

Nursing interventions
• After establishing that the patient has no drug allergies, administer antibiotics and analgesics, as ordered.
• Monitor vital signs for fever and fluid intake and output for signs of dehydration. Watch for abdominal rigidity and distention, possible signs of developing peritonitis.
• Provide frequent perineal care if vaginal drainage occurs.
• Use meticulous hand-washing technique; follow wound and skin precautions, if necessary.
• Encourage the patient to discuss her feelings, offer emotional support, and help her develop effective coping strategies.

Patient teaching
• To prevent recurrence, encourage compliance with treatment, and explain the disease and its severity.
• Stress the need for the patient's sexual partner to be examined and, if necessary, treated for infection.
• Discuss the use of condoms to prevent the spread of sexually transmitted diseases.

• Because PID may cause dyspareunia, advise the patient to consult with her doctor about sexual activity.
• To prevent infection after minor gynecologic procedures, such as dilatation and curettage, tell the patient to immediately report any fever, increased vaginal discharge, or pain. After such procedures, instruct her to avoid douching or intercourse for at least 7 days.

DISORDERS OF PREGNANCY

Many obstetric disorders—including spontaneous abortion, ectopic pregnancy, pregnancy-induced hypertension, placenta previa, abruptio placentae, and premature labor—require emergency care. These disorders and others, such as premature rupture of the membranes and puerperal infection, may threaten the life of the mother, the fetus, or both.

ABORTION
In spontaneous abortion (miscarriage) or induced (therapeutic) abortion, the products of conception are expelled from the uterus before fetal viability (fetal weight of less than 17½ oz [about 500 g] and gestation of less than 20 weeks). Up to 15% of all pregnancies and about 30% of first pregnancies end in miscarriage. (See *Types of spontaneous abortion*, page 1066.) At least 75% of miscarriages occur during the first trimester. The incidence of legal induced abortions is rising in the United States.

Causes
Spontaneous abortion may result from fetal, placental, or maternal factors:
• *Fetal factors* usually cause such abortions between 9 and 12 weeks of gestation and include defective embry-

TYPES OF SPONTANEOUS ABORTION

Depending on clinical findings, a spontaneous abortion (miscarriage) may be threatened or inevitable; incomplete or complete; or missed, habitual, or septic. Here's how the seven types compare.

Threatened abortion
Bloody vaginal discharge occurs during the first half of pregnancy. About 20% of pregnant women have vaginal spotting or actual bleeding early in pregnancy; of these, about 50% abort.

Inevitable abortion
The membranes rupture and the cervix dilates. As labor continues, the uterus expels the products of conception.

Incomplete abortion
The uterus retains part or all of the placenta. Before the 10th week of gestation, the fetus and placenta usually are expelled together; after the 10th week, separately. Because part of the placenta may adhere to the uterine wall, bleeding continues. Hemorrhage is possible because the uterus doesn't contract and seal the large vessels that fed the placenta.

Complete abortion
The uterus passes all the products of conception. Minimal bleeding usually accompanies complete abortion because the uterus contracts and compresses the maternal blood vessels that fed the placenta.

Missed abortion
The uterus retains the products of conception for 2 months or more after the death of the fetus. Uterine growth ceases; uterine size may even seem to decrease. Prolonged retention of the dead products of conception may cause coagulation defects, such as disseminated intravascular coagulation.

Habitual abortion
Spontaneous loss of three or more consecutive pregnancies constitutes habitual abortion.

Septic abortion
Infection accompanies abortion. This may occur with spontaneous abortion but usually results from an illegal abortion or from the presence of an intrauterine device.

ologic development due to abnormal chromosome division (most common cause of fetal death), faulty implantation of fertilized ovum, and failure of the endometrium to accept the fertilized ovum.

• *Placental factors* usually cause abortion around the 14th week of gestation when the placenta takes over the hormone production necessary to maintain the pregnancy. Factors include premature separation of the normally implanted placenta, abnormal placental implantation, and abnormal platelet function.

• *Maternal factors* usually cause abortion between 11 and 19 weeks of gestation and include maternal infection, severe malnutrition, and abnormalities of the reproductive organs.

Other maternal factors include endocrine problems, such as thyroid gland dysfunction or lowered estriol secretion; trauma, including any type of surgery that necessitates manipulation of the pelvic organs; blood group incompatibility and Rh isoimmunization (still under investigation as a possible cause); and recreational drug use and environmental toxins.

Therapeutic abortion is performed to preserve the mother's mental or physical health in cases of rape, unplanned pregnancy, or medical conditions, such as cardiac dysfunction or fetal abnormality.

Complications
Possible complications of abortion may include infections (if the products of conception are not completely expelled), hemorrhage and anemia (if the bleeding is excessive and not controlled), and coagulation defects, such as disseminated intravascular coagulation (if the products of conception are retained for a long period).

Assessment findings
A patient who has experienced a spontaneous abortion may report a pink discharge for several days or a scant brown discharge for several weeks before onset of cramps and increased vaginal bleeding. She may describe cramps that appear for a few hours, intensify, and occur more frequently.

If the patient has expelled the entire contents of the uterus, the cramps and bleeding may subside. However, if any contents remain, cramps and bleeding will continue.

Diagnostic tests
• Human chorionic gonadotropin (HCG) in the blood or urine confirms pregnancy; *decreased HCG levels* suggest spontaneous abortion.

• *Cytologic analysis* indicates evidence of products of conception.

• *Laboratory tests* reflect decreased hematocrit and hemoglobin levels due to blood loss.

• *Ultrasound examination* confirms the presence or absence of fetal heart tones or an empty amniotic sac. The newer vaginal probe technique enables earlier visualization of the gestational sac.

Treatment

An accurate evaluation of uterine contents is necessary before planning treatment.

The progression of spontaneous abortion can't be prevented, except in those cases caused by an incompetent cervix. Hospitalization is necessary to control severe hemorrhage. Severe bleeding requires transfusion with packed red blood cells or whole blood. Initially, I.V. administration of oxytocin stimulates uterine contractions. If remnants remain in the uterus, dilatation and curettage (D&C) or dilatation and evacuation (D&E) should be performed.

D&E is also used in first-trimester induced abortions. In second-trimester induced abortions, an injection of hypertonic saline solution or of prostaglandin into the amniotic sac or insertion of a prostaglandin vaginal suppository induces labor and expulsion of uterine contents.

After an abortion, spontaneous or induced, an Rh-negative female with a negative indirect Coombs' test should receive $Rh_o(D)$ immune globulin (RhoGAM) to prevent future Rh isoimmunization.

In a habitual aborter, spontaneous abortion can result from an incompetent cervix. Treatment, therefore, involves surgical reinforcement of the cervix (cerclage, Shirodkar-Barter procedure) about 14 to 16 weeks after the last menstrual period. A few weeks before the estimated delivery date, the sutures are removed, and the patient waits for the onset of labor. An alternative procedure, especially for the woman who wants to have more children, is to leave the sutures in place, and to deliver the infant by cesarean section.

Nursing diagnoses

• Anxiety
• Dysfunctional grieving
• Ineffective family coping
• Ineffective individual coping
• Knowledge deficit
• Risk for infection

Nursing interventions

Before possible abortion:

• Do *not* allow bathroom privileges because the patient may expel uterine contents without knowing it. After she uses the bedpan, inspect the contents carefully for intrauterine material.

After spontaneous or elective abortion:

• Note the amount, color, and odor of vaginal bleeding. Save all pads the patient uses, for evaluation.
• Administer analgesics and oxytocin, as ordered.
• Check the patient's blood type and administer RhoGAM, as ordered.
• Provide good perineal care.
• Monitor vital signs every 4 hours for 24 hours.
• Monitor urine output.

After spontaneous abortion:

• Provide emotional support and counseling during the grieving process. Encourage the patient and her partner to express their feelings. Some couples may want to talk to a member of the clergy or, depending on their religion, may wish to have the fetus baptized.
• Help the patient to develop effective coping strategies.

After elective abortion:

• Encourage the patient to verbalize her feelings. Remember, she may feel ambivalent about the procedure; intellectual and emotional acceptance of abortion are not the same. Refer her for counseling, if necessary.

Patient teaching

• Explain all procedures thoroughly.
• Tell the patient to expect vaginal bleeding or spotting and to report immediately any bleeding that lasts longer than 8 to 10 days or excessive, bright red blood.
• Advise the patient to watch for signs of infection, such as a temperature higher than 100° F (37.8° C) and foul-smelling vaginal discharge.
• Encourage the gradual increase of daily activities to include whatever tasks the patient feels comfortable doing if these activities don't increase vaginal bleeding or cause fatigue. Most patients return to work within 1 to 4 weeks.
• Urge 2 to 3 weeks' abstinence from intercourse, and encourage the use of a contraceptive when the patient resumes intercourse.
• Instruct the patient to avoid using tampons for 2 to 4 weeks.
• Tell the patient to see her doctor in 2 to 4 weeks for a follow-up examination.

For elective abortion:

• Be sure to inform the patient of all the available alternatives. She needs to know what the procedure involves,

IMPLANTATION SITES OF ECTOPIC PREGNANCY

In roughly 95% of patients with ectopic pregnancy, the ovum implants in the fallopian tube—in the fimbria, ampulla, or isthmus. Other possible abnormal sites of implantation include the interstitium, tubo-ovarian ligament, ovary, abdominal viscera, and internal cervical os.

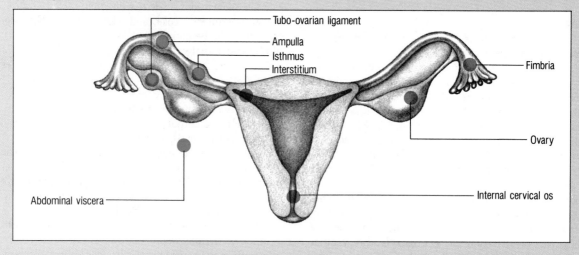

what the risks are, and what to expect during and after the procedure, both emotionally and physically. Be sure to ascertain whether the patient is comfortable with her decision to have an elective abortion. Encourage her to verbalize her thoughts when the procedure is performed and at a follow-up visit, usually 2 weeks later. If you identify an inappropriate coping response, refer the patient for professional counseling.
• To reduce the risks associated with repeated elective abortion, provide the patient with contraceptive information.

ECTOPIC PREGNANCY

Implantation of the fertilized ovum outside the uterine cavity, ectopic pregnancy most commonly occurs in the fallopian tube, but other sites are possible. (See *Implantation sites of ectopic pregnancy*.)

In whites, ectopic pregnancy occurs in about 1 in 200 pregnancies; in nonwhites, in about 1 in 120. The prognosis for the woman is good with prompt diagnosis, appropriate surgical intervention, and control of bleeding; rarely, in cases of abdominal implantation, the fetus may survive to term. Usually, only 1 in 3 women who experience an ectopic pregnancy give birth to a live neonate in a subsequent pregnancy.

Causes

Conditions that prevent or retard the passage of the fertilized ovum through the fallopian tube and into the uterine cavity include:
• *endosalpingitis,* an inflammatory reaction that causes folds of the tubal mucosa to agglutinate, narrowing the tube
• *diverticula,* the formation of blind pouches that cause tubal abnormalities
• *tumors* pressing against the tube
• *previous surgery* (tubal ligation or resection, or adhesions from previous abdominal or pelvic surgery)
• *transmigration of the ovum* (from one ovary to the opposite tube), resulting in delayed implantation.

Ectopic pregnancy may also result from congenital defects in the reproductive tract or ectopic endometrial implants in the tubal mucosa. The increased prevalence of sexually transmitted tubal infection may also be a factor as may the use of an intrauterine device (IUD), which causes irritation of the cellular lining of the uterus and the fallopian tubes.

Complications

Rupture of the tube causes life-threatening complications, including hemorrhage, shock, and peritonitis. Infertility results if the uterus or both fallopian tubes or both ovaries are removed.

Assessment findings

Ectopic pregnancy sometimes produces symptoms of normal pregnancy or no symptoms other than mild abdominal pain (the latter is especially likely in abdominal pregnancy), making diagnosis difficult.

Typically, the patient reports amenorrhea or abnormal menses (after fallopian tube implantation), followed by slight vaginal bleeding and unilateral pelvic pain over the mass.

If the tube ruptures, the patient may complain of sharp lower abdominal pain, possibly radiating to the shoulders and neck. She may indicate that this pain is often precipitated by activities that increase abdominal pressure, such as a bowel movement.

During a pelvic examination, the patient may report extreme pain when the cervix is moved and the adnexa is palpated. The uterus feels boggy and is tender.

Diagnostic tests

• *Serum pregnancy (human chorionic gonadotropin [HCG]) test* shows an abnormally low level of HCG and, when repeated in 48 hours, the level remains lower than the levels found in a normal intrauterine pregnancy.
• *Real-time ultrasonography* determines intrauterine pregnancy or ovarian cyst (performed if serum pregnancy test results are positive).
• *Culdocentesis* (aspiration of fluid from the vaginal cul-de-sac) detects free blood in the peritoneum (performed if ultrasonography detects absence of a gestational sac in the uterus).
• *Laparoscopy* may reveal pregnancy outside the uterus (performed if culdocentesis is positive).

Treatment

If culdocentesis shows blood in the peritoneum, laparotomy and salpingectomy are indicated, possibly preceded by laparoscopy, to remove the affected fallopian tube and control bleeding. Patients who wish to have children can undergo microsurgical repair of the fallopian tube. The ovary is saved, if possible; however, ovarian pregnancy requires oophorectomy.

Interstitial pregnancy may require hysterectomy; abdominal pregnancy requires a laparotomy to remove the fetus, except in rare cases, when the fetus survives to term or calcifies undetected in the abdominal cavity.

Supportive treatment includes transfusion with whole blood or packed red blood cells to replace excessive blood loss, administration of broad-spectrum I.V. antibiotics for sepsis, administration of supplemental iron (given orally or I.M.), and institution of a high-protein diet.

Nursing diagnoses

• Anxiety
• Dysfunctional grieving
• Fear
• Fluid volume deficit
• Ineffective individual coping
• Knowledge deficit

Nursing interventions

• Assess vital signs and monitor vaginal bleeding. Prepare the patient with excessive blood loss for emergency surgery. Administer blood transfusions (for replacement), as ordered, and provide emotional support.
• Record the location and character of the pain, and administer analgesics, as ordered.
• Check the amount, color, and odor of vaginal bleeding.
• Monitor vital signs and fluid intake and output for signs of hypovolemia and impending shock.
• Determine if the patient is Rh-negative. If she is, administer $Rh_o(D)$ immune globulin (RhoGAM), as ordered. Ask the patient the date of her last menstrual period, and have her describe the character of this period.
• Provide a quiet, relaxing environment, and encourage the patient and her partner to express their feelings of fear, loss, and grief. Help the patient to develop effective coping strategies. Refer her to a mental health professional for additional counseling, if necessary.

Patient teaching

• Teach the patient about the anatomic structures and reproductive processes involved in this disorder. Explain all procedures and treatment options. Prepare her for surgery, and discuss what to expect postoperatively.
• To prevent recurrent ectopic pregnancy, advise prompt treatment of pelvic infections to prevent diseases of the fallopian tube. Inform patients who have undergone surgery involving the fallopian tubes or those with confirmed pelvic inflammatory disease that they are at increased risk for another ectopic pregnancy.

HYPEREMESIS GRAVIDARUM

Unlike the transient nausea and vomiting normally experienced until about the 12th week of pregnancy, hyperemesis gravidarum is severe and unremitting nausea and vomiting that persists after the first trimester. It usually occurs with the first pregnancy and commonly affects pregnant women with conditions that produce high levels of human chorionic gonadotropin, such as hydatidiform mole or multiple pregnancy.

This disorder occurs among blacks in about 7 in 1,000 pregnancies and among whites in about 1·6 in 1,000 pregnancies. The prognosis is good.

Causes

Although the specific cause of hyperemesis gravidarum is unknown, possible causes include pancreatitis (elevated serum amylase levels are common), biliary tract disease, decreased secretion of free hydrochloric acid in the stomach, decreased gastric motility, drug toxicity, inflammatory obstructive bowel disease, and vitamin deficiency (especially of B_6). In some patients, this disorder may be related to psychological factors.

Complications

If untreated, hyperemesis gravidarum produces substantial weight loss; starvation, with ketosis and acetonuria; dehydration, with subsequent fluid and electrolyte imbalance (hypokalemia); and acid-base disturbances (acidosis and alkalosis). Retinal, neurologic, and renal damage may also occur.

Assessment findings

The patient typically complains of unremitting nausea and vomiting, the cardinal symptoms of hyperemesis gravidarum. The vomitus initially contains undigested food, mucus, and small amounts of bile; later, it contains only bile and mucus; and finally, blood and material that resembles coffee grounds. The patient may report substantial weight loss and eventual emaciation caused by persistent vomiting, thirst, hiccups, oliguria, vertigo, and headache.

Inspection may reveal pale, dry, waxy, and possibly jaundiced skin, with decreased skin turgor; a dry and coated tongue; subnormal or elevated temperature; rapid pulse; and a fetid, fruity breath odor from acidosis. The patient may appear confused and delirious. Lassitude, stupor and, possibly, coma may occur.

Diagnostic tests

Diagnosis must rule out other disorders, such as gastroenteritis, cholecystitis, and peptic ulcer, which produce similar clinical effects. The following test results support a diagnosis of hyperemesis gravidarum:
• Serum analysis shows decreased protein, chloride, sodium, and potassium levels and increased blood urea nitrogen levels.

• Other laboratory tests reveal ketonuria, slight proteinuria, elevated hemoglobin levels, and an elevated white blood cell count.

Treatment

The patient with hyperemesis gravidarum may require hospitalization to correct electrolyte imbalance and prevent starvation. I.V. infusions maintain nutrition until she can tolerate oral feedings. She progresses slowly to a clear liquid diet, then a full liquid diet, and finally, small, frequent meals of high-protein solid foods. A midnight snack helps stabilize blood glucose levels.

Parenteral vitamin supplements and potassium replacements help correct deficiencies.

When persistent vomiting jeopardizes health, antiemetic medications are administered. Currently, only meclizine and diphenhydramine are known to have a low risk for teratogenicity.

When vomiting stops and electrolyte balance has been restored, the pregnancy usually continues without recurrence of hyperemesis gravidarum. Most patients feel better as they begin to regain normal weight, but some continue to vomit throughout the pregnancy, requiring extended treatment. If appropriate, some patients may benefit from consultations with clinical nurse specialists, psychologists, or psychiatrists.

Nursing diagnoses

• Altered nutrition: Less than body requirements
• Altered protection
• Anxiety
• Fluid volume deficit
• Ineffective individual coping
• Knowledge deficit

Nursing interventions

• Maintain I.V. fluids, as ordered, until the patient can tolerate oral feedings.
• Monitor fluid intake and output, vital signs, weight, serum electrolyte levels, and urine for ketones.
• Provide frequent mouth care.
• Consult a dietitian to provide a diet high in dry, complex carbohydrates. Suggest decreased liquid intake during meals. Company and diversionary conversation at mealtime may be beneficial.
• Provide reassurance and a calm, restful atmosphere. Encourage the patient to discuss her feelings about her pregnancy and the disorder.
• Help the patient to develop effective coping strategies. Refer her to a mental health professional for additional counseling, if necessary. Also refer her to the social ser-

vice department for help in caring for other children at home, if appropriate.

Patient teaching

• Instruct the patient to remain upright for 45 minutes after eating to decrease reflux.
• Suggest that the patient eat two or three dry crackers upon awakening in the morning before getting out of bed to alleviate nausea.
• Teach the patient protective measures to conserve energy and promote rest. Include relaxation techniques; fresh air and moderate exercise, if tolerated; and activities scheduled to prevent fatigue.

PREGNANCY-INDUCED HYPERTENSION

A potentially life-threatening disorder, pregnancy-induced hypertension usually develops after the 20th week of pregnancy. It most often occurs in nulliparous women and may be nonconvulsive or convulsive.

Preeclampsia, the nonconvulsive form of the disorder, is marked by the onset of hypertension after 20 weeks' gestation. It develops in about 7% of pregnancies and may be mild or severe. The incidence is significantly higher in low socioeconomic groups.

Eclampsia, the convulsive form, occurs between 24 weeks' gestation and the end of the first postpartal week. The incidence increases among women who are pregnant for the first time, have multiple fetuses, and have a history of vascular disease.

About 5% of women with preeclampsia develop eclampsia; of these, about 15% die of eclampsia or its complications. Fetal mortality is high because of the increased incidence of premature delivery.

Pregnancy-induced hypertension and its complications represent the current most common cause of maternal death in developed countries.

Causes

The cause of pregnancy-induced hypertension is unknown. However, geographic, ethnic, racial, nutritional, immunologic, and familial factors may contribute to preexisting vascular disease, which, in turn, may contribute to its occurrence. Age is also a factor. Adolescents and primiparas over age 35 are at higher risk for preeclampsia.

Other theories postulate a long list of potential toxic sources, such as autolysis of placental infarcts, autoin-toxication, uremia, maternal sensitization to total proteins, and pyelonephritis.

Complications

Generalized arteriolar vasoconstriction is thought to produce decreased blood flow through the placenta and maternal organs. This can result in intrauterine growth retardation, placental infarcts, and abruptio placentae. Severe eclampsia is marked by hemolysis, elevated liver enzyme levels, and a low platelet count (HELLP syndrome). A unique form of coagulopathy is also associated with this disorder.

Other possible complications include stillbirth of the neonate, seizures, coma, premature labor, renal failure, and hepatic damage in the mother.

Assessment findings

A patient with mild preeclampsia typically reports a sudden weight gain of more than 3 lb (1.36 kg) a week in the second trimester or more than 1 lb (0.45 kg) a week during the third trimester.

The patient's history reveals hypertension, as evidenced by elevated blood pressure readings: 140 mm Hg or more systolic, or a rise of 30 mm Hg or more above the patient's normal systolic pressure, measured on two occasions, 6 hours apart; and 90 mm Hg or more diastolic, or a rise of 15 mm Hg or more above the patient's normal diastolic pressure, measured on two occasions, 6 hours apart.

Inspection detects generalized edema, especially of the face. Palpation may reveal pitting edema of the legs and feet. Deep tendon reflexes may indicate hyporeflexia or hyperreflexia.

As preeclampsia worsens, the patient may demonstrate oliguria (urine output of 400 ml/day or less), blurred vision caused by retinal arteriolar spasms, epigastric pain or heartburn, irritability, and emotional tension. She may complain of a severe frontal headache.

In severe preeclampsia, blood pressure readings rise to 160/110 mm Hg or higher on two occasions, 6 hours apart, during bed rest. Also, ophthalmoscopic examination may reveal vascular spasm, papilledema, retinal edema or detachment, and arteriovenous nicking or hemorrhage.

Preeclampsia can suddenly progress to eclampsia with the onset of seizures. The patient with eclampsia may appear to cease breathing, then suddenly take a deep, stertorous breath and resume breathing. The patient may then lapse into a coma, lasting a few minutes to several hours. Awakening from the coma, the patient may have no memory of the seizure. Mild eclampsia may involve more than one seizure; severe eclampsia up to 20 seizures.

In eclampsia, physical examination findings are similar to those in preeclampsia but more severe. Systolic blood pressure may rise to 180 mm Hg and even to 200 mm Hg. The patient may have a fever (50% of cases). Inspection may reveal marked edema, but some patients exhibit no visible edema.

Diagnostic tests
Laboratory test findings reveal proteinuria (more than 300 mg/24 hours [1+] with preeclampsia, and 5 g/24 hours [5+] or more with severe eclampsia). Test results may suggest the HELLP syndrome.

Ultrasonography, stress and nonstress tests, and biophysical profiles evaluate fetal well-being.

Treatment
Therapy for preeclampsia is designed to halt the disorder's progress — specifically, the early effects of eclampsia, such as seizures, residual hypertension, and renal shutdown — and to ensure fetal survival. Some doctors advocate the prompt induction of labor, especially if the patient is near term; others follow a more conservative approach. Therapy may include:
• *complete bed rest* in the preferred left lateral lying position to enhance venous return
• *antihypertensive drugs,* such as methyldopa and hydralazine
• *magnesium sulfate* to promote diuresis, reduce blood pressure, and prevent seizures if the patient's blood pressure fails to respond to bed rest and antihypertensives and persistently rises above 160/100 mm Hg, or if central nervous system irritability increases.

If these measures fail to improve the patient's condition, or if fetal life is endangered (as determined by stress or nonstress tests and biophysical profiles), cesarean section or oxytocin induction may be required to terminate the pregnancy.

Emergency treatment of eclamptic seizures consists of immediate administration of magnesium sulfate (I.V. drip), oxygen administration, and electronic fetal monitoring. After the patient's condition stabilizes, cesarean section may be performed.

Adequate nutrition, good prenatal care, and control of preexisting hypertension during pregnancy decrease the incidence and severity of preeclampsia. Early recognition and prompt treatment of preeclampsia can prevent progression to eclampsia.

Nursing diagnoses
• Activity intolerance
• Altered cerebral or peripheral tissue perfusion
• Altered urinary elimination
• Anxiety
• Fear
• Fluid volume excess
• Ineffective family coping
• Ineffective individual coping
• Knowledge deficit
• Risk for injury
• Sensory or perceptual alterations (visual)

Nursing interventions
• Monitor the patient regularly for changes in blood pressure, pulse rate, respiratory rate, fetal heart rate, vision, level of consciousness, and deep tendon reflexes and for headache unrelieved by medication. Report changes immediately. Assess these signs before administering medications.
• Monitor the extent and location of edema. Elevate affected extremities to promote venous return. Avoid constricting hose, slippers, or bed linens.
• Assess fluid balance by measuring intake and output and by checking daily weight. Insert an indwelling urinary catheter, if necessary.
• Observe for signs of fetal distress by closely monitoring the results of stress and nonstress tests.
• Keep emergency resuscitative equipment and anticonvulsants available in case of seizures and cardiac or respiratory arrest. Carefully monitor the administration of magnesium sulfate. Signs of toxicity include absence of patellar reflexes, flushing, and muscle flaccidity. Keep calcium gluconate at the bedside to counteract the toxic effects of magnesium sulfate.
• Prepare for emergency cesarean section, if indicated. Alert the anesthesiologist and pediatrician.
• To protect the patient from injury, maintain seizure precautions. Don't leave an unstable patient unattended. Keep an airway and oxygen available.
• Provide a quiet, darkened room until the patient's condition stabilizes, and enforce absolute bed rest.
• Provide emotional support for the patient and family. Encourage them to verbalize their feelings. If the patient's condition necessitates premature delivery, point out that infants of mothers with pregnancy-induced hypertension are usually small for gestational age but sometimes fare better than other premature babies of the same weight, possibly because they have developed adaptive responses to stress in utero.

• Help the patient and family to develop effective coping strategies.

Patient teaching

• Teach the patient and family to identify and report signs of preeclampsia and eclampsia, such as headache, weight gain, edema, and oliguria.
• Instruct the patient to maintain bed rest, as ordered. Advise her to lie in a left lateral position to increase venous return, cardiac output, and renal blood flow.
• Stress the importance of adequate nutrition in the prenatal period. Advise the patient to avoid foods high in sodium.
• Emphasize the importance of scheduling and keeping prenatal visits.

GESTATIONAL TROPHOBLASTIC DISEASE

Depending on histopathologic changes that occur in the trophoblast cells of the chorionic villi, gestational trophoblastic disease takes one of three forms. The first is *hydatidiform mole,* a nonmalignant neoplasm that forms on the chorion (the outer layer of the membrane containing amniotic fluid). The second form, commonly called *invasive mole* (chorioadenoma destruens), is a self-limiting, malignant tumor that occurs when trophoblastic tissue continues to grow and locally invades the uterine myometrium and pelvic blood supply. The third category is *choriocarcinoma,* a serious, rapidly developing, but rare, carcinoma. Neoplastic trophoblasts proliferate without cystic villi and may metastasize profusely throughout the body.

Gestational trophoblastic disease is reported to occur in about 1 in every 2,000 pregnancies. Recent research indicates, however, that the incidence would be much higher if all cases of the disorder were identified. Some cases are not recognized because the pregnancy is aborted early, and the products of conception are not available for analysis. The incidence is increased in women from low socioeconomic groups, older women, and multiparous women. The incidence is highest in Oriental women, especially those from southeast Asia.

With prompt diagnosis and appropriate treatment, the prognosis is usually excellent for patients with hydatidiform or invasive mole; however, about 10% of patients with hydatidiform mole develop choriocarcinoma. Recurrence is possible in about 2% of patients.

Causes

The cause of hydatidiform mole is unknown, although several theories relate gestational trophoblastic disease to a nutritional deficit, specifically an insufficient intake of protein and folic acid; chromosomal abnormalities; or hormonal imbalances. These theories, however, remain unsubstantiated. About half the patients with choriocarcinoma have had a preceding molar pregnancy. In the remaining half, the disease is usually preceded by a spontaneous or induced abortion, ectopic pregnancy, or normal pregnancy.

Complications

Possible complications of hydatidiform and invasive moles include anemia, infection, spontaneous abortion, uterine rupture, and hemorrhage.

Complications of invasive mole and choriocarcinoma include metastasis to all body structures. In invasive mole, metastasis occurs occasionally to the vagina and lungs. (This lesion accounts for the majority of women who have persistently high human chorionic gonadotropin [HCG] levels after the evacuation of a molar pregnancy.)

Choriocarcinoma disseminates hematogenously, particularly to the lungs, brain, liver, kidneys, and GI tract.

Assessment findings

A patient with hydatidiform mole may report vaginal bleeding, ranging from brownish red spotting to bright red hemorrhage. She may even report passing tissue that resembles grape clusters. Her history may also include lower abdominal cramps, such as those that accompany spontaneous abortion, hyperemesis, and signs and symptoms of preeclampsia.

On inspection, you'll detect a uterus that's exceptionally large for the patient's gestational date. On pelvic examination, you may discover grapelike vesicles in the vagina. Palpation may find ovarian enlargement due to theca-lutein cysts. Auscultation of the uterus may reveal the absence of fetal heart tones normally noted during a previous visit.

A patient with choriocarcinoma typically reports vaginal bleeding. If the disease has metastasized, she may also report hemoptysis, cough, dyspnea, headache, dizzy spells, weakness, paralysis, and rectal bleeding.

Occasionally, a patient with choriocarcinoma may exhibit an acute abdomen due to rupture of the uterus, liver, or theca-lutein cyst. On inspection, the uterus may be enlarged, with blood coming through the os. A tumor may be visible within the vagina.

Diagnostic tests

• *Radioimmunoassay of HCG levels,* performed frequently, can achieve early and accurate diagnosis. HCG levels that are extremely elevated for early pregnancy indicate gestational trophoblastic disease.

• *Histologic examination* of possible hydatid vesicles confirms the diagnosis.

• *Ultrasonography* performed after the third month shows grapelike clusters rather than a fetus.

• *Aminography,* a procedure that introduces a water-soluble dye into the uterus, may reveal the absence of a fetus (performed only when the diagnosis is in question).

• *Doppler ultrasonography* demonstrates the absence of fetal heart tones.

• *Hemoglobin and hematocrit levels, red blood cell count, prothrombin time, partial thromboplastin time, fibrinogen levels,* and *hepatic and renal function findings* are abnormal.

• *White blood cell count* and *erythrocyte sedimentation rate* are increased.

• *Chest X-rays, computed tomography scan,* and *magnetic resonance imaging* may identify choriocarcinoma metastasis.

• *Lumbar puncture* may detect early cerebral metastasis if HCG is in the cerebrospinal fluid.

Treatment

Gestational trophoblastic disease requires uterine evacuation by dilatation and curettage, abdominal hysterectomy, or instrument or suction curettage, depending on uterine size. I.V. oxytocin may be used to promote uterine contractions.

Postoperative treatment varies, depending on the amount of blood lost and complications. If no complications develop, hospitalization is usually brief, and normal activities can be resumed quickly, as tolerated.

Because of the possibility of choriocarcinoma development following hydatidiform mole, scrupulous follow-up care is essential. Such care includes monitoring HCG levels once weekly until titers are negative for 3 consecutive weeks; then once monthly for 6 months; then every 2 months for 6 months. It also includes chest X-rays to check for lung metastasis once monthly until HCG titers are negative, then once every 2 months for 1 year.

Another pregnancy should be postponed until at least 1 year after all titers and X-ray findings are negative. An oral contraceptive is indicated to prevent pregnancy.

Prophylactic chemotherapy with either methotrexate or actinomycin D after evacuation of the uterus has been successful in preventing malignant gestational trophoblastic disease. Chemotherapy with combination therapy and irradiation are used for metastatic choriocarcinoma.

Nursing diagnoses

• Anxiety
• Dysfunctional grieving
• Ineffective family coping
• Ineffective individual coping
• Knowledge deficit
• Risk for infection

Nursing interventions

• Preoperatively, observe for signs of complications, such as hemorrhage and uterine infection, and vaginal passage of hydatid vesicles. Save any expelled tissue for laboratory analysis.

• Postoperatively, monitor vital signs, fluid intake and output, and for signs of hemorrhage.

• Encourage the patient and family to express their feelings about the disorder. Offer emotional support, and help them through the grieving process for their lost infant.

• Help the patient and family to develop effective coping strategies. Refer them to a mental health professional for additional counseling, if needed.

Patient teaching

• Stress the need for regular monitoring (HCG levels and chest X-rays) to detect any malignant changes.

• Instruct the patient to report promptly any new symptoms (for example, hemoptysis, cough, suspected pregnancy, nausea, vomiting, and vaginal bleeding).

• Explain to the patient that she must use contraceptives to prevent pregnancy for at least 1 year after HCG levels return to normal and her body reestablishes regular ovulation and menstrual cycles.

PLACENTA PREVIA

In this disorder, the placenta implants in the lower uterine segment, where it encroaches on the internal cervical os. Placenta previa, one of the most common causes of bleeding during the second half of pregnancy, occurs in about 1 in 200 pregnancies, more commonly in multigravidas than in primigravidas.

The placenta may cover all, part, or a fraction of the internal cervical os. (See *Three types of placenta previa.*)

Among patients who develop placenta previa in the second trimester of pregnancy, less than 15% will have a persistent previa at term. The elongation of the upper and lower uterine segments causes the placenta to be located higher on the uterine wall.

THREE TYPES OF PLACENTA PREVIA

The degree of placenta previa depends largely on the extent of cervical dilation at the time of examination because the dilating cervix gradually uncovers the placenta, as shown below.

Marginal placenta previa
If the placenta covers just a fraction of the internal cervical os, your patient has marginal, or low-lying placenta previa.

Partial placenta previa
Your patient has the partial, or incomplete, form of the disorder if the placenta caps a larger part of the internal os.

Total placenta previa
If the placenta covers all of the internal os, your patient has total, complete, or central placenta previa.

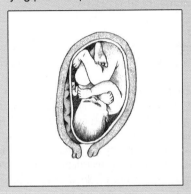

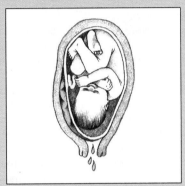

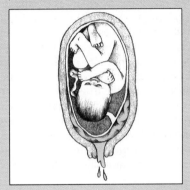

Generally, termination of pregnancy is necessary when placenta previa is diagnosed in the presence of heavy maternal bleeding. The maternal prognosis is good if hemorrhage can be controlled; the fetal prognosis depends on gestational age and the amount of blood lost.

Causes

Although the specific cause of placenta previa is unknown, factors that may affect the site of the placenta's attachment to the uterine wall include:
• defective vascularization of the decidua
• multiple pregnancy (the placenta requires a larger surface for attachment)
• previous uterine surgery
• multiparity
• advanced maternal age.

Complications

Possible complications of placenta previa include anemia, hemorrhage, disseminated intravascular coagulation, shock, renal damage, cerebral ischemia, and maternal or fetal death.

Assessment findings

Typically, a patient with placenta previa reports the onset of painless, bright red, vaginal bleeding after the 20th week of pregnancy. Such bleeding, beginning before the onset of labor, tends to be episodic; it starts without warning, stops spontaneously, and resumes later.

About 7% of all patients with placenta previa are asymptomatic; in these women, ultrasound examination reveals the disorder incidentally.

Palpation may reveal a soft, nontender uterus. Abdominal examination using Leopold's maneuvers reveals various malpresentations due to interference with the descent of the fetal head caused by the placenta's abnormal location. Minimal descent of the fetal presenting part may indicate placenta previa. The fetus remains active, however, with good heart tones audible on auscultation.

Diagnostic tests

• *Ultrasound examination* determines placental position. Vaginal and rectal examinations are *never* performed unless delivery is imminent. If the placenta is located on the posterior wall of the uterus, its lower margin may be obscured. In this case, a vaginal examination is performed with a double setup (preparations for an immediate emergency cesarean section) to confirm the diagnosis. Usually, only the cervix is visualized.

• *Amniocentesis* determines fetal lung maturity before cesarean section.

• *Laboratory studies* may reveal decreased maternal hemoglobin levels (due to blood loss).

Treatment

Medical management of placenta previa is designed to assess, control, and restore blood loss; to deliver a viable infant; and to prevent coagulation disorders.

Immediate therapy includes starting an I.V. infusion using a large-bore catheter; drawing blood for hemoglobin and hematocrit levels and for typing and cross matching; initiating external electronic fetal monitoring; monitoring maternal blood pressure, pulse rate, and respirations; and assessing the amount of vaginal bleeding.

If the fetus is premature (following determination of the degree of placenta previa and necessary fluid and blood replacement), treatment consists of careful observation to allow the fetus more time to mature.

If clinical evaluation confirms complete placenta previa, the patient is usually hospitalized due to the increased risk of hemorrhage. As soon as the fetus is sufficiently mature, or in case of intervening severe hemorrhage, immediate delivery by cesarean section may be necessary.

Vaginal delivery is considered only when the bleeding is minimal and the placenta previa is marginal or when the labor is rapid.

Because of possible fetal blood loss through the placenta, a pediatric team should be on hand during such delivery to immediately assess and treat neonatal shock, blood loss, and hypoxia.

Nursing diagnoses

• Anxiety
• Dysfunctional grieving
• Fear
• Fluid volume deficit
• Ineffective family coping
• Ineffective individual coping
• Knowledge deficit
• Pain
• Risk for injury

Nursing interventions

• If the patient with placenta previa shows active bleeding, continuously monitor her blood pressure, pulse rate, respirations, central venous pressure, intake and output, amount of vaginal bleeding, and the fetal heart rate. Electronic monitoring of fetal heart tones is recommended.
• If the patient is Rh-negative, administer $Rh_o(D)$ immune globulin (RhoGAM) after every bleeding episode.

• Provide emotional support during labor. Because of the infant's prematurity, the patient may not be given analgesics, so labor pain may be intense. Reassure her of her progress throughout labor, and keep her informed of the fetus's condition.
• During the postpartum period, monitor the patient for signs of hemorrhage and shock caused by the uterus's diminished ability to contract.
• Encourage the patient and her family to verbalize their feelings. Help them to develop effective coping strategies. Refer them for counseling, if necessary.

Patient teaching

• Teach the asymptomatic patient to identify and report signs of placenta previa (bleeding, cramping) immediately.
• Prepare the patient and her family for the possibility of an emergency cesarean section, the birth of a premature infant, and the physical and emotional changes of the postpartum period.
• Tactfully discuss the possibility of neonatal death. Tell the mother that the infant's survival depends primarily on gestational age, the amount of blood lost, and associated hypertensive disorders. Assure her that frequent monitoring and prompt management greatly reduce the risk of death.

ABRUPTIO PLACENTAE

Also called placental abruption, abruptio placentae occurs when the placenta separates from the uterine wall prematurely, usually after the 20th week of gestation, producing hemorrhage. This disorder may be classified according to the degree of placental separation and the severity of maternal and fetal symptoms. (See *Degrees of placental separation in abruptio placentae.*)

Abruptio placentae is most common in multigravidas — usually in women over age 35 — and is a common cause of bleeding during the second half of pregnancy. Firm diagnosis, in the presence of heavy maternal bleeding, generally necessitates termination of pregnancy. The fetal prognosis depends on gestational age and amount of blood lost; the maternal prognosis is good if hemorrhage can be controlled.

Causes and pathophysiology

The cause of abruptio placentae is unknown. Predisposing factors include traumatic injury (such as a direct blow to the uterus), placental site bleeding from a needle puncture during amniocentesis, chronic or pregnancy-induced hypertension (which raises pressure on the ma-

DEGREES OF PLACENTAL SEPARATION IN ABRUPTIO PLACENTAE

Placental abruption is classified according to the degree of placental separation from the uterine wall and the extent of hemorrhage.

Mild separation
Internal bleeding between the placenta and uterine wall characterize mild separation.

Moderate separation
In moderate separation, external hemorrhage occurs through the vagina.

Severe separation
External hemorrhage is also characteristic in severe separation.

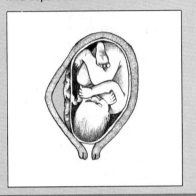
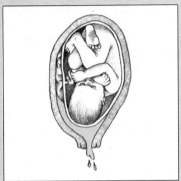
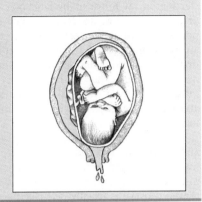

ternal side of the placenta), multiparity, short umbilical cord, dietary deficiency, smoking, advanced maternal age, and pressure on the vena cava from an enlarged uterus.

The spontaneous rupture of blood vessels at the placental bed may be due to lack of resiliency or to abnormal changes in the uterine vasculature. The condition may be complicated by hypertension or by an enlarged uterus that can't contract sufficiently to seal off the torn vessels. Consequently, bleeding continues unchecked, possibly shearing off the placenta partially or completely.

Complications
Besides hemorrhage and shock, possible complications of abruptio placentae include renal failure, disseminated intravascular coagulation (DIC), and maternal and fetal death.

Assessment findings
Abruptio placentae produces a wide range of clinical effects, depending on the extent of placental separation and the amount of blood lost from maternal circulation.

A patient with *mild abruptio placentae* (marginal separation) may report mild to moderate vaginal bleeding, vague lower abdominal discomfort, and mild to moderate abdominal tenderness. Fetal monitoring may indicate uterine irritability. Auscultation reveals strong and regular fetal heart tones.

A patient with *moderate abruptio placentae* (about 50% placental separation) may report continuous abdominal pain and moderate dark red vaginal bleeding. Onset of symptoms may be gradual or abrupt.

Vital signs may indicate impending shock. Palpation reveals a tender uterus that remains firm between contractions. Fetal monitoring may reveal barely audible or irregular and bradycardic fetal heart tones. Labor usually starts within 2 hours and often proceeds rapidly.

A patient with *severe abruptio placentae* (70% placental separation) will report abrupt onset of agonizing, unremitting uterine pain (described as tearing or knifelike) and moderate vaginal bleeding.

Vital signs indicate rapidly progressive shock. Fetal monitoring indicates an absence of fetal heart tones.

Palpation reveals a tender uterus with boardlike rigidity. Uterine size may increase in severe concealed abruptions.

Diagnostic tests
Pelvic examination under double setup (preparations for an emergency cesarean) and ultrasonography are performed to rule out placenta previa. Decreased hemoglobin levels and platelet counts support the diagnosis. Periodic assays for fibrin split products aid in monitoring

the progression of abruptio placentae and in detecting DIC.

Treatment

Medical management of abruptio placentae is designed to assess, control, and restore the amount of blood lost; to deliver a viable infant; and to prevent coagulation disorders.

Immediate measures for abruptio placentae include starting an I.V. infusion (by large-bore catheter) of appropriate fluids (lactated Ringer's solution) to combat hypovolemia; inserting a central venous pressure line and an indwelling urinary catheter to monitor fluid status; drawing blood for hemoglobin and hematocrit determination and coagulation studies and for typing and cross matching; starting external electronic fetal monitoring; and monitoring maternal vital signs and vaginal bleeding.

After determining the severity of placental abruption and appropriate fluid and blood replacement, prompt delivery by cesarean section is necessary if the fetus is in distress. If the fetus is not in distress, monitoring continues; delivery is usually performed at the first sign of fetal distress. (If placental separation is severe with no signs of fetal life, vaginal delivery may be performed unless uncontrolled hemorrhage or other complications contraindicate it.)

Because of possible fetal blood loss through the placenta, a pediatric team should be ready at delivery to assess and treat the neonate for shock, blood loss, and hypoxia.

Complications of abruptio placentae require appropriate treatment. With a complication, such as DIC, for example, the patient will need immediate intervention with heparin, platelets, and whole blood, as ordered, to prevent exsanguination.

Nursing diagnoses

• Altered tissue perfusion
• Anxiety
• Dysfunctional grieving
• Fear
• Ineffective family coping
• Ineffective individual coping
• Pain

Nursing interventions

• Monitor maternal blood pressure, pulse rate, respirations, central venous pressure, intake and output, and amount of vaginal bleeding every 10 to 15 minutes.
• Monitor fetal heart rate electronically.

• If vaginal delivery is elected, provide emotional support during labor. Because of the neonate's prematurity, the mother may not receive analgesics during labor and may experience intense pain. Reassure the patient of her progress through labor, and keep her informed of the fetus's condition.
• Encourage the patient and her family to verbalize their feelings. Help them to develop effective coping strategies. Refer them for counseling, if necessary.

Patient teaching

• Teach the patient to identify and report signs of placental abruption, such as bleeding and cramping.
• Explain all procedures and treatments to allay anxiety.
• Prepare the patient and her family for the possibility of an emergency cesarean section, the delivery of a premature infant, and the changes to expect in the postpartum period. Offer emotional support and an honest assessment of the situation.
• Tactfully discuss the possibility of neonatal death. Tell the mother that the neonate's survival depends primarily on gestational age, the amount of blood lost, and associated hypertensive disorders. Assure her that frequent monitoring and prompt management greatly reduce the risk of death.

PREMATURE LABOR

Also known as preterm labor, premature labor is the onset of rhythmic uterine contractions that produce cervical changes after fetal viability but before fetal maturity. It usually occurs between the 20th and 37th week of gestation. About 5% to 10% of pregnancies end prematurely; about 75% to 85% of neonatal deaths, and many birth defects, result from this disorder.

Fetal prognosis depends on birth weight and length of gestation: Neonates weighing under 1 lb 10 oz (737 g) and of less than 26 weeks' gestation have a survival rate of about 10%; neonates weighing 1 lb 10 oz to 2 lb 3 oz (737 to 992 g) and of 27 to 28 weeks' gestation have a survival rate of more than 50%; those weighing 2 lb 3 oz to 2 lb 11 oz (992 to 1,219 g) and of more than 28 weeks' gestation have a 70% to 90% survival rate.

Causes

Premature labor may result from premature rupture of the membranes (occurs in 30% to 50% of premature labors), pregnancy-induced or chronic hypertension, hydramnios, multiple pregnancy, placenta previa, abruptio placentae, incompetent cervix, abdominal surgery, trauma, structural uterine anomalies, infections, hormonal imbalance, genetic defects, and fetal death.

Numerous maternal risk factors also increase the incidence of premature labor. (See *Reviewing risk factors for premature labor.*)

Complications

Premature labor is a major cause of perinatal morbidity and mortality. Respiratory distress syndrome and intracranial bleeding are the primary neonatal complications.

Assessment findings

The patient reports the onset of rhythmic uterine contractions, possible rupture of membranes, passage of the cervical mucus plug, and a bloody discharge. Her history indicates that she's in the 20th to 37th week of pregnancy. Inspection during vaginal examination shows cervical effacement and dilation.

Diagnostic tests

Premature labor is confirmed by the combined results of prenatal history, physical examination, and presenting signs and symptoms. The following diagnostic studies support the diagnosis:
• *Ultrasonography* identifies the position of the fetus in relation to the mother's pelvis, documents the gestational age, and estimates the fetal weight.
• *Vaginal examination* confirms progressive cervical effacement and dilation.
• *Electronic fetal monitoring* confirms rhythmic uterine contractions and monitors fetal well-being. Ambulatory home monitoring with a tocodynamometer may identify preterm contractions.

Treatment

Medical management focuses on suppressing premature labor when tests show immature fetal pulmonary development, cervical dilation of less than 4 cm, and factors that warrant continuation of pregnancy. Treatment includes the following measures.

Primary interventions include bed rest and hydration. If the patient doesn't respond, tocolytic therapy is instituted unless contraindicated. Beta-adrenergic stimulants (terbutaline, isoxsuprine, or ritodrine) stimulate the $beta_2$ receptors, inhibiting the contractility of uterine smooth muscle.

Magnesium sulfate may be used to relax the myometrium. After successful tocolysis, oral therapy is maintained until 36 weeks' gestation. Some patients successfully deliver at term after this treatment. Glucocorticoid administration to the mother at less than 33

REVIEWING RISK FACTORS FOR PREMATURE LABOR

The following factors may increase a pregnant patient's risk of premature labor:
• diethylstilbestrol (DES) exposure
• habitual abortion
• heavy work and long travel to work
• history of cone biopsy of the cervix
• history of genitourinary infections or renal disease
• history of induced abortion, preterm delivery, or perinatal death
• low socioeconomic class
• maternal undernutrition and inadequate weight gain during pregnancy
• multiple gestation
• multiple or large uterine leiomyomas
• single parenthood
• smoking
• substance abuse
• uterine or cervical abnormalities.

---

weeks' gestation enhances fetal pulmonary maturation and reduces the incidence of respiratory distress syndrome.

Ideally, treatment for active premature labor should take place in a regional perinatal intensive care center, where the staff is specially trained to handle this situation. Regardless of where treatment and delivery take place, they require intensive team effort, focusing on:
• continuous fetal monitoring
• avoidance of amniotomy, if possible, to prevent cord prolapse or damage to the fetus's soft skull
• maintenance of adequate hydration through I.V. fluids
• avoidance of sedatives and narcotics that might harm the fetus. (*Note:* Morphine or meperidine may be required to minimize maternal pain. These drugs have little effect on uterine contractions; but because they depress the central nervous system (CNS), they may cause fetal respiratory depression. They should be given in the smallest dose possible and only when needed.)

Prevention of premature labor requires good prenatal care, adequate nutrition, and proper rest. Insertion of a purse-string suture (cerclage) to reinforce an incompetent cervix at 14 to 18 weeks' gestation may prevent premature labor in patients with histories of this disorder.

Nursing diagnoses
• Altered family processes
• Anxiety
• Dysfunctional grieving
• Fear

- Ineffective breathing pattern
- Ineffective family coping
- Ineffective individual coping
- Pain

Nursing interventions

- During attempts to suppress premature labor, maintain bed rest and administer medications, as ordered. Give sedatives and analgesics sparingly, mindful of their potentially harmful effect on the fetus. Minimize the need for these drugs by providing comfort measures, such as frequent repositioning and good perineal and back care.
- When giving beta-adrenergic stimulants, sedatives, and narcotics, monitor blood pressure, pulse rate, respirations, fetal heart rate, and uterine contraction pattern. Minimize adverse effects by keeping the patient in a lateral recumbent position as much as possible. Provide adequate hydration.
- When giving magnesium sulfate, monitor neurologic reflexes and be alert for maternal adverse effects, such as tachycardia and hypotension. Keep calcium gluconate at the bedside. Watch the neonate for signs of magnesium toxicity, including neuromuscular, respiratory, and CNS depression, and decreased sucking reflex.
- During active premature labor, remember that the premature infant has a lower tolerance for the stress of labor and is much more likely to become hypoxic than the term infant. If necessary, give oxygen to the patient through a nasal cannula. Encourage her to lie on her left side or sit up during labor; this position prevents caval compression, which can cause supine hypotension and subsequent fetal hypoxia. Observe fetal response to labor through continuous fetal monitoring. Fetal heart rate patterns that are relatively innocuous in term infants may prove ominous in preterm infants.
- Prevent maternal hyperventilation; use a rebreathing bag, if necessary. Continually reassure the patient throughout labor to help reduce her anxiety.
- Help the patient get through labor with as little analgesic and anesthetic as possible. To minimize fetal CNS depression, avoid administering analgesics when delivery seems imminent. Monitor fetal and maternal response to local and regional anesthetics.
- During delivery, instruct the patient to push only during the contractions and only as long as instructed. Pushing between contractions is not only ineffective but can damage the premature infant's soft skull.
- Notify an anesthesiologist or anesthetist and a pediatrician to be in attendance to care for the premature infant immediately after delivery. Prepare resuscitation equipment and notify the neonatal intensive care unit.

- Encourage the patient and family to discuss their feelings. Offer emotional support and help them to develop effective coping strategies.
- If possible, arrange for the parents to see and hold the infant soon after delivery to facilitate bonding.

Patient teaching

- After delivery, inform the parents of their child's condition. Describe his appearance, and explain the purpose of any supportive equipment. Help them gain confidence in their ability to care for their child. Provide privacy, and encourage them to hold and feed the infant, when possible.
- As necessary, before the parents leave the hospital with the infant, refer them to a home health nurse who can help them adjust to caring for a premature infant. Encourage them to contact and join community support groups for premature infants and their families.

PREMATURE RUPTURE OF THE MEMBRANES

A common abnormality of parturition, premature rupture of the membranes is a spontaneous break or tear in the amniotic sac before onset of regular contractions, resulting in progressive cervical dilation. This disorder occurs in nearly 10% of all pregnancies over 20 weeks' gestation, and labor usually starts within 24 hours; more than 80% of these infants are mature.

The latent period (between membrane rupture and onset of labor) is generally brief when the membranes rupture near term; when the infant is premature, this period is prolonged, which increases the risk of mortality from maternal infection (amnionitis, endometritis), fetal infection (pneumonia, septicemia), and prematurity.

Causes

Although the cause of premature rupture is unknown, malpresentation and contracted pelvis commonly accompany the rupture. Predisposing factors may include poor nutrition and hygiene and lack of prenatal care; incompetent cervix; increased intrauterine tension due to hydramnios or multiple pregnancies; defects in the amniotic membrane; and uterine, vaginal, and cervical infections (most commonly group B streptococci, gonococci, chlamydiae, and anaerobic organisms).

Complications

Maternal complications associated with premature rupture of the membranes include cesarean delivery, endometritis, amnionitis and, if untreated, septic shock and death. Neonatal complications include an increased incidence of respiratory distress syndrome, asphyxia, pulmonary hypoplasia, congenital anomalies, malpresentation, and cord prolapse. Severe fetal distress may result in neonatal death.

Assessment findings
Typically, a patient who has experienced premature rupture will report gushing or leaking of blood-tinged amniotic fluid containing vernix particles. Inspection during sterile speculum examination shows amniotic fluid in the vagina.

Diagnostic tests
Characteristic passage of amniotic fluid confirms the rupture. Slight fundal pressure or Valsalva's maneuver may expel fluid through the cervical os. The following diagnostic tests support the diagnosis:
• Alkaline pH of fluid collected from the posterior fornix turns nitrazine paper deep blue. (The presence of blood can give a false-positive result.)
• A smear of fluid, placed on a slide and allowed to dry, takes on a fernlike pattern (because of the high sodium and protein content of amniotic fluid). This positive ferning identifies the substance as amniotic fluid.
• Vaginal probe ultrasonography may be done to visualize the amniotic sac.

Treatment
Fetal age and the risk of infection determine the course of treatment for premature rupture of the membranes.

In a term pregnancy, if spontaneous labor and vaginal delivery aren't achieved within 24 hours after the membranes rupture, induction of labor with oxytocin is usually required; if induction fails, cesarean delivery is usually necessary. Cesarean hysterectomy is recommended with gross uterine infection.

Management of a preterm pregnancy of less than 34 weeks is controversial. However, with advanced technology, a conservative approach may prove effective. With a preterm pregnancy of 28 to 34 weeks, treatment includes hospitalization and observation for signs of infection (maternal leukocytosis or fever and fetal tachycardia) while awaiting fetal maturation. If clinical status suggests infection, baseline cultures and sensitivity tests are appropriate. If these tests confirm infection, labor must be induced, followed by I.V. administration of antibiotics. A culture should also be made of gastric aspirate or a swabbing from the neonate's ear because antibiotic therapy may be indicated for him as well.

During delivery, resuscitative equipment and anesthesia should be available. A pediatrician should be present to treat neonatal distress.

Nursing diagnoses
• Anxiety
• Dysfunctional grieving
• Ineffective family coping
• Ineffective individual coping
• Knowledge deficit
• Risk for infection

Nursing interventions
• During the examination, stay with the patient and offer reassurance. Provide sterile gloves and sterile lubricating jelly. Don't use iodophor antiseptic solution; it discolors nitrazine paper and makes pH determination impossible.
• After the examination, provide proper perineal care.
• Send fluid specimens to the laboratory promptly because bacteriologic studies need immediate evaluation.
• If labor starts, observe the mother's contractions, and monitor vital signs every 2 hours. Watch for signs of maternal infection (fever, abdominal tenderness, and changes in amniotic fluid, such as purulence or foul odor) and fetal tachycardia. (Fetal tachycardia may precede maternal fever.) Report such signs immediately.
• Encourage the patient and family to express their feelings and concerns for the infant's health and survival.

Patient teaching
• Teach the patient in the early stages of pregnancy how to recognize premature rupture of the membranes. Make sure she understands that amniotic fluid doesn't always gush; it sometimes leaks slowly.
• Stress that she *must* report premature rupture immediately because prompt treatment may prevent dangerous infection.
• Warn the patient not to engage in sexual intercourse, douche, or take tub baths after the membranes rupture.

PUERPERAL INFECTION
A common cause of childbirth-related death, puerperal infection is an inflammation of the birth canal after birth or abortion. It can occur as localized lesions of the perineum, vulva, and vagina, or it may spread, causing endometritis, parametritis, pelvic and femoral thrombophlebitis, peritonitis, and life-threatening endomyoparametritis. In the United States, puerperal infection

PREDISPOSING FACTORS FOR PUERPERAL INFECTION

The following factors increase the risk of puerperal infection:
• anemia
• cesarean section
• frequent vaginal examinations during labor
• intercourse after rupture of membranes
• invasive techniques, such as midforceps delivery
• manual removal of the placenta
• poor maternal nutrition
• poor hygiene
• premature or prolonged rupture of membranes
• prolonged internal fetal monitoring
• prolonged labor
• retained placental fragments.

develops in about 6% of maternity patients. The prognosis is good with treatment.

Causes

Causative microorganisms include streptococci, coagulase-negative staphylococci, *Clostridium perfringens*, *Bacteroides fragilis*, and *Escherichia coli*. Most of these organisms are considered normal vaginal flora but are known to cause puerperal infection in the presence of certain predisposing factors. (See *Predisposing factors for puerperal infection*.)

Complications

Any puerperal infection can lead to systemic infection, resulting in septicemia, bacteremic shock, and death. Other complications include pulmonary embolus, cardiac arrest, and cerebrovascular accident.

Assessment findings

Typically, the history reveals a temperature of at least 100.4° F (38° C) developing 2 to 3 days postpartum, or on any 2 consecutive days up to the 11th day, exclusive of the first 24 hours. (Fever during the first 24 hours postpartum may be from dehydration.) The fever can rise as high as 105° F (40.6° C). The patient may also report chills, headache, malaise, restlessness, and anxiety.

With local lesions of the perineum, vulva, and vagina, the patient may complain of pain and dysuria. Inspection may show inflammation and edema of the affected area and profuse purulent discharge.

A patient with endometritis may present with a backache and severe uterine contractions that persist after childbirth. Inspection finds heavy, sometimes foul-smelling lochia. Palpation reveals a tender, enlarged uterus.

With parametritis (pelvic cellulitis), the history may include vaginal tenderness and abdominal pain and tenderness (pain may become more intense as infection spreads). In pelvic thrombophlebitis, the history may reveal severe, repeated chills and dramatic swings in body temperature. The patient may complain of lower abdominal or flank pain. Palpation may reveal a tender mass over the affected area, which usually develops near the second postpartum week.

A patient with femoral thrombophlebitis may report pain, stiffness, or swelling in a leg or the groin. Malaise, fever, and chills usually begin 10 to 20 days postpartum. Inspection reveals inflammation or a shiny, white appearance of the affected leg. Palpation detects Rielander's sign (palpable veins inside the calf and thigh). Examination also may provoke Payr's sign (pain in the calf when pressure is applied to the inside of the foot) and Homans' sign (pain on dorsiflexion of the foot with the knee extended). These signs may precede pulmonary embolism.

In peritonitis, fever accompanies tachycardia (over 140 beats/minute) and a weak pulse. The patient may complain of hiccups, nausea, vomiting, and diarrhea, as well as constant, possibly excruciating, abdominal pain.

Diagnostic tests

Development of the typical clinical features, especially fever within 48 hours after delivery, suggests a puerperal infection. Extrapelvic causes of fever (breast engorgement, mastitis, pneumonia, pyelonephritis, wound infection) should be ruled out in the initial evaluation.
• *Culture of lochia, blood, incisional exudate (from cesarean incision or episiotomy), uterine tissue,* or *material collected from the vaginal cuff,* revealing the causative organism, confirms the diagnosis.
• *White blood cell count* 36 to 48 hours postpartum usually reveals leukocytosis (15,000 to 30,000/mm³) and an increased erythrocyte sedimentation rate.
• *Pelvic examination* shows induration without purulent discharge in parametritis.
• *Culdoscopy* shows pelvic adnexal induration and thickening. Red, swollen abscesses on the broad ligaments are even more serious, since rupture leads to peritonitis.
• *Venography* and *Doppler ultrasonography* help to confirm pelvic or femoral thrombophlebitis.

Treatment

Therapy usually begins with I.V. infusion of a broad-spectrum antibiotic to control the infection while awaiting culture results. After identification of the infecting organism, a more specific antibiotic should be administered. (An oral antibiotic may be prescribed after discharge.)

Ancillary measures include analgesics for pain; anticoagulants, such as I.V. heparin, for thrombophlebitis and endometritis (after clotting time and partial thromboplastin time determine dosage); antiseptics for local lesions; and antiemetics for nausea and vomiting from peritonitis. Isolation or transfer from the maternity unit also may be indicated.

Supportive care includes bed rest, adequate fluid intake, I.V. fluids when necessary, and measures to reduce fever. Sitz baths and heat lamps may relieve discomfort from local lesions. Surgery may be needed to remove any remaining products of conception or to drain local lesions, such as an abscess in parametritis.

Management of femoral thrombophlebitis requires warm soaks, elevation of the affected leg to promote venous return, and observation for signs of pulmonary embolism.

Nursing diagnoses
• Altered parenting
• Anxiety
• Fluid volume deficit
• Infection
• Knowledge deficit
• Pain
• Risk for impaired skin integrity

Nursing interventions
• Monitor vital signs every 4 hours (more frequently if peritonitis has developed) plus intake and output. Enforce strict bed rest.
• Frequently inspect the perineum. Assess the fundus, and palpate for tenderness (subinvolution may indicate endometritis). Note the amount, color, and odor of vaginal drainage, and document your observations.
• Administer antibiotics and analgesics, as ordered. Assess and document the type, degree, and location of pain, as well as the patient's response to analgesics. Give antiemetics to relieve nausea and vomiting, as necessary.
• Provide sitz baths and a heat lamp for local lesions. Change bed linens and perineal pads frequently. Keep the patient warm.
• Elevate a thrombophlebitic leg about 30 degrees. *Don't* rub or manipulate it or compress it with bed linens. Provide warm soaks for the leg. Watch for such signs of pulmonary embolism as dyspnea and chest pain.

• Offer reassurance and emotional support. Encourage the patient and her family to express their concerns, and help them develop effective coping strategies.
• If the mother is separated from her infant, keep her informed about his progress. Also encourage the father to reassure the mother about the infant's condition.

To prevent puerperal infection:
• Maintain aseptic technique when performing a vaginal examination. Limit the number of vaginal examinations performed during labor.
• Use meticulous hand-washing technique after each patient contact.
• Keep the episiotomy site clean, and provide good perineal hygiene and skin care.
• Screen personnel and visitors to keep persons with active infections away from the patient.

Patient teaching
• Instruct all pregnant patients to call their doctors immediately when their membranes rupture. Warn them to avoid intercourse after rupture or leak of the amniotic sac.
• Teach patients good hand-washing technique and perineal hygiene to prevent infection.

BREAST DISORDERS

Some breast disorders, such as mastitis, stem from infection and usually affect lactating women. Others, such as galactorrhea, result from hormonal dysfunction unrelated to lactation.

MASTITIS

Parenchymatous inflammation of the mammary glands, or mastitis, occurs postpartum in about 1% of lactating women, mainly in primiparas who are breast-feeding. It occurs occasionally in nonlactating women and rarely in men. The prognosis is good.

Causes
Mastitis develops when a pathogen that typically originates in the nursing infant's nose or pharynx invades breast tissue through a fissured or cracked nipple and disrupts normal lactation. The most common pathogen is *Staphylococcus aureus;* less frequently, it's *S. epidermidis* or beta-hemolytic streptococci. Rarely, mastitis may result from disseminated tuberculosis or the mumps virus.

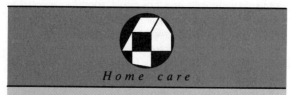

Home care

PREVENTING MASTITIS

To help your patient prevent mastitis from recurring, follow these guidelines:
Stress the importance of emptying the breasts completely because milk stasis can cause infection and mastitis.
• Teach the patient to alternate feeding positions and to rotate pressure areas on the nipples.
• Remind the patient to position the infant properly on the breast with the entire areola in his mouth.
• Advise her to expose sore nipples to the air as often as possible.
• Teach the patient proper hand-washing technique and personal hygiene.
• Instruct her to get plenty of rest and consume sufficient fluids and a balanced diet to enhance breast-feeding.
• Suggest applying a warm, wet towel to the affected breast or taking a warm shower to relax and improve breast-feeding.

Predisposing factors include a fissure or abrasion of the nipple, blocked milk ducts, and an incomplete let-down reflex. Blocked milk ducts can result from a tight bra or prolonged intervals between breast-feedings.

Complications
An untreated breast infection can lead to abscess.

Assessment findings
Usually, the patient reports a fever of 101° F (38.3° C) or higher in acute mastitis, malaise, and flulike symptoms that develop 2 to 4 weeks postpartum, although they may develop anytime during lactation. Inspection and palpation may uncover redness, swelling, warmth, hardness, tenderness, nipple cracks or fissures, and enlarged axillary lymph nodes.

Diagnostic tests
Cultures of expressed milk confirm generalized mastitis; cultures of breast skin confirm localized mastitis. Such cultures also determine antibiotic therapy.

Treatment
Antibiotic therapy, the primary treatment, usually consists of penicillin G to combat staphylococci; erythro-

mycin or kanamycin is used for penicillin-resistant strains. A cephalosporin or dicloxacillin is also used. Symptoms usually subside in 2 to 3 days, but antibiotics should continue for 10 days. Other measures include analgesics and, rarely, breast abscess incision and drainage.

Nursing diagnoses
• Ineffective breast-feeding
• Infection
• Knowledge deficit
• Pain
• Risk for impaired skin integrity

Nursing interventions
• Give analgesics, as needed. Provide comfort measures, such as warm soaks.
• Use meticulous hand-washing technique and provide good skin care.

Patient teaching
• Tell the patient to take the antibiotic *exactly* as prescribed, even if her symptoms subside.
• Reassure the mother that breast-feeding won't harm her infant because he's the source of the infection.
• If only one breast is affected, advise the patient to offer the infant that breast first to promote complete emptying and prevent clogged ducts. However, if an open abscess develops, she must stop breast-feeding with this breast and use a breast pump until the abscess heals. She should continue to breast-feed on the unaffected side.
• Show how to position the infant properly to prevent cracked nipples. (See *Preventing mastitis.*)

GALACTORRHEA
Inappropriate breast milk secretion, or galactorrhea, may occur 3 to 6 months after the discontinuation of breast-feeding (usually after a first delivery). Also known as hyperprolactinemia, this disorder may follow an abortion or may develop in a female who hasn't been pregnant; it rarely occurs in males. (Some degree of galactorrhea normally occurs for 3 weeks after weaning.)

Causes
Galactorrhea usually develops in a person with increased prolactin secretion from the anterior pituitary gland, with possible abnormal patterns of secretion of growth, thyroid, and adrenocorticotropic hormones and disruption of the menstrual cycle. However, increased serum prolactin doesn't always cause galactorrhea. Additional precipitating factors include the following:

- *endogenous factors,* including pituitary, ovarian, or adrenal gland tumors and hypothyroidism. In males, galactorrhea usually results from pituitary, testicular, or pineal gland tumors.
- *idiopathic factors,* possibly from stress or anxiety, which cause neurogenic depression of the prolactin-inhibiting factor.
- *exogenous factors,* such as breast stimulation, genital stimulation, or drugs (such as oral contraceptives, meprobamate, and phenothiazines).

Complications
When galactorrhea stems from a pituitary gland tumor, possible complications may include increased intracranial pressure, central nervous system (CNS) disturbances, or visual field disturbances.

Assessment findings
Usually, a woman with galactorrhea reports that her breast milk continues to flow after the 21-day period that is normal after weaning. The flow may be spontaneous and unrelated to normal lactation, or it may stem from manual expression. Typically, she reports that both breasts are affected. She may also report amenorrhea.

Diagnostic tests
Galactorrhea is determined by palpating the breast from the periphery toward the nipple in an attempt to express any secretion. The diagnosis is confirmed by microscopically observing multiple fat droplets in the fluid. (A computed tomography scan and, possibly, a mammogram may be ordered to rule out tumors.)

Treatment
The underlying cause determines the course of treatment, which ranges from simple avoidance of precipitating exogenous factors, such as drugs, to treatment of tumors with surgery, radiation, or chemotherapy.

The choice of therapy for idiopathic galactorrhea depends on whether the patient plans to have more children. If she does, treatment usually consists of bromocriptine; if she doesn't, oral estrogens (such as ethinyl estradiol) and progestins (such as progesterone) effectively treat this disorder. After treatment with bromocriptine, milk secretion usually stops in 1 to 2 months, and menstruation recurs after 6 to 24 weeks. Idiopathic galactorrhea may recur after discontinuation of drug therapy.

Nursing diagnoses
- Body image disturbance
- Ineffective individual coping
- Knowledge deficit

Nursing interventions
- Monitor for CNS abnormalities, such as headache, failing vision, and dizziness, which may indicate enlarging microadenoma of the pituitary gland.
- Maintain adequate fluid intake, especially if the patient has a fever. However, advise her to avoid tea, coffee, and certain tranquilizers that may aggravate engorgement.
- Encourage the patient to express her feelings about the disorder. Offer emotional support and reassurance.
- Help her develop effective coping strategies.

Patient teaching
- Instruct the patient to keep her breasts and nipples clean. Teach her meticulous hand-washing technique.
- Tell the patient who is taking bromocriptine to report nausea, vomiting, dyspepsia, loss of appetite, dizziness, fatigue, numbness, and hypotension. To prevent GI upset, advise her to eat small meals frequently and to take this drug with dry toast or crackers.

SELECTED REFERENCES
Haley, J. "Welcome to the Antenatal Day Unit," *Modern Midwife* 5(6):27-30, June 1995.
Illustrated Manual of Nursing Practice, 2nd ed. Springhouse, Pa.: Springhouse Corp., 1994.
Pillitteri, A. *Maternal and Child Health Nursing: Care of the Childbearing and Childrearing Family,* 2nd ed. Philadelphia: J.B. Lippincott Co., 1995.
Rakel, R.E., ed. *Conn's Current Therapy 1996.* Philadelphia: W.B. Saunders Co., 1996.
Scott, J., et al. *Danforth's Obstetrics and Gynecology,* 7th ed. Philadelphia: J.B. Lippincott Co., 1994.
Sexually Transmitted Diseases Treatment Guidelines. Seattle: University of Washington School of Medicine, January 1995.
Taylor, C.M., and Sparks, S.M. *Nursing Diagnosis Reference Manual,* 3rd ed. Springhouse, Pa.: Springhouse Corp., 1995.
Tierney, L., et al. *Current Medical Diagnosis and Treatment 1995.* East Norwalk, Conn.: Appleton & Lange, 1995.
Thyland, S., et al. "Endometriosis May Develop after Menopause," *Nurse Practitioner* 20(4):15-16, April 1995.

16 EYE DISORDERS

INTRODUCTION

When you consider that humans receive about 70% of all sensory information visually, you can understand why health care professionals urge their patients to seek routine ophthalmologic examination and early treatment to correct impaired vision and avoid blindness. (See *Leading causes of blindness*, page 1088.)

The ocular system consists of the bony orbit that houses the eye; the contents of the orbit, including the eyeball, optic nerve, extraocular muscles, cranial nerves (III, IV, and VI), blood vessels, orbital fat, and lacrimal system; and the eyelid that protects and covers the eye.

The *orbit* (or socket) encloses the eyeball in a protective recess in the skull. Its seven bones—frontal, sphenoid, zygomatic, maxilla, palatine, ethmoid, and lacrimal—form a cone, the apex of which points toward the brain; the cone's base forms the orbital rim. The periorbita covers the orbital bones. The thinness of the orbital wall makes this area particularly vulnerable to fractures.

Various extraocular muscles hold the eyeball in place and control its movement. These muscles include the following:
• *superior rectus*, which rotates the eye upward as well as adducts and rotates it inward
• *inferior rectus*, which rotates the eye downward as well as adducts and rotates it outward
• *lateral rectus*, which turns the eye outward (laterally)
• *medial rectus*, which turns the eye inward (medially)
• *superior oblique*, which turns the eye downward as well as abducts and rotates it inward
• *inferior oblique*, which turns the eye upward as well as abducts and turns it outward.

The actions of these muscles are mutually antagonistic. As one contracts, its opposing muscle relaxes.

Ocular layers

The eye has three structural layers: the cornea and sclera, the uveal tract, and the retina.

Corneoscleral layer

A dense, white, fibrous protective tissue, the *sclera* surrounds the eyeball and continues as the cornea at the limbus (corneoscleral junction) anteriorly and into the dural sheath of the optic nerve posteriorly. In this area, a sievelike structure (the lamina cribrosa) composed of a few strands of scleral tissue makes a passage for the ganglionic cell axons. (On examination, this area appears as the optic disk.) The episclera, a thin layer of fine elastic tissue, covers the sclera.

Continuous with the sclera, the *cornea* is transparent, avascular, and curved. It has five layers:

• the epithelium, which contains sensory nerves
• Bowman's membrane, which is the basement membrane for the epithelial cells
• the stroma, which constitutes the supporting tissue (90% of the cornea)
• Descemet's membrane, which provides elasticity
• the endothelium, which acts as a pump to maintain proper intraocular pressure, thereby preventing corneal turgescence (or distention).

Bathing the posterior surface of the cornea, aqueous humor maintains intraocular pressure by its volume and flow rate. Tears bathe and moisten the anterior cornea. The cornea's only function is to refract light.

Uveal layer

Known as the *uveal tract,* the middle layer of the eye is pigmented and vascular. It contains the iris and the ciliary body in the anterior portion and the choroid in the posterior portion.

The *iris* is a circular contractile disk. Centered in the iris is the pupil, through which light enters the eye. Sphincter and dilator muscles of the iris control the amount of light entering the eye. The pupil itself controls the flow of aqueous humor from the posterior to the anterior chamber.

The anterior iris joins the posterior corneal surface at an angle. Here, many tiny collecting channels form the trabecular meshwork. Aqueous humor drains through these channels into an encircling venous system called the canal of Schlemm.

Extending from the root of the iris to the ora serrata, the *ciliary body* produces aqueous humor and controls lens shape (accommodation) by its action on the zonular fibers.

The *choroid,* the largest part of the uveal tract, is made of blood vessels bound externally by the suprachoroid and internally by Bruch's membrane. Extending from the ora serrata to the optic nerve and attached to Bruch's membrane are the retina and the retinal pigment epithelium (RPE).

Retinal layer

The *retina* receives visual images and transmits them to the brain for interpretation. Although it holds no pain fibers, the retina is a multilayered sheet of neural tissue. It attaches to a layer of pigmented epithelial cells: the RPE, which adheres lightly to the choroid. Beside and beneath the RPE are rods and cones. These light receptors perceive light but process it in different ways. Rods, scattered throughout the retina, respond to low light levels and detect moving objects; cones, located in the fovea

LEADING CAUSES OF BLINDNESS

In the United States, blindness has been defined by law. A person who has optimal visual acuity of 20/200 or less in the better eye after best correction, or who has a visual field not exceeding 20 degrees in the better eye, is legally blind.

The most common causes of acquired blindness include glaucoma, age-related macular degeneration, and diabetic retinopathy. Encouragingly, the incidence of blindness from glaucoma is decreasing, most likely a result of early detection and treatment.

Rare causes of acquired blindness include herpes simplex keratitis, cataracts, and retinal detachment.

Worldwide causes

The most common causes of preventable blindness worldwide are trachoma, cataracts, onchocerciasis (microfilarial infection transmitted by a blackfly and other species of *Simulium*), and xerophthalmia (dryness of conjunctiva and cornea from vitamin A deficiency).

centralis, function best in brighter light and perceive finer details.

Three types of cones contain different visual pigments and react to specific light wavelengths: One type reacts to red light, one to green, and one to blue-violet. The eye mixes these colors into various shades; the cones can detect 150 shades.

The lens and accommodation

The *lens* of the eye is biconvex, avascular, and transparent; the lens capsule is a semipermeable membrane that can admit water and electrolytes. The lens changes shape for both near and far vision. For near vision, the ciliary body contracts and relaxes the zonular fibers, the lens becomes spherical, the pupil constricts, and the eyes converge. For far vision, the ciliary body relaxes, the zonular fibers tighten, the lens becomes flatter, the pupils dilate, and the eyes straighten. The lens refines the refraction necessary to focus a clear image on the retina.

The *vitreous body*, which is 99% water and a small amount of insoluble protein, constitutes two-thirds of the volume of the eye. This gelatinous body gives the eye its shape and contributes to the refraction of light rays. The vitreous is firmly attached anteriorly to the ora serrata of the ciliary body and posteriorly to the optic disk. The vitreous face contacts the lens; the vitreous gel rests against the retina.

Lacrimal network and eyelids

Tears are secreted by the lacrimal apparatus, which consists of the lacrimal gland, upper and lower canaliculi, lacrimal sac, and nasolacrimal duct. The tear gland, located in a shallow fossa beneath the superior temporal orbital rim, secretes fluid to keep the cornea and conjunctiva moist. These tears flow through 8 to 12 excretory ducts and contain lysozyme, an enzyme that protects the conjunctiva from bacteria. With every blink, the eyelids direct the flow to the inner canthus, where the tears pool and then drain through a tiny opening called the punctum. The tears then pass through the canaliculi and lacrimal sac and down the nasolacrimal duct, which opens into the nasal cavity.

The eyelids (palpebrae) consist of tarsal plates that are composed of dense connective tissue. The orbital septum — the fascia behind the orbicularis oculi muscle — acts as a barrier between the lids and the orbit. The levator palpebrae muscle elevates the upper lid. The eyelids contain three types of glands:

• *Meibomian glands* are sebaceous glands in the tarsal plates that secrete an oily substance to prevent evaporation of the tear film. The upper eyelid holds about 25 of these glands; the lower lid, about 20.

• *Glands of Zeis* are modified sebaceous glands connected to the follicles of the eyelashes.

• *Moll's glands* are ordinary sweat glands.

The *conjunctiva* is the thin mucous membrane that lines the eyelids (palpebral conjunctiva), folds over at the fornix, and covers the surface of the eyeball (bulbar conjunctiva). The ophthalmic and lacrimal arteries supply blood to the lids. The space between the open lids is the palpebral fissure; the juncture of the upper and lower lids is the canthus. The junction near the nose is called the nasal, medial, or inner canthus; the junction on the temporal side, the lateral or external canthus.

Depth perception

In normal binocular vision, a perceived image is projected onto the two foveae. Impulses then travel along the optic pathways to the occipital cortex, which perceives a single image. However, the cortex receives two images — each from a slightly different angle — giving the images perspective and depth.

Patient history and physical examination

Begin by asking the patient to describe any current eye problems. Ask specifically if he's had blurred vision, floaters, halos, or infection. Ask whether he wears, or has worn, eyeglasses or contact lenses. If so, when was his prescription last changed?

Find out whether he has health problems, such as hypertension or diabetes. Ask whether he takes any prescription medications. Has he had eye surgery? Also investigate the family history for cataracts, glaucoma, or blindness.

Finally, explore the patient's social and work environments to detect potential causes of eye disorders. For example, extensive reading or the use of video display terminals may strain the eyes and cause dryness. Exposure to cigarette smoke, chemicals, or glues can irritate the eyes.

Throughout the interview, observe the patient's eye movements and ability to focus for clues to eye muscle coordination and visual acuity. Note the appearance of the eyelids, eyelashes, eyeballs, and lacrimal apparatus. Do the eyelids close completely over the sclera? Is eyelid color consistent with the patient's complexion? Are the eyelashes equally distributed along the upper and lower eyelid margins, and do they curve appropriately? Do the eyes tear normally, or does the patient complain of dryness or excessive tearing? Is the punctum free of inflammation or swelling?

Examine the conjunctiva and sclera. The conjunctiva should be clear and the sclera white, although small, dark-pigmented spots occur normally on the sclera of dark-skinned persons, such as those of African or Mediterranean ancestry.

Inspect the iris, noting shape and color. Check the anterior chamber and cornea to determine if they're clear and transparent. Is the cornea shiny and bright, free of scars and other irregularities?

Check both pupils for equality of size and shape. Note pupillary reaction to light and accommodation.

After completing your inspection, gently palpate the eyelids, noting any swelling or complaints of tenderness. Extend the palpation to include the eyeballs, which should feel equally firm.

Palpate the lacrimal sac while observing the punctum. Excessive tearing or regurgitation of purulent material may indicate a blockage of the nasolacrimal duct.

Diagnostic tests

Several tests assess visual acuity and identify defects:

• *Color vision testing* may be performed to identify color blindness. The test involves showing the patient a series of pseudoisochromatic cardlike plates, such as *Ishihara's* or *Hardy-Rand-Rittler* plates. These test cards have a variegated, colored background and contain a letter, number, or pattern of a slightly different color in the center of each plate. The patient with deficient color perception can't perceive the differences in hue or, consequently, the designs formed by the color contrasts.

• *Snellen chart* or other eye charts evaluate visual acuity. Such charts use progressively smaller letters or symbols to determine central vision on a numerical scale.

• *Ophthalmoscopy* allows examination of the interior of the eye after the pupil has been dilated with a mydriatic agent.

• *Refraction tests* may be performed with or without cycloplegic agents. In cycloplegic refraction, eyedrops temporarily paralyze the ciliary muscle, thereby causing the pupil to dilate. This dilation lets the examiner identify the error of refraction more accurately.

• *Maddox rod test* assesses muscle dysfunction; it's especially useful to disclose and measure heterophoria (the tendency of the eyes to deviate).

• *Duction test* checks eye movement in all directions. While one eye is covered, the other eye follows a moving light. This test detects any weakness of rotation caused by muscle paralysis or structural dysfunction.

• *Test for convergence* locates the breaking point of fusion. For this test, the examiner holds a small object in front of the patient's nose and slowly brings it closer to the patient. Normally, the patient can maintain convergence until the object reaches the bridge of the nose. The point at which the eyes "break" is termed the near point of convergence and is measured in centimeters.

• *Cover-uncover test* assesses muscle deviation. The patient stares at a small, fixed object—first from a distance of 20' (6 m), then from 1' (30.5 cm). The examiner covers the patient's eyes one at a time, noting any movement of the uncovered eye, the direction of any deviation, and the rate at which the eyes recover normal binocular vision when latent heterophoria is present.

• *Slit-lamp examination* allows a well-illuminated microscopic examination of the eyelids and the anterior segment of the eyeball.

• *Visual field tests* examine the function of the peripheral retina, outline the blind spot (which corresponds to the optic nerve), and define the field defects resulting from lesions along the optic pathways.

• *Schiøtz tonometry* and *applanation tonometry* measure intraocular pressure. After instilling a local anesthetic in the patient's eye, the examiner places the Schiøtz tonometer lightly on the corneal surface and measures the indentation of the cornea produced by a given weight. Applanation tonometry gauges the force required to flatten, rather than indent, a small area of central cornea.

• *Gonioscopy* allows for direct visualization of the anterior chamber angle through the use of a goniolens; the slit lamp is the light source and microscope.

INSTILLING AN OPHTHALMIC OINTMENT

Follow these directions to administer an ophthalmic ointment cleanly and quickly:
• Tilt the patient's head backward, and ask him to look toward the ceiling.
• Gently pull the lower eyelid down, and apply ointment directly onto the exposed conjunctiva from the inner to the outer canthus.
• Take care to avoid touching the eye with the tip of the ointment tube.
• Repeat this procedure for the other eye.

• *Fluorescein angiography* evaluates blood vessels in the choroid and the retina after I.V. injection of fluorescein dye; images of the dye-enhanced vasculature are recorded by rapid-sequence photographs of the fundus.
• *Ocular ultrasonography* involves transmitting high-frequency sound waves into the eye and measuring their echo from ocular structures. A-scan ultrasonography measures axial eye length. B-scan ultrasonography evaluates eye structures and helps diagnose abnormalities.

DISORDERS OF THE EYELIDS AND LACRIMAL DUCTS

Caused by a range of factors from infection to congenital deformity, disorders of the eyelid and lacrimal duct are commonly apparent upon examination. They include blepharitis, ptosis, orbital cellulitis, dacryocystitis, chalazion, and stye.

BLEPHARITIS

A common inflammation of eyelash follicles and meibomian glands of the upper or lower eyelids, blepharitis gives a red-rimmed appearance to the eyelid margins. The disorder, which may affect both eyes (and both upper and lower eyelids), tends to recur and may become chronic. Seborrheic (nonulcerative) blepharitis is more common in elderly persons but may also affect persons with red hair. Staphylococcal (ulcerative) blepharitis may coexist with seborrheic blepharitis. Both types can be controlled if treatment begins before the onset of ocular involvement.

Causes

Seborrheic blepharitis generally results from seborrhea of the scalp, eyebrows, and ears; ulcerative blepharitis, from a *Staphylococcus aureus* infection. (Chalazia and styes are likely to develop with this infection.)

Complications

Without adequate treatment, blepharitis may lead to keratitis.

Assessment findings

The patient typically complains that his eyelids itch, burn, or feel like they have a foreign body in them. He may also complain that his eyelids are crusty and stick together when he awakens in the morning.

Inspection may reveal that the patient unknowingly rubs his eyes (causing the red rims) or continually blinks. You may also note waxy scales along the eyelids, indicating seborrheic blepharitis. Flaky scales on the eyelashes, missing eyelashes, or ulcerations on eyelid margins suggest ulcerative blepharitis.

Diagnostic tests

A culture of the ulcerated eyelid margin may detect *S. aureus* in ulcerative blepharitis.

Treatment

Early treatment is essential to prevent recurrence or complications. For seborrheic blepharitis, treatment includes daily shampooing (using a mild shampoo on a cotton-tipped applicator or a washcloth) to remove scales from the eyelid margins. The patient should also shampoo the scalp and eyebrows and follow up with warm eye compresses.

Ulcerative blepharitis requires the same treatment in addition to a sulfonamide or an appropriate antibiotic eye ointment. (See *Instilling an ophthalmic ointment.*)

Nursing diagnoses

• Altered health maintenance
• Body image disturbance
• Impaired skin integrity
• Risk for injury

Nursing interventions

• Provide eyelid care at least twice daily. To do so, dip a cotton-tipped applicator in baby shampoo, and then shake the applicator to remove any excess shampoo. Using a downward motion from the eyelid margin to the tips of the eyelashes, gently clean the upper eyelid margin. Repeat on the lower eyelid margin. Use a warm, wet washcloth to rinse the shampoo away.

Patient teaching
• Encourage the patient to participate in eyelid care.
• Show him how to use a cotton-tipped applicator or a clean washcloth to remove the scales from his eyelids. Instruct him to do this daily.
• Demonstrate how to apply warm compresses: First, run warm water into a clean bowl. Then, immerse a clean cloth in the water and wring the water from the cloth. Next, place the warm cloth against the closed eyelid. (Be careful not to use hot water, which could burn the skin.) Hold the compress in place until it cools. Continue this procedure for 15 minutes.

PTOSIS

A congenital or acquired disorder, ptosis is a drooping upper eyelid that remains lowered despite the patient's effort to raise it. The condition may be unilateral or bilateral, continuous or intermittent. Severe ptosis usually responds well to treatment; slight ptosis may require no treatment at all.

Causes and pathophysiology

Congenital ptosis is transmitted as an autosomal dominant trait, or it results from a congenital anomaly in which the levator muscles of the eyelids fail to develop. Although this condition is usually unilateral, it can be bilateral.

Acquired ptosis may result from any of the following:
• *age* (senile ptosis), which causes loss of levator muscle tone and usually produces bilateral ptosis.
• *mechanical factors* that make the eyelid heavy, such as swelling caused by a foreign body on the eyelid's palpebral surface. Other mechanical factors include edema, inflammation produced by a tumor or pseudotumor, or an extra fatty fold.
• *myogenic factors,* such as muscular dystrophy or myasthenia gravis (in which the defect may involve humoral transmission at the myoneural junction).
• *neurogenic (paralytic) factors* from interference in eyelid innervation by the oculomotor nerve (cranial nerve III). This usually results from trauma, diabetes mellitus, or carotid aneurysm. Or it may result from an interruption of sympathetic innervation to the eye (resulting in Horner's syndrome with ipsilateral miosis and ptosis).
• *nutritional factors,* such as a thiamine deficiency caused by chronic alcoholism or other malnutrition-producing states, such as hyperemesis gravidarum.

RECOGNIZING PTOSIS

A drooping upper eyelid—typically apparent on visual examination—is the hallmark of ptosis. The disorder may affect one or both eyelids.

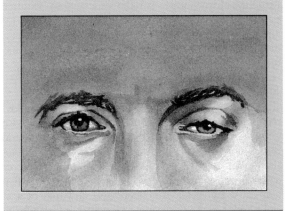

Complications
Ptosis may disturb normal vision.

Assessment findings
In ptosis, your findings will vary, depending on the patient's age. Inspection of the infant with congenital ptosis may reveal a smooth, flat upper eyelid without the tarsal fold normally caused by the pull of the levator muscle. You may also note an associated weakness of the superior rectus muscle. (See *Recognizing ptosis.*)

The child with unilateral ptosis that covers the pupil may experience amblyopia, possibly from disuse or lack of eye stimulation. If the child has bilateral ptosis, his eyebrow may be elevated or his forehead wrinkled because of attempts to raise the upper eyelid. You may also observe the child tilt his head backward to see objects straight ahead.

The adult patient with ptosis may have a history of chronic alcoholism or excessive vomiting. Upon inspection, you may see that one eyelid either covers the patient's iris completely or covers more of the iris than the other eyelid. If the patient has myasthenia gravis, inspection may reveal ptosis that occurs during the evening. You may also observe a fixed, dilated pupil; divergent strabismus; and slight depression of the eyeball.

Diagnostic tests

Measuring palpebral fissure widths and checking the range of eyelid movement help determine the severity of ptosis. Other tests determine the underlying cause of the disorder. For instance, the glucose tolerance test may detect diabetes mellitus. The edrophonium test can confirm myasthenia gravis (in the patient with acquired ptosis and no history of trauma). Ophthalmologic examination may disclose foreign bodies. Magnetic resonance imaging or digital subtraction angiography may reveal an aneurysm.

Treatment

Slight ptosis that doesn't produce deformity or vision loss requires no treatment. Severe ptosis that interferes with vision or disfigures appearance may require surgery to resection weak levator muscles. To correct congenital ptosis, the patient may undergo surgery at age 3 or 4, or earlier if ptosis is unilateral and if pupillary occlusion may cause amblyopia. An option to surgery may be special eyeglasses with an attached suspended crutch on the frame to elevate the eyelid.

Effective management also includes treatment of the underlying cause. For example, in myasthenia gravis, neostigmine may be prescribed to enhance innervation to the muscles.

Nursing diagnoses
• Altered health maintenance
• Risk for infection
• Risk for injury
• Sensory or perceptual alterations (visual)

Nursing interventions
• Provide a safe environment by removing excess equipment and furniture from the patient's room.
• Report postoperative bleeding immediately.
• Apply ointment to sutures, as prescribed.
• Apply ice compresses to decrease swelling.

Patient teaching
• After surgery, emphasize the need to protect the surgical site during healing (usually 6 weeks). Explain that injury at the suture line can precipitate recurrent ptosis. Review the signs of infection.
• If the patient is a young child, encourage his parents to review safety measures with him.
• Provide oral and written instructions for using medications, including ophthalmic ointment.

ORBITAL CELLULITIS

An acute infection, orbital cellulitis involves the fatty orbital tissues and eyelids but not the eyeball itself. With treatment, the prognosis is good.

Causes

Orbital cellulitis usually results from infection of nearby structures—typically by streptococcal, staphylococcal, and pneumococcal organisms. In children, orbital cellulitis may follow *Haemophilus influenzae* infection. These organisms invade the orbit, commonly by direct extension through the sinuses (especially the ethmoid sinus), the bloodstream, or the lymphatic ducts.

Primary orbital cellulitis results from orbital injury (such as an insect bite) that permits bacterial entry. Although this disease form is common in young children, it also affects people with poor dental hygiene and those who snort cocaine.

Complications

The infection may extend posteriorly, causing cavernous sinus thrombosis, meningitis, or brain abscess and, possibly, death. If the disease leads to optic neuritis, atrophy and subsequent vision loss may occur.

Assessment findings

The patient typically complains of severe orbital pain. He may also report chills, fever, and malaise.

Inspection may reveal chemosis (excessive conjunctival edema) and unilateral eye edema. You may also observe impaired eye movement, hyperemia of the orbital tissue, reddened eyelids, and a purulent ocular discharge that mats the lashes. In advanced orbital cellulitis, examination may reveal proptosis caused by edematous tissues within the bony orbit.

Diagnostic tests

Wound culture and sensitivity testing may identify the infecting organism. A white blood cell count typically reveals leukocytosis.

Treatment

To prevent complications, treatment should begin promptly. Primary treatment consists of systemic oral or I.V. antibiotics and eyedrops or ointment. Supportive treatment consists of bed rest, fluids, and warm, moist eye compresses. If cellulitis fails to respond to antibiotics after 3 days, incision and drainage may be necessary.

Nursing diagnoses
• Altered health maintenance
• Fear
• Pain
• Risk for infection
• Risk for injury

Nursing interventions
• Monitor vital signs, fluid and electrolyte balance, and visual acuity every 4 hours.
• Assess the patient's pain level, and administer analgesics as prescribed. Monitor their effectiveness.
• Apply warm compresses every 3 to 4 hours to the inflamed area to relieve discomfort.

Patient teaching
• Help the patient to identify avoidable hazards that may cause eye injury.
• Teach him how to apply warm eye compresses.
• Explain the actions, dosages, routes, and adverse effects of prescribed medications.
• Before discharge, instruct the patient to complete the full prescribed antibiotic regimen. To prevent recurrent orbital cellulitis, teach him to maintain good general hygiene and to carefully clean abrasions and cuts that occur near the eye. Urge early treatment of orbital cellulitis to prevent spreading infection.

DACRYOCYSTITIS
A common infection, dacryocystitis may be acute or chronic. In adults, this infection of the lacrimal sac may follow an obstruction (dacryostenosis) of the nasolacrimal duct (most prevalent in women over age 40) or trauma. In infants, it results from congenital atresia of the nasolacrimal duct. Usually unilateral, dacryocystitis can also be bilateral.

Causes and pathophysiology
The most common infecting organism in acute dacryocystitis is *Staphylococcus aureus* or, occasionally, beta-hemolytic streptococcus. In chronic dacryocystitis, *Streptococcus pneumoniae* or, sometimes, a fungus—such as *Candida albicans*—is responsible for the infection.

In infants, atresia of the nasolacrimal ducts results from failure of canalization or, in the first few weeks of life, from blockage when the membrane between the lower nasolacrimal duct and the inferior nasal meatus fails to open spontaneously before tear secretion.

Complications
Untreated dacryocystitis may result in skin perforation and fistulas.

Assessment findings
The patient typically complains of constant tearing—the hallmark of both acute and chronic dacryocystitis—and tenderness over the lacrimal sac.

In acute disease, pressure applied to the lacrimal sac causes the punctum to produce a purulent discharge. In chronic dacryocystitis, the tear sac produces a mucoid discharge.

Diagnostic tests
• *Cultures* of exudate identify the pathogen, typically *Staphylococcus aureus* and, occasionally, beta-hemolytic streptococcus in acute dacryocystitis; *Streptococcus pneumoniae* or *C. albicans* in chronic disease.
• *White blood cell (WBC) count* may rise in acute disease; it's usually normal in chronic dacryocystitis.
• *Dacryocystography* can locate the site of congenital atresia.

Treatment
Topical and systemic antibiotics and warm compresses may relieve acute dacryocystitis. Chronic dacryocystitis may eventually require dacryocystorhinostomy.

For nasolacrimal duct obstruction in an infant, treatment consists of carefully massaging the lacrimal sac area four times daily until the infant is 8 or 9 months old. At that time, the obstruction commonly resolves spontaneously. If massage fails to open the duct, dilating the punctum and probing the duct may be necessary.

Nursing diagnoses
• Altered health maintenance
• Altered tissue perfusion
• Anxiety
• Impaired gas exchange
• Impaired tissue integrity

Nursing interventions
• If the patient will have surgery, encourage him to express any fears related to the procedure.
• Monitor the postoperative patient for bleeding—a rare complication.
• Apply ice compresses postoperatively to the affected area.
• After surgery, assist the patient with pulmonary hygiene to prevent atelectasis.

A LOOK AT A CHALAZION

A chalazion typically appears as a nontender bump on one of the eyelids. Here, a chalazion affects the upper eyelid.

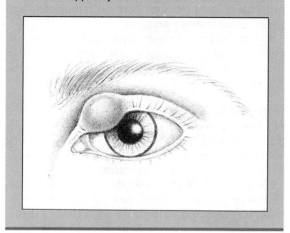

Patient teaching
• Instruct the patient with acute dacryocystitis to complete the prescribed course of antibiotic therapy. Give instructions concerning the medication's purpose, dosage, and possible adverse effects.
• Teach the patient how to apply warm compresses before instilling antibiotic eyedrops.
• Review reportable signs of worsening infection.
• If the patient is having surgery for chronic dacryocystitis, tell him to expect blood to ooze from his nose after surgery. To reduce this blood flow, he may have an ice compress applied over the pressure bandage at the incision site. Inform him that he'll lie on the affected side for up to 24 hours after surgery until the bleeding stops. Explain that this position will prevent him from swallowing blood.
• Advise the patient not to drink hot beverages for the first 3 days after surgery and to avoid alcohol for 2 weeks postoperatively. Warn him not to blow his nose for 1 week after surgery.

CHALAZION

A common eye disorder, a chalazion is a granulomatous inflammation of a meibomian (sebaceous) gland in the upper or lower eyelid. This disorder usually develops slowly over several weeks. A large chalazion seldom subsides spontaneously. Because the upper eyelid holds 25 meibomian glands and the lower eyelid holds 20, more than one gland can be infected at the same time. Generally benign and chronic, a chalazion can occur at any age.

Causes
Obstruction of the meibomian gland duct causes a chalazion.

Complications
Untreated, a chalazion may press on the cornea and cause a vision disturbance, such as astigmatism.

Assessment findings
The patient may complain of a small bump or lump on the eyelid. Inspection may reveal a small nodule pointing toward the eyelid's conjunctival side. The area may look inflamed. However, if the chalazion has grown large, inflammation may have subsided. (See *A look at a chalazion.*) Upon eversion of the eyelid, you'll see a red or red-yellow elevated area on the conjunctival surface. Palpation of the eyelid may disclose a small bump or nodule. The bump isn't tender initially, but it may become tender in later stages.

Diagnostic tests
Recurrent chalazions, especially in an adult, necessitate a biopsy to rule out meibomian gland cancer.

Treatment
Initial therapy consists of applying warm compresses to open the glandular lumen and, occasionally, instilling sulfonamide eyedrops. If this therapy fails, if the chalazion presses on the eyeball, or if the swelling causes a cosmetic problem, incision and curettage under local anesthesia may be necessary. Afterward, a pressure patch is applied to the eye for 8 to 12 hours to control bleeding and swelling. When the patch is removed, treatment again involves warm eye compresses applied for 10 to 15 minutes, two to four times daily. Antimicrobial eyedrops or eye ointment may be ordered to prevent secondary infection.

Nursing diagnoses
• Altered health maintenance
• Anxiety
• Body image disturbance
• Risk for injury
• Sensory or perceptual alterations (visual)

Nursing interventions

• Instill antimicrobial eyedrops or ointment, as ordered.
• Provide a safe environment by removing excess equipment from the patient's room. Orient him to the room, and show him how to use the call button.
• Assess the patient's visual acuity preoperatively and at the first postoperative visit.

Patient teaching

• Teach the patient about any antimicrobial drugs used to treat the chalazion. Name the drug and its desired actions, and discuss its dosage and possible adverse effects. Also, show the patient or a family member how to instill eyedrops. Reinforce your instruction with written information.
• Teach proper eyelid hygiene to the patient predisposed to chalazia. Show him how to wash his eyelid with water and mild baby shampoo applied with a cotton-tipped applicator.
• Instruct the patient how to properly apply *warm* compresses. Caution him not to use hot water that may burn his skin. Advise him to use a clean compress. Direct him to apply warm compresses at the first sign of eyelid irritation. Explain that this will increase circulation in the area and keep the lumen open.
• Urge him to keep follow-up appointments.

STYE

Also called a hordeolum, a stye is a localized infection that can occur externally (in the lumen of the smaller glands of Zeis or in Moll's glands) or internally (in the larger meibomian gland). A stye can occur in any patient at any age. Generally, the infection responds well to treatment but tends to recur.

Causes

A staphylococcal organism causes a stye.

Complications

If untreated, a stye may lead to cellulitis of the eyelid.

Assessment findings

The patient typically complains of a painful swelling of the eyelid. Inspection of the eyelid may reveal a red, swollen area. At the eyelid margin, you may also observe an abscess that displaces the eyelash, making the eyelash point straight outward from the abscess center. (See *Inspecting a stye.*)

INSPECTING A STYE

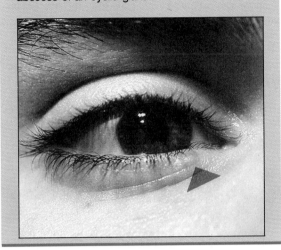

Visual examination alone usually confirms a stye. This infection appears as a localized red, swollen abscess of an eyelid gland.

Diagnostic tests

A culture of the purulent material from the abscess usually reveals a staphylococcal organism.

Treatment

Warm compresses applied for 10 to 15 minutes, four times daily for 3 to 4 days, facilitate drainage of the abscess. This treatment also relieves pain and inflammation and promotes suppuration. Drug therapy includes a topical sulfonamide or antibiotic eyedrops or ointment and, occasionally, a systemic antibiotic. If conservative treatment fails, incision and drainage may be necessary.

Nursing diagnoses

• Altered health maintenance
• Impaired skin integrity
• Pain
• Risk for infection
• Risk for injury
• Sensory or perceptual alterations (visual)

Nursing interventions

• Administer antibiotics as ordered.
• Apply warm compresses to help drain infection and relieve pain. Use a sterile bowl and gauze and warm tap water.

Patient teaching

• Instruct the patient to use a clean cloth for each warm compress application and to dispose of it or launder it separately to prevent spreading infection to family members. For the same reason, the patient should avoid sharing towels and washcloths.
• Caution the patient to avoid squeezing the stye or rubbing the eye; this spreads the infection and may cause cellulitis.
• Teach the patient or a family member how to instill eyedrops or ointment into the cul-de-sac of the lower eyelid.
• Warn that ophthalmic ointment may blur vision.
• Teach proper eye hygiene to prevent recurrent infections.

DISORDERS OF THE CONJUNCTIVA

Conjunctival disorders typically cause obvious inflammation. Although some are self-limiting, others may lead to blindness if left untreated.

INCLUSION CONJUNCTIVITIS

A fairly common, acute ocular inflammation, inclusion conjunctivitis results from infection by *Chlamydia trachomatis*. Also known as inclusion blennorrhea, the disease develops 5 to 10 days after contamination and may persist for weeks or months. Occasionally it becomes chronic, but the prognosis is usually good.

Causes and pathophysiology

The microorganism *C. trachomatis* causes inclusion conjunctivitis. This pathogen, which usually infects the urethra in males and the cervix in females, may be transmitted during sexual activity. (Because contaminated cervical secretions can infect the eyes of the neonate during birth, the organism that causes inclusion conjunctivitis may contribute to some cases of ophthalmia neonatorum.) Rarely, inclusion conjunctivitis may result from autoinfection (when a person transfers the virus from his genitourinary tract to his own eyes).

Complications

Children and adults may develop otitis media secondary to preauricular lymphadenopathy. In the neonate, pseudomembranes may form, which can lead to conjunctival scarring. Untreated infection may result in blindness.

Assessment findings

In a neonate, you'll notice swollen, reddened lower eyelids, excessive tearing, and a moderately purulent discharge. In a child or an adult, you may hear complaints of photosensitivity, which may indicate uveitis. The patient may also report sexual contact with an infected individual. Additionally, you may observe swollen eyelids.

Diagnostic tests

Examination of Giemsa-stained conjunctival scrapings reveals cytoplasmic inclusion bodies in conjunctival epithelial cells and many polymorphonuclear leukocytes. Culture results are usually negative for bacteria.

Treatment

In infants, treatment consists of instilling eyedrops of 1% tetracycline in oil, erythromycin ophthalmic ointment, or sulfonamide eyedrops five or six times daily for 2 weeks. To prevent ophthalmia neonatorum, neonates receive tetracycline or erythromycin ophthalmic ointment as a one-time dose 1 hour after birth.

For adults, treatment calls for administering oral tetracycline or erythromycin for 3 weeks. Severe disease may require concomitant systemic sulfonamide therapy. If the patient has associated uveitis, treatment may include corticosteroids and cycloplegic eyedrops.

Nursing diagnoses

• Altered health maintenance
• Pain
• Risk for infection
• Sensory or perceptual alterations (visual)

Nursing interventions

• Keep the patient's eyes clean. Using aseptic technique, clean the eyes from the inner to the outer canthus. Record the amount and color of drainage. Apply warm compresses as needed.
• If the patient's eyes are sensitive to light, keep the room dark or suggest that he wear dark glasses. Provide appropriate diversional activities.
• To prevent further spread of inclusion conjunctivitis, wash your hands thoroughly before and after instilling eye medications.

Patient teaching

• Remind the patient not to rub his eyes, which can irritate them. Teach proper hand-washing techniques and disposal of facial tissues.

• Inform the patient about his prescribed medication, including its desired actions, dosage, possible adverse effects, and necessary duration of therapy.
• Review the signs of *C. trachomatis* infections. Discuss ways to prevent infection; for example, with barrier contraceptives.
• Advise genital examination of the mother of an infected neonate, or of any adult with inclusion conjunctivitis.
• Recommend that the patient alert recent sexual partners to the possibility of chlamydial infection.

CONJUNCTIVITIS

Whether caused by an allergen, a viral or bacterial infection, or a chemical reaction, conjunctivitis is characterized by hyperemia of the conjunctiva. The disorder is transmitted by contaminated towels, washcloths, or the patient's own hand, and it usually spreads rapidly from one eye to the other. Commonly benign and self-limiting, it seldom affects vision. Chronic conjunctivitis may signal degenerative changes or damage from repeated acute attacks.

Acute bacterial conjunctivitis—or pinkeye—usually lasts about 2 weeks. Some viral conjunctival infections may last 2 to 3 weeks, whereas others follow a chronic course and may produce severe disability. In the Western hemisphere, conjunctivitis is probably the most common eye disorder.

Causes

Among the substances and organisms that cause conjunctivitis are:
• allergens, such as pollen, grass, cosmetics, topical medications, air pollutants, smoke, or seasonal allergens. Vernal conjunctivitis apparently results from various, unidentified allergens, although it's sometimes associated with grass or pollen sensitivity. This form of conjunctivitis affects both eyes, usually begins before puberty, and may persist intermittently for about 10 years.
• bacteria, such as *Staphylococcus aureus, Streptococcus pneumoniae, Neisseria gonorrhoeae,* and *N. meningitidis*
• chlamydia, such as *Chlamydia trachomatis* (which causes inclusion conjunctivitis)
• viruses, such as herpes simplex virus type 1 and adenovirus types 3, 7, and 8 (type 8 is primarily responsible for epidemic keratoconjunctivitis).

An idiopathic form of conjunctivitis may be associated with certain systemic diseases, such as erythema multiforme, chronic follicular conjunctivitis, and thyroid disease. Conjunctivitis may also be secondary to pneu-mococcal dacryocystitis or canaliculitis caused by a candidal infection.

Complications

Untreated, allergic conjunctivitis may lead to a tic; epidemic keratoconjunctivitis may result in corneal infiltrates; and herpes simplex conjunctivitis may lead to corneal ulcers and subsequent eye loss.

Assessment findings

The patient may complain of eye pain and sensitivity to light (photophobia). He may also report burning, itching, and the sensation of a foreign body in the eye (which suggests bacterial conjunctivitis). If the patient is a child, he may complain of a sore throat and fever as well.

Inspection typically discloses conjunctival hyperemia, discharge, and tearing. You may also see a crust of sticky, mucopurulent discharge, which indicates bacterial conjunctivitis. Or you may see a profuse, purulent discharge, which indicates gonococcal conjunctivitis. Copious tearing and minimal discharge suggest viral conjunctivitis.

In vernal conjunctivitis, inspection of the conjunctiva of the upper eyelid may reveal bumps, or conjunctival papillae. (See *Conjunctival papillae,* page 1098.) Palpation of the preauricular lymph node on the affected side may uncover an enlargement, suggesting viral conjunctivitis.

Diagnostic tests

• *Stained smears* of conjunctival scrapings show mostly monocytes if a virus causes conjunctivitis. Polymorphonuclear cells (neutrophils) predominate if bacteria causes conjunctivitis, and eosinophils if an allergen causes conjunctivitis.
• *Culture and sensitivity tests* can identify a bacterial pathogen and indicate appropriate antibiotic therapy.

Treatment

Bacterial conjunctivitis requires an appropriate topical antibiotic. Although viral conjunctivitis resists treatment, broad-spectrum antibiotic eyedrops may prevent secondary infection. Herpes simplex infection generally responds to treatment with trifluridine drops, vidarabine ointment, or oral acyclovir, but the infection may persist for 2 to 3 weeks. Treatment of vernal conjunctivitis includes instillation of corticosteroid drops followed by cromolyn, cold compresses to relieve itching and, occasionally, oral antihistamines.

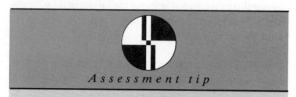

A s s e s s m e n t   t i p

CONJUNCTIVAL PAPILLAE

If you see papillae in the conjunctiva of the upper eyelid, your patient may have vernal (allergic) conjunctivitis. These cobblestone bumps are the telltale sign. They result from swollen lymph tissue within the conjunctival membrane.

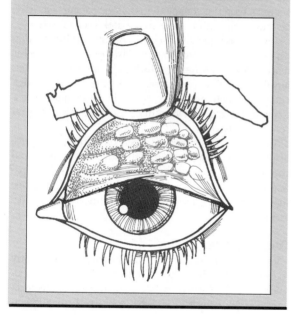

Instillation of a one-time dose of tetracycline or erythromycin ointment in the eyes of neonates prevents gonococcal and chlamydial conjunctivitis.

Nursing diagnoses
• Altered health maintenance
• Anxiety
• Risk for infection
• Sensory or perceptual alterations (visual)

Nursing interventions
• Apply warm compresses and therapeutic ointment or eyedrops, as ordered. Don't irrigate the eye because this will spread the infection.
• Notify public health officials if culture results identify *N. gonorrhoeae.*

• Obtain culture specimens before antibiotic therapy.

Patient teaching
• Show the patient proper hand-washing techniques. Because some forms of conjunctivitis are highly contagious, urge the patient and family members to avoid sharing washcloths, towels, and pillows.
• Caution the patient against rubbing his infected eye. This can spread the infection to the other eye and to other persons.
• Warn the patient with "cold sores" to avoid kissing others on the eyelids to prevent the spread of the disease.
• Demonstrate how to instill eyedrops and ointments correctly—without touching the bottle tip to the eye or eyelashes.
• Explain the purpose, dosage, and possible adverse effects of drug therapy. Emphasize the importance of completing the prescribed course.
• If conjunctivitis results from a sexually transmitted organism, such as *N. gonorrhoeae,* review the methods for preventing disease transmission.
• Stress the importance of wearing safety glasses if the patient works near chemical irritants.

DISORDERS OF THE CORNEA

Some corneal disorders, such as abrasions, may be mild and seldom cause complications. Others, such as ulcers, may be severe and lead to blindness.

KERATITIS
Acute or chronic, this corneal inflammation usually affects only one eye. The inflammation may be deep or superficial. Superficial keratitis is fairly common and may develop at any age. The prognosis depends on the cause.

Causes
Keratitis most commonly results from infection by herpes simplex virus type 1. It may also result from exposure—from the patient's inability to close his eyelids—or from congenital syphilis (interstitial keratitis). Less commonly, it stems from bacterial and fungal infections.

Complications
Untreated, recurrent keratitis may lead to blindness.

Assessment findings

The history may reveal a recent upper respiratory tract infection, accompanied by cold sores. The patient with keratitis may complain of eye pain, central vision loss, and sensitivity. He may also report the sensation of a foreign body in his eye. A complaint concerning blurred vision indicates an infection in the center of the cornea.

Inspection may reveal a cornea without its normal luster. If only the lower portion of the cornea is affected, the inflammation may result from exposure.

Diagnostic tests

Slit-lamp examination of the eye stained with sodium fluorescein may show a portion of the cornea retaining the dye. This indicates that the patient has a corneal inflammation or abrasion. If the fluorescein-stained area shows small branchlike (dendritic) lesions, the keratitis may be caused by a herpes simplex virus.

Treatment

Acute dendritic keratitis may respond to trifluridine eyedrops or vidarabine ophthalmic ointment, and a broad-spectrum antibiotic may prevent secondary bacterial infection. Oral acyclovir—under clinical investigation in the United States—is used extensively in Europe and Canada.

Chronic dendritic keratitis may respond more quickly to vidarabine therapy, and long-term topical therapy may be necessary. (Corticosteroid therapy is usually contraindicated in dendritic keratitis or any other viral or fungal disease of the cornea.) For fungal keratitis, natamycin is the treatment of choice.

Keratitis caused by exposure requires applying a moisturizing ointment and a plastic bubble eye shield or eye patch over the exposed cornea. Treatment for severe corneal scarring may include keratoplasty (cornea transplantation).

Nursing diagnoses

- Altered health maintenance
- Pain
- Risk for infection
- Risk for injury (corneal)
- Sensory or perceptual alterations (visual)

Nursing interventions

- Watch for keratitis in patients predisposed to cold sores.
- Wear gloves when in contact with the eyes or ocular drainage of the patient with keratitis from herpes simplex virus.
- Apply warm compresses to the patient's eye to help relieve pain.
- Dim the lights if the patient has photophobia.

Patient teaching

- Review drug action, dosage, instillation techniques, and possible adverse effects.
- Explain that stress, traumatic injury, fever, colds, and overexposure to the sun may trigger a flare-up of keratitis.
- Recommend wearing sunglasses to minimize the effects of photophobia.
- If the keratitis is contagious, teach meticulous hand washing and explain other ways to prevent spreading infection.

CORNEAL ABRASION

A scratch on the epithelial surface of the cornea is called a corneal abrasion. With appropriate treatment for this common eye injury, the prognosis is usually good.

Causes

A corneal abrasion usually results from a foreign object, such as a cinder or dirt speck, that becomes embedded under the eyelid. Even if tears wash away the object, the cornea may still sustain injury. Other corneal abrasions may occur in the workplace, especially if a worker doesn't wear safety glasses. Tiny metal fragments may fly in the worker's eyes and quickly rust on the cornea. Similar abrasions commonly affect the eyes of people who fall asleep wearing hard contact lenses.

Complications

A corneal scratch produced by a fingernail, a piece of paper, or other organic substance may cause a persistent lesion. If the epithelium doesn't heal properly, recurrent corneal erosion and ulceration may develop, which can lead to permanent vision loss.

Assessment findings

Patient history may include eye trauma or contact lenses worn for a prolonged period. The patient typically reports a sensation of "something in the eye," sensitivity to light, decreased visual acuity (if the abrasion occurs in the pupillary region), and pain. Discomfort develops because the cornea is richly endowed with nerve endings from the trigeminal nerve (cranial nerve V). This results in pain that's disproportionate to the injury size.

Inspection may reveal redness, increased tearing and, possibly, a foreign body on the cornea. Eversion of the eyelid may uncover a foreign object embedded under the eyelid.

Diagnostic tests
After staining with fluorescein, the cornea's injured area appears green when illuminated by a flashlight. Slit-lamp examination discloses the abrasion's depth.

Treatment
A deeply embedded foreign body requires removal with a foreign body spud after anesthetizing the cornea with a topical agent. A rust ring on the cornea can be removed with an ophthalmic burr after applying a topical anesthetic. When only partial removal of the rust ring is possible, the eye is left alone to allow reepithelialization, which lifts the rust ring to the surface, allowing complete removal the next day.

Additional treatment includes instilling broad-spectrum antibiotic eyedrops in the affected eye every 3 to 4 hours.

Nursing diagnoses
• Altered health maintenance
• Fear
• Pain
• Risk for injury
• Sensory or perceptual alterations (visual)

Nursing interventions
• Use a flashlight to inspect the patient's cornea. Check his visual acuity before treatment begins. This provides a medical baseline and a legal safeguard.
• If you see a foreign body in the patient's eye, irrigate the eye with 0.9% sodium chloride solution.
• Administer prescribed antibiotics and cycloplegics as ordered.
• Instill a topical anesthetic, as ordered, to ensure comfort and cooperation. (However, never give the patient topical anesthetic drops for self-administration. Abuse of this medication can delay healing—especially if the patient rubs the numb eye and further injures it.)

Patient teaching
• Reassure the patient that the corneal epithelium usually heals in 24 to 48 hours.
• Teach proper instillation of antibiotic eyedrops, as ordered. Explain that an untreated corneal infection can lead to ulceration and permanent vision loss.
• Emphasize wearing safety glasses in the workplace, if appropriate.

• If the patient wears contact lenses, review instructions for wear and care to prevent future injury.

CORNEAL ULCERS
A major cause of blindness worldwide, corneal ulcers produce scarring or perforation. They occur in the central or marginal cornea, vary in shape and size, and may be singular or multiple. Prompt treatment (within hours of onset) can prevent visual impairment.

Causes
Corneal ulcers usually result from bacterial, viral, or fungal infections. Common bacterial sources include *Staphylococcus aureus, Staphylococcus epidermis, Pseudomonas aeruginosa, Streptococcus pneumoniae,* and *Moraxella liquefaciens.* Viral causes include herpes simplex type 1, variola, vaccinia, and varicella-zoster viruses. Common fungal infections result from *Candida albicans, Fusarium, Cephalosporium,* and *Aspergillus* organisms.

Other causes include traumatic injury, reactions to toxins and allergens, and corneal exposure. Tuberculoprotein causes a classic phlyctenular (blistering) keratoconjunctivitis; a vitamin A deficiency may lead to xerophthalmia; and fifth cranial nerve lesions produce neurotropic ulcers.

Complications
Corneal ulcers may produce scarring and blindness.

Assessment findings
Patient history may include a traumatic injury or the use of contact lenses (hard or soft). The patient usually reports pain (aggravated by blinking), photophobia, and increased tearing. He may also complain of pronounced blurred vision (suggesting central corneal ulceration).

On inspection, you may observe eye congestion and, if the patient has a bacterial ulcer, a purulent discharge. Examination of the cornea may also disclose a sterile hypopyon (an accumulation of white blood cells in the anterior chamber). Resembling a white crescent moon, the hypopyon moves as the patient tilts his head.

Diagnostic tests
Fluorescein dye, instilled in the conjunctival sac, stains the outline of the ulcer, making it visible to the naked eye. Then a slit-lamp examination helps to assess the ulcer's depth. Additionally, culture and sensitivity testing of a corneal scraping may help to identify the causative bacterium or fungus.

TREATING CORNEAL ULCERS

For corneal ulcers caused by bacterial, viral, or fungal infection, the main treatment consists of drug therapy to destroy the infection. Drug choices depend on the infecting organism. Steroid preparations are contraindicated because they can encourage microorganism growth.

Bacterial infections

Medications typically include broad-spectrum antibiotics. If the corneal ulcer results from infection with *Pseudomonas aeruginosa*—the most common infecting organism in contact lens wearers—typical medications include tobramycin and piperacillin. I.V. ticarcillin may be used when the infection involves the corneoscleral limbus, or fortified tobramycin may be given alternately with fortified cefazolin eyedrops every 30 minutes around the clock.

An infection with *P. aeruginosa* spreads rapidly and can cause corneal perforation and eye loss within 24 hours. To prevent this, treatment should begin immediately. If the patient is hospitalized, he should be isolated.

Viral infections

If corneal ulceration results from herpes simplex type 1 virus, treatment includes topical applications of trifluridine drops or vidarabine ointment. Corneal ulcers resulting from herpes infection typically recur, requiring further trifluridine treatment.

If tests identify a varicella-zoster viral infection, treatment includes oral acyclovir to stem the primary infection and topical sulfonamide ointment three to four times daily to prevent secondary infection. In this painful infection, corneal lesions are unilateral and follow the fifth cranial nerve pathway. Analgesics are given for pain relief and cycloplegic eyedrops for associated anterior uveitis.

Fungal infections

For corneal ulcers caused by *Fusarium, Cephalosporium,* or *Candida* organisms, the treatment of choice is topical instillation of natamycin.

Treatment

For infection-related ulcers, therapy calls for systemic and topical broad-spectrum antibiotics until culture results identify the organism responsible for corneal ulcers. Treatment goals include eliminating the ulcer's underlying cause and providing pain relief. (See *Treating corneal ulcers.*)

For corneal ulcers related to hypovitaminosis A, treatment aims to correct dietary deficiency or GI malabsorption of vitamin A.

Treatment for neurotropic ulcers or for corneal ulcers resulting from exposure keratitis may include frequent instillation of artificial tears or lubricating ointments or application of a plastic bubble eye shield. Even tarsorrhaphy (suturing the eyelids closed) may be necessary until the eye heals.

Nursing diagnoses

• Pain
• Risk for infection
• Sensory or perceptual alterations (visual)

Nursing interventions

• Use gloves when caring for a patient who has an ocular discharge.
• Instill eyedrops as ordered. Clean and medicate the noninfected eye and put on new gloves before treating the infected eye.
• Administer pain medication, as ordered.
• Keep the patient's room darkened, and orient him as necessary.
• If the patient receives cycloplegic drugs, watch for signs of secondary glaucoma, such as transient vision loss or the perception of halos around lights.
• Encourage the patient to discuss his fears and concerns about potential vision loss.

Patient teaching

• Provide diversional activities as appropriate, and reassure the patient who must be in isolation.
• Emphasize the importance of prompt treatment for corneal ulcers to prevent complications and avoid vision impairment.
• Teach the patient about his medication. Explain its purpose, dosage, and possible adverse effects.
• Teach the patient to dispose of contaminated facial tissues properly. Caution him not to use the same tissue on both eyes because doing so may spread the infection.
• Explain all tests and procedures before performing them.

DISORDERS OF THE UVEAL TRACT, RETINA, AND LENS

These disorders may be acute or chronic and may cause visual disturbances or even vision loss. They include uveitis, retinal detachment, vascular retinopathies, cataract, age-related macular degeneration, and retinitis pigmentosa.

UVEITIS

An inflammation of one uveal tract, uveitis may occur as anterior uveitis, which affects the iris (iritis) or the iris and the ciliary body (iridocyclitis); as posterior uveitis, which affects the choroid (choroiditis) or the choroid and the retina (chorioretinitis); or as panuveitis, which affects the entire uveal tract.

Although clinical distinction is not always possible, anterior uveitis occurs in two forms—granulomatous and nongranulomatous. Granulomatous uveitis was once thought to result from tuberculosis bacilli; nongranulomatous uveitis, from streptococci. Though these pathogens are known now not to cause the disease forms, the names remain in use. The onset of anterior uveitis may be acute or insidious. Posterior uveitis begins insidiously and may be acute or chronic.

Causes

Typically an idiopathic inflammation, uveitis can result from allergy, bacteria, viruses, fungi, chemicals, trauma, surgery, or systemic diseases (such as rheumatoid arthritis and ankylosing spondylitis).

Complications

Untreated, anterior uveitis progresses to posterior uveitis, which may lead to scarring, cataracts, glaucoma, or retinal detachment. Posterior uveitis usually produces some residual vision loss and markedly blurred vision.

Assessment findings

The patient with anterior uveitis may complain of a dull ache in one eye, blurred vision, and sensitivity to light. With posterior uveitis, he may report slightly blurred vision or floating spots.

Inspection of the external eye may disclose severe ciliary congestion, tearing, and a small pupil that doesn't react to light. Iris color may change.

Diagnostic tests

• *Slit-lamp examination* findings both in anterior and posterior uveitis reveal milkiness of the aqueous humor and inflammatory cell particles on the back of the cornea. This pattern resembles light passing through smoke. With a special lens, slit-lamp examination and ophthalmoscopy can also identify active inflammatory fundal lesions involving the retina or the choroid or both.
• *Serologic tests* can detect toxoplasmosis as the cause of posterior uveitis.

Treatment

Uveitis requires vigorous and prompt management, which includes treatment of any known underlying cause and application of a topical cycloplegic, such as 1% atropine sulfate. Additional therapy may involve applying topical and subconjunctival corticosteroids.

For severe uveitis, the patient may receive oral systemic corticosteroids. Because long-term corticosteroid therapy can increase intraocular pressure (IOP) and cause cataracts, the patient will need IOP monitoring during the active inflammatory stage. If IOP rises, therapy includes an antiglaucoma drug, such as the beta blocker timolol, or acetazolamide, a carbonic anhydrase inhibitor.

Nursing diagnoses

• Altered health maintenance
• Anxiety
• Pain
• Risk for infection
• Risk for injury
• Sensory or perceptual alterations (visual)

Nursing interventions

• Encourage rest during the acute phase of uveitis.
• Administer prescribed drugs, including analgesics.

Patient teaching

• Teach the patient how to instill eyedrops.
• Explain the prescribed drug's purpose, dosage, and adverse effects. Instruct him to report adverse effects of systemic corticosteroids—edema and weakness, for example.
• Suggest wearing sunglasses to relieve photophobia.
• Urge the patient to seek follow-up care because of the strong likelihood of recurrence. Instruct him to seek treatment at the first sign of uveitis.

RETINAL DETACHMENT

In this disorder, separation of the retinal layers creates a subretinal space that fills with fluid. Twice as common in men as in women, retinal detachment may be primary or secondary. The disorder usually involves only one eye but may occur in the other eye later. Rarely healing spontaneously, a detached retina can usually be reattached successfully with surgery. The prognosis depends on the area of the retina affected.

Causes and pathophysiology

A retinal detachment may be primary or secondary. A *primary detachment* occurs spontaneously because of a change in the retina or the vitreous, whereas a *secondary detachment* results from another problem, such as intraocular inflammation or trauma. The most common cause of retinal detachment is a hole or tear in the retina. This hole allows the liquid vitreous to seep between the retinal layers and separate the sensory retinal layer from its choroidal blood supply. In adults, retinal detachment usually results from degenerative changes related to aging (which cause a spontaneous tear). Predisposing factors include myopia, cataract surgery, and trauma.

Additionally, retinal detachment may result from fluid seeping into the subretinal space as an effect of inflammation, tumors, or systemic disease. (See *Understanding retinal detachment,* page 1104.) Or detachment may result from traction placed on the retina by vitreous bands or membranes (resulting from proliferative diabetic retinopathy, posterior uveitis, or a traumatic intraocular foreign body, for example).

The disorder may occasionally develop in a child from retinopathy of prematurity, tumors (retinoblastomas), or trauma. Retinal detachment can also be inherited, usually in association with myopia.

Complications

Retinal detachment may result in severe vision impairment and possible blindness.

Assessment findings

Initially, the patient may complain that he sees floating spots and recurrent light flashes. As detachment progresses, he may report gradual, painless vision loss described as looking through a veil, curtain, or cobweb. He may relate that the "veil" obscures objects in a particular visual field.

Diagnostic tests

• *Direct ophthalmoscopy,* after full pupil dilation, shows folds or discoloration in the usually transparent retina.

• *Indirect ophthalmoscopy* can detect retinal tears.
• *Ocular ultrasonography* may be performed to examine the retina if the patient has an opaque lens.

Treatment

Depending on the detachment's location and severity, treatment may include restricting eye movements to prevent further separation until surgical repair can be made.

A hole in the peripheral retina may be treated with cryotherapy. A hole in the posterior retina may respond to laser therapy.

To reattach the retina, scleral buckling may be performed. In this procedure, the surgeon places a silicone plate or sponge over the reattachment site and secures it in place with an encircling band. The pressure exerted gently pushes the choroid and retina together. Scleral buckling may be followed by replacement of the vitreous with silicone, oil, air, or gas.

Nursing diagnoses

• Altered health maintenance
• Anxiety
• Diversional activity deficit
• Risk for infection
• Sensory or perceptual alterations (visual)

Nursing interventions

• Provide encouragement and emotional support to decrease anxiety caused by vision loss.
• Prepare the patient for surgery by cleaning his face with a mild (no-tears) shampoo. Give antibiotics and cycloplegic or mydriatic eyedrops, as ordered.
• In macular involvement, keep the patient on bed rest (with or without bathroom privileges) to prevent further retinal detachment.
• Postoperatively, position the patient as directed (the position will vary according to the surgical procedure). To prevent increasing intraocular pressure (IOP), administer antiemetics as indicated. Discourage any activities that would raise IOP.
• Observe for slight localized corneal edema and perilimbal congestion, which may follow laser therapy. To reduce edema and discomfort, apply ice packs, and administer acetaminophen, as ordered, for headache.
• If the patient receives a retrobulbar injection, apply a protective eye patch because the eyelid will remain partially open.
• After removing the protective patch, give cycloplegic and steroidal or antibiotic eyedrops, as ordered. Apply cold compresses to decrease swelling and pain, but avoid putting pressure on the eye.

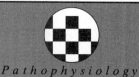

Pathophysiology

UNDERSTANDING RETINAL DETACHMENT

Traumatic injury or degenerative changes may cause retinal detachment by allowing the retina's sensory tissue layers to separate from the retinal pigment epithelium. This permits fluid—from the vitreous, for example—to seep into the space between the retinal pigment epithelium and the rods and cones of the tissue layers.

The pressure, which results from the fluid entering the space, balloons the retina into the vitreous cavity away from choroidal circulation. Separated from its blood supply, the retina can't function. Without prompt repair, the detached retina may cause permanent vision loss.

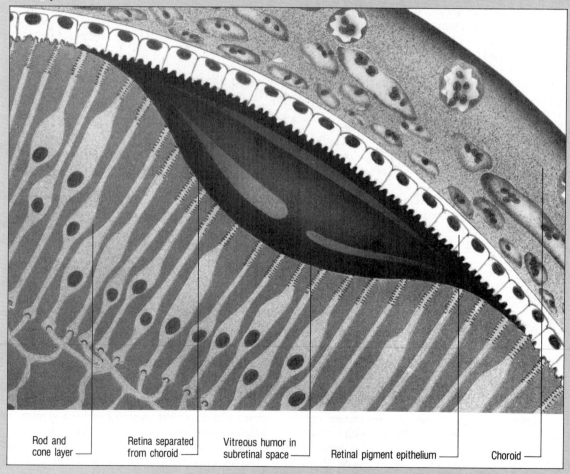

Rod and cone layer —

Retina separated from choroid —

Vitreous humor in subretinal space —

Retinal pigment epithelium —

Choroid —

• Give analgesics as needed, and report persistent pain.

Patient teaching
• Encourage leg and deep-breathing exercises to prevent complications of immobility.
• Explain to the patient undergoing laser therapy that the procedure may be done in same-day surgery. Forewarn him that he may have blurred vision for several days afterward.
• Instruct him to rest and to avoid driving, bending, heavy lifting, or any other activities that affect intraocular pressure for several days after eye surgery. Discourage activities that may cause the patient to bump his eye.
• Show the patient having scleral buckling surgery how to instill eyedrops properly. After surgery, remind him to lie in the position recommended by the doctor.
• Advise the patient to wear sunglasses if photosensitivity occurs.
• Instruct the patient to take acetaminophen as needed for headaches and to apply ice packs to his eye to reduce swelling and alleviate discomfort.
• Review the signs of infection, emphasizing those requiring immediate attention.

VASCULAR RETINOPATHIES
An interruption in blood supply to the eye can produce a vascular retinopathy—a noninflammatory retinal disorder. Common vascular retinopathies include central retinal artery occlusion, central retinal vein occlusion, diabetic retinopathy, and hypertensive retinopathy.

Central retinal artery occlusion occurs unilaterally and affects elderly patients. The prognosis is poor—in 5% to 20% of patients, secondary glaucoma develops rapidly 3 to 4 months after occlusion.

Central retinal vein occlusion, most prevalent in elderly patients, causes vision loss more slowly than central retinal artery occlusion.

Diabetic retinopathy is the leading cause of blindness among people ages 20 to 44. About 40% of patients with insulin-dependent (Type I or juvenile-onset) diabetes and about 25% of those with non-insulin-dependent (Type II or adult-onset) diabetes for 10 years develop retinopathy. In 15 years, the disorder develops in about 95% of people with Type I diabetes and in about 50% of those with Type II diabetes. At additional risk are pregnant patients, blacks (who have a 20% higher risk than whites), and women (who have a 23% higher risk than men).

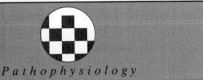

Pathophysiology

PROGRESSION OF DIABETIC RETINOPATHY
The patient with diabetic retinopathy needs careful vision monitoring because the disorder can accelerate without warning, progressing from a nonproliferative condition to a proliferative disease.

Nonproliferative diabetic retinopathy
Initially, the retinal blood vessel linings undergo changes. These changes cause the vessels to leak plasma or fatty substances that decrease or block blood flow (nonperfusion) within the retina. Diabetic retinopathy may also produce microaneurysms and small hemorrhages.

Proliferative diabetic retinopathy
Later, in a process called neovascularization, fragile new blood vessels form and proliferate on the optic disk and elsewhere on the fundus. These vessels can grow into the vitreous and then rupture, causing vitreous hemorrhage and subsequent blindness. What's more, scar tissue may form along the new blood vessels and pull on the retina, causing macular distortion and possible retinal detachment.

Causes and pathophysiology
When a retinal vessel becomes obstructed, the diminished blood flow causes visual deficits. *Central retinal artery occlusion* may be idiopathic or may result from embolism, atherosclerosis, infection, or conditions that retard blood flow, such as temporal arteritis, carotid occlusion, and heart failure.

Central retinal vein occlusion may result from external compression of the retinal vein, trauma, diabetes, thrombosis, granulomatous diseases, generalized and localized infections, glaucoma, and atherosclerosis.

Diabetic retinopathy results from diabetes, which causes microcirculatory changes. These changes occur more rapidly when diabetes is poorly controlled. (See *Progression of diabetic retinopathy.*)

Hypertensive retinopathy results from prolonged hypertension, which produces retinal vasospasm and consequent damage to and narrowing of the arteriolar lumen.

DIAGNOSTIC TESTS IN VASCULAR RETINOPATHIES

In vascular retinopathies, diagnostic tests vary, depending on the type of retinopathy; for example, central retinal artery occlusion, central retinal vein occlusion, diabetic retinopathy, or hypertensive retinopathy.

Central retinal artery occlusion
• *Ophthalmoscopy (direct or indirect)* shows emptying of retinal arterioles.
• *Slit-lamp examination* within 2 hours of occlusion reveals clumps or segmentation in the artery. Later examination shows a milky white retina around the optic disk (resulting from swelling and necrosis of ganglion cells caused by reduced blood supply). Other findings include a cherry-red spot in the macula. (This spot subsides after several weeks.)
• *Ophthalmodynamometry* approximately measures relative pressures in the central retinal arteries and indirectly assesses internal carotid artery blockage.
• *Ultrasonography* reveals blood vessel conditions in the neck.
• *Digital subtraction angiography* evaluates carotid occlusion with no need for arteriography.
• *Magnetic resonance imaging* displays the reason for obstruction.
• *Contrast-enhanced computed tomography scan* discloses the diseased carotid artery.

Central retinal vein occlusion
• *Ophthalmoscopy (direct or indirect)* reveals retinal hemorrhage, retinal vein engorgement, white patches among hemorrhages, and edema around the optic disk.
• *Ultrasonography* can confirm or rule out occluded blood vessels.

Diabetic retinopathy
• *Slit-lamp examination* shows thickening of retinal capillary walls.
• *Indirect ophthalmoscopy* demonstrates retinal changes, such as microaneurysms (earliest change), retinal hemorrhages and edema, venous dilation and beading, exudates, vitreous hemorrhage, proliferation of fibrin into vitreous from retinal holes, growth of new blood vessels, and microinfarctions of nerve fiber layer.
• *Fluorescein angiography* highlights leakage of fluorescein from dilated vessels and differentiates between microaneurysms and true hemorrhages.

Hypertensive retinopathy
• *Ophthalmoscopy (direct or indirect)* performed in early disease discloses hard and shiny deposits, tiny hemorrhages, narrowed arterioles, nicking of the veins where arteries cross them (referred to as arteriovenous nicking), and elevated arterial blood pressure.
  The same test in later disease shows cotton wool patches, exudates, retinal edema, papilledema caused by ischemia and capillary insufficiency, hemorrhages, and microaneurysms.

Complications
In many patients, central retinal artery occlusion causes permanent blindness. Central retinal vein occlusion may result in secondary glaucoma. Diabetic retinopathy may end in blindness or cranial nerve neuropathy. Hypertensive retinopathy may also lead to blindness.

Assessment findings
The patient with central retinal artery occlusion may complain of transient vision loss in one eye. The episode may last from a few seconds to 10 minutes. As the disorder progresses, however, the patient may report sudden, painless, partial or complete vision loss in the eye. (Note: Although this condition typically causes permanent blindness, some patients experience spontaneous resolution within hours and regain partial vision.) If central retinal artery occlusion results in secondary neurovascular glaucoma (uncontrolled proliferation of weak blood vessels), the patient typically complains of eye pain.

In central retinal vein occlusion, the patient usually complains of diminished visual acuity. He may perceive only hand movement and light.

Some patients with diabetic retinopathy may report no symptoms. Complaints in hypertensive retinopathy depend on the location of retinopathy. For example, retinopathy near the macula may cause only blurred vision. Patients with prolonged severe disease may report headaches and severe vision loss—even blindness. In the pregnant patient, hypertensive retinopathy may occur with eclampsia.

Diagnostic tests
Appropriate tests depend on the type of vascular retinopathy. Evaluation needs to include visual acuity findings and ophthalmoscopic examination. (See *Diagnostic tests in vascular retinopathies.*)

Treatment
No particular treatment is known to control central retinal artery occlusion. However, an attempt is made to

release the occlusive plaque or emboli into the peripheral retinal circulation. To reduce intraocular pressure, therapy includes acetazolamide 500 mg I.V.; eyeball massage with a Goldman-type goniolens; and, possibly, anterior chamber paracentesis. Therapy also includes inhalation of carbogen (95% oxygen and 5% carbon dioxide) to improve retinal oxygenation. Because inhalation therapy may be given hourly for up to 48 hours, the patient requires hospitalization for close monitoring of vital signs.

Therapy for central retinal vein occlusion may include aspirin, which acts as a mild anticoagulant. Laser photocoagulation may reduce the risk of neovascular glaucoma for some patients whose eyes have widespread capillary nonperfusion.

Treatment of early-stage, nonproliferative diabetic retinopathy is prophylactic. Careful control of the patient's blood glucose levels during the first 5 years of diabetes may decrease the severity of retinopathy or delay its onset. For the patient with microaneurysms, therapy should include frequent eye examinations (three or four times yearly) to monitor the condition. For a child with diabetes, therapy should include an annual eye examination by an ophthalmologist.

The treatment choice for proliferative diabetic retinopathy is laser photocoagulation. This process cauterizes the weak, leaking blood vessels. Laser treatment may be focal (aimed directly at new blood vessels) or panretinal (placing as many as 2,000 burns throughout the peripheral retina). Despite such treatment, neovascularization doesn't always regress, and vitreous hemorrhage, with or without retinal detachment, may follow. If the leaked blood isn't absorbed in 3 to 6 months, vitrectomy may be performed to restore partial vision.

Treatment for hypertensive retinopathy includes controlling blood pressure with appropriate drugs, diet, and exercise. Adherence to this regimen typically resolves ocular signs and symptoms.

Nursing diagnoses
• Altered health maintenance
• Anxiety
• Fear
• Impaired adjustment
• Risk for injury
• Sensory or perceptual alterations (visual)

Nursing interventions
• Arrange for *immediate* ophthalmologic evaluation when a patient complains of sudden vision loss. Blindness may be permanent if treatment is delayed.

• Encourage the patient to express his fears about vision loss.
• Monitor the patient's blood pressure if he complains of occipital headache and blurred vision.
• Administer acetazolamide I.V. as ordered. During inhalation therapy, monitor vital signs before and after treatment. Continue this therapy if the patient's blood pressure fluctuates markedly, if an arrhythmia develops, or if the patient becomes disoriented.

Patient teaching
• Urge the patient with hypertensive retinopathy to comply with antihypertensive therapy and to have regular blood pressure checks.
• Teach the diabetic patient about care procedures, as necessary. Explain home glucose monitoring, insulin therapy, dietary modifications, and exercise regimens. Urge the patient to comply with the prescribed regimen. Encourage regular eye examinations.
• Review ways to modify the environment for safety, especially if the patient has vision loss.

CATARACT

A common cause of gradual vision loss, a cataract is an opacity of the lens or the lens capsule of the eye. Light shining through the cornea is blocked by the clouded lens. This, in turn, blurs the image cast onto the retina. As a result, the brain interprets a hazy image.

Cataracts commonly affect both eyes, but each cataract progresses independently. Exceptions are traumatic cataracts, which are usually unilateral, and congenital cataracts, which may remain stationary. Cataracts are most prevalent in persons over age 70. Surgery restores vision in about 95% of patients.

Causes
Cataracts are classified by their causes:
• *Senile cataracts* develop in elderly people, probably because of chemical changes in lens proteins.
• *Congenital cataracts* occur in neonates from inborn errors of metabolism or from maternal rubella infection during the first trimester. These cataracts may also result from a congenital anomaly or from genetic causes. Transmission is usually autosomal dominant; however, recessive cataracts may be sex-linked.
• *Traumatic cataracts* develop after a foreign body injures the lens with sufficient force to allow aqueous or vitreous humor to enter the lens capsule.
• *Complicated cataracts* occur secondary to uveitis, glaucoma, retinitis pigmentosa, or retinal detachment. They

can also occur with systemic disease, such as diabetes, hypoparathyroidism, or atopic dermatitis, or from ionizing radiation or infrared rays.

• *Toxic cataracts* result from drug or chemical toxicity with ergot, dinitrophenol, naphthalene, and phenothiazines.

Complications
Without surgery, a cataract eventually leads to complete vision loss.

Assessment findings
Typically, the patient complains of painless, gradual vision loss. He may also report a blinding glare from headlights when he drives at night, poor reading vision, and an annoying glare and poor vision in bright sunlight. If he has a central opacity, the patient may report seeing better in dim light than in bright light. That's because this cataract is nuclear, and as the pupil dilates, the patient can see around the opacity.

Inspection with a penlight may reveal a milky white pupil and, with an advanced cataract, a grayish white area behind the pupil.

Diagnostic tests
• *Indirect ophthalmoscopy* reveals a dark area in the normally homogeneous red reflex.
• *Slit-lamp examination* confirms the diagnosis of a lens opacity.
• *Visual acuity test* confirms the degree of vision loss.

Treatment
Surgical lens extraction and implantation of an intraocular lens to correct the visual deficit is the treatment for cataract. The surgery is usually performed as a same-day, or outpatient, procedure. (See *Planning care for the patient having cataract surgery.*)

Surgical procedures include the following:
• *Extracapsular cataract extraction,* the most common procedure, involves removing the anterior lens capsule and cortex and leaving the posterior capsule intact. In this procedure, the surgeon implants a posterior chamber intraocular lens (IOL) where the patient's own lens used to be. This procedure is used for patients of all ages.
• *Intracapsular cataract extraction* involves removing the entire lens within the intact capsule by cryoextraction (the moist lens sticks to an extremely cold metal probe for easy and safe removal with gentle traction). Once the surgeon removes the lens, he implants an IOL in either the anterior or posterior chamber. If the patient doesn't

receive an IOL, he'll use contact lenses or aphakic glasses to correct vision.
• *Phacoemulsification* relies on ultrasonic vibrations to fragment the lens. The broken pieces are removed by aspiration.
• *Discission and aspiration,* a technique used for children with soft cataracts, has largely been replaced by other procedures.

Possible complications of surgery include loss of vitreous (during surgery), wound dehiscence from loosening of sutures and flat anterior chamber or iris prolapse into the wound, hyphema, pupillary block glaucoma, retinal detachment, and infection.

A patient with an IOL implant may experience improved vision almost immediately; however, the IOL corrects distance vision only. The patient also needs either corrective reading glasses or a corrective contact lens, which can be fitted 4 to 8 weeks after surgery.

If the patient did not receive an IOL, he may receive temporary aphakic cataract glasses. Then, sometime between 4 and 8 weeks after surgery, he'll have a refraction examination for permanent glasses.

Some patients who have an extracapsular cataract extraction develop a secondary membrane in the posterior lens capsule (which has been left intact), and that causes decreased visual acuity. This membrane can be removed by the Nd:YAG laser, which cuts an area from the membrane center, thus restoring vision. However, laser surgery alone cannot remove a cataract.

Nursing diagnoses
• Anxiety
• Risk for infection
• Risk for injury
• Sensory or perceptual alterations (visual)

Nursing interventions
• Postoperatively, monitor the patient until he recovers from the effects of the anesthetic. Keep the bed's side rails up, monitor vital signs, and assist him with early ambulation.
• Apply an eye shield or an eye patch postoperatively as ordered.

Patient teaching
• Because the patient will be discharged after he recovers from the anesthetic, remind him to return for a checkup the next day. Caution him to avoid activities that increase intraocular pressure, such as straining with coughing, bowel movements, or lifting.

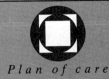

Plan of care

PLANNING CARE FOR THE PATIENT HAVING CATARACT SURGERY

Typically, you have more time to devise an effective plan of care for a hospitalized patient than for a patient undergoing same-day surgery. But for many patients with cataracts, surgery doesn't involve an overnight stay. To prepare for giving care to such patients, assume that you've just met Henry Navarro, age 77, who is scheduled for cataract surgery today. His wife, Mercedes, is with him.

Patient history

Mr. Navarro, a retired jeweler, is meticulously groomed and congenial. He tells you that a cataract has dimmed the vision in his left eye. He adds that his doctor told him that he was nearsighted with 150/20 vision in his right eye.

About 2 years ago, Mr. Navarro learned that he had a cataract. Soon he began seeing "shadows" in the periphery of his left visual field. He also had difficulty distinguishing color and reading newsprint even when he wore his eyeglasses. When his sight grew hazier and he began bumping into furniture, he went back to his doctor, who recommended surgery. Without hesitation, Mr. Navarro tells you that he feels somewhat apprehensive. He wonders if the surgery could leave him completely blind.

Mr. Navarro reports that he's had generally excellent physical and emotional health, which he attributes to hard work, a positive outlook, and an excellent marriage of 52 years.

Assessment findings

Your physical examination begins with Mr. Navarro's vital signs: temperature, 97.6° F (36.4° C); pulse rate, 74 beats/minute and regular; respiratory rate, 16 unlabored breaths/minute; and blood pressure, 132/66 mm Hg.

Your inspection reveals an opaque left lens, with the left pupil appearing grayish white. The right eye appears normal, with slight postmovement tremors when his gaze shifts from side to side.

On auscultation, his lungs sound clear. He states that he has no symptoms of an upper respiratory tract infection (which could complicate his impending surgery).

Routine preadmission testing detected no condition that would preclude performing an intracapsular cataract extraction and an intraocular lens implant.

Nursing diagnoses

After reviewing Mr. Navarro's history and his doctor's reports, you select these nursing diagnoses:
• Anxiety related to impending surgery, transient loss of vision, and unfamiliarity with surgical procedures
• Knowledge deficit related to postoperative eye care and activity limitations
• Risk for eye injury related to vision deficit after discharge
• Sensory or perceptual alterations (visual) related to a new lens.

Expected outcomes

Keeping in mind that Mr. Navarro will be discharged soon after surgery — barring complications — you define goals that require Mr. Navarro's participation in postoperative care. Mr. Navarro will be able to:
• express minimal anxiety about surgery
• demonstrate knowledge of postoperative eye care and name activity restrictions related to surgery
• adopt measures to reduce the risk of injury to his left eye
• adjust to temporary visual alterations.

Implementation

Taking the following steps, you implement Mr. Navarro's plan of care.

To minimize anxiety
• Allow Mr. Navarro ample opportunity to express his concerns about eye surgery. Offer reassurance, and answer his questions.
• Encourage him to identify and use previously successful coping mechanisms to relieve his stress.
• Preview surgery and care procedures. Discuss preoperative sedation, anesthesia, duration of the operation, sounds and smells of the operating room, and postoperative monitoring and eye patching procedures.
• Provide analgesics as needed.
• Encourage Mrs. Navarro's participation in all demonstrations and explanations. Include both Navarros in discharge instructions.

To understand postoperative care and activity restrictions
• As soon as possible, show the Navarros how to properly instill eyedrops. If possible, ask for a return demonstration.
• List activities to avoid, such as rubbing the affected eye, straining during bowel movements, and bending at the waist.
• Recommend sedentary activities that do not include riding in or driving a vehicle for about 2 weeks after surgery.

To reduce the risk of eye injury
• Move and position Mr. Navarro's head carefully and slowly after surgery.
• As Mr. Navarro recovers, help him to keep his fingers, tissues, and handkerchiefs away from his left eye. If the eye tears, tell him to "pat" absorbent, soft gauze under the left lower eyelid.
• Before giving eye care, such as instilling eyedrops or ointment or ap-

(continued)

PLANNING CARE FOR THE PATIENT HAVING CATARACT SURGERY *(continued)*

plying a patch, wash your hands to avoid transmitting infection. Remind Mr. Navarro to do this at home.
• Review written instructions:
—Avoid lifting objects weighing more than 15 lb (6.8 kg).
—Protect the affected eye with an eye shield at night.
—Recognize and report signs of infection, including increased eye discharge, decreasing vision, or pain.
—When in bed, lie on the side or the back.
—Wear dark glasses to relieve glare from harsh light.
—Watch television only for brief periods.

—Keep the affected eye dry when showering or washing hair.
—Clean eyes gently upon rising in the morning when the eyelids stick together.

To adjust to changes in vision
• Consult an occupational therapist to reorient Mr. Navarro to home traffic patterns and furniture arrangements. Advise the Navarros to remove barriers to unobstructed passage.
• Tell Mr. Navarro to keep traffic areas well lighted, especially at night.
• Direct Mr. Navarro to follow instructions for medication use. Remind him to allow time for adjustment to the new corrective lenses, which will be prescribed when appropriate after surgery.

• Encourage strict adherence to the follow-up care schedule.
• Encourage the Navarros to prearrange clothing and toiletries to help Mr. Navarro perform self-care easily.
• Offer referrals to organizations for the visually impaired. Suggest audiotapes of books, music, or dialogues for listening pleasure and diversion until Mr. Navarro's sight improves.

Evaluation
The goals for Mr. Navarro are met if he feels less anxiety about cataract surgery and if he can explain and perform proper eye care, state desirable activity limitations and safety behaviors, and adapt safely to temporary visual alterations.

• Advise the patient to abstain from sex until he receives his doctor's approval.
• Teach the patient or family member how to instill ophthalmic ointment or drops.
• If the patient has increased eye discharge, sharp eye pain (unrelieved by analgesics), or a deterioration in vision, instruct him to notify his doctor immediately.

AGE-RELATED MACULAR DEGENERATION

At least 10% of elderly Americans have irreversible central vision loss from age-related macular degeneration. Two primary forms include the atrophic (also called the involutional or dry) form, which accounts for about 70% of cases, and the exudative (also called the hemorrhagic or wet) form of macular degeneration.

Commonly affecting both eyes, macular degeneration is a leading cause of blindness in the United States.

Causes
Age-related macular degeneration results from hardening and obstruction of the retinal arteries, usually associated with age-related degenerative changes. As a result, new blood vessels form (neovascularization) in the macular area and totally obscure central vision. The disorder may also be genetic in origin, or it may result from an injury, inflammation, or infection.

Complications
Age-related macular degeneration may result in blindness. Bilateral macular lesions may lead to nystagmus.

Assessment findings
The patient may complain of seeing a blank spot in the center of a page (scotoma) while reading. He may tell you that his central vision blurs intermittently and has gradually worsened. He may also report that straight lines appear distorted.

Diagnostic tests
• *Indirect ophthalmoscopy* through a dilated pupil discloses changes in the macular region of the fundus.
• *Fluorescein angiography* may identify (in sequential photographs) leaking vessels in the subretinal neovascular net.
• *Amsler grid tests* can detect visual distortion (metamorphopsia) on a daily basis, if appropriate.

Treatment
No cure currently exists for the atrophic form of macular degeneration. In patients with the exudative form, argon laser photocoagulation may slow the progression of severe visual loss in 5% to 10% of cases.

Nursing diagnoses
- Fear
- Risk for injury
- Sensory or perceptual alterations (visual)
- Social isolation

Nursing interventions
- Help the patient obtain optical aids for low vision—magnifiers and special lamps, for example.
- Offer emotional support, and encourage the patient to express his fears and concerns.

Patient teaching
- Point out ways to modify the patient's home environment for safety.
- Explain that macular degeneration usually doesn't affect peripheral vision, which should be adequate for performing routine activities.
- If the patient likes to read, refer him to an agency such as the American Foundation for the Blind or Associated Services for the Blind. Agencies like these offer classes in braille and reading alternatives, such as books and other materials on audiocassettes.

RETINITIS PIGMENTOSA
A genetically transmitted, progressive destruction of the retinal rods, retinitis pigmentosa results in atrophy of the retinal pigment epithelium and eventual blindness. As degeneration progresses from the rods to the cones, central vision loss occurs.

The incidence of disease ranges from 1 in 2,000 to 1 in 7,000 live births. Retinitis pigmentosa commonly accompanies other hereditary disorders in several distinct syndromes, most commonly the Laurence-Moon-Biedl syndrome typified by visual destruction (from retinitis pigmentosa), obesity, mental retardation, polydactyly, and hypogonadism.

Causes
About 80% of children with retinitis pigmentosa inherit it as an autosomal recessive trait. Onset occurs before age 20, initially affecting night and peripheral vision. The disease progresses inevitably—sometimes rapidly—to blindness before age 50. Retinitis pigmentosa may also be transmitted as an X-linked trait, which leads to the least common but most severe form of the disease and which usually causes blindness before age 40.

Complications
Retinitis pigmentosa ultimately results in total blindness.

Assessment findings
Patient history may include additional eye disorders, such as cataracts, choroidal sclerosis, macular degeneration, glaucoma, keratoconus, or scotoma (blind spots). The patient's family history may include other members with retinitis pigmentosa.

The patient generally complains of night blindness beginning in his teenage years. As the disease progresses, he typically reports a gradually narrowing visual field described as tunnel or "gun-barrel" vision. Blindness ultimately results.

Diagnostic tests
- *Electroretinography* shows an absent or slower than normal retinal response time.
- *Visual field testing* (using a tangent screen) detects ring scotomata.
- *Ophthalmoscopy* may initially disclose a normal fundus and later show characteristic black pigmentary disturbances.

Treatment
Although extensive research continues, no cure exists for retinitis pigmentosa.

Nursing diagnoses
- Body image disturbance
- Dysfunctional grieving
- Fear
- Powerlessness
- Risk for injury
- Sensory or perceptual alterations (visual)

Nursing interventions
- Allow the patient to express his feelings about impending blindness. Offer emotional support, and refer the patient to an appropriate clinical specialist as necessary.
- Accept the patient's perception of self. Assess his readiness for decision making. Then, as appropriate, involve him in making choices and decisions related to his care.
- Encourage participation in self-care. Provide reinforcement for the patient's positive efforts and activities.

Patient teaching
- Teach the patient and his family about retinitis pigmentosa. Explain that it's hereditary, and suggest genetic

counseling for adults who risk transmitting it to future offspring.

• Point out ways of modifying the environment for safety. Orient the patient to the layout of his room and the location of the furniture. Tell the patient's family to keep walkways clear of obstruction.

• Forewarn the patient about driving a car at night, explaining that eventually poor vision will impede safety. If appropriate, provide information about special eyeglasses that may help patients with retinitis pigmentosa see at night. (These lenses are expensive.)

• Refer the patient to a social service agency or to the National Retinitis Pigmentosa Foundation for additional information and counseling.

MISCELLANEOUS DISORDERS

These disorders include extraocular motor nerve palsies, strabismus, and glaucoma.

EXTRAOCULAR MOTOR NERVE PALSIES

In extraocular motor nerve palsies, dysfunction affects the third, fourth, and sixth cranial nerves. These nerves are responsible for innervating eye movement. The superior branch of the oculomotor (cranial III) nerve innervates the levator superioris muscle of the upper eyelid and the superior rectus muscle of the eye itself; the inferior branch innervates the interior rectus, the medial rectus, and the inferior oblique muscles. It also supplies the intrinsic pupillary and ciliary body muscles, which control lens shape and accommodation. The trochlear (cranial IV) nerve innervates the superior oblique muscles, which control downward rotation, intorsion, and abduction of the eye. The abducens (cranial VI) nerve innervates the lateral rectus muscles, which control inward movement of the eye.

Causes

The most common causes of extraocular motor nerve palsies include diabetic neuropathy, trauma, and pressure from an aneurysm or a brain tumor. Other causes vary, depending on the cranial nerve involved.

Oculomotor (third nerve) palsy, also known as acute ophthalmoplegia, also results from brain stem ischemia or from other cerebrovascular disorders; poisoning (lead, carbon monoxide, botulism); alcohol abuse; infections (measles, encephalitis); trauma to the extraocular muscles; myasthenia gravis; or tumors in the cavernous sinus area.

Trochlear (fourth nerve) palsy also may result from closed-head trauma (a blowout fracture, for example) or sinus surgery.

Abducens (sixth nerve) palsy also results from increased intracranial pressure, brain abscess, cerebrovascular accident, meningitis, arterial brain occlusion, infections of the petrous bone (rare), lateral sinus thrombosis, myasthenia gravis, and thyrotropic exophthalmos.

Complications

In extraocular motor nerve palsies, the complications are those problems that accompany the disease, including diplopia, ptosis, strabismus, nystagmus, and ocular torticollis.

Assessment findings

The patient characteristically reports the recent onset of diplopia, which varies in different fields of gaze, depending on the eye muscles affected. Additionally, the patient with fourth or sixth nerve palsy may complain of torticollis (wry neck) from repeatedly turning his head to compensate for visual field deficits.

If the patient has third nerve palsy, inspection may uncover ptosis, exotropia (eye positioned outward), pupillary dilation, and unresponsiveness to light and accommodation. What's more, the patient cannot move the eye.

If the patient has fourth nerve palsy, you may observe that he can't rotate his eye downward or upward. The patient with sixth nerve palsy may have esotropia (inward deviation of the eye).

Diagnostic tests

A patient with extraocular motor nerve palsy needs to supply a full health history and undergo a complete neuro-ophthalmologic examination before his diagnosis is confirmed. Differential diagnosis of third, fourth, or sixth nerve palsy depends on the specific motor defect exhibited by the patient.

Depending on the patient's symptoms, the following tests may be ordered: blood studies to detect diabetes; a computed tomography scan, magnetic resonance imaging, or skull X-rays to rule out intracranial tumors; and cerebral angiography to evaluate possible vascular abnormalities, such as aneurysm. If sixth nerve palsy results from an infection, culture and sensitivity tests may identify the causative organism and determine therapy.

Treatment

Appropriate treatment may vary, depending on the cause. For instance, neurosurgery may be necessary for a brain tumor or an aneurysm. For infection, massive doses of I.V. antibiotics may be appropriate. After treatment of the primary condition, the patient may need to perform exercises that stretch the neck muscles to correct acquired torticollis. Other care and treatments depend on residual symptoms.

Nursing diagnoses

• Anxiety
• Body image disturbance
• Fear
• Risk for injury
• Sensory or perceptual alterations (visual)

Nursing interventions

• Provide emotional support to help minimize the patient's anxiety about the cause of the motor nerve palsy.

Patient teaching

• Show the patient with acquired torticollis how to perform neck-stretching and range-of-motion exercises.
• Teach the patient to be alert for factors that may contribute to injury; for example, the patient with diplopia lacks depth perception. Instruct him to navigate stairs cautiously.

STRABISMUS

Also known as heterotropia — or called by such slang terms as squint, cross-eye, or walleye — strabismus results from eye misalignment, which produces nonparallel, uncoordinated eye movement that impairs vision.

The prognosis for correction varies with the timing of treatment and the onset of the disease. Depending on the cause, eye muscle imbalances may be corrected by eyeglasses, patching, or surgery. However, residual defects in vision and extraocular muscle alignment may persist even after treatment.

Strabismus affects about 2% of the population. The incidence is higher in patients with central nervous system (CNS) disorders, cerebral palsy, and mental retardation.

The disorder takes many forms and is described in various ways. In children, strabismus may be termed as follows:
• concomitant — the degree of deviation doesn't vary with the direction of gaze
• nonconcomitant — the degree of deviation varies with the direction of gaze

• congenital — apparent at birth or during the first 6 months
• acquired — present during the child's first 30 months.

In children and adults, strabismus that occurs periodically may be considered latent (phoria) or apparent; for example, when the child is tired or sick. Constant strabismus is considered manifest (tropia). Additional descriptive terms signify strabismic direction, for example:
• esotropia or esophoria — eyes deviate inward
• exotropia or exophoria — eyes deviate outward
• hypertropia or hyperphoria — eyes deviate upward
• hypotropia or hypophoria — eyes deviate downward.

Other classifications describe paralytic and nonparalytic deviations. Both types may be congenital or acquired. The nonparalytic type is typically intermittent (as in latent strabismus, the gaze doesn't deviate all the time), variable (the amount of deviation varies throughout the day), or alternating (the eyes alternate fixation with the nonfixing eye deviating).

Causes and pathophysiology

In adults, strabismus may result from trauma. In children, controversy continues over whether amblyopia (lazy eye) causes or results from strabismus. Possibly caused by hyperopia (farsightedness) or from anisometropia (unequal refractive power), strabismic amblyopia is characterized by a loss of central vision in one eye. This typically results in esotropia (from fixation by the dominant eye and suppression of images by the deviating eye).

Esotropia itself (either congenital or acquired) may result from muscle imbalance. In accommodative esotropia, the child's attempt to compensate for farsightedness affects the convergent reflex, and the eyes cross. This subsequent misalignment of the eyes leads to vision suppression in one eye, which, in turn, causes amblyopia (if misalignment develops early in life before bifoveal fixation is established).

Complications

Strabismus complications are limited to diplopia, amblyopia, and other vision disturbances.

Assessment findings

Parents of a child with strabismus typically describe the child as clumsy, frequently stumbling and bumping into furniture. This description suggests diplopia and lack of depth perception — usually the first indication of strabismus in a child.

RECOGNIZING STRABISMUS

This patient with strabismus has medial deviation of the left eye.

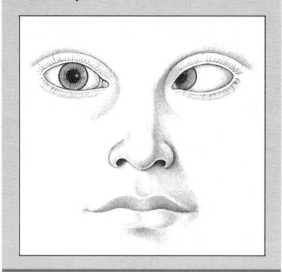

Simple observation may disclose apparent eye misalignment. (See *Recognizing strabismus*.) Ophthalmoscopic observation of the corneal light reflex in the pupillary center can detect strabismus that's less obvious. Other findings may include ptosis, abnormal head position (tilted to one side), nystagmus, and eye deviation.

During inspection you may also notice an overhanging epicanthus. This hallmark of Down's syndrome may give a child the appearance of having strabismus (pseudostrabismus). In such a patient, pinch the skin over the bridge of the nose into a fold; if the epicanthal fold disappears, then the child may have pseudostrabismus.

In older patients, chief complaints include double vision and unhappiness with appearance.

Diagnostic tests

If the onset of strabismus is sudden or if the CNS is involved, neurologic examination may determine the condition's origin (muscular or neurologic). Other diagnostic procedures can help determine the best treatment.
• *Visual acuity test* evaluates macular vision by determining the patient's vision from a 20′ (6 m) distance.
• *Hirschberg's method* measures the degree of deviation. As the patient gazes at a light about 13″ (33 cm) away, the examiner notes how the cornea reflects light.

• *Retinoscopy* determines refractive error (usually with the pupils dilated).
• *Maddox rods test* assesses specific muscle involvement.
• *Convergence test* shows distance at which convergence is sustained.
• *Duction test* reveals eye movement limitations.
• *Cover-uncover test* demonstrates eye deviation and the rate of recovery to original alignment.
• *Alternate cover test* shows intermittent or latent deviation.

Treatment

Therapy on the type of strabismus. For amblyopia, it includes patching the normal eye and prescribing corrective glasses to keep the eye straight and to counteract farsightedness (as in accommodative esotropia).

Or surgery may correct strabismus related to basic esotropia or residual accommodative esotropia after correction with glasses. This may be done to correct misalignment and improve the patient's appearance.

The timing of surgery varies. For example, at age 6 months, an infant with equal visual acuity and obvious esotropia will have the deviation corrected surgically. But a child with unequal visual acuity and an acquired deviation will have the affected eye patched until visual acuity is equal. *Then* he may undergo surgery.

Surgical correction includes recession (moving the muscle posteriorly from its original insertion) or resection (shortening the muscle). In some patients, combination surgery, such as the resection of one muscle and the recession of its antagonist, is required.

Other procedures involve transplanting a muscle to improve rotation of a paralyzed muscle or using adjustable sutures. Complications may include overcorrection, undercorrection, slipped muscle, and globe perforation.

Postoperative therapy may include patching the affected eye and applying combination antibiotic and corticosteroid eyedrops. Corrective glasses may still be necessary, and surgery may have to be repeated.

Nursing diagnoses
• Anxiety
• Body image disturbance
• Knowledge deficit
• Risk for injury
• Sensory or perceptual alterations (visual)

Nursing interventions
• Encourage the patient and family to discuss their feelings about the patient's appearance. Offer emotional support and referrals to appropriate specialists if desired.

• After surgery, gently wipe the patient's tears, which will be serosanguineous. Reassure the patient and his parents that this kind of tearing is normal after surgery.
• Administer antiemetics, if necessary.
• Apply antibiotic ointment, as ordered.

Patient teaching
• Explain all medications and procedures, especially those related to eye surgery.
• Postoperatively, discourage the patient from rubbing his eyes, and prepare him for discharge. (See *Dealing with strabismus.*)

GLAUCOMA

A group of disorders, glaucoma is characterized by high intraocular pressure (IOP) that damages the optic nerve. Glaucoma may occur as a primary or congenital disease or secondary to other causes, such as injury, infection, surgery, or prolonged topical corticosteroid use.

Primary glaucoma has two forms: *open-angle* (also known as chronic, simple, or wide-angle glaucoma) and *angle-closure* (also known as acute or narrow-angle) glaucoma. Angle-closure glaucoma attacks suddenly and may cause permanent vision loss in 48 to 72 hours.

One of the leading causes of blindness, glaucoma affects about 2% of Americans over age 40 and accounts for about 12% of newly diagnosed blindness in the United States. The incidence is highest among blacks. In the United States, early detection and effective treatment contribute to the good prognosis for preserving vision.

Causes and pathophysiology
Open-angle glaucoma results from degenerative changes in the trabecular meshwork. These changes block the flow of aqueous humor from the eye, which causes IOP to increase. The result is optic nerve damage. Affecting about 90% of all patients who have glaucoma, open-angle glaucoma commonly occurs in families.

Angle-closure glaucoma results from obstruction to the outflow of aqueous humor caused by an anatomically narrow angle between the iris and the cornea. This causes IOP to increase suddenly. Angle-closure glaucoma attacks may be triggered by trauma, pupillary dilation, stress, or any ocular change that pushes the iris forward (a hemorrhage or a swollen lens, for example).

Secondary glaucoma can proceed from such conditions as uveitis, trauma, drug use (such as corticosteroids), venous occlusion, or diabetes. In some instances, new blood vessels (neovascularization) may form, blocking the passage of aqueous humor.

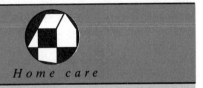

Home care

DEALING WITH STRABISMUS
When a patient is being treated for strabismus, follow these guidelines for home care:
• Help the parents look for and eliminate environmental hazards.
• Suggest that the parents keep pathways clear of objects and assist the patient whenever necessary.
• Teach the parents or patient how to instill eye medications properly.
• Teach the parents to recognize adverse drug reactions, emphasizing those that require immediate care.
• Instruct the parents or patient to blot tears from the cheek, not to wipe them from the eye.
• Stress the importance of complying with follow-up care.

Complications
If untreated, glaucoma can progress from gradual vision loss to total blindness.

Assessment findings
Because open-angle glaucoma begins insidiously and progresses slowly, the patient may have no symptoms. Later, he may complain of a dull, morning headache; mild aching in the eyes; loss of peripheral vision; seeing halos around lights; and reduced visual acuity (especially at night) that's uncorrected by glasses.

In contrast, angle-closure glaucoma typically has a rapid onset and constitutes an emergency. The patient may complain of pain and pressure over the eye, blurred vision, decreased visual acuity, seeing halos around lights, and nausea and vomiting (from increased IOP).

Inspection may reveal unilateral eye inflammation, a cloudy cornea, and a moderately dilated pupil that's nonreactive to light. Palpation may also disclose increased IOP discovered by applying gentle fingertip pressure to the patient's closed eyelids. With angle-closure glaucoma, one eye may feel harder than the other.

Diagnostic tests
• *Tonometry* (with an applanation, Schiøtz, or pneumatic tonometer) measures IOP and provides a baseline for reference. Normal IOP ranges from 8 to 21 mm Hg. How-

ever, patients whose pressures fall within the normal range can develop signs and symptoms of glaucoma, and patients who have abnormally high pressure may have no clinical effects.

• *Slit-lamp examination* allows the examiner to see the effects of glaucoma on the anterior eye structures, including the cornea, iris, and lens.

• *Gonioscopy* determines the angle of the eye's anterior chamber. This enables the examiner to distinguish between open-angle and angle-closure glaucoma. The angle is normal in open-angle glaucoma. In older patients, however, partial closure of the angle may occur (allowing two forms of glaucoma to coexist).

• *Ophthalmoscopy* facilitates visualization of the fundus. In open-angle glaucoma, cupping of the optic disk may be seen earlier than in angle-closure glaucoma.

• *Perimetry or visual field tests* determine the extent of peripheral vision loss, which helps evaluate deterioration in open-angle glaucoma.

• *Fundus photography* monitors and records optic disk changes.

Treatment

For open-angle glaucoma, initial treatment aims to reduce pressure by decreasing aqueous humor production with medications. These include beta blockers, such as timolol (used cautiously in asthmatics or patients with bradycardia) or betaxolol. Other drug treatments include epinephrine to dilate the pupil (contraindicated in angle-closure glaucoma) and miotic eyedrops, such as pilocarpine, to promote aqueous humor outflow.

Patients who don't respond to drug therapy may benefit from argon laser trabeculoplasty or from a surgical filtering procedure called trabeculectomy. This procedure creates an opening for outflowing aqueous humor.

To perform *argon laser trabeculoplasty,* the ophthalmologist focuses an argon laser beam on the trabecular meshwork of an open angle. This produces a thermal burn that changes the meshwork surface and facilitates the outflow of aqueous humor.

To perform a *trabeculectomy,* the surgeon dissects a flap of sclera to expose the trabecular meshwork. He removes a small tissue block and performs a peripheral iridectomy, which produces an opening for aqueous outflow under the conjunctiva and creates a filtering bleb. Postoperatively, subconjunctival injections of fluorouracil may be given to maintain the fistula's patency.

An emergency, angle-closure glaucoma requires immediate treatment to lower high IOP. Initial preoperative drug therapy aims to lower IOP with acetazolamide, pilocarpine (which constricts the pupil, forces the iris

away from the trabeculae, and allows fluid to escape), and I.V. mannitol or oral glycerin (which forces fluid from the eye by making the blood hypertonic). If these medications fail to decrease the pressure, laser iridotomy or surgical peripheral iridectomy must be performed promptly to save the patient's vision.

An *iridectomy* relieves pressure by excising part of the iris to reestablish the outflow of aqueous humor. A few days later, the surgeon performs a prophylactic iridectomy on the other eye. This prevents an episode of acute glaucoma in the normal eye.

If the patient has severe pain, treatment may include narcotic analgesics. After peripheral iridectomy, treatment includes cycloplegic eyedrops to relax the ciliary muscle and to decrease inflammation and thereby prevent adhesions.

Nursing diagnoses
• Anxiety
• Fear
• Knowledge deficit
• Pain
• Risk for injury
• Sensory or perceptual alterations (visual)

Nursing interventions
• For the patient with angle-closure glaucoma, give medications, as ordered, and prepare him physically and psychologically for laser iridotomy or surgery.

• Remember to administer cycloplegic eyedrops *in the affected eye only.* In the unaffected eye, these drops may precipitate an attack of angle-closure glaucoma and threaten the patient's residual vision.

• After trabeculectomy, give medications, as ordered, to dilate the pupil. Also apply topical corticosteroids, as ordered, to rest the pupil.

• After surgery, protect the affected eye by applying an eye patch and shield, positioning the patient on his back or unaffected side, and following general safety measures.

• Administer pain medication, as ordered.

• Encourage ambulation immediately after surgery.

• Encourage the patient to express his concerns related to having a chronic condition.

Patient teaching
• Stress the importance of meticulous compliance with prescribed drug therapy to maintain low IOP and prevent optic disk changes that cause vision loss.

• Explain all procedures and treatments, especially surgery, to help reduce the patient's anxiety.

• Inform the patient that lost vision cannot be restored but that treatment can usually prevent further loss.

• Instruct the family how to modify the patient's environment for safety. For example, suggest keeping pathways clear and reorienting the patient to room layouts, if necessary.

• Teach the patient the signs and symptoms that require immediate medical attention, such as sudden vision change or eye pain.

• Discuss the importance of glaucoma screening for early detection and prevention. Point out that all persons over age 35 should have an annual tonometric examination.

SELECTED REFERENCES

Freeman, R.S., et al. "Cloudy Lenses and Issues: A Pedigree of Unoperated Congenital Cataracts," *Journal of Ophthalmic Nursing & Technology* 14(3):118-23, May-June 1995.

Ignatavicius, D.D., *Medical-Surgical Nursing: A Nursing Process Approach,* 2nd ed. Philadelphia: W.B. Saunders Co., 1995.

Isselbacher, K., et al., eds. *Harrison's Principles of Internal Medicine,* 13th ed. New York: McGraw-Hill Book Co., 1995.

Phipps, W.J., et al. *Medical-Surgical Nursing: Concepts and Clinical Practice,* 5th ed. St. Louis: Mosby–Year Book Inc., 1995.

Rakel, R.E., ed. *Conn's Current Therapy 1996.* Philadelphia: W.B. Saunders Co., 1996.

Semes, L. "Primary Care Update: Diagnosis and Primary Care Management of Tear Film Deficiencies," *Optometry Clinics* 4(3):87-104, 1995.

Spires, R. "Aspergillus-induced Endophthalmitis," *Journal of Ophthalmic Nursing & Technology* 14(3):124-26, May-June 1995.

Taylor, C.M., and Sparks, S.M. *Nursing Diagnosis Reference Manual,* 3rd ed. Springhouse, Pa.: Springhouse Corp., 1995.

Tierney, L.M., et al. *Current Medical Diagnosis and Treatment 1995.* East Norwalk, Conn.: Appleton & Lange, 1995.

17   EAR, NOSE, AND THROAT DISORDERS

INTRODUCTION

Although ear, nose, and throat disorders seldom prove fatal, they may cause serious social, cosmetic, and communication problems. When left untreated, ear disorders can impair equilibrium and cause hearing loss that drastically impairs communication. Nasal disorders can change facial features and interfere with breathing and taste. Throat disorders may threaten airway patency and interfere with speech.

The ear

A sensory organ that allows hearing and maintains equilibrium, the ear consists of three main parts: the external ear, the middle ear, and the inner ear. The skin-covered cartilaginous auricle and the external auditory canal compose the external ear.

Separating the external ear and the middle ear at the proximal portion of the auditory canal is the tympanic membrane (eardrum), a structure made of layered skin, fibrous tissue, and mucous membrane. The eustachian tube (which connects the middle ear to the nasopharynx) equalizes pressure between the inner and outer surfaces of the tympanic membrane.

On the inner side of the tympanic membrane lies the middle ear, a small, air-filled cavity in the temporal bone. Within the middle ear are three small bones—the malleus, the incus, and the stapes (which sits in an opening called the oval window). These bones link together to transmit sound. The middle ear leads to the inner ear, a bony and membranous labyrinth consisting of the vestibule, the cochlea (containing the organ of Corti), and the semicircular canals.

Hearing and equilibrium

The auricle picks up sound waves and channels them into the auditory canal. There, they strike the tympanic membrane, which vibrates and causes the malleus to vibrate also. These vibrations travel from the malleus to the incus to the stapes, through the oval window and the fluid in the cochlea, to the round window, which opens to the inner ear. The membrane covering the round window shakes the delicate hair cells in the organ of Corti, which stimulates the sensory endings of the cochlear branch of the acoustic nerve (cranial nerve VIII). The nerve sends the impulses to the auditory area of the brain's temporal lobe, which then interprets the sound.

Inner ear structures also maintain equilibrium and balance by means of the fluid in the semicircular canals. This fluid is set in motion by body movement and stimulates nerve cells that line the canals. These cells, in turn, transmit impulses to the brain by way of the vestibular branch of the acoustic nerve.

Although the ear can respond to sounds with frequencies of 20 to 20,000 hertz (Hz), the range of normal speech is 250 to 4,000 Hz, with 70% of it falling between 500 and 2,000 Hz. The decibel (dB), a measure of sound intensity, is the lowest volume at which any given sound can be heard. A faint whisper registers 10 to 15 dB; average conversation, 50 to 60 dB; a shout, 85 to 90 dB. Hearing damage may follow exposure to sounds louder than 90 dB.

Assessing the ear

After obtaining a thorough history of ear disease, ask whether the patient has experienced episodes of vertigo, blurred vision, or ear pain. To test for vertigo, have the patient stand on one foot with his eyes closed, or have him walk a straight line with his eyes closed. Ask if he always falls to the same side and if the room seems to be spinning.

Examine ear color and size. The ears should be similarly shaped, colored the same as the face, and sized in proportion to the head. Inspect the auricle and surrounding tissue for deformities, nodules, lumps, skin lesions, and drainage. Check the ear canal for discharge, foreign bodies, and excessive cerumen (some ears normally drain large amounts of cerumen). Also check behind the ear for inflammation, masses, and lesions. If you see inflammation, check for tenderness by moving the auricle and pressing on the tragus and the mastoid process.

Palpate the external ear and the mastoid process (the bony structure beneath and behind the ear) to discover any areas of tenderness or swelling, nodules, or lesions, then gently pull the helix of the ear backward to determine if the patient feels tenderness or pain.

Perform an otoscopic examination to help assess the auditory canal and the tympanic membrane.

Inspect and palpate the temporomandibular joints. Evaluate them for movability, approximation (drawing of the bones together), and discomfort. This process should be smooth and painless for a normal patient.

Audiometric testing

To evaluate hearing and determine the type and extent of hearing loss, perform an audiometric test. The simplest but least reliable method for judging hearing acuity consists of covering one of the patient's ears, standing 18″ to 24″ (45 to 60 cm) from the uncovered ear, and whispering a short phrase or series of numbers. (Block the patient's vision to prevent lip reading.) Then ask the patient to repeat the phrase or series of numbers. To test hearing at both high and low frequencies, repeat the test in a normal speaking voice. (As an alternative, hold a ticking watch to the patient's ear.)

If you identify a hearing loss, do further testing to determine if the loss is conductive or sensorineural. A conductive loss can result from faulty bone conduction (inability of the acoustic nerve to respond to sound waves traveling through the skull) or faulty air conduction (impaired transmission of sound through ear structures to the acoustic nerve and, ultimately, the brain). A sensorineural loss results from nerve damage.

The following tests assess bone and air conduction:
• *Weber test* (used to test unilateral hearing loss). To perform this test, place the base of a lightly vibrating tuning fork on the midline of the patient's forehead or firmly in the middle of the patient's head. Normally, the patient should hear sounds equally in both ears. In conductive hearing loss, sound lateralizes (localizes) to the ear with the poorest hearing. In sensorineural loss, sound lateralizes to the better functioning ear.
• *Rinne test* (used to compare bone conduction with air conduction). To assess bone conduction, place the base of a vibrating tuning fork on the mastoid process, noting how many seconds pass before the patient can no longer hear it. Then, to assess air conduction, place the still-vibrating tuning fork near the ear canal, with the tines parallel to the patient's auricle. Hold the tuning fork in this position until the patient no longer hears the tone.

In patients with normal hearing and in those with sensorineural loss, the air-conducted tones are heard longer than the bone-conducted tones (positive Rinne test). In conductive loss, the patient hears a bone-conducted tone for as long as or longer than he hears an air-conducted tone (negative Rinne test).

After the hearing loss is identified as conductive, sensorineural, or mixed, further audiometric testing determines the extent of the loss. These audiometric tests include pure tone audiometry, speech audiometry, impedance audiometry, and tympanometry.

The nose, sinuses, mouth, and throat

The sensory organ for smell, the nose also warms, filters, and humidifies inhaled air. Consisting of bone and cartilage, it is separated into nostrils (nares) by the nasal septum. Lining the vestibule at the nostril entrance are cilia (tiny hairs). As air filters past the cilia and over mucosa-lined passages to bony structures called turbinates, it is warmed, filtered, and humidified. The nose ends at the posterior air passages known as the choanae, which lead to the oropharynx.

The sinuses lie within the facial bones. Hollow, air-filled cavities, they include the frontal, sphenoid, ethmoid, and maxillary sinuses. The same mucous membrane lines the sinuses and the nasal cavity. Consequently, the same viruses and bacteria that cause upper respiratory tract infections also infect the sinuses. Besides aiding voice resonance, the sinuses may help warm, filter, and humidify inhaled air, although this role hasn't been firmly established.

The sensory organ for taste, the mouth begins externally at the lips and continues with the tongue, gingivae, teeth, and salivary glands. The frenulum (a restraining band of tissue) attaches the tongue to the floor of the mouth. The gingivae cover the necks and roots of the teeth. Near the beginning of the throat, the anterior and posterior pillars form a cavity that houses the tonsils. Located nearby, three pairs of salivary glands — parotid (near the ear), sublingual (under the tongue), and submandibular (adjacent to the parotid glands) — keep the mouth moist. Bordering the mouth posteriorly are the soft palate and the uvula. Other boundaries include the mandibular bone forming the floor of the mouth and the hard palate that forms the roof of the mouth.

Located in the anterior part of the neck, the throat includes the pharynx, epiglottis, and larynx. Food travels through the pharynx to the esophagus. Air travels through it to the larynx. The epiglottis diverts material away from the glottis during swallowing. By vibrating expired air through the vocal cords, the larynx produces sounds. Changes in vocal cord length and air pressure affect the voice's pitch and intensity. The larynx also stimulates the vital cough reflex when a foreign body touches its sensitive mucosa.

Assessing the nose

Inspect the external nose for symmetry and contour, noting any areas of deformity, swelling, and discoloration. Check for redness, edema, lumps, tumors, and poor alignment. Marked septal cartilage depression may indicate saddle deformity due to septal destruction from trauma or congenital syphilis. Extreme lateral deviation may mean septal destruction from injury. Red nostrils may indicate frequent nose blowing caused by allergies or infectious rhinitis. Dilated, engorged blood vessels may suggest alcoholism or constant exposure to the elements. A bulbous, discolored nose may be a sign of rosacea.

With a nasal speculum and adequate lighting, check the nasal mucosa for pallor and edema, redness and inflammation, dried mucus plugs, furuncles, and polyps. Also look for abnormal appearance of capillaries and a deviated or perforated septum. Check for nasal discharge (assess its color, consistency, and odor) and blood. A profuse, thin, watery discharge may stem from an allergy or a cold; a profuse, thin, purulent discharge may indicate a cold or a chronic sinus infection.

Palpate the nose, checking for any painful or tender areas, swelling, and deformities. Evaluate nostril patency by gently occluding one nostril with your finger and having the patient exhale through the other.

Assessing the sinuses
To assess the paranasal sinuses, inspect, palpate, and percuss the frontal and maxillary sinuses (location of the other sinuses precludes assessment). First, inspect the external skin surfaces above and to the side of the nose for inflammation and edema. Then palpate and percuss the sinuses.

Pain after pressure is applied above the upper orbital rims indicates frontal sinus irritation; pain after pressure is applied to the cheeks, maxillary sinus irritation.

Assessing the mouth and the throat
Using a bright light, gloves, and a tongue blade, inspect the patient's mouth and throat. Note any unusual breath odors. Look for inflammation, white patches, and any irregularities on the tongue and throat.

Assess vital signs and respiratory status. Make sure the patient's airway isn't compromised. Watch for and immediately report signs of respiratory distress (dyspnea, tachycardia, tachypnea, inspiratory stridor, restlessness) and changes in voice or skin color, such as circumoral or nail bed cyanosis.

Assess the symmetry of the tongue and the function of the soft palate. To assess the underside of the tongue, have the patient touch the roof of his mouth with the tip of his tongue. Inspect the hard and soft palates. Note any deformities, lesions, areas of tenderness or inflammation, and other abnormalities.

Observe the tonsils for unilateral or bilateral enlargement. Inspect the maxillary mucobuccal fold and the labial frenulum for irritation and inflammation. Palpate the upper and lower lips and the tongue to evaluate muscle tone and surface structure.

EXTERNAL EAR DISORDERS

Disorders of the external ear are fairly common and are typically caused by routine daily activities, such as ear piercing and the use of cotton-tipped applicators and hair-care products. Although seldom life-threatening, these disorders can result in hearing loss and other complications if left untreated.

OTITIS EXTERNA
An acute or chronic inflammation of the skin of the external ear canal and auricle, otitis externa occurs most commonly during the summer, although it can occur throughout the year.

With treatment, acute otitis externa usually subsides within 7 days; however, it may become chronic and tends to recur. Severe, chronic otitis externa may reflect underlying diabetes mellitus, hypothyroidism, or nephritis.

Other names for this disorder are external otitis and swimmer's ear.

Causes
Otitis externa usually results when a traumatic injury or an excessively moist ear canal predisposes the area to infection. Common infecting organisms include bacteria, such as *Pseudomonas*, *Proteus vulgaris*, streptococci, *Staphylococcus aureus*, *Escherichia coli*, *Proteus mirabilis*, and *Klebsiella*; less commonly, fungi, such as *Aspergillus niger* and *Candida albicans* (fungal otitis externa is most common in the tropics). Occasionally, chronic otitis externa results from dermatologic conditions, such as seborrhea or psoriasis.

Predisposing factors include:
• swimming in contaminated water (cerumen creates a culture medium for the water-borne organism)
• cleaning the ear canal with a cotton-tipped applicator, bobby pin, finger, or other object, which irritates the ear canal and may introduce the infecting microorganism
• exposure to dust, hair-care products, or other irritants, which causes the patient to scratch the ear, excoriating the auricle and canal
• regular use of earphones, earplugs, or earmuffs, which trap moisture in the ear canal, creating a culture medium for infection
• chronic drainage from a perforated tympanic membrane.

Complications
Without effective treatment, otitis externa can lead to a complete closure of the ear canal, causing significant hearing loss. The infection may progress to the middle ear, resulting in otitis media. In severe otitis externa, cellulitis may develop, requiring oral or parenteral antibiotic therapy.

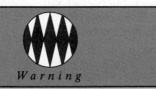

Warning

NEOMYCIN ALERT

Commonly used to treat otitis externa, neomycin may itself be the cause of contact dermatitis. Worsening of otitis externa 1 to 3 days after starting neomycin drops, along with itching and burning in a reddened area below the ear, may indicate contact dermatitis.

Malignant otitis externa, most common in patients with Type I diabetes mellitus, may develop as a result of a fulminant *Pseudomonas* infection.

Assessment findings
A review of the patient history usually shows repeated exposure to ear trauma, water, use of earphones, or allergic response to hair spray, dye, or other hair-care products. The patient also may relate a history of mild to severe ear itching or pain (or both) that is aggravated by jaw motion, clenching the teeth, opening the mouth, or chewing.

Inspection may reveal a swollen, inflamed ear canal and an ear discharge that may be foul-smelling. In chronic otitis externa, inspection shows a thick red epithelium in the ear canal. The patient may complain of increased pain or itching on palpation or manipulation of the pinna or tragus.

Otoscopy reveals a swollen external ear canal (sometimes to the point of complete closure), periauricular lymphadenopathy (tender nodes in front of the tragus, behind the ear, or in the upper neck) and, occasionally, regional cellulitis.

Fungal otitis externa may be asymptomatic, although *A. niger* may appear on otoscopy as a black or gray, ink-blot-like growth in the ear canal.

Diagnostic tests
• *Audiometric testing* may detect a partial hearing loss.
• *Microscopic examination* or *culture and sensitivity tests* can identify the causative organism and determine antibiotic treatment. In fungal otitis externa, removal of the growth reveals thick, red epithelium.

Treatment
Emphasizing site care and drug therapy, treatment includes:
• cleaning debris from the ear canal with suction and small cotton-tipped applicators under direct visualization through an ear speculum
• instilling antibiotic or anti-inflammatory drops—a combination of polymyxin B, neomycin, and hydrocortisone (Cortisporin Otic Solution) to manage gram-negative and gram-positive organisms and to decrease inflammation
• inserting an ear wick or a piece of medicine-soaked cotton into the ear (when the canal is moderately or severely swollen) for 24 to 48 hours (see *Neomycin alert*).
• administering analgesics, as appropriate
• administering systemic antibiotics to combat systemic signs, such as fever.

For the patient with a *fungal infection,* treatment includes:
• thorough cleaning of the external ear canal
• instilling an acetic acid with propylene glycol solution or an antifungal medication.

Fungal infections are more difficult to treat than simple bacterial infections. Therefore patients with such infections need to be referred to an ear, nose, and throat specialist.

In *chronic otitis externa,* treatment involves:
• cleaning the ear and removing debris
• instilling antibiotic eardrops or applying antibiotic ointment or cream (neomycin, bacitracin, or polymyxin B, possibly combined with hydrocortisone). An ointment containing phenol, salicylic acid, precipitated sulfur, and petroleum jelly, which produces exfoliative and antipruritic effects, also may be used.

For *mild chronic otitis externa,* treatment includes:
• instilling antibiotic eardrops once or twice weekly
• wearing specially fitted earplugs while showering, shampooing, or swimming.

Nursing diagnoses
• Fear
• Impaired verbal communication
• Knowledge deficit
• Pain
• Risk for infection
• Sensory alteration (auditory)

Nursing interventions
• Answer the patient's questions, encourage him to discuss concerns about hearing loss, and offer reassurance when appropriate.

• If the patient has difficulty understanding procedures because of hearing loss, give clear, concise explanations of treatments and procedures. Face him when speaking; enunciate words clearly, slowly, and in a normal tone; and allow adequate time for him to grasp what you have said. Provide a pencil and paper to aid communication, and alert the staff to his communication problem.

• If the patient has chronic otitis externa, clean the ear thoroughly. Use wet soaks intermittently on oozing or infected skin.

• If the patient has a chronic fungal infection, clean the ear canal well and then apply an exfoliative ointment.

If the patient has *acute otitis externa*:

• Monitor vital signs, particularly temperature. Watch for and record the type and amount of aural drainage.

• Remove debris, and gently clean the ear canal with mild Burow's solution (aluminum acetate). Place a wisp of cotton soaked with solution into the ear, and apply a saturated compress directly to the auricle. Afterward, dry the ear gently but thoroughly. (In severe otitis externa, such cleaning may be delayed until after initial treatment with antibiotic eardrops.)

• To instill eardrops in an adult, pull the pinna upward and backward to straighten the canal. To ensure that the drops reach the epithelium, insert a wisp of cotton moistened with eardrops.

Patient teaching

• Instruct the patient in proper hand washing and daily cleaning of the ear.

• Caution the patient to take antibiotics on time, to finish the prescription, and to report any adverse reactions.

• To prevent recurrence, tell the patient to avoid potential irritants, such as hair-care products and earrings.

• Advise the patient to use lamb's wool earplugs coated with petroleum jelly to keep water out of the ears when showering or shampooing.

• Inform parents of a young child that modeling clay makes a tight seal and prevents water from getting into the external canal.

• Tell the patient to wear earplugs or to keep his head above water when swimming, and to instill two or three drops of 3% boric acid solution in 70% alcohol into the ear before and after swimming to toughen the skin of the external ear canal.

• Warn against cleaning the ears with cotton-tipped applicators or other objects.

BENIGN TUMORS OF THE EAR CANAL

Capable of developing anywhere in the ear canal, common benign tumors include keloids, osteomas, and sebaceous cysts. Blacks and young women are most susceptible to keloids, which tend to recur. Osteomas are three times more common in males than in females.

These tumors seldom become malignant; with proper treatment, the prognosis is excellent.

Causes

Keloids result from an overgrowth of collagenous scar tissue at the site of a wound or traumatic injury, such as ear piercing. Osteomas are of idiopathic origin. Sebaceous cysts result from obstruction of a sebaceous gland.

Complications

Benign tumors may cause hearing loss.

Assessment findings

The patient usually doesn't report any symptoms unless the tumor becomes infected, in which case he may complain of pain and fever or inflammation. A patient history of pain commonly is a symptom of a malignant tumor.

On otoscopic examination, a keloid appears as elevated tissue that is round and firm, with irregular margins.

Osteomas usually occur bilaterally and in multiples (exostoses) and appear as bony outgrowths from the wall of the external auditory meatus.

A sebaceous cyst usually is palpated behind the ear near the lobule or meatus within the skin and appears as a small cyst with a black dot in the center. The cheese-like contents of the cyst have a rancid odor.

Diagnostic tests

When otoscopic examination confirms a tumor, a biopsy rules out cancer.

Treatment

A benign tumor usually requires surgical excision if it obstructs the ear canal, is cosmetically undesirable, or becomes malignant.

Treatment of a keloid may include surgery, followed by repeated injections of long-acting steroids into the suture line. Excision must be complete, but even this may not prevent recurrence.

Surgical excision of an osteoma consists of elevating the skin from the surface of the bony growth and shaving the osteoma with a mechanical burr or drill.

Before surgery, a sebaceous cyst requires preliminary treatment with antibiotics to reduce inflammation. To prevent recurrence, excision must be complete, including the sac or capsule of the cyst.

Nursing diagnoses
• Anxiety
• Knowledge deficit
• Pain
• Risk for infection

Nursing interventions
• Answer the patient's questions, encourage him to express his concerns, and offer reassurance when appropriate.

Patient teaching
• After surgery, instruct the patient in good aural hygiene. Until the ear is completely healed, advise the patient not to insert anything into it or to allow water into it. Suggest that he cover the ears with a cap when showering.
• Tell the patient to report immediately any signs of infection, such as pain, fever, localized redness, and swelling.
• Counsel the patient to take antibiotics at the times prescribed and to finish the prescription. Alert him to watch for and report any signs of an adverse reaction.

MIDDLE EAR DISORDERS

Most commonly resulting from viral or bacterial infections, disorders of the middle ear also may be genetic in origin. Some of these disorders can easily become chronic, causing irreparable hearing loss. However, proper treatment with antibiotics, surgery, or both usually produces a good prognosis.

OTITIS MEDIA
An inflammation of the middle ear associated with fluid accumulation, otitis media may be acute or chronic, suppurative or secretory.

Acute otitis media is most common in infants and children because they have a shorter and more horizontal eustachian tube than adults, which predisposes them to middle ear infections. The incidence peaks between ages 6 and 24 months and subsides after age 3 years. It occurs most frequently during the winter months, paralleling the seasonal rise in nonbacterial respiratory tract infections.

With prompt treatment, the prognosis for acute otitis media is excellent. However, prolonged accumulation of fluid in the middle ear cavity can cause chronic otitis media, with possible perforation of the tympanic membrane. Chronic suppurative otitis media may lead to scarring, adhesions, and severe structural or functional ear damage; chronic secretory otitis media, with its persistent inflammation and pressure, may cause conductive hearing loss.

Causes
Acute otitis media results from disruption of eustachian tube patency.

Suppurative otitis media usually results from bacterial infection with pneumococci, *Haemophilus influenzae* (the most common cause in children under age 6), beta-hemolytic streptococci, staphylococci (the most common cause in children age 6 or older), and gram-negative bacteria. In this disorder, respiratory tract infections, allergic reactions, and position changes (such as holding an infant supine during feeding) allow reflux of nasopharyngeal flora through the eustachian tube and colonization in the middle ear.

Chronic suppurative otitis media results from inadequate treatment of acute otitis episodes or from infection by resistant strains of bacteria.

Secretory otitis media stems from a viral infection, an allergy, or barotrauma (pressure injury from an inability to equalize pressures between the environment and the middle ear), such as that experienced during rapid aircraft descent or rapid underwater ascent in scuba diving (barotitis media). In this disorder, obstruction of the eustachian tube promotes transudation of sterile serous fluid from blood vessels in the middle ear membrane.

Chronic secretory otitis media is caused by adenoidal tissue overgrowth that obstructs the eustachian tube, edema resulting from allergic rhinitis, chronic sinus infection, or inadequate treatment of acute suppurative otitis media.

Complications
Spontaneous rupture of the tympanic membrane may cause persistent perforation that may develop into chronic otitis media. Other complications are mastoiditis, meningitis, cholesteatomas (cystlike masses in the middle ear), and permanent hearing loss.

Assessment findings
The patient history may reveal an upper respiratory tract infection. (See *Planning care for the patient with otitis media.*) The patient may complain of severe, deep, throbbing

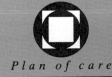

Plan of care

PLANNING CARE FOR THE PATIENT WITH OTITIS MEDIA

Before you develop nursing diagnoses and a plan of care for a patient with otitis media, consider how you would care for Jimmy Thompson, age 6, who arrives at the clinic with his mother.

Patient history
Jimmy's ear and throat have hurt for 2 days. Mrs. Thompson has noted a progressively rising temperature, irritability, an attention deficit, and loss of appetite since yesterday morning. She reports that her daughter has an upper respiratory tract infection and that the children play together when Jimmy comes home from school.

She says that Jimmy has had a long history of otitis media. Tympanostomy tubes were placed in both ears when he was age 4.

He had little sleep last night, and this morning he refused to eat his breakfast, stating that when he swallows, "it hurts and my ears pop." Mrs. Thompson has not noticed any drainage from his ears. Immunizations are current.

Assessment findings
Jimmy's temperature is 102.8° F (39.3° C); pulse, 132 beats/minute; and respirations, 22 breaths/minute. His blood pressure is normal at 98/56 mm Hg.

Otoscopic examination reveals the tympanic membranes bilaterally translucent and gray, secondary to scar formation, and a new, concealed infection indicated by minimal eardrum movement and a slight bulging.

You also note cervical neck glands enlarged bilaterally, especially the left, and a reddened oropharynx and uvula with white patches on both lateral walls. Jimmy's lungs are clear. The Rinne test discloses that air conduction is less than bone conduction bilaterally and that he can't hear above a whisper at 12" (30.5 cm).

Tests reveal a white blood cell count of 11,200/mm³ and a throat culture positive for streptococci. Jimmy will be discharged on amoxicillin and acetaminophen.

Nursing diagnoses
Based on Jimmy's history and your assessment findings, you formulate these nursing diagnoses:
• Sensory alteration (auditory) related to middle ear suppuration
• Sleep pattern disturbance related to fever and ear pain
• Altered nutrition: Less than body requirements, related to swallowing difficulty
• Pain related to accumulation of excess fluid in the middle ears.

Expected outcomes
Carefully, you define these goals for Jimmy. He will:
• improve perception and hearing as infection subsides and drainage is facilitated
• sleep through the night and take naps without waking to discomfort
• improve nutritional and fluid status
• have decreased pain.

Implementation
What instructions will you give Mrs. Thompson to help her care for Jimmy?

To improve perception and hearing
• Advise Mrs. Thompson to use effective communication techniques while the infection is causing transient hearing loss. Suggest that she first gain Jimmy's attention, speak in a normal tone while directly facing him, and repeat her words calmly and directly.
• Tell Mrs. Thompson to keep radio, television, video games, and general environmental noise to a minimum.
• Instruct her to have Jimmy's hearing retested if the hearing loss persists after the infection clears.
• Stress the importance of avoiding practices that can lead to further ear damage, such as swimming.

To promote sleep and rest
• Advise Mrs. Thompson to provide a quiet, nonstimulating environment and to dress Jimmy in lightweight but warm clothing.
• Suggest giving Jimmy a warm bath and fresh pajamas at bedtime.
• Tell her to give acetaminophen to reduce fever and promote comfort.
• Instruct her to help Jimmy pace his activities throughout the day and evening to allow adequate rest.

To improve nutritional and fluid status
• Suggest that Mrs. Thompson offer Jimmy his favorite foods and liquids and prepare them so that he won't aggravate his condition while eating. She may offer frozen juice pops, pudding pops, sherbet, and jello if he won't drink adequate fluids.

To decrease pain
• Instruct her to give acetaminophen as ordered and when needed.
• Encourage her to offer diversional activities to keep up Jimmy's spirits.
• Tell her to place a cotton ball on the external ear canal to decrease cold air flow to the area.
• Have her apply ice packs to Jimmy's neck and give him ice chips to suck on, to relieve sore throat.

Evaluation
Your interventions will have succeeded when Jimmy is free of ear pain, has a normal temperature, can rest comfortably and sleep during the night, consumes adequate amounts of food and fluids, and has a normal hearing test.

MYRINGOTOMY

Also called tympanocentesis, myringotomy is the surgical puncture of the tympanic membrane for removal of fluid from the middle ear. The semicircular incision is made along the bottom arc of the membrane (shown, with other landmarks).

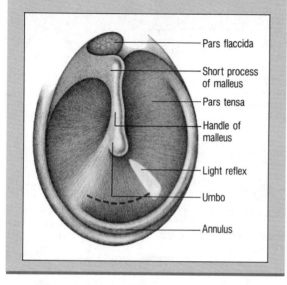

- Pars flaccida
- Short process of malleus
- Pars tensa
- Handle of malleus
- Light reflex
- Umbo
- Annulus

ear pain (from pressure behind the tympanic membrane) and dizziness, nausea, and vomiting. With acute secretory otitis media, the patient may describe a sensation of fullness in the ear and popping, crackling, or clicking sounds on swallowing or moving the jaw. The patient with an accumulation of fluid may describe hearing an echo when speaking and experiencing a vague feeling of top-heaviness.

If the tympanic membrane has ruptured, the patient may state that the pain has suddenly stopped. A history of recent air travel or scuba diving suggests barotitis media.

Inspection may reveal sneezing and coughing due to an upper respiratory tract infection. Vital sign assessment may detect a mild to very high fever. In chronic suppurative otitis media, inspection may reveal a painless, purulent discharge.

In acute suppurative otitis media, otoscopic examination may show obscured or distorted bony landmarks of the tympanic membrane. In acute secretory otitis media, otoscopy reveals tympanic membrane retraction, which causes the bony landmarks to appear more prominent. Otoscopy also detects clear or amber fluid behind the tympanic membrane, possibly with a meniscus and bubbles. If hemorrhage into the middle ear has occurred, as in barotrauma, otoscopy will expose a blue-black tympanic membrane.

In chronic otitis media, otoscopic examination may show thickening and scarring of the tympanic membrane, decreased or absent tympanic membrane mobility, or cholesteatoma. If a tympanic perforation is present, a pulsating discharge may be visible.

In acute secretory otitis media, audiometric tests may reveal severe conductive hearing loss varying from 15 to 35 dB, depending on the thickness and amount of fluid in the middle ear cavity. In chronic suppurative otitis media, the associated conductive hearing loss varies with the size and type of tympanic membrane perforation and ossicular destruction.

Diagnostic tests

- *Pneumatoscopy* shows decreased tympanic membrane mobility. (This procedure is painful when the tympanic membrane is obviously bulging and erythematous.)
- *Tympanometry* assesses hearing loss and evaluates the condition of the middle ear. It measures how well the tympanic membrane functions.
- *Culture and sensitivity tests* of exudate identify the causative organism.
- *Radiographic studies* depict mastoid involvement.
- *Audiometry* detects and measures the degree of hearing loss.

Treatment

In acute suppurative otitis media, antibiotic therapy includes ampicillin or amoxicillin, and amoxicillin-clavulanate (Augmentin) for infants, children, and adults. Therapy for patients allergic to penicillin derivatives may include sulfonamides, erythromycin, tetracycline, and other broad-spectrum antibiotics. Aspirin or acetaminophen controls pain and fever.

Severe, painful bulging of the tympanic membrane usually requires myringotomy. (For more information, see *Myringotomy*.)

Broad-spectrum antibiotics can help prevent acute suppurative otitis media in high-risk patients, such as children with recurring episodes of otitis. However, in these patients, antibiotics must be used sparingly and with discretion to prevent development of resistant bacteria.

In acute secretory otitis media, performing Valsalva's maneuver several times a day to inflate the eustachian tube may be the only treatment required. If this isn't successful, nasopharyngeal decongestant therapy may be helpful; it should continue for at least 2 weeks and sometimes indefinitely, with periodic evaluation. If decongestant therapy fails, myringotomy and aspiration of middle ear fluid are necessary, followed by insertion of a polyethylene tube into the tympanic membrane to equalize pressure. This pressure-equalizing tube, called a tympanostomy tube, remains in place for 6 to 12 months, although it may fall out on its own. Concomitant treatment of the underlying cause (such as allergen elimination or adenoidectomy) also may be helpful.

Treatment of chronic otitis media may include antibiotics for exacerbations of acute otitis media, elimination of eustachian tube obstruction, treatment of otitis externa (when present), myringoplasty (tympanic membrane graft), tympanoplasty to reconstruct middle ear structures when thickening and scarring are present, mastoidectomy, or cholesteatoma excision.

Nursing diagnoses
• Impaired verbal communication
• Knowledge deficit
• Pain
• Risk for infection
• Sensory alteration (auditory)

Nursing interventions
• Answer the patient's or his parents' questions. Encourage them to discuss concerns about hearing loss, and offer reassurance when appropriate.
• If the patient has difficulty understanding procedures because of hearing loss, provide clear, concise explanations. Face him when speaking; enunciate clearly, slowly, and in a normal tone; and allow time for him to grasp what you have said. Provide a pencil and paper, and alert the staff to his communication problem.
• After myringotomy, maintain the drainage flow. Don't place cotton or plugs deep in the ear canal; you may place sterile cotton loosely in the external ear to absorb drainage. To prevent infection, change the cotton when it gets damp, and wash your hands before and after ear care. As prescribed, give codeine and aspirin for pain and antiemetics for nausea and vomiting.
• After tympanoplasty, reinforce dressings and observe for excessive bleeding from the ear canal. Administer analgesics, as needed.
• Identify and treat allergies.

Patient teaching
• Advise the patient with acute secretory otitis media or his parents to watch for and immediately report pain and fever, which indicate secondary infection.

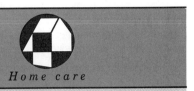

Home care

PREVENTING OTITIS MEDIA
For a patient recovering from otitis media at home, follow these guidelines to help prevent a recurrence:
• Teach the patient how to recognize upper respiratory tract infections, and encourage early treatment of them.
• Instruct parents not to feed an infant in a supine position and not to put him to bed with a bottle. Explain that doing so could cause reflux of nasopharyngeal flora.
• Teach the patient to promote eustachian tube patency by performing Valsalva's maneuver several times a day, especially during airplane travel.
• After tympanoplasty, advise the patient not to blow his nose or get his ear wet when bathing.
• Explain all adverse reactions to the prescribed medication, emphasizing those that require immediate medical attention.

• If nasopharyngeal decongestants are ordered, teach correct instillation.
• Tell the patient that some doctors require fitted ear plugs for swimming after myringotomy and tympanostomy tube insertion. Advise the patient to notify the doctor if the tube falls out and if any ear pain, fever, or pus-filled ear discharge occurs.
• Explain how to prevent recurrence. (See *Preventing otitis media*.)

MASTOIDITIS
A bacterial infection and inflammation of the air cells of the mastoid antrum, mastoiditis was much more common as a sequela to ear infections in the preantibiotic era. When it occurs now, it usually results from suboptimal antibiotic selection or poor patient compliance with drug therapy.

Mastoiditis is usually a complication of chronic otitis media and, less frequently, of acute otitis media. An accumulation of pus under pressure in the middle ear cavity results in necrosis of adjacent tissue and extension of the infection into the mastoid cells. Chronic systemic diseases or immunosuppression may also lead to mastoiditis. The prognosis is good with early treatment.

Causes

Bacteria that cause mastoiditis include pneumococci (usually in children under age 6), *Haemophilus influenzae*, beta-hemolytic streptococci, staphylococci, and gram-negative organisms.

Complications

The infection may spread, leading to facial paralysis, suppurative labyrinthitis, meningitis, epidural abscess, brain abscess, or venous sinus thrombosis.

Assessment findings

The patient may complain of a dull ache and tenderness in the area of the mastoid process, and a thick, purulent discharge that gradually becomes more profuse, possibly leading to otitis externa.

The auricle may appear pushed away from the head (from postauricular erythema and edema). Otoscopy may show swelling and obstruction of the external ear canal, caused by pressure within the edematous mastoid antrum. The patient may also have a low-grade fever.

Diagnostic tests

• *X-rays* confirm the diagnosis and demonstrate clouding of the air cells and decalcification of the bony wall between the cells.
• *Culture and sensitivity tests* may determine the causative agent.
• *Audiometric testing* may reveal a conductive hearing loss.

Treatment

Intense parenteral antibiotic therapy is the primary treatment for mastoiditis. If bone damage is minimal, myringotomy is performed to drain purulent fluid and to provide a specimen for culture and sensitivity testing.

Recurrent or persistent infection or signs of intracranial complications necessitate simple mastoidectomy. This procedure involves removing the diseased bone and cleaning the affected area, then inserting a drain.

A chronically inflamed mastoid requires radical mastoidectomy—excision of the posterior wall of the ear canal, remnants of the tympanic membrane, and the malleus and incus (although these bones are usually destroyed by infection before surgery). The stapes and facial nerve remain intact. In some patients, grafts of skin, fascia, or muscle are created to facilitate closure of the space.

After radical mastoidectomy, the patient may be able to hear with a hearing aid or may lose hearing permanently in the operated ear. With either surgical procedure, the patient continues oral antibiotic therapy for several weeks after surgery and hospital discharge.

Nursing diagnoses

• Anxiety
• Impaired verbal communication
• Knowledge deficit
• Pain
• Risk for infection
• Risk for injury
• Sensory alteration (auditory)

Nursing interventions

• After simple mastoidectomy, give pain medication as needed. Check wound drainage, and reinforce dressings (the surgeon usually changes the dressing daily and removes the drain in 72 hours). Check the patient's hearing, and watch for signs of complications, especially infection (either localized or extending to the brain), facial nerve paralysis with unilateral facial drooping, bleeding, and vertigo (especially when the patient stands). Position the patient on the affected side after simple mastoidectomy to facilitate drainage.
• After radical mastoidectomy, you'll find the wound packed with petroleum gauze or gauze treated with an antibiotic ointment. Administer pain medication before the packing is removed on the fourth or fifth postoperative day.
• Because of stimulation to the inner ear during surgery, the patient may feel dizzy and nauseated for several days afterward. Keep the bed's side rails up, and assist the patient with ambulation. Also, give prescribed antiemetics as needed. If a graft was taken from the arm or leg, check the donor site for infection, and monitor the healing process.
• Answer the patient's questions, encourage him to express his concerns about hearing loss, and offer reassurance when appropriate.
• If the patient has difficulty understanding procedures because of hearing loss, give clear, concise explanations of treatments and procedures. Face him when speaking; enunciate clearly, slowly, and in a normal tone; and allow adequate time for him to grasp what you have said.
• Provide a pencil and paper to aid communication, and alert the staff to the patient's communication problem.

Patient teaching

• Before surgery, give preoperative and postoperative instructions to the patient. Advise him that vertigo is normal after surgery, as well as some hearing loss because of the packing.
• Tell the patient and family how to reinforce the dressing and to avoid getting it wet. After the first dressing change by the surgeon, teach proper dressing change technique.

- Emphasize the necessity of taking antibiotics as prescribed until therapy is completed. Caution the patient to report any adverse reactions.
- Because hearing loss from the packing and dressings is common, teach safety measures in the home. Teach the patient and family alternate methods of communication.
- Encourage regular follow-up care.

OTOSCLEROSIS

The most common cause of conductive hearing loss, otosclerosis is the slow formation of spongy bone in the otic capsule, particularly at the oval window. This otosclerotic bone growth eventually causes the footplate of the stapes to become locked or fixed in position, disrupting the conduction of vibrations from the tympanic membrane to the cochlea.

Otosclerosis occurs in at least 10% of whites, is twice as common in women as in men, and usually occurs between ages 15 and 50. With surgery, the prognosis is good.

Causes
Otosclerosis may result from a genetic factor transmitted as an autosomal dominant trait. Many patients with this disorder report family histories of hearing loss (excluding presbycusis). Pregnancy may trigger the onset of this condition.

Complications
Unilateral at first, this disorder may advance to bilateral conductive hearing loss.

Assessment findings
The patient may report a history of slow, progressive hearing loss in one ear, which may have progressed to both ears, without middle ear infection. She may also describe tinnitus and the ability to hear a conversation better in a noisy environment than in a quiet one (paracusis of Willis).

Otoscopic examination usually reveals a tympanic membrane that appears normal. Occasionally, however, you may see a faint pink blush through the membrane from the vascularity of the active otosclerotic bone (Schwartze's sign).

Diagnostic tests
- *Rinne test* demonstrates that the bone-conducted tone is heard longer than the air-conducted tone (normally,

the reverse is true). As otosclerosis progresses, bone conduction also deteriorates.
- *Weber's test* detects sound lateralizing to the more damaged ear.
- *Audiometric testing* reveals hearing loss, ranging from 60 dB in early stages to total loss as the disease advances.

Treatment
In most cases, treatment consists of stapedectomy (removal of the stapes) and insertion of a prosthesis to restore partial or total hearing. This procedure is performed on one ear at a time, beginning with the ear that has sustained greater damage. Postoperative treatment includes hospitalization for 2 to 3 days and antibiotics to prevent infection. (See *Types of stapedectomy*, page 1130.)

Other surgical procedures include fenestration and stapes mobilization; all require normal cochlear function.

Sometimes further hearing loss can be prevented by giving the patient sodium fluoride and calcium supplements to promote recalcification and to arrest spongy bone formation.

Hearing aids enable the patient to hear conversation in normal surroundings.

Nursing diagnoses
- Anxiety
- Fear
- Impaired verbal communication
- Knowledge deficit
- Risk for infection
- Sensory alteration (auditory)

Nursing interventions
- Address the patient's questions, encourage her to discuss her concerns about hearing loss, and offer reassurance when appropriate.
- If the patient has difficulty understanding procedures because of hearing loss, give clear, concise explanations of treatments and procedures. Face her when speaking; enunciate clearly, slowly, and in a normal tone; and allow adequate time for her to grasp what you have said. Provide a pencil and paper to aid communication, and alert the staff to her communication problem.
- Follow the doctor's orders regarding specific postoperative positioning for the patient—on the unaffected side to prevent graft displacement or on the affected side to facilitate drainage. Some doctors allow any position that doesn't cause vertigo.

TYPES OF STAPEDECTOMY

Surgery may remove part or all of the stapes, depending on the extent of otosclerotic growth. It may be performed using various techniques. Two techniques used to implant a prosthesis are shown below.

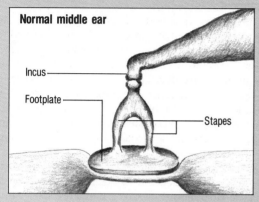

Normal middle ear

Incus

Footplate

Stapes

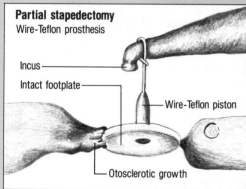

Partial stapedectomy
Wire-Teflon prosthesis

Incus

Intact footplate

Wire-Teflon piston

Otosclerotic growth

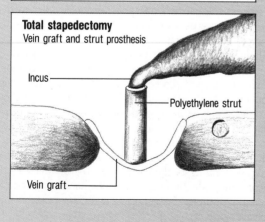

Total stapedectomy
Vein graft and strut prosthesis

Incus

Polyethylene strut

Vein graft

• After surgery, keep the bed's side rails up, and help the patient walk.

• Administer prescribed medication for pain and assess the patient's response. Meperidine may be given initially, followed by milder analgesics.

Patient teaching

• For a patient undergoing surgery, provide preoperative and postoperative teaching. After surgery, advise her to move slowly to prevent vertigo.

• Stress the importance of protecting the ears against cold. Advise the patient to avoid any activities that provoke dizziness, such as straining, bending, or heavy lifting, and to avoid contact with anyone with an upper respiratory tract infection.

• Teach the patient and family how to change the external ear dressing (eye or gauze pad) and care for the incision. Emphasize the need to complete the prescribed antibiotic regimen and to return for scheduled follow-up care, which includes removing the packing.

• Point out that hearing may be masked by packing and dressing as well as swelling from the operation. Inform the patient that hearing may not be noticeably improved for 1 to 4 weeks after surgery.

• Before discharge, instruct the patient to avoid loud noises and sudden pressure changes (such as those that occur while diving or flying) until healing is complete (usually within 6 months). Advise her against blowing her nose for at least 1 week to prevent contaminated air and bacteria from entering the eustachian tube.

• Advise the patient to avoid sudden movements, which may result in dizziness. Also caution against wetting her head in the shower or swimming for about 6 weeks. Tell her to postpone washing her hair for 2 weeks and to avoid getting water in the ear for an additional 4 weeks.

• Instruct the patient not to strain while defecating and to avoid constipation.

INFECTIOUS MYRINGITIS

Characterized by inflammation, hemorrhage, and effusion of fluid into the tissue at the end of the external ear canal and the tympanic membrane, acute infectious myringitis is a self-limiting disorder that resolves spontaneously within 3 days to 2 weeks.

This disorder commonly follows acute otitis media or upper respiratory tract infection and frequently occurs epidemically in children. Chronic granular myringitis is a rare inflammation of the squamous layer of the tympanic membrane.

Causes

Acute infectious myringitis usually follows viral infection but may result from infection with bacteria (pneumococci, *Haemophilus influenzae*, beta-hemolytic streptococci, and staphylococci) or any other organism that may cause acute otitis media. Myringitis is a rare sequela of atypical pneumonia caused by *Mycoplasma pneumoniae*.

The cause of chronic granular myringitis is unknown.

Complications

Chronic granular myringitis may lead to stenosis of the ear canal and gradual hearing loss.

Assessment findings

The patient with acute infectious myringitis may complain of severe ear pain, commonly accompanied by tenderness over the mastoid process. In chronic granular myringitis, the patient history may reveal pruritus, purulent discharge, and gradual hearing loss.

Otoscopic examination will show small, reddened, inflamed blebs in the ear canal, on the tympanic membrane and, with bacterial invasion, in the middle ear. Spontaneous rupture of these blebs may cause a bloody discharge. In chronic granular myringitis, examination may reveal granulation extending from the tympanic membrane to the external ear.

Fever and hearing loss are rare unless fluid accumulates in the middle ear or a large bleb completely obstructs the external auditory meatus.

Diagnostic tests

Culture and sensitivity testing of exudate identifies secondary infection.

Treatment

Hospitalization usually isn't required for acute infectious myringitis. Treatment consists of:
• analgesics, such as aspirin or acetaminophen, to relieve pain
• application of heat to the external ear
• codeine for severe pain
• systemic or topical antibiotics to prevent or treat secondary infection
• incision of blebs and evacuation of serum and blood to relieve pressure and help drain exudate. However, these measures don't speed recovery.

Treatment of chronic granular myringitis consists of systemic antibiotics or local anti-inflammatory antibiotic combination eardrops, and surgical excision and cautery. If stenosis is present, surgical reconstruction is necessary.

Nursing diagnoses

• Anxiety
• Impaired verbal communication
• Knowledge deficit
• Pain
• Sensory alteration (auditory)

Nursing interventions

• Answer the patient's questions, encourage him to express his concerns about hearing loss, and offer reassurance when appropriate.
• If the patient has difficulty understanding procedures because of hearing loss, give clear, concise explanations of treatments and procedures. Face him when speaking; enunciate words clearly, slowly, and in a normal tone; and allow adequate time for him to grasp what's expected. Provide a pencil and paper to aid communication, and alert the staff to his communication problem.
• Assess the patient's level of pain, and give analgesics as needed. Also give antibiotic eardrops, as ordered. Monitor his response to these medications.
• To instill eardrops in an adult, pull the pinna upward and backward to straighten the canal. To ensure that the drops reach the epithelium, insert a wisp of cotton moistened with eardrops.

Patient teaching

• Explain all procedures, such as bleb incision.
• Stress the importance of completing the prescribed antibiotic therapy. Advise the patient to report any adverse reactions.
• Teach the patient or his family how to instill antibiotic eardrops.
• Explain the signs and symptoms of infectious myringitis and the necessity for prompt treatment of otitis media.

INNER EAR DISORDERS

Because the inner ear controls balance and hearing, disorders affecting it commonly produce loss of equilibrium, vertigo, nausea and vomiting, and hearing loss. Treatment varies with the disorder and may include drug therapy, surgery, and use of amplification devices.

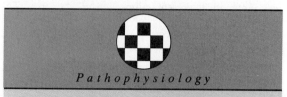

Pathophysiology

WHAT HAPPENS IN MÉNIÈRE'S DISEASE

In a person with normal hearing, the inner ear's two fluid-filled structures make hearing possible and maintain balance. The snail-shaped cochlea transduces sound waves into nerve impulses, which then continue on to the brain. The loop-shaped semicircular canals detect changes in balance and body orientation. Together, these two structures form the labyrinth, named for its complicated twists, bends, and turns.

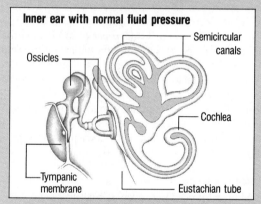

Inner ear with normal fluid pressure

Ossicles

Semicircular canals

Cochlea

Tympanic membrane

Eustachian tube

In Ménière's disease, the fluid pressure in the labyrinth increases, perhaps because of an overproduction or underabsorption of fluid. The resultant swelling causes hearing loss, dizziness, and related symptoms.

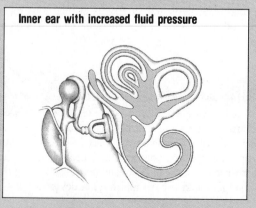

Inner ear with increased fluid pressure

MÉNIÈRE'S DISEASE

An inner ear problem stemming from a labyrinthine dysfunction, Ménière's disease is associated with increased fluid pressure within the labyrinth. Although it usually affects adults between the ages of 30 and 60, it may begin at any age. It occurs in both sexes.

Also called endolymphatic hydrops, the disease involves only one ear at first, but about 20% of patients eventually develop problems in both ears. Even with proper treatment, this chronic disease may cause hearing loss.

Causes and pathophysiology

Ménière's disease may result from an overproduction or decreased absorption of endolymph, the fluid within the cochlea and semicircular canals. Pressure from this excess fluid disturbs and damages the sensory cells that transmit hearing and balance perception to the brain. (See *What happens in Ménière's disease.*)

The cause of this overproduction (or underabsorption) is unknown. Various theories attribute the problem to excess sodium retention, an allergic reaction to certain foods, or vascular spasms that constrict blood vessels supplying the inner ear.

Complications

This disorder leads to residual tinnitus and hearing loss.

Assessment findings

In taking the patient history, you'll hear about the cardinal symptom of Ménière's disease: vertigo. The patient may complain that the symptom has a sudden onset and lasts up to several hours. If the disorder has progressed, the patient may relate that attacks occur more frequently, as often as every 2 or 3 days. The dizziness may be so severe that the patient loses his balance and falls to the affected side.

The patient may also complain about tinnitus that occurs as a low, fluctuating buzzing, hissing, or humming sound in the ear that's often louder preceding and during an attack. In fact, this may be the only symptom the patient notices between attacks. He may report a distortion in sound, hearing loss, and a feeling of pressure or fullness in the affected ear.

Diagnostic tests

• *Electronystagmography* measures the electropotential of eye movements when nystagmus is produced and provides a graphic recording of labyrinth function.
• *Audiometric tests* reveal sensorineural loss and loss of discrimination and recruitment.

• *Magnetic resonance imaging* evaluates the structure of the brain and rules out brain lesions or tumors.
• *Auditory brain stem response test* helps determine if a cochlear or retrocochlear lesion is causing hearing loss.

Treatment

Management of Ménière's disease aims to eliminate vertigo and prevent further hearing loss. For an acute attack, the patient may assume whatever position is comfortable. Atropine may stop the attack in 20 to 30 minutes. Dimenhydrinate, meclizine, diphenhydramine, or diazepam may relieve a mild attack. A severe attack may respond to epinephrine or diphenhydramine.

Long-term management includes the use of diuretics or vasodilators and restricted sodium intake. Prophylactic antihistamines or mild sedatives may also help. Three-fourths of patients respond to a salt-free diet and the use of diuretics. However, diuretic efficacy hasn't been proven.

If Ménière's disease persists after more than 2 years of treatment or produces incapacitating vertigo, the patient may require surgery. Some patients benefit from endolymphatic sac decompression (endolymphatic shunt). This procedure creates an opening in the labyrinth to drain excess fluid from the ear. A more complex procedure resects the vestibular nerve, which carries impulses from the mechanisms involved with position sense in the inner ear to the brain. If the patient has severe hearing loss in one ear, radical labyrinthectomy may be helpful.

Nursing diagnoses

• Altered nutrition: More than body requirements
• Anxiety
• Fear
• Fluid volume deficit
• Knowledge deficit
• Risk for injury
• Sensory alteration (auditory)

Nursing interventions

• If the patient experiences an attack in the hospital, keep the bed's side rails up to prevent falls. Don't let the patient rise or walk without help.
• Answer the patient's questions, encourage him to express his concerns about hearing loss, and offer reassurance when appropriate.
• If the patient has difficulty understanding procedures due to hearing loss, give clear, concise explanations of treatments and procedures. Face him when speaking; enunciate words clearly, slowly, and in a normal tone;

and allow adequate time for him to grasp what's expected. Provide a pencil and paper to aid communication, and alert the staff to his communication problem.
• Before surgery, if the patient is vomiting, record fluid intake and output and characteristics of emesis. Administer antiemetics, as ordered, and give small amounts of fluid frequently.
• After surgery, record intake and output carefully.
• Give prophylactic antibiotics and antiemetics, as ordered, and monitor the patient's response.

Patient teaching

• Review with the patient a low-sodium diet. Discuss foods and nonprescription medications that contain sodium.
• Instruct the patient about prescribed diuretics and vasodilators. Tell him to report any adverse reactions.
• Advise against reading and exposure to glaring lights, to reduce dizziness.
• Instruct the patient to avoid sudden position changes and any tasks that vertigo makes hazardous because an attack can begin quite rapidly.
• Because stress and fatigue can trigger attacks, teach the patient relaxation techniques. Review ways of modifying the patient's life-style, including making adequate time for rest and relaxation.

After surgery:
• Tell the patient to expect dizziness and nausea for 1 to 2 days after surgery.
• Because Bell's palsy is a complication of surgery, instruct the patient to be alert for possible signs, such as facial numbness and tingling and incomplete eye closure.

LABYRINTHITIS

An inflammation of the labyrinth of the inner ear (which controls both hearing and balance), labyrinthitis typically produces severe vertigo with head movement and sensorineural hearing loss. Vertigo begins gradually but peaks within 48 hours. Because it may last 3 to 5 days, causing loss of balance and falling in the direction of the affected ear, it often incapacitates the patient. Symptoms gradually subside over 3 to 6 weeks. Prevention is possible through early and vigorous treatment of predisposing conditions, such as otitis media and any local or systemic infection.

Causes

Labyrinthitis results from the same organisms that cause acute febrile diseases, such as pneumonia, influenza and, especially, chronic otitis media. In chronic otitis media, cholesteatoma formation erodes the labyrinth bone, allowing bacteria to enter from the middle ear. Drug toxicity also may cause labyrinthitis.

Complications
Meningitis may develop, although it's uncommon.

Assessment findings
The patient with labyrinthitis may complain of severe vertigo from any movement of the head, nausea and vomiting, and a hearing loss. Questioning may uncover a recent upper respiratory tract infection.

On inspection, you'll note spontaneous nystagmus, with jerking movements of the eyes toward the unaffected ear. The patient may also demonstrate excessive giddiness. To minimize these symptoms, he may assume a characteristic posture — lying on the side of the unaffected ear and looking in the direction of the affected ear. Examination of the affected ear may reveal purulent drainage.

Diagnostic tests
Evaluation of labyrinthitis relies on:
• *culture and sensitivity tests,* to identify the infecting organism, if purulent drainage is present
• *audiometric testing,* to reveal any sensorineural hearing loss
• *computed tomography scan,* to rule out a brain lesion.

Treatment
Essentially based on relieving the patient's symptoms, treatment includes bed rest, with the head immobilized between pillows, meclizine orally to relieve vertigo, and massive doses of antibiotics to combat diffuse purulent labyrinthitis. Oral fluids can prevent dehydration from vomiting; I.V. fluids may be needed for severe nausea and vomiting.

When conservative management fails, treatment necessitates surgical excision of the cholesteatoma and drainage of the infected areas of the middle and inner ear.

Nursing diagnoses
• Anxiety
• Fear
• Knowledge deficit
• Risk for fluid volume deficit
• Risk for injury
• Sensory alteration (auditory)

Nursing interventions
• Answer the patient's questions, encourage him to express his concerns about hearing loss, and offer reassurance when appropriate.
• If the patient has difficulty understanding procedures due to hearing loss, give clear, concise explanations of treatments and procedures. Face him when speaking; enunciate words clearly, slowly, and in a normal tone; and allow adequate time for him to grasp what's expected. Provide a pencil and paper to aid communication, and alert the staff to his communication problem.
• Keep the bed's side rails up to ensure the patient's safety. Assist with ambulation, as needed, to prevent falls.
• Maintain the patient on bed rest in a darkened room with his head immobile to reduce symptoms.
• Give antiemetics, as ordered, and monitor the patient's response.
• Provide the patient with oral fluids to prevent dehydration from vomiting. If vomiting precludes oral intake, administer I.V. fluids, as ordered, and monitor the patient's intake and output.

Patient teaching
• Caution the patient to limit activities, such as driving a motor vehicle or operating machinery, to avoid danger from vertigo.
• Reassure the patient that recovery is certain but may take as long as 6 weeks.
• Encourage the patient to seek prompt treatment for upper respiratory tract and systemic infections, particularly for otitis media.
• Stress the importance of controlling the use of salicylates and other potentially toxic substances.
• Instruct the patient to complete the medication regimen as prescribed. Warn him to discontinue the drug and notify his doctor if any adverse reactions occur.
• If surgery is required, give the patient preoperative and postoperative instructions.

HEARING LOSS
Mechanical or nervous impediment to the transmission of sound waves can produce hearing loss. The major forms are classified as conductive, sensorineural, or mixed.

In conductive hearing loss, sound is interrupted as it travels from the external canal to the inner ear (the junction of the stapes and the oval window). In sensorineural hearing loss, sound wave transmission is interrupted between the inner ear and the brain. The most common type of sensorineural hearing loss, presbycusis, is prevalent in adults over age 50 and cannot be reversed or corrected. Mixed hearing loss combines dysfunction of conduction and sensorineural transmission.

Congenital hearing loss can be conductive or sensorineural. Premature or low-birth-weight infants with congenital hearing loss are most likely to have structural or functional hearing impairments; those infants with serum bilirubin levels greater than 20 mg/dl also risk hearing impairment from the toxic effects of these high levels on the brain.

Sudden hearing loss, which can occur in a patient with no previous hearing loss, can be conductive, sensorineural, or mixed, and usually affects only one ear. Depending on the cause, prompt treatment (within 48 hours) may restore hearing.

Noise-induced hearing loss may be transient or permanent. Such hearing loss is common in workers subjected to constant industrial noise and in military personnel, hunters, and rock musicians.

Hearing loss may be partial or total and is calculated from the American Medical Association formula: Hearing is 1.5% impaired for every decibel (dB) that the pure tone average exceeds 25 dB.

Causes and pathophysiology

The most common cause of conductive hearing loss is cerumen (wax) impaction, which occurs in patients with small or hairy ear canals. Other causes include otitis media, which is common in children and may accompany an upper respiratory tract infection; otitis externa, which results from a gram-negative bacterial infection of the external ear canal; and otosclerosis, which produces ossification of the stapediovestibular joint.

Sensorineural hearing loss is caused by impairment of the cochlea and the eighth cranial or acoustic nerve. The most common form of this type of hearing loss, presbycusis, results from loss of hair cells and nerve fibers in the cochlea or from drug toxicity. Sensorineural hearing loss may also follow prolonged exposure to loud noise (85 to 90 dB) or brief exposure to extremely loud noise (greater than 90 dB). Occasionally, sensorineural hearing loss results from an acoustic neuroma (a benign tumor that can be life-threatening).

Congenital hearing loss, which may be sensorineural or conductive, may be transmitted as a dominant, autosomal dominant, autosomal recessive, or sex-linked recessive trait. Hearing loss in neonates may also result from trauma, toxicity, or infection during pregnancy or delivery.

Predisposing factors include a family history of hearing loss or known hereditary disorders (otosclerosis, for example); maternal exposure to rubella or syphilis during pregnancy; use of ototoxic drugs during pregnancy; prolonged fetal anoxia during delivery; and congenital abnormalities of the ears, nose, or throat. In addition, trauma during delivery may cause intracranial hemorrhage and damage the cochlea or acoustic nerve.

The cause of sudden hearing loss is unknown. However, the possibilities include occlusion of the internal auditory artery by spasm or thrombosis; subclinical mumps and other bacterial and viral infections; acoustic neuroma; or a single episode of Ménière's disease.

Sudden hearing loss also may be caused by metabolic disorders, such as hypothyroidism, diabetes mellitus, and hyperlipoproteinemia; vascular disorders, such as hypertension and arteriosclerosis; neurologic disorders, such as multiple sclerosis and neurosyphilis; blood dyscrasias, such as leukemia and hypercoagulation; and ototoxic drugs, such as tobramycin, streptomycin, quinine, gentamicin, furosemide, and ethacrynic acid. (See *Common ototoxic substances*, page 1136.)

Complications

If untreated, conductive hearing loss resulting from otitis media can lead to tympanic membrane perforation, cholesteatoma, and permanent hearing loss.

Assessment findings

Although congenital hearing loss may produce no obvious signs of hearing impairment at birth, the infant generally will demonstrate deficient response to auditory stimuli within 2 to 3 days. In an older child, the patient history may describe a hearing loss that impairs speech development. The Rinne and Weber tests may indicate if the hearing loss is conductive or sensorineural.

In conductive hearing loss, the history may uncover a recent upper respiratory tract infection. The Weber test will be positive, and the Rinne test also may be positive (although a positive Rinne test also may indicate sensorineural hearing loss).

A patient with sudden deafness may report recent exposure to loud noise or brief exposure to an extremely loud noise. The patient may complain of persistent tinnitus and transient vertigo. Audiometric tests will indicate that the patient has a loss of perception of certain frequencies (around 4,000 Hz) or, if he's experienced lengthy exposure, loss of perception of all frequencies. The Weber and Rinne tests may indicate conductive or sensorineural hearing loss.

COMMON OTOTOXIC SUBSTANCES

Certain drugs and other substances can seriously damage the auditory function of the inner ear. Hearing loss from these substances may occur suddenly during short-term use or exposure, or it may be delayed.

The patient may notice only tinnitus, but audiometric tests will show a progressive, high-tone, sensorineural hearing loss. If the patient has renal disease, the potential for ototoxicity increases.

Patients taking these drugs should report tinnitus, vertigo, or hearing loss immediately. Routine blood tests may be used to monitor the drug level in the patient's blood.

Common ototoxic substances include the following antibiotics, diuretics, and miscellaneous agents.

Antibiotics

Aminoglycosides, such as amikacin, gentamicin, kanamycin, neomycin, netilmicin, streptomycin, and tobramycin, can cause permanent hearing loss.

Other antibiotics that have the potential for ototoxicity include capreomycin, erythromycin, minocycline, polymyxin B, and vancomycin.

These antibiotics cause deafness by destroying the hair cells of the cochlea.

Diuretics

Ethacrynic acid and furosemide are ototoxic drugs. These diuretics affect the stria vascularis (the layer of fibrous tissue covering the cochlear duct). Inform the patient that discontinuing these drugs usually restores hearing.

Miscellaneous agents

Anticancer drugs, such as bleomycin, carmustine, and cisplatin; chloroquine; quinidine gluconate; and quinine have toxic effects on the inner ear. So do salicylates. And although their action isn't known, stopping these drugs usually restores hearing.

Poisons, such as arsenic, cadmium, disulfide, carbon monoxide, lead, mercury, and phosphorus are also toxic to the inner ear. Poisons and other miscellaneous agents usually affect the nerve pathway. Hearing loss associated with these agents may be temporary or permanent.

In sensorineural hearing loss due to presbycusis, the patient history is probably the most valuable assessment tool because the patient may not have noticed the hearing loss or may deny it. The history also may expose the use of ototoxic substances. Hearing tests will reveal a loss that's usually in the high-frequency tones. The patient may report a history of tinnitus. A positive Rinne test may indicate sensorineural hearing loss. (See *Detecting hearing loss*.)

Diagnostic tests

• *Auditory brain response* measures activity in the auditory nerve and brain stem. If the test results are positive or inconclusive, additional tests may be ordered.
• *Computed tomography scan* helps to evaluate vestibular and auditory pathways.
• *Pure tone audiometry* assesses the presence and degree of hearing loss.
• *Magnetic resonance imaging* evaluates brain condition and helps detect acoustic tumors or lesions.
• *Electronystagmography* evaluates vestibular function.

Treatment

Varying with the type and cause of impairment, treatment for hearing loss may include medication to treat infections and dissolve cerumen; surgery (stapedectomy,

tympanoplasty, cochlear implant, and myringotomy); hearing aids or other effective means of aiding communication; and antibiotics and decongestants for hearing loss due to otitis media.

Treatment for sudden deafness requires prompt identification of the underlying cause.

For noise-induced hearing loss, overnight rest usually restores normal hearing in patients who have been exposed to noise levels greater than 90 dB for several hours, but not in those who have been exposed to such noise repeatedly. As hearing deteriorates, treatment must include speech and hearing rehabilitation because hearing aids rarely help.

Presbycusis may require a hearing aid.

Dietary measures can help prevent further hearing loss. Studies suggest that people with high cholesterol levels have greater hearing loss as they age than people with low cholesterol levels.

Nursing diagnoses

• Altered nutrition: More than body requirements
• Anxiety
• Fear
• Impaired verbal communication
• Knowledge deficit
• Risk for injury

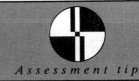

Assessment tip

DETECTING HEARING LOSS

As you take a history, question your patient and his family about the following signs and symptoms of hearing loss.

In adults
Signs of conductive or sensorineural hearing loss include:
• inattentiveness
• inappropriate responses to questions or environmental sounds
• irrelevant comments
• requests for speaker to repeat statements
• cocking one ear toward sound
• unusually loud speech or unusual voice quality.
  Other signs and symptoms of sensorineural hearing loss are:
• diminished ability to hear high-pitched voices
• hypersensitivity to loud sounds
• tinnitus
• difficulty discriminating between speech and background noise
• inability to follow or participate adequately in a conversation.

In toddlers
Signs of hearing loss include:
• failure to talk clearly by age 2
• habitual yelling or shrieking when playing or communicating
• greater response to facial expressions than to speech
• shyness or withdrawal; playing alone preferred over socializing
• inattentiveness, dreaminess, or stubbornness
• air of confusion or puzzlement
• disinterest in being read to or playing word games.

In infants
Signs of hearing loss include:
• failure to blink or startle at a loud noise
• sleeping through a loud noise
• failure to turn the head toward familiar sounds
• greater response to loud noises than to voices
• failure to babble, coo, or squeal often or in response to voice; monotonal babbling.

• Self-esteem disturbance
• Sensory alteration (auditory)

Nursing interventions
• Answer the patient's questions, encourage him to discuss his concerns about hearing loss, and offer reassurance when appropriate.
• If the patient has difficulty understanding procedures due to hearing loss, give clear, concise explanations of treatments and procedures. Face him when speaking; enunciate words clearly, slowly, and in a normal tone; and allow adequate time for him to grasp what's expected. Provide a pencil and paper to aid communication, and alert the staff to his communication problem.
• To speak to a patient who can read lips, approach within his visual range and elicit attention by raising your arm or waving. (Touching him may be unnecessarily startling.) Then stand directly in front of him, with the light on your face, and speak slowly and distinctly.
• Place the patient with a hearing loss in a place where he can observe unit activities and persons approaching because such a patient depends totally on visual clues.

• Encourage the patient who's learning to use a hearing aid because he may experience periods of self-doubt and apprehension about wearing the aid.
• Refer children with suspected hearing loss to an audiologist or otolaryngologist for further evaluation.

Patient teaching
• Explain all tests and procedures. For the patient who requires surgery, give preoperative and postoperative instructions.
• For the patient requiring a hearing aid, demonstrate how to operate and maintain the device, and suggest carrying extra batteries at all times. Remind him that the aid won't restore hearing to a normal level and that it makes speech louder but not necessarily clearer. Encourage him to experiment with the controls for best results. Advise him that lessons in lipreading may increase the effectiveness of the aid. Tell him that if the hearing aid requires repair, he may borrow one from the repair agency.

• For the patient with temporary hearing loss, emphasize the danger of excessive exposure to noise, and encourage the use of protective devices in a noisy environment.

• If the patient is pregnant, stress the danger of exposure to drugs, chemicals, and infection (especially rubella).

• Encourage the patient to maintain a low-cholesterol diet. Teach the patient about foods that are low in cholesterol.

• If the patient's hearing loss stems from cerumen buildup and the doctor has advised ear cleaning or irrigation, demonstrate the proper technique for this and for instilling medication.

• If the patient has hearing loss due to otitis media, discuss the antibiotics and decongestants ordered, and tell him to report any adverse reactions.

NASAL DISORDERS

Although seldom life-threatening, disorders of the nose can severely impair breathing and occasionally cause serious complications. Many nasal disorders are more common in children than adults. Treatment includes drug therapy, surgery, and measures to control bleeding and improve breathing.

SEPTAL PERFORATION AND DEVIATION

Septal perforation, a hole in the nasal septum between the two air passages, usually occurs in the anterior cartilaginous septum but also may occur in the bony septum. Septal deviation is a shift from the midline, common in adults, that may be severe enough to obstruct the passage of air through the nostrils. With surgical correction, the prognosis for either disorder is good.

Causes
Septal perforation can result from several factors, including a traumatic irritation, excessive nose picking, perichondritis, syphilis, tuberculosis, untreated septal hematoma, inhalation of irritating chemicals, cocaine snorting, chronic nasal infections, nasal carcinoma, granuloma, and chronic sinusitis. Less frequently, it results from repeated cauterization for epistaxis.

Septal deviation may develop during growth as the septum shifts from one side to the other. It also can result from nasal trauma due to a fall, a blow to the nose,

or surgery that further exaggerates the deviation. Congenital deviation is rare.

Complications
Hemorrhage, infections, and deformity are possible complications of both septal perforation and deviation.

Assessment findings
Although a small septal perforation usually produces no symptoms, the patient may complain of hearing a whistling noise upon inspiration. A patient with a large perforation may report a history of rhinitis and epistaxis. The patient's history also may reveal a possible cause of the perforation, such as chronic sinusitis, tuberculosis, or inhalation of irritating chemicals. Inspection may reveal nasal crusting and a watery discharge. Inspection with a nasal speculum may also reveal the septal perforation.

The patient with a deviated septum may report a recent traumatic injury to the nose or a history of nasal obstruction. He may complain of a sensation of fullness in the face, shortness of breath, nasal discharge, recurring epistaxis, infection, sinusitis, and headache. Inspection may disclose a crooked nose as the midline deflects to one side.

Diagnostic tests
Clinical inspection confirms septal perforation or deviation. No specific diagnostic tests exist.

Treatment
Based on the patient's symptoms, treatment of a perforated septum includes decongestants to reduce nasal congestion by local vasoconstriction, local application of lanolin or petroleum jelly to prevent ulceration and crusting, and antibiotics to combat infection. Surgery may be necessary to graft part of the perichondrial layer over the perforation. Also, a plastic or Silastic "button" prosthesis may be used to close the perforation.

Treatment of a deviated septum is also based on the patient's symptoms. It usually includes analgesics to relieve headache, decongestants to minimize secretions, and vasoconstrictors, nasal packing, or cauterization as needed to control hemorrhage. Manipulation of the nasal septum at birth can correct congenital deviated septum.

Corrective surgery may consist of reconstruction of the nasal septum by submucous resection to reposition the nasal septal cartilage and relieve nasal obstruction. Other surgical procedures include rhinoplasty to correct nasal structure deformity by intranasal incisions and septoplasty to relieve nasal obstruction and enhance cosmetic appearance. Surgical complications include possible hemorrhage, infection, and deformity.

Nursing diagnoses
• Altered oral mucous membrane
• Anxiety
• Ineffective airway clearance
• Knowledge deficit
• Risk for infection

Nursing interventions
• Answer the patient's questions, and encourage him to express his concerns. Include the patient and his family in care decisions.
• For the patient with a perforated septum, use a cotton applicator to apply petroleum jelly to the nasal mucosa to minimize crusting and ulceration.
• To relieve nasal congestion, instill 0.9% sodium chloride solution, and provide a humidifier. Give decongestants, as ordered.
• If the patient experiences epistaxis, elevate the head of the bed, provide an emesis basin, and instruct the patient to expectorate any blood. Compress the outer nose portion against the septum for 10 to 15 minutes, and apply ice packs. If bleeding persists, notify the doctor.

After surgery:
• To prevent or reduce edema and promote drainage, place the patient in semi-Fowler's position and use a cool-mist vaporizer to liquefy secretions and facilitate normal breathing. To lessen facial edema and pain, place crushed ice in a rubber glove or a small ice bag and apply over the eyes and nose intermittently for 24 hours.
• Because the patient is breathing through the mouth, provide frequent and meticulous mouth care.
• Change the mustache dressing or drip pad, as needed. Record the color, consistency, and amount of drainage. While nasal packing is in place, expect slight, bright-red drainage, with clots. After the packing is removed, watch for purulent discharge, an indication of infection.
• Watch for and report excessive swallowing, hematoma, or a falling or flapping septum (depressed or soft and unstable septum). Perform intranasal examination to detect hematoma formation. These complications require surgical correction, so notify the doctor immediately.
• Administer sedatives and analgesics, as ordered, and monitor the patient's response to these medications.

Patient teaching
• If corrective surgery is scheduled, prepare the patient to expect postoperative facial edema, periorbital bruising, and nasal packing, which will remain in place for

12 to 24 hours and force the patient to breathe through the mouth. Tell the patient that a splint may be placed on the nose after surgery. Also tell him to remain in an upright position after surgery.
• Explain the anticoagulant properties of aspirin, products containing aspirin and its derivatives, and alcohol, and advise the patient to avoid these items.
• Warn the patient with perforation or severe deviation against nose blowing, even after nasal packing is removed, because it may cause bruising and swelling. After surgery, advise the patient to limit physical activity for 2 or 3 days. If he smokes, advise him to stop smoking for at least 2 days.
• Explain to the patient that his sense of smell may be decreased and that he may feel anorexic for a while after surgery.

CLEFT LIP AND PALATE
These deformities originate in the second month of gestation when the front and sides of the face and the palatine shelves fuse imperfectly. They fall into four categories: clefts of the lip (unilateral or bilateral); clefts of the palate (along the midline); unilateral clefts of the lip, alveolus (gum pad), and palate (twice as common on the left side as the right); and bilateral clefts of the lip, alveolus, and palate. Another cleft disorder, Pierre Robin syndrome, occurs when micrognathia and glossoptosis coexist with cleft palate.

Cleft lip and palate deformities occur in about 1 in 800 births. Cleft lip with or without cleft palate is more common in males. Cleft palate alone is more common in females.

Because the palate is essential to speech, structural changes—even in a repaired cleft—can permanently affect speech patterns. Furthermore, children with cleft palates commonly experience hearing difficulties because of middle ear damage or infection.

Causes
Cleft lip and palate are genetic, resulting from multifactorial (polygenic) errors. (See *How cleft lip and palate develop,* page 1140.)

Complications
Speech difficulties and a failure to thrive (due to inadequate oral intake) are possible complications of unrepaired clefts.

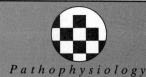

Pathophysiology

HOW CLEFT LIP AND PALATE DEVELOP

Although cleft lip and cleft palate are common birth defects, their precise cause is unknown.

Cleft lip

Cleft lip occurs around the 7th week of gestation. Normal fetal development at 5 weeks shows two horseshoe-shaped swellings on each side of the face (as shown in the 5th-week illustration). By 7 weeks' gestation, these swellings slowly move toward the middle of the face (7th-week illustration). When this fusion doesn't take place, a cleft lip results. Eventually (around 9 weeks' gestation) these swellings form the nostrils. Tissue just below the nostrils also moves together to form the upper lip (12th-week illustration).

Cleft palate

Cleft palate may occur a few weeks later in gestation. As the neck and jaws of the fetus take form, the tongue separates the two sides of the palate. Normally, the tongue moves downward and the two sides of the secondary palate fuse together above it. If this movement is delayed, or if the tongue doesn't descend, the palate won't fuse.

Various manifestations

Because the lip and the palate develop separately, a child can have a cleft lip, a cleft palate, or both.

Clefts of the lip can appear on one side of a child's mouth (unilateral), or on both sides (bilateral). The severity varies; the cleft may involve only the vermilion (darkened) tissue of the lip, or it may extend into the nose.

Cleft palate also varies in severity. It may affect only the uvula and the soft palate (the rear of the mouth), or it may extend from the soft palate into the hard palate. A cleft that stretches into only one nasal cavity is called a unilateral cleft palate; a bilateral cleft palate affects both nasal cavities.

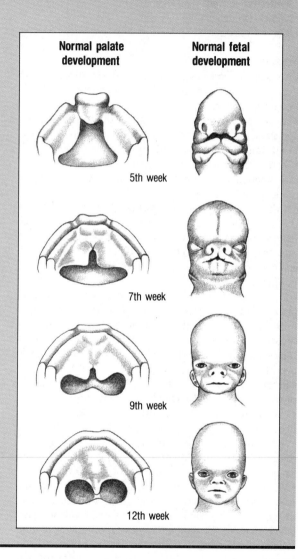

Normal palate development   **Normal fetal development**

5th week

7th week

9th week

12th week

Assessment findings

Inspection findings range from a simple notch to a complete cleft that extends from the lip through the floor of the nostril, on either side of the midline. A cleft palate may be partial or complete; if complete, inspection may show involvement of the soft palate, the bones of the max-illa, and the alveolus on one or both sides of the premaxilla.

In a double cleft, the most severe of all cleft deformities, inspection may disclose a cleft that runs from the soft palate forward to either side of the nose, separating the maxilla and the premaxilla into free-moving segments. The tongue and other muscles can displace these segments, enlarging the cleft.

Diagnostic tests
No specific tests exist for cleft lip and palate.

Treatment
Cleft deformities must be treated with a combination of speech therapy and surgery, although the timing of surgery varies.

When a wide horseshoe defect makes surgery impossible, a contoured speech bulb attached to the posterior of a denture, to occlude the nasopharynx, helps the child develop intelligible speech.

Nursing diagnoses
• Altered nutrition: Less than body requirements
• Anxiety
• Fear
• Knowledge deficit
• Risk for altered parent/infant/child attachment
• Risk for aspiration
• Risk for injury

Nursing interventions
• The parents of a neonate with cleft lip or palate often feel shock, disappointment, and guilt when they first see their baby. Help them by staying calm and directing their attention to their child's assets, emphasizing what is "right" about the baby. To encourage normal bonding, immediately include them in the infant's care and feeding. Answer their questions, encourage them to express their concerns, and stay with them during anxious periods. Refer them to a social worker who can guide them to community resources.
• Never place the infant with Pierre Robin syndrome on his back because the tongue can fall back and obstruct the airway. Train such an infant to sleep on one side. All other infants with cleft palate can sleep on their backs without difficulty.
• Maintain adequate nutrition for normal growth and development. Experiment with feeding devices. An infant with cleft palate has an excellent appetite, but often has trouble feeding due to nasal regurgitation and air leaks around the cleft. Usually, such an infant feeds better from a nipple with a flange that occludes the cleft, a lamb's nipple (a big, soft nipple with large holes), or a regular nipple with enlarged holes.

After surgery:
• Restrain the infant to prevent self-injury. Elbow restraints allow the infant to move his hands while keeping them away from the mouth. When necessary, use an infant seat to keep the infant in a comfortable position. Hang toys within reach of his restricted hands.
• If the doctor has placed a curved metal Logan bow over a repaired cleft lip to minimize tension on the suture line, check institutional policy about follow-up care. You may need to remove the gauze before feedings, replace it frequently, and moisten it with 0.9% sodium chloride solution until the sutures are removed.

Patient teaching
• Stress to parents that surgery can repair the cleft. Provide instructions, so they can take proper care of the infant at home.
• Encourage the mother of an infant with cleft lip to breast-feed if the cleft doesn't impede effective sucking. Tell the mother of an infant who has cleft palate or has just had corrective surgery that breast-feeding is impossible (postoperatively, the infant cannot suck for up to 6 weeks). However, if the mother desires, suggest that she use a breast pump to express her milk for bottle feedings.
• Teach the mother to hold the infant in a near-sitting position when feeding, with the flow directed to the side or back of the infant's tongue. Tell her to burp the infant frequently because he may tend to swallow a lot of air.

SINUSITIS

Inflammation of the paranasal sinuses may be acute, subacute, chronic, allergic, or hyperplastic. Acute sinusitis usually results from the common cold; in about 10% of patients, it lingers in subacute form. Chronic sinusitis follows persistent bacterial infection, generally occurring when a cold spreads to the sinuses.

Allergic sinusitis accompanies allergic rhinitis. Hyperplastic sinusitis is a combination of purulent acute sinusitis and allergic sinusitis or rhinitis. For all types, the prognosis is good.

Causes
Sinusitis usually results from a bacterial infection (*Haemophilus influenzae*, anaerobes) or, less frequently, from a viral infection.

Acute sinusitis most commonly is caused by *Staphylococcus aureus*, *Streptococcus pneumoniae*, and *Streptococcus pyogenes*. Predisposing factors include any condition that interferes with sinus drainage and ventilation, such as chronic nasal edema, a deviated septum, or viscous mucus. Bacterial invasion also may result from swimming in contaminated water. Generalized debilitating conditions, including chemotherapy, malnutri-

LOCATING THE PARANASAL SINUSES

The location of a patient's sinusitis pain indicates the affected sinus. For example, an infected maxillary sinus may cause tooth pain. (*Note:* The sphenoid sinus, which lies under the eye and above the soft palate, isn't shown here.)

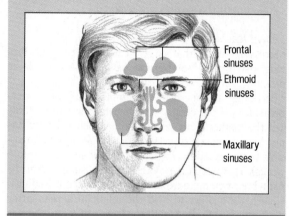

Frontal sinuses

Ethmoid sinuses

Maxillary sinuses

tion, diabetes, blood dyscrasias, long-term steroids, and immunodeficiency, also may predispose an individual to sinusitis.

Complications

Typically resulting from inadequate therapy during the acute phase or from a delay in treatment, complications may include meningitis, frontal lobe abscess, osteomyelitis, mucocele, and orbital cellulitis.

Assessment findings

The patient with acute sinusitis typically complains of nasal congestion that preceded a gradual buildup of pressure in the affected sinus. He may state that for 24 to 48 hours after onset, a nasal discharge was present and later became purulent. He may also list a sore throat, a localized headache, and a general feeling of malaise.

The patient may point to pain specific to the affected sinus: in the cheeks and upper teeth (maxillary sinusitis); over the eyes (ethmoid sinusitis); over the eyebrows (frontal sinusitis); or behind the eyes, over the occiput, or at the top of the head (sphenoid sinusitis, a rare condition).

The patient also may report purulent nasal drainage that continues longer than 3 weeks after an acute infection subsides, which usually suggests subacute sinusitis. The patient with chronic sinusitis may report continuous

and mucopurulent discharge. In the acute form, the patient may complain of a stuffy nose, vague facial discomfort, fatigue, and a nonproductive cough.

Vital signs assessment may detect a low-grade fever of 99° to 99.5° F (37.2° to 37.5° C).

The areas over the sinuses may appear swollen (caused by bacterial growth on diseased tissue in *hyperplastic sinusitis*). Inspection also may reveal enlarged turbinates and thickening of the mucosal lining and mucosal polyps (*hyperplastic sinusitis*). Palpation may cause the patient pain and pressure over the affected sinus areas. Transillumination may expose diminished areas of light. This indicates areas of purulent drainage that prevent the passage of light. (See *Locating the paranasal sinuses.*)

Diagnostic tests

• *Sinus X-rays* reveal cloudiness in the affected sinus, air-fluid levels, or thickened mucosal lining.
• *Ultrasonography* and *computed tomography scan* may uncover suspected complications, recurrent or chronic sinusitis, or unresolved and serious sinusitis.
• *Antral puncture* promotes drainage and removal of purulent material. It also may provide a specimen for culture and sensitivity identification of the infecting organism, but this test is rarely performed.

Treatment

Antibiotics represent the primary treatment for acute sinusitis. Analgesics may be prescribed to relieve pain. Other appropriate measures include vasoconstrictors, such as epinephrine or phenylephrine, to decrease nasal secretions. Steam inhalation also promotes vasoconstriction and encourages drainage.

Antibiotic therapy—usually with amoxicillin or ampicillin—combats persistent infection. Local heat applications may help to relieve pain and congestion.

In subacute sinusitis, antibiotic therapy also is the primary treatment. As in acute sinusitis, vasoconstrictors may lessen nasal secretions.

Severe allergic symptoms may require treatment with corticosteroids and epinephrine.

In both chronic sinusitis and hyperplastic sinusitis, antibiotics and a steroid nasal spray may relieve pain and congestion. Antihistamines may be judiciously prescribed for relief of symptoms but are administered cautiously because they may thicken nasal secretions and prevent effective sinus drainage.

If a subacute infection persists, the maxillary sinus may be irrigated. The ethmoid and sphenoid sinuses can be drained indirectly with the Poetz displacement method—a technique that uses gravity to displace thick, purulent material with thin irrigating fluid. If these irrigating techniques fail to relieve symptoms, one or more sinuses may require surgery. (See *Surgery for chronic and hyperplastic sinusitis.*)

Nursing diagnoses
- Altered oral mucous membrane
- Anxiety
- Fear
- Ineffective breathing pattern
- Knowledge deficit
- Pain
- Risk for infection

Nursing interventions
- Enforce bed rest, and encourage the patient to drink plenty of fluids to promote drainage. Don't elevate the head of the bed more than 30 degrees.
- Encourage the patient to express his concerns, and answer his questions. Include the patient and his family in planning and implementing the patient's care.
- To relieve pain and promote drainage, apply warm compresses continuously or four times daily at 2-hour intervals. Administer analgesics and antihistamines as ordered and as needed, monitoring the patient's response.
- Watch for and report vomiting, chills, fever, edema of the forehead or eyelids, blurred or double vision, and personality changes, which could indicate complications.
  After surgery:
- Monitor for excessive drainage or bleeding.
- To prevent edema and promote drainage, place the patient in semi-Fowler's position. To relieve edema and pain and minimize bleeding, apply ice compresses or a rubber glove filled with ice chips over the nose and iced saline gauze over the eyes. Continue these measures for 24 hours.
- Frequently change the mustache dressing or drip pad, recording the consistency, amount, and color of drainage (expect scant, bright-red drainage with some clots).
- Because the patient is breathing through the mouth, provide meticulous and frequent mouth care.

Patient teaching
- Inform the patient about prescribed medications, including action, dosage, and adverse effects. For antihistamines or analgesics including narcotics, caution against driving a motor vehicle or consuming alcohol. Tell the patient to complete the full course of therapy for prescribed antibiotics, even if symptoms disappear.

SURGERY FOR CHRONIC AND HYPERPLASTIC SINUSITIS

When drug therapy and irrigation fail to relieve infection, surgery may be necessary to correct chronic and hyperplastic sinusitis. The following procedures are common.

For maxillary sinusitis
- *Nasal window procedure* creates an opening in the sinus, allowing secretions and pus to drain through the nose.
- *Caldwell-Luc procedure* removes diseased mucosa in the maxillary sinus through an incision under the upper lip.

For chronic ethmoid sinusitis
- *Ethmoidectomy* removes all infected tissue through an external or intranasal incision into the ethmoid sinus.

For sphenoid sinusitis
- *External ethmoidectomy* removes infected ethmoid sinus tissue through a crescent-shaped incision, beginning under the inner eyebrow and extending along the side of the nose.

For chronic frontal sinusitis
- *Fronto-ethmoidectomy* removes infected frontal sinus tissue through an extended external ethmoidectomy.
- *Osteoplastic flap* drains the sinuses through an incision across the skull, behind the hairline.

- If surgery is necessary, tell the patient that nasal packing will be in place for 12 to 24 hours following surgery. He'll have to breathe through the mouth; refrain from nose blowing, which may cause bleeding and swelling; and try not to sneeze.
- If the patient is a smoker, instruct him to refrain for at least 2 to 3 days after surgery.
- Inform the patient undergoing a Caldwell-Luc procedure that the operative area may be numb for several weeks. Advise him against wearing dentures for several weeks or nose blowing for 2 weeks following packing removal.
- Reinforce the patient's understanding of sinusitis, review signs and symptoms of complications, and emphasize the importance of medical follow-up.
- Discuss proper disposal of tissues, and review handwashing technique to prevent the spread of infection.

NASAL POLYPS

Benign and edematous growths, nasal polyps usually are multiple, mobile, and bilateral. They may become large and numerous enough to cause nasal distention and enlargement of the bony framework, possibly occluding the airway. More common in adults than in children, nasal polyps tend to recur.

Causes

Nasal polyps usually are produced by continuous pressure, resulting from a chronic allergy that causes prolonged mucous membrane edema in the nose and sinuses. Other predisposing factors include chronic sinusitis, chronic rhinitis, and recurrent nasal infections.

Complications

Nasal polyps may result in airway obstruction.

Assessment findings

Patient history may detail chronic allergic rhinitis, chronic sinusitis, and recurrent nasal infections. The patient may describe nasal obstruction, loss of smell, a sensation of fullness in the face, a nasal discharge, and shortness of breath.

Inspection of the intranasal area finds a dry, red surface, with pale, clear, or gray soft growths. Large growths may resemble tumors. In contrast to normal nasal tissue, these growths don't elicit pain upon probing or manipulation.

Diagnostic tests

X-rays of the sinuses and nasal passages reveal soft-tissue shadows over the affected areas. Nasal polyps in children require further testing to rule out cystic fibrosis.

Treatment

Treatment usually consists of corticosteroids (either by direct injection into the polyps or by local spray) to temporarily reduce the polyp. Treatment of the underlying cause may include antihistamines to control allergy and antibiotic therapy if infection is present. Local application of an astringent shrinks hypertrophied tissue.

Such therapies alone rarely are effective; consequently, the treatment of choice is polypectomy (intranasal removal of the polyp with a wire snare), usually performed under local anesthesia. Continued recurrence may require surgical opening of the ethmoid and maxillary sinuses and evacuation of diseased tissue.

Nursing diagnoses
• Ineffective breathing pattern
• Knowledge deficit
• Pain
• Risk for injury

Nursing interventions
• For the patient with allergies, administer antihistamines, as ordered, and monitor his response.
   After surgery:
• Monitor for excessive bleeding or other drainage, and promote patient comfort. Give pain medications, as ordered, and monitor the patient's response.
• Elevate the head of the bed to facilitate breathing, reduce swelling, and promote adequate drainage. Change the mustache dressing or drip pad as needed, recording the consistency, amount, and color of nasal drainage.
• Intermittently apply ice compresses over the nostrils to lessen swelling, prevent bleeding, and relieve pain.
• If nasal bleeding occurs—most likely after packing is removed—elevate the head of the bed, monitor vital signs, and advise the patient not to swallow blood. Compress the outside of the nose against the septum for 10 to 15 minutes. If bleeding persists, notify the doctor immediately; nasal packing may be necessary.

Patient teaching
• Prepare the patient for surgery by explaining what to expect postoperatively, such as nasal packing for 1 to 2 days after surgery.
• To prevent recurrence of polyps, instruct the patient with allergies to avoid exposure to allergens and to take antihistamines at the first sign of an allergic reaction. Teach him to identify potential triggers to allergic reactions and to avoid them, if possible.
• Advise the patient to avoid overuse of nose drops and sprays. Teach him the proper use of nasal sprays.
• Caution the patient to report any adverse reactions to his prescribed medications.

NASAL PAPILLOMAS

A benign epithelial tissue overgrowth within the intranasal mucosa, a nasal papilloma may be inverted or exophytic. Inverted papillomas grow into the underlying tissue, usually at the junction of the antrum and the ethmoid sinus; they generally occur unilaterally and sometimes are associated with squamous cell carcinoma. Exophytic papillomas, which tend to occur singly, arise from epithelial tissue, commonly on the surface of the nasal septum. Both types are most prevalent in males. Recurrence is likely, even after surgical excision.

Causes
A papilloma may arise as a benign precursor of a neoplasm or as a response to tissue injury or viral infection, but its cause is unknown.

Complications
Rarely, nasal papillomas result in severe respiratory distress, nasal drainage, and infection.

Assessment findings
The patient with inverted or exophytic papillomas typically complains of nasal stuffiness, postnasal drip, headache, shortness of breath, dyspnea, and occasionally, with exophytic papillomas, epistaxis.

With inverted papillomas, inspection of the nasal mucosa usually reveals large lesions that are bulky, highly vascular, and edematous, with a color and consistency that varies from dark red to gray and firm to friable. Exophytic papillomas are commonly raised, firm, and rubbery, pink to gray in color. They are securely attached by a broad or pedunculated base to the mucous membrane.

Diagnostic tests
Tissue biopsy for histologic examination confirms the diagnosis.

Treatment
The most effective treatment is wide surgical excision or diathermy with careful inspection of adjacent tissues and sinuses to rule out extension. Aspirin or acetaminophen and decongestants may relieve symptoms.

Nursing diagnoses
• Altered oral mucous membrane
• Anxiety
• Fear
• Ineffective breathing pattern
• Knowledge deficit
• Risk for injury

Nursing interventions
• Answer the patient's questions, encourage him to express concerns, and stay with him during anxious periods. Include the patient and his family in all phases of care.
• If bleeding occurs, raise the head of the bed and have the patient expectorate blood into an emesis basin. Compress the sides of the nose against the septum for 10 to 15 minutes and, if necessary, apply ice compresses to the nose.
• Check for airway obstruction by placing your hand under the patient's nostrils, or use a mirror to assess air exchange. Watch for signs of mild shortness of breath.

After surgery:
• Monitor vital signs and respiratory status.
• As needed, administer analgesics and monitor the patient's response.
• Because the patient with nasal packing is unable to breathe through the nose, provide frequent and meticulous mouth care.
• To reduce or prevent edema and promote drainage, place the patient in semi-Fowler's position, and use a cool-mist vaporizer to liquefy secretions and facilitate normal breathing. To lessen facial edema and pain, place crushed ice in a rubber glove or a small ice bag, and apply the glove or ice bag intermittently over the eyes and nose for 24 hours.
• To ensure proper absorption of drainage, frequently change the mustache dressing or drip pad, recording the type and amount of drainage. While the nasal packing is in place, expect scant, usually bright-red drainage that contains some clots. Remember that the amount of drainage often increases for a few hours after the packing is removed.

Patient teaching
• If surgery is scheduled, review what to expect postoperatively: that nostrils probably will be packed and that it will be necessary to breathe through the mouth. Instruct the patient not to blow the nose. (Packing usually is removed 12 to 24 hours after surgery.)
• Because papillomas tend to recur, tell the patient to seek medical attention at the first sign of nasal discomfort, discharge, or congestion that doesn't subside with conservative treatment.
• Encourage regular follow-up visits to detect early signs of recurrence.

ADENOID HYPERPLASIA
A fairly common childhood condition, adenoid hyperplasia (adenoid hypertrophy) is enlargement of the lymphoid tissue of the nasopharynx. Normally, adenoidal tissue is small at birth ($\frac{3}{4}$" to $1\frac{1}{4}$" [1.9 to 3.2 cm]), grows until the child reaches adolescence, and then slowly begins to atrophy. In adenoid hyperplasia, however, this tissue continues to grow.

Warning

ASSESSING FOR BLEEDING

After adenoidectomy, bleeding can be a serious complication. To assess the patient for bleeding, frequently check the throat for blood, and observe for continuous swallowing of blood. While the patient is asleep, note the frequency of swallowing. Be alert for vomiting of old, partially digested blood (coffee-ground vomitus). If bleeding persists, notify the doctor immediately.

Causes

Although the precise cause of adenoid hyperplasia is unknown, contributing factors may include heredity, repeated infection, chronic nasal congestion, persistent allergy, insufficient aeration, and inefficient nasal breathing. Inflammation resulting from repeated infection increases the patient's risk of respiratory obstruction.

Complications

Adenoid hyperplasia can obstruct the eustachian tube and predispose the patient to otitis media, which in turn can lead to fluctuating conductive hearing loss. Stasis of nasal secretions from adenoidal inflammation can lead to sinusitis.

Adenoid hyperplasia in children may cause sleep apnea, transient breathing difficulties that may result in acidosis and pulmonary arterial hypertension.

Assessment findings

Typically, adenoid hyperplasia produces symptoms of respiratory obstruction. The parents may report that the child breathes through the mouth; snores at night; experiences frequent, prolonged nasal congestion; and has a history of chronic otitis media with some hearing loss. The child may mention a decrease in appetite due to alteration in taste and smell.

Inspection confirms mouth breathing. The child's voice may sound nasal and muffled. You may also detect foul breath and dry oral mucous membranes. If the child experienced persistent mouth breathing during the formative years, inspection may show distinctive facial features changes, including a slightly elongated face, open mouth, highly arched palate, shortened upper lip, and vacant expression. Signs of nocturnal respiratory insuf-

ficiency may be apparent, including intercostal retractions and nasal flaring.

Cervical posterior lymph nodes may feel enlarged on palpation.

Diagnostic tests

• *Nasopharyngoscopic or rhinoscopic visualization* of abnormal tissue mass confirms adenoid hyperplasia.
• *X-rays* (lateral pharyngeal films) show obliteration of the nasopharyngeal air column.

Treatment

Adenoidectomy, the treatment of choice for adenoid hyperplasia, commonly is recommended for the patient with recurrent or prolonged mouth breathing, nasal speech, adenoid facies, recurrent otitis media, constant nasopharyngitis, and nocturnal respiratory distress. This procedure usually eliminates recurrent nasal infections and ear complications and reverses any secondary hearing loss.

Adenoidectomy should be performed in conjunction with tympanotomy tube placement when the adenoidal hypertrophy contributes to ear disorders.

Nursing diagnoses

• Anxiety
• Fear
• Ineffective breathing pattern
• Knowledge deficit
• Pain
• Risk for aspiration

Nursing interventions

• Answer questions from the patient and his family, encourage them to express their concerns, and stay with the patient during anxious periods. Include the patient and his family in all phases of care.
  After surgery:
• Maintain a patent airway. Position the child on his side, with his head down, to prevent aspiration of draining secretions. Frequently assess the child for bleeding. (See *Assessing for bleeding.*)
• Closely monitor vital signs and report excessive bleeding, a rise in pulse rate, a drop in blood pressure, tachypnea, restlessness, and a fever above 101° F (38.3° C).
• If no bleeding occurs, offer ice chips or water when the patient is fully awake.
• Provide analgesics for pain relief. Crying may irritate the operative site, so keep the child comfortable.
• Keep suction equipment at the bedside.

Patient teaching

• Before surgery, describe the hospital routine, and arrange for the child and parents to tour relevant hospital areas.
• Explain adenoidectomy to the child and his family, using illustrations if necessary. Detail the recovery process. Explain that surgery may be performed on an outpatient basis with about 6 hours of postoperative observation, provided no complications require inpatient hospitalization. Tell them that the child's voice may sound nasal temporarily after surgery.
• After surgery, discuss normal postoperative findings, including halitosis, low-grade fever, and a slight earache. Tell the patient and his family that a heating pad may be used for local comfort.
• Review signs and symptoms of bleeding, and instruct the family how to assess the child for possible bleeding.
• Discuss signs and symptoms requiring medical intervention, including severe earache, fever above 101° F, or cough.
• Emphasize the importance of not smoking and of avoiding aspirin.

THROAT DISORDERS

Characterized by a sore throat, dysphagia, hoarseness, and airway obstruction, throat disorders may be caused by bacterial or viral infections, an aneurysm, surgical trauma, cancer, smoking, and overuse of the vocal cords. These disorders include pharyngitis, tonsillitis, throat abscesses, vocal cord paralysis, vocal cord nodules and polyps, laryngitis, and juvenile angiofibroma.

PHARYNGITIS

The most common throat disorder, pharyngitis is an acute or chronic inflammation of the pharynx. It's widespread among adults who live or work in dusty or dry environments, use their voices excessively, habitually use tobacco or alcohol, or suffer from chronic sinusitis, persistent coughs, or allergies. Uncomplicated pharyngitis usually subsides in 3 to 10 days.

Acute pharyngitis may precede the common cold or other communicable diseases. Chronic pharyngitis commonly is an extension of nasopharyngeal obstruction or inflammation.

Causes

In 90% of cases, pharyngitis occurs as a result of a virus. In children, streptococcal bacteria often cause pharyngitis.

Complications

If pharyngitis is caused by a bacterial infection, complications may include otitis media, sinusitis, mastoiditis, rheumatic fever, and nephritis.

Assessment findings

Typically, the patient complains of a sore throat and slight difficulty in swallowing; swallowing saliva hurts more than swallowing food. The patient also may complain of a sensation of a lump in the throat, a constant and aggravating urge to swallow, a headache, and muscle and joint pain (especially in bacterial pharyngitis). Vital signs assessment may detect a mild fever.

On inspection, you'll find the posterior pharyngeal wall a fiery red color with swollen, exudate-flecked tonsils and lymphoid follicles. If the patient has bacterial pharyngitis, his throat will be acutely inflamed, with patches of white and yellow follicles. The tongue may be strawberry red in color.

Neck palpation may detect enlarged, tender cervical lymph nodes.

Diagnostic tests

• *Throat culture* may identify the bacterial organisms causing the inflammation but may not detect other causative organisms.
• *Rapid strep tests* generally detect streptococcal infections with group A, but they miss the fairly common streptococcal groups C and G.

Treatment

Based on the patient's symptoms, treatment for acute viral pharyngitis consists mainly of rest, warm saline gargles, throat lozenges containing a mild anesthetic, plenty of fluids, and analgesics, as needed. If the patient can't swallow fluids, he may need hospitalization for I.V. hydration.

Bacterial pharyngitis requires rigorous treatment with penicillin (or another broad-spectrum antibiotic, if the patient is allergic to penicillin) because streptococcus is the chief infecting organism. Antibiotic therapy should continue for 48 hours after visible signs of infection have disappeared or for at least 7 to 10 days.

Chronic pharyngitis requires the same supportive measures as acute pharyngitis but with greater emphasis on eliminating the underlying cause, such as an allergen.

Preventive measures include adequate humidification and avoiding excessive exposure to air conditioning. In addition, the patient should be urged to stop smoking (if appropriate).

Nursing diagnoses
• Altered nutrition: Less than body requirements
• Altered oral mucous membrane
• Fatigue
• Knowledge deficit
• Pain
• Risk for fluid volume deficit

Nursing interventions
• Administer analgesics and warm saline gargles, as ordered and as appropriate.
• Encourage the patient to drink plenty of fluids (up to 2,500 ml/day). Monitor intake and output scrupulously, and watch for signs of dehydration (cracked lips, dry mucous membranes, low urine output). Provide meticulous mouth care to prevent dry lips and oral pyoderma, and maintain a restful environment.
• Obtain throat cultures and administer antibiotics, as ordered.
• Maintain the patient on bed rest, especially while febrile, to conserve energy.
• Encourage a soft, light diet with plenty of liquids to combat the commonly experienced anorexia. Antiemetics can be given before eating, if ordered.
• Examine the skin twice a day for possible drug sensitivity rashes or for rashes indicating a communicable disease.
• Administer antitussives, as ordered, if the patient has a cough.

Patient teaching
• If the patient has acute bacterial pharyngitis, emphasize the importance of completing the full course of antibiotic therapy. Tell him to call the doctor if any adverse reactions develop.
• Advise the patient with chronic pharyngitis how to minimize sources of throat irritation in the environment, such as using a bedside humidifier. Refer him to a self-help group to stop smoking, if appropriate.
• Inform the patient and his family that in the case of a positive streptococcal infection, all family members should undergo throat cultures, regardless of the presence or absence of symptoms. Individuals with positive cultures require penicillin therapy.

TONSILLITIS
Inflammation of the tonsils can be acute or chronic. The uncomplicated acute form usually lasts 4 to 6 days and commonly affects children between ages 5 and 10. Tonsils tend to hypertrophy during childhood and atrophy after puberty.

Causes
Tonsillitis generally results from infection with beta-hemolytic streptococci but also can result from other bacteria or viruses.

Complications
Chronic tonsillitis may result in chronic upper airway obstruction, causing sleep apnea or sleep disturbances, cor pulmonale, failure to thrive, eating or swallowing disorders, and speech abnormalities. Febrile seizures, otitis media, cardiac valvular disease, and abscessed cervical lymph nodes also may occur.

Assessment findings
The patient with acute tonsillitis may complain of a mild to severe sore throat. In a child too young to complain about throat pain, the parents may report that the child has stopped eating. The patient or his parents also may report muscle and joint pain, chills, malaise, headache, and pain that's frequently referred to the ears. Because of excess secretions, the patient may complain of a constant urge to swallow and a constricted feeling in the back of the throat. Such discomfort usually subsides after 72 hours.

Fever may be present, and palpation may detect swollen, tender lymph glands in the submandibular area.

Inspection of the throat may discover generalized inflammation of the pharyngeal wall, with swollen tonsils that project from between the pillars of the fauces and exude white or yellow follicles. Purulent drainage becomes apparent when you apply pressure to the tonsillar pillars. The uvula may also be edematous and inflamed.

In chronic tonsillitis, the patient may report recurrent sore throats and attacks of acute tonsillitis. Inspection may expose purulent drainage in the tonsillar crypts.

Diagnostic tests
• *Throat culture* may determine the infecting organism and indicate appropriate antibiotic therapy.
• *White blood cell count* usually reveals leukocytosis.

Treatment
Emphasizing relief of symptoms, management of acute tonsillitis requires rest, adequate fluid intake, aspirin or

acetaminophen and, for bacterial infection, antibiotics. For Group A beta-hemolytic streptococcus, penicillin is the drug of choice (erythromycin or another broad-spectrum antibiotic may be given if the patient is allergic to penicillin). To prevent complications, antibiotic therapy should continue for 10 days.

Chronic tonsillitis or complications may require tonsillectomy but only after the patient has been free of tonsillar or respiratory tract infections for 3 to 4 weeks.

Nursing diagnoses
• Anxiety
• Ineffective breathing pattern
• Knowledge deficit
• Risk for aspiration
• Risk for fluid volume deficit

Nursing interventions
• Despite dysphagia, urge the patient to drink plenty of fluids, especially if fever is present. Offer a child ice cream and flavored drinks and ices.
• Suggest gargling to soothe the throat.
• Before surgery, assess for bleeding abnormalities.
  After surgery:
• Maintain a patent airway. To prevent aspiration, place the patient on his side. Keep suction equipment nearby.
• Monitor vital signs frequently and check for bleeding. Immediately report excessive bleeding, increased pulse rate, or dropping blood pressure.
• When the patient is fully alert and the gag reflex has returned, give him water. Later, encourage nonirritating fluids. Avoid milk products; they coat the throat, causing throat clearing and increasing the risk of bleeding.
• Provide analgesics for pain relief. Because crying irritates the operative site, keep the child comfortable.
• Encourage deep-breathing exercises to prevent pulmonary complications.

Patient teaching
• Before surgery, explain tonsillectomy to the pediatric patient in a simple, nonthreatening way. Show him the operating and recovery rooms, and briefly explain the hospital routine. Note if a parent may stay with him.
• Explain to the adult patient that a local anesthetic prevents pain but allows a sensation of pressure during surgery. Warn the patient to expect considerable throat discomfort and some bleeding postoperatively.
• Before discharge, provide written home-care instructions. Tell the family to expect a white scab to form in the throat 5 to 10 days postoperatively and to report

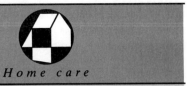

Home care

PROMOTING RECOVERY FROM TONSILLITIS

For a patient recovering from tonsillitis, give him these guidelines:
• Make sure the patient or his parents understand the importance of completing the prescribed course of antibiotics.
• Explain adverse reactions to the prescribed medications, especially those that demand medical attention.
• Instruct the patient or his parents to avoid spicy, irritating foods; to eat primarily soft, nutritious foods; and to avoid using straws or forks.
• Advise the patient or his parents to restrict activities for 7 to 10 days postoperatively and to avoid aspirin or aspirin-containing products during that time.

bleeding, ear discomfort, or a fever for 3 days or more. (See *Promoting recovery from tonsillitis.*)

THROAT ABSCESSES

Affecting patients of all ages, throat abscesses may be peritonsillar (quinsy) or retropharyngeal.

A peritonsillar abscess forms in the connective tissue space between the tonsil capsule and constrictor muscle of the pharynx. It's more common in adolescents and young adults than in children.

A retropharyngeal abscess forms between the posterior pharyngeal wall and prevertebral fascia. Because these lymph glands begin to atrophy after age 2, acute retropharyngeal abscess commonly affects children under age 2. Chronic retropharyngeal abscess can occur at any age. With treatment, the prognosis for both types of abscesses is good.

Causes
Peritonsillar abscess forms as a complication of acute tonsillitis, usually after streptococcal or staphylococcal infection. Acute retropharyngeal abscess results from infection in the retropharyngeal lymph glands, which may follow an upper respiratory tract bacterial infection. Chronic retropharyngeal abscess results from tuberculosis of the cervical spine (Pott's disease).

Complications

A very large abscess may press on the larynx, producing edema, or may erode into major vessels, causing sudden death from asphyxia, aspiration, or hemorrhage.

Assessment findings

The patient with a peritonsillar abscess may complain of severe throat pain, occasional ear pain on the same side as the abscess, tenderness of the submandibular gland, and swallowing difficulty that may produce drooling. Additionally, the patient may report a history of chills, malaise, rancid breath, and nausea. A vital signs assessment may reveal fever. On inspection, you may discover a prolonged tonic spasm of the jaw muscles (trismus) as a result of edema and the spread of infection from the peritonsillar space to the pterygoid muscles. The patient's speech may sound muffled. Palpation may reveal cervical adenopathy.

In retropharyngeal abscess, the patient history may reveal an episode of staphylococcal or streptococcal infection. The patient may complain of pain and dysphagia. A vital signs assessment may reveal fever.

When the abscess is located in the upper pharynx, clinical findings include nasal obstruction; with a low-positioned abscess, findings include dyspnea, progressive inspiratory stridor (from laryngeal obstruction), neck hyperextension, and, in children, drooling and muffled crying. Examination of the throat shows swelling of the soft palate on the abscessed side, with displacement of the uvula to the opposite side; red, edematous mucous membranes; tonsil displacement toward the midline; and a soft, red, and bulging posterior pharyngeal wall.

Diagnostic tests

• *X-rays* show the larynx to be pushed forward and a widened space between the posterior pharyngeal wall and vertebrae.
• *Throat culture and sensitivity testing* isolates the causative organism and determines the appropriate antibiotic.

Treatment

For early-stage peritonsillar abscess, large doses of penicillin or another broad-spectrum antibiotic are necessary. For late-stage abscess with cellulitis of the tonsillar space, primary treatment usually consists of incision and drainage under local anesthesia, followed by I.V. antibiotic therapy for 7 to 10 days. Tonsillectomy, scheduled no sooner than 1 month after healing, prevents recurrence but is recommended only after several episodes.

In acute retropharyngeal abscess, the primary treatment is incision and drainage through the pharyngeal wall. In chronic retropharyngeal abscess, drainage is performed through an external incision behind the sternomastoid muscle. During incision and drainage, strong, continuous mouth suction is necessary to prevent aspiration of pus. Postoperative drug therapy includes I.V. antibiotics (usually penicillin) and analgesics.

Nursing diagnoses

• Altered oral mucous membrane
• Anxiety
• Fear
• Impaired gas exchange
• Knowledge deficit
• Pain
• Risk for aspiration
• Risk for fluid volume deficit

Nursing interventions

• Be alert for signs of respiratory obstruction (inspiratory stridor, dyspnea, increasing restlessness, or cyanosis), and keep emergency airway equipment nearby.
• Answer the patient's questions, and encourage him and his family to discuss their concerns. Include the patient and his family in all phases of care.
• Because the procedure generally is performed under local anesthesia, the patient may be apprehensive. Offer reassurance as necessary.
• Assist with incision and drainage. To allow easy expectoration and suction of pus and blood, place the patient in a semi-recumbent or sitting position.
• After incision and drainage, give antibiotics, analgesics, and antipyretics as ordered, and monitor the patient's response.
• Monitor vital signs, and report any significant changes or bleeding.
• If the patient can't swallow, ensure adequate hydration with I.V. therapy. Monitor fluid intake and output, and watch for dehydration.
• Provide meticulous mouth care. Apply petroleum jelly to the patient's lips. Promote healing with warm saline gargles or throat irrigations for 24 to 36 hours after incision and drainage.
• Use an ice collar to promote comfort and help reduce swelling and bleeding.

Patient teaching

• Explain the procedure to the patient and his family. Include a description of local anesthesia, positioning during incision and drainage, and post-procedure care.

• After the procedure and before discharge, stress the importance of completing the full course of prescribed antibiotic therapy. Tell the patient to report any adverse reactions.
• Teach the patient and his family the signs and symptoms of possible complications, and remind them to report these to the doctor.
• Instruct the patient in the effective use of saline gargles.

VOCAL CORD PARALYSIS

Resulting from disease of or injury to the superior or, most often, the recurrent laryngeal nerve, vocal cord paralysis may be unilateral or bilateral. Unilateral paralysis is most common.

Causes

Vocal cord paralysis commonly results from the accidental severing of the recurrent laryngeal nerve or one of its extralaryngeal branches during thyroidectomy or cardiac or thoracic surgery. Other causes include pressure from an aortic aneurysm or from an enlarged atrium (in patients with mitral stenosis), bronchial or esophageal carcinoma, hypertrophy of the thyroid gland, trauma (such as neck injuries), and neuritis due to infections or metallic poisoning.

Vocal cord paralysis also can result from hysteria and, rarely, lesions of the central nervous system. Ten percent of vocal cord paralysis cases are idiopathic in nature with a possible viral etiology.

Complications

Respiratory failure resulting from airway obstruction is a major complication of bilateral vocal cord paralysis.

Assessment findings

Signs and symptoms of vocal cord paralysis depend on whether the paralysis is unilateral or bilateral and on the position of the cord or cords when paralyzed. A patient with unilateral paralysis, the most common form, may complain of vocal weakness and hoarseness. A patient with bilateral paralysis typically reports vocal weakness and may have incapacitating airway obstruction if the cords become paralyzed in the adducted position.

Diagnostic tests

• *Indirect laryngoscopy* shows one or both cords fixed in an adducted or partially abducted position.
• *Bronchoscopy* and *esophagoscopy* (fiber-optic techniques used to visualize the larynx) also may be used.

Treatment

Unilateral vocal cord paralysis is treated under direct laryngoscopy with injection of Teflon into the paralyzed cord. This procedure enlarges the cord and brings it closer to the other cord, usually strengthening the voice and protecting the airway from aspiration.

Bilateral cord paralysis can be a surgical emergency and generally requires a tracheotomy to restore a patent airway. Alternative treatments for adult patients include arytenoidectomy to open the glottis and lateral fixation of the arytenoid cartilage through an external neck incision. Lateralization of the vocal cords negates the need for a tracheostomy. Excision or fixation of the arytenoid cartilage improves airway patency but produces residual voice impairment. Many patients with bilateral cord paralysis prefer to keep a tracheostomy instead of having an arytenoidectomy; their voices generally are better with a tracheostomy alone than after corrective surgery.

Treatment of hysterical aphonia may include psychotherapy and, for some patients, hypnosis.

Nursing diagnoses

• Anxiety
• Fear
• Impaired verbal communication
• Ineffective breathing pattern
• Knowledge deficit
• Risk for aspiration

Nursing interventions

• For the patient choosing direct laryngoscopy and Teflon injection, provide humidified oxygen postoperatively, and encourage the patient to remain mute for 24 hours.
• Give the patient nothing by mouth for 3 to 4 hours to avoid aspiration.
• Monitor the patient's respiratory status closely for airway obstruction.
• Administer antibiotics and corticosteroids, as ordered, and monitor the patient's response to these medications.
• Answer the patient's questions, and encourage him to discuss his concerns, offering reassurance when appropriate.
• If the patient has difficulty understanding procedures due to impaired communication, give clear, concise explanations of treatments and procedures, and allow adequate time for him to grasp what's expected. Provide a pencil and paper to aid communication, and alert the staff to his communication problem.
• Because the tracheotomy is performed under local anesthesia, the patient may be apprehensive. Provide emo-

HOW NODULES CAUSE HOARSENESS

Nodules that erupt on the vocal cords prevent the cords from closing properly (approximating) during phonation. The result: hoarseness. The most common site of vocal cord nodules is the point of maximal vibration and impact (the junction of the anterior one-third and the posterior two-thirds of the vocal cord), as seen in the illustration.

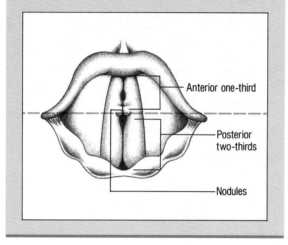

tional support and reassurance during the procedure and throughout hospitalization.

Patient teaching
• Explain all procedures. If the patient is scheduled to undergo a tracheotomy, offer reassurance. If the patient chooses direct laryngoscopy and Teflon injection, inform him that these measures will improve his voice but won't restore it to normal. If the patient elects arytenoidectomy, explain that the tracheostomy will remain in place until the edema has subsided and the airway is patent.
For a tracheostomy patient:
• Teach him how to suction, clean, and change the tracheostomy tube.
• Explain that he can still speak by covering the lumen of the tracheostomy tube with a finger or a tracheostomy plug.
• Advise the patient to wear a medical identification necklace or bracelet, indicating the presence of the tracheostomy.
• Suggest that he wear a loose weave scarf or closed shirt to cover the stoma to warm and filter the inspired air.

• Instruct him to avoid swimming or showering, to prevent aspiration.

VOCAL CORD NODULES AND POLYPS
Teachers, singers, sports fans, and energetic children who continuously shout while playing are prone to vocal cord nodules and polyps. Vocal cord nodules, resulting from hypertrophy of fibrous tissue, form at the point where the cords come together forcibly. (See *How nodules cause hoarseness.*)

Vocal cord polyps are chronic, subepithelial, edematous masses that also are common in adults who smoke, live in dry climates, or have allergies. Both nodules and polyps have good prognoses unless continued voice abuse causes recurrence with subsequent scarring and permanent hoarseness.

Causes
Vocal cord nodules and polyps usually result from voice abuse, sinusitis, upper respiratory tract infections, and allergies.

Complications
Permanent hoarseness is the primary complication of vocal cord nodules and polyps.

Assessment findings
The patient may report painless hoarseness and may display a breathy or husky voice.

Diagnostic tests
Indirect (mirror) or direct laryngoscopy enables visualization of nodules and shows small, red nodes that eventually become white, solid nodes on one or both cords. In the patient with polyps, laryngoscopy reveals unilateral or, occasionally, bilateral sessile or pedunculated polyps of varying sizes, anywhere on the vocal cords.

Treatment
Conservative management of small vocal cord nodules and polyps includes humidification, speech therapy (voice rest and training to reduce the intensity and duration of voice production), and treatment of any underlying allergies.

When conservative treatment fails to relieve hoarseness, nodules or polyps require removal under direct laryngoscopy. Microlaryngoscopy may be performed for small lesions to avoid injuring the vocal cord surface. For bilateral nodules or polyps, excision may be performed in two stages to allow one cord to heal before surgery on the other cord. Two-stage excision prevents laryngeal web, which occurs when epithelial tissue is removed from adjacent cord surfaces and these surfaces grow together.

For children, treatment consists of speech therapy. If possible, surgery should be delayed until the child is old enough to benefit from voice training or until the child can understand the need to abstain from voice abuse.

Nursing diagnoses
- Anxiety
- Fear
- Impaired verbal communication
- Knowledge deficit
- Risk for injury

Nursing interventions
- Answer the patient's questions, and encourage him to discuss his concerns. Include the patient and his family in all phases of care.

After surgery:
- Provide the patient with an alternative means of communication—a Magic Slate, pad and pencil, or an alphabet board. Place a sign over the bed to remind visitors that the patient shouldn't talk. Mark the intercom so other staff members are aware that the patient can't answer. Minimize the patient's urge to speak by trying to anticipate his needs.
- Use a vaporizer to increase humidity and decrease throat irritation.
- Make sure the patient receives speech therapy after healing, if necessary, because continued voice abuse causes recurrence of growths.

Patient teaching
- Postoperatively, stress the importance of resting the voice for 10 days to 2 weeks while the vocal cords heal. Encourage the patient who is a smoker to stop smoking entirely or, at the very least, to refrain from smoking during recovery from surgery.
- Teach the patient the relationship between voice abuse and vocal cord nodules and polyps. Emphasize the importance of follow-up speech therapy.

LARYNGITIS

A common disorder, laryngitis is an acute or chronic inflammation of the vocal cords. Acute laryngitis may occur as an isolated infection or as part of a generalized bacterial or viral upper respiratory tract infection. Repeated attacks of acute laryngitis cause inflammatory changes associated with chronic laryngitis.

Causes
Acute laryngitis usually results from infection or excessive use of the voice, an occupational hazard in certain vocations (teaching, public speaking, and singing, for example). It also may result from overuse of voice (such as cheering at a sports event), inhalation of smoke or fumes, or aspiration of caustic chemicals. Causes of chronic laryngitis include chronic upper respiratory tract disorders (sinusitis, bronchitis, nasal polyps, allergy), mouth breathing, smoking, constant exposure to dust or other irritants, and alcohol abuse.

Complications
Chronic laryngitis may result in permanent laryngeal tissue changes, accompanied by hoarseness. Severe, acute laryngitis may occasionally result in airway obstruction.

Assessment findings
In acute laryngitis, the patient typically complains of hoarseness, ranging from mild to complete loss of voice. The patient also may report pain (especially when swallowing or speaking), a dry cough, and malaise.

In chronic laryngitis, hoarseness may be the patient's only complaint. Obtain a detailed patient history to help determine the disorder's cause.

Diagnostic tests
Indirect laryngoscopy confirms the diagnosis by revealing red, inflamed, and, occasionally, hemorrhagic vocal cords with rounded rather than sharp edges, and exudate. Bilateral swelling that restricts movement but doesn't cause paralysis also may be apparent.

Treatment
Resting the voice is the primary treatment. For viral infection, care is based on the patient's symptoms and includes analgesics and throat lozenges for pain relief. Bacterial infection requires antibiotic therapy. Severe, acute laryngitis may necessitate hospitalization. Occasionally, when laryngeal edema results in airway obstruction, a tracheotomy may be necessary. In chronic laryngitis, effective treatment must eliminate the underlying cause.

Nursing diagnoses
- Fear
- Impaired verbal communication

- Ineffective breathing pattern
- Knowledge deficit

Nursing interventions

- Encourage the patient to discuss his concerns about his impaired communication. Answer questions as best you can.
- In severe, acute laryngitis, monitor the patient for signs and symptoms of airway obstruction (tachycardia, use of accessory muscles, anxiety, stridor). Keep a tracheotomy tray at the bedside.
- If the patient has chronic laryngitis, encourage modification of habits that predispose him to the disorder.
- Place a sign over the bed to remind others of the patient's restrictions on verbal communication. Provide a Magic Slate, pad and pencil, or alphabet board for communication. Mark the intercom panel so that other staff members are aware that the patient can't answer. Minimize the patient's urge to talk by trying to anticipate his needs.
- Provide analgesics, as needed, and monitor the patient's response.

Patient teaching

- Explain to the patient why he shouldn't talk, and teach alternate methods of communication, such as flash cards. If he must talk, speak softly rather than whisper.
- Suggest that the patient maintain adequate humidification by using a vaporizer or humidifier during the winter, by avoiding air conditioning during the summer (because it dehumidifies), by using medicated throat lozenges, and by not smoking.
- Urge completion of prescribed antibiotics, and tell the patient to report any adverse reactions.

JUVENILE ANGIOFIBROMA

An uncommon disorder, juvenile angiofibroma is a highly vascular, nasopharyngeal tumor made up of masses of fibrous tissue containing many thin-walled blood vessels. These tumors are found primarily in adolescent males and are extremely rare in females. Incidence is higher in Egypt, India, Southeast Asia, and Kenya than in the United States and Europe. The prognosis is good with treatment.

Causes

Although its cause is unknown, juvenile angiofibroma has been identified as a type of hemangioma.

Complications

Juvenile angiofibroma may result in secondary anemia due to tumor bleeding.

Assessment findings

Usually between the ages of 7 and 21, the patient reports a history of unilateral or bilateral nasal obstruction and severe recurrent epistaxis. The patient also may reveal a history of purulent rhinorrhea and serous otitis media, with resultant hearing loss from eustachian tube obstruction. Inspection may reveal facial deformity and nasal speech.

Diagnostic tests

- Examination with a nasopharyngeal mirror or nasal speculum permits visualization of the tumor, which appears as a blue mass in the nose or nasopharynx.
- *X-rays* show a bowing of the posterior wall of the maxillary sinus.
- *Angiography* determines the size and location of the tumor and source of vascularization. Biopsy is contraindicated because of the danger of hemorrhage.

Treatment

Several surgical methods, ranging from avulsion to cryosurgical techniques, are used to treat juvenile angiofibroma. Whichever surgical method is used, the tumor must be removed in its entirety and not in pieces. Surgical excision is preferred after embolization with Teflon or absorbable gelatin sponge, to decrease vascularization. Blood transfusions may be necessary during avulsion. Preoperative hormonal therapy may decrease the tumor's size and vascularity.

Although radiation therapy produces only a temporary regression in an angiofibroma, it remains the treatment of choice if the tumor has expanded into the cranium or ocular orbit. Because the tumor is multilobular and locally invasive, recurrent symptoms are common (occurring in about 30% of patients) during the first year after treatment but are uncommon after 2 years.

Nursing diagnoses

- Altered oral mucous membrane
- Altered tissue perfusion
- Anxiety
- Fear
- Knowledge deficit
- Risk for injury
- Sensory alteration (auditory)

Nursing interventions

• If the patient has experienced hearing loss, provide a means to facilitate communication. Face the patient when speaking; speak in a slow, calm voice; and alert other staff to his communication problem.

• Answer questions, and encourage the patient and his family to discuss their concerns. Include the patient and his family in all phases of care.

After surgery:

• Report excessive bleeding immediately. Check hemoglobin levels and hematocrit for anemia. Make sure an adequate supply of typed and cross-matched blood is available for transfusion.

• Monitor for any change in vital signs.

• Provide meticulous and frequent mouth care, and use a bedside vaporizer to raise humidity.

• During blood transfusion, watch for transfusion reactions, such as fever, chills, or a rash. If any of these reactions occur, discontinue the transfusion and notify the doctor immediately.

Patient teaching

• Explain all diagnostic and surgical procedures. Provide emotional support because severe epistaxis frightens many patients and family members to the point of panic.

• Instruct the patient and his family to seek immediate medical attention if bleeding occurs after discharge, and teach them how to apply pressure over the affected area.

• Stress the importance of providing adequate humidification at home to keep nasal mucosa moist.

SELECTED REFERENCES

Baber, W.J.M. "Ménière's Disease," *New Zealand Practical Nurse,* 49-51, September 1994.

Kitahara, M., et al. "Pressure Test for the Diagnosis of Ménière's Disease," *ACTA Otolaryngology* 114(suppl 510):107-10, 1994.

Phipps, W.J., et al. *Medical-Surgical Nursing: Concepts and Clinical Practice,* 5th ed. St. Louis: Mosby–Year Book, Inc., 1995.

Rakel, R.E., ed. *Conn's Current Therapy 1996.* Philadelphia: W.B. Saunders Co., 1996.

Smeltzer, S., and Bare, B. *Brunner and Suddarth's Textbook of Medical-Surgical Nursing,* 8th ed. Philadelphia: J.B. Lippincott Co., 1996.

Wong, D. *Whaley and Wong's Nursing Care of Infants and Children,* 5th ed. St. Louis: Mosby–Year Book, Inc., 1995.

18 SKIN DISORDERS

INTRODUCTION

The largest and heaviest body system, the skin and its appendages (the hair, nails, and certain glands) perform many vital functions. They protect the inner organs, bones, muscles, and blood vessels, help to regulate body temperature, and provide sensory information. They also prevent body fluids from escaping and eliminate body wastes through more than 2 million pores.

Two layers of skin (integument), the epidermis and dermis, lie above a third layer of subcutaneous tissue. Numerous epidermal appendages exist throughout the skin, including hair, nails, sebaceous glands, and two types of sweat glands: eccrine glands (located over most of the body except the lips) and apocrine glands (found in the axilla and groin near hair follicles). The integumentary system covers an area of 10¾ to 21½ ft² (1 to 2 m²) and accounts for about 15% of body weight.

Epidermis

This outermost skin layer varies in thickness from less than 0.1 mm on the eyelids to more than 1 mm on the palms and soles. It's composed of avascular, stratified squamous (scaly or platelike) epithelial tissue that contains multiple layers: a superficial, keratinized, horny layer of cells (stratum corneum) — composed of several layers of cells in various stages of change as they migrate upward — and a deeper, germinal (basal cell) layer.

Stratum corneum

After mitosis occurs in the basal cell layer, epithelial cells undergo a series of changes as they migrate to the outermost part of the stratum corneum, made up of tightly arranged layers of cellular membranes and keratin. Interspersed among the keratinized cells below the stratum corneum are the specialized Langerhans' cells. These cells have a function in the immune response and assist in the initial processing of antigens that enter the epidermis. Epidermal cells usually are shed from the surface as epidermal dust. Differentiation of cells from the basal cell layer to the stratum corneum takes up to 28 days.

Basal cell layer

This layer produces new cells to replace the superficial keratinized cells that are continuously shed or worn away. The layer's deepest part contains melanocytes, which produce the brown pigment melanin and disperse it to the surrounding epithelial cells. Melanin primarily serves to filter ultraviolet radiation (light). Exposure to ultraviolet light can stimulate melanin production.

Dermis

Also called the corium, this second layer of skin is an elastic system that contains and supports blood vessels, lymphatic vessels, nerves, and epidermal appendages (hair, nails, and eccrine and apocrine glands). The dermis itself consists of two layers: the superficial papillary dermis and the reticular dermis.

The papillary dermis is studded with fingerlike projections (papillae) that nourish the epidermal cells. The epidermis lies over these papillae and bulges downward to fill the spaces. A collagenous membrane known as the basement membrane lies between the epidermis and dermis, holding them together.

The reticular dermis covers a layer of subcutaneous tissue (adipose layer, or panniculus adiposus), a specialized layer primarily composed of fat cells. It insulates the body to conserve heat, acts as a mechanical shock absorber, and provides energy.

Intercellular material called matrix makes up most of the dermis. Matrix contains connective tissue fibers called collagen, elastin, and reticular fibers. Collagen, a protein, gives strength to the dermis; elastin makes the skin pliable; and reticular fibers bind the collagen and elastin together.

The matrix and connective tissue fibers are produced by spindle-shaped connective tissue cells (dermal fibroblasts), which become part of the matrix as it forms. Fibers are loosely arranged in the papillary dermis but more tightly packed in the deeper reticular dermis.

Epidermal appendages

These include hair, nails, sebaceous glands, eccrine glands, and apocrine glands.

Hair

These long, slender shafts are composed of keratin. Each hair has an expanded lower end (bulb or root) indented on its undersurface by a cluster of connective tissue and blood vessels called a hair pilus. Each lies within an epithelium-lined sheath called a hair follicle. A bundle of smooth-muscle fibers (arrector pili) extends through the dermis to attach to the base of the hair follicle. Contraction of these muscle fibers causes the hair to stand on end. Hair follicles also have a rich blood and nerve supply.

Nails

Like hair, nails are composed mainly of keratin. They're situated over the distal surface of the end of each digit. The nail plate, surrounded on three sides by the nail folds (cuticles), lies on the nail bed; the germinative nail matrix, which extends proximally for about 5 mm beneath the nail fold, forms the plate. The distal portion of the matrix shows through the nail as a pale, semilunar area (the lunula). The translucent nail plate distal to the lunula exposes the nail bed. The vascular bed imparts the characteristic pink appearance under the nails.

Sebaceous glands
These glands are found on all skin parts except for the palms and the soles. They occur predominantly on the scalp, face, upper torso, and anogenital region. Sebum, a lipid substance, is produced by the sebaceous glands and secreted in the hair follicle by way of the excretory duct and then exits through the hair follicle opening to reach the skin surface. Sebum may help waterproof the hair and skin and promote the absorption of fat-soluble substances into the dermis. It may also be involved in the production of vitamin D_3 and have some antibacterial function.

Eccrine glands
These widely distributed, coiled glands produce an odorless, watery fluid with a sodium concentration equal to that of plasma. A duct from the secretory coils passes through the dermis and epidermis and opens into the skin surface. Eccrine glands in the palms and soles secrete fluid primarily in response to emotional stress (such as taking a test). The remaining 3 million eccrine glands respond primarily to thermal stress, effectively regulating temperature.

Apocrine glands
Located primarily in the axillary and anogenital areas, apocrine glands have a coiled secretory portion that lies deeper in the dermis than the eccrine glands. A duct connects the apocrine glands to the upper portion of the hair follicle. Apocrine glands, which begin to function at puberty, have no known biological function. Bacterial decomposition of the fluid produced by these glands causes body odor.

Skin functions
The skin performs many functions: protection of underlying structures, sensory perception, temperature and blood pressure regulation, vitamin synthesis, and excretion.

Protection
The epidermis protects against trauma, noxious chemicals, and invasion by microorganisms.

Sensory perception
To perform this function, sensory nerve fibers carry impulses to the central nervous system. Autonomic nerve fibers carry impulses to smooth muscles in the walls of the dermal blood vessels, to the muscles around the hair roots, and to the sweat glands. Sensory nerve fibers originate in the dorsal nerve roots and supply specific skin areas, known as dermatomes. Through these fibers, the skin can transmit various sensations, including temperature, touch, pressure, pain, and itching.

Temperature and blood pressure regulation
Abundant nerves, blood vessels, and eccrine glands within the dermis assist with thermoregulation. When the skin is exposed to cold or a drop in internal body temperature, the blood vessels constrict in response to stimuli from the autonomic nervous system. This action decreases blood flow through the skin and conserves body heat.

When the skin is too hot or internal body temperature rises, the small arteries in the dermis dilate. Increased blood flow through these vessels reduces body heat. If this doesn't adequately lower temperature, the eccrine glands act to increase sweat production; subsequent evaporation cools the skin. Dermal blood vessels also help regulate systemic blood pressure by vasoconstriction.

Vitamin synthesis
When stimulated by ultraviolet light, the skin synthesizes vitamin D_3 (cholecalciferol).

Excretion
The skin also is an excretory organ: The sweat glands excrete sweat, which contains water, electrolytes, urea, and lactic acid. The skin maintains body surface integrity by cell migration and by shedding, and can repair surface wounds by intensifying normal cell replacement mechanisms. However, regeneration won't occur if the dermal layer is destroyed. The sebaceous glands produce sebum, a mixture of keratin, fat, and cellulose debris. Combined with sweat, sebum forms a moist, oily, acidic film that is mildly antibacterial and antifungal and protects the skin surface.

Vascular influence
The skin contains a vast arteriovenous network, extending from subcutaneous tissue to the dermis. These blood vessels provide oxygen and nutrients to sensory nerves (which control touch, temperature, and pain), motor nerves (which control the activities of sweat glands, ar-

ASSESSING SKIN COLOR VARIATIONS

Skin color variations in certain areas of the body may indicate a particular condition, as shown below.

Color	Distribution	Possible cause
Absent	Small circumscribed areas Generalized	Vitiligo Albinism
Blue	Around lips (circumoral pallor) Generalized	Cyanosis Cyanosis
Deep red	Generalized	Polycythemia vera (increased red blood cell count)
Pink	Local or generalized	Erythema (superficial capillary dilation and congestion)
Tan to brown	Face patches	Chloasma of pregnancy; birthmark
Tan to brown-bronze	Generalized	Addison's disease (not related to sun exposure)
Yellow	Sclera Generalized	Jaundice from liver dysfunction Jaundice from liver dysfunction
Yellow-orange	Palms, soles, and face; not sclera	Carotenemia (carotene in the blood)

terioles, and smooth muscles of the skin), and skin appendages. Blood flow also influences skin coloring because the amount of oxygen carried to capillaries in the dermis can produce transient changes in color. For example, decreased oxygen supply can turn the skin pale or bluish; increased oxygen can turn it pink or ruddy.

Assessing the skin
Assessment includes a thorough history to determine whether a skin disorder is an acute flare-up, a recurrent problem, or a chronic condition and a physical examination.

Patient history
Ask the patient how long the problem has been present, how a typical flare-up or attack begins, whether or not pruritus occurs, and which medications—systemic or topical—he has used to treat it. Ask whether any family members, friends, or other contacts have the same problem and if the patient lives or works in an environment that could cause the condition.

Physical examination
• *Inspection.* Carefully examine the patient's body: mucous membranes, hair, scalp, axillae, groin, palms, soles, and nails. Because abnormal skin variations require identification and description, note changes in pigmentation (light or dark areas compared to the rest of the skin), freckles, moles (nevi), and tanning (usually considered a normal variation). Next, note the color of healthy skin as well as problem areas. Rashes or lesions may range from red to brown or may be hypopigmented (as in vitiligo). (See *Assessing skin color variations.*)

Look for skin lesions. If you find any, record the color, size, shape and configuration, elevation or depression, texture, and location, and if they are pedunculated (connected to the skin by a stem or a stalk). (See *Differentiating among skin lesions,* pages 1160 and 1161.)

If more than one lesion is evident, try to determine which is the primary lesion (the one that appeared first); the patient may be able to point it out. Note the pattern of distribution. Lesions can be localized (isolated), regional, generalized, or universal (total), involving the entire skin, hair, and nails. Observe whether the lesions are unilateral or bilateral and symmetrical or asym-

DIFFERENTIATING AMONG SKIN LESIONS

The illustrations below depict the most common primary and secondary skin lesions.

Primary lesions

Bulla
Fluid-filled lesion more than ¾" (2 cm) in diameter (also called a blister), as occurs in severe poison oak or ivy dermatitis, bullous pemphigoid, and second-degree burns

Comedo
Plugged, exfoliative pilosebaceous duct formed from sebum and keratin—for example, blackhead (open comedo) and whitehead (closed comedo)

Cyst
Semisolid or fluid-filled encapsulated mass extending deep into dermis—for example, acne

Macule
Flat, pigmented, circumscribed area less than ⅜" (1 cm) in diameter—for example, freckle or rash that occurs in rubella

Nodule
Firm, raised lesion, ¼" to ¾" (0.6 to 2 cm) in diameter, that is deeper than a papule and extends into dermal layer—for example, intradermal nevus

Papule
Firm, inflammatory, raised lesion up to ¼" (0.6 cm) in diameter that may be same color as skin or pigmented—for example, acne papule and lichen planus

Patch
Flat, pigmented, circumscribed area more than ⅜" (1 cm) in diameter—for example, herald patch (pityriasis rosea)

Plaque
Circumscribed, solid, elevated lesion more than ⅜" (1 cm) in diameter that is elevated above skin surface and that occupies larger surface area in comparison with height, as occurs in psoriasis

Pustule
Raised, circumscribed lesion, usually less than ⅜" (1 cm) in diameter, that contains purulent material, making it a yellow-white color—for example, acne or impetiginous pustule and furuncle

Tumor
Elevated, solid lesion larger than ¾" (2 cm) in diameter that extends into dermal and subcutaneous layers—for example, dermatofibroma

Vesicle
Raised, circumscribed, fluid-filled lesion less than ¼" (0.6 cm) in diameter, as occurs in chicken pox or herpes simplex infection

Wheal
Raised, firm lesion with intense localized skin edema that varies in size, shape, and color (from pale pink to red) and that disappears in hours—for example, hives and insect bites

Secondary lesions

Atrophy
Thinning of skin surface at site of disorder—for example, striae and aging skin

Crust
Dried sebum or serous, sanguineous, or purulent exudate, overlying an erosion or a weeping vesicle, bulla, or pustule, as occurs in impetigo

Erosion
Circumscribed lesion that involves loss of superficial epidermis—for example, abrasion

Excoriation
Linear scratched or abraded areas, often self-induced—for example, abraded acne lesions or eczema

DIFFERENTIATING AMONG SKIN LESIONS (continued)

Secondary lesions (continued)

Fissure
Linear cracking of the skin that extends into the dermal layer—for example, hand dermatitis (chapped skin)

Lichenification
Thickened, prominent skin markings caused by constant rubbing, as occurs in chronic atopic dermatitis

Scale
Thin, dry flakes of shedding skin, as occurs in psoriasis, dry skin, or neonatal desquamation

Scar
Fibrous tissue caused by trauma, deep inflammation, or surgical incision, which can be red and raised (recent), pink and flat (6 weeks), or pale and depressed (old)—for example, a healed surgical incision

Ulcer
Epidermal and dermal destruction that may extend into subcutaneous tissue and that usually heals with scarring—for example, pressure ulcer or stasis ulcer

metrical, and note the arrangement of lesions (a clustered or linear configuration, for example).
• *Palpation.* Use palpation to assess skin texture, consistency, temperature, moisture, and turgor and to evaluate changes in or tenderness of particular lesions. Wear gloves when palpating moist lesions.

Diagnostic tests
Several tests may help identify skin disorders.
• *Diascopy,* in which a lesion is covered with a microscopic slide or piece of clear plastic, helps to determine whether dilated capillaries or extravasated blood is causing a lesion's redness.
• *Microscopic immunofluorescence* identifies immunoglobulins and elastic tissue in manifestations of immune disorders.
• *Phototesting* exposes small areas of the patient's skin to ultraviolet-A (UVA) or ultraviolet-B (UVB) light to detect

photosensitivity. Phototesting in combination with patch testing evaluates a patient's photosensitivity with compounds placed on the skin (photopatch testing).
• *Tzanck test* requires smearing vesicular fluid or exudate from an ulcer on a glass slide and then staining it with Papanicolaou's, Wright's, Giemsa, or methylene blue stain. When the slide is examined microscopically, the presence of multinucleated giant cells, intranuclear inclusion bodies, and ballooning degeneration confirms herpesvirus infection.
• *Potassium hydroxide (KOH) test* helps to identify fungal skin infections. It requires removing scales from the skin by scraping and then mixing the scales with a few drops of 10% to 25% KOH on a glass slide. After heating the slide, skin cells will dissolve, leaving fungal elements visible on microscopic examination.
• *Gram stains and exudate cultures* help to identify the organism responsible for an underlying infection by separating bacteria into two classifications—gram-negative and gram-positive. Although staining provides rapid, valuable diagnostic leads, firm identification must be made by culturing the organisms.
• *Patch tests* identify the cause of allergic contact sensitization.
• *Skin biopsy* determines the histology of cells and may be diagnostic, confirmatory, or inconclusive, depending on the disease.

BACTERIAL INFECTIONS

Skin disorders caused by bacterial infection include impetigo; folliculitis, furunculosis, and carbunculosis; and staphylococcal scalded skin syndrome. They're commonly treated with oral or topical antibiotics or both. The prognosis usually is good.

IMPETIGO
A contagious, superficial skin infection, impetigo (impetigo contagiosa) occurs in nonbullous and bullous forms. This vesiculopustular eruptive disorder spreads most easily among infants, young children, and elderly people. It appears most commonly on the face and other exposed areas, usually around the nose and mouth.

Infants and young children may develop aural impetigo or otitis externa. These lesions usually clear without treatment in 2 to 3 weeks unless an underlying disorder, such as eczema, is present. Lesions in the diaper area may be complicated by candidal organisms, additional

COMPARING ECTHYMA AND IMPETIGO

Ecthyma is a superficial skin infection that usually causes scarring. It generally results from infection by beta-hemolytic streptococci.

Ecthyma differs from impetigo in that its characteristic ulcer results from deeper penetration of the skin by the infecting organism (involving the lower epidermis and dermis) and the overlying crust tends to be raised (⅜" to 1¼" [1 to 3 cm]). These lesions usually are found on the legs after a scratch or an insect bite. Autoinoculation can transmit ecthyma to other parts of the body, especially to sites that have been scratched open.

Therapy is basically the same as for impetigo, beginning with removal of the crust, but the patient's response may be slower. Parenteral antibiotics also are used.

bacteria, fungi, or viruses. In addition, impetigo may complicate chicken pox, eczema, and other skin disorders marked by open lesions.

Causes

Bullous impetigo, which starts as a blister, is caused by coagulase-positive *Staphylococcus aureus*. Beta-hemolytic streptococci produce the nonbullous form of impetigo, which later also may harbor staphylococci, producing a mixed-organism infection.

Predisposing factors, such as poor hygiene, anemia, malnutrition, and a warm climate, favor outbreaks of this infection, which most often occur during the late summer and early fall. The most common transmitters appear to be biting insects, such as mosquitoes and flies, and autoinoculation through scratching.

Complications

A rare but serious complication of streptococcal impetigo is glomerulonephritis, caused by a nephritogenic strain of beta-hemolytic streptococci.

Ecthyma, an ulcerative form of impetigo, may result from deeper skin penetration by the infecting organism. (See *Comparing ecthyma and impetigo.*)

Assessment findings

The patient history discloses exposure to insect bites or other predisposing factors. Additionally, the patient may relate a history of painless pruritus and burning.

In streptococcal impetigo, inspection typically reveals a small, red macule that has turned into a vesicle, becoming pustular within a few hours. When the vesicle

breaks, a characteristic thick, honey-colored crust forms from the exudate. Autoinoculation may cause satellite lesions to appear.

In staphylococcal impetigo, a thin-walled vesicle opens. Inspection finds a thin, clear crust forming from the exudate and a lesion that appears as a central clearing circumscribed by an outer rim—much like a ringworm lesion. Observation commonly reveals these lesions on the face or other exposed areas.

Both forms may appear simultaneously and can be clinically indistinguishable.

Diagnostic tests

• *Gram stain* of vesicular fluid and visualization under a microscope usually confirms *S. aureus* infection.
• *Culture and sensitivity testing* of fluid or denuded skin may indicate the most appropriate antibiotic, but therapy should not be delayed for laboratory results, which can take 3 days.
• *White blood cell count* may be elevated in infection.

Treatment

Measures include broad-spectrum systemic antibiotics (usually a penicillinase-resistant penicillin, or erythromycin for patients who are allergic to penicillin). Treatment also includes the removal of the exudate by washing the lesions two to three times a day with soap and water or, for stubborn crusts, using warm soaks or compresses of 0.9% sodium chloride or a diluted soap solution.

Topical agents, such as neomycin, polymyxin B, polymyxin B with bacitracin, mupirocin, clioquinol, and tetracycline, have been used successfully in combination with crust removal with each application.

Antihistamines to alleviate itching and daily bathing with bactericidal soaps as a preventive measure are additional treatments.

Nursing diagnoses

• Body image disturbance
• Impaired skin integrity
• Impaired tissue integrity
• Risk for infection

Nursing interventions

• Use meticulous hand-washing technique and universal precautions to prevent spreading the infection.
• Cut the patient's fingernails short to prevent scratching, which can cause autoinoculation and new skin breaks.
• Remove the crusts by gently washing with bactericidal soap and water. Soften stubborn crusts with cool com-

presses; scrub gently to aid crust removal before applying a topical antibiotic.

• Give medications, as ordered, and monitor the patient's response. Remember to check for penicillin allergy.

• Encourage the patient to verbalize his feelings about his body image, and acknowledge the importance of body image.

Patient teaching

• To prevent contagion, emphasize to the patient and family the importance of meticulous hand-washing technique. Advise parents to cut their child's fingernails short. Encourage frequent bathing with a bactericidal soap. Tell the patient not to share towels, washcloths, and bed linens, which should be kept separate and laundered in hot water before reuse.

• Teach family members how to identify characteristic lesions. Encourage regular inspections, especially of children, to identify new lesions. If the patient is a schoolchild, notify the school of his condition.

• Stress the need to continue prescribed medications for 7 to 10 days, even after lesions have healed. Instruct the patient and family to notify the doctor if adverse reactions occur.

• Provide written instructions for the care of impetiginous lesions, including crust removal, application of topical medications, and dressing change technique.

FOLLICULITIS, FURUNCULOSIS, AND CARBUNCULOSIS

A bacterial infection of the hair follicle, folliculitis causes the formation of a pustule. The infection can be superficial (follicular impetigo or Bockhart's impetigo) or deep (sycosis barbae). Folliculitis also may lead to the development of furuncles (furunculosis), commonly known as boils, or carbuncles (carbunculosis). These disorders may be recurrent and are particularly troublesome to healthy young adults. The prognosis depends on the severity of the infection and on the patient's physical condition and ability to resist infection.

Causes

The most common cause of folliculitis, furunculosis, or carbunculosis is coagulase-positive *Staphylococcus aureus*. Predisposing factors include an infected wound elsewhere on the body, poor personal hygiene, debilitation, diabetes mellitus, occlusive cosmetics, tight clothes, friction, exposure to chemicals (cutting oils), and management of skin lesions with tar or with occlu-

sive therapy, using steroids. Folliculitis may be caused by bacteria other than *S. aureus*, especially as a sequela to erythromycin and tetracycline therapy.

Furunculosis commonly follows folliculitis that is exacerbated by irritation, pressure, friction, or perspiration. Carbunculosis develops more slowly and usually follows persistent *S. aureus* infection and furunculosis.

Complications

Untreated furunculosis may lead to cellulitis, which in turn may progress to septicemia if the infection reaches the dermal vascular plexus. This condition occurs most commonly in infants and others with impaired immune status.

In severe cases, these disorders may result in residual scarring.

Assessment findings

The patient history recounts predisposing factors. The patient may complain of pain, erythema, and edema of several days' duration.

In folliculitis, inspection usually reveals pustules on the scalp, arms, and legs in children; on the face of bearded men (sycosis barbae); and on the eyelids (styes). (See *Bacterial skin infection: A question of degree,* page 1164.)

Folliculitis may progress to furunculosis, in which the patient complains of hard, painful nodules, usually on the neck, face, axillae, and buttocks. If nodules enlarge and rupture, inspection will reveal discharged pus and necrotic material on the skin surface. Erythema may persist for days or weeks after nodule rupture.

In severe cases of systemic infection and in carbunculosis, vital sign assessment may reveal fever, and the patient may complain of malaise. Inspection reveals lesions that range from tiny, white-topped pustules to large, yellow pus-filled lesions. The patient with carbunculosis will complain of extremely painful, deep abscesses that drain through multiple openings onto the skin surface, usually around several hair follicles. Palpation detects pain, tenderness, and edema around the pustule sites; in both furunculosis and carbunculosis, it also reveals hard nodules under the skin surface.

A systemic response to the infection may include localized lymphadenopathy.

Diagnostic tests

• *Wound culture* shows *S. aureus*.

• *Complete blood count* may reveal an elevated white blood cell count (leukocytosis).

BACTERIAL SKIN INFECTION: A QUESTION OF DEGREE

The degree of hair follicle involvement in bacterial skin infection ranges from superficial folliculitis (erythema and a pustule in a single follicle) to deep folliculitis (extensive follicle involvement), to furunculosis (red, tender nodules that surround follicles with a single draining point) and, finally, to carbunculosis (deep abscesses that involve several follicles with multiple draining points).

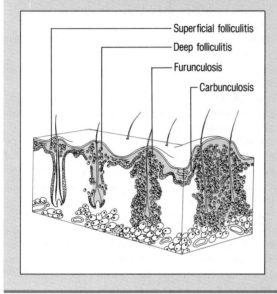

- Superficial folliculitis
- Deep folliculitis
- Furunculosis
- Carbunculosis

Treatment

Emphasizing site care and drug therapy, treatment includes:
- cleaning the infected area thoroughly with soap and water
- applying hot, wet compresses to promote vasodilation and drainage from the lesions
- administering topical antibiotics, such as bacitracin with polymyxin B
- administering systemic antibiotics (erythromycin or dicloxacillin) in extensive infection and in carbunculosis.

Furunculosis also may require incision and drainage of ripe lesions after application of hot, wet compresses, and topical antibiotics after drainage.

Nursing diagnoses

- Body image disturbance
- Impaired skin integrity
- Pain
- Risk for infection

Nursing interventions

- Be alert for possible reactions to systemic antibiotic therapy, which may include gastric disturbances, sensitivity reactions, and tooth discoloration in young children.
- Change the dressing frequently and maintain aseptic technique; to prevent the spread of infection, properly dispose of contaminated dressings and use universal precautions.
- Assess for patient discomfort and apply warm, moist compresses to assist suppuration.
- Encourage the patient to verbalize his feelings about his appearance. Recognize the importance of body image.
- Assist with general hygiene and comfort measures as needed.
- Administer pain medications and antibiotics, as ordered, and monitor the patient's response.

Patient teaching

- Teach the patient and family meticulous hand-washing technique, and encourage the patient to take daily baths with bactericidal soap to prevent the spread of infection.
- Teach the patient and family how to apply warm compresses, change dressings with aseptic technique, and properly dispose of contaminated dressings.
- Stress the importance of not squeezing lesions to prevent the spread of infection to surrounding areas and to minimize scarring.
- To avoid spreading bacteria among family members, urge the patient not to share clothes, towels, washcloths, or bed linens and to launder these items in hot water before reusing. Tell him to change his clothes and bedsheets daily.
- Instruct the patient and family to continue the entire antibiotic regimen until completed, even if the lesions appear to have healed. Advise them to notify the doctor if adverse reactions to systemic antibiotic therapy occur.
- Advise the patient with recurrent furunculosis to have a physical examination because an underlying disease, such as diabetes mellitus, may be present.

STAPHYLOCOCCAL SCALDED SKIN SYNDROME

A severe skin disorder, staphylococcal scalded skin syndrome is marked by epidermal erythema, peeling, and necrosis that give the skin a scalded appearance. This disorder is most prevalent in infants ages 1 to 3 months but may develop in children under age 5; it's uncommon in adults. It follows a consistent pattern of progression, and most patients recover fully.

Causes
Group 2 *Staphylococcus aureus,* primarily phage type 71, is the causative organism in staphylococcal scalded skin syndrome. This penicillinase-producing organism releases epidermolytic toxins that are widely disseminated from a systemic site.

Predisposing factors may include impaired immunity and renal insufficiency—present to some extent in the normal neonate because of immature development of these systems. Rarely, this disorder may affect adults undergoing immunosuppressive therapy.

Complications
In 2% to 3% of cases, staphylococcal scalded skin syndrome results in death because of complications of fluid and electrolyte loss, sepsis, and involvement of other body systems. Septicemia and secondary infections from *Candida* species and gram-negative bacteria also may occur.

Assessment findings
The patient history includes a prodromal upper respiratory tract infection, possibly with concomitant purulent conjunctivitis. Usually, the patient appears profoundly ill. Inspection reveals characteristic lesions. Exfoliation may appear within 24 to 48 hours of onset. Assessment of vital signs typically reveals a fever. Palpation may reveal tenderness over the lesions.

Visible cutaneous changes progress through the following three stages:
• *Erythema.* Becoming visible usually around the mouth and other orifices, erythema may spread in widening circles over the entire body surface.
• *Exfoliation* (24 to 48 hours later). In the more common, localized disease form, superficial erosions and minimal crusting occur, usually around body orifices, and may spread to exposed skin areas. In the more severe disease forms, large, flaccid bullae erupt and may spread to cover extensive body areas. Once ruptured, these bullae expose sections of tender, oozing, denuded skin. Intact lesions may not be found because the bullae are fragile; only the erosions may be visible.

At first, the patient with this disorder may appear to be sunburned or to have scarlet fever, but inspection of the mouth shows that he lacks the oral lesions characteristic of scarlet fever.

• *Desquamation.* In this final stage, affected areas dry up and powdery scales form. Normal skin replaces these scales in 5 to 7 days. Residual scarring is rare.

During the initial disease stages, palpation of the affected areas results in Nikolsky's sign (sloughing of the skin when friction is applied). Bullae are so fragile that minimal palpation produces very tender, red, moist areas.

Diagnostic tests
Diagnosis requires careful observation of the three-stage progression of this disease as well as the following tests:
• *Exfoliative cytology and biopsy* aid in differential diagnosis, ruling out erythema multiforme and drug-induced toxic epidermal necrolysis, both of which are similar to staphylococcal scalded skin syndrome. Isolation of group 2 *S. aureus* on cultures of skin lesions confirms the diagnosis. However, skin lesions sometimes appear sterile.
• *Blood cultures* may recover some causative organisms in a very ill patient. If this disorder occurs in a nursery setting, cultures from the nose, throat, and any skin breaks of nursing personnel can identify potential carriers of the organism.

Treatment
Systemic antibiotics (usually penicillinase-resistant penicillin) to prevent secondary infections and replacement measures to maintain fluid and electrolyte balance are the most common treatments.

Nursing diagnoses
• Body image disturbance
• Impaired skin integrity
• Ineffective thermoregulation
• Pain
• Risk for fluid volume deficit
• Risk for infection

Nursing interventions
• Provide special care for the neonate, if required, including placement in an Isolette to maintain body temperature and provide isolation.
• Carefully monitor intake and output to assess fluid and electrolyte balance. In severe cases, provide I.V. fluid replacement, as ordered.
• Check vital signs. Be especially alert for a sudden rise in temperature, indicating sepsis, which requires prompt, aggressive treatment.
• Maintain skin integrity. Use strict aseptic technique to preclude secondary infection, especially during the ex-

foliation stage, because of open lesions. To prevent friction and sloughing of the skin, leave affected areas uncovered or loosely covered. Place cotton between severely affected fingers and toes to prevent webbing.
• Administer warm baths and soaks during the recovery period. Gently debride exfoliated areas.

Patient teaching
• Reassure the parents that complications are rare and residual scars are unlikely.
• Instruct the parents to use meticulous hand-washing and aseptic techniques when changing dressings and providing comfort measures, such as warm soaks or baths.
• Stress the importance of avoiding friction on the skin surface during the exfoliation stage and avoiding picking or rubbing scales during the desquamation stage.
• Instruct the parents to contact the doctor if adverse reactions to antibiotic therapy occur. Also explain the importance of completing the entire regimen of antibiotic therapy, even after the lesions appear to have healed.

FUNGAL INFECTIONS

Varying in appearance and severity, fungal infections include tinea versicolor and dermatophytosis. Complications are minor, and drug therapy, most commonly with topical antifungal agents, usually produces good results.

TINEA VERSICOLOR
A chronic, superficial fungal infection, tinea versicolor (pityriasis versicolor) may produce a multicolored rash, commonly on the upper trunk. Primarily a cosmetic defect, it usually affects young people, especially during warm weather, and is most prevalent in tropical countries. Recurrence is common.

Causes
Pityrosporum orbiculare (Microsporum furfur) causes tinea versicolor. Whether this condition is infectious or merely a proliferation of normal skin fungi is uncertain.

Complications
Rarely, skin breaks caused by scratching may result in secondary bacterial infections.

Assessment findings
The patient may report seeking medical help because some areas of the body don't tan when exposed to sunlight, causing a cosmetic defect.

Inspection and palpation usually reveal raised or macular, round or oval, slightly scaly lesions on the upper trunk. The lesions may extend to the lower abdomen, neck, arms and, rarely, the face. They usually appear tawny but may range from white (hypopigmented) patches in dark-skinned patients to brown (hyperpigmented) patches in fair-skinned patients. Itching, burning, and inflammation are unusual.

Diagnostic tests
• Wood's light examination strongly suggests tinea versicolor.
• Potassium hydroxide test of skin scrapings confirms tinea versicolor by showing hyphae and clusters of yeast.

Treatment
The most economical and effective treatment is selenium sulfide lotion 2.5% applied once a day for 7 days. The lotion remains on the skin for 10 minutes and then is rinsed off thoroughly. In persistent cases, therapy may require a single 12-hour application of this lotion, followed by weekly washing with an antifungal soap.

More expensive treatments include topical antifungals, such as tolnaftate, and oral antifungals, such as griseofulvin and ketoconazole.

Nursing diagnoses
• Body image disturbance
• Impaired skin integrity
• Risk for infection

Nursing interventions
• Have the patient's fingernails cut short to prevent skin breaks caused by scratching, if necessary.
• Recognize the importance of body image. Encourage the patient to verbalize his feelings about his appearance, if appropriate.

Patient teaching
• Teach the patient meticulous hand-washing technique, and encourage good personal hygiene.
• Stress the importance of not scratching or picking lesions to avoid the risk of skin breaks and secondary bacterial infections.
• Provide written instructions for using ordered medications. Tell the patient to contact the doctor if adverse reactions occur.

• Assure the patient that once the fungal infection is cured, discolored areas will gradually blend in after exposure to the sun or ultraviolet light.
• Because recurrence of tinea versicolor is common, advise the patient to watch for new areas of discoloration.

DERMATOPHYTOSIS

A group of superficial fungal infections usually classified according to their anatomic location, dermatophytosis (tinea) may affect the scalp (tinea capitis), the bearded skin of the face (tinea barbae), the body (tinea corporis, occurring mainly in children), the groin (tinea cruris, or jock itch), the nails (tinea unguium, also called onychomycosis), and the feet (tinea pedis, or athlete's foot). These disorders vary from mild inflammations to acute vesicular reactions.

Tinea infections are prevalent in the United States and are usually more common in males than in females. Although remissions and exacerbations are common, with effective treatment, the cure rate is very high. About 20% of infected people develop chronic conditions.

Causes
Tinea infections result from dermatophytes (fungi) of the genera *Trichophyton*, *Microsporum*, and *Epidermophyton*. Transmission can occur directly (through contact with infected lesions) or indirectly (through contact with contaminated articles, such as shoes, towels, or shower stalls). Warm weather and tight clothing encourage fungus growth.

Complications
Hair or nail loss and secondary bacterial or candidal infections, resulting in inflammation, itching, tenderness, and maceration, are common complications of tinea infections.

Assessment findings
Tinea lesions vary in appearance and duration. Inspection of the patient with *tinea capitis* may expose small, spreading papules on the scalp that may progress to inflamed, pus-filled lesions (kerions). Patchy hair loss with scaling may be visible.

Tinia barbae appears as pustular folliculitis in the bearded area.

In *tinea corporis,* inspection and palpation reveal flat skin lesions at any site except the scalp, bearded skin, or feet. These lesions may be dry and scaly or moist and crusty; as they enlarge, their centers heal, producing the classic ring-shaped appearance.

DERMATOPHYTOSIS OF THE FEET

Popularly called athlete's foot, dermatophytosis of the feet (tinea pedis) causes macerated, scaling lesions that may spread from the interdigital spaces to the sole. Diagnosis must rule out other possible causes of signs and symptoms, including eczema, psoriasis, contact dermatitis, and maceration caused by tight, ill-fitting shoes.

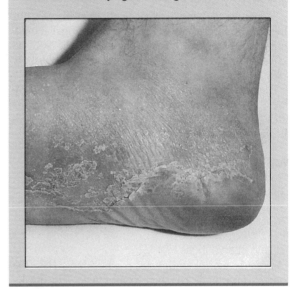

In *tinea cruris,* inspection and palpation find raised, sharply defined, itchy red lesions in the groin that may extend to the buttocks, inner thighs, and external genitalia.

Tinea unguium starts at the tip of one or more toenails (fingernail infection is less common). Inspection will reveal gradual thickening, discoloration, and crumbling of the nail, with accumulation of subungual debris. Eventually, the nail may be completely destroyed.

A patient with severe *tinea pedis* may complain of extreme itching and pain on walking. Inspection findings include scaling and blisters between the toes and, possibly, a dry, squamous inflammation that affects the entire sole. (See *Dermatophytosis of the feet.*)

Diagnostic tests
• *Potassium hydroxide test* and microscopic examination of lesion scrapings usually confirm tinea infection.
• *Wood's light examination* may confirm some types of tinea capitis.

• *Culture* of the affected area may help identify the infecting organism.

Treatment

Local tinea infections usually respond to topical antifungal agents, such as clotrimazole, miconazole, haloprogin, or tolnaftate. Tinea capitis and other persistent tinea infections require treatment with oral griseofulvin for 6 to 8 weeks. Treatments should continue for 2 weeks after lesions resolve.

Supportive measures include application of open wet dressings, the removal of scabs and scales, and the administration of keratolytics, such as salicylic acid, to soften and remove hyperkeratotic lesions of the heels or soles.

The patient with tinea capitis should use selenium sulfide 2.5% shampoo during treatment and for 6 months after griseofulvin therapy ends to decrease fungal shedding and prevent recurrence.

Nursing diagnoses

• Body image disturbance
• Impaired skin integrity
• Pain
• Risk for infection

Nursing interventions

• Assess the patient for discomfort and itching. Have the patient's fingernails cut short to minimize skin breaks and the spread of infection from scratching.
• Be alert for possible adverse reactions to griseofulvin therapy, including sensitivity reactions, GI disturbances, headaches, photosensitivity and, possibly, liver damage. Monitor liver function.
• For the patient with tinea capitis, discontinue medications and notify the doctor if the condition worsens. Use careful hand-washing technique.
• For the tinea corporis patient with excessive abdominal girth, use abdominal pads between skin folds, and change the pads frequently. Check the patient daily for excoriated, newly denuded skin areas. Apply open wet dressings two or three times daily to decrease inflammation and help remove scales.
• For tinea unguium, keep the patient's nails short and straight, and gently remove the debris under the nails. Prepare the patient for prolonged therapy, and explain possible adverse reactions to griseofulvin.
• For the patient with tinea cruris, provide sitz baths, as ordered, to relieve itching.

Patient teaching

• Teach the patient and family about transmission and recurrence of the infection. Teach them to identify environmental conditions that encourage fungal growth or aggravate the disorder.
• Advise the patient not to share clothing, hats, towels, bed linens, or pillows with other family members and to keep the lesions covered.
• Instruct the patient to wear loose-fitting, cotton clothing, which should be changed frequently and laundered in hot water to avoid aggravating the condition.
• Stress the importance of good hand washing and personal hygiene in preventing the spread of infection.
• Teach the patient and family about prescribed medications and preparations. Stress the importance of completing the entire treatment regimen, even after the lesions appear to have healed. Tell them to notify the doctor if adverse reactions occur.
• Advise the patient to avoid scratching because scarring and secondary infection may occur.
• If the patient has tinea capitis, suggest that other family members be checked for the disorder.
• Instruct the patient with tinea cruris to dry the affected area thoroughly after bathing and to dust evenly with antifungal powder. Suggest sitz baths to relieve itching.
• Recommend that the patient with tinea barbae let his beard grow and trim his whiskers with scissors, not a razor. If he insists that he must shave, advise him to use an electric razor instead of a blade.
• Encourage the patient with tinea pedis to expose his feet to air whenever possible and to wear sandals or leather shoes and clean cotton socks. Tell him to wash his feet twice daily and, after drying them thoroughly, to dust evenly with an antifungal powder to absorb perspiration and prevent excoriation. In severe infection, the patient may need to disinfect his socks in boiling water.

PARASITIC INFESTATIONS

Highly contagious and rapidly spreading, parasitic infestations are fairly common and respond well to drug therapy. They include scabies, cutaneous larva migrans, and pediculosis.

SCABIES

An age-old, highly transmissible skin infestation, scabies is characterized by burrows, pruritus, and excoriations with secondary infections. It occurs worldwide, is associated with overcrowding and poor hygiene, and can be endemic. The mites that cause this disorder can live their entire life cycles in human skin, causing chronic infection. The female mite burrows into the skin to lay eggs, from which larvae emerge to copulate and then re-burrow under the skin.

Although scabies can occur in anyone, children under age 15 have the highest incidence and usually are the first family members to contract the disease. In the United States, up to 4% of patients seen by dermatologists have scabies.

Causes

Infestation with *Sarcoptes scabiei* var. *hominis* (itch mite) causes scabies. (See *Scabies: Cause and effect.*)

Transmission of scabies occurs through skin contact or venereally. Schoolchildren, family members, and intimate contacts of those with scabies are at greatest risk for spreading the infection. The adult mite can live for 2 to 3 days without a human host; therefore, inanimate objects cannot be ruled out as a means of transmission.

Complications

Persistent pruritus caused by secondary mite sensitization is a complication of scabies. Intense scratching can lead to severe excoriation, tissue trauma, and secondary bacterial infection.

Assessment findings

The history may uncover predisposing factors. The patient may first present with asymptomatic lesions. The patient who has been infected for several weeks will complain of intense itching that becomes more severe at night.

Inspection may reveal characteristic gray-brown burrows, which may appear as erythematous nodules when excoriated. These threadlike lesions, about ⅜" (1 cm) long, occur between the fingers, on flexor surfaces of the wrists, on the elbows, in axillary folds, at the waistline, on the nipples in females, and on the genitalia in males. In infants, the burrows (lesions) may appear on the head and neck. Secondary infection may develop, resulting in the formation of papules and vesicles and in crusting.

Diagnostic tests

• *Potassium hydroxide test* of burrow scraping may reveal adults, larvae, and eggs.
• *Punch biopsy* may help confirm the diagnosis.

If scabies is strongly suspected but diagnostic tests offer no positive identification of the mite, skin clearing

SCABIES: CAUSE AND EFFECT

Infestation with *Sarcoptes scabiei*—the itch mite—causes scabies. This mite (shown enlarged below) has a hard shell and measures a microscopic 0.1 mm. The second illustration shows the erythematous nodules with excoriation that appear in patients with scabies.

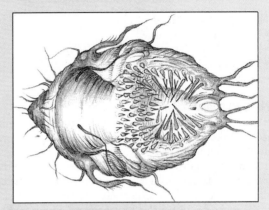

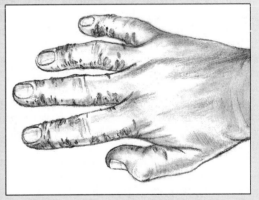

with a therapeutic trial of a pediculicide confirms the diagnosis.

Treatment

Scabies treatment consists of bathing with soap and water, followed by application of a pediculicide. Lindane cream should be applied in a thin layer over the entire skin surface, left on for 8 to 12 hours, and then thoroughly washed off. Because this cream is not ovicidal, application must be repeated in 1 week. Another pediculicide, crotamiton cream, is massaged into the skin and a second dose can be applied in 24 hours. Benzyl benzoate (25%) is applied in a similar manner.

Because about 10% of a pediculicide is absorbed systemically, a less toxic 6% to 10% sulfur solution may be applied for 3 consecutive days as an alternative therapy for infants and pregnant women. Secondary bacterial infections may require systemic antibiotics. An antipruritic emollient can reduce itching. Topical steroids, which may potentiate the infection, shouldn't be used.

Nursing diagnoses
• Body image disturbance
• Impaired skin integrity
• Risk for infection
• Situational low self-esteem

Nursing interventions
• Have the patient's fingernails cut short to minimize skin breaks from scratching, which may lead to secondary bacterial infections.
• To prevent transmission to family members or other patients, isolate the patient until treatment is completed; use meticulous hand washing; observe wound and skin precautions for 24 hours after treatment with a pediculicide; sterilize blood pressure cuffs in a gas autoclave before using them on other patients; isolate linens, towels, clothing, and personal articles until the patient is noninfectious; thoroughly disinfect the patient's room after discharge; and have all contaminated clothing and personal articles washed and disinfected.
• Suggest that the patient's family and other close personal contacts be checked for symptoms. Have the patient notify sexual contacts. If the patient is a schoolchild, notify the school of his condition.
• Be alert for complications associated with treatment, including contact dermatitis and hypersensitivity reactions from repeated use of pediculicides. Remember that prolonged use of pediculicides may lead to excessive central nervous system stimulation and seizures.
• Encourage the patient to verbalize his feelings about the infestation, including embarrassment, fear of rejection by others, and body image disturbance.

Patient teaching
• Teach the patient and his family to identify characteristic lesions and the modes of transmission. Assure the patient and his family that the infestation can be treated successfully with good hygiene and the use of pediculicides. Stress the importance of meticulous hand washing to prevent the infection's spread and recurrence.

• Instruct the patient to apply lindane cream from the neck down, covering the entire body. (He may need assistance to reach all body areas.) Tell him to wait about 15 minutes after application before dressing and to avoid bathing for 24 hours.
• Tell the patient not to apply lindane cream to raw or inflamed skin. Teach him the signs of skin irritation and hypersensitivity reaction. Advise him to notify the doctor immediately, to discontinue using the drug, and to wash the drug from the skin if these signs develop.

CUTANEOUS LARVA MIGRANS
Also known as creeping eruption, cutaneous larva migrans is a skin reaction to infestation by the nematodes (hookworms or roundworms) that usually infect dogs and cats. This parasitic infection most often affects people who come in contact with infected soil or sand, such as children and farmers.

Eruptions associated with cutaneous larva migrans clear completely with treatment.

Causes
Ancylostoma braziliense, the larvae of dog and cat hookworm, is responsible for cutaneous larva migrans. The other dog hookworms *A. caninum* and *Uncinaria stenocephala,* as well as the human parasites *Strongyloides stercoralis* and *Necator americanus,* also may produce the disease.

Under favorable conditions—warmth, moisture, and sandy soil—hookworm or roundworm ova are present in the feces of affected animals (such as dogs and cats) and hatch into larvae, which can then burrow into human skin on contact. After penetrating its host, the larva becomes trapped under the skin, unable to reach the intestines to complete its normal life cycle. It then begins to move around, producing peculiar, tunnel-like, alternately meandering and linear lesions that reflect the nematode's persistent and unsuccessful attempts to escape its host.

Complications
The persistent and intense itching associated with this infestation may lead to tissue trauma, excoriation, crusting, and secondary bacterial infections. In areas with inadequate water and sewage treatment, ingestion of the parasite leads to a more serious condition that involves major body systems.

Assessment findings

The patient history shows contact with warm, moist soil in the past several months.

Inspection finds a transient rash or, possibly, a small vesicle at the penetration point. Penetration usually occurs on an exposed area that has come in contact with the ground, such as the feet, legs, or buttocks. The incubation period may be weeks or months, or the parasite may be active almost as soon as it enters the skin.

Palpation reveals a thin, raised, red line on the skin, which becomes visible as the parasite migrates. This may become vesicular and encrusted as pruritus develops and scratching occurs. The larva's apparently random path can cover from 1 mm to 1 cm a day. Penetration of more than one larva may involve a much larger skin area, marking it with many tracks.

Diagnostic tests

Patient history and clinical observation of the characteristic lesions are diagnostic. No specific diagnostic test exists for this disorder.

Treatment

Cutaneous larva migrans infections may require administration of 50 mg/kg thiabendazole given orally for 2 or 3 days or a single dose of pyrantel pamoate, 11 mg/kg of body weight. Alternatively, a 10% aqueous suspension may be applied topically to avoid systemic toxicity. Treatment may also include antihistamines to alleviate itching.

Nursing diagnoses

• Body image disturbance
• Impaired skin integrity
• Risk for infection
• Situational low self-esteem

Nursing interventions

• Have the patient's nails cut short to prevent skin breaks and secondary bacterial infection from scratching.
• Apply cool, moist compresses to alleviate itching.
• Be alert for possible adverse reactions associated with systemic thiabendazole treatment, including nausea, vomiting, abdominal pain, and dizziness.
• Encourage the patient to verbalize feelings about the infestation, including embarrassment, fear of rejection by others, and body image disturbance. Give reassurance that larva migrans lesions usually clear within 1 to 2 weeks after treatment.

Patient teaching

• Teach the patient about the existence of the parasites, sanitation of beaches and sandboxes, and proper pet care.
• Instruct the patient and his family in good hand washing, and stress the importance of preventing the spread of the infection among family members.
• Explain the importance of adhering to the treatment regimen exactly as ordered. Tell the patient about the possible adverse effects of treatment and to notify the doctor if these occur.

PEDICULOSIS

Any human infestation of parasitic forms of lice is known as pediculosis. It can occur anywhere on the body; the most common species, *pediculosis capitis,* feeds on the scalp and, rarely, in the eyebrows, eyelashes, and beard. *Pediculosis corporis* (body lice) lives next to the skin in clothing seams, leaving only to feed on blood. *Pediculosis pubis* is found primarily in pubic hairs but also may extend to the eyebrows, eyelashes, and axillary or body hair.

All of these types of lice feed on human blood and lay eggs (nits) in body hairs or clothing fibers. After the nits hatch, the lice must feed within 24 hours or die; they mature in about 2 to 3 weeks. When a louse bites, it injects a toxin into the skin that produces mild irritation and a purpuric spot. Repeated bites cause sensitization to the toxin, leading to more serious inflammation. In severe cases, wheals or a rash may appear on the trunk caused by sensitization to the parasite. Headache, fever, and malaise also may occur, along with the cutaneous changes.

Treatment can effectively eliminate lice.

Causes

Pediculosis capitis (head lice) is caused by *Pediculus humanus* var. *capitis. P. humanus* var. *corporis* causes pediculosis corporis (body lice). *Phthirus pubis* causes pediculosis pubis (crab lice). (See *Types of lice,* page 1172.)

Usually due to overcrowded conditions and poor personal hygiene, pediculosis capitis commonly affects children, especially girls. It spreads through shared clothing, hats, combs, and hairbrushes.

Pediculosis corporis is commonly associated with prolonged wearing of the same clothing (which might occur in cold climates), overcrowding, and poor personal hygiene. It spreads through shared clothing and bedsheets.

TYPES OF LICE

Head louse
Pediculus humanus var. *capitis* (head louse) has an appearance similar to that of *P. humanus* var. *corporis*.

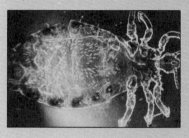

Body louse
Pediculus humanus var. *corporis* (body louse) has a long abdomen, and all its legs are about the same length.

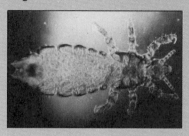

Pubic louse
Phthirus pubis (pubic, or crab, louse) is slightly translucent; its first set of legs is shorter than its second and third sets.

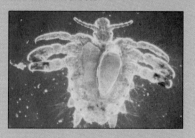

Pediculosis pubis is transmitted through sexual intercourse or by contact with clothing, bed sheets, or towels harboring lice.

Complications

Excoriation and secondary bacterial infections from scratching are common complications of pediculosis. Left untreated, pediculosis may result in dry, hyperpigmented, thickly encrusted, scaly skin with residual scarring.

Assessment findings

The patient history discloses predisposing factors. In a patient with pediculosis capitis, inspection notes excoriation (with severe itching); matted, foul-smelling, lusterless hair (in severe cases); occipital and cervical lymphadenopathy; and a rash on the trunk, probably caused by sensitization. Hair shafts display oval, gray-white nits, which can't be shaken off like dandruff.

Inspection of a patient with pediculosis corporis initially exposes red papules (usually on the shoulders, trunk, or buttocks), which change to urticaria from scratching. Nits are found on clothing.

Inspection of the pediculosis pubis patient finds skin irritation from scratching that's usually more obvious than the bites. Small, gray-blue spots (maculae caeruleae) may appear on the thighs or upper body. The nits, attached to pubic hairs, feel coarse and grainy.

Diagnostic tests

• *Wood's light examination* achieves fluorescence of the adult lice.

• *Microscopic examination* shows nits visible on the hair shaft.

Treatment

For pediculosis capitis, treatment consists of 0.3% pyrethrin and piperonyl butoxide (RID), 1% gamma benzene hexachloride (lindane, Kwell), or 1% permethrin (Nix). If applied inappropriately, Kwell may be absorbed through the skin, resulting in central nervous system (CNS) toxicity. It shouldn't be used on infants and pregnant women.

RID is rubbed into the hair for at least 10 minutes, Kwell for 4 minutes; Nix is a cream rinse applied for 10 minutes after regular shampooing. Then, the hair is rinsed, dried, and combed with a fine-toothed comb to remove the nits. If RID or Kwell have been used, the process should be repeated in 7 to 10 days to remove any eggs that were left behind. Clothes and bed linens must be laundered to prevent reinfestation.

Pediculosis corporis requires lathering the patient's body for 10 minutes with RID or 4 minutes with Kwell and then rinsing thoroughly. Lice may be removed from clothes by heat sterilization or by washing, ironing, or dry cleaning. Storing clothes for more than 30 days or placing them in dry heat of 140° F (60° C) kills lice. If clothes can't be washed or changed, application of 10% lindane powder is effective.

Treatment of pediculosis pubis includes application of Kwell or RID cream or lotion. It should be left on for 24 hours, and treatment should be repeated in 1 week. Clothes and bed linens must be laundered to prevent reinfestation.

Nursing diagnoses
• Body image disturbance
• Impaired skin integrity
• Risk for impaired skin integrity
• Risk for infection
• Situational low self-esteem

Nursing interventions
• Isolate the patient until treatment is complete to prevent spreading the infection.
• Have the patient's fingernails cut short to prevent skin breaks and secondary bacterial infections caused by scratching.
• Be alert for possible adverse reactions associated with treatment with antiparasitics, including sensitivity reactions and, in some cases, CNS toxicity.
• To prevent self-infestation, avoid prolonged contact with the patient's hair, clothing, and bed sheets. Use gloves, gown, and a protective head covering when administering delousing treatment.
• Ask the patient with pediculosis pubis for the names of recent sexual contacts, so that they can be examined and treated. If the infestation occurs in a schoolchild, notify the school.
• To prevent the spread of pediculosis to other hospitalized patients, examine all high-risk patients on admission, especially elderly patients who depend on others for care, those admitted from nursing homes, people living in crowded conditions, and homeless people.
• Encourage the patient to verbalize his feelings about the infestation, including embarrassment, fear of rejection by others, and body image disturbances. Assure the patient and his family that pediculosis can be treated successfully.

Patient teaching
• Teach the patient and his family how to inspect for and identify lice, eggs, and lesions. Teach them how to decontaminate infestation sources, and stress the importance of not borrowing personal articles. Tell parents that if the child's stuffed animals can't be washed, they can be closed in a plastic bag for at least 30 days until all the nits and eggs have died.
• Instruct the patient and his family on the use of the creams, lotions, powders, and shampoos that can eliminate lice. Teach them how to remove nits from the hair with a fine-toothed comb and how to use a cotton-tipped applicator to remove lice from eyelashes.
• Instruct the patient in the proper application of lindane, which can be absorbed by the skin and cause CNS complications. Tell the patient to be alert for possible adverse

reactions to treatment and to notify the doctor if these occur.

FOLLICULAR AND GLANDULAR DISORDERS

Because they affect appearance, follicular and glandular disorders can cause extreme anxiety. Treating patients with these disorders, which include acne vulgaris, alopecia, and rosacea, means providing reassurance and supportive care.

ACNE VULGARIS
An inflammatory disease of the skin glands and hair follicles, acne vulgaris is characterized by comedones, pustules, nodules, and nodular lesions. This disorder affects nearly 75% of adolescents, although lesions can appear as early as age 8. Boys are affected more often and more severely, but acne occurs in girls at an earlier age and tends to affect them for a longer time, sometimes into adulthood. It tends to run in families. With treatment, the prognosis is good.

Causes
Many factors cause acne. Research now centers on hormonal dysfunction and oversecretion of sebum as possible primary causes.

Acne flare-ups may be associated with the monthly menstrual cycle, stress, trauma, tropical climates, and rubbing from tight clothing. Flare-ups also may be associated with environmental exposure to coal tar derivatives, certain chemicals, cosmetics, or hair pomades.

Certain medications are linked to acne. These include oral contraceptives containing norethindrone and norgestrel; testosterone; anabolic agents; corticotropin; gonadotropins; corticosteroids (prolonged use); iodine- or bromine-containing drugs; trimethadione; phenytoin; isoniazid; lithium; and halothane.

Theories regarding dietary influences (including the nearly universally held "chocolate causes acne" theory) appear to be groundless.

Complications
In severe cases, acne may develop into a deep cystic process with interconnecting channels, gross inflammation, abscess formation, and secondary bacterial infections. Chronic recurring lesions produce distinctive acne scars.

Assessment findings

Patient history may disclose predisposing factors and seasonal or monthly eruption patterns. Additionally, the history may include pain and tenderness around the area of the infected follicle.

Inspection reveals acne lesions, most commonly on the face, neck, shoulders, chest, and upper back. The area around the infected follicle may appear red and swollen. The acne plug itself may appear as a closed comedo, or whitehead (if it doesn't protrude from the follicle and is covered by the epidermis), or as an open comedo, or blackhead (if it does protrude and isn't covered by the epidermis). A blackhead's coloration results from the melanin or pigment of the follicle.

The rupture or leakage of an enlarged plug into the dermis produces inflammation and characteristic acne pustules, papules or, in severe forms, acne cysts or abscesses. If the patient has previously picked or squeezed the lesions, scars may be visible.

Diagnostic tests

The presence of characteristic lesions, predisposing factors, and scarring confirms the diagnosis of acne vulgaris.

Treatment

Common therapy for acne includes benzoyl peroxide (a powerful antibacterial), either alone or in combination with isotretinoin (retinoic acid or topical vitamin A), a keratolytic. Topical antibiotics, such as erythromycin, meclocycline sulfosalicylate, co-trimoxazole, and tetracycline, have antibacterial and anti-inflammatory effects. Systemic antibiotics, such as tetracycline, minocycline, clindamycin, and systemic retinoids, are used to decrease bacterial growth until the patient is in remission; a lower dose is used for long-term maintenance. Exacerbation of pustules or abscesses during either type of antibiotic therapy requires a culture to identify a possible secondary bacterial infection.

Oral isotretinoin combats acne by inhibiting sebaceous gland function and keratinization. Because of severe adverse reactions, however, the 16- to 20-week course of isotretinoin is limited to patients with severe papulopustular or cystic acne or to those who don't respond to conventional therapy. Because this drug is known to cause birth defects, the manufacturer, with Food and Drug Administration approval, recommends the following precautions: pregnancy testing before dispensing; dispensing only a 30-day supply; repeat pregnancy testing throughout the treatment period; effective contraception during treatment; and informed consent of the patient or parents regarding the danger of the drug. A serum triglyceride level should be drawn before therapy with isotretinoin begins and at intervals throughout its course.

Female patients may benefit from the administration of estrogens to inhibit androgen activity. Improvement rarely occurs before 2 to 4 months, and exacerbations may follow discontinuation of the therapy. Nevertheless, this treatment is preferred to the use of isotretinoin.

Other treatments for acne vulgaris include intralesional corticosteroid injections, exposure to ultraviolet light (but never when a photosensitizing agent, such as isotretinoin, is being used), cryotherapy, and surgery.

Nursing diagnoses

- Body image disturbance
- Impaired skin integrity
- Knowledge deficit
- Risk for infection
- Situational low self-esteem

Nursing interventions

- Assist the patient in identifying and eliminating predisposing factors.
- Encourage good personal hygiene and the use of oil-free skin care products. Discourage picking or squeezing the lesions, to eliminate secondary bacterial infections and scarring.
- Monitor liver function studies and serum triglyceride levels.
- Be alert for possible complications associated with treatment with systemic antibiotics (such as tetracycline), including sensitivity reactions, GI disturbances, and liver dysfunction.
- Remember that tetracycline is contraindicated during pregnancy because it will discolor the fetus's unerupted teeth.
- Be alert for possible adverse reactions associated with the use of isotretinoin, including possible skin irritation, dry skin and mucous membranes, and elevated triglyceride levels.
- Encourage the patient with acne to verbalize his feelings, including embarrassment, fear of rejection by others, and body image disturbances. Note the importance of body image in growth and development. Encourage him to develop interests that support a positive self-image and de-emphasize appearance.

Patient teaching

• Explain the causes of acne to the patient and his family. Encourage the patient to seek medical treatment when acne develops.

• Make sure the patient and his family understand that the prescribed treatment will improve acne more than a strict diet or fanatic scrubbing with soap and water. Dispel myths concerning the influence of diet and sexual activity on the development of acne.

• Provide written instructions regarding treatment. Instruct the patient receiving isotretinoin to apply it at least 30 minutes after washing the face and at least 1 hour before bedtime. Warn against using it around the eyes or lips. Explain that after treatments, the skin should look pink and dry, and that some amount of peeling is normal in the morning when isotretinoin has been applied at night. Tell the patient that if the skin appears irritated, the preparation may have to be weakened or applied less often. Advise the patient to avoid exposure to sunlight while wearing the solution or to use a sunscreen.

• If the prescribed regimen includes isotretinoin and benzoyl peroxide, advise the patient to avoid skin irritation by using one preparation in the morning and the other at night. Also advise the patient that acne commonly flares up during the early course of treatment, probably because of the uncovering of early, developing lesions.

• Instruct the patient to take tetracycline on an empty stomach. Advise him not to take tetracycline with antacids or milk because it interacts with their metallic ions and then is poorly absorbed.

• Tell the patient taking isotretinoin to avoid vitamin A supplements, which can worsen any adverse effects. Warn the patient against giving blood during treatment with this drug and to avoid alcohol ingestion. Also teach him how to deal with the dry skin and mucous membranes that usually occur during treatment. Instruct the female patient on the severe risk of teratogenicity. Encourage the patient to schedule and follow up with the necessary laboratory studies.

• Teach the patient and his family techniques to maintain a well-balanced diet, get adequate rest, and manage stress.

• Inform the patient that acne takes a long time—in some cases, years—to clear. Encourage continued local skin care even after acne clears.

ALOPECIA

More commonly known as hair loss, alopecia typically occurs on the scalp; hair loss elsewhere on the body is less common and less conspicuous. In the nonscarring form of this disorder (noncicatricial alopecia), the hair follicle can generally regrow hair. Scarring alopecia usually destroys the hair follicle, making hair loss irreversible.

The most common form of nonscarring alopecia is male-pattern alopecia. Female-pattern alopecia involves diffuse thinning over the top of the scalp. Genetic predisposition commonly influences the time of onset, the degree of baldness, the speed with which it spreads, and the pattern of hair loss.

Other forms of nonscarring alopecia include:

• *physiologic alopecia,* a sudden (usually temporary) hair loss in infants, a loss of straight hairline in adolescents, and a diffuse hair loss in women after childbirth

• *alopecia areata* (idiopathic form), a generally reversible and self-limiting disorder most prevalent in young and middle-aged adults of both sexes

• *trichotillomania,* the compulsive pulling out of one's own hair, most commonly found in children and adolescents.

Causes

Male-pattern alopecia appears to be related to androgen levels and to aging. Predisposing factors of nonscarring alopecia also include radiation, chemotherapy, many types of drug therapies and drug reactions, bacterial and fungal infections, psoriasis, seborrhea, and endocrine disorders, such as thyroid, parathyroid, and pituitary dysfunctions. (See *Cancer drugs that cause alopecia,* page 1176.) Excessive vitamin A can also cause alopecia.

Scarring alopecia may result from physical or chemical trauma, radiation or chemotherapy, or chronic tension on a hair shaft, such as braiding or rolling the hair. Diseases that produce scarring alopecia include destructive skin tumors, granulomas, lupus erythematosus, scleroderma, follicular lichen planus, and severe bacterial or viral infections, such as folliculitis and herpes simplex.

Complications

Although hair loss has no physiologic complications, it can impair the patient's self-image.

Assessment findings

In male-pattern alopecia, the history reveals predisposing factors and a family history. It also usually reveals a gradual onset of hair loss. The male patient typically describes his hairline as receding and his crown becoming bald. The female patient describes a widening of her part and increasing visibility of her front scalp or crown.

CANCER DRUGS THAT CAUSE ALOPECIA

In cancer chemotherapy, certain drugs can cause hair loss, ranging from sporadic thinning to complete baldness. Some drugs damage hair follicles and cause hair roots to atrophy.

Mild alopecia
- bleomycin (Blenoxane)
- carmustine (BiCNU)
- fluorouracil (5-FU)
- hydroxyurea (Hydrea)
- melphalan (Alkeran)

Moderate alopecia
- busulfan (Myleran)
- etoposide (VP-16)
- floxuridine (FUDR)
- methotrexate (Folex)
- mitomycin (Mutamycin)

Severe alopecia
- cyclophosphamide (Cytoxan)
- daunorubicin (Cerubidine)
- doxorubicin (Adriamycin)
- vinblastine (Velban)
- vincristine (Oncovin)

In alopecia areata, the history includes a sudden loss of hair. Inspection may reveal small patches of visible scalp or may show the entire scalp affected (alopecia totalis) or the entire body (alopecia universalis). Although mild erythema may occur initially, affected areas of scalp or skin appear normal. "Exclamation point" hairs (loose hairs with dark, rough, brushlike tips on narrow, less pigmented shafts) occur at the periphery of new patches. Regrowth initially appears as fine, white, downy hair, which is replaced by normal hair.

In trichotillomania, patchy and incomplete areas of hair loss with many broken hairs appear on the scalp but also may occur on other areas, such as the eyebrows.

Diagnostic tests
• *Pluck or pull test* may confirm alopecia. (In this test, the doctor firmly and smoothly tugs a group of 8 to 10 hairs; if more than 4 hairs come out, the patient probably has alopecia.)
• *Microscopic analysis,* performed if the pluck or pull test is positive, determines structural abnormalities or signs of infection.
• *Wood's lamp examination* identifies fungal infection. If infected areas glow or fluoresce, the test is positive. The scalp may then be scraped lightly and the scraping viewed under a microscope.
• *Trichogram* determines the ratio of anagen to telogen hairs to evaluate the severity and predict the course of hair loss.
• *Biopsy* helps to determine the cause of alopecia by pinpointing hair phase and the extent of structural damage.

Diagnosis also must identify any underlying disorder.

Treatment
Topical application of minoxidil has limited success in treating male-pattern and female-pattern alopecia. An alternate treatment is surgical redistribution of hair follicles by autografting. In alopecia areata, minoxidil is more effective, although treatment often is unnecessary because spontaneous regrowth is common.

Corticosteroids, such as betamethasone dipropionate, halcinonide, and triamcinolone acetonide, in topical form or by intralesional injections, may help to stimulate hair growth if hair loss is confined to small patches; this therapy may produce regrowth in 4 to 6 weeks. Hair loss that persists for more than 1 year has a poor prognosis for regrowth.

Other drug therapy may include photochemotherapy with methoxsalen and ultraviolet light; dermatomucosal agents, such as anthralin; antibiotics for bacterial infections; and antifungal agents for fungal infections.

Chemotherapy patients may benefit from procedures that reduce the blood supply to the scalp and thereby preserve more hair structure. These procedures — cold cap application and scalp tourniquet — aren't appropriate for patients with leukemia, lymphoma, or highly metastatic tumors because cancer drugs must be allowed to perfuse the scalp area to irradiate these neoplastic cells.

For some patients, hair transplantation and tunnel grafting or cosmetic interventions (hairpieces, weaving, or bonding) are beneficial.

In trichotillomania, an occlusive dressing promotes normal hair growth by protecting the site of hair loss. The treatment for other types of alopecia varies according to the underlying cause.

Nursing diagnoses
• Body image disturbance
• Risk for impaired skin integrity
• Risk for infection
• Situational low self-esteem

Nursing interventions

• Reassure the patient with female-pattern alopecia that hair thinning doesn't lead to total baldness. Suggest that she use a wig or hairpiece.
• For the patient undergoing radiation therapy or chemotherapy with drugs that cause alopecia, suggest selecting a hair replacement before treatment.
• Encourage the patient to express his feelings. Help him develop interests that contribute to a positive self-image.

Patient teaching

• Remember to explain the familial link in male-pattern alopecia.
• Inform the patient that a well-balanced diet with adequate protein promotes healthy hair. If alopecia results from excessive vitamin A, advise the patient to avoid vitamin A supplements.
• Tell the patient that commercial preparations won't restore or promote hair growth.
• If the patient is receiving topical minoxidil, inform him that 40% of patients report moderate to dense hair growth after 1 year of regular treatment. Caution him that results may not become apparent for 4 or more months. Explain the proper use of the drug, and point out that increasing the dose or the frequency of treatment won't increase the rate of hair growth. Describe possible adverse reactions, and advise him to notify the doctor if they occur.
• Instruct the patient receiving corticosteroids to report signs and symptoms of skin infection, such as redness; pus-filled blisters; pain, burning, itching, or peeling; numbness in the fingers; weight gain, facial puffiness; thinning skin with bruising; and any new hair loss.
• Advise the patient with alopecia caused by chemotherapy that hair may grow back in a different color or type, such as curly or straight.

ROSACEA

A chronic skin eruption, rosacea produces flushing and dilation of small blood vessels in the face, especially the nose and cheeks. Papules and pustules also may appear, but without the characteristic comedones of acne vulgaris.

Rosacea is most common in white women between ages 30 and 50. However, when the disorder affects men, it strikes with greater severity and is commonly associated with rhinophyma, which is characterized by dilated follicles and thickened, bulbous skin on the nose. Rosacea usually spreads slowly and seldom subsides spontaneously.

Causes

Rosacea's cause is unknown, but stress, infection, vitamin deficiency, and endocrine abnormalities can aggravate this condition. Anything that produces flushing—for example, hot beverages, such as tea or coffee; tobacco; alcohol; spicy foods; physical activity; sunlight; and extreme heat or cold—also can aggravate rosacea.

Complications

Ocular involvement may result in blepharitis, conjunctivitis, uveitis, or keratitis.

Assessment findings

The patient history reveals predisposing factors or exposure to conditions that aggravate rosacea. On inspection, you'll see a blush area on the cheeks, nose, forehead, and chin, usually beginning across the central oval of the face. Redness, intermittent at first, later becomes permanent. Telangiectasia may be present, along with pustules and papules.

Although rhinophyma commonly accompanies severe rosacea, it may occur alone. It usually appears first on the lower half of the nose and produces red, thickened skin and follicular enlargement.

Diagnostic tests

Rosacea is confirmed by the presence of typical vascular and acneiform lesions without the comedones characteristically associated with acne vulgaris and, in severe cases, by rhinophyma.

Treatment

Oral tetracycline in gradually decreasing doses as symptoms subside treats the acneiform component of rosacea. Topical application of 1% hydrocortisone cream reduces erythema and inflammation. Other treatment may include electrolysis to destroy large, dilated blood vessels and removal of excess tissue in patients with rhinophyma.

Nursing diagnoses

• Body image disturbance
• High risk for infection
• Impaired skin integrity
• Knowledge deficit
• Situational low self-esteem

Nursing interventions

• Be alert for possible sensitivity reactions and GI disturbances that may accompany treatment with systemic antibiotics.

• Encourage the patient to express her feelings. Offer emotional support and reassurance.

Patient teaching
• Assist the patient in identifying and eliminating aggravating factors. If stress and anxiety seem to trigger the disease, teach relaxation techniques and encourage her to use them often.
• Instruct the patient to use meticulous hand washing and personal hygiene to avoid irritating and aggravating the condition. To prevent infection, stress the importance of not picking or squeezing the lesions.
• Provide directions for antibiotic therapy, and tell the patient to report any adverse reactions.

DISORDERS OF PIGMENTATION

Characterized by a loss or change of skin pigment, disorders of pigmentation include albinism, vitiligo, melasma, and photosensitivity reactions.

ALBINISM
An inherited disorder, albinism results from a defect in melanin metabolism of the skin and eyes (oculocutaneous albinism) or just the eyes (ocular albinism). Ocular albinism impairs visual acuity. Oculocutaneous albinism also causes severe intolerance to sunlight and heightens susceptibility to skin cancer in exposed areas.

Causes and pathophysiology
Oculocutaneous albinism results from an autosomal recessive trait; ocular albinism from an X-linked recessive trait that causes hypopigmentation only in the iris and the ocular fundus.

Normally, melanocytes (pigment cells) synthesize melanin. Melanosomes, melanin-containing granules within melanocytes, diffuse and absorb the sun's ultraviolet light, thus protecting the skin and eyes from its dangerous effects.

In tyrosinase-negative oculocutaneous albinism (most common), melanosomes don't contain melanin because they lack tyrosinase, the enzyme that stimulates melanin production. In tyrosinase-positive oculocutaneous albinism, melanosomes contain tyrosine, a tyrosinase substrate, but a defect in the tyrosine transport system impairs melanin production. In tyrosinase-variable albinism (rare), an unidentified enzyme defect probably impairs synthesis of a melanin precursor.

Tyrosinase-negative albinism affects about 1 in every 34,000 persons in the United States and strikes whites and blacks equally. Tyrosinase-positive albinism strikes more blacks than whites. Native Americans have a high incidence of both forms.

Complications
Lack of pigmentation in the eyes may result in nystagmus, photosensitivity, and errors of refraction. Some patients develop pigmented nevi, which require surgical removal. Other complications include actinic keratosis and increased susceptibility to skin cancer.

Assessment findings
The family history will reveal albinism. In light-skinned white patients with tyrosinase-negative albinism, inspection shows pale skin, hair that's white to yellow, and pupils that appear red because of translucent irides. Blacks with the same disorder have hair that may be white, faintly tinged with yellow, or yellow-brown. Both whites and blacks with tyrosinase-positive albinism grow darker as they age. For instance, their hair may become straw-colored or light brown and their skin cream-colored or pink. Inspection of patients with tyrosinase-positive albinism may reveal freckles and pigmented nevi that may require excision.

Diagnostic tests
• *Microscopic examination* of the skin and of hair follicles determines the amount of pigment present.
• *Pigmentation testing* of plucked hair roots by incubating them in tyrosinase distinguishes tyrosinase-negative albinism from tyrosinase-positive albinism. Tyrosinase-positive hair bulbs will develop color.

Treatment
No treatment exists. Therapy consists of preventive measures to avoid skin damage from sunlight and supportive measures to help the patient and family cope with social and emotional problems.

Nursing diagnoses
• Body image disturbance
• Defensive coping
• Knowledge deficit
• Risk for impaired skin integrity
• Situational low self-esteem

Nursing interventions
• Encourage the patient to express his concerns about body image. Answer his questions, and stay with him

during periods of anxiety. Discuss his embarrassment and fear of rejection by others.

• Offer emotional support and reassurance. Help the patient develop interests that support a positive self-image and de-emphasize appearance.

• If the patient and family experience difficulty adjusting to the patient's appearance, advise them to seek counseling to develop effective coping strategies.

Patient teaching

• Advise the patient to wear full-spectrum sunblocks, dark glasses, and appropriate protective clothing when exposed to sunlight.

• Inform him of cosmetic measures (glasses with tinted lenses, makeup) that can alter his appearance.

• Stress the need for frequent refractions and eye examinations to correct visual defects.

• Advise the family that genetic counseling can provide information about the probability of albinism's recurrence in future offspring.

VITILIGO

Marked by stark-white skin patches that may cause a serious cosmetic problem, vitiligo results from the destruction and loss of melanocytes (pigment cells). This condition affects about 1% of the U.S. population, usually people between ages 10 and 30, with peak incidence around age 20. It shows no racial preference, but the distinctive patches are most prominent in blacks. Vitiligo doesn't favor either sex; however, women tend to seek treatment more often than men. Repigmentation therapy may necessitate several summers of exposure to sunlight; the effects of this treatment may be temporary.

Causes

The cause of vitiligo is unknown; however, one theory implicates an autoimmune process that destroys existing melanocytes. Even at the periphery of lesions, melanocytes appear abnormal and in various stages of cell demise. However, melanocytes may migrate from residual areas, such as hair follicles, and repigment lesions.

Other theories implicate enzymatic self-destructing mechanisms and abnormal neurogenic stimuli. Heredity may play a role: About 30% of patients with vitiligo have family members with the same condition.

Some link exists between vitiligo and several other disorders that it commonly accompanies—thyroid dysfunction, pernicious anemia, Addison's disease, aseptic meningitis, diabetes mellitus, photophobia, hearing defects, alopecia areata, and halo nevi.

The most common precipitating factor is a stressful physical or psychological event, such as severe sunburn, surgery, pregnancy, loss of a job, or bereavement. Chemical agents, such as phenols and catechols, may also cause this condition.

Complications

Common complications include extreme photosensitivity in depigmented areas. Patients may also develop hypersensitivity reactions to therapeutic agents and to the dyes or cosmetics used to camouflage the lesions.

Assessment findings

The family history may reveal vitiligo as well as a precipitating factor. Inspection may find depigmented or stark-white skin patches that are almost imperceptible on fair-skinned whites. These patches usually are bilaterally symmetrical, with distinct borders that may be raised and hyperpigmented. You'll probably note these patches over bony prominences, around orifices (eyes, mouth), within body folds, and at sites of traumatic injury. The hair within these lesions may also be white. Because hair follicles and certain eye parts also contain melanocytes, your inspection may reveal prematurely gray hair and ocular pigment changes.

Diagnostic tests

In fair-skinned patients, Wood's light examination in a darkened room detects vitiliginous patches: Depigmented skin reflects the light, whereas pigmented skin absorbs it. If autoimmune or endocrine disorders are suspected, laboratory studies are appropriate. Other skin disorders, such as tinea versicolor, must be ruled out.

Treatment

Repigmentation therapy combines systemic or topical psoralen compounds, or both, with exposure to sunlight or artificial ultraviolet-A (UVA) light. New pigment rises from hair follicles and appears on the skin as small freckles, which gradually enlarge and coalesce. Body parts that contain few hair follicles (such as the fingertips) may resist this therapy.

Because psoralens and UVA affect the entire skin surface, systemic therapy enhances the contrast between normal skin, which turns darker than usual, and white, vitiliginous skin. The use of sunscreen on normal skin may minimize the contrast while preventing sunburn.

Depigmentation therapy is suggested for patients with vitiligo that affects more than 50% of the body surface. A cream containing 20% monobenzone permanently destroys melanocytes in unaffected skin areas and produces a uniform skin tone. This medication is applied initially to a small area of normal skin once daily to test for unfavorable reactions. If no such reactions occur, the patient begins applying the cream twice daily to those areas he wants to depigment first. Eventually, the entire skin may be depigmented to achieve a uniform color. Depigmentation is permanent and results in extreme photosensitivity.

Commercial cosmetics may help de-emphasize vitiliginous skin. Some patients prefer dyes because these remain on the skin for several days.

Nursing diagnoses
• Body image disturbance
• Knowledge deficit
• Risk for impaired skin integrity
• Situational low self-esteem

Nursing interventions
• Encourage the patient to express his feelings about his appearance. Offer emotional support and reassurance, but avoid promoting unrealistic hope for a total cure.

Patient teaching
• Explain the disorder to the patient and answer his questions.
• In repigmentation therapy, instruct the patient to use psoralen medications three or four times weekly. (*Note:* Systemic psoralens should be taken 2 hours before exposure to sun; topical solutions should be applied 30 to 60 minutes before exposure.)
• Remind patients undergoing repigmentation therapy that exposure to sunlight also darkens normal skin. After being exposed to UVA for the prescribed amount of time, the patient should apply a sunscreen if he plans to be exposed to sunlight also. If sunburn occurs, advise the patient to discontinue the therapy temporarily and to apply open wet dressings (using thin sheeting) to affected areas for 15 to 20 minutes, four or five times daily or as necessary for comfort. After applying wet dressings, the patient should allow the skin to air dry. Suggest that he apply a soothing lubricating cream or lotion while the skin is still slightly moist.
• Suggest that the patient receiving depigmentation therapy wear protective clothing and use a sunscreen (SPF 15). Explain the therapy thoroughly, and allow the patient plenty of time to decide whether to undergo this treatment. Make sure he understands that the results of depigmentation are permanent and that he must thereafter protect his skin from the adverse effects of sunlight.

• Warn the patient to use a sunscreen (no less than SPF 8) to protect both affected and normal skin during exposure to sun and to wear sunglasses after taking the medication. If periorbital areas require exposure, tell the patient to keep his eyes closed during treatment.
• Caution the patient about buying commercial cosmetics or dyes without trying them first because some may not be suitable.

MELASMA
A patchy, hypermelanotic skin disorder, melasma poses a serious cosmetic problem. Although it tends to occur equally in all races, the light-brown color characteristic of melasma is most visible on dark-skinned whites. Also called chloasma or mask of pregnancy, melasma affects women more often than men; it may be chronic but is never life-threatening.

Causes
The cause of melasma is unknown. Histologically, hyperpigmentation results from increased melanin production, although the number of melanocytes remains normal. Melasma may be related to the increased hormonal levels associated with pregnancy, ovarian cancer, and the use of oral contraceptives. Progestational agents, phenytoin, and mephenytoin may also contribute to this disorder. Exposure to sunlight stimulates melasma, but the condition may develop without any apparent predisposing factor.

Complications
Untreated melasma produces no complications.

Assessment findings
The patient history may reveal predisposing factors. Inspection may show large, brown, irregular patches symmetrically distributed on the forehead, cheeks, and sides of the nose. You may also note patches on the patient's neck, upper lip, and temples, although these occur less commonly.

Diagnostic tests
Observation of characteristic dark patches on the face usually confirms melasma.

Treatment
The primary treatment is the application of a bleaching agent containing 2% to 4% hydroquinone to inhibit melanin synthesis. This medication is applied twice daily for up to 8 weeks. Adjunctive measures include avoiding

exposure to sunlight, using sunscreens, and discontinuing oral contraceptives.

Nursing diagnoses
• Body image disturbance
• Knowledge deficit
• Situational low self-esteem

Nursing interventions
• Help the patient identify and eliminate predisposing factors.
• Encourage the patient to express her feelings about her body image, including any feelings of embarrassment or fear of rejection. Offer reassurance when appropriate.

Patient teaching
• Advise the patient to avoid exposure to the sun by using sunscreens and wearing protective clothing.
• Inform the patient that bleaching agents may help mask melasma but may require repeated treatments to maintain the desired effect.
• Mention that cosmetics also may help mask deep pigmentation.
• Make sure the patient knows the proper method of applying bleaching agents and the possible adverse effects associated with them (erythema, stinging, or other sensitivity reactions). Advise her to call the doctor if such reactions occur and persist.
• Reassure the patient that melasma is treatable. It may fade spontaneously with protection from sunlight, postpartum, and after discontinuing oral contraceptives. Serial photographs help show the patient that patches are improving.

PHOTOSENSITIVITY REACTIONS
An adverse reaction to natural or artificial light or to light and certain chemicals (including some medications) characterizes photosensitivity reactions. The most common reaction is sunburn, which is dose-related. The other two types include phototoxic reactions, which are also dose-related, and photoallergic reactions, which are uncommon and not dose-related — even slight exposure can cause a severe reaction.

Causes
Sunburn results from unprotected exposure to the sun's ultraviolet rays. (See *How ultraviolet rays damage the skin.*)

A phototoxic reaction results from exposure to sunlight teamed with certain medications — such as anti-

HOW ULTRAVIOLET RAYS DAMAGE THE SKIN

Unprotected exposure to the sun's rays can damage the skin in several ways.

Superficial skin damage
The sun's UVB rays penetrate superficial skin, causing the outermost layer to burn, blister, dry, and peel. These rays also change and darken the protective melanin in epidermal cells. In response to the damage, blood volume in the area increases, resulting in red, swollen, sore skin that's painful to the touch.

Connective tissue damage
Meanwhile, UVA rays penetrate deeper into connective tissue, damaging the proteins that keep the skin flexible and youthful looking. These rays may also inhibit the enzymes necessary to repair the cells damaged by UVB rays, contributing to skin cancer.

Further damage
Eventually, ultraviolet rays cause further skin changes, including loss of elasticity and a diminished vascular network. The result: thick, wrinkled skin at best and skin cancer at worst.

histamines and antimicrobials — or chemicals — such as dyes, coal tar, and furocoumarin compounds found in plants. Even certain foods (such as celery, parsnips, carrots, and limes) that touch the patient's skin while he's in the sun can cause a phototoxic reaction. Berlock dermatitis, a specific photosensitivity reaction, results from the use of oil of bergamot — a common component of perfumes, colognes, and pomades.

A photoallergic reaction is an immune response that can arise after even slight exposure to light.

Risk factors associated with photosensitivity include:
• outdoor occupation
• outdoor life-style
• youth or age
• certain environmental factors (high altitude or proximity to equator)
• decreased ozone layer density.

Complications
Repeated photosensitivity reactions, mainly sunburn, may eventually cause premature aging of the skin (wrinkling and a dry, leathery appearance) and skin cancer. The burning and itching that accompany a photosensi-

CATEGORIZING PHOTOSENSITIVITY

The American Academy of Dermatology categorizes photosensitivity by skin types that range from I to VI. A patient with fair, sensitive skin has skin type I; a patient with dark, insensitive skin has skin type VI. Use the following chart to estimate your patient's photosensitivity. Then follow this rule of thumb for choosing sunscreens with numbered sun protection factors: The fairer the patient's skin, the higher the sun protection factor needed.

Skin type	Sun exposure history
I	Always burns, never tans; extremely sensitive skin
II	Always burns easily, tans slightly; very sensitive skin
III	Sometimes burns, tans gradually to light brown; sensitive skin
IV	Burns slightly, always tans to moderate brown; minimally sensitive skin
V	Rarely burns, tans well; insensitive skin
VI	Never burns, deep pigmentation; insensitive skin

tivity reaction may cause scratching, which can lead to skin breaks and secondary bacterial infections.

Assessment findings

The sunburned patient typically reports recent exposure to ultraviolet rays and may complain of burning and itching in sun-exposed areas. Inspection may reveal skin redness, swelling, blistering, and peeling.

In a phototoxic reaction, the patient may report that immediately after exposure to an allergen or toxic compound, he felt a burning sensation followed by erythema, edema, desquamation, and hyperpigmentation. In Berlock dermatitis, the patient may describe an acute reaction that produced erythematous vesicles that later became hyperpigmented.

Photoallergic reactions may take one of two forms. In polymorphous light eruption, the patient may report that he began developing signs and symptoms 2 to 5 hours after sun exposure. Inspection of the skin may reveal erythema, papules, vesicles, urticara, and eczematous lesions; pruritus may persist for 1 to 2 weeks. In solar urticaria, the patient may report that his skin began to itch and burn after only a few minutes' exposure to the sun and that the symptoms lasted about an hour. Inspection of the skin after that time may reveal erythema and wheals.

Diagnostic tests

• *Photopatch test* for ultraviolet-A and -B (UVA and UVB) rays may aid diagnosis and identify the causative light wavelength.
• *Skin punch biopsy* will help to diagnose skin damage resulting from the sun.

Other studies must rule out connective tissue disease, such as lupus erythematosus and porphyrias.

Treatment

For many photosensitive patients, treatment focuses on prevention by using a sunscreen, wearing protective clothing, and limiting exposure to sunlight. (See *Categorizing photosensitivity*.) For other patients, progressive exposure to sunlight can thicken the skin and produce a tan that interferes with photoallergens and prevents further eruptions.

PUVA (psoralen and UVA) may be used to treat polymorphous light eruption. Treatment for solar urticaria may also require PUVA. Although hyperpigmentation usually fades in several months, hydroquinone preparations can hasten the process.

Nursing diagnoses

• Body image disturbance
• Knowledge deficit
• Risk for fluid volume deficit
• Risk for impaired skin integrity
• Risk for infection

Nursing interventions

• Help the patient identify possible causative agents.
• Discourage picking, squeezing, or scratching of skin lesions to prevent secondary bacterial infection.
• Apply cool, moist compresses to provide relief from itching and burning.
• Be alert for adverse reactions associated with PUVA treatment, such as localized burning, pruritus, nausea, and squamous cell epitheliomas. Applying hydroquinone preparations to hyperpigmented areas may also cause skin irritation and burning.

• Encourage the patient to express his feelings about his body image and other concerns.

Patient teaching
• Teach the patient to check his skin frequently for signs of skin cancer. Tell him to report any mole that has changed in color, size, or shape; any mole with irregular borders; any persistent, waxy lumps or rough, red patches; or any sore that won't heal.
• Encourage the patient to drink plenty of fluids whenever he's in the sun and anytime he has a sunburn to replenish fluid lost through perspiration and dehydration.
• Provide written instructions for the use of PUVA and hydroquinone preparations.
• Explain the different types of sunscreens and their degree of protection, and help the patient choose an appropriate sunscreen. Advise him to pick one that protects against both UVA and UVB radiation and that contains para-aminobenzoic acid (PABA) or a PABA substitute (benzophenone, cinnamate, and salicylate). Explain that this ingredient offers the best protection against skin damage and skin cancer.
• Encourage the patient to limit his amount of sun exposure between 10 a.m. and 3 p.m. If he must be in the sun during these hours, suggest that he wear protective clothing, such as long-sleeved shirts and long pants of tightly woven, dark fabrics.

INFLAMMATORY REACTION

Characterized by redness, swelling, and itching of the skin, an inflammatory reaction may be short-lived or may lead to scarring and other permanent skin changes.

DERMATITIS
Marked by inflammation of the skin, dermatitis can be acute or chronic and occurs in several forms, including contact, seborrheic, nummular, exfoliative, and stasis dermatitides. (See *Types of dermatitis,* pages 1184 to 1186.)

Atopic dermatitis (discussed here), also commonly referred to as atopic or infantile eczema, neurodermatitis constitutionalis, or Besnier's prurigo, is a chronic inflammatory response often associated with other atopic diseases, such as bronchial asthma, allergic rhinitis, and chronic urticaria. It usually develops in infants and toddlers between ages 6 months and 2 years, commonly in

those with strong family histories of atopic disease. These children typically acquire other atopic disorders as they grow older. In most cases, this form of dermatitis subsides spontaneously by age 3 and remains in remission until prepuberty (ages 10 to 12), when it flares up again. The disorder affects about 9 out of every 1,000 persons.

Causes
Although the exact cause of atopic dermatitis is unknown, several theories attempt to explain its pathogenesis. One theory suggests an underlying metabolically or biochemically induced skin disorder, genetically linked to elevated serum immunoglobulin E (IgE) levels. Another theory suggests defective T-cell function.

Atopic dermatitis is exacerbated by certain irritants, infections (commonly *Staphylococcus aureus*), and allergens. Common allergens include pollen, wool, silk, fur, ointment, detergent, perfume, and certain foods, particularly wheat, milk, and eggs. Flare-ups may occur in response to temperature extremes, humidity, sweating, and stress.

Complications
Without proper treatment, dermatitis can cause permanent skin damage, including lichenification (thickening and hardening of the skin with exaggerated normal markings), altered pigmentation, and scarring. Uncontrolled atopic dermatitis increases the patient's susceptibility to bacterial, fungal, and viral infections. In turn, certain viral infections, such as vaccinia and herpes simplex, can lead to Kaposi's varicelliform eruption, which can be fatal.

Assessment findings
The patient history typically reveals a family history of atopic dermatitis as well as exposure to an allergen or irritant. The patient typically complains of intense itching.

Early in the course of atopic dermatitis, inspection of the skin may reveal erythematous patches in excessively dry areas. In children, look for these lesions on the forehead, cheeks, and extensor surfaces of the arms and legs; in adults, look at flexion points (antecubital fossa, popliteal area, and neck). During a flare-up, you may note edema, scaling, and vesiculation because of scratching; the vesicles may be pus-filled. In chronic disease, you may observe multiple areas of dry, scaly skin, with white dermatographism, blanching, and lichenification.

The distribution of skin lesions in atopic dermatitis rules out other inflammatory skin lesions, such as diaper

(Text continues on page 1186.)

TYPES OF DERMATITIS

Type	Causes	Assessment findings	Diagnosis	Treatment and intervention
Chronic dermatitis Characterized by inflammatory eruptions of the hands and feet	• Usually unknown but may result from progressive contact dermatitis • Secondary factors: trauma, infections, redistribution of normal flora, photosensitivity, and food sensitivity, which may perpetuate this condition	• Thick, lichenified, single or multiple lesions on any part of the body (commonly on the hands) • Inflammation and scaling • Recurrence after long remissions	• No characteristic pattern or course; diagnosis based on detailed history and physical findings	• Elimination of known allergens and decreased exposure to irritants; wearing protective clothing, such as gloves; and washing immediately after contact with irritants or allergens • Antibiotics for secondary infection • Avoidance of excessive washing and drying of hands, and of accumulation of soaps and detergents under rings • Use of emollients with topical steroids
Contact dermatitis Often sharply demarcated skin inflammation and irritation due to contact with concentrated substances to which the skin is sensitive, such as perfumes or chemicals	• Mild irritants: chronic exposure to detergents or solvents • Strong irritants: damage on contact with acids or alkalis • Allergens: sensitization after repeated exposure	• Mild irritants and allergens: erythema and small vesicles that ooze, scale, and itch • Strong irritants: blisters and ulcerations • Classic allergic response: clearly defined lesions, with straight lines following points of contact • Severe allergic reaction: marked edema of affected areas	• Patient history • Patch testing to identify allergens • Shape and distribution of lesions	• Same as for chronic dermatitis • Topical anti-inflammatory agents (including steroids), systemic steroids for edema and bullae, antihistamines, and local applications of Burow's solution (for blisters) • Other nursing interventions similar to those for atopic dermatitis
Exfoliative dermatitis Severe, chronic skin inflammation characterized by redness and widespread erythema and scaling	• Progression of preexisting skin lesions to exfoliative stage, as in contact dermatitis, drug reaction, lymphoma, or leukemia	• Generalized dermatitis, with acute loss of stratum corneum, and erythema and scaling • Sensation of tight skin • Hair loss • Possibly fever, sensitivity to cold, shivering, gynecomastia, and lymphadenopathy	• Identification of the underlying cause	• Hospitalization, with protective isolation and hygienic measures to prevent secondary bacterial infection • Open wet dressings, with colloidal baths • Bland lotions over topical steroids • Maintenance of constant environmental temperature to prevent chilling or overheating • Careful monitoring of renal and cardiac status • Systemic antibiotics and steroids • Other nursing interventions similar to those for atopic dermatitis

TYPES OF DERMATITIS *(continued)*

Type	Causes	Assessment findings	Diagnosis	Treatment and intervention
Localized neuro-dermatitis (essential pruritus) Superficial skin inflammation characterized by itching and papular eruptions that appear on thickened, hyperpigmented skin	• Chronic scratching or rubbing of a primary lesion or insect bite, or other skin irritation	• Intense, sometimes continual scratching • Thick, sharp-bordered, possibly dry, scaly lesions, with raised papules • Usually affects easily reached areas, such as ankles, lower legs, anogenital area, back of neck, and ears	• Physical findings	• Fixed dressing or Unna's boot to cover affected area • Topical steroids (occlusive dressings or intralesional injections) • Antihistamines and open wet dressings • Emollients
Nummular dermatitis Chronic form of dermatitis characterized by coin-shaped, vesicular, crusted scales and, possibly, pruritic lesions	• Possibly precipitated by stress; or dryness, irritants, or scratching	• Round, nummular (coin-shaped) lesions, usually on arms and legs, with distinct borders of crusts and scales • Possibly oozing and severe itching • Summertime remissions common, with wintertime recurrence	• Physical findings and patient history; history of atopic dermatitis in middle-aged or older patient • Exclusion of fungal infections, atopic or contact dermatitis, and psoriasis	• Elimination of known irritants • Measures to relieve dry skin: increased humidification; limited frequency of baths and use of bland soap and bath oils; and application of emollients • Wet dressings in acute phase • Topical steroids (occlusive dressings or intralesional injections) for persistent lesions • Tar preparations and antihistamines for itching and antibiotics for secondary infection • Other interventions similar to those for atopic dermatitis
Seborrheic dermatitis An acute or subacute disease that affects the scalp, face, and occasionally other areas and is characterized by lesions covered with yellow or brownish gray scales	• Unknown; stress and neurologic conditions may be predisposing factors	• Eruptions in areas with many sebaceous glands (usually scalp, face, and trunk) and in skin folds • Itching, redness, and inflammation of affected areas; lesions that may appear greasy; possibly fissures • Indistinct, occasionally yellowish scaly patches from excess stratum corneum (dandruff may be a mild seborrheic dermatitis)	• Patient history and physical findings, especially distribution of lesions in sebaceous gland areas • Exclusion of psoriasis	• Removal of scales by frequent washing and shampooing with selenium sulfide suspension (most effective), zinc pyrithione, or tar and salicylic acid shampoo • Application of fluorinated steroids to nonhairy areas

(continued)

TYPES OF DERMATITIS *(continued)*

Type	Causes	Assessment findings	Diagnosis	Treatment and intervention
Stasis dermatitis Condition usually caused by impaired circulation and characterized by eczema of the legs with edema, hyperpigmentation, and persistent inflammation	• Secondary to peripheral vascular diseases affecting legs, such as recurrent thrombophlebitis and resultant chronic venous insufficiency	• Varicosities and edema common, but obvious vascular insufficiency not always present • Usually affects the lower leg, just above internal malleolus, or sites of trauma or irritation • Early signs: dusky red deposits of hemosiderin in skin, with itching and dimpling of subcutaneous tissue; later signs: edema, redness, and scaling of large area of legs • Possibly fissures, crusts, and ulcers	• Positive history of venous insufficiency and physical findings, such as varicosities	• Measures to prevent venous stasis: avoidance of prolonged sitting or standing, use of support stockings, and weight reduction for obese patients • Corrective surgery for underlying cause • After ulcer develops, rest periods with legs elevated; open wet dressings; Unna's boot (provides continuous pressure to affected areas); and antibiotics for secondary infection after wound culture

rash (lesions confined to the diapered area), seborrheic dermatitis (no pigmentation changes or lichenification in chronic lesions), and chronic contact dermatitis (lesions affecting hands and forearms, sparing antecubital fossa and popliteal areas).

Diagnostic tests
• *Firm stroking of the patient's skin with a blunt instrument* will cause a white — not reddened — dermatographism (hive) to appear on the skin of 70% of patients with atopic dermatitis.
• *Patch testing* and *inspecting the distribution of lesions* helps pinpoint the provoking allergen.
• *Food elimination diet,* although seldom revealing the primary cause of atopic dermatitis, may help identify at least one allergen.
• *Serum analysis* shows elevated IgE levels.
• *Tissue cultures* may be done to rule out bacterial, viral, or fungal superinfections.
• *Allergy testing* may also be done to identify allergic rhinitis or asthma.

Treatment
Effective treatment of atopic lesions consists of eliminating allergens and avoiding irritants, extreme temperature changes, and other precipitating factors. Local and systemic measures relieve itching and inflammation.

Systemic antihistamines, such as hydroxyzine hydrochloride and diphenhydramine, relieve pruritus, and topical application of a corticosteroid cream, especially after bathing, often alleviates inflammation. A typical medication routine may include a systemic antihistamine, a topical corticosteroid, and a bland emollient. Between steroid doses, application of petroleum jelly can help retain moisture.

Systemic corticosteroid therapy should be used only during extreme exacerbations. Weak tar preparations and ultraviolet-B light therapy are used to increase the thickness of the stratum corneum. Antibiotics are appropriate if a bacterial agent has been cultured; antifungal or antiviral medications may be prescribed to fight a fungal or viral infection.

Nursing diagnoses
• Altered oral mucous membrane
• Body image disturbance
• Impaired skin integrity
• Knowledge deficit
• Risk for infection

Nursing interventions
• Assist the patient in scheduling daily skin care. Keep his fingernails short to limit excoriation and secondary infections caused by scratching.

• Be alert for possible adverse reactions associated with corticosteroid use: sensitivity reactions, gastric disturbances, musculoskeletal weakness, neurologic disturbances, and cushingoid symptoms.
• To help clear lichenified skin, apply occlusive dressings (such as a plastic film) intermittently. This treatment requires a doctor's order and experience in dermatologic treatment.
• Apply cool, moist compresses to relieve itching and burning.
• Encourage the patient to verbalize his feelings about his appearance, including embarrassment and fear of rejection. Offer him emotional support and reassurance, and arrange for counseling if necessary.

Patient teaching
• Provide written instructions for skin care and treatment with corticosteroids. Teach the patient and family to recognize signs of corticosteroid overdose and to notify the doctor immediately if they occur.
• If the patient experiences an excessively dry mouth because of antihistamine use, advise him to drink water or suck ice chips.
• Warn that drowsiness is possible with the use of antihistamines to relieve daytime itching. If nocturnal itching interferes with sleep, suggest methods for inducing natural sleep, such as drinking a glass of warm milk, to prevent overuse of sedatives.
• Stress the importance of meticulous hand washing and good personal hygiene.
• Caution the patient to avoid bathing in hot water because heat causes vasodilation, which induces pruritus. Instruct him to use plain, tepid water (96° F [35.6° C]) with a nonfatty, nonperfumed soap but to avoid using any soap when lesions are acutely inflamed. Advise him to shampoo frequently and to apply corticosteroid solution to the scalp afterward. Suggest using a lubricating lotion after a bath.
• In severe dermatitis, show the patient how to apply occlusive dressings. For example, hands with severe contact dermatitis may require a topical corticosteroid and occlusion with gloves to increase drug absorption and skin hydration.
• Teach the patient how to apply wet-to-dry dressings to soothe inflammation, itching, and burning; remove crusting and scales from dry lesions; and help dry up oozing lesions.
• Help the patient identify and avoid aggravating factors and allergens associated with atopic dermatitis. Suggest that he investigate his daily life for possible irritants.

MISCELLANEOUS DISORDERS

Many other disorders can affect the skin. They range from common, benign disorders, such as warts, to rare and potentially fatal disorders, such as toxic epidermal necrolysis.

TOXIC EPIDERMAL NECROLYSIS
A rare, severe skin disorder, toxic epidermal necrolysis causes epidermal erythema, superficial necrosis, and skin erosions. The skin appears to be scalded; hence the alternate name of scalded skin syndrome. Mortality is high (30%), especially among debilitated and elderly patients. Reepithelialization is slow, and residual scarring is common. The disorder primarily affects adults.

Causes
Toxic epidermal necrolysis usually results from a drug reaction—most commonly to butazones, sulfonamides, penicillins, barbiturates, hydantoins, allopurinol, phenolphthalein, and phenylbutazone, but it may be associated with other drugs as well. This disorder may reflect an immune response or may be related to overwhelming physiologic stress (coexisting sepsis, neoplastic diseases, and drug treatment). Airborne toxins, such as carbon monoxide, have also been linked to toxic epidermal necrolysis.

Complications
Patients with toxic epidermal necrolysis commonly develop secondary bacterial and candidal infections. Systemic complications include bronchopneumonia, pulmonary edema, GI and esophageal hemorrhage, shock, renal failure, sepsis, and disseminated intravascular coagulation. These conditions markedly increase mortality.

Assessment findings
The patient with early symptoms complains of a burning sensation in the conjunctiva, malaise, fever, and generalized skin tenderness. Inspection may reveal inflamed mucous membranes. If such prodromal symptoms have passed, observation of the skin may disclose one of the next three phases of toxic epidermal necrolysis:
• diffuse, erythematous rash
• vesiculation and blistering
• large-scale epidermal necrolysis and desquamation.
 You may also note large, flaccid bullae that rupture easily, as well as extensive areas of denuded skin. Slight

rubbing over erythematous areas will cause skin to slough (Nikolsky's sign).

Diagnostic tests

Serum analysis shows leukocytosis, elevated levels of alanine aminotransferase and aspartate aminotransferase, and evidence of fluid and electrolyte imbalance. Urinalysis indicates albuminuria. A culture and Gram stain of lesions help rule out infection, and exfoliative cytology and biopsy help rule out erythema multiforme and exfoliative dermatitis.

Treatment

Appropriate treatment consists of high-dose systemic corticosteroids and maintenance of fluid and electrolyte balance with I.V. fluid replacement. Prophylactic antibiotics may also be needed.

Nursing diagnoses

- Anxiety
- Body image disturbance
- Impaired skin integrity
- Ineffective thermoregulation
- Knowledge deficit
- Pain
- Risk for fluid volume deficit
- Risk for infection

Nursing interventions

- Monitor hematocrit and hemoglobin, electrolyte, serum protein, and arterial blood gas levels.
- Monitor vital signs, central venous pressure, and urine output. Watch for signs of renal failure (decreased urine output) and bleeding. Report temperature elevations immediately, and obtain blood samples for culture and sensitivity tests promptly. Maintain protective isolation.
- Be alert for possible adverse reactions associated with high-dose corticosteroid therapy, including gastric and neurologic disturbances, weakness, and cushingoid symptoms.
- Maintain skin integrity as much as possible. The patient shouldn't wear clothing and should be covered loosely to prevent friction and sloughing of skin. A turning frame and other pressure relief aids are helpful.
- Administer analgesics, as needed, and monitor the patient's response. Apply cool, sterile compresses to help alleviate discomfort.
- Because ocular lesions are common, provide frequent eye care to remove exudate.

- Provide emotional support for the patient and his family. Encourage the patient to express his feelings about his body image and other concerns.

Patient teaching

- Stress the importance of avoiding friction on the skin surface during the blistering and desquamation stages of the disorder. Discourage picking or rubbing the lesions.
- Offer the patient and his family a realistic assessment of the patient's condition. Determine their level of knowledge, and correct any misconceptions to prevent false hope for recovery.

EPIDERMOLYSIS BULLOSA

A heterogeneous group of disorders that affect the skin and mucous membranes, epidermolysis bullosa produces blisters in response to normally harmless heat and frictional trauma. As many as 16 scarring and nonscarring forms may exist, including an acquired form (epidermolysis bullosa acquisita) that develops after childhood and is not genetically inherited.

All nonscarring forms produce a split *above* the basement membrane, the layer between the epidermis and dermis. The scarring forms — except for dominant dystrophic epidermolysis bullosa — produce a split *below* the basement membrane in the upper part of the dermis. Children with dystrophic epidermolysis bullosa have been found to have fewer — and abnormal — anchoring fibrils securing the epidermis to the dermis. These children also have more — and abnormal — collagenase, an enzyme that may destroy the anchoring fibrils. Some patients with epidermolysis bullosa simplex also have deficiencies of other enzymes involved in collagen synthesis.

The prognosis depends on the severity of the disease. In the nonscarring forms of epidermolysis bullosa, the blisters become less severe and less frequent as the patient matures. But the severe scarring forms commonly cause disability or disfigurement and may be fatal during infancy or childhood.

Epidermolysis bullosa occurs in about 1 per 50,000 births; the more severe scarring forms, in about 1 per 500,000 births. The Dystrophic Epidermolysis Bullosa Research Association of America estimates that 25,000 to 50,000 Americans have this disorder.

Causes

The nonscarring forms of epidermolysis bullosa result from autosomal dominant inheritance — except for junctional epidermolysis bullosa (epidermolysis bullosa Herlitz or epidermolysis bullosa letalis), which is recessively inherited.

Except for dominant dystrophic epidermolysis bullosa, the scarring forms result from autosomal recessive inheritance. Sometimes, this disorder occurs as a mutation in families with no history of blistering disorders.

Complications

In all scarring forms and some nonscarring forms, parturition causes widespread blistering and occasional sloughing of large areas of a neonate's skin. Neonates can develop sucking blisters as well as blistering in the GI, respiratory, or genitourinary tract that may lead to strictures or adhesions. Death may occur from fluid and electrolyte imbalance, heat loss, sepsis, and extensive scarring and mucocutaneous erosions.

Ocular complications may include eyelid blisters, conjunctivitis, blepharitis, adhesions, and corneal opacities. Other complications include fusion of fingers and toes with accompanying loss of function, delayed tooth eruption, malformed or carious teeth, alopecia, abnormal nails, retarded growth, anemia, constipation, malnutrition, infection, squamous cell carcinoma, and pyloric atresia.

Assessment findings

The patient history may reveal that tense, clear bullae first appeared in infancy, or they may not appear until early adulthood. Skin inspection may find lesions on any area exposed to friction—such as from footwear, crawling, or bed linens—or to warm weather. However, some forms of epidermolysis bullosa develop in areas not exposed to trauma. Common lesion sites include the feet, extensor surfaces of the extremities, and the knees and elbows.

If the patient has the simple form of epidermolysis bullosa, the lesions will be superficial; these usually heal without scarring. In the dystrophic form of the disease, you may see large eroded areas, hypertrophic scars, and adhesions on the upper dermis. On further inspection, you may note that the patient's fingers and toes have fused.

Differential diagnosis of epidermolysis bullosa should rule out other chronic, nonhereditary bullous diseases, such as juvenile bullous pemphigus, chronic bullous disease of childhood, and congenital herpes infection.

Diagnostic tests

Skin biopsy using immunofluorescence and electron microscopy of a freshly induced blister will identify the type of epidermolysis bullosa. Fetoscopy and biopsy at 20 weeks' gestation will identify the severe scarring forms. (Diagnosis cannot be confirmed by amniocentesis alone.)

Treatment

Phenytoin may be used to treat recessive dystrophic forms of epidermolysis bullosa; corticosteroids and retinoids may be used in other forms. Supportive treatment consists of guarding the skin from trauma and friction through application of protective dressings and skin lubricants. A high-calorie diet containing vitamin and mineral supplements helps combat chronic malnutrition, and iron supplements or transfusions help counteract anemia. Occupational and physical therapy help prevent contractures and deformities.

Nursing diagnoses

- Altered oral mucous membrane
- Body image disturbance
- Fluid volume deficit
- Impaired physical mobility
- Impaired skin integrity
- Impaired tissue integrity
- Ineffective thermoregulation
- Risk for infection

Nursing interventions

- Use meticulous hand washing and hygiene to prevent secondary infection. Have the patient's fingernails cut short to minimize tissue trauma from scratching. Avoid friction from bed linens, dressings, and clothing. If necessary, maintain protective isolation.
- Be alert for complications associated with the use of corticosteroids, retinoids, and antibiotics. Possible adverse effects include GI disturbances, neurologic dysfunction, musculoskeletal weakness, and cushingoid symptoms.
- Inspect and assess the lesions on mucous membranes. Provide frequent mouth care, avoid astringent or acidic fluids, and provide the patient with a bland, soft diet to prevent infection and promote comfort.
- If the patient is a critically ill infant, use an Isolette to maintain body temperature and provide isolation. Carefully monitor intake and output and laboratory test results to assess fluid and electrolyte balance. Maintain I.V. fluid replacement as necessary. Check vital signs, being especially alert for temperature spikes, which indicate sepsis.
- Maintain the patient's skin integrity and promote circulation. Assess the extent of scarring and adhesions.

• Preserve joint mobility and prevent contractures with passive and active range-of-motion (ROM) exercises. In severe cases, place the patient in a Stryker frame or CircOlectric bed, and arrange for physical and occupational therapy.
• Encourage the patient and his family to express their feelings. Discuss embarrassment, fear of rejection by others, loss of function, and the potential loss of the infant.
• Refer the patient and his family to a mental health professional for additional counseling, if necessary, and to any local support groups.

Patient teaching
• Emphasize the importance of meticulous hand washing, and teach the patient to use aseptic technique when changing dressings to prevent secondary infection.
• Stress the importance of avoiding trauma and friction. Encourage the use of protective clothing, such as properly fitted shoes, nonrestrictive long-sleeved shirts and long pants, and knee pads for crawling infants.
• Teach the patient and his family active and passive ROM exercises to minimize disability from scarring and joint immobility.
• Provide written instructions about the patient's diet and treatment regimen. Warn the patient and his family about possible adverse drug reactions, and instruct them to notify the doctor if any occur.
• Help the patient identify his strengths, and reinforce effective coping behaviors. Provide a realistic assessment of the patient's condition, and avoid giving false hope for a complete recovery.

WARTS

Also called verrucae, warts are common, benign infections of the skin and adjacent mucous membranes. Although warts may occur at any age, common warts (verrucae vulgaris) are most prevalent in children and young adults. Flat warts usually occur in children but can also affect adults. Genital warts may be transmitted through sexual contact; however, they're not always venereal in origin.

The prognosis varies: Some warts disappear readily with treatment; others necessitate vigorous, prolonged treatment. About 8% to 10% of the population have warts.

Causes
Warts are caused by infection with the human papillomavirus, a group of ether-resistant, deoxyribonucleic acid–containing papovaviruses. The mode of transmis-

sion is probably through direct contact, but autoinoculation is possible.

Complications
Common complications include secondary infection and scarring.

Assessment findings
Clinical signs depend on the type of wart:
• *Common.* This wart is usually found on the extremities, particularly the hands and fingers. Inspection and palpation reveal rough, elevated, rounded surfaces.
• *Filiform.* Inspection exposes a single, thin, threadlike projection, commonly around the face and neck.
• *Periungual.* Inspection of the patient's fingernails and toenails discloses rough, irregularly shaped, elevated surfaces around the nail edges. If the wart has extended under the nail and lifted it off the nail bed, the patient may complain of pain.
• *Flat.* Inspection and palpation reveal multiple groupings of up to several hundred slightly raised lesions with smooth, flat, or slightly rounded tops. You may notice the lesions on the patient's face, neck, chest, knees, dorsa of the hands, wrists, and flexor surfaces of the forearms. The distribution is often linear because these warts can spread from scratching or shaving.
• *Plantar.* The patient may complain of pain in his feet with pressure. Inspection of the pressure points of the patient's feet finds slightly elevated or flat lesions appearing singly or in large clusters (mosaic warts). The warts may obliterate the natural skin lines.
• *Digitate.* Inspection of the scalp and hairline shows a fingerlike, horny projection, arising from a pea-shaped base.
• *Moist.* Inspection of the penis, scrotum, vulva, or anus reveals small pink to red warts, known also as condyloma acuminatum. Moist and soft, the warts may appear singly or in large cauliflowerlike clusters.

Diagnostic tests
Visual examination usually confirms the diagnosis. Recurrent anal warts require sigmoidoscopy to rule out internal involvement, which may necessitate surgery. To distinguish plantar warts from corns and calluses, gently shave down the lesion with a scalpel; plantar warts will exhibit red or black capillary dots.

Treatment
Effective treatment varies with the location, size, and number of warts. It also depends on the patient's age, pain level (current and projected), history of therapy, and

compliance with treatment. Most people develop an immune response that causes warts to disappear spontaneously and require no treatment.

Treatment may include:

• *electrodesiccation and curettage*. High-frequency electric current destroys the wart and is followed by surgical removal of dead tissue at the base. After application of an antibiotic ointment, the area is covered with a bandage for 48 hours.

• *cryotherapy*. Liquid nitrogen kills the wart; the resulting dried blister is peeled off several days later. If initial treatment isn't successful, it can be repeated at 2- to 4-week intervals. This method is useful for either periungual warts or for common warts on the face, extremities, penis, vagina, or anus.

• *acid therapy (primary or adjunctive)*. The patient applies acid-impregnated plaster patches (such as 40% salicylic acid plasters) or acid drops (such as 5% to 20% salicylic and lactic acid in flexible collodion [Duofilm]) every 12 to 24 hours for 2 to 4 weeks. This method is not recommended for areas in which perspiration is heavy or that are likely to get wet, or for exposed body parts on which patches are cosmetically undesirable.

• *25% podophyllum resin in compound with tincture of benzoin (for venereal warts)*. The podophyllum solution is applied on moist warts. The patient must lie still while it dries, leave it on for 4 hours, and then wash it off with soap and water. The treatment may be repeated every 3 to 4 days and, in some cases, must be left on a maximum of 24 hours, depending on the patient's tolerance. The use of this drug is contraindicated in pregnant patients.

The use of antiviral drugs is under investigation. Suggestion and hypnosis are occasionally successful, especially with children. Carbon dioxide laser treatment has successfully been used to remove genital warts.

Nursing diagnoses
• Body image disturbance
• Impaired skin integrity
• Pain
• Risk for infection

Nursing interventions
• To protect adjacent unaffected skin during acid or podophyllum treatment, cover it with petroleum jelly or sodium bicarbonate.
• Encourage the patient to verbalize his feelings about his appearance. Discuss any embarrassment or fear of rejection he may have. Offer emotional support, and assure him that warts respond to treatment.

• Be alert for possible adverse effects of acid therapy, such as burning and irritation of surrounding tissues.

Patient teaching
• Teach the patient and family that warts are contagious and can be spread by shaving, sharing personal articles, scratching, and sexual contact. Help the patient identify all contacts, and tell him that he should encourage them to seek medical treatment. Advise him that warts commonly recur.
• If the patient is receiving acid therapy, make sure he knows how to apply the plaster patches. Instruct him to leave the patches on for 12 to 24 hours. Stress the importance of protecting healthy tissue and avoiding picking, rubbing, or scratching lesions. Emphasize that compliance with the treatment regimen is essential to successful wart removal and prevention of scarring.
• If the patient is receiving electrosurgery to remove warts, explain the procedure and give any preoperative and postoperative instructions.

PSORIASIS
Characterized by recurring remissions and exacerbations, psoriasis is a chronic skin disease marked by epidermal proliferation. Its lesions, which appear as erythematous papules and plaques covered with silvery scales, vary widely in severity and distribution.

Psoriasis affects about 2% of the U.S. population, and the incidence is higher among whites than among people of other races. The disease affects men and women equally and, although it may occur at any age, it occurs less frequently after age 40.

Flare-ups are often related to specific systemic and environmental factors but may be unpredictable; they can usually be controlled with therapy.

Causes and pathophysiology
The tendency to develop psoriasis is genetically determined. Researchers have discovered a significantly higher than normal incidence of certain histocompatibility antigens (HLA) in patients with psoriasis, suggesting a possible autoimmune process.

The onset of the disease is also influenced by environmental factors. Trauma can trigger the isomorphic effect, or Koebner's phenomenon, in which lesions develop at injury sites. Infections, especially those resulting from beta-hemolytic streptococci, may cause a flare of guttate (drop-shaped) lesions. Other contributing factors include pregnancy, endocrine changes, climatic conditions (cold

IDENTIFYING TYPES OF PSORIASIS

Psoriasis occurs in various forms, ranging from one or two localized plaques that seldom require long-term medical attention to widespread lesions and crippling arthritis.

Erythrodermic psoriasis
This type is marked by extensive flushing all over the body, which may or may not result in scaling. The rash may begin rapidly, signaling new psoriasis; it may develop gradually, in chronic psoriasis; or it may occur as an adverse reaction to a drug.

Guttate psoriasis
This type typically affects children and young adults. Erupting in drop-sized plaques over the trunk, arms, legs and, sometimes, the scalp, this rash of plaques generalizes in several days. It's commonly associated with upper respiratory tract streptococcal infections.

Inverse psoriasis
Smooth, dry, bright red plaques characterize inverse psoriasis. Located in skin folds (the armpits and groin, for example), the plaques fissure easily.

Psoriasis vulgaris
This is the most common type of psoriasis. It begins with red, dotlike lesions that gradually enlarge and produce dry, silvery scales. The plaques usually appear symmetrically on the knees, elbows, extremities, genitalia, scalp, and nails.

Pustular psoriasis
This type features an eruption of local or extensive small, raised, pus-filled plaques. Precursors include emotional stress, sweat, infections, and adverse drug reactions.

weather tends to exacerbate psoriasis), and emotional stress.

A skin cell normally takes 14 days to move from the basal layer to the stratum corneum where, after 14 days of normal wear and tear, it's sloughed off. In contrast to this 28-day cycle, the life cycle of a psoriatic cell is only 4 days. This markedly shortened cycle doesn't allow time for the cell to mature. Consequently, the stratum corneum becomes thick and flaky, producing the cardinal manifestations of psoriasis.

Complications
If the patient doesn't comply with prescribed treatment, infection may result. Also, altered self-image may lead to social isolation and depression.

Assessment findings
The patient history may reveal a family history of psoriasis as well as predisposing factors. The patient complains of skin lesions that itch and burn and may be painful. He may also describe arthritic symptoms — "morning stiffness" — usually in one or more finger or toe joints, sometimes in the sacroiliac joints. In some patients, this progresses to spondylitis. Joint symptoms show no consistent linkage to the course of the cutaneous manifestation of psoriasis; they demonstrate remissions and exacerbations similar to those of rheumatoid arthritis.

On inspection, you'll see erythematous, well-defined plaques covered with characteristic silver scales. In mild

psoriasis, plaques are scattered over a small skin area. The patient with moderate psoriasis displays more and larger plaques, up to several centimeters in diameter. Severe psoriasis involves at least half the body.

Plaques usually appear on the scalp, chest, elbows, knees, back, and buttocks. Palpation may cause the scales to flake off easily, or you may note that the scales have thickened and covered the lesion. Attempting to remove the psoriatic scales may produce fine bleeding points (Auspitz sign). You may also see small guttate lesions, either alone or with plaques; these lesions are typically thin and erythematous, with few scales. (See *Identifying types of psoriasis.*)

In about 30% of patients, you'll find that psoriasis has spread to the fingernails or, more often, the toenails, producing small indentations or pits, and yellow or brown discoloration. In severe cases, the accumulation of thick crumbly debris under the nail causes the nail to separate from the nail bed.

Diagnostic tests
The patient history and lesion appearance guide the diagnosis. A skin biopsy will help rule out other diseases. The serum uric acid level is elevated because of accelerated nucleic acid degradation, but indications of gout are absent. HLA 13 and 17 may be present.

Treatment
Treatment depends on the type of psoriasis, the extent of the disease, and the disease's effect on the patient's

life-style. No permanent cure exists; all treatments are palliative.

Lukewarm baths and the application of occlusive ointment bases, such as petroleum jelly, or preparations that contain urea or salicylic acid may soften and help remove psoriatic scales. Steroid creams are also useful.

Methods to retard rapid cell production include exposure to ultraviolet-B (UVB) light or natural sunlight to the point of minimal erythema. Coal tar preparations retard skin cell growth and relieve inflammation, itching, and scaling.

Topical corticosteroids are the treatment of choice for mild to moderate psoriasis of the trunk, arms, and legs. These drugs decrease epidermal cell growth and reduce inflammation. They may also reduce symptoms by inducing vasoconstriction. Treatment commonly combines topical corticosteroids with emollients, coal tar preparations, and UV light therapy. For many patients, this is an inexpensive regimen that minimizes adverse reactions.

Mild psoriasis involving the extremities may be relieved by 0.025% triamcinolone acetonide ointment. Facial, groin, or axillary plaques may respond to 1% desonide cream or alclometasone dipropionate. More potent topical preparations, such as 0.1% betamethasone valerate or 0.1% triamcinolone acetonide, may be prescribed for moderate psoriasis.

Anthralin may help large plaques that don't respond to coal tar or topical corticosteroid preparations. Methotrexate, a drug that inhibits cell replication, may relieve severe, unresponsive psoriasis. Etretinate is a potent retinoic acid derivative that may be used for psoriasis that's resistant to other drugs or treatments. It's especially effective·for treating pustular and erythrodermic psoriasis and may also relieve extensive plaque-type psoriasis. However, the disease commonly recurs within 2 months after the cessation of therapy.

Patients with severe chronic psoriasis may use the Goeckerman treatment, which combines topical coal tar treatment with ultraviolet-A (UVA) or UVB light therapy. The regimen is used monthly during flare-ups; it may also be used to treat chronic, resistant plaques for extended periods. The Ingram technique is a variation of this treatment, using anthralin instead of coal tar. A modified Goeckerman treatment combines UVB light therapy with topical drugs, such as coal tar preparations, corticosteroids, or kerolytic agents. This therapy may relieve psoriasis more quickly than the standard Goeckerman treatment, but remission may be briefer. A photochemotherapy program called PUVA combines ad-

ministration of psoralen, either orally or topically, with exposure to UVA light.

Low-dose antihistamine therapy, oatmeal baths, emollients (perhaps with phenol and menthol), and open wet dressings may help relieve pruritus. Aspirin and local heat help alleviate the pain of psoriatic arthritis; severe cases may require nonsteroidal anti-inflammatory drugs.

Therapy for psoriasis of the scalp typically consists of a coal tar shampoo, followed by the application of a steroid lotion while the hair is still wet. No effective treatment exists for psoriasis of the nails. The nails usually improve as skin lesions improve.

Nursing diagnoses
• Body image disturbance
• Impaired skin integrity
• Knowledge deficit
• Pain
• Powerlessness
• Social isolation

Nursing interventions
• Your care will include careful monitoring for adverse reactions to therapy, patient teaching, and sympathetic support. (See *Planning care for the patient with psoriasis*, pages 1194 and 1195.)
• Apply all topical medications, especially those that contain anthralin and coal tar, with a downward motion, to avoid rubbing them into the follicles. Wear gloves because anthralin stains and injures the skin. After application, allow the patient to dust himself with powder to help prevent anthralin from rubbing off on his clothes.
• Watch for adverse reactions to therapeutic agents. These may include allergic reactions to anthralin; atrophy and acne from steroids; and burning, itching, nausea, and squamous cell epitheliomas from PUVA.
• Initially evaluate the patient on methotrexate weekly and then monthly for red blood cell, white blood cell, and platelet counts because cytotoxins may cause hepatic or bone marrow toxicity. Liver biopsy may be done to assess the effects of methotrexate.
• Encourage the patient to verbalize his feelings about his appearance; his feelings of embarrassment, frustration, or powerlessness; or his fear of rejection. Involve family members in the treatment regimen to lessen the patient's feelings of social isolation. Help the patient build a positive self-image by encouraging his participation in activities that de-emphasize appearance.

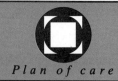

Plan of care

PLANNING CARE FOR THE PATIENT WITH PSORIASIS

Comprehensive management of psoriasis means providing the care needed to ameliorate the disease and help the patient cope with his condition. The following is a plan you might develop for Elliott Russell, a 21-year-old college student on his first visit to the dermatology clinic.

Patient history
Elliott begins by describing his chief complaint: sore, itchy, scaling lesions on his hands, arms, elbows, scalp, and knees that have gradually worsened. He also admits to having constant irritation from above his anus extending into the sacral area. He tells you that sometimes some of the scalp lesions erode and bleed.

Elliott says that he keeps his skin very clean—taking two showers daily with antibacterial soaps—and wears only clothing with a high-cotton content. He tells you that he has used nonprescription topical hydrocortisone ointments on his lesions but without any great relief. "The patches feel better for a few minutes at the most, but they never go away."

Elliott appears timid, speaking in a low voice and describing his symptoms haltingly. With encouragement, he admits that he's been under a great deal of stress for the past 2 years, which he attributes to taking an overload of college courses.

Assessment findings
You take Elliott's vital signs and find an oral temperature of 98.4° F (36.9° C), a pulse rate of 72 beats/minute, and respirations unlabored at 18 breaths/minute. His blood pressure reading is 134/82 mm Hg.

Inspecting Elliott's scalp and extremities, you note varying degrees of scales, red or silvery patches, lesions, and "normal-looking" dry skin. The lesions have irregular borders and are randomly scattered. You also notice three pustular lesions on his right palm and several scabs of dried blood and exudate on his parietal scalp. When you examine his fingernails, you see that the nail beds are pitted and discolored. The nails themselves are thin, with each plate peeling away from the layer below.

Using a graphic anatomic figure chart to document your findings, you carefully describe the location, morphology, color, and exudate of every involved area.

The dermatologist examines Elliott and diagnoses him as having psoriasis. After ordering a culture of the pustular drainage from the right hand, the doctor prescribes a group of topical treatments.

Nursing diagnoses
Based on your assessment findings, you devise the following nursing diagnoses for Elliott:
• Knowledge deficit related to the disease process and treatment
• Impaired skin integrity and high risk for infection related to decreased protection from the skin
• Pain related to sensitive lesions and skin excoriation
• Body image disturbance related to perceived unsightliness.

Expected outcomes
Being sensitive to Elliott's emotional and physical needs, you set several goals. For example, you decide that Elliot needs to:
• learn about psoriasis and exhibit an understanding of the disease
• improve skin integrity and protection by controlling new lesions and smoothing existing patches

• relieve pain by treating lesions and patches topically
• improve his body image and relieve his embarrassment about his appearance.

Implementation
To help Elliott reach his goals, you intervene as follows.

To improve understanding of psoriasis
• Assess what Elliott already knows about the integumentary system, its protective elements, skin cleanliness, psoriasis treatments, and long-term disease effects.
• Explain and demonstrate how to apply the topical medications that have been prescribed.

To improve skin protection and integrity
• Encourage Elliott to be meticulous in caring for his skin and in following his treatment regimen.
• Instruct him to drink plenty of fluids and use prescribed emollients to keep his skin moist and smooth.
• Encourage him to eat a balanced diet and to exercise.
• Caution him to always wear sunscreen when in the sun.
• Tell him to avoid wearing clothing or using soaps that irritate his skin.

To decrease pain
• Instruct Elliott to take tepid baths; to avoid using bubble bath, drying soaps, or perfumes; and to pat himself dry.
• Advise him to apply prescribed emollients immediately after bathing.
• Caution him to avoid using nonprescription creams and lotions that claim to relieve skin irritation.
• Tell him to cover as much of his affected skin as possible with soft, breathable clothing.

PLANNING CARE FOR THE PATIENT WITH PSORIASIS
(continued)

• Encourage him to decrease stressors that heighten the pain response to psoriasis and to obtain adequate rest.

To improve body image
• Encourage Elliott to be patient and persistent with his skin care.
• Tell him that following his prescribed treatment regimen and keeping his skin as soft as possible will produce less fissuring and decrease lesion formation.

• Keep your expression free of any sign of revulsion when caring for the lesions.
• Encourage Elliott to join a local chapter of the National Psoriasis Foundation and to attend group meetings and functions.
• Offer to refer him to a mental health professional, if necessary, to help him cope with his illness.

Evaluation
If your plan of care has been successful, Elliott will exhibit an understanding of psoriasis, describing its cause and stating, realistically, his

chances for improvement. He'll describe his treatment regimen and demonstrate correctly how to apply the prescribed topical medications. He'll also identify clothing that may irritate his skin.

On his next visit, Elliott will report decreased discomfort as a result of following his skin care program, and you'll see no evidence of secondary skin infection. He'll also report that he has lightened his school course load, attended a meeting of the local chapter of the National Psoriasis Foundation, and feels more optimistic about himself.

Patient teaching
• Explain the causes, predisposing factors, and course of psoriasis to the patient and his family. Stress that psoriasis is not communicable. Advise them that exacerbations and remissions commonly occur, but that they can usually control the disorder by adhering to the treatment regimen.
• Make sure the patient understands his prescribed therapy; provide written instructions to avoid confusion. Teach correct application of prescribed ointments, creams, and lotions.
• Instruct the patient to avoid scratching the plaques. Suggest that he wear gloves to help protect his skin from unconscious scratching. Tell him that pressing ice cubes against the lesions or applying a mentholated shaving cream may provide relief. Recommend using a humidifier in the winter to avoid dry skin, which may increase itching.
• Caution the patient to avoid scrubbing his skin vigorously. If a medication has been applied to the scales to soften them, suggest that the patient use a soft brush to remove them.
• Warn the patient never to put an occlusive dressing over anthralin. Suggest the use of mineral oil and then soap and water to remove anthralin.
• Caution the patient receiving PUVA therapy to stay out of the sun on the treatment day and to protect his eyes with sunglasses that screen UVA for 24 hours after treatment. Tell him to wear goggles during exposure to this light.
• If the patient is using etretinate, inform him that the drug may remain in his body for up to 3 years after the treatment ends. For this reason, discourage female pa-

tients who may want to become pregnant from using this drug.
• Caution the patient using methotrexate not to drink alcoholic beverages; explain that alcohol ingestion increases the risk of hepatotoxicity.
• Warn the patient and his family about possible adverse reactions associated with the therapeutic agents. Tell them to notify the doctor if any occur.
• Teach the patient stress-reduction techniques and injury-prevention strategies to prevent exacerbations.
• Explain the relation between psoriasis and arthritis, but point out that psoriasis causes no other systemic disturbances.
• Refer the patient to the National Psoriasis Foundation.

CORNS AND CALLUSES
Usually located on areas of repeated trauma (most often the feet), corns and calluses are acquired skin conditions. A corn is marked by hyperkeratosis of the stratum corneum and is classified as soft or hard. A callus is an area of thickened skin, generally on the foot or hand. People whose activities produce repeated trauma (for example, manual laborers or guitarists) commonly develop calluses. The severity of a corn or callus depends on the degree and duration of trauma. The prognosis for both is good with proper hand or foot care.

Causes
A corn usually results from external pressure, such as that from ill-fitting shoes or, less commonly, from internal pressure, such as that caused by a protruding un-

derlying bone (resulting from arthritis, for example). A callus is produced by external pressure or friction.

Complications
Secondary infections may occur when patients try to cut away corns or calluses with sharp instruments.

Assessment findings
The patient may complain of pain when pressure is applied to the area. A thorough history discloses chronic friction or pressure.

On inspection, you'll be able to differentiate corns from calluses: Corns contain a central keratinous core, are smaller and more clearly defined than calluses, and are usually more painful. Soft corns appear as whitish thickenings and are commonly found between the toes, most often in the fourth interdigital web. Hard corns are sharply delineated and conical and appear most frequently over the dorsolateral aspect of the fifth toe. In contrast, if the patient has a callus, you'll note that the lesion, which may be quite large, has an indefinite border. Although calluses commonly appear over plantar warts, normal skin markings distinguish them from the warts.

Palpation of a corn may elicit a complaint of dull and constant, or even sharp, pain. Palpation of a callus usually produces dull pain on pressure, rather than constant pain.

Diagnostic tests
No tests are needed because examination identifies corns and calluses.

Treatment
Surgical debridement may be performed, usually under a local anesthetic, to remove the nucleus of a corn. In intermittent debridement, keratolytics — usually 40% salicylic acid plasters — are applied to affected areas. Injections of corticosteroids beneath the corn may be necessary to relieve pain. However, the simplest and best treatment is essentially preventive — avoidance of trauma. Corns and calluses disappear after the source of trauma has been removed. Metatarsal pads may redistribute the weight-bearing areas of the foot; corn pads may prevent painful pressure.

Patients with persistent corns or calluses require referral to a podiatrist or dermatologist; those with corns or calluses caused by a bony malformation, as in arthritis, require an orthopedic consultation.

Nursing diagnoses
• Impaired physical mobility
• Impaired skin integrity
• Knowledge deficit
• Pain

Nursing interventions
• Promote progressive mobilization to the maximum allowable within the patient's pain limitation.
• When applying salicylic acid plasters, make sure the plaster is large enough to cover the affected area. Place the sticky side against the patient's skin, and cover the plaster with adhesive tape.
• Watch for sensitivity reactions associated with salicylic acid plasters.

Patient teaching
• Teach the patient how to apply salicylic acid plasters. Tell him that the plasters are usually taken off after an overnight application but may be left in place for as long as 7 days. After removing the plaster, the patient should soak the area in water and abrade the soft, macerated skin with a towel or pumice stone. He should then reapply the plaster and repeat the entire procedure until he has removed all the hyperkeratotic skin.
• Warn the patient against removing corns or calluses with a sharp instrument, such as a razor blade.
• Advise him to wear properly fitted shoes. Suggest the use of metatarsal or corn pads to relieve pressure. Refer him to a podiatrist, a dermatologist, or an orthopedist, if necessary.
• Assure him that good foot care can correct these conditions.
• If the patient is to have his corns or calluses debrided, give preoperative and postoperative instructions.

PITYRIASIS ROSEA
An acute, self-limiting, inflammatory skin disease, pityriasis rosea produces a "herald" patch — which usually goes undetected — followed by a generalized eruption of papulosquamous lesions. Although this noncontagious disorder may develop at any age, it's most apt to occur in adolescents and young adults. The incidence rises in the spring and fall. Secondary syphilis, dermatophytosis, or a drug reaction may mimic the condition.

Causes
In pityriasis rosea, the cause is unknown, but the disease's brief course and the virtual absence of recurrence suggest a viral agent or an autoimmune disorder.

Complications

Pruritus and scratching may lead to secondary bacterial infections.

Assessment findings

The patient with pityriasis may initially complain of a slightly raised, oval, erythematous lesion anywhere on his body. (However, although this lesion is ¾″ to 2⅜″ [2 to 6 cm] in diameter, many patients don't notice this herald patch.) After a few days to several weeks, the patient may note lesions on his trunk and extremities; if he's an adolescent, the lesions may also appear on his face, hands, and feet. Most patients report only slight itching; sometimes, though, the itching may be severe.

Inspection of the patient's skin may reveal red-to-brown patches with an erythematous border and trailing scales. The lesions are oval, ¼″ to ⅜″ (0.5 to 1 cm) in diameter, and arranged along body cleavage lines, producing a pattern similar to that of a pine tree. The patches may be macular, vesicular, or urticarial.

On further questioning, the patient may disclose that the eruptions have continued for 7 to 10 days. The patches may persist for 2 to 6 weeks.

Diagnostic tests

Serologic testing will rule out secondary syphilis.

Treatment

Focusing on relief of pruritus, treatment involves emollients, oatmeal baths, antihistamines and, occasionally, exposure to ultraviolet light or sunlight. Topical steroids in a hydrophilic cream base may be beneficial. Rarely, if inflammation is severe, systemic corticosteroids may be required.

Nursing diagnoses

• Body image disturbance
• Impaired skin integrity
• Knowledge deficit
• Risk for infection

Nursing interventions

• Have the patient's fingernails cut short to prevent secondary bacterial infection from scratching.
• Give antihistamines, as ordered, to relieve pruritus.
• Encourage the patient to verbalize his feelings about his appearance. Reassure him that pityriasis rosea is noncontagious, that spontaneous remission usually occurs in 2 to 6 weeks, and that lesions generally don't recur.

Patient teaching

• Explain the disease and all procedures.
• Provide written instructions for the treatment regimen. Make sure the patient understands his prescribed treatment and medication routine. Warn him that antihistamines may cause drowsiness.
• Encourage good hand washing and personal hygiene. Advise the patient to avoid hot baths or showers, which intensify itching. Encourage him to use lubricating lotions after bathing.

PRESSURE ULCERS

Localized areas of cellular necrosis, pressure ulcers occur most often in the skin and subcutaneous tissue over bony prominences, particularly the sacrum, ischial tuberosities, greater trochanter, heels, malleoli, and elbows. These ulcers—also called decubitus ulcers, pressure sores, or bedsores—may be superficial, caused by local skin irritation with subsequent surface maceration, or deep, originating in underlying tissue. Deep lesions often go undetected until they penetrate the skin, but by then, they've usually caused subcutaneous damage.

Causes and pathophysiology

Pressure, particularly over bony prominences, interrupts normal circulatory function and causes most pressure ulcers. The intensity and duration of such pressure govern the severity of the ulcer; pressure exerted over an area for a moderate period (1 to 2 hours) produces tissue ischemia and increased capillary pressure, leading to edema and multiple small-vessel thromboses. An inflammatory reaction gives way to ulceration and necrosis of ischemic cells. In turn, necrotic tissue predisposes the body to bacterial invasion and infection. (See *Pressure points: Common sites of pressure ulcers,* page 1198.)

Shearing force, the force applied when tissue layers move over one another, can also cause ulcerations. This force stretches the skin, compressing local circulation. As an example, if the head of the patient's bed is raised, gravity tends to pull the patient downward and forward, creating a shearing force. The friction of the patient's skin against the bed, such as occurs when a patient slides himself up in bed rather than lifting his hips, compounds the problem.

Moisture, whether from perspiration or incontinence, can also cause pressure ulcers. Such moisture softens skin layers and provides an environment for bacterial growth, leading to skin breakdown.

Other factors that can predispose a patient to pressure ulcers and also delay healing include poor nutrition, dia-

PRESSURE POINTS: COMMON SITES OF PRESSURE ULCERS

Pressure ulcers may develop at any of these pressure points. To prevent sores, reposition the patient frequently, and check carefully for any skin changes.

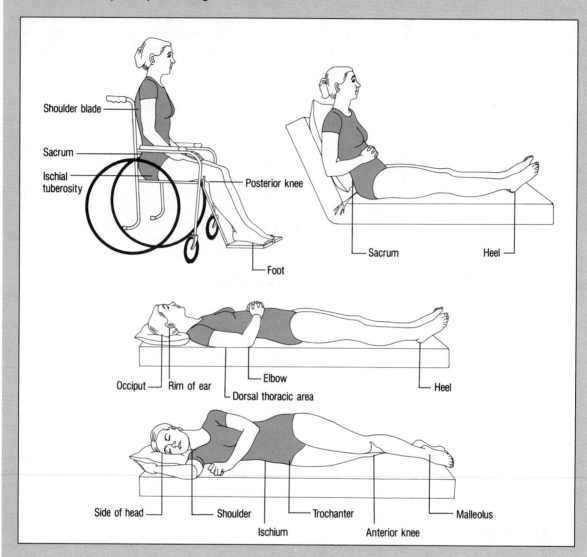

Complications

betes mellitus, paralysis, cardiovascular disorders, and aging. Added risks include obesity, insufficient weight, edema, anemia, poor hygiene, and exposure to chemicals.

Bacterial invasion and secondary infection, possibly leading to bacteremia and septicemia, are common complications of pressure ulcers. If the ulcer is large, a continuous loss of serum may deplete the body of its normal circulating fluids and essential proteins. In severe cases, ulcers may extend through subcutaneous fat layers, fibrous tissue, and muscle until reaching the bone.

Assessment findings

The patient with a pressure ulcer will have a history of one or more predisposing factors. Inspection of an early, superficial lesion notes shiny, erythematous changes over the compressed area, caused by localized vasodilation when pressure is relieved. If the superficial erythema has progressed, you'll see small blisters or erosions and, ultimately, necrosis and ulceration.

In underlying damage from pressure between deep tissue and bone, you'll note an inflamed skin surface area. Bacteria in a compressed site cause inflammation and, eventually, infection, which leads to further necrosis. You may detect a foul-smelling, purulent discharge seeping from a lesion that has penetrated the skin from beneath. A black eschar may develop around and over the lesion because infected, necrotic tissue prevents healthy granulation of scar tissue. (See *Four stages of pressure ulcers,* page 1200.)

Diagnostic tests

Wound culture and sensitivity testing of the ulcer exudate identify infecting organisms. Serum protein and serum albumin studies may be ordered to determine severe hypoproteinemia.

Treatment

Prevention is most important in pressure ulcers by such means as movement and exercise to improve circulation and adequate nutrition to maintain skin health. When pressure ulcers do develop, successful management involves relieving pressure on the affected area, keeping the area clean and dry, and promoting healing. To relieve pressure, devices such as pads, mattresses, and special beds may be used. Bear in mind that turning and repositioning are still necessary. (See *Pressure-relief devices,* page 1201.) In addition, a diet high in protein, iron, and vitamin C will help promote healing.

Other treatments depend on the ulcer stage. Stage 1 treatment aims to increase tissue pliability, stimulate local circulation, promote healing, and prevent skin breakdown. Specific measures include the use of lubricants (such as Lubriderm), clear plastic dressings (Op-Site), gelatin-type wafers (DuoDerm), vasodilator sprays (Proderm), and whirlpool baths.

For Stage 2 ulcers, additional treatments include cleaning the ulcer with 0.9% sodium chloride solution or water and hydrogen peroxide. This removes ulcer debris and helps prevent further skin damage and infection.

Therapy for Stage 3 or 4 ulcers aims to treat existing infection, prevent further infection, and remove necrotic tissue. Specific measures include cleaning the ulcer with hydrogen peroxide and povidone-iodine solution and applying granular and absorbent dressings. These dressings promote wound drainage and absorb any exudate. In addition, enzymatic ointments (such as Elase or Travase) break down dead tissue, whereas healing ointments clean deep or infected ulcers and stimulate new cell growth.

Debridement of necrotic tissue may be necessary to allow healing. One method is to apply open wet dressings and allow them to dry on the ulcer. Removal of the dressings mechanically debrides exudate and necrotic tissue. On occasion, the ulcer may require debridement using surgical, mechanical, or chemical techniques. In severe cases, skin grafting may be necessary.

Nursing diagnoses

- Altered nutrition: Less than body requirements
- Altered protection
- Impaired physical mobility
- Impaired skin integrity
- Impaired tissue integrity
- Risk for infection

Nursing interventions

- During each shift, check the bedridden patient's skin for changes in color, turgor, temperature, and sensation. Examine an existing ulcer for any change in size or degree of damage.
- Reposition the bedridden patient at least every 2 hours around the clock. Minimize the effects of shearing force by using a footboard and not raising the head of the bed to an angle that exceeds 60 degrees. Keep the patient's knees slightly flexed for short periods.
- Perform passive range-of-motion (ROM) exercises, or encourage the patient to do active exercises, if possible.
- To prevent pressure ulcers in an immobilized patient, use pressure-relief aids on his bed.
- Give the patient meticulous skin care. Keep his skin clean and dry without using harsh soaps. Gently massaging the skin around the affected area (not on it) promotes healing. Rub moisturizing lotions into the skin thoroughly to prevent maceration of the skin surface. Change bed linens frequently for a diaphoretic or incontinent patient.
- If the patient is incontinent, offer him a bedpan or commode frequently. Use only a single layer of padding for urine and fecal incontinence because excessive padding increases perspiration, which leads to maceration. Ex-

FOUR STAGES OF PRESSURE ULCERS

To protect the patient from pressure ulcer complications, learn to recognize the four stages of ulcer formation.

Stage 1
In this stage, the skin stays red for 5 minutes after removal of pressure and may develop an abrasion of the epidermis. (A black person's skin may look purple.) The skin also feels warm and firm. The sore is usually reversible if you remove pressure.

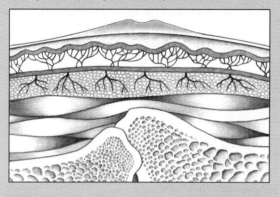

Stage 3
A hole develops that oozes foul-smelling yellow or green fluid. Extending into the muscle, the ulcer may develop a black leathery crust or eschar at its edges and, eventually, at the center. The ulcer isn't painful, but healing may take months.

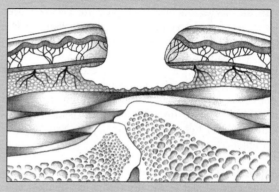

Stage 2
Breaks appear in the skin, and discoloration may occur. Penetrating to the subcutaneous fat layer, the sore is painful and visibly swollen. If pressure is removed, the sore may heal within 1 to 2 weeks.

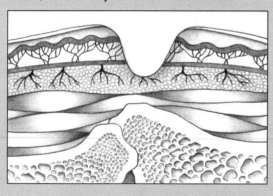

Stage 4
The ulcer destroys tissue from the skin to the bone and becomes necrotic. Findings include foul drainage and deep tunnels that extend from the ulcer. Months or even a year may elapse before the ulcer heals.

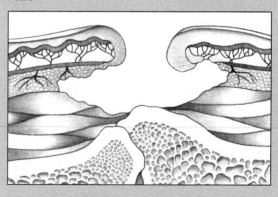

cessive padding also may wrinkle, irritating the skin.
• Clean open lesions with a 0.9% sodium chloride solution. If possible, expose the lesions to air and sunlight to promote healing. Dressings, if needed, should be porous and lightly taped to healthy skin.

• Encourage adequate food and fluid intake to maintain body weight and promote healing. Consult the dietitian to provide a diet that promotes granulation of new tissue. Encourage the debilitated patient to eat frequent, small meals that include protein- and calorie-rich supplements. Assist the weakened patient with meals.

PRESSURE-RELIEF DEVICES

Special pads, mattresses, and beds can help relieve pressure for the patient who is confined to one position for long periods and in danger of developing pressure ulcers.

Gel flotation pads
These wide pads disperse pressure over a wide surface area.

Alternating-pressure mattress
Alternating deflation and inflation of mattress tubes change areas of pressure.

Convoluted foam mattress or pads
Elevated foam areas cushion the skin, minimizing pressure. Depressed areas relieve pressure.

Foam rubber
Cut to just the right size and shape, foam rubber cushions individual areas on the patient.

Clinitron bed
This bed contains beads that move under an air-flow to support the patient, thus eliminating shearing force and friction.

Stryker or Foster frame or CircOlectric bed
These devices ease turning of immobile patients to relieve pressure.

Comfortex DeCube mattress
Inside mattress has a matrix of 15 removable square foam cubes from the shoulder area to the midthigh area and two rectangular cubes at the head and foot areas. Cubes can be removed under areas of pressure.

Padding
Pillows, towels, and soft blankets in the patient's body hollows can reduce pressure on nearby pressure points.

Foot cradle
This device lifts the bedclothes to relieve pressure over the patient's feet.

• Because anemia and elevated blood glucose levels may lead to skin breakdown, monitor hemoglobin and blood glucose levels and hematocrit.

Patient teaching
• Explain the function of pressure-relief aids and topical agents, and demonstrate their proper use.
• Teach the patient and his family position-changing techniques and active and passive ROM exercises.
• Stress good hygiene. Teach the patient to avoid skin-damaging agents, such as harsh soaps, alcohol-based products, tincture of benzoin, and hexachlorophene.
• As indicated, explain debridement procedures, and prepare the patient for skin graft surgery.
• Teach the patient and his family to recognize and record signs of healing. Explain that treatment typically varies according to the stage of healing.
• Encourage the patient to eat a well-balanced diet and consume an adequate amount of fluids, explaining their importance for skin health. Point out dietary sources rich in vitamin C, which aids wound healing, promotes iron absorption, and helps in collagen formation.

SELECTED REFERENCES

Friedman-Jimenez, G., et al. "Work-related Illness: Lung and Skin Disorders," *Patient Care* 28(16):48-50,55, 58+, October 15, 1994.

Ignatavicius, D.D., et al. *Medical-Surgical Nursing: A Nursing Process Approach,* 2nd ed. Philadelphia: W.B. Saunders Co., 1995.

Isselbacher, K., et al., eds. *Harrison's Principles of Internal Medicine,* 13th ed. New York: McGraw-Hill Book Co., 1995.

Rakel, R.E., ed. *Conn's Current Therapy 1996.* Philadelphia: W.B. Saunders Co., 1996.

Rosen, T., et al. "Bacterial Skin Infections: Diagnostic Clues and Treatment Choices, " *Consultant* 34(11)1525-28, 1531, 1535-81, November 1994.

Stein, J.H., et al. *Internal Medicine,* 4th ed. St. Louis: Mosby–Year Book, Inc., 1994.

Taylor, C.M., and Sparks, S.M. *Nursing Diagnosis Reference Manual,* 3rd ed. Springhouse, Pa.: Springhouse Corp., 1995.

Tierney, L., et al. *Current Medical Diagnosis and Treatment 1995.* East Norwalk, Conn.: Appleton & Lange, 1995.

Wysocki, A.B., "A Review of the Skin and Its Appendages," Part 1. *Advanced Wound Care* 8(2)53-54, 56-62, 64+, March-April 1995.

Young, D. "Dermatology: Contact Dermatitis," *New Zealand Practical Nurse,* 41-42, September 1994.

APPENDIX: NUTRITIONAL DISORDERS

This appendix provides a summary of nutritional disorders. It briefly describes each disorder's characteristics, possible causes, signs and symptoms, and treatment.

Hypervitaminoses A and D • Accumulation of excessive amounts of vitamin A or D.

This accumulation occurs because these vitamins aren't dissolved and excreted in urine. These conditions are most prevalent in infants and children and commonly result from accidental or misguided overdose of supplemental vitamin preparations. In chronic hypervitaminosis A, signs and symptoms include anorexia, irritability, headache, hair loss, malaise, itching, vertigo, and bone pain. In hypervitaminosis D, anorexia, headache, nausea, vomiting, weight loss, polyuria, and polydipsia occur. Withholding vitamin supplements usually corrects hypervitaminoses A and D.

Iodine deficiency • Lack of sufficient levels of iodine to satisfy daily metabolic requirements.

This deficiency may lead to hypothyroidism and thyroid hypertrophy (endemic goiter). Other effects range from dental caries to cretinism in infants born to iodine-deficient mothers. Insufficient ingestion of dietary iodine or increased metabolic demands during pregnancy, lactation, and adolescence may cause this deficit. Signs and symptoms vary. Treatment consists of iodine supplements.

Obesity • Body weight exceeding the norm by 20% or more.

This condition results when caloric intake consistently exceeds metabolic demands. Theories to explain this condition include psychological factors, hypothalamic dysfunction of hunger and satiety centers, genetic predisposition, abnormal absorption of nutrients, and impaired action of GI and growth hormones and of hormonal regulators, such as insulin. An inverse relationship between socioeconomic status and the prevalence of obesity has been documented, especially in women. Obesity in parents increases the probability of obesity in children.

Weight reduction and maintenance of weight loss are the goals of treatment, which includes a low-calorie diet, behavior modification, aerobic exercise, and social support.

Protein-calorie malnutrition • Occurs as marasmus (protein-calorie deficiency) and as kwashiorkor (protein deficiency despite adequate calories).

Both depletion disorders commonly affect infants in underdeveloped countries. In industrialized countries, these disorders most commonly affect hospitalized patients. Infants with marasmus suffer from growth retardation and wasting, physical inactivity, apathy, frequent infections, anorexia, weakness, irritability, hunger, diarrhea, nausea, and vomiting. In kwashiorkor, the child may be severely lethargic, irritable, and anorexic. Growth retardation may be less pronounced than in marasmus. Treatment involves providing high-quality protein foods and protein-calorie supplements.

Vitamin A deficiency • Decreased serum levels that commonly result from inadequate dietary intake of foods high in vitamin A, which maintains epithelial tissue and retinal function. Other causes are malabsorption, massive urinary excretion caused by other disorders, and decreased storage and transport of vitamin A in hepatic disease.

Night blindness and mild conjunctival changes may be reversed with oral or parenteral doses of vitamin A. Dry and scaly skin responds to cream- or petroleum jelly–based products. Corneal damage requires emergency treatment.

Vitamin B deficiencies • Marked by low urine or serum levels of B-complex vitamins, water-soluble vitamins essential to normal metabolism, cell growth, and blood formation.

Thiamine (B_1) deficiency results from malabsorption or inadequate dietary intake of thiamine. Early complaints include anorexia, irritability, muscle cramps, and paresthesia. Advanced deficiency may result in complaints related to heart disease or the nervous system.

Riboflavin (B₂) deficiency results from a diet deficient in milk, meat, fish, green leafy vegetables, and legumes. Signs and symptoms include sore throat and mouth, weakness, and eye involvement (burning, itching, light sensitivity, and tearing).

Niacin deficiency predominantly affects those who subsist mainly on corn and consume minimal animal protein. It also is associated with alcoholism and nutrient-drug interactions. Early-stage complaints include fatigue, anorexia, muscle weakness, headache, indigestion, weight loss, and backache. Advanced deficiency (pellagra) may produce skin eruptions, mouth soreness, GI distress, and dementia.

Uncommon in adults, *pyridoxine (B₆) deficiency* usually occurs from pyridoxine destruction by autoclaving infant formulas. Signs and symptoms include sore mouth, weakness, abdominal pain, irritability, dermatitis, vomiting, and central nervous system disturbances.

Cobalamin (B₁₂) deficiency, causing anorexia, weight loss, abdominal discomfort, sore mouth, diarrhea, and constipation, commonly results from an absence of intrinsic factor in gastric secretions or an absence of receptor sites after ileal resection.

Diet and supplementary vitamins can prevent or correct vitamin B deficiencies.

Vitamin C deficiency • Insufficient serum levels of ascorbic acid (vitamin C) primarily caused by a diet lacking foods rich in vitamin C.

The deficiency is characterized by weakness, malaise, anorexia, limb and joint pain, and capillary fragility. Advanced deficiency can lead to scurvy, bone fractures, and psychological disturbances. Signs and symptoms subside in a few days to 3 weeks with adequate vitamin C intake.

Vitamin D deficiency • Nutritional deficit that interferes with normal bone calcification, resulting in rickets in infants and young children and osteomalacia in adults.

Rare today, this deficiency results from inadequate dietary intake of preformed vitamin D, malabsorption of vitamin D, or too little exposure to sunlight. Early signs and symptoms include profuse sweating, restlessness, and irritability. If bone deformity occurs, patients may have difficulty in walking and in climbing stairs, leg and lower back pain, bowed legs, knock-knee, poorly developed muscles, and infantile tetany. For osteomalacia and rickets—except when due to malabsorption—treatment consists of massive oral doses of vitamin D or cod liver oil. Rickets refractory to vitamin D or accompanied by hepatic or renal disease requires 25-hydroxycholecalciferol, 1,25-dihydroxycholecalciferol, or a synthetic analogue of active vitamin D.

Vitamin E deficiency • Manifests as hemolytic anemia in low-birth-weight or premature infants.

In infants, this deficiency commonly results from formulas high in polyunsaturated fatty acids that are fortified with iron but not vitamin E. It also develops in conditions associated with fat malabsorption. Signs and symptoms include edema and skin lesions; adults may display muscle weakness, intermittent claudication, and gait disturbances. Replacement of vitamin E with a supplement is the only appropriate treatment.

Vitamin K deficiency • Deficit of the element necessary for the formation of prothrombin and other clotting factors.

This deficiency is common in neonates in the first few days postpartum, because of poor placental transfer of vitamin K and inadequate production of vitamin K–producing intestinal flora. Other causes are prolonged use of certain drugs, decreased bile flow to the small intestine, malabsorption of vitamin K, chronic hepatic disease, and cystic fibrosis. The cardinal sign is an abnormal bleeding tendency. Treatment consists of administration of vitamin K with continued monitoring of prothrombin time to guide therapy.

Zinc deficiency • Low serum levels of zinc, an essential trace element present in the bones, teeth, hair, skin, testes, liver, and muscles.

This deficiency usually results from excessive intake of foods that bind zinc to form insoluble chelates, which prevent its absorption. Other causes include malabsorption disorders and malnutrition. Typically, the patient exhibits sparse hair growth; soft, misshapen nails; and dry, scaling skin. Treatment consists of correcting the underlying cause and administering supplements.

INDEX

A

ABCs, assessment of, 221
Abdominal and pelvic neoplasms, 318-342
Abdominal aneurysm, **591-594**
Abdominal injuries, blunt and penetrating, **240-242**
  removal of penetrating object in, 242
Abdominal X-ray, 869
Abducens nerve, testing, 692
Abducens palsy, 1112. *See also* Extraocular motor nerve palsies.
ABO blood typing, 455
ABO incompatibility, 504t
Abortion, **1065-1068**
  types of, 1065-1066
Abortive poliomyelitis, 729. *See also* Myelitis.
Abruptio placentae, **1076-1078**
Abscess. *See specific type.*
Abscesses, throat, 1149-1151
Absolute T₄ helper count, 455
Absolute T4 helper count, 455
Absorbable gelatin sponges, 487
Acceleration-deceleration injuries, 233-234
Accessory muscles of respiration, 609
Accommodation, lens and, 1088
Acetazolamide, 994
Achilles tendon contracture, **801-802**
Acid-base balance, 955
  assessing, 955
  disorders of, 992-995
Acid-fast bacillus isolation, 99t
Acidosis. *See* Respiratory acidosis.
Acid perfusion test, 869
Acne vulgaris, **1173-1175**
Acoustic nerve, testing, 692-693
Acoustic neurinoma. *See* Schwannoma.
Acquired adrenal virilism, 1032. *See also* Adrenogenital syndrome.
Acquired agammaglobulinemia. *See* Common variable immunodeficiency.
Acquired immunodeficiency syndrome, 439-443
Acral-lentiginous melanoma, 370, 372. *See also* Melanoma, malignant.
Acromegaly. *See* Hyperpituitarism.
Actinic keratosis, 369t
Actinomycosis, 114
Activated partial thromboplastin time, 455
Acute aneurysmal thrombosis, 594. *See also* Femoral and popliteal aneurysms.
Acute febrile juvenile rheumatoid arthritis. *See* Systemic juvenile rheumatoid arthritis.
Acute febrile respiratory illness, 158t. *See also* Adenoviral infections.
Acute follicular conjunctivitis, 158t. *See also* Adenoviral infections.
Acute glomerulonephritis. *See* Acute poststreptococcal glomerulonephritis.

Acute herpetic stomatitis, 869, 871. *See also* Stomatitis.
Acute idiopathic polyneuritis. *See* Guillain-Barré syndrome.
Acute infective tubulointerstitial nephritis. *See* Acute pyelonephritis.
Acute intermittent porphyria, 971t, 972. *See also* Porphyrias.
Acute leukemia, 381-383
Acute lymphoblastic (lymphocytic) leukemia, 381, 382. *See also* Acute leukemia.
Acute monoblastic (monocytic) leukemia, 381, 382. *See also* Acute leukemia.
Acute myeloblastic (myelogenous) leukemia, 381, 382. *See also* Acute leukemia.
Acute ophthalmoplegia. *See* Oculomotor palsy.
Acute pharyngoconjunctival fever, 158t. *See also* Adenoviral infections.
Acute poststreptococcal glomerulonephritis, **820-822**
Acute pyelonephritis, **818-820**
Acute renal disorders, 815-829
Acute renal failure, **815-818**
  classifying, 815
  phases of, 815
Acute respiratory disease, 158t. *See also* Adenoviral infections.
Acute respiratory disorders, 624-667
Acute respiratory failure in COPD, 624-629
  caring for patient with, 627-628
  identifying, 626
  mechanics of, 625i
Acute sequestration crisis, 471
Acute transverse myelitis, 728, 729. *See also* Myelitis.
Acute tubular necrosis, **822-824**
Acute tubulointerstitial nephritis. *See* Acute tubular necrosis.
Acute vulvitis, 1055, 1056. *See also* Vulvovaginitis.
Acyclovir, 179
Adaptive Behavior Scale, 9-10
Addison's anemia. *See* Pernicious anemia.
Addison's disease. *See* Adrenal hypofunction.
Addisonian crisis, 1024, 1025i
Adenoidectomy, 1146
Adenoid hyperplasia, **1145-1147**
Adenoid hypertrophy. *See* Adenoid hyperplasia.
Adenoma, toxic, 1015
Adenoviral infections, **157-159**
Adenovirus pneumonia, 652t. *See also* Pneumonia.
Adolescence, mental disorders of, 12-18
Adoptive transfer of immunity, 290
Adrenal cortex, function of, 997-998
Adrenal crisis, 1024, 1025i
Adrenal disorders, **1023-1036**

Adrenal hypofunction, **1023-1027**
Adrenal insufficiency. *See* Adrenal hypofunction.
Adrenal medulla, function of, 998
Adrenal virilism, 1032. *See also* Adrenogenital syndrome.
Adrenalectomy, aftercare for, 1029, 1035
Adrenogenital syndrome, **1031-1034**
Adult chorea. *See* Huntington's disease.
Adult respiratory distress syndrome, **629-633**
  stages of, 631
Adventitious breath sounds, 612
Afferent neurons, 687
Agammaglobulinemia
  acquired, 436-437
  Bruton's 435-436
  common variable, 436-437
  X-linked infantile, 435-436
Aganglionic megacolon. *See* Hirschsprung's disease.
Agglutination tests, 455
Agoraphobia, 54-55. *See also* Phobias.
Agranulocytosis, 507. *See also* Granulocytopenia.
AIDS. *See* Acquired immunodeficiency syndrome.
AIDS dementia, 442
Air in pleural cavity. *See* Pneumothorax.
Airway, establishing, 614
Airway crisis, preparing for, 623
Airway patency, assessing, 221
Akathisia, drug-induced, 40
Albinism, **1178-1179**
Alcohol abuse, 33t. *See also* Alcoholism.
Alcohol dependence. *See* Alcoholism.
Alcoholism, **26-30**
  diagnostic criteria for, 27-29
Alcohol withdrawal, signs and symptoms of, 28t
Aldosterone, 807, 997-998
  excessive secretion of, 1030i
Alglucerase, 968
Alkalosis. *See* Respiratory alkalosis.
ALL. *See* Acute lymphoblastic (lymphocytic) leukemia.
Allergens. *See* Antigens.
Allergic angiitis, 432t
Allergic disorders, 393, 394i, 398-407
Allergic purpuras, **481-482**
Allergic rhinitis, **398-400**
Allergic shiners, 399
Allergic transfusion reaction, 406. *See also* Blood transfusion reaction.
Alopecia, **1175-1177**
  cancer drugs that cause, 1176
Alpha-fetoprotein as tumor marker, 286
Alpha-thalassemia, 473. *See also* Thalassemia.
ALS. *See* Amyotrophic lateral sclerosis.
Alveolar hypoventilation, 625i
Alveolocapillary membrane, 609
Alzheimer's disease, **730-733**
  stages of, 732

i refers to an illustration; t refers to a table

i refers to an illustration; t refers to a table

i refers to an illustration; t refers to a table

i refers to an illustration; t refers to a table

i refers to an illustration; t refers to a table